Atlas on Cornea

Berthold Seitz · Elias Flockerzi · Loay Daas
Editors

Atlas on Cornea

Diagnostics, Diseases and Therapies

Springer

Editors
Berthold Seitz
Department of Ophthalmology Saarland
University Medical Center
Homburg, Germany

Elias Flockerzi
Department of Ophthalmology Saarland
University Medical Center
Homburg, Germany

Loay Daas
Department of Ophthalmology Saarland
University Medical Center
Homburg, Germany

ISBN 978-3-031-65421-3 ISBN 978-3-031-65422-0 (eBook)
https://doi.org/10.1007/978-3-031-65422-0

This Springer imprint is published by the registered company Springer Nature Switzerland AG
The registered company address is: Gewerbestrasse 11, 6330 Cham, Switzerland

Foreword

"In the fields of observation chance favors only the prepared mind"

- Louis Pasteur, 1854

Early in their careers, many young clinicians are struck by the beauty and functionality of the cornea and choose this tissue to be the focus of their subsequent careers as physicians and surgeons. In addition to its key role in the optics of the eye, this avascular and transparent cornea provides us with a unique opportunity to study many remarkable aspects of human biology.

Renal transplant surgeons can only infer the status of their grafts and the behavior of their patients' immune systems on the basis of serum chemistry tests, while corneal surgeons can directly observe the presence and behavior of immune cells and the response to our therapeutic interventions. Infectious disease "specialists" can only envy our ability to directly observe the infectious processes and use tell-tale morphologic features to make educated guesses as to the responsible pathogen, inform our therapeutic decision-making, and assess the response to therapy. Students of stem cell biology are able to monitor the status and health of the limbal stem cell population, while those of us interested in neoplasia can observe the morphology and growth of malign and benign lesions that, if located elsewhere in the body, would not be detectable until they had enlarged by an order of magnitude or more and achieved a much later stage of disease.

Trauma, autoimmune disease, inherited degenerations, and connective tissue disorders—the list of pathologic conditions that manifest and are directly observable within the special tissue that is the cornea goes on and on.

As Louis Pasteur so famously pointed out, the mind that is prepared to logically analyze what it sees is the mind that will garner the best insights and make the most logical decisions. This atlas beautifully illustrates the key morphologic features of the cornea in health and disease and will prepare the minds of those who wish to master the diagnosis and management of corneal pathology.

The many experts in the field of cornea and external disease and corneal surgery whose collective tremendous efforts have produced this valuable work are to be congratulated, as this atlas covers the spectrum of corneal pathology and (very helpfully) the major surgical procedures. It is a valuable tool for the instruction of our young trainees and an excellent resource for not-so-young physicians who have decided to become lifelong students of the cornea.

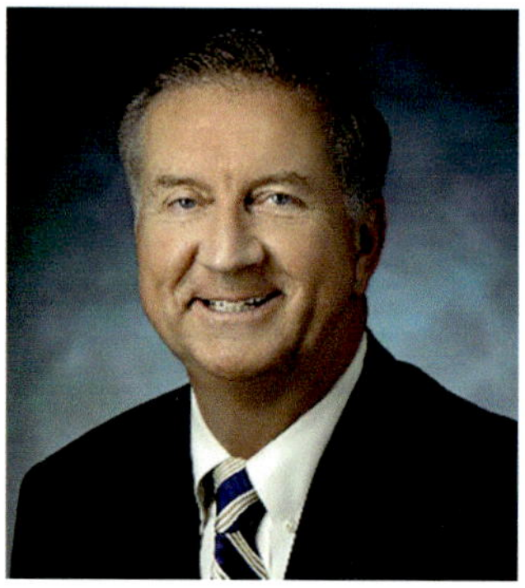

Peter J. McDonnell MD
Professor of Ophthalmology
Johns Hopkins University School of Medicine
Director of the Wilmer Eye Institute at Johns Hopkins Hospital
Baltimore, USA

Foreword

It is with great pleasure for me to introduce this comprehensive Cornea Atlas and Mini Textbook from my esteemed cornea colleagues in Germany. Reflecting on my own experience as a young university professor in the '80s, I hold fond memories of my time in Bonn. The German ophthalmic community has undoubtedly left an indelible mark on my personal and professional growth.

Looking back over the past few decades, there has likewise been a remarkable evolution in the field of Cornea and External Disease. Advances in the pathogenesis of these conditions, coupled with the development of sophisticated diagnostic techniques, have paved the way for a wealth of effective medical and surgical treatments for various corneal diseases. This progress is vividly reflected in the pages of this atlas.

Throughout the atlas, readers will find clear explanations and visually engaging content, showcasing the authors' deep knowledge and passion for the subject. The work is easy to read, brief but complete, including excellent images and well-documented pathologic features.

Notably, the genesis of this atlas was spearheaded by Berthold Seitz, a dear friend and worldwide respected colleague. His leadership and vision have brought together a team of experts to create a resource that will undoubtedly influence the future of corneal research and clinical practice. I commend the authors for their collaborative efforts in compiling this invaluable resource.

Herzlichen Glückwunsch zu diesem herausragenden Werk!

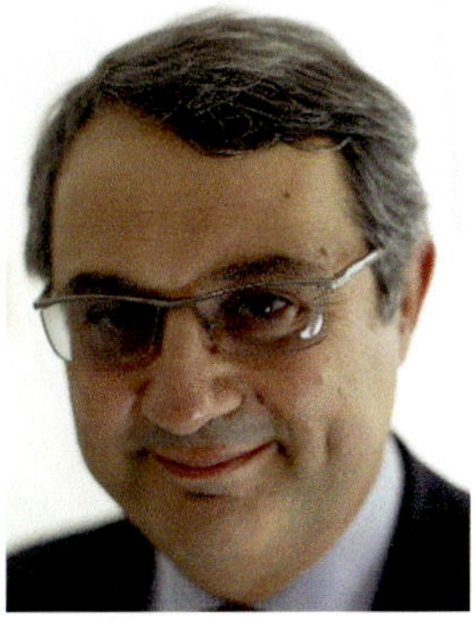

Massimo Busin MD
Professor of Ophthalmology at University of Ferrara
Clinical Director Ospedali Privati Forlì
Department of Ophthalmology
Forlì, Italy

Foreword

It is a great honor for me to write this foreword to this new atlas and "mini-textbook" on corneal diseases and therapies.

Over the past decades, several textbooks on the cornea have been published, a few ophthalmic color atlases have been available as well, and several dedicated books on specific topics related to corneal surgical procedures are accessible.

The current atlas seems to cover all aspects needed for ophthalmologists with a broad focus on all clinical aspects related to corneal structure, diagnostics, diseases, and therapy. On top, the atlas is abundantly illustrated with superb illustrations, making it a real comprehensive piece of work.

The atlas is edited by Prof. Dr. Berthold Seitz, Direktor der Klinik für Augenheilkunde und Hochschulambulanz at the Universitätsklinikum des Saarlandes UKS in Homburg/Saar, Germany. The editor has managed to recruit contributing experts from the clinic in Homburg/Saar and many other authorities from mainly German institutions. The 6 parts with a total of 64 individual chapters are well organized. Fortunately, the atlas is published in English language, and this will possibly make it a global reference work for residents and specialists with an interest in patients with corneal diseases.

Image recognition and analysis is an important skill when examining the cornea. Today artificial intelligence is the new "smart" technology with the goal to be able to recognize patterns, make decisions, and judge like humans. We are not there now, and it may take several decades before corneal examinations and decision-making can be automated. Until then, this atlas is an indispensable source of information, which without doubt will improve our care for patients with corneal diseases.

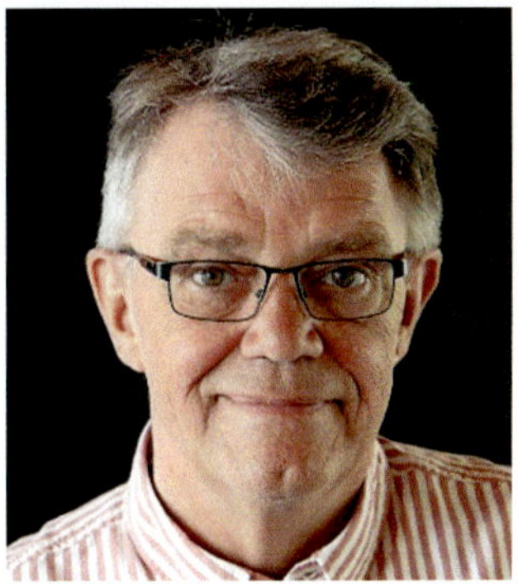

Jesper Hjortdal MD
Clinical Professor
Chief Physician, DMSc, PhD
Head of Corneal & Refractive Surgery
Medical Director and Responsible Person for The Danish Cornea Bank
Department of Ophthalmology
University Hospital Aarhus
Aarhus, Denmark

Preface

Viva Corneophilia

Dear Readers,

it was an honor when Ms. Elizabeth Pope from Springer Publishers, London, approached me in June 2021 to contribute "a book project." It was indisputably clear to me that it must be dedicated to CORNEA, or not at all.

In which other medical specialty can clinicians witness a disease entity, its gradual progression, and its response to treatment so vividly, only with the help of 40x magnification of our biomicroscope in daily use, the slit lamp?

While retinologists believe that the clear cornea is only necessary for a good insight into the eye for vitreoretinal surgery, most corneal specialists are sure that the human cornea is not only essential to sight but also is the most accessible part of the eye in terms of diagnostics and effective therapy.

This color atlas and mini-textbook is aimed at presenting an updated summary of corneal diseases as well as new techniques regarding diagnostics and therapy to assist fellow ophthalmologists and corneal surgeons in their counseling and selection of patients for the correct diagnosis and the best conservative and/or micro-surgical procedures, considering benefits and risks. Our intention is not for our color atlas to be used in isolation but we sincerely hope that it will prove useful in combination with the comprehensive (albeit often scarcely illustrated) textbooks on corneal diseases that are already available and help resolve some of the diagnostic and therapeutic difficulties.

We are well aware that there are excellent books referring to some individual topics of this atlas, for example, on corneal diseases (Reinhard & Larkin: "Cornea and External Eye Disease"), keratoconus (Das: "Keratoconus"), aniridia (Ponzin et al.: "Aniridia"), corneal infections (Das & Jhanji: "Infections of the Cornea and Conjunctiva"), corneal surgery (Brightbill, McDonnell, McGhee, Farjo & Serdarevic: "Corneal Surgery" or Linke & Katz: "Complications in Corneal Laser Surgery"), eye banking and corneal transplantation (Hjortdal: "Corneal Transplantation" or Alió & Alió del Barrio: "Modern Keratoplasty"), and so on.

Nevertheless, we wanted to compile an *Atlas on Cornea* with many large-format (not in "stamp size"), high-quality color pictures with excellent legends. Each author was given the liberty to add as much text as he/she considered appropriate on an individual basis of estimation for his/her chapter. As a multi-authored text, there are multiple literary styles. We, as editors, have worked to provide a certain level of conformity and scientific balance without sacrificing the originality and style of the individual authors. A distinctive and attractive feature of this *Atlas on Cornea* is the diversity of its many outstanding contributors in addition to their leadership in the field. Each chapter has been written by a true expert in the field, who not only deals with the cornea from a theoretical point of view but also applies this knowledge for the best possible treatment of our patients on a daily practical basis.

It has been my good fortune to come across many fine people during my travels throughout my professional life. A significant number of them are contributors to this book. Moreover, many authors are indirectly linked to the tradition of our great teacher Professor Dr. Dr. h.c. mult. Gottfried Otto Helmut Naumann, Head of the Department of

Ophthalmology in Erlangen, Germany, from 1980 to 2003. Prof. Naumann sadly passed away on 5 June 2021 in Erlangen but has left a legacy which inspires ophthalmologists around the globe. His great two-volume book "Pathology of the Eye" dating back to 1997 is in the hand of all of our young colleagues who absorb the "special taste of corneology" with all their senses from the first day of their residency here in Homburg, just as I did back in Erlangen from 1989 to 2005.

Fritz Naumann shaped an entire generation of ophthalmologists through his outstanding research, extensive teaching activities, and countless original papers and standard works. His remarkable clinical and scientific ophthalmological competence has had a pioneering and lasting impact on German as well as international ophthalmology—especially in the field of cornea and corneal transplantation. "No effect without affect!"

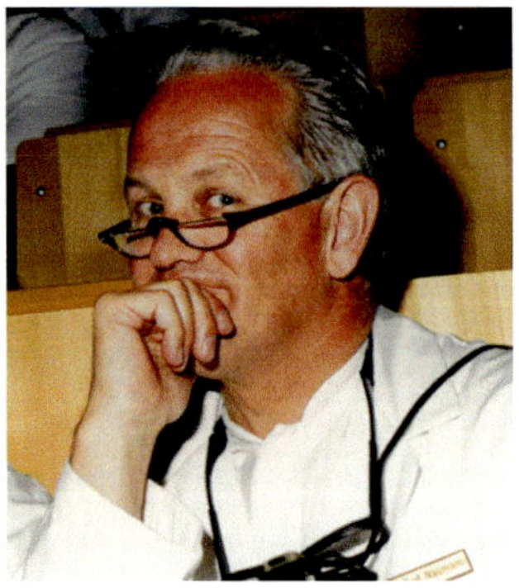

Additionally, for more than 30 years, I share mutual admiration and respect with Peter J. McDonnell, Massimo Busin, and Jesper Hjortdal who are internationally renowned specialists in the field of cornea. Therefore, I am very proud that they have accepted to each contribute a short foreword to our atlas.

Especially Peter J. McDonnell and I share a friendship going back to the year 1995, where I joined the Doheny Eye Institute, USC School of Medicine in Los Angeles, USA, as a research fellow in corneal and refractive surgery. "Stop talking – start writing!"

I am glad that my fellow editors, Dr. Loay Daas and PD Dr. Elias Flockerzi, supported this project with their knowledge and comments regarding the content and realization of this atlas. Dr. Daas and PD Dr. Flockerzi are both outstanding ophthalmologists and micro-surgeons here in Homburg and it has been a pleasure to work on this atlas together.

This project could not have been successfully finalized without the incredible support of Ms. Christina Turner, who not only helped collect the chapters for this atlas but also kept track of all the details that were required formally. She has also added great value with her native speaker quality concerning the English language.

The variety of pictures is clearly an integral part of this atlas. In this respect, we sincerely thank our photographer Mr. Marc Müller who provides us daily with a vast amount of excellent, high-quality pictures during patients' visits for diagnosis, procedures, and follow-ups and, therefore, Marc Müller is an indispensable part in the making of this atlas.

We also thank the publishers, particularly Ms. Elizabeth Pope, for the encouragement to start this project and for her great assistance in finalizing the project with an unlimited number of large-format color photographs and being a valuable point of contact for us during the process.

Moreover, the editors gratefully acknowledge the support of the faculties and staff of the Department of Ophthalmology at Saarland University Medical Center who contributed greatly to the completion of this project.

It has been an immense effort to realize the publication of this atlas but as a team, we have been able to make it a reality. Thanks to all of them, we hope that this *Homburg Cornea Color Atlas* will find a meaningful and valued place in the libraries of ophthalmology today and in the future as a welcome source of reference.

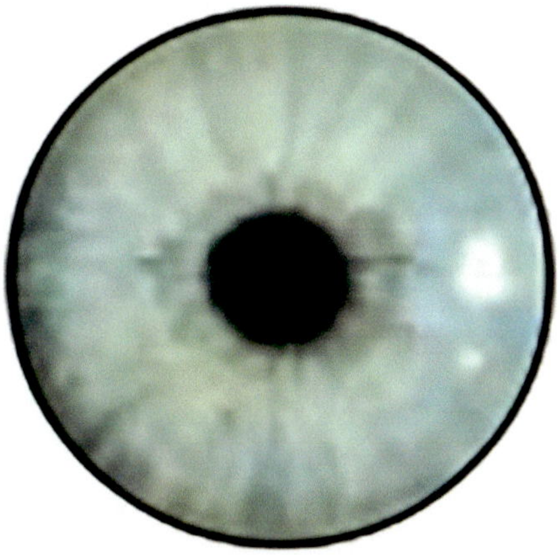

Prof. Dr. Berthold Seitz
also on behalf of:

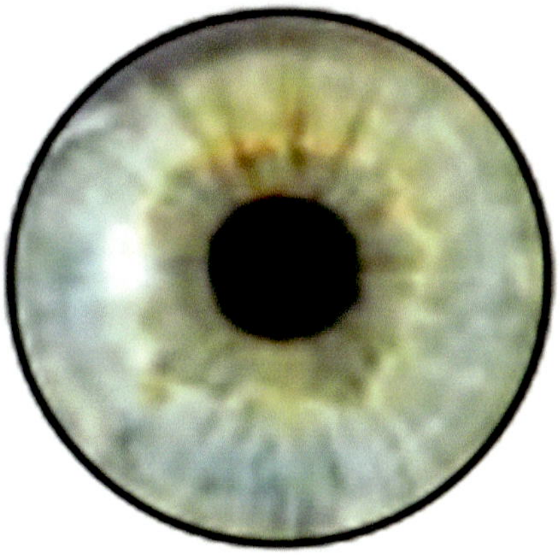

PD Dr. Elias Flockerzi

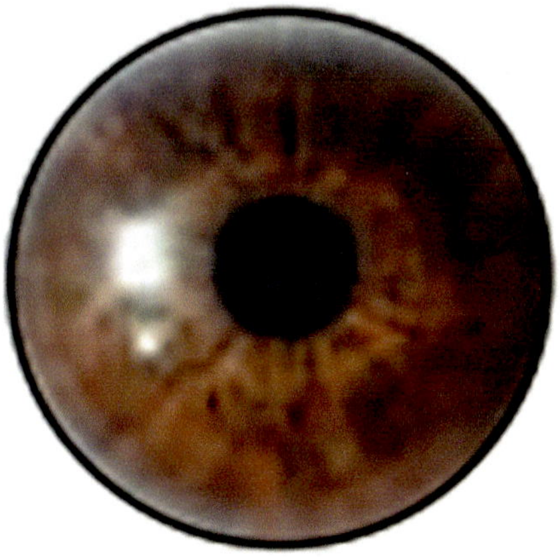

Dr. Loay Daas

Homburg/Saar, Germany, April 2025

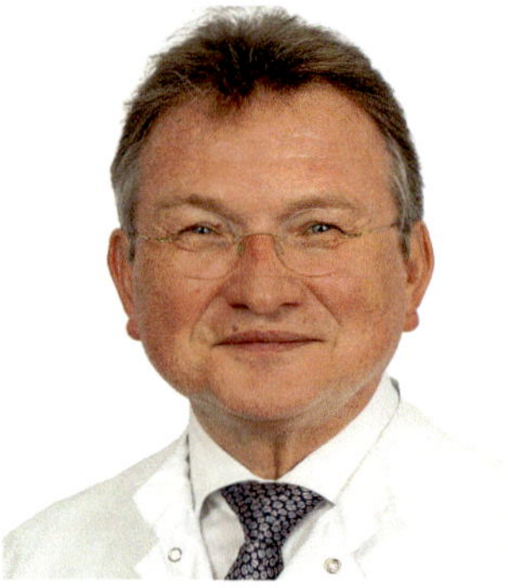

Prof. Dr. Berthold Seitz ML FEBO
Professor and Chairman
Department of Ophthalmology
Saarland University Medical Center
Homburg/Saar, Germany

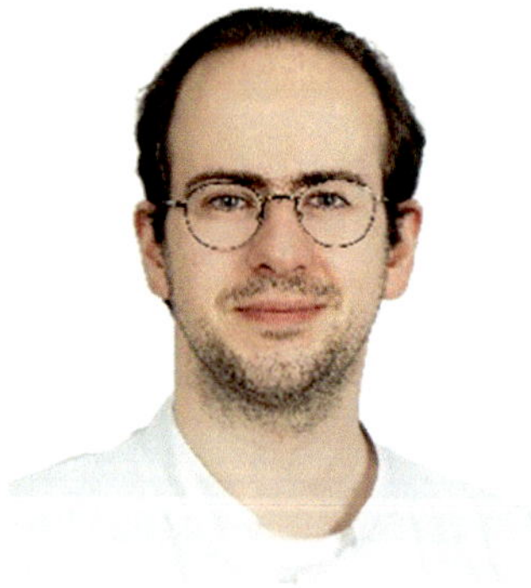

PD Dr. Elias Flockerzi FEBO MHBA
Senior physician
Department of Ophthalmology,
Saarland University Medical Center
Homburg/Saar, Germany

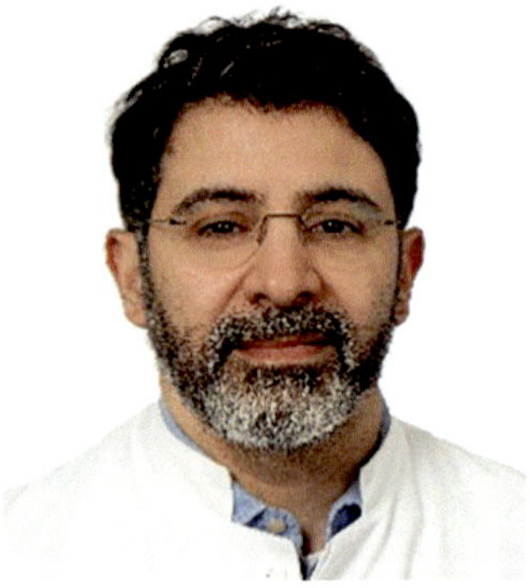

Dr. Loay Daas
Head physician
Department of Ophthalmology,
Saarland University Medical Center
Homburg/Saar, Germany

Contents

Diseases

The Human Cornea

Morphology of the Human Cornea as Displayed by in Vivo and Ex Vivo Imaging Techniques

Rudolf F. Guthoff, Sebastian Bohn, Oliver Stachs, Ursula Schlötzer-Schrehardt, and Thomas Stahnke

Abstract

From a functional perspective, the complex anatomical structure of the cornea acts more like an organ than a tissue. Different highly specialized cells interact to fulfill these duties. The multilayered epithelium, with its regenerative capacity (total replacement every week), acts in conjunction with the microvilli-covered surface with the tear film as a high-precision optical interface and a barrier against pathogens. Bowman layer represents the most anterior, acellular portion of the corneal stroma with high mechanical stability. In addition to the stabilization function, it provides the lead structure for the subbasal nerve plexus, making it easily accessible by in vivo confocal microscopy due to its surface parallelism as well as for Langerhans cells in the case of injuries or inflammations. The stroma, in total, is composed of regularly arranged bundles of collagen fibrils embedded in a glycosaminoglycan-rich extracellular matrix, which are interspersed with flattened fibroblast-like cells termed keratocytes. The boundary to the anterior chamber is formed by the Descemet membrane, which represents the thickened (10–12 μm), specialized basement membrane of the corneal endothelium. The endothelium, which is the only non-regenerative cell population of the cornea, provides the stable water balance and, thus, the transparency of the stroma by means of the pump function. The overall concept of this chapter is to describe the morphology of the human cornea by building bridges between findings of conventional clinical examination techniques and information delivered by confocal in vivo-, light-, and electron-microscopy. This may stimulate the clinician to seek deeper insights into corneal physiology and pathophysiology and stimulate interest in further research.

Keywords

In vivo confocal laser scanning microscopy (CLSM) · Keratocyte density · Subbasal nerve plexus (SNP) · Epithelial cell layers · Corneal immune response · Langerhans cells

1 Gross Anatomy and Physiology

In adults, the cornea has a horizontal diameter of 11.0–12.0 mm, a vertical diameter of 10.0–11.0 mm, and a thickness of approximately 500–550 μm at the center, which gradually increases to 600–800 μm toward the periphery [1]. The cornea has an aspheric anterior surface that is steeper in the center and flatter in the periphery. The average refractive power is 43.25 diopters, the average radius of curvature is 7.8 mm, and the corneal index of refraction is 1.376. It is composed of five anatomical layers, i.e., corneal epithelium, Bowman layer, corneal stroma, Descemet membrane, and corneal endothelium (Fig. 1).

Besides these conventional layers of the cornea, an additional pre-Descemet stromal layer has been recently

R. F. Guthoff (✉) · S. Bohn · O. Stachs · T. Stahnke
Department of Ophthalmology, Rostock University Medical Center, Rostock, Germany
e-mail: rudolf.guthoff@med.uni-rostock.de

S. Bohn
e-mail: sebastian.bohn@uni-rostock.de

O. Stachs
e-mail: oliver.stachs@med.uni-rostock.de

T. Stahnke
e-mail: Thomas.stahnke@med.uni-rostock.de

U. Schlötzer-Schrehardt
Department of Ophthalmology, University of Erlangen-Nurnberg, Erlangen, Germany
e-mail: ursula.schloetzer-schrehardt@uk-erlangen.de

B. Seitz et al. (eds.), *Atlas on Cornea*, https://doi.org/10.1007/978-3-031-65422-0_1

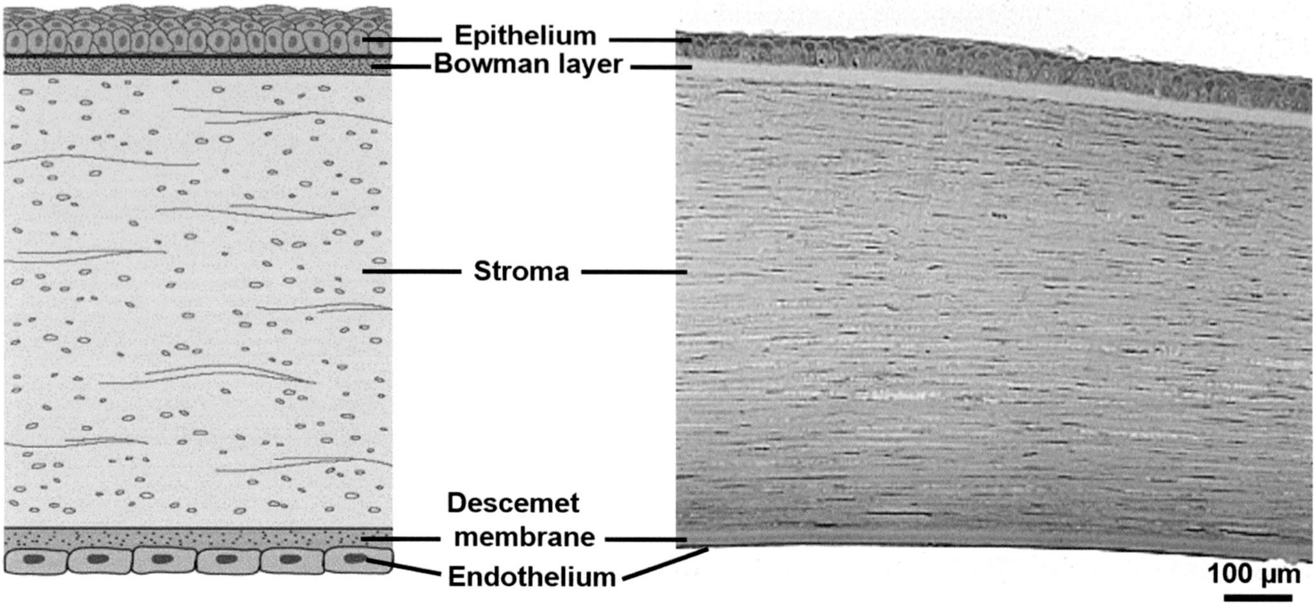

Fig. 1 Schematic illustration (left) and light micrograph (right) of anatomical corneal layers

described [2], which has, however, been subsequently disproved by a multicenter study [3]. A more detailed insight into the structural configuration of the individual corneal tissues can be obtained by means of electron microscopy ex vivo (Fig. 2).

In vivo confocal laser scanning microscopy (CLSM) with the Heidelberg retina tomograph (HRT) II and Rostock Cornea Module can be used for in vivo imaging of all anatomical layers and corneal cell types including nerve plexus and immune cells (Fig. 3E).

2 Corneal Epithelium

The epithelial surface of the cornea represents the physical barrier to the outer environment and an integral part of the smooth tear film–cornea interface that is critical for the refractive power of the eye. It is responsible for protecting the eye against loss of fluid and invasion of foreign bodies and pathogens and for absorbing oxygen and nutrients from the tear film. The corneal surface is covered by a stratified, nonkeratinizing, squamous epithelium, about 50 µm in thickness, comprising 5–7 cell layers. It can be structured into three layers: the superficial or squamous cell layer, the suprabasal wing cell layer, and the basal columnar cell layer (Fig. 2A) [1, 5]. This complex structure can be displayed in vivo by confocal laser scanning microscopy (Fig. 3).

A detailed view of the various epithelial structures and the anterior stroma (magnification approximately 800×) are shown to a depth of approximately 120 µm. The substructures of the epithelium are easily distinguished and are bounded by the superficial cells and the surface of Bowman layer. Figure 3B shows the roof tile-like overlap of the superficial cells with a maximum diameter of about 50 µm and sometimes clearly visible nuclei. The most superficial of the cells about to desquamate exhibit signal-intensive cytoplasm. The mean cell density there is about 1000 cells per mm^2.

In the wing cell layer shown in Fig. 3C, the cell boundaries are particularly well visible as highly reflective structures, which can be explained morphologically by the scattered light properties of the desmosomes connecting the individual epithelial cells (see also Fig. 2A). In contrast, the cytoplasm of the wing cells exhibits a uniform mean scattered light intensity, and cell nuclei are not discernible. The mean cell density there is about 1000 cells per mm^2. In the wing cell layer shown in Fig. 3C, the cell borders are particularly well visible as highly reflective structures, and the cytoplasm has a medium to low intensity. In the wing cell layer shown in Fig. 3C, the cell boundaries are particularly well seen as highly reflective structures, the cytoplasm exhibits uniform medium to low intensity, and cell nuclei are not visible. The cell density is about 3000 cells per mm^2.

The basal cell layer (Fig. 3D) is characterized by cells whose cytoplasm has different scattered light characteristics. The cell borders and the cell nuclei are easily recognizable so that a high cell density of up to 8000 cells per mm^2 can be reliably determined. Figure 3E shows an inconspicuous subbasal nerve plexus (SNP) with few dendritic

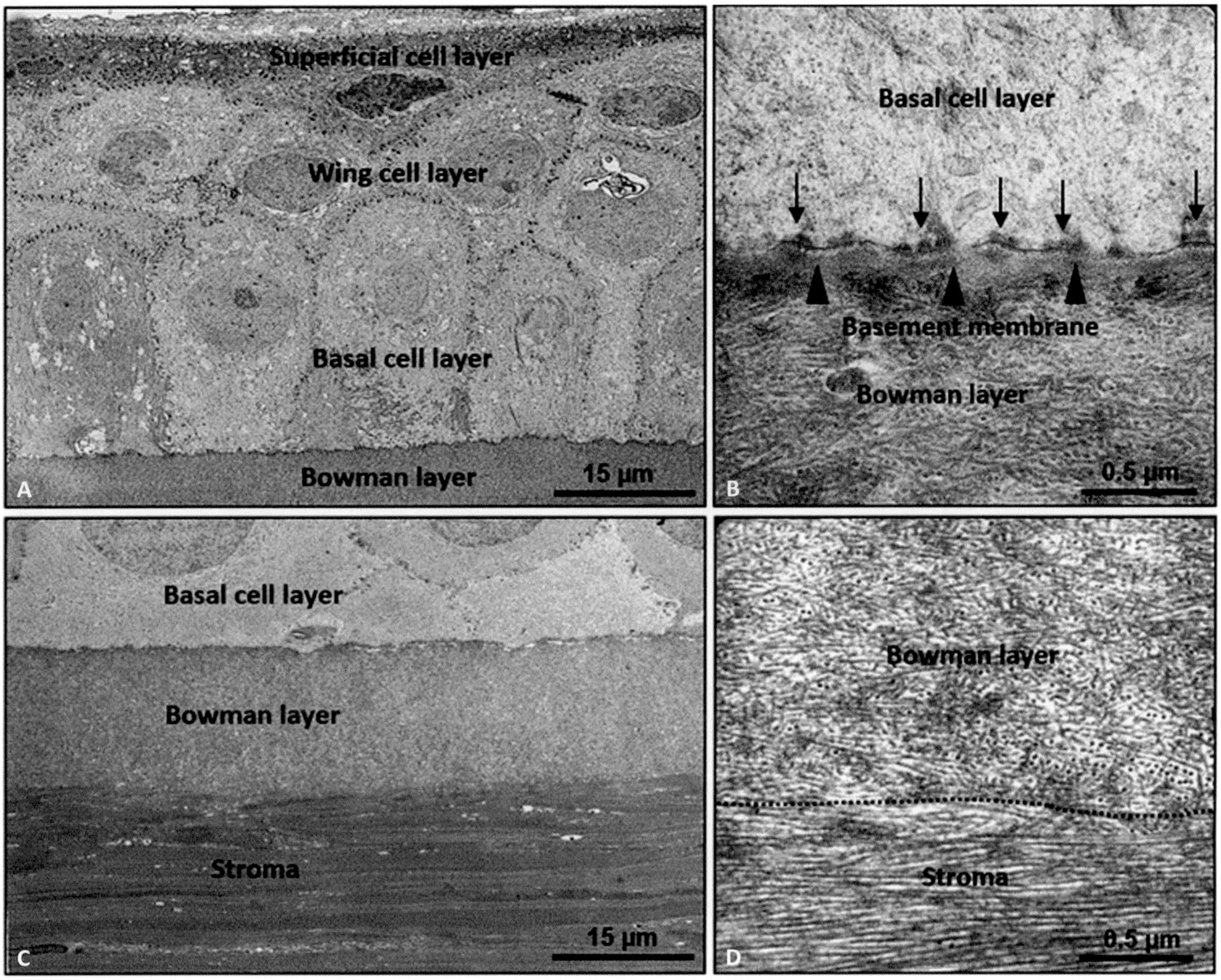

Fig. 2 Transmission electron micrographs of anatomical corneal layers. (**A**) Corneal epithelium shows three layers: the superficial or squamous cell layer, the suprabasal wing cell layer, and the basal columnar cell layer resting on Bowman layer. (**B**) Anchoring complexes formed by hemidesmosomes (arrows) and anchoring fibrils (arrowheads) mediate the attachment of basal epithelial cells to the basement membrane and Bowman layer. (**C**) Bowman layer represents the most anterior portion of the corneal stroma. (**D**) The interface (dotted line) between Bowman layer and corneal stroma shows differing arrangement of collagen fibrils. (**E**) Keratocyte between collagen lamellae of the corneal stroma. (**F**) Collagen fibril organization in adjacent collagen lamellae. **G**) Descemet membrane, the basement membrane of the corneal endothelium, is composed of the interfacial matrix (IFM), anterior banded layer (ABL), and posterior nonbanded layer (PNBL). (**H**) "Bowman-like layer" (BL) is a meshwork of randomly arranged collagen fibrils at the interface between Descemet membrane and stroma. (**A–C, G–H**) Reproduced from Schlötzer-Schrehardt and Kruse [4], with permission from Springer

cells. Figure 3F shows a surface-parallel cross-sectional image of the largely low-contrast Bowman layer, which has a thickness of approximately 10 µm, as seen in slit-lamp comparable Fig. 3A. The distance between the superficial epithelial cells and the SNP is approximately 50 µm in our example and can be used as a measure of epithelial thickness. Figures 3G–I show sections through the anterior stromal regions characterized in Fig. 3A, showing the well-identifiable nuclei of keratocytes. In some stromal layers of this example, particularly at a depth of 121 µm (Fig. 3I), discrete cytoplasmic elements of the complex keratocyte plexus can be identified as fine granular structures of less than 2 µm. These elements may play a role in assessing the transformation of keratocytes to an activated state [6].

The CLSM-generated image data, using piezo-based focus shifting controls, can produce data sets that allow 3D reconstruction of in vivo image data from the cornea (Fig. 4) [7].

Desmosomes promote strong adhesion between cells of all epithelial layers. The superficial layer of the cornea is formed by 2–3 layers of flat polygonal cells, which form intercellular tight junctions to provide an effective barrier

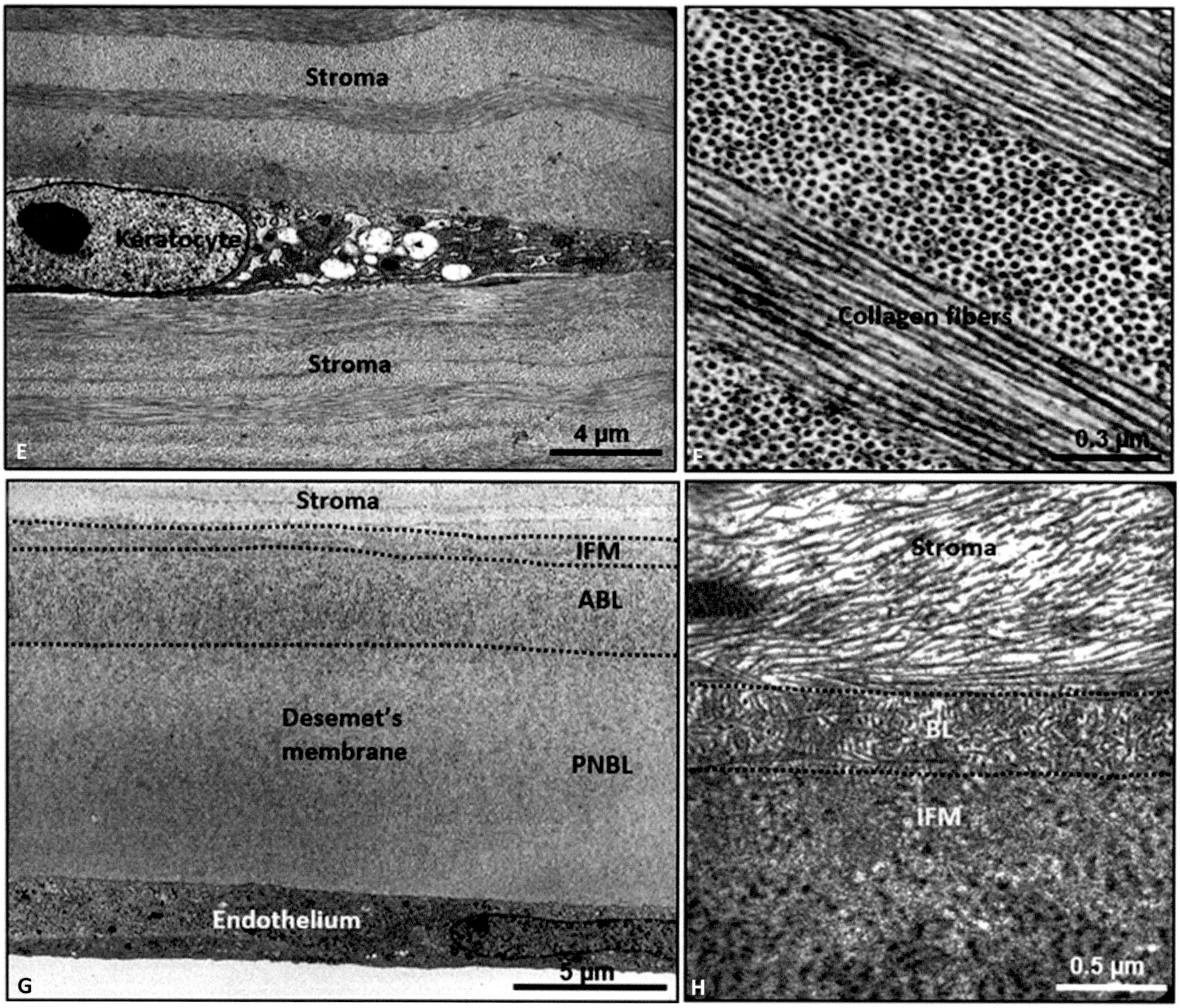

Fig. 2 continued

against the entry of macromolecules, microorganisms, and nanoparticles into the intercellular space (extracellular matrix). Superficial cells are characterized by numerous surface microvilli, which increase the cellular surface area and enhance oxygen and nutrient uptake from the tear film. The cell membrane of the microvilli is formed by a lipid bilayer that is coated by a matrix of closely packed transmembrane mucins MUC1, MUC4, and MUC16, all expressed at the tips of the epithelial microvilli. These membrane-bound mucins form the glycocalyx, which accounts for the water-binding, lubricative, and antiadhesive function of the corneal epithelium. Cross-linking of MUC1 and MUC16 by galectin 3 reinforces the barrier function against entry across the apical epithelial cell membrane.

The precorneal tear film is composed of a muco-aqueous layer covered by a superficial lipid layer. Within the muco-aqueous layer, the concentration of gel-forming mucin MUC5AC secreted by the goblet cell of the conjunctiva increases from the lipid layer toward the glycocalyx. Whereas, in the past, it had been postulated that the main function of the lipid layer is protection from evaporation, it is now recognized that the lipid layer only provides a minor barrier against evaporation but is essential for the spreading of the tears during blinking and their stability between blinks [8–12].

The tear film also supplies immunological and growth factors that are critical for epithelial health, proliferation, and repair, and defects in the tear film, e.g., in neurotrophic keratopathy after corneal surgery, can cause epithelial wound healing problems and surface inflammation. The

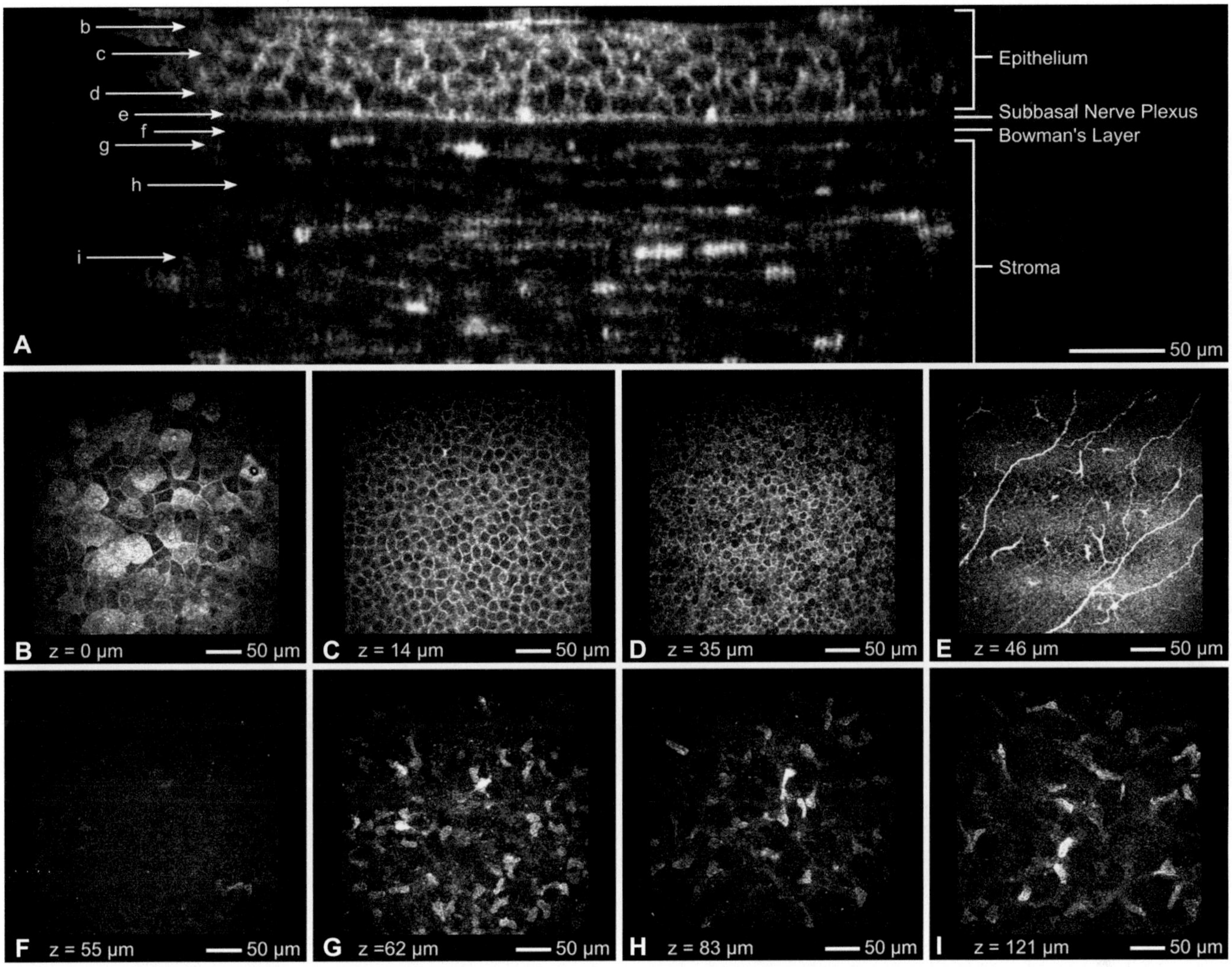

Fig. 3 (**A**) In vivo confocal laser scanning microscopy (CLSM)-based detailed view of normal findings of epithelium and anterior stroma of the human cornea. (**B–I**) Images from the stack parallel to the surface as the depths given in (**A**)

wing cell layer is formed by 2–3 layers of wing-shaped cells that have laterally interdigitated cell membranes with numerous desmosomes (Fig. 2A). The basal layer consists of a single layer of columnar cells (Fig. 2A), which are attached to the underlying basement membrane by hemidesmosomes (Fig. 2B). The epithelial basement membrane has a critical role in corneal wound healing, because defects in this delicate layer allow penetration of growth factors from the epithelium into the stroma [13]. Corneal epithelial adhesion to Bowman layer is maintained by an anchoring complex, including anchoring fibrils (type VII collagen) and anchoring plaques (type VI collagen) (Fig. 2B) [14]. Abnormalities in these anchoring complexes may result clinically in recurrent corneal erosions or nonhealing epithelial defects. Besides epithelial cells, there are numerous nerve endings in between the cells, which exert important trophic influences on the corneal epithelium and have been estimated to amount to a density of 7000 nociceptors per mm^2, which is 400 times more than in the skin [15]. Mechanical stress to these nerves, such as in bullous keratopathy, can therefore cause tremendous pain. Furthermore, resident MHC class II-expressing cells, i.e., CD11c+-dendritic cells and CD207+-Langerhans cells, were identified in the human basal epithelium and anterior stroma, which are capable of rapidly mobilizing to the site of epithelial trauma and viral infection within the cornea [16]. The corneal epithelium itself exerts strong anti-inflammatory and antiangiogenic properties.

Corneal epithelial cells routinely undergo apoptosis and desquamation from the surface. This process results in complete turnover of the corneal epithelial layer every 5–7 days as deeper cells replace the desquamating superficial cells in an orderly, apically directed fashion. Two populations of cells, the basal epithelial cells and limbal stem cells, help renew the epithelial surface [17]. The epithelial stem cells and their progenitors are located at the bottom of the

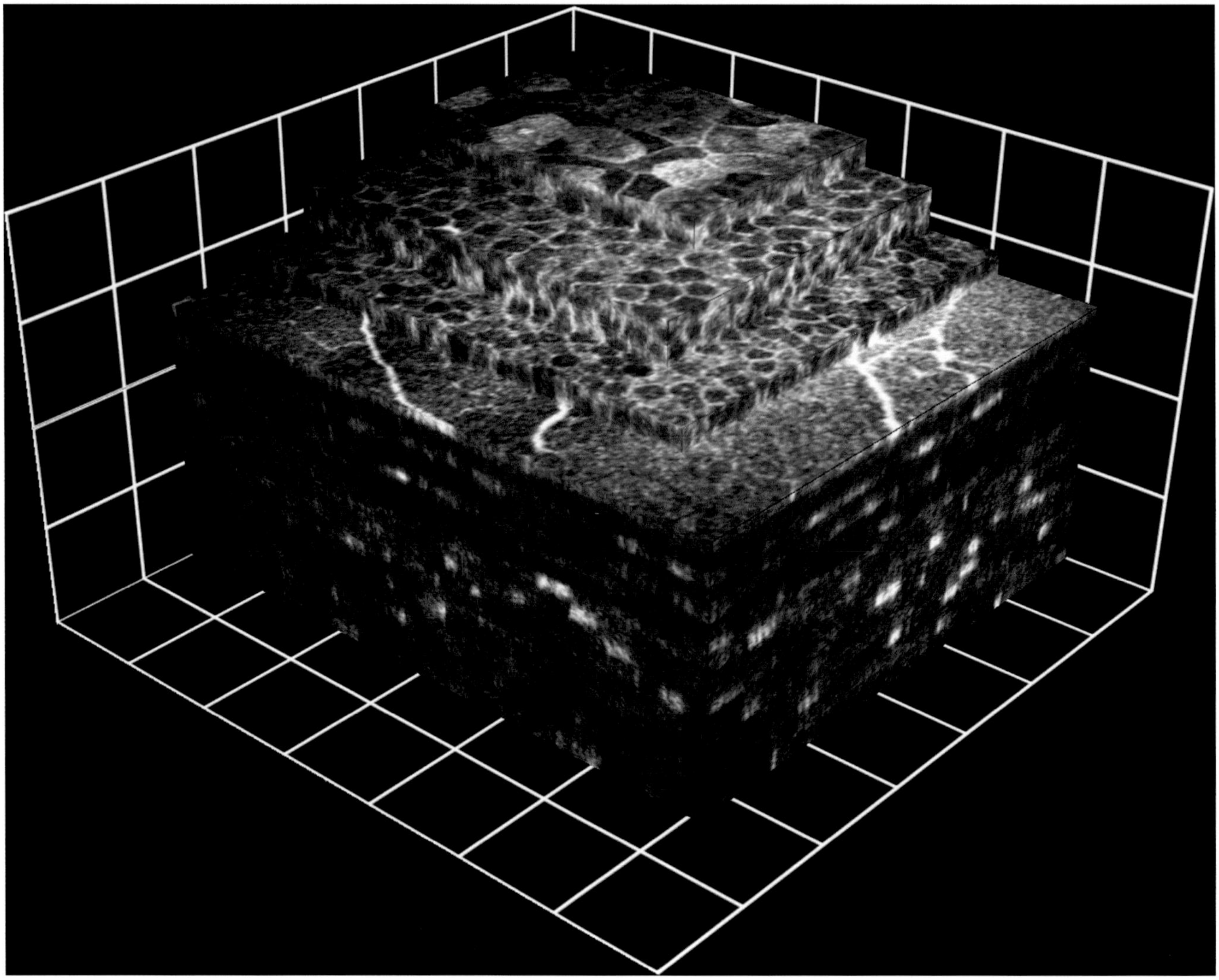

Fig. 4 3D reconstruction and segmentation of the corneal epithelial and anterior stromal cell layers. Edge length of a box: 50 μm

palisades of Vogt at the corneoscleral limbus [18]. Depletion of this stem cell reservoir, e.g., after chemical burns, can cause severe ocular surface disease and significant visual deterioration, a condition known as limbal stem cell deficiency [19]. In these cases, the epithelium of conjunctival phenotype may replace the corneal surface. Transplantation of limbal autografts or allografts [20] and ex vivo expanded limbal epithelial stem cells are established therapeutic strategies to regenerate the damaged corneal surface [21].

3 Bowman Layer

Bowman layer represents the most anterior, acellular portion of the corneal stroma (Fig. 2C). It is approximately 8–12 μm thick and structurally composed of randomly oriented collagen fibrils, 20–25 nm in diameter, consisting of collagen types I, III, V, and VI (Fig. 2D) [22]. Its thickness has been reported to decline with age by 0.06 μm per year, thus losing one-third of its thickness between 20 and 80 years of age [23].

Unmyelinated nerve axons penetrate Bowman layer to terminate within the epithelium. The functional role of Bowman layer is not completely known, but it is believed to serve as a barrier that protects corneal stroma and nerves from traumatic injury. In addition, it has been suggested that it ensures epithelial anchorage to the corneal stroma and helps to maintain the shape and tensile strength of the cornea. Bowman layer also functions as an important UV shield protecting the inner eye and a nearly insurmountable barrier against the invasion of epithelial tumors into the corneal stroma [5].

4 Corneal Stroma

The stroma is the thickest layer of the cornea, measuring approximately 500 μm in width, and represents a dense avascular connective tissue of remarkable and unique regularity. It is composed of regularly arranged bundles of collagen fibrils embedded in a glycosaminoglycan-rich extracellular matrix, which are interspersed with flattened fibroblast-like cells termed keratocytes (Fig. 2E) [1].

Collagen organization in the stroma is crucial to corneal functions such as light transmission and maintenance of corneal curvature, tensile strength, and rigidity [24]. The individual collagen fibrils, being mainly composed of collagen types I and V, are extremely uniform in diameter, measuring about 25–30 nm [25, 26], and are organized into approximately 250–300 sheets or lamellae of 2 μm thickness (Fig. 2F). Regular spacing of fibrils within these lamellae is maintained by interactions of collagens with proteoglycans forming bridges between the fibrils [27]. The major proteoglycans of the stroma are keratan sulfate proteoglycans, such as keratocan and lumican, and chondroitin/dermatan sulfate proteoglycans, such as decorin [24, 28], which also regulate stromal hydration by means of their ability to bind water molecules. The collagenous lamellae form a highly organized tissue layer, with adjacent lamellae being oriented at right angles, although there are organizational differences in the collagen bundles between anterior and posterior stroma [29]. In the anterior third of the stroma, lamellae are oriented more obliquely, mediating a tighter cohesive strength and rigidity, which appears particularly important in maintaining corneal curvature [30], whereas, in the posterior two-thirds, lamellae run in parallel to the corneal surface. These differences in stromal collagen organization may also explain why the anterior stroma resists changes to stromal hydration much better [29] and why surgical dissection in a particular plane is easier in the posterior depths of the stroma, e.g., in DALK. Moreover, the peripheral stroma is thicker than the central stroma, and the collagen fibrils may change direction to form a circumferentially oriented network, which is thought to be pivotal in maintaining corneal stability and curvature as they approach the limbus [29]. Any disturbance of this fine-tuned arrangement, either by deposition of abnormal extracellular matrix, e.g., deposition of mucopolysaccharides in macular corneal dystrophy, or the irregular arrangement of collagen fibrils in stromal scars, can cause corneal opacity. The collagen lamellae are interspersed with flattened stellate keratocytes, which are interconnected by gap junctions and arranged in a circular, corkscrew pattern forming a coherent network [31, 32]. The density of keratocytes in the anterior stroma is 20,000–24,000 cells/mm^2, and the density decreases posteriorly. It has been demonstrated, using a 3-D reconstruction technique, that by volume, keratocytes occupy more than 20% of the stroma [33]. Keratocytes are metabolically active cells involved in the synthesis and turnover of extracellular matrix components, i.e., collagen molecules and glycosaminoglycans. They contain water-soluble proteins, corneal "crystallins", which appear to be responsible for reducing the backscatter of light from the keratocytes and for maintaining corneal transparency [34]. In addition, sensory nerve fibers are present in the anterior stroma, which are cut during PKP, leading to a mild neurotrophic keratopathy [35], and MHC class II antigen-presenting cells, which seem to migrate out of the cornea during organ preservation, thereby explaining the reduced rates of immune rejections of longer organ-cultured grafts [36].

Recently, the existence of a novel, previously unrecognized layer of the pre-Descemet corneal stroma, which can be separated by air injection into the stroma during DALK using big-bubble technique, has been reported [2]. This distinct layer was reported to measure about 10 μm in width and was characterized to lack any keratocytes and to show a pronounced immunostaining for collagen types III, IV, and VI [37].

However, the description of this hypothesized new anatomic layer was critically commented on in the literature and eventually refuted by a detailed ultrastructural reinvestigation of the human corneal stroma [3]. The findings of this three-center study provided evidence that there is no distinctive acellular pre-Descemet stromal zone justifying the term "layer" apart from a thin (0.5–1.0 μm) intermediary "Bowman-like zone" of randomly arranged collagen fibers at the Descemet membrane–stromal interface (Fig. 2H). The collagen fibers of this intermediary layer partly extend into Descemet membrane serving a connecting function. Stromal keratocytes were found to approach Descemet membrane up to 1.5 μm (mean 4.97 ± 2.19 μm) in the central regions and up to 4.5 μm (mean 9.77 ± 2.90 μm) in the peripheral regions of the cornea. The intrastromal cleavage plane after pneumodissection, which seemed to occur at multiple stromal levels along rows of keratocytes offering the least resistance to mechanical forces, was obviously determined by the variable distances of keratocytes to Descemet membrane.

5 Descemet Membrane

Descemet membrane represents the thickened (10–12 μm), specialized basement membrane of the corneal endothelium consisting of collagen types IV, VIII, and XVIII and non-collagenous components, including fibronectin, laminin, nidogen, and perlecan as well as dermatan, keratan, heparan, and chondroitin sulfate proteoglycans [4]. Apart from providing the structural integrity of the cornea, the Descemet membrane has been suggested to play a role in several important physiological processes, including corneal hydration, endothelial cell differentiation and proliferation, and maintenance of the corneal curvature. It is composed of an anterior banded (fetal) layer, approx. 3 µm in thickness, and a posterior non-banded (postnatal) layer that gradually thickens with age, reaching up to 10 µm in elderly individuals (Fig. 2G) [38, 39]. In the periphery, the Descemet membrane forms wartlike excrescences (Hassall–Henle warts) and merges into the trabecular meshwork beams. The thickened fusion site, known as Schwalbe line, is a gonioscopic landmark that defines the end of Descemet membrane and the beginning of the trabecular meshwork.

The Descemet membrane is attached to the corneal stroma by a narrow (about 1 µm thick) transitional zone of amorphous extracellular matrix termed the "interfacial matrix," which contains increased amounts of adhesive glycoproteins such as fibronectin (Fig. 2G,H) [4]. Connecting collagen fibers projecting from the "Bowman-like" stromal layer into this interfacial matrix zone further promotes anchorage. Extracellular matrix complexes formed by keratoepithelin (transforming growth factor β-induced) and collagen type VI are also involved in maintaining adherence at Descemet membrane–stroma interface. Adhesive forces appear to be slightly stronger in the central than in the peripheral parts of the cornea.

6 Corneal Endothelium

The innermost layer of the cornea, the corneal endothelium, is a single layer of cuboidal cells, which have a critical role in maintaining corneal hydration and, thus, transparency (Fig. 2G). The cells, which form a hexagonal honeycomb-like mosaic when viewed from the posterior surface, are 5–6 µm in height and 18–20 µm in diameter. Some cells have apical cilia, which play a role in morphogenesis and repair of the endothelial monolayer [40]. Their lateral surfaces are highly interdigitated and possess apical junctional complexes comprising both gap and tight junctions, forming a leaky barrier and allowing paracellular movement of fluid and substances from the aqueous into the cornea. The basal surface of the endothelium contains hemidesmosomes that promote adhesion to Descemet membrane. The endothelial layer is responsible for the dehydration of the cornea and maintenance of corneal transparency by pumping water out of the corneal stroma [41]. The dehydration process is described by the "pump-leak hypothesis," in which leakage of solutes and nutrients from aqueous humor to superficial layers of the cornea is counteracted by pumping water in the opposite direction. This passive bulk fluid movement is fueled by the energy-requiring processes of transporting ions to generate the osmotic gradient. The most important ion transport systems are the membrane-bound sodium/potassium ATPase and the intracellular carbonic anhydrase, producing a net flux of ions from the stroma to the aqueous humor [42]. The number of endothelial cells decreases with age, trauma, inflammation, surgery, and disease processes such as Fuchs' endothelial dystrophy. Endothelial cell density at birth is approximately 3500–4000 cells/mm^2, decreasing gradually at an average rate of 0.6% per year to 2500 cells/mm^2 at age 50 and 2000 cells/mm^2 at age 80 [43]. Endothelial cells of the human cornea have a low proliferative capacity, and lost cells are replaced by the spreading of adjacent cells, resulting in an increase in cell size (polymegethism) and an increase in variation of cell shape (pleomorphism). With increasing cell loss, the pump and barrier functions of the endothelium may be compromised. A density lower than 400–500 cells/mm^2 may lead to endothelial decompensation and corneal edema with concomitant loss of transparency [44].

CLSM using long-stroke piezo-based control elements is now capable of imaging and evaluating the entire human cornea from epithelium to endothelium during one single examination procedure. These studies confirmed former findings that keratocyte density in the anterior stroma is significantly higher than that of the middle and posterior stroma [45]. In Fig. 5, an exemplarily result is demonstrated (Fig. 5). The idea that there is a keratocyte-free layer in front of the Descemet membrane could be disproved, confirming light and electron microscopic multicenter studies [3].

Figure 5A shows the sagittal section of a subject along its optical axis calculated from the volume data set. Inconspicuous wing cells (z = 20 µm) are found in Fig. 5B, an unremarkable SNP without dendritic cells (z = 45 µm) in Fig. 5C, and the structureless Bowman layer (z = 55 µm) in Fig. 5D. The highly reflective keratocyte nuclei with a maximum diameter of 20 µm are much more densely packed in the anterior layers of the stroma (e) than in the intermediate and posterior stroma (Figs. 5F–H). There, the nuclear shapes are generally elongated with a length-to-width ratio of about 1:4 to 1:6 (Fig. 5E–H). The nuclei can be seen up to about 10 µm in front of the Descemet membrane, which itself has no scattering light sources (Fig. 5I). The endothelial cells appear similar to those seen in specular microscopy and have in this individual a cell density of approximately 2200 cells per mm^2 (Fig. 5J). In the present example, the central corneal thickness is 464 µm, which corresponds to the position of the superficial up to the endothelial cells.

The dataset used in Fig. 5 allows 3D reconstruction of the central area of the cornea (Fig. 6). This figure displays a tissue cuboid of 464 × 225 × 125 µm.

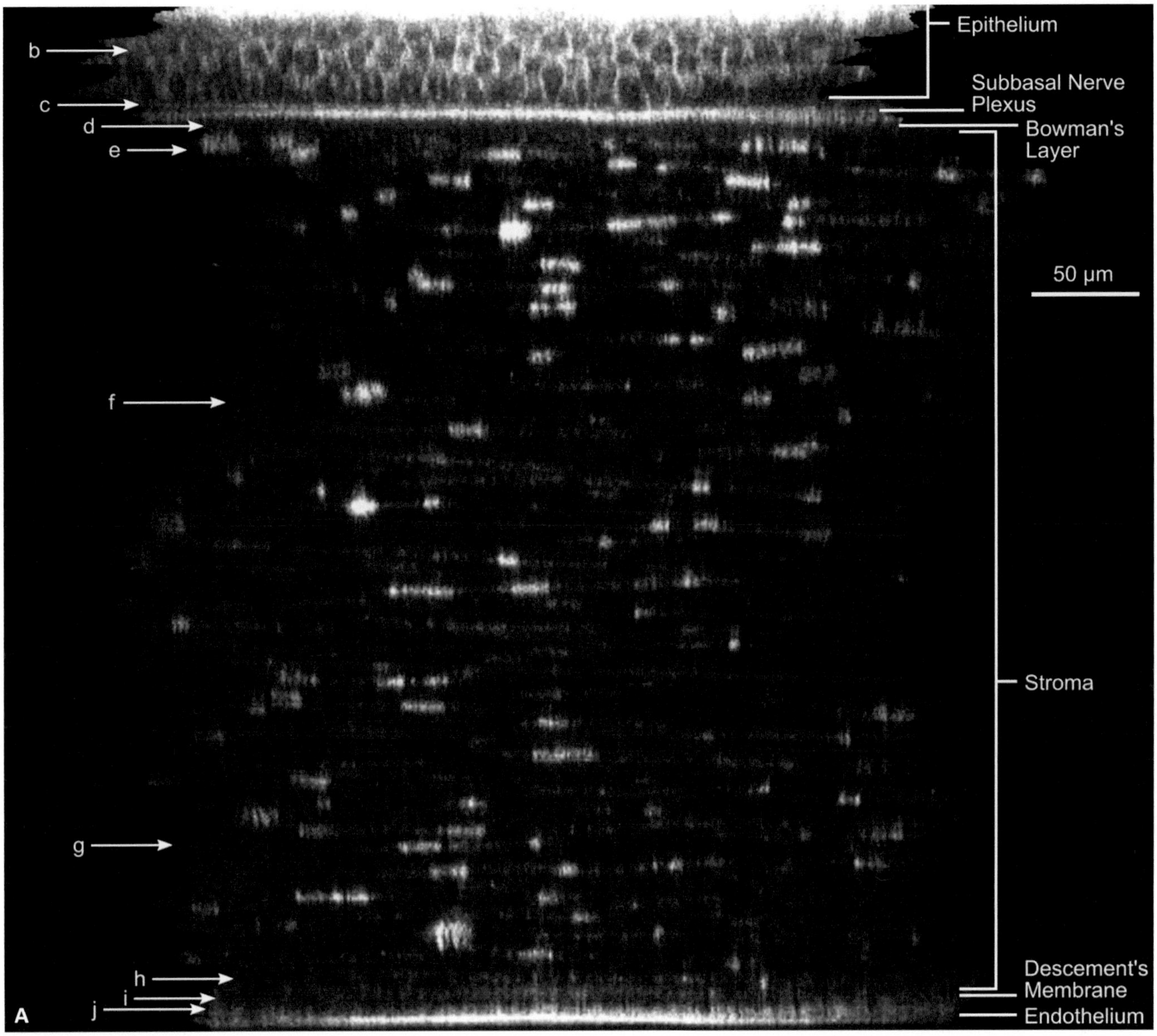

Fig. 5 (**A**) In vivo confocal laser scanning microscopy (CLSM)-based imaging of a 54-year-old healthy volunteer

7 Corneal Innervation

The cornea is densely innervated by unmyelinated sensory nerve fibers derived from the trigeminal nerve, mainly via the long ciliary nerves. About 70 main nerve bundles enter the peripheral cornea in a radial manner and move centrally in the anterior one-third of the stroma. They divide into smaller branches and penetrate Bowman layer to form the subepithelial or SNP at the interface between the Bowman layer and the corneal epithelium [46] (Fig. 7).

The complex morphology and dynamics of this SNP are now, since confocal microscopy are freely available for clinicians, a matter of intensive research [4, 48]. It could be demonstrated for the first time by Patel and McGhee [49] that "with the recent application of laser scanning in vivo confocal microscopy, the micromorphological pattern of the SNP could be fully identified for the first time highlighting a previously unknown orientation towards a whirl-like complex, 1–2 mm inferior to the apex. This differs significantly from the nerve pattern in keratoconus patients. It is

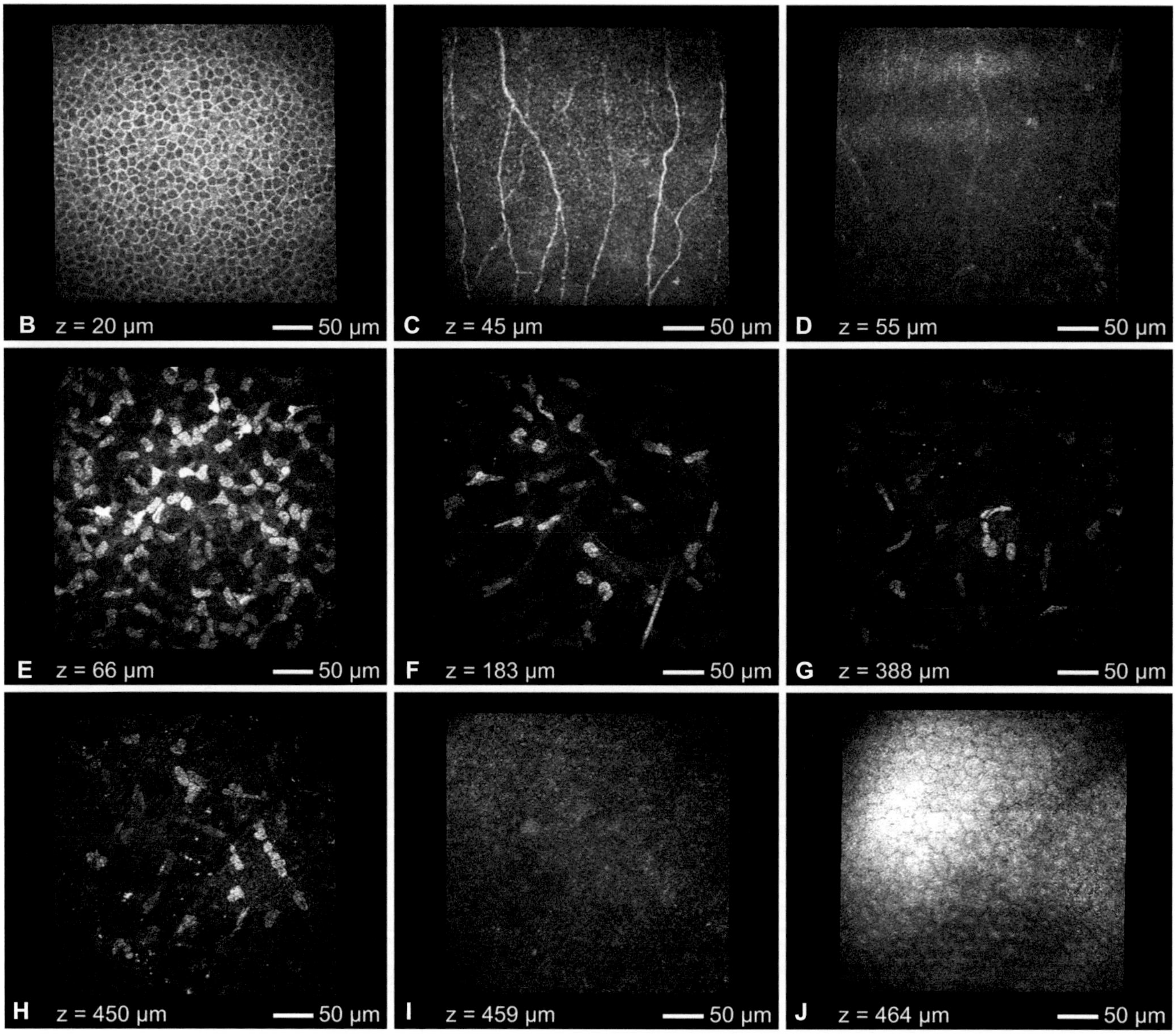

Fig. 5 Figures (**B–J**) show sections parallel to the surface at the depths indicated in a. Please note the obvious difference in the density of keratocyte nuclei between the anterior stroma (**E**) and deeper stromal layers (**F–H**)

our challenge to identify the variations of this previously unknown configuration to possibly subclassify diseases with related abnormalities in corneal innervation [50]."

A large-scale CLSM-generated representation of the SNP (approximately 12 mm^2 of the central corneal surface) is shown in Fig. 8.

Individual fibers penetrate all epithelial layers and terminate in the superficial layers. It is estimated that there are approx. 7000 nociceptors per mm^2 in the human corneal epithelium [15]. The density of nerve endings per unit area is 400 times higher than in the skin, making the cornea one of the most densely innervated tissues in the body. In conformity with the density of nerve endings, corneal sensitivity increases from the limbus to the central cornea. Corneal nerves release neuropeptides, such as substance P and calcitonin gene-related peptide (CGRP), which have important trophic functions on the corneal epithelium and stimulate epithelial wound healing [51]. Loss of corneal sensory innervation can lead to neurotrophic keratopathy, involving epithelial defects, poor wound healing, and ulcers [52].

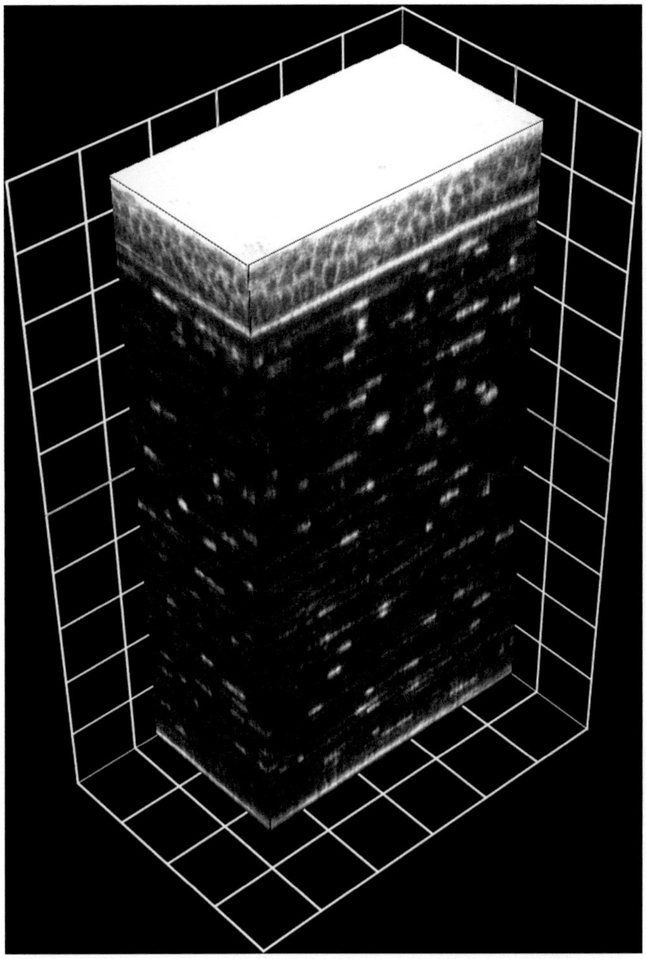

Fig. 6 3D reconstruction of a tissue cuboid of a healthy central human cornea based on the dataset from Fig. 5. Edge length of a box: 50 μm

8 Corneal Immune Privilege

Since corneal avascularity is an essential factor for corneal transparency, the cornea has developed strategies to maintain avascularity, a phenomenon termed "corneal antiangiogenic privilege" [36, 53]. Several antiangiogenic factors have been shown to contribute to corneal avascularity, including pigment epithelium-derived factor (PEDF), thrombospondins, and receptors binding and inactivating angiogenic growth factors like vascular endothelial growth factor (VEGF). The strong expression of VEGF receptor 3 on the corneal epithelium, which is normally expressed on vascular endothelial cells, seems to be especially potent. The cornea has also developed strategies to minimize inflammatory reactions, a phenomenon termed "corneal immune privilege." The success of allogeneic corneal transplantation benefits from this property, which is attributed to multiple anatomical, physiological, and immunoregulatory factors [54]. For instance, the absence of blood and lymph vessels in the graft bed is essential for graft survival. Thus, the molecular mechanisms of immune privilege are similar to those mediating avascularity, e.g., thrombospondin-1 is involved in both processes. Corneal epithelial and stromal cells secrete soluble factors, including VEGFR-2 and endostatin, which inhibit lymphangiogenesis and hemangiogenesis, thereby maintaining immune privilege [55]. The corneal endothelium also expresses membrane-bound molecules, such as Fas ligand (FasL), which defend against immune effector cells, including T-cells and components of the complement cascade. Another mechanism contributing to the success of allogeneic corneal transplantation is "anterior chamber associated immune deviation (ACAID)," which is defined as the systemic downregulation of an immune response against antigens injected into the anterior chamber of the eye [54]. As a consequence, immune reactions against, e.g., donor endothelial antigens are less destructive.

Nevertheless, the central corneal stroma and epithelium are endowed with significant numbers of resident MHC class II-negative inflammatory and antigen-presenting cells, including dendritic cells and epithelial Langerhans cells as well as macrophages [56, 57]. These cells become activated and increase in numbers after contact lens use and inflammation (Fig. 2.2d), causing higher injection rates in inflamed high-risk recipient beds [48].

Previously elusive antigen-presenting dendritic cells (Langerhans cells) have now become a well-recognized clinical phenomenon in the human cornea [58]. They present as bright corpuscular particles with characteristic dendritic cell morphology. Moreover, in vivo confocal microscopy possibly permits differentiation between 'immature' and 'mature' types, the latter being more frequently observed in patients treated long-term with topical eye drops containing preservatives [50].

In Fig. 9, Langerhans cell clusters are demonstrated as they were detected in an inconspicuous cornea in a patient after starting chemotherapy for breast cancer (Fig. 9). Similar findings could be observed in a patient with rheumatoid arthritis and keratitis, where slit lamp examination only demonstrated a mild anterior stroma opacification (Fig. 10). Sections parallel to the surface show normal wing cells at a depth of 25 μm (Fig. 10B), between 44 μm and 53 μm there are massive infiltrates with dendritic cells (Fig. 10C). In the anterior and intermediate stroma, a dense network of keratocyte structures is found, some with high reflective cytoplasm (Fig. 10D).

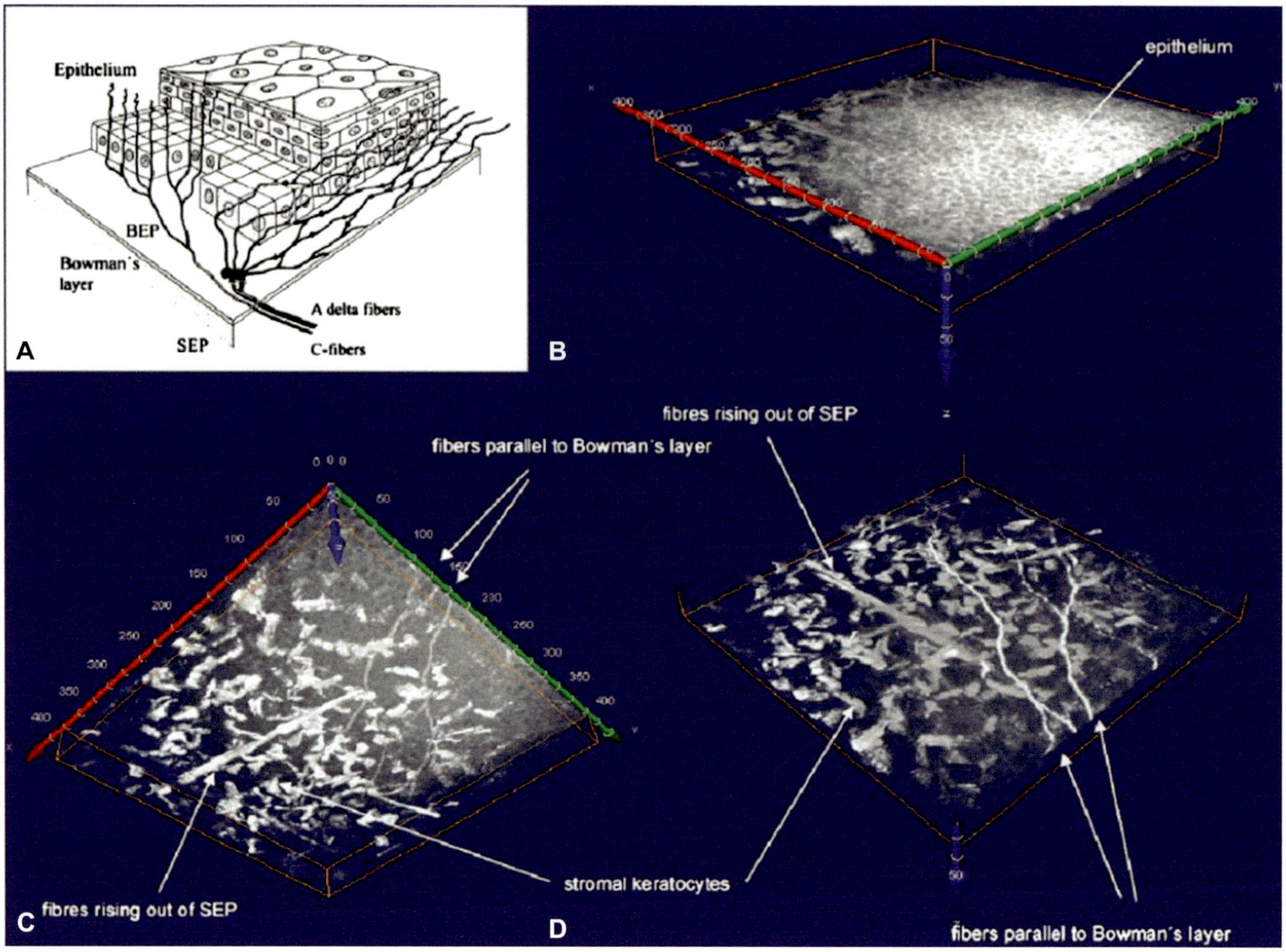

Fig. 7 (**A**) Schematic drawing according to Guthoff et al. [47]; (**B–D**) 3D-reconstruction of the corneal epithelium with anterior stroma and nerves: (**B**) anterior view; (**C**) posterior view; (**D**) anterior view with virtual removal of the epithelium (100 pixels = 78 μm)

Sections parallel to the surface show normal wing cells at a depth of 25 μm (Fig. 10B), and massive infiltrates are found between 40 μm and 50 μm (Fig. 10C) with dendritic cells, which can also be identified on the Bowman layer with markedly reduced SNP. In the anterior and intermediate stroma, there is a dense network of keratocyte structures, some with extremely highly reflective cytoplasm, and cell nuclei can no longer be demarcated in the deeper stroma (Fig. 10D).

In Fig. 11, which displays a 3D reconstruction of this opacified cornea, the localization of Langerhans cells and their relation to the anterior keratocytes is illustrated (Fig. 11).

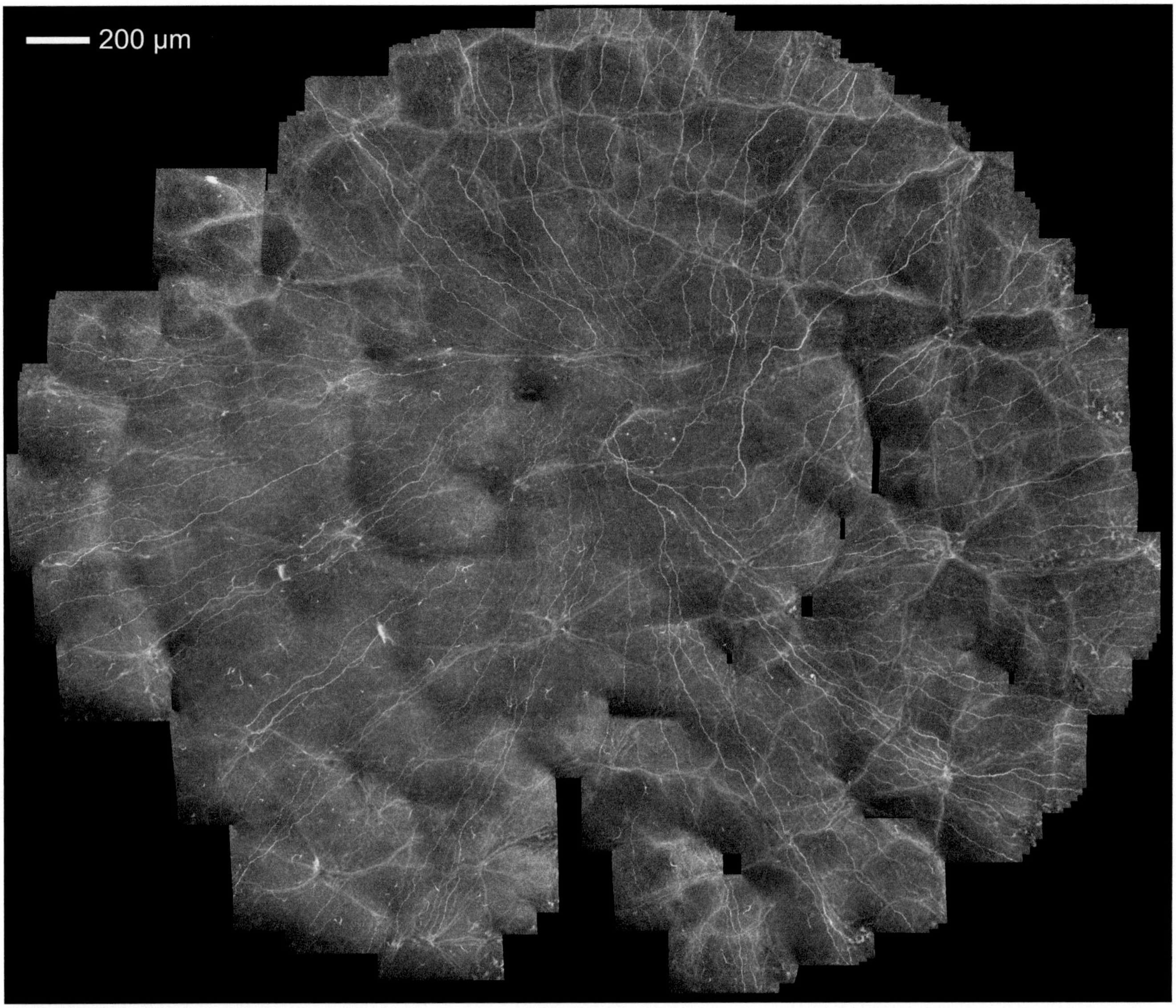

Fig. 8 In vivo large-area confocal laser scanning microscopy (CLSM) of the subbasal nerve plexus (SNP) of a human cornea. The so-called whirl of the nerve fibers is displayed visibly in the center of the image

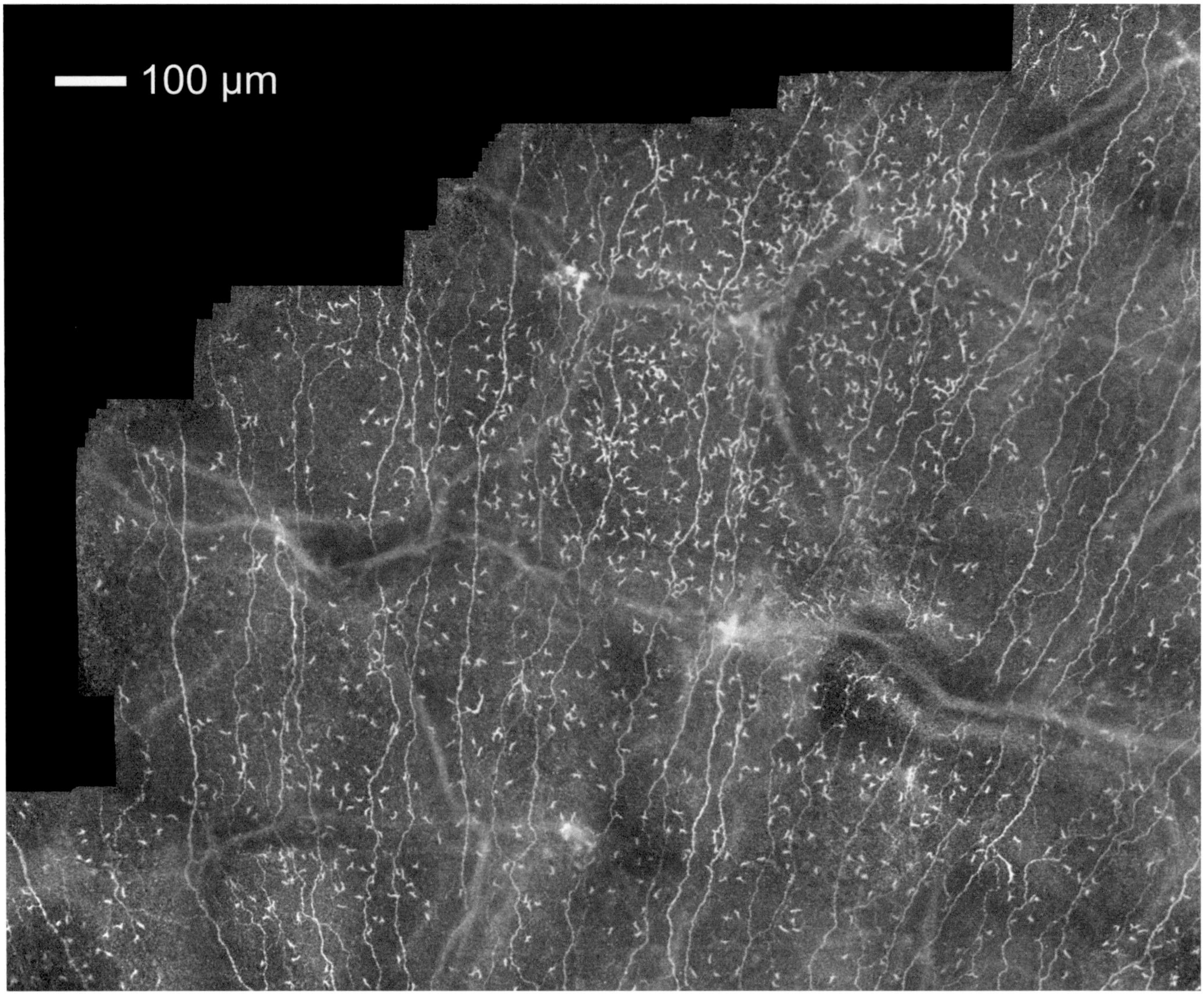

Fig. 9 Image section of in vivo large-area confocal laser scanning microscopy (CLSM) of the subbasal nerve plexus (SNP) of a human epidermal growth factor receptor (HER)-2 positive breast cancer patient during paclitaxel and trastuzumab therapy. Local differences in dendritic cell (DC) density could be observed 11 weeks after the start of therapy [59, 60]

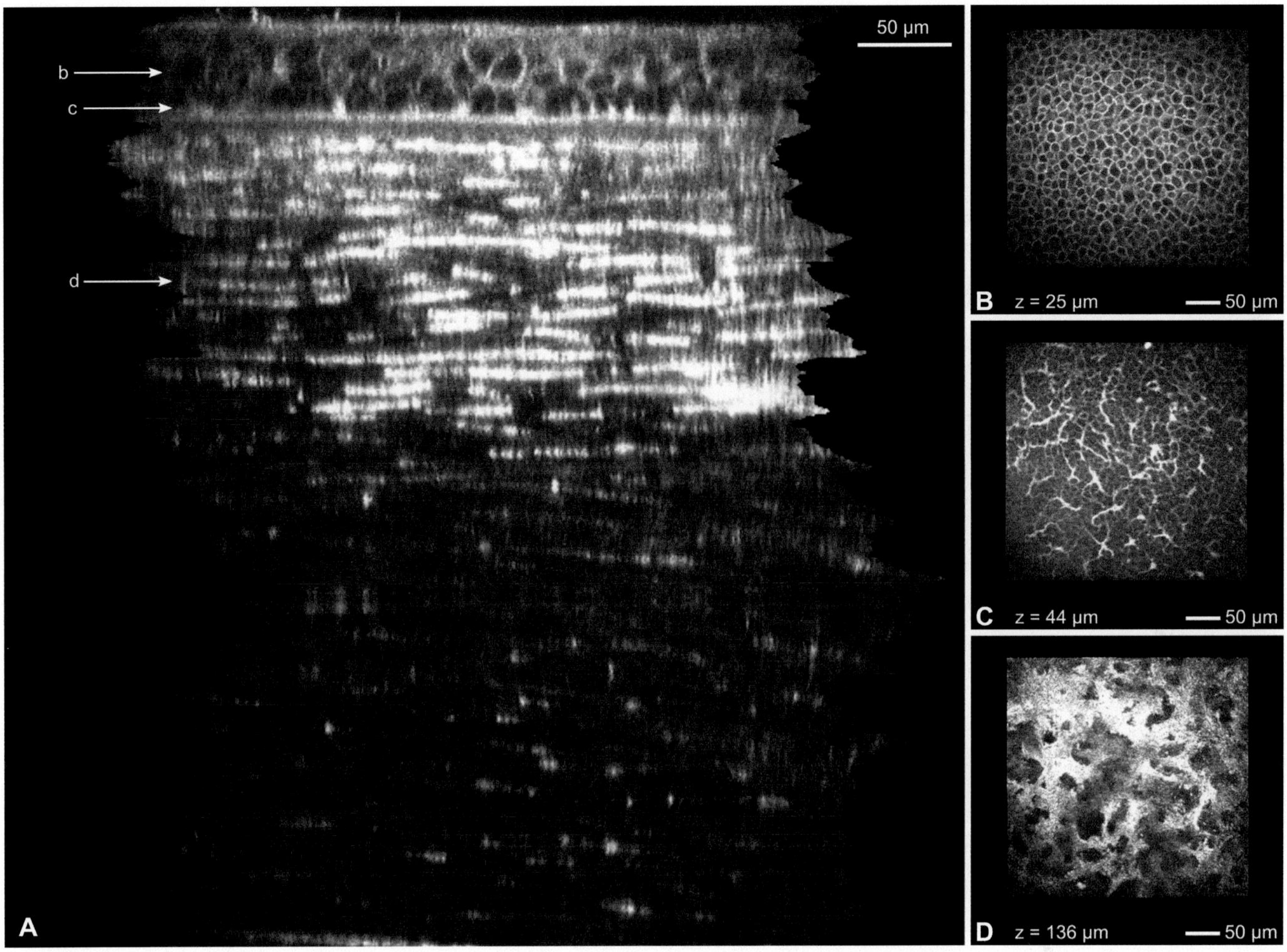

Fig. 10 Confocal microscopy of the cornea of a 49-year-old patient with chronic rheumatoid arthritis (**A**). Sections of the epithelium parallel to the surface show normal wing cells (**B**). Compared to slit lamp microscopy (mild diffuse opacity of the anterior stroma), in vivo confocal laser scanning microscopy (CLSM) displays dense infiltration on Bowman layer with Langerhans cells (**C**) and opacities of the adjacent corneal layers limited to the keratocytes (**A**). The opacifying elements in the stroma can be assigned with high probability to the cytoplasmic structures of the keratocyte (**D**). Deeper stromal layers demonstrate inconspicuous keratocyte structures

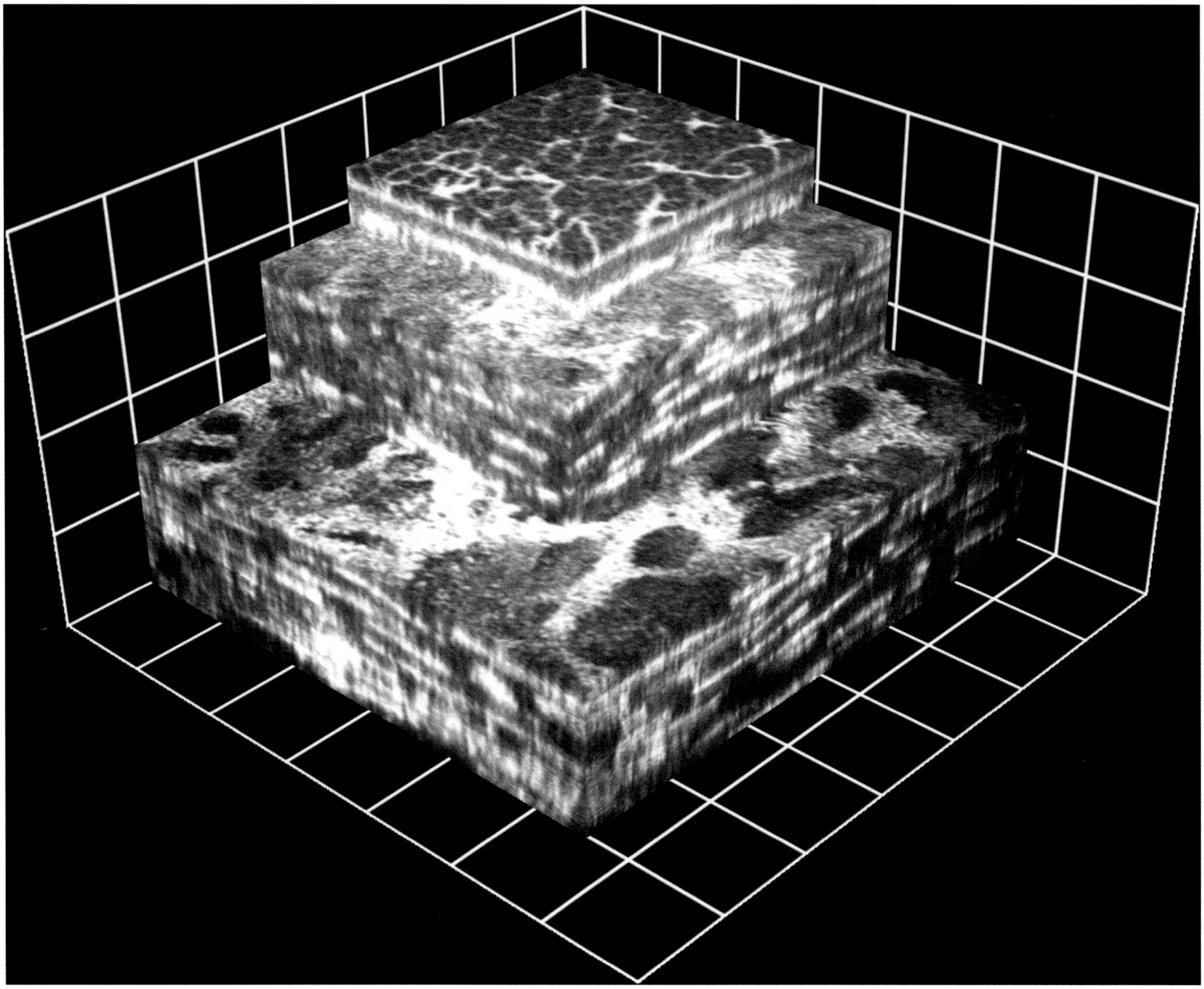

Fig. 11 3D reconstruction of the full data set of Fig. 10. In the upper part of the cuboid, Langerhans cells are visible on the Bowman layer. In the middle and lower block, highly reflective keratocytes with cytoplasmic extensions that appear to be in contact with their neighboring cells (syncytium) are visible. Edge length of a box: 50 μm

9 Conclusion

The high magnification of in vivo CLSM (approximately 800 fold) allows clinically a sub-differentiation of the complex structure of the cornea. Taking into account that its anatomical structure can, for the first time, be differentiated, displaying single cells in vivo, this technique gives rise to new questions for a deeper understanding of the pathogenesis of corneal diseases. It already found its place in the management of fungal and acanthamoebae infections. New insights have been achieved in recent years for the understanding of diabetic neuropathy, which can be first noticed by changes in the corneal SNP. This precedes any other morphological or functional change of the disease complex of diabetes mellitus. Corneal Langerhans cells, before the introduction of laser scanning in vivo microscopy, had been totally hidden from the clinician. The inclusion of Langerhans cell density and its irregular distribution at the level of the Bowman layer now enables a more precise description of immunological processes, offering new data for diagnosis and follow-up.

As we better define the morphology and functional relationships of Langerhans cells to surrounding tissues, the timing of surgical procedures such as corneal transplantation and refractive surgery may possibly be influenced by the presence and even shape or absence of such dendritic cells in the central and peripheral cornea.

The authors of the chapter hope that readers will enjoy and gain new stimuli addressing clinical and scientific challenges.

References

1. DelMonte DW, Kim T. Anatomy and physiology of the cornea. J Cataract Refract Surg. 2011;37:588–98. https://doi.org/10.1016/j.jcrs.2010.12.037.
2. Dua HS, Faraj LA, Said DG, Gray T, Lowe J. Human corneal anatomy redefined: a novel pre-Descemet's layer (Dua's layer). Ophthalmology. 2013;120:1778–85. https://doi.org/10.1016/j.ophtha.2013.01.018.
3. Schlötzer-Schrehardt U, Bachmann BO, Tourtas T, Torricelli AA, Singh A, Gonzalez S, Mei H, Deng SX, Wilson SE, Kruse FE. Ultrastructure of the posterior corneal stroma. Ophthalmology. 2015;122:693–9. https://doi.org/10.1016/j.ophtha.2014.09.037.
4. Schlötzer-Schrehardt U, Bachmann BO, Laaser K, Cursiefen C, Kruse FE. Characterization of the cleavage plane in Descemet's membrane endothelial keratoplasty. Ophthalmology. 2011;118:1950–7. https://doi.org/10.1016/j.ophtha.2011.03.025.
5. Poothullil AM, Gipson IK. Cornea: structural features and wound healing. In: John T, editor. Lamellar corneal surgery. New York: The McGraw-Hill Companies;2008. p. 3–14. ISBN-13: 9780071601924.
6. Hovakimyan M, Falke K, Stahnke T, Guthoff R, Witt M, Wree A, Stachs O. Morphological analysis of quiescent and activated keratocytes: a review of ex vivo and in vivo findings. Curr Eye Res. 2014;39(12):1129–44. https://doi.org/10.3109/02713683.2014.902073.
7. Bohn S, Sperlich K, Allgeier S, Bartschat A, Prakasam R, Reichert KM, Stolz H, Guthoff R, Mikut R, Köhler B, Stachs O. Cellular in vivo 3D imaging of the cornea by confocal laser scanning microscopy. Biomed Opt Express. 2018;9(6):2511–25. https://doi.org/10.1364/BOE.9.002511.
8. Georgiev GA, Yokoi N, Ivanova S, Tonchev V, Nencheva Y, Krastev R. Surface relaxations as a tool to distinguish the dynamic interfacial properties of films formed by normal and diseased meibomian lipids. Soft Matter. 2014;10(30):5579–88. https://doi.org/10.1039/c4sm00758a.
9. King-Smith PE, Hinel EA, Nichols JJ. Application of a novel interferometric method to investigate the relation between lipid layer thickness and tear film thinning. Invest Ophthalmol Vis Sci. 2010;51(5):2418–23. https://doi.org/10.1167/iovs.09-4387.
10. King-Smith PE, Ramamoorthy P, Braun RJ, Nichols JJ. Tear film images and breakup analyzed using fluorescent quenching. Invest Ophthalmol Vis Sci. 2013;54(9):6003–11. https://doi.org/10.1167/iovs.13-12628.
11. King-Smith PE, Reuter KS, Braun RJ, Nichols JJ, Nichols KK. Tear film breakup and structure studied by simultaneous video recording of fluorescence and tear film lipid layer images. Invest Ophthalmol Vis Sci. 2013;54(7):4900–9. https://doi.org/10.1167/iovs.13-11878.
12. Millar TJ, Schuett BS. The real reason for having a meibomian lipid layer covering the outer surface of the tear film-A review. Exp Eye Res. 2015;137:125–38. https://doi.org/10.1016/j.exer.2015.05.002.
13. Torricelli AA, Wilson SE. Cellular and extracellular matrix modulation of corneal stromal opacity. Exp Eye Res. 2014;129:151–60. https://doi.org/10.1016/j.exer.2014.09.013.
14. Gipson IK. Adhesive mechanisms of the corneal epithelium. Acta Ophthalmol Suppl. 1992;202:13–7. https://doi.org/10.1111/j.1755-3768.1992.tb02162.x.
15. Müller LJ, Marfurt CF, Kruse F, Tervo TM. Corneal nerves: structure, contents and function. Exp Eye Res. 2003;76:521–42. https://doi.org/10.1016/s0014-4835(03)00050-2.
16. Knickelbein JE, Buela KA, Hendricks RL. Antigen-presenting cells are stratified within normal human corneas and are rapidly mobilized during ex vivo viral infection. Invest Ophthalmol Vis Sci. 2014;55:1118–23. https://doi.org/10.1167/iovs.13-13523.
17. Beebe DC, Masters BR. Cell lineage and the differentiation of corneal epithelial cells. Invest Ophthalmol Vis Sci. 1996;37:1815–25 PMID: 8759349.
18. Cotsarelis G, Cheng SZ, Dong G, Sun TT, Lavker RM. Existence of slow-cycling limbal epithelial basal cells that can be preferentially stimulated to proliferate: implications on epithelial stem cells. Cell. 1989;57:201–9. https://doi.org/10.1016/0092-8674(89)90958-6.
19. Ahmad S. Concise review: limbal stem cell deficiency, dysfunction, and distress. Stem Cells Transl Med. 2012;1:110–5. https://doi.org/10.5966/sctm.2011-0037.
20. Kenyon KR, Tseng SC. Limbal autograft transplantation for ocular surface disorders. Ophthalmology. 1989;96:709–22. https://doi.org/10.1016/s0161-6420(89)32833-8.
21. Shortt AJ, Secker GA, Notara MD, Limb GA, Khaw PT, Tuft SJ, Daniels JT. Transplantation of ex vivo cultured limbal epithelial stem cells: a review of techniques and clinical results. Surv Ophthalmol. 2007;52:483–502. https://doi.org/10.1016/j.survophthal.2007.06.013.
22. Wilson SE, Hong JW. Bowman's layer structure and function: critical or dispensable to corneal function? A hypothesis Cornea. 2000;19:417–20.https://doi.org/10.1097/00003226-200007000-00001.
23. Germundsson J, Karanis G, Fagerholm P, Lagali N. Age-related thinning of Bowman's layer in the human cornea in vivo. Invest Ophthalmol Vis Sci. 2013;54:6143–9. https://doi.org/10.1167/iovs.13-12535.
24. Hassell JR, Birk DE. The molecular basis of corneal transparency. Exp Eye Res. 2010;91:326–35. https://doi.org/10.1016/j.exer.2010.06.021.
25. Komai Y, Ushiki T. The three-dimensional organization of collagen fibrils in the human cornea and sclera. Invest Ophthalmol Vis Sci. 1991;32:2244–58 PMID: 2071337.
26. Meek KM, Leonard DW. Ultrastructure of the corneal stroma: a comparative study. Biophys J. 1993;64:273–80. https://doi.org/10.1016/S0006-3495(93)81364-X.
27. Müller LJ, Pels E, Schurmans LR, Vrensen GF. A new three-dimensional model of the organization of proteoglycans and collagen fibrils in the human corneal stroma. Exp Eye Res. 2004;78:493–501. https://doi.org/10.1016/s0014-4835(03)00206-9.
28. Michelacci YM. Collagens and proteoglycans of the corneal extracellular matrix. Braz J Med Biol Res. 2003;36:1037–46. https://doi.org/10.1590/s0100-879x2003000800009.
29. Meek KM, Boote C. The organization of collagen in the corneal stroma. Exp Eye Res. 2004;78:503–12. https://doi.org/10.1016/j.exer.2003.07.003.
30. Müller LJ, Pels E, Vrensen GF. The specific architecture of the anterior stroma accounts for maintenance of corneal curvature. Br J Ophthalmol. 2001;85:437–43. https://doi.org/10.1136/bjo.85.4.43.
31. Müller LJ, Pels L, Vrensen GF. Novel aspects of the ultrastructural organization of human corneal keratocytes. Invest Ophthalmol Vis Sci. 1995;36:2557–67 PMID: 7499078.
32. Poole CA, Brookes NH, Clover GM. Confocal imaging of the human keratocyte network using the vital dye 5-chloromethylfluorescein diacetate. Clin Experiment Ophthalmol. 2003;31:147–54. https://doi.org/10.1046/j.1442-9071.2003.00623.x.

33. Chen S, Mienaltowski MJ, Birk DE. Regulation of corneal stroma extracellular matrix assembly. Exp Eye Res. 2015;133:69–80. https://doi.org/10.1016/j.exer.2014.08.001.
34. Jester JV, Moller-Pedersen T, Huang J, Sax CM, Kays WT, Cavangh HD, Petroll WM, Piatigorsky J. The cellular basis of corneal transparency: evidence for 'corneal crystallins.' J Cell Sci. 1999;112:613–22. https://doi.org/10.1242/jcs.112.5.613.
35. Stachs O, Zhivov A, Kraak R, Hovakimyan M, Wree A, Guthoff R. Structural-functional correlations of corneal innervation after LASIK and penetrating keratoplasty. J Refract Surg. 2010;26:159–67. https://doi.org/10.3928/1081597X-20100224-01.
36. Cursiefen C, Kruse FE, Naumann GOH. Special anatomy and pathology in intraocular microsurgery: cornea and limbus. In: Naumann GOH, Holbach L, Kruse FE, editors. Applied pathology for ophthalmic microsurgeons. Berlin/Heidelberg: Springer; 1st ed. 2008;97–130. ISBN-13: 978–3642063381.
37. Dua HS, Faraj LA, Branch MJ, Yeung AM, Elalfy MS, Said DG, Gray T, Lowe J. The collagen matrix of the human trabecular meshwork is an extension of the novel pre-Descemet's layer (Dua's layer). Br J Ophthalmol. 2014;98(5):691–7. https://doi.org/10.1136/bjophthalmol-2013-304593.
38. Johnson DH, Bourne WM, Campbell RJ. The ultrastructure of Descemet's membrane. I. Changes with age in normal corneas. Arch Ophthalmol. 1982;100:1942–1947. https://doi.org/10.1001/archopht.1982.01030040922011.
39. Murphy C, Alvarado J, Juster R. Prenatal and postnatal growth of the human Descemet's membrane. Invest Ophthalmol Vis Sci. 1984;25:1402–15 PMID: 6511224.
40. Blitzer AL, Panagis L, Gusella GL, Danias J, Mlodzik M, Iomini C. Primary cilia dynamics instruct tissue patterning and repair of corneal endothelium. Proc Natl Acad Sci USA. 2011;108:2819–24. https://doi.org/10.1073/pnas.1016702108.
41. Geroski DH, Matsuda M, Yee RW, Edelhauser HF. Pump function of the human corneal endothelium. Effects of age and cornea guttata. Ophthalmology. 1985;92:759–763. https://doi.org/10.1016/s0161-6420(85)33973-8.
42. Bonanno JA. Molecular mechanisms underlying the corneal endothelial pump. Exp Eye Res. 2012;95:2–7. https://doi.org/10.1016/j.exer.2011.06.004.
43. Bahn CF, Glassman RM, MacCallum DK, Lillie JH, Meyer RF, Robinson BJ, Rich NM. Postnatal development of corneal endothelium. Invest Ophthalmol Vis Sci. 1986;27:44–51 PMID: 3941037.
44. Vaiciuliene R, Rylskyte N, Baguzyte G, Jasinskas V. Risk factors for fluctuations in corneal endothelial cell density (Review). Exp Ther Med. 2022;23(2):129. https://doi.org/10.3892/etm.2021.11052.
45. Berlau J, Becker HH, Stave J, Oriwol C, Guthoff RF. Depth and age-dependent distribution of keratocytes in healthy human corneas: a study using scanning-slit confocal microscopy in vivo. J Cataract Refract Surg. 2002;28(4):611–6. https://doi.org/10.1016/s0886-3350(01)01227-5. PMID: 11955900.
46. Stachs O, Zhivov A, Kraak R, Stave J, Guthoff R. In vivo three-dimensional confocal laser scanning microscopy of the epithelial nerve structure in the human cornea. Graefes Arch Clin Exp Ophthalmol. 2007;245(4):569–75. https://doi.org/10.1007/s00417-006-0387-2.
47. Guthoff RF, Wree A, Wienss H, Hahnel C. Epithelial innervation of human cornea: a three-dimensional study using confocal laser scanning fluorescence microscopy. Cornea. 2005;24(5):608–13. https://doi.org/10.1097/01.ico.0000154384.05614.8f
48. Cruzat A, Witkin D, Baniasadi N, Zheng L, Ciolino JB, Jurkunas UV, Chodosh J, Pavan-Langston D, Dana R, Hamrah P. Inflammation and the nervous system: the connection in the cornea in patients with infectious keratitis. Invest Ophthalmol Vis Sci. 2011;52:5136–43. https://doi.org/10.1167/iovs.10-7048.
49. Patel DV, McGhee CNJ. Mapping the corneal sub-basal nerve plexus in keratoconus by in vivo laser scanning confocal microscopy. Invest Ophthalmol Vis Sci. 2006;47(4):1348–51. https://doi.org/10.1167/iovs.05-1217
50. Guthoff RF, Stachs O, Stave J. From bench to bedside–in vivo confocal imaging on its way to a clinical decision-making tool. Clin Exp Ophthalmol. 2007;35:1–2. https://doi.org/10.1111/j.1442-9071.2007.01431.x.
51. Garcia-Hirschfeld J, Lopez-Briones LG, Belmonte C. Neurotrophic influences on corneal epithelial cells. Exp Eye Res. 1994;59:597–605. https://doi.org/10.1006/exer.1994.1145.
52. De Clerck EE, Schouten JS, Berendschot TT, Kessels AG, Nuijts RM, Beckers HJ, Schram MT, Stehouwer CD, Webers CA. New ophthalmologic imaging techniques for detection and monitoring of neurodegenerative changes in diabetes: a systematic review. Lancet Diabetes Endocrinol. 2015;3(8):653–63. https://doi.org/10.1016/S2213-8587(15)00136-9.
53. Azar DT. Corneal angiogenic privilege: angiogenic and antiangiogenic factors in corneal avascularity, vasculogenesis, and wound healing (an American Ophthalmological Society thesis). Trans Am Ophthalmol Soc. 2006;104:264–302 PMID: 17471348.
54. Niederkorn JY. Corneal transplantation and immune privilege. Int Rev Immunol. 2013;32:57–67. https://doi.org/10.3109/08830185.2012.737877.
55. Albuquerque RJ, Hayashi T, Cho WG, Kleinman ME, Dridi S, Takeda A, Baffi JZ, Yamada K, Kaneko H, Green MG, Chappell J, Wilting J, Weich HA, Yamagami S, Amano S, Mizuki N, Alexander JS, Peterson ML, Brekken RA, Hirashima M, Capoor S, Usui T, Ambati BK, Ambati J. Alternatively spliced vascular endothelial growth factor receptor-2 is an essential endogenous inhibitor of lymphatic vessel growth. Nat Med. 2009;15:1023–30. https://doi.org/10.1038/nm.2018.
56. Chinnery HR, Leong CM, Chen W, Forrester JV, McMenamin PG. TLR9 and TLR7/8 activation induces formation of keratic precipitates and giant macrophages in the mouse cornea. J Leukoc Biol. 2015;97:103–10. https://doi.org/10.1189/jlb.3AB0414-216R.
57. Hamrah P, Liu Y, Zhang Q, et al. The corneal stroma is endowed with a significant number of resident dendritic cells. Invest Ophthalmol Vis Sci. 2003;44:581–9. https://doi.org/10.1167/iovs.02-0838.
58. Zhivov A, Stave J, Vollmar B, Guthoff RF. In-vivo confocal microscopic evaluation of Langerhans cell density and distribution in the normal human corneal epithelium. Graefes Arch Clin Exp Ophthalmol. 2005;243:1056–61. https://doi.org/10.1007/s00417-004-1075-8.
59. Sterenczak KA, Stache N, Bohn S, Allgeier S, Köhler B, Bartschat A, George C, Guthoff RF, Stachs O, Stachs A. Burst of corneal dendritic cells during Trastuzumab and paclitaxel treatment. Diagnostics (Basel). 2021;11(5):838. https://doi.org/10.3390/diagnostics11050838.
60. Bohn S, Stache N, Sperlich K, Allgeier S, Köhler B, Bartschat A, Do HV, George C, Guthoff RF, Stachs A, Stachs O, Sterenczak KA. In Vivo monitoring of corneal dendritic cells in the subbasal nerve plexus during Trastuzumab and paclitaxel breast cancer therapy-A one-year follow-up. Diagnostics (Basel). 2022;12(5):1180. https://doi.org/10.3390/diagnostics12051180.

Optics and Surgery

Optics and Impact on IOL Power Calculation

Achim Langenbucher, Alan Cayless, and Jens Schrecker

Abstract

For more than 70 years, implantable intraocular lenses have been used in cataract surgery as a routine replacement for the opaque crystalline lens, preventing postoperative aphakia. Intraocular lenses can also be implanted into the phakic eye to adjust refraction in cases where corneal refractive surgery is contraindicated. IOLs as supplementary lenses can also be an option for pseudophakic eyes to correct for residual refractive error. Such lenses must be selected carefully for each individual patient. There are different options for calculating the refractive power of intraocular lenses for a given patient, based on biometric measures and intended target refraction. These options include empirical calculation strategies (using a big data approach), formula based calculations (with formulae based on simplified linear Gaussian optics), and (numerical) raytracing. In this chapter we summarise the available strategies for calculating standard stigmatic lenses, toric lenses for correction of corneal astigmatism, and supplementary lenses. The relevant input parameters will be discussed and the fundamentals for extracting formula constants outlined, using methods based on clinical datasets of preoperative biometric measures and postoperative outcome data to tune the results and reduce the calculation prediction error for future cataract surgeries.

A. Langenbucher (✉) · J. Schrecker
Department of Experimental Ophthalmology, Saarland University, Homburg/Saar, Germany
e-mail: achim.langenbucher@uni-saarland.de

A. Cayless
School of Physical Sciences, The Open University, Milton Keynes, UK

J. Schrecker
Department of Ophthalmology, Rudolf-Virchow-Clinics, Glauchau, Germany

Keywords

IOL power calculation · Prediction of residual refraction · Vergence formulae · Paraxial Gaussian optics · Raytracing · Toric lenses · IOL calculation after LASIK

1 Introduction to IOL Power Calculation

Intraocular lenses (IOLs) as replacements for the natural crystalline lens in the eye were first introduced to ophthalmology by Harold Ridley in 1949. Prior to this, cataract surgeries were performed using intracapsular or extracapsular surgical techniques without a replacement lens, with the consequence of excessive postoperative hyperopia of around 12 dpt. At that time no ocular biometry or lens power calculation methods were available. The lenses used by Harold Ridley, made from polymethyl methacrylate, aimed to replicate the natural lens, but the larger refractive index of the lens material tended to result in high myopia following surgery. In 1967, when ultrasound biometry was already established in ophthalmology, the first calculation formula for determining the power of an intraocular lens was introduced by Fyodorov and independently in 1970 by Gernet, Ostholt and Werner, both using basic eye measures such as axial length, anterior chamber depth, central thickness of the crystalline lens, or vitreous depth together with the measurement of the corneal front surface radius.

Determining the appropriate artificial lens for implantation is as crucial to the success of cataract surgery as the surgery itself. Based on the biometry performed in advance, the surgeon first chooses the type of intraocular lens (IOL) to be implanted in the patient's eye, taking into account the patient's needs and expectations. At this point it is also determined whether a lens with spherical or aspherical base curve should be used and whether the lens should

B. Seitz et al. (eds.), *Atlas on Cornea*, https://doi.org/10.1007/978-3-031-65422-0_2

implement additional properties such as bi- or multifocality, astigmatism correction or a colour filter effect. The appropriate haptic geometry is also determined at this time. For calculation of the lens power, typically only the selected lens type is taken into account using appropriate adjustment factors (in general formula constants). If necessary, an extended calculation scheme is applied in the case of a toric IOL lens; the asphericity of the basic geometry and additional functionalities such as multifocality or colour filter effect are usually not taken into account. Techniques used in the early days of cataract surgery aimed only to replicate the geometry of the crystalline lens with a replacement artificial lens [1]. When calculations for IOL power were introduced, these were initially based on ultrasound biometry. Optical biometry subsequently replaced ultrasound techniques, having several advantages including significantly higher reproducibility, easier handling and noncontact measurement [2]. Furthermore, optical biometry enabled the simultaneous measurement of all relevant distances along the patient's fixation line, together with the corneal front surface radius, in a single acquisition [3]. The models on which the lens calculations are based have increased in complexity as the numbers of measurable parameters have increased. Models have been developed still further with the introduction of anterior segment tomography, which provides many thousands of measured data points for both corneal surfaces, and even deeper structures such as the anterior and posterior lens surfaces. The availability of high resolution tomographic data has laid the cornerstone for ray tracing through the whole eye to determine the refractive power of an IOL [3, 4]. In raytracing, a bundle of rays is projected onto the cornea starting from an object and successively transformed through all optical interfaces and optical media of the pseudophakic eye model, enabling the expected retinal image to be assessed depending on the lens type and the lens refractive power [5]. For raytracing to be most effective, detailed geometrical data of each respective lens type and for every possible refractive power of the lens are needed, in addition to the basic optical material properties. These requirements go far beyond the level of information typically available on the packaging of the lens, such as the overall IOL power [5]. The labelling alone generally does not provide sufficient information for raytracing.

In standard procedures for IOL calculation, a distinction is made between empirical and theoretical-optical approaches [6–9]. In the case of empirical methods, the calculation is not based on a pseudophakic eye model [10]. Instead, the target value, the 'refractive power of the IOL', is determined on the basis of a simple regression approach (e.g. SRK and SRK2 formulas) or complex prediction models (e.g. Hill-RBF calculator) using modern artificial intelligence methods. As no data from a pseudophakic model eye (considering anatomy, physiology or optical properties and interactions) are used, such empirical methods rely on the availability of large quantities of highly reliable results from previous measurements. To make reliable predictions of the required lens power for a given case awaiting surgery, measurement data from a significant number of previous cataract operations involving implantation of the same type of IOL are needed. Conversely, both theoretical-optical calculation strategies and raytracing use a pseudophakic eye model which is then combined with measurement data as far as possible. However, we have to be aware that in all IOL power calculation strategies based on a pseudophakic model eye, the axial position of the lens can only be estimated with any empirical (linear or nonlinear) prediction model before applying simplified linear Gaussian optics (vergence calculation) or raytracing.

2 Optical Model for IOL Power Calculation

Where theoretical-optical approaches are used to determine the refractive power of the IOL, they are based on a pseudophakic eye model. Depending on which biometric measurements are to be taken into account for the calculation, a simplified model is used [11, 12]. For the classical calculation formulae such as SRK/T, Hoffer Q [6, 7, 13], Holladay 1 [14] or Haigis [2], a pseudophakic eye model consisting of 3 thin lenses is used. These consist of: a spectacle lens having the post-cataract surgery target refraction (TR)—this is located at the spectacle plane (defined in terms of the vertex distance (VD) from the front of the cornea); the cornea itself (C); and the intraocular lens (IOL), modelled as a thin lens located at the effective lens position (ELP) behind the cornea. The refractive indices of the optical media ($n = 1$ for the air in front of the spectacles and between the spectacles and the cornea, n_A for the aqueous humour between the cornea and the lens and n_V for the vitreous humour between the lens and the retina) are specified in the model. Where available, the parameters in the model are replaced by measured variables. In the simplest form, this applies to the refractive power of the cornea (PC) and the axial length of the eye (AL). The target refraction is then specified by the surgeon in consultation with the patient, and the axial position of the lens is determined using an empirical approach (Fig. 1A).

This initial simplified eye model as shown in Fig. 1A can be further developed and extended if necessary and where the appropriate data are available. For example, where geometry data for the corneal anterior and posterior surfaces (as shown in Fig. 1 a and b: (C_a, radius RC_a, power PC_a), (C_p, radius RC_p, power PC_p) respectively), and the central corneal thickness (CCT) are available from a tomographic measurement of the anterior segment of the

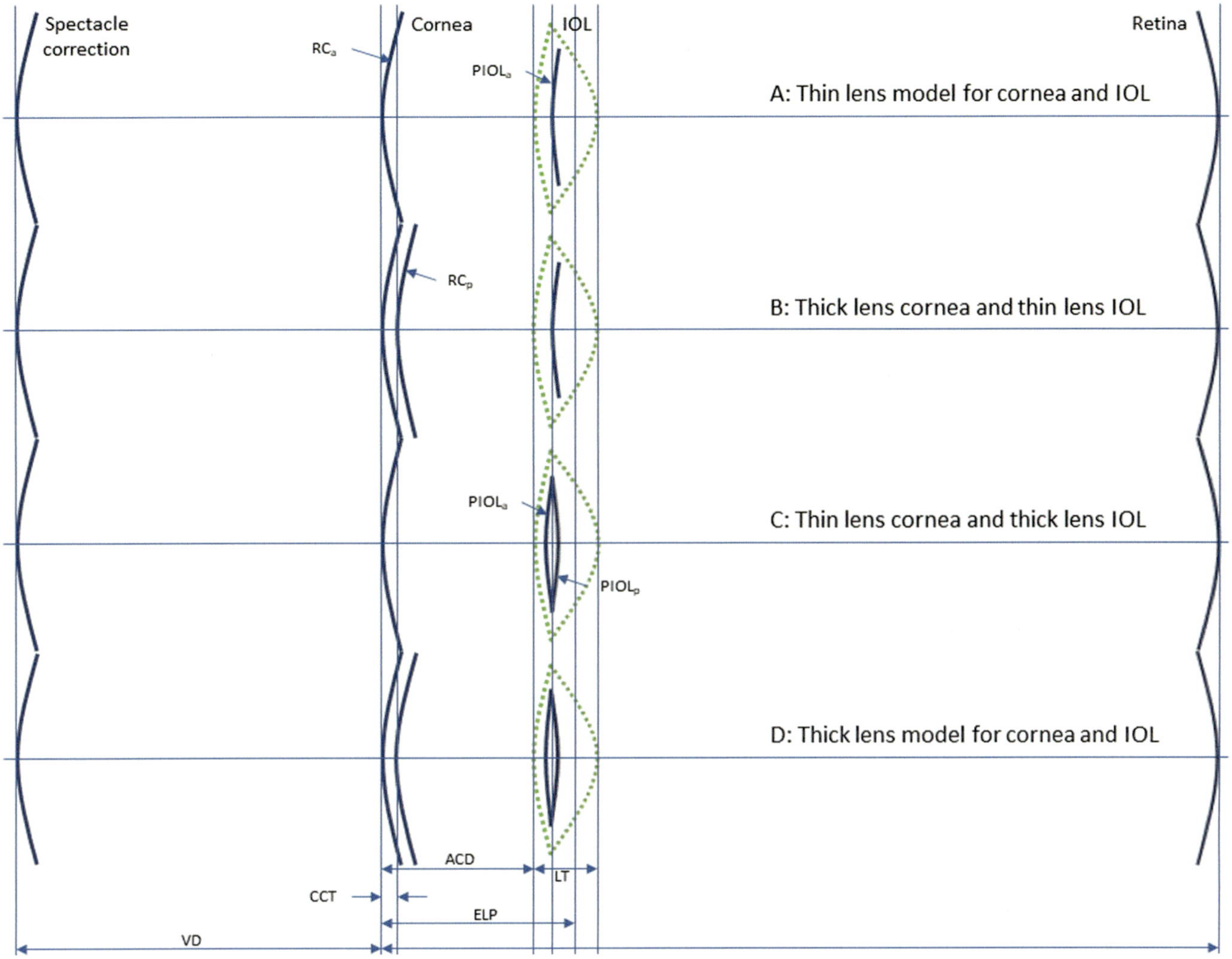

Fig. 1 Pseudophakic eye models used for intraocular lens power calculation. In the simplest form only 3 refractive surfaces are considered with a pseudophakic spectacle correction, a thin lens cornea and lens (**A**). This model can be upgraded to a thick lens cornea (**B**), a thick lens IOL (**C**), or a thick lens model for both the cornea and the IOL (**D**). (VD…vertex distance, CCT…central corneal thickness, ELP…estimated lens position, ACD…anterior chamber depth, RCa…anterior corneal radius, RCp…posterior corneal radius, $PIOL_a$…IOL anterior surface power, $PIOL_p$…IOL posterior surface power)

eye, then the pseudophakic eye model could be upgraded or generalised to a thick lens model of the cornea provided the refractive index of the cornea (n_C) is also known (Fig. 1B) [15–17]. Where the IOL manufacturer, in addition to the IOL power (PIOL) labelled on the package, has also disclosed the design data of the IOL to be implanted, including data of the anterior and posterior surfaces ((IOL_a, radius $RIOL_a$, surface power $PIOL_a$) and (IOL_p, radius $RIOL_p$, surface power $PIOL_p$) respectively), together with the central thickness (IOLT) and the refractive index (n_{IOL}), the pseudophakic eye model can be further extended to take these parameters into account in the calculation (Fig. 1C,D).

3 Required Parameters for IOL Power Calculation

Cataract surgery where an IOL is implanted to replace the crystalline lens involves the removal of an optically effective element from the eye. Therefore, the AL measurement is essential [18]. As a minimum requirement, and in addition to the target refraction (TR) defined by the surgeon, the length of the eye and the curvature of the anterior corneal surface RC_a must be measured [19]. The refractive power of the cornea PC_a can be estimated using the keratometric equation and the measured value of RC_a [20]. Furthermore, the AL and the corneal curvature are used in the lens calculation scheme to estimate the axial position of the lens in the eye. In the first generation calculation schemes such as SRK/T, Hoffer Q, Holladay 1 these two parameters supplemented by a formula constant are sufficient for the lens calculation. For the Haigis formula, in addition to the AL, the phakic anterior chamber depth ACD is taken into account when estimating the axial lens position and for the Olsen or the Castrop formula, this estimation is also based on the phakic anterior chamber depth ACD and the central thickness of the natural lens (LT) [12, 21–23]. Some modern calculation formulae such as Holladay 2, Kane, K6, Hoffer QST, T2 or Barrett use additional biometric parameters to calculate the refractive power of the IOL [24]. In these formulae, measurements such as the horizontal corneal diameter (CD), the age or gender of the patient or the refractive status of the phakic eye are also taken into account.

By contrast, the AL is not required for the calculation of phakic or pseudophakic supplementary lenses in the context of refractive surgery, as no optically effective element is removed from the eye. The aim here is to transfer some or all of the required correction from the spectacle plane into the eye (to the IOL plane) [25, 26]. Thus, the existing refraction must be known for the calculation, in addition to the target refraction TR defined by the surgeon. Since there is often a large ametropia preoperatively, especially with phakic supplementary lenses, the corresponding back vertex distance of the original corrective lenses (VD) should also always be determined during refractometry [27].

Where toric cataract replacement lenses or phakic/pseudophakic supplementary lenses are to be implanted, we have to deal with spherocylindrical vergences instead of spherical vergences, meaning that the flat and steep meridians (and their orientations) of all refractive surfaces in our pseudophakic eye model have to be determined. As a minimum requirement, the flat and steep meridian (together with the respective axes) of the corneal front surface should be provided for calculation of cataract replacement lenses, and additionally the preoperative spherocylindrical refraction (in terms of VD, sphere (REF_S, cylinder (REF_C) and cylinder axis (REF_A)) together with the (spherocylindrical) target refraction (if not plano) should be recorded [28–30].

4 The Axial IOL Position

The estimated lens position or effective lens position ELP is a fictitious plane in the eye where the thin reference lens is located according to the lens calculation formula [16, 31, 32]. It is not directly related to the physical/geometrical lens position, which can be measured in the pseudophakic eye after cataract surgery [31]. In the simplified pseudophakic model eye containing 3 refractive surfaces (Fig. 1A), then assuming that the keratometer index represents a proper conversion of the corneal front surface radius RC_a to PC, and that all refractive indices (n_A and n_V) are appropriate, and that the distance from the anterior corneal vertex to the photoreceptor layer is correctly described by the AL and further that the cornea as well as the IOL both can be simplified by a thin lens model, then the ELP coincides with the physical lens position. In the theoretical-optical formulae, the ELP is the parameter by means of which the refractive power of the IOL can be adjusted, since all other parameters in the calculation model are assumed as given (e.g. the measured AL or the corneal power PC determined from the radius of curvature of the corneal anterior surface RC_a). However, since the assumptions on which the formulae are based are sometimes incorrect or at least not generally valid for all eyes, the modulation of the ELP serves to adjust the IOL power [31, 33]. If the ELP is adjusted to higher/lower values, this results in a higher/lower IOL power with the consequence of a refractive shift of the eye towards myopia/hyperopia respectively. In addition to some preoperative biometric parameters, the ELP is mostly influenced by the formula constants, which adjust the 'one size fits all' lens calculation formula to the specific conditions of an IOL type in terms of geometry of the optic and haptic part, the central thickness or optic edge thickness, or the refractive index. In some formulae (e.g. the Haigis formula) the ELP can be extracted directly from the formula definition and the formula constants, whereas in other formulae the ELP is not explicitly mentioned and must be extracted by formula inversion [2]. If a systematic deviation between the achieved refraction after cataract surgery and the intended target refraction is noticed in a representative set of patient eyes, the ELP is systematically adjusted by optimising the formula constants—downwards in the case of negative refraction values (myopic eye) or upwards in the case of positive refraction values (hyperopic eye) [31, 34]. If the ELP prediction derived from the IOL calculation formula is compared with the actual physical position of the IOL in the pseudophakic eye (e.g. with the equatorial plane of the IOL), the IOL is generally positioned towards the anterior as compared to the ELP.

5 Keratometer Index and Corneal Power

The corneal refractive power cannot be determined by in situ measurement. As a rough approximation, the corneal front surface radius of curvature RC_a is usually measured using a keratometer or a Placido topographer [11, 14, 35, 36]. Previously with ultrasound biometry the corneal power had to be determined separately using a keratometer, but keratometry is integrated into modern optical biometers meaning that the relevant distances in the eye together with RC_a can be determined simultaneously along the same fixation axis. Only the mean corneal power is required for determination of stigmatic (non-toric) IOLs, while for toric IOLs the corneal refraction is processed in both cardinal meridians, the flat (RC_a1) as well as the steep main section (RC_a2). Modern anterior segment tomographers based on Scheimpflug imaging or high-resolution OCT are not restricted to corneal front surface measurement and also derive CCT and corneal back surface measurement (mean radius RC_p or meridional radii RC_p1/RC_p2 for stigmatic or toric lens power calculation) [37–39]. If only the corneal front surface radius is determined, it must be converted to corneal power PC using the keratometer equation (with a characteristic keratometer index n_K) based on certain simplifying assumptions. The model assumptions on which the conversion is based are as follows:

- Fixed radius ratio of anterior surface to posterior cornea surface, taken from a schematic eye model,
- Fixed corneal thickness, taken from a schematic eye model,

The thin lens reference plane for the cornea could be located either at the corneal front vertex (PC as front vertex power), the corneal back vertex (PC as back vertex power) or the image-sided principal plane (PC as equivalent power):

$$\frac{n_K-1}{RC_a} = \frac{n_C-1}{RC_a} + \frac{n_A-n_C}{RC_p} - \frac{n_C-1}{RC_a} \cdot \frac{n_A-n_C}{RC_p} \cdot \frac{CCT}{n_C} = PC_{EQ} \text{ (PC as equivalent power)}$$

$$\frac{n_K-1}{RC_a} = \frac{\frac{n_C-1}{RC_a}}{\left(1-\frac{n_C-1}{RC_a}\cdot\frac{CCT}{n_C}\right)} + \frac{n_A-n_C}{RC_p} = PC_{BV} \text{ (PC as back vertex power)}$$

$$\frac{n_K-1}{RC_a} = \frac{PC_{BV}}{\left(1+PC_{BV}\cdot\frac{CCT}{n_A}\right)} = PC_{FV} \text{ (PC as front vertex power)}$$

The keratometer index n_K used for the conversion, implicitly commits us to a corneal front to back surface ratio and a central corneal thickness CCT, and to a reference plane. E.g., with the Zeiss/Javal keratometer index $n_K = 1.332/1.3375$ we are bound to the Gullstrand front to back surface ratio of 7.7 mm to 6.8 mm (and CCT = 0.5 mm) and the corneal front/back vertex plane as a reference. Using the data of the Gullstrand schematic model eye results in a corneal power value of PC = 43.05 dpt with the Zeiss/43.83 with the Javal keratometer index, both for a corneal front surface radius of $RC_a = 7.7$ mm (difference around 0.75 dpt). If modern schematic model eyes such as the Liou–Brennan model eye are used instead of the Gullstrand model, we obtain different keratometer indices to convert RC_a to PC (keratometer index $n_K = 1.3287/PC_{EQ} = 42.692$ dpt for the image sided principal plane, $n_K = 1.3295/PC_{FV} = 42.788$ dpt for the front vertex plane and $n_K = 1.3347/PC_{BV} = 43.463$ dpt for the back vertex plane). Lens calculation formulae use different conversions to derive corneal power from the radius of curvature. These differences must be compensated for by optimising the formula constants or by corrections elsewhere to eliminate the overall mean error in a patient dataset, ultimately affecting the formula constants used in the ELP prediction.

6 Calculation of Standard Lenses

Today, theoretical-optical formulae are used for the majority of IOL calculations. The empirical regression formulae SRK or SRK2 were declared obsolete by the formula authors Sanders, Retzlaff and Kraff decades ago [40–44]. The classical formulae such as SRK/T, Hoffer-Q, Holladay1, Haigis, and also many modern formulae such as the Olsen, Castrop, Holladay2, Barrett or Kane formulae are based on the simplified eye model with a thin (Fig. 1A) or thick lens (Fig. 1B) for the cornea and a thin lens model for the IOL [22, 32, 45–47]. These calculation strategies are based on a 'master formula' as published independently by Fyodorov in 1967 and by Gernet, Ostholt and Walter in 1970 [1, 48]. The derivation of this formula can be explained in terms of a simple vergence transformation by assuming a vergence of 0 in front of the intended pseudophakic spectacle refraction and successively following the vergence through the TR, the cornea and the aqueous humour through to the fictitious plane where the thin lens IOL is located (the ELP). If, in a second step, the vergence in the ELP plane behind the thin lens IOL is calculated in order to achieve an image on the retina, the refractive power of the lens is defined as the difference between the two vergences. The IOL must therefore compensate the vergence deficit (vergence directly behind the ELP plane minus the vergence directly in front of the ELP plane) as the IOL power PIOL:

$$PIOL = \frac{n_V}{AL-ELP} - \frac{1}{\frac{1}{\frac{TR}{1-TR\cdot VD}+\frac{n_K-1}{RC_a}} - \frac{ELP}{n_A}} \text{ (cornea as thin lens)}$$

$$PIOL = \frac{n_V}{AL-ELP} - \frac{1}{\frac{1}{\frac{1}{\frac{1}{\frac{TR}{1-TR\cdot VD}+\frac{n_C-1}{RC_a}} - \frac{CCT}{n_C}} + \frac{n_A-n_C}{RC_p}} - \frac{ELP-CCT}{n_A}} \text{ (cornea as thick lens)}$$

Conversely, the expected refraction at the spectacle plane (TR) when an IOL is specified can be derived directly by converting this 'master formula':

$$TR = \frac{1}{\frac{1}{\frac{1}{\frac{1}{\frac{n_V}{AL-ELP}-PIOL}+\frac{ELP}{n_A}} - \frac{n_K-1}{RC_a}} + VD} \text{ (cornea as thin lens)}$$

$$TR = \frac{1}{\frac{1}{\frac{1}{\frac{1}{\frac{1}{\frac{1}{\frac{n_V}{AL-ELP}-PIOL}+\frac{ELP-CCT}{n_A}} - \frac{n_A-n_C}{RC_p}} + \frac{CCT}{n_C}} - \frac{n_C-1}{RC_a}} + VD} \text{ (cornea as thick lens)}$$

The Haigis formula, for example, directly uses this 'master formula' with the cornea modelled as a thin lens, together with an empirical estimation of the ELP from a bivariate linear regression with the predictor variables AL and ACD. The keratometer index $n_K = 1.3315$ used in the Haigis formula refers to the Gullstrand schematic model eye and corneal power referenced to the principal plane PC_{EQ}.

Other established formulae such as the SRK/T, Hoffer Q and Holladay 1 use the conversion from the radius of curvature of the cornea to the refractive power of the cornea according to the Javal keratometer index for the lens calculation [9, 13, 29, 49, 50]. Since the distances in the eye (ELP and AL) are referenced to the corneal front vertex (and not to the back vertex) the Javal keratometer index typically overestimates the corneal power PC, with the consequence that the PIOL is underestimated. To compensate for this PIOL under-correction, the IOL must be shifted backwards (ELP increased to a value behind the physical IOL position) to obtain a higher PIOL value from the IOL calculation scheme.

Additionally, in most of the theoretical-optical formulae various correction terms are introduced at different points in the formulae (e.g. an offset value of 0.2 mm to account for retinal thickness in the Holladay1 formula) or parameter limitations may be imposed (on the AL (SRK/T, Hoffer Q and Holladay 1) or corneal power (Holladay 1)) to account for model errors in long/short eyes or eyes with an unusual corneal radius [10, 14].

Some of the modern calculation formulae such as Holladay 2, Olsen, Barrett or Kane are unpublished, or at least not fully disclosed, making analysis of the characteristics of these formulae difficult or even impossible. This also means that the corresponding formula constants cannot be optimised directly either. Most of these formulae are also based on a simplified pseudophakic eye model as shown in Fig. 1 but, in addition to the AL and the PC, other biometric variables such as the horizontal diameter of the cornea CD, the patient's age or gender, the ACD (Haigis, Olsen or Castrop formula) or the crystalline lens thickness LT (Olsen or Castrop formula) are taken into account for the estimation of the ELP [34, 46, 51]. The Castrop formula uses a pseudophakic model with a thick lens cornea (with RC_a/RC_p, CCT and n_C instead or RC_a and n_K) and a thin lens IOL (as typically no design data for the IOL are provided by the IOL manufacturers). The clear advantage of such lens power calculation concepts that model the cornea as a thick lens is that by entering the corneal front and back surface radii (together with the CCT), the calculation is independent of a keratometer index (since the refractive index of cornea n_C is used) and situations with unusual front to back surface ratio values (e.g. eyes with a history of corneal laser surgery) where the conversion from corneal front surface radius to corneal power would fail can instead be easily calculated without any further correction [16, 17, 21].

7 Calculation of Toric Lenses

Unlike the calculation of standard lenses, the calculation of toric intraocular lenses is not feasible in a closed form [52, 53]. Most of the manufacturers of toric intraocular lenses provide a dedicated toric IOL calculation service or WEB applications for toric lenses in which the characteristics and delivery ranges are already considered. However, the concepts of such WEB based toric calculators are not disclosed.

Provided that the principal meridians of all refractive surfaces are aligned (coincide in axis), standard lens power calculation strategies can be used to calculate toric IOLs. Because this is unlikely in most cases, it is important to ensure that the ELP does not depend on the corneal power in these strategies, otherwise different values would be obtained for the ELP for the steep and the flat meridians. As soon as the principal meridians of the target refraction, the corneal astigmatism and the IOL are no longer aligned, theoretical-optical formulae fail and instead we need to resort to solutions with cylindrical vergences or matrix methods [39, 51, 54]. When calculating toric lenses, astigmatism induced during cataract surgery is often taken into account. This so-called ‘Surgical Induced Astigmatism’ (SIA) is an estimated value derived from the results of previous cataract surgeries using a vector calculation [55, 56]. Typically, the SIA represents a statistical measure (such as the arithmetic or geometric mean) of the change in corneal astigmatism that the surgeon documents by comparing the postoperative with the preoperative corneal astigmatism findings. However, we should be aware that this does not necessarily reflect the individually induced astigmatism as we typically observe a large scatter in the vector change from preoperative to postoperative.

For the general case of crossed cylinders, the tracing of spherocylindrical vergences through the eye offers a simple and consistent option for calculating toric IOLs or estimating the expected refraction at the spectacle plane when using a toric IOL. Assuming that the axial position of the principal meridians does not change when a beam passes through a homogeneous optical medium, the so-called standard notation consisting of the two power values in the principal meridians and the corresponding axial positions is used for the vergence transformation. This transformation through a homogeneous optical medium is comparable to the conversion of refraction from the spectacle plane to the corneal plane (contact lens refraction). When a ray passes through a refractive interface, the ray is bent (ray angles change), but the beam height will remain unchanged. Here, a complementary representation of the vergences is used, consisting of the equivalent refraction value and the projection of the cylinder onto the straight and oblique meridians based on the double angle representation. Here, the respective components of the refractive surface (equivalent and both projections) can be added to the corresponding values of the vergence in front of the interface to obtain the corresponding components of the vergence behind the interface.

Such a calculation scheme can be very easily transferred into a calculation template as shown below in Table 1 as an example for the simplified pseudophakic eye model with a thin lens cornea and IOL described above. The iatrogenic vector change at the cornea is assumed as the SIA with 0.3 dpt at 90° without changing the corneal equivalent power:

The example describes a situation where a toric IOL is to be calculated for a target refraction of 0.0–0.5 dpt/90° (line 4 in the table). The vergence immediately behind the target refraction (line 5, calculated by adding the corresponding components of the Humphrey notation) is transferred into the standard notation, then both main sections are corrected by the VD (here 12 mm) (line 7). Back in the Humphrey notation, the vergence behind the cornea is determined by adding the corresponding components of the corneal refractive index (RHHa1 = 7.9 mm in 10°, RHHa2 = 7.5 mm in 100°, n_K = 1.332, line 8) as well as the SIA (line 9) (line 10) and transferred back into the standard notation. After correcting the vergence by the distance between the cornea and the estimated lens position (ELP = 5.1 mm, n_A = 1.336, reduced distance ELP/n_A), the vergence immediately in front of the IOL is determined (line 12). By subtracting the vergence immediately behind the IOL in the Humphrey notation (vergence = n_V/(AL-ELP) with AL = 23.8 and n_V = 1.336, line 14), the refractive power of the lens is obtained, either in the Humphrey notation or, after recalculation, also in the standard notation (line 13, lens refractive power 18.40 + 3.47 dpt/99°, equivalent refractive power 20.14 dpt).

This calculation scheme can be easily generalised to a pseudophakic eye model with a thick lens cornea and/or IOL or to a back-calculation of residual refraction when a toric IOL is specified (calculation path from bottom to top). It can be seen directly from the table that the toric IOL with the implantation axis (flat meridian of the IOL) at 99° is able to correct for the crossed cylinders of the target refraction (minus cylinder at 90°), the cornea (plus cylinder at 10°) and the SIA (plus cylinder at 90°).

8 Calculation of Supplementary Phakic or Pseudophakic Lenses

The calculation of supplementary lenses (SIOL) in the eye is based on subjective refraction results (in contrast to replacement lenses based on ocular biometry) (Fig. 2) [25, 57, 58]. As opposed to IOLs which are considered to be located at the ELP, the axial position of the SIOL could be determined using high resolution anterior segment tomography. Based on the manufacturer's experience and recommendation, the SIOL will be located at a specific distance (vault) in front of the crystalline lens (Fig. 2A) or the already implanted IOL (Fig. 2B). A typical value for this vault is 0.4 mm (0.25–0.60 mm). This means that the axial SIOL position in the eye with respect to the corneal front vertex (SELP) will be the measured phakic or pseudophakic anterior chamber depth ACD minus the vault.

The calculation formula for a stigmatic (non-toric) SIOL was first described by van der Heijde. This vergence-based

Table 1 Calculation example for a toric IOL based on a vergence calculation scheme. The 2 complementary forms of representation of a spherocylindrical vergence allow tracing through a homogeneous optical medium (standard notation) as well as the consideration of spherocylindrical surfaces (Humphrey or component notation) even in the presence of crossed cylinders

		Standard notation				Humphrey (component) notation			1
	Geometrical distance in mm	Meridian 1 in dpt	Axis 1 in °	Meridian 2 in dpt	Cylinder in dpt	Equivalent in dpt	Projection 0/90° in dpt	Projection 45/135° in dpt	2
		0.00	0	0.00	0.00	0.00	0.00	0.00	3
Target refraction		−0.50	0	0.00	0.50	−0.25	0.5	0.0	4
		−0.50	0	0.00	0.50	−0.25	0.5	0.0	5
	12.0								6
		−0.49	0	0.0	0.49	−0.25	0.49	0.00	7
Cornea		42.03	10	44.27	2.24	43.15	2.11	0.77	8
SIA		−0.15	90	0.15	0.30	0.00	−0.30	0.00	9
		41.68	9	44.11	2.43	42.90	2.30	0.77	10
I	5.1								11
		49.57	9	53.04	3.47	51.30	3.29	1.10	12
IOL		**18.40**	**99**	**21.87**	**3.47**	**20.14**	**−3.29**	**1.10**	13
	18.7	71.44	0	71.44	90	71.44	0	0	14

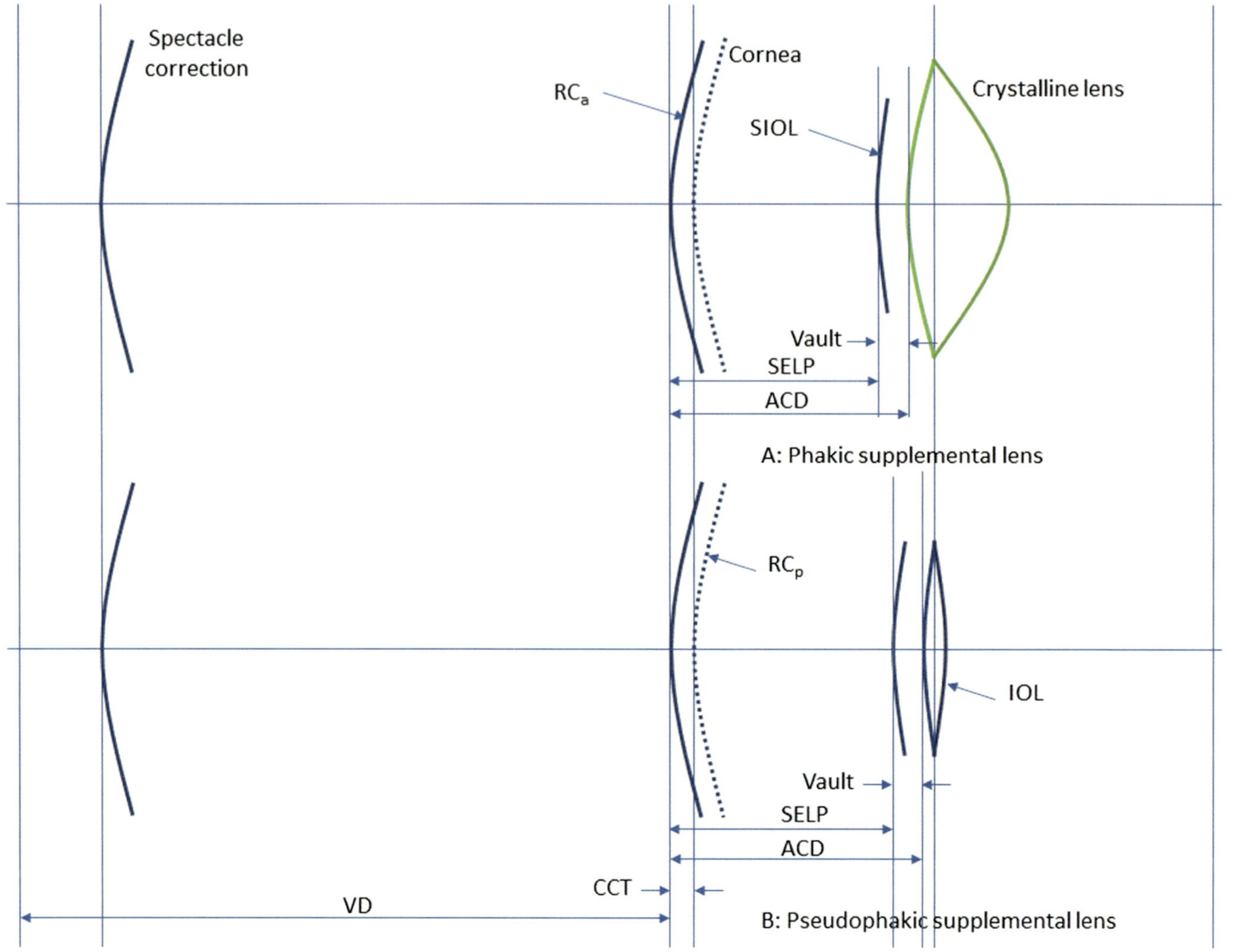

Fig. 2 Model of the anterior eye segment used for calculation of phakic (**A**) or pseudophakic (**B**) supplemental lenses. As the calculation is based on refraction, the posterior eye segment or the axial length measurement is not required

formula is derived by comparing the vergence in the implantation plane (SELP) of the supplementary lens after implantation (V_{post}) with the vergence before implantation V_{pre}. The preoperative refraction at the spectacle plane (REF) could be fully or partially corrected by the SIOL (shift from the spectacle plane to the SELP plane) to achieve a postoperative refraction TR. In analogy to the basic formula for IOL calculation (as shown before), the following vergences for the simplest case of a pseudophakic eye model with a thin lens cornea and SIOL result as follows for the preoperative and postoperative situation:

$$V_{pre} = \frac{1}{\frac{1}{\frac{REF}{1-REF\cdot VD}+\frac{n_K-1}{RC_a}}-\frac{SELP}{n_A}}$$

$$V_{post} = \frac{1}{\frac{1}{\frac{TR}{1-TR\cdot VD}+\frac{n_K-1}{RC_a}}-\frac{ELP}{n_A}}$$

The difference between the two vergences defines the refractive power (PSIOL) of the required SIOL:

$$PSIOL = V_{pre} - V_{post}$$

For calculation of a toric SIOL, the calculation scheme for toric cataract lenses (as shown in Table 1) can be used, with some modifications [52, 53, 59]. As with the van der Heijde formula, the preoperative situation and the postoperative situation are taken into account and the IOL is calculated as the difference between the two vergences in the SELP plane (Table 2). The following table shows an example of the procedure for calculating a phakic toric IOL. The current refraction is assumed to be -5.0–2.5 dpt /15°. Values for the target refraction, the corneal refractive index and the SIA are taken from Table 1. The SELP was derived in this example from a ACD value of 3.6 mm and a vault prediction of 0.4 mm to be SELP = 3.2 mm.

The upper part of the calculation scheme (lines 3–11) describes the preoperative situation with the current refraction REF (line 4), the refraction converted to the corneal

Table 2 Calculation example for a phakic toric supplementary lens based on a vergence calculation. The 2 complementary forms of representation of a spherocylindrical vergence allow tracing through a homogeneous optical medium (standard notation) as well as consideration of spherocylindrical surfaces (Humphrey or component notation) even in the presence of crossed cylinders

		Standard notation				Humphrey (component) notation			1
	Distance in mm	Meridian 1 in dpt	Axis 1 in °	Meridian 2 in dpt	Cylinder in dpt	Equivalent in dpt	Projection 0/90° in dpt	Projection 45/135° in dpt	2
		0.00	0	0.00	0.00	0.00	0.00	0.00	3
Current refraction REF		–7.50	1050	–5.00	2.50	–6.25	–2.17	–1.25	4
		–7.50	1050	–5.00	2.50	–6.25	–2.17	–1.25	5
	12.0								6
		–6.88	105	–4.72	2.16	–5.80	–1.87	–1.08	7
Cornea		42.03	10	44.27	2.24	43.15	2.11	0.77	8
		37.15	153	37.54	0.39	37.35	0.23	–0.32	9
I	3.2								10
V_{pre}		40.90	153	41.38	0.48	41.14	0.28	–0.38	11
		0.00	0	0.00	0.00	0.00	0.00	0.00	12
Target refraction TR		–0.50	0	0.00	0.50	–0.25	0.5	0.0	13
		–0.50	0	0.00	0.50	–0.25	0.5	0.0	14
	12.0								15
		–0.49	0	0.0	0.49	–0.25	0.49	0.00	16
Cornea		42.03	10	44.27	2.24	43.15	2.11	0.77	17
SIA		–0.15	90	0.15	0.30	0.00	–0.30	0.00	18
		41.68	9	44.11	2.43	42.90	2.30	0.77	19
I	3.2								20
V_{post}		46.47	9	49.51	3.04	47.99	2.88	0.96	21
SIOL		**–8.31**	**104**	**–5.38**	**2.92**	**–6.84**	**–2.60**	**–1.34**	**22**

plane (line 7) up to the vergence in the SELP plane (proposed implantation plane of the supplementary lens) (line 11). The postoperative situation is presented in the following lines (12–21), characterised by the target refraction at the spectacle plane TR (line 13) and at the corneal plane (line 15). In the postoperative situation, the SIA (line 18) is taken into account and the vergence in the SELP plane of the lens is shown in line 21. The power of the toric supplementary lens (line 22; –5.38—2.92 dpt/14°, equivalent power -6.84 dpt) results from the comparison of the preoperative with the postoperative vergence (lines 11 and 21).

9 Calculation in Patients with a History of Laser Refractive Surgery

It is well known from the literature that standard lens power calculations may fail in patients with a history of laser refractive surgery. The main reason for this is that the corneal front surface curvature is modulated by laser tissue ablation during refractive surgery procedures, and consequently the ratio between corneal front-to-back surface curvature (and corneal thickness) is changed. Even when the corneal front surface curvature is subsequently measured properly, the conversion from corneal front surface radius to corneal power using a keratometer index will no longer be correct, systematically underestimating/overestimating the corneal power after myopic/hyperopic refractive correction respectively. Additionally, in the early years of laser corneal refractive surgery, surgeons typically used small optical zones and since keratometers (either standalone or integrated in a biometer) measure the corneal front surface curvature at a distance of 1.2 to 1.8 mm from the centre, small or slightly decentered optical zones could affect the measurement of corneal radius with the consequence of overestimating/underestimating corneal power in situations after myopic/hyperopic corneal refractive surgery. Furthermore, some lens power calculation formulae consider the corneal front surface radius or corneal power in predicting the axial IOL position in the pseudophakic eye (e.g. SRK/T, Hoffer Q and Holladay 1 formula), with the consequence that the iatrogenic flattening or steepening of the cornea affects the ELP prediction.

This misinterpretation of corneal power from the keratometer measured corneal front surface radius is not restricted to situations after laser refractive surgeries such as PRK,

LASIK, LASEK, SMILE or FLEX. The ratio of corneal front to back surface curvature and/or corneal thickness might likewise be changed after posterior lamellar keratoplasty (e.g. DSAEK/DMEK), with corneal ectasia (e.g. keratoconus or pellucide marginal degeneration, even in a mild form), or with a corneal oedema which cannot be considered by a keratometer.

There are two concepts for calculating the power of an IOL after laser refractive surgery: firstly, where 'historical data' of the eye in terms of keratometry/topography or refraction before and after laser surgery are available, then the corneal power and IOL power could be derived from the actual measurements, taking the change of corneal power or refraction during laser surgery into account using 'clinical history methods' as described in the literature. If no (reliable) 'clinical history' data are available, the corneal front and back surface curvature together with corneal thickness could be measured by modern corneal tomographers using Scheimpflug or optical coherence tomography techniques. Having these measurement data of both corneal surfaces available would make it possible to use IOL power calculation concepts based on a thick lens model for the cornea (e.g. the Castrop formula) or on composite indices provided by the tomographer considering the cornea as thick lens (e.g. TK, RealPower, TotalPower, TrueNet or TCRP value). Where tomographic data of the cornea are unavailable, calculation concepts based on statistical models for corneal power (e.g. the Haigis-L formula) could be used. However, we should be aware that such statistical models are designed to correct the radius of curvature to corneal power conversion error of keratometers after laser refractive surgery only on average in a patient cohort, and do not fully consider the individual situation of an eye.

The American Society of Cataract and Refractive Surgery (ASCRS) provides a WEB based platform with implementations of several calculation concepts published in the literature (https://iolcalc.ascrs.org/). Biometric data, together with clinical history data before and after laser refractive surgery, can be entered on this platform and the results both with and without consideration of data before and after laser refractive surgery are listed.

10 Customisation of Formula Constants

The optimisation of formula constants serves to minimise or eliminate the systematic part of the formula prediction error, expressed as the difference between the formula predicted refraction and the achieved refraction measured after cataract surgery [60, 61]. In this way, the optical characteristics of an IOL type are generally taken into account. In addition, the material-specific characteristics and the design of the haptics (such as haptic angulation or step vault as an offset between optic edge plane and haptic plane) are included in the optimization [50, 62–65]. The following parameters are required for the optimisation of formula constants:

- All biometric parameters required for the lens calculation,
- The power of the implanted IOL (PIOL),
- The postoperative refraction.

The postoperative refraction should be collected at the earliest 4 weeks, and preferably 3 months, after cataract surgery, to ensure that the lens has stabilised in the eye and no further drift of the refraction can be observed. In any case, the refraction should be determined manually using a phoropter or trial glasses in a trial frame. Special attention should be paid to determination of refraction after implantation of multifocal lenses or EDOF lenses. In this case, additional fogging with plus lenses (and minus lenses) should be carried out in order to determine the defocus curve and the correction lens at which visual acuity begins to deteriorate. With EDOF IOLs in particular, the plateau in the defocus curve can otherwise lead to the formula constants not being optimised for correction with maximum plus glasses without loss of visual acuity, but e.g. to any other refraction in the plateau, with the consequence that pseudophakic pseudo-accommodation response would be partially reduced if these formula constants were used in future cataract surgeries. It should also be noted that with IOLs with partial or complete chromatic correction (achromat or apochromat e.g. realised by combinations of refractive surface and a superimposed diffractive structure) a red-green fine adjustment is no longer effective.

For the selection of a proper optimisation strategy we have to distinguish between calculation formulae with a single formula constant (e.g. SRK/T, Hoffer Q, Holladay 1, Holladay 2) or with more than one constant (e.g. the Haigis or Castrop formula with 3 constants) [66–69]. If only one constant is used, the formula (provided that it is fully disclosed) can usually be inverted directly according to the formula constant, so that an individual formula constant results for each eye, taking into account the PIOL and the postoperative refraction [8, 21, 70]. If the mean or median of the individually determined formula constants is derived from a representative number of clinical cases treated with one IOL type, this statistical value can be used as the optimised constant. If an optimisation of the 3 Haigis formula constants a0, a1 and a2 or 3 Castrop formula constants C, H, and R is carried out, it is not possible to determine a unique triplet of constants individually for each clinical case. Rather, there are numbers of triplets that fulfil this condition. In this way, a triplet of constants is determined over a representative data set based on minimising the overall mean squared formula prediction error [63–65]. Either a multiple regression approach (applicable only in some special configurations of formula constants) or in a general case a non-linear iterative approach or AI based data driven approach could be used.

However, in addition to the IOL type, the formula constant also reflects the composition of the patient population, the biometer (with its calibration), the surgical technique (e.g. the corneal incision) and the postoperative refraction technique (including the measurement lane distance). This implies that, if the data are sufficient and reliable, the formula constants should be personalised whenever possible. Only the personalisation of the constants for a surgeon together with the diagnostic and surgical environment will make it possible to eliminate the systematic position of the formula prediction error for future cataract surgeries. However, the optimisation of formula constants cannot compensate for individual formula prediction errors [21, 64, 71, 72].

Surgeons have the option of using WEB platforms to optimise formula constants. The IOLCon platform (www.IOLCon.org) offers the possibility of entering clinical data sets consisting of biometric data, the type and refractive power of the implanted lens and the postoperative refraction (preferably specifying the biometer used, the keratometer index for the case of entry with corneal power values as well as the measurement lane distance) into a template. This template could be sent on request or directly downloaded after registration. In addition, the technical specifications of all common lenses together with their manufacturer recommended/IOLCon optimized formula constants and delivery ranges of the lenses are available with IOLCon. A direct data export from IOLCon to some modern optical biometers is available via an open interface for direct data transfer.

11 Raytracing for IOL Power Calculation

Full aperture ray tracing (numerical raytracing) offers the possibility of both calculating IOLs and simulating the imaging properties of the IOLs prior to cataract surgery. In this method, a representative pencil of rays is projected onto the cornea and successively traced through the eye from one optical surface to the next until reaching the retina [5, 73, 74]. Raytracing is not restricted to the simplifications of linear Gaussian optics, as the refraction law published by Snell van Royen (Snell's law) is applied for each ray surface intersection. The prerequisite for a raytracing application is that all refractive surfaces in the eye are known with sufficient accuracy. This includes measurements of the anterior and posterior surface of the cornea (together with the central corneal thickness) made with a high precision tomographer, and also requires that the geometry of the pupil (under different illumination conditions) is known and that the IOL design data (complete geometry data together with the refractive index and central thickness) of the lens model are disclosed for all refractive power steps [4, 75]. In addition, the alignment of all refractive surfaces and the aperture with respect to the visual axis must be known.

Nevertheless, even with ray tracing, the axial and lateral position of the IOL within the pseudophakic eye has to be predicted using any empirical prediction model. Assuming that all the above data are available with sufficient accuracy, different lens types or refractive power values can be examined with regard to the expected retinal image and the surgeon can assess in advance which visual performance can be achieved at best (if no other pathologies are present). There are currently various tomographers available to the clinician capable of analysing the anterior segment of the eye with sufficient accuracy. The difficulty lies in obtaining reliable geometry and material data for each lens type for all power steps. With Okulix (www.okulix.de), a comprehensive software solution is available that stores the corresponding lens data for many IOL types so that surgeons can analyse the expected retinal images in addition to calculating the appropriate lens refractive power.

12 Conclusion

In this chapter we have shown how to calculate intraocular lenses based on preoperative biometric measures. Different techniques for deriving the power of standard lenses, toric lenses, and supplementary lenses have been summarised, and the relevance of the input parameters as predictors for calculation of the appropriate intraocular lens power discussed. In a clinical situation the plug-in calculation modules built in to most biometers can be used to determine the lens power in most cases. However, in 'special cases' with uncommon biometric values or combinations of values it is worthwhile to perform calculations 'outside the standard environment' using calculation concepts such as considering both corneal surfaces (thick lens model for the cornea). This can be helpful for lens power calculation in situations such as patients with a history of corneal refractive surgery.

References

1. van der Feltz van der Sloot D, van der Heijde GL, Hoogesteger MF. Evaluation of the value of preoperatively determined IOL power. Doc Ophthalmol. 1987;67(1–2):69–72. https://doi.org/10.1007/BF00142699.
2. Haigis W, Lege B, Miller N, Schneider B. Comparison of immersion ultrasound biometry and partial coherence interferometry for intraocular lens calculation according to Haigis. Graefes Arch Clin

Exp Ophthalmol. 2000;238(9):765–73. https://doi.org/10.1007/s004170000188.
3. Fişuş AD, Hirnschall ND, Findl O. Comparison of 2 swept-source optical coherence tomography-based biometry devices. J Cataract Refract Surg. 2021;47(1):87–92. https://doi.org/10.1097/j.jcrs.0000000000000373.
4. Langenbucher A, Viestenz A, Viestenz A, Brünner H, Seitz B. Ray tracing through a schematic eye containing second-order (quadric) surfaces using 4 x 4 matrix notation. Ophthalmic Physiol Opt. 2006;26(2):180–8. https://doi.org/10.1111/j.1475-1313.2006.00346.x.
5. Olsen T, Hoffmann P. C constant: new concept for ray tracing-assisted intraocular lens power calculation. J Cataract Refract Surg. 2014;40(5):764–73. https://doi.org/10.1016/j.jcrs.2013.10.037.
6. Hoffer KJ. J Steps for IOL power calculation. Am Intraocul Implant Soc. 1980;6(4):370.
7. Hoffer KJ. The Hoffer Q formula: a comparison of theoretic and regression formulas. J Cataract Refract Surg. 1993;19(6):700–12. https://doi.org/10.1016/s0886-3350(13)80338-0.
8. Langenbucher A, Szentmáry N, Cayless A, Röggla V, Leydolt C, Wendelstein J, Hoffmann P. Similarity of eyes in a cataractous population-How reliable is the biometry of the fellow eye for lens power calculation? PLoS ONE. 2022;17(6): e0269709. https://doi.org/10.1371/journal.pone.0269709.
9. Sanders DR, Retzlaff JA, Kraff MC, Gimbel HV, Raanan MG. Comparison of the SRK/T formula and other theoretical and regression formulas. J Cataract Refract Surg. 1990;16(3):341–6. https://doi.org/10.1016/s0886-3350(13)80706-7. PMID: 2355322.
10. Olsen T, Thim K, Corydon L. Theoretical versus SRK I and SRK II calculation of intraocular lens power. J Cataract Refract Surg. 1990;16(2):217–25. https://doi.org/10.1016/s0886-3350(13)80734-1. PMID: 2329481.
11. Cooke DL, Cooke TL, Suheimat M, Atchison DA. Standardizing sum-of-segments axial length using refractive index models. Biomed Opt Express. 2020;11(10):5860–70. https://doi.org/10.1364/BOE.400471.
12. Langenbucher A, Schwemm M, Eppig T, Schröder S, Cayless A, Szentmáry N. Optimal dataset sizes for constant optimization in published theoretical optical formulae. Curr Eye Res. 2021;46(10):1589–96. https://doi.org/10.1080/02713683.2021.1900272.
13. Hoffer KJ. Intraocular lens calculation: the problem of the short eye. Ophthalmic Surg. 1981;12(4):269–72. PMID: 7254770 No abstract available.
14. Holladay JT, Prager TC, Chandler TY, Musgrove KH, Lewis JW, Ruiz RS. A three-part system for refining intraocular lens power calculations. J Cataract Refract Surg. 1988;14(1):17–24. https://doi.org/10.1016/s0886-3350(88)80059-2.
15. Debellemanière G, Dubois M, Gauvin M, Wallerstein A, Brenner LF, Rampat R, Saad A, Gatinel D. The PEARL-DGS formula: the development of an open-source machine learning-based thick IOL calculation formula. Am J Ophthalmol. 2021;232:58–69. https://doi.org/10.1016/j.ajo.2021.05.004.
16. Gatinel D, Debellemanière G, Saad A, Dubois M, Rampat R. Determining the theoretical effective lens position of thick intraocular lenses for machine learning-based IOL power calculation and simulation. Transl Vis Sci Technol. 2021;10(4):27. https://doi.org/10.1167/tvst.10.4.27.
17. Langenbucher A, Hoffmann P, Cayless A, Gatinel D, Debellemanière G, Wendelstein J, Szentmáry N. Considerations of a thick lens formula for intraocular lens power calculation. Z Med Phys. 2022;S0939–3889(22):00124–6. https://doi.org/10.1016/j.zemedi.2022.11.007.
18. Cooke DL, Cooke TL. A comparison of two methods to calculate axial length. J Cataract Refract Surg. 2019;45(3):284–92. https://doi.org/10.1016/j.jcrs.2018.10.039.
19. Cooke DL, Cooke TL. Approximating sum-of-segments axial length from a traditional optical low-coherence reflectometry measurement. J Cataract Refract Surg. 2019;45(3):351–4. https://doi.org/10.1016/j.jcrs.2018.12.026.
20. Langenbucher A, Szentmáry N, Cayless A, Wendelstein J, Hoffmann P. Formula constant optimisation techniques including variation of keratometer or corneal refractive index and consideration for classical and modern IOL formulae. PLoS ONE. 2023;18(2): e0282213. https://doi.org/10.1371/journal.pone.0282213.
21. Langenbucher A, Szentmáry N, Cayless A, Müller M, Eppig T, Schröder S, Fabian E. IOL Formula constants: strategies for optimization and defining standards for presenting data. Ophthalmic Res. 2021;64(6):1055–67. https://doi.org/10.1159/000514916.
22. Langenbucher A, Szentmáry N, Cayless A, Weisensee J, Fabian E, Wendelstein J, Hoffmann P. Considerations on the Castrop formula for calculation of intraocular lens power. PLoS ONE. 2021;16(6): e0252102. https://doi.org/10.1371/journal.pone.0252102.
23. Olsen T, Corydon L, Gimbel H. Intraocular lens power calculation with an improved anterior chamber depth prediction algorithm. J Cataract Refract Surg. 1995;21(3):313–9. https://doi.org/10.1016/s0886-3350(13)80140-x.
24. Olsen T, Cooke DL, Findl O, Gatinel D, Koch D, Langenbucher A, Melles RB, Yeo TK. Surgeons need to know more about IOL design for accurate power calculation. J Cataract Refract Surg. 2023. https://doi.org/10.1097/j.jcrs.0000000000001159.
25. Eppig T, Gillner M, Walter S, Viestenz A, Langenbucher A. [Calculation of phakic intraocular lenses]. Klin Monbl Augenheilkd. 2011;228(8):690–7. https://doi.org/10.1055/s-0031-1281598. Epub 2011 Aug 11. PMID: 21837583 Review. German.
26. Gernet H, Ostholt H & Werner H. Die präoperative Berechnung intraocularer Binkhorst-Linsen. 122. Vers. d. Ver. Rhein.-Westfäl. Augenärzte. Balve 1970, Verlag Zimmermann, Germany, pp. 54–55.
27. Fechner PU, van der Heijde GL, Worst JG. The correction of myopia by lens implantation into phakic eyes. Am J Ophthalmol. 1989;107(6):659–63. https://doi.org/10.1016/0002-9394(89)90264-x. PMID: 2729412.
28. Langenbucher A, Szentmáry N, Cayless A, Weisensee J, Wendelstein J, Hoffmann P. Prediction of CW chord as a measure for the eye's orientation axis after cataract surgery from preoperative IOLMaster 700 measurement data. Acta Ophthalmol. 2022;100(6):e1232–9. https://doi.org/10.1111/aos.15071.
29. Elliott M, Callender MG, Elliott DB. Accuracy of Javal's rule in the determination of spectacle astigmatism. Optom Vis Sci. 1994;71(1):23–6.
30. Langenbucher A, Hoffmann P, Cayless A, Wendelstein J, Bolz M, Szentmáry N. Meridional ocular magnification after cataract surgery with toric and non-toric intraocular lenses. Graefes Arch Clin Exp Ophthalmol. 2022;260(12):3869–82. https://doi.org/10.1007/s00417-022-05740-4.
31. Langenbucher A, Szentmáry N, Cayless A, Wendelstein J, Hoffmann P. Prediction of the axial lens position after cataract surgery using deep learning algorithms and multilinear regression. Acta Ophthalmol. 2022;100(7):e1378–84. https://doi.org/10.1111/aos.15108.
32. Olsen T. J Prediction of the effective postoperative (intraocular lens) anterior chamber depth. Cataract Refract Surg. 2006;32(3):419–24. https://doi.org/10.1016/j.jcrs.2005.12.139.
33. Norrby NE, Koranyi G. Prediction of intraocular lens power using the lens haptic plane concept. J Cataract Refract Surg. 1997;23(2):254–9. https://doi.org/10.1016/s0886-3350(97)80350-1.
34. Abulafia A, Barrett GD, Rotenberg M, Kleinmann G, Levy A, Reitblat O, Koch DD, Wang L, Assia EI. Intraocular lens

power calculation for eyes with an axial length greater than 26.0 mm: comparison of formulas and methods. J Cataract Refract Surg. 2015 Mar;41(3):548–56. https://doi.org/10.1016/j.jcrs.2014.06.033. Epub 2015 Feb 21.
35. Langenbucher A, Cayless A, Szentmáry N, Weisensee J, Wendelstein J, Hoffmann P. Prediction of total corneal power from measured anterior corneal power on the IOLMaster 700 using a feedforward shallow neural network. Acta Ophthalmol. 2022;100(5):e1080–7. https://doi.org/10.1111/aos.15040.
36. Langenbucher A, Eppig T, Cayless A, Gatzioufas Z, Wendelstein J, Hoffmann P, Szentmáry N. Simulation of corneal imaging properties for near objects. Ophthalmic Physiol Opt. 2021;41(5):1152–60. https://doi.org/10.1111/opo.12861.
37. Langenbucher A, Szentmáry N, Cayless A, Münninghoff L, Wortmann R, Wendelstein J, Hoffmann P. Translation model for anterior segment tomographic data to corneal spherical aberration derived from a Monte-Carlo simulation based on raytracing. Acta Ophthalmol. 2022;100(8):e1665–74. https://doi.org/10.1111/aos.15125. Epub 2022 Mar 1.
38. Langenbucher A, Szentmáry N, Cayless A, Weisensee J, Wendelstein J, Hoffmann P. Prediction of corneal back surface power—deep learning algorithm versus multivariate regression. Ophthalmic Physiol Opt. 2022;42(1):185–94. https://doi.org/10.1111/opo.12909.
39. Savini G, Næser K, Schiano-Lomoriello D, Ducoli P. Optimized keratometry and total corneal astigmatism for toric intraocular lens calculation. J Cataract Refract Surg. 2017;43(9):1140–8.
40. Hoffer KJ, Savini G. Update on intraocular lens power calculation study protocols: the better way to design and report clinical trials. Ophthalmology. 2021;128(11):e115–20. https://doi.org/10.1016/j.ophtha.2020.07.005.
41. Langenbucher A, Szentmáry N, Cayless A, Wendelstein J, Hoffmann P. Bootstrap outlier identification in clinical datasets for lens power formula constant optimization. Curr Eye Res. 2023;48(3):263–9. https://doi.org/10.1080/02713683.2022.2108457.
42. Melles RB, Kane JX, Olsen T, Chang WJ. Update on intraocular lens calculation formulas. Ophthalmology. 2019;126(9):1334–5. https://doi.org/10.1016/j.ophtha.2019.04.011. Epub 2019 Apr 11 PMID: 30980854.
43. Savini G, Taroni L, Hoffer KJ. Recent developments in intraocular lens power calculation methods-update 2020. Ann Transl Med. 2020;8(22):1553. https://doi.org/10.21037/atm-20-2290.
44. Shammas HJ. Intraocular lens power calculations. Slack Inc. 2004, USA, ISBN-13: 978–1556426520.
45. Hill W. https://doctor-hill.com/iol-power-calculations/extreme_axial_myopia/ (access 26.05.2020)
46. Langenbucher A, Szentmáry N, Cayless A, Weisensee J, Wendelstein J, Hoffmann P. The Castrop formula for calculation of toric intraocular lenses. Graefes Arch Clin Exp Ophthalmol. 2021;259(11):3321–31. https://doi.org/10.1007/s00417-021-05287-w.
47. Olsen T. Calculation of intraocular lens power: a review. Acta Ophthalmol Scand. 2007;85(5):472–85. https://doi.org/10.1111/j.1600-0420.2007.00879.x.
48. Fyodorov SN, Galin MA, Linksz A. Calculation of the optical power of intraocular lenses. Invest Ophthalmol. 1975;14:625–8.
49. Retzlaff JA, Sanders DR, Kraff MC. Development of the SRK/T intraocular lens implant power calculation formula. J Cataract Refract Surg. 1990;16(3):333–40. https://doi.org/10.1016/s0886-3350(13)80705-5. PMID: 2355321.
50. Simpson MJ. Pre-clinical estimation of the intraocular lens A-constant, and its relationship to power, shape factor, and asphericity. Appl Opt. 2021;60(19):5662–8. https://doi.org/10.1364/AO.426155.
51. Abulafia A, Koch DD, Wang L, Hill WE, Assia EI, Franchina M, Barrett GD. New regression formula for toric intraocular lens calculations. J Cataract Refract Surg. 2016;42(5):663–71. https://doi.org/10.1016/j.jcrs.2016.02.038.
52. Langenbucher A, Schrecker J, Cayless A, Hoffmann P, Wendelstein J, Szentmáry N. Calculation of equivalent and Toric power in AddOn lenses based on a Monte Carlo simulation. Ophthalmic Res. 2022;65(3):300–9. https://doi.org/10.1159/000521702.
53. Langenbucher A, Schrecker J, Eppig T, Schröder S, Cayless A, Schwemm M, Nagy Z, Szentmáry N. Ratio of torus and equivalent power to refractive cylinder and spherical equivalent in phakic lenses—a Monte-Carlo simulation study. Acta Ophthalmol. 2022;100(1):58–67. https://doi.org/10.1111/aos.14902.
54. Langenbucher A, Viestenz A, Szentmáry N, Behrens-Baumann W, Viestenz A. Toric intraocular lenses–theory, matrix calculations, and clinical practice. J Refract Surg. 2009;25(7):611–22. https://doi.org/10.3928/1081597X-20090610-07.
55. Cooke DL, Cooke TL, Atchison DA. Effect of cataract-induced refractive change on intraocular lens power formula predictions. Biomed Opt Express. 2021;12(5):2550–6. https://doi.org/10.1364/BOE.422190.
56. Langenbucher A, Szentmáry N, Cayless A, Casaza M, Weisensee J, Hoffmann P, Wendelstein J. Surgically Induced Astigmatism after Cataract Surgery—A Vector Analysis. Curr Eye Res. 2022;47(9):1279–87. https://doi.org/10.1080/02713683.2022.2052108.
57. Langenbucher A, Szentmáry N, Leydolt C, Cayless A, Schwarzenbacher L, Zsolt Nagy Z, Menapace R. Calculation of ocular magnification in phakic and pseudophakic eyes based on anterior segment OCT data. Ophthalmic Physiol Opt. 2021;41(4):831–41. https://doi.org/10.1111/opo.12822.
58. Schrecker J, Langenbucher A. Clinical results of a multifocal pseudophakic additional lens. Ophthalmologe. 2015;112(2):148–54. https://doi.org/10.1007/s00347-014-3102-4.
59. Langenbucher A, Szentmáry N, Seitz B. Calculating the power of toric phakic intraocular lenses. Ophthalmic Physiol Opt. 2007;27(4):373–80. https://doi.org/10.1111/j.1475-1313.2007.00487.x.
60. Cooke DL, Cooke TL. Comparison of 9 intraocular lens power calculation formulas. J Cataract Refract Surg. 2016;42(8):1157–64. https://doi.org/10.1016/j.jcrs.2016.06.029.
61. Wendelstein J, Hoffmann P, Hirnschall N, Fischinger IR, Mariacher S, Wingert T, Langenbucher A, Bolz M. Project hyperopic power prediction: accuracy of 13 different concepts for intraocular lens calculation in short eyes. Br J Ophthalmol. 2022;106(6):795–801. https://doi.org/10.1136/bjophthalmol-2020-318272.
62. Cooke DL, Cooke TL. Effect of altering lens constants. J Cataract Refract Surg. 2017;43(6):853. https://doi.org/10.1016/j.jcrs.2017.05.001.
63. Langenbucher A, Szentmáry N, Cayless A, Wendelstein J, Hoffmann P. Evaluating intraocular lens power formula constant robustness using bootstrap algorithms. Acta Ophthalmol. 2022. https://doi.org/10.1111/aos.15277. Epub ahead of print.
64. Langenbucher A, Szentmáry N, Cayless A, Wendelstein J, Hoffmann P. Particle swarm optimisation strategies for IOL formula constant optimisation. Acta Ophthalmol. 2023. https://doi.org/10.1111/aos.15664. Epub ahead of print.
65. Langenbucher A, Szentmáry N, Cayless A, Wendelstein J, Hoffmann P. Strategies for formula constant optimisation for intraocular lens power calculation. PLoS ONE. 2022;17(5): e0267352. https://doi.org/10.1371/journal.pone.0267352.
66. Taroni L, Hoffer KJ, Pellegrini M, Lupardi E, Savini G. Comparison of the New Hoffer QST with 4 modern accurate

formulas. J Cataract Refract Surg. 2022. https://doi.org/10.1097/j.jcrs.0000000000001126.
67. Turnbull AMJ, Hill WE, Barrett GD. Accuracy of intraocular lens power calculation methods when targeting low myopia in monovision. J Cataract Refract Surg. 2020. https://doi.org/10.1097/j.jcrs.0000000000000187.
68. Wang L, Holladay JT, Koch DD. Wang-Koch axial length adjustment for the Holladay 2 formula in long eyes. J Cataract Refract Surg. 2018;44(10):1291–2.
69. Wang L, Koch DDJ. Modified axial length adjustment formulas in long eyes. Cataract Refract Surg. 2018;44(11):1396–7.
70. Langenbucher A, Szentmáry N, Cayless A, Wendelstein J, Hoffmann P. Preconditioning of clinical data for intraocular lens formula constant optimisation using random forest quantile regression trees. Z Med Phys. 2023;S0939–3889(22):00129–35. https://doi.org/10.1016/j.zemedi.2022.11.009.
71. Wang L, Shirayama M, Ma XJ, Kohnen T, Koch DD. Optimizing intraocular lens power calculations in eyes with axial lengths above 25.0 mm. J Cataract Refract Surg. 2011;37(11):2018–27
72. Langenbucher A, Szentmáry N, Cayless A, Wendelstein J, Hoffmann P. Prediction of ocular magnification and aniseikonia after cataract surgery. Acta Ophthalmol. 2022;100(8):e1675–84. https://doi.org/10.1111/aos.15190.
73. Langenbucher A, Szentmáry N, Weisensee J, Wendelstein J, Cayless A, Menapace R, Hoffmann P. Prediction model for best focus, power, and spherical aberration of the cornea: raytracing on a large dataset of OCT data. PLoS ONE. 2021;16(2): e0247048. https://doi.org/10.1371/journal.pone.0247048.
74. Liou HL, Brennan NA. Anatomically accurate, finite model eye for optical modelling. J Opt Soc Am A Opt Image Sci Vis. 1997;14(8):1684–95. https://doi.org/10.1364/josaa.14.001684.
75. Langenbucher A, Szentmáry N, Weisensee J, Cayless A, Menapace R, Hoffmann P. Back-calculation of keratometer index based on OCT data and raytracing—a Monte Carlo simulation. Acta Ophthalmol. 2021;99(8):843–9. https://doi.org/10.1111/aos.14794.

Repair and Regeneration

Wound Healing

Tobias Brockmann, Thomas A. Fuchsluger, and Uwe Pleyer

Abstract

This chapter gives an overview on the basic understanding of corneal wound healing and fibrogenesis. On the one hand, the cornea forms the anterior barrier of the eye and it is particularly exposed to various external influences, such as those caused by injuries or pathogens. On the other hand, the cornea significantly contributes to a crisp optical image on the retina by its transparency, avascularity and specific curvature. In this context, due to its multifunctional role and as a border to the environment, proper wound healing, especially without the formation of light-scattering scars, is essential to preserve the integrity and function of the cornea; and the eye itself. Misdirected wound healing is of great clinical relevance, as it can lead to corneal fibrosis with subsequent visual loss. Corneal fibrosis may result in permanent opacification, which can lead to blindness. Physiologic wound healing is a complex process and involves numerous tissue processes. At the cellular level, it occurs in a sequence of migration or transformation, proliferation, and modulation of the extracellular matrix. Understanding the pathophysiological mechanisms of wound healing and fibrogenesis is of great importance for diagnostics, therapy, and the classification of healing processes of corneal wounds to counteract a permanent corneal damage at an early stage in the future.

Keywords

Pathophysiology · Corneal fibrosis · Myofibroblast activation · Innate immune response · Inflammation · Pathophysiologic modulation and therapy

T. Brockmann (✶) · T. A. Fuchsluger
Department of Ophthalmology, Universitätsmedizin Rostock, Rostock, Germany
e-mail: tobias.brockmann@med.uni-rostock.de

T. Brockmann
Faculty of Science and Technology (SciTec), Ernst-Abbe-University of Applied Sciences Jena, Jena, Germany

U. Pleyer
Department of Ophthalmology, Charité—Universitätsmedizin, Berlin, Germany

U. Pleyer
Freie Universität Berlin, Humboldt-Universität Zu Berlin, Berlin Institute of Health, Berlin, Germany

1 Introduction

Ocular diseases associated with massive vision loss are often the result of misled wound healing or fibrogenesis and represent reactions to ischemic or inflammatory processes [1]. Misdirected wound healing is of utmost clinical relevance, especially in the cornea [1]. Corneal fibrosis results in a loss of optical transparency, significantly reducing the visual acuity, which may lead to blindness of the affected eye. Stromal corneal scarring can result from corneal herpes infection (metaherpetic), microbial keratitis, mechanical or chemical affection, stromal keratopathy, and chronic corneal edema, e.g., in bullous keratopathy or graft failure. In many cases, the penetrating keratoplasty still is the only option for visual rehabilitation. Worldwide, close to 200,000 corneal transplants are performed annually, and the number is increasing (German Keratoplasty Register 2018 and Flockerzi, et al. 2018) [2, 3]. In addition, the number of corneal complications with scarring is increasing due to the high prevalence of contact lenses and laser refractive corneal surgery. Furthermore, the risk of ocular trauma, with possible corneal involvement, cannot be ignored: the lifetime incidence is 20% [4]! Against this background, therapeutic strategies to support corneal wound healing and against corneal fibrosis are of increasing importance.

In the following, the pathophysiology and basics of corneal wound healing will be reviewed on clinical cases.

B. Seitz et al. (eds.), *Atlas on Cornea*, https://doi.org/10.1007/978-3-031-65422-0_3

2 Pathogenesis and Basics

Physiological wound healing engages a number of tissue processes and occurs in a sequence of cell migration or transformation, proliferation, and modulation of the extracellular matrix, as outlined in Fig. 1 [4]. During regular wound healing, protein deposition in the extracellular matrix is reversible [5]. In contrast, irreversible deposition of collagens, fibronectin, and matrix proteins occurs during fibrotic remodeling processes due to dysregulation of inflammatory responses. This process is a consequence of severe or chronic tissue damage, tissue stress or dysfunction [6]. Myofibroblasts are the key mediators in this process [7]. The transformation of keratocytes to activated fibroblasts and myofibroblasts, as well as the modulation of the extracellular matrix, is regulated by inflammatory and fibrogenic growth factors, as well as by cytokines and factors of the complement system [8, 9]. The following signaling pathways are involved in the processes of stromal wound healing in the cornea [4, 5]:

1. Transformation of Keratocytes to Fibroblasts and Myofibroblasts.

Resting keratocytes are activated by specific growth factors (TGFβ, FGF-2, PDGF-AB) to form fibroblasts, capable of division [10]. These can proliferate and are able to fill or close a wound. In addition, keratocyte-specific proteins, such as transketolase and aldehyde dehydrogenase 1A1, are downregulated and proteins of the extracellular matrix and matrix metalloproteinases are increasingly expressed. Under the further influence of growth factors, fibroblasts transform into myofibroblasts. These motile cells are

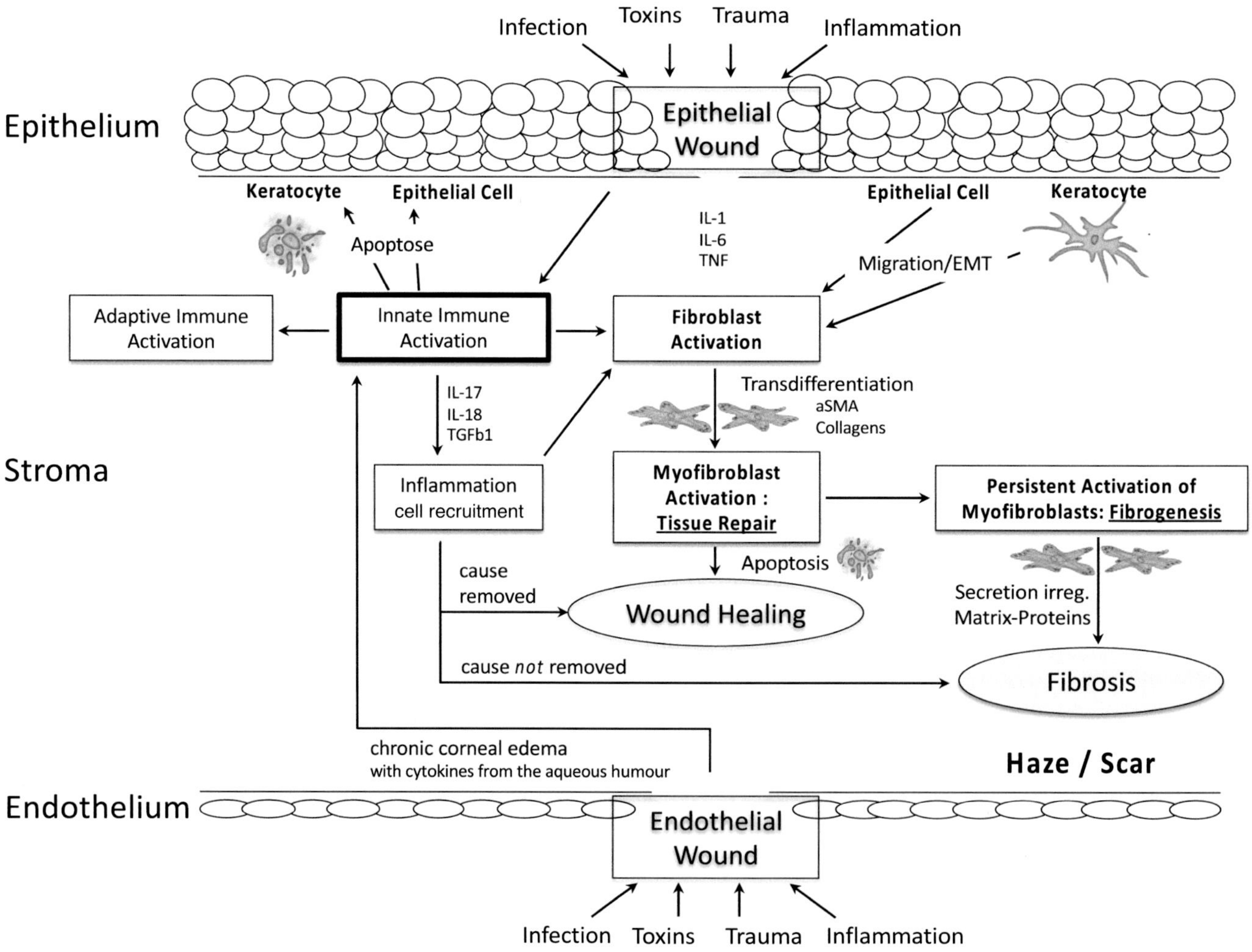

Fig. 1 Scheme of corneal wound healing mechanisms (modified from Wynn TA et al. 2012 Nat. Med. and Chaurasia SS et al. 2015 J. Funct. Biomater). The eye, and more specifically the cornea, possesses an immune privilege characterized by avascularity, low lymphatic activity, and reduced numbers of antigen-presenting cells (compared to other tissues). Because of these conditions, innate immune responses (cellular and humoral) are of primary importance in the context of corneal pathologies. Wound healing results from a sequence of cell migration/transformation, proliferation, and extracellular matrix production/modulation

characterized by the expression of vimentin, α-Smooth Muscle Actin (α-SMA) and desmin, which enable them to contract. They significantly contribute to the irreversible remodeling of the extracellular matrix through the excessive expression of matrix proteins [11].

2. Coagulation System and Innate Humoral Immune Response.

Rapid protein cascades, especially those of hemostasis, play an important role in the initiation and support of wound healing [12]. This involves von Willebrand factor-and prothrombin-mediated conversion of fibrinogen to fibrin [13]. In addition, the innate humoral immune response, starting from the complement system, contributes to further fibrosis [9, 14]. Complement cleavage products have been found in corneal wound healing and significantly influence pathophysiological processes likewise [9, 15–17].

3. Innate Cellular Immune Response

Activated fibroblasts secrete chemotactic cytokines such as monocyte chemotactic protein-1 (MCP-1), whereupon inflammatory cells migrate into the wound [18]. Innate immune defense cells, such as monocytes, macrophages, neutrophils, and eosinophils, may exert pro-inflammatory effects on fibroblasts and myofibroblasts through secretion of tumor necrosis factor-α (TNF-α) and interleukin-1β (IL-1β) and contribute to IL-6-mediated fibrosis [19, 20]. Alternatively-activated macrophages (M2, IL-4/IL-1), which also express arginase-1 (Arg1), assume a special function by inducing collagen synthesis by myofibroblasts. They support the healing process and contribute to the resolution of inflammatory processes through anti-inflammatory effects [21].

3 Causes of Stromal Corneal Opacity

Mild corneal opacification can already be induced by activated corneal fibroblasts. In contrast to resting keratocytes, activated corneal fibroblasts have a lower intracellular concentration of water-soluble crystallin proteins [22, 23]. Crystallins are particularly present in the cornea and lens. They provide UV absorption, serve to protect from reactive oxygen species (ROS) and maintain optical transparency by reducing scattered light by allowing the cytoplasm of keratocytes to achieve a refractive index similar to that of the stromal extracellular matrix [24]. Thus, a reduced concentration of cytoplasmic crystallins, as in activated corneal fibroblasts or myofibroblasts, leads to visible corneal opacity by an increase in light scattering, as it may occur as 'haze' after corneal crosslinking (Fig. 2).

With further transdifferentiation of fibroblasts to myofibroblasts, the increase in focal contraction forces within the cornea results in an alteration of the corneal surface with the development of higher order aberrations and associated light scattering, as shown in the presentation of a metaherpetic corneal scar in Fig. 3 [25].

In addition, myofibroblasts induce a remodeling of the corneal fiber structure by the excessive deposition of disorganized extracellular matrix, which lead to corneal opacification by its back-scattering of light, as typically present in focal scars after corneal ulceration (Fig. 4) [26]. The major components of myofibroblast-produced extracellular matrix are: Type I-VI and XVIII collagens, laminin, nidogen-1 and -2, fibronectin, tenascin, thrombospondin, glycosaminoglycans, hyaluronic acid, heparin sulfate, and chondroitin [27–29]. Here, the deposits of collagen I and III were quantitatively most significant [30].

4 Causes of Misdirected Wound Healing and Fibrogenesis

Myofibroblasts are the directional agents of wound healing or fibrogenesis. They can fill or close wounds by cellular contraction and they can remodel corneal tissue by secretion of extracellular matrix and proteases to achieve or restore mechanical stability. Evolutionarily, in this way, the integrity of the eye, by closing an open corneal wound with the associated risk of intraocular carriage of pathogens—under the frequent loss of vision due to scarring—could be maintained. Physiologically, the shape and function of the corneal stroma are restored by the degradation of extracellular matrix products and myofibroblast apoptosis, or their reversion to fibroblasts [18].

Thus, the crucial switch for the transition to aberrant wound healing and fibrogenesis is the failure of myofibroblasts to undergo an orderly transition to apoptosis, as depicted in Fig. 5.

Myofibroblasts require specific growth factors (the most important: TGFβ, FGF-2, PDGF-AB) for their ongoing survival. While keratocytes, monocytes/macrophages, fibroblasts and myofibroblasts can produce TGFβ1 and TGFβ2, these cells do not reach the necessary effective concentrations and localizations to ensure sustained autocrine activation of mature myofibroblasts [31–34].

Accordingly, continuous supplementation of the specific growth factors, especially TGFβ1 and/or TGFβ2, from other sources is necessary to maintain myofibroblast vitality [35]. The most important sources of growth factors are the corneal epithelium, endothelium and tear film [36, 37]. In this respect, a corneal wound healing disorder is often associated with persistent corneal epithelial defects that is a main driver of fibrosis and scarring, as shown in Fig. 6.

In addition to restoring corneal epithelial or endothelial defects, the integrity of the anatomical barrier, i.e., the

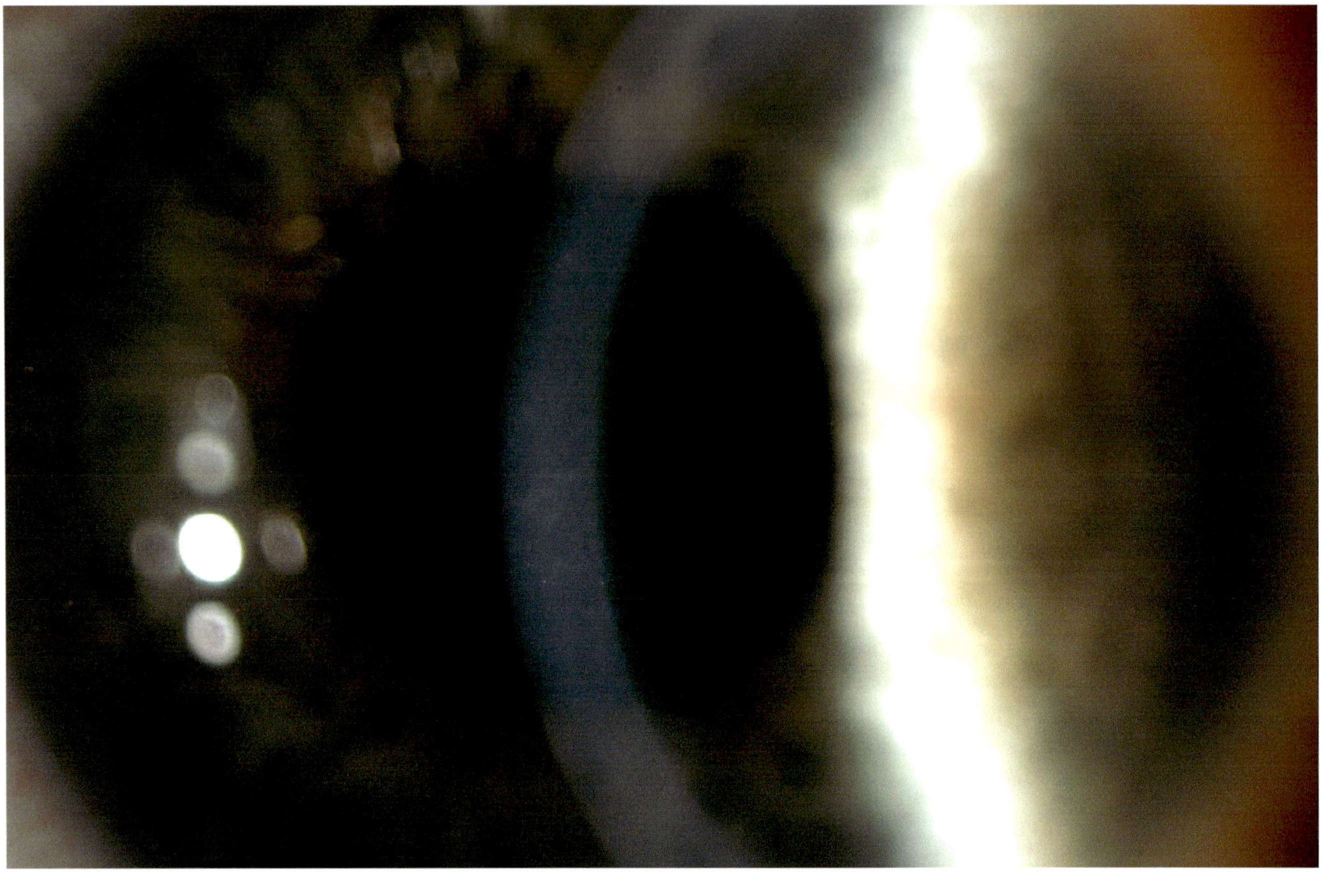

Fig. 2 Residual persistent corneal 'haze' 5 years after UV-crosslinking with riboflavin in the left eye of a 30-year-old man with keratoconus. Hazy opacity, especially of the anterior corneal stroma generally occurs immediately after crosslinking procedure as a sign of keratocyte activation. The hazy opacification usually vanishes over time within weeks under corticosteroidal treatment but may individually last longer or persist in a mild form, as shown

epithelial basement membrane or Descemet membrane, is essential to prevent the accumulation of growth factors [38, 39]. In this context, specific components of the basement membrane (perlecan, nidogen, and collagen IV) are responsible for binding TGFβ or PDGF to neutralize them before they enter the corneal stroma [38, 40]. Therefore, the progression of misled wound healing and the onset of fibrogenesis can be often seen due to the inability to restore the basement membranes. In case the reestablishment of the barrier membranes fails, fibrogenesis continues due to persisting underlying cause, as shown in Fig. 7.

While the epithelial basement membrane can be rebuilt by an intact epithelial layer, the mechanisms of regeneration of the endothelial barrier on the layer of Descemet membrane are insufficiently understood so far. Descemet membrane defects usually result in an inflow of aqueous humor into the corneal stroma, along with its cytokines and growth factors, causing stromal fibrosis, as shown in Fig. 8.

In accordance with this understanding, several etiologic mechanisms exist that may lead to corneal fibrogenesis, as listed below:

5 Etiology

Infectious (viral (Fig. 3), bacterial (Fig. 4), mycotic, parasitic (acanthamoebae, Fig. 9)).

Mechanical (entropion, ectropion (Fig. 7), exposure keratopathy, traumatic (Fig. 6)).

Physical (UV-light exposure (Fig. 2), thermal burns, traumatic).

Chemical (chemical burn (Fig. 5), toxins).

Immunologic (rheumatogenic, e.g., Mooren ulcer, ocular pemphigoid, Stevens–Johnson syndrome, marginal corneal ulceration (Fig. 10), ocular rosacea-associated blepharokeratoconjunctivitis (Fig. 12)).

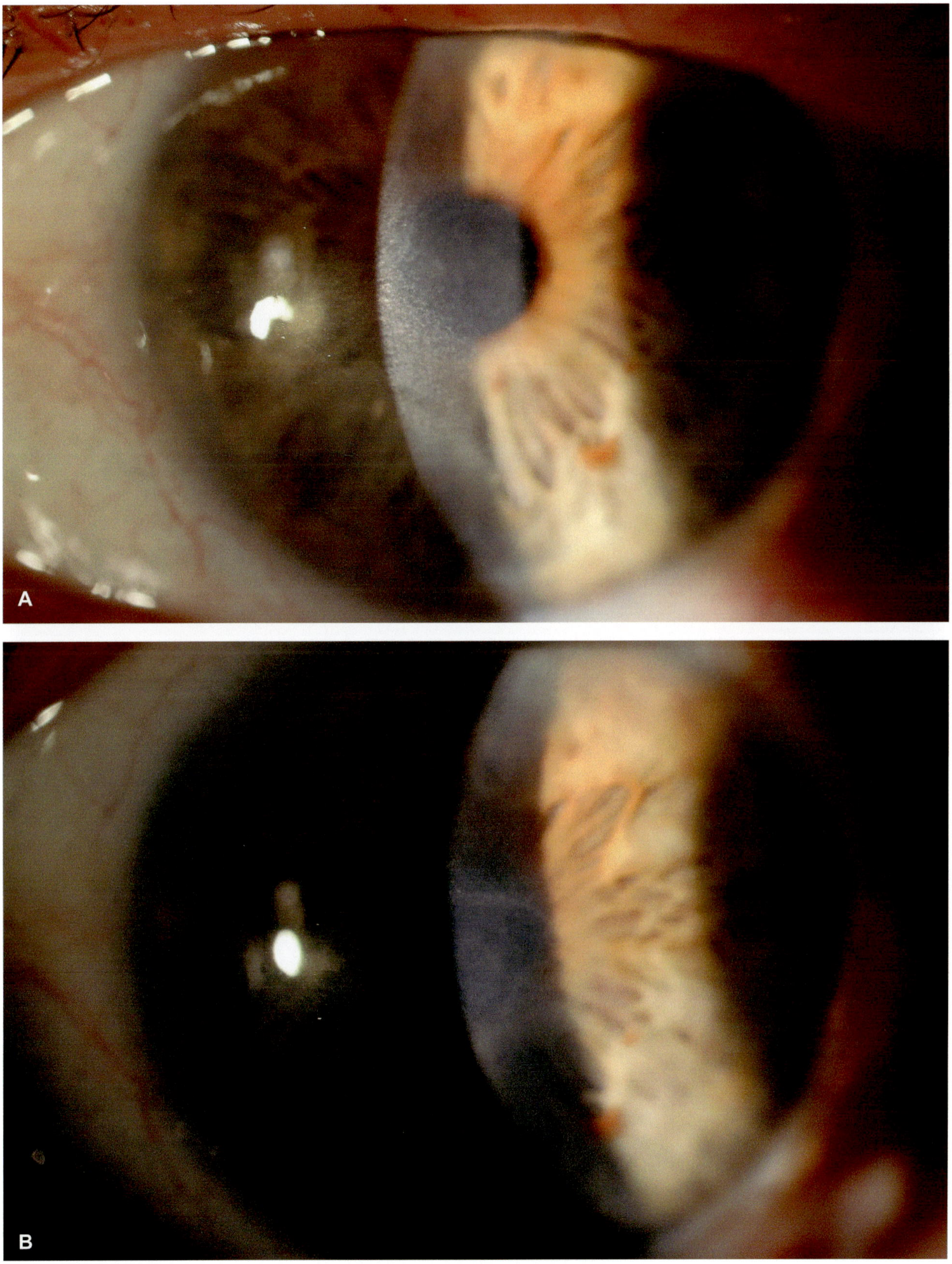

Fig. 3 (**A**) Mild subepithelial corneal opacification one year after herpetic keratitis in the left eye of a 77-year-old man. (**B**) The patient presented with a reduced visual acuity to 20/100 and disturbing photophobia, especially due to the persistent scar-inducing irregular corneal surface

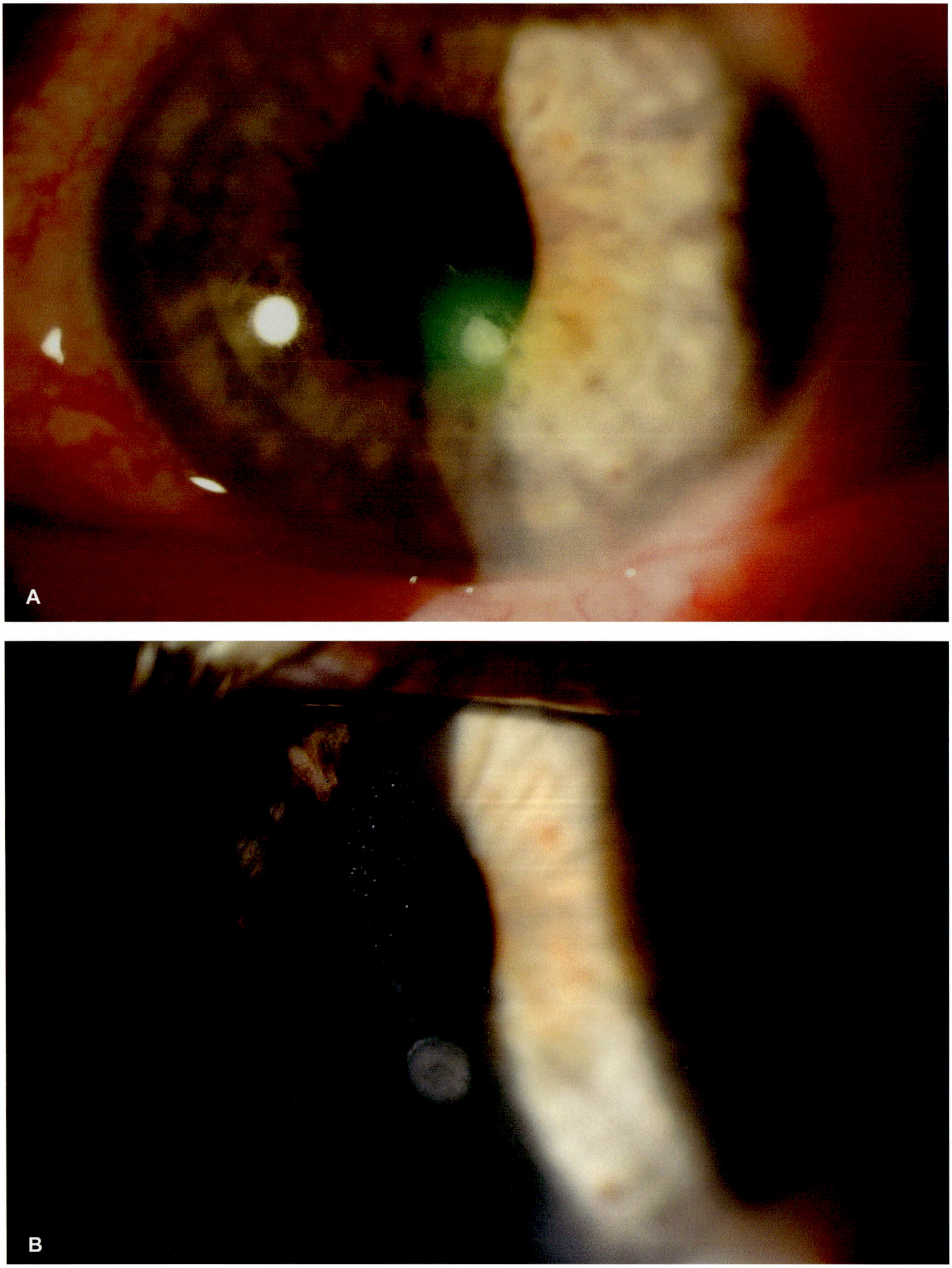

Fig. 4 (**A**) Presentation of a mid-peripheral focal bacterial ulcer after foreign body injury by a pine needle in the left eye of a 70-year-old man. (**B**) Persistent corneal stroma scar after 5 months, despite a timely anti-inflammatory co-treatment, as presentation of the permanent and excessive deposition of disorganized extracellular matrix proteins. Yet, the patients' visual acuity increased from 20/40 (**A**) to 20/20 Snellen (**B**)

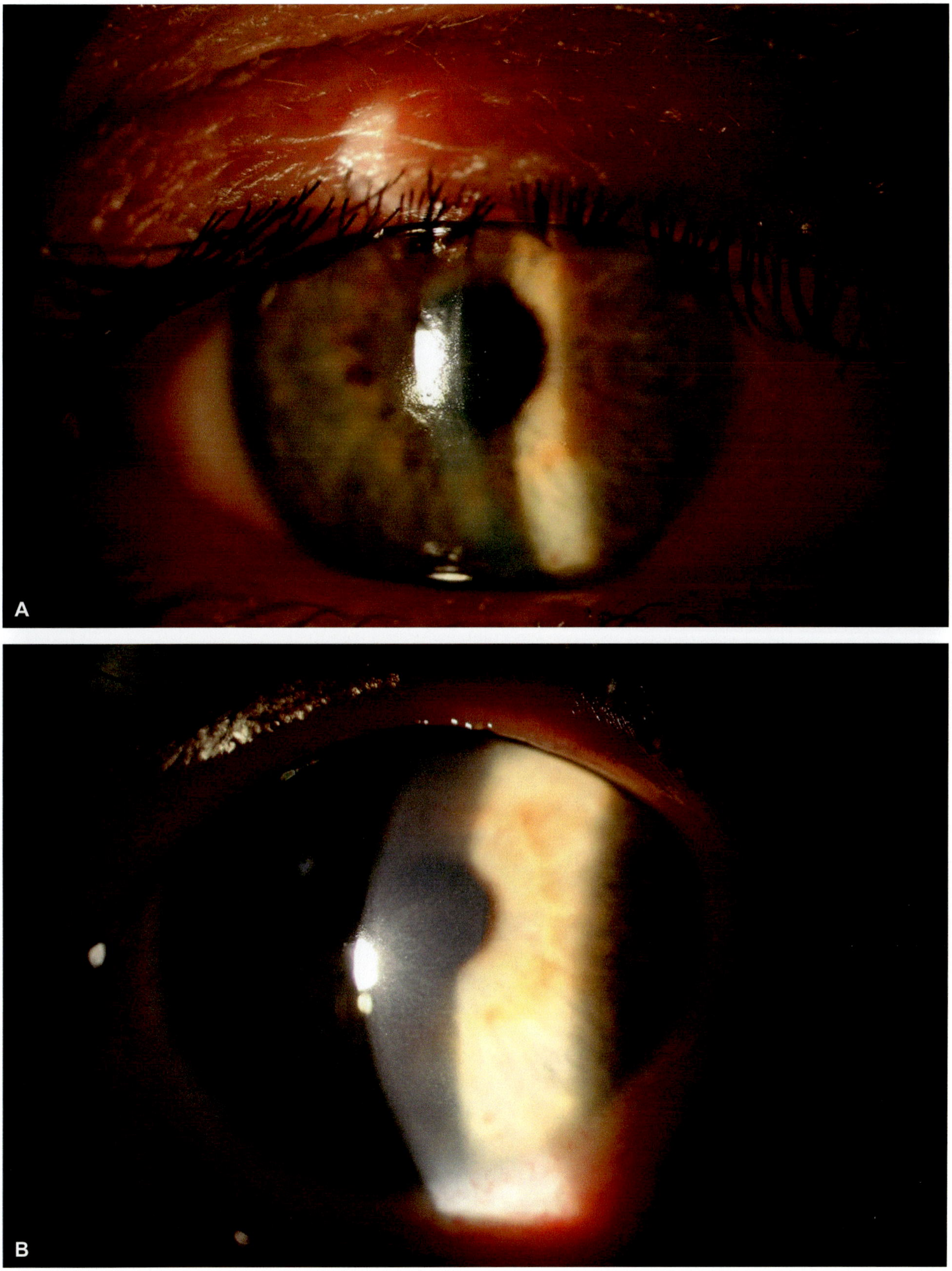

Fig. 5 (**A**) A 37-year-old man suffered from a corneal burn in the right eye by acidic chemicals of epoxy resin and initially presented with a severe corneal burn, subtotal corneal erosion and ischemic limbal conjunctiva. (**B**) Two weeks after incidence, after initial peritomy and amniotic membrane transplantation, a general corneal opacity has formed while the corneal epithelium has healed

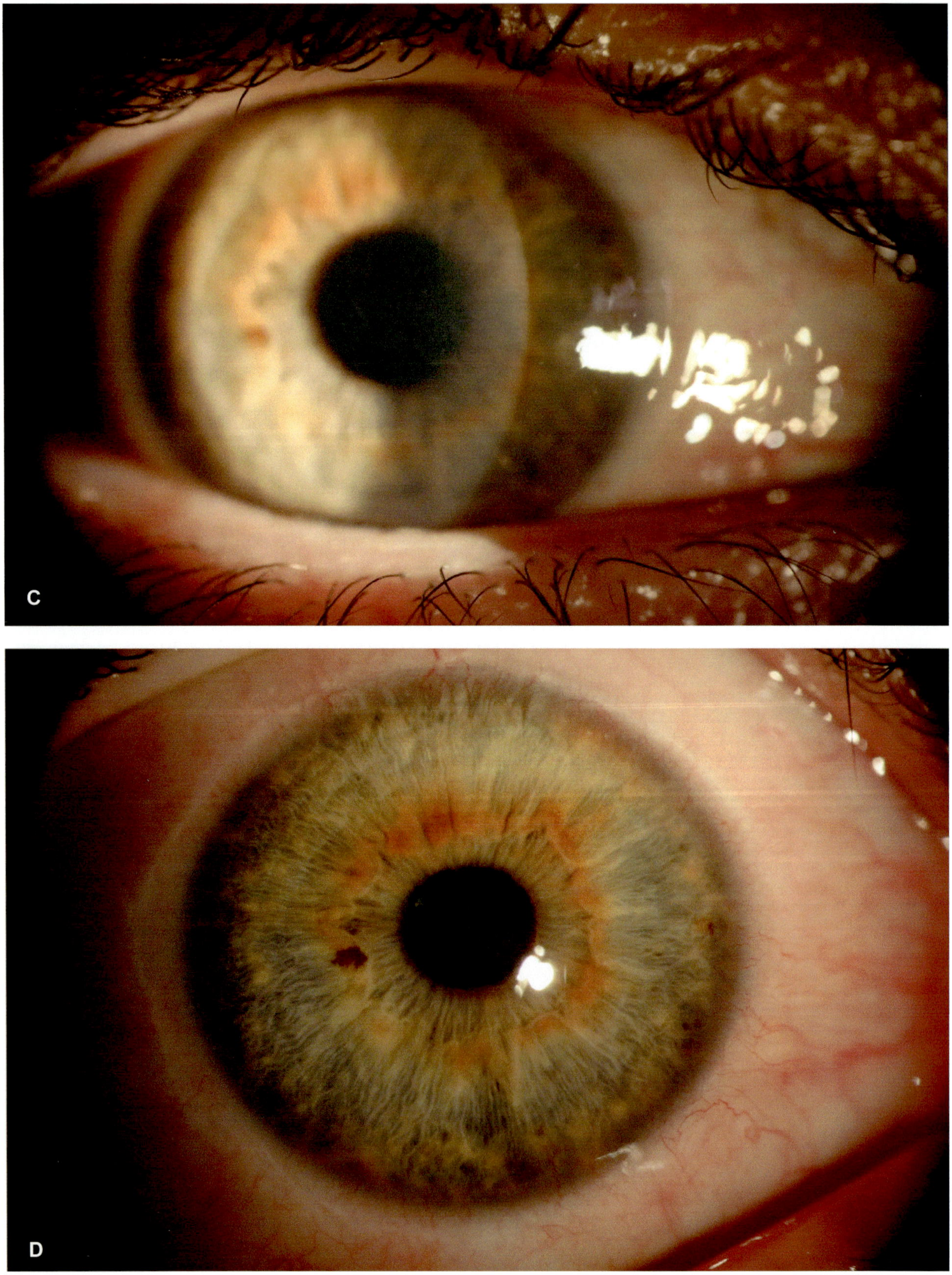

Fig. 5 (**C**) In the follow-up curse, 6 weeks after incidence, after a mild resolution of the corneal opacity—still with persistent stomal haze—is present. (**D**) Finally, 7 months after incidence and continuous intensive anti-inflammatory topical treatment a full resolution of the corneal opacification and a visual acuity of 20/20 was reattained

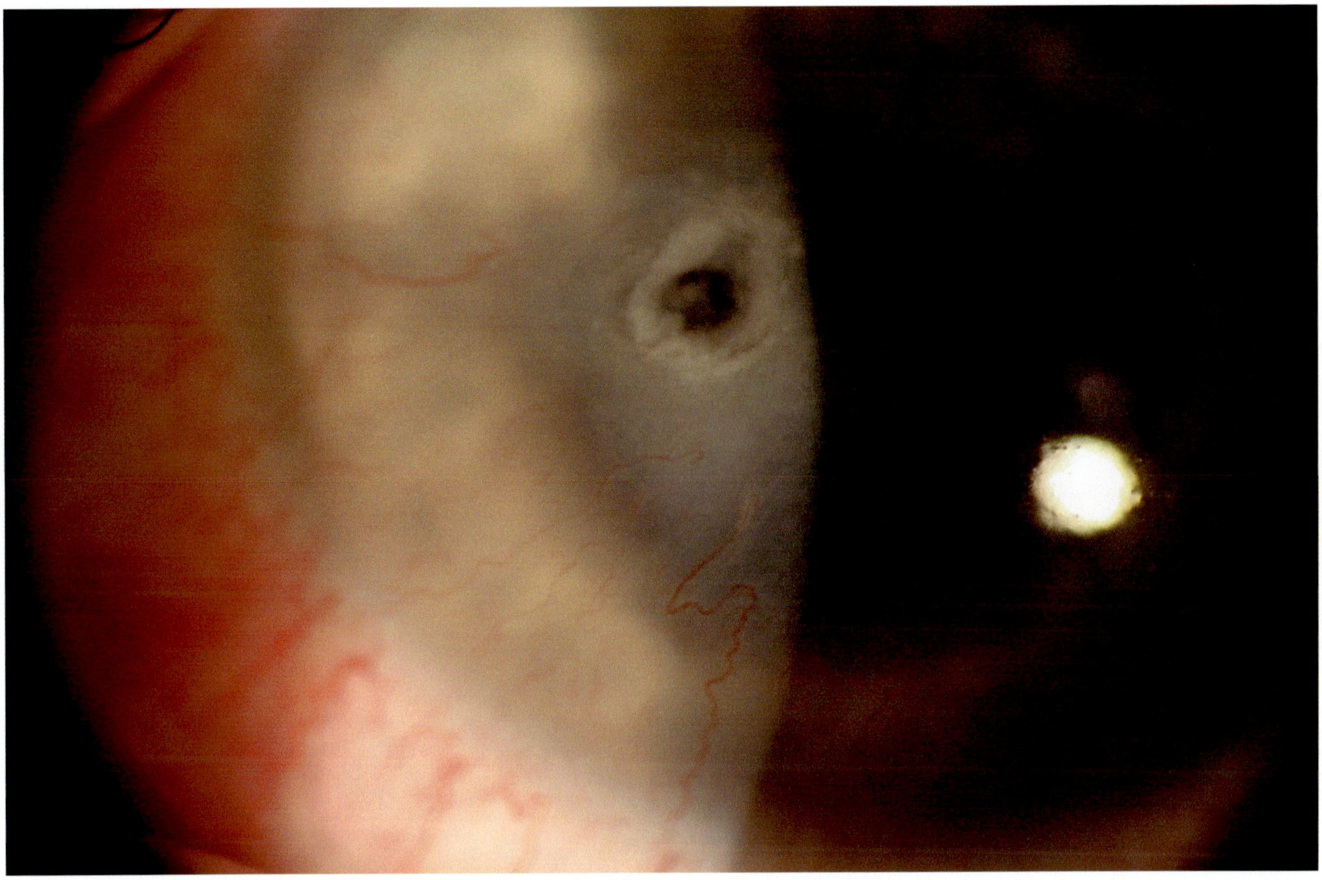

Fig. 6 Deep corneal stroma defect with associated areal fibrosis and vascularization in the left eye of a 15-year-old girl due to recurrent corneal erosions since the 6th year of life

Neurogenic (neurotrophic keratitis (Fig. 11), corneal sensitivity disorder, lagophthalmos in facial nerve palsy).

Genetic (corneal dystrophies).

Senescent: crocodile shagreen, corneal keloids, Salzmann nodular degeneration (Fig. 14).

Varia: chronic corneal edema e.g. in graft failure, hydrops in keratoconus (Fig. 8), Fuchs endothelial dystrophy, bullous keratopathy, iatrogenic (Fig. 13).

6 Modulation and Treatment Options

A variety of pharmacological and surgical options are available for the treatment of corneal wound healing disorders. The decision, appropriate selection and indication for the optimal therapy mainly depends on the clinical presentation of the corneal wound or fibrosis/scar. While the treatment of epithelial healing disorders can mostly be addressed by topical surface care, if necessary, under the protection of local antibiotics. Newer concepts of pharmacological stimulation of epithelial wound healing exist. These include the topical application of autologous serum, albumin or specific growth factors, e.g. for corneal nerve regeneration in neurotropic ulcers by using a recombinant nerve growth factor (NGF). Topical application of anti-inflammatory agents represents an essential component in the treatment of chronic corneal wound healing disorders and for modulation of stromal wound healing. These can be conventional corticosteroids with different pharmacokinetics (surface- or deep-acting formulations), or immunomodulating agents (e.g., ciclosporin A and tacrolimus). Pharmacologic manipulation of corneal wound healing is still limited. In particular, the specific modulation of the innate humoral immune response would be useful in this regard and should be within the focus of further developments. In case of insufficient efficacy of a pharmacological therapy, surgical procedures are useful. In this context, amniotic membrane transplantation is a cornerstone in the treatment of conservatively refractory epithelial and stromal defects. In this way, supportive growth factors are also applied to the wound. In addition to the possible surgical correction of the underlying cause of a wound healing disorder, such as exposure keratopathy due to ectropion, by reconstructive eyelid surgery, the temporary closure of the eyelid can also be an effective option. In this case, eyelid closure can be achieved temporarily by suturing or pharmacologically by botulism

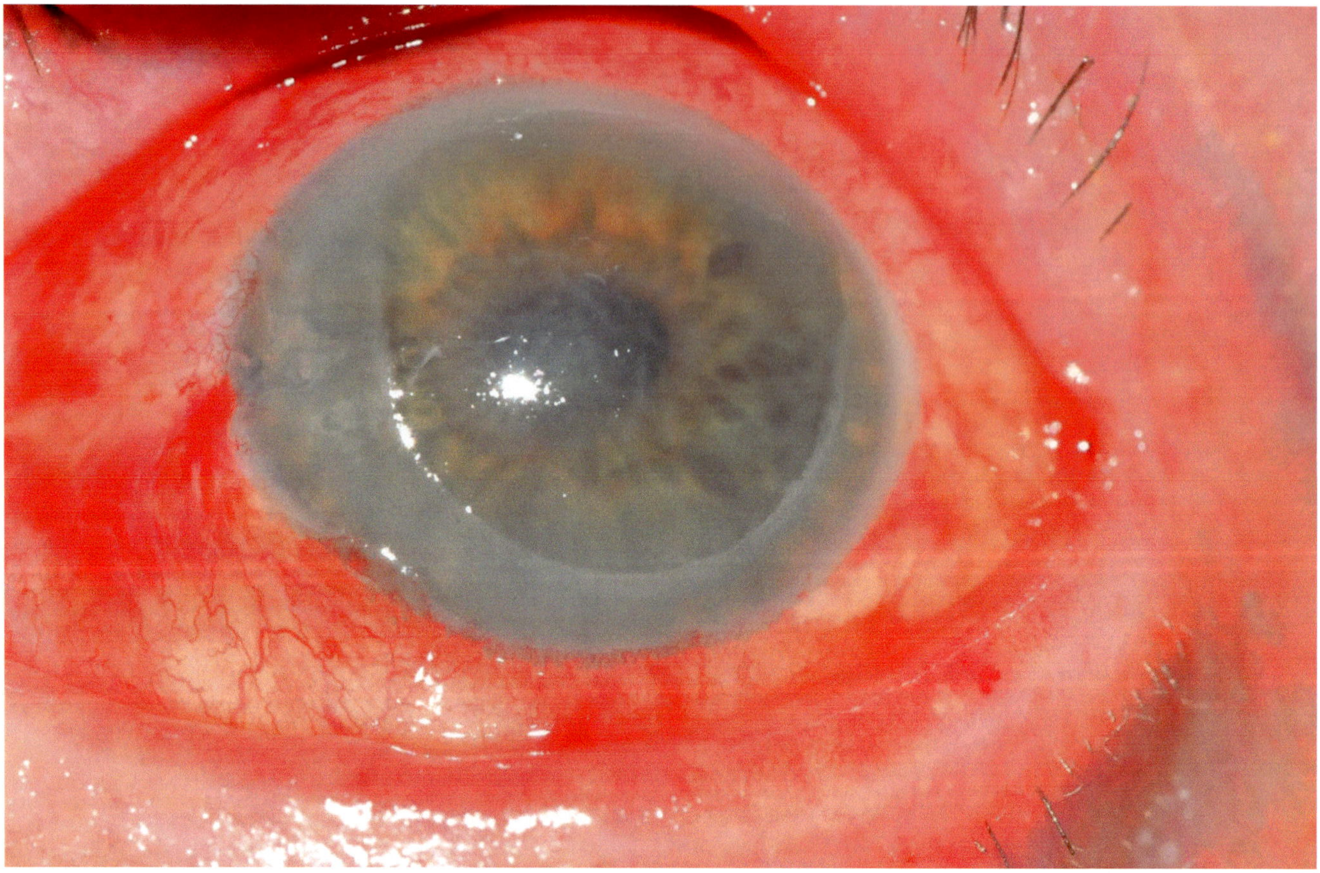

Fig. 7 Subtotal persistent corneal epithelial erosion with an epithelial rim and corneal fibrosis by prolonged decompensation caused due to a surface disturbance due to lower lid ectropium in the left eye of a 84-year-old man

toxin injections. Another option is a temporary or permanent narrowing of the palpebral fissure by tarsorrhaphy.

Regarding the further treatment of chronic wound healing disorders especially in cases of limbal stem cell insufficiency, autologous limbal stem cell transplantation can also be performed in different surgical variants. Finally, in advanced wound healing disorders with loss of ocular integrity or in findings with pronounced fibrotic remodeling and significantly reduced vision due to corneal scars, lamellar or penetrating corneal transplantation is the adequate treatment option to restore visual prognosis. The results of these various treatment options are promising and in particular often successful. Nevertheless, the treatment of corneal wound healing disorders is still often limited by the need for further optimization—pharmacologically and surgically.

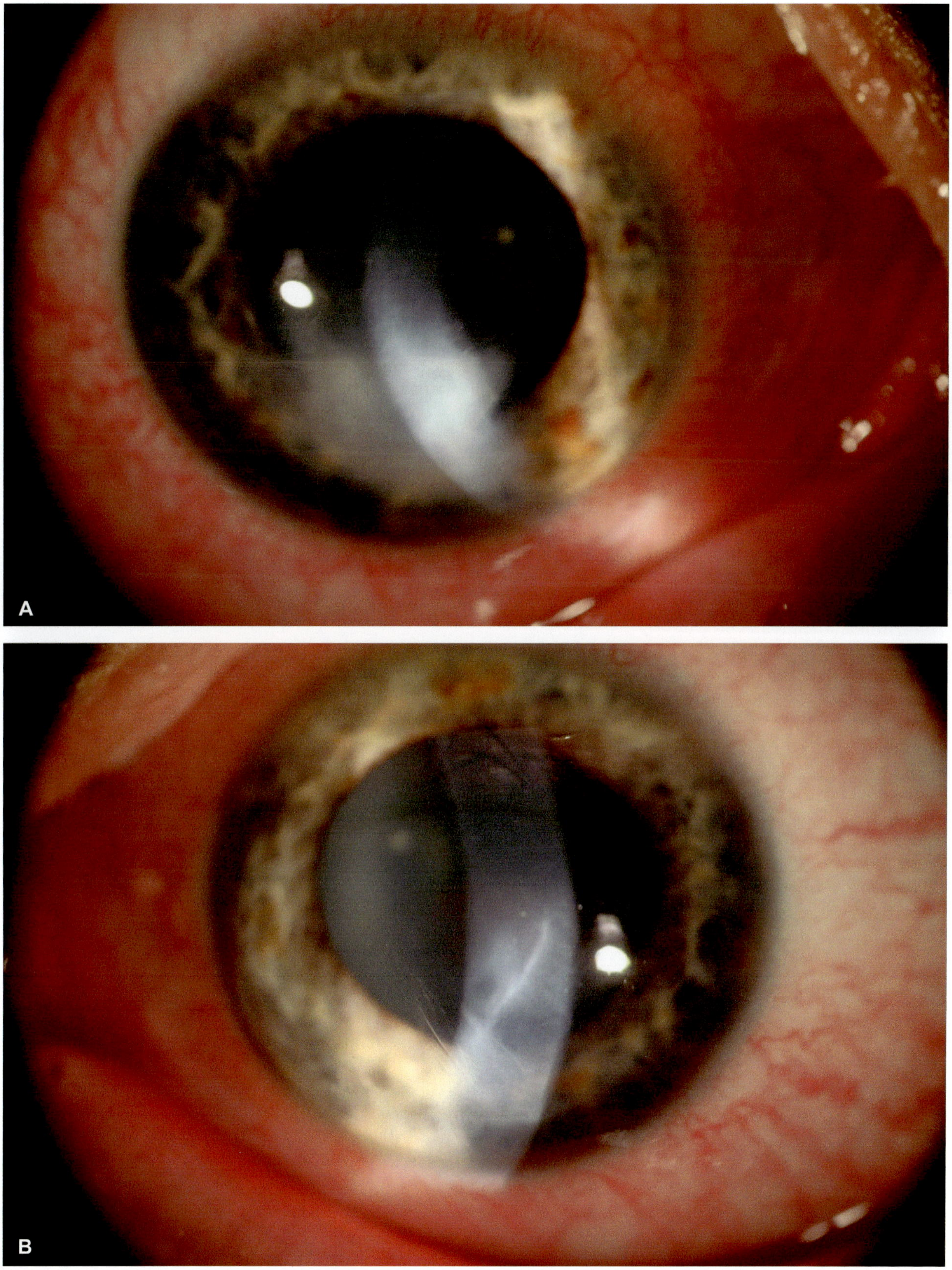

Fig. 8 (**A**) An extensive avascular and thorough stromal scar of the lower corneal hemisphere in the right eye of a 47-year-old man after corneal hydrops due to keratoconus one year ago. (**B**) Evident rupture of the Descemet membrane in the inferior paracentral cornea with accompanied stromal scaring in the left eye of the same patient, also after corneal hydrops due to keratoconus

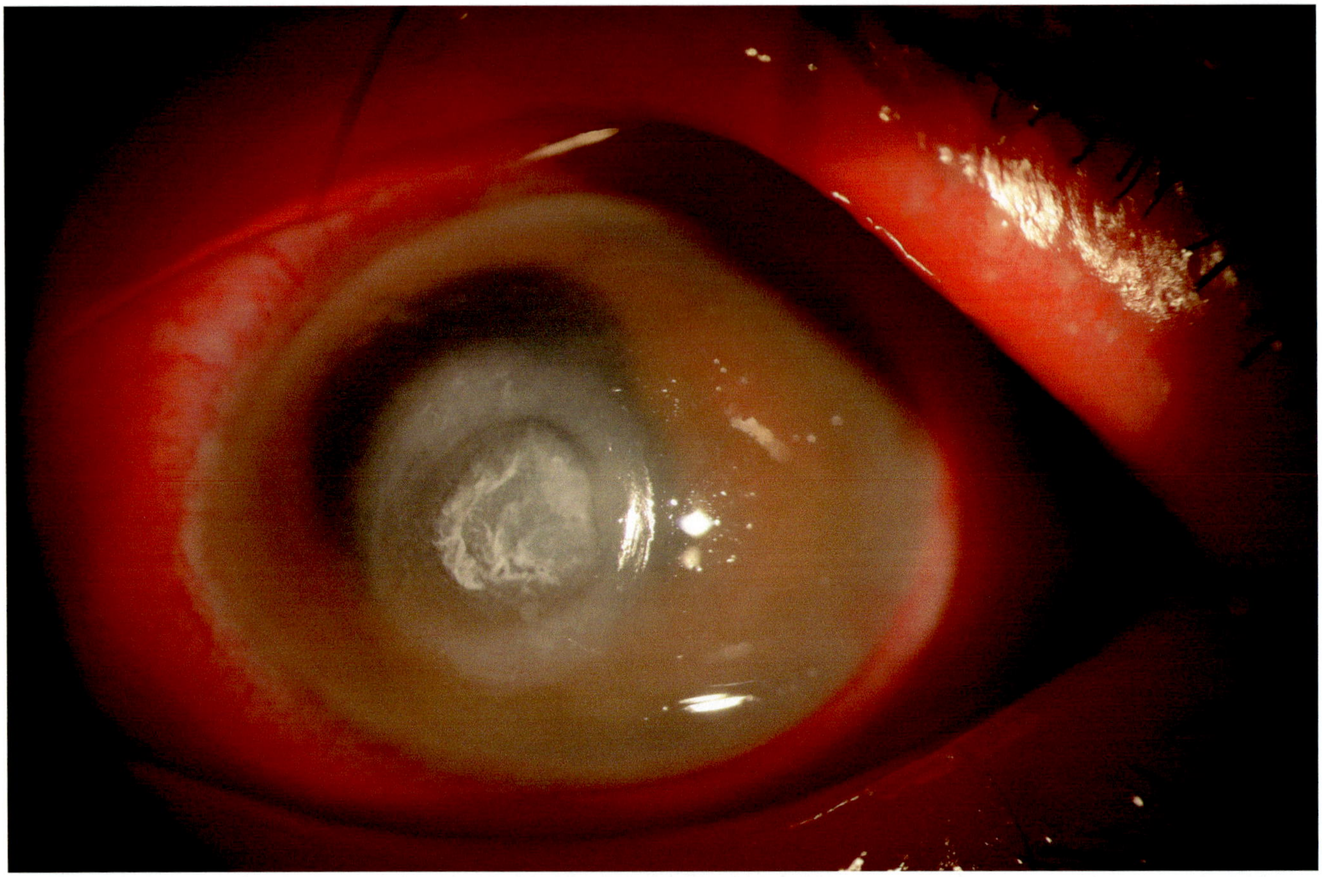

Fig. 9 Central deep corneal ulcer with surrounding ring infiltrate and anterior chamber inflammation with posterior synechiae in the right eye of a 40-year-old man. The microbial screening revealed a fungal and acanthamoeba co-infection after an ocular incidence during dirt work with wastewater

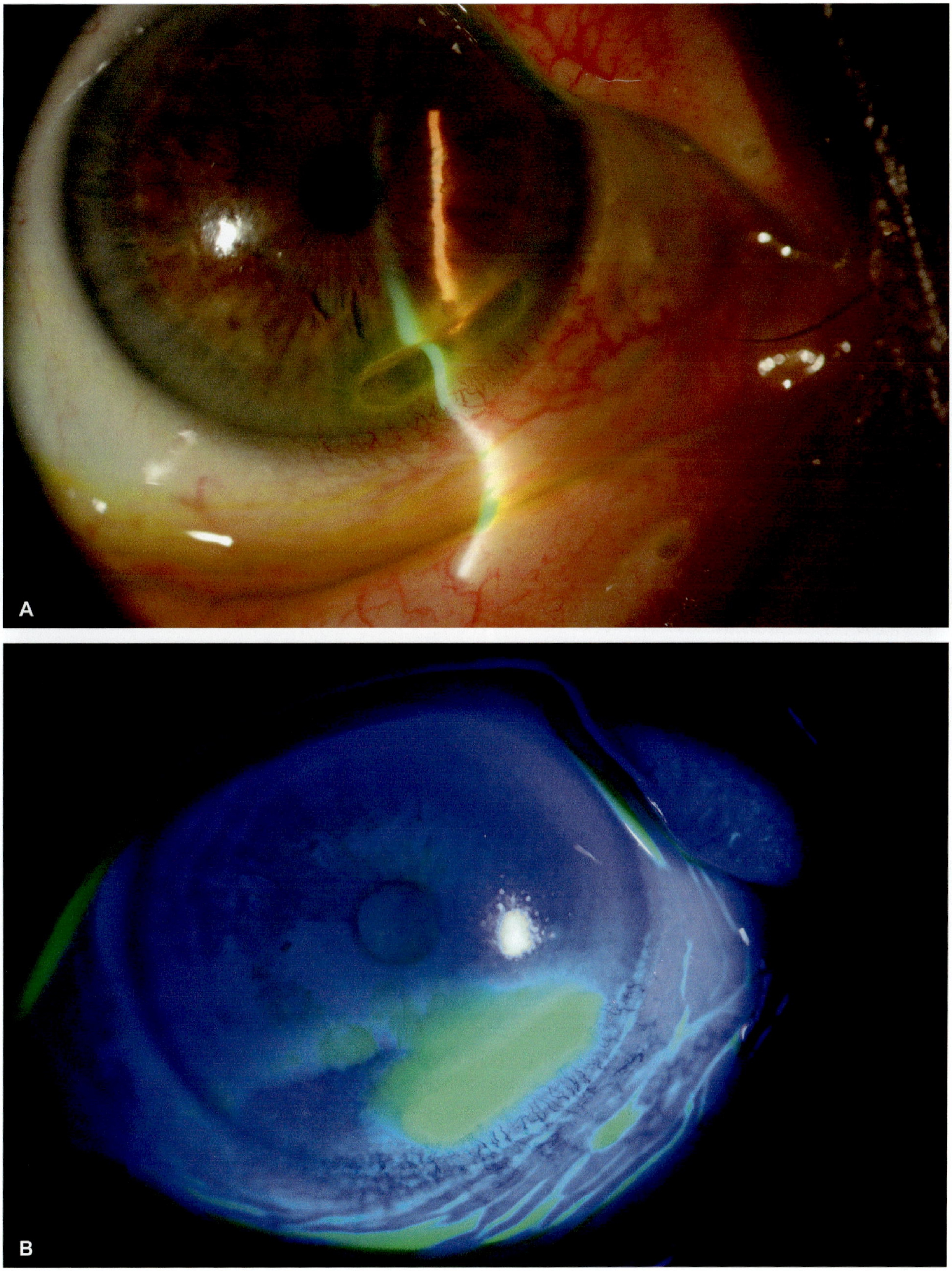

Fig. 10 Marginal corneal ulceration in the right eye of a 69-year-old woman with deep stromal thinning (**A**) with circumferential epithelial erosion and central fluorescein pooling (**B**)

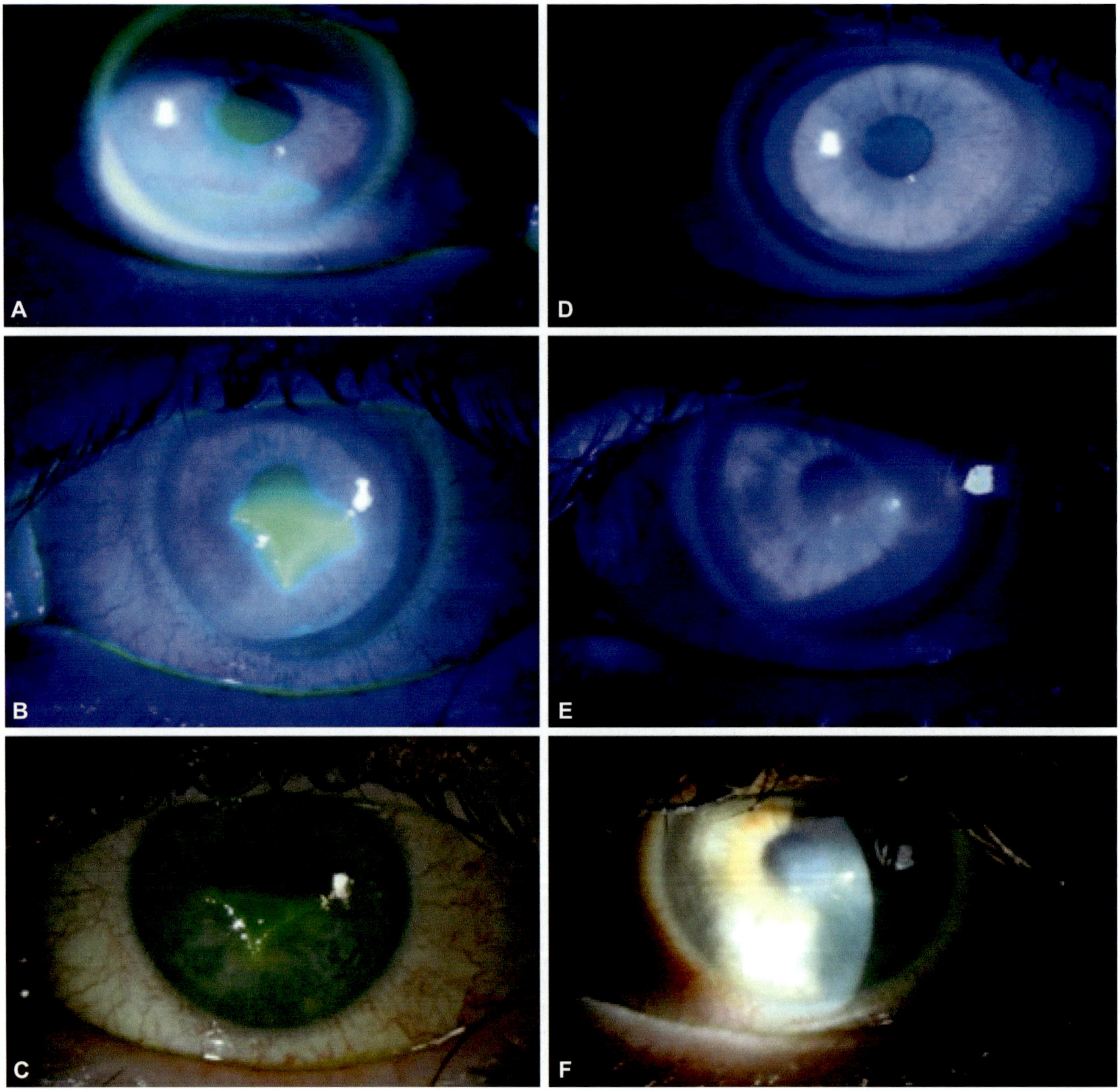

Fig. 11 Epithelial defects of the cornea in a patient with neurotrophic keratitis after chemotherapy and autologous stem cell transplantation for multiple myeloma. Staining with fluorescein of the right (**A**) and left eye (**B, C**). (**D–F**) Closed epithelium after 8 weeks of therapy with nerve growth factor (NGF, Cenegermin) eye drops. *Photo* Department of Ophthalmology, Charité, Universitätsmedizin Berlin)

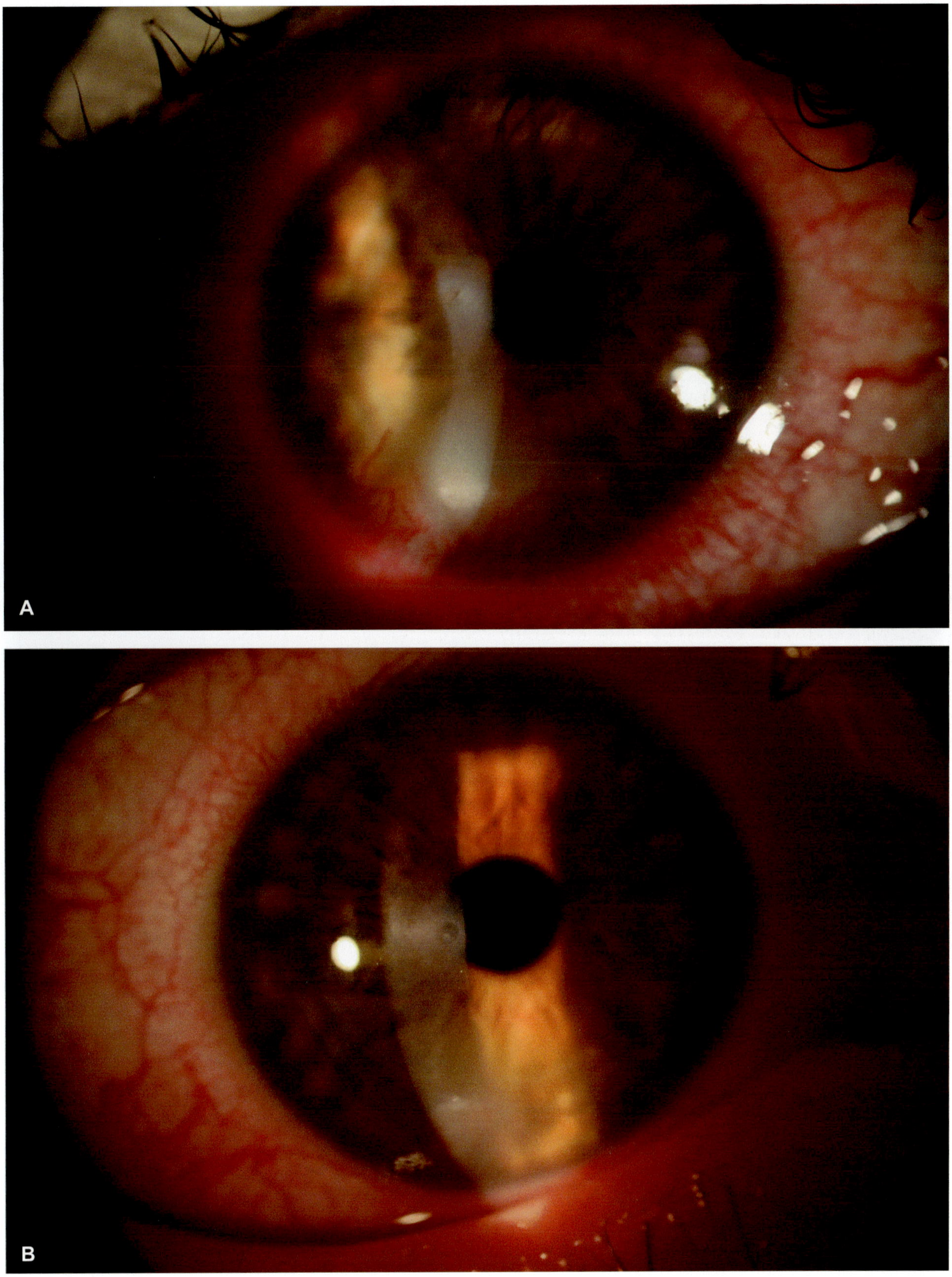

Fig. 12 (**A**) Initial presentation of a deep sterile corneal ulcus and deep vascularization in the 6'o clock position in a right eye of a 24-year-old man with distinctive ocular rosacea-associated blepharitis and keratitis. (**B**) Presentation of the same eye 10 days after conventional intensified topical antibiotic and anti-inflammatory treatment, and consequent eyelid care. A reduction of the ocular surface inflammation and less perfusion of the deep corneal vascularization was attained

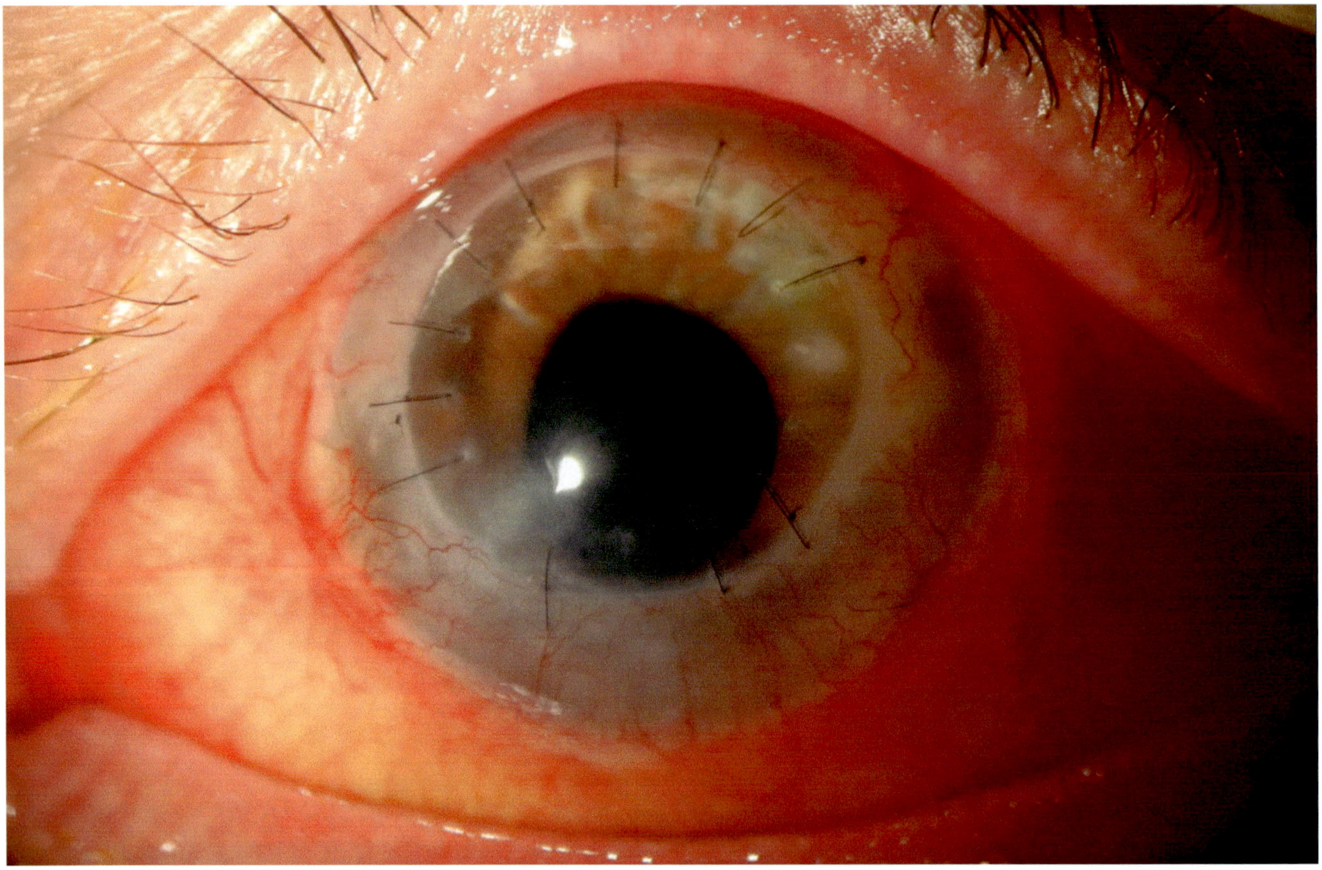

Fig. 13 Infiltrate of the corneal suture at 2'o clock position and residuals of a suture infiltrate at 3'o clock position in the left eye of a 64-year-old man after repeated penetrating keratoplasty (initially due to a perforated corneal ulcer on the basis of a decompensated corneal graft after penetrating keratoplasty for keratoglobus 20 years ago) and wound healing disorder

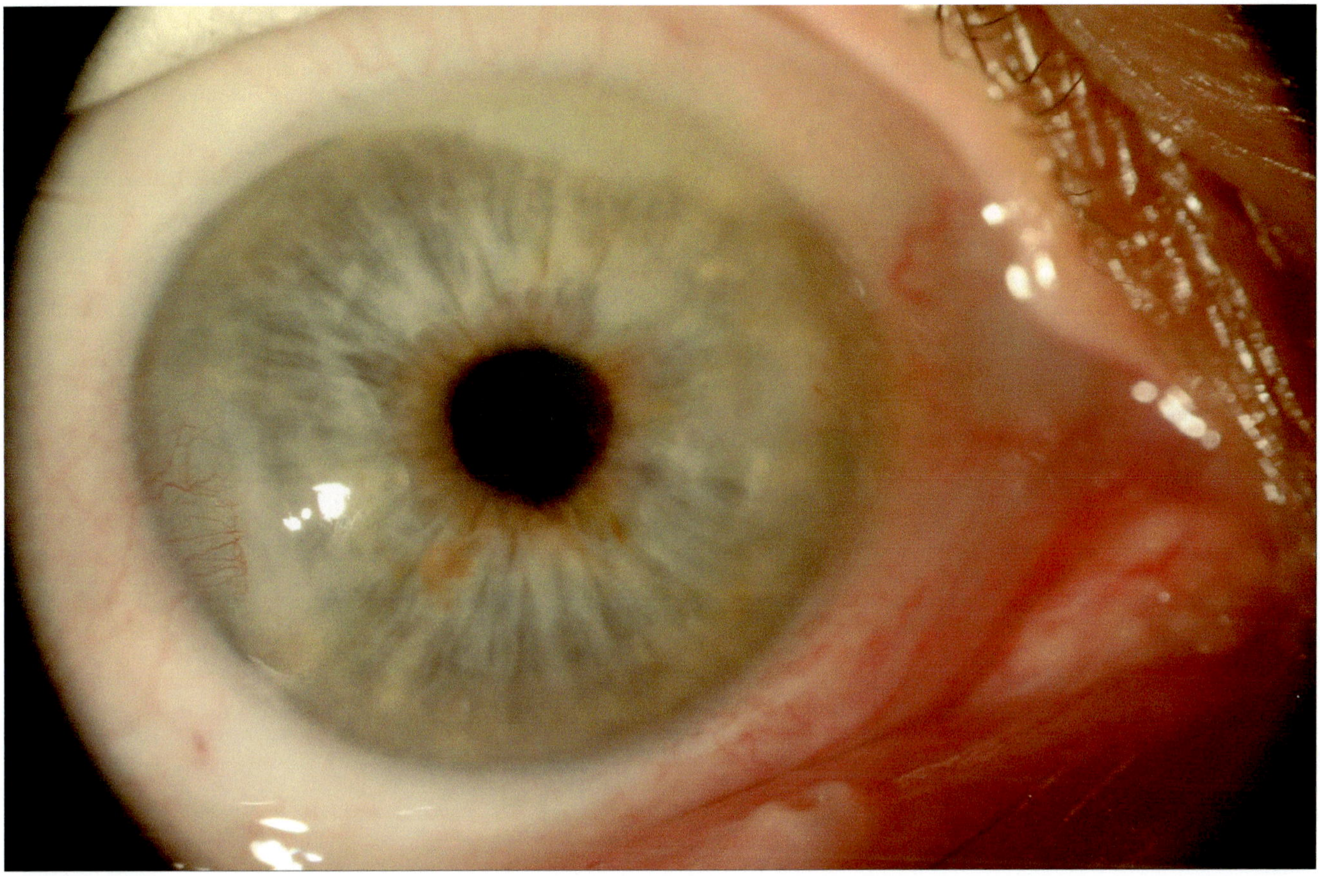

Fig. 14 Pronounced superficial corneal fibrosis and vascularization in the 9'o clock position in the right eye of a 64-year-old women with long-standing Salzmann nodular degeneration. Despite the beginning central fibrosis, reaching from the 3'o clock nodulus, the corrected visual acuity still attained 20/25 Snellen

7 Conclusion

A thorough understanding of the pathomechanisms of corneal wound healing and fibrogenesis allows the differentiation of misdirection from regular wound healing and can help to identify and eliminate the underlying cause of the corresponding disease as early as possible. Similarly, it provides a better basis for action on the necessary timing and means to modulate misled wound healing.

References

1. Friedlander M. Fibrosis and diseases of the eye. J Clin Invest. 2007;117(3):576–86.
2. Gain P, Jullienne R, He Z, Aldossary M, Acquart S, Cognasse F, et al. Global survey of corneal transplantation and eye banking. JAMA Ophthalmol. 2016;134(2):167–73.
3. Flockerzi E, Maier P, Böhringer D, Reinshagen H, Kruse F, Cursiefen C, et al. Trends in corneal transplantation from 2001 to 2016 in Germany: a report of the DOG-section cornea and its keratoplasty registry. Am J Ophthalmol. 2018.
4. Ljubimov AV, Saghizadeh M. Progress in corneal wound healing. Prog Retin Eye Res. 2015.
5. Wynn TA, Ramalingam TR. Mechanisms of fibrosis: therapeutic translation for fibrotic disease. Nat Med. 2012;18(7):1028–40.
6. Medzhitov R. Inflammation 2010: new adventures of an old flame. Cell. 2010;140(6):771–6.
7. Gabbiani G. The myofibroblast in wound healing and fibrocontractive diseases. J Pathol. 2003;200(4):500–3.
8. Saika S, Yamanaka O, Sumioka T, Miyamoto T, Miyazaki K, Okada Y, et al. Fibrotic disorders in the eye: targets of gene therapy. Prog Retin Eye Res. 2008;27(2):177–96.
9. Brockmann T. Influence of the complement system on corneal wound healing. Acta Ophthalmologica. 2019;97(S263).
10. West-Mays JA, Dwivedi DJ. The keratocyte: corneal stromal cell with variable repair phenotypes. Int J Biochem Cell Biol. 2006;38(10):1625–31.
11. Chaurasia SS, Kaur H, de Medeiros FW, Smith SD, Wilson SE. Dynamics of the expression of intermediate filaments vimentin and desmin during myofibroblast differentiation after corneal injury. Exp Eye Res. 2009;89(2):133–9.
12. Kao WW, Kao CW, Kaufman AH, Kombrinck KW, Converse RL, Good WV, et al. Healing of corneal epithelial defects in plasminogen-and fibrinogen-deficient mice. Invest Ophthalmol Vis Sci. 1998;39(3):502–8.
13. Esmon CT. The interactions between inflammation and coagulation. Br J Haematol. 2005;131(4):417–30.
14. Vasel M, Rutz R, Bersch C, Feick P, Singer MV, Kirschfink M, et al. Complement activation correlates with liver necrosis and fibrosis in chronic hepatitis C. Clin Immunol. 2014;150(2):149–56.

15. Gardner BP, Pleyer U, Mondino BJ, Sumner HL, Frieberg ML, Imperia PS. Complement-derived anaphylatoxins in human donor corneas treated with excimer laser. Ophthalmic Surg Lasers. 1995;26(6):568–71.
16. Pleyer U, Mondino BJ, Sumner HL. The effect of systemic decomplementation with cobra venom factor on corneal complement levels in guinea pigs. Invest Ophthalmol Vis Sci. 1992;33(7):2212–5.
17. Mondino BJ, Sumner HL. Generation of complement-derived anaphylatoxins in normal human donor corneas. Invest Ophthalmol Vis Sci. 1990;31(10):1945–9.
18. Wilson SE, Mohan RR, Ambrósio R, Hong J, Lee J. The corneal wound healing response: cytokine-mediated interaction of the epithelium, stroma, and inflammatory cells. Prog Retin Eye Res. 2001;20(5):625–37.
19. Zhang Y, Lee TC, Guillemin B, Yu MC, Rom WN. Enhanced IL-1 beta and tumor necrosis factor-alpha release and messenger RNA expression in macrophages from idiopathic pulmonary fibrosis or after asbestos exposure. J Immunol. 1993;150(9):4188–96.
20. Wynn TA, Barron L. Macrophages: master regulators of inflammation and fibrosis. Semin Liver Dis. 2010;30(3):245–57.
21. Hesse M, Modolell M, La Flamme AC, Schito M, Fuentes JM, Cheever AW, et al. Differential regulation of nitric oxide synthase-2 and arginase-1 by type 1/type 2 cytokines in vivo: granulomatous pathology is shaped by the pattern of L-arginine metabolism. J Immunol. 2001;167(11):6533–44.
22. Jester JV, Moller-Pedersen T, Huang J, Sax CM, Kays WT, Cavangh HD, et al. The cellular basis of corneal transparency: evidence for 'corneal crystallins.' J Cell Sci. 1999;112(Pt 5):613–22.
23. Marino GK, Santhiago MR, Santhanam A, Torricelli AAM, Wilson SE. Regeneration of defective epithelial basement membrane and restoration of corneal transparency after photorefractive keratectomy. J Refract Surg. 2017;33(5):337–46.
24. Chen Y, Thompson DC, Koppaka V, Jester JV, Vasiliou V. Ocular aldehyde dehydrogenases: protection against ultraviolet damage and maintenance of transparency for vision. Prog Retin Eye Res. 2013;33:28–39.
25. Bühren J, Nagy L, Swanton JN, Kenner S, MacRae S, Phipps RP, et al. Optical effects of anti-TGFbeta treatment after photorefractive keratectomy in a cat model. Invest Ophthalmol Vis Sci. 2009;50(2):634–43.
26. Meek KM, Knupp C. Corneal structure and transparency. Prog Retin Eye Res. 2015;49:1–16.
27. Powell DW, Mifflin RC, Valentich JD, Crowe SE, Saada JI, West AB. Myofibroblasts. I. Paracrine cells important in health and disease. Am J Physiol. 1999;277(1):C1–9.
28. Powell DW, Mifflin RC, Valentich JD, Crowe SE, Saada JI, West AB. Myofibroblasts. II. Intestinal subepithelial myofibroblasts. Am J Physiol. 1999;277(2):C183–201.
29. Wilson SE. Corneal myofibroblasts and fibrosis. Exp Eye Res. 2020;201: 108272.
30. Saikia P, Crabb JS, Dibbin LL, Juszczak MJ, Willard B, Jang GF, et al. Quantitative proteomic comparison of myofibroblasts derived from bone marrow and cornea. Sci Rep. 2020;10(1):16717.
31. Kay EP, Lee MS, Seong GJ, Lee YG. TGF-beta s stimulate cell proliferation via an autocrine production of FGF-2 in corneal stromal fibroblasts. Curr Eye Res. 1998;17(3):286–93.
32. Wilson SE, Schultz GS, Chegini N, Weng J, He YG. Epidermal growth factor, transforming growth factor alpha, transforming growth factor beta, acidic fibroblast growth factor, basic fibroblast growth factor, and interleukin-1 proteins in the cornea. Exp Eye Res. 1994;59(1):63–71.
33. Wahl SM, McCartney-Francis N, Allen JB, Dougherty EB, Dougherty SF. Macrophage production of TGF-beta and regulation by TGF-beta. Ann N Y Acad Sci. 1990;593:188–96.
34. Wang JF, Jiao H, Stewart TL, Shankowsky HA, Scott PG, Tredget EE. Fibrocytes from burn patients regulate the activities of fibroblasts. Wound Repair Regen. 2007;15(1):113–21.
35. Singh V, Santhiago MR, Barbosa FL, Agrawal V, Singh N, Ambati BK, et al. Effect of TGFβ and PDGF-B blockade on corneal myofibroblast development in mice. Exp Eye Res. 2011;93(6):810–7.
36. Mohan RR, Hutcheon AE, Choi R, Hong J, Lee J, Ambrósio R, et al. Apoptosis, necrosis, proliferation, and myofibroblast generation in the stroma following LASIK and PRK. Exp Eye Res. 2003;76(1):71–87.
37. Medeiros CS, Lassance L, Saikia P, Santhiago MR, Wilson SE. Posterior stromal cell apoptosis triggered by mechanical endothelial injury and basement membrane component nidogen-1 production in the cornea. Exp Eye Res. 2018;172:30–5.
38. Medeiros CS, Marino GK, Santhiago MR, Wilson SE. The corneal basement membranes and stromal fibrosis. Invest Ophthalmol Vis Sci. 2018;59(10):4044–53.
39. Medeiros CS, Saikia P, de Oliveira RC, Lassance L, Santhiago MR, Wilson SE. Descemet's membrane modulation of posterior corneal fibrosis. Invest Ophthalmol Vis Sci. 2019;60(4):1010–20.
40. Kim WJ, Mohan RR, Wilson SE. Effect of PDGF, IL-1alpha, and BMP2/4 on corneal fibroblast chemotaxis: expression of the platelet-derived growth factor system in the cornea. Invest Ophthalmol Vis Sci. 1999;40(7):1364–72.

Diagnostics

Slit Lamp Biomicroscopy

Tim Berger and Berthold Seitz

Abstract

The slit lamp is a specialized stereoscopic biomicroscope that uses a high intensity light source to illuminate and magnify the structures of the eye. It allows for a detailed evaluation of the cornea, including its shape, thickness, and transparency. This chapter describes the principles and different techniques of examining the cornea with the slit lamp biomicroscope, as a comprehensive understanding is essential for accurate diagnosis and treatment of various corneal diseases.

Keywords

Slit lamp · Biomicroscopy · Corneal examination · Examination techniques · Cornea

1 Principles and Components

The slit lamp is a highly advanced stereoscopic biomicroscope that emits a focused beam of light with adjustable height, width, and angle. It enables a three-dimensional visualization and allows for a detailed examination of the anterior and posterior segments of the eye [1, 2].

A slit lamp biomicroscope consists of three main components: the viewing arm, which includes the eyepieces/oculars and magnifying elements, the illumination arm, which contains the light source and its regulating elements, and the patient positioning frame. Viewing and illumination arm are connected to a base that can be moved using a joystick to shift both components forward, backward, laterally, or diagonally [1, 2]. The different parts of a slit lamp are shown in Fig. 1.

2 Examination and Illumination Techniques

Establishing a general routine for examination is a crucial aspect of effectively using the slit lamp. This involves starting with a large field of view, using different illumination techniques and gradually zooming in on specific details using higher magnification as needed [3, 4].

For examination of the cornea, it is essential to determine the horizontal extent of corneal changes (e.g. focal or total affection, shape and border), which is usually done with a wide slit setting. The sagittal extension is equally important for further differentiation of corneal changes in order to show whether it is a prominent lesion (e.g. Salzmann nodular degeneration), a tissue reduction (e.g. corneal ulcer, scarring) and to detect the affected layers (depth of the lesion). It is always recommended to examine the cornea of both eyes (e.g. corneal dystrophy) with a dilated pupil [5, 6].

Illumination techniques can be divided into direct and indirect forms. For the direct illumination method (diffuse or focal), the structure to be examined is directly illuminated by the light beam, whereas in the indirect method a secondary surface reflects or transmits the light onto the structure to be examined. Each of the different illumination methods offers distinct characteristics, advantages, disadvantages and applications depending on the clinical setting [3, 4].

The following illumination techniques for examination of the cornea can be distinguished:

The authors have no funding or conflicts of interest to disclose.

T. Berger (✉) · B. Seitz
Department of Ophthalmology, Saarland University Medical Center, Homburg, Germany
e-mail: tim.berger@uks.eu

B. Seitz et al. (eds.), *Atlas on Cornea*, https://doi.org/10.1007/978-3-031-65422-0_4

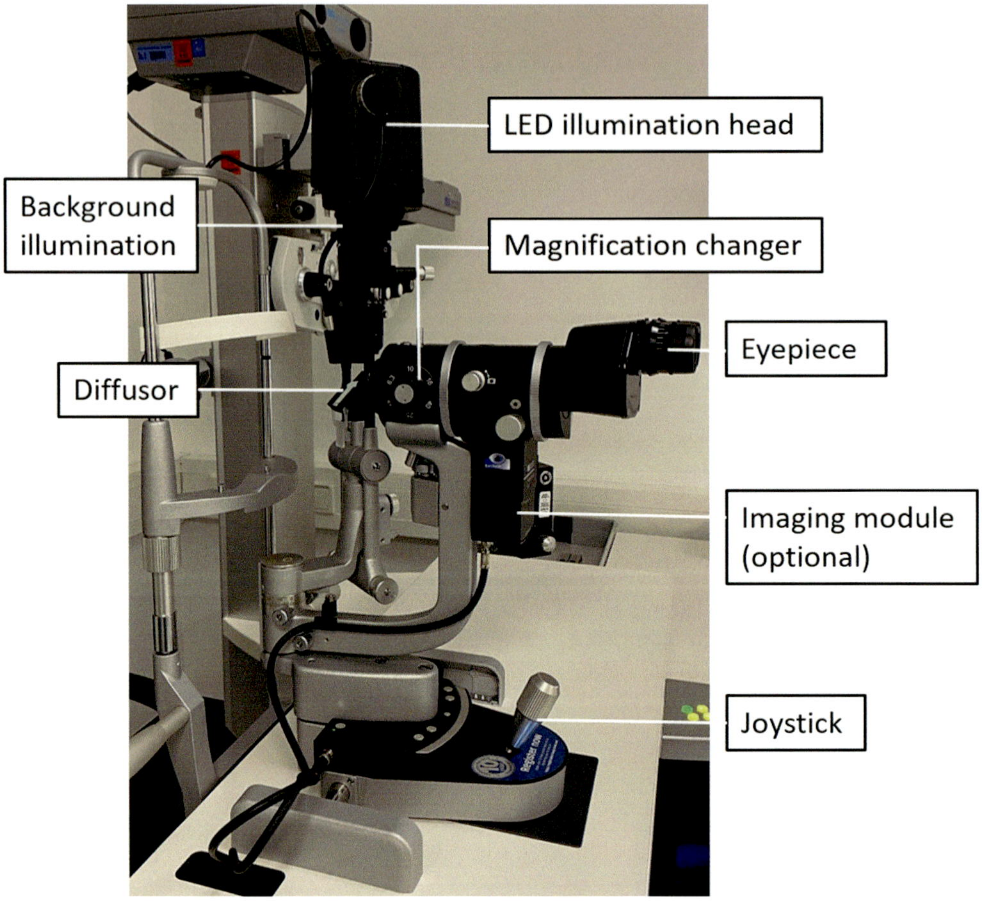

Fig. 1 Overview of the most important components of a slit lamp (Model: BQ 900, Haag-Streit, Köniz, Switzerland)

Diffuse illumination: This setting (Fig. 2) is primarily used to obtain an overview of the ocular surface tissues and the intraocular structures such as the iris and lens. It is particularly helpful to get a first overview of the cornea.

The use of a cobalt blue filter after instillation of sodium fluorescein eye drops (Fig. 3) is essential for the evaluation of superficial corneal disorders up to corneal perforation (epithelial defects, Seidel test, loose sutures, "late fluorescein staining") [7].

Besides sodium fluorescein, other common vital dyes for the cornea and conjunctiva are Rose Bengal (Fig. 4) and lissamine green, each of them having their own characteristics, advantages, and disadvantages for the diagnosis of ocular surface diseases.

Direct focal illumination (moderate slit): A full-height, medium-width and medium-bright beam of light is obliquely directed into the eye, focussing on the cornea to generate a square-shaped block of light (Fig. 5). This illumination

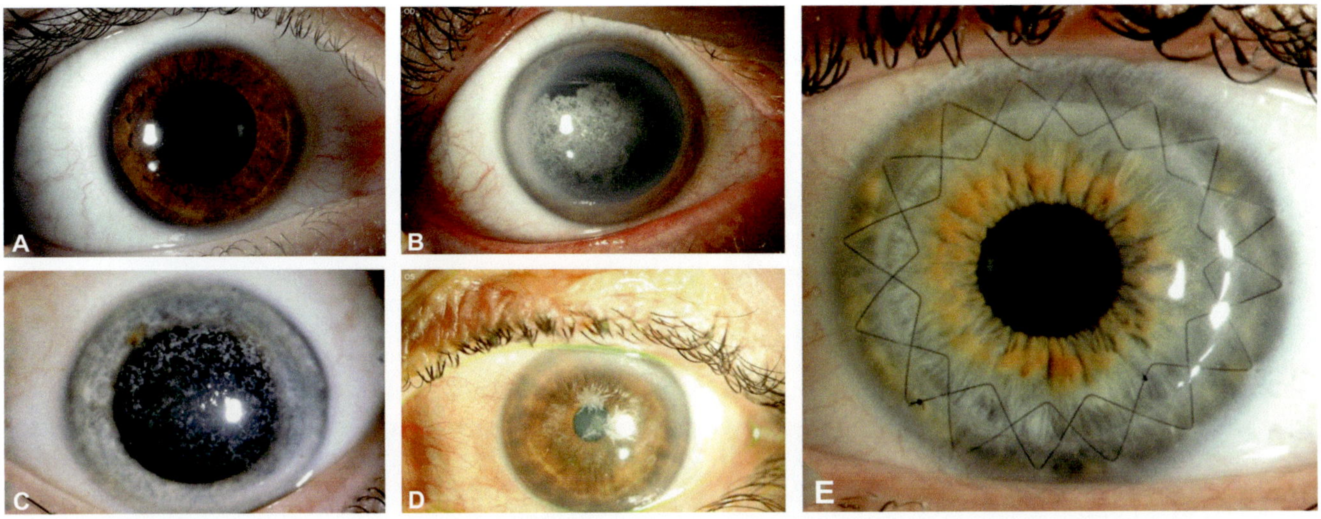

Fig. 2 Overview photographs of various corneal conditions with diffuse illumination. (**A**) Normal cornea. (**B**) Schnyder's corneal dystrophy: Cornea with cholesterol crystals and arcus lipoides. (**C, D**) Granular dystrophy: Based on the appearance a distinction of different subtypes of corneal dystrophies is feasible. (C: Type 1—snowflake appearance, D: Type 2—star-shaped/finger-shaped appearance). (**E**) Corneal graft with a double running cross-stich suture after penetrating keratoplasty

method produces two different layers of illumination, one on the epithelium and one on the endothelium [3, 4].

Direct focal illumination (narrow slit): Using a narrow slit beam is an effective illumination method to obtain a cross sectional view of the cornea (Fig. 6 and 7). By setting the light intensity to a maximum and adjusting the slit beam to a width just before the optical section loses its structural integrity, a finer delineation of the information within that section is obtained to locate the layer of the pathological changes [3, 4].

Specular reflection: Specular reflection is the mirror-like reflection of light from a surface and its most important application is the evaluation of the corneal endothelium. A narrow (thicker than an optical section) to medium-sized beam of light is directed towards the eye from the temporal side using an angle of illumination of 50°–60° relative to the examiner's observation axis (slightly nasal to the visual axis of the patient). This technique will reveal a bright zone of specular reflection of the tear film layer and by observing the adjacent area on the side

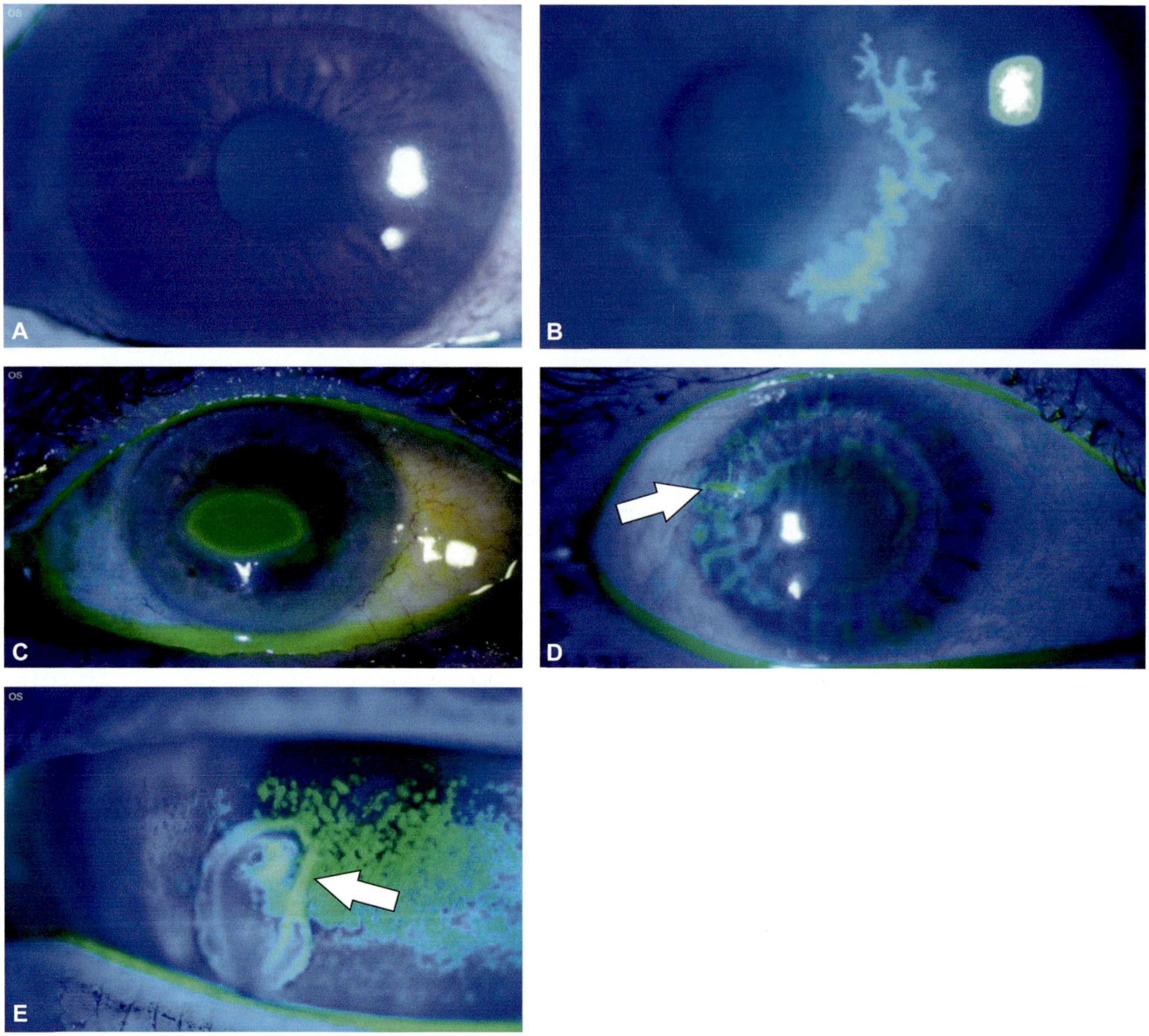

Fig. 3 Vital stain with fluorescein. (**A**) Normal staining with uniform fluorescein distribution. (**B**) Herpetic keratitis with dendritic lesion. (**C**) Neurotrophic ulcer (oval shaped). (**D**) Suture staining (arrow) due to loosening after penetrating keratoplasty. (**E**) Corneal perforation with positive Seidel test (arrow)

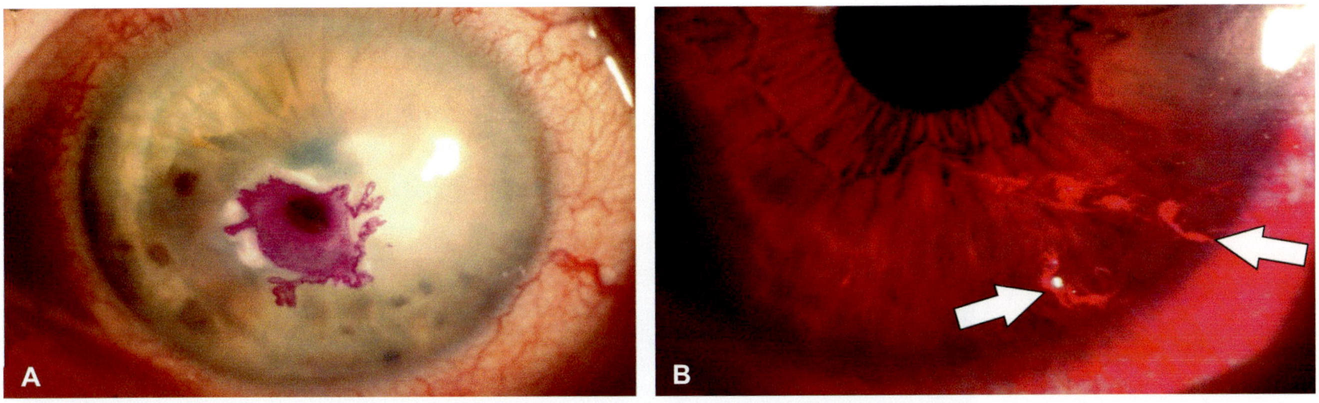

Fig. 4 Vital stain with Rose Bengal. (**A**) Descemetocele in diffuse illumination. (**B**) Filamentary keratitis (arrows) stains best with Rose Bengal

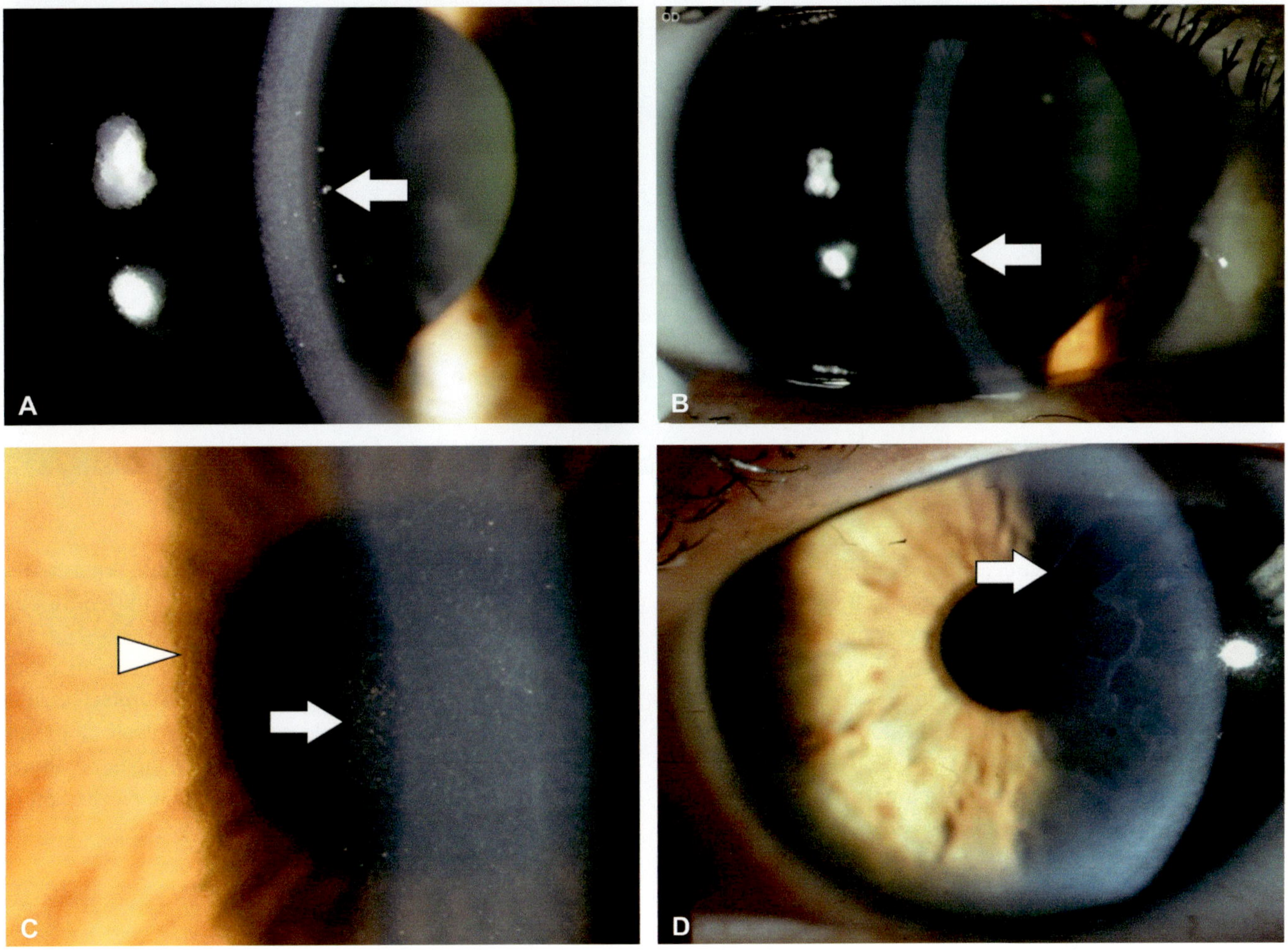

Fig. 5 Direct focal illumination using a moderate slit. (**A**) Pseudoexfoliation (PEX) syndrome: Focal illumination reveals white PEX flakes (arrow) on the posterior surface of the cornea. (**B**) Krukenberg spindle: Pigment (arrow) on the posterior surface of the cornea. (**C**) Cornea guttata: Guttae visible on the posterior surface of the cornea in direct (arrow) and indirect (arrowhead) illumination. (**D**) Map-dot fingerprint dystrophy: Superficial illumination demonstrates the characteristic map-like patterns (arrow)

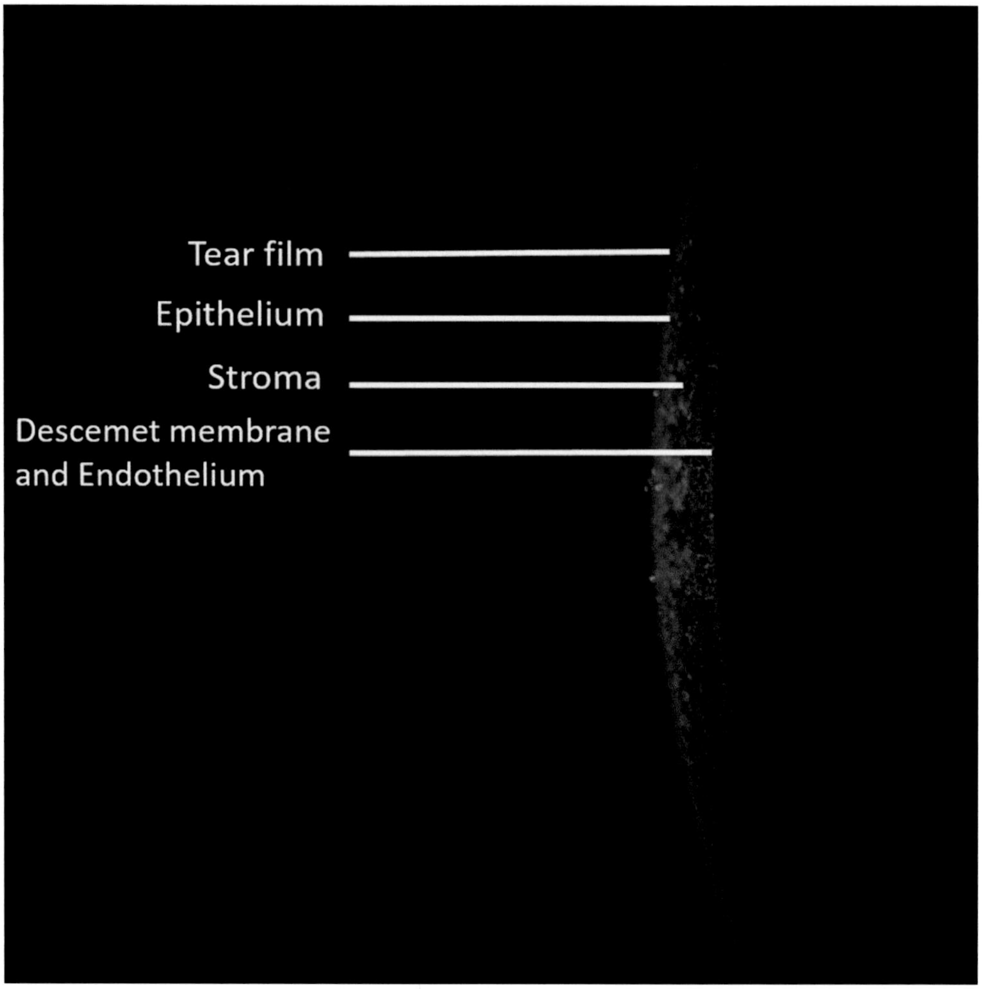

Fig. 6 Narrow slit image of a healthy cornea

opposite of the light source, an endothelial reflection can be examined in more detail by moving the biomicroscope anteriorly to obtain more focus (recommended magnification of 40×) [3, 4, 8].

Retroillumination: This technique is suitable for detection of corneal dystrophies, edema, scars and fine corneal vascularization (Figs. 8, 9, 10, 11) [3, 4, 6]. A light beam of medium width is projected onto a part of the eye deeper than the area to be examined (e.g. iris, fundus).

Sclerotic scatter: This technique (Fig. 12) allows illumination of the entire cornea against a largely unilluminated background by placing a slit beam of moderate width at the corneoscleral junction. Light passes through the entire cornea by total reflection.

In normal corneas, the passage of light is undisturbed and is only visible as a ring of light at the limbus as it is reflected by the sclera, while the cornea itself does not appear illuminated. In contrast, corneal changes or abnormalities can be visualized through the axially reflected or refracted light [3, 4].

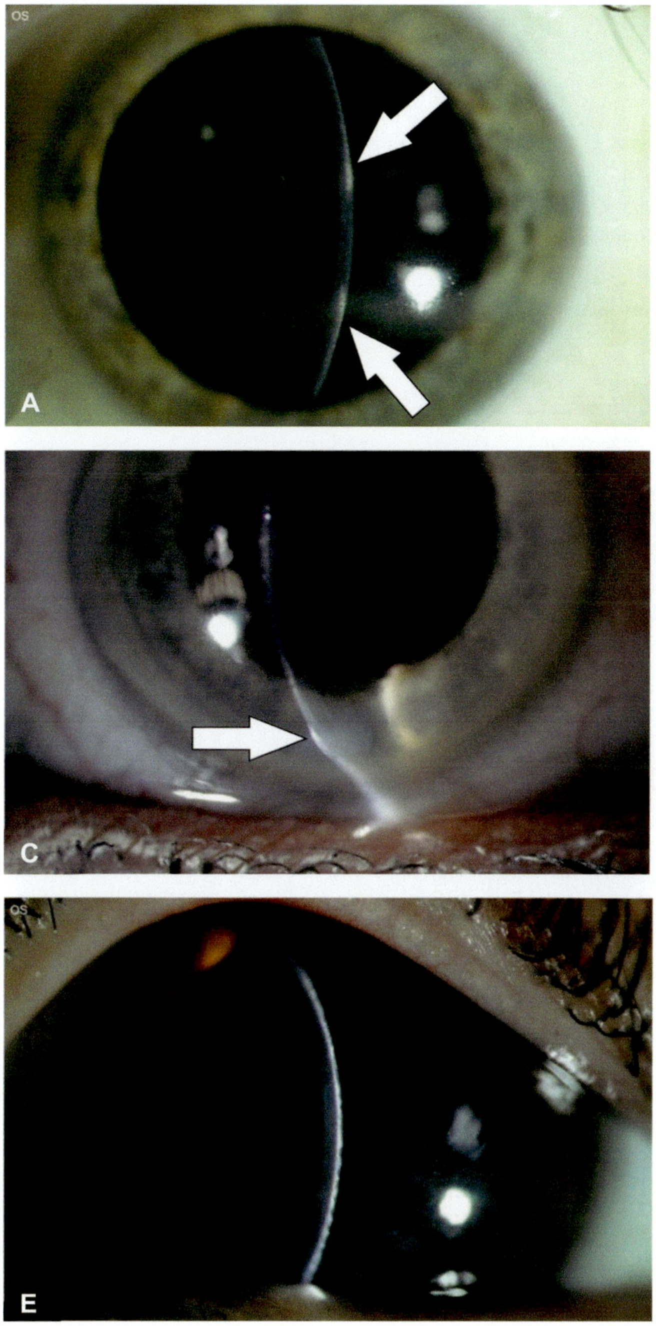

Fig. 7 Direct focal illumination using a narrow slit. (**A**) Superficial anterior stromal corneal scarring (arrows). (**B**) Full-thickness corneal scar. (**C**) Salzmann nodular degeneration: Elevated slit beam (arrow) at the Salzmann nodule. (**D**) Corneal ulcer: depth evaluation by using a narrow slit setting. (**E**) Thiel Behnke corneal dystrophy: superficial (Epithelium and Bowman layer) dystrophic deposits in "saw-tooth" appearance

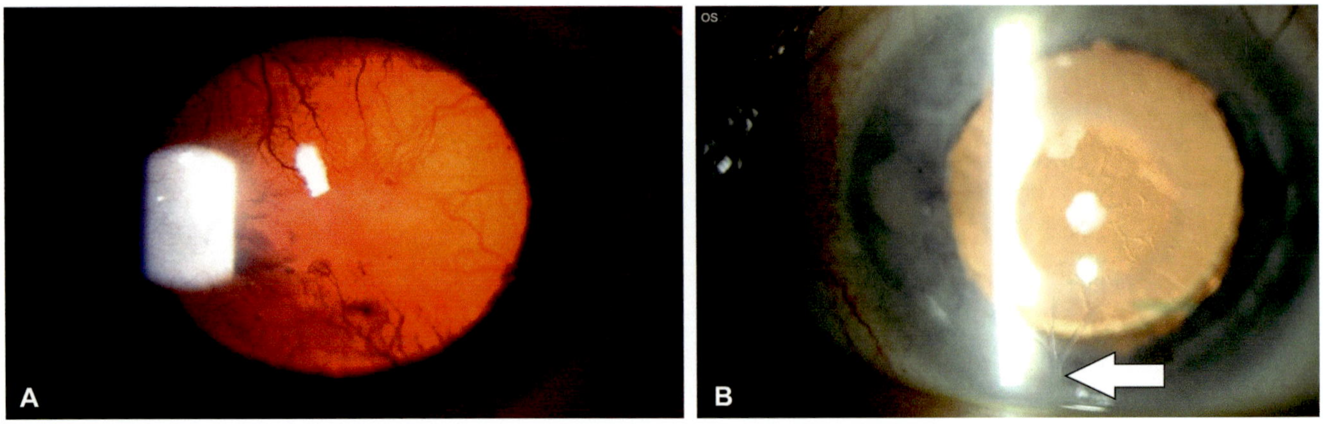

Fig. 8 Retroillumination for corneal vascularization. (**A**) Circular superficial and deep stromal corneal vascularization. (**B**) Clear, non-perfused corneal vascularization ("ghost vessels") (arrow)

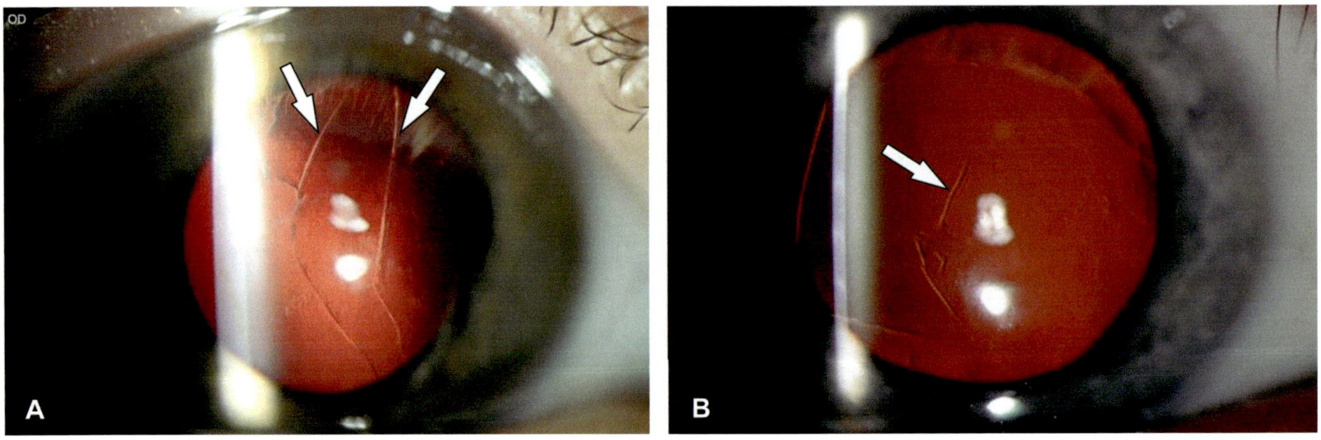

Fig. 9 Retroillumination for demonstrating defects of Descemet membrane. (**A**) Rupture of Descemet membrane (arrows) after corneal hydrops in keratoglobus. (**B**) Intraoperative iatrogenic injury of Descemet membrane (arrow) after penetrating keratoplasty

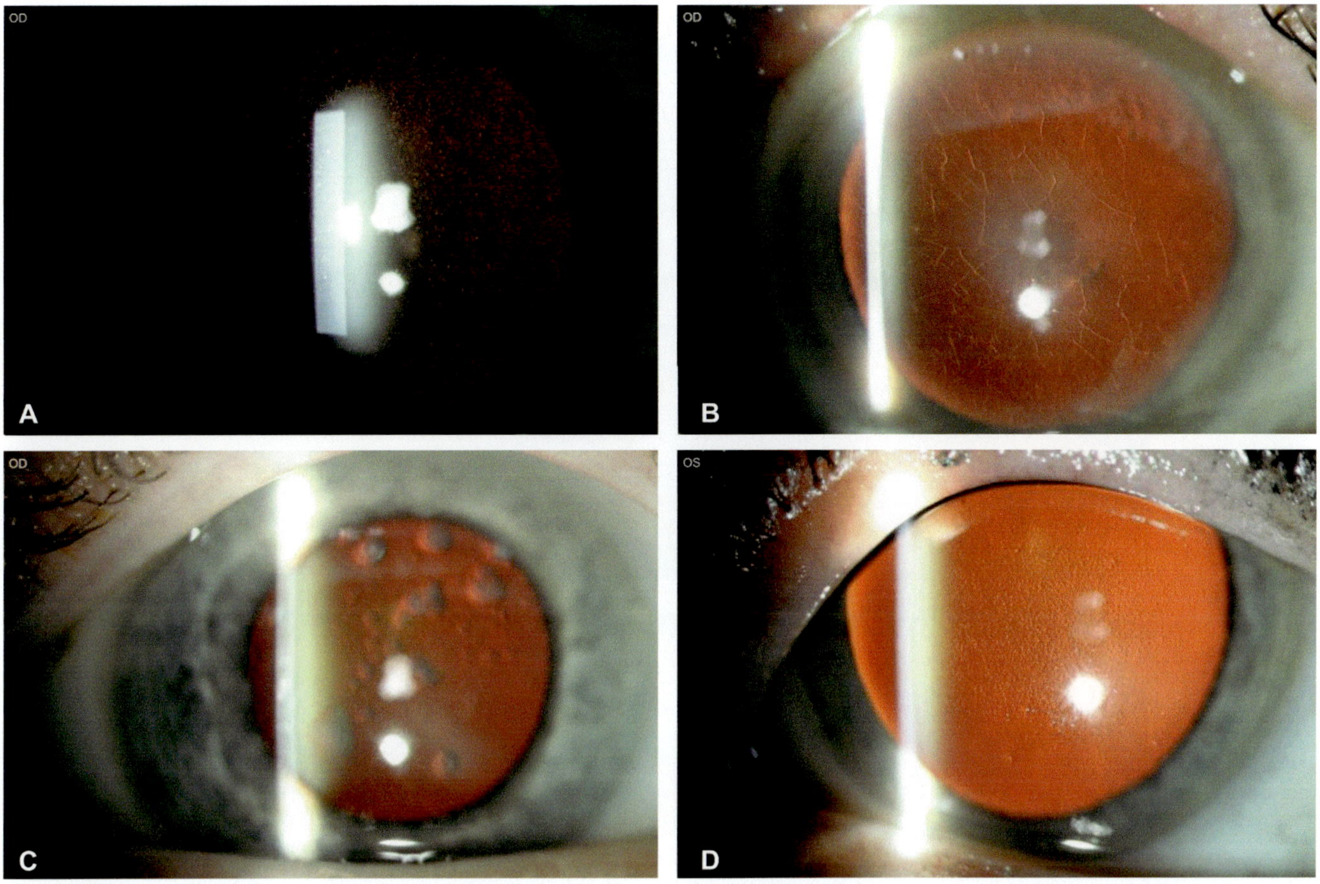

Fig. 10 Retroillumination for various corneal dystrophies. (**A**) Meesmann corneal dystrophy with small intraepithelial cysts. (**B**) Lattice corneal dystrophy with branching lattice lines. (**C**) Posterior polymorphous corneal dystrophy with severe verrucous lesions [9]. (**D**) Fuchs' endothelial corneal dystrophy with corneal guttae

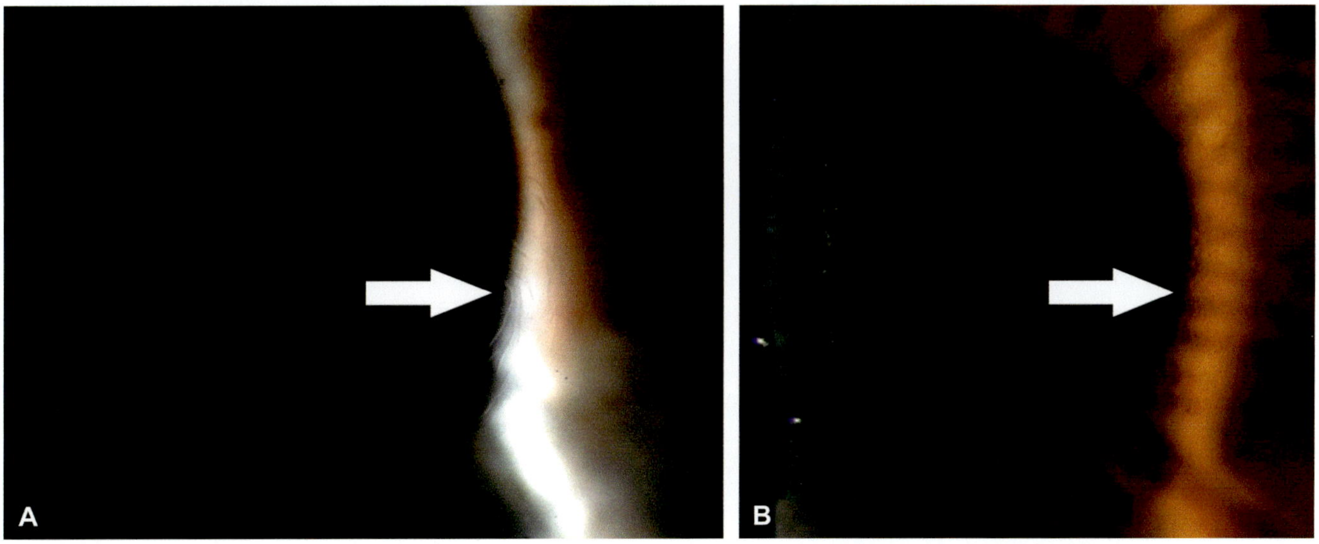

Fig. 11 Indirect retroillumnation of the iris for evaluation of the cornea. (**A**) Map-Dot Fingerprint Dystrophy with fingerprint lesions (arrow). (**B**) Fuchs endothelial corneal dystrophy with corneal guttae next to the reflected slit (arrow)

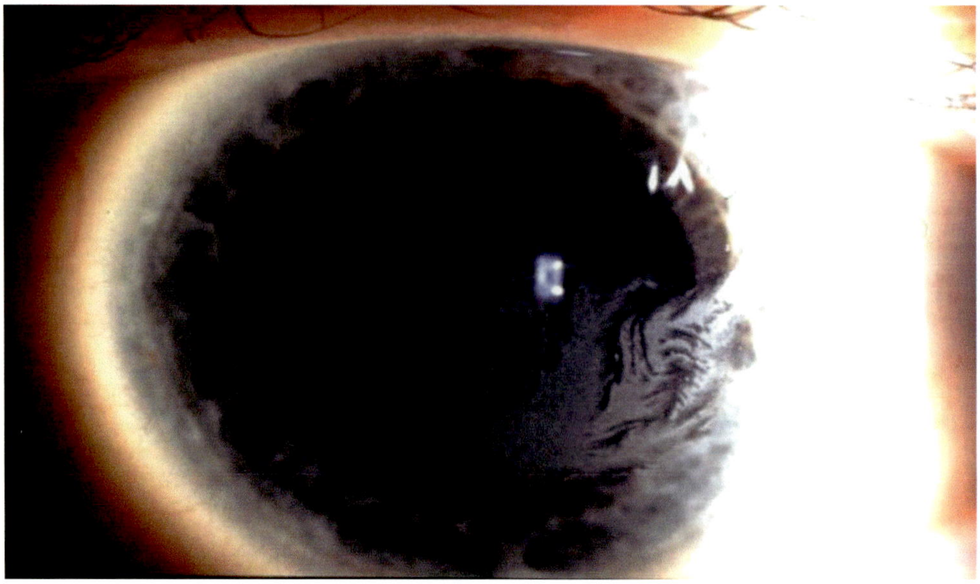

Fig. 12 Sclerotic scatter for the visualization of superficial whorl-like opacities in Lisch epithelial corneal dystrophy

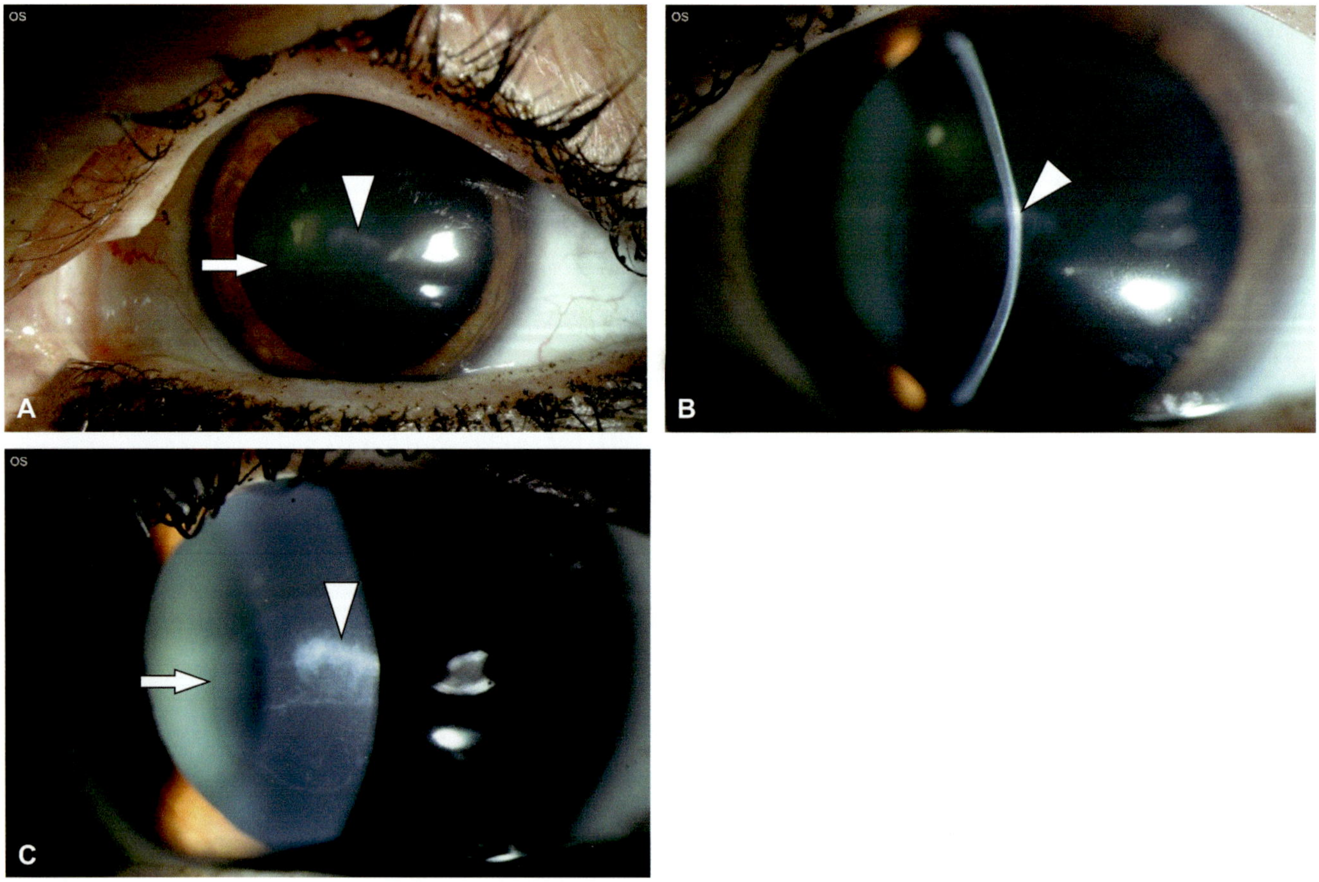

Fig. 13 Exemplary overview of different illumination techniques for a cornea with keratoconus. (**A**) Diffuse illumination: Complete Fleischer ring (arrow) and a central corneal scarring (arrowhead). The shape of the cornea and the depth of the corneal scar cannot be assessed by using this illumination technique. (**B**) Focal illumination (narrow slit): The narrow slit demonstrates paracentral thinning with mid-stromal scarring (arrowhead). The cornea is conically protruded. (**C**) Focal illumination (broad slit): This illumination technique allows a better view of the Fleischer ring (arrow) and the horizontal extension of the corneal scar (arrowhead)

3 Conclusion

Slit lamp biomicroscopy is an essential tool for ophthalmologists in diagnosing and monitoring corneal diseases [10]. Different illumination techniques offer varying degrees of visualization and can help identify specific corneal abnormalities. Knowledge of the precise examination methods and their interpretation is therefore of utmost importance. In order to be capable of making an accurate diagnosis, it is particularly important to always evaluate the combination of all available illumination techniques (Fig. 13).

References

1. Gellrich MM. History of the slit lamp. Slit Lamp, Springer-Verlag, Berlin;2014, p. 189–210. https://doi.org/10.1007/978-3-642-39793-6_6.
2. Gellrich MM. Basics. Slit Lamp, Springer-Verlag, Berlin;2014, p. 1–20. https://doi.org/10.1007/978-3-642-39793-6_1.
3. Krachmer JH, Mannis MJ, Holland EJ. Slit lamp examination and photography. Cornea, Elsevier-Verlag, Amsterdam;2021, p. 53–80.
4. Gellrich MM. Biomicroscopy. Slit Lamp, Springer-Verlag, Berlin;2014, p. 21–74. https://doi.org/10.1007/978-3-642-39793-6_2.
5. Weiss JS, Møller HU, Aldave AJ, Seitz B, Bredrup C, Kivelä T, et al. IC3D classification of corneal dystrophies-edition 2. Cornea. 2015;34:117–59. https://doi.org/10.1097/ICO.0000000000000307.
6. Seitz B, Lisch W, Weiss J. The revised newest IC^{3}D classification of corneal dystrophies. Klin Monbl Augenheilkd. 2015;232:283–94. https://doi.org/10.1055/s-0041-100774.
7. Efron N. Putting vital stains in context. Clin Exp Optom. 2013;96:400–21. https://doi.org/10.1111/j.1444-0938.2012.00802.x.
8. Ong Tone S, Jurkunas U. Imaging the corneal endothelium in Fuchs corneal endothelial dystrophy. Semin Ophthalmol. 2019;34:340–6. https://doi.org/10.1080/08820538.2019.1632355.
9. Berger T, Seitz B, Löw U, Flockerzi F, Schlötzer-Schrehardt U, Daas L. Descemet membrane endothelial keratoplasty (DMEK) for severe verrucous posterior polymorphous corneal dystrophy with uncommon clinical and ultrastructural findings. Klin Monbl Augenheilkd 2022. epub ahead of print. https://doi.org/10.1055/a-1862-8403.
10. Berger T, Flockerzi E, Daas L, Hamon L, Khattabi Z, Berger M, Seitz B. Modern corneal diagnostics as the key for the correct classification of the disease and optimal treatment decisions. Ophthalmologie. 2023;120:1238–50. https://doi.org/10.1007/s00347-023-01919-0.

Endothelial Cell Analysis

Tarek Safi, Loïc Hamon, Loay Daas, and Berthold Seitz

Abstract

The first microscopes created allowing the examination of the endothelial layer date back to the year 1968. Since then, many advances were made until reaching the non-contact specular microscopy, currently considered as the method of choice for examining the endothelial layer. This microscope allows the objective assessment of the endothelial layer using 4 important parameters: Endothelial cell density (ECD), cell area, pleomorphism and polymegethism. Hereby, endothelial integrity and vitality can be assessed and many diseases of the endothelial layer can be detected such as cornea guttata, corneal decompensation, posterior polymorphous corneal dystrophy or iridocorneal endothelial (ICE) syndrome. Further advancement in this diagnostic modality is currently incorporating artificial intelligence as an image analysis tool providing automatic segmentation and analysis of the endothelial images.

Keywords

Endothelial cell density · Specular microscopy · Endothelial layer · Cornea guttata · Endothelial disease · Polymegethism and pleomorphism

1 Introduction

The first documented direct visualization of the endothelial layer using slit lamp microscopy was demonstrated by Vogt in 1918 [1]. Afterwards, the first attempt to examine and analyze the corneal endothelial layer dates back to 1968, when David Maurice designed a laboratory contact specular microscope to enable to see the endothelial cells [2]. This microscope was further developed and improved by others such as Laing et al. [3], and later Bourne and Kaufman [4]. Thereafter, with the development of the non-contact specular microscopy, the assessment of the endothelial layer and the determination of the endothelial cell density (ECD) with both contact and non-contact microscopes were possible with comparable and reproducible results for both microscopes [5, 6]. Currently, the non-contact specular microscopy has become the method of choice in visualizing and analyzing the corneal endothelial layer (Fig. 1) [7].

2 Concept of Specular Microscopy

The optical principle of this microscope is based on the specular reflex that occurs at the interface of two surfaces with different refractive indices, with the light from the subject having an angle of incidence equal to the angle of reflection to the observer [8]. In other words, light is projected onto the posterior corneal surface at nearly normal incidence, with most of this light being transmitted into the aqueous humor. However, a small fraction of this light, around 0.02%, is reflected from the aqueous humor–endothelial cell interface back into the cornea. This specularly reflected light is collected by the objective lens of the photomicroscope and forms an image of the corneal endothelium [9], as shown in Fig. 2.

T. Safi (✉) · L. Hamon · L. Daas · B. Seitz
Department of Ophthalmology, Saarland University Medical Center, Homburg, Germany
e-mail: tarek.safi@outlook.com

B. Seitz et al. (eds.), *Atlas on Cornea*, https://doi.org/10.1007/978-3-031-65422-0_5

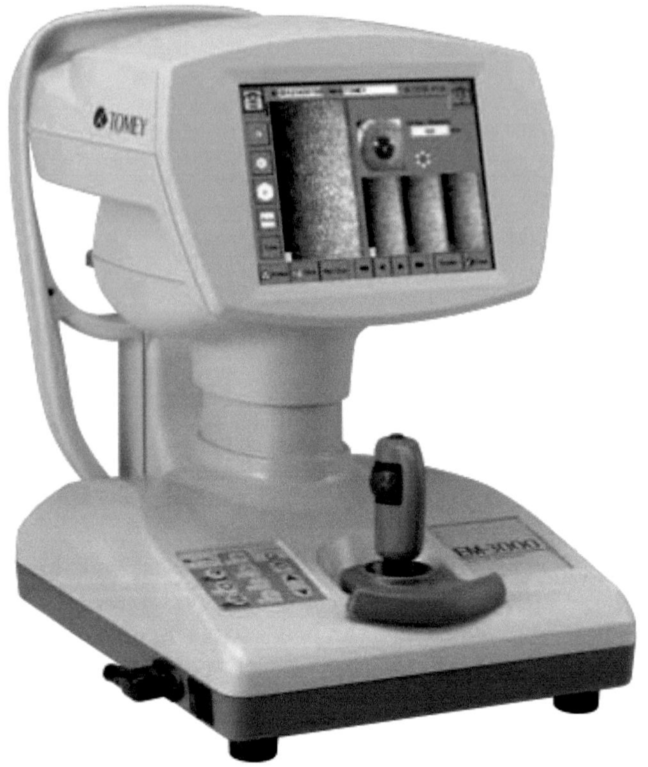

Fig. 1 Non-contact specular microscopy. Specular microscope EM-3000 from Tomey. (From Tomey Inc., used under a creative commons CC–BY-NC-ND license)

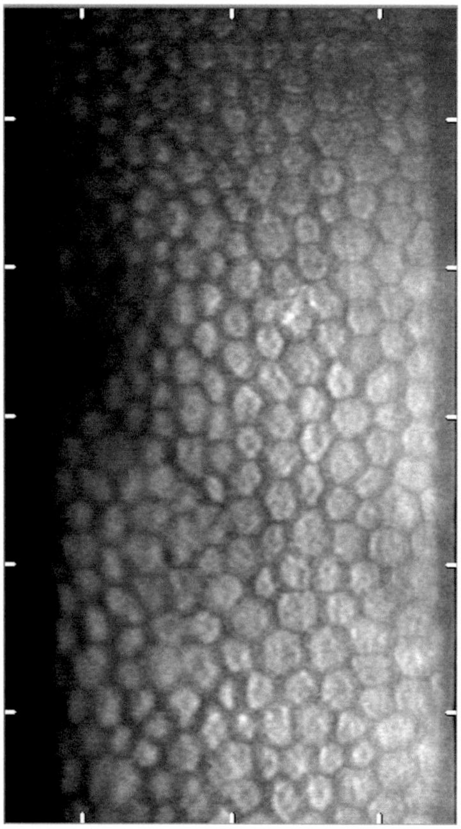

Fig. 2 A typical image of the endothelial layer of a healthy cornea

3 Endothelial Layer Assessment Using Specular Microscopy

Since using specular microscopy, a better illustration and understanding of the endothelial layer and its diseases was achieved. The corneal endothelium is formed by single-layered hexagonal endothelial cells measuring 5 µm in height and between 18 and 20 µm in width and are connected at their apical pole by tight junctions. This layer plays a critical role in keeping the cornea clear and transparent by pumping out water from the corneal stroma to the anterior chamber through an active transport system of electrolytes and liquids [10]. Through a membrane-bound Na^+-K^+-ATPases, the endothelium regulates the aqueous humor outflow from the stroma into the anterior chamber and also forms a barrier to prevent "inflow" into the corneal stroma [11].

Since the endothelial cells are mostly non regenerative, their density decreases gradually and constantly throughout life at an average rate of 0,6% per year, starting from 5000–6000 cells/mm^2 in newborns and reaching 2000–3000 cells/mm^2 in a normal adult eye [12, 13]. It has been shown that a minimal density of around 500 cells/mm^2 is needed to maintain the function of the endothelial layer, and values below this number are associated with corneal decompensation and bullous keratopathy [14]. Therefore, a minimum of 2000 cells/mm^2 in the donor corneas are generally required in most eye banks around the world for elective keratoplasty [15, 16]. The ECD is calculated as the reciprocal of the average cell area.

Not only the quantity of endothelial cells but also their morphology are important indicators of the functional capacity and vitality of the endothelial layer. The corneal endothelium consists ideally of hexagonal cells, a configuration that is the most energy-efficient as it confers the greatest surface area relative to its circumference [17]. Using specular microscopy, the morphology of the endothelial layer can be objectively assessed, quantitatively as well as qualitatively, using the following 3 parameters:

1. **Cell area** ± SD (µm^2). A normal cell area varies between 200 und 400 µm^2 depending on the patients' age [1].
2. **Polymegethism**. Defined as the differences in size of the endothelial cells, this parameter is measured as a coefficient of variation (CV) which is calculated as the standard deviation of the average cell area/average cell area. A normal CV for healthy endothelial layer ranges between 0.2 and 0.3 [18]. Corneas with high CV have large differences in endothelial cells size and are therefore usually less stable and resistant to physiological and pathological stress [19]. Nevertheless, studies have shown that a high CV does not affect the permeability of the endothelium or its ability to maintain stromal transparency [18]. Severe polymegethism has been found in

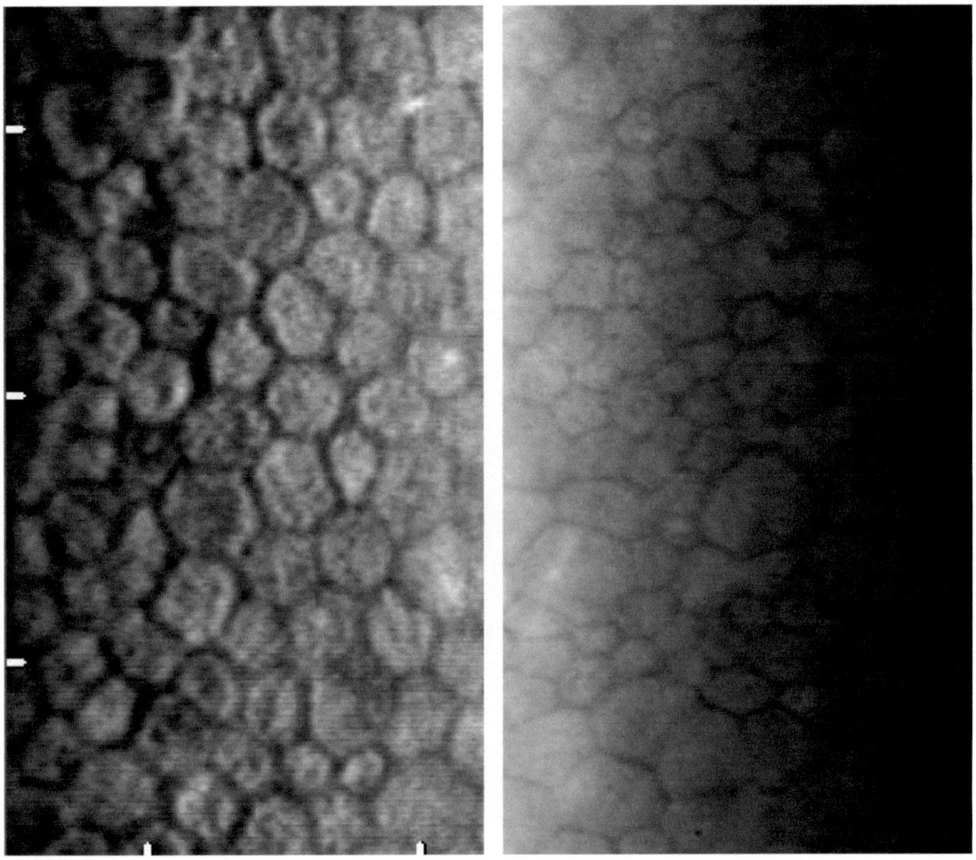

Fig. 3 Corneal endothelium with moderate polymegethism (left), and severe polymegethism (right) [22]

the corneas of donors using contact lenses, donors with diabetes, keratoconus, inflammation or infection, and donors with a previous history of anterior chamber surgery (Fig. 3) [20]. It has been assumed that polymegethism could result of endothelial cell wound repair mechanisms. It is also worth noting that the accuracy of the estimated ECD decreases as the polymegethism increases. Polymegethism represented by CV is calculated using the following equation [21]:

$$\mathrm{CV} = \frac{\text{Standard deviation of the average cell area}}{\text{Average cell area}}$$

3. **Pleomorphism**. It is defined as the shape of the individual cells and expressed in terms of polygonality or hexagonality. The percentage of hexagonal cells in the endothelial layer is an important parameter of corneal vitality, which is expected to be around 48–90% in normal corneas, with 25–38% of the cells being heptagonal and 15–38% being pentagonal [6, 23]. Low percentages of hexagonality are more frequently found in older corneas, after trauma, or due to the repair mechanisms of the endothelium, in which dead endothelial cells are replaced by their neighbors [24, 25]. High pleomorphism is frequently associated with high polymegethism and indicates poor endothelial vitality (Fig. 4).

A typical image of endothelial layer analysis is displayed in Fig. 5.

4 Endothelial Diseases and Specular Microscopy

Several diseases and dystrophies affecting the endothelial layer can be detected or confirmed using specular microscopy. Cornea guttata (CG), which are excrescences of the Descemet membrane made by accumulations of basement membrane and fibrillary collagens that disrupt the endothelial mosaic leading to endothelial cell loss, are easily detectable and quantifiable using specular microscopy (Fig. 6) [10].

There are several grading scales for the severity of cornea guttata, among them the recently published Homburg CG grading system which take into account the clinical severity of the disease. According to this grading system, Grade 0 (G0) described a healthy cornea in which no CG is detected. In grade 1 (G1), less than 40% of the observed area

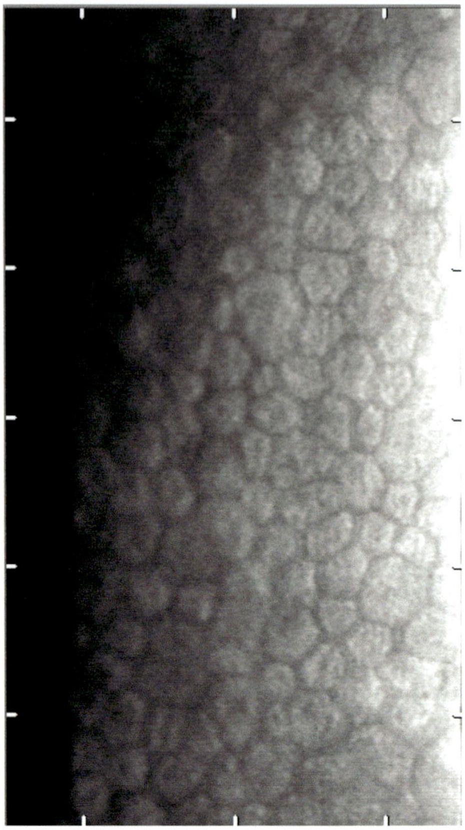

Fig. 4 Corneal endothelium with high pleomorphism (low percentage of hexagonal cells)

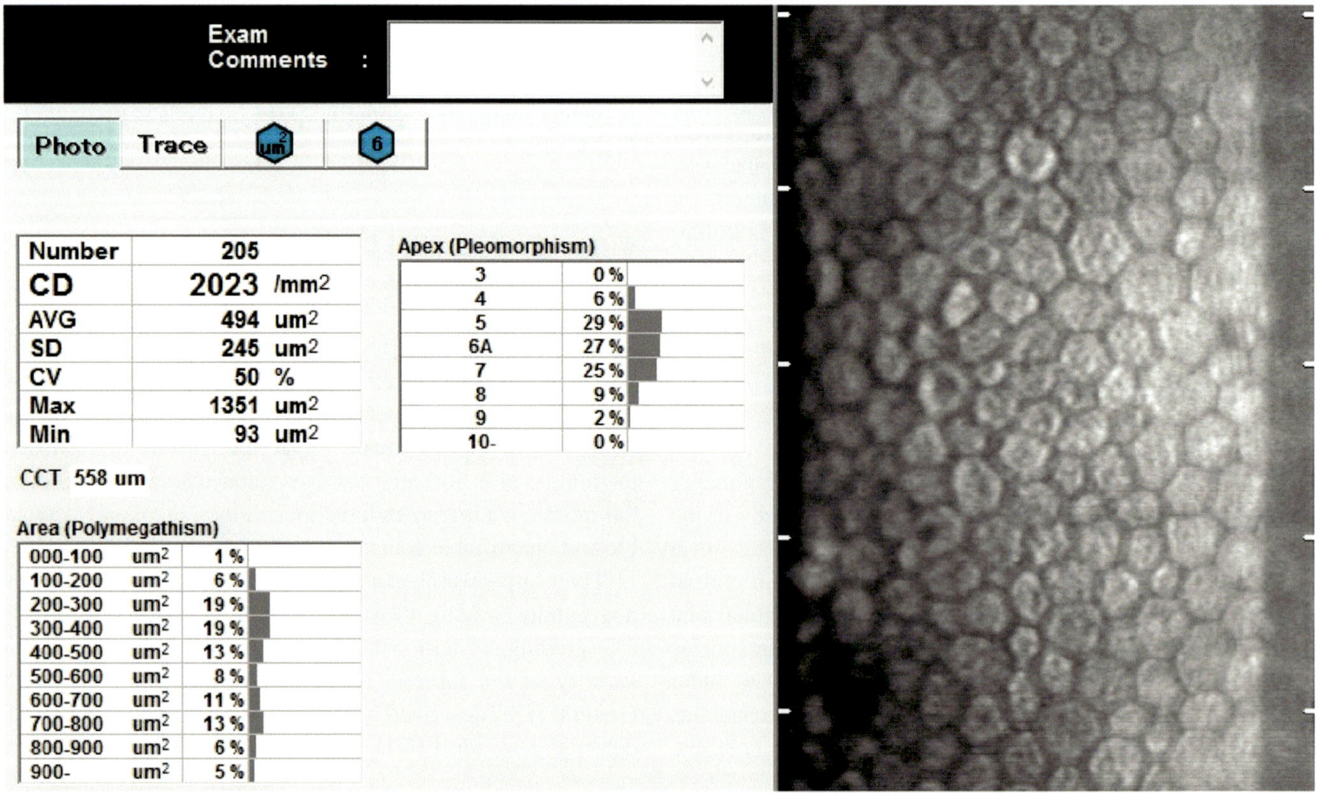

Fig. 5 Typical display from the cell analysis software EM 1100 after endothelial cell measurements (Number = Number of endothelial cells, CD = endothelial cell density, AVG = average cell area, SD = standard deviation of the AVG, CV = cell variation coefficient, Max./Min. = maximal/minimal cell area, Apex = Pleomorphic histogram, Area = polymorphic Histogram)

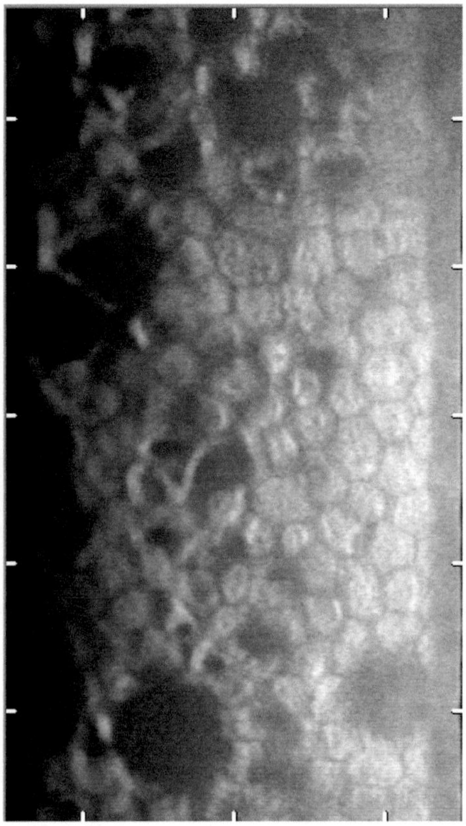

Fig. 6 Guttae appearing as black rounded cell depleted areas

is affected by CG. G1 generally represents only a mild form of the disease with no clinical significance. Grade 2 (G2) presents a CG affected area of 40%–80% and is considered clinically significant with negative impact on the visual acuity, and Grade 3 (G3) describes the highest grade with a CG affected area of more than 80%. Grade 3 represents a total decompensation of the endothelial layer (Fig. 7) [26, 27].

Two other abnormalities can be detected using non-contact specular microscopy:

– Posterior polymorphous corneal dystrophy (PPCD), in which a thickening of the Descemet basement membrane is present. Vesicular, band-like or diffuse groupings of blister-like vesicles and gray-white plaques lead to opacification of the posterior cornea [28] (Fig. 8).
– Iridocorneal endothelial (ICE) syndrome is a rare hereditary disorder characterized by structural and proliferative abnormalities affecting the posterior cornea, the anterior chamber angle, and the iris. An important diagnostic method of this rare disease is the detection of 'ICE cells' on the corneal endothelium using specular microscopy. As illustrated in Fig. 9, these ICE cells are typically abnormal, rounded, large, and pleomorphic, with specular reflex showing a typical "light–dark reversal" consisting in a dark surface, with occasional central light spot, and intercellular light borders [30].

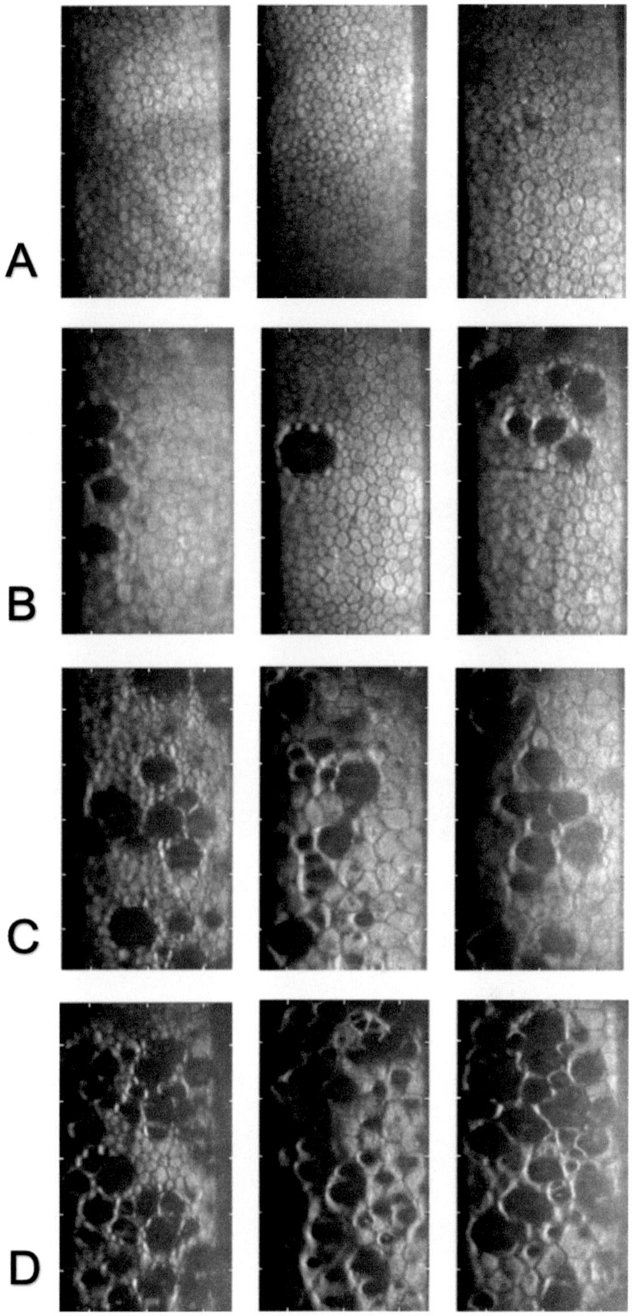

Fig. 7 Homburg classification of cornea guttata based on the affected area using non-contact specular microscopy images from grade 0 to grade 3. (**A**). Cornea guttata Grade 0. (**B**). Cornea guttata Grade 1. (**C**). Cornea guttata Grade 2. (**D**). Cornea guttata Grade 3 [26, 27]

5 Advances in Specular Microscopy

Currently, image analysis including cell recognition is performed through a semi-automated process, where the software marks and delineates the individual endothelial cells in the image and a manual inspection and correction follows. Nevertheless, much effort is now dedicated to

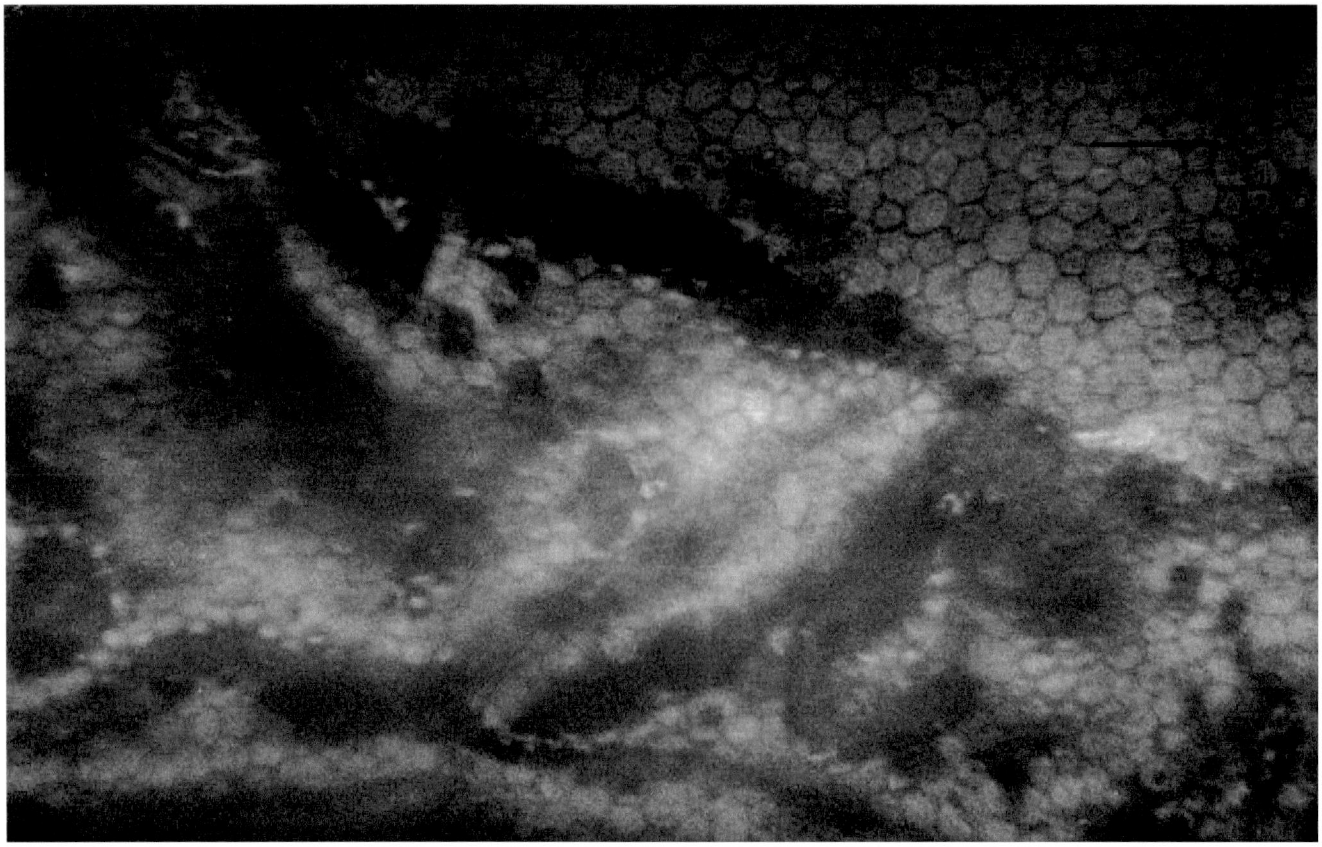

Fig. 8 Specular photomicrograph of posterior polymorphous corneal dystrophy band showing endothelium on a strip of roughened Descemet membrane delineated by dark borders. Endothelial cells 'within' and 'without' the band are clear, in focus and greatly enlarged; many 'within' and on the borders are masked (Bar on the top right = 0,1 mm.) [29]

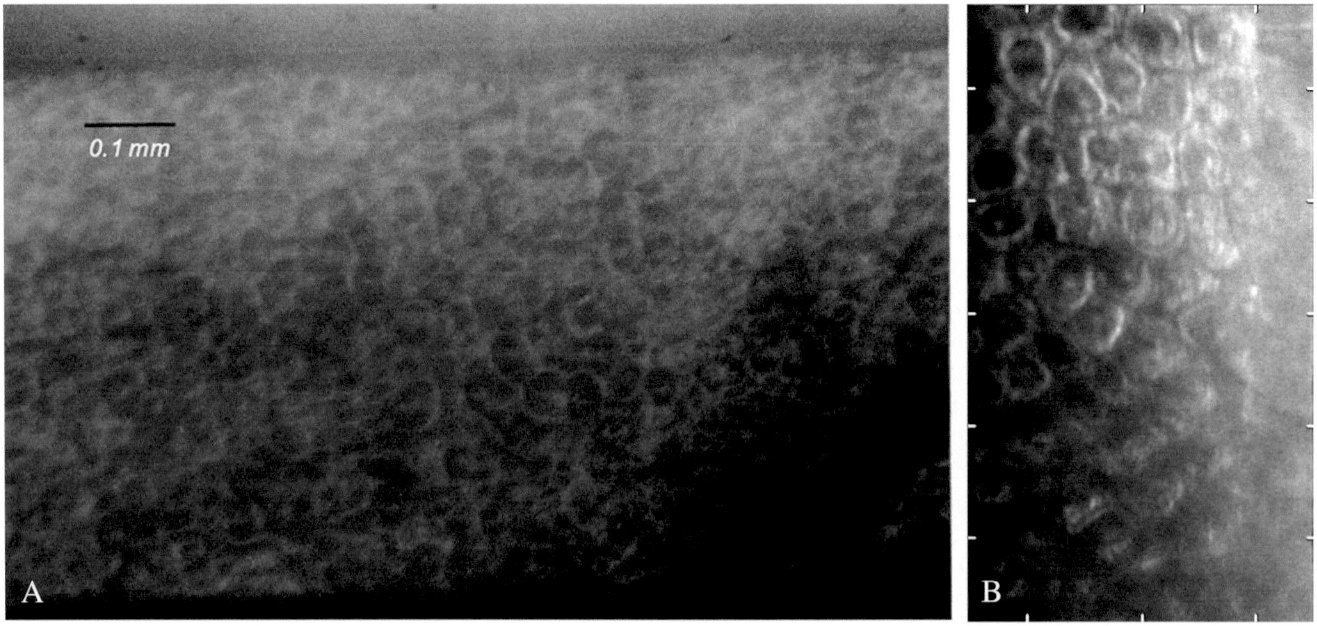

Fig. 9 (**A, B**) Specular microscopy of typical iridocorneal endothelial (ICE) cells, presenting dark center and a bright intercellular border, in opposition to the normal endothelium [29]. (**B**) ICE cells showing central light spots surrounded by dark cellular area and bright intercellular border

providing a fully automated software for the segmentation and analysis of the endothelial images using artificial intelligence. Creating such a software would increase the precision of the image analysis and reduce the working time per image [31, 32]. Some of these instruments have also the function of measuring the central corneal thickness [33].

6 Conclusion

This chapter summarizes the important diagnostic modalities of the corneal endothelial cell analysis using specular microscopy. A detailed examination and assessment of the endothelial cells can be performed through specular microscopy which can measure the ECD and provide a qualitative morphological assessment by estimating levels of pleomorphism and polymegethism. Several endothelial diseases, such as cornea guttata, PPCD and ice syndromes, can be diagnosed or specified using specular microscopy. Further automatization using artificial intelligence is currently underway in order to segment and analyze endothelial cells with a higher precision and accuracy.

References

1. Yee RW. Widefield clinical specular microscopy and computerized morphometric analysis. In: Chandler JW, Sugar J, Edelhauser HF, editors. External diseases: cornea, conjunctiva, sclera eyelids, lacrimal system. Mosby-Year Book Europe Ltd.; 1994.
2. Masters BR. David Maurice's contributions to optical ophthalmic instrumentation: roots of the scanning slit clinical confocal microscope. Exp Eye Res. 2004;78(3):315–26.
3. Laing RA, Sandstrom MM, Leibowitz HM. In vivo photomicrography of the corneal endothelium. Arch Ophthalmol. 1975;93(2):143–5.
4. Bourne WM, Kaufman HE. Specular microscopy of human corneal endothelium in vivo. Am J Ophthalmol. 1976;81(3):319–23.
5. Seitz B, Müller EE, Langenbucher A, Kus MM, Naumann GOH. Reproducibility and validity of a new automatic method of specular microscopy analysis of corneal endothelium. Ophthalmologe. 1997;94(2):127–35.
6. Módis L, Langenbucher A, Seitz B. Corneal endothelial cell density and pachymetry measured by contact and noncontact specular microscopy. J Cataract Refract Surg. 2002;28(10):1763–9.
7. Ong Tone S, Jurkunas U. Imaging the corneal endothelium in Fuchs corneal endothelial dystrophy. Semin Ophthalmol. 2019;34(4):340–6.
8. McCarey BE, Edelhauser HF, Lynn MJ. Review of corneal endothelial specular microscopy for FDA clinical trials of refractive procedures, surgical devices, and new intraocular drugs and solutions. Cornea. 2008;27(1):1–16.
9. Laing RA, Sandstrom MM, Leibowitz HM. Clinical specular microscopy I. Optical principles. Arch Ophthalmol. 1979;97(9):1714–9.
10. Giasson CJ, Solomon LD, Polse KA. Morphometry of corneal endothelium in patients with corneal guttata. Ophthalmology. 2007;114(8):1469–75.
11. Bonanno JA. Molecular mechanisms underlying the corneal endothelial pump. Exp Eye Res. 2012;95(1):2–7.
12. Bourne WM. Biology of the corneal endothelium in health and disease. Eye (Lond). 2003;17(8):912–8.
13. Bourne WM, Nelson LR, Hodge DO. Central corneal endothelial cell changes over a ten-year period. Invest Ophthalmol Vis Sci. 1997;38(3):779–82.
14. Sobottka Ventura AC, Wälti R, Böhnke M. Corneal thickness and endothelial density before and after cataract surgery. Br J Ophthalmol. 2001;85(1):18–20.
15. Wykrota AA, Weinstein I, Hamon L, Daas L, Flockerzi E, Suffo S, Seitz B. Approval rates for corneal donation and the origin of donor tissue for transplantation at a university-based tertiary referral center with corneal subspecialization hosting a LIONS Eye Bank. BMC Ophthalmol. 2022;22(1):1–12.
16. Safi T, Seitz B, Berg K, Schulz K, Langenbucher A, Daas L. Reproducibility of non-invasive endothelial cell loss assessment of the pre-stripped DMEK roll after preparation and storage. Am J Ophthalmol. 2021;221:17–26.
17. Chaurasia S, Vanathi M. Specular microscopy in clinical practice. Indian J Ophthalmol. 2021;69(3):517.
18. Bourne WM, Hodge D, Mclaren JW. Estimation of corneal endothelial pump function in long-term contact lens wearers. Invest Ophthalmol Vis Sci. 1999;40(3):603–11.
19. Harper CL, Boulton ME, Marcyniuk B, Tullo AB, Ridgway AE. Endothelial viability of organ-cultured corneas following penetrating keratoplasty. Eye (Lond). 1998;12(5):834–8.
20. Bourne WM, Kaufman HE. Cataract extraction and the corneal endothelium. Am J Ophthalmol. 1976;82(1):44–7.
21. Jirsova K. Light and specular microscopy of the cornea. Springer International Publishing; 2017.
22. Abib FC, Hida RY, dos Santos RM. Corneal endothelium: histology, physiology and in-vivo examination with specular microscope. JSM Ophthalmol. 2017;5(4):1063.
23. Rao GN, Aquavella J V, Goldberg SH, Berk SL. Pseudophakic bullous keratopathy. relationship to preoperative corneal endothelial status. Ophthalmology. 1984;91(10):1135–1140.
24. Treffers WF. Human corneal endothelial wound repair in vitro and in vivo. Ophthalmology. 1982;89(6):605–13.
25. Doughman DJ, Van Horn D, Rodman WP, Byrnes P, Lindstrom RL. Human corneal endothelial layer repair during organ culture. Arch Ophthalmol. 1976;94(10):1791–6.
26. Schmitz LM, Safi T, Munteanu C, Seitz B, Daas L. Prevalence and severity of cornea Guttata in the graft following Descemet Membrane Endothelial Keratoplasty (DMEK). Acta Ophthalmol. 2022;100(8):e1737–45.
27. Schönit S, Maamri A, Zemova E, Munteanu C, Safi T, Daas L, Seitz B. Prevalence and impact of cornea Guttata in the graft after penetrating Keratoplasty in Germany. Cornea. 2022;41(12):1495–502.
28. Lisch W, Seitz B. New international classification of corneal dystrophies (CD). Ophthalmologe. 2011;108(9):883–97.
29. Laganowski HC, Sherrard ES, Kerr Muir MG, Buckley RG. Distinguishing features of the iridocorneal endothelial syndrome and posterior polymorphous dystrophy: value of endothelial specular microscopy. Br J Ophthalmol. 1991;75(4):212–6.
30. Sacchetti M, Mantelli F, Marenco M, Macchi I, Ambrosio O, Rama P. Diagnosis and management of iridocorneal endothelial syndrome. Biomed Res Int. 2015;2015: 763093.
31. Daniel MC, Atzrodt L, Bucher F, Wacker k, Böhringer S, Reinhard T, Böhringer D. Automated segmentation of the corneal endothelium in a large set of 'real-world' specular microscopy images using the U-Net architecture. Scientific Reports. 2019;9(1):1–7.
32. Nurzynska K. Deep learning as a tool for automatic segmentation of corneal endothelium images. Symmetry. 2018;10(3):60.
33. Tam ES, Rootman DS. Comparison of central corneal thickness measurements by specular microscopy, ultrasound pachymetry, and ultrasound biomicroscopy. J Cataract Refract Surg. 2003;29(6):1179–84.

Corneal Pachymetry

Loïc Hamon and Max Bofferding

Abstract

Pachymetry is a cardinal parameter in corneal evaluation. Already appreciable with the slit lamp, current technologies allow a complete mapping of the cornea and a selective pachymetry of the distinct corneal segments or layers. Multiple pathologies can alter the corneal thickness. This chapter explores the clinical applications of pachymetry.

Keywords

Pachymetry · Corneal thickness · Correction factor · Misinterpretation

1 Introduction

The pachymetry is the measurement of the **corneal thickness**. It is an important element to evaluate the integrity and function of the cornea. Usually the central corneal thickness (CCT) is taken as a reference measurement point. Other points such as corneal apex thickness (CAT), corneal thinnest location (CTL), mid-peripheral corneal thickness (MPCT) or pupil corneal thickness (PCT) can be used to monitor the corneal thickness variations in various contexts [1]. Healthy adult corneal thickness varies physiologically between 450 and 632 µm, with mean CCT of 551 µm [1], without significant difference between the left and right eye [2]. The CTL is often localized in the infratemporal quadrant of the cornea [2]. The corneal thickness increases gradually towards the periphery up to a value of 785 ± 47 µm [1]. After birth, the corneal thickness grows to reach its maximal thickness at the age of 5–9 years [3]. During adulthood, the cornea gets progressively thinner again, especially in the periphery [4] (Table 1). In addition to normal diurnal and physiological variations during life, systemic changes can induce a thickening of the cornea. For example, a temporary corneal thickening can be observed during the second trimester of pregnancy [5]. In addition, diabetes type 1 and 2 can induce a global thickening of the cornea [6]. On the other hand, local changes such as dry eyes or regular wear of contact lenses can reduce the corneal thickness up to 50 µm [7].

2 Types of Measurement

The measurement of the pachymetry can be evaluated with a slit lamp (Fig. 1) [8]. A medium zoom allows to evaluate the global corneal thickness and its increasing enlargement from the center to the periphery. The use of a higher zoom (e.g. 40x) allows to detect and evaluate localized thickness anomalies (Fig. 2).

Manual pachymetry is performed with an ultrasound sensor (Fig. 3). The accuracy of the measurements is excellent but not easily reproducible, as the measurement must always be performed at the exact same position (with the same pressure on the eye). This measurement has the limitation of measuring only one precise point of the cornea and must therefore be performed several times at the center and at different locations in the periphery to obtain a global overview of the corneal thickness.

The pachymetry can also be assessed on tomographic corneal elevation maps, where pachymetry is estimated by the difference between the anterior and posterior corneal

L. Hamon (✉) · M. Bofferding
Department of Ophthalmology, Saarland University Medical Center (UKS), Homburg, Saar, Germany
e-mail: hamon.loic@outlook.com

M. Bofferding
e-mail: max.bofferding@uks.eu

L. Hamon
Department of Ophthalmology, Clinique Notre-Dame de Grâce, Charleroi, Belgium

B. Seitz et al. (eds.), *Atlas on Cornea*, https://doi.org/10.1007/978-3-031-65422-0_6

Table 1 Evolution of mean central corneal thickness related to age

Age [years]	2–4[a]	5–9[a]	10–18[b]	18–29[b]	30–39[b]	40–49[b]	50–59[b]	60–69[b]	70–79[b]	≥80[b]
Central corneal thickness (CCT) [μm]	546	566	554	550	557	551	544	544	535	530

[a]Hussein et al. [3]
[b]Galgauskas et al. [25]

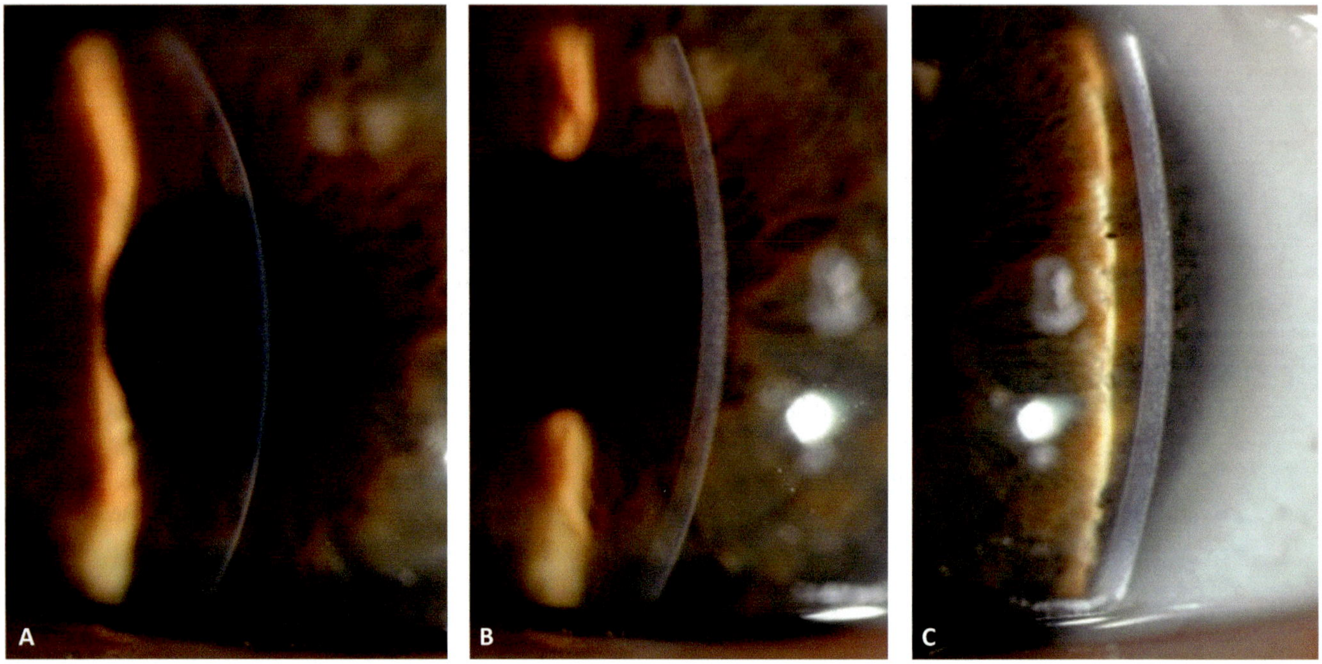

Fig. 1 **Appreciation of corneal thickness using slit lamp on healthy subject**. The increase in corneal thickness from the center (**A**) through the mid-periphery (**B**) to the periphery (**C**) can be discerned by using a thin slit

elevations (indirect measurement) [2]. Anterior segment optical coherence tomography (AS-OCT) also allows accurate and reproducible corneal thickness mapping. Depending on the equipment and software, the pachymetry appears on mapping images (Fig. 4) or can also be measured manually at specific points (Fig. 5).

3 Clinical Applications

The pachymetry can be locally or globally altered in multiple corneal pathologies. These changes are either **thickening**, usually associated with corneal edema (Fig. 6) or **thinning** due to a loss of corneal tissue, retractions (stromal scars) or corneal ectasias such as keratoconus (Fig. 7). Other characteristics like the mono-and bilateral symmetricity or enantiomorphism (mirror image of both corneas) of the thickening or thinning are helpful criteria for the differential diagnosis.

Central corneal thickness also plays an important role in classical intraocular pressure (IOP) measurement by Goldmann applanation tonometry. Applanation tonometry will be underestimated for thin corneas and overestimated for thick corneas [9, 10]. The IOP can be approximately adjusted by a correction factor, e.g. the Dresden correction table (Table 2), or using more complex algorithms [11]. New tonometers, such as the dynamic contour tonometer, seem to be less dependent on corneal properties [12]. Exceptions to this rule are edematous corneas, which are thickened but also "softer" than normal corneas, leading to an IOP underestimation [13, 14]. In the field of glaucoma, ocular hypertension has been associated with higher values for central corneal thickness [15]. Therefore, it is advisable to perform corneal pachymetry in glaucoma patients to correct the IOP values with central corneal thickness [16].

Corneal thickness also plays an important role in planning ablative keratorefractive surgery. According to current recommendations, the percentage of tissue alterated (PTA) should not exceed 40% of the total corneal thickness in order to prevent the risk of iatrogenic ectasia [17].

In the field of eye banking, ex-vivo pachymetry of the graft is possible and can be useful to evaluate the thickness of the graft and/or to confirm graft deswelling before keratoplasty. For those purposes, "sterile donor tomography" allows an

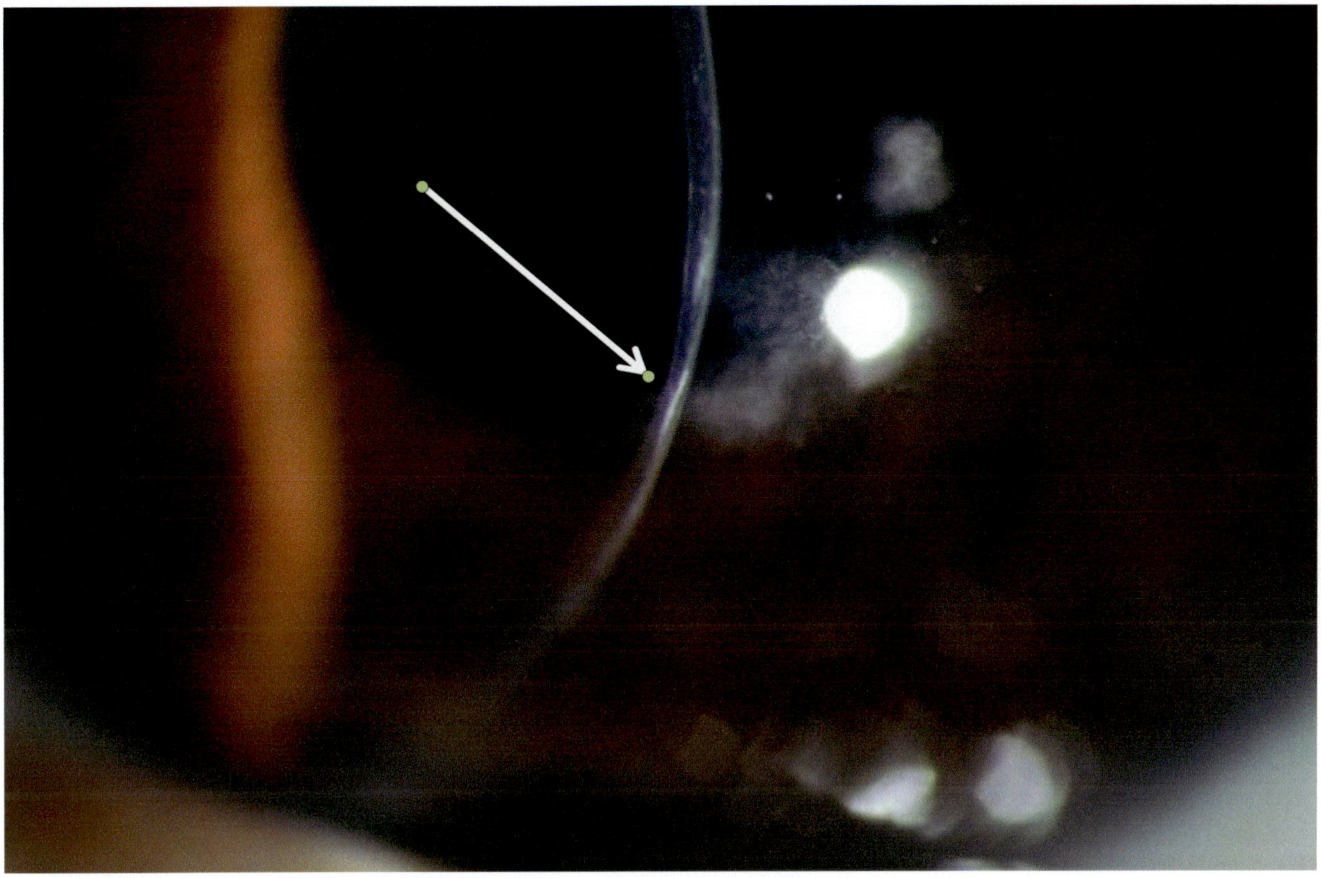

Fig. 2 **Slit lamp photography (Zoom × 40).** Pronounced central corneal thinning with superficial avascular scaring (**arrow**) due to keratoconus

analysis of the graft including a mapping of the corneal thickness [18] (Fig. 8). This reproducible measurement represents an interesting tool in addition to the current examinations in order to improve graft selection in the eye bank [19].

4 Artefacts and Frequent Mistakes

Many factors can influence the measurement or lead to a false interpretation of corneal pachymetry. A classic error is to measure the pachymetry of a patient, who is still wearing his/her contact lens(es), thus greatly overestimating the pachymetry value of the eye(s) concerned. The existence of a pterygium or a pannus, such as in aniridia associated keratopathy, also leads to an overestimation of the corneal pachymetry of the area where the lesion is located. In addition, corneal deposits or accumulations, typically glycosaminoglycans, can interfere with the Scheimpflug camera and cause artifacts, thus rendering the measurement uninterpretable (Figs. 9 and 10). Finally, the association of a pathology causing corneal thinning with another causing corneal thickening can mask one or even both pathologies on the pachymetry analysis (erroneous healthy appearance of the cornea despite for example keratoconus and Fuchs endothelial corneal dystrophy) (Fig. 11).

5 Further Perspectives

Independent of the advances in terms of measurement techniques, new applications of pachymetry have emerged in recent years. One of them is the use of AS-OCT in the operating theatre allowing the surgeon to determine its localization in the cornea (depth) as well as a monitoring of the pachymetry values. This tool is particularly used for anterior lamellar surgeries to avoid endothelial perforation [20].

The measurement of epithelial layer thickness has also been of great interest in recent years, particularly in the preoperative screening of keratorefractive surgery (Fig. 12). Indeed, alterations in epithelial thickness have been correlated with the presence of keratoconus and with an increased risk of developing iatrogenic keratectasia [21].

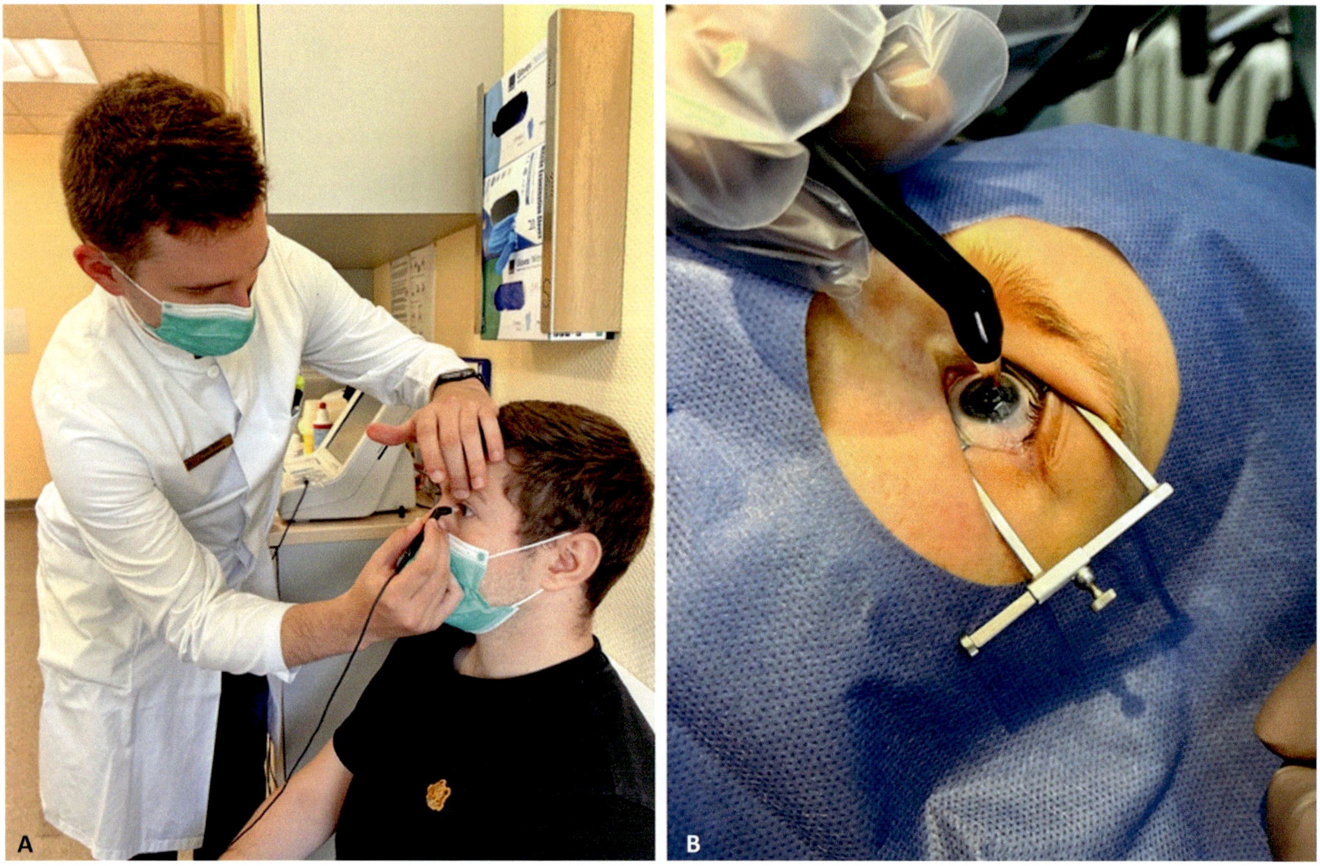

Fig. 3 Pachymetry using ultrasound. (**A**) Measurement of the central corneal thickness in combination with eye length. (**B**) Intraoperative monitoring of pachymetry during riboflavin A accelerated corneal collagen crosslinking

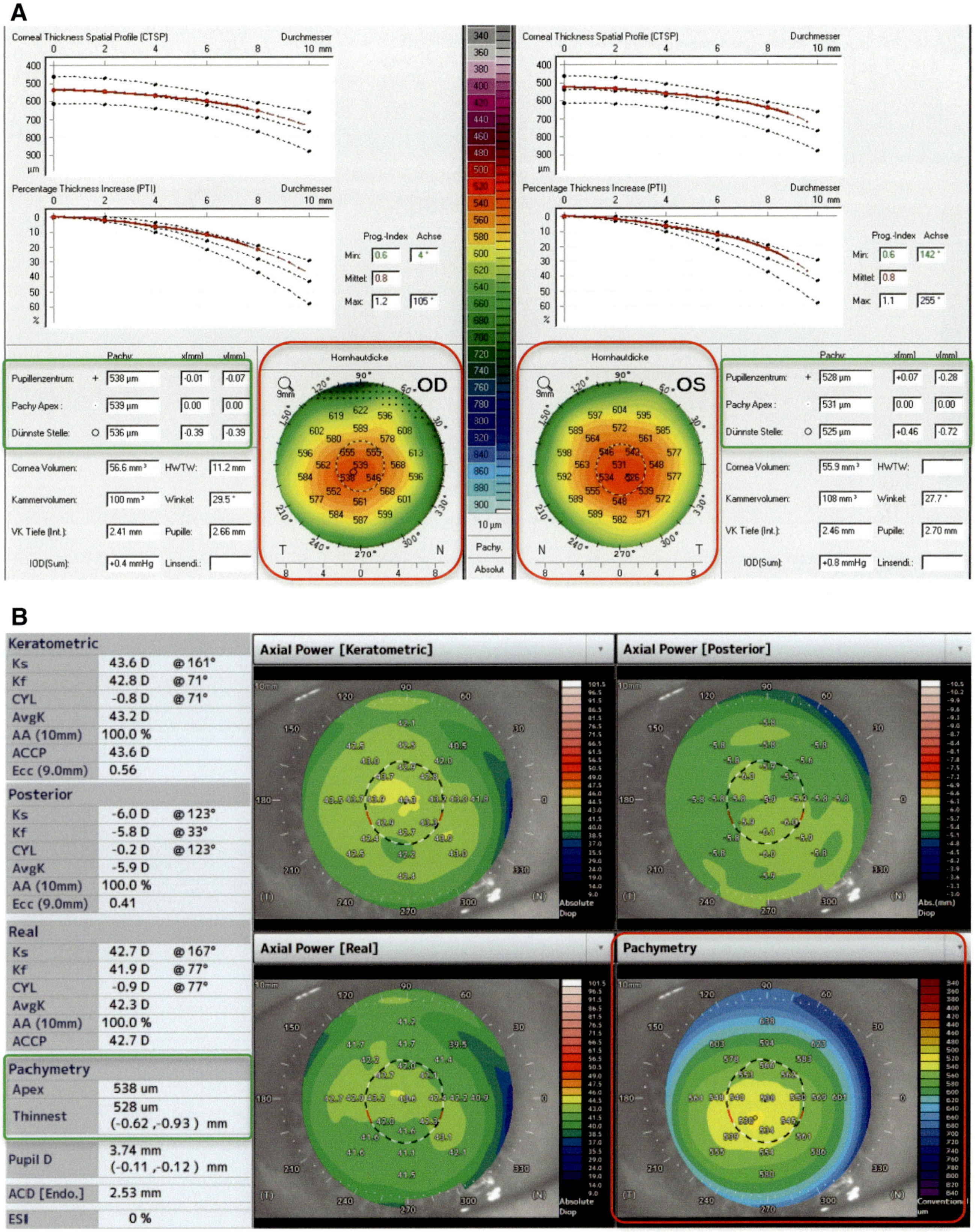

Fig. 4 Pachymetry using currently available tomographs. **(A)** Corneal mapping incl. pachymetry (**red frames**) performed with the Scheimpflug camera Pentacam HR (OCULUS GmbH, Wetzlar, Germany). The corneal thickness spatial profile and percentage thickness increase describe the variation of corneal thickness towards the periphery (up to 10 mm). The mostly used parameters (corneal apex thickness (CAT), corneal thinnest location (CTL) and pupil corneal thickness (PCT)) are displayed (**green frames**). **(B)** Corneal mapping incl. pachymetry with anterior segment optical coherence tomograph (AS-OCT) Casia 2 (Tomey, Nagoya, Japan). In addition to the corneal thickness map (**red frame**), corneal apex thickness and corneal thinnest location (CTL) are displayed (**green frame**)

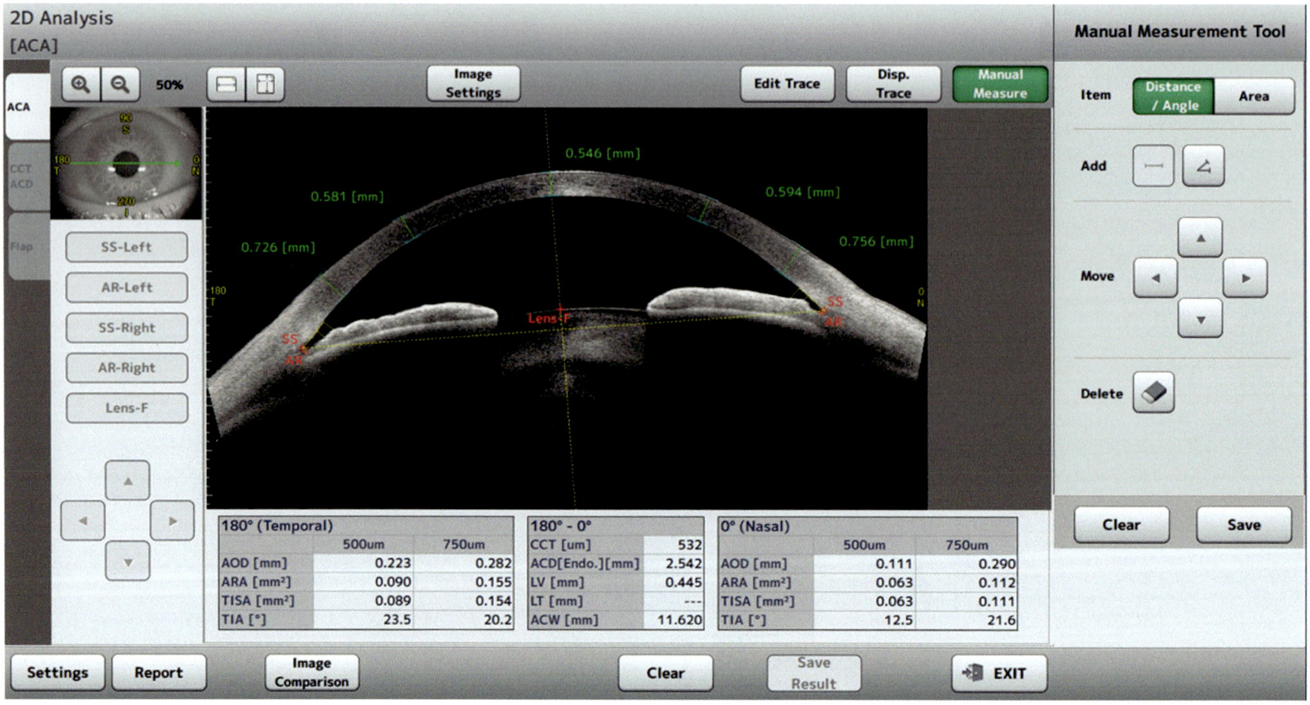

Fig. 5 **Manual pachymetry** using anterior segment optical coherence tomograph (AS-OCT) Casia 2 (Tomey, Nagoya, Japan). Manual measurement tool of AS-OCT software enables to measure distances or angles between two selected points. Represented green measures are distances between manually selected endothelium and epithelium, representing the full corneal thickness at chosen segments central and peripheral. This type of measurement could also be used to examine scars diameter or thickness (not represented)

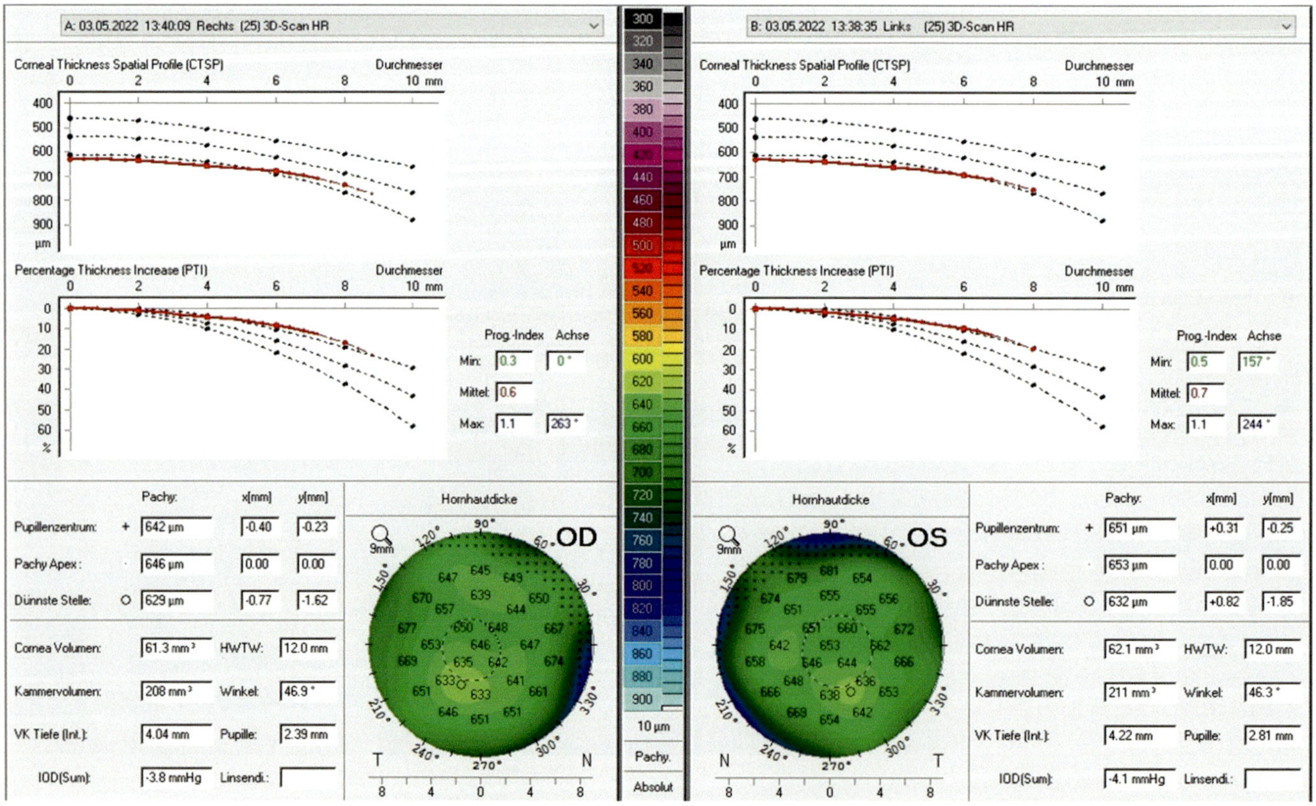

Fig. 6 Typical image of a patient with **Fuchs endothelial corneal dystrophy (FECD)** using corneal tomography (Pentacam HR—OCULUS GmbH, Wetzlar, Germany). Pachymetry allows indirect evaluation of the loss of endothelial function by measuring progressive, bilateral and diffuse corneal **thickening** related to edema. The corneal thickening is often associated with a reduction of visual acuity, photophobia and halos

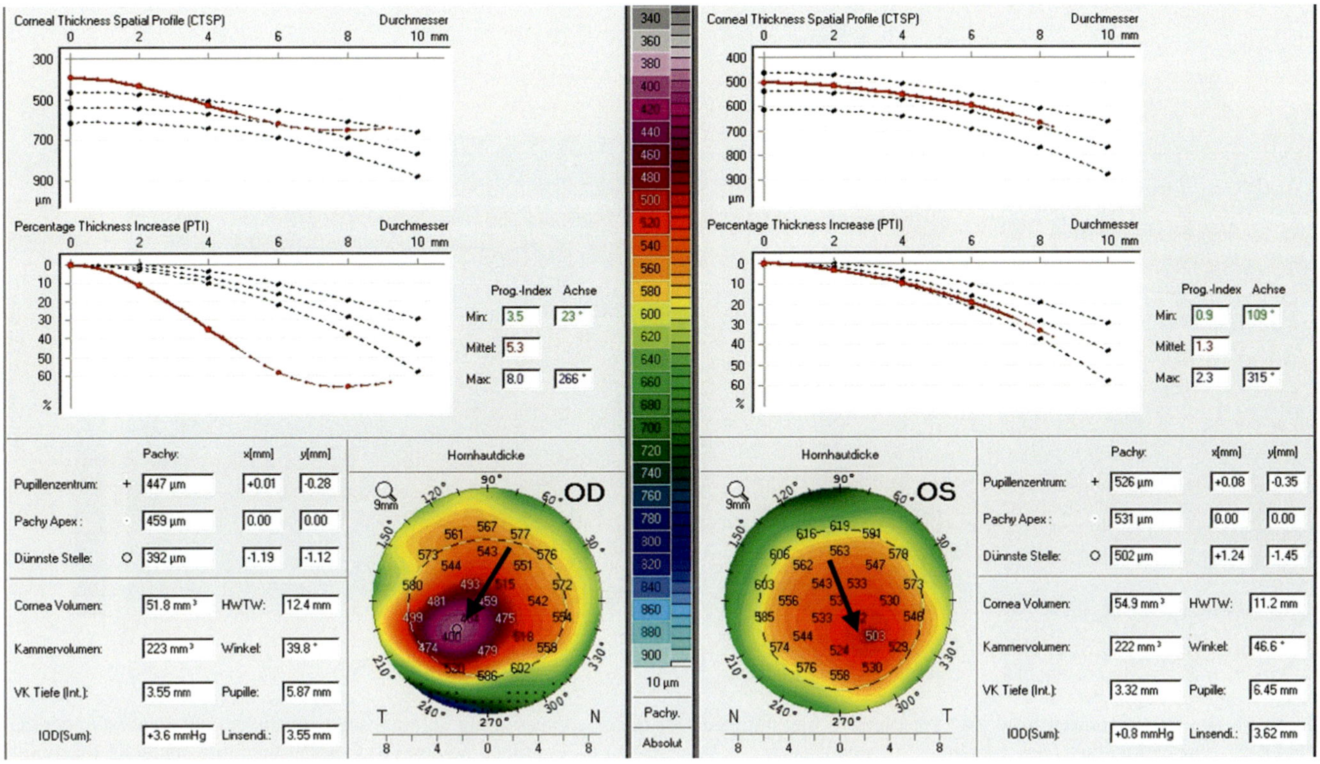

Fig. 7 Typical image of a patient presenting **keratoconus** using corneal tomography (Pentacam HR—OCULUS GmbH, Wetzlar, Germany). The pathology presents with a localized paracentral asymmetrical corneal **thinning** (arrows). Typically, both eyes are affected in different severity stages (in this case right>left). The corneal thinning is associated with an irregular astigmatism, reduction of visual acuity and optical phenomena like halos

Table 2 **Dresden correction table**. Simplified version of the original table by Kohlhaas et al. [9]. Adjustment of intraocular pressure (IOP) after Goldmann applanation tonometry in adult corneas with no history of eye surgery or corneal pathology

Central corneal thickness (CCT) [µm]	475	500	525	550	575	600	625	650	675
Correction factor [mmHg]	+3	+2	+1	0	−1	−2	−3	−4	−5

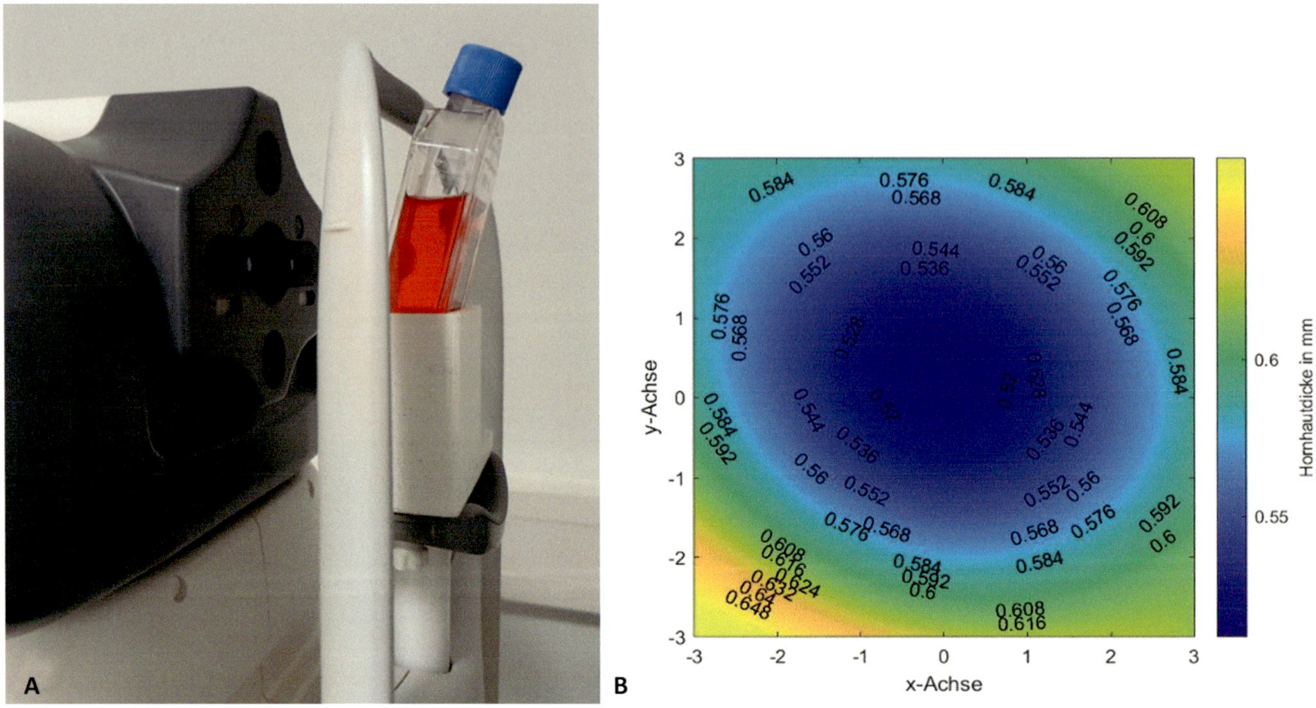

Fig. 8 **Sterile donor tomography**. (**A**) Preoperative measurements of donor corneas using anterior segment optical coherence tomography (AS-OCT). The cell culture flask containing the donor cornea is mounted on a 3D-printed holder. (**B**) Corneal thickness mapping (in millimeters) of the donor cornea, generated with a self-made MATLAB program according to the method of Mäurer, Damian and Langenbucher [18, 22–24]

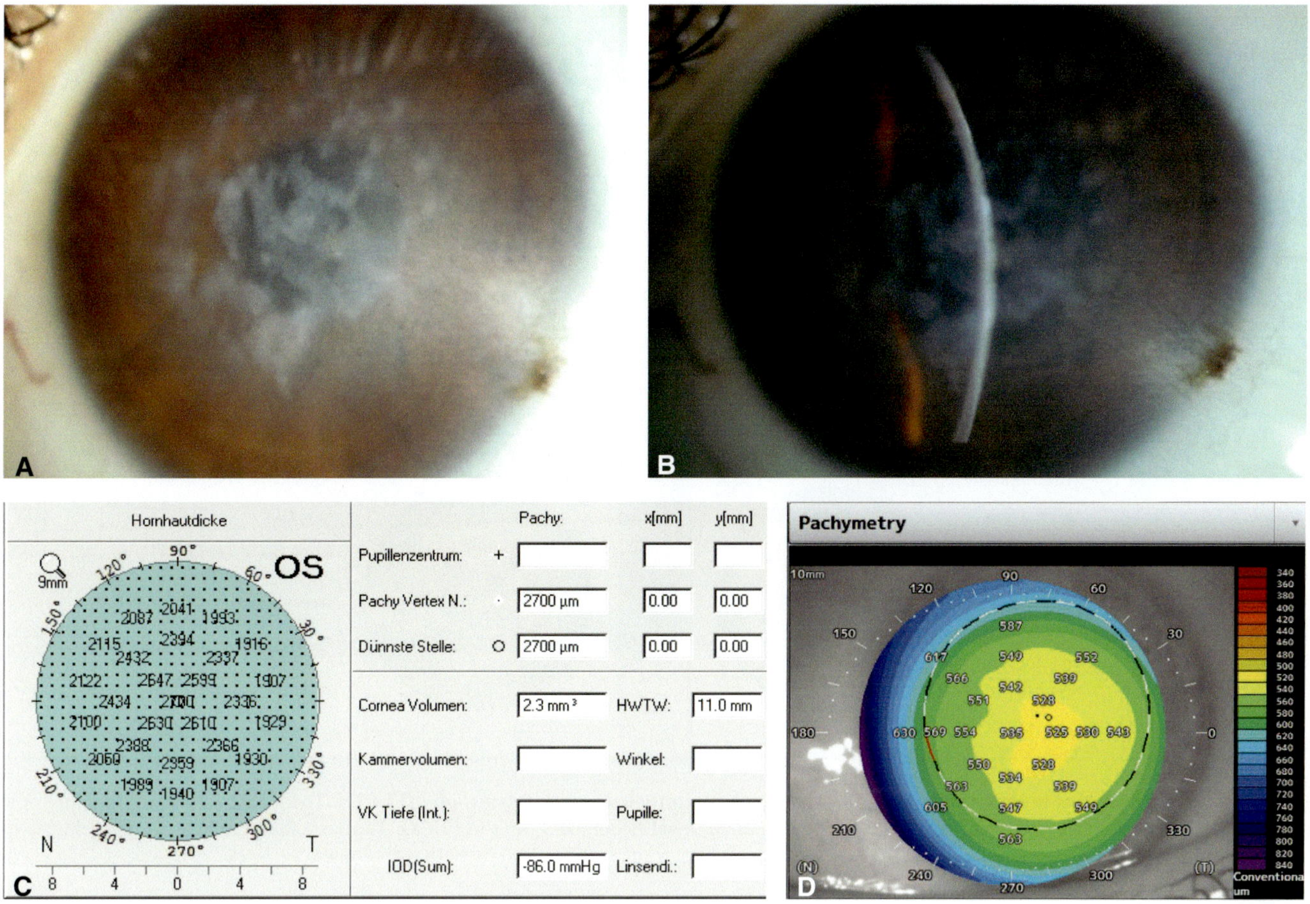

Fig. 9 **Pachymetry on cornea with macular dystrophy**. (**A**) Clinical findings, presenting with typical anterior stromal, irregular whitish fleck-like opacities caused by intra- and extracellular accumulation of glycosaminoglycans (GAG). (**B**) Thin slit. Central corneal thickness (CCT) appears normal. (**C**) Pachymetry using a Scheimpflug camera (Pentacam HR—OCULUS GmbH, Wetzlar, Germany). **Artifacts** are caused by light reflections related to dense GAG accumulation, causing an extreme false overestimation of corneal thickness (CCT 2700 µm). A pachymetry with Scheimpflug camera is not interpretable in this case. (**D**) Pachymetry using anterior segment OCT (CASIA 2—Tomey, Nagoya, Japan) (CCT 525 µm). This measurement technique is not affected by GAG deposits and should be preferred in such cases of corneal dystrophies

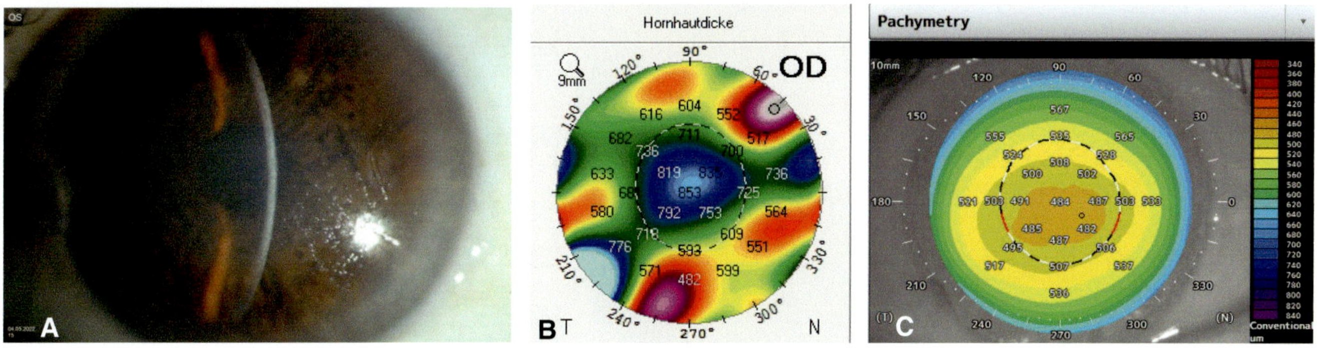

Fig. 10 **Pachymetry on cornea with Schnyder dystrophy**. (**A**) Clinical findings, with a ring-like corneal opacity and superficial cloudy aspect. (**B**) Pachymetry using a Scheimpflug camera (Pentacam HR—OCULUS GmbH, Wetzlar, Germany). **Artifacts** are caused by light reflections due to phospholipids, also causing an overestimation of corneal thickness (central corneal thickness (CCT) 853 µm). (**C**) Pachymetry using and anterior segment OCT (CASIA 2—Tomey, Nagoya, Japan) results in a valid measurement (CCT 484 µm)

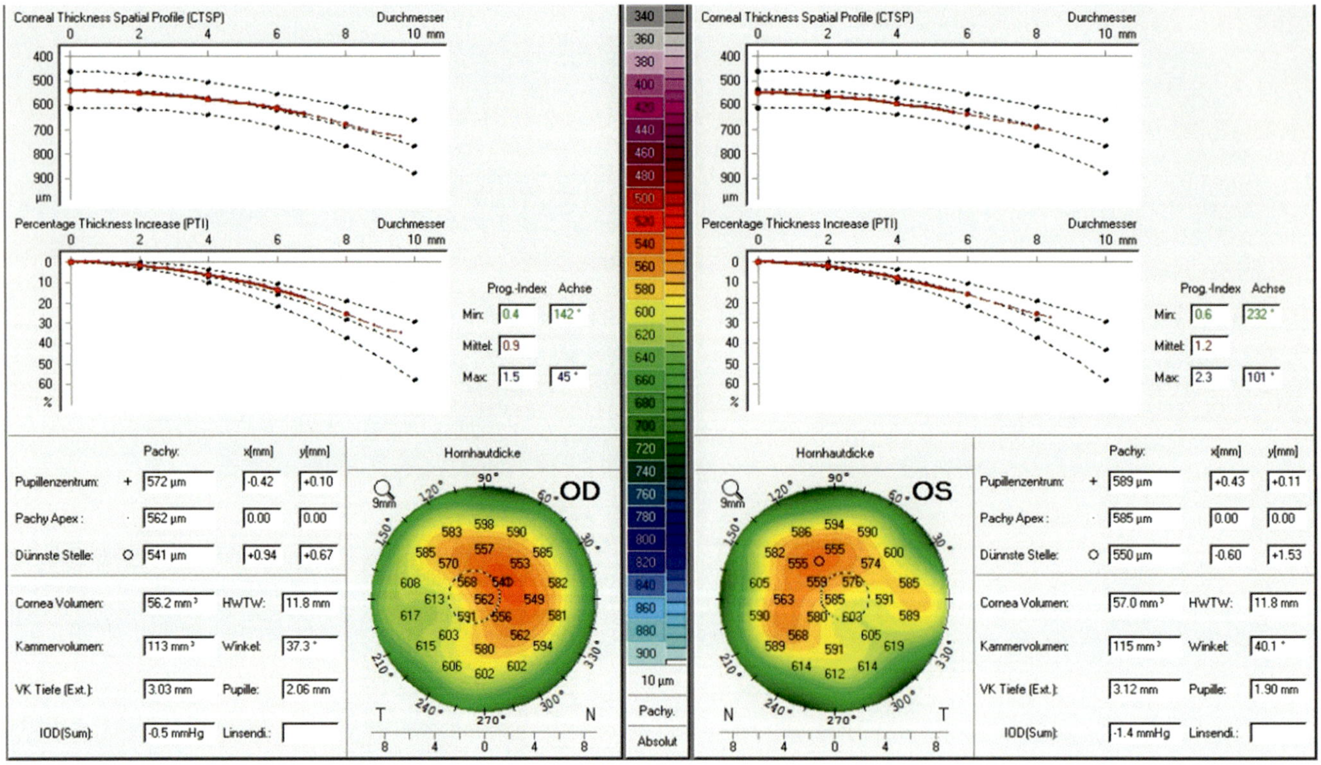

Fig. 11 **Patient presenting both keratoconus (KC) and Fuchs endothelial corneal dystrophy (FECD)**. The localized corneal thinning of the KC is balanced by the diffuse corneal thickening caused by endothelial decompensation in FECD. The association of the two pathologies can give an erroneously healthy appearance of the cornea on the pachymetry mapping caused by both pathologies

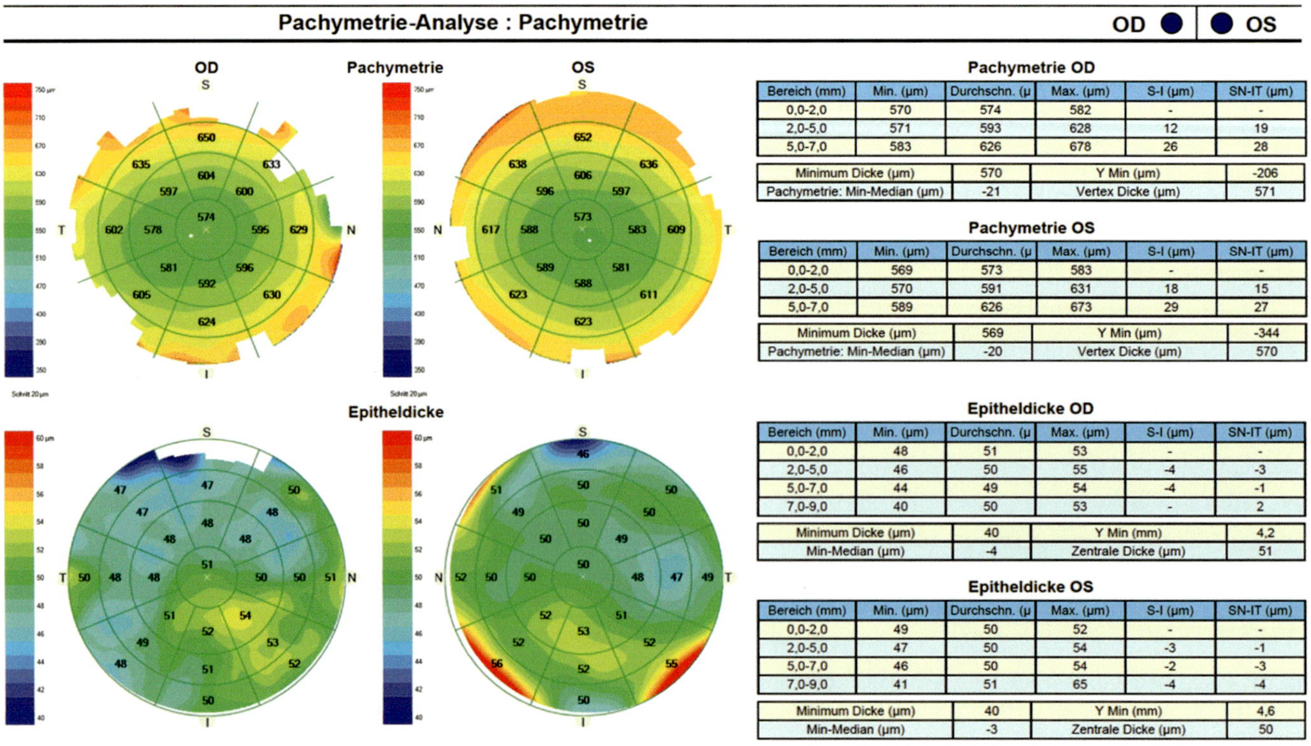

Fig. 12 **Epithelial thickness map** from the pachymetry analysis of the tomograph Cirrus HD (Carl Zeiss Meditech, Oberkochen, Germany)

6 Conclusion

Corneal pachymetry can be evaluated with a multitude of different instruments and is influenced by many factors and pathologies. Independent of the purpose of the measurements, a prior clinical examination is essential to choose the right device and thus obtaining the most accurate measurements.

References

1. Fares U, Otri AM, Al-Aqaba MA, Dua HS. Correlation of central and peripheral corneal thickness in healthy corneas. Cont Lens Anterior Eye. 2012;35:39–45. https://doi.org/10.1016/j.clae.2011.07.004.
2. Módis L Jr, Langenbucher A, Seitz B. Evaluation of normal corneas using the scanning-slit topography/pachymetry system. Cornea. 2004; 23:689–94. https://doi.org/10.1097/01.ico.0000126315.05519.0b.
3. Hussein MA, Paysse EA, Bell NP, Coats DK, Brady McCreery KM, Koch DD, Orengo-Nania S, Baskin D, Wilhelmus KR. Corneal thickness in children. Am J Ophthalmol. 2004;138:744–8. https://doi.org/10.1016/j.ajo.2004.06.030.
4. Ma R, Liu Y, Zhang L, Ma J, Cui T, Lei Y, Hou J, Shen Z, Yi X, Liang G, Wang Y. Changes in corneal morphology with age in asian population: a multicenter study of 30,618 cases. Adv Ther. 2021;38:5763–76. https://doi.org/10.1007/s12325-021-01922-4.
5. Wang C, Li AL, Pang Y, Lei YQ, Yu L. Changes in intraocular pressure and central corneal thickness during pregnancy: a systematic review and Meta-analysis. Int J Ophthalmol. 2017;10:1573–9. https://doi.org/10.18240/ijo.2017.10.15.
6. Amador-Muñoz DP, Conforti V, Matheus LM, Molano-Gonzalez N, Payán-Gómez C. Diabetes mellitus type 1 has a higher impact on corneal endothelial cell density and pachymetry than diabetes mellitus type 2, independent of age: a Meta-regression model. Cornea. 2022;41:965–73. https://doi.org/10.1097/ICO.0000000000002841.
7. Liu Z, Pflugfelder SC. Corneal thickness is reduced in dry eye. Cornea. 1999;18:403–7. https://doi.org/10.1097/00003226-199907000-00002.
8. Gellrich MM, Hufendiek K. Pachymetry with a video slit lamp. Ophthalmologe. 2021;118:162–8. https://doi.org/10.1007/s00347-020-01108-3.
9. Kohlhaas M, Boehm AG, Spoerl E, Pürsten A, Grein HJ, Pillunat LE. Effect of central corneal thickness, corneal curvature, and axial length on applanation tonometry. Arch Ophthalmol. 2006;124:471–6. https://doi.org/10.1001/archopht.124.4.471.
10. Knauf D, Seitz B, Schießl G, Zemova E, Flockerzi E. Analysis of various modalities for intraocular pressure measurement in relation to keratoconus severity in 246 eyes of the Homburg Keratoconus Center. Cornea 2023;42:829–36. https://doi.org/10.1097/ICO.0000000000003170.
11. Chan MP, Grossi CM, Khawaja AP, Yip JL, Khaw KT, Patel PJ, Khaw PT, Morgan JE, Vernon SA, Foster PJ. UK biobank eye and vision consortium. Associations with intraocular pressure in a large cohort: Results from the UK biobank. Ophthalmology 2016;123:771–782. https://doi.org/10.1016/j.ophtha.2015.11.031.
12. ElMallah MK, Asrani SG. New ways to measure intraocular pressure. Curr Opin Ophthalmol. 2008;19:122–6. https://doi.org/10.1097/ICU.0b013e3282f391ae.
13. Simon G, Small RH, Ren Q, Parel JM. Effect of corneal hydration on Goldmann applanation tonometry and corneal topography. Refract Corneal Surg. 1993;9:110–7.
14. Marx W, Madjlessi F, Reinhard T, Althaus C, Sundmacher R. More than 4 years' experience with electronic intraocular needle tonometry. Ophthalmologe 1999;96:498–502. https://doi.org/10.1007/s003470050444.
15. Brandt JD, Beiser JA, Kass MA, Gordon MO. Central corneal thickness in the Ocular Hypertension Treatment Study (OHTS). Ophthalmology. 2001;108:1779–88.
16. Rüfer F. Sources of error in Goldmann applanation tonometry. Ophthalmologe. 2011;108:546–52. https://doi.org/10.1007/s00347-011-2370-5.
17. Santhiago MR. Percent tissue altered and corneal ectasia. Curr Opin Ophthalmol. 2016;27:311–5. https://doi.org/10.1097/ICU.0000000000000276.
18. Seitz B, Asi F, Mäurer S, Hamon L, Quintin A, Langenbucher A. Anterior segment OCT: application to improve graft selection for corneal transplantation. Atlas of anterior segment optical coherence tomography. Springer 2021, Cham, pp. 223–236.
19. Hamon L, Quintin A, Mäurer S, Weinstein I, Langenbucher A, Seitz B, Daas L. Reliability and efficiency of corneal thickness measurements using sterile donor tomography in the eye bank. Cell Tissue Bank. 2021. https://doi.org/10.1007/s10561-021-09980-2.
20. Lang SJ, Heinzelmann S, Böhringer D, Reinhard T, Maier P. Indications for intraoperative anterior segment optical coherence tomography in corneal surgery. Int Ophthalmol. 2020;40:2617–25. https://doi.org/10.1007/s10792-020-01442-0.
21. Reinstein DZ, Archer TJ, Vida RS. Epithelial thickness mapping for corneal refractive surgery. Curr Opin Ophthalmol. 2022;33:258–68. https://doi.org/10.1097/ICU.0000000000000867.
22. Janunts E, Langenbucher A, Seitz B. In vitro corneal tomography of donor cornea using anterior segment OCT. Cornea. 2016;35:647–53. https://doi.org/10.1097/ICO.0000000000000761.
23. Damian A, Seitz B, Langenbucher A, Eppig T. Optical coherence tomography-based topography determination of corneal grafts in eye bank cultivation. J Biomed Opt. 2017;22:16001. https://doi.org/10.1117/1.JBO.22.1.016001.
24. Mäurer S, Asi F, Rawer A, Damian A, Seitz B, Langenbucher A, Eppig T. Concept for 3D measurement of corneal donor tissue using a clinical OCT. Ophthalmologe. 2019;116:640–6. https://doi.org/10.1007/s00347-018-0801-2.
25. Galgauskas S, Juodkaite G, Tutkuvienė J. Age-related changes in central corneal thickness in normal eyes among the adult Lithuanian population. Clin Interv Aging. 2014;9:1145–51. https://doi.org/10.2147/CIA.S61790.

Scheimpflug Tomography

Elias Flockerzi and Berthold Seitz

Abstract

This chapter is not intended to be a handbook nor can it present all the diagnostic features provided by the Pentacam®—for this, please refer to the interpretation guide provided by the manufacturer (Oculus, Wetzlar, Germany). However, it presents typical Scheimpflug imaging findings (as raised with the Pentacam HR®) from daily practice in a university-based outpatient department with a focus on recognizing typical patterns of keratectasia and their possible differential diagnoses.

Keywords
Scheimpflug · Keratoconus · Keratoglobus · Pellucid Marginal Degeneration

1 Introduction

Scheimpflug imaging was patented by the Austrian Theodor Scheimpflug in 1904, who tilted the lens plane so that there was an intersection with both the film and focal plane and used this method to correct perspective distortion in aerial photographs [1]. The Pentacam® (Oculus, Wetzlar, Germany) was introduced in 2002 and was the first instrument that used a rotational Scheimpflug camera to enable non-contact and three-dimensional imaging of the anterior segment of the human eye [2]. It uses a blue light source of 475 nm and two cameras. The first camera is static and monitors eye fixation and pupil size, whilst the second camera is a rotational Scheimpflug camera, that captures 100 cross-sectional images with 138,000 data points on an angle from 0 to 180 degrees in two seconds (Pentacam HR (high resolution), technical data from the manufacturer). Afterwards, a three-dimensional model of the anterior segment of the examined eye is calculated. The Pentacam® offers multiple displays and presents the captured data in anterior and posterior sagittal and tangential curvature maps, refractive power maps, anterior and posterior elevation maps [1], data about anterior chamber angle, volume, depth and both cornea and lens densitometry. In general, the Pentacam® uses a reference sphere with a diameter of eight or nine millimeters (selection in the settings), which is approximated to the examined human cornea. Deviations from the reference sphere are presented color-coded as height and curvature data and can be interpreted clinically. Currently, there exist four generations of the Pentacam® reaching from the (1) Pentacam® that captures 25,000 data points in two seconds to the (2) Pentacam HR® (high resolution) capturing 138,000 data points in the same time to the (3) Pentacam AXL® that includes axial length measurement of the eye and intraocular lens calculation and the (4) Pentacam AXL Wave® that provides objective refraction measurement and wavefront aberrometry of the entire eye as additional features. A fifth generation including anterior segment optical coherence tomography imaging has recently been presented. This chapter aims to provide a short overview about some functions of the Pentacam® that may be relevant for ophthalmologists working in an outpatient department specialized on cornea.

2 Clinical Application

The Pentacam® Fast Screening Report shows 15 key parameters of one eye examination including in this example the (1) anterior chamber angle ("Chamber Angle"), (2) thinnest corneal pachymetry ("Pachy Min"), (3) maximal pachymetric progression index ("Pachy Prog.-Index Max."), (4) posterior corneal elevation ("Elevation (Back)"), (5) anterior chamber depth ("A. C. Depth"), (6) apex pachymetry ("Pachy Apex"), (7) maximal anterior keratometry ("K Max

E. Flockerzi (✉) · B. Seitz
Department of Ophthalmology, Saarland University Medical Center, Homburg, Germany
e-mail: elias.flockerzi@uks.eu

B. Seitz et al. (eds.), *Atlas on Cornea*, https://doi.org/10.1007/978-3-031-65422-0_7

(Front)"), (8) averaged cornea densitometry for posterior 60 µm, annulus 0–2 mm ("Cornea Densito Avg."), (9) anterior chamber volume ("Chamber Volume"), (10) averaged pachymetric progression index ("Pachy Prog.-Index Av."), (11) anterior corneal elevation ("Elevation (Front)"), (12) averaged cornea densitometry for posterior 60 µm, annulus 2–6 mm, (13) Belin/Ambrósio Deviation Index ("BAD-D") indicating keratectasia severity, (14) Topographic Keratoconus Classification ("TKC") and (15) Pentacam® Nucleus Staging ("PNS") providing a lens opacity staging (Fig. 1).

The pachymetric Pentacam® display shows corneal thickness measurements for both the right ("OD") and the left ("OS") eye of one patient. First, there is the "Corneal Thickness Spatial Profile", which shows a sloping curve in normal corneas, as it begins in the center of the cornea (0 mm diameter) and thickness increases towards the periphery of the cornea (diameter 2–4–6–8–10 mm, Fig. 2). Whilst the first curve deals with absolute thickness values in µm (400–500–600–700–800–900), the "Percentage Thickness Increase" indicates the percentual thickness increase from the center towards the periphery of the cornea in the same intervals as the "Corneal Thickness Spatial Profile". Below, there are different pachymetric values displayed such as pachymetry at the pupil center, apex pachymetry and thinnest corneal pachymetry. Those are followed by the cornea volume and diameter, the anterior chamber volume, angle and depth, the pupil diameter and the pachymetry-based intraocular pressure correction factor in mmHg. The corneal thickness map is color-coded (with warm colors representing areas of thinning and cold colors representing areas of thickening) and displays multiple thickness values over the corneal surface as measured by the Pentacam® (Fig. 2).

Specular microscopy of the corneal endothelium of the eyes shown in Fig. 2 revealed a dysmorphic endothelium in the thickened cornea of the right and a normal endothelium in the left eye (Fig. 3).

The topometric Pentacam® display (Fig. 4) shows anterior ("Cornea front") and posterior ("Cornea back") curvature and keratometry data. The "True Net Power" display indicates corneal refractive power based on the refractive

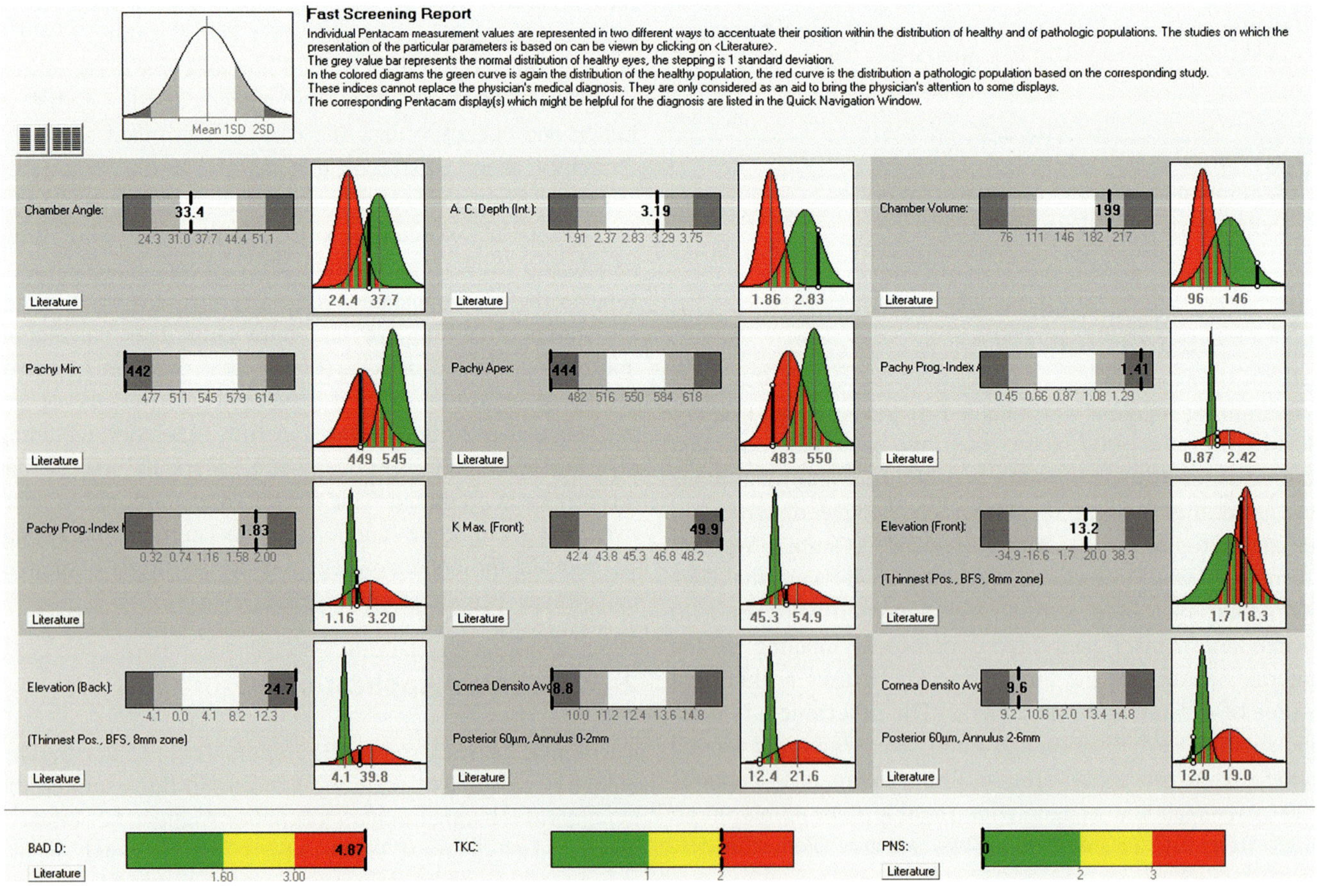

Fig. 1 Fast Screening Report providing a short overview of different Pentacam® parameters. Different grey scales showing whether the examined eye ranges within the normal distribution of healthy eyes or within one or two standard deviations. Colored diagrams showing a healthy population in green and a pathologic population in red. Results of a 24-year-old male patient with keratoconus (topographic keratoconus classification TKC stage 2). BAD-D, Belin/Ambrósio Deviation Index 4.87

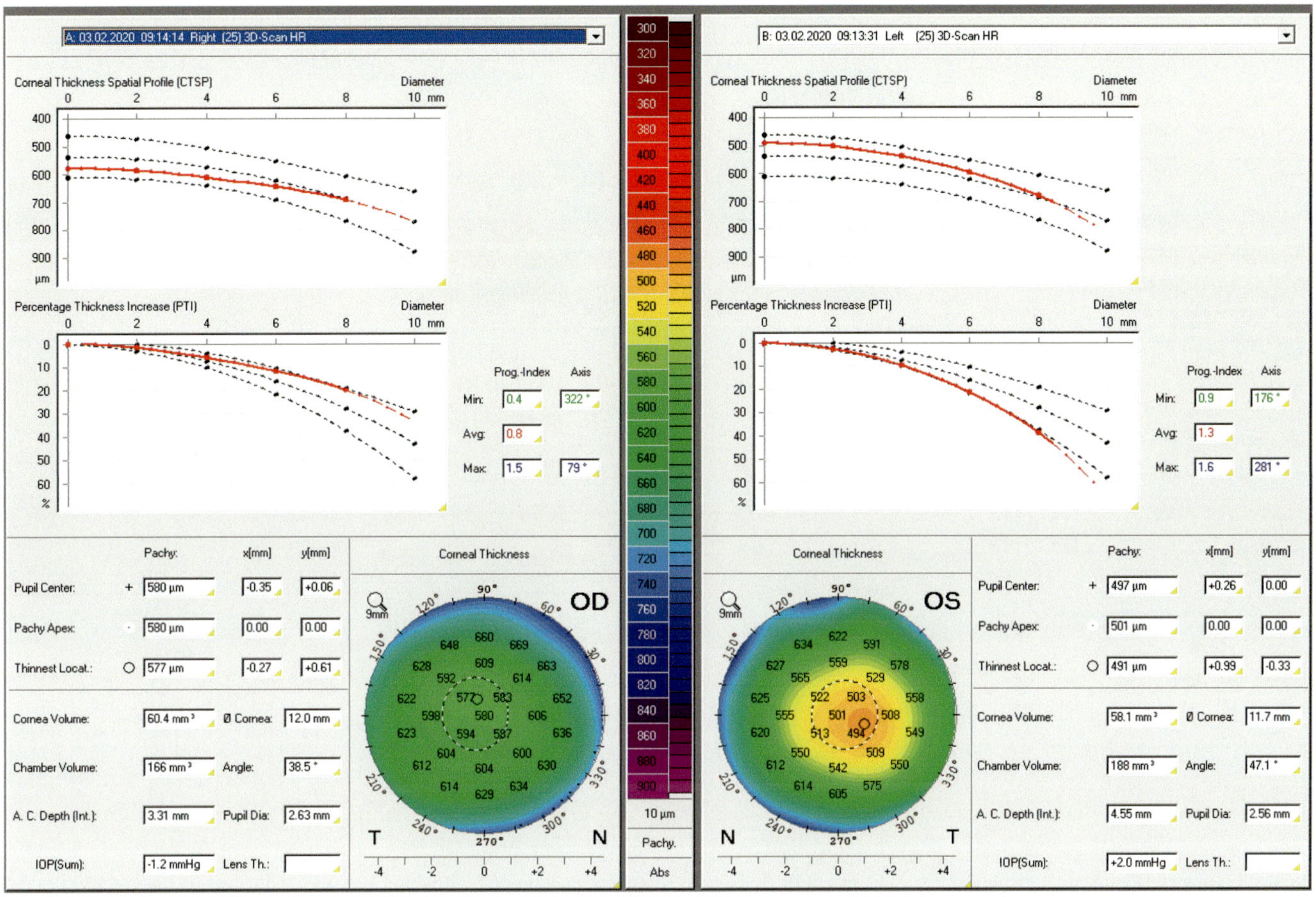

Fig. 2 Pachymetric Pentacam® display of a right (OD) and left (OS) eye. Cold-colored thicker pachymetry values in OD as opposed to warm-colored thinner pachymetry values in OS. Thinnest pachymetry OD: 577 µm and OS: 491 µm

Fig. 3 Specular microscopy of the corneal endothelium of the eyes shown in Fig. 2 revealing dysmorphic endothelium in the right and normal endothelium in the left eye

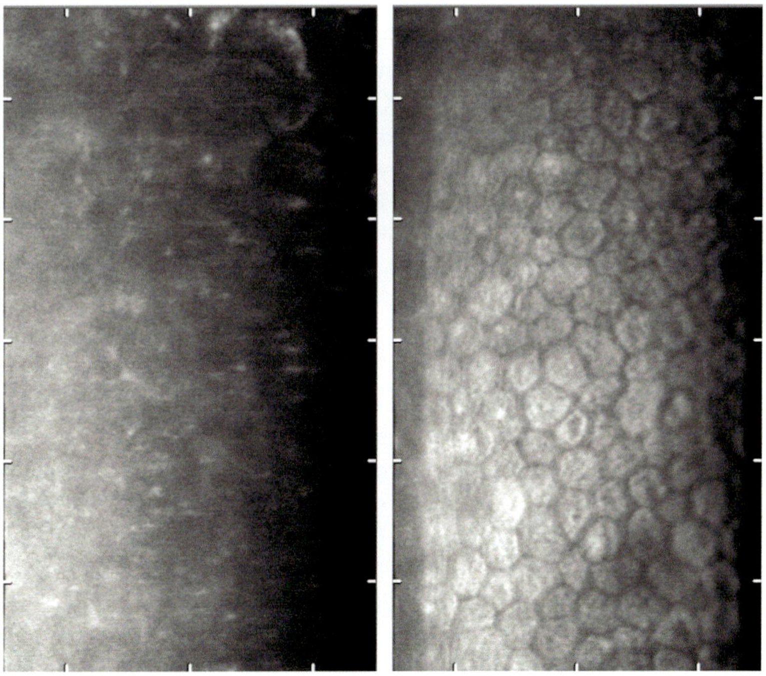

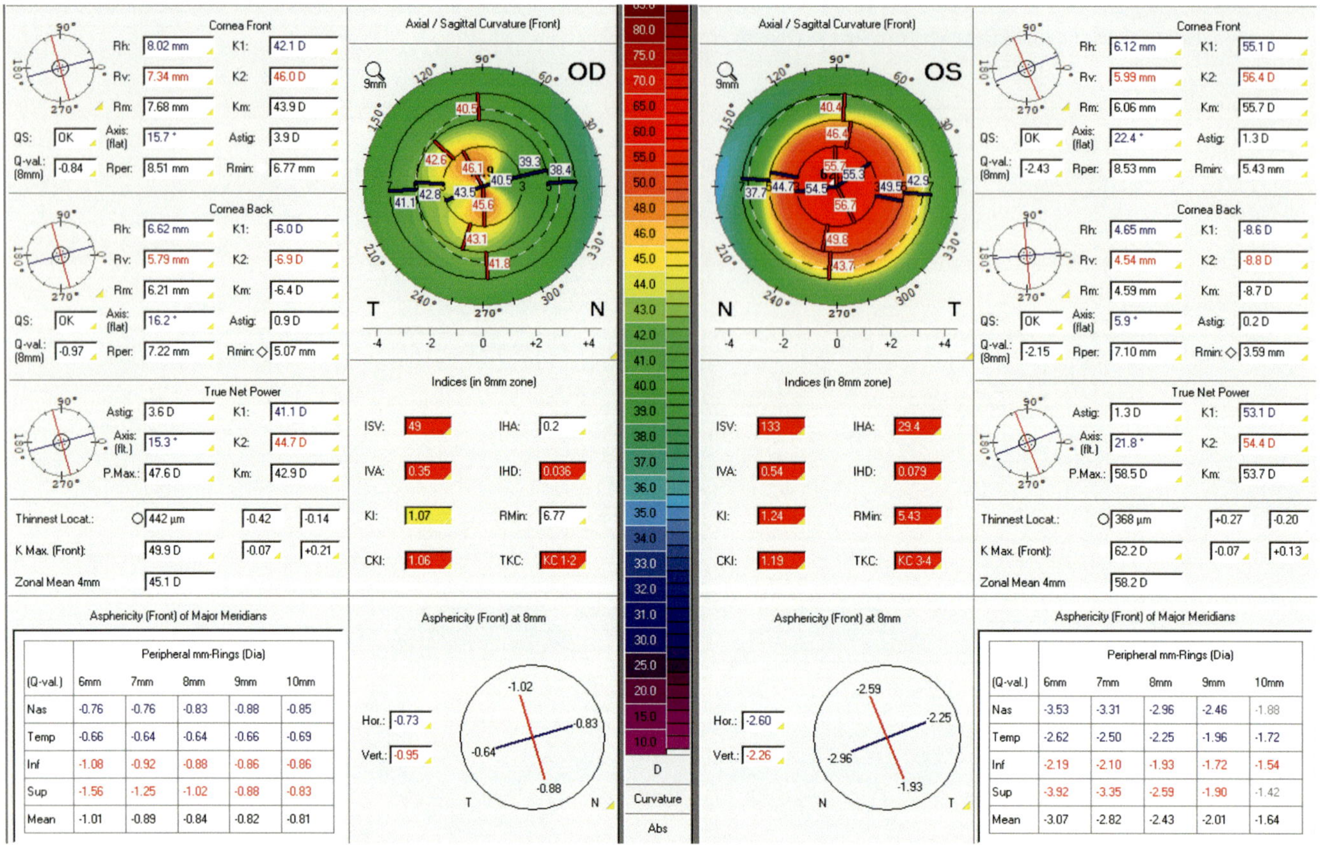

Fig. 4 Topometric Pentacam® display (OD: right eye, OS: left eye). Keratectasia indices highlighted red and indicating keratoconus in stages TKC1-2 (OD) and TKC3-4 (OS). Right eye with paracentral steepening (yellow), left eye with central keratoconus (higher degree of steepening, red)

indices of air, cornea and aqueous and considering anterior and posterior radii of curvature. The different indices (ISV: Index of Surface Variance, IHA: Index of Height Asymmetry, IVA: Index of Vertical Asymmetry, IHD: Index of Height Decentration, KI: Keratoconus Index, Rmin: Minimum Sagittal Curvature, CKI: Central Keratoconus Index, TKC: Topographic Keratoconus Classification) have a white background in normal eyes and are highlighted yellow in borderline or red in clearly ectatic corneas. The anterior axial / sagittal curvature of the cornea is displayed in color with warm colors indicating areas of corneal steepening. The two meridians are also color-coded (steep: red, flat: blue).

Besides the Topographic Keratoconus Classification (TKC) that serves for keratectasia severity staging, the Pentacam® also includes the recently introduced tomographic Belin ABCD Keratoconus Staging System [3, 4]. This staging system is based on the individual staging of anterior ("A") and posterior ("B") radius of curvature, thinnest corneal thickness ("C") and best-corrected distance visual acuity with spectacles ("D"). In contrast to punctually measured values like maximal anterior keratometry (Kmax), both "A" and "B" are measured over a 3.0 mm optical zone centered on the thinnest pachymetry ("C"). Each parameter is individually staged (0 to 4) so that the result is a combination of letters and numbers for each eye. The staging is performed automatically by the Pentacam® software in the topometric keratoconus staging Pentacam® display (Fig. 5). The example shows the same eyes as shown in Fig. 4, with "A", "B" and "C" calculated by the Pentacam®. "D" has to be added manually by the physician after visual acuity testing.

Early keratectasia may be diagnosed based on the color-coded inferior area of steepening (Fig. 6). Some of the keratectasia indices show normal values (white background), borderline results are highlighted in yellow and clearly abnormal values in red (Fig. 6).

Very early cases and subtle changes indicative of keratectasia can be revealed by the Belin/Ambrósio Enhanced Ectasia Screening Pentacam® display (Fig. 7). It displays anterior and posterior elevation data of the cornea examination (Fig. 7, upper left). Then, it excludes the 3.0 or 3.5 mm zone (selection in the settings) around the thinnest corneal pachymetry. Consequently, the reference sphere of the Pentacam® approximates more the periphery of the cornea which enables an enhanced detection of ectatic regions (Fig. 7, center left). In a third step, the Pentacam® generates for each anterior and posterior elevation data the difference

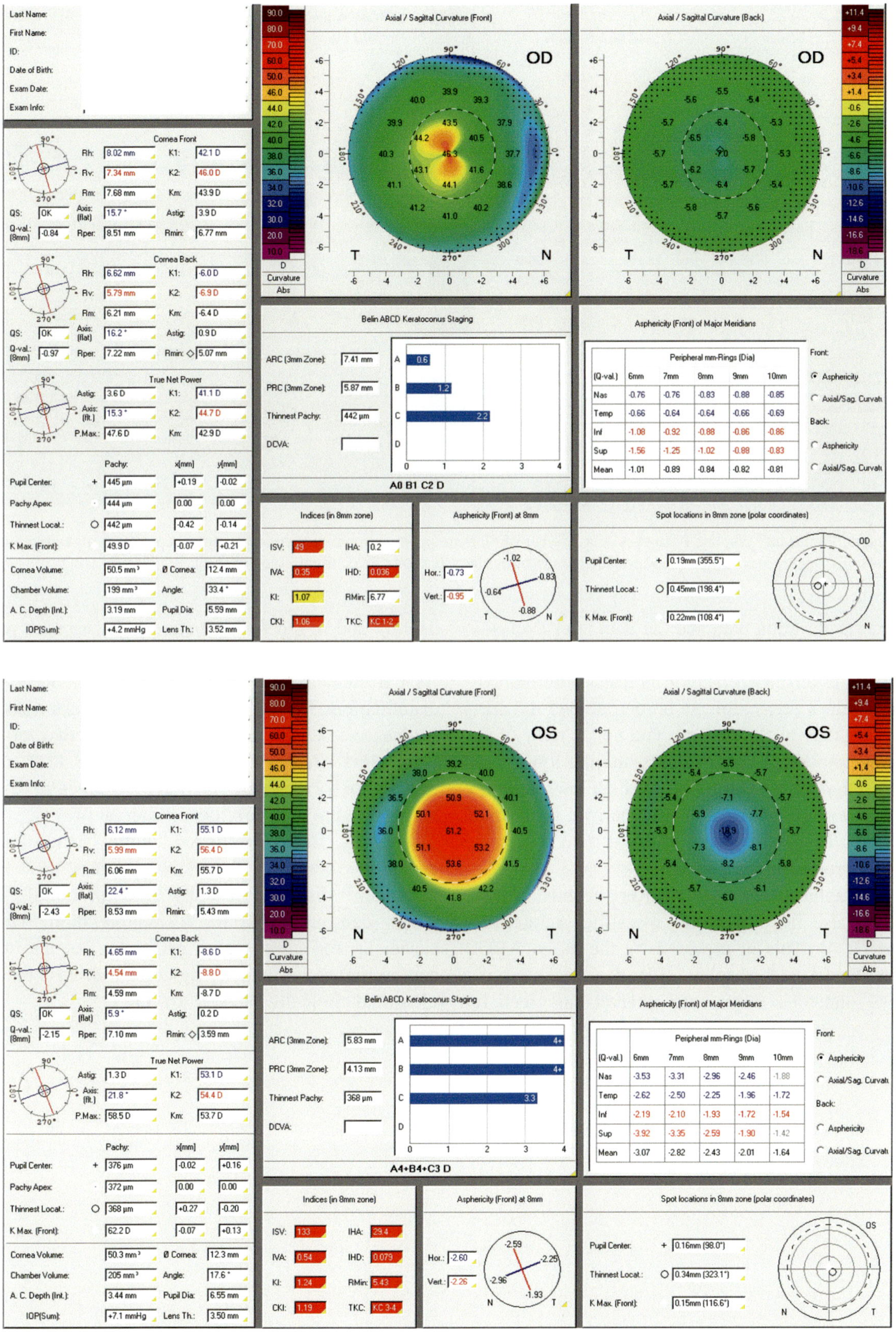

Fig. 5 Topometric keratoconus staging Pentacam® display. Belin ABCD Keratoconus Staging indicating stages 0 to 4 for "A"—anterior radius of curvature, "B"—posterior radius of curvature (both measured over a 3.0 mm zone) centered at "C"—thinnest corneal thickness. OD: A0B1C2, OS: A4B4C3 – same eyes as in Fig. 4

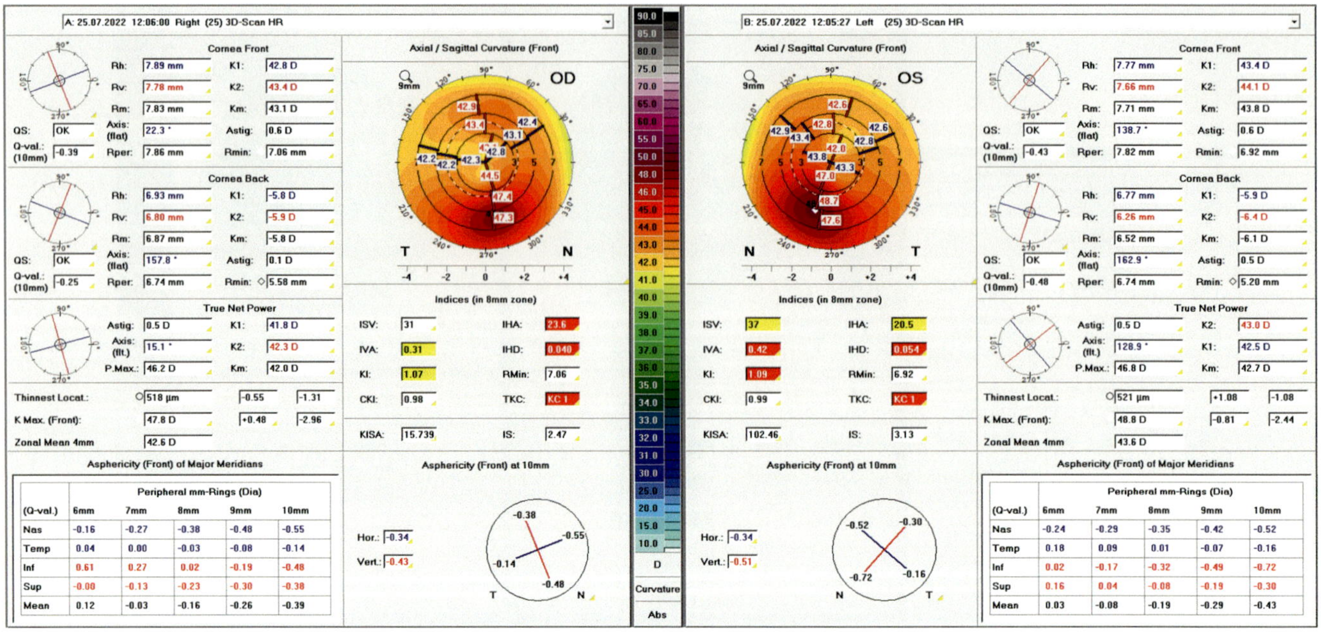

Fig. 6 Topometric Pentacam® display. Both eyes of a 35-year-old female patient showing inferior corneal steepening with keratoconus topography and keratoconus stage 1 according to topographic keratoconus classification (TKC, highlighted in red)

between general elevation data and the data after exclusion of the 3.0 or 3.5 mm zone which results in the difference map (Fig. 7, lower left): Green color indicates a normal cornea, whereas yellow areas indicate borderline and red areas clearly ectatic areas of the cornea. The upper right of the display shows tomographic parameters and the lower right shows the pachymetric progression data. Below, there are different deviation indices that are summarized in the final Belin/Ambrósio Deviation Index, which is also a measure for keratectasia severity [5].

The tomographic Belin ABCD Keratoconus Staging System may also be used for assessing keratectasia progression [3, 4]. This is provided by the Belin ABCD Progression Pentacam® display (Fig. 8), which shows defined 80% and 95% confidence intervals in green for healthy and in red for an ectatic population. A progression assessment is performed individually for each parameter "A"|"B"|"C" based on several color-coded follow-up examinations (Fig. 8) and it has been proposed to define progressive keratectasia based on (1) two of the three parameters "A"|"B"|"C" surpassing the 80% confidence interval or (2) one of the three parameters "A"|"B"|"C" surpassing the 95% confidence interval [4].

Despite being equipped with such sophisticated detection systems for keratectasia, the topometric Pentacam® display is usually used for initial assessment, which can also lead to misinterpretation. This applies especially for cases with a pseudokeratoconic topography caused by another underlying corneal disease that has to be identified clinically (Figs. 9, 10, 11, 12).

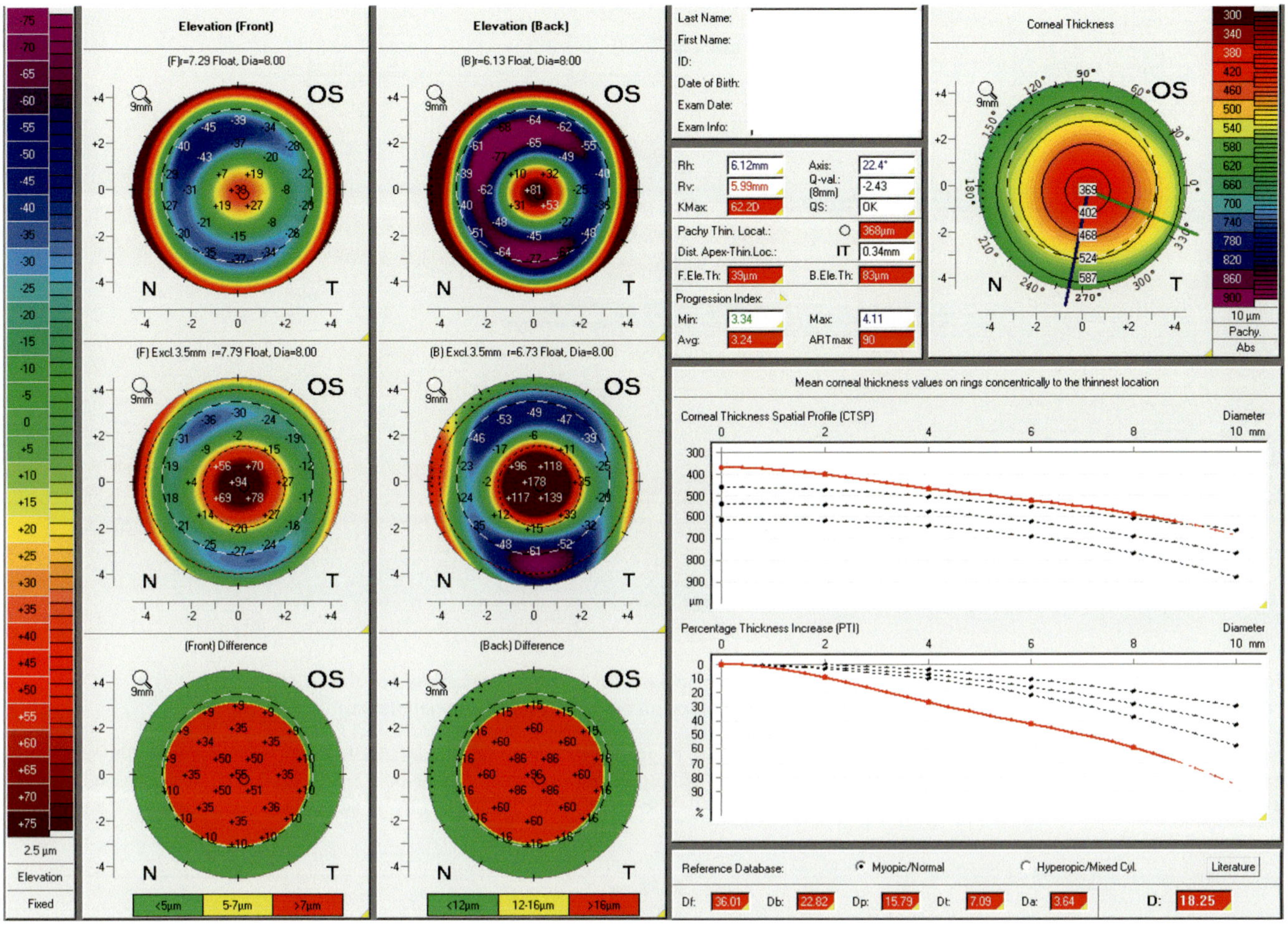

Fig. 7 Belin/Ambrósio Enhanced Ectasia Screening Pentacam® display. Left, front elevation data. Center, back elevation data. By excluding the 3.0/3.5 mm zone around thinnest pachymetry, the reference sphere approaches the periphery of the cornea and the elevation of the ectatic region is detected earlier. Yellow, suspect, ≥ 1.6 standard deviations from the mean. Red, abnormal, ≥ 2.6 standard deviations from the mean

Right inferior part: Pachymetric progression in absolute thickness values and percentages. In ectatic corneal diseases, (para-) central corneal thickness is reduced and increases faster towards the periphery than in healthy corneas. Therefore, the red curve is steeper in ectatic than in healthy corneas. Deviation values for front ("Df") and back elevation ("Db"), pachymetric progression ("Dp"), thinnest corneal thickness ("Dt") and maximal Ambrósio relational thickness (ARTmax, "Da") resulting in a combined Belin/Ambrósio Deviation Index "BAD-D"

With-the-rule astigmatism itself is also another differential diagnosis of keratoconus (Figs. 13–16).

Pellucid Marginal Degeneration (PMD) is another differential diagnosis of keratoconus and it has been overdiagnosed in the past based on anterior curvature pattern such as "kissing bird", "lobster claw" or "crab claw" [6] (Fig. 17). However, many of these corneas classified formerly as PMD turn out to be actually cases of inferior keratoconus (Fig. 18).

The major criterion for diagnosing true PMD is the inferior band of thinning located one to two millimeters away from the limbus with excessive flattening and a sharp transition above the band of thinning [6]. Because of the peripheral location, it can only be differentiated from inferior keratoconus by a full corneal thickness map that reveals the inferior band of thinning parallel to the corneal limbus [6] (Fig. 19).

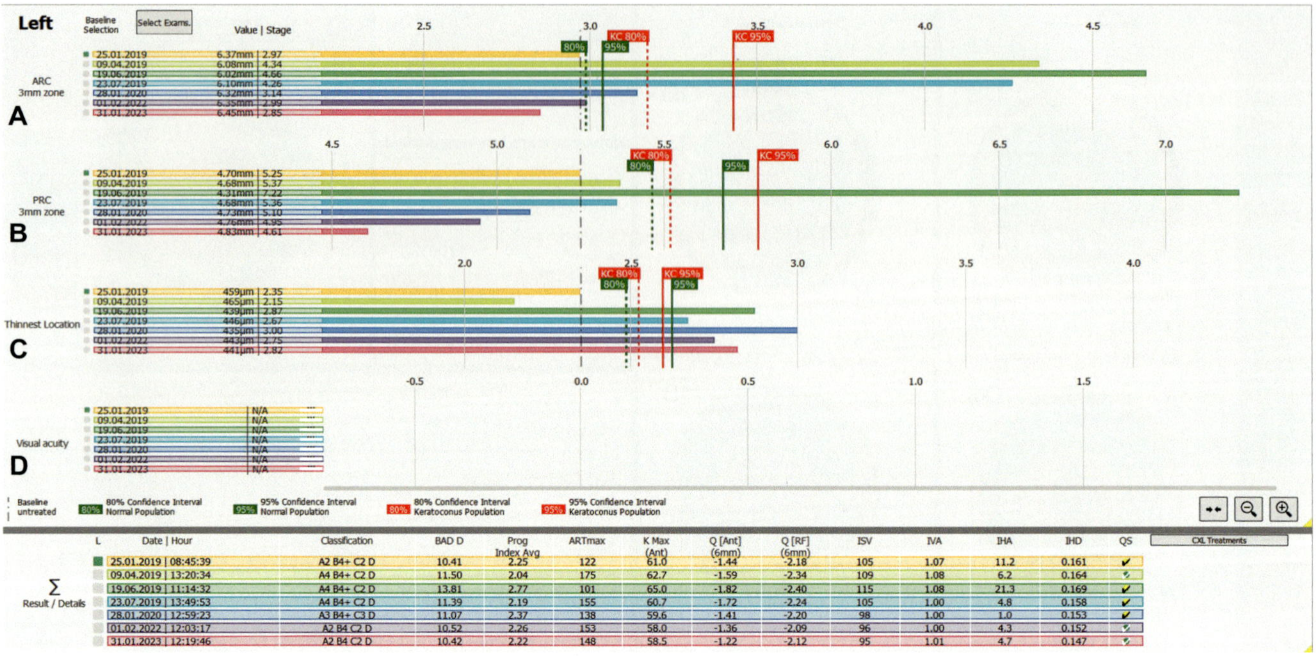

Fig. 8 Belin ABCD Progression Pentacam® Display. Progression analysis for corneal ectasia based on the (**ABCD**) staging system. Defined 80 and 95% confidence intervals in green for a healthy normal population and in red for an ectatic population

Different colors representing different follow-up examinations. Bright green, first follow-up (09.04.2019) with ("A") surpassing the 95% confidence interval for keratectasia. Accelerated corneal crosslinking with epithelial debridement was performed (06.05.2019) with pseudoprogression ("A, B") in the next follow-up examination (green, 19.06.2019). Subsequent stabilization of ("A") and ("B")

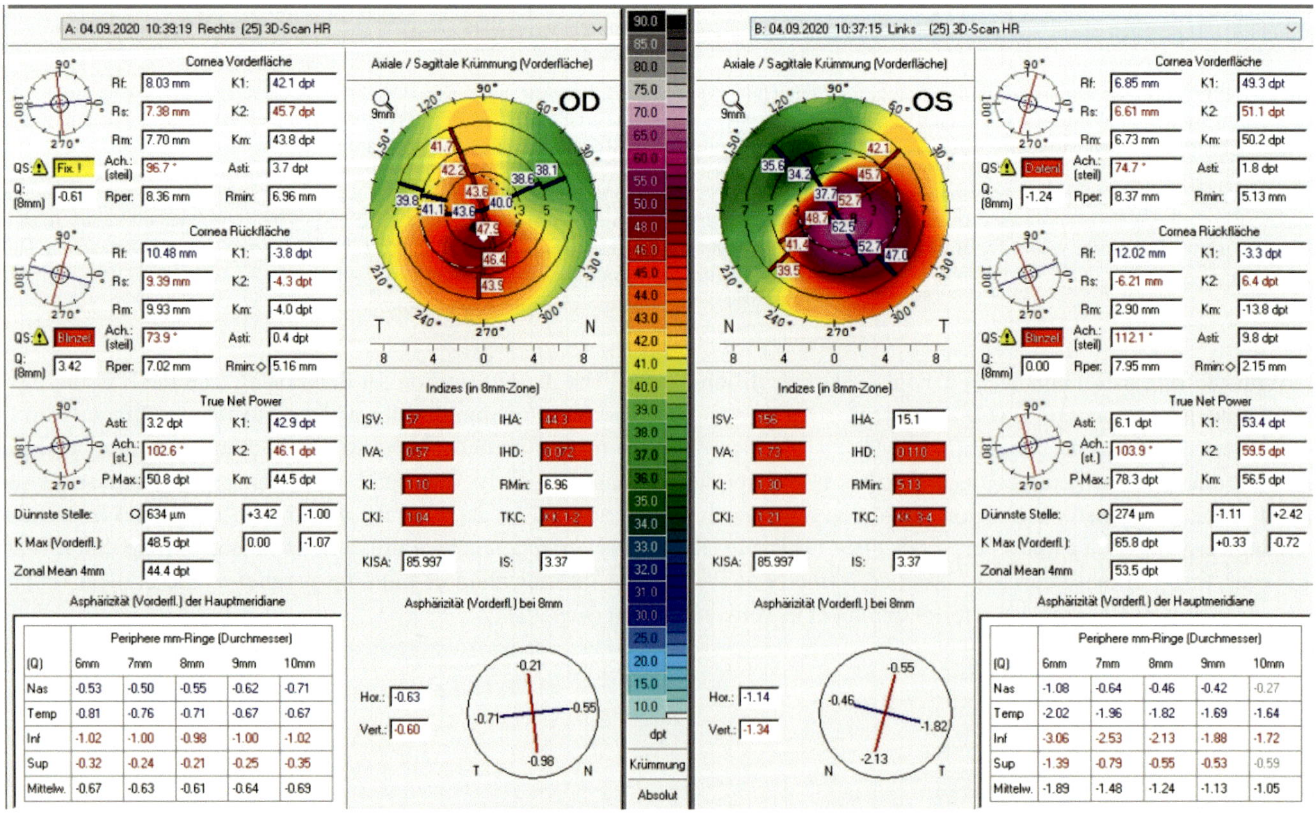

Fig. 9 Topometric Pentacam® display. Inferior corneal steepening in the right eye and temporally inferior steepening in the left eye. Classification as keratoconus in stages TKC1-2 (OD) and TKC3-4 (OS). Note thinnest corneal thickness 634 µm (OD), 274 µm (OS), and the limited quality scores. Slit lamp examination led to diagnosis of Fuchs endothelial corneal dystrophy with centrally swollen–thus steepened–cornea !

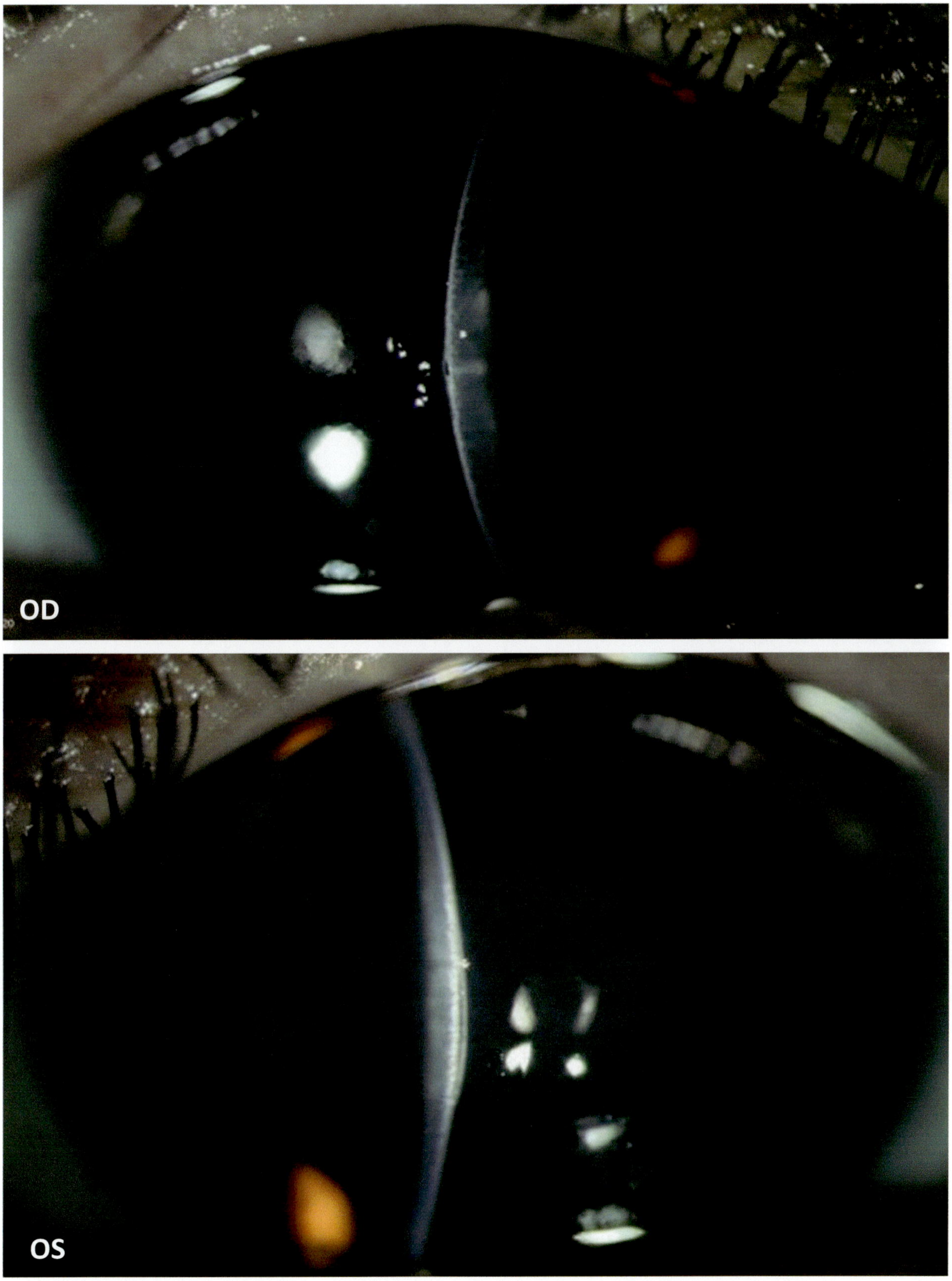

Fig. 10 Slit lamp imaging OD, OS of the eyes from Fig. 9 showing Fuchs endothelial corneal dystrophy with central endothelium-epithelium decompensation

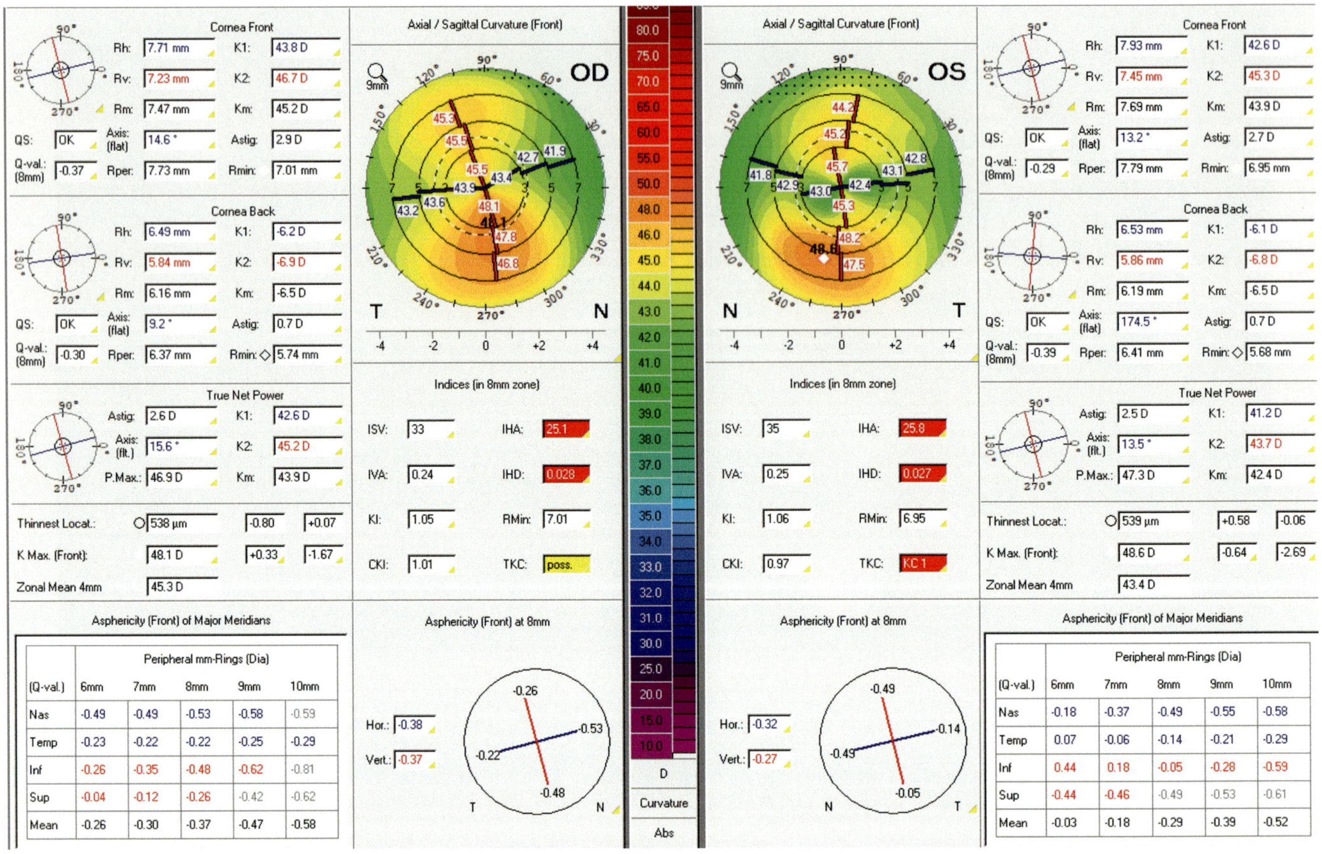

Fig. 11 Topometric Pentacam® display showing with-the-rule astigmatism in OD and OS with inferior steepening and suspect of beginning keratoconus—note the Topographic Keratoconus Classification assessment OD: possible and OS: keratoconus stage TKC1

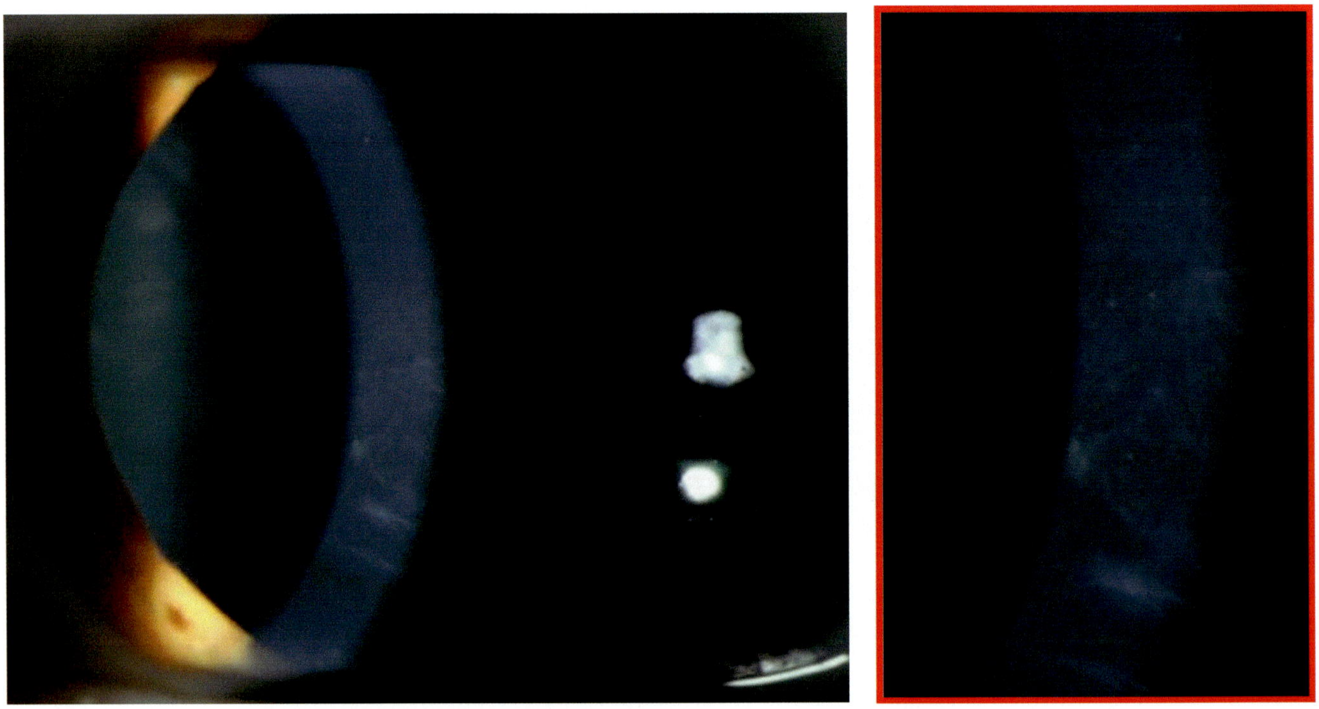

Fig. 12 Slit lamp image with magnification (right) of the left eye as shown in Fig. 11 revealing epithelial basement membrane dystrophy (map-dot-fingerprint dystrophy) causing inferior corneal steepening and resulting in a pseudokeratoconic topography

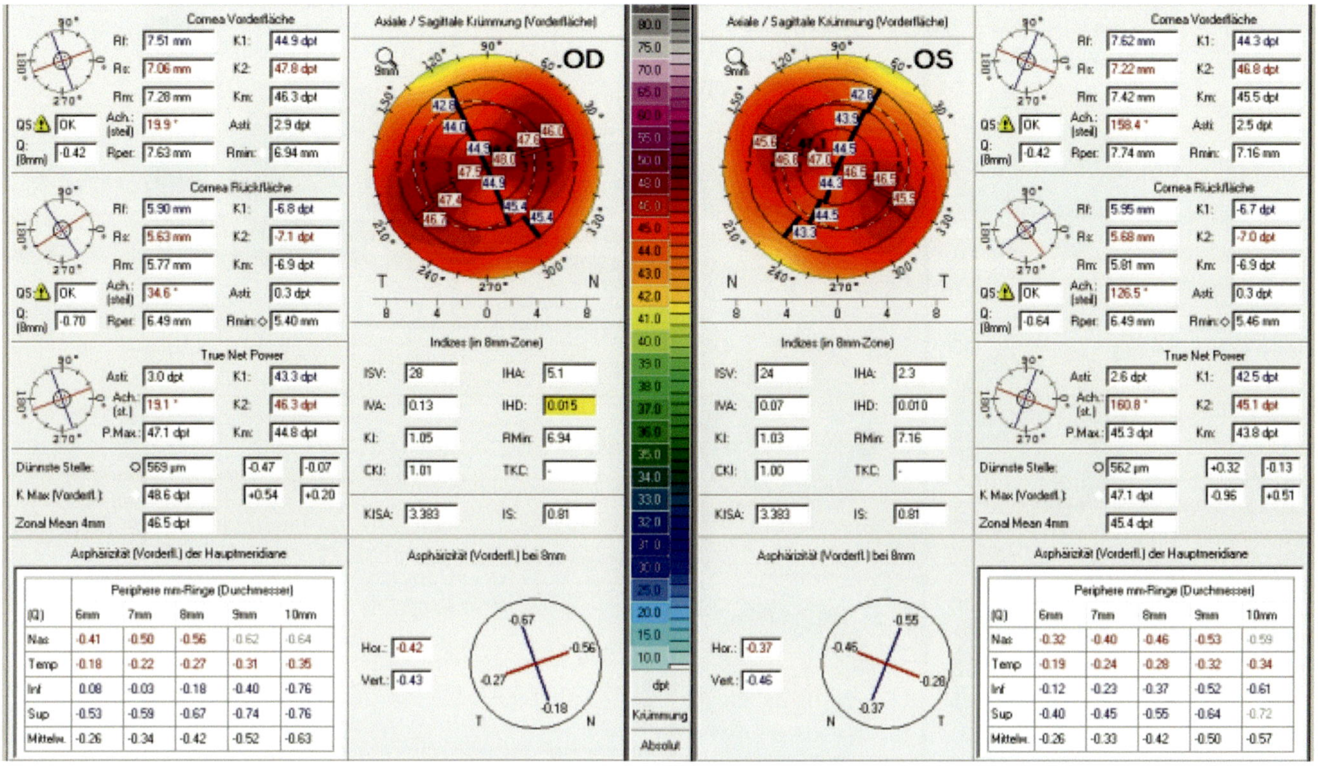

Fig. 13 Topometric Pentacam® exam of a 48-year-old female patient referred with suspect of keratoconus presenting oblique astigmatism (red: steep meridian, blue: flat meridian). With the exception of the Index of Height Decentration in the right eye, all the keratoconus indices show normal values

Besides keratoconus and Pellucid Marginal Degeneration, keratoglobus is another rare differential diagnosis of keratectasia, which is characterized by a globally thinned and steepened cornea (Fig. 20).

Keratectasia after Laser In Situ Keratomileusis (LASIK) is characterized by an ectatic configuration of the cornea that resembles to that of keratoconus (Fig. 21).

There exist some case reports about superior keratoconus [7–9] (Fig. 22), however this diagnosis has to be critically questioned, because early cases of epithelial basement membrane dystrophy or Salzmann nodular degeneration may present with a superior steepening of the cornea.

The topometric Pentacam® display may also be used clinically for the assessment of both pachymetry and astigmatism after penetrating keratoplasty (Fig. 23).

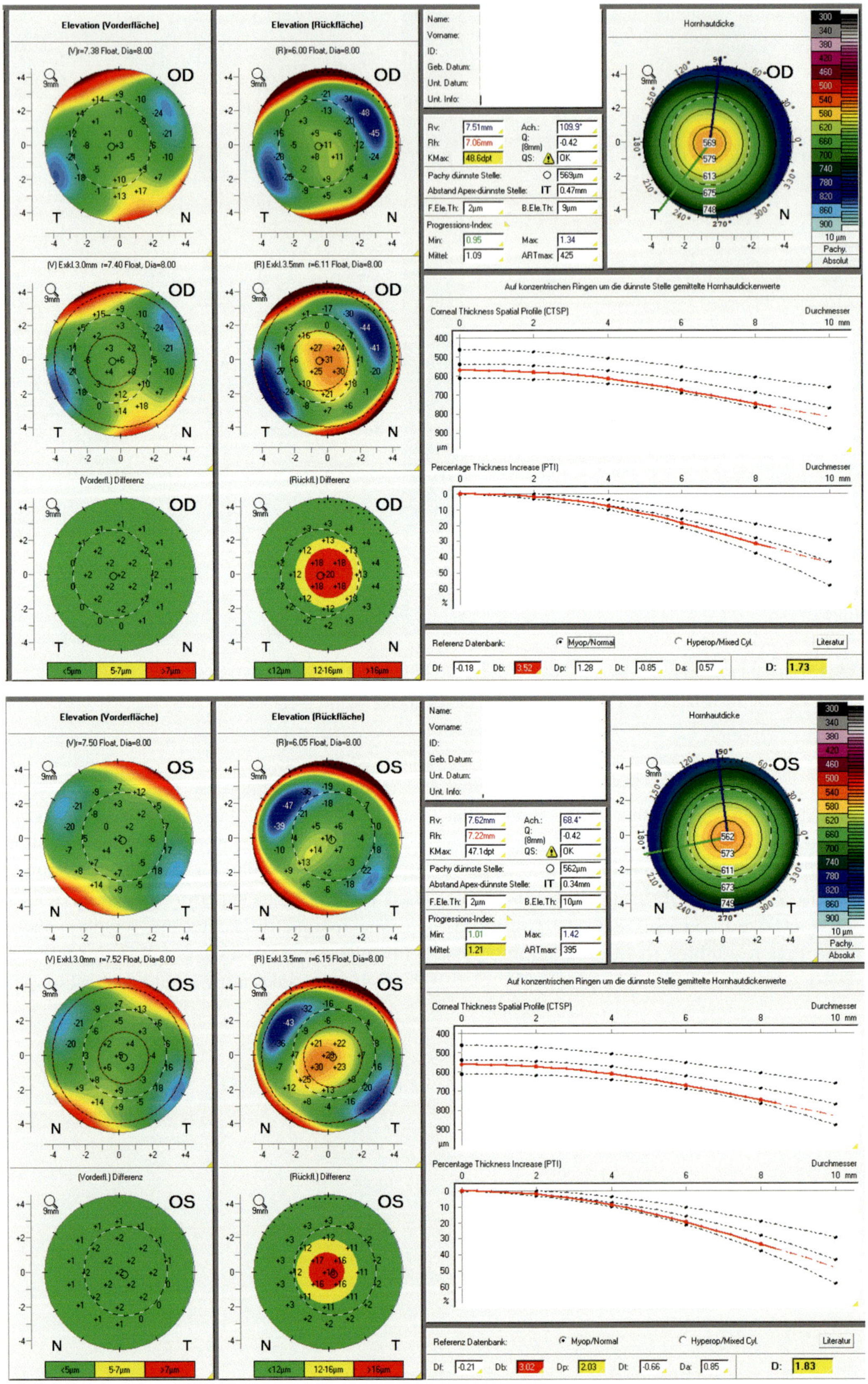

Fig. 14 Belin/Ambrósio Enhanced Ectasia Screening Pentacam® display of the same eyes as in Fig. 13 showing abnormal posterior elevation data and borderline Belin/Ambrósio Deviation Index—indicating that there may be more than just with-the-rule astigmatism in these eyes

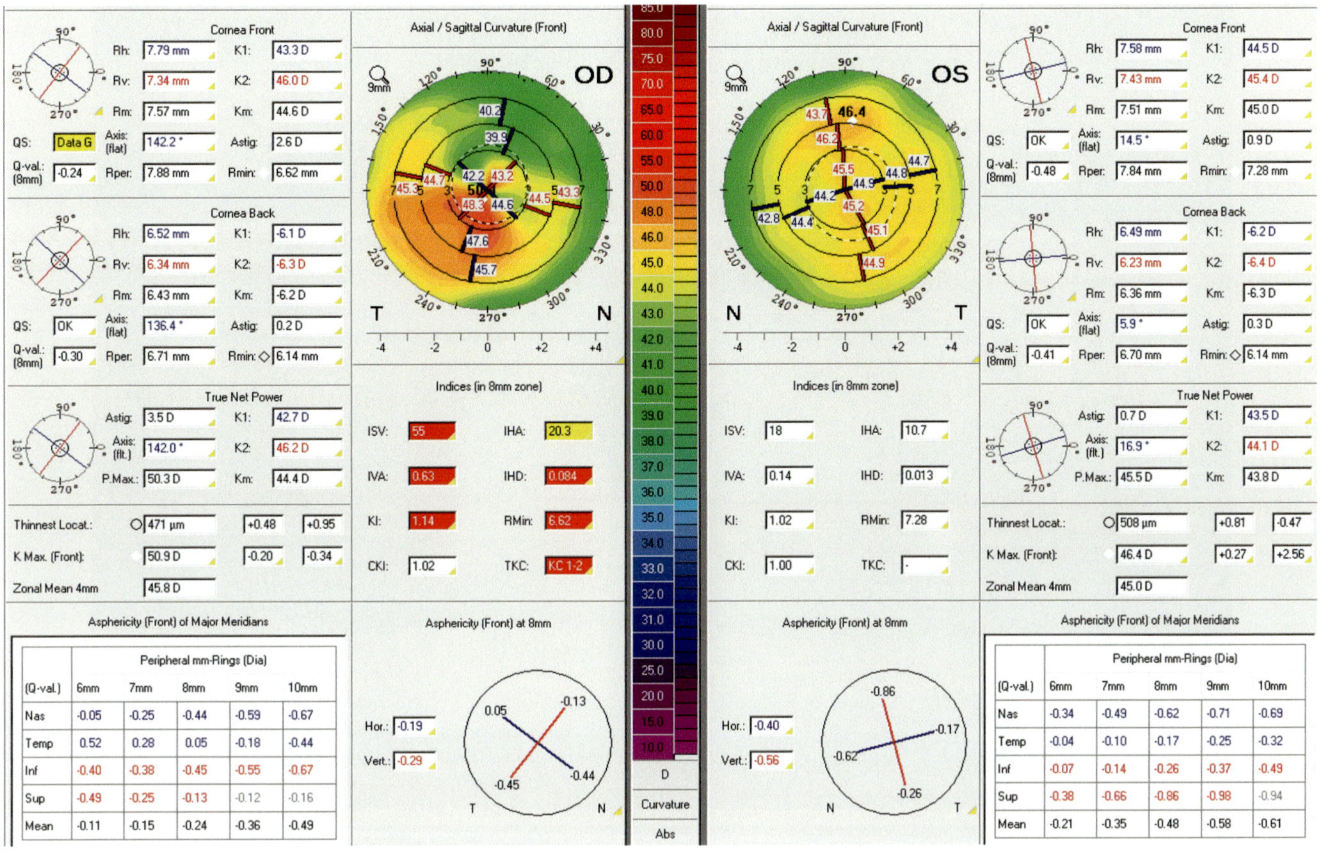

Fig. 15 Topometric Pentacam® display showing against-the-rule astigmatism in OD with inferior steepening and with-the-rule astigmatism OS with superior steepening (red: steep meridian, blue: flat meridian)

When considering the surgical treatment options of high postoperative astigmatism after penetrating keratoplasty such as incisions and compression sutures or the implantation of a toric intraocular lens, the Fourier Analysis Pentacam® display may be helpful, because it shows even more clearly the configuration and extent of the astigmatism (Fig. 24, bottom center).

The pachymetric Pentacam® display provides pachymetric information as shown in Fig. 2, but also information about anterior chamber volume, angle and depth. It has been reported that a normal anterior chamber depth in a healthy population is about 3.1 mm [10]. The example shows a reduced anterior chamber depth of 1.57 mm with a slightly thickened, almost normal corneal thickness profile

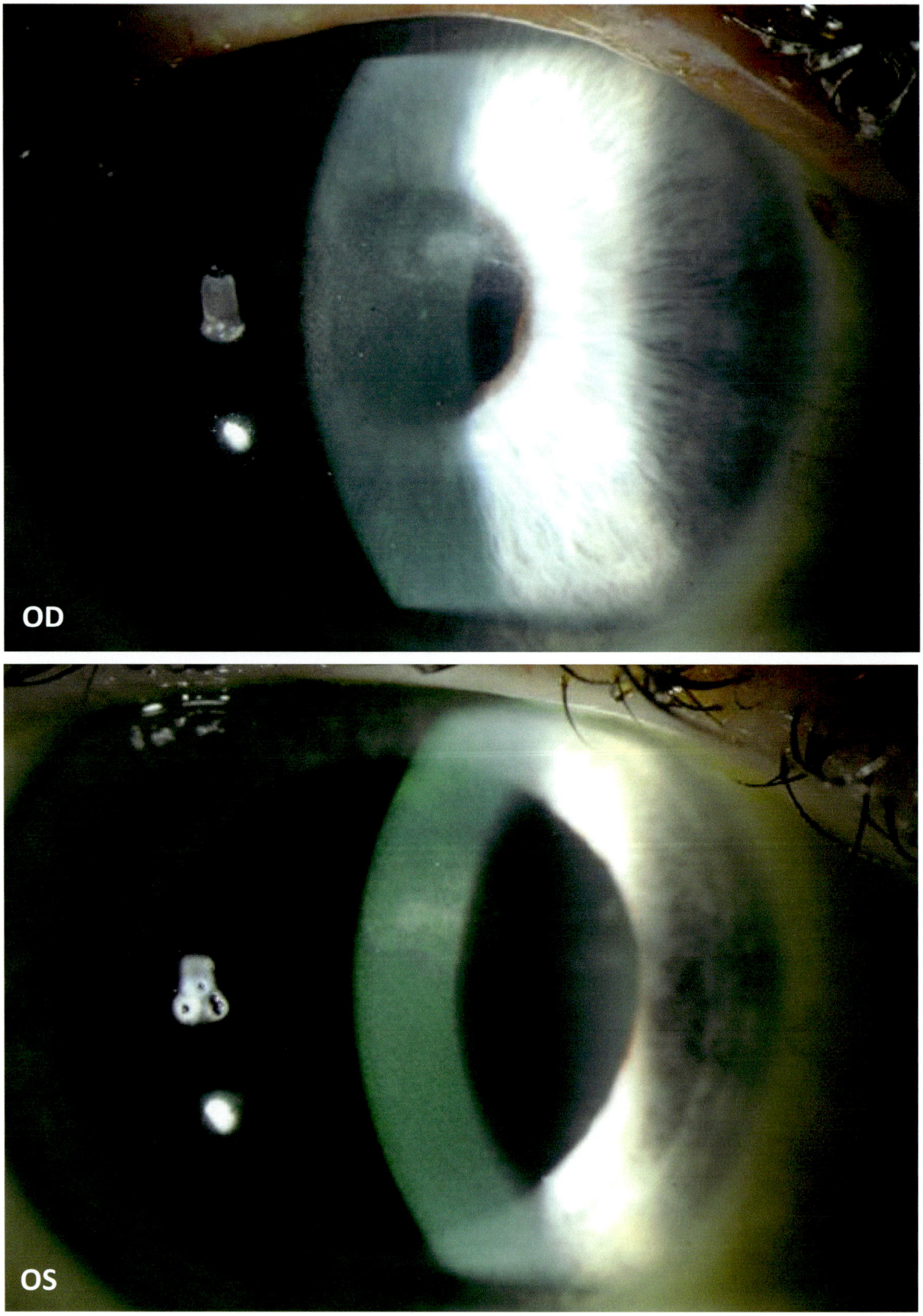

Fig. 16 Slit lamp images of the right (OD) and left (OS) eye as shown in Fig. 15 revealing subepithelial-stromal avascular corneal scars causing inferior and superior steepening

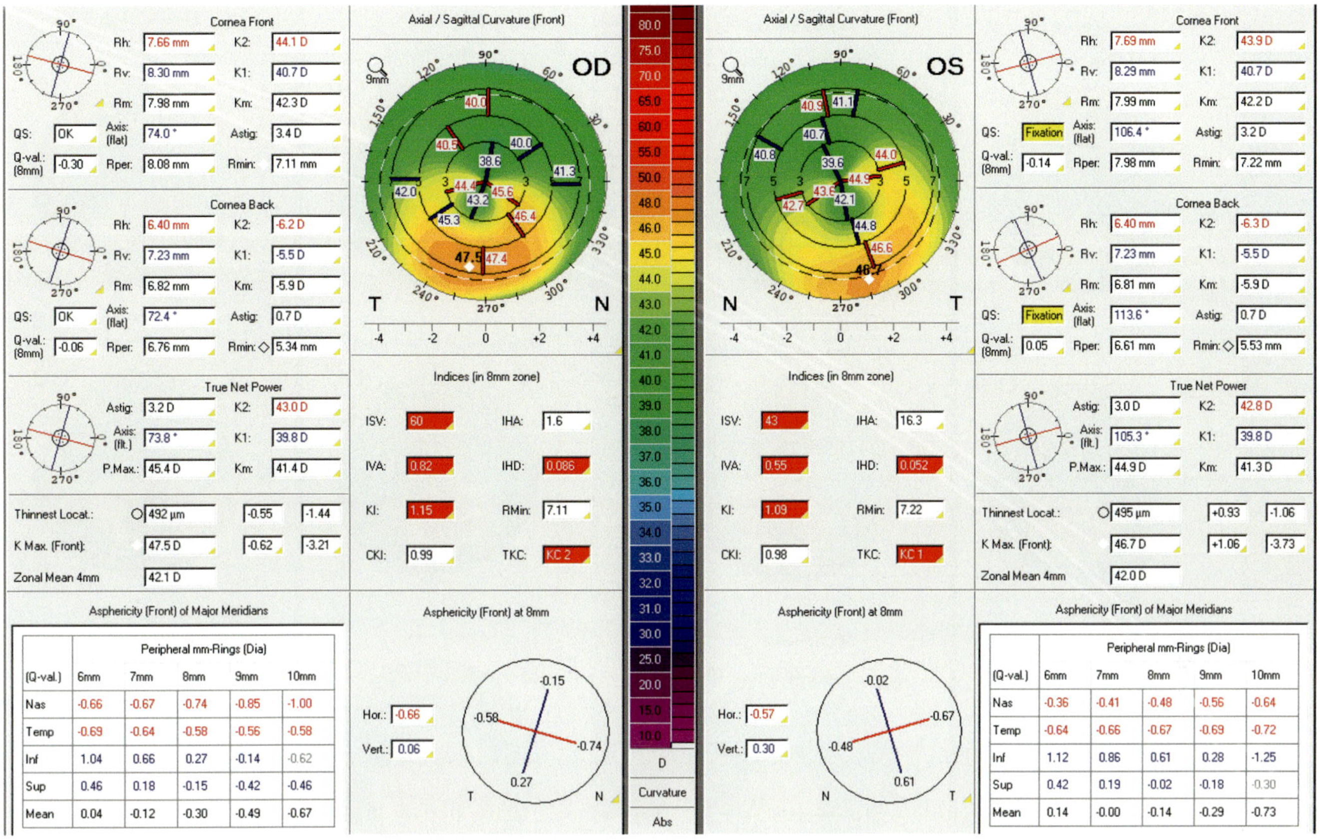

Fig. 17 Topometric Pentacam® display showing "kissing bird" or "crab claw" pattern in OD and OS formerly supposed to be indicative of pellucid marginal degeneration

in the right eye and 1.11 mm with an abnormally thickened cornea in the left eye (Fig. 25).

As it is a Scheimpflug imaging device, the Pentacam® visualizes the anterior segment and the different image sections may be viewed and examined in the Pentacam® Scheimpflug imaging display (Fig. 26).

Another Scheimpflug imaging based staging system implemented within the Pentacam® software is the Pentacam Nucleus Staging which is also shown in the Fast Screening Report (Fig. 1). It serves as a lens opacity staging, aiming to quantitatively assess a cataract stage (Fig. 27).

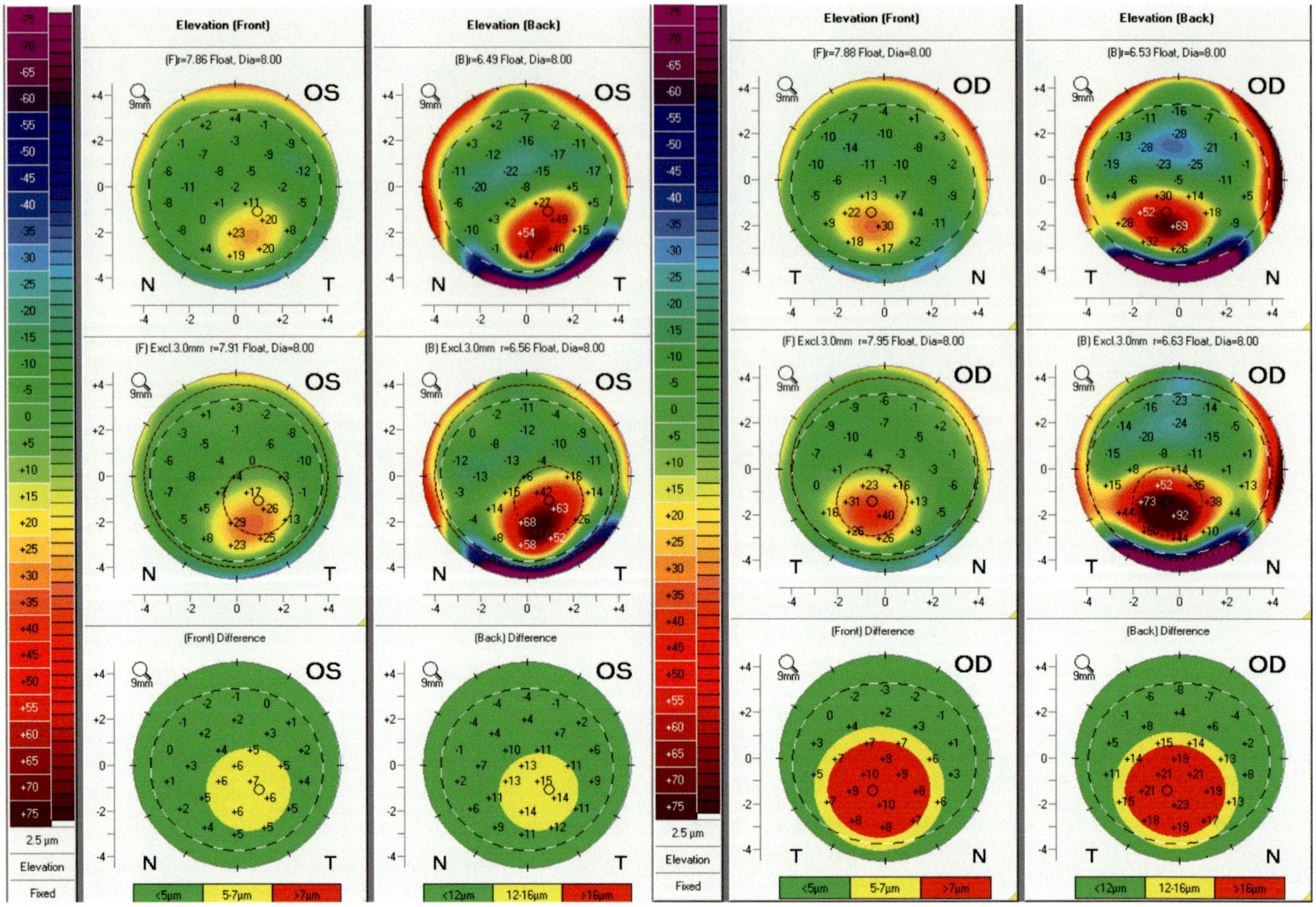

Fig. 18 Belin/Ambrósio Enhanced Ectasia Screening Pentacam® display of the same eyes as shown in Fig. 17 showing an inferior elevation island indicative of inferior keratoconus instead of pellucid marginal degeneration (which should show a peripheral thinning band parallel to the limbus)

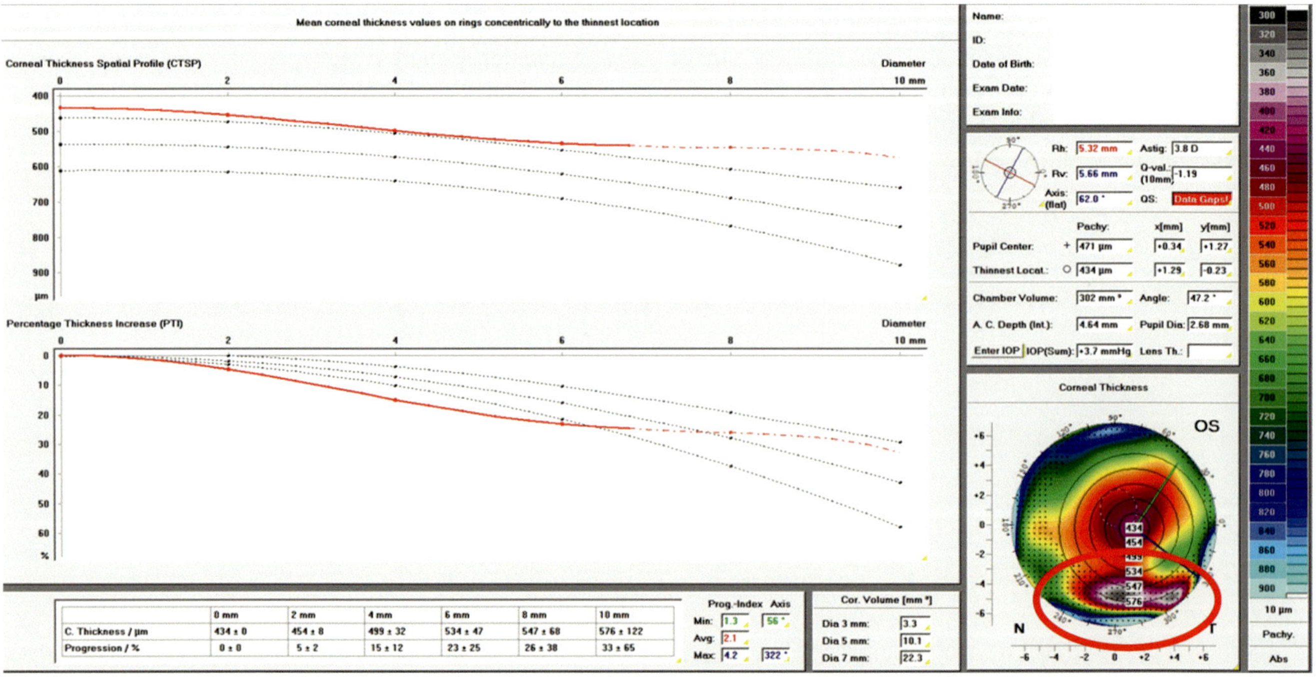

Fig. 19 Full-thickness pachymetric Pentacam® display revealing inferior thinning band parallel to the limbus (lower right, red circle) typical for pellucid marginal degeneration

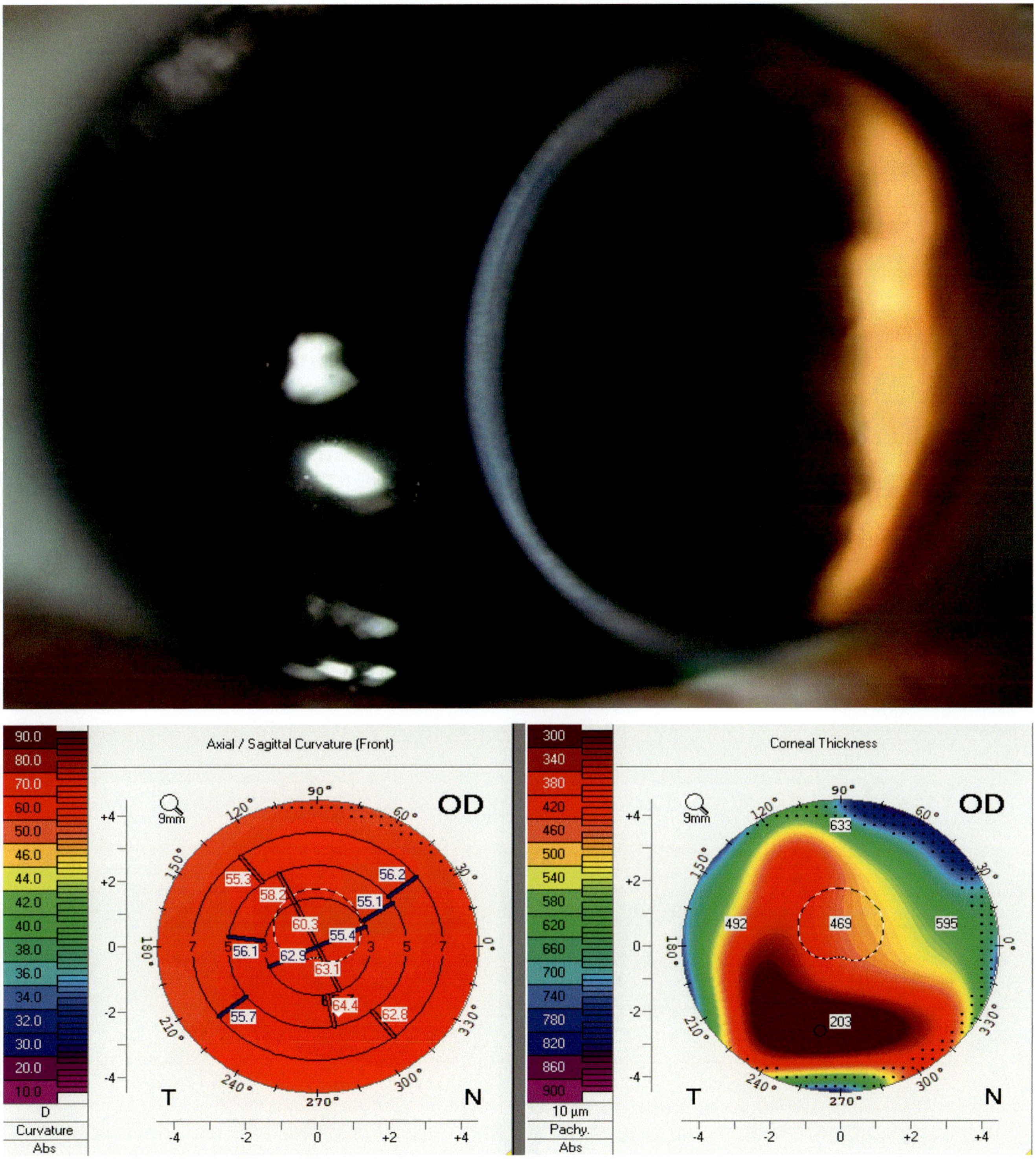

Fig. 20 Front axial/sagittal curvature and pachymetric Pentacam® display revealing globally thinned and steepened cornea indicative of keratoglobus

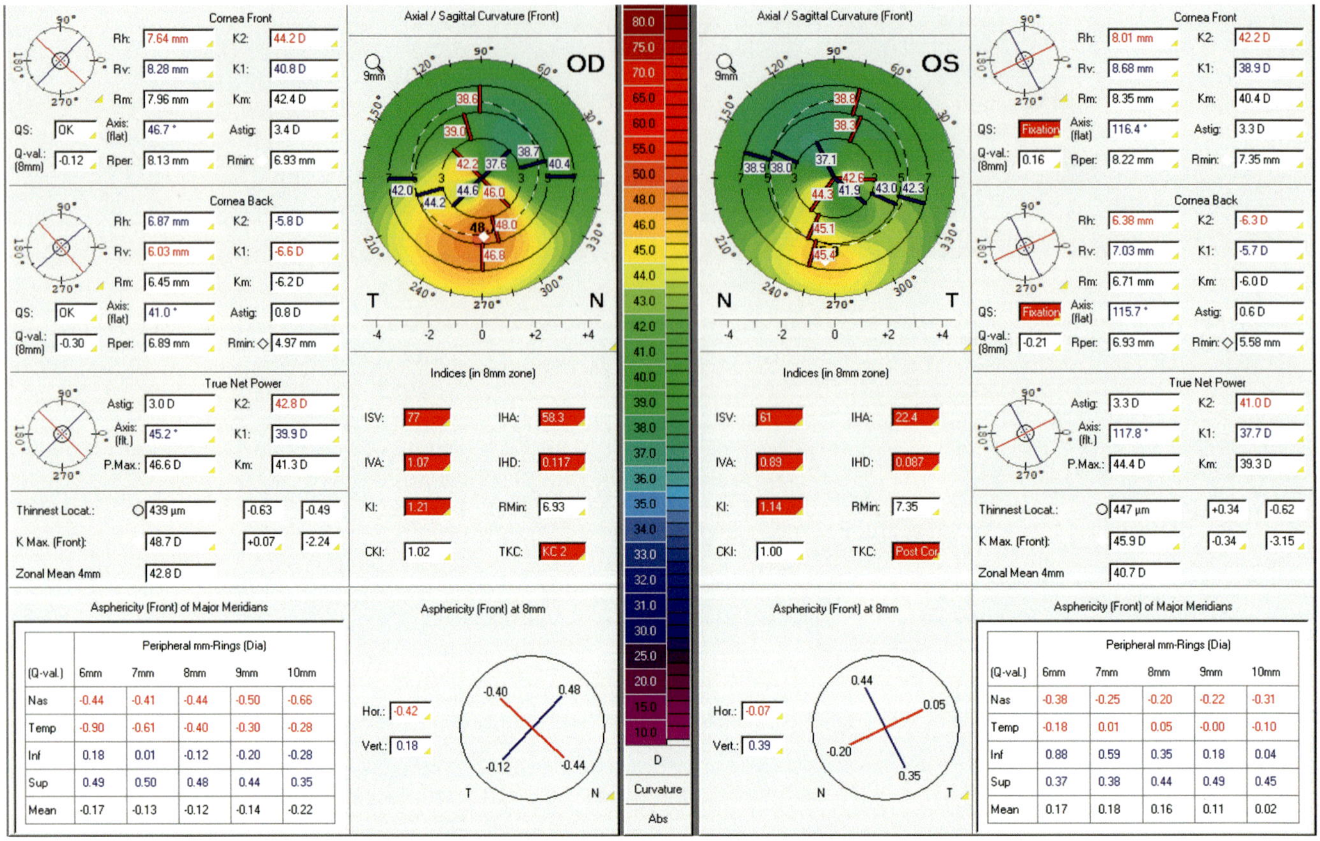

Fig. 21 Topometric Pentacam® display showing inferior steepening more in OD than OS in a case of keratectasia after Laser In Situ Keratomileusis (LASIK)

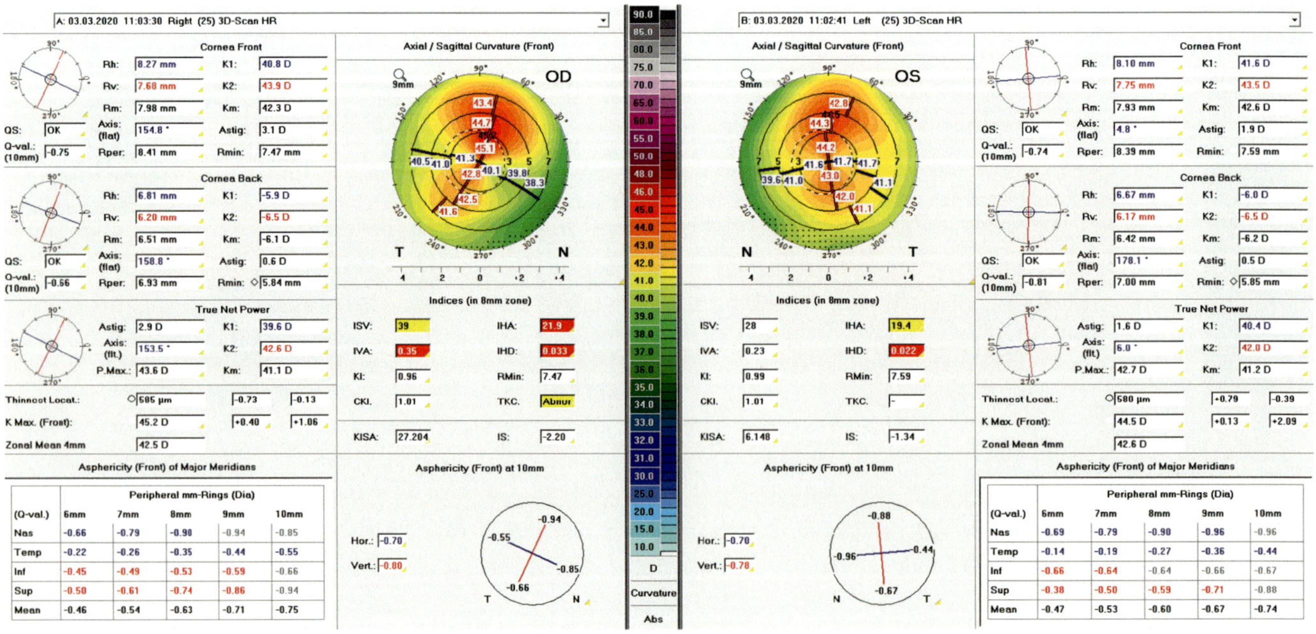

Fig. 22 Topometric Pentacam® display showing a case of superior corneal steepening (orange-colored superior elevation) without clinically visible abnormalities possibly representing a case of "superior keratoconus"

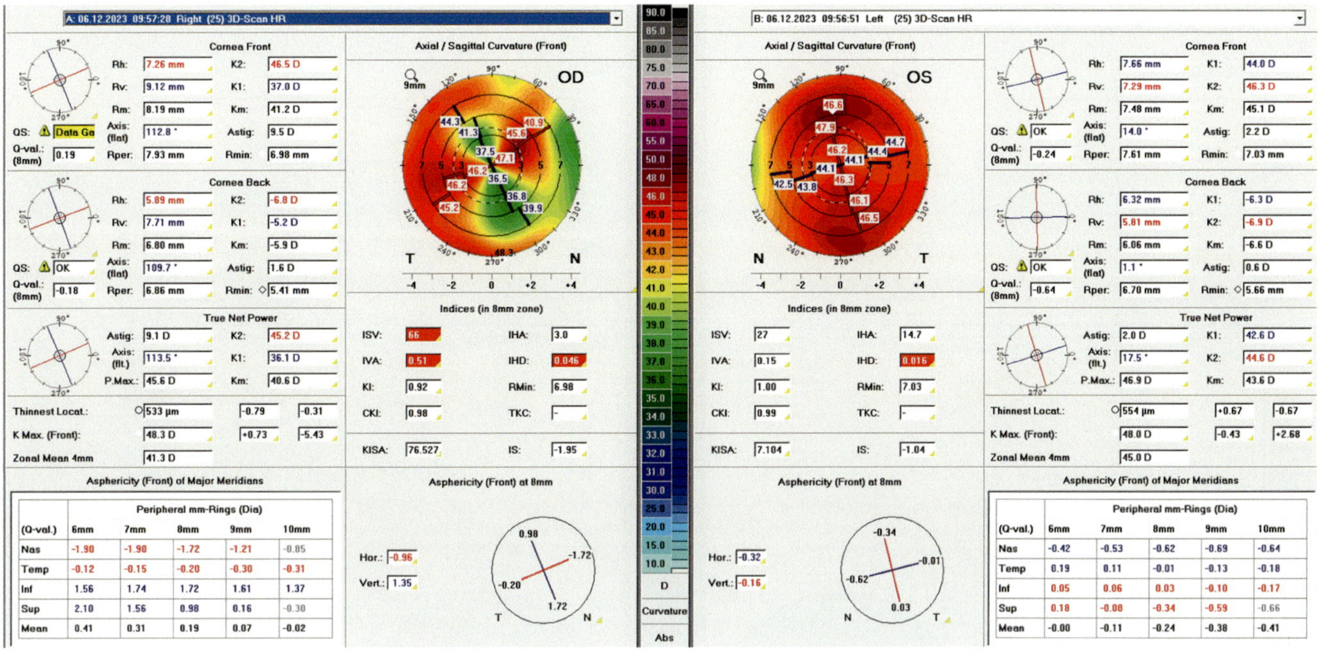

Fig. 23 Topometric Pentacam® display of a right (OD) and left (OS) eye after penetrating keratoplasty because of underlying keratoconus. With-the-rule astigmatism in both eyes with OD: 9.5 diopters, OS: 2.2 diopters. Thinnest corneal pachymetry OD: 533 µm, OS: 554 µm

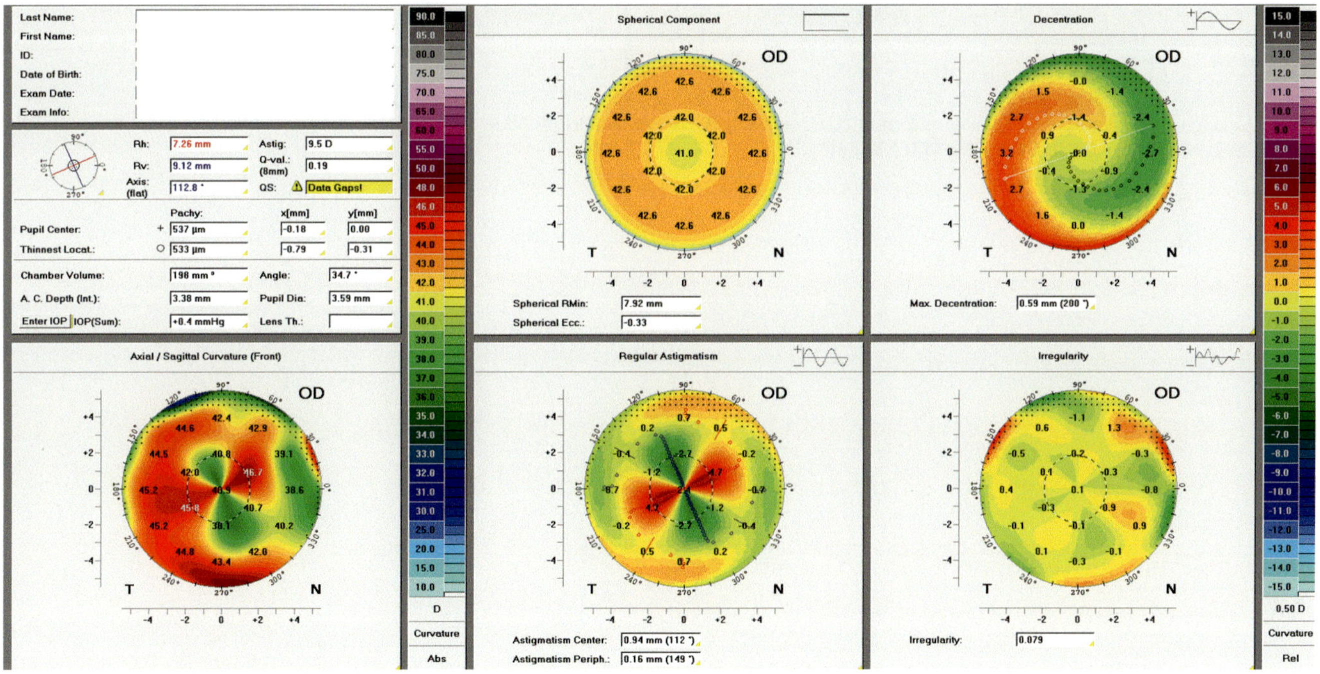

Fig. 24 Fourier analysis Pentacam® display of the right eye (OD) shown in Fig. 23 (lower left). Regular astigmatism (bottom center) on the graft that can be treated with incisions and compression sutures or toric intraocular lens implantation

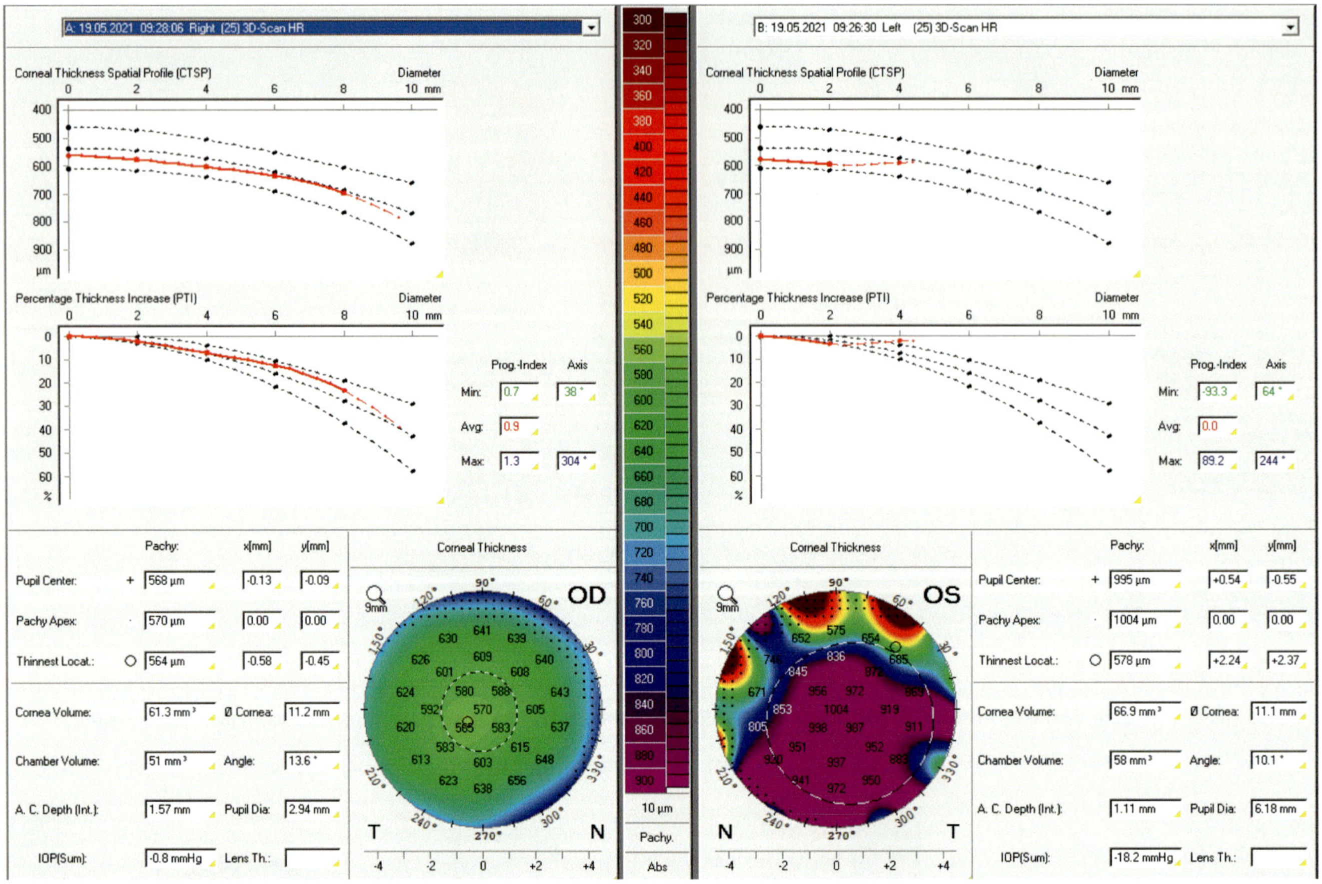

Fig. 25 Pachymetric Pentacam® display of a right (OD) and left (OS) eye. Anterior chamber depth OD: 1.57 mm and OS: 1.11 mm with thinnest corneal pachymetry OD: 564 µm and OS: 578 µm

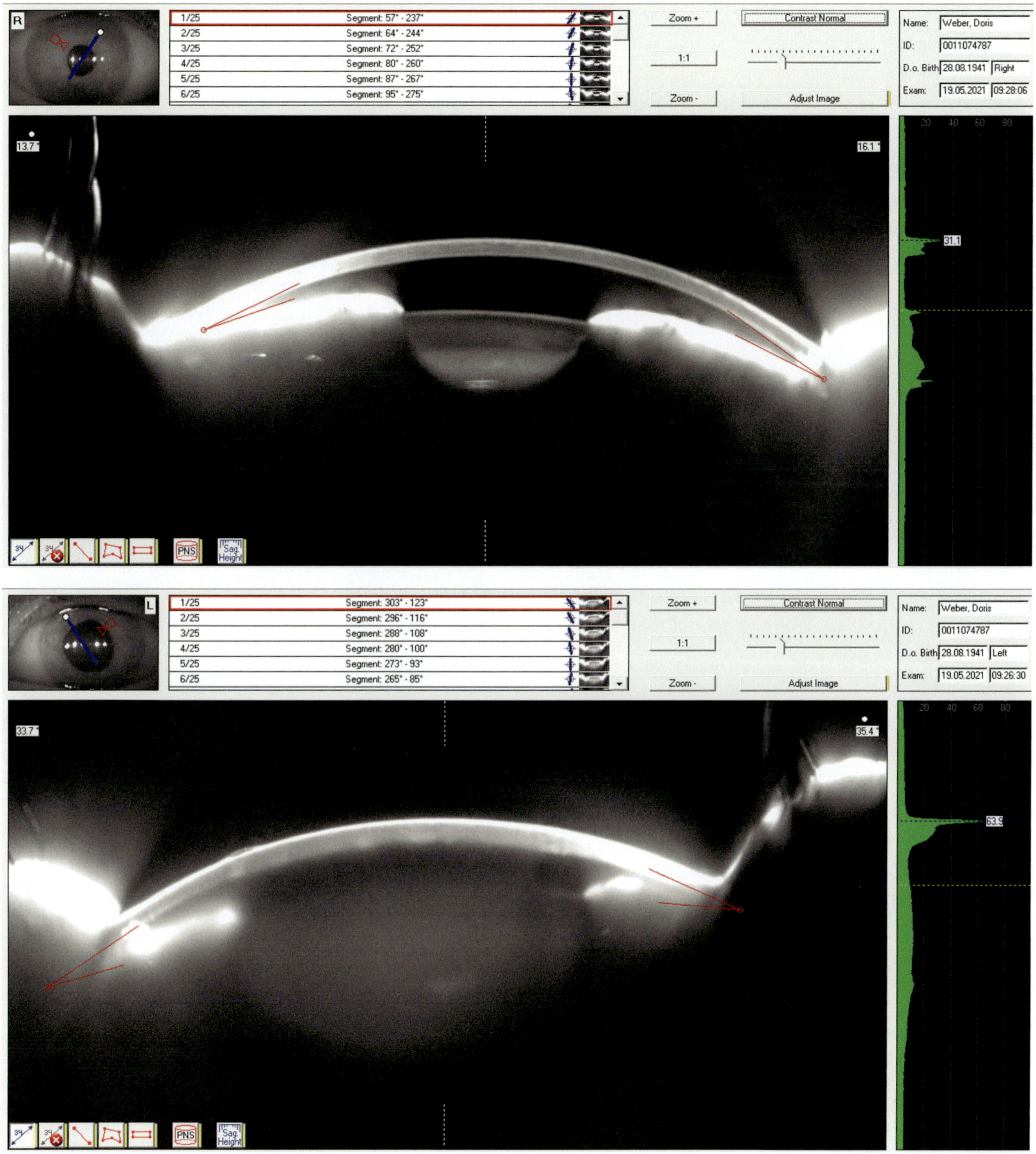

Fig. 26 Pentacam® Scheimpflug imaging display of the eyes shown in Fig. 25. Right eye with shallow anterior chamber and clear cornea. Left eye with shallower anterior chamber, iridocorneal contact and corneal decompensation in a case of acute raise of intraocular pressure because of pupillary block

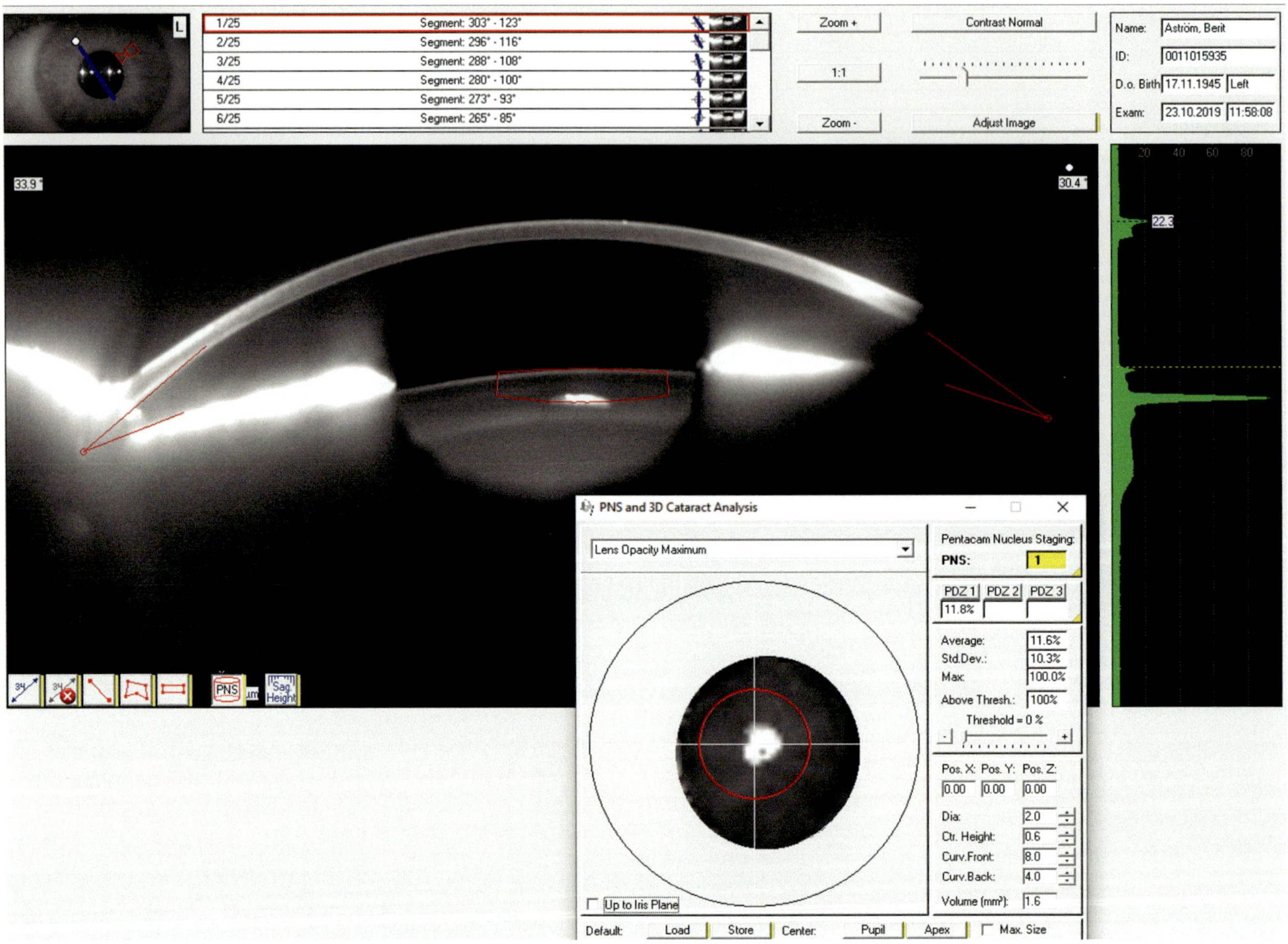

Fig. 27 Pentacam® Nucleus Staging (PNS) providing a lens opacity staging

3 Conclusion

The Pentacam® does not only provide a myriad of individual measurement values, but also independently diagnoses corneal diseases such as keratectasia. It includes several classification or staging systems that can be used clinically. Even if automated diagnoses must always be critically scrutinized, the Pentacam® has become an invaluable tool for the practicing ophthalmologist.

References

1. Jones LW, Srinivasan S, Ng A, et al. Diagnostic Instruments. Contact Lens Practice. Elsevier. 2018:327–345.e5. https://doi.org/10.1016/B978-0-7020-6660-3.00036-8.
2. Ambrósio R, Valbon BF, Faria-Correia F, et al. Scheimpflug imaging for laser refractive surgery. Curr Opin Ophthalmol. 2013;24(4):310–20.
3. Belin MW, Duncan JK. Keratoconus: the ABCD grading system. Klin Monbl Augenheilkd. 2016;233(6):701–7.
4. Belin MW, Meyer JJ, Duncan JK, et al. Assessing progression of keratoconus and cross-linking efficacy: the Belin ABCD progression display. Int J Kerat Ect Cor Dis. 2017;6:1–10.
5. Belin M, Ambrósio R. Scheimpflug imaging for keratoconus and ectatic disease. Indian J Ophthalmol. 2013;61(8):401–6.
6. Belin MW. Keratoconus and ectatic disease: evolving criteria for diagnosis. Klin Monbl Augenheilkd. 2020;237(6):740–4.
7. Weed KH, McGhee CNJ, MacEwen CJ. Atypical unilateral superior keratoconus in young males. Cont Lens Anterior Eye. 2005;28(4):177–9.
8. Tananuvat N, Leeungurasatien P, Wiriyaluppa C. Superior keratoconus with hydrops. Int Ophthalmol. 2009;29(5):419–21.
9. Prisant O, Legeais JM, Renard G. Superior keratoconus. Cornea. 1997;16(6):693–4.
10. Feng MT, Belin MW, Ambrósio R, et al. Anterior chamber depth in normal subjects by rotating scheimpflug imaging. Saudi J Ophthalmol. 2011;25(3):255–9.

Anterior Segment OCT

Elias Flockerzi, Marc Müller, and Berthold Seitz

Abstract

The focus of this chapter is to point out which structures of the human eye can be visualized using anterior segment optical coherence tomography. The devices that were used for imaging (Casia SS-1000® and Casia2®, Tomey, Nagoya, Japan) are exemplary for those of other manufacturers. In particular, there shall be findings presented, that could potentially be overlooked with a purely slit-lamp-based clinical examination. The examinations are presented as both anterior segment optical coherence tomography captures and clinical slit lamp images from the outside to the inside: first the ocular surface and cornea, then the anterior chamber and iris, and finally the (artificial) lens and the vitreous. This shall highlight the diagnostic value of anterior segment optical coherence tomography in the human eye.

Keywords

Anterior segment optical coherence tomography · AS-OCT · OCT imaging

1 Introduction

The predecessor of anterior segment optical coherence tomography (OCT) of the human eye is ultrasound biomicroscopy, which still has its role in diagnostics today when the question is about diagnosing tumors of the iris and ciliary body [1]. For analysis of the cornea, the anterior chamber, the iris and even the lens, it has been replaced by anterior segment OCT of the human eye because it provides a faster image acquisition time and a non-contact in-depth assessment of the anterior segment of the human eye. Anterior segment OCT was introduced in 1994 [2] and provides two- and three-dimensional cross-sectional tissue imaging by conglomerating multiple axial scans into a composite B-scan image [3]. It measures the echo time delay of light that is back scattered from tissue structures by splitting light from a low coherence light source into (1) a reference arm with a mirror reflecting the light and (2) the sample arm with light being back scattered by the tissue [4]. Existing anterior segment OCT devices provide cross-sections of the cornea with 5–20 μm axial resolution at a variety of widths from 6 to 16 mm and depths from 2 to 6 mm [4]. The findings shown in this chapter present the anterior segment OCT finding and the corresponding clinical slit lamp image captured by the swept-source anterior segment OCT devices Casia SS-1000® (30,000 A-scans per second, horizontal scan width of 16 mm and scan depth of 6 mm) and Casia2® (50,000 A-scans per second, horizontal scan width of 16 mm and scan depth of 13 mm (both Tomey, Nagoya, Japan)).

Besides topo- and tomographic analysis, a main area of anterior segment OCT application in clinical practice is the examination of complex anterior segment pathologies because it provides

(1) an in-depth assessment of conjunctival, scleral, epi- or intracorneal lesions, scars, deposits or implants,
(2) an insight into the anterior chamber and the chamber angle even if the cornea lacks transparency,
(3) visualization of both the iris configuration and iris lesions,
(4) visualization of the lens status reaching from the position of anterior chamber intraocular lenses to implantable collamer lenses and sclera-fixated intraocular lenses and

E. Flockerzi (✉) · M. Müller · B. Seitz
Department of Ophthalmology, Saarland University Medical Center, Homburg, Germany
e-mail: elias.flockerzi@uks.eu

B. Seitz et al. (eds.), *Atlas on Cornea*, https://doi.org/10.1007/978-3-031-65422-0_8

(5)a comparably fast image acquisition time, that results in useful images even with nystagmus.

Each new generation of anterior segment OCT devices results in an improvement in terms of image depth, resolution and acquisition speed and it has been proposed that anterior segment OCT will provide an "optical tissue biopsy" of ocular structures in the future, when it becomes capable of imaging nerves and vessels at a cellular level [1].

2 Ocular Surface and Cornea

Anterior segment optical coherence tomography may be helpful in glaucoma surgery when selecting blebs for needling and analysis after laser-assisted suture lysis [5] (Fig. 1).

Ocular surface neoplasia is characterized by a hyperreflective, thickened abrupt transition (arrow) from normal to abnormal epithelium and solid masses spreading onto the cornea which remains intact below [6] (Figs. 2 and 3).

Anterior segment OCT also enables the visualization and measurement of areas of focal corneal thinning such as in Fuchs–Terrien marginal degeneration (Fig. 4).

Pterygia (only the head is attached to the cornea, Fig. 5) can be distinguished from pseudopterygia (the overlying membrane remains detached from the cornea [7]) and pinguecula (respecting the limbus [8]).

Anterior segment OCT also provides a visualization and depth assessment of intra- and epicorneal deposits (Figs. 6, 7, 8).

Anterior segment OCT is helpful in visualizing anterior segment pathology when dealing with cloudy, scarred and vascularized corneas that impede insight into the anterior chamber (Fig. 9).

Even subtle pathologies at the innermost layer of the cornea may be detected and visualized, such as Haab striae (Fig. 10).

A clinical and tomographic assessment of ectatic corneal conditions such as keratoconus is possible and provides additional information about the depth of corneal scarring (Figs. 11–15).

Corneal layers can be clearly delineated and decisions can be taken for surgical techniques to remove epithelial ingrowth, corneal deposits in corneal dystrophies or scar tissue [4] (Figs. 16–28).

Anterior segment OCT also provides intra- and postoperative visualization and measurement of the implantation depth of intracorneal implants such as intracorneal ring segments Figs. 29–32).

The different techniques of corneal transplantation may be visualized and recapitulated (Figs. 33–36) and the anterior segment OCT images may help in deciding which transplantation technique should be applied in the individual patient (Fig. 37).

With the advent of lamellar corneal transplantation techniques, the visualization of lamellar detachments has gained increasingly importance (Figs. 38–40).

Especially in cases of corneal scarring or edema, Descemet tears or detachments can be visualized that may have been overlooked upon sole slit lamp-based examination (Fig. 41).

Presumed corneal hydrops can be distinguished from other pathologies presenting with similar clinical findings (Figs. 42, 43).

Both the corneal thinning and depth of corneal ulcers can be assessed (Figs. 44–46).

Anterior segment pathology that remains nearly unvisible in slit lamp examination may be revealed based on anterior segment OCT (Fig. 47).

Visualization of the anterior segment remains possible even after complex anterior segment surgery such as keratoprosthetics (Fig. 48) or double anterior chamber formation after deep anterior lamellar keratoplasty (Fig. 49).

3 Iris

Besides corneal findings, the anterior segment OCT also enables visualization of the missing iris (Fig. 50), iris details (Fig. 51) or pathologic iris configurations (Figs. 52–54) even if the cornea lacks transparency.

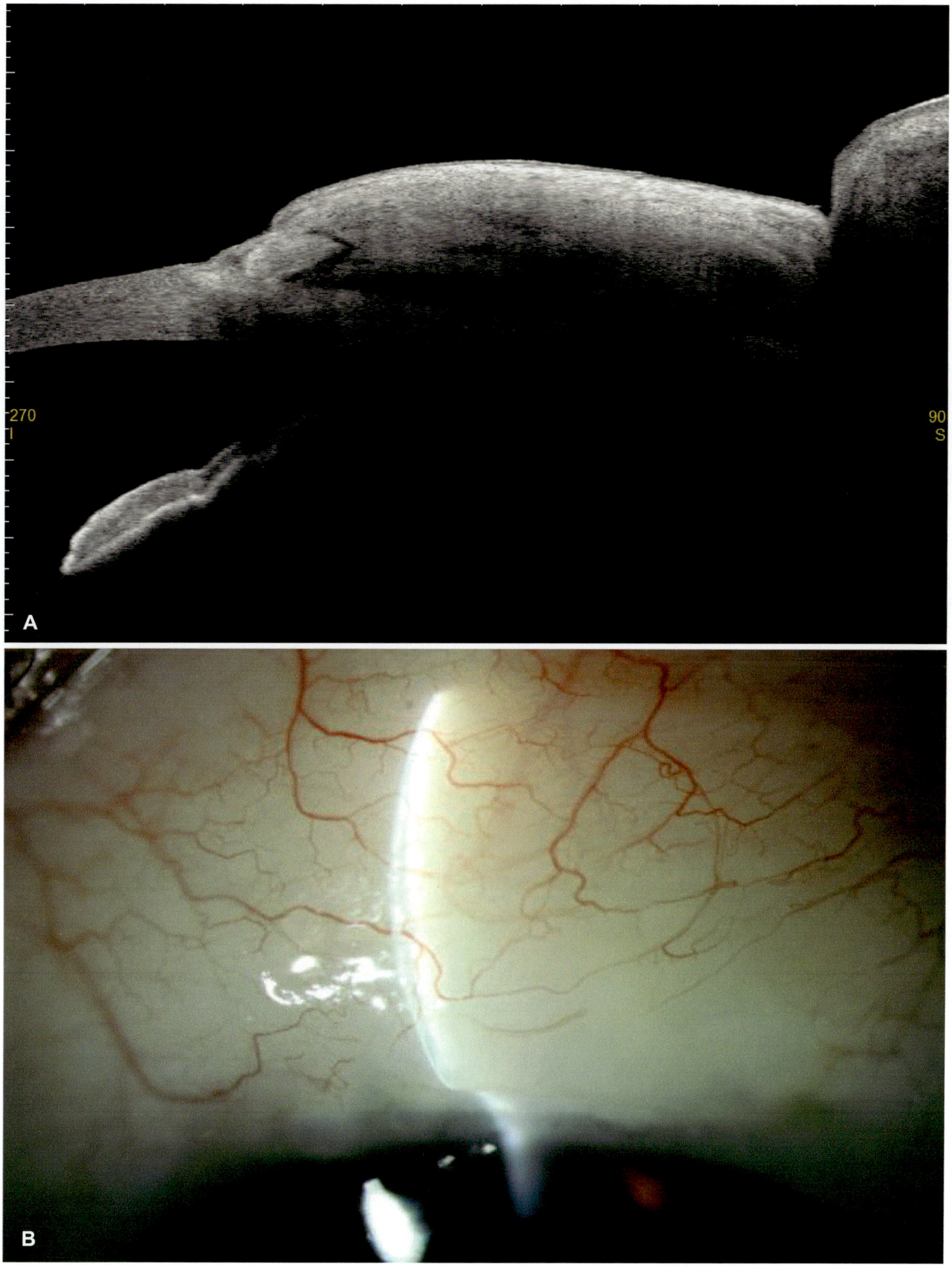

Fig. 1 (**A, B**) Trabeculectomy bleb. (**A**) anterior segment optical coherence tomography. (**B**) slit lamp imaging

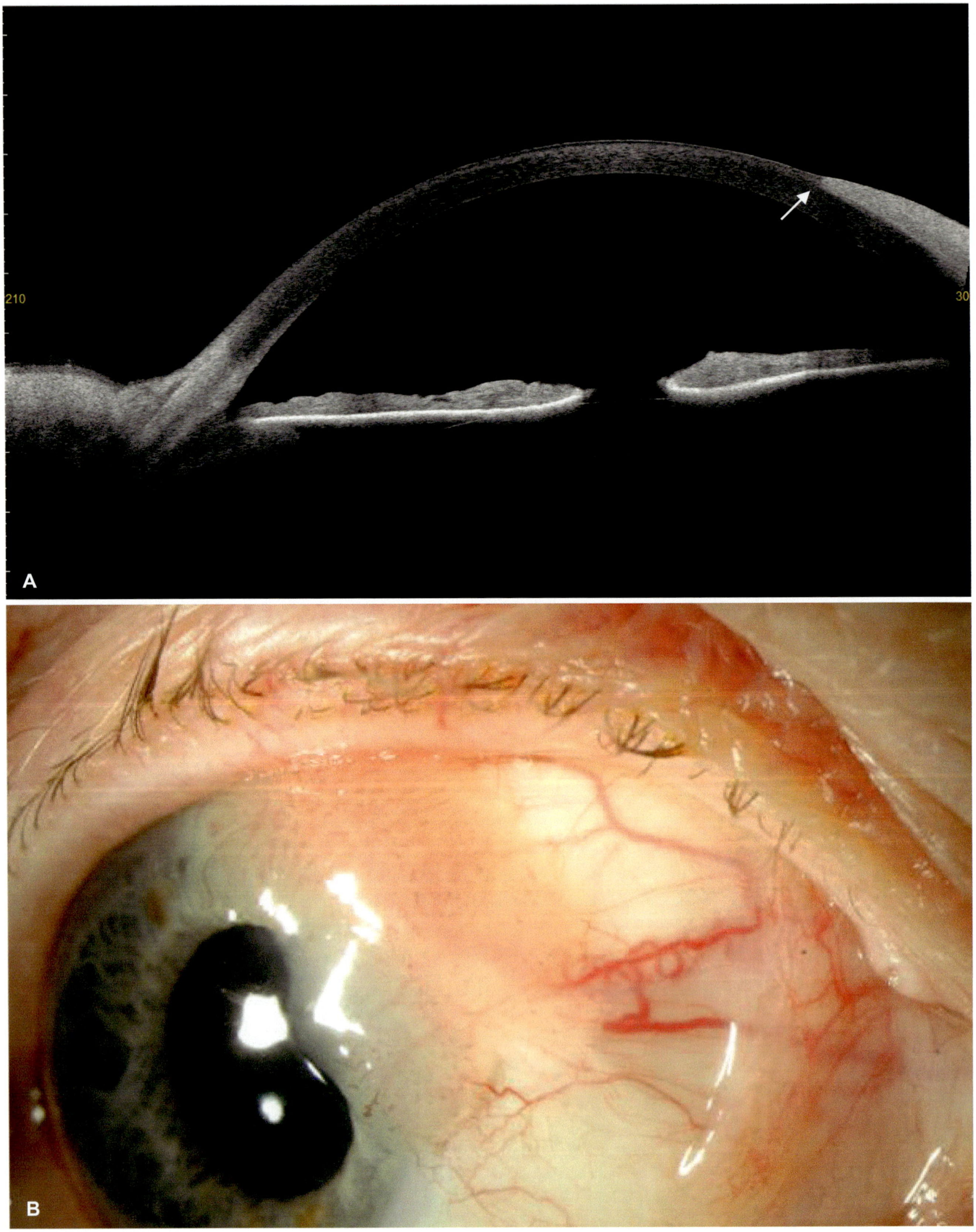

Fig. 2 (**A, B**) Mucosal papilloma with moderate squamous dysplasia. (**A**) anterior segment optical coherence tomography, white arrow showing intact cornea below the lesion. (**B**) slit lamp imaging

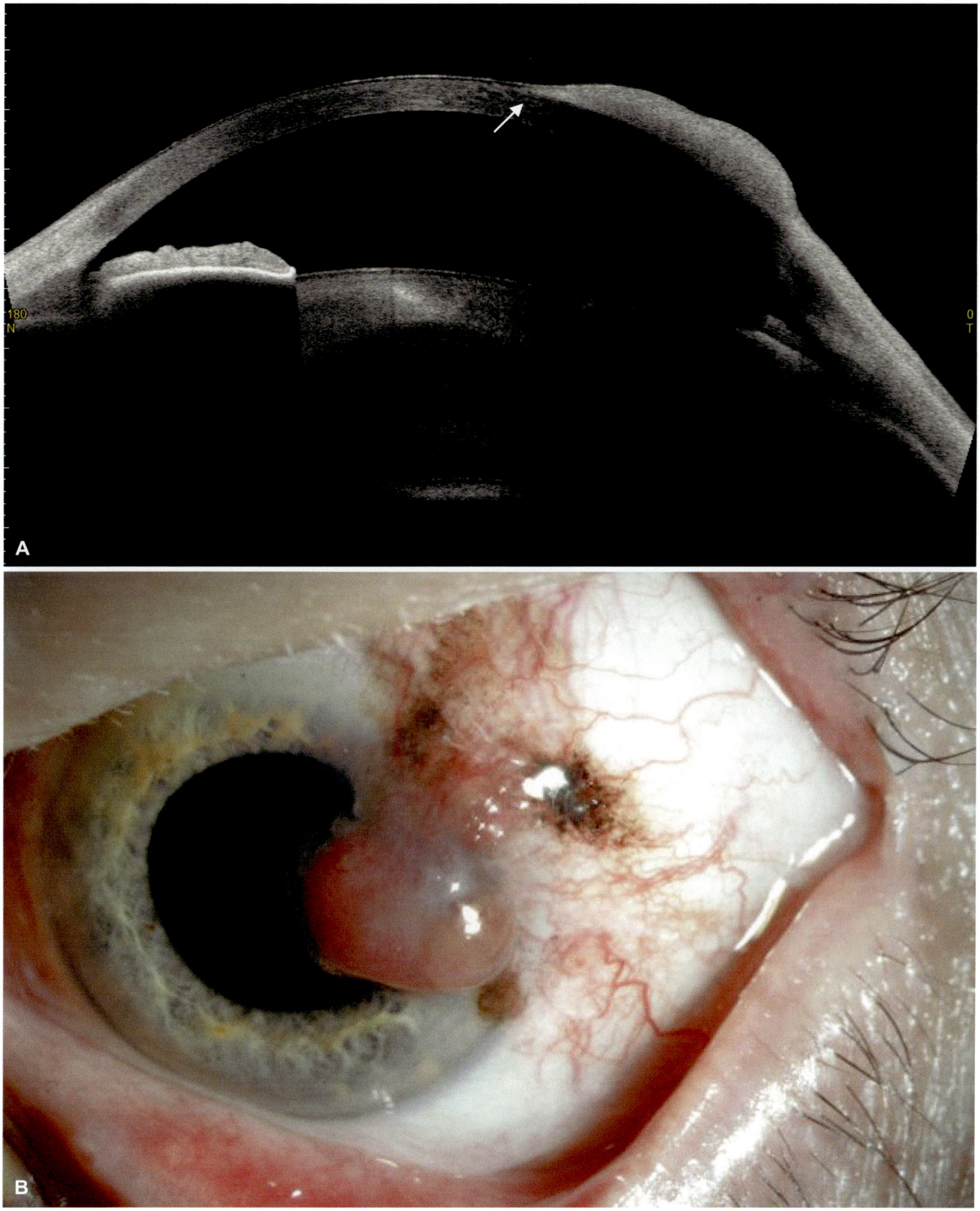

Fig. 3 (**A, B**) Conjunctival melanoma spreading onto the cornea. (**A**) anterior segment optical coherence tomography, white arrow showing intact cornea below the lesion. (**B**) slit lamp imaging

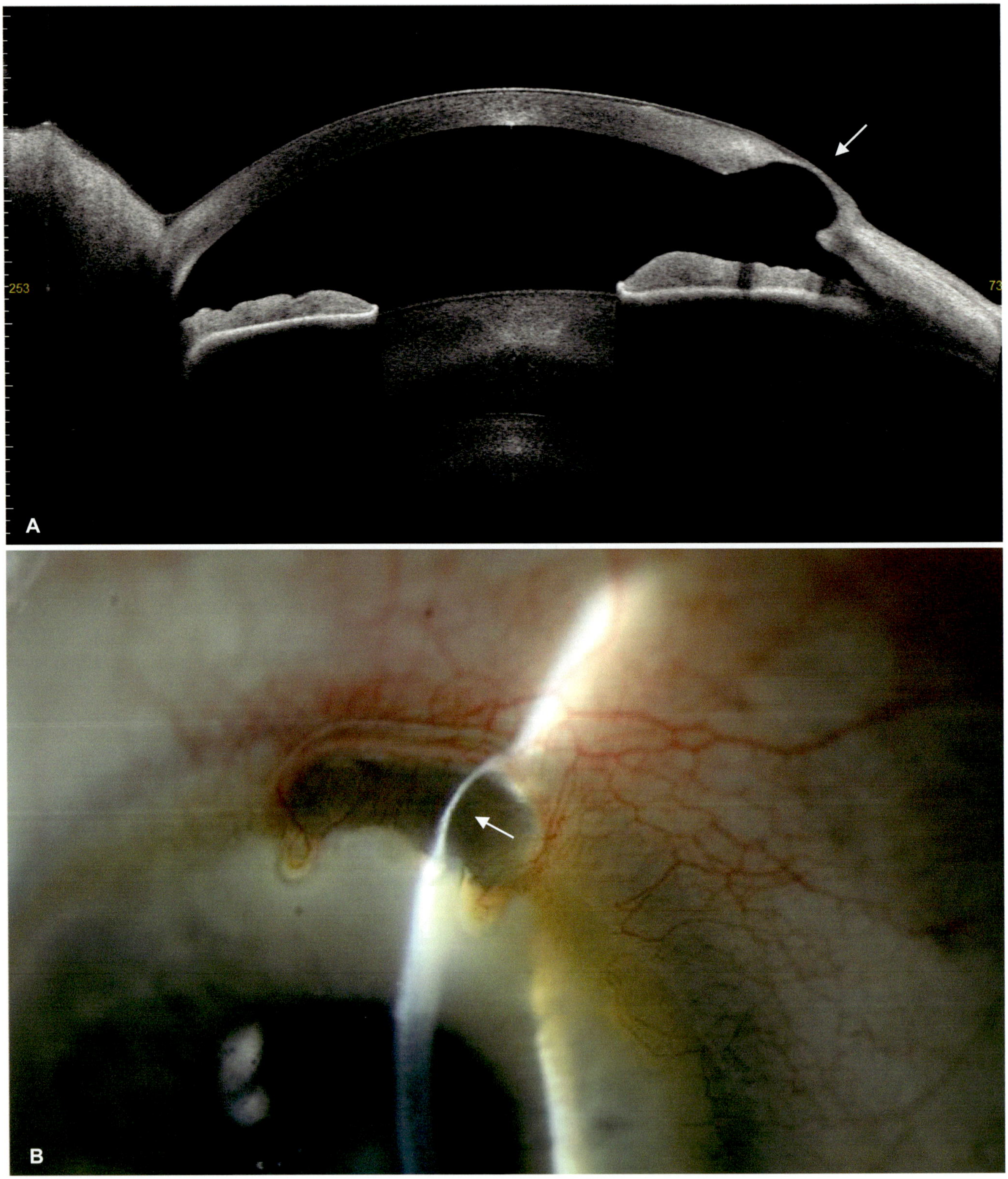

Fig. 4 (**A, B**) Fuchs–Terrien marginal corneal degeneration. (**A**) anterior segment optical coherence tomography. (**B**) slit lamp imaging. White arrow indicating the peripheral paralimbal thinning of the cornea typically in a superior position

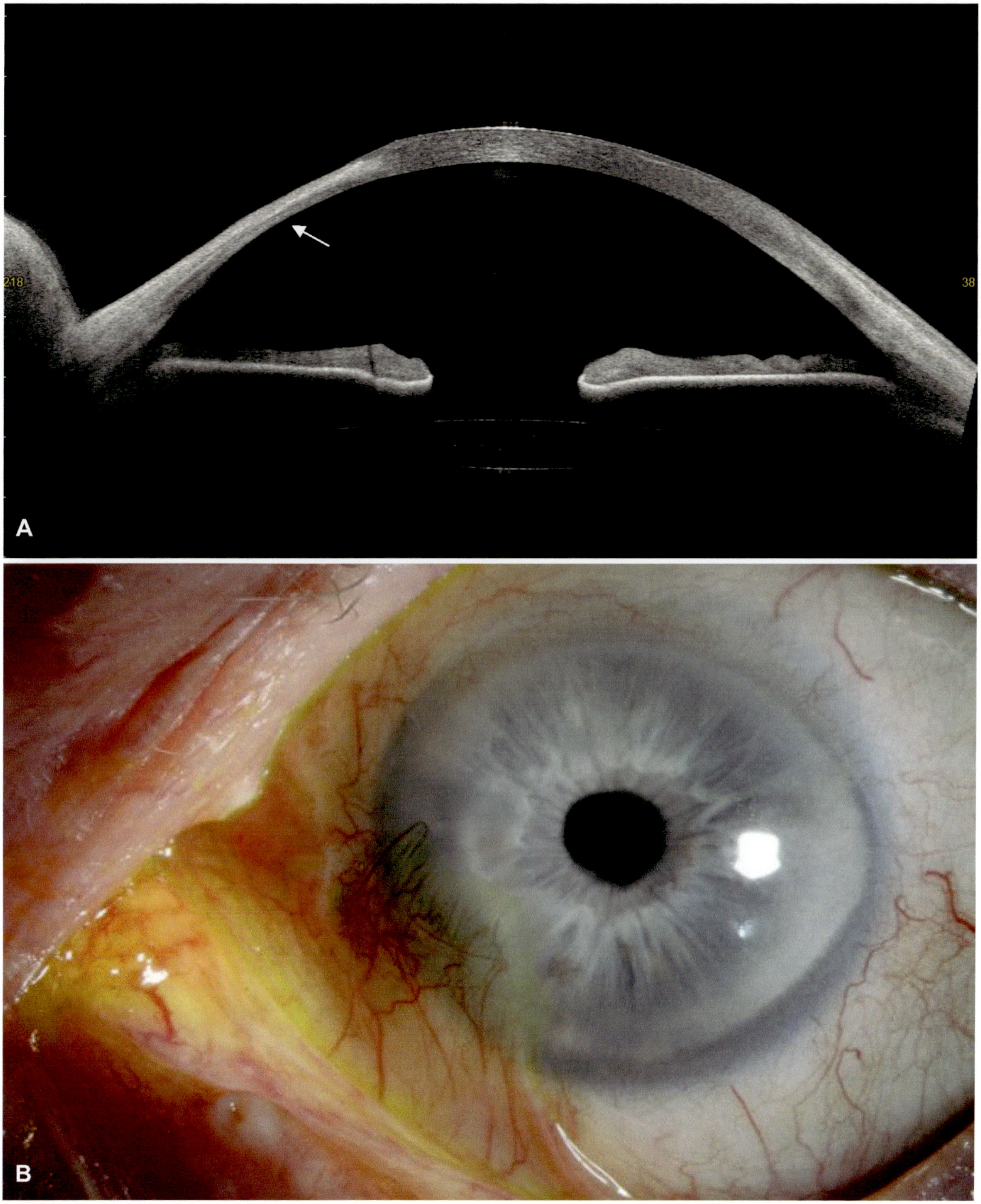

Fig. 5 (**A, B**) Recurrence of a pterygium after excision with free conjunctival flap. (**A**) anterior segment optical coherence tomography. (**B**) slit lamp imaging. White arrow indicating a thinned cornea with deep stromal scarring

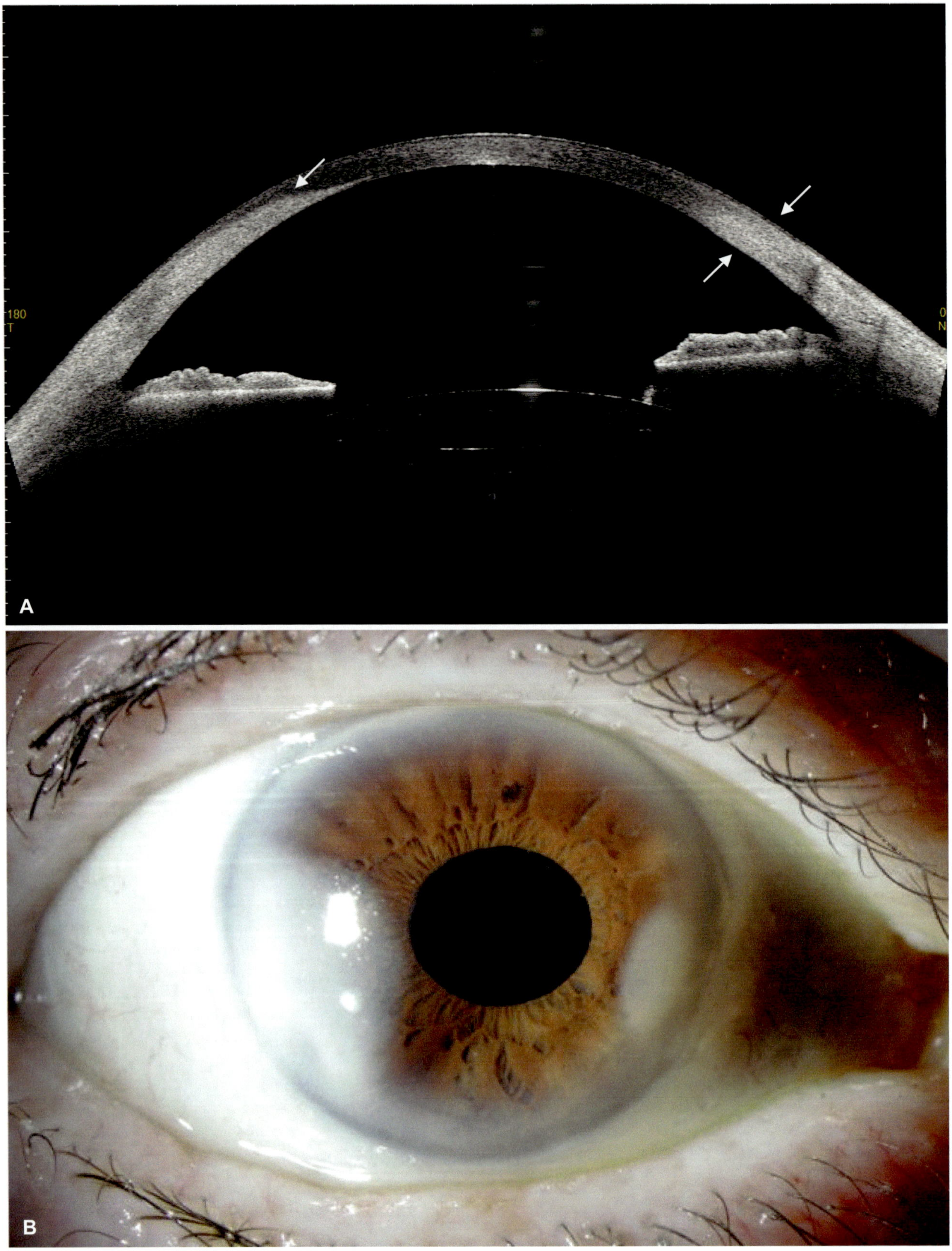

Fig. 6 (**A, B**) Early stage of calcareous corneal degeneration with deep stromal calcifications (arrows). (**A**) anterior segment optical coherence tomography. (**B**) slit lamp imaging

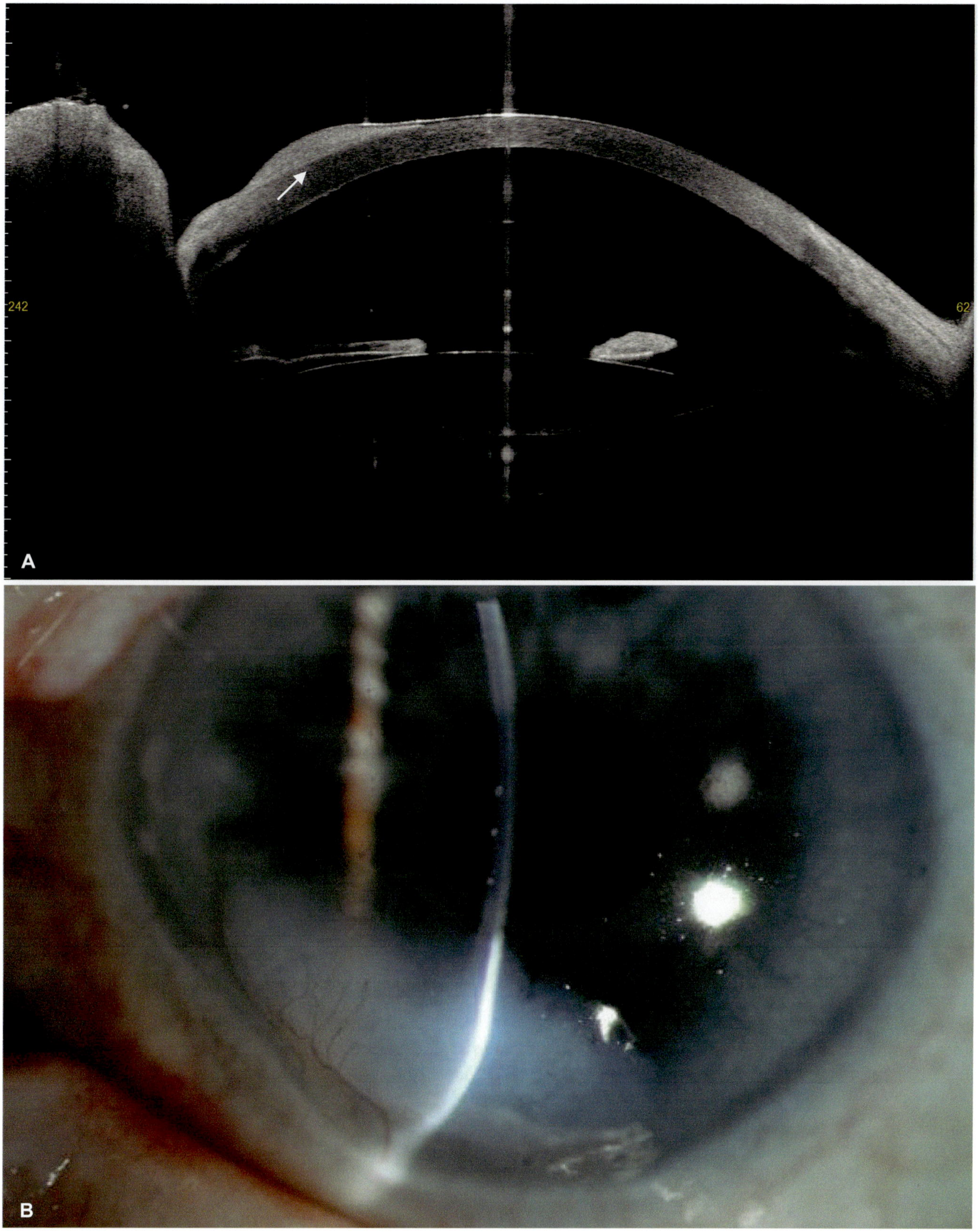

Fig. 7 (**A, B**) Salzmann nodular degeneration from 06 to 08.00 o'clock position. (**A**) anterior segment optical coherence tomography. (**B**) slit lamp imaging

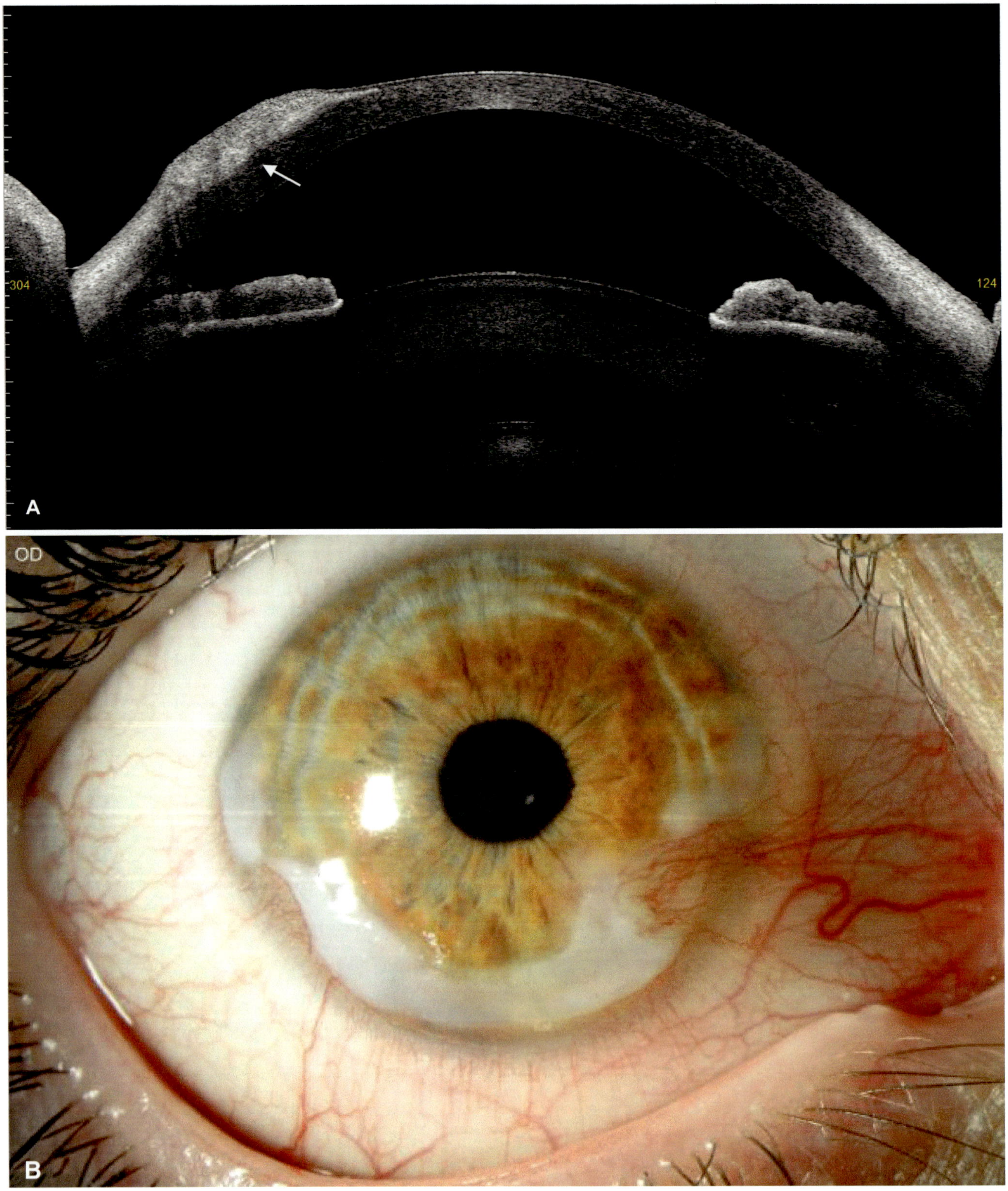

Fig. 8 (**A, B**) Peripheral hypertrophic subepithelial corneal degeneration (PHSCD) with typical sausage- or banana-like shape as opposed to Salzmann nodular degeneration. Small pterygium at the 04 o'clock position. (**A**) anterior segment optical coherence tomography. (**B**) slit lamp imaging

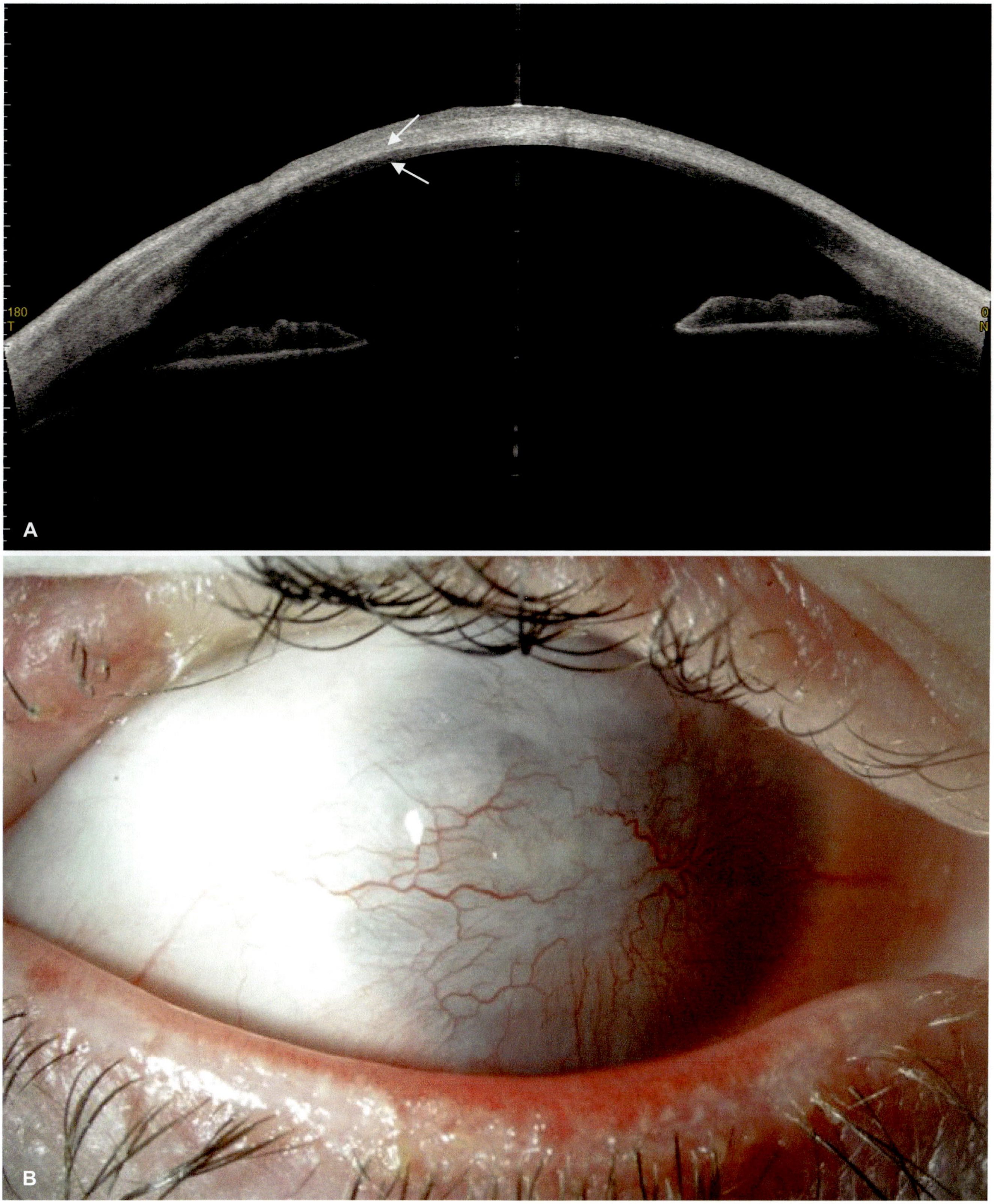

Fig. 9 (**A, B**) Total conjunctivalization because of circular limbal stem cell defiency after firework burn. (**A**) anterior segment optical coherence tomography. (**B**) slit lamp imaging. Arrows indicating the very thin remaining part of clear stroma within the cornea. See chapter "Surgical Treatment Options of Limbal Stem Cell Deficiency" for surgical treatment

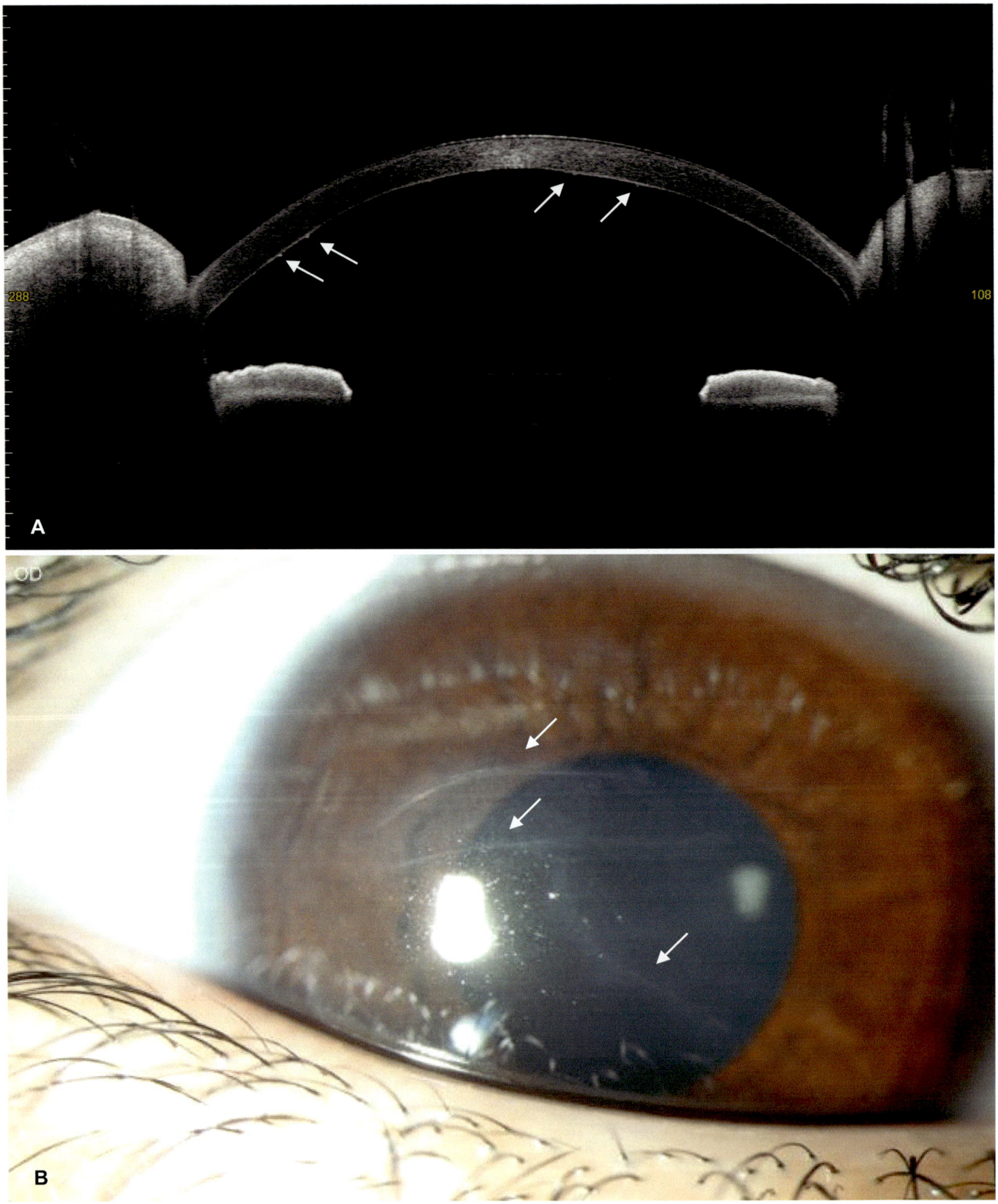

Fig. 10 (**A, B**) Haab striae (arrows) in buphthalmus. (**A**) anterior segment optical coherence tomography. (**B**) slit lamp imaging

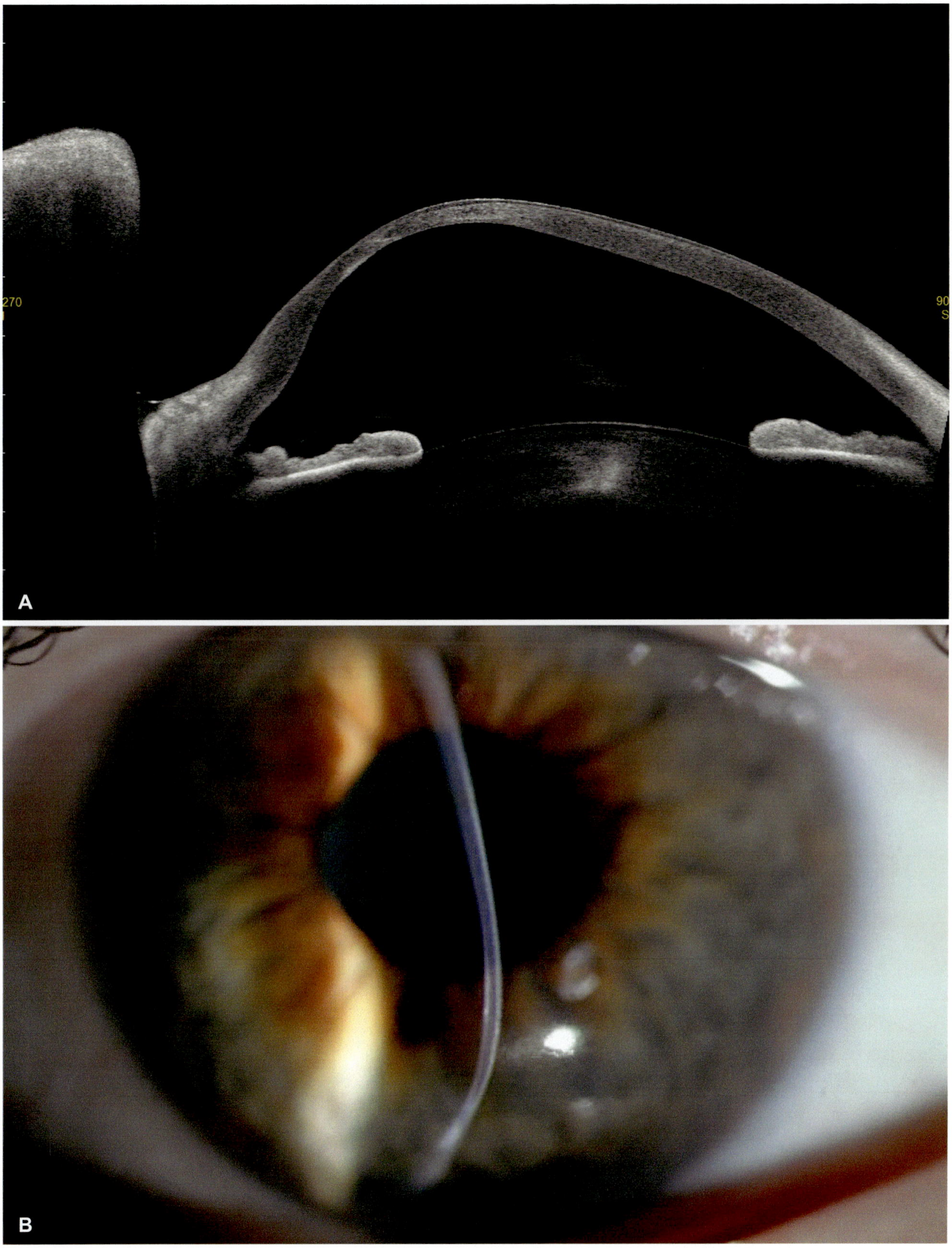

Fig. 11 (**A, B**) Paracentral thinning and inferior steepening in severe keratoconus. (**A**) anterior segment optical coherence tomography. (**B**) slit lamp imaging

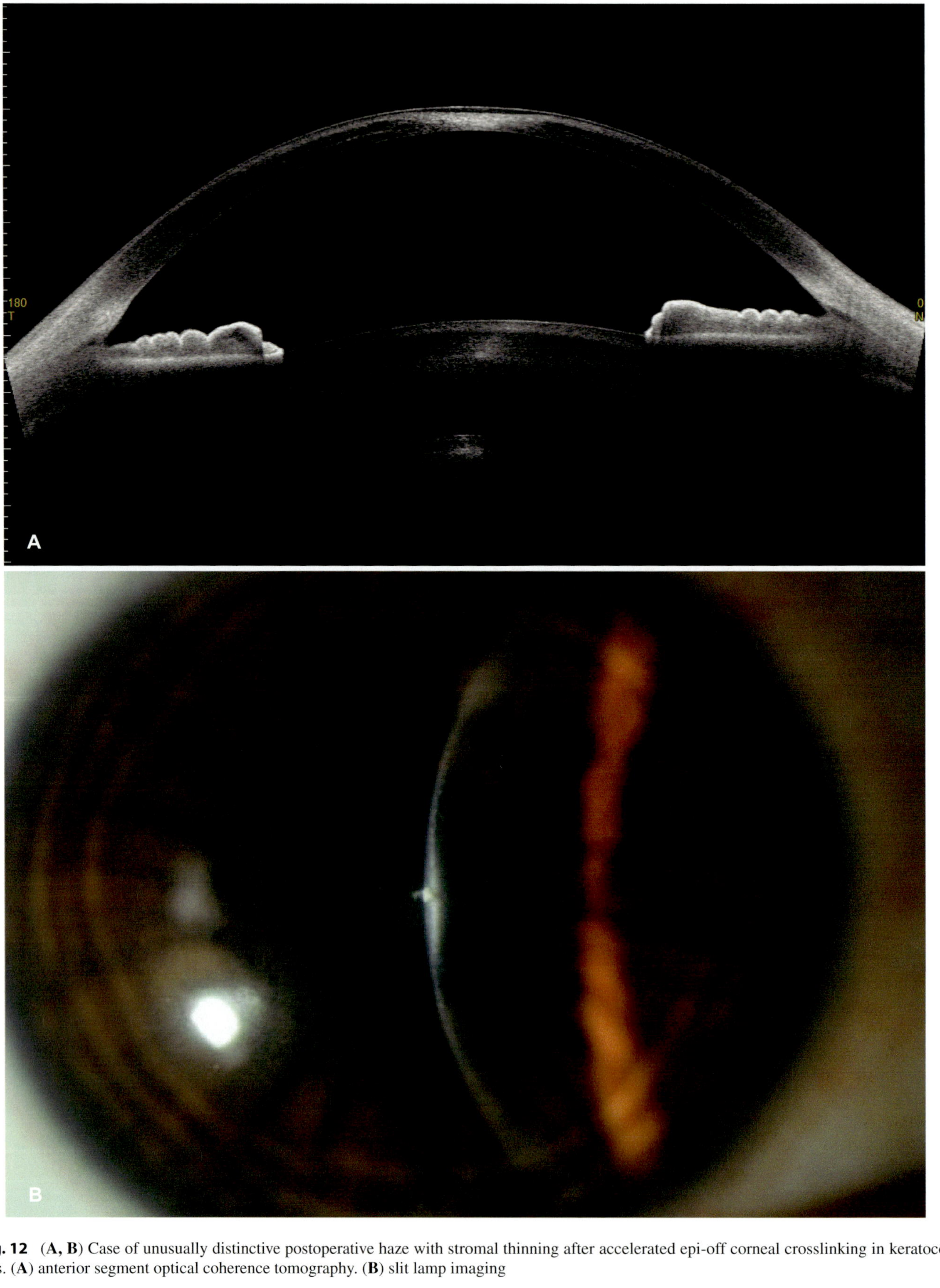

Fig. 12 (**A, B**) Case of unusually distinctive postoperative haze with stromal thinning after accelerated epi-off corneal crosslinking in keratoconus. (**A**) anterior segment optical coherence tomography. (**B**) slit lamp imaging

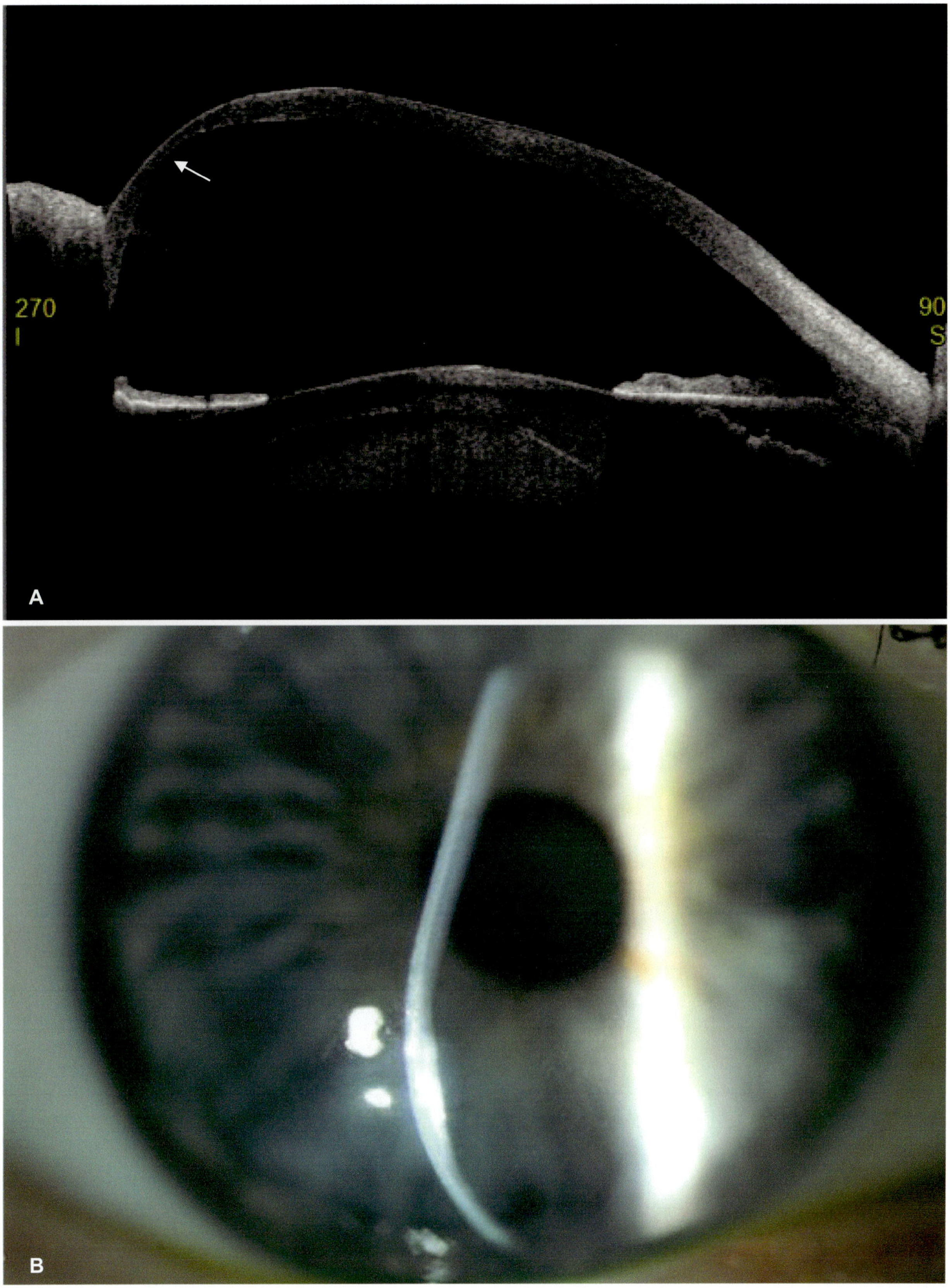

Fig. 13 (**A, B**) Pellucid marginal degeneration (PMD) with inferior limbus-parallel band of thinning. (**A**) anterior segment optical coherence tomography. (**B**) slit lamp imaging

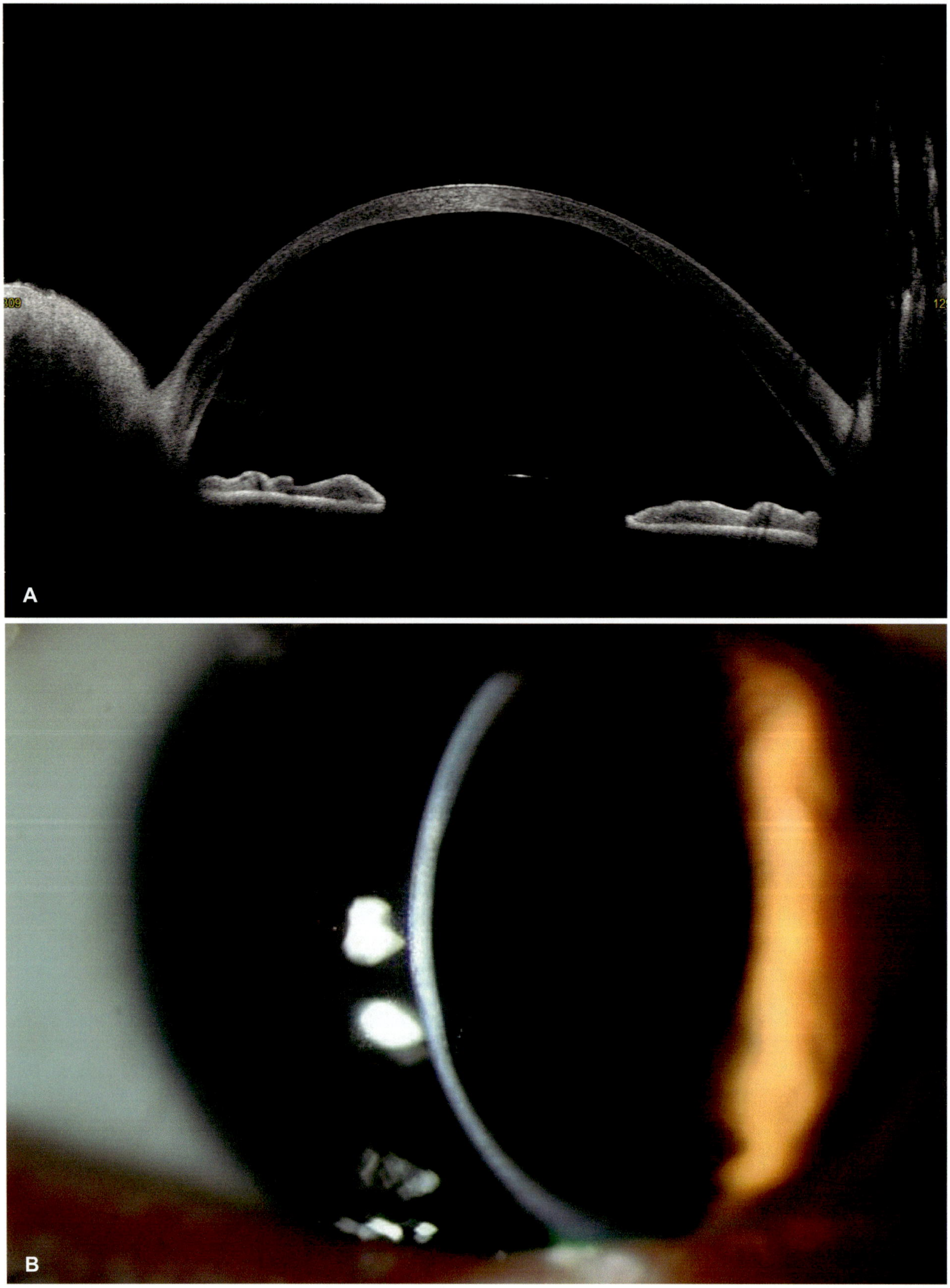

Fig. 14 (**A, B**) Keratoglobus with globally thinned and steepened cornea (thinnest corneal thickness 223 µm as opposed to megalocornea). (**A**) anterior segment optical coherence tomography. (**B**) slit lamp imaging

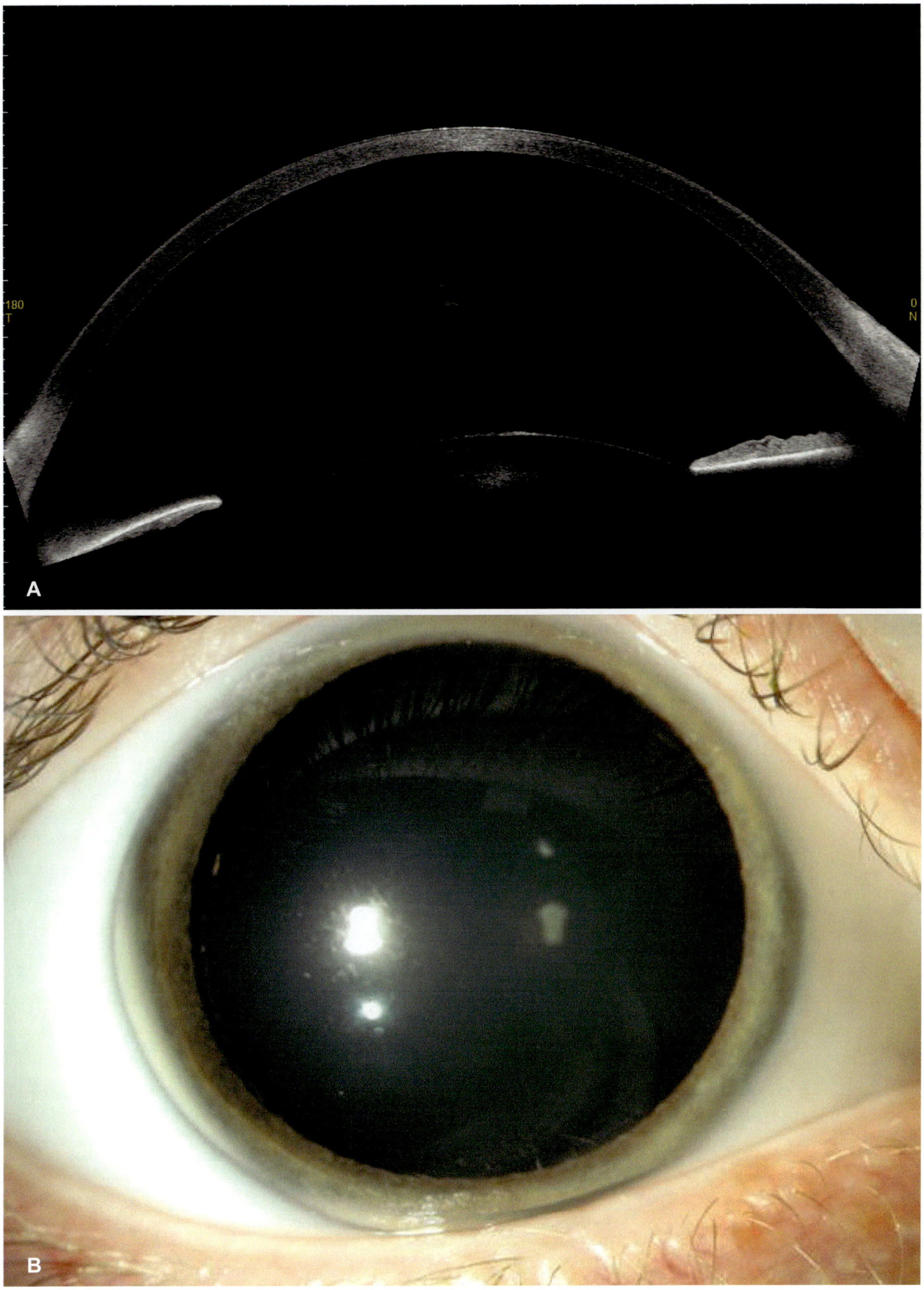

Fig. 15 (**A, B**) Megalocornea with globally thinned and steepened cornea (thinnest corneal thickness 413 μm as opposed to keratoglobus, diameter 14 × 15 mm). (**A**) anterior segment optical coherence tomography. (**B**) slit lamp imaging

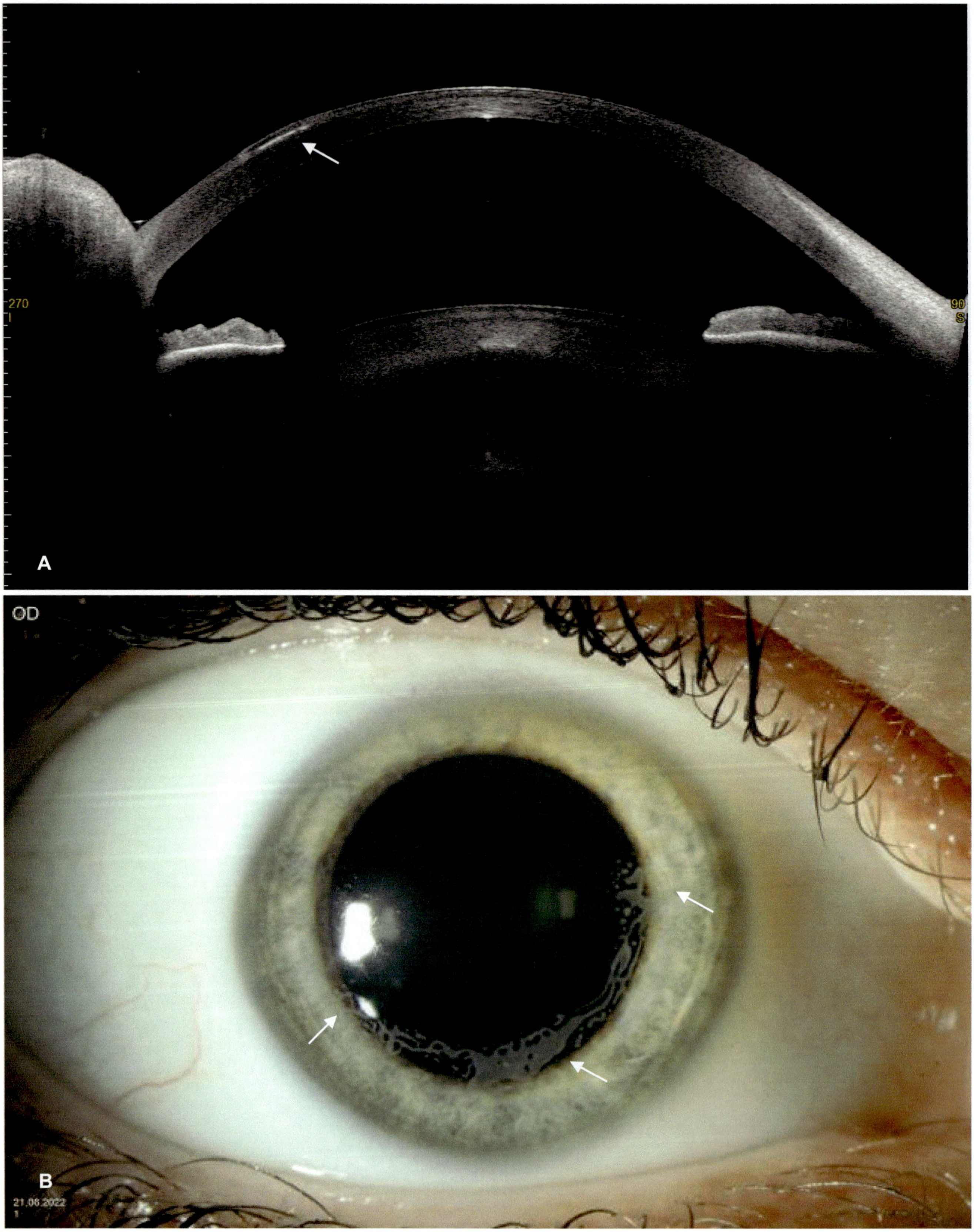

Fig. 16 (**A, B**) Epithelial ingrowth below the flap after Laser-in-situ-keratomileusis (arrows). (**A**) anterior segment optical coherence tomography. (**B**) slit lamp imaging

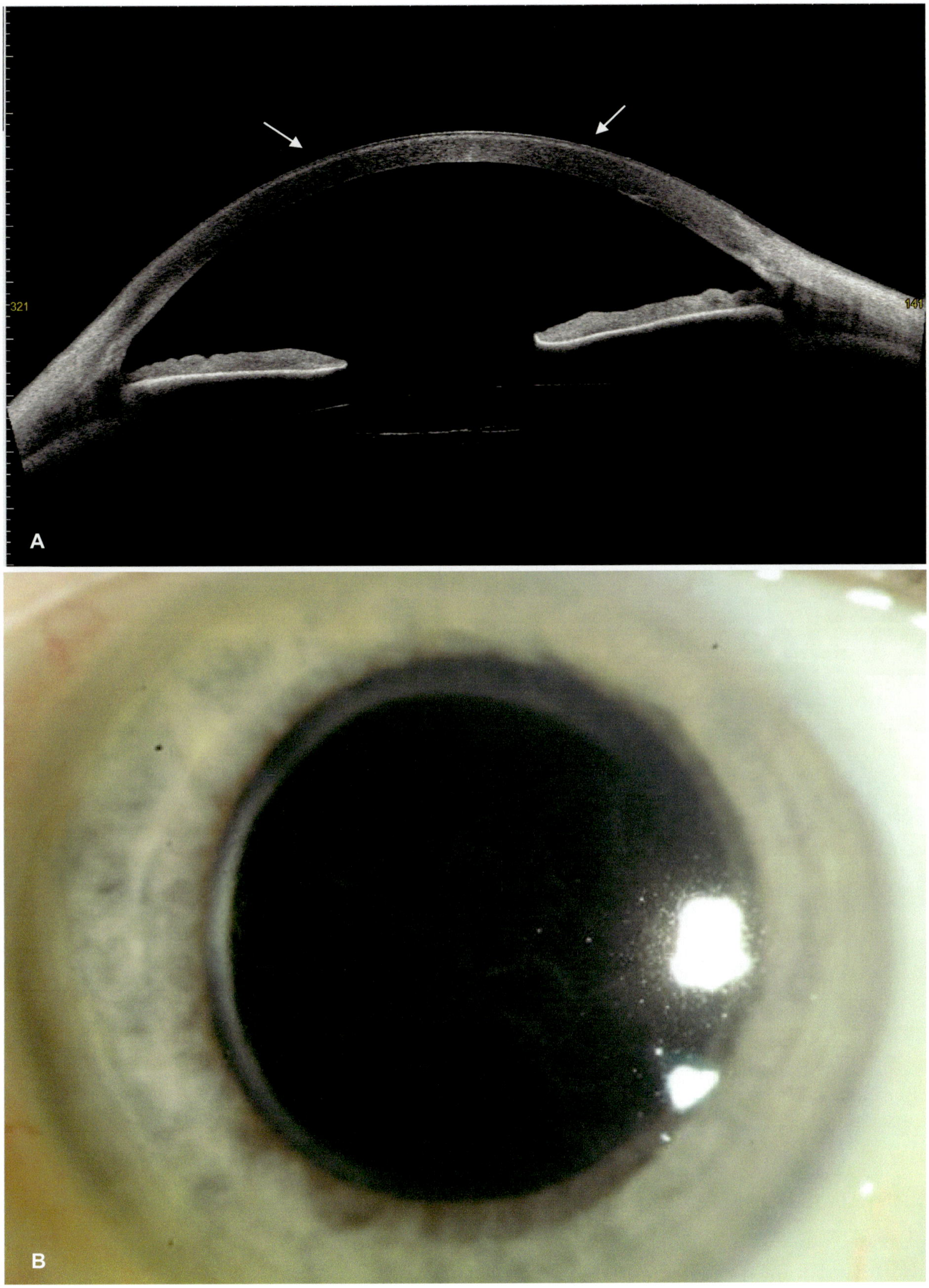

Fig. 17 (**A, B**) Map-Dot-Fingerprint Dystrophy (epithelial and subepithelial dystrophy). (**A**) anterior segment optical coherence tomography. (**B**) slit lamp imaging

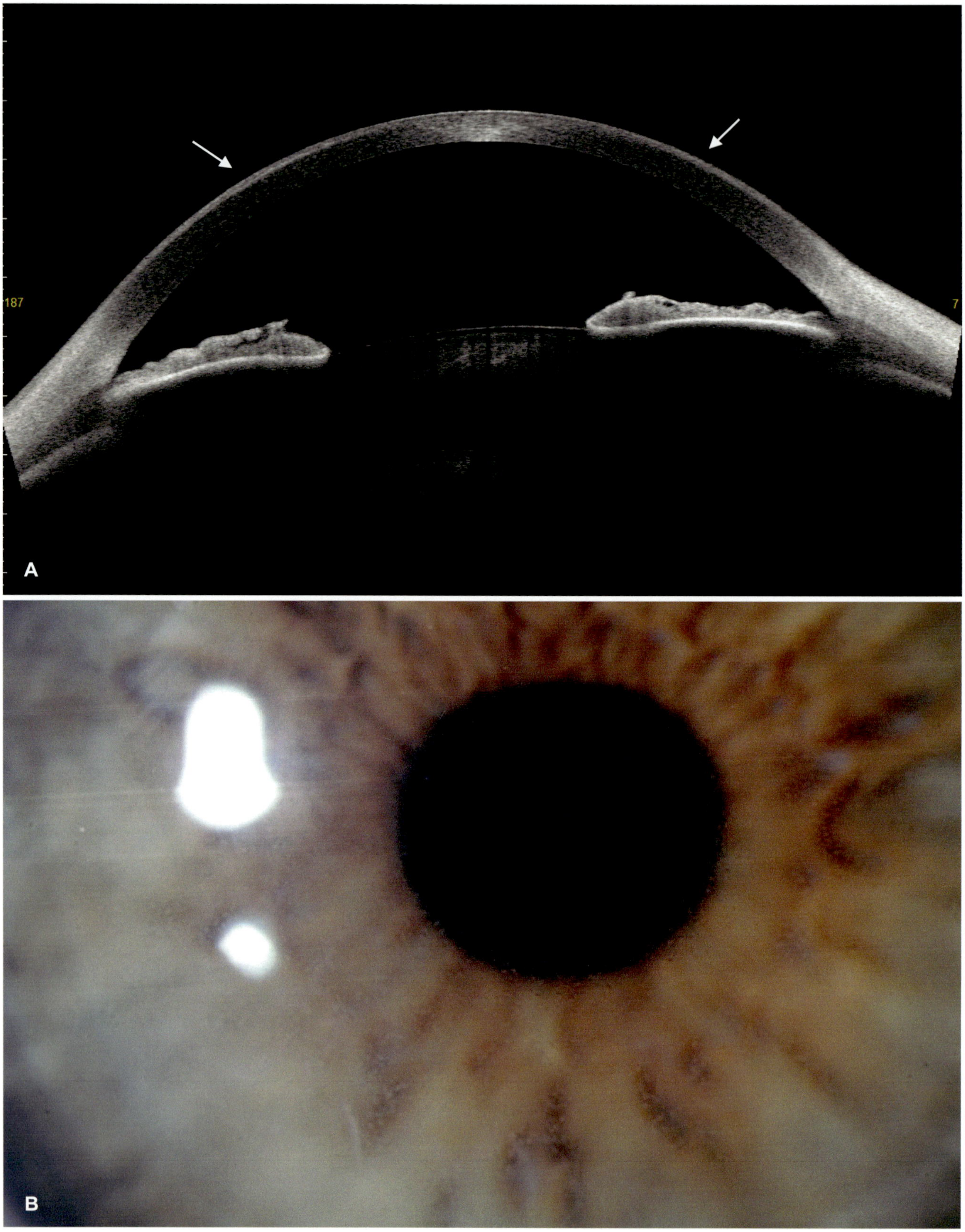

Fig. 18 (**A, B**) Meesmann corneal dystrophy (epithelial and subepithelial dystrophy). Diffuse greyish opacities (arrows) and round clear microcysts. (**A**) anterior segment optical coherence tomography. (**B**) slit lamp imaging

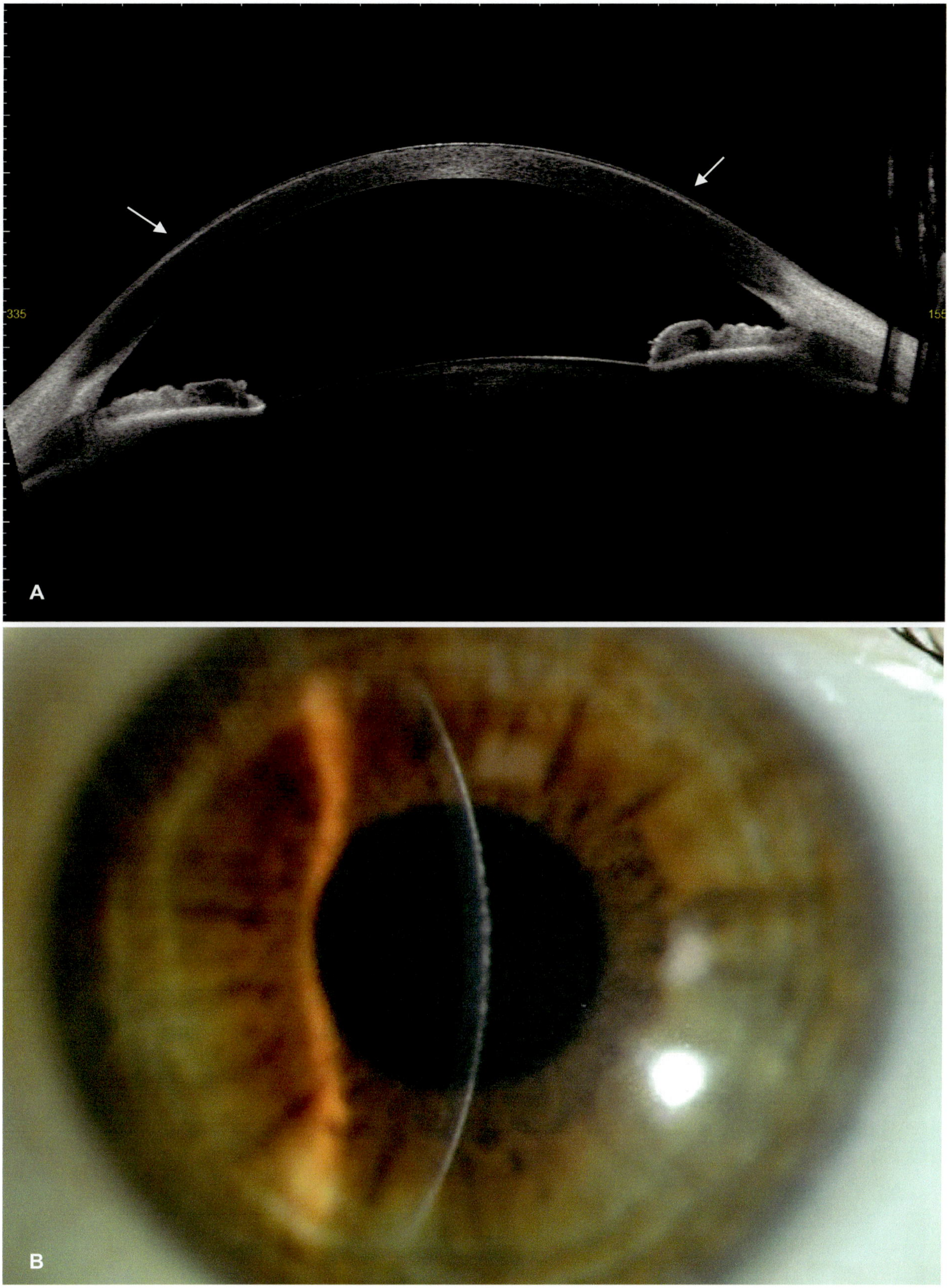

Fig. 19 (**A, B**) Thiel–Behnke corneal dystrophy (epithelial-stromal TGFβ dystrophy). Subepithelial honeycomb opacities, fibrillary subepithelial layer replacing Bowman layer. (**A**) anterior segment optical coherence tomography. (**B**) slit lamp imaging

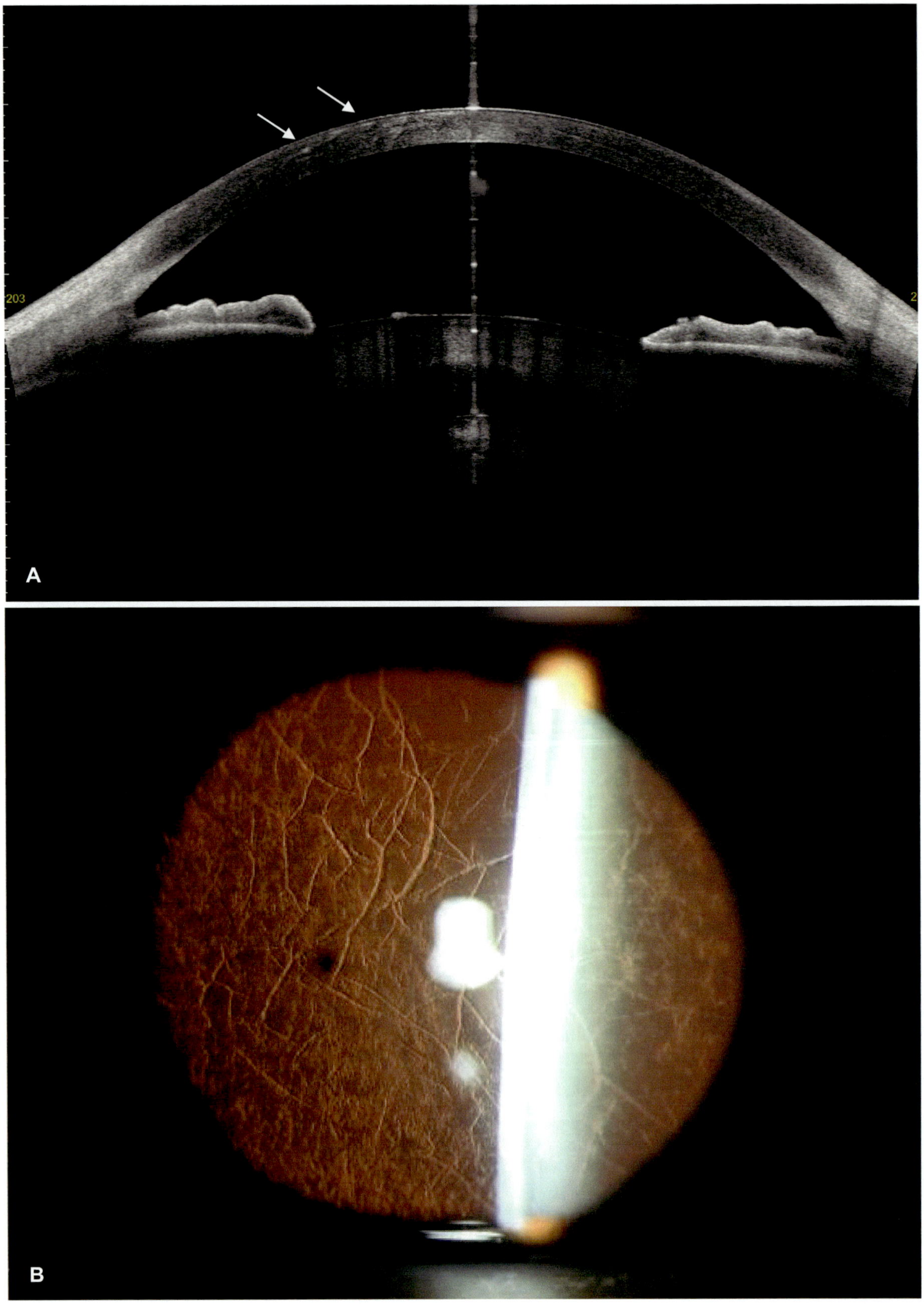

Fig. 20 (**A, B**) Lattice corneal dystrophy (epithelial-stromal TGFβ dystrophy). Subepithelial and midstromal amyloid deposits (arrows). (**A**) anterior segment optical coherence tomography. (**B**) slit lamp imaging

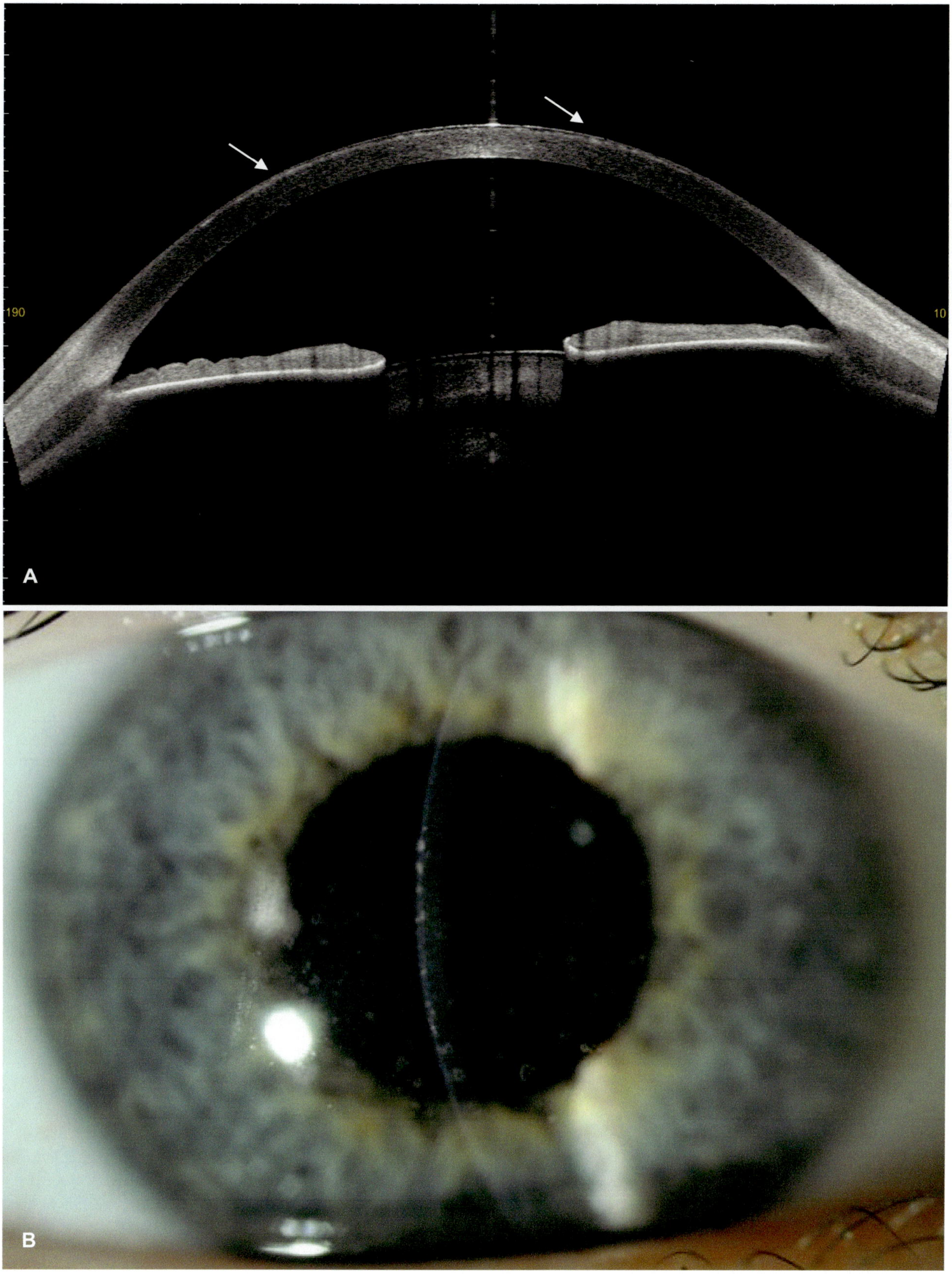

Fig. 21 (**A**, **B**) Early stage of granular corneal dystrophy type I (epithelial-stromal TGFβ dystrophy). Subepithelial hyaline deposits (arrows). (**A**) anterior segment optical coherence tomography. (**B**) slit lamp imaging

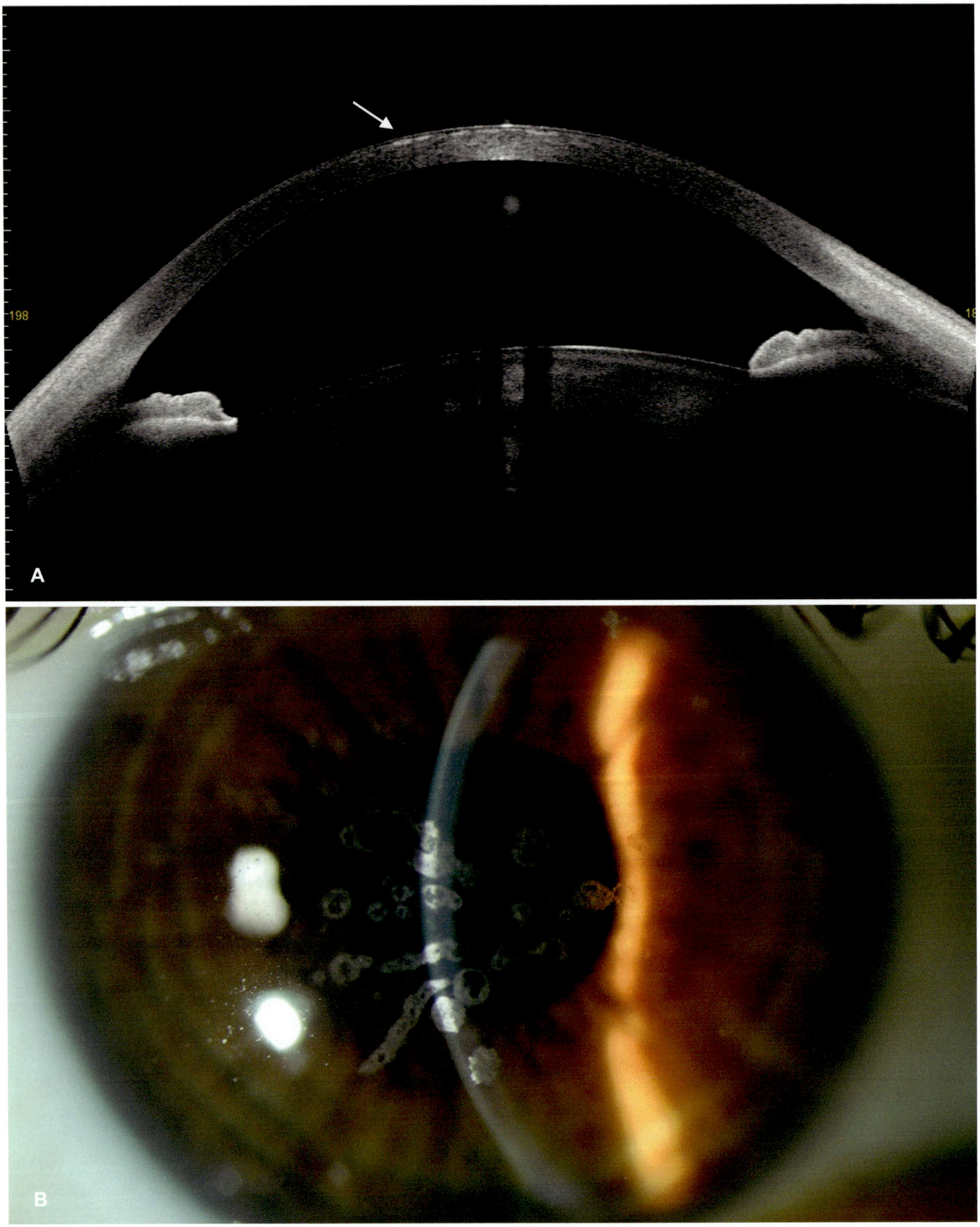

Fig. 22 (**A, B**) Granular corneal dystrophy type IIa (epithelial-stromal TGFβ dystrophy). Subepithelial hyaline deposits (arrows). (**A**) anterior segment optical coherence tomography. (**B**) slit lamp imaging ("rings and stars")

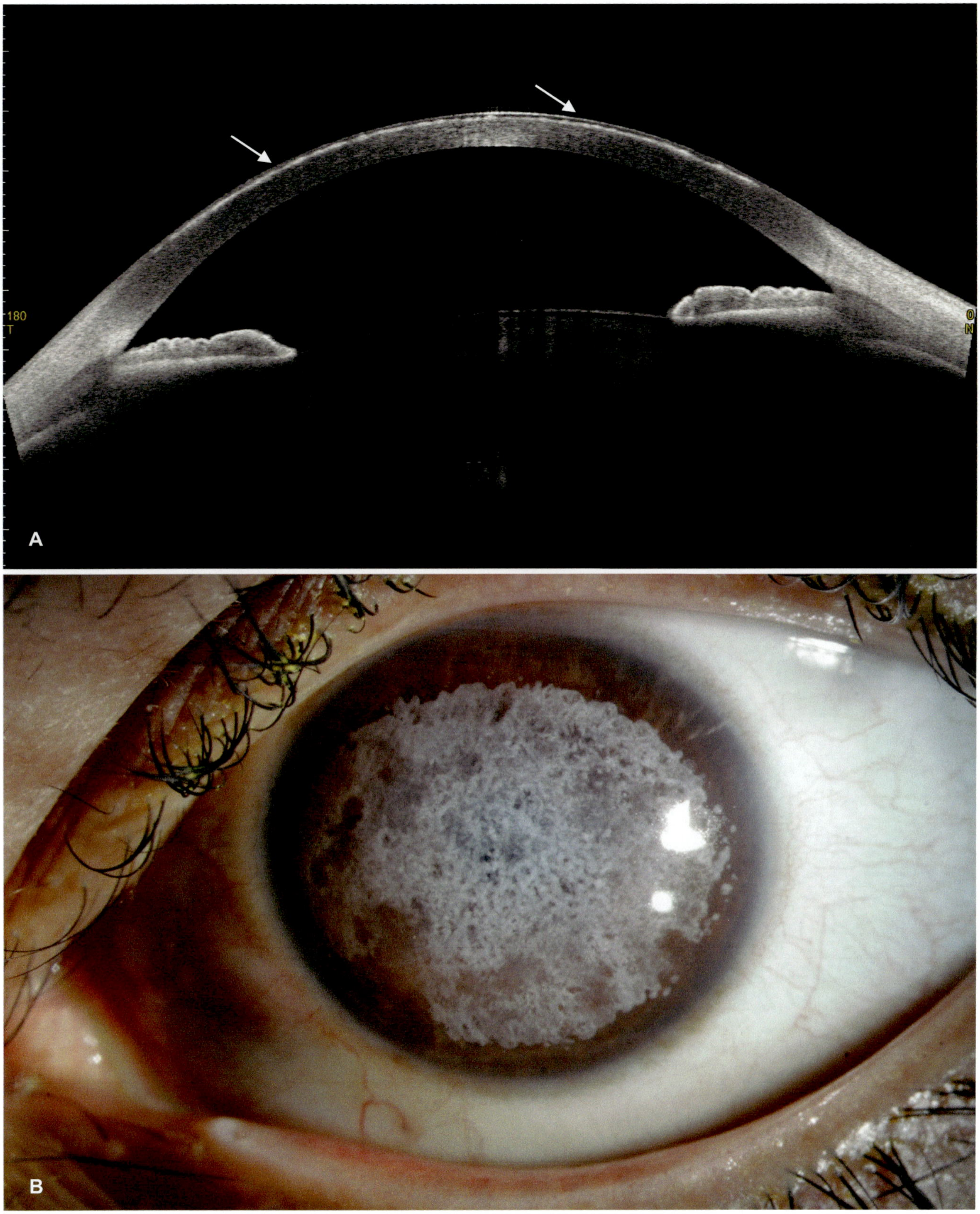

Fig. 23 (**A, B**) Granular corneal dystrophy type IIb (epithelial-stromal TGFβ dystrophy). Subepithelial hyaline deposits (arrows). (**A**) anterior segment optical coherence tomography. (**B**) slit lamp imaging

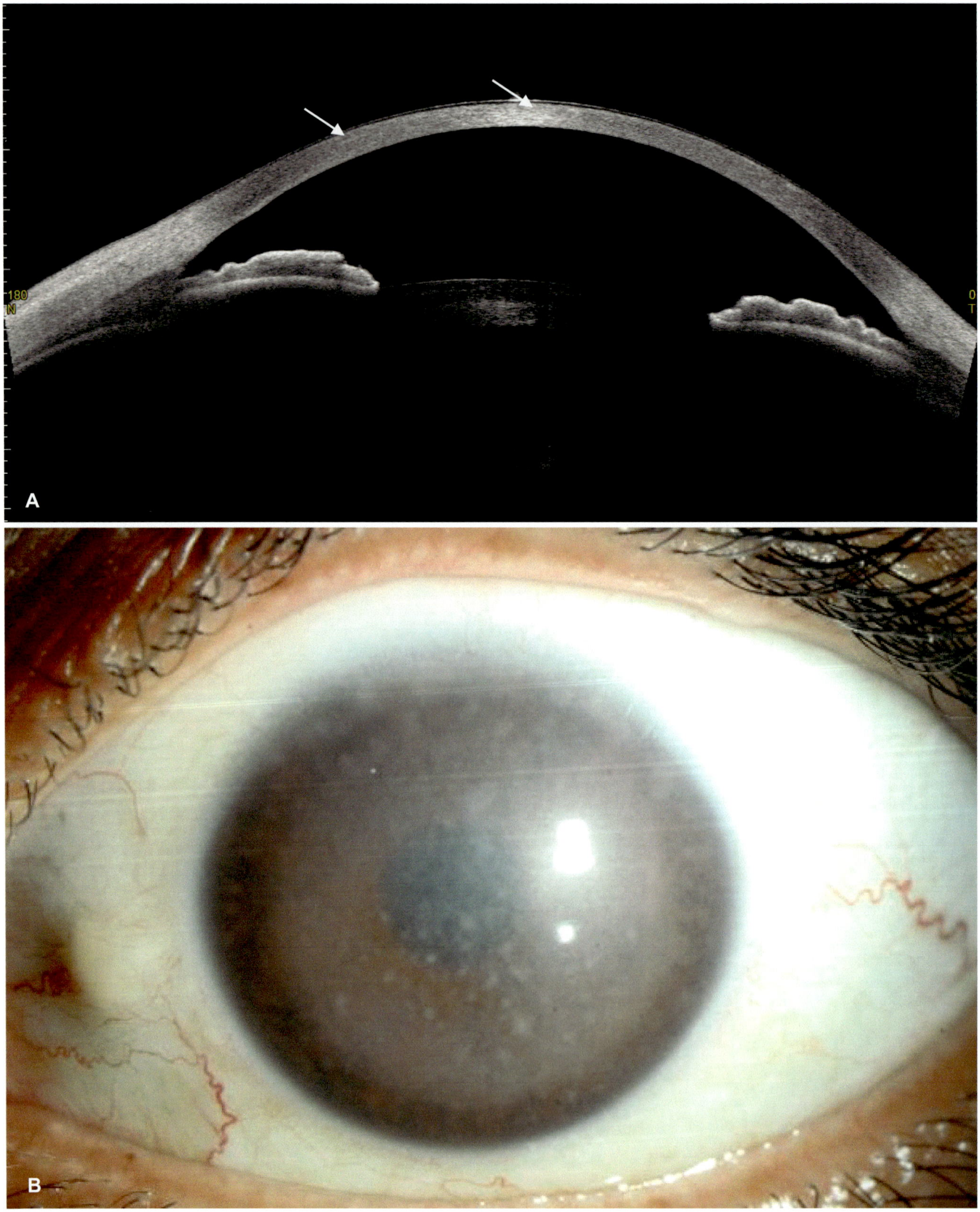

Fig. 24 (**A, B**) Macular corneal dystrophy (stromal dystrophy). Stromal mucopolysaccharide deposits (arrows). (**A**) anterior segment optical coherence tomography. (**B**) slit lamp imaging

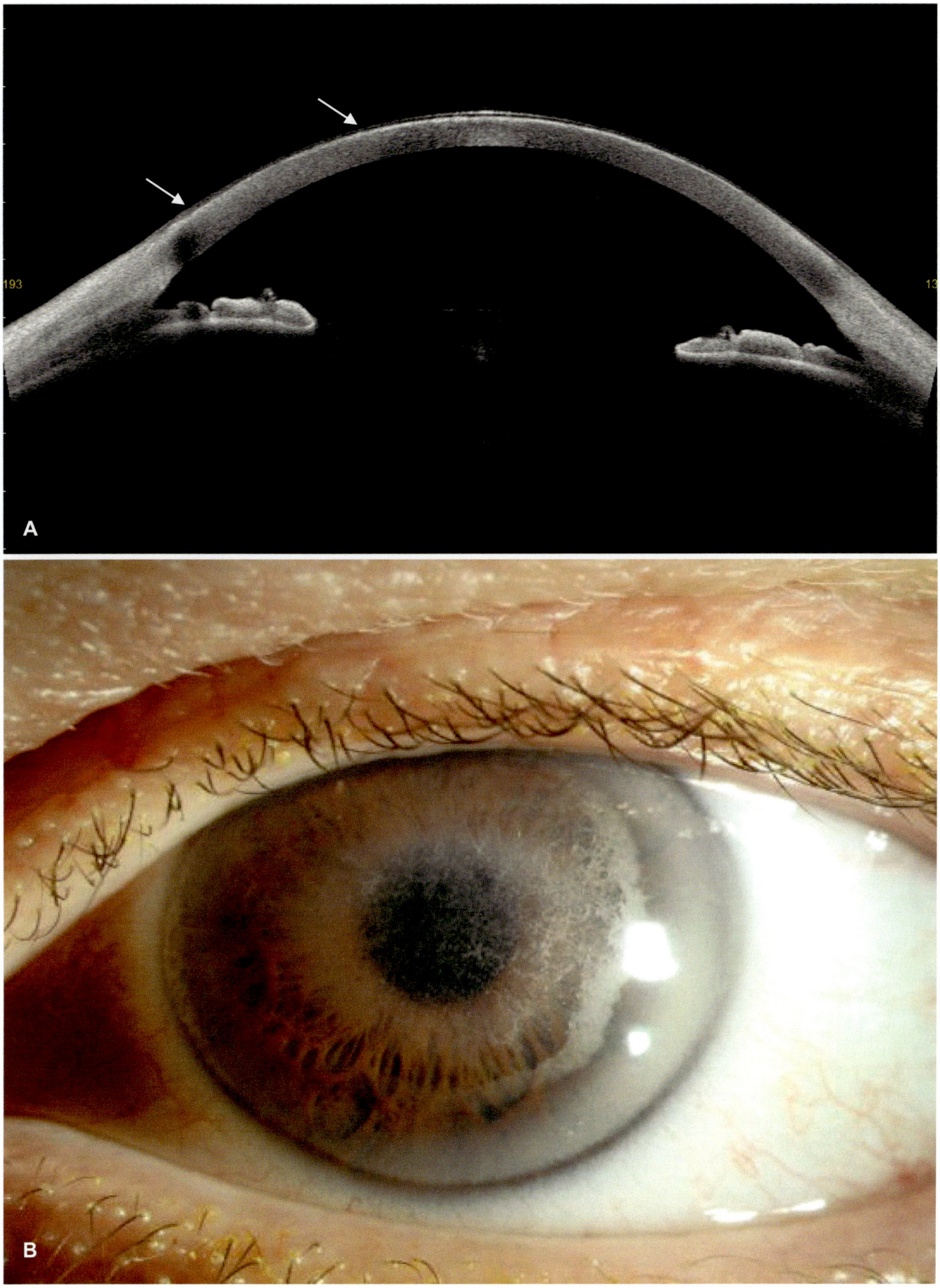

Fig. 25 (**A, B**) Schnyder corneal dystrophy with crystals (stromal dystrophy). Peripheral arcus lipoides and central crystalline deposits (arrows). (**A**) anterior segment optical coherence tomography. (**B**) slit lamp imaging

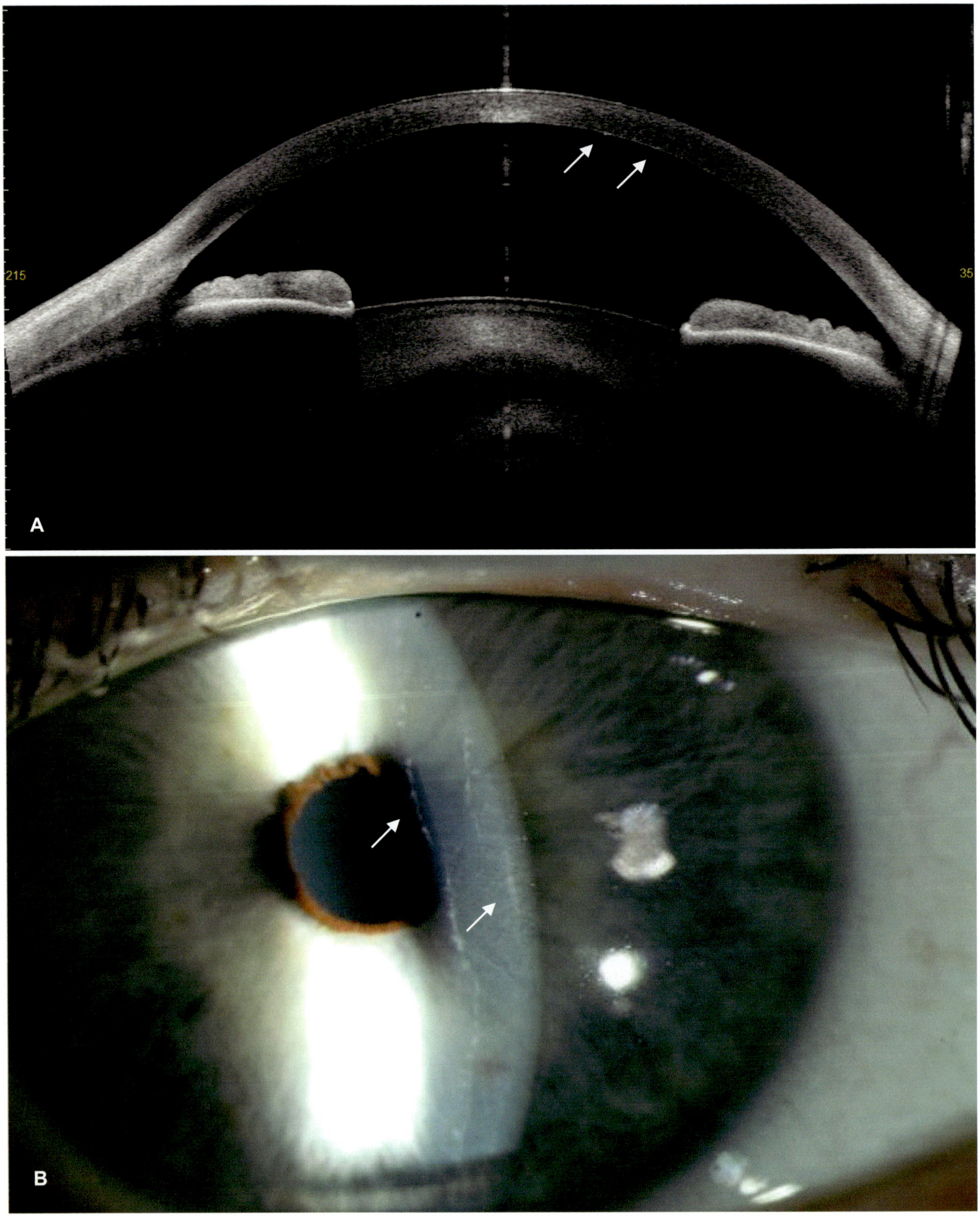

Fig. 26 (**A, B**) Posterior polymorphous corneal dystrophy (endothelial dystrophy). "Railroad track sign"—common finding. (**A**) anterior segment optical coherence tomography. (**B**) slit lamp imaging

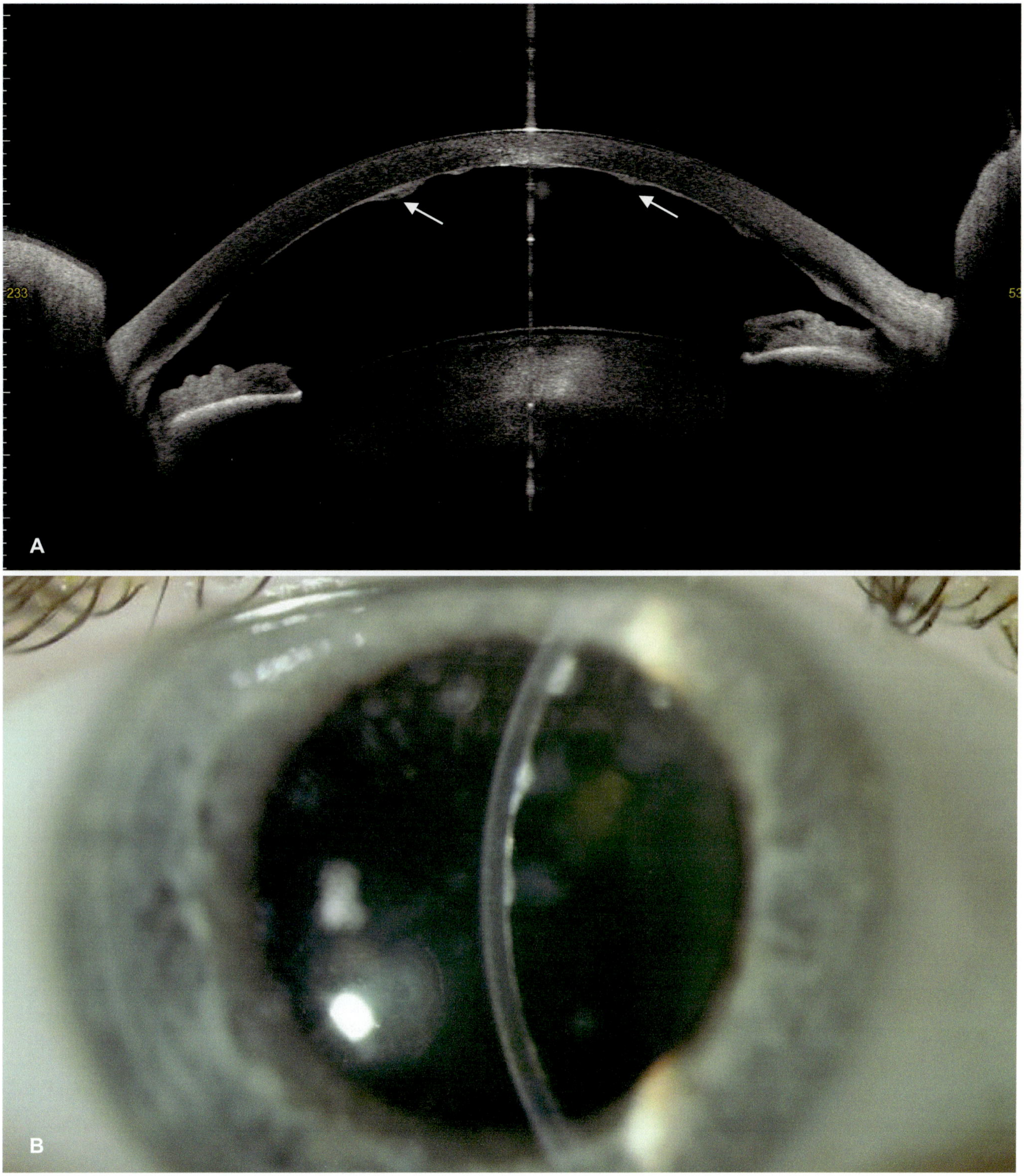

Fig. 27 (**A, B**) Posterior polymorphous corneal dystrophy (endothelial dystrophy). Rare case with extensive retrocorneal deposits [9]. (**A**) anterior segment optical coherence tomography. (**B**) slit lamp imaging

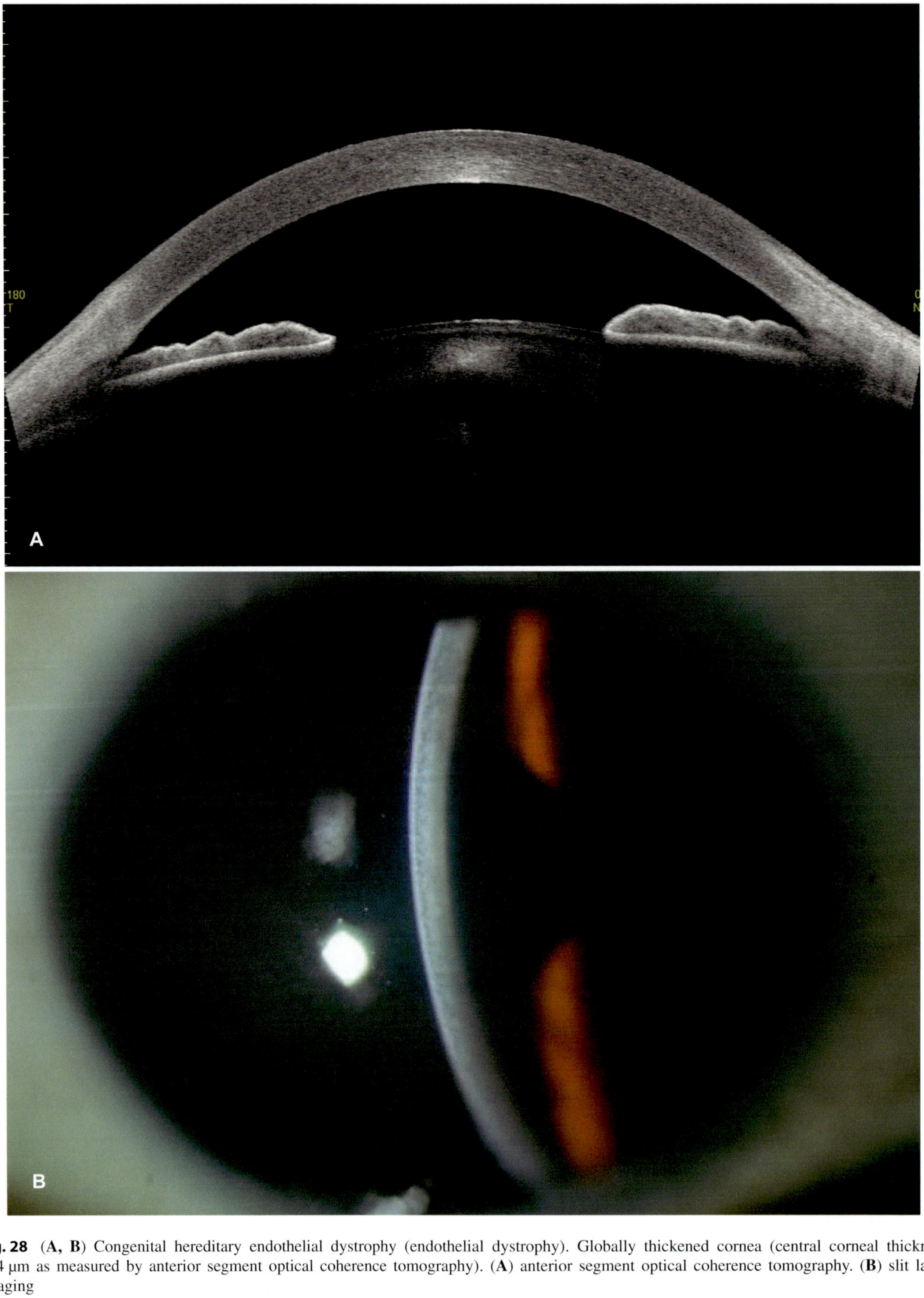

Fig. 28 (**A, B**) Congenital hereditary endothelial dystrophy (endothelial dystrophy). Globally thickened cornea (central corneal thickness 924 µm as measured by anterior segment optical coherence tomography). (**A**) anterior segment optical coherence tomography. (**B**) slit lamp imaging

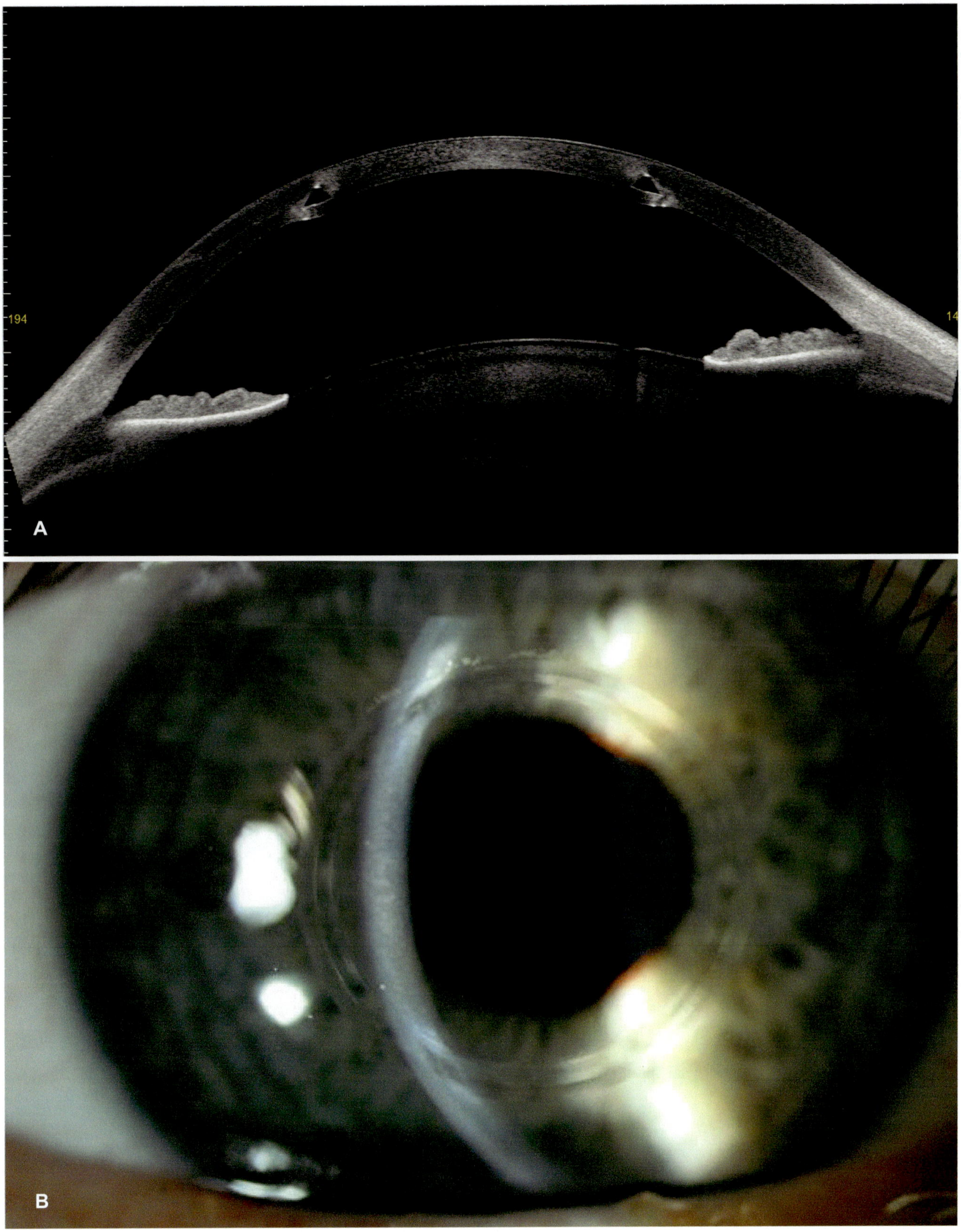

Fig. 29 (**A, B**) Myoring® (complete ring according to Daxer [10], triangular) in keratoconus. (**A**) anterior segment optical coherence tomography. (**B**) slit lamp imaging

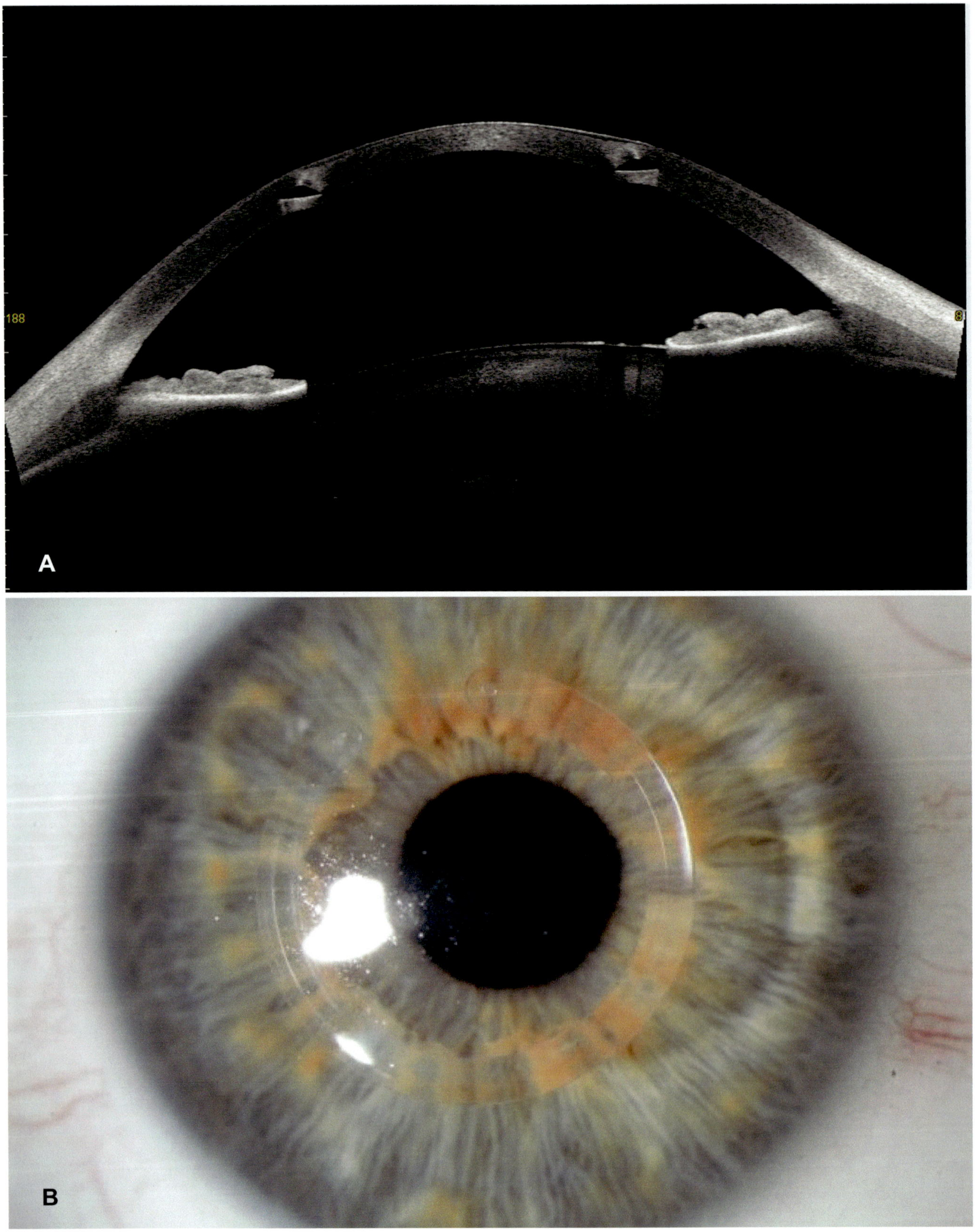

Fig. 30 (**A, B**) Ferrara ring® (gap between 11–12 o'clock position, triangular) in keratoconus. (**A**) anterior segment optical coherence tomography. (**B**) slit lamp imaging

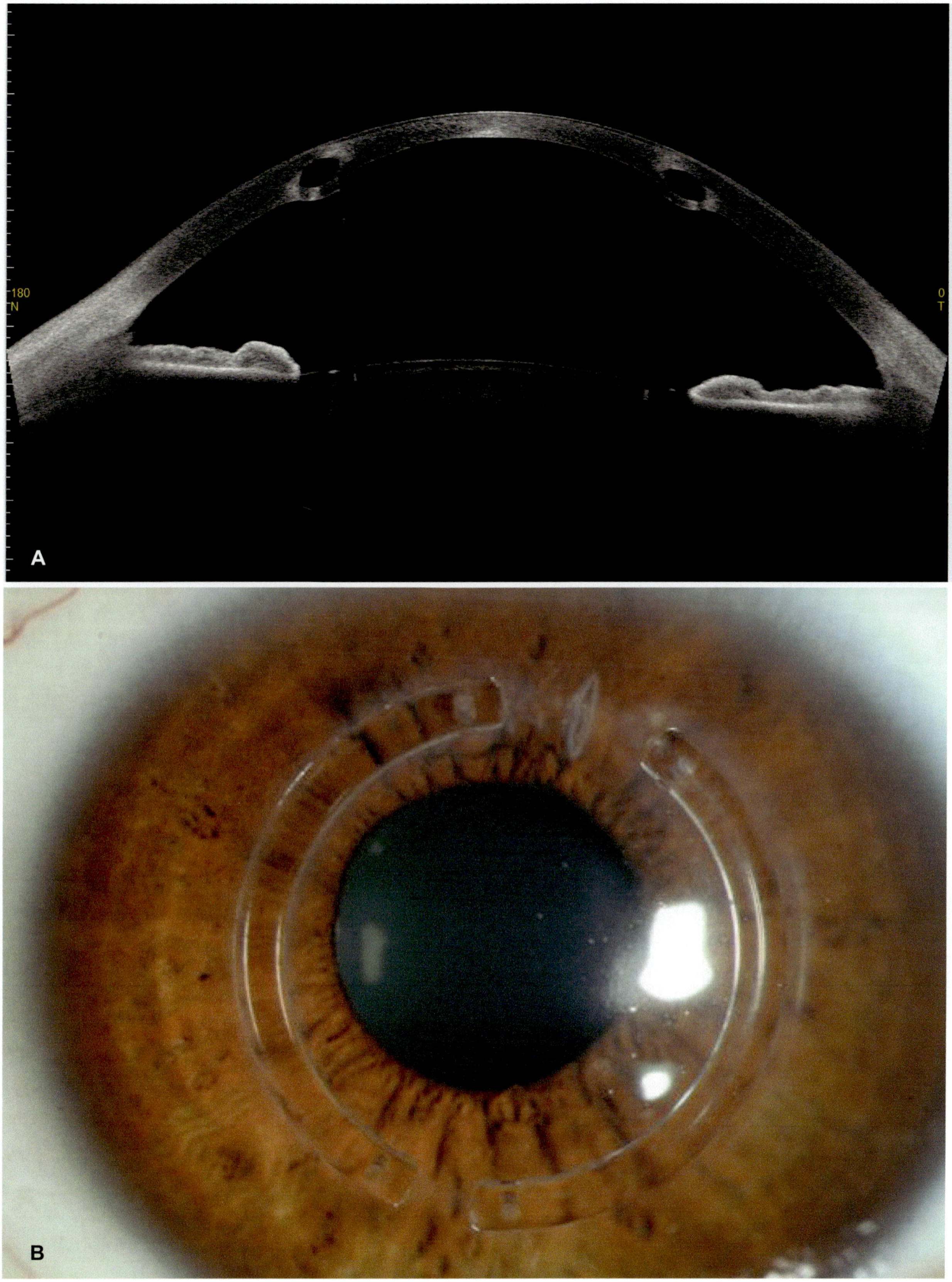

Fig. 31 (**A, B**) INTACS SK® ring segments (hexagonal) in keratoconus. (**A**) anterior segment optical coherence tomography. (**B**) slit lamp imaging

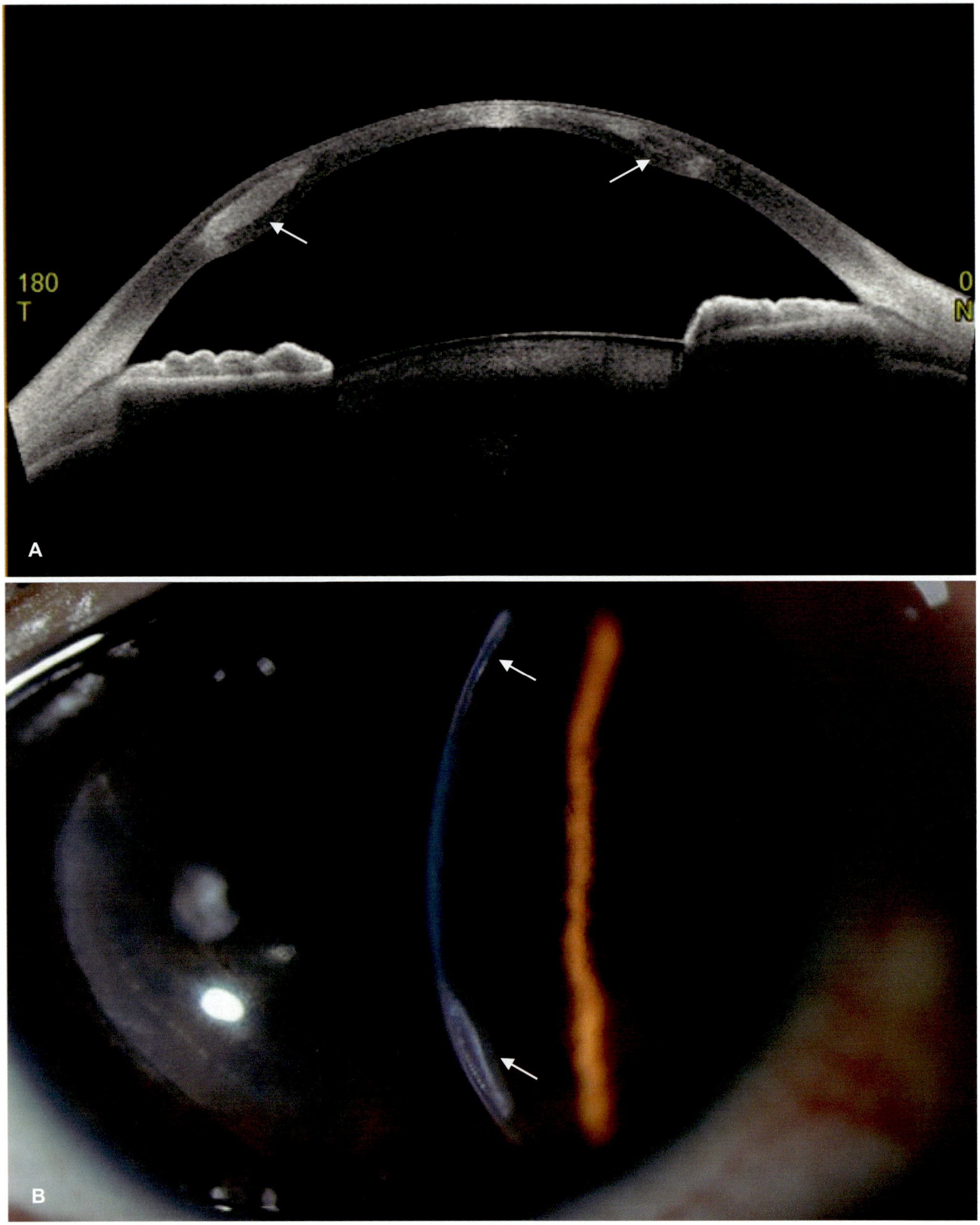

Fig. 32 (**A, B**) Asymmetric Corneal Allogenic Intrastromal Ring Segments (CAIRS) in keratoconus. (**A**) anterior segment optical coherence tomography. (**B**) slit lamp imaging

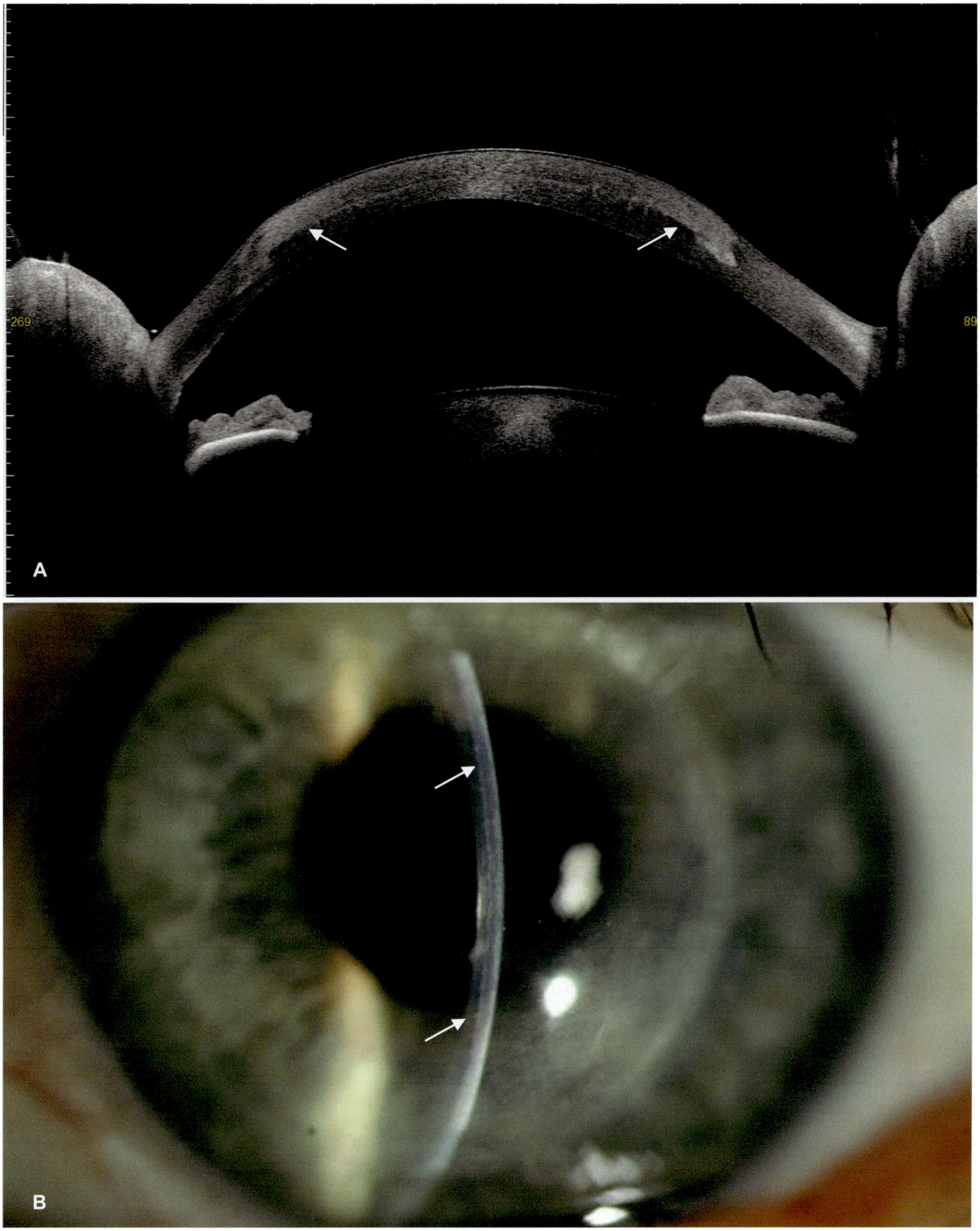

Fig. 33 (**A, B**) Epikeratophakia in keratoconus with the aim of restoring a normal corneal thickness by suturing a corneal donor lenticule (arrows) onto the thinned cornea. (**A**) anterior segment optical coherence tomography. (**B**) slit lamp imaging

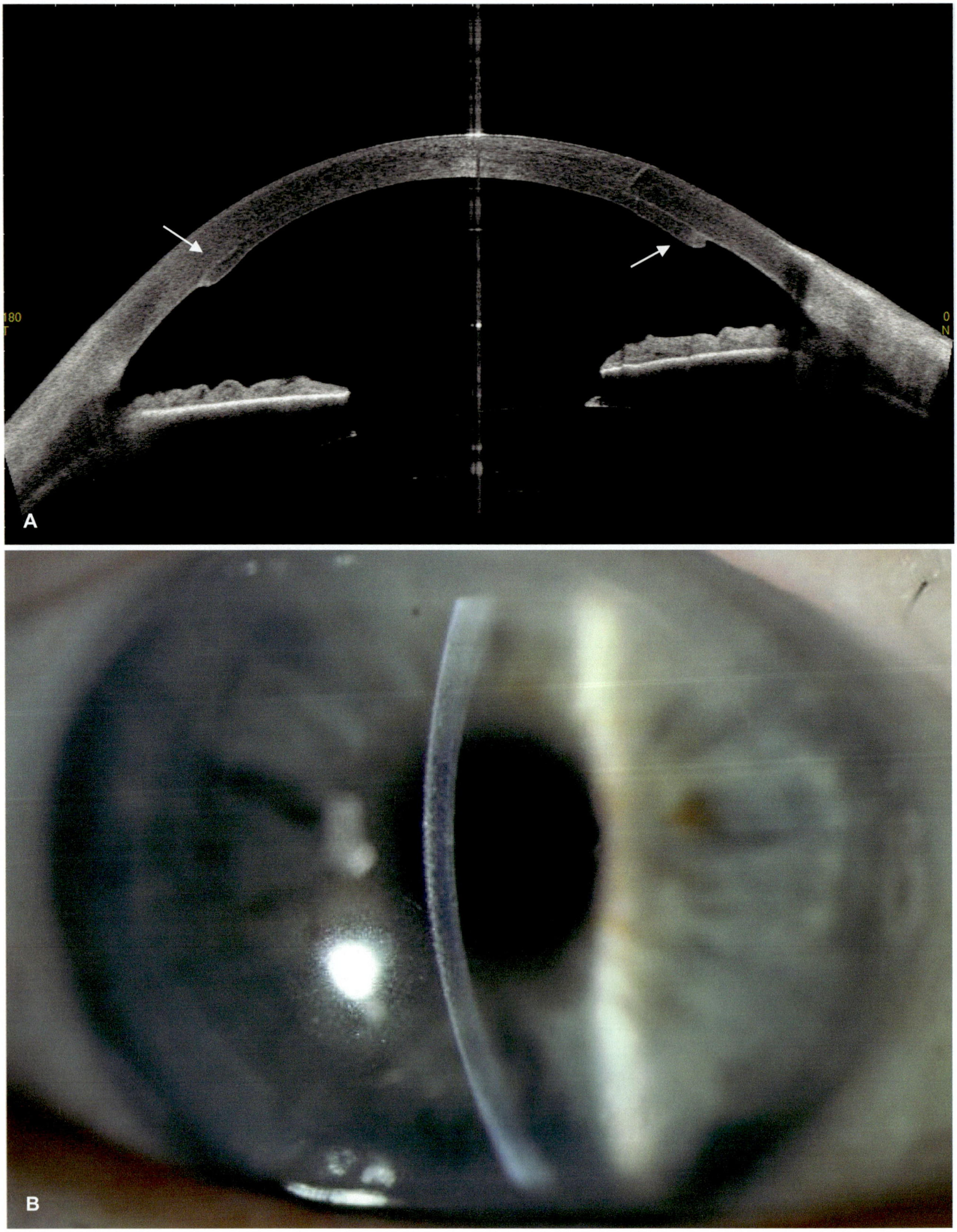

Fig. 34 (**A, B**) Descemet Stripping (Automated) Endothelial Keratoplasty (DSAEK, arrows) in Fuchs endothelial dystrophy. (**A**) anterior segment optical coherence tomography. (**B**) slit lamp imaging

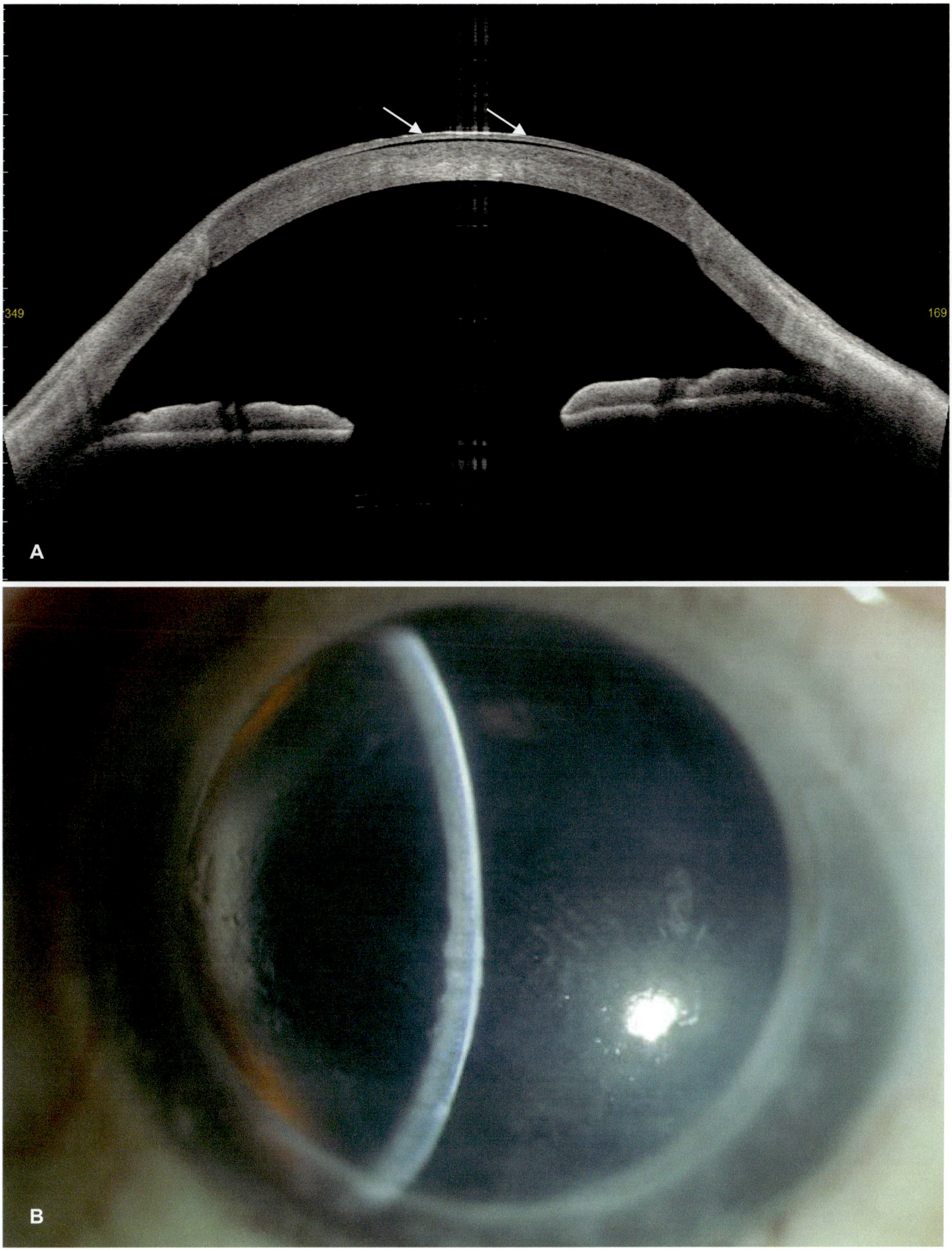

Fig. 35 (**A, B**) Interface fluid syndrome in a penetrating keratoplasty graft presumably treated with refractive surgery prior to transplantation. (**A**) anterior segment optical coherence tomography. (**B**) slit lamp imaging

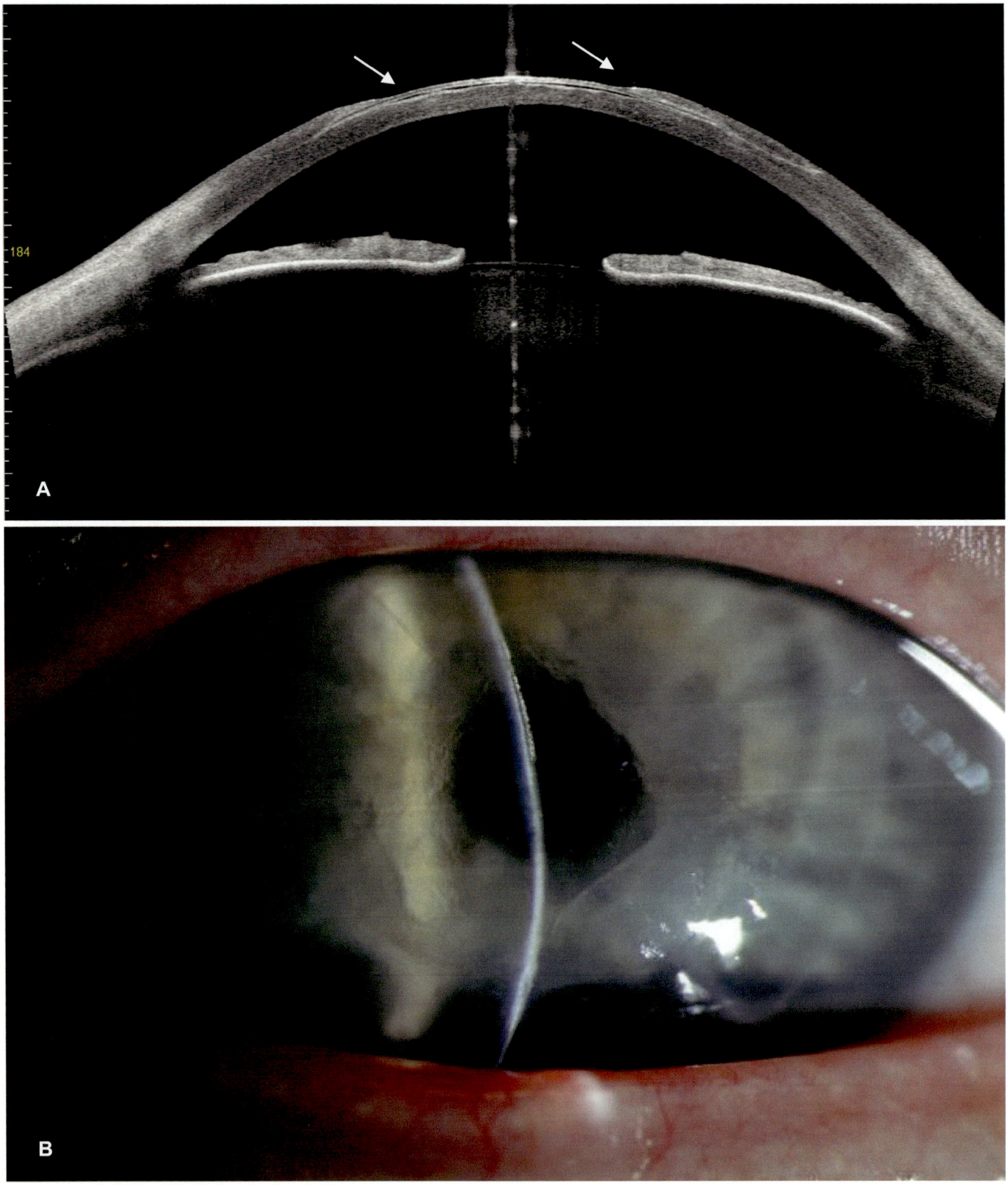

Fig. 36 (**A, B**) Corneal melting after porcine corneal lenticule implantation in a human keratoconus cornea with intention to improve topography and visual acuity (arrows [11]). (**A**) anterior segment optical coherence tomography. (**B**) slit lamp imaging

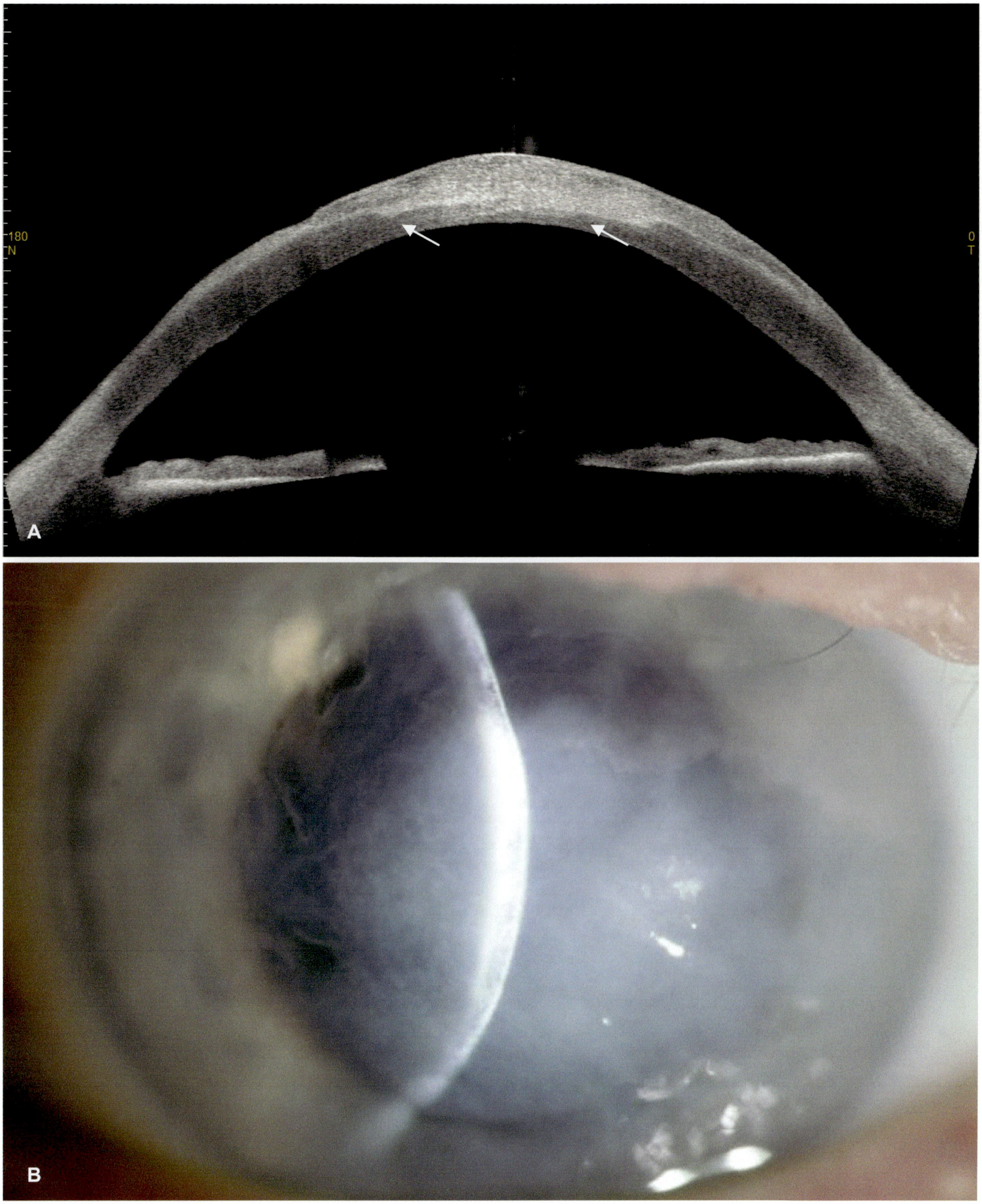

Fig. 37 (**A, B**) Giant Salzmann nodular degeneration after deep stromal corneal ulceration (arrows). Treatment consisted of pannectomy and excimerlaser-assisted penetrating keratoplasty. (**A**) anterior segment optical coherence tomography. (**B**) slit lamp imaging

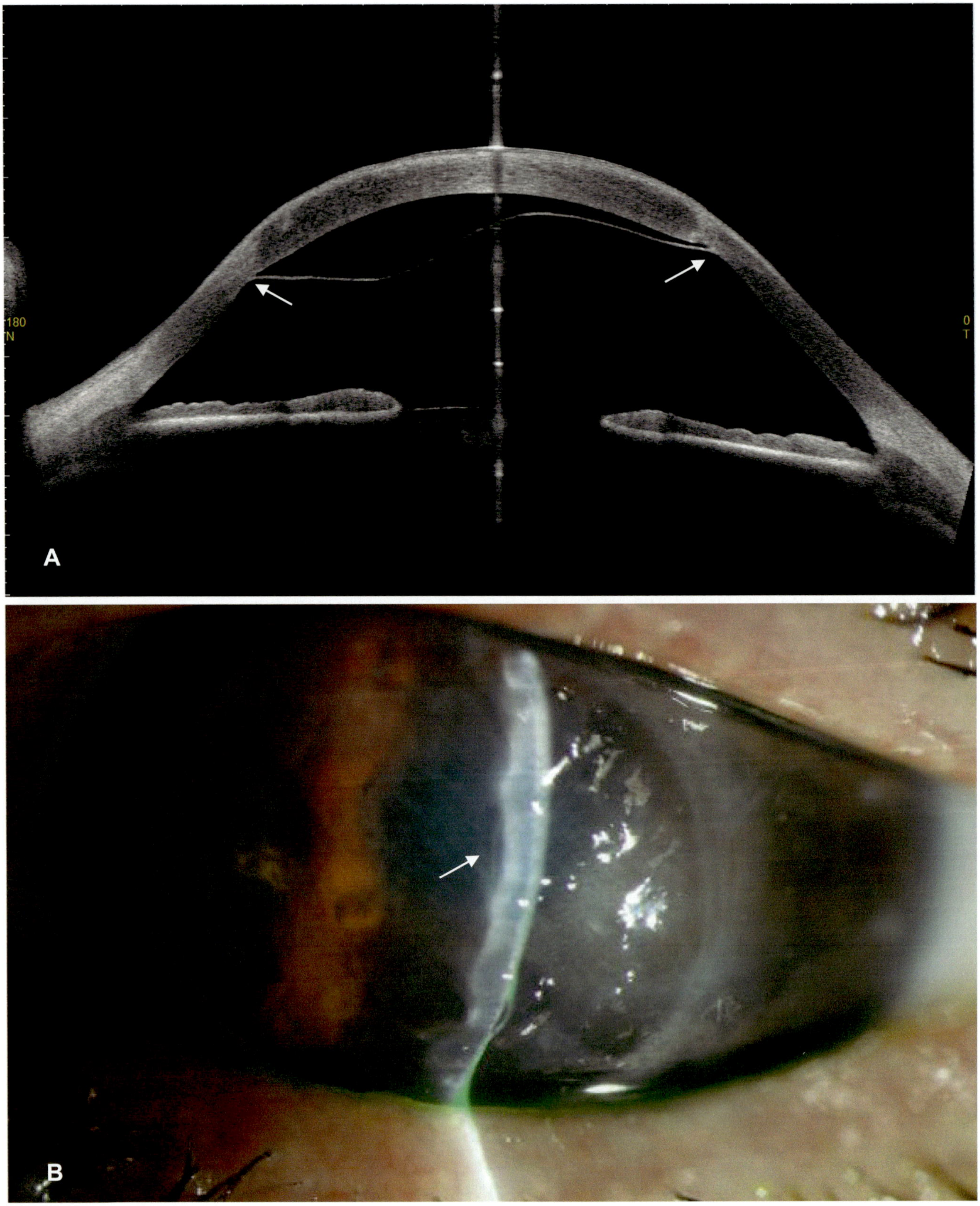

Fig. 38 (**A, B**) Chronic descemetolysis after penetrating keratoplasty, presumably because of secondary graft ectasia. Descemet membrane still attached at the host-graft interface (arrows). (**A**) anterior segment optical coherence tomography. (**B**) slit lamp imaging

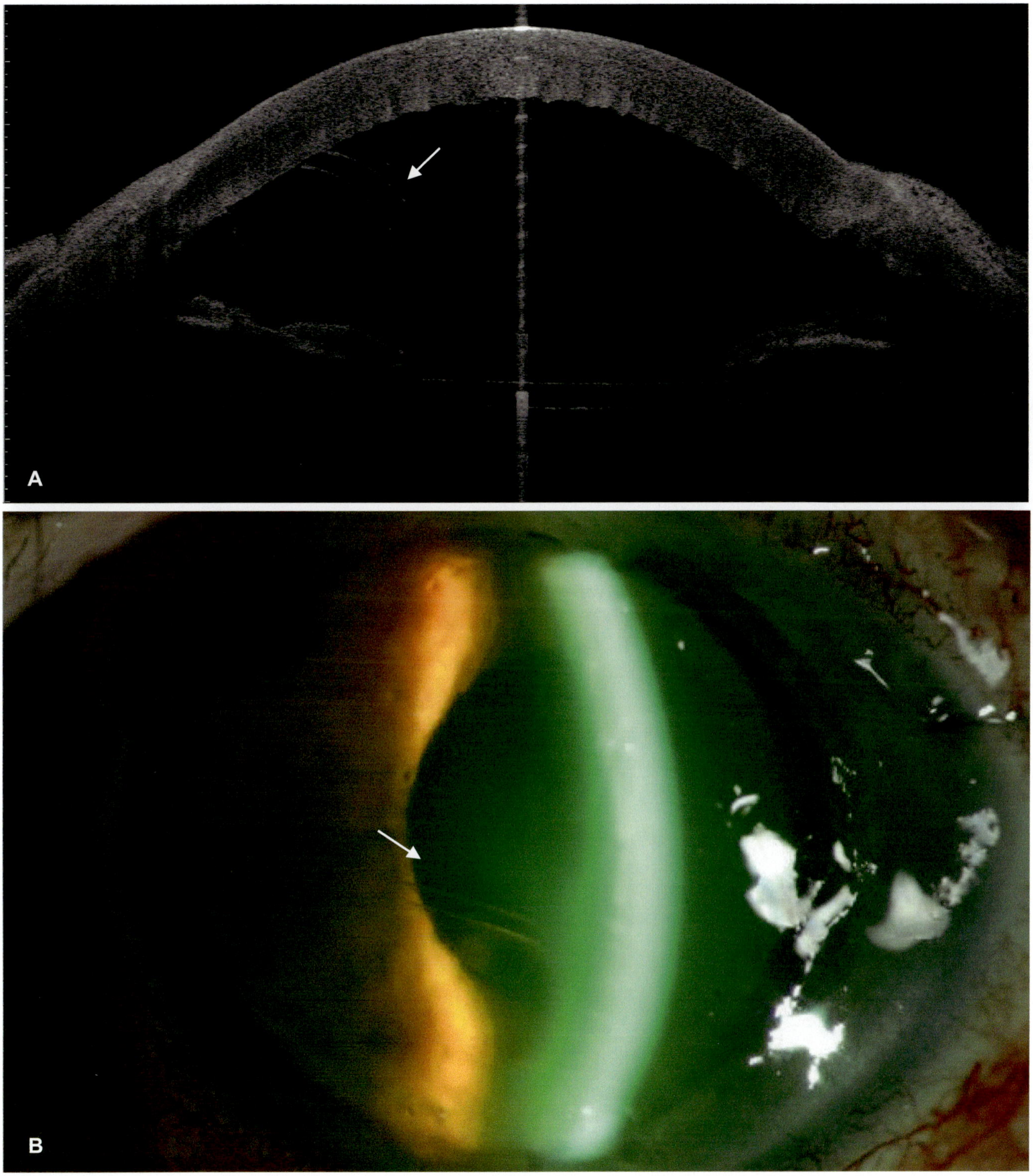

Fig. 39 (**A, B**) Completely detached and rolled Descemet-endothelium-lamella after Descemet membrane endothelial keratoplasty (DMEK, arrows). (**A**) anterior segment optical coherence tomography. (**B**) slit lamp imaging

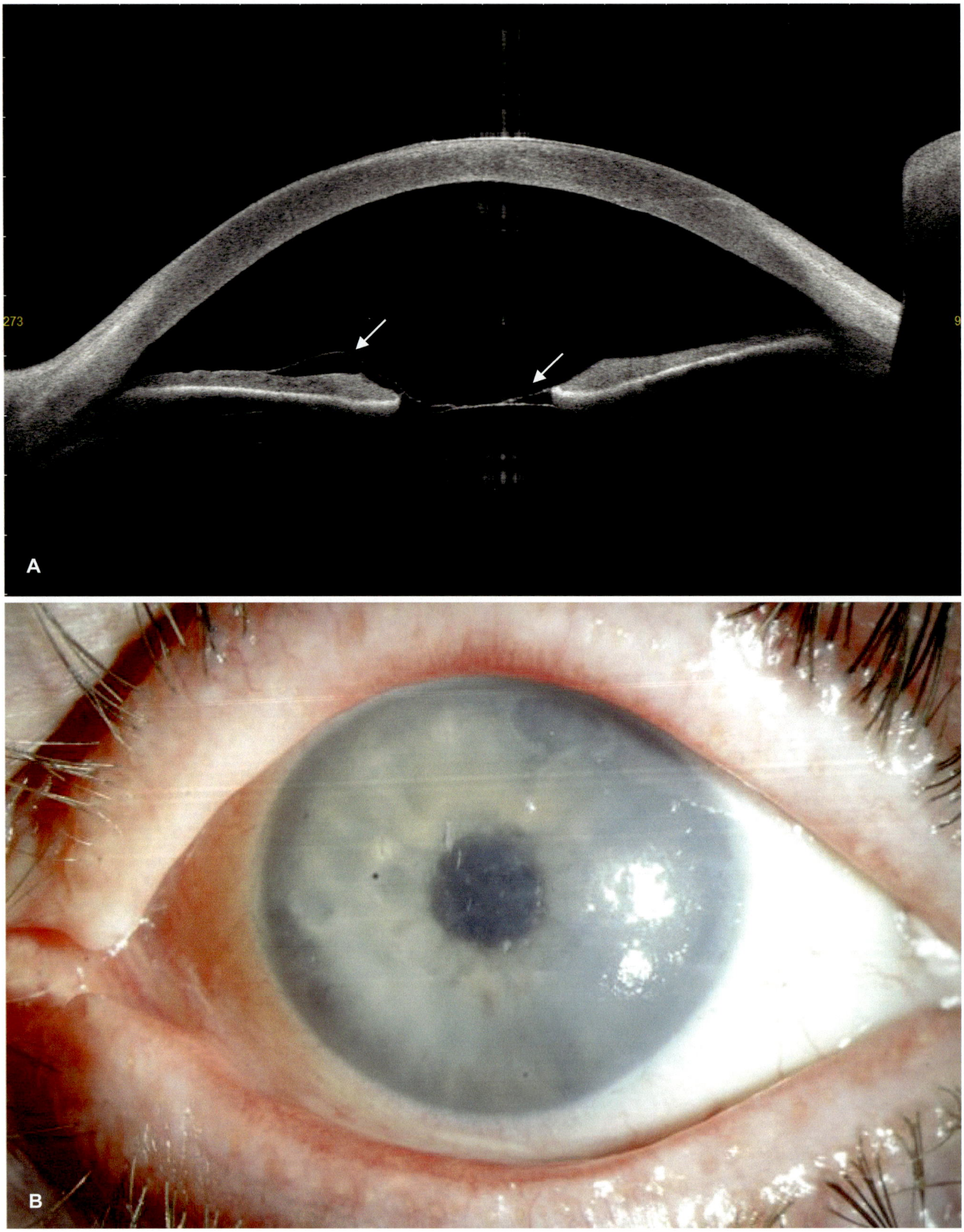

Fig. 40 (**A, B**) Completely detached Descemet-endothelium-lamella adhering to the iris and intraocular lens after Descemet membrane endothelial keratoplasty (DMEK, arrows). (**A**) anterior segment optical coherence tomography. (**B**) slit lamp imaging

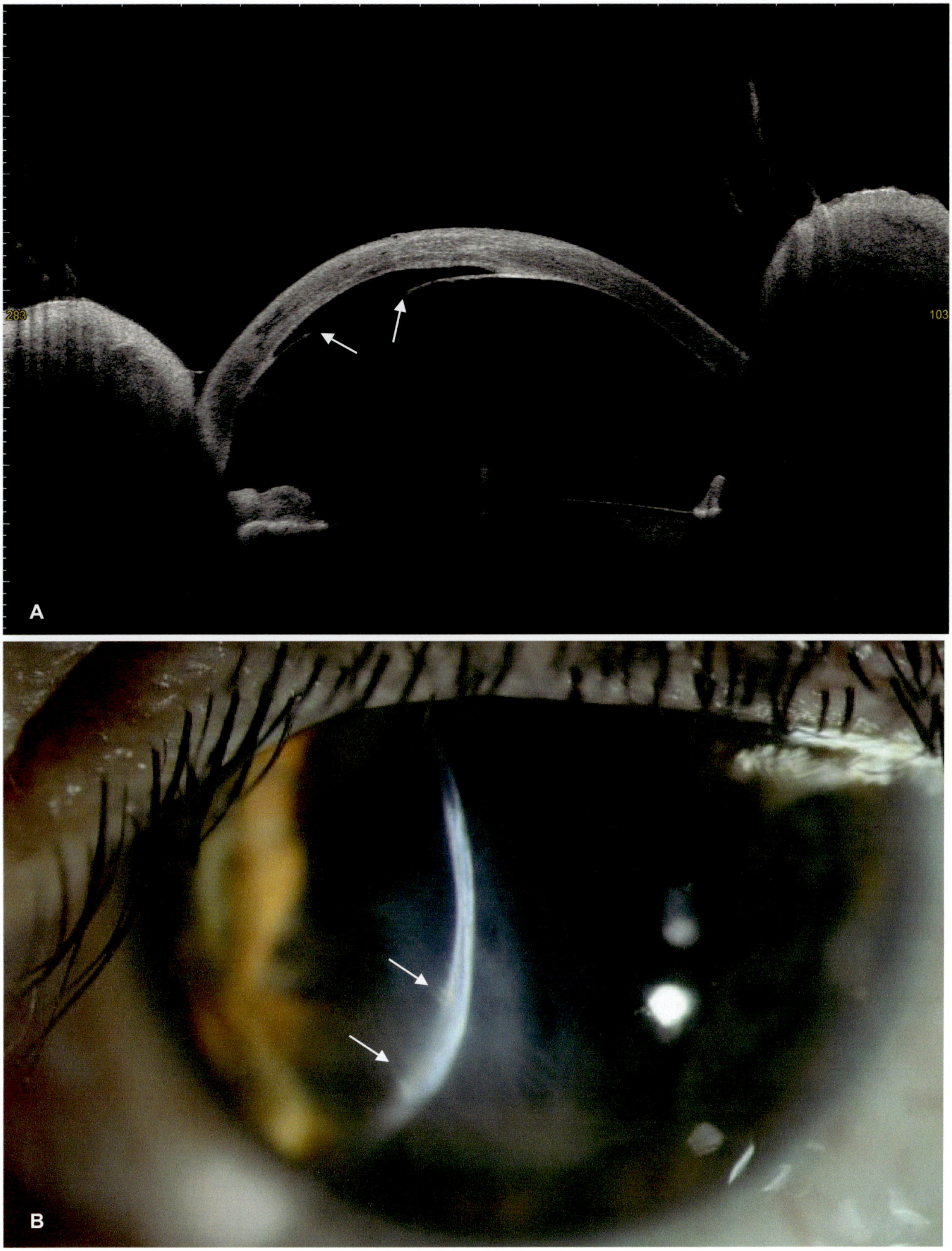

Fig. 41 (**A, B**) Descemet tear with previous hydrops in advanced keratoconus (arrows) with deep stromal scarring. (**A**) anterior segment optical coherence tomography. (**B**) slit lamp imaging

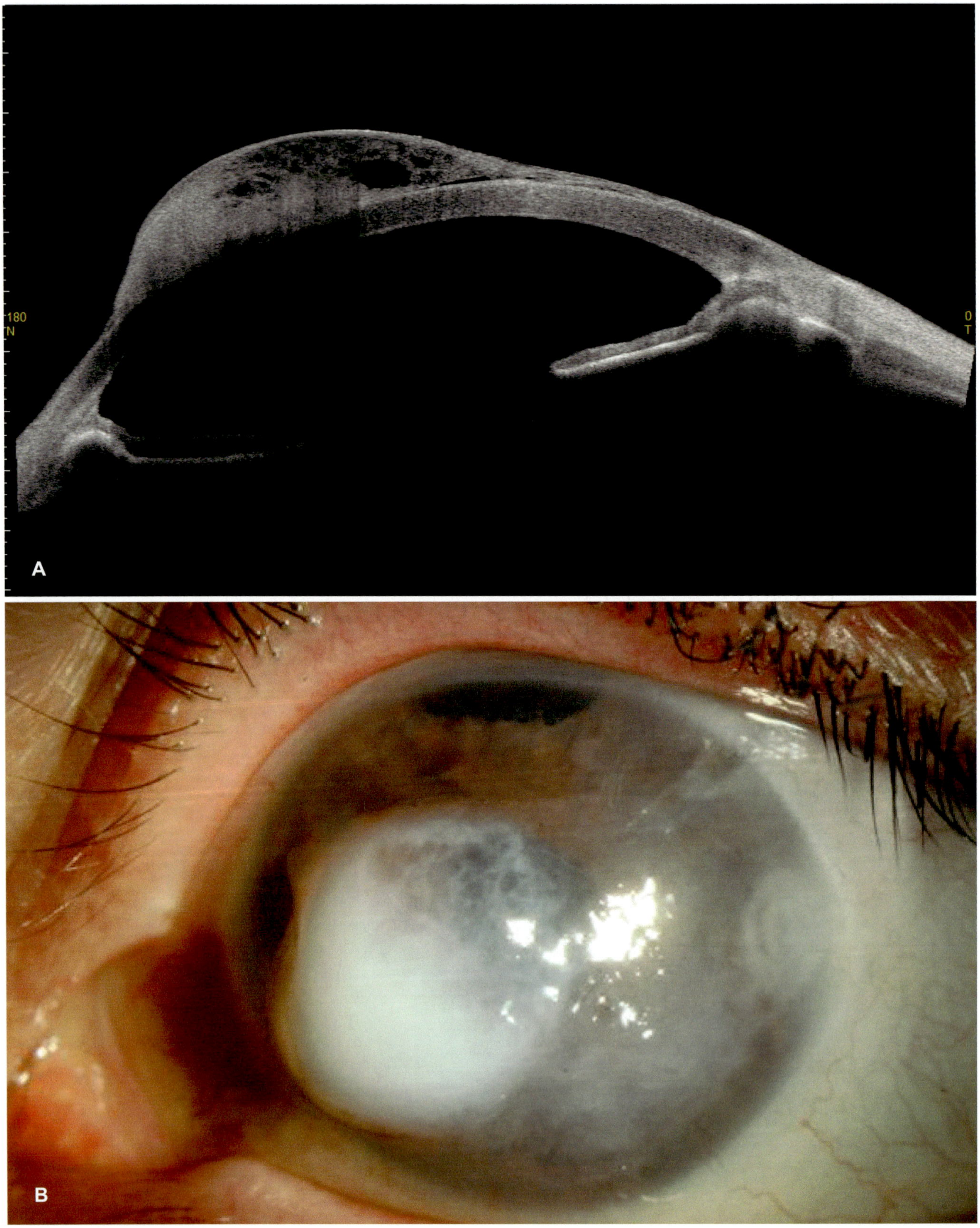

Fig. 42 (**A, B**) Suspected corneal hydrops—anterior segment optical coherence tomography revealing a giant Salzmann nodular degeneration [12]. (**A**) anterior segment optical coherence tomography. (**B**) slit lamp imaging

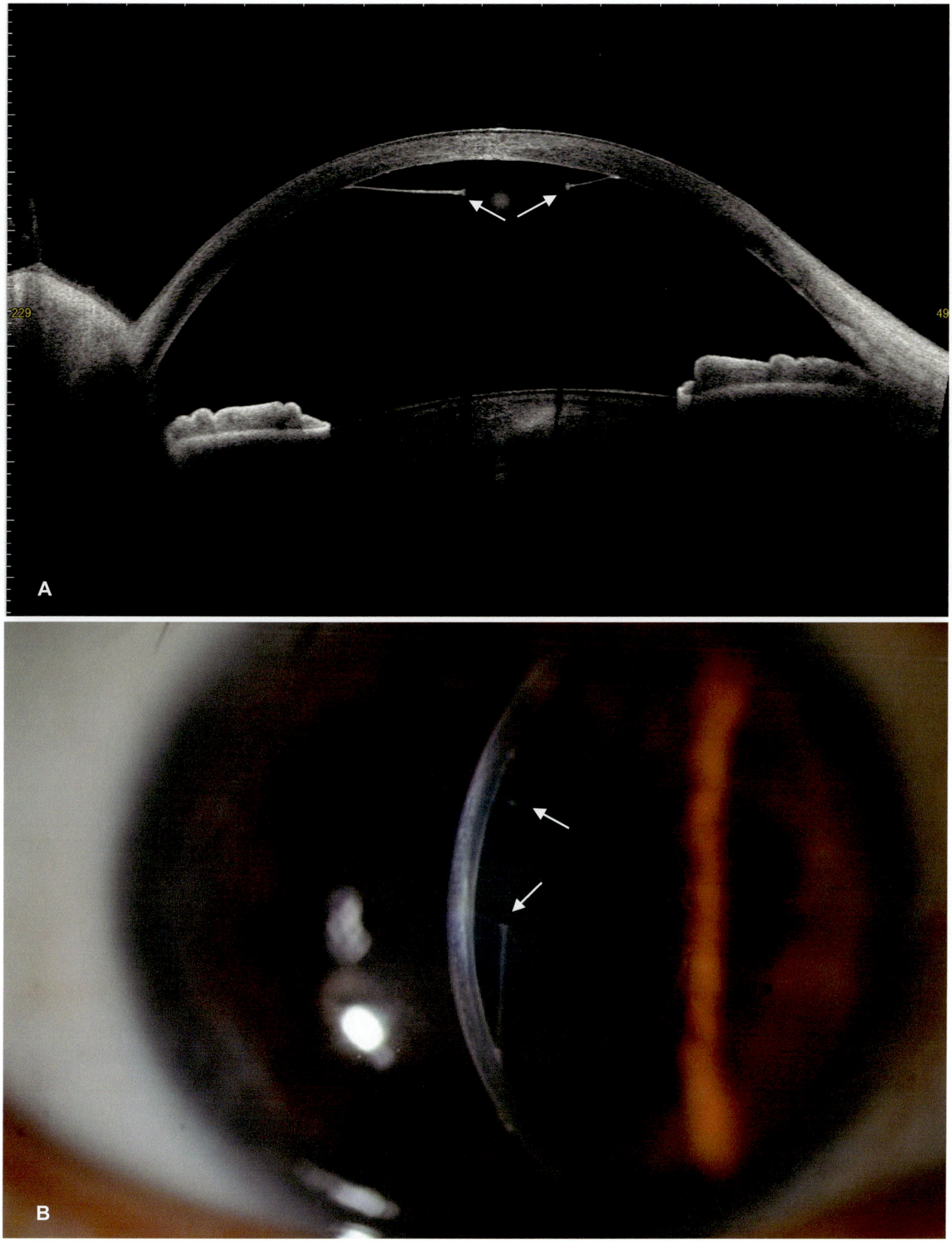

Fig. 43 (**A, B**) Persisting descemetolysis with Descemet tear presumably in juvenile keratoconus (arrows) because of keratoconus in the fellow eye. (**A**) anterior segment optical coherence tomography. (**B**) slit lamp imaging

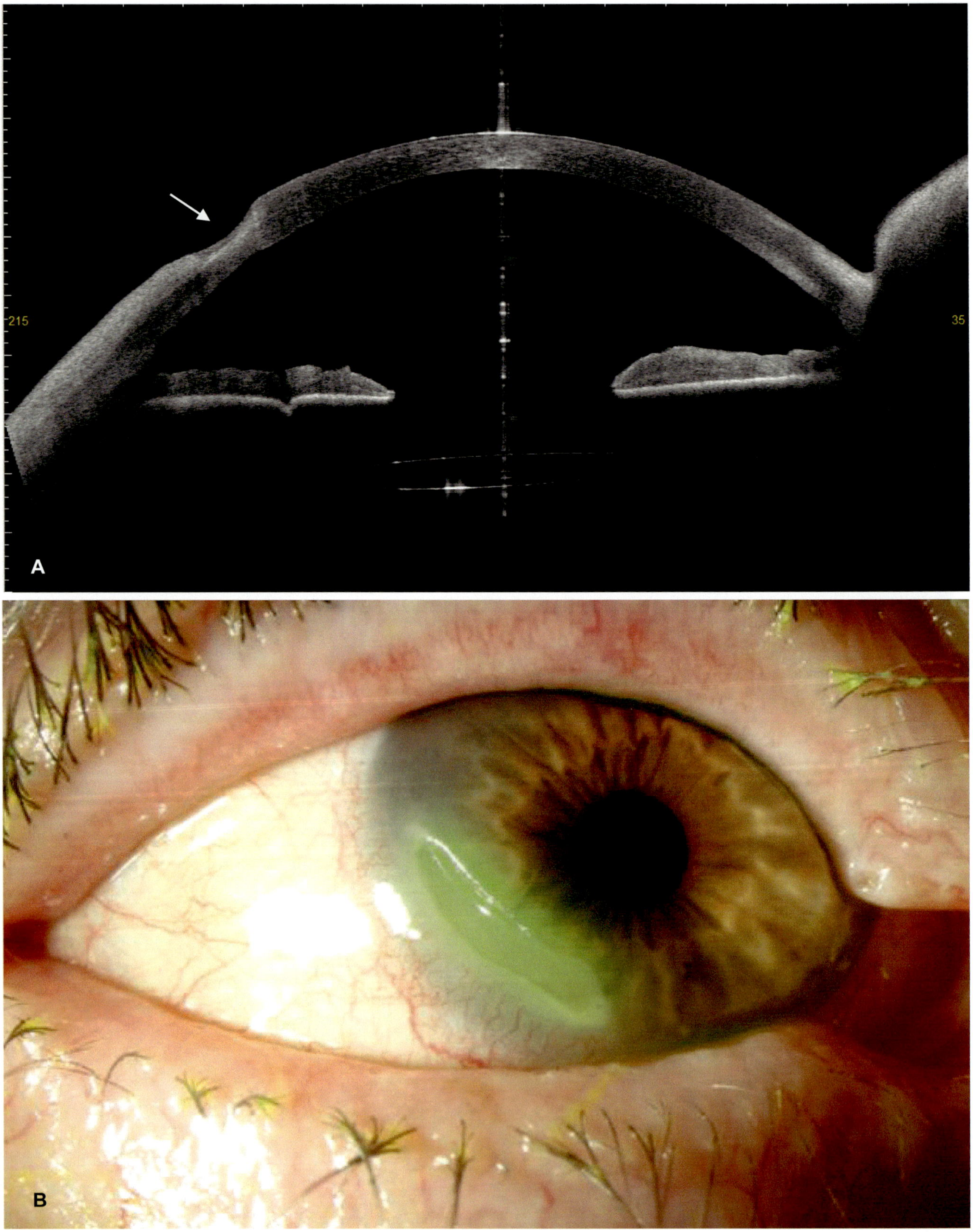

Fig. 44 (**A, B**) Sterile rheumatic corneal ulcer (arrow) in case of Peripheral Ulcerative Keratitis (PUK). (**A**) anterior segment optical coherence tomography. (**B**) slit lamp imaging

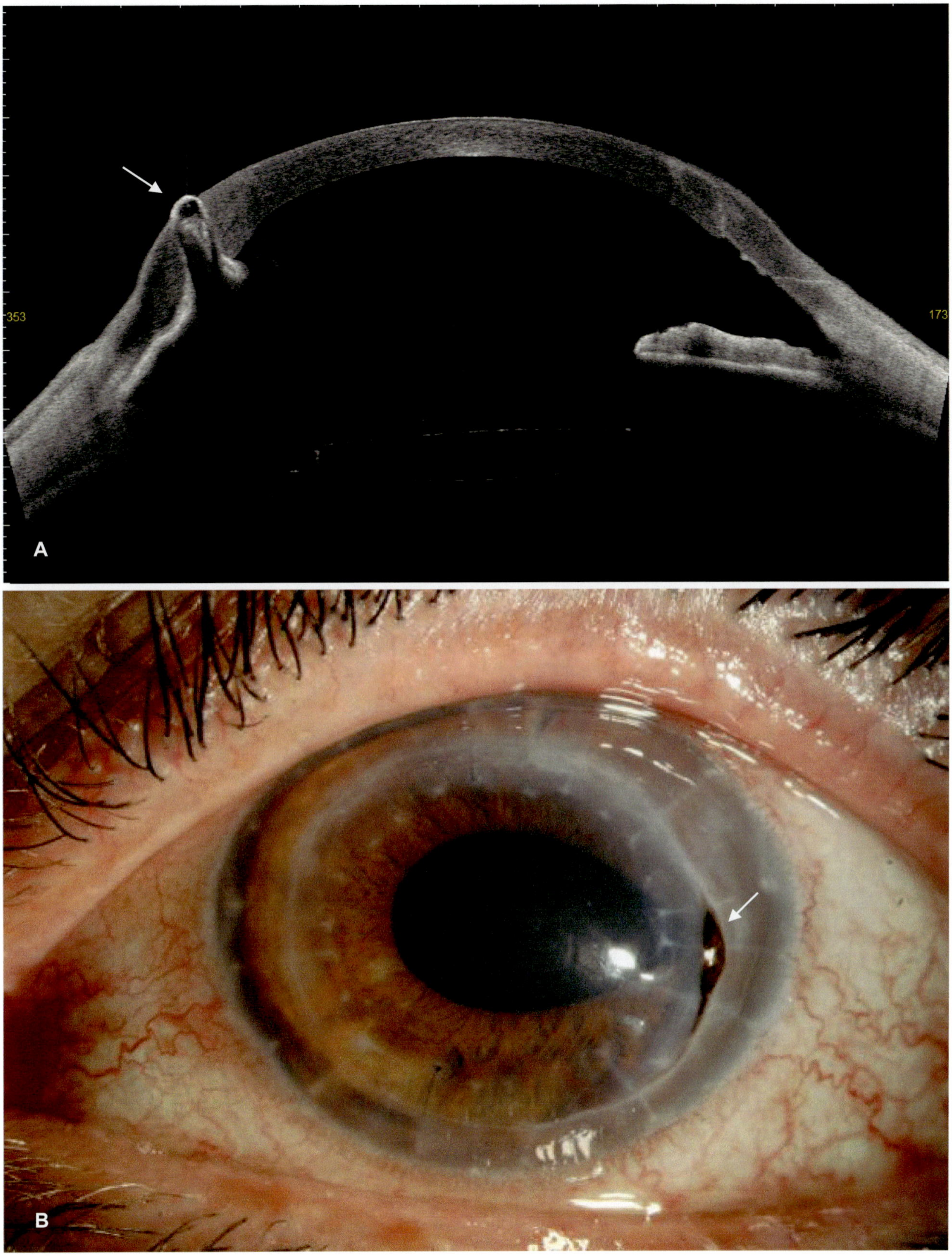

Fig. 45 (**A, B**) Graft dehiscence after forced eye rubbing with iris prolapse after PKP (arrows). (**A**) anterior segment optical coherence tomography. (**B**) slit lamp imaging

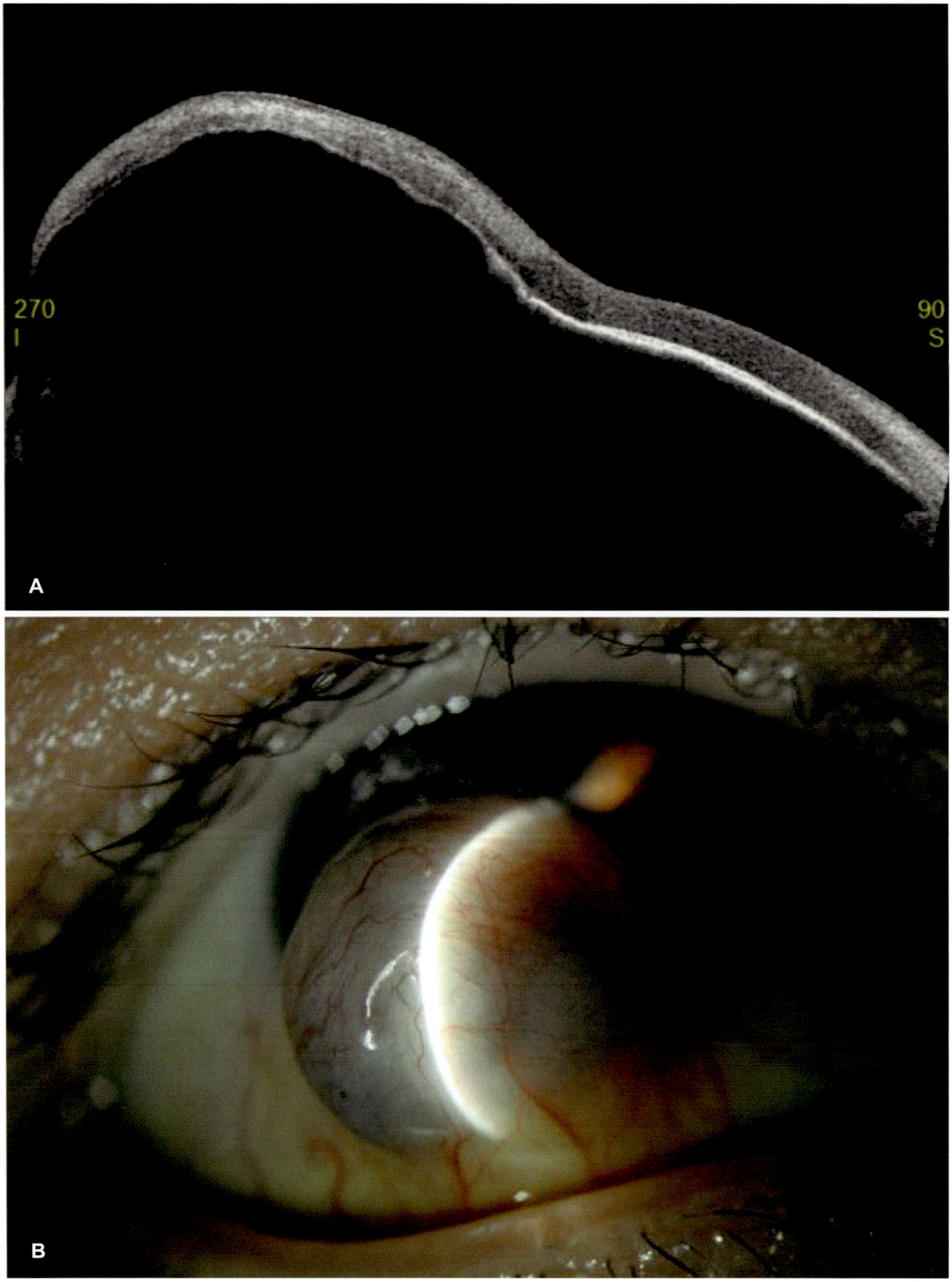

Fig. 46 (**A, B**) Anterior chamber herniation after covering a corneal perforation with multiple amniotic membrane grafts. (**A**) anterior segment optical coherence tomography. (**B**) slit lamp imaging

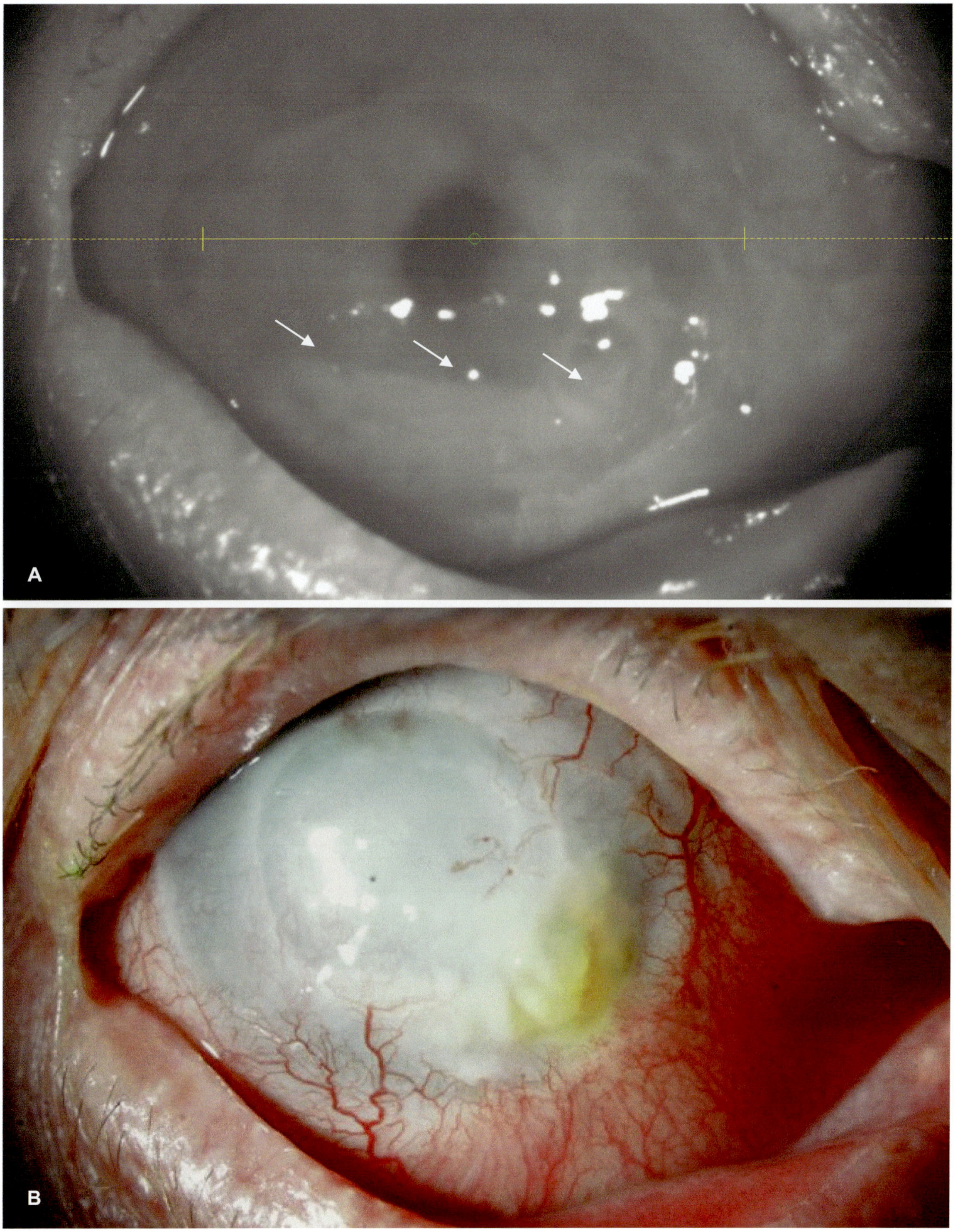

Fig. 47 (**A, B**) Anterior segment optical coherence tomography may help in diagnosing hypopyon in cases of opaque corneas (arrows). (**A**) anterior segment optical coherence tomography. (**B**) slit lamp imaging

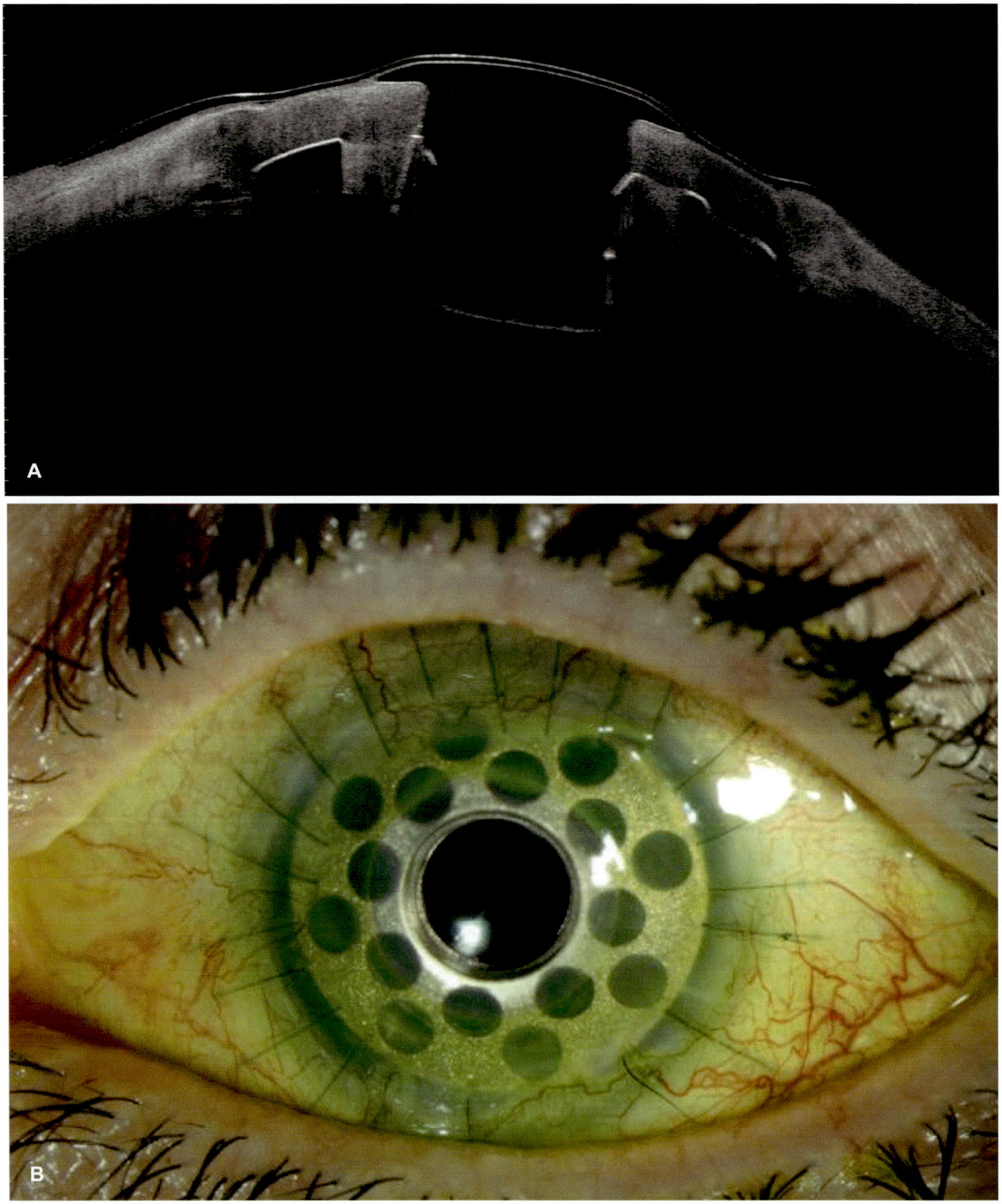

Fig. 48 (**A, B**) Boston keratoprosthesis type I: Bandage contact lens, central optical cylinder surrounded by a human corneal graft, followed by a back plate with holes and a locking ring. (**A**) anterior segment optical coherence tomography. (**B**) slit lamp imaging

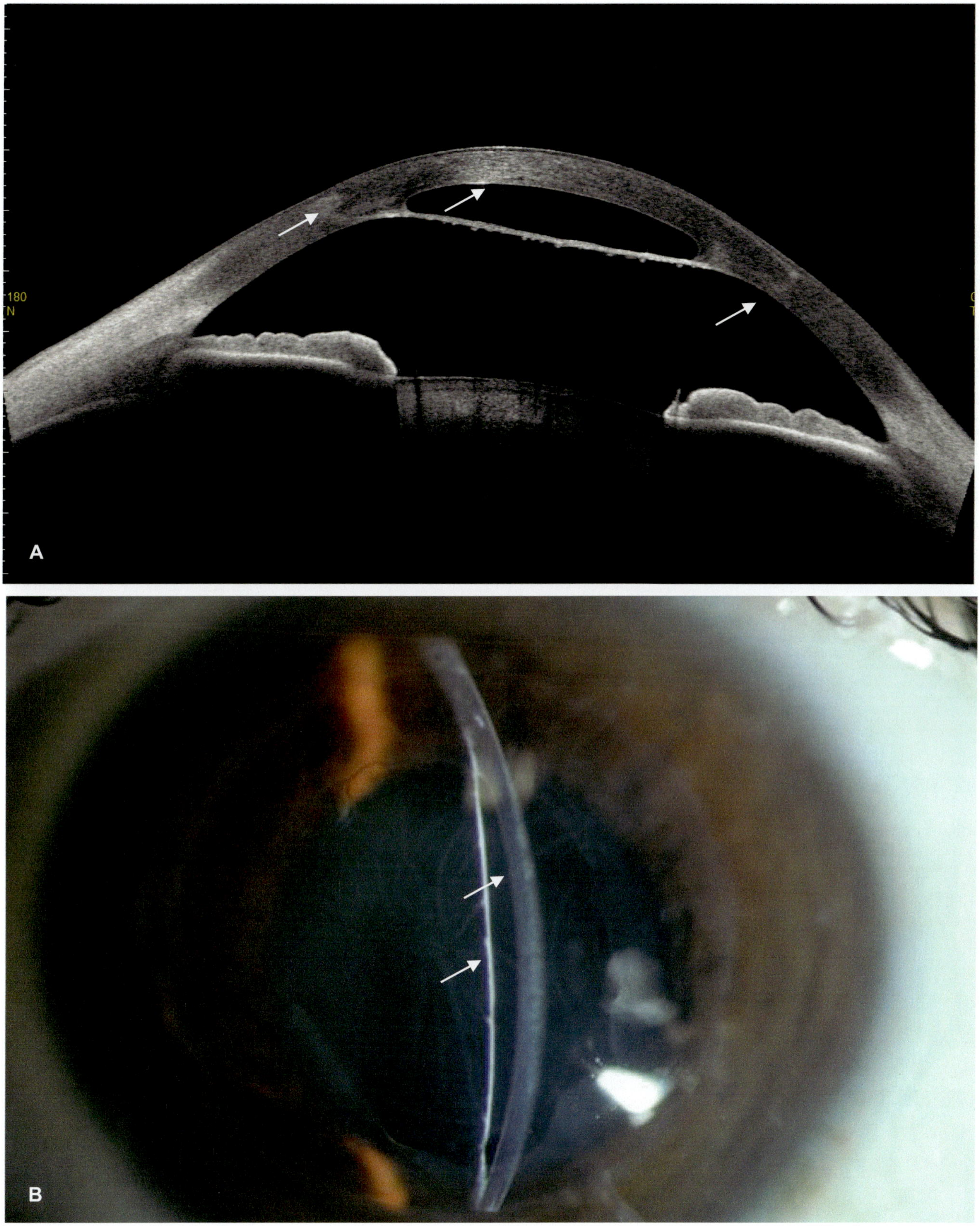

Fig. 49 (**A, B**) Persisting double anterior chamber after central small deep anterior lamellar keratoplasty (DALK) without removing the donor endothelial layer (arrows). (**A**) anterior segment optical coherence tomography. (**B**) slit lamp imaging

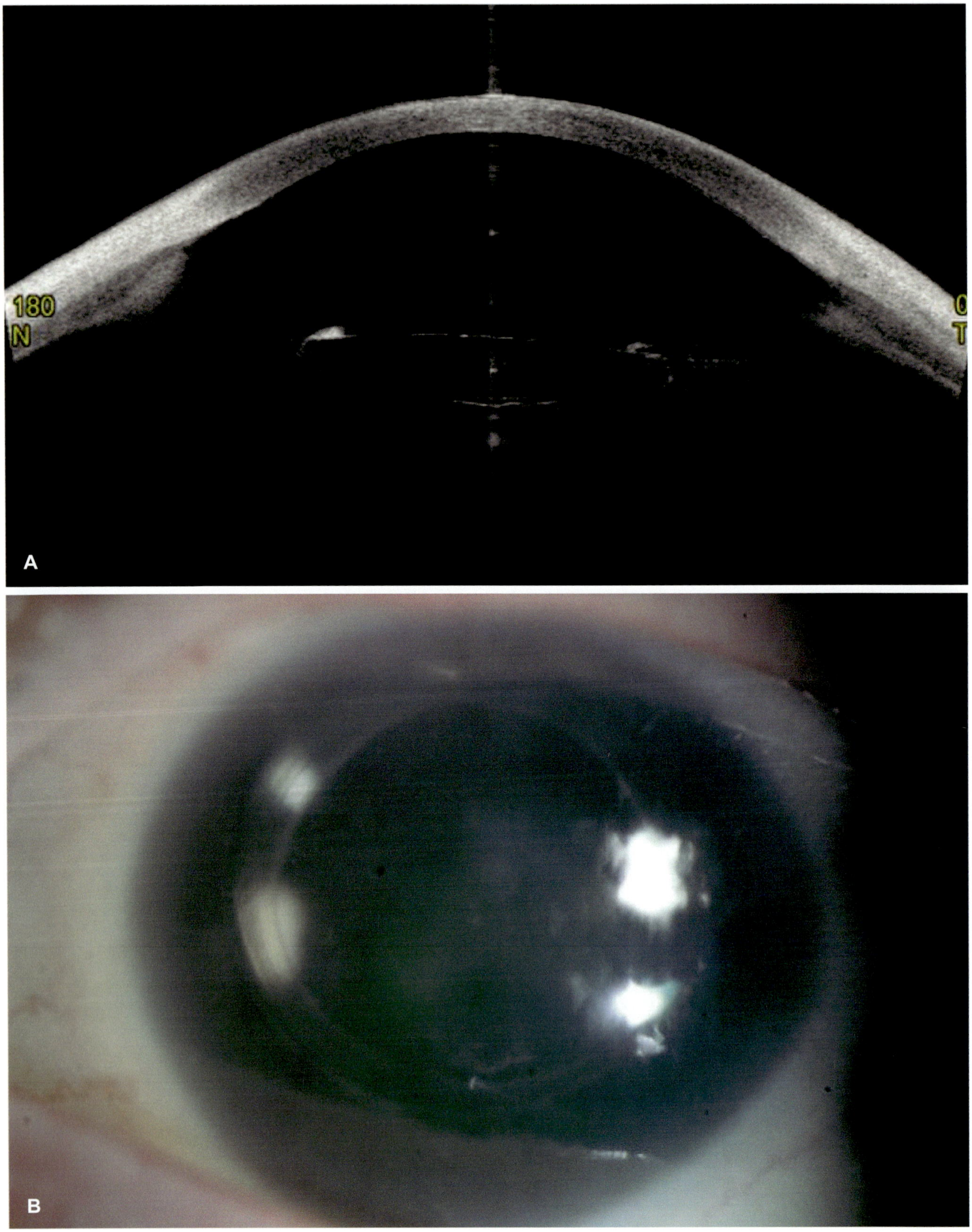

Fig. 50 (**A, B**) Congenital aniridia without limbal stem cell insufficiency and clear cornea. Anterior segment OCT revealing total aniridia with the intraocular lens centered in the bag. (**A**) anterior segment optical coherence tomography. (**B**) slit lamp imaging

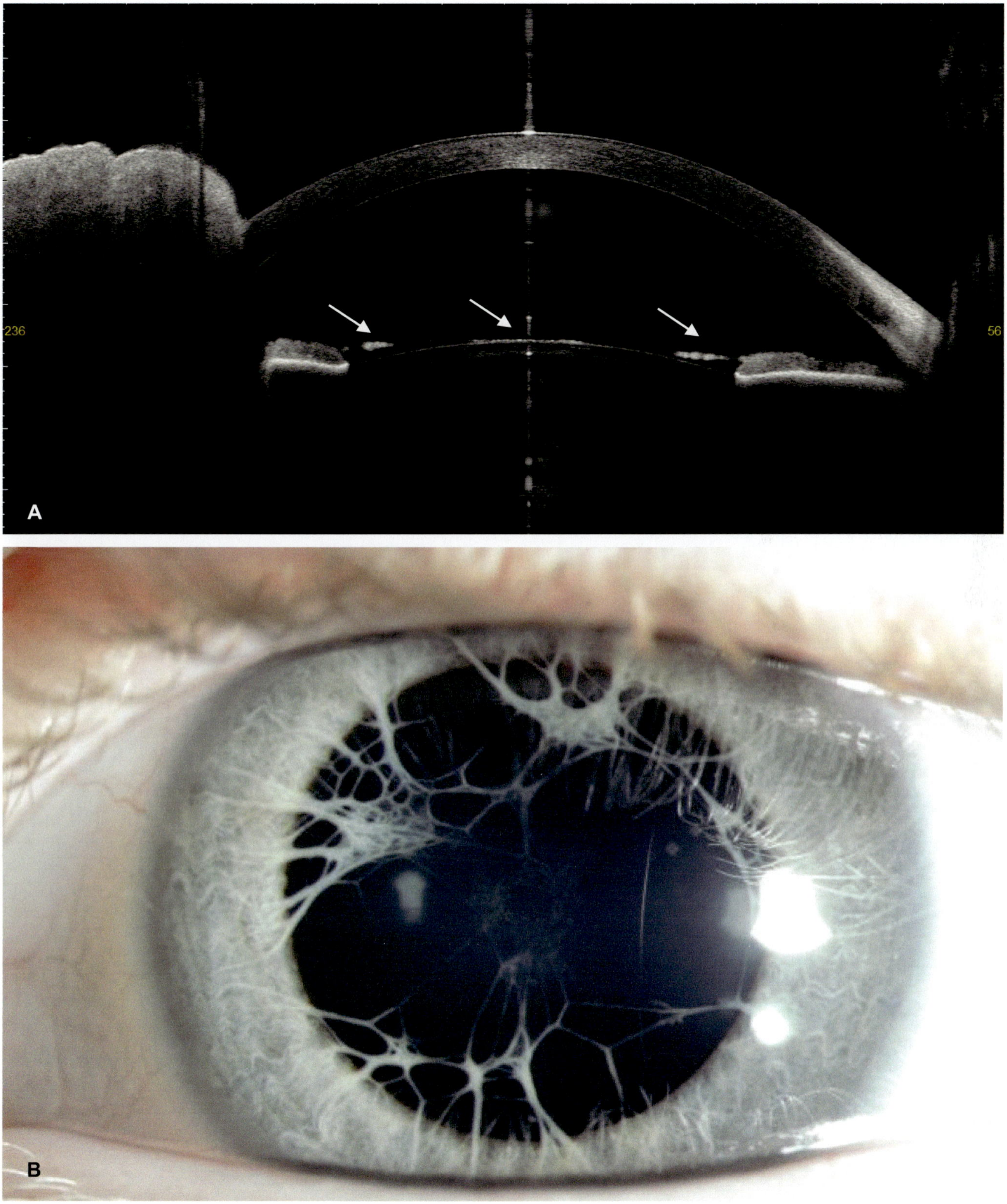

Fig. 51 (**A, B**) Maximally persistent pupillary filaments with central adhesions on the anterior lens capsule (arrows). (**A**) anterior segment optical coherence tomography. (**B**) slit lamp imaging

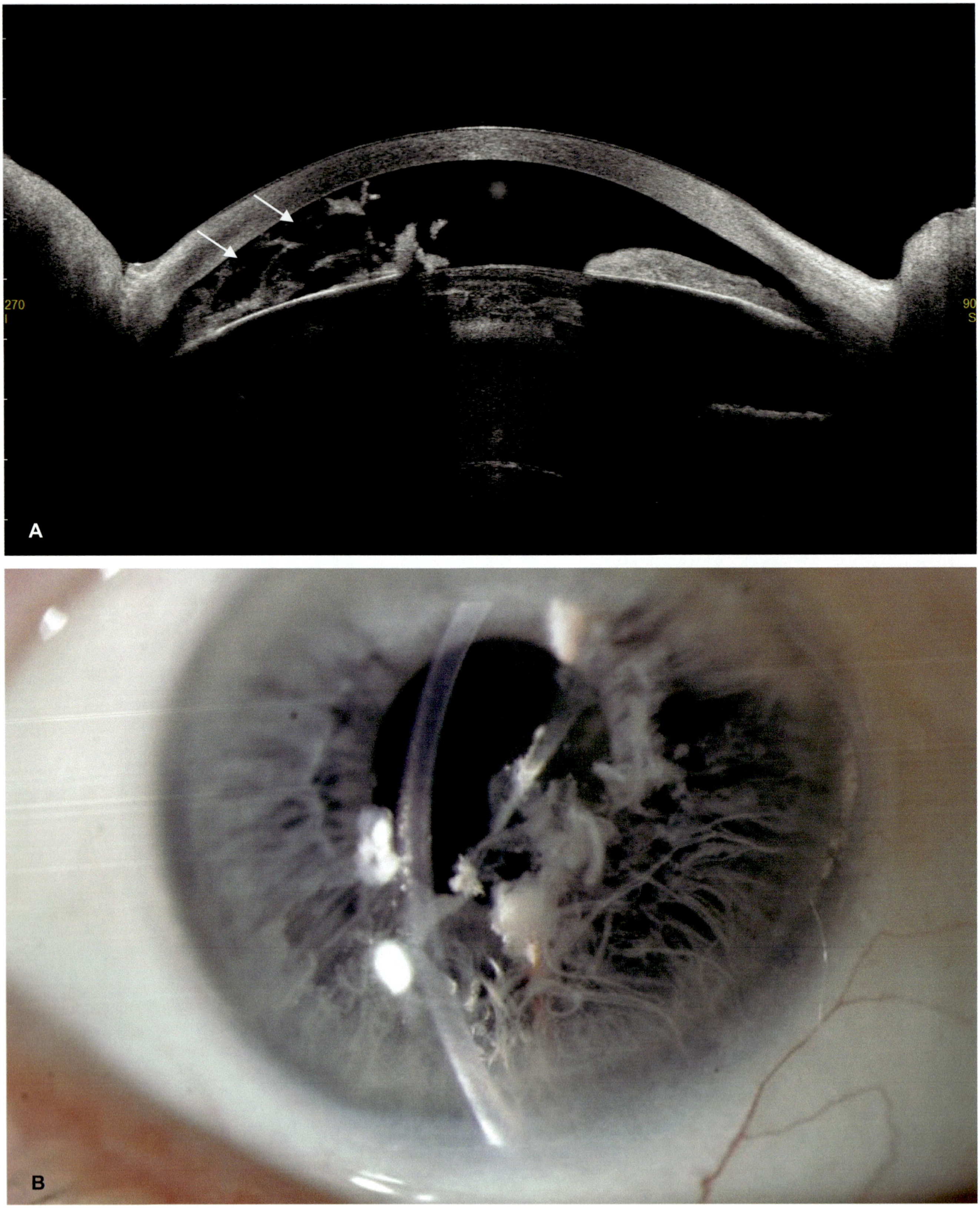

Fig. 52 (**A, B**) Atrophic iris filaments fluctuating in the anterior chamber (arrows) in a phakic eye. (**A**) anterior segment optical coherence tomography. (**B**) slit lamp imaging

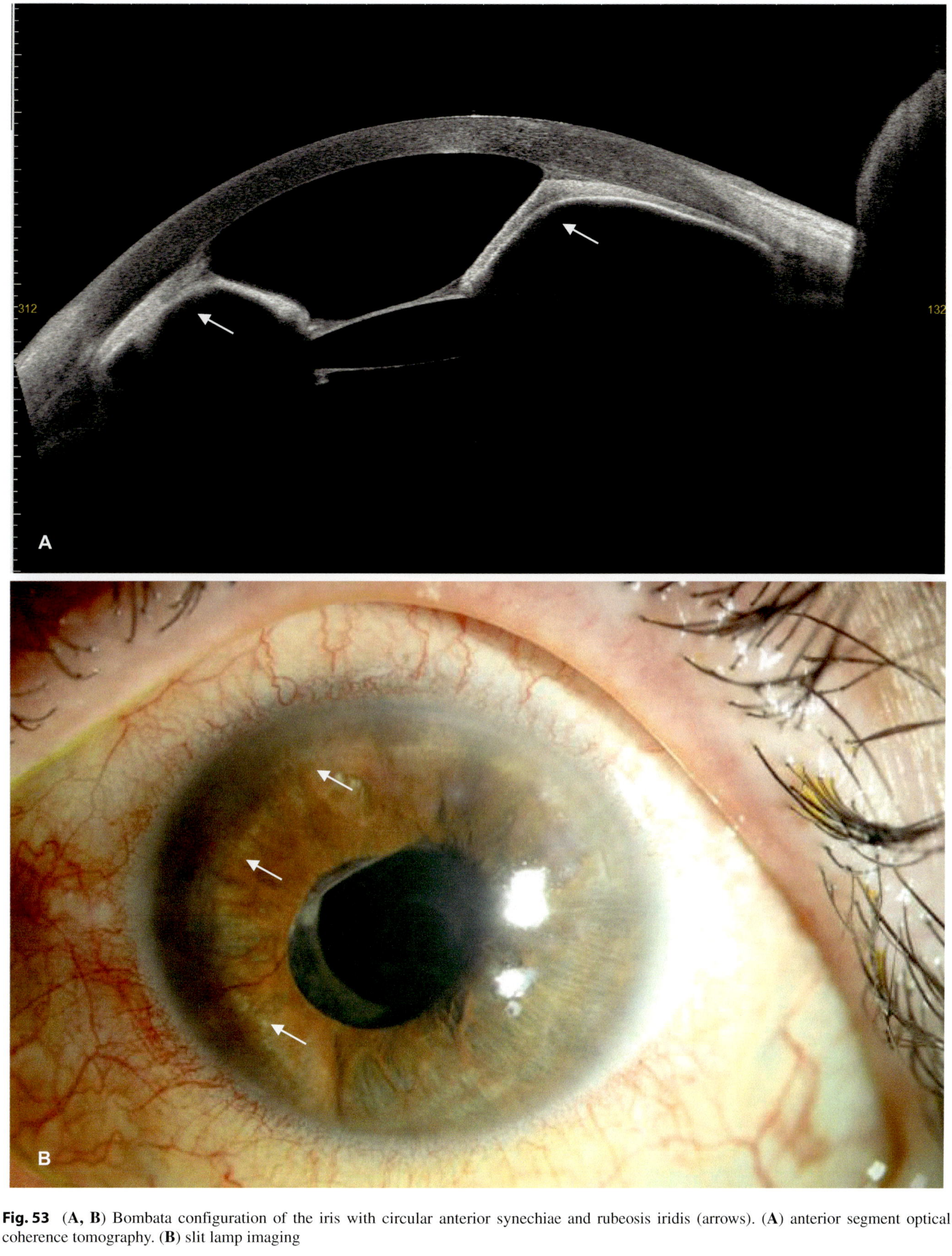

Fig. 53 (**A, B**) Bombata configuration of the iris with circular anterior synechiae and rubeosis iridis (arrows). (**A**) anterior segment optical coherence tomography. (**B**) slit lamp imaging

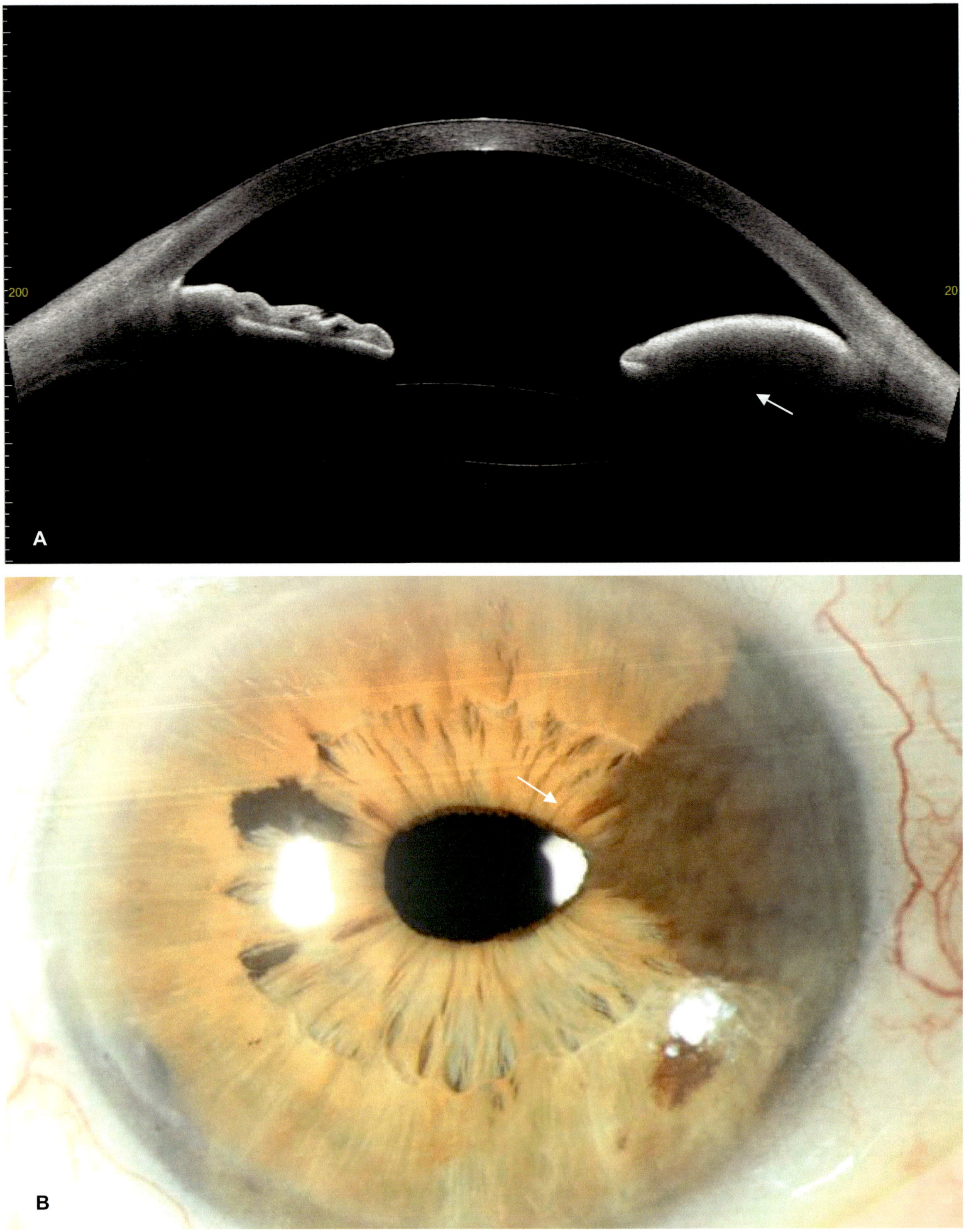

Fig. 54 (**A, B**) Iris melanoma with distorted pupil (arrows). (**A**) anterior segment optical coherence tomography. (**B**) slit lamp imaging

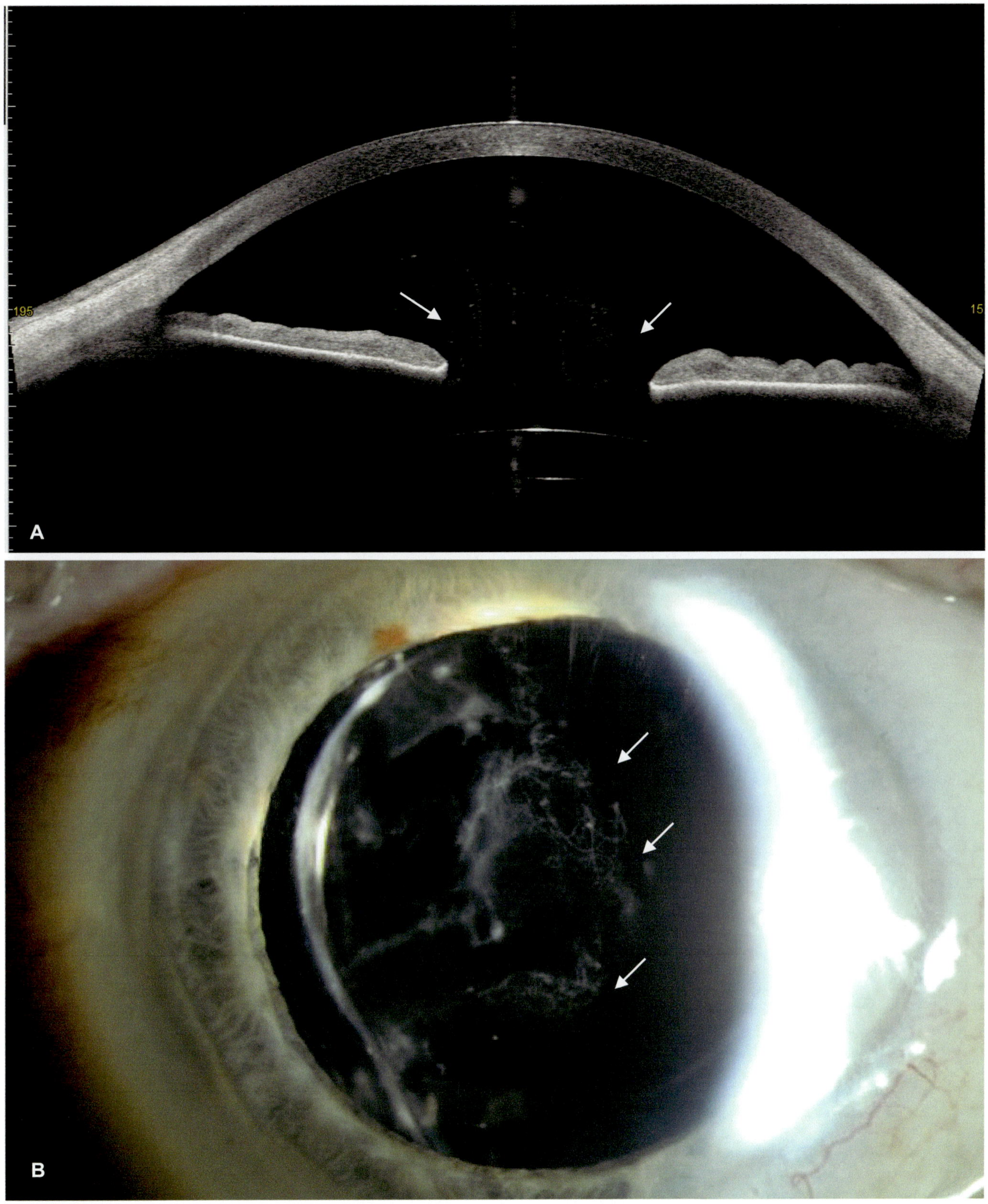

Fig. 55 (**A, B**) Vitreous prolapse into the anterior chamber (arrows). (**A**) anterior segment optical coherence tomography. (**B**) slit lamp imaging

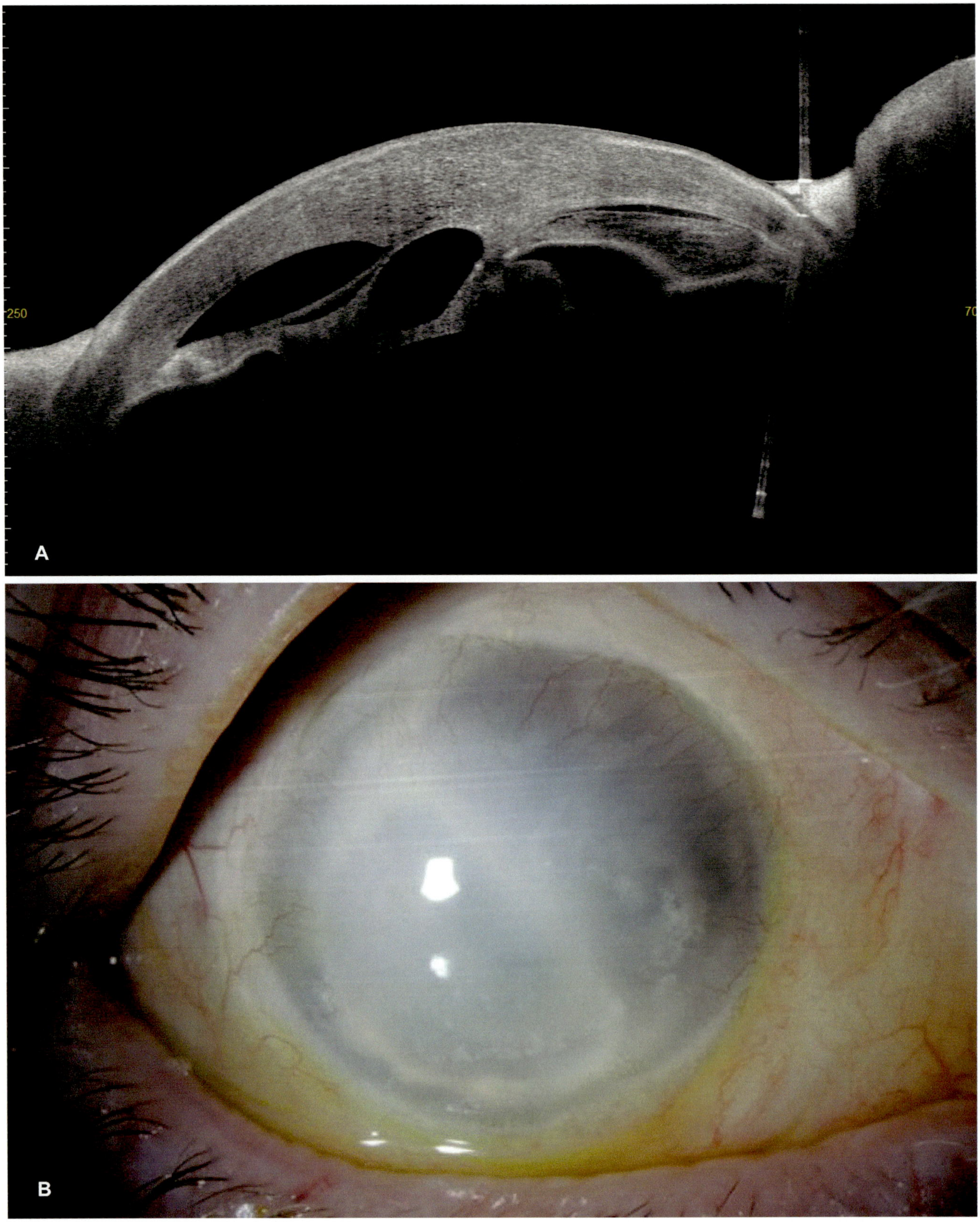

Fig. 56 (**A, B**) Anterior segment optical coherence tomography revealing thick retrocorneal membranes and synechiae invisible in slit lamp examination because of corneal loss of transparency. (**A**) anterior segment optical coherence tomography. (**B**) slit lamp imaging

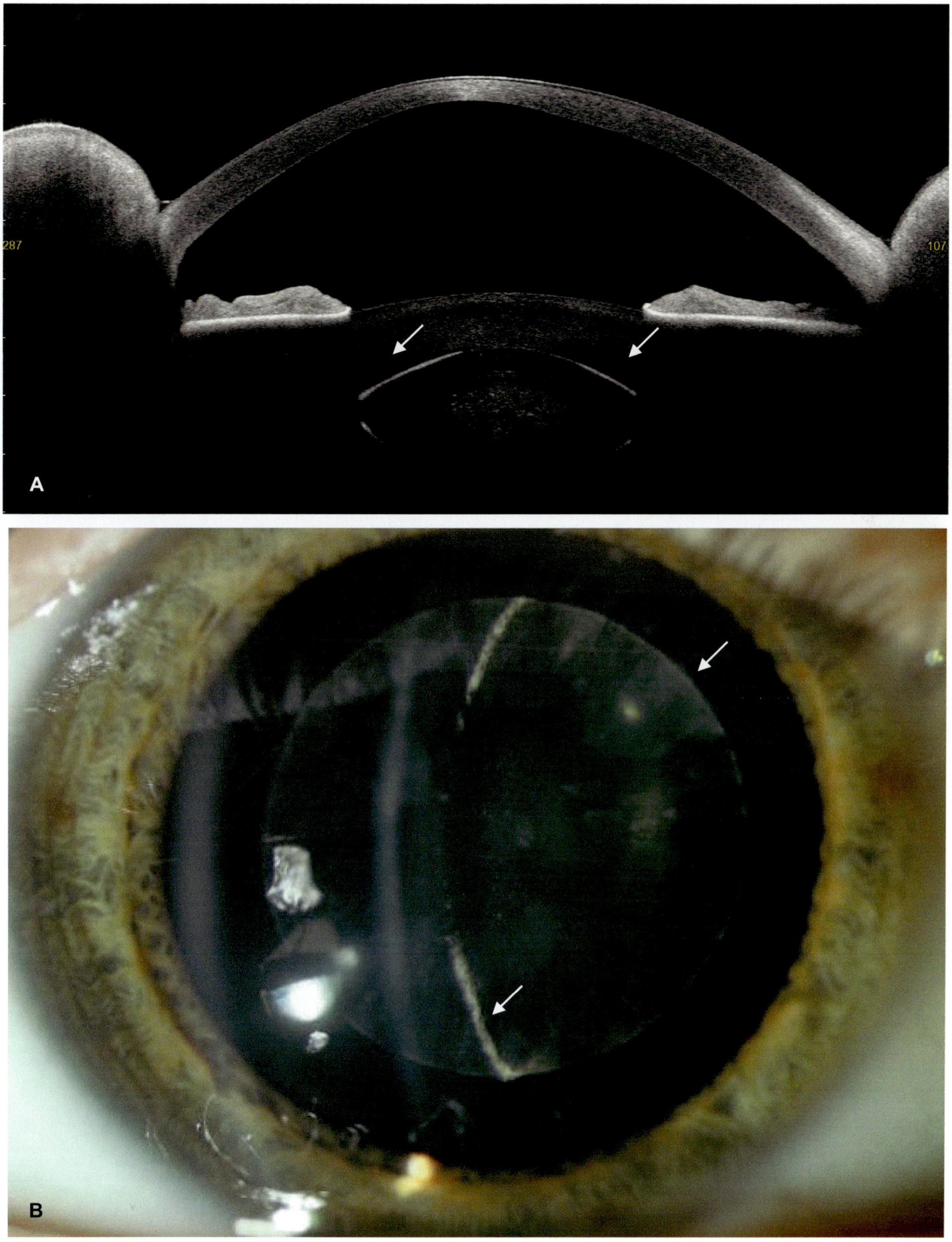

Fig. 57 (**A, B**) Cataracta zonularis congenita ("Reiterchen") with clear cortex (arrows). (**A**) anterior segment optical coherence tomography. (**B**) slit lamp imaging

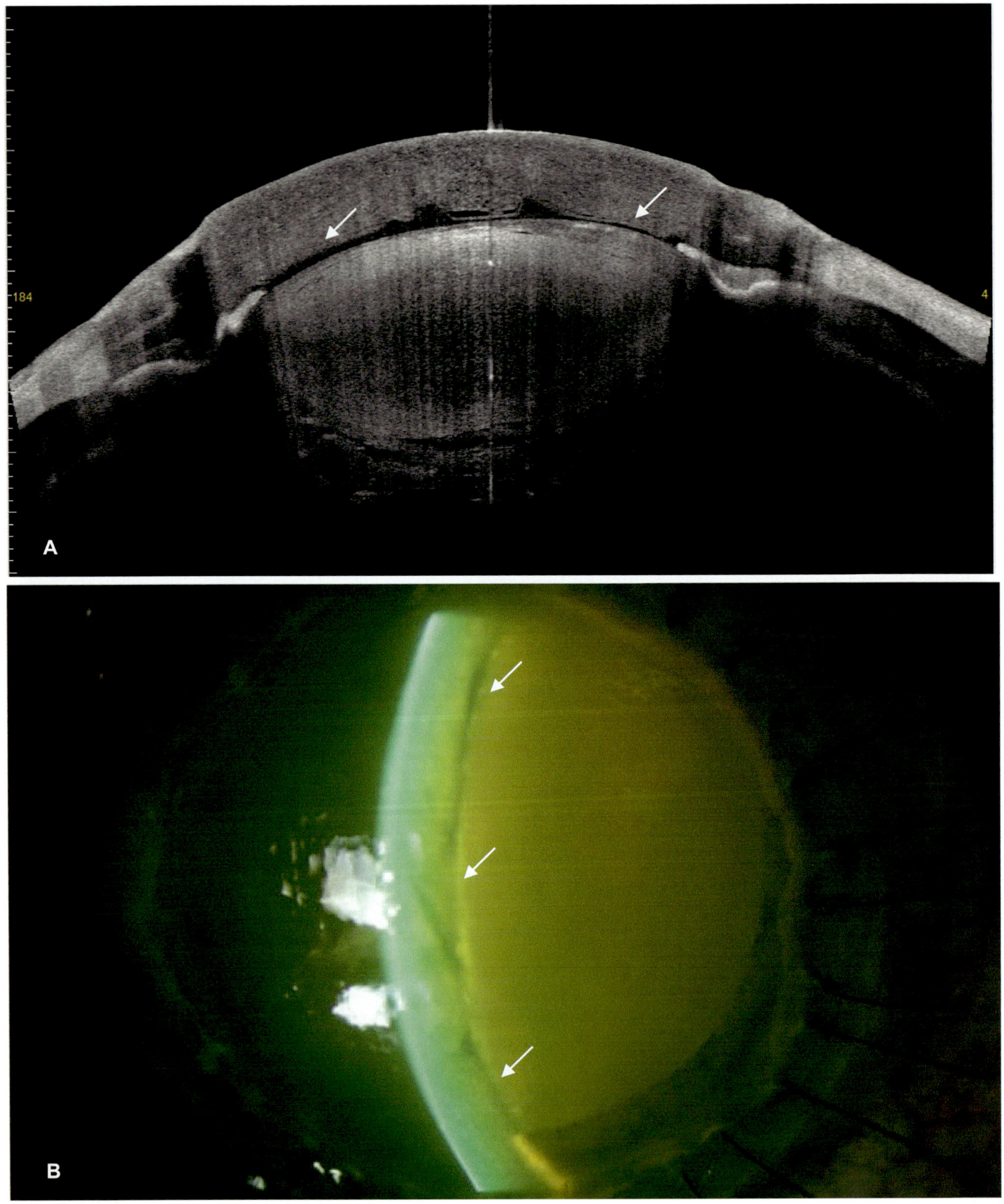

Fig. 58 (**A, B**) Intumescent cataract protruding in the anterior chamber after corneal graft because of acanthamoeba keratitis (arrows). (**A**) anterior segment optical coherence tomography. (**B**) slit lamp imaging

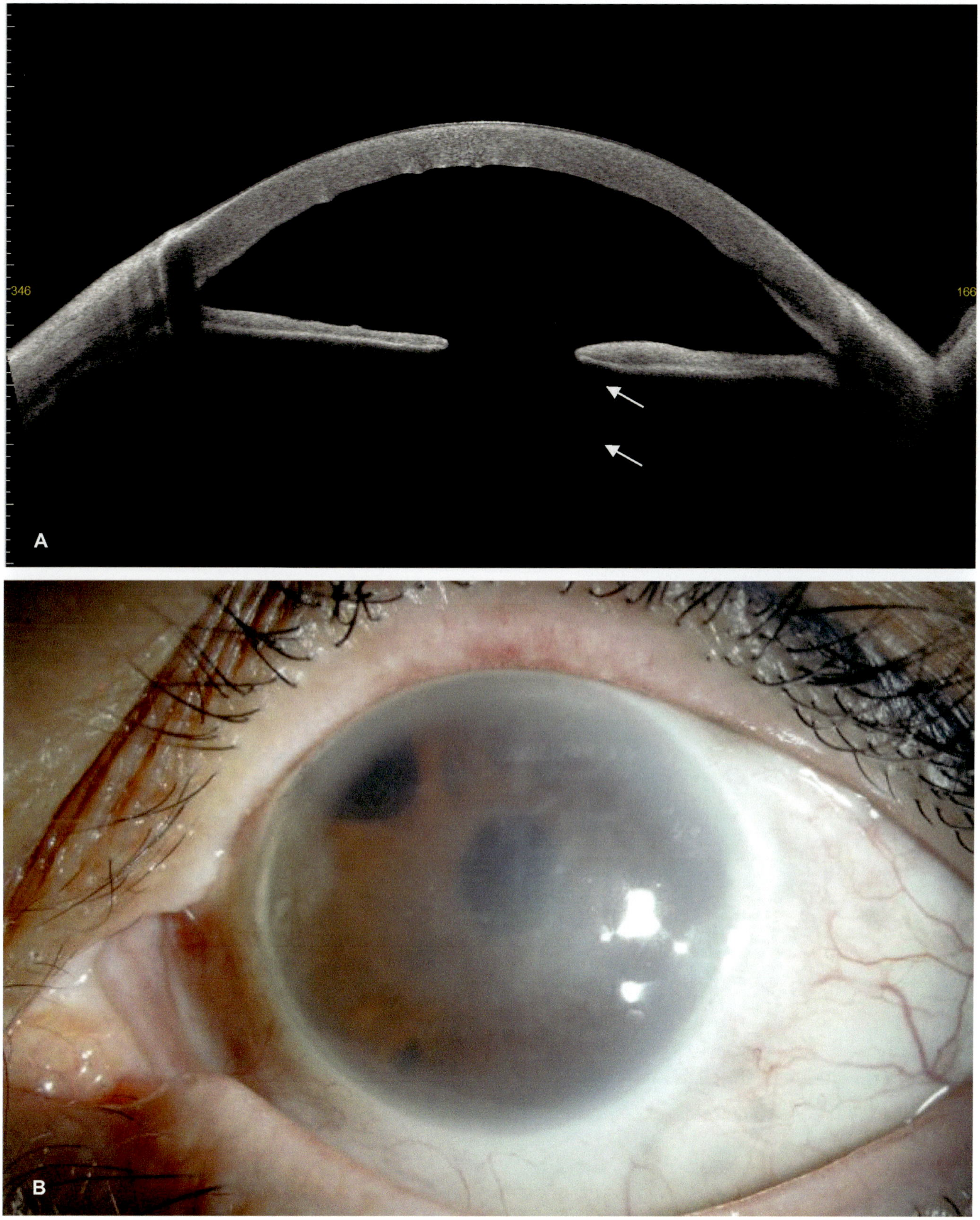

Fig. 59 (**A, B**) Aphakia revealed by anterior segment optical coherence tomography in a case of corneal decompensation with reduced iris motility (arrows). (**A**) anterior segment optical coherence tomography. (**B**) slit lamp imaging

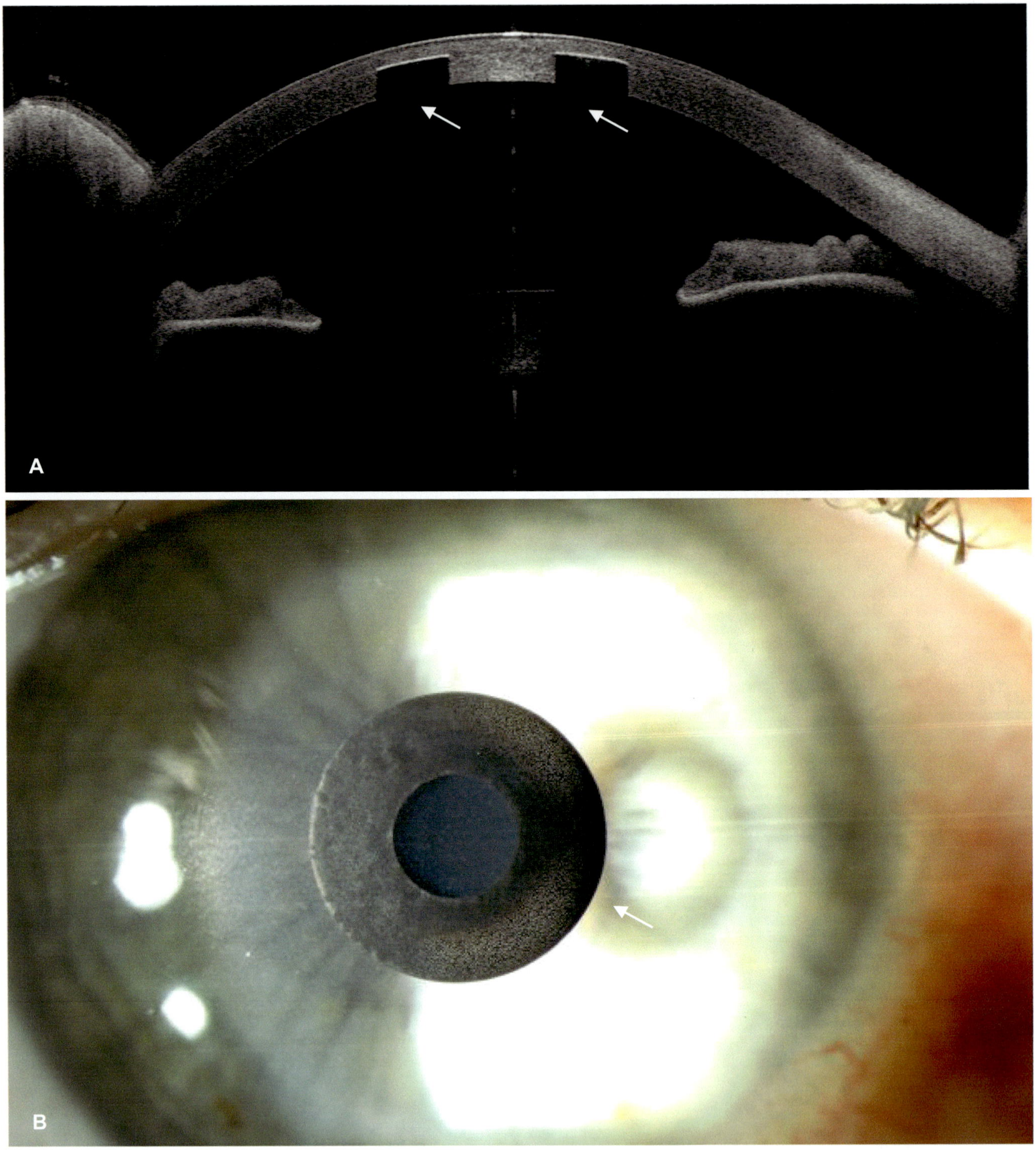

Fig. 60 (**A, B**) Intracorneal KAMRA® implant to increase depth of focus in presbyopia (arrows). (**A**) anterior segment optical coherence tomography. (**B**) slit lamp imaging

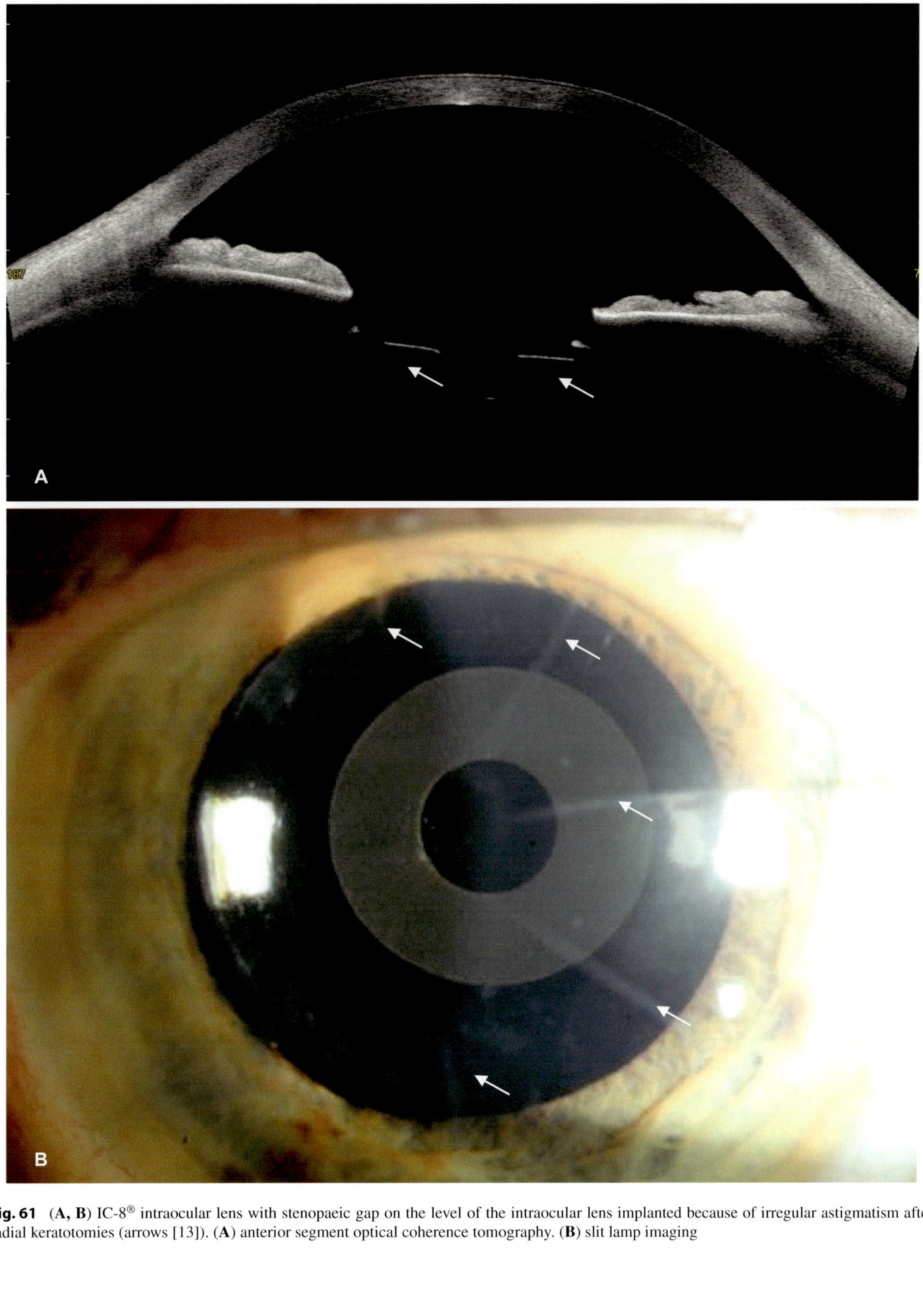

Fig. 61 (**A, B**) IC-8® intraocular lens with stenopaeic gap on the level of the intraocular lens implanted because of irregular astigmatism after radial keratotomies (arrows [13]). (**A**) anterior segment optical coherence tomography. (**B**) slit lamp imaging

Anterior segment OCT safely diagnoses whether there is a vitreous prolapse into the anterior chamber and, if present, assesses its extent and whether it draws to the paracentesis (Fig. 55).

Structures such as membranes in the anterior chamber may be visualized even if the cornea does not provide an insight at slit lamp examination (Fig. 56).

4 Lens

Even without dilation of the pupil, the anterior segment OCT enables an assessment of the intraocular lens status (Figs. 57–61).

5 Conclusion

Anterior segment optical coherence tomography has nowadays a leading role in diagnosing anterior segment pathologies in clinical practice. Additionally, its use is not limited to corneal topography and tomography, but also extends to glaucoma surgery, refractive surgery and the calculation of intraocular lenses in cataract surgery.

References

1. Wang SB, Cornish EE, Grigg JR, et al. Anterior segment optical coherence tomography and its clinical applications. Clin Exp Optom. 2019;102:195–207.
2. Izatt JA. Micrometer-scale resolution imaging of the anterior eye in vivo with optical coherence tomography. Arch Ophthalmol. 1994;112:1584.
3. Ramos JLB, Li Y, Huang D. Clinical and research applications of anterior segment optical coherence tomography—a review. Clin Exp Ophthalmol. 2009;37:81–9.
4. Ang M, Baskaran M, Werkmeister RM, et al. Anterior segment optical coherence tomography. Prog Retin Eye Res. 2018;66:132–56.
5. Guthoff R, Guthoff T, Hensler D, et al. Bleb needling in encapsulated filtering blebs: evaluation by optical coherence tomography. Ophthalmologica. 2010;224(4):204–8.
6. Nanji AA, Sayyad FE, Galor A, et al. High-resolution optical coherence tomography as an adjunctive tool in the diagnosis of corneal and conjunctival pathology. Ocul Surf. 2015;13(3):226–35.
7. Lim S-H. Clinical applications of anterior segment optical coherence tomography. J Ophthalmol. 2015;2015:1–12.
8. Soliman W, Mohamed TA. Spectral domain anterior segment optical coherence tomography assessment of pterygium and pinguecula. Acta Ophthalmol. 2012;90(5):461–5.
9. Berger T, Seitz B, Löw U, Flockerzi F, Schlötzer-Schrehardt U, Daas L. Descemet membrane endothelial keratoplasty (DMEK) for severe verrucous posterior polymorphous corneal dystrophy with uncommon clinical and ultrastructural findings. Klin Monbl Augenheilkd. 2024;241:1081–90.
10. Daxer A, Ettl A, Hörantner R. Long-term results of MyoRing treatment of keratoconus. J Optom. 2017;10(2):123–9.
11. Berger T, Schlötzer-Schrehardt U, Flockerzi F, Daas L, Flockerzi E, Seitz B. Severe ulcerative keratopathy following implantation of an acellular porcine corneal stromal lenticule in a patient with keratoconus. Cont Lens Anterior Eye. 2024;47:102145.
12. Paoletti T, Maamri A, Zemova E, et al. Large Salzmann's nodules or acute keratoconus? Ophthalmologie. 2022;119(8):841–4.
13. Hartmann M, Hamon L, Flockerzi E, et al. Implantation of a small-aperture intraocular lens (IOL) in two patients with irregular astigmatism after keratorefractive surgery. Ophthalmologe. 2021;118(12):1264–6.

Placido-Based Topography

Tim Berger, Loay Daas, and Berthold Seitz

Abstract

The anterior cornea is the most important refractive surface of the eye, responsible for more than two-thirds of the total dioptric power. Even very small changes in corneal curvature might have dramatic effects on visual acuity. Topography is the science that describes the characteristics of a specific location in detail. As clinical demands continue to evolve, new techniques for corneal topography have been developed over time, making it an indispensable tool in clinical practice today. This section provides an overview of the features of Placido-based corneal topography measured with the Topographic Modelling System 5 (TMS-5, Tomey Corp., Nagoya, Japan).

Keywords

Corneal topography · Cornea · Placido-based corneal topography · Corneal curvature · Astigmatism

1 Corneal Topography

The anterior corneal surface is subdivided into four areas. The central (apical) surface (4 mm area, important for optical properties), the paracentral area (4 mm to 7–8 mm, flatter radius of curvature), the periphery (flattest radius of curvature) and the limbal zone (0.5–1 mm, focal slope to form the scleral sulcus). The latter is usually not detected by topographic measurements [1].

There are two main methods for measuring corneal topography.

Reflection-based methods such as Placido rings, keratometer, and videokeratoscopy measure the slope of the corneal surface to calculate radius of curvature and corneal power. However, no information about the elevation are provided by reflection-based methods [2].

In contrast, projection-based methods such as the Scheimpflug tomography measure the elevation from which slope, curvature and power are calculated [2].

Placido-based corneal topography (videokeratoscopy) projects a series of concentric rings (black and white) on the anterior corneal surface. The number of rings can vary between different manufacturers. However, a larger number of rings provide more values. The reflected image is captured by a digital camera to determine the location of each mire and convert them into curvature at each measuring point, which is then analyzed by the software to generate a colour-coded map of the corneal surface. This map can be used to identify irregularities in corneal shape and curvature that might be associated with various corneal diseases such as keratoconus, iatrogenic corneal ectasia and corneal scars. The objective data provided by corneal topography is also useful in monitoring changes over time and evaluating disease progression or success of treatment [3, 4].

2 Indications

1. Ectatic disorders
2. Contact lens fitting
3. Pre- and postoperative assessment after keratoplasty and refractive procedures [5–7]
4. Astigmatism (regular / irregular)
5. Corneal degenerations and dystrophies
6. Corneal scarring
7. Any case of visual impairment

T. Berger (✉) · L. Daas · B. Seitz
Department of Ophthalmology, Saarland University Medical Center, Homburg, Germany
e-mail: tim.berger@uks.eu

B. Seitz et al. (eds.), *Atlas on Cornea*, https://doi.org/10.1007/978-3-031-65422-0_9

3 Limitations of Placido-Based Corneal Topography

The reflection occurs at the air–tear interface and might be disturbed by severe irregularities (corneal opacities, scarring) or abnormal tear film thickness (dry eye, delayed image capture). Artifacts might be caused by shadowing (eyelashes, nose trichiasis), by ptosis/non-sufficient eye opening, or by too short working distance of a small Placido disk cone. Since the area of corneal coverage (about 60% of the corneal surface) is limited, important data for early detection of peripheral diseases (e.g. pellucid marginal degeneration) might be missing. Placido-based topography does not provide information about the posterior corneal surface, making it ineffective for early diagnosis of keratectasia. In addition, there is no data about the corneal thickness. The evaluation of the rings (keratoscopic raw image) provides qualitative information on the acceptance or rejection of the measurement (Fig. 1).

4 Interpretation

When interpreting corneal topography, there are several important factors to consider. First, it is important to confirm the patient's name, the date of the measurement, and which eye the measurement was conducted on.

In addition, a careful examination of the colour-coded topographic map is necessary. Visual representation of local corneal dioptric power values is achieved through a colour-coded topographic map using warmer (red) colours to indicate higher dioptric powers (steeper curvatures) and cooler (blue) colours to represent lower dioptric powers (flatter curvatures).

It is also important to review previous measurements, as well as the corresponding data from the partner eye.

The adjustment of scale (step interval, type of measurement e.g. height, curvature, power) to display topographic changes is crucial for diagnostic purposes and to accurately identify features that might impair vision. Smaller dioptric intervals might lead to an excessive amount of noise, while broader intervals might mask irregularities [8].

The topographic maps can be displayed with different scales (Fig. 2), partly depending on the manufacturer. The absolute scale uses the same scale in each map (for TMS-5: 26 different colours with a narrower graduation of colour changes in the range of 43 diopters, Min: 9.5 Diopters, Max: 100 Diopters) and is suitable for direct comparison between different maps.

In contrast, the normalized scale is different for each map. The software determines the minimum and maximum curvature for the map and automatically sets the colour range, which is best for viewing variations for a particular cornea (for TMS-5: 11 colours with equal intervals, minimum interval of 0.4 Diopters). The greater the difference between the minimum and maximum refractive power, the greater the colour change, while a smaller difference results in a smaller colour range.

A normal topography of a cornea with minimal astigmatism shows a fairly uniform colour pattern in the center with natural flattening in the periphery.

Regular corneal astigmatism (Fig. 3) is a condition characterized by a uniform steepening along a single meridian. The corneal topographic image illustrates a symmetrical

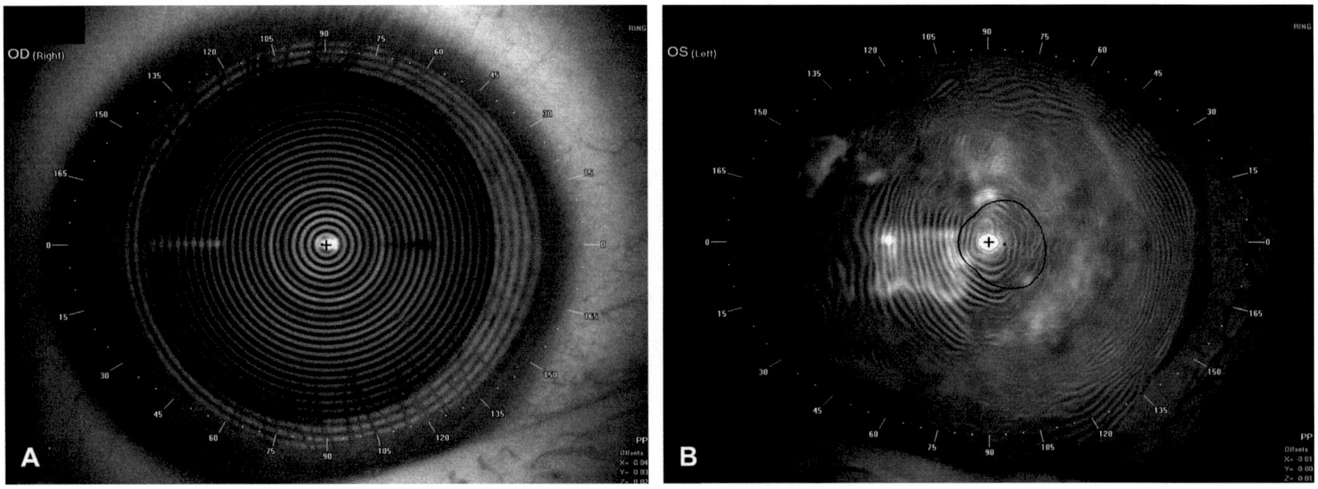

Fig. 1 Keratoscopic raw image. (**A**) Normal configuration of the rings in a healthy cornea. (**B**) Irregular configuration of the rings in case of severe corneal scarring. The measurable rings detected by the device are marked in green

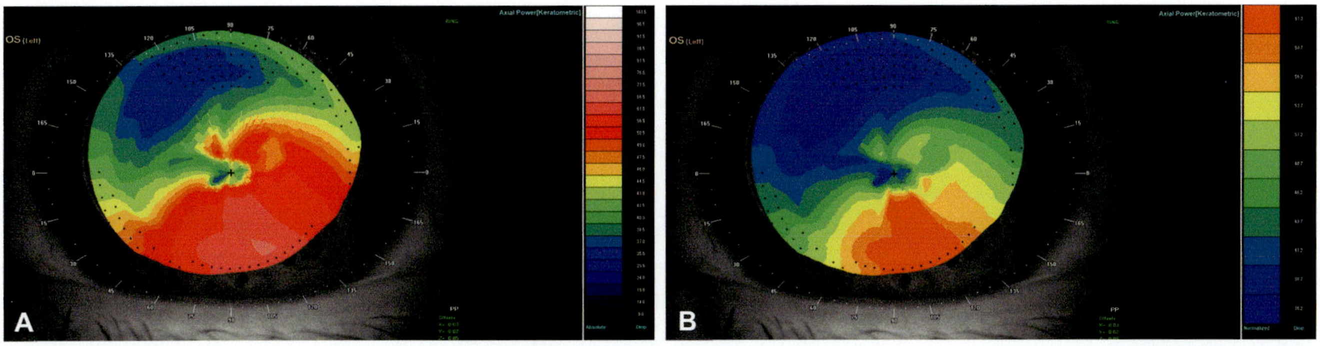

Fig. 2 Colour-coded topographic maps of the same cornea using different scales. (**A**) Absolute scale: it divides the range between 9 and 100 diopters into 26 sub-ranges and assigns specific colours to them. This scale shows the same refractive power for all measured eyes in all ranges with the same colour and provides a good comparison with other measurements. (**B**) Normalized scale: the refractive power is divided into 11 intervals. If there is a significant difference between the highest and the lowest refractive power, the colour range representing this range becomes large. In the opposite case, it becomes small. The minimum interval is 0.4 diopters

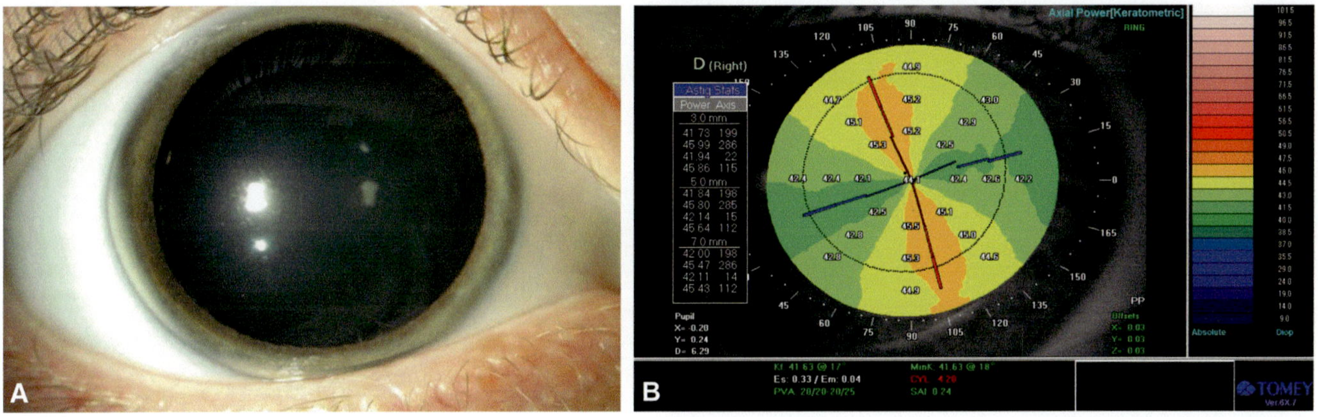

Fig. 3 Megalocornea with a diameter of 13.5 mm (**A**) demonstrating high regular with-the-rule astigmatism of 4.2 diopters (**B**)

bow tie pattern along a single meridian, with a straight axis on both sides of the center.

However, the bow tie pattern is an artifact as Placido-based imaging is not able to detect the curvature at the corneal center. Therefore, the meridional steepening of the cornea appears to attenuate at the center and becomes more pronounced with increasing distance from the center.

Astigmatic axes (Fig. 4) include orthogonal axes (represent major and minor meridians by averaging power from rings within the central 3 mm), zonal axes (steepest and flattest meridian within the 3, 5 and 7 mm zones) and instantaneous axes (true major and minor axes, continuous lines connecting the points of maximum and minimum power on each ring) [9].

The topographic classification of different patterns (Fig. 5) is beneficial in facilitating the identification and comprehension of unique features and characteristics associated with various corneal conditions resulting in a faster and more accurate diagnosis [10]. In order to develop a comprehensive understanding of what constitutes a normal cornea, it is equally important to be able to distinguish between abnormalities caused by artifacts and those caused by the cornea itself.

5 Common Corneal Maps

The most common corneal maps used in clinical practice are described in the following text passage [11]. All figures represent the same eye (Figs. 6–8).

5.1 Axial Map

The axial curvature map (concept of axial distance) is a reference-based measurement and the most common method in clinical setting for diagnostic and screening purposes (Fig. 6).

This method calculates the radius of curvature at each reflected mire assuming that the cornea is spherical and

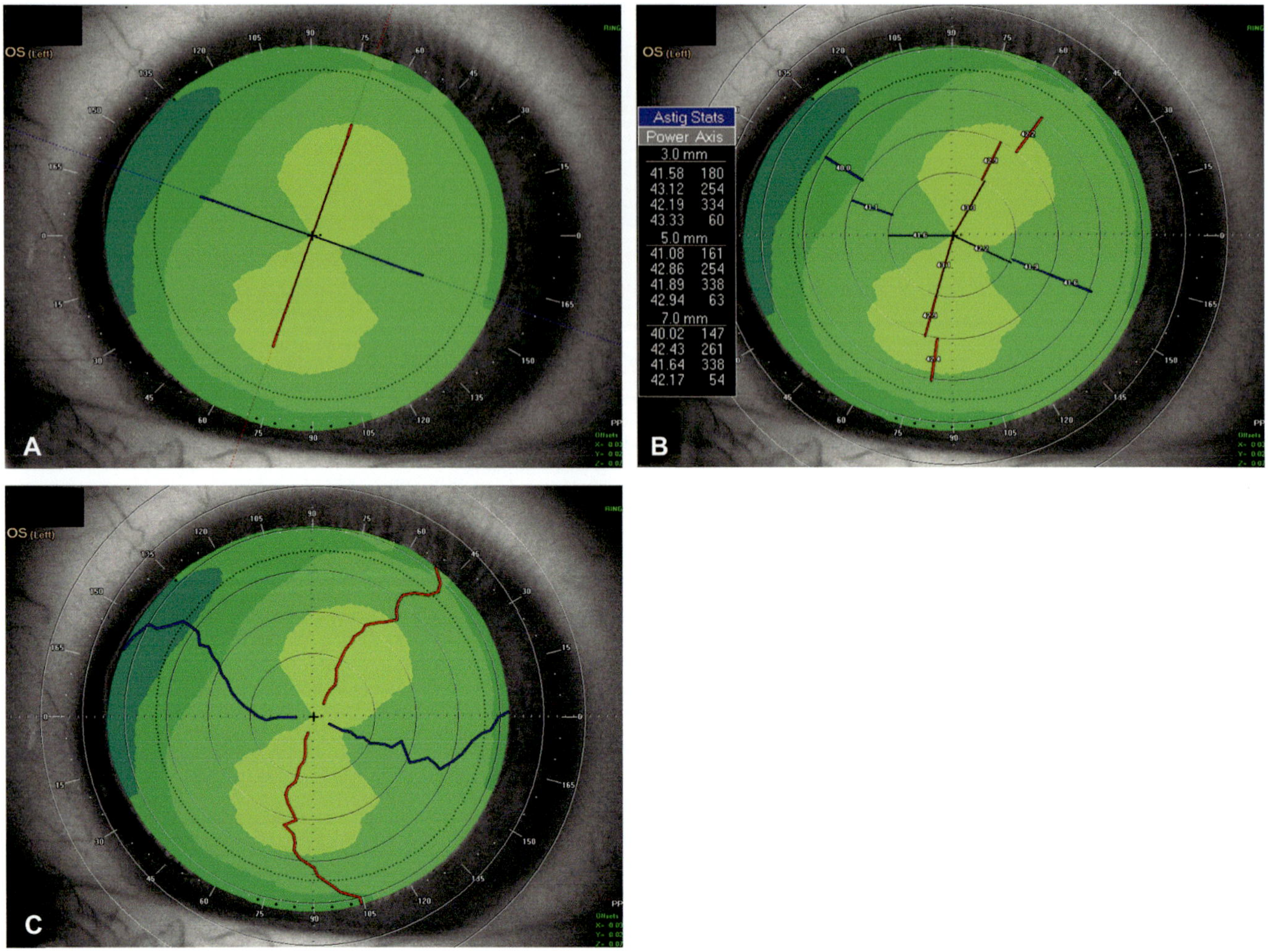

Fig. 4 Different astigmatic axes. (**A**) Orthogonal: this mode is demonstrating the axis with the greatest mean power in the 3 mm zone and the orthogonal axis to it. This setting is only useful for regular astigmatism. Since they simulate the axis measured by the keratometer, the amount of information is limited. (**B**) Zonal: this setting is displaying the steepest and flattest axes in the 3, 5 and 7 mm zones. (**C**) Instantaneous: continuous lines connecting the points of maximum and minimum power on each ring representing the "true axis" and is especially useful in irregular astigmatism. It provides more detailed information than the orthogonal or zonal axes

that the angle of incidence of the instrument is normal to the cornea. The healthy cornea is typically prolate or more curved in the center than in the periphery. However, axial maps can sometimes obscure details, as they tend to average the corneal curvature and underestimate steep curvatures and overestimate flat curvatures [9, 12].

The assumption that the cornea is a sphere causes spherical bias with decreasing accuracy towards the periphery. Furthermore, an identical corneal shape might have many different curvatures based on the axis used for the measurement, leading to further spherical bias as each measurement is referred to the optical axis. The curvature and refractive power of the central 1–2 mm of the cornea are generally not well represented by Placido disc techniques, which are extrapolated by the software and therefore potentially inaccurate. Axial power maps provide an intuitive sense of the physiologic flattening but do not represent the true refractive power or the true curvature of peripheral regions of the cornea [9, 12].

5.2 Refractive Power Map

The refractive power map (Fig. 7) is calculated according to Snell's law and converts curvature values into refractive power values. As the angle of incidence of the rays in

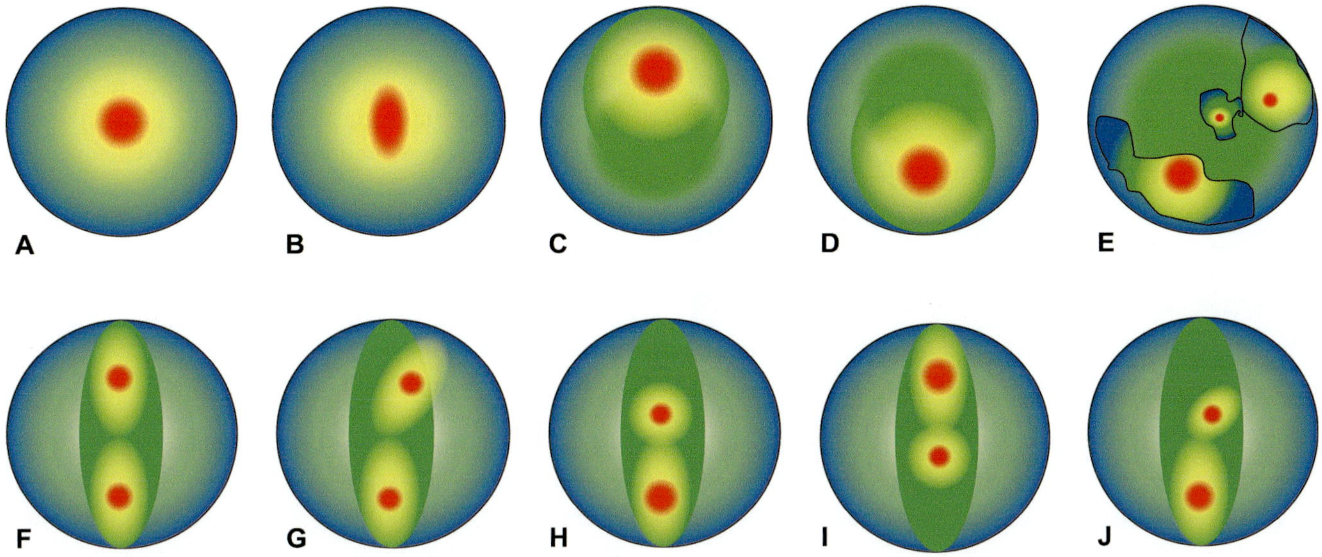

Fig. 5 Topographic patterns according to the proposed classification of Rabinowitz et al. [10]. (**A**) Round. (**B**) Oval. (**C**) Superior steepening. (**D**) Inferior steepening. (**E**) Irregular. (**F**) Symmetric bow-tie. (**G**) Symmetric bow-tie with skewed radial axes. (**H**) Asymmetric bow-tie with inferior steepening. (**I**) Asymmetric bow-tie with superior steepening. (**J**) Asymmetric bow-tie with skewed radial axes

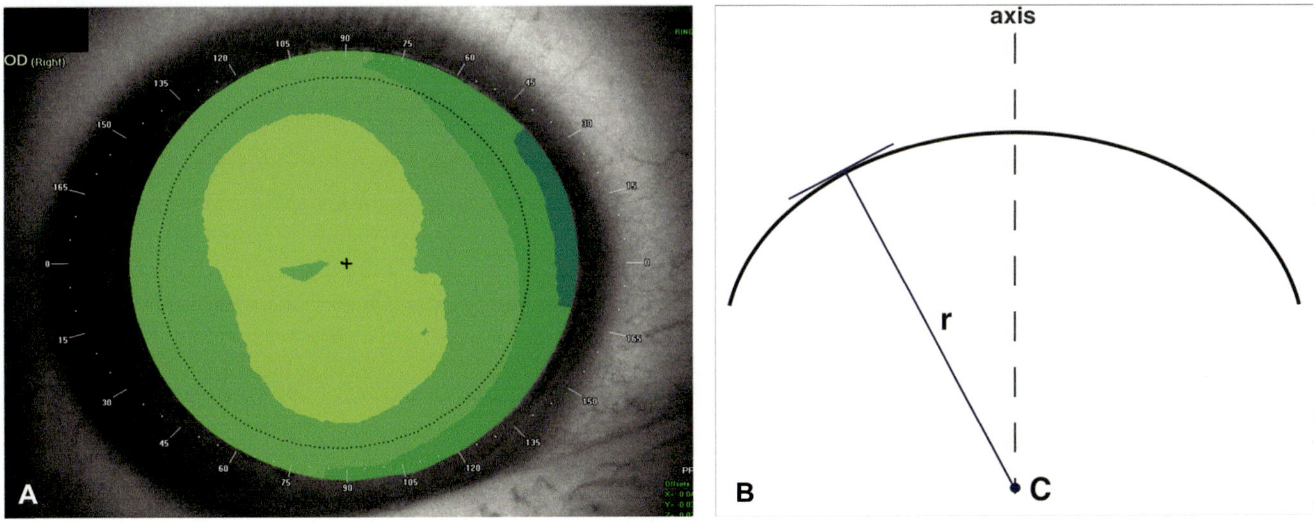

Fig. 6 Axial map. (**A**) Colour-coded axial map of a normal cornea. (**B**) The radius of curvature is the perpendicular distance (r) from a tangent at a point to the optical axis. The centre of curvature (C) is always located on the optical axis

the periphery of the cornea is higher, the refractive power increases [11]. This setting does not provide any information about curvature and shape of the cornea.

In normal corneas, this results in a higher calculated power in the periphery than in the center representing the natural spherical aberrations of the cornea. The peripheral increase of corneal power might hide pathologies such as early keratoconus.

5.3 Instantaneous or Tangential Curvature Map

Another method of describing the corneal curvature is the instantaneous map (Fig. 8), in which the radius of curvature applies to a sphere that best fits the shape of a small area surrounding each point. This map has less spherical

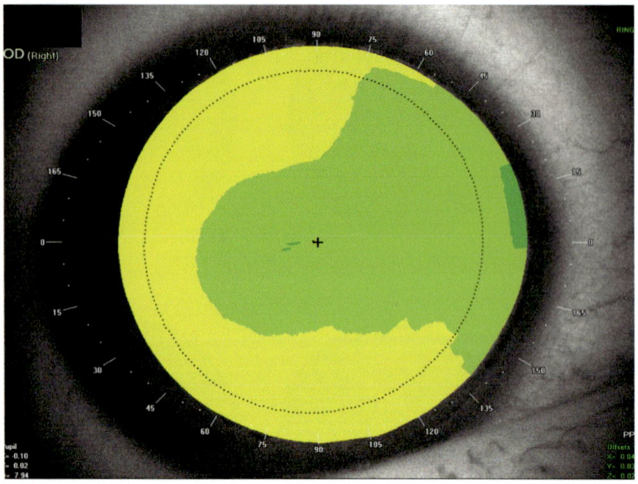

Fig. 7 Colour-coded refractive map of a normal cornea

bias as the curvature is calculated for a small single group of points, without reference to the visual axis or the overall shape of the cornea [13, 14].

It offers a better sensitivity and accuracy for detecting irregular astigmatism and for peripheral changes with less smoothing of the curvature compared to the axial map, but cause mathematical noise and fluctuations in the curvature values (excessive details without clinical relevance). Diopters in instantaneous maps are relative units of curvature and not a direct measure of corneal power in diopters [13, 14].

A difference map (Fig. 9) is able to demonstrate changes in corneal power over time and allows evaluation of changes in corneal refractive power caused by surgery, contact lens wear, or other conditions [15].

5.4 Statistical Indices

Statistical indices are numerical values that represent a summary of specific corneal features to quantify topographic characteristics, monitor changes over time and evaluate the effectiveness of treatment. Each of these values is compared to a normal range or grouped together to summarize the topography of multiple patients. Even though various manufacturers use different terms for those indices, they are calculated in a similar way and fulfil the same function [12].

The most important indices for TMS-5 include:

1. **Simulated keratometry (SimK)**: Obtained from the greatest power observed in the corneal surface from an average of rings 6–8 along every meridian. The power and axis orthogonal (90°) to the highest power are also reported as they are in traditional keratometry.
2. **Simulated keratometric cylinder (Cyl)**: Obtained from the SimK readings by calculating the difference between the major and minor axes.
3. **Minimum Keratometry (MinK)**: As the meridians of highest and lowest power are often not orthogonal, the MinK Value is useful to identify the meridian for which the actual minimum power occurs.
4. **Surface Asymmetry Index (SAI)**: Measures the difference in corneal powers at every ring (180° apart) over the entire corneal surface with more importance given to the central points.
5. **Surface Regularity Index (SRI)**: This is a correlate to potential visual acuity and compares the power of each point in this area with that of the points surrounding it, evaluating the local regularity of the surface as it is

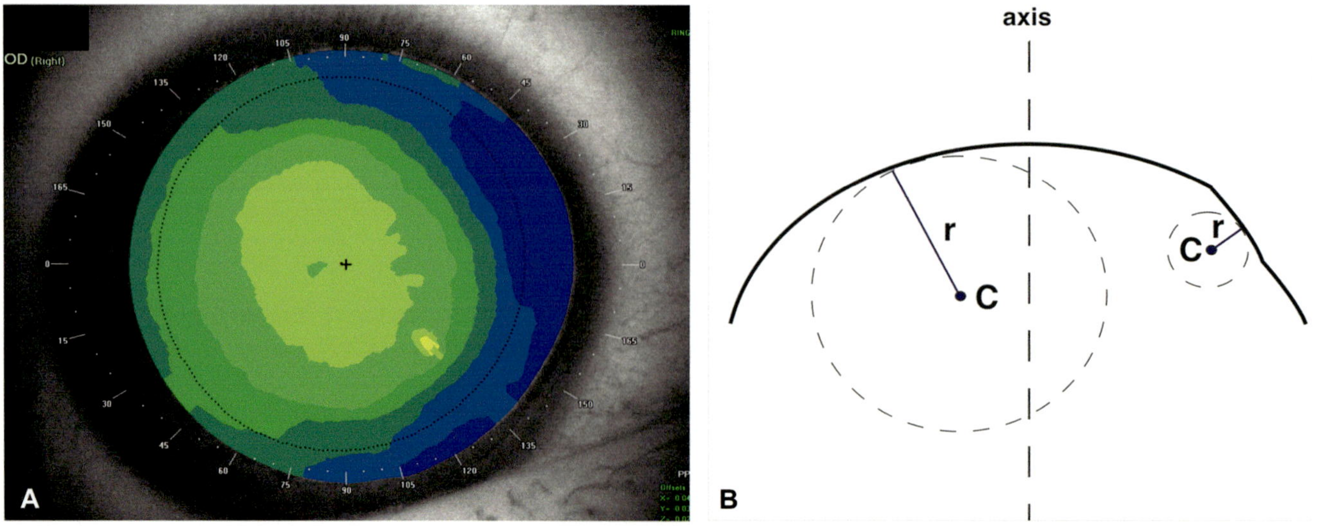

Fig. 8 Instantaneous or tangential curvature map. (**A**) Colour-coded map of a normal cornea. (**B**) The radius of curvature (r) applies to a sphere that best fits the shape of a small area surrounding each point. The centre of curvature (C) is not referring to the optical axis

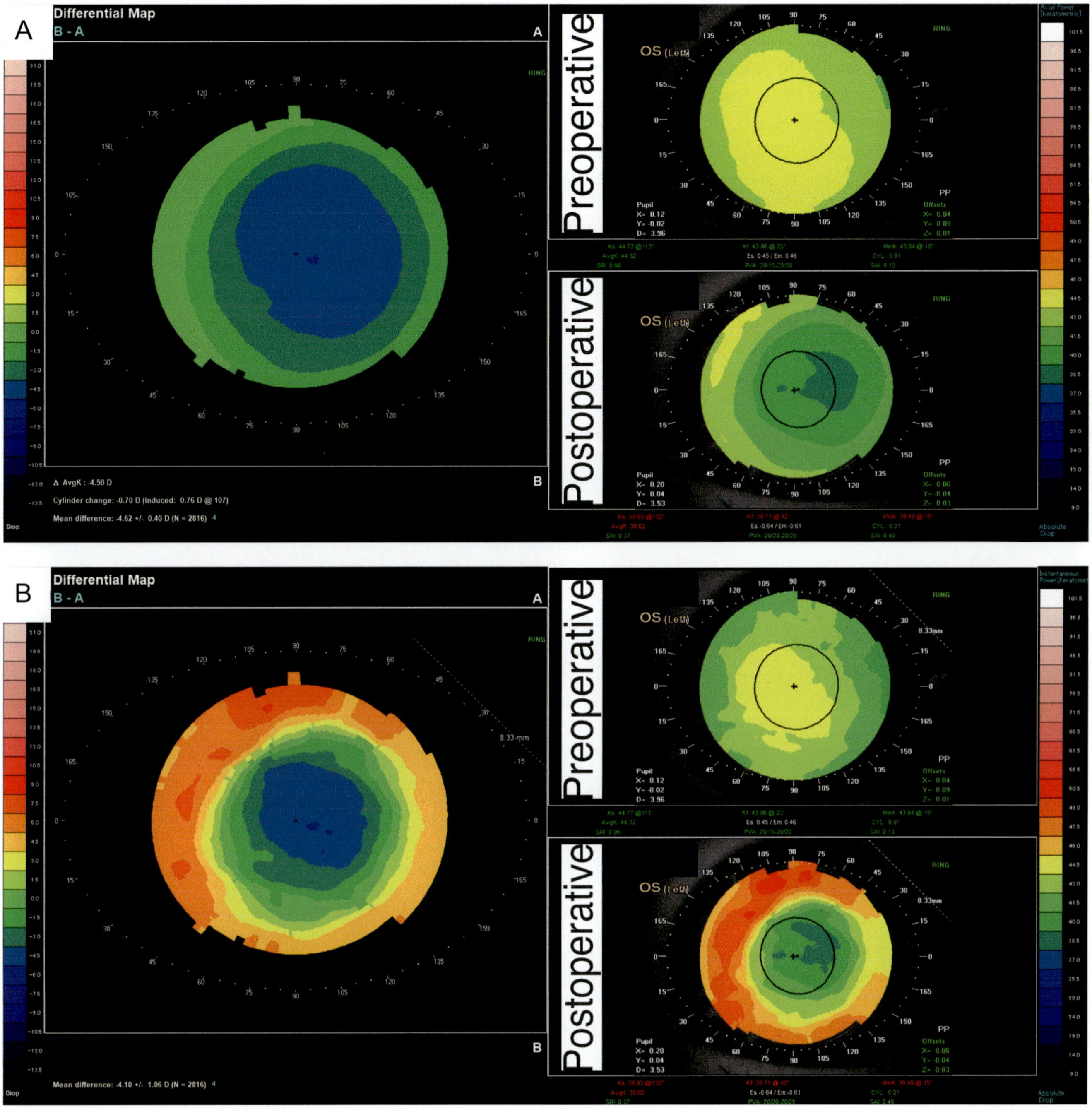

Fig. 9 Differential map of a cornea after myopic Laser in situ Keratomileusis (LASIK). (**A**) Axial curvature map: preoperative (top right) and postoperative (bottom right) corneal topography after LASIK. Postoperative topography demonstrating a central flattening of the cornea. The differential map (left) displays the greatest difference in corneal power in the center. (**B**) Instantaneous curvature map: the differential instantaneous map of the same patient increases the detail of curvature changes, especially in the periphery of the cornea, and is useful for evaluation of corneal topography after refractive surgery

a measure of local fluctuations in central corneal power within a diameter of 4.5 mm.

6. **Average Corneal Power (ACP)**: Area-corrected average of the corneal power ahead of the entrance pupil.
7. **Corneal Eccentricity Index (CEI)**: CEI is a global shape factor. A positive (normal) value represents a prolate surface, a nil value a sphere and a negative value an oblate surface.
8. **Irregular Astigmatism Index (IAI)**: Area-compensated average summation of inter-ring power variations along every meridian for the entire corneal surface (Fig. 10).

6 Clinical Applications of Corneal Topography

There are many corneal diseases that can be detected through corneal topography, but some of the most important ones include:

6.1 Keratectasia (Keratoconus, Pellucid Marginal Degeneration, Keratoglobus)

Keratoconus (Figs. 11–14) is a bilateral, progressive ectatic corneal disease, which results in a cone-shaped protrusion of the cornea due to the thinning of the corneal stroma. These morphological changes are associated with reduced visual acuity, progressive myopia, and irregular astigmatism [16–18].

The apex of the cone is characteristically displaced towards the lower mid-peripheral region in the temporal quadrant, although in rare cases the ectatic changes may occur in other regions (e.g. central or superior) of the cornea [12, 19].

Various conditions can mimic a keratoconus-like topography ("pseudokeratoconus"), such as map-dot-fingerprint dystrophy or keratokonjunctivitis sicca [20].

The so-called kissing- or crab-claw sign has often been associated with pellucid marginal degeneration, but is predominantly seen in inferior keratoconus. Therefore

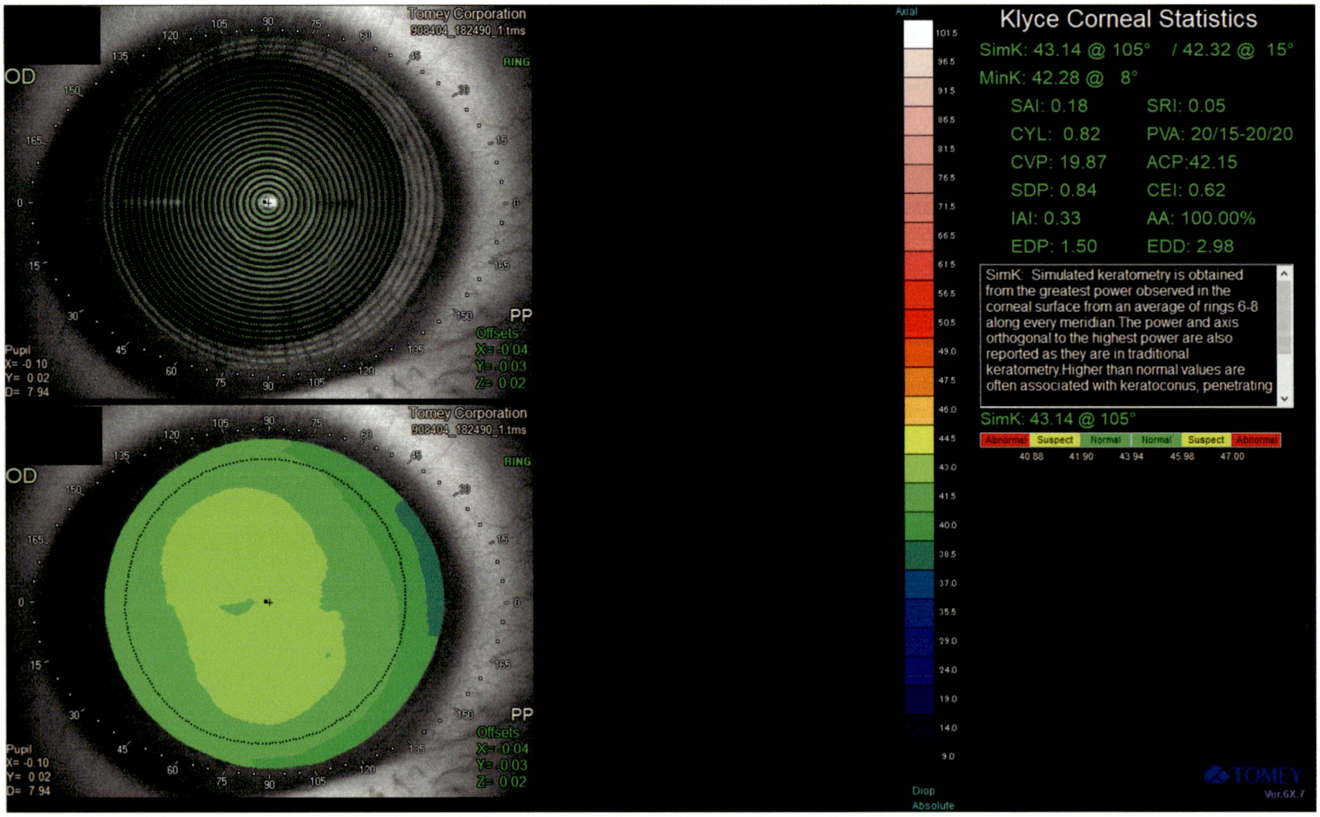

Fig. 10 KIyce corneal statistics of a normal cornea providing an overview of different topographic indices. All values are depicted in green color ("normal"), yellow means "suspicious", red means "abnormal"

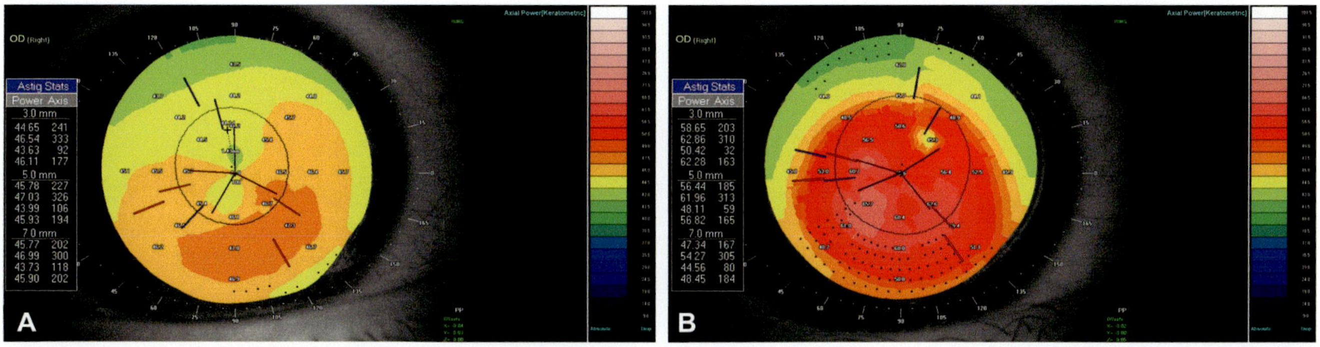

Fig. 11 Corneal topography in keratoconus. (**A**) Mild keratoconus with focal steepening of the inferior cornea. (**B**) Advanced keratoconus with a well-defined area of high dioptric power surrounded by zones of progressively decreasing curvature

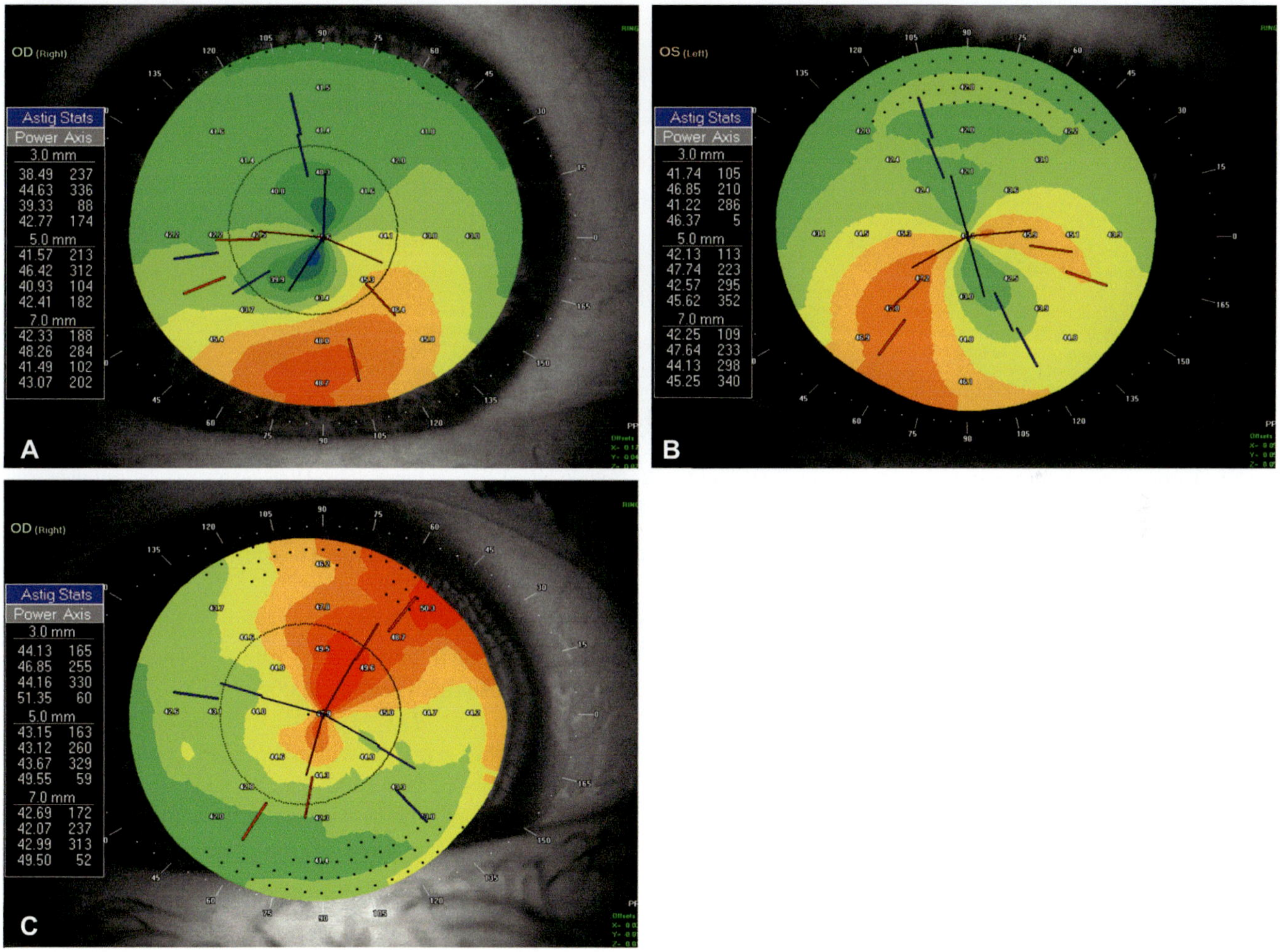

Fig. 12 Inferior and superior keratoconus. (**A**), (**B**) Inferior keratoconus with focal steepening (a) or crab-claw/kissing-bird sign (b). (**C**) Superior keratoconus demonstrating a predominant steepening in the upper hemisphere

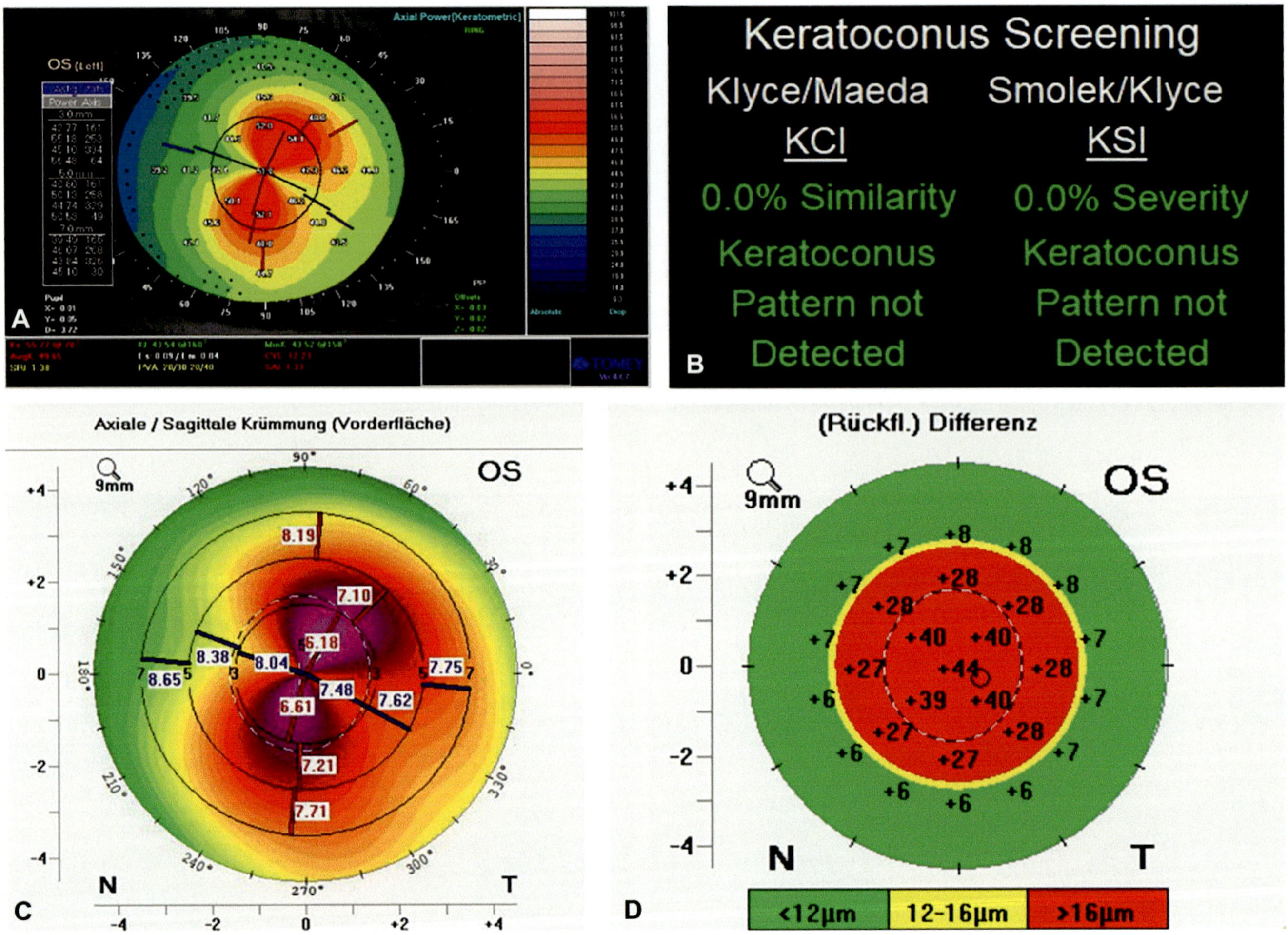

Fig. 13 Topo- and tomographic analysis of a central keratoconus (**A, B**) Placido-based corneal topography. High central regular astigmatism is visible (**A**). However, device-specific keratoconus indices (**B**) are unremarkable and do not detect the central keratoconus. (**C, D**) Scheimpflug tomography (OCULUS Optikgeräte GmbH, Wetzlar, Germany): An hourglass-shaped configuration is present in the sagittal curvature map of the anterior surface (**C**). The diagnosis in this case can be made by pathological posterior surface elevation (**D**) and abnormal biomechanics (not shown). Tomography is clearly superior to topography in such cases

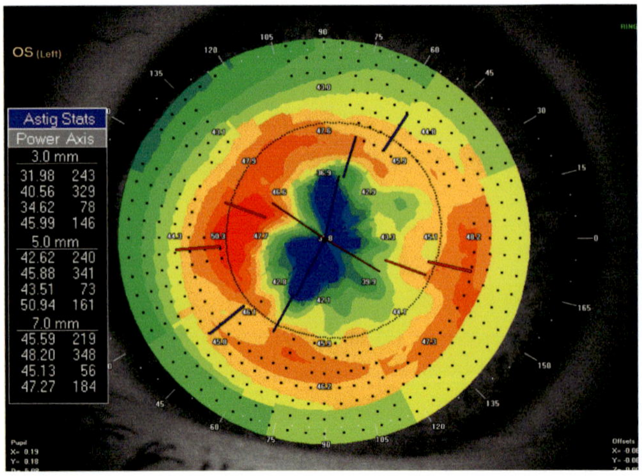

Fig. 14 Keratoconus with central predescemetal corneal scarring: corneal topography shows a central flattening induced by a predescemetic scarring surrounded by a "ring-shaped" corneal steepening

additional corneal tomography might facilitate the differential diagnosis between keratoconus and pellucid marginal degeneration [21, 22].

Topographic patterns with suspected keratoconus often present as subtle asymmetry in corneal power. Since all corneas have some degree of asymmetry, it is important to distinguish between these normal variations and changes indicative of keratoconus.

There are two methods for keratoconus screening available for the TMS-5 (Fig. 15).

The Klyce/Maeda method uses a discriminant analysis and a decision tree to report the similarity in percent of a corneal topography to clinical keratoconus (sensitivity = 89%, specificity = 99%, accuracy = 96%) [23].

The Smolek/Klyce method utilises a neural network that was trained to distinguish among keratoconus suspect patterns, clinical keratoconus patterns, and other patterns (sensitivity = 100%, specificity = 100%, accuracy = 100%) [24].

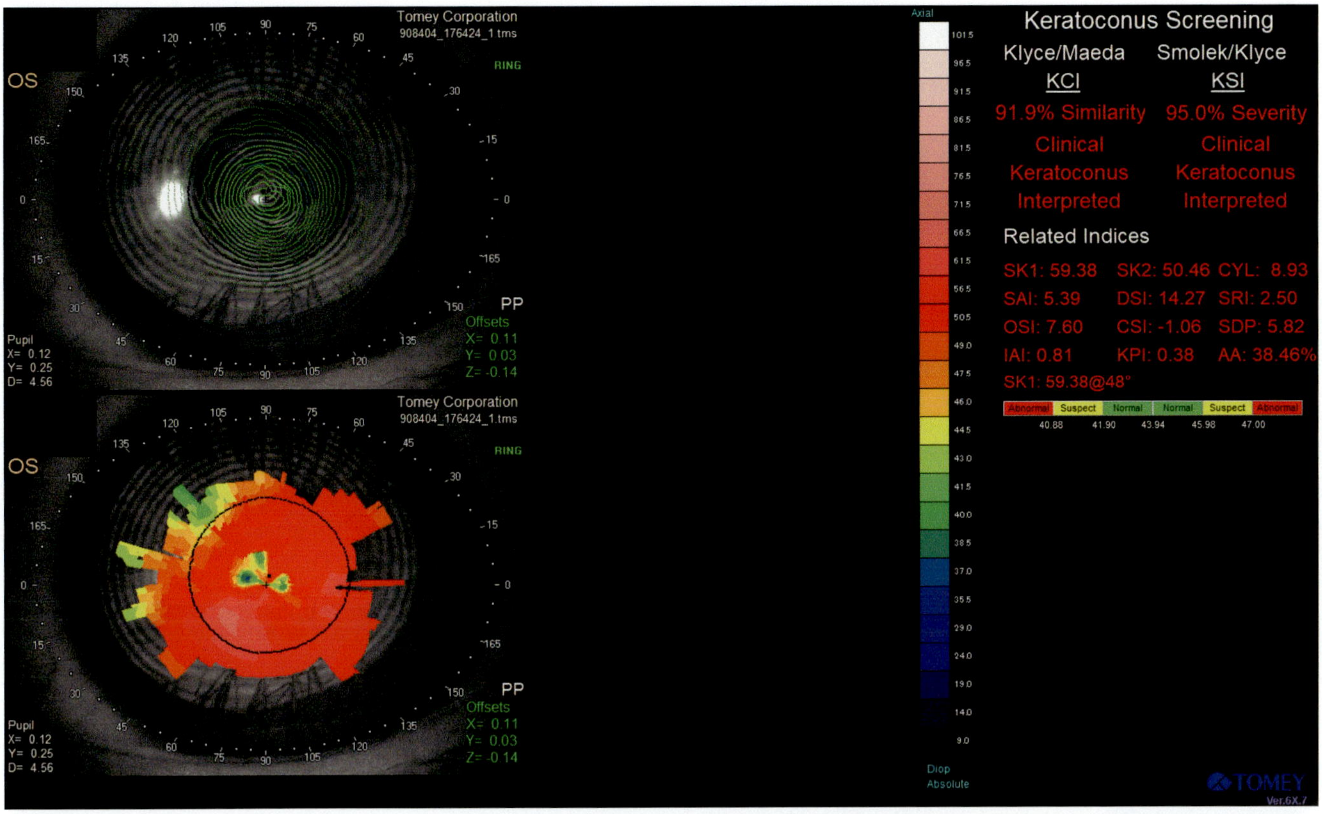

Fig. 15 TMS-5 keratoconus screening tool using different keratoconus indices (Klyce/Maeda and Smolek/Klyce)

Pellucid marginal degeneration (PMD) is a non-inflammatory and progressive ectatic disease that typically affects the inferior peripheral cornea and results in corresponding steepening and thinning. The characteristic finding is a 1–2 mm wide narrow band of corneal thinning parallel to the inferior limbus. The area between the thinned section and the limbus is usually unaffected until severe stages. High against-the-rule astigmatism is typical for PMD and a consequence of corneal protrusion above the thinned area (Fig. 16) [25].

Keratoglobus (Fig. 17) is a bilateral generalized thinning and global protrusion of the cornea, which is often more pronounced in the periphery. In severe stages, the cornea shows a high irregular astigmatism [22, 26, 27].

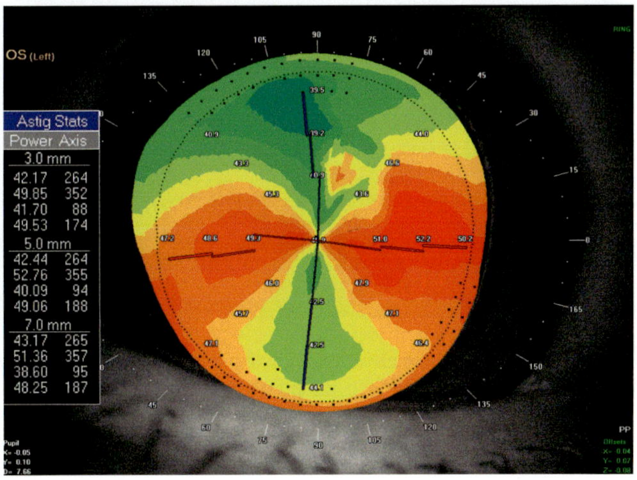

Fig. 16 Pellucid marginal degeneration corneal topography shows inferior steepening and high against-the-rule astigmatism (crab-claw pattern)

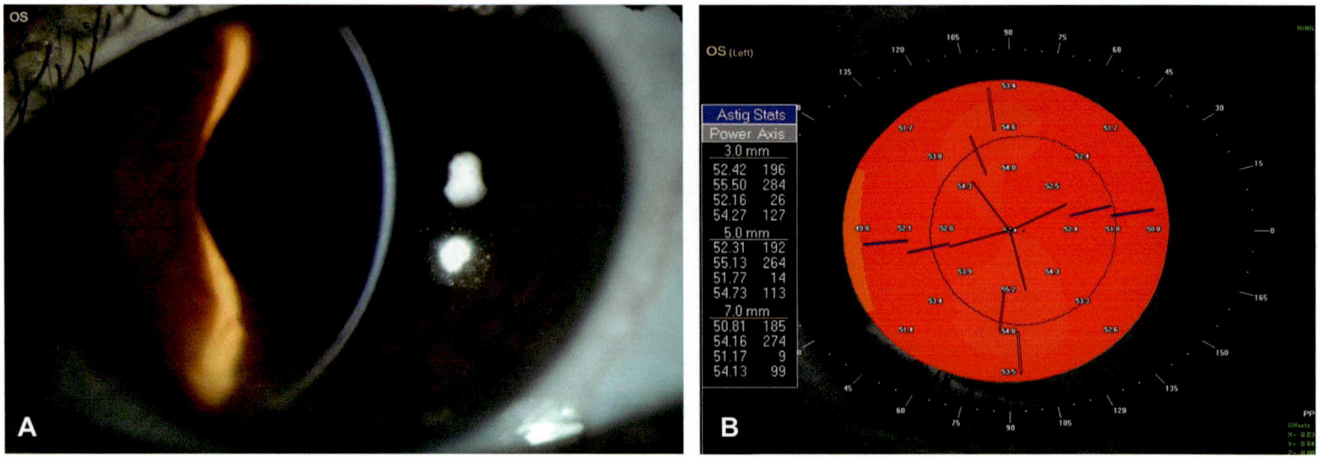

Fig. 17 Keratoglobus. (**A**) Narrow slit-illumination showing a generally thinned and steep cornea. (**B**) The corresponding topography demonstrates high corneal power of the measured area with regular astigmatism (Average Keratometry 53.5 Diopters)

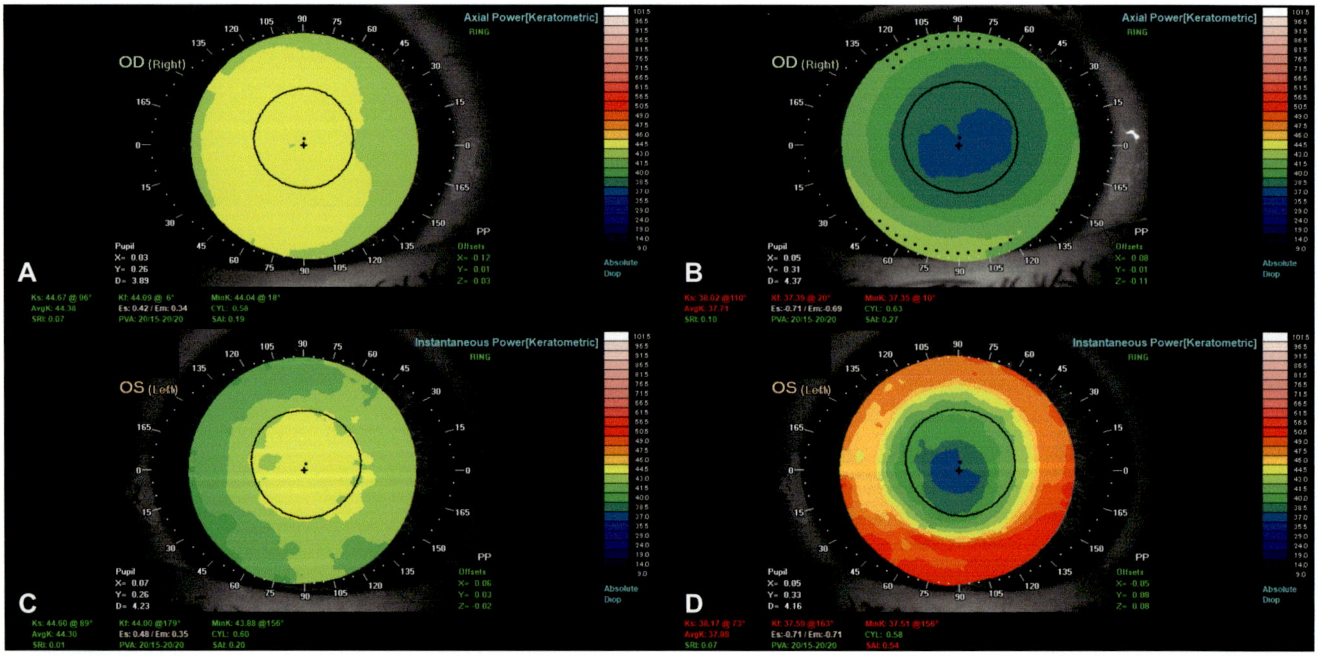

Fig. 18 Pre- and postoperative maps after photorefractive keratectomy with flattening of the corneal center. (**A**, **B**) Axial map: this map does not provide much information as the periphery is not well represented (**A**: preoperative, **B**: postoperative). (**C**, **D**) Instantaneous map: peripheral changes are better highlighted using this setting (**C**: preoperative, **D**: postoperative)

6.2 Refractive Surgery

Corneal topography is essential for planning refractive surgery and for follow-up care. Topographic changes after refractive surgery are best visible by using an instantaneous (Fig. 18) and difference map (Fig. 9).

In the past, radial keratotomy was performed for myopia treatment by placing radial corneal incisions leading to steepening of the periphery and compensatory flattening of the corneal center (Fig. 19). Because of the high complication risk, radial keratotomy is nowadays considered as obsolete [28].

Iatrogenic keratectasia (Fig. 20) is a rare but serious complication following refractive surgery in which the cornea becomes unstable and bulges, leading to deterioration of vision. Corneal topography can help to detect early signs of ectasia and initiate appropriate treatment [29, 30].

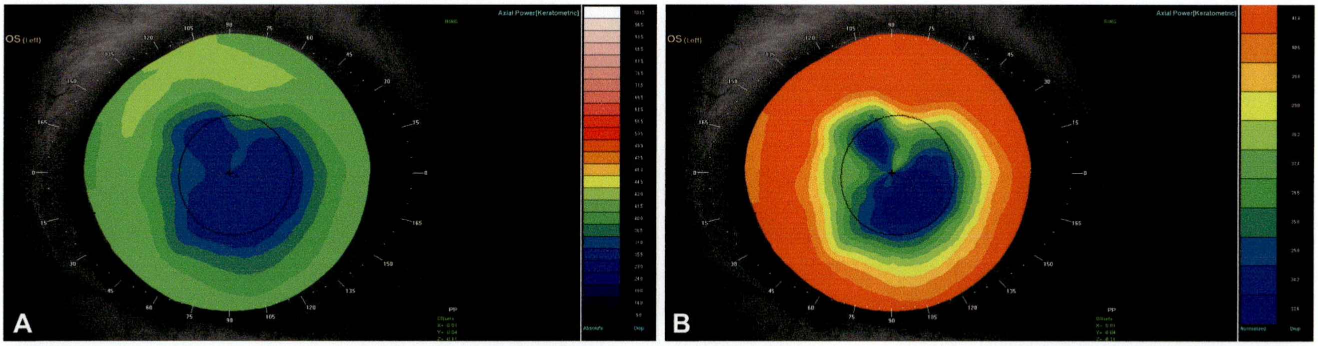

Fig. 19 Topographic steepening of the corneal periphery with compensatory flattening of the corneal center ("coupling effect") after radial keratotomies (a: absolute scale, b: normalized scale)

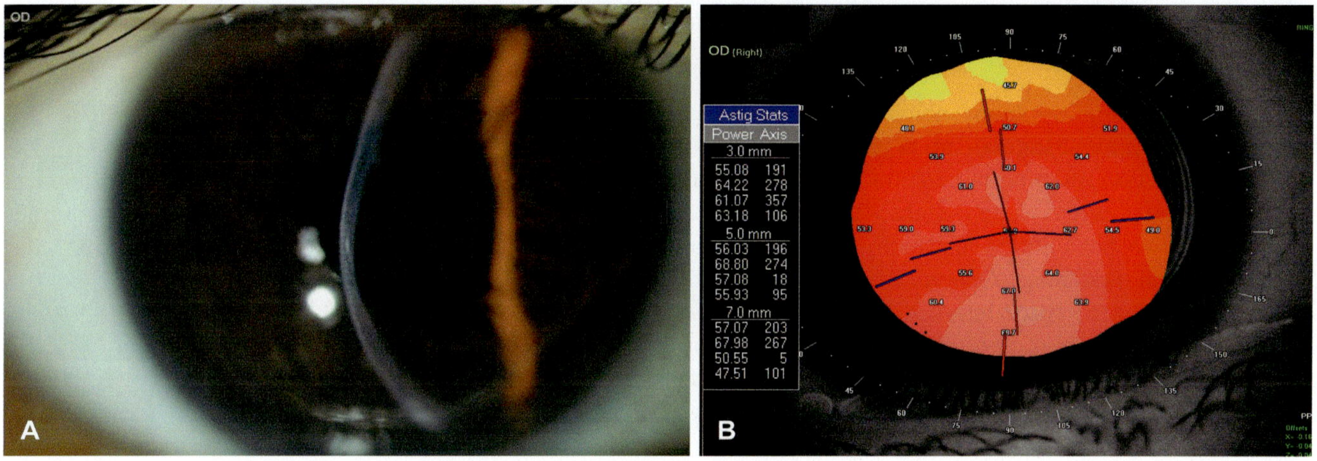

Fig. 20 Iatrogenic keratectasia after after myopic Laser in situ Keratomileusis (LASIK). (**A**) The cornea displays a conical protrusion. (**B**) Corneal topography is characterized by a keratoconus-like pattern with severe steepening

6.3 Corneal Dystrophies and Degenerations

Corneal dystrophies and degenerations may cause high irregular astigmatism, among other refractive changes of the cornea.

Map-dot-fingerprint dystrophy (Figs. 21, 22) is a common corneal disorder, which can lead to irregular astigmatism and affect vision. Although the cornea is clear, Excimerlaser-assisted phototherapeutic keratectomy is recommended for severe topographic changes and better adhesion of the epithelium [31, 32].

Other degenerative corneal diseases such as Salzmann nodular degeneration (Fig. 23) might lead to high and/or irregular astigmatism among other refractive errors (e.g. hyperopia by "optical cornea plana" due to asymmetric tear film distribution) [33, 34].

6.4 Pterygium

Pterygia (Fig. 24) result in structural abnormalities that occur at the level of the epithelium and also affect the overlying tear film and underlying stroma [35].

Progressive clinical findings might induce high (irregular) astigmatism. The type and extent of astigmatism is controversial, as some studies found a higher prevalence of horizontal steepening, while other studies described

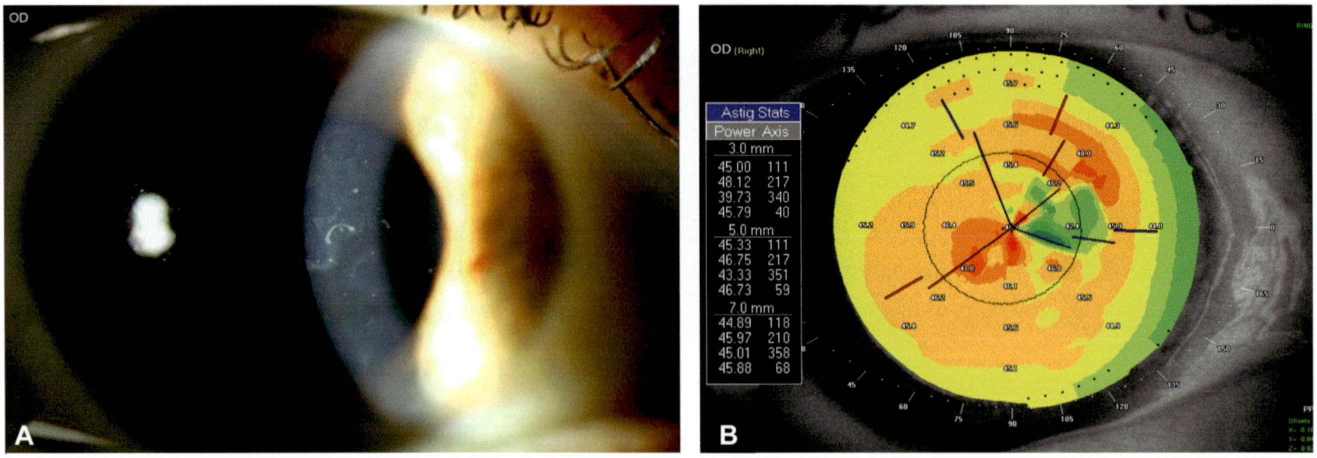

Fig. 21 Map-dot-fingerprint dystrophy leading to irregular astigmatism. (**A**) Dystrophic changes are best seen using a broader slit illumination. (**B**) Irregular astigmatism secondary to the dystrophic surface alterations

horizontal flattening as more common. The average induced topographic astigmatism is usually less pronounced and vision often remains good until the pterygium invades the pupillary zone (height > 2.5 mm) [36].

There are two possibilities in which a pterygium can cause horizontal flattening. One mechanism is that the tear meniscus fills the space between the pterygium head and the paracentral cornea. Secondly, subepithelial fibrosis beneath the pterygium might induced local flattening with steepening of the adjacent cornea [37].

6.5 Fuchs Terrien Marginal Degeneration

Corneal thinning in Fuchs-Terrien marginal degeneration typically begins superiorly and results in flattening of the vertical meridian and inducing against-the-rule astigmatism, which has been reported in previous studies [38, 39] (Fig. 25).

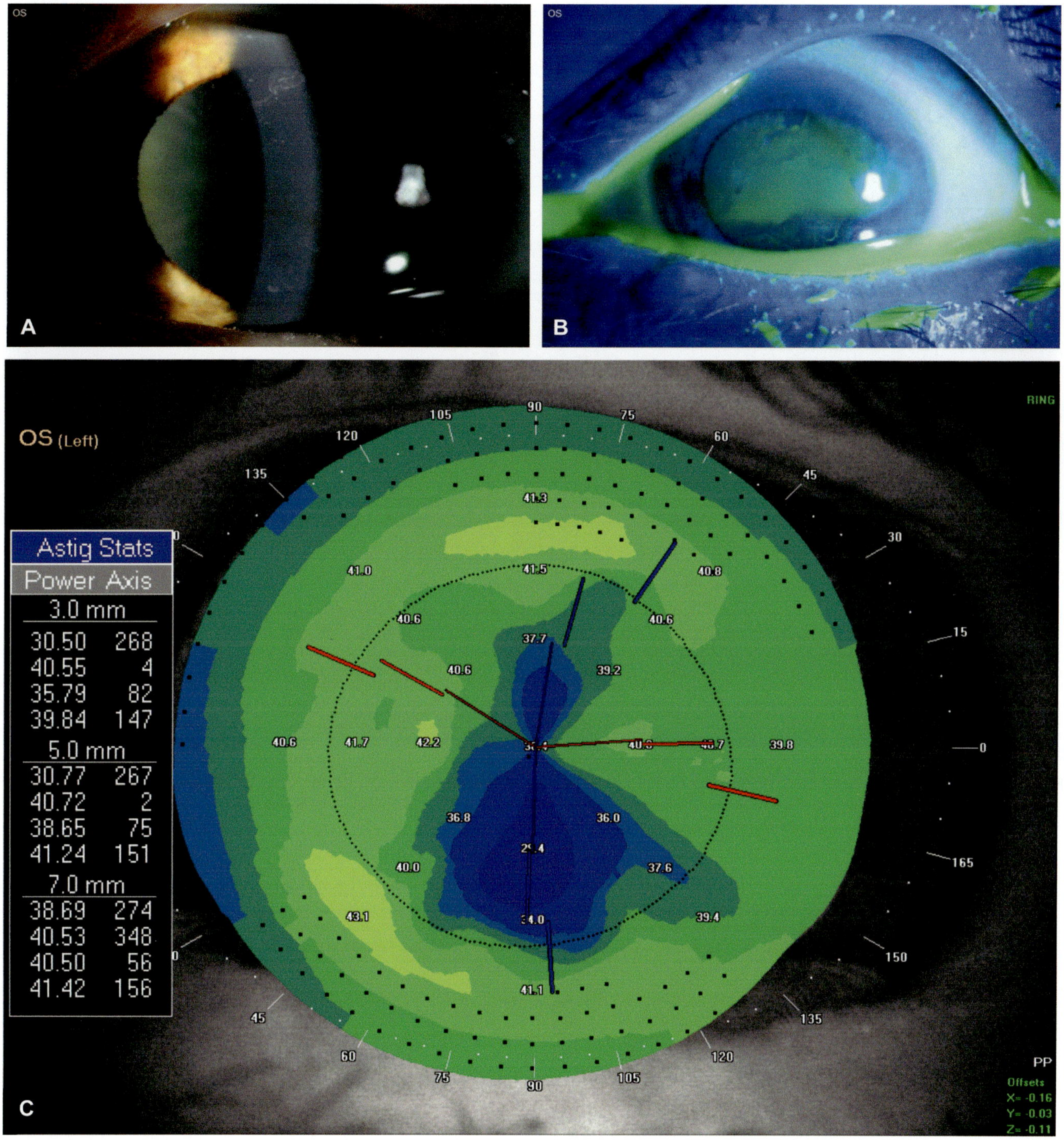

Fig. 22 Map-dot-fingerprint dystrophy inducing corneal flattening. (**A, B**) Dystrophic changes are seen on corneal midperiphery (**A**) leading to a asymmetric tear film distribution (**B**). (**C**) The dystrophic changes induce corneal flattening with high irregular astigmatism

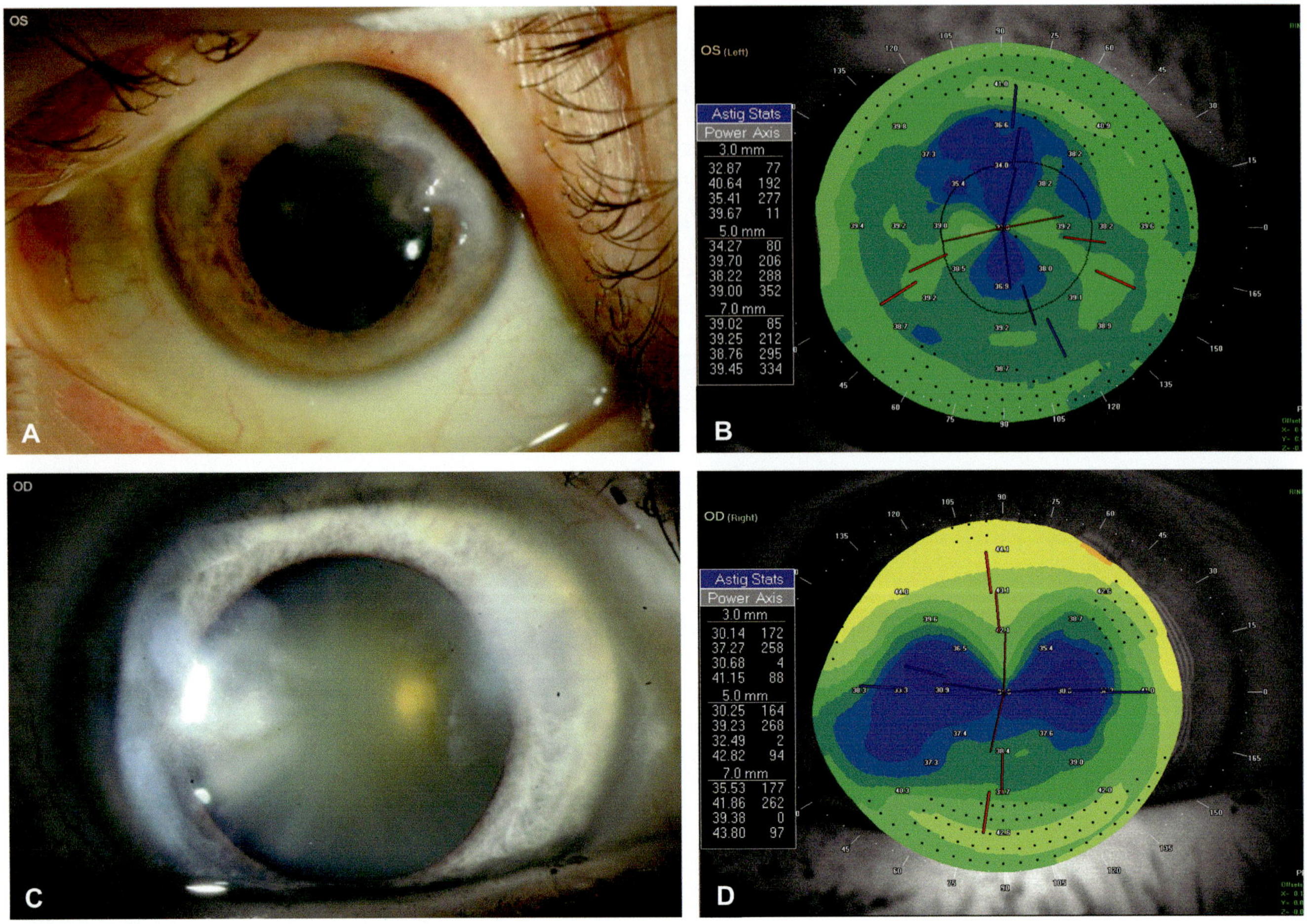

Fig. 23 Clinical photographs of Salzmann nodular degeneration with corresponding corneal topography. (**A, B**) Large Salzmann nodular degeneration (**A**) leading to a flattening of corneal curvature (Mean keratometry 37.4 Diopters) (**B**). (**C, D**) Salzmann nodules are located nasally and temporally (**C**) causing a high with-the-rule astigmatism with optical cornea plana (**D**)

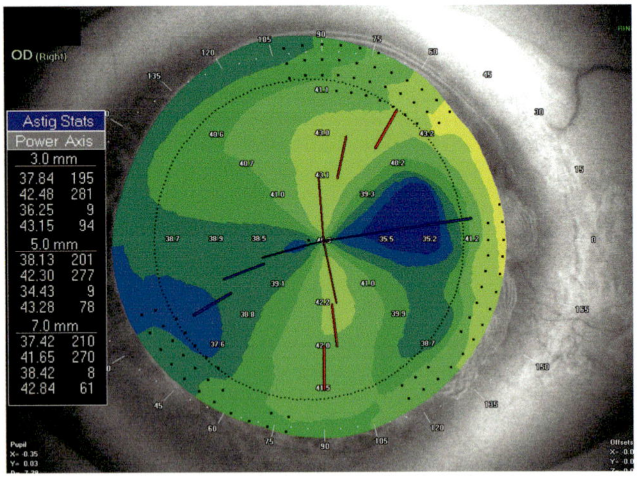

Fig. 24 Corneal topography of a large nasal pterygium inducing horizontal flattening and high regular with-the-rule astigmatism

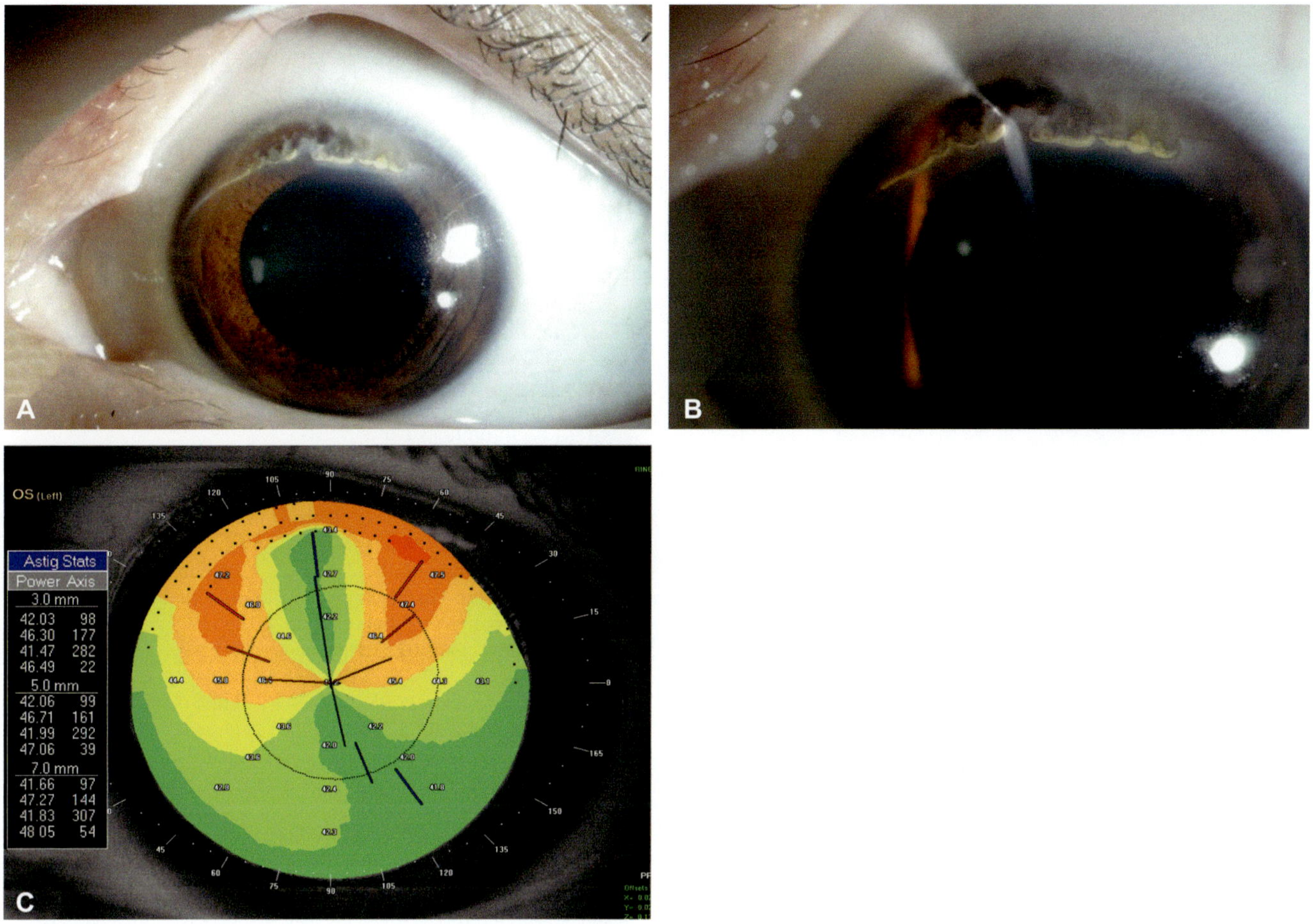

Fig. 25 Fuchs-Terrien marginal degeneration. (**A**) and (**B**) Clinical photograph of advanced Fuchs-Terrien marginal degeneration with superior thinning and lipid deposits due to stromal vascularization (**A**: diffuse illumination, **B**: narrow slit illumination). (**C**) Corneal topography demonstrating against-the-rule astigmatism with inverse crab-claw pattern

7 Conclusion

Corneal topography is a valuable tool for detecting a wide range of corneal curvature anomalies. It allows for early detection, accurate diagnosis, and effective treatment of corneal diseases. However, corneal topography has its limitations and should be supplemented by other imaging techniques to enable accurate classification of corneal diseases.

References

1. Corbett MC, O'Brart DPS, Saunders DC, Rosen ES. The topography of the normal cornea. Eur J Implant Refract Surg. 1994;6:286–97. https://doi.org/10.1016/S0955-3681(13)80229-8.
2. Kanclerz P, Khoramnia R, Wang X. Current developments in corneal topography and tomography. Diagnostics. 2021;11:1466. https://doi.org/10.3390/diagnostics11081466.
3. Martin R. Cornea and anterior eye assessment with placido-disc keratoscopy, slit scanning evaluation topography and scheimpflug imaging tomography. Indian J Ophthalmol. 2018;66:360. https://doi.org/10.4103/ijo.IJO_850_17.
4. Seitz B, Behrens A, Langenbucher A. Corneal topography. Curr Opin Ophthalmol. 1997;8:8–24. https://doi.org/10.1097/00055735-199708000-00003.
5. Langenbucher A, Seitz B, Kus M, Vilchis E, Naumann GOH. Regularity of corneal topography after penetrating keratoplasty—nonmechanical trephination with the excimer laser 193 nm vs mechanical trephination. Klin Monbl Augenheilkd. 1996;208:450–8. https://doi.org/10.1055/s-2008-1035263.
6. Vilchis E, Seitz B, Langenbucher A, Küchle M, Kus M, Naumann GOH. Arcuate keratotomies and compression sutures for treatment of high astigmatism after penetrating keratoplasty: a vector analysis and topographic study. Klin Monbl Augenheilkd. 1997;211:151–8. https://doi.org/10.1055/s-2008-1035115.
7. Das S, Langenbucher A, Seitz B. Excimer laser phototherapeutic keratectomy for granular and lattice corneal dystrophy: a comparative study. J Refract Surg. 2005;21:727–31. https://doi.org/10.3928/1081-597X-20051101-12.
8. Wilson SE, Klyce SD, Husseini ZM. Standardized color-coded maps for corneal topography. Ophthalmology. 1993;100:1723–7. https://doi.org/10.1016/S0161-6420(93)31410-7.
9. Corbett M, Maycock N, Rosen E, O'Brart D. Presentation of topographic information. Corneal topogr, Cham: Springer International Publishing; 2019, p. 51–82. https://doi.org/10.1007/978-3-030-10696-6_5

10. Rabinowitz YS, McDonnell PJ. Computer-assisted corneal topography in keratoconus. Refract Corneal Surg. 1989;5:400–8.
11. Budak K, Hamed AM, Friedman NJ, Koch DD. Corneal topography classification in myopic eyes based on axial, instantaneous, refractive, and profile difference maps. J Cataract Refract Surg. 1999;25:1069–79. https://doi.org/10.1016/S0886-3350(99)00130-3.
12. Cavas-Martínez F, De la Cruz SE, Nieto Martínez J, Fernández Cañavate FJ, Fernández-Pacheco DG. Corneal topography in keratoconus: state of the art. Eye Vis. 2016;3:5. https://doi.org/10.1186/s40662-016-0036-8.
13. Chan JS, Mandell RB, Burger DS, Fusaro RE. Accuracy of videokeratography for instantaneous radius in keratoconus. Optom Vis Sci. 1995;72:793–9. https://doi.org/10.1097/00006324-199511000-00004.
14. Klein SA, Mandell RB. Shape and refractive powers in corneal topography. Investig Ophthalmol Vis Sci. 1995;36:2096–109.
15. Yoshida T, Miyata K, Tokunaga T, Tanabe T, Oshika T. Difference map or single elevation map in the evaluation of corneal forward shift after LASIK. Ophthalmology. 2003;110:1926–30. https://doi.org/10.1016/S0161-6420(03)00621-3.
16. Seitz B, Daas L, Hamon L, Xanthopoulou K, Goebels S, Spira-Eppig C, et al. Stage-appropriate treatment of keratoconus. Ophthalmologie. 2021;118:1069–88. https://doi.org/10.1007/s00347-021-01410-8.
17. Belin MW, Jang HS, Borgstrom M. Keratoconus: diagnosis and staging. Cornea. 2022;41:1–11. https://doi.org/10.1097/ICO.0000000000002781.
18. Santodomingo-Rubido J, Carracedo G, Suzaki A, Villa-Collar C, Vincent SJ, Wolffsohn JS. Keratoconus: an updated review. Contact Lens Anterior Eye. 2022;45:101559. https://doi.org/10.1016/j.clae.2021.101559.
19. Wilson SE, Lin DT, Klyce SD. Corneal topography of keratoconus. Cornea. 1991;10:2–8.
20. De Paiva CS, Harris LD, Pflugfelder SC. Keratoconus-like topographic changes in keratoconjunctivitis sicca. Cornea. 2003;22:22–4. https://doi.org/10.1097/00003226-200301000-00006.
21. Koc M, Tekin K, Inanc M, Kosekahya P, Yilmazbas P. Crab claw pattern on corneal topography: pellucid marginal degeneration or inferior keratoconus? Eye. 2018;32:11–8. https://doi.org/10.1038/eye.2017.198.
22. Sideroudi H, Flockerzi E, Seitz B. Differential diagnosis of keratoconus based on new technologies. Klin Monbl Augenheilkd. 2023;240:57–72. https://doi.org/10.1055/a-1920-6929.
23. Maeda N, Klyce SD, Smolek MK, Thompson HW. Automated keratoconus screening with corneal topography analysis. Investig Ophthalmol Vis Sci. 1994;35:2749–57.
24. Smolek MK, Klyce SD. Current keratoconus detection methods compared with a neural network approach. Investig Ophthalmol Vis Sci. 1997;38:2290–9.
25. Martínez-Abad A, Piñero DP. Pellucid marginal degeneration: detection, discrimination from other corneal ectatic disorders and progression. Contact Lens Anterior Eye. 2019;42:341–9. https://doi.org/10.1016/j.clae.2018.11.010.
26. Wallang BS, Das S. Keratoglobus. Eye. 2013;27:1004–12. https://doi.org/10.1038/eye.2013.130.
27. El Halabi M, Daas L, Flockerzi F, Seitz B. Penetrating excimer laser keratoplasty after acute keratoglobus in osteogenesis imperfecta. Ophthalmologie. 2023;120:771–75. https://doi.org/10.1007/s00347-023-01827-3.
28. Waring GO III, Lynn MJ, McDonnell PJ. Results of the prospective evaluation of radial keratotomy (PERK) study 10 years after surgery. Arch Ophthalmol. 1994;112:1298–308. https://doi.org/10.1001/archopht.1994.01090220048022.
29. Winkler von Mohrenfels C, Salgado J, Khoramnia R. Keratectasia after refractive surgery. Klin Monbl Augenheilkd 2011; 228:704–11. https://doi.org/10.1055/s-0029-1245754.
30. Seitz B, Torres F, Langenbucher A, Behrens A, Suárez E. Posterior corneal curvature changes after myopic laser in situ keratomileusis. Ophthalmology. 2001;108:666–72. https://doi.org/10.1016/S0161-6420(00)00581-9.
31. Pogorelov P, Langenbucher A, Kruse F, Seitz B. Long-term results of phototherapeutic keratectomy for corneal map-dot-fingerprint dystrophy (Cogan-Guerry). Cornea. 2006;25:774–7. https://doi.org/10.1097/01.ico.0000214801.02195.d4.
32. Adams C, Mahler SBC, Daas L, Langenbucher A, Seitz B. Phototherapeutic keratectomy for epithelial basement membrane dystrophy. Ophthalmologie. 2022;119:945–51. https://doi.org/10.1007/s00347-022-01610-w.
33. Das S, Link B, Seitz B. Salzmann's nodular degeneration of the cornea. Cornea. 2005;24:772–7. https://doi.org/10.1097/01.ico.0000153100.74033.ef.
34. Viestenz A, Bischoff-Jung M, Langenbucher A, Eppig T, Seitz B. Phototherapeutic keratectomy in Salzmann nodular degeneration with optical cornea plana. Cornea. 2016;35:843–6. https://doi.org/10.1097/ICO.0000000000000816.
35. Rokohl AC, Heindl LM, Cursiefen C. Pterygium: pathogenesis, diagnosis and treatment. Ophthalmologe. 2021;118:749–63. https://doi.org/10.1007/s00347-021-01366-9.
36. Seitz B, Gütay A, Küchle M, Kus MM, Langenbucher A. Impact of pterygium size on corneal topography and visual acuity - a prospective clinical cross-sectional study. Klin Monbl Augenheilkd. 2001;218:609–15. https://doi.org/10.1055/s-2001-17639.
37. Corbett M, Maycock N, Rosen E, O'Brart D. Corneal surface disease. Corneal topography, Cham: Springer International Publishing; 2019, p. 125–36. https://doi.org/10.1007/978-3-030-10696-6_8.
38. Chan AT, Ulate R, Goldich Y, Rootman DS, Chan CC. Terrien marginal degeneration: clinical characteristics and outcomes. Am J Ophthalmol 2015;160:867–72.e1. https://doi.org/10.1016/j.ajo.2015.07.031.
39. Wilson SE, Lin DT, Klyce SD, Insler MS. Terrien's marginal degeneration: corneal topography. Refract Corneal Surg. 1990;6:15–20.

In Vivo Confocal Microscopy

Albéric Sneyers, Loay Daas, and Berthold Seitz

Abstract

In this chapter, we discuss the basic principles of confocal microscopy and the benefits of this technique to evaluate the human cornea. Starting with the morphology of a normal cornea and its in vivo confocal microscopic properties, we assess its clinical use in a tertiary reference hospital. We review the use of in vivo confocal microscopy as a diagnostic tool in infectious corneal pathologies more in-depth.

Keywords

In vivo confocal microscopy · Corneal morphology · Confocal microscopy principles · Clinical applications of in vivo confocal microscopy · Infectious keratitis

1 Introduction: Basic Principles

The principle of laser scanning confocal microscopy was first described by Marvin Minsky in 1955, who proposed the concept of combining the observation (objective) and illumination (condenser) system to a single focal point. Once this is achieved, the principle of confocality is accomplished [16].

The light of a laser passes through a collimating lens, which forms a beam of light in which all of the light waves are traveling in the same direction. The light is reflected by a dichroic mirror to the objective lens, which focuses the collimated beam of light into a point source at the focal plane (Figs. 1 and 3). Focused illumination restricts the excitation of fluorophores to a small portion of the field of view. Nevertheless, light traveling through the sample, both above and below the focal plane, excites fluorophores, which generate out-of-focus fluorescence. This is resolved by the second feature of the confocal principle: a pinhole at the image plane [34].

The light emitted by the fluorophore follows the emission light path and the tube lens focuses the light onto a plane within the microscope, called the image plane, where the pinhole resides. Fluorescence emitted by objects in the sample that reside within the focal plane of the objective lens passes through the pinhole to the detector, which collects the photons and generates a digital image of the sample (Figs. 2 and 3). Any objects outside the focal plane of the objective that are excited by the laser, are also collected by the objective lens, but are focused outside of the image plane. Such that the image is out-of-focus when passing through the pinhole, blocking the majority of the light emitted by these out-of-focus objects, thereby preventing this light from reaching the detector. This greatly improves image resolution and contrast. It is important to note that the pinhole is not able to block all of the emitted light of out-of-focus objects, therefore the out-of-focus fluorescence can only be largely reduced instead of being completely eliminated (Fig. 4) [34].

The size of the pinhole affects image quality and is, therefore, an important parameter in confocal microscope performance. If the size of the pinhole matches the size of the image focused on the image plane, the maximum amount of out-of-focus fluorescence is blocked by the pinhole. As the diameter of the pinhole increases, more out-of-focus light is able to pass through and thus reduces the contrast and resolution of the image [34].

The backward and forward movement (along the z-axis) of the objective lens permits the scanning of the different layers of the cornea. A transparent, viscous, sterile gel is

A. Sneyers (✉) · L. Daas · B. Seitz
Department of Ophthalmology, Saarland University Medical Center, Homburg, Germany
e-mail: alberic.sneyers@uks.eu

B. Seitz et al. (eds.), *Atlas on Cornea*, https://doi.org/10.1007/978-3-031-65422-0_10

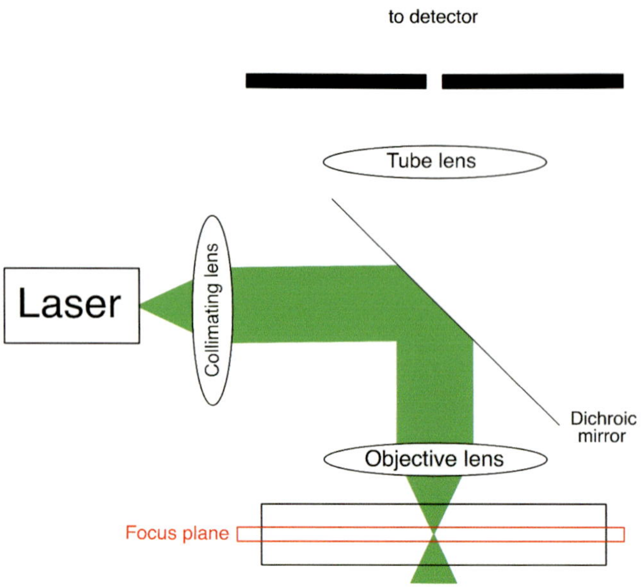

Fig. 1 **Basic principles of confocal microscopy.** The laser is the source of light. A collimating lens forms a beam of light in which all of the light waves are traveling in the same direction. A dichroic mirror (or dual-wavelength mirror) is a mirror with significantly different reflection or transmission properties at two different wavelengths and redirects the light from our light source to the specimen. The objective lens or objective lenses focus the parallel light ray into a point source at the focal plane

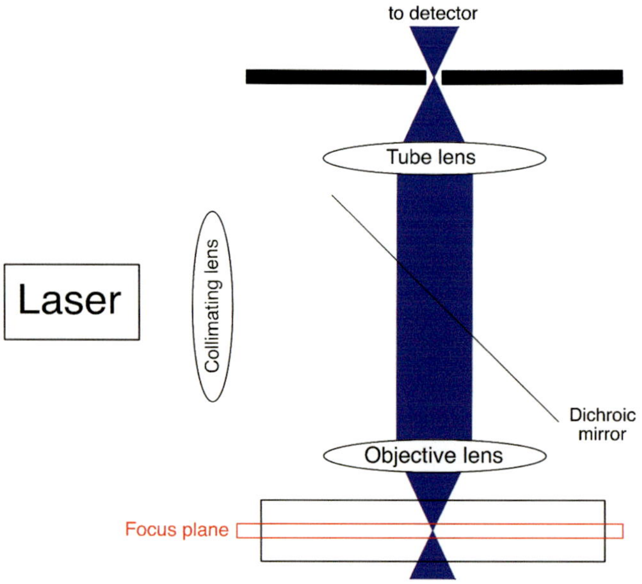

Fig. 2 **Basic principles of confocal microscopy.** The fluorophore emits after excitation due to the laser light source. The emitted light passes through the dichroic mirror, instead of being reflected back to the laser source. The tube lens focusses the emitted light onto a plane within the microscope, called the image plane, where the pinhole resides. Fluorescence emitted by objects in the sample that reside within the focal plane of the objective lens passes through the pinhole to the detector, which collects the photons and generates a digital image of the sample. Any objects outside the focal plane of the objective that are excited by the laser, are also collected by the objective lens, but are focused outside of the image plane

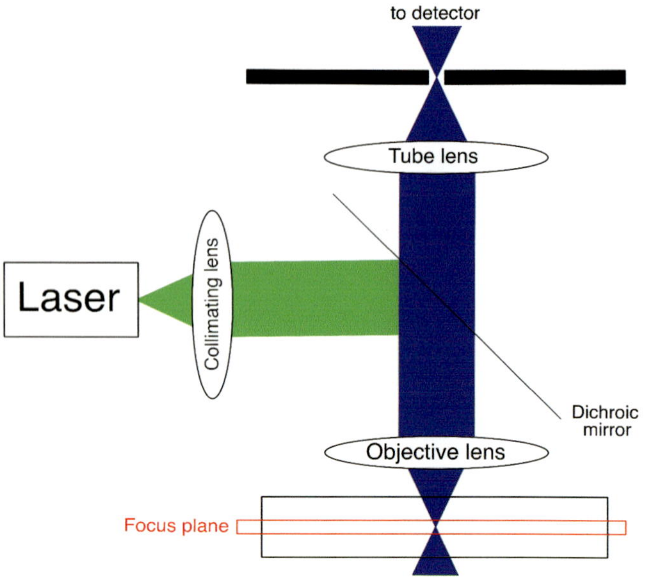

Fig. 3 **Basic principles of confocal microscopy.** The complete trajectory of the light from the laser, reflected by the dichroic mirror to the objective lens (green). The emission light path to the detector is represented by the blue color

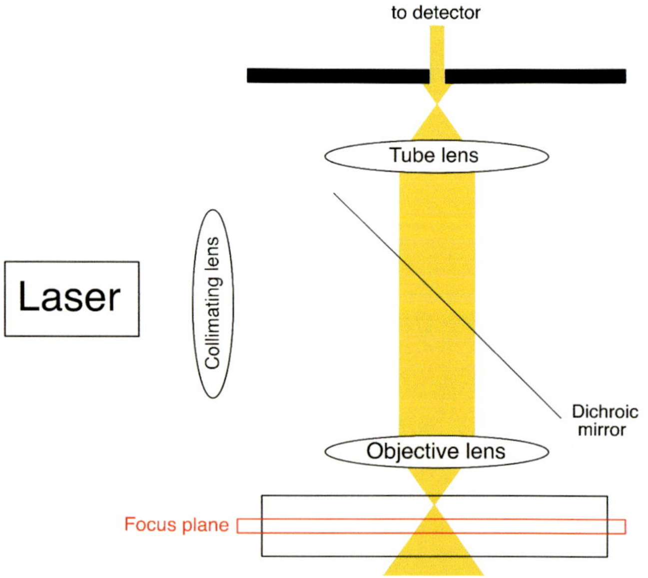

Fig. 4 **Basic principles of confocal microscopy.** Light emitted by a fluorophore anterior or posterior to the focal plane will be partially blocked by the pinhole at the image plane. This greatly reduces the out-of-focus fluorescence instead of eliminating it

interposed between the apex of the objective and the cornea to avoid optical interference by eliminating extremely different refractive indices and maintaining the required focal length. The acquisition of the mean reflectance recorded with each image, combined with the position along the

Z-axis, allows the corneal tissue to be graphically represented as a Z-scan curve or profile. Considering a normal transparent cornea, it is clear that corneal layers intrinsically have a different reflectivity. The endothelium has the highest reflectivity, while the posterior stroma has the lowest. The epithelium shows intermediate values. This clarifies the morphology of a Z-scan profile in normal corneas: a high endothelial peak, followed by a decrease in reflectivity toward the anterior layers and an intermediate superficial epithelial peak. Based on the reflectivity of the individual corneal layers, it is thus possible to follow the pachymetry of the entire cornea or a specific layer (dynamic optical pachymetry). The movement of the eye and the ocular blood pulse set limits to this approach [34].

A confocal microscope is therefore able to visualize separate layers of transparent organic structures and tissues of the human cornea in high magnification, resolution and contrast.

2 Morphology of the Normal Cornea

In vivo confocal microscopy can provide real-time noninvasive serial imaging with high resolution and contrast of most layers of the cornea: the epithelium (superficial, intermediate, and basal), the stroma (anterior to posterior), and the endothelium. The Bowman layer and Descemet membrane, both acellular layers, cannot be visualized directly in patients with normal corneas. However, abnormal features of these structures can be visualized if they are involved in pathological processes, e.g. in Fuchs endothelial dystrophy.

2.1 Epithelium

The human corneal epithelium consists of five to seven cell layers that can be subdivided into three different types: superficial, intermediate and basal cells. The latter, which lies on the basal membrane, is the only one capable of mitotic activity. Epithelial stem cells are located at the corneal limbus [15]. Corneal stem cells divide and differentiate into basal corneal epithelial cells (transiently amplifying), which differentiate into wing cells (post-mitotic), and finally into superficial squamous cells (terminally differentiated).

The superficial cells appear polygonal in shape and generally have distinct nuclei, well-defined cell borders and homogeneous density (Fig. 5). Due to the brighter appearance of the nuclei, a typical perinuclear hyporeflective dark ring can be seen. Superficial cells often show a wide variation in the reflectivity of the cytoplasm, which is thought to represent different stages in the progression toward cell death [12]. The average cell density in the cornea varies, being lower centrally (approximately 600 cells/mm^2) and higher in the periphery (around 1200 cells/mm^2) [18, 32].

The epithelial cells of the intermediate layer, the so-called wing cells, form a regular mosaic with sharp and reflective cell borders (Fig. 6). These wing cells are smaller and exhibit a regular shape. They can be classified into upper and lower wing cells, with the lower wing cells being smaller. Also these cells are less abundant in the center than in the periphery of the cornea, respectively 5000 cells/mm^2 and 5500 cells/mm^2 [5–10].

The basal epithelial cells are smaller than the upper layers and appear as cylindrical cells with reflective borders in

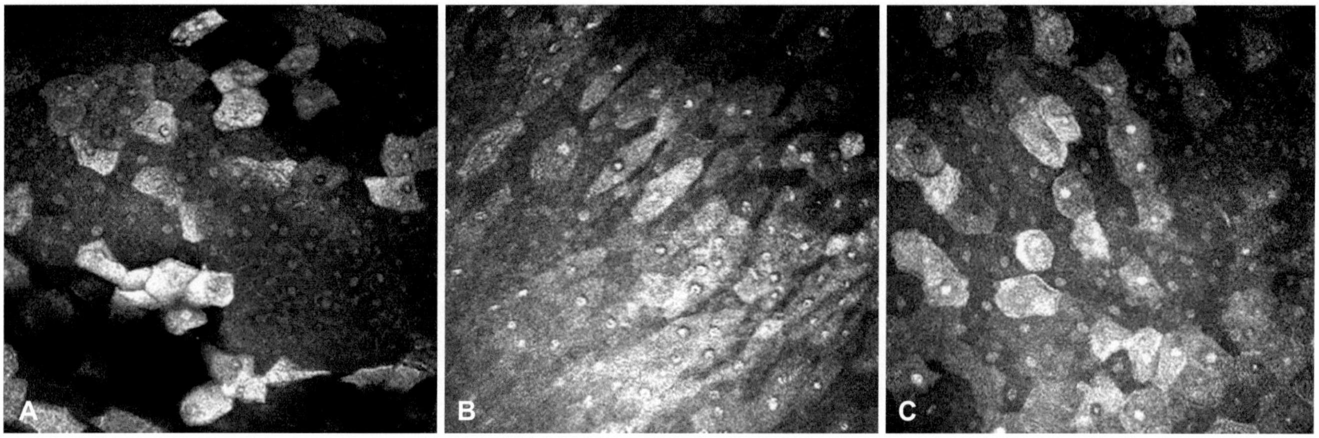

Fig. 5 Superficial epithelium layer. These cells have well-defined cell borders and a polygonal shape. Distinct bright nuclei with darker homogeneous cytoplasm and a perinuclear hyporeflective dark ring are visible. Superficial cells often display a large variation in cytoplasmic reflectivity

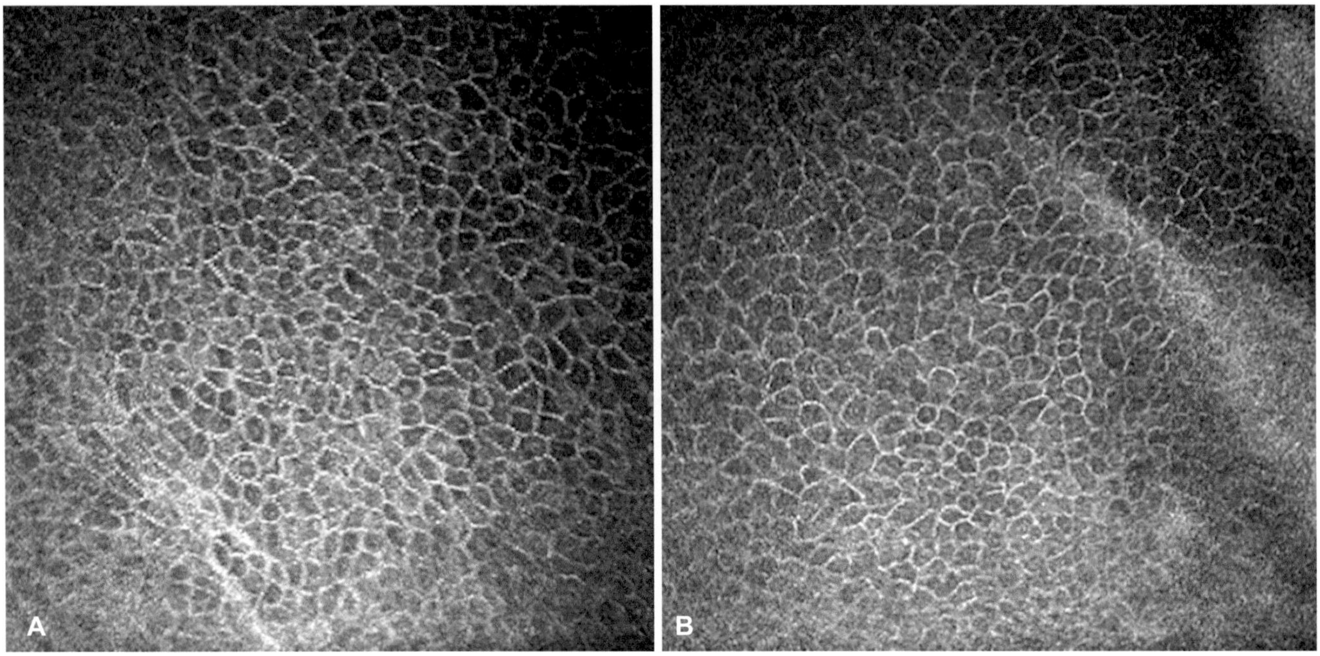

Fig. 6 **Intermediate epithelium layer.** These so-called wing cells are defined by sharp, reflective cell borders and form a regular mosaic. The nuclei are not as distinct as in the superficial layer but are visible compared to the basal layer. The cytoplasm appears dark with nearly no variety in cytoplasmatic reflectivity

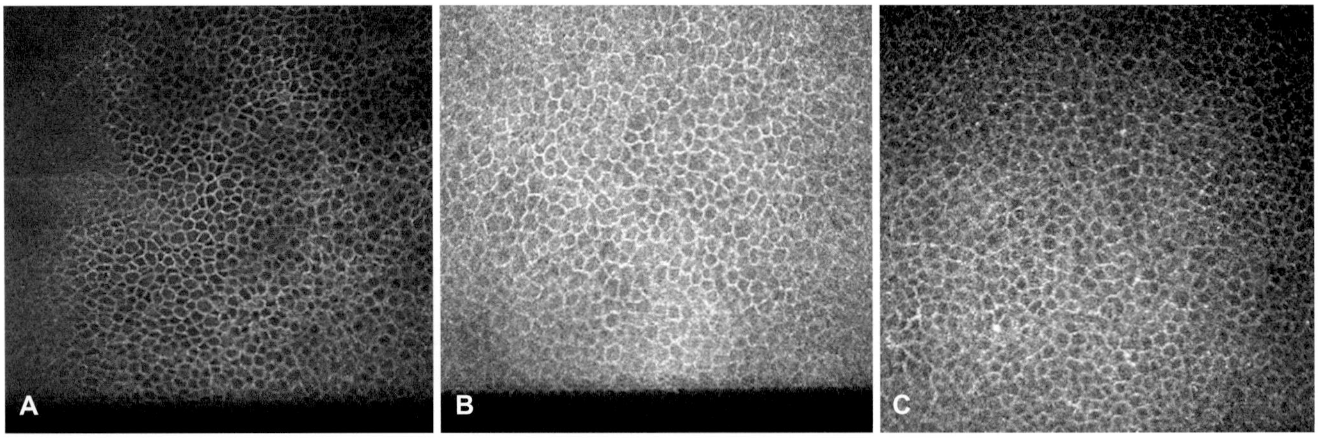

Fig. 7 **Basal epithelium layer.** The cylindrical cells have reflective borders with no visible nuclei and a homogeneous dark cytoplasmic mass

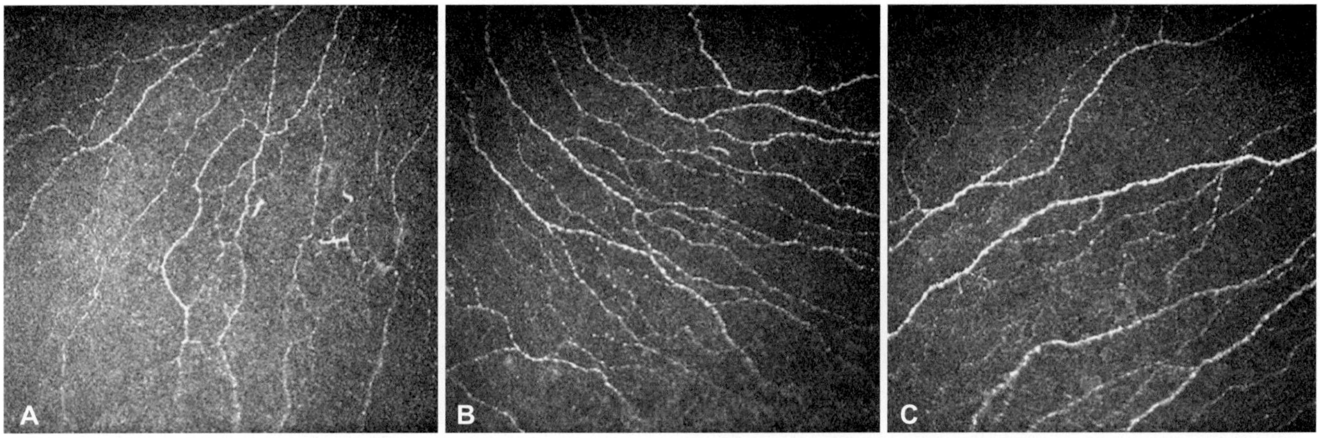

Fig. 8 **Subbasal nerve plexus.** The nerve fibers have a bright, well-contrasted and uniform appearance against a dark background. They run parallel and have interconnecting bundles

which no nuclei are distinguishable (Fig. 7). The average cell density varies from 6000 to 9000 cells/mm^2 centrally and 10.000 cells/mm^2 peripherally [5–25].

2.2 Subepithelial and Subbasal Nerve Plexus

The subbasal nerve plexus, which runs between the basal cell layer and the most anterior portion of the Bowman layer, and the subepithelial nerve plexus, which is located beneath the Bowman layer, are clearly visible in healthy corneas (Fig. 8). This corneal innervation originates from the long ciliary nerves, which are connected to the ophthalmic branch of the fifth cranial nerve (CN V1), the trigeminal nerve. At the sclerocorneal limbus, the nerve fibers originating from the long ciliary nerves are arrayed in a circular plexus from which further fibers emanate. These fibers run radially with several anastomoses within the posterior stroma and form the deep corneal plexus. Thin vertical fibers emanate from this plexus and form the subepithelial nerve plexus. They penetrate the Bowman layer at the level of the basal epithelium and form the subbasal nerve plexus. Its fibers run superficially, innervating the basal epithelial cells and terminating in the superficial epithelial layers. The nerve fibers can be observed as long, parallel-running interconnected bundles. These appear bright, well-contrasted and homogenous against a dark background. The thickness of a subbasal nerve fiber ranges from 2 to 4 μm, whereas the subepithelial fibers are on average 3–7 μm in width [21].

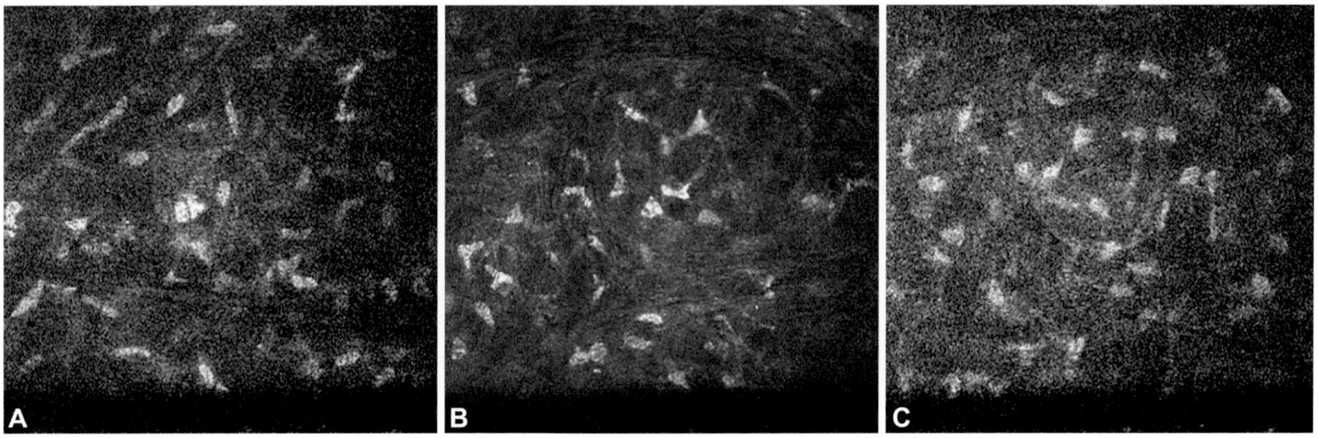

Fig. 9 **Keratocytes at different levels of the stroma.** Keratocyte nuclei are observed as ovoid, reflective light bodies. Keratocytes are more abundant in the anterior stroma (**A**) The density of keratocytes is lower in the middle stroma (**B**) and increases slightly in the posterior stroma (**C**)

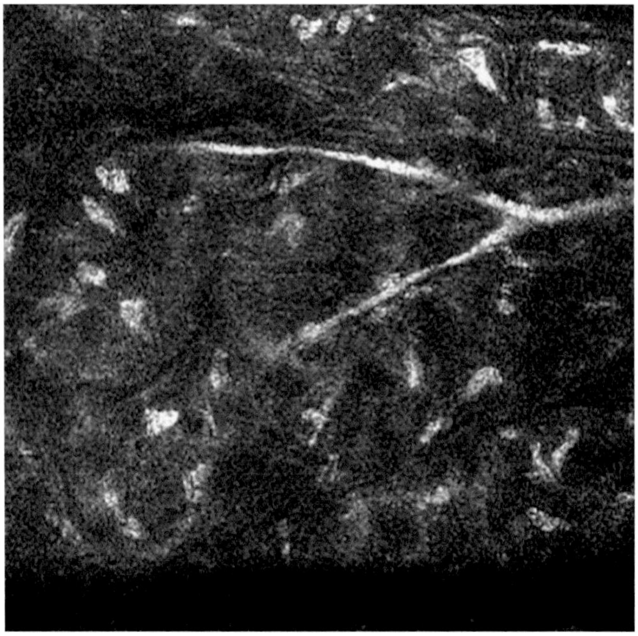

Fig. 10 **Y-shaped bifurcation of the stromal nerve plexus.** A well-defined stromal nerve single fiber surrounded by keratocytes in a Y-shaped branching pattern

2.3 Stroma

The total corneal volume consists of 80–90% of corneal stroma. It is characterized by three main histological components: cellular, acellular and neurosensory.

The cellular component predominantly consists of keratocytes and accounts for about 5% of the total stromal volume. The keratocyte nuclei are observable as ovoid, reflective light bodies (Fig. 9). Keratocyte density follows a gradient, being highest in the anterior stroma, significantly decreasing towards the central stroma, and then slightly increasing in the posterior stroma. As age increases, keratocyte density decreases [23, 24]. In the anterior stroma the density of keratocytes varies between 600 and 1600 cells/mm^2, whereas posteriorly it resides between 500 and 1100 cells/mm^2 [18].

The acellular part, which accounts for 90–95% of the stromal volume, comprises regular collagen lamellar structures (mainly type I collagen, but also type III and V) and interstitial substance [19]. The connective tissue lamellae appear dark (transparent) due to their optical properties [10].

The neurosensory apparatus of the stroma is formed by the stromal nerve plexus (Fig. 10). The stromal nerve fibers appear thicker (3- to 5-fold) than their subepithelial counterparts and have a straight course, although dichotomous branches in a T or Y shape are sometimes seen. In addition, they generally run as single fibers and not in a plexus like the subepithelial and subbasal nerves. These nerve fibers of the deep corneal plexus are mostly visible in the anterior to mid-stroma and absent in the posterior stroma [21].

2.4 Endothelium

The rearmost layer of the cornea is the endothelium. It consists of a single layer of cells arranged like a honeycomb and derived from the neural crest. The endothelium, as well as the Descemet membrane are not innervated in the human cornea [11].

The endothelial cell density (ECD) is the highest at birth with up to 7500 cells/mm^2. It declines rapidly in the first years of life and reaches mean values of 2700 cells/mm^2 in adulthood [20, 33]. The normal range in healthy adults lies

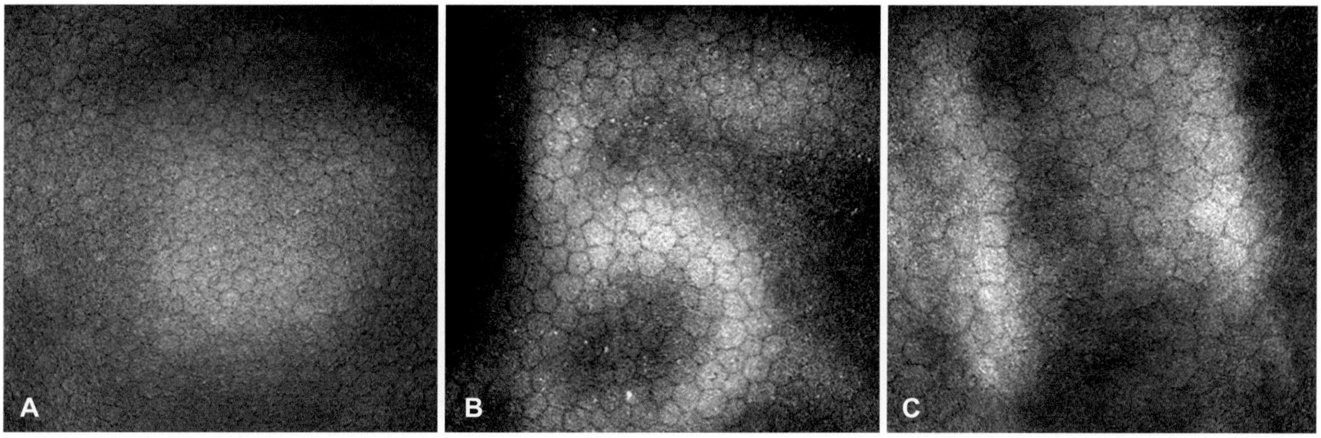

Fig. 11 **Endothelial layer**. Endothelial cells are easily recognized by their non-reflecting thin cell borders and bright homogeneous cytoplasm without visible nuclei. Depending on the density of the endothelial cells, the size (polymegethism) and shape (pleomorphism) of the cells change

between 1600 and 3200 cells/mm^2. If the ECD approaches the critical threshold of 500 cells/mm^2 as a result of pathological conditions, corneal endothelial epithelial decompensation is likely to occur [17]. The ECD progressively declines with age [36].

In childhood, the endothelial cells appear to be uniformly hexagonal in shape and homogeneous in size. Due to the continuous loss of endothelial cells over the years, the shape and size of the endothelial cells change, which is respectively described as pleomorphism and polymegethism [36].

Polymegethism, a term to describe the variation in size in the endothelial monolayer, derived from the Greek prefix *poly*, meaning "many", and *megethos*, meaning "size", was first used by Rao et al. [26]. *Megethos* should be distinguished from the Greek word *megalos*, meaning "large" [22]. Polymegethism is caused by ageing, contact lens wear, anterior uveitis, glaucoma, eye surgery, trauma and damage [3, 8].

Due to the properties of the endothelial cells, they are easy to recognize by in vivo confocal microscopy. The cell nuclei are not visible and the cell body is generally homogeneously bright and white. The borders of the endothelial cells are identifiable as thin, regular, non-reflective lines (Fig. 11). However, in the case of corneal decompensation, the endothelial cells cannot be visualized well.

3 Clinical Use

The most important limiting factor when observing a microstructure with light microscopy is that reflected light from surrounding microstructures obscures the observed image, reducing contrast and resolution. Therefore, ophthalmic instruments such as the slit lamp cannot provide details of corneal structures at the cellular level. Thus, in vivo laser scanning confocal microscopy is a complementary diagnostic tool to differentiate pathologies at the cellular and subcellular levels.

In clinical practice, real-time in vivo cellular assessment is of utmost therapeutic importance mainly in infectious pathologies, since successful treatment of infectious keratitis depends on timely and accurate diagnosis followed by appropriate management. In vivo confocal microscopy is able to differentiate microorganisms and cell types based on morphology. However, the implementation and interpretation of in vivo confocal microscopy heavily depends on the experience of the user. Since gaining experience with in vivo confocal microscopy in infectious keratitis is difficult as a novice ophthalmologist, alternative ways of learning to differentiate between pathogens should be explored. Roth et al. demonstrated that by practicing with an in vivo confocal microscopy simulator using infected human corneal cadavers and a database of in vivo confocal microscopy images, a novice can acquire the skills necessary to differentiate pathologies when dealing with real patients [27].

In vivo confocal microscopy can also be used to visualize almost all other morphological changes of the cornea, such as corneal dystrophies, degenerations, micro-deposits, loss of corneal innervation, etc. As an example, corneal confocal microscopy reveals subtle changes within the subbasal nerve plexus in keratoconus. These changes include a significantly lower corneal nerve fiber length and an increased tortuosity of the subbasal nerve plexus [9]. Since these diseases involve chronic processes, a cellular in vivo real-time examination is less clinically relevant, which is why we will not discuss it further in this chapter.

4 Infectious Keratitis

4.1 Bacterial Keratitis

In a temperate climate, bacteria are predominately the causative organism of infectious keratitis. This may vary geographically due to epidemiological and microbiological characteristics of bacteria [13]. As the size of most bacteria (usually < 5 μm) is smaller than the resolution limit (5–7 μm) of in vivo confocal microscopy, the literature on the characteristics of bacterial keratitis with in vivo confocal microscopy is limited. The current in vivo confocal microscopy resolution is most likely not able to distinguish between bacteria, inflammatory cells and cell debris based on morphological features [14]. As leucocytes (6–8 μm), lymphocytes and granulocytes (7–10 μm) are large enough to be visualized and are present during bacterial keratitis, it is possible to monitor the inflammatory processes during treatment. In most clinical cases this would be too time consuming and difficult to quantify objectively as it depends on the user and the visualized part of the cornea.

4.2 Viral Keratitis

Similar to bacterial keratitis, the clinical relevance of in vivo confocal microscopy for diagnosing viral keratitis is limited due to the current resolution limit (5–7 μm) and the size of the viruses (nanometers). However, in vivo confocal microscopy can be utilized to evaluate structural and corneal changes after viral infections, for example stromal scarring after herpetic keratitis caused by herpes simplex virus (HSV).

4.3 Fungal Keratitis

Due to the nonspecific clinical manifestations in the early phase of fungal keratitis, the diagnosis is often not established until a first line treatment for bacterial, viral or amoebic keratitis is unsuccessful. As an example, cornea specialists were only able to distinguish bacterial from fungal keratitis in 66% of cases based on corneal photographs [6]. Conventional microbiological diagnostics, such as direct microscopy of smears, fungal culture or PCR have variable degrees of sensitivity and are time consuming. According to the literature, the overall sensitivity and specificity of in vivo confocal microscopy for detecting fungal pathogens, particularly filamentous fungi, is estimated at 66.7%–85.7% and 81.4%–100% respectively [28, 31].

4.3.1 Filamentous Fungi

Fusarium and Aspergillus are the most important causative organisms of fungal keratitis [29]. Aspergillus consists of septate hyphae with dichotomous branches orientated at a 45° angle, 5–10 μm in diameter and 200–400 μm in length (Fig. 12). Fusarium is also a septate filamentous fungus similar to Aspergillus but with hyphae that branch at a 90° angle and a somewhat shorter length of 200–300 μm (Fig. 13). Filamentous fungi are observed as hyperreflective filaments and can be distinguished from the subbasal and subepithelial nerve plexus based on the branching pattern.

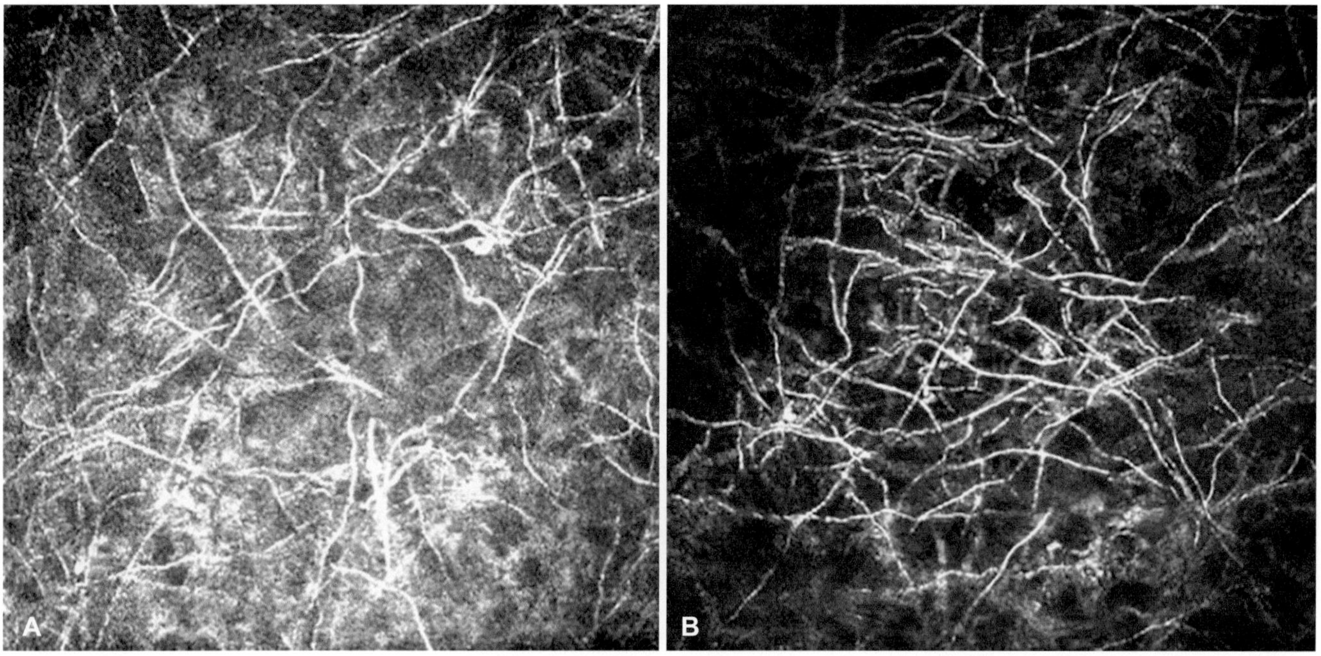

Fig. 12 Filamentous fungi, Aspergillus spp. In vivo confocal microscopy images of a microbiologically confirmed case of Aspergillus spp. showing well-defined, hyperreflective, linear, dichotomous hyphae. Clinical differentiation between filamentous species was not possible based on the branching pattern in these images

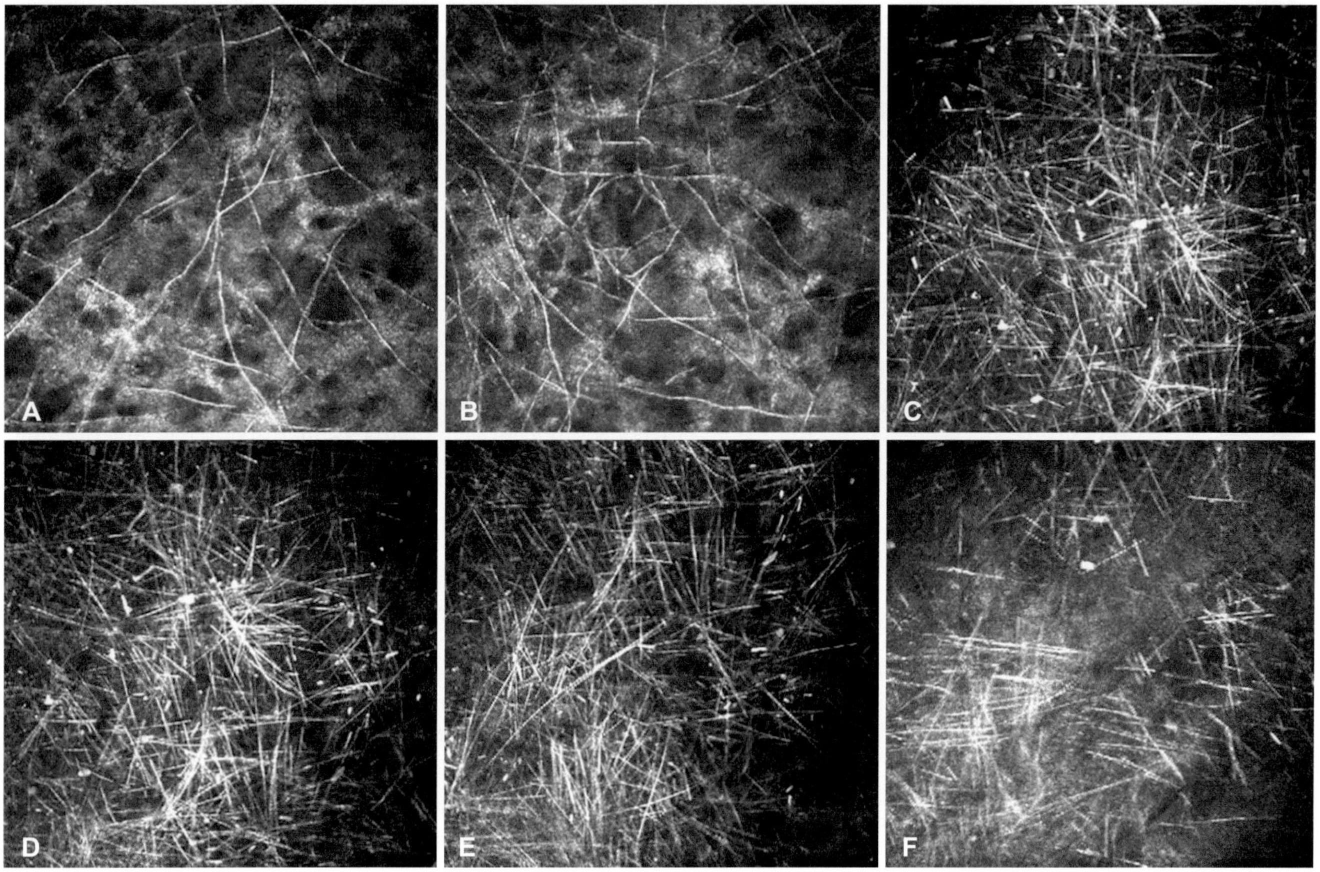

Fig. 13 Filamentous fungi, Fusarium spp. In vivo confocal microscopy images of a microbiologically confirmed case of Fusarium spp. showing well-defined, hyperreflective, linear, dichotomous hyphae. Railroad tracks are a pathognomic sign for filamentous fungi. Clinical differentiation between filamentous species was not possible based on the branching pattern in these images

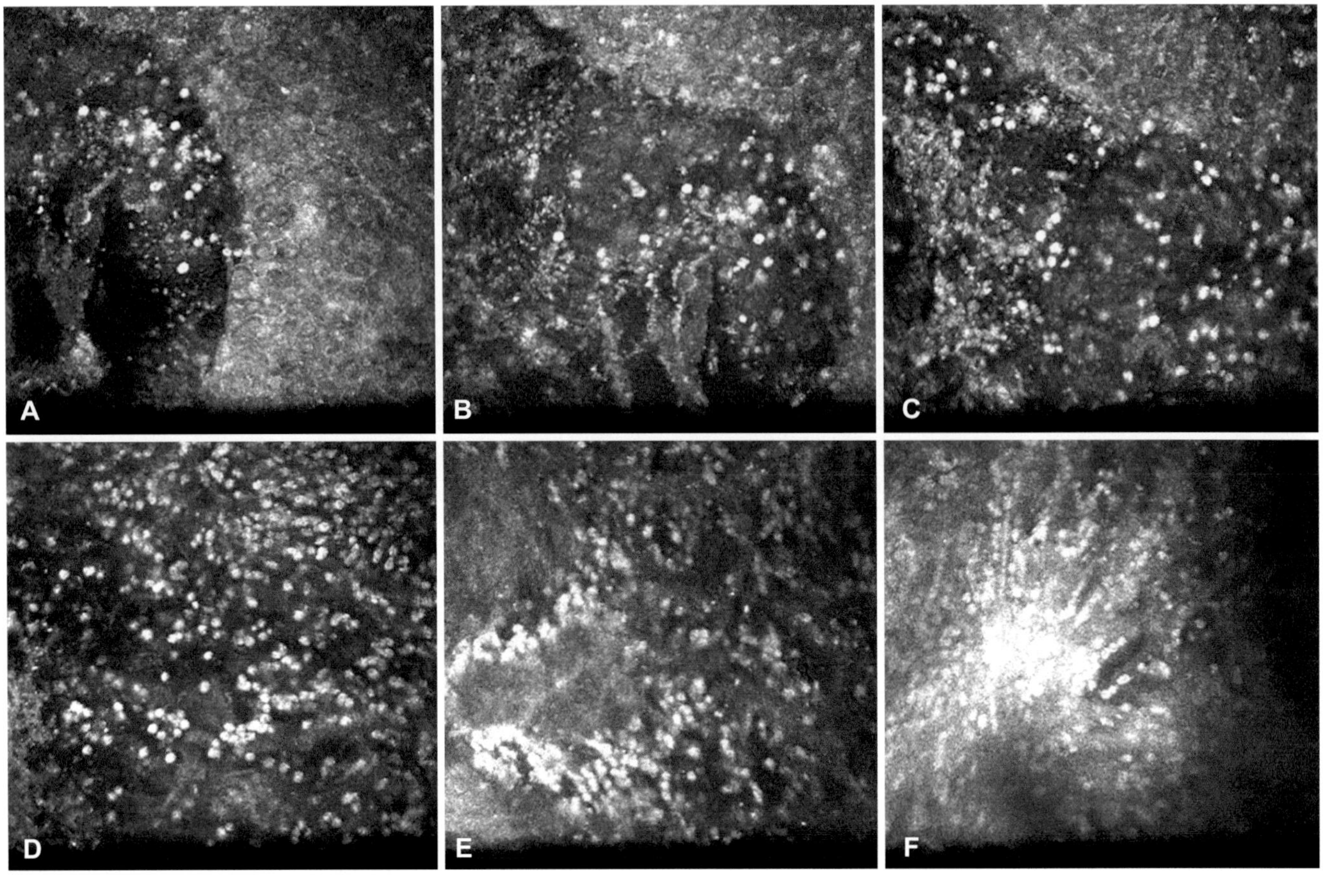

Fig. 14 **Yeast, Candida spp.** In vivo confocal microscopy images of a microbiologically confirmed case of Candida spp. showing round budding bodies (**A–F**) which often clump. Pseudohyphae (**F**) are occasionally observed

Although morphological differences between fusarium and aspergillus have been described in the literature in vivo confocal microscopy, in reality they are difficult to distinguish. While the subbasal and subepithelial nerve plexus have relatively moderate branching, filamentous fungi are characterized by its numerous and chaotic branching. In the deeper stromal layers, the nerve fibers are much larger in diameter (25–50 μm) [35].

4.3.2 Yeast

Candida, in particular, is known to be an eminent cause of fungal keratitis. It is characterized by round, budding bodies that may develop pseudohyphae. They measure 5–10 μm in diameter and 10–40 μm in length [2]. Due to its shorter length, this organism is more difficult to visualize in comparison to its filamentous counterparts (Fig. 14).

4.4 Acanthamoeba Keratitis

Acanthamoeba is an ubiquitous protozoan found in water, air, and soil with a life cycle consisting of two stages: active trophozoites and quiescent cysts. Due to the increasing use of contact lenses, about 5% of contact lens-associated keratitis is nowadays caused by acanthamoeba [4, 32, 33]. Acanthamoeba keratitis is disproportionally painful compared to clinical observations and is a vision-threatening infection [4, 30]. As with fungal keratitis, conventional microbiological diagnostics vary in sensitivity and are time-consuming. In vivo confocal microscopy has superior diagnostic performance in detecting Acanthamoeba keratitis, with overall sensitivity and specificity of 80.0%–100% and 84.0%–100%, respectively [30, 31]. Additionally, it can be used to identify the early signs of relapse after keratoplasty in patients with Acanthamoeba keratitis, but also as an additional follow-up tool after antimicrobial crosslinking [5].

Acanthamoeba spp. may present itself in various morphological appearances when using in vivo confocal microscopy. At first as double walled cysts (the dormant form) with a 15–30 μm in diameter, usually in the epithelium and/or stroma, which is the most commonly reported in vivo confocal microscopy feature of Acanthamoeba keratitis. They are observed as spherical, round, ovoid, or pear- or egg-shaped hyperreflective structures (Fig. 15).

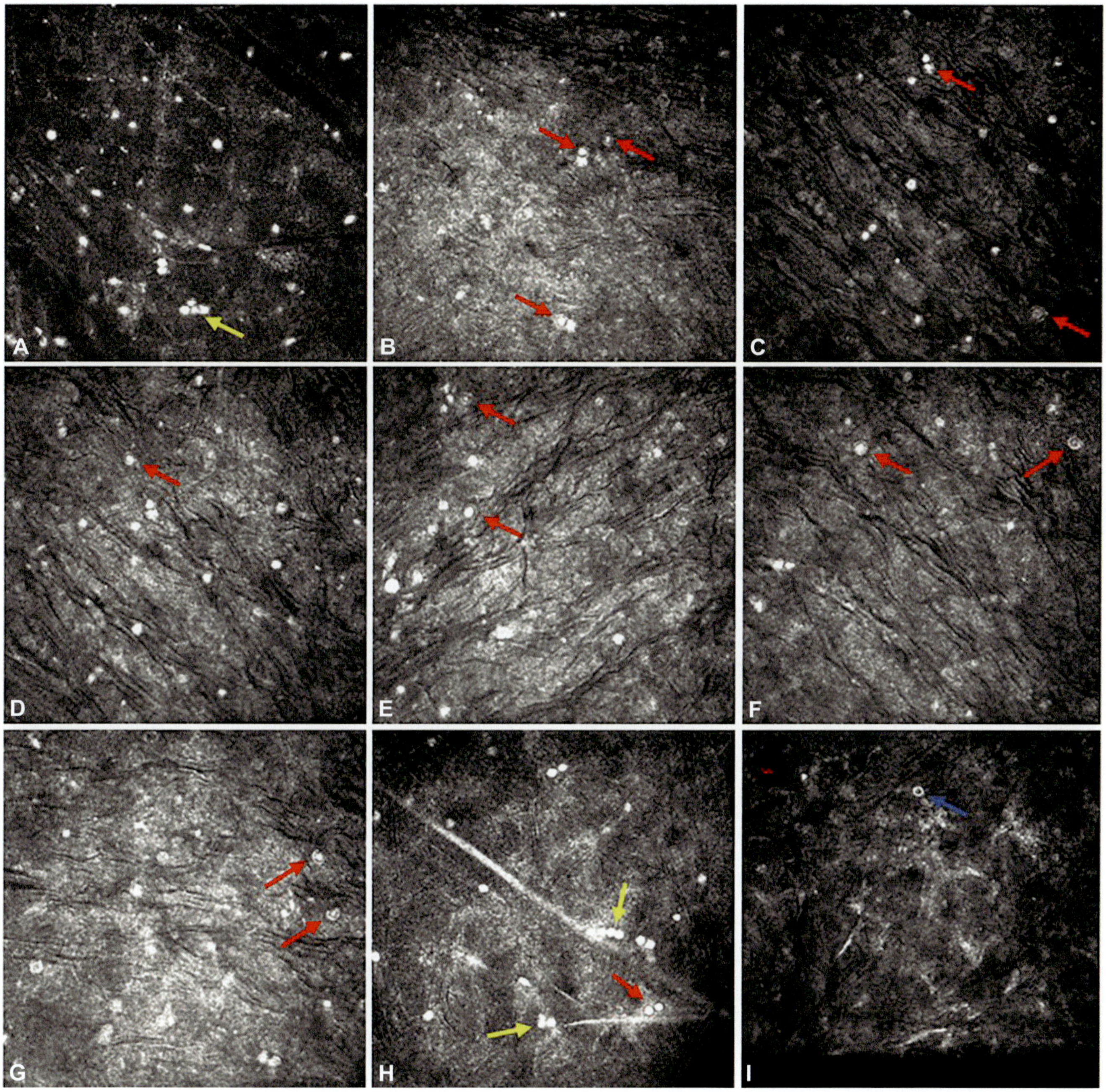

Fig. 15 **Acanthamoeba cysts.** In vivo confocal microscopy images of a microbiologically confirmed case of Acanthamoeba spp. showing well-defined, spherical, round, hyperreflective structures. They mostly appear as single cysts, but can sometimes be clustered (**A** & **H**, yellow arrow). A pathognomonic sign is the double-walled appearance ((**B**–**H**), red arrow) or a signet ring appearance ((**I**), blue arrow) of the cysts. Perineural infiltration of Acanthamoeba with double-walled appearance and clusters in hyperreflective spindle-shaped material (**H**)

The differentiation between cysts, leukocytes, lymphocytes, epithelial cells, or even cellular debris may be difficult in the absence of the characteristic double-walled appearance [14]. Interestingly, cyst accumulation was observed after treatment with topical steroids, which was associated with a poor prognosis [37]. Secondly, Acanthamoeba spp. appear as trophozoites (the active form) with a size of 25–40 μm, described as hyperreflective structures but they are even more difficult to distinguish from other hyperreflective infectious changes. A pathognomonic feature of Acanthamoeba keratitis is perineural infiltrates, which appear as reflective patchy lesions with surrounding hyperreflective spindle-shaped material. Acanthamoeba may also appear as bright spots or signet rings [14].

5 Conclusion

As a non-invasive imaging technique, in vivo confocal microscopy is a low-threshold diagnostic instrument that provides high-resolution images of all the corneal layers. For the treatment and outcome of infectious keratitis, an accurate and rapid diagnosis is crucial and, therefore, in vivo confocal microscopy is one of the most important clinical applications. Due to the limited availability of this device, an accurate and thorough anamnesis to assess the risk of possible fungal or Acanthamoeba keratitis is a key factor in deciding whether to refer the patient to a tertiary center. The value of in vivo confocal microscopy has been demonstrated for the diagnosis and management of Acanthamoeba and fungal keratitis. However, the resolution of imaging limits its applicability in viral and bacterial keratitis.

References

1. Acharya NR, Lietman TM, Margolis TP. Parasites on the rise: a new epidemic of Acanthamoeba keratitis. Am J Ophthalmol. 2007;144:292–3. https://doi.org/10.1016/j.ajo.2007.06.026.
2. Brasnu E, Bourcier T, Dupas B, Degorge S, Rodallec T, Laroche L, Borderie V, Baudouin C. In vivo confocal microscopy in fungal keratitis. Br J Ophthalmol. 2007;91:588–91. https://doi.org/10.1136/bjo.2006.107243.
3. Connor CG, Zagrod ME. Contact lens-induced corneal endothelial polymegathism: functional significance and possible mechanisms. Am J Optom Physiol Opt. 1986;63:539–44. https://doi.org/10.1097/00006324-198607000-00007.
4. Daas L, Szentmáry N, Eppig T, Langenbucher A, Hasenfus A, Roth M, Saeger M, Nölle B, Lippmann B, Böhringer D, Reinhard T, Kelbsch C, Messmer E, Pleyer U, Roters S, Zhivov A, Engelmann K, Schrecker J, Zumhagen L, Thieme H, Darawsha R, Meyer-Ter-Vehn T, Dick B, Görsch I, Hermel M, Kohlhaas M, Seitz B. The German acanthamoeba keratitis register: Initial results of a multicenter study. Ophthalmologe. 2015;112:752–63. https://doi.org/10.1007/s00347-014-3225-7.
5. Daas L, Viestenz A, Schnabel PA, Fries FN, Hager T, SzentmÁry N, Seitz B. Confocal microscopy as an early relapse marker for acanthamoeba keratitis. Clin Anat. 2018;31:60–3. https://doi.org/10.1002/ca.22925.
6. Dalmon C, Porco TC, Lietman TM, Prajna NV, Prajna L, Das MR, Kumar JA, Mascarenhas J, Margolis TP, Whitcher JP, Jeng BH, Keenan JD, Chan MF, McLeod SD, Acharya NR. The clinical differentiation of bacterial and fungal keratitis: a photographic survey. Invest Ophthalmol Vis Sci. 2012;53:1787–91. https://doi.org/10.1167/iovs.11-8478.
7. Eckard A, Stave J, Guthoff RF. In vivo investigations of the corneal epithelium with the confocal rostock laser scanning microscope (RLSM). Cornea. 2006;25:127–31. https://doi.org/10.1097/01.ico.0000170694.90455.f7.
8. Esgin H, Erda N. Corneal endothelial polymegethism and pleomorphism induced by daily-wear rigid gas-permeable contact lenses. CLAO J. 2002;28:40–3.
9. Flockerzi E, Daas L, Seitz B. Structural changes in the corneal subbasal nerve plexus in keratoconus. Acta Ophthalmol 2020;98. https://doi.org/10.1111/aos.14432.
10. Guthoff RF, Zhivov A, Stachs O. In vivo confocal microscopy, an inner vision of the cornea—a major review. Clin Exp Ophthalmol. 2009;37:100–17. https://doi.org/10.1111/j.1442-9071.2009.02016.x.
11. Hogan M, Alvarado J, Weddell J. Histology of the human eye: an atlas and textbook. Philadelphia: WB Saunders; 1971.
12. Jalbert I. In vivo confocal microscopy of the human cornea. Br J Ophthalmol. 2003;87:225–36. https://doi.org/10.1136/bjo.87.2.225.
13. Keay L, Edwards K, Naduvilath T, Taylor HR, Snibson GR, Forde K, Stapleton F. Microbial keratitis predisposing factors and morbidity. Ophthalmology. 2006;113:109–16. https://doi.org/10.1016/j.ophtha.2005.08.013.
14. Labbé A, Khammari C, Dupas B, Gabison E, Brasnu E, Labetoulle M, Baudouin C. Contribution of In Vivo Confocal Microscopy to the Diagnosis and Management of Infectious Keratitis. Ocul Surf. 2009;7:41–52. https://doi.org/10.1016/S1542-0124(12)70291-4.
15. Mastropasqua L, Nubile M. Confocal microscopy of the cornea. Thorofare: SLACK incoporated; 2002.
16. Minsky M. Memoir on inventing the confocal scanning microscope. Scanning. 1988;10:128–38. https://doi.org/10.1002/sca.4950100403.
17. Mishima S. Clinical investigations on the corneal endothelium. Ophthalmology. 1982;89:525–30. https://doi.org/10.1016/s0161-6420(82)34755-7.
18. Mustonen RK, McDonald MB, Srivannaboon S, Tan AL, Doubrava MW, Kim CK. Normal human corneal cell populations evaluated by in vivo scanning slit confocal microscopy. Cornea. 1998;17:485–92. https://doi.org/10.1097/00003226-199809000-00005.
19. Nakayasu K, Tanaka M, Konomi H, Hayashi T. Distribution of types I, II, III, IV and V collagen in normal and keratoconus corneas. Ophthalmic Res. 1986;18:1–10. https://doi.org/10.1159/000265406.
20. Nucci P, Brancato R, Mets MB, Shevell SK. Normal endothelial cell density range in childhood. Arch Ophthalmol. 1990;108:247–8. https://doi.org/10.1001/archopht.1990.01070040099039.
21. Oliveira-Soto L, Efron N. Morphology of corneal nerves using confocal microscopy. Cornea. 2001;20:374–84. https://doi.org/10.1097/00003226-200105000-00008.
22. Panton RW. Etymology of polymegethism. Arch Ophthalmol. 1991;109:318. https://doi.org/10.1001/archopht.1991.01080030020011.
23. Patel S, McLaren J, Hodge D, Bourne W. Normal human keratocyte density and corneal thickness measurement by using confocal microscopy in vivo. Invest Ophthalmol Vis Sci. 2001;42:333–9.
24. Patel DV, McGhee CN. Contemporary in vivo confocal microscopy of the living human cornea using white light and laser scanning techniques: a major review. Clin Exp Ophthalmol 2007;35:71–88. https://doi.org/10.1111/j.1442-9071.2007.01423.x.
25. Popper M, Morgado AM, Quadrado MJ, van Best JA. Corneal cell density measurement in vivo by scanning slit confocal microscopy: method and validation. Ophthalmic Res. 2004;36:270–6. https://doi.org/10.1159/000081207.
26. Rao GN, Shaw EL, Arthur EJ, Aquavella JV. Endothelial cell morphology and corneal deturgescence. Ann Ophthalmol 1979;11:885–99.
27. Roth M, Daas L, MacKenzie CR, Balasiu A, Stachon T, Neumann I, Steindor F, Seitz B, Geerling G. Development and assessment of a simulator for in vivo confocal microscopy in fungal and acanthamoeba keratitis. Curr Eye Res. 2020;45:1484–9. https://doi.org/10.1080/02713683.2020.1772830.
28. Sourlis C, Seitz B, Roth M, Hamon L, Daas L. Outcomes of severe fungal keratitis using in vivo confocal microscopy and early therapeutic penetrating keratoplasty. Clin Ophthalmol. 2022;16:2245–54. https://doi.org/10.2147/OPTH.S358709.
29. Srinivasan M. Fungal keratitis. Curr Opin Ophthalmol. 2004;15:321–7. https://doi.org/10.1097/00055735-200408000-00008.
30. Szentmáry N, Daas L, Shi L, Laurik KL, Lepper S, Milioti G, Seitz B. Acanthamoeba keratitis—clinical signs, differential diagnosis and treatment. J Curr Ophthalmol. 2019;31:16–23. https://doi.org/10.1016/j.joco.2018.09.008.

31. Ting DSJ, Gopal BP, Deshmukh R, Seitzman GD, Said DG, Dua HS. Diagnostic armamentarium of infectious keratitis: a comprehensive review. Ocul Surf. 2022;23:27–39. https://doi.org/10.1016/j.jtos.2021.11.003.
32. Tomii S, Kinoshita S. Observations of human corneal epithelium by tandem scanning confocal microscope. Scanning. 1994;16:305–6.
33. Tuft SJ, Coster DJ. The corneal endothelium. Eye (Lond). 1990;4(Pt 3):389–424. https://doi.org/10.1038/eye.1990.53.
34. Webb RH. Confocal optical microscopy. Rep Prog Phys. 1996;59:427–71. https://doi.org/10.1088/0034-4885/59/3/003.
35. Winchester K, Mathers WD, Sutphin JE. Diagnosis of aspergillus keratitis in vivo with confocal microscopy. Cornea. 1997;16:27–31.
36. Yee RW, Matsuda M, Schultz RO, Edelhauser HF. Changes in the normal corneal endothelial cellular pattern as a function of age. Curr Eye Res. 1985;4:671–8. https://doi.org/10.3109/02713688509017661.
37. Zhang X, Sun X, Jiang C, Wang Z, Zhang Y, Deng S, Labbé A. A new in vivo confocal microscopy prognostic factor in acanthamoeba keratitis. J Fr Ophtalmol. 2014;37:130–7. https://doi.org/10.1016/j.jfo.2013.09.004.

Corneal Biomechanics and the Ocular Response Analyzer ORA

Faady Yahya and Zisis Gkatzioufas

Abstract

Corneal biomechanics is a modern field in ophthalmology, which studies the corneal capability to deform reversibly. The Ocular Response Analyzer is a non-contact technique to measure the corneal biomechanical properties in vivo. Corneal biomechanical assessment plays an important role in the screening, diagnosis, prognosis and clinical follow-up for ectatic corneal diseases such as keratoconus or pellucid marginal degeneration. Furthermore, it could be used to predict and determine the impact of corneal refractive surgery and laser refractive procedures such as LASIK, PRK and SMILE on the biomechanical properties of the cornea. However, to date there is no gold standard measurement technique of corneal biomechanical characteristics. We explain the measurement technique and the data analysis of the Ocular Response Analyzer and discuss its clinical application for the diagnosis of keratoconus, keratoconus suspect and pellucid marginal degeneration. Furthermore, we evaluate measurable changes of corneal biomechanics after corneal crosslinking and after intrastromal corneal ring segment implantation. We acknowledge the growing important role of the Ocular Response Analyzer in the management of corneal ectasias and in the pre- and postoperative assessment for refractive procedures and we encourage an implementation of corneal biomechanical testing into the clinical setting. Nevertheless, further research and validation are indispensable for establishing the Ocular Response Analyzer as a standard screening technique to evaluate biomechanical strength and stability in the context of corneal refractive surgery.

F. Yahya · Z. Gkatzioufas (✉)
Department of Ophthalmology, University Hospital Basel USB, Basel, Switzerland
e-mail: zisis.gkatzioufas@usb.ch

Abbreviations

CH	Corneal Hysteresis
CRF	Corneal resistance factor
ORA	Ocular Response analyzer
KMI	Keratoconus Match Index
KMP	Keratoconus Match Probabilities
KC	Keratoconus
sKC	Subclinical Keratoconus
IOPcc	Corneal Compensated Intraocular Pressure, cornea-adjusted
IOPg	Goldmann correlated IOP, not cornea-adjusted
WS	Waveform Score

1 Introduction to Corneal Biomechanics

The investigation of corneal biomechanics has gained momentum in modern ophthalmology, because relatively new technologies are now able to provide in vivo information about the biomechanical properties of the cornea. Whereas corneal thickness and topography rather represent geometrical features, biomechanical parameters characterize elastic and viscoelastic features, i.e., describe the capability of the cornea to deform reversibly to the application of stress.

The corneal elastic property derives from the explicit collagen fiber architecture in the cornea and represents the static response to mechanical stress applied on the cornea [1]. In contrast, the viscous property is regarded as a dynamic time-dependent deformation response originating from the arrangement of the extracellular matrix scaffold of the cornea [1]. Corneal hysteresis is a parameter defined by corneal elasticity and viscosity and describes the degree of corneal capacity to absorb and dissipate energy applied on the cornea [2].

B. Seitz et al. (eds.), *Atlas on Cornea*, https://doi.org/10.1007/978-3-031-65422-0_11

To date, several non-contact measurement techniques have been developed, out of which the Ocular Response Analyzer (ORA, Reichert Ophthalmic Instruments, Buffalo, NY) is the first device to analyze corneal biomechanical properties in vivo and thereby it is commonly used in clinical practice.

2 Ocular Response Analyzer

Commercially introduced in 2005, the ORA device provides in vivo information about corneal biomechanics by the fully-automated measurement of corneal hysteresis (CH) as well as corneal resistance factor (CRF), Goldmann correlated IOP (IOPg) and corneal-compensated intraocular pressure (IOPcc). Additionally, a waveform score (WS), generated from algorithms by a calculation software, is utilized to enhance the reliability and repeatability of these measurements [3].

2.1 Measurement Setting

The following simplified image visualizes the key components in the setting of an ORA measurement: the ORA device with its three-piece sensor system consisting of an infrared light emitter, a light collimation detector and a pneumatic tool for air blast release and tonometry. An even-shaped corneal surface is positioned as target object on the opposite side (Fig. 1).

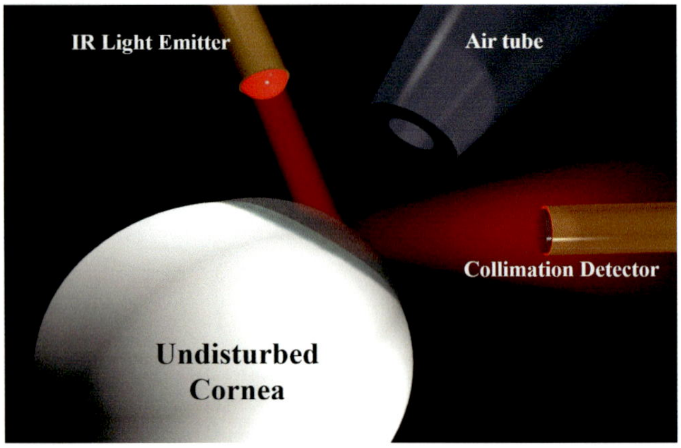

Fig. 1 Measurement setting
An air tube directs an air blast towards the opposing cornea. Changes in curvature are detected by fluctuations in collimated infrared light rays.
(The image is courtesy of Reichert Ophthalmic Instruments, Inc.)

2.2 Measurement Technique

In a pressure-controlled, dynamic bi-directional applanation process, the change in corneal curvature by a rapid air blast is recorded in real time for the duration of 20 ms using an electro-optical infrared light detector (Fig. 2). In order to understand this measurement technique, it is useful to divide the applanation process in its two phases: First the air blast pushes the convex cornea inwardly and flattens it into an even plane and beyond into a concave state. The air blast sists and initiates the second phase. The cornea moves outwardly back to its original state, passing through a moment of a second applanation before it becomes convex-shaped again.

2.3 Measurement Signal Analysis

The measurement explained above is repeated 3–4 times automatically. Displayed signals are based on the best-obtained waveform score (WS), graded on a scale of 0–10 (0 being lowest, 10 being highest). The higher the waveform score, the more reliable the measurement data.

Figure 3 illustrates two graphs: The green curve represents the air pressure applied on the cornea. The red curve indicates the signal amplitude of the infrared light beam detector when applanating the cornea. First, the cornea is applanated inward, then undergoes a short concave phase and returns finally to its original shape after the air blast is switched off. This applanation process takes place normally within 20–25 ms, and the corresponding deformation of the cornea is detected with an electro-optical system (the infrared light collimation detector).

The pressure required for inward applanation is called "pressure 1" or "P1", the second outward applanation pressure is called "pressure 2" or "P2". In each of these two applanated states, a focused light reflection occurs towards the detector, which is shown in the two peaks of the measurement signal (red curve): one during the inward movement of the cornea ("In" signal peak) and the other during the return of the cornea to its normal configuration ("Out" signal peak).

Due to its viscoelastic damping properties, the cornea absorbs some of the applied air pulse energy, which causes a delay between inward and outward movement. The difference between the pressure values of the applanation points during inward (P1) and the lower outward (P2) movement is called corneal hysteresis (CH). The average of P1 and P2 provides the Goldmann-correlated intraocular pressure (IOPg). Corneal applanation signals from normal eyes appear symmetrical and relatively free of "noise".

In addition, the corneal resistance factor (CRF) is determined, which characterizes the overall resistance of the cornea to deformation. This factor is defined by the viscous

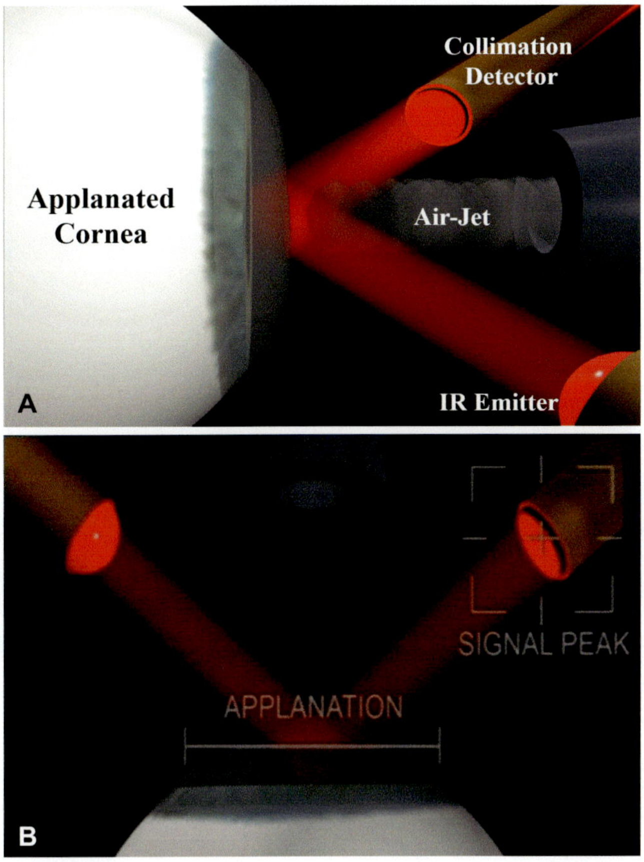

Fig. 2 **Phases of the applanation process.** (**A**) phase 1: the air jet pushes the cornea inwardly, intermittent applanation causes a signal peak by focused reflection of infrared light from the cornea to the collimation detector. (**B**) phase 2: after the air jet stops, the cornea is moving outwardly back to its convex curvature, undergoing another applanated state that causes a second signal peak
(The image is courtesy of Reichert Ophthalmic Instruments, Inc.)

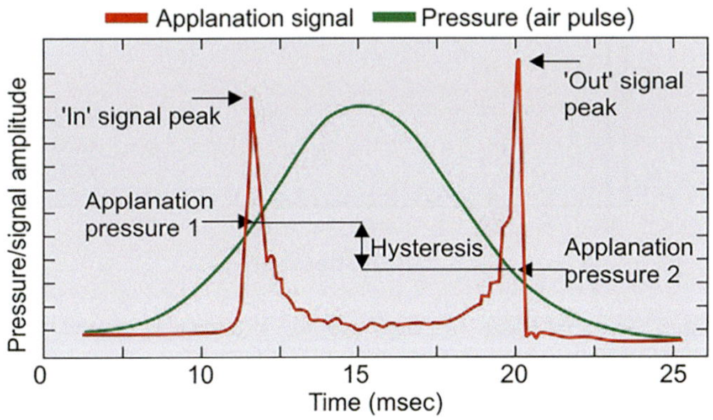

Fig. 3 ORA generated signals displaying the air pulse curve (green) and its corresponding corneal applanation response curve (red). Corneal hysteresis is calculated by the difference of the applanation pressures 1 and 2. (Picture taken with permission from the publishers from Kaushik et al. 2012 [2])

damping and the elastic resistance of corneal tissue. It is expressed by the following equation:

$$\text{CRF} = \text{k1} \times (\text{P1} - 0.7 \times \text{P2}) + \text{k2}$$

(k1and k2 resemble constants) [4, 5]. Corneal compensated intraocular pressure ("IOPcc") is a parameter derived from air puff tonometry and corneal hysteresis calculation. It provides an indication of intraocular pressure that is less influenced by biomechanical properties in contrast to other measurement methods, such as the Goldmann applanation tonometer [6].

2.4 Clinical Applications

The Ocular Response Analyzer is primarily used in the early diagnosis of corneal ectatic disease (keratoconus, pellucid marginal degeneration, post-LASIK ectasia, etc.), as well as in the assessment of the therapeutic effect of corneal crosslinking and intracorneal ring segment implantation for corneal ectasia. Moreover, ORA enables the evaluation of the impact of laser refractive procedures such as LASIK, PRK and SMILE on the biomechanical properties of the cornea.

2.4.1 Diagnosis of Keratoconus

Several studies have demonstrated that keratoconus is associated with significantly decreased corneal stiffness and attenuated tissue damping capacity [3, 7–9], The modified viscoelastic properties of the cornea are reflected in the reduced CH and CRF values in ORA measurements [3]. In ORA signal analysis, keratoconus shows a significant reduction of P1 and P2 amplitudes, increased noise between P1 and P2, and multiple spikes on P2 [3, 7]. However, CH and CRF taken alone revealed only insufficient sensitivity and specificity for the diagnosis of KC, especially for the detection of keratoconus suspect (KCS) [8, 10, 11].

The updated software program ORA 3.01 allows biomechanical classification of keratoconus by waveform analysis of the ORA signal. This signal analysis includes the evaluation of the individual signal parameters, which show a strong differentiation ability between the normal cornea and the cornea with keratoconus. According to this classification system, the value 1.0 ± 0.37 (mean ± standard deviation) corresponds to the normal cornea, and the value -0.46 ± 0.32 corresponds to advanced keratoconus. In between are the values characterizing the different threshold degrees of keratoconus (-0.25 ± 0.35 for moderate keratoconus, $+0.11 \pm 0.43$ for mild keratoconus, and $+0.62 \pm 0.37$ for form-fruste keratoconus). These indices are referred to as the keratoconus match index (KMI) and derive from 7 waveform scores representing the similarity of the waveform in the examined eye to the mean waveform scores in ectatic eyes in the machine's database. When plotted as percentages, these indices generate the keratoconus match probabilities (KMP). KMP indicate the probability of keratoconus diagnosis for each severity level. According to Labiris et al. the receiver operating curves (ROC) curve analysis indicated an overall predictive accuracy of 97.7% for KMI in keratoconus (Fig. 4) [12]. The cutoff point was 0.512, with sensitivity of 91.18% and specificity of 94.34%. However, KMP was less accurate because it misidentified nearly a quarter of the examined keratoconic eyes only as suspect keratoconus [12]. Goebels et al. confirm the diagnostic value of KMI for the detection of keratoconus, yet introduce varying thresholds for the classification of KMI indices into keratoconus grades: The cut-off point was found to be 0.77 and the other thresholds for grades 2–4 were 0.32/−0.08/−0.3, respectively [13].

The development of this biomechanical grading of keratoconus is based on data analysis of patients with keratoconus at different international centers ("data bank analysis"). After extensive validation of these indices, a high sensitivity as well as a high specificity of the KMI and KMP in the diagnosis of keratoconus and especially in the detection of form-fruste keratoconus could be proven [12]. The detection of subclinical keratoconus might be more challenging. According to Labiris et al. the KMI seems to be a valid diagnostic index, whereas the KMP revealed low sensitivity and therefore provides only limited clinical significance [14]. The ROC analysis of the KMI indicated a predictive accuracy of 94% (cutoff point 0.72) (Fig. 5). However, the KMP index identified about one-fourth (27.65%) of the control eyes false positively as keratoconus suspect while about one-third (32.14%) of keratoconus-suspect eyes were classified wrongly as definite keratoconus [14]. Galletti et al. concludes similarly, that sensitivity and specificity of indices measured with ORA to detect subclinical ectasia are lower as for keratoconus [15].

Figure 6 illustrates exemplarily measurement results with the ORA device comparing the KMI and KMP values of normal vs. keratoconus suspect vs. keratoconus corneas.

2.4.2 Diagnosis of Pellucid Marginal Degeneration

With regard to pellucid marginal degeneration (PMD), a typically bilateral inferior corneal ectatic disease, ORA measurements seem to add only limited diagnostic value. Labiris et al. have analyzed the ORA parameters (CH, CRF, and CH-CHF) and the sensitivity of the KMI and KMP [17]. CH

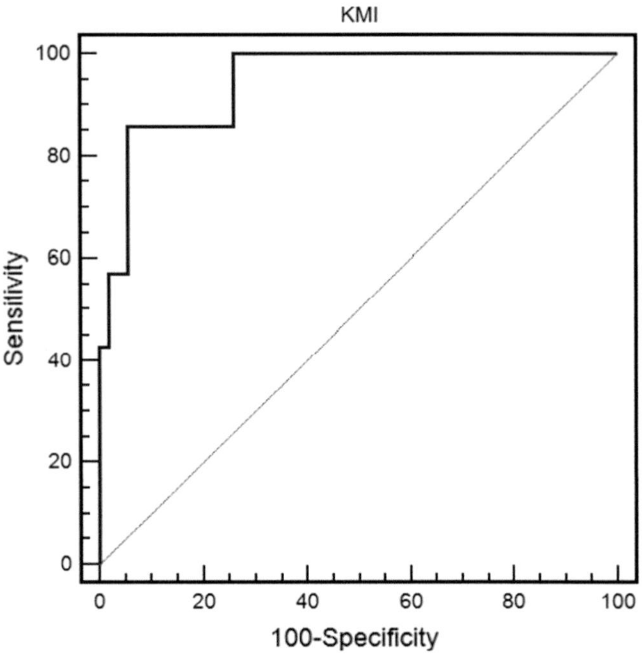

Fig. 4 Receiver operating characteristic (ROC) curve analysis of keratoconus match index (KMI) in keratoconus [12]

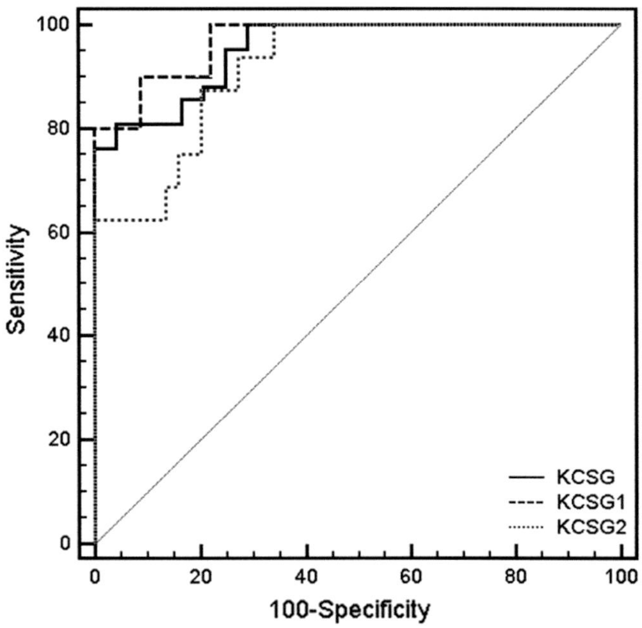

Fig. 5 ROC analysis of the KMI in keratoconus-suspect eyes (KCSG = keratoconus suspect group; KCSG1 = keratoconus suspect subgroup 1; KCSG2 = keratoconus suspect subgroup 2). The division into subgroups was based on thinnest corneal thickness (TCT) measurements: KCSG1 with TCT < 520 μm, KCSG1 with TCT > 520 μm [14]

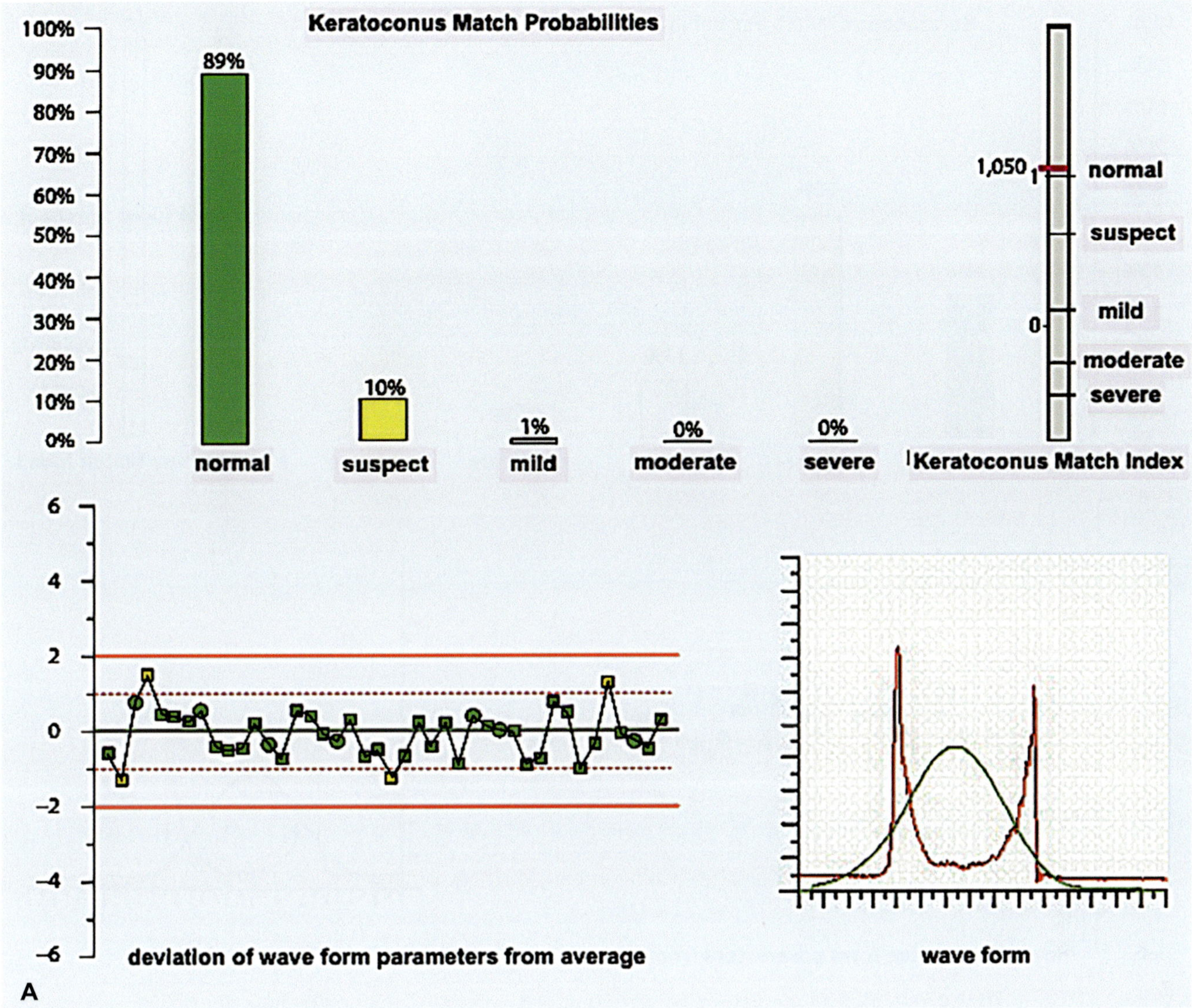

Fig. 6 Measurement examples with the ocular response analyzer. (**A**) Keratoconus match index and keratoconus match probabilities in a normal cornea

and CRF values were lower in the PMD study group when compared to the control group in accordance with a more recent study by Sedaghat et al. [18]. The KMI showed a good prediction accuracy of 94,8% in the ROC curve analyses with a sensitivity of 85.71% and specificity of 90.1% (Fig. 7). In contrast, the KMP revealed a poor diagnostic ability due to a relatively high percentage of false-positive and false-negative results. However, it is important to note that the calculation of both, KMI and KMP parameters, are based on the ORA device's reference population of patients with keratoconus and not with pellucid marginal degeneration.

2.4.3 Evaluation of the Therapeutic Effect of Corneal Crosslinking for Corneal Ectasia

Corneal collagen cross-linking (CXL) with UV-A light is nowadays a standard procedure in the management of progressive keratoconus in order to stabilize the corneal tissue and prevent further progression. Up to date, there is only inconclusive evidence in the literature regarding the question whether the ORA device is able to reliably detect and monitor the impact of CXL on the corneal biomechanics.

According to some authors, the biomechanical parameters CH and CRF remain mostly unchanged after CXL.

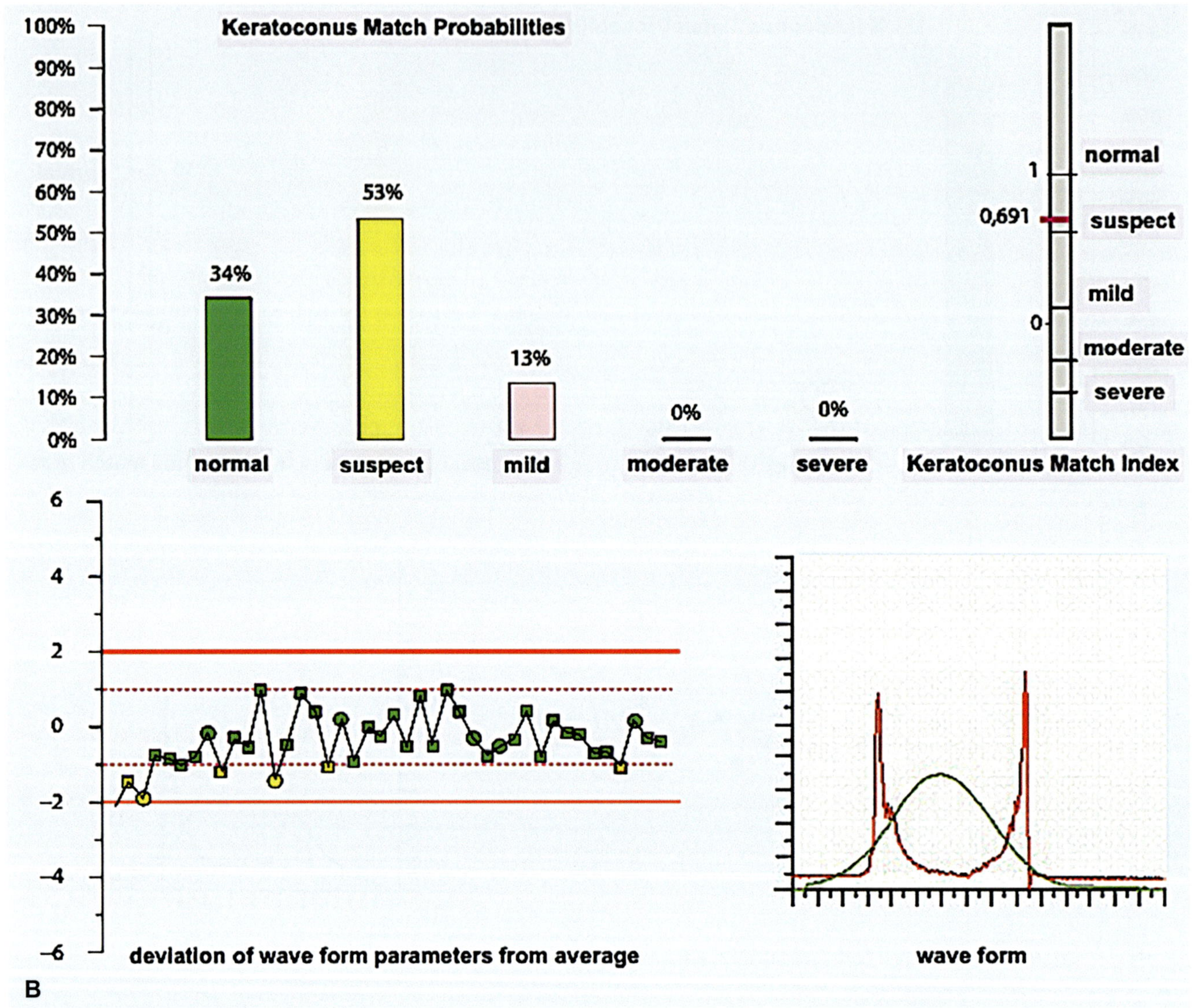

Fig. 6 (**B**) Keratoconus match index and keratoconus match probabilities in a cornea with forme fruste keratoconus

Their studies showed no statistically relevant long-lasting differences in neither of these parameters when comparing pre- and post-CXL results [19–22]. This could be partially explained by the relatively large measurement zone of the ORA device, thus providing information about the averaged general corneal response instead of subtle localized changes. In contrast, later studies performed by Salouti et al. and De Bernardo et al. describe a decrease in measured CRF, but not CH, post-CXL in keratoconic corneas [23, 24].

Hallahan et al. argue that these parameters are not as sensitive as other newer custom ORA variables, for example the applied pressure peak or the impulse intensity, which primarily characterize the elastic property of the cornea [25]. The authors describe a significant increase of these parameters 3 months after CXL for post-refractive surgery ectasia as evidence for an enhanced stiffing effect of the CXL treatment [25]. However, these results could not be reproduced in keratoconic eyes. Spoerl et al. present "the area under peak 2" (p2area) as a potential sensitive parameter to evaluate biomechanical changes after CXL in keratoconic eyes [21]. In accordance, Uzel et al. reported significant post-CXL increase in p1 area and p2 area among other values and no relevant changes in CRF and CH one year postoperatively after applying accelerated CXL to eyes with progressive keratoconus [26].

However, further research with larger sample sizes has to be performed to confirm and evaluate these data. Furthermore, corneal ectatic diseases might be responsible for a disturbed waveform quality leading to inadequate calculation of the waveform-derived parameters CRF and CH.

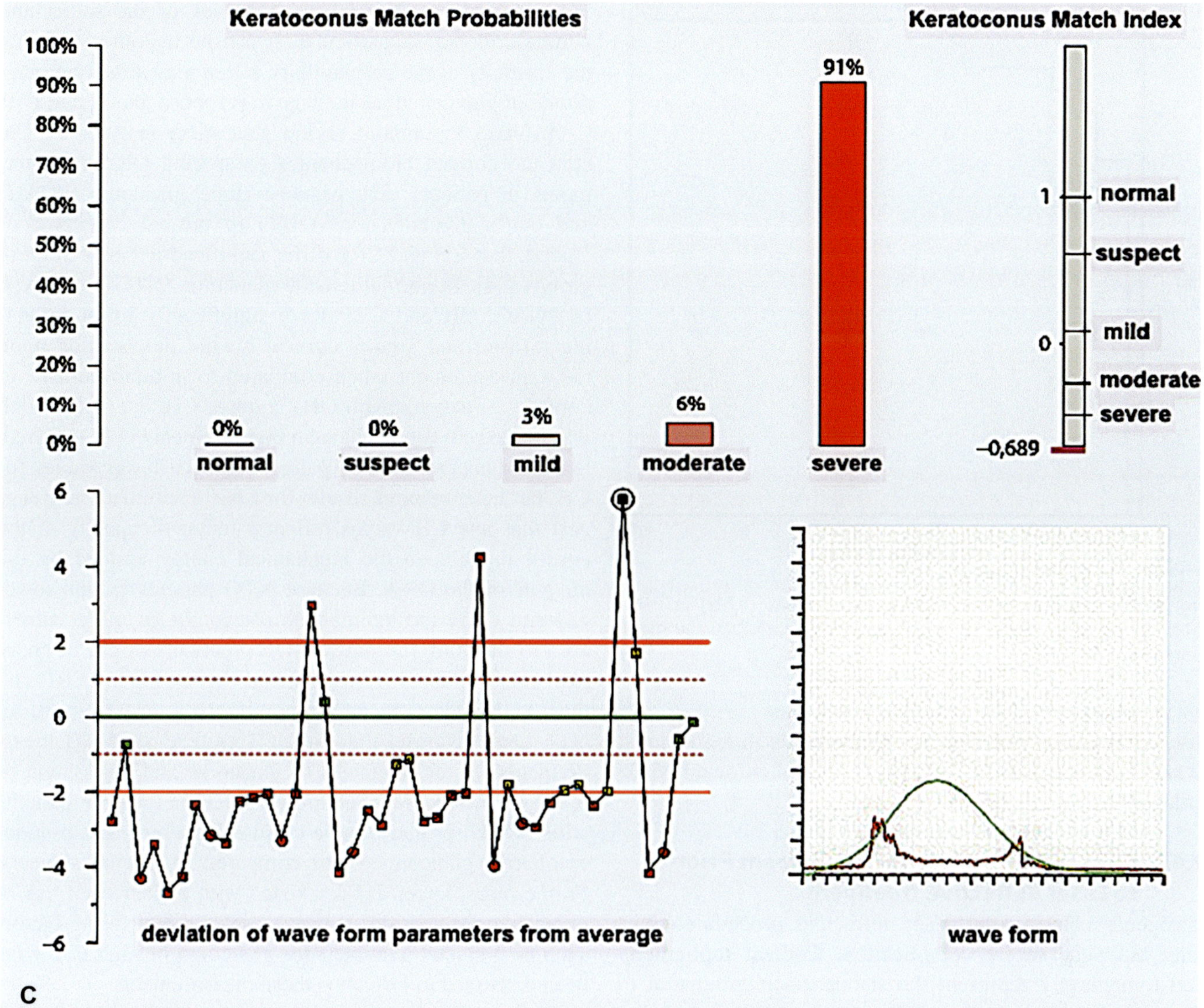

C

Fig. 6 (C) Keratoconus match index and keratoconus match probabilities in a cornea with advanced keratoconus. (Adopted and modified with authors' permission from: Gatzioufas Z, Seitz B. New aspects on biomechanics of the cornea in keratoconus. Ophthalmologe. 2013;110(9):810–817. [16])

2.4.4 Corneal Biomechanical Changes After Intrastromal Corneal Ring Segment Implantation

The implantation of Intrastromal Corneal Ring Segments (ICRS) into the corneal mid-periphery is a modern, minimally-invasive surgical method for visual improvement in primary, e.g., keratoconus, or secondary, e.g., post-refractive surgery, corneal ectasia [27, 28]. ICRS modify the corneal geometry in a manner that enhances its refractive properties and thereby, they improve visual acuity. It is well-documented that implantation of ICRS decreases the keratometric readings, spherical equivalent and cylinder, reduces high-order aberrations and improves uncorrected distance visual acuity (UDVA) and best-corrected distance visual acuity (BCDVA) in patients with keratoconus [29]. However, it is still controversial, whether this alteration of corneal geometry influences the corneal viscoelasticity or not.

Dauwe et al. evaluated 18 keratoconic eyes and found no significant change in CH and CRF pre- and 6-months postoperatively after the implantation of Intacs® ICRS [30]. Similarly, Salgado-Borges et al. examined 20 keratoconic eyes for CH and CRF before and after manual implantation of Ferrara® ICRS and observed no significant changes after an average of 18 months [31]. Peris-Martinez et al. reported unaltered CH and CRF values after femtosecond laser-assisted KeraRing® IRCS implantation in cases with post-LASIK corneal ectasia during a 12-month follow-up [32].

In contrast, Pinero et al. measured significant changes in CH and CRF 3 and 6 months after femtosecond

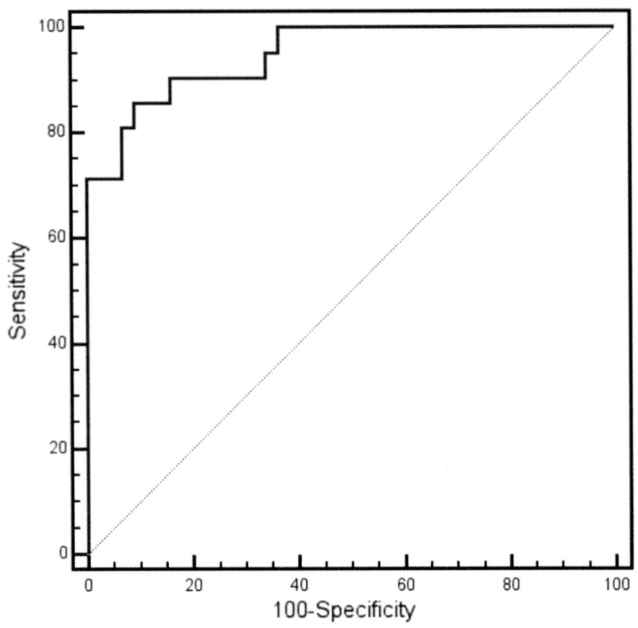

Fig. 7 ROC analysis of Keratoconus match index (KMI) in PMD eyes. The cutoff point is 0.626 with a sensitivity of 85.71% and specificity of 90.1% [17]

laser-assisted KeraRing® IRCS implantation in keratoconic eyes, which correlated with the reduction of corneal higher-order aberrations [33].

2.4.5 Corneal Biomechanical Assessment Prior to Laser Refractive Treatment

Iatrogenic ectasia after laser refractive procedures is a rare, but very severe complication. Corneal topography and tomography represent the standard screening tool to detect and exclude pathologic corneas with high risk for postoperative corneal ectasia. ORA provides an additional tool to enhance the patient selection process, by identifying corneal with 'biomechanical weakness', which could be prone to ectasia or by delivering useful information on corneas with topographical alterations, which require further evaluation. Although corneal biomechanical assessment is not an absolute requirement in preoperative screening for corneal laser refractive procedures, it could be of great value in certain cases and increase safety in patient selection.

2.4.6 Corneal Biomechanical Analysis for the Diagnosis of Glaucoma and Assessment of Progression Risk

The role of corneal biomechanical analysis for the assessment of glaucomatous damage has gained increased research interest in recent times. Due to the fact, that corneal stroma and the sclera have the same mesodermal origin, it is discussed whether corneal biomechanics could indirectly reflect the elastic properties of the sclera and lamina cribrosa, in particular. It can be hypothesized, that the elasticity of the peripapillary sclera may affect the magnitude of glaucomatous damage in response to elevated IOP.

A broad systematic review and meta-analysis by Liu et al. on corneal biomechanics comparing ORA measurements in patients with primary angle glaucoma (POAG) and ocular hypertension (OHT) to normal cohorts concluded, that CH and CRF differ significantly between these groups [34]. In normal tension glaucoma (NTG), a subtype of POAG, CH and CRF were significantly lower reflecting a faster and greater corneal inward deformation upon ORA measurement when compared to normal corneas. In contrast, in patients with OHT a lower CH, but higher CRF was measured. Biomechanical measurements in POAG high tension glaucoma (HTG) patients showed lower values for CH, but heterogenous results for CRF. These data may suggest that low CH values reflect a reduced capacity of the cornea to dampen the mechanical energy applied by the air puff of the ORA. Because NTG patients exhibit lower CH and CRF, the lamina cribrosa might be more vulnerable to the IOP. In contrast, OHT patients might be more resilient to glaucomatous damage due to higher CRF and thus, higher elasticity of the cornea. In a recent report, Sit et al. have reviewed the clinical significance of CH measurements for the diagnosis of glaucoma and assessment of progression risk [35]. Accordingly, CH is lower in patients with POAG, primary angle-closure glaucoma and pseudoexfoliative glaucoma when compared to normal subjects. Furthermore, lower CH correlated with an increased risk of glaucoma progression. However, several interfering factors such as previous treatment for glaucoma or high IOP have been discussed to influence these measurements.

We conclude, that the measurement of corneal hysteresis provides relevant complementary evidence for the diagnosis and the progression risk of glaucoma in addition to structural and functional glaucoma assessments.

3 Conclusion

The assessment of corneal biomechanical properties in vivo with the Ocular Response Analyzer is a useful tool, which enhances the diagnosis of corneal ectatic disease and contributes to evaluation of the therapeutic effect of CXL and/or ICRS implantation in the management of corneal ectasias. Furthermore, it enables a reliable patient screening and selection in the preoperative assessment prior to corneal laser procedures by increasing the capacity of identifying cases with 'high-risk' for corneal ectasia. By implementing this technology into the clinical setting for patient screening and monitoring, the ORA measurement may provide valuable information regarding the individual corneal ectasia susceptibility in undiagnosed corneal ectatic disorders. In addition, recent findings support the ORA as a beneficial tool for complementary analyses in context of glaucoma. However, further research and validation are required in order to establish ORA as a standard screening procedure to evaluate biomechanical strength and stability in the context of corneal refractive surgery.

References

1. Kling S, Hafezi F. Corneal biomechanics—a review. Ophthalmic Physiol Opt. 2017;37(3):240–52.
2. Kaushik S, Pandav SS. Ocular response analyzer. J Curr Glaucoma Pract. 2012;6(1):17–9.
3. Luce DA. Determining in vivo biomechanical properties of the cornea with an ocular response analyzer. J Cataract Refract Surg. 2005;31(1):156–62.
4. Spörl E, Terai N, Haustein M, Böhm AG, Raiskup-Wolf F, Pillunat LE. Biomechanical condition of the cornea as a new indicator for pathological and structural changes. Ophthalmologe. 2009;106(6):512–20.
5. Terai N, Raiskup F, Haustein M, Pillunat LE, Spoerl E. Identification of biomechanical properties of the cornea: the ocular response analyzer. Curr Eye Res. 2012;37(7):553–62.
6. Bayer A, Sahin A, Hürmeriç V, Ozge G. Intraocular pressure values obtained by ocular response analyzer, dynamic contour tonometry, and goldmann tonometry in keratokonic corneas. J Glaucoma. 2010;19(8):540–5.
7. Shah S, Laiquzzaman M, Bhojwani R, Mantry S, Cunliffe I. Assessment of the biomechanical properties of the cornea with the ocular response analyzer in normal and keratoconic eyes. Invest Ophthalmol Vis Sci. 2007;48(7):3026–31.
8. Fontes BM, Ambrósio R Jr, Jardim D, Velarde GC, Nosé W. Corneal biomechanical metrics and anterior segment parameters in mild keratoconus. Ophthalmology. 2010;117(4):673–9.
9. Piñero DP, Alio JL, Barraquer RI, Michael R, Jiménez R. Corneal biomechanics, refraction, and corneal aberrometry in keratoconus: an integrated study. Invest Ophthalmol Vis Sci. 2010;51(4):1948–55.
10. Fontes BM, Ambrosio Junior R, Jardim D, Velarde GC, Nose W. Ability of corneal biomechanical metrics and anterior segment data in the differentiation of keratoconus and healthy corneas. Arq Bras Oftalmol. 2010;73(4):333–7.
11. Saad A, Lteif Y, Azan E, Gatinel D. Biomechanical properties of keratoconus suspect eyes. Invest Ophthalmol Vis Sci. 2010;51(6):2912–6.
12. Labiris G, Gatzioufas Z, Sideroudi H, Giarmoukakis A, Kozobolis V, Seitz B. Biomechanical diagnosis of keratoconus: evaluation of the keratoconus match index and the keratoconus match probability. Acta Ophthalmol. 2013;91(4):e258–62.
13. Goebels S, Eppig T, Wagenpfeil S, Cayless A, Seitz B, Langenbucher A. Staging of keratoconus indices regarding tomography, topography, and biomechanical measurements. Am J Ophthalmol. 2015;159(4):733–8.
14. Labiris G, Giarmoukakis A, Gatzioufas Z, Sideroudi H, Kozobolis V, Seitz B. Diagnostic capacity of the keratoconus match index and keratoconus match probability in subclinical keratoconus. J Cataract Refract Surg. 2014;40(6):999–1005.
15. Galletti JD, Ruiseñor Vázquez PR, Fuentes Bonthoux F, Pförtner T, Galletti JG. Multivariate analysis of the ocular response analyzer's corneal deformation response curve for early keratoconus detection. J Ophthalmol. 2015;2015: 496382.
16. Gatzioufas Z, Seitz B. New aspects on biomechanics of the cornea in keratoconus. Ophthalmologe. 2013;110(9):810–7.
17. Labiris G, Giarmoukakis A, Sideroudi H, Song X, Kozobolis V, Seitz B, Gatzioufas Z. Diagnostic capacity of biomechanical indices from a dynamic bidirectional applanation device in pellucid marginal degeneration. J Cataract Refract Surg. 2014;40(6):1006–12.
18. Sedaghat MR, Ostadi-Moghadam H, Jabbarvand M, Askarizadeh F, Momeni-Moghaddam H, Narooie-Noori F. Corneal hysteresis and corneal resistance factor in pellucid marginal degeneration. J Curr Ophthalmol. 2017;30(1):42–7.
19. Vinciguerra P, Albè E, Mahmoud AM, Trazza S, Hafezi F, Roberts CJ. Intra-and postoperative variation in ocular response analyzer parameters in keratoconic eyes after corneal cross-linking. J Refract Surg. 2010;26(9):669–76.
20. Sedaghat M, Naderi M, Zarei-Ghanavati M. Biomechanical parameters of the cornea after collagen crosslinking measured by waveform analysis. J Cataract Refract Surg. 2010;36(10):1728–31.
21. Spoerl E, Terai N, Scholz F, Raiskup F, Pillunat LE. Detection of biomechanical changes after corneal cross-linking using ocular response analyzer software. J Refract Surg. 2011;27(6):452–7.
22. Gkika M, Labiris G, Giarmoukakis A, Koutsogianni A, Kozobolis V. Evaluation of corneal hysteresis and corneal resistance factor after corneal cross-linking for keratoconus. Graefes Arch Clin Exp Ophthalmol. 2012;250(4):565–73.
23. De Bernardo M, Capasso L, Lanza M, Tortori A, Iaccarino S, Cennamo M, Borrelli M, Rosa N. Long-term results of corneal collagen crosslinking for progressive keratoconus. J Optom. 2015;8(3):180–6.
24. Salouti R, Khalili MR, Zamani M, Ghoreyshi M, Nowroozzadeh MH. Assessment of the changes in corneal biomechanical properties after collagen cross-linking in patients with keratoconus. J Curr Ophthalmol. 2019;31(3):262–7.
25. Hallahan KM, Rocha K, Roy AS, Randleman JB, Stulting RD, Dupps WJ Jr. Effects of corneal cross-linking on ocular response analyzer waveform-derived variables in keratoconus and postrefractive surgery ectasia. Eye Contact Lens. 2014;40(6):339–44.
26. Uzel MM, Koc M, Can C, Polat S, Yılmazbaş P, Ileri D. Effect of accelerated corneal crosslinking on ocular response analyzer waveform-derived parameters in progressive keratoconus. Arq Bras Oftalmol. 2019;82(1):18–24.
27. Piñero DP, Alio JL, Uceda-Montanes A, Kady BE, Pascual I. Intracorneal ring segment implantation in corneas with post-laser in situ keratomileusis keratectasia. Ophthalmology. 2009;116(9):1665–74.
28. Piñero DP, Alio JL, Teus MA, Barraquer RI, Uceda-Montañés A. Modeling the intracorneal ring segment effect in keratoconus using refractive, keratometric, and corneal aberrometric data. Invest Ophthalmol Vis Sci. 2010;51(11):5583–91.
29. Sakellaris D, Balidis M, Gorou O, Szentmary N, Alexoudis A, Grieshaber MC, Sagri D, Scholl H, Gatzioufas Z. Intracorneal ring segment implantation in the management of keratoconus: an evidence-based approach. Ophthalmol Ther. 2019;8(Suppl 1):5–14.
30. Dauwe C, Touboul D, Roberts CJ, Mahmoud AM, Kérautret J, Fournier P, Malecaze F, Colin J. Biomechanical and morphological corneal response to placement of intrastromal corneal ring segments for keratoconus. J Cataract Refract Surg. 2009;35(10):1761–7.
31. Salgado-Borges JM, Costa-Ferreira C, Monteiro M, et al. Refractive, tomographic and biomechanical outcomes after implantation of ferrara ICRS in keratoconus patients. Int J Keratoconus Ectatic Corneal Diseases. 2012;1(1):16–21.
32. Peris-Martínez C, Bueno-Gimeno I, Alvarez-Arana I, Piñero DP, Gené-Sampedro A. Characterization of the effect of intracorneal ring segment in corneal ectasia after laser refractive surgery. Eur J Ophthalmol. 2020;30(1):125–31.

33. Piñero DP, Alio JL, Barraquer RI, Michael R. Corneal biomechanical changes after intracorneal ring segment implantation in keratoconus. Cornea. 2012;31(5):491–9.
34. Liu MX, Zhou M, Li DL, Dong XX, Liang G, Pan CW. Corneal biomechanics in primary open angle glaucoma and ocular hypertension: a systematic review and meta-analysis. J Glaucoma. 2023;32(3):e24–e32.
35. Sit AJ, Chen TC, Takusagawa HL, Rosdahl JA, Hoguet A, Chopra V, Richter GM, Ou Y, Kim SJ, WuDunn D. Corneal hysteresis for the diagnosis of glaucoma and assessment of progression risk: a report by the American Academy of Ophthalmology. Ophthalmology. 2023;130(4):433–42.

Corneal Visualization Scheimpflug Technology CORVIS ST

Elias Flockerzi and Berthold Seitz

Abstract

This chapter is not intended to be a handbook nor can it present all the diagnostic features provided by the Corvis ST® (Oculus, Wetzlar, Germany)—for this, we recommend the use of the software which provides explanations when clicking on the yellow flag in the lower right of each field or the recently published interpretation guide provided by the manufacturer. The Corvis ST® is a pneumotonometer that analyzes the biomechanical characteristics of the human cornea and differentiates between (1) healthy versus ectatic corneas, (2) normal corneas versus keratectasia after keratorefractive surgery and (3) healthy eyes versus normal tension glaucoma. Additionally, it provides the biomechanical E-Staging as a supplement to the tomographic ABCD keratectasia staging system, thus enabling a biomechanical staging, monitoring and progression assessment for keratectasia.

1 Introduction

Initially based on the principle of non-contact pneumotonometers, the analysis of corneal biomechanics has nowadays become an established part of the diagnostic armamentarium for ectatic corneal diseases. A deformation response results, when the human cornea is exposed to a standardized air puff indentation. The deformation analysis is suitable for differentiating between ectatic corneas, that are biomechanically weakened and healthy human corneas [1, 2]. Keratoconus (KC) as the most common ectatic corneal disease is biomechanically characterized by less resistance against deformation, thus resulting in a larger deformation response than healthy corneas [3, 4]. Biomechanical analysis of the human cornea has gained increasing importance in the early keratectasia detection in recent years, because the biomechanical destabilization of the cornea in keratectasia may even precede changes of corneal curvature [2, 5].

2 Biomechanical In Vivo Analysis of the Human Cornea

One of the devices that is able to measure and analyze the deformation reponse of the human cornea to a standardized air puff indentation is the Corneal Visualization Scheimpflug Technology (Corvis ST®, CST, Oculus, Wetzlar, Germany), which is able to detect biomechanical abnormalities in normal tension glaucoma [6] and even in early or subclinical KC [5, 7, 8]. It uses an ultra-high-speed Scheimpflug camera, which is combined with a non-contact pneumotonometer and captures 140 images within 31 ms and covers eight millimeters of the central cornea in a single horizontal meridian [7, 9]. Besides measuring and interpreting a myriad of individual biomechanical parameters, the CST also imports and incorporates tomographic data from the Pentacam® (Oculus, Wetzlar, Germany), thus resulting in a combined tomographic biomechanical assessment of the human cornea. The most common and clinically useful parameters will be presented in this chapter, because they may be helpful in diagnosing keratoconus or even other ectatic corneal diseases [10, 11].

As there exist different systems to stage and classify KC tomographically [12, 13], the question arose how to biomechanically stage KC [14–16] and how to combine tomographic and biomechanical staging information. A possible answer is the combined ABCDE-Staging system based on

E. Flockerzi (✉) · B. Seitz
Department of Ophthalmology, Saarland University Medical Center, Homburg, Germany
e-mail: elias.flockerzi@uks.eu

B. Seitz et al. (eds.), *Atlas on Cornea*, https://doi.org/10.1007/978-3-031-65422-0_12

Belin's tomographic ABCD keratoconus staging system [13] and the Homburg Biomechanical E-Staging [17–19], that has been introduced recently and enables staging and progression assessment of keratectasia.

The biomechanical/tomographic assessment CST display shows biomechanical CST data on the left and tomographic Pentacam® data on the right side (Fig. 1). Considering the biomechanical measurements, single values are presented in front of the background of a normal population (green color) and an ectatic population (red color). Below, the display shows the deformation video, that has been captured during the examination (Fig. 1). Finally, the device generates the Corvis Biomechanical Index (CBI) which distinguishes in a quasi-binary manner between a healthy cornea (green, value "0") and a KC cornea (red, value "1") [7, 9, 20]. The tomographic assessment of the Pentacam® includes corneal curvature and thickness measurements, maximal anterior keratometry (Kmax), inferior-superior value, Pentacam Random Forest Index, Topographic Keratoconus Classification and the final Belin/Ambrósio Deviation Index (BAD-D, Fig. 1). Then, the combined Tomographic Biomechanical Index (TBI) is calculated which can also assume values between "0" (green, healthy) and "1" (red, ectatic, Fig. 1) [5].

When the CST detects prior Laser Vision Correction (LVC), a warning "Post-LVC recognized!" pops up and asks the physician to confirm and specify, whether the examined eye is "post-Photorefractive Keratectomy (PRK)", "post-Laser Assisted In Situ Keratomileusis (LASIK)" or "post-Small Incision Lenticule Extraction (SMILE)" (Fig. 2). In unclear cases, the physician can choose between "post-LVC" and "no LVC" (Fig. 2). If confirmed, the CST does not calculate the CBI, but the CBI-LVC instead [21].

The CBI-LVC is a purely biomechanical parameter [21] that also behaves in a quasi-binary manner similar to the CBI. When the CBI-LVC is applied, the reference groups change from normal versus keratoconus population (Fig. 1) to post-LASIK versus ectasia population and the CBI-LVC separates between eyes with post-LVC keratectasia (Fig. 3) and stable eyes after keratorefractive surgery (Figs. 3, 4).

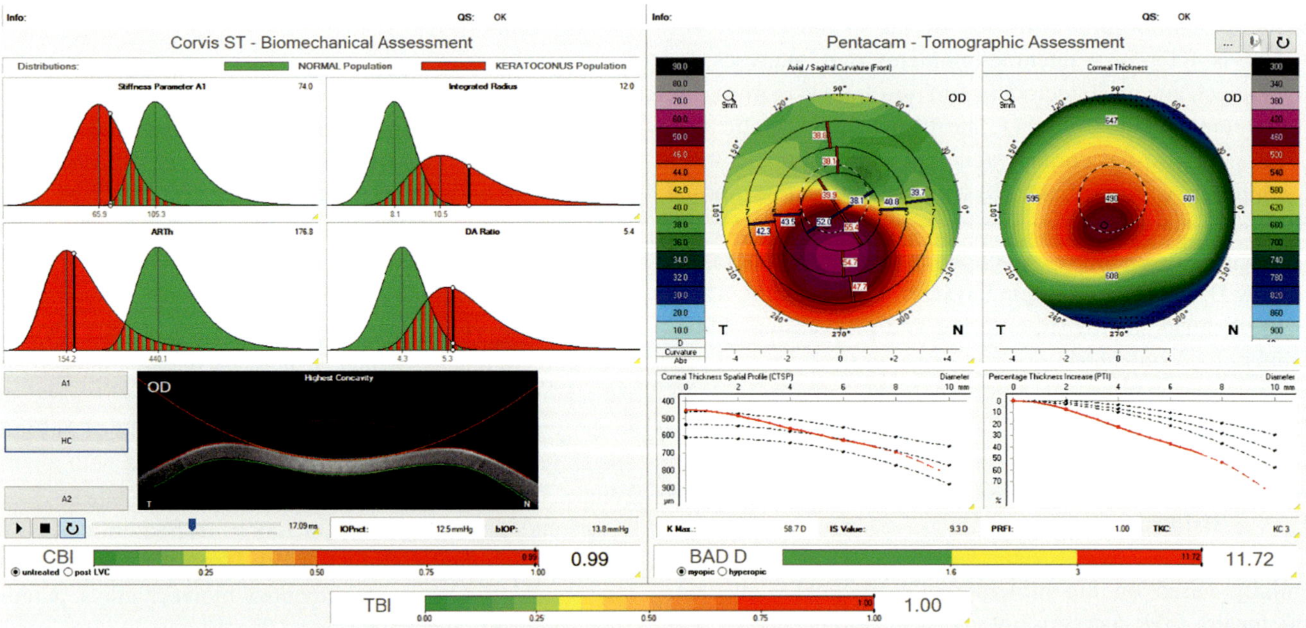

Fig. 1 Biomechanical/Tomographic Assessment Corvis ST® display of a right eye of a 22-year-old male keratoconus patient. Upper left: "Corvis ST—biomechanical assessment": Individual biomechanical parameters are displayed including stiffness parameter A1 (stiffness parameter on inward applanation), integrated inverse radius (sum of the inverse radii of the concave state between in- and outward applanation), ARTh (ratio of thinnest corneal pachymetry to the pachymetric progression index), and DA ratio 2mm (ratio between central deformation and deformation two millimeters from the center). "Keratoconus population" highlighted in red, "normal population" in green. Black vertical line marking the patient's value, thus indicating to which group the patient belongs. Lower left: deformation curve of the cornea after application of an air puff indentation. Corvis Biomechanical Index (CBI) with quasi-binary decision between a healthy cornea (green, value zero) and keratoconus (red, value one)—in this example, the value is 0.99. Right: "Pentacam—tomographic assessment" showing anterior radius of curvature, corneal thickness, pachymetric progression, maximal anterior keratometry (Kmax), inferior-superior value, Pentacam Random Forest Index (PRFI), Topographic Keratoconus Classification (TKC) and final Belin/Ambrósio Deviation index (BAD-D). Quasi-binary Tomographic Biomechanical Index (TBI) resulting of combined data. Intraocular pressure measurement results displayed as the non-corrected intraocular pressure (IOPnct) and biomechanically corrected intraocular pressure (bIOP) corrected for corneal pachymetry, age and biomechanical response

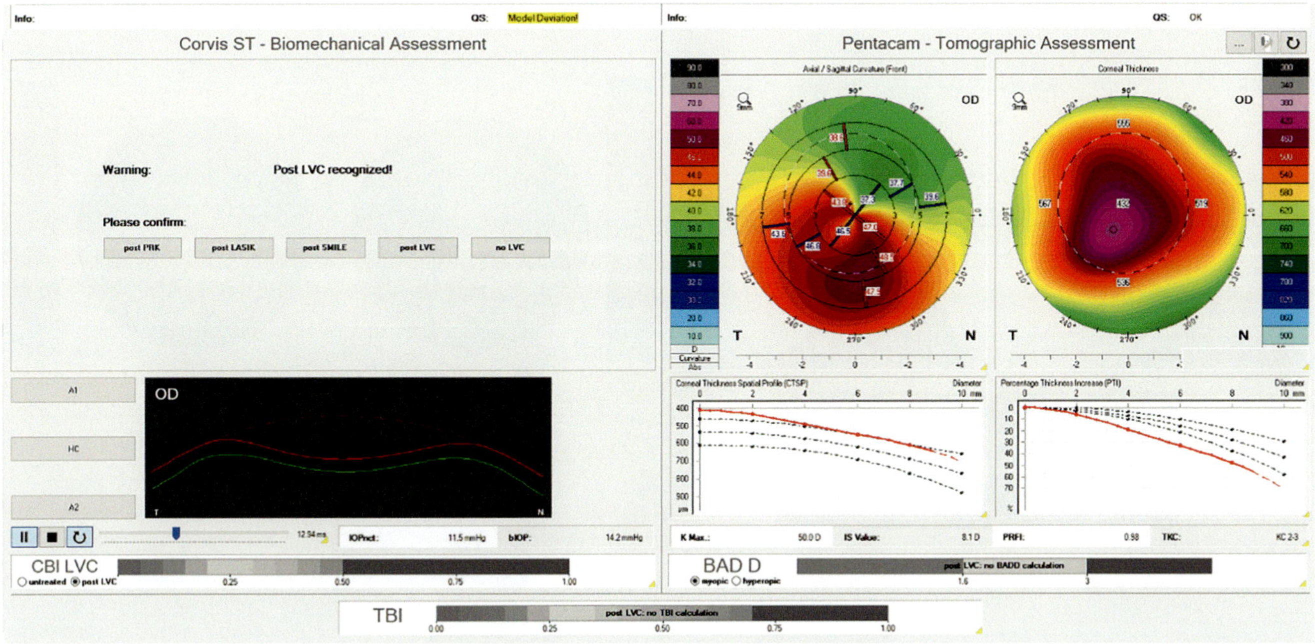

Fig. 2 Biomechanical/tomographic assessment Corvis ST® display of a right eye of a 29-year-old male patient with keratectasia after Laser-in-situ-keratomileusis (LASIK). When prior laser vision correction (LVC) is detected, a "warning: post-LVC recognized" pops up and asks for confirmation with the options "post-Photorefractive Keratectomy (PRK)", "post-Laser-in-situ-keratomileusis (LASIK)", "post-Small Incision Lenticule Extraction (SMILE)", "post-LVC" or "no LVC"

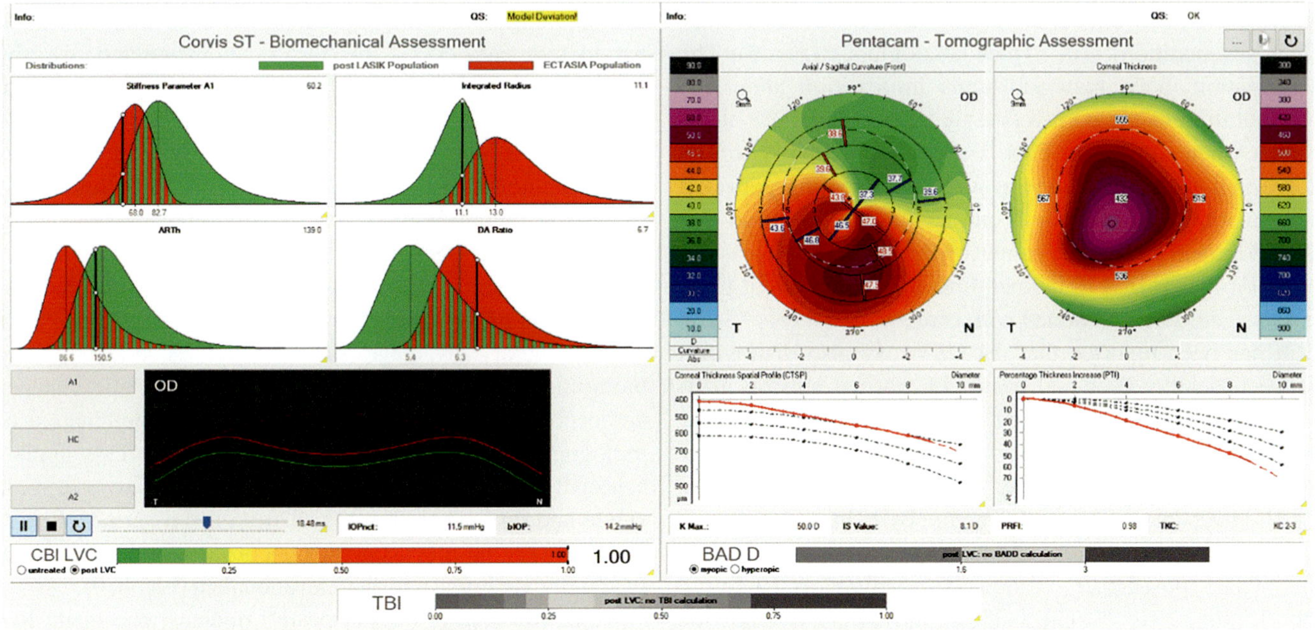

Fig. 3 Biomechanical/Tomographic Assessment Corvis ST® display. Same eye as in Fig. 2 after confirming "post-LASIK". The CBI-LVC (Laser Vision Correction) is displayed instead of the CBI and indicates biomechanical detection of keratectasia (value 1.00, red). Note also the change of the reference populations to normal "post-LASIK population" (green) and abnormal "ectasia population" (red)

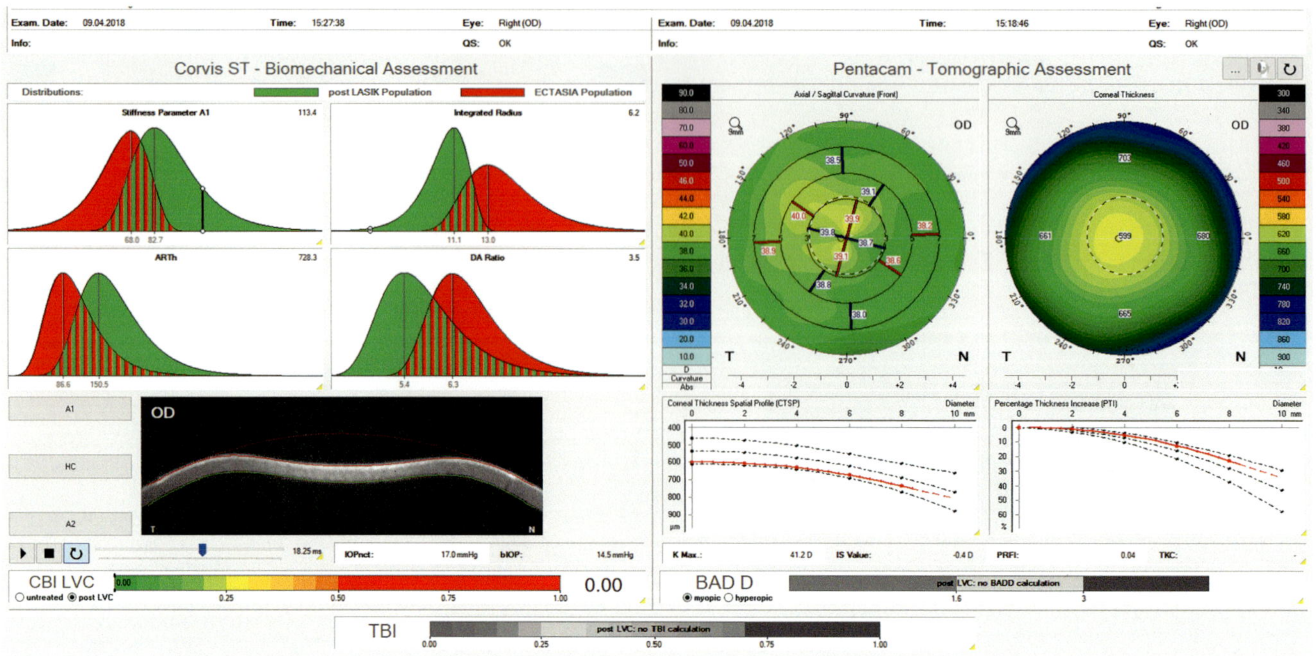

Fig. 4 Biomechanical/tomographic assessment Corvis ST® display. Right eye of a 60-year-old male patient examined several years after uneventful Laser-in-situ-keratomileusis (LASIK). Laser vision correction detected by the device and confirmation by the physician led to the CBI-LVC, here with biomechanical characteristics of a normal "post-LASIK population" (value 0, green)

The CST may also be used to examine keratectasia other than keratoconus like keratotorus (= pellucid marginal degeneration) [10, 11] or keratoglobus (Fig. 5). The deformation video may add some information about the configuration of the cornea (see thickness difference of the cornea when comparing Figs. 1 and 5 and larger deformation amplitude in Fig. 5). However, when dealing with pellucid marginal degeneration, one has to keep in mind that the CST measures in the center of the cornea, whereas the pathology is located in the paralimbal region, so that these results should be interpreted with care.

It has been reported that the CST may also distinguish between healthy eyes and eyes with normal tension glaucoma based on biomechanical measurements [6]. For this purpose, the CST offers the Glaucoma screening display including different intraocular pressure measurements and the Biomechanical Glaucoma Factor (BGF, Fig. 6) [6].

Whereas the Corvis Biomechanical Index (CBI), the CBI post-Laser Vision Correction (CBI-LVC), the Tomographic Biomechanical Index (TBI) and the Biomechanical Glaucoma Factor (BGF) aim to clearly separate between healthy and abnormal eyes (0 or 1, green or red), the Homburg Biomechanical E-Staging has been developed with the aim of providing a biomechanical staging system for KC and other ectatic corneal diseases (Fig. 7). The Homburg Biomechanical E-Staging display may show up to four different color-coded examinations of one eye at the same time. Two deformation videos may be presented in single windows and superimposed (Fig. 7, upper part). The CST also shows standard deviations and absolute values for some individual biomechanical parameters introduced in Fig. 1 supplemented by the stress–strain index, which is a measure for material stiffness. The Homburg Biomechanical E-Staging is displayed in the right part (Fig. 7) and indicates biomechanical keratectasia severity [17–19]. Below the individual biomechanical parameters and the Homburg Biomechanical E-Staging, the CST summarizes, whether the findings are stable or there has been a biomechanical keratectasia progression (Fig. 7).

The major advantage of the CST is not only the biomechanical analysis, which may detect ectatic changes earlier than tomography [2, 5], but also the combination of tomographic and biomechanical information. This applies especially, when tomographic abnormalities are still very subtle and difficult to distinguish from norm variants like in cases of with-the-rule astigmatism and suspected KC because of slightly abnormal anterior elevation data (Fig. 8, 9).

After considering the Pentacam® findings, one might like to add some biomechanical diagnostics and begin with the CST biomechanical/tomographic assessment. Even in cases with minor tomographic abnormalities, the CBI may indicate abnormal corneal biomechanics and, thus, impending corneal destabilization (Fig. 10). The TBIv1, however, may not be as clear in separating between healthy and ectatic corneas in these early cases, because it combines abnormal corneal biomechanics with almost normal tomography (Fig. 10, OS, TBI: 0.55).

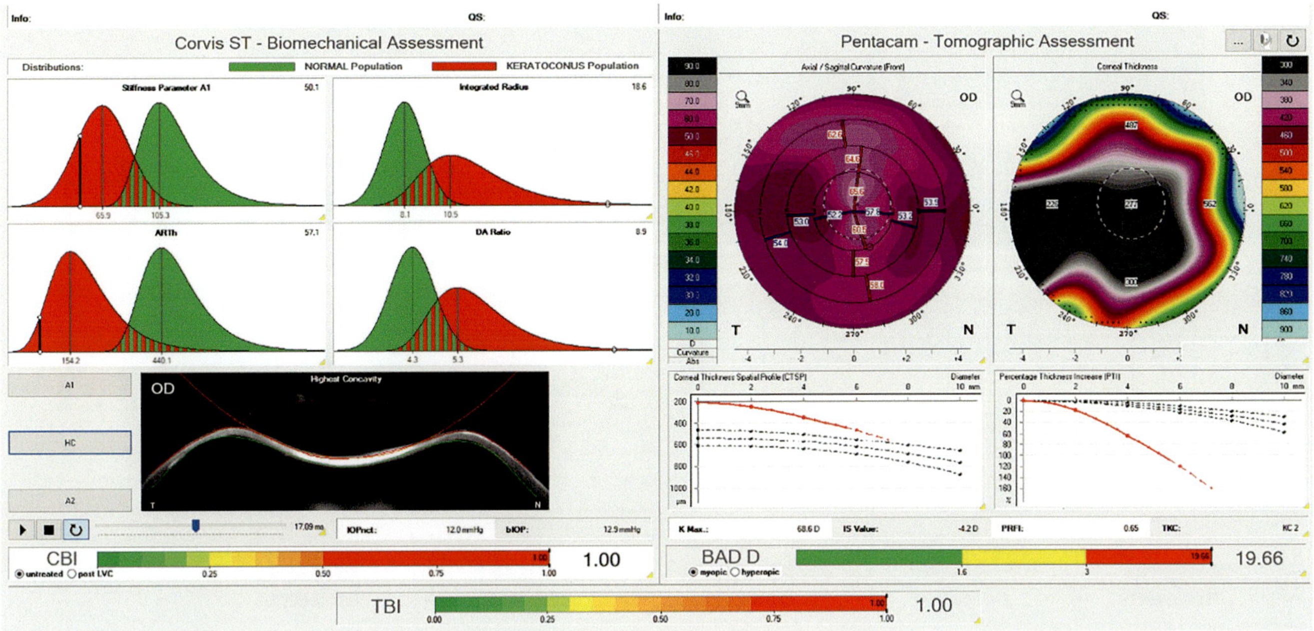

Fig. 5 Biomechanical/tomographic assessment Corvis ST® display. Right eye of a 40-year-old male patient with keratoglobus. Corvis Biomechanical Index (CBI) and tomographic biomechanical index (TBI) detecting keratectasia (value 1.00, red). Lower left, note the markedly thinned cornea with larger deformation in the Scheimpflug images when compared to the findings in Fig. 1 (keratoconus)

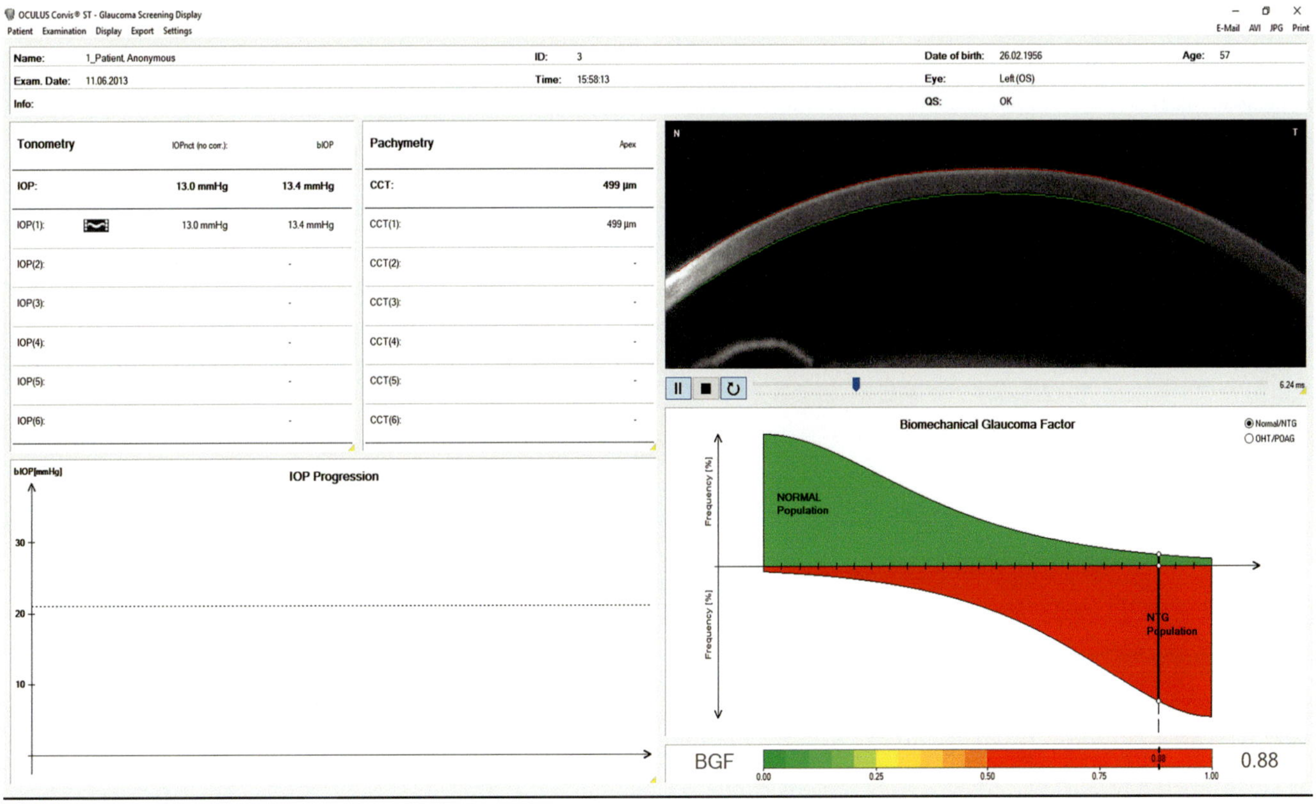

Fig. 6 Glaucoma screening Corvis ST® display. Left eye of a 57-year-old patient with suspect of normal tension glaucoma (NTG), an intraocular pressure of 13.4 mmHg (bIOP) and a cup–disc ratio of 0.7. The Biomechanical Glaucoma Factor (BGF) reveals abnormal biomechanics, indicating the presence of normal tension glaucoma (NTG)

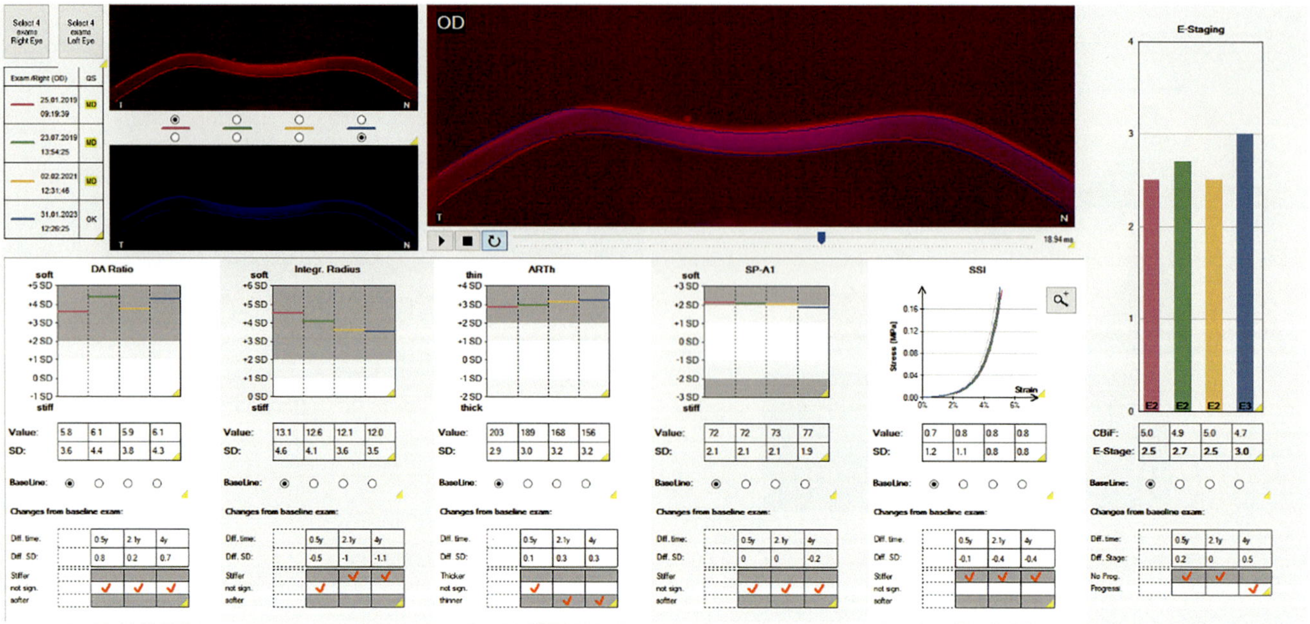

Fig. 7 Homburg Biomechanical E-Staging Corvis ST® display. Right eye of a male, 38-year-old patient with keratoconus and follow-up examinations from 2019 to 2023. Top left: data from the four separate examinations presented at the same time (red, green, yellow, and blue), visualization of the baseline corneal deformation (red), and corneal deformation in the final examination (blue). Upper center: Superimposed display of corneal deformation visualizations. Below: absolute values and number of standard deviations from the mean value in healthy patients for (1) deformation amplitude ratio 2.0 mm (DA ratio), (2) integrated inverse radius, (3) Ambrósio relational thickness horizontal (ARTh), and (4) stiffness parameter SP-A1. SSI, stress–strain index; left-shift of the curve corresponds to a higher, and right shift to a lower material stiffness. Right part: Biomechanical E-Staging for the four examination time points. No progression from red (25.01.2019) to green (23.07.2019) to yellow (02.02.2021). Progression four years after initial presentation (blue, 31.01.2023). Progression assessment displayed below the individual biomechanical parameters. Progression assessment also displayed below the biomechanical E-Staging indicating progression at last follow-up examination (blue)

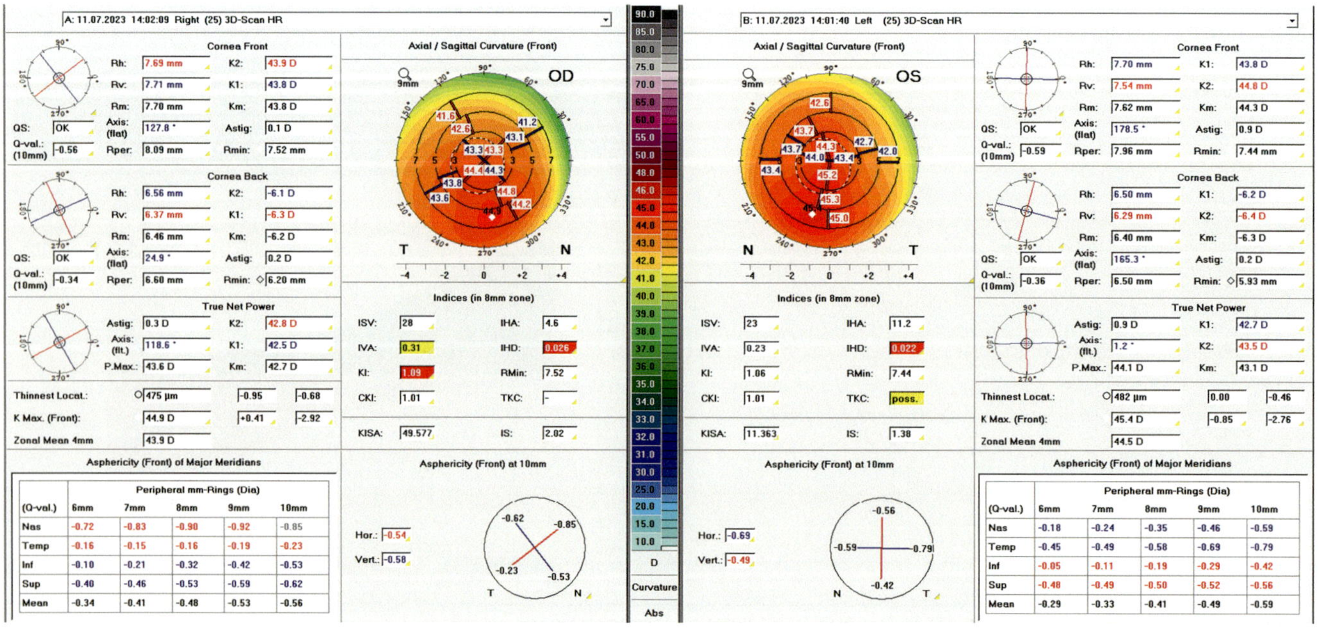

Fig. 8 Topometric Pentacam® display. Both eyes of a 26-year-old female patient with suspect of keratoconus. With-the-rule astigmatism with inferior corneal steepening and partially suspicious keratoconus indices in both eyes

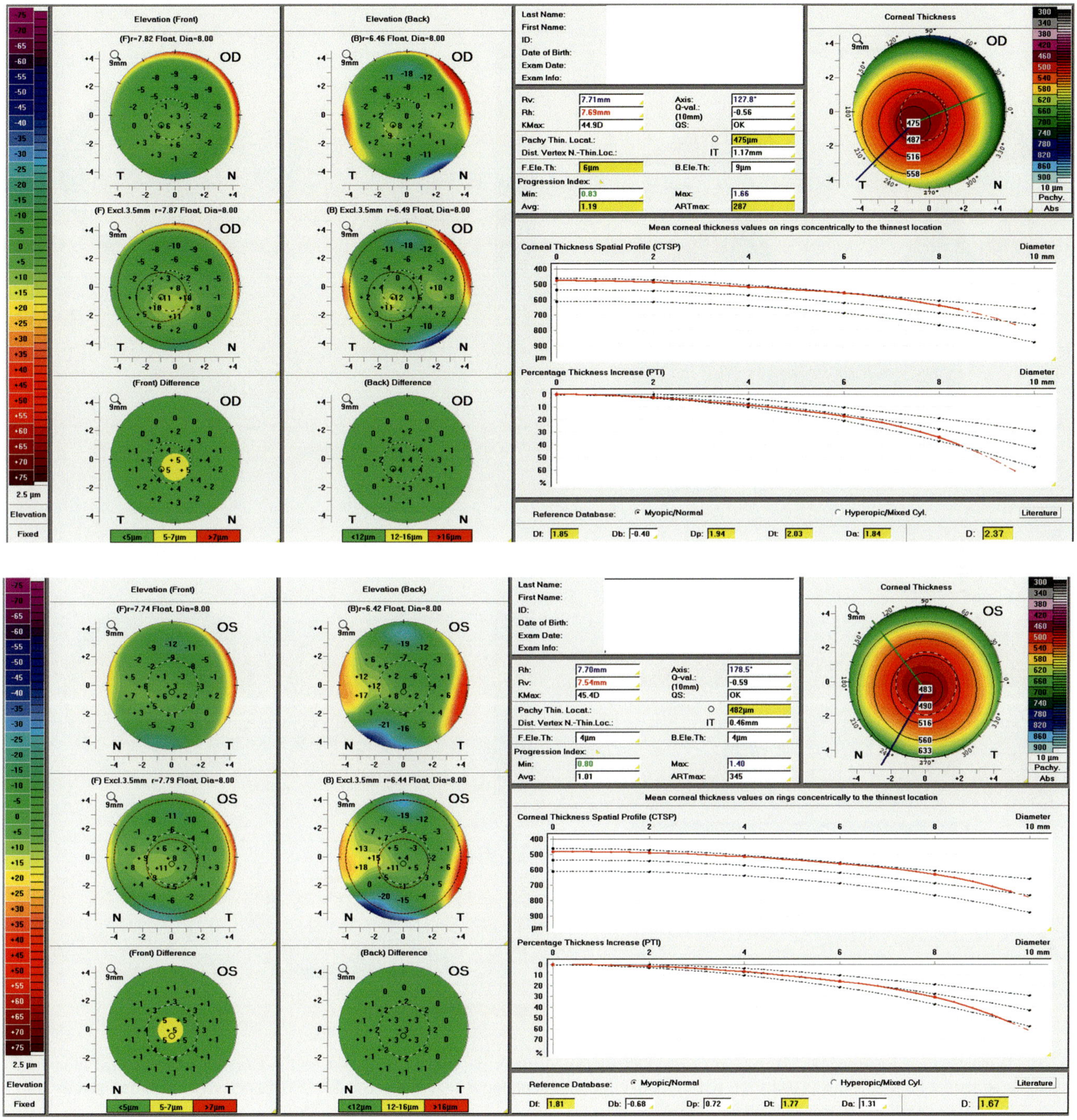

Fig. 9 Belin/Ambrósio enhanced ectasia screening Pentacam® display. Same eyes as shown in Fig. 8 with slightly abnormal anterior elevation data shown in the difference chart (lower left for each eye). Note abnormal Belin/Ambrósio deviation indices for both eyes (OD: 2.37, OS: 1.67)

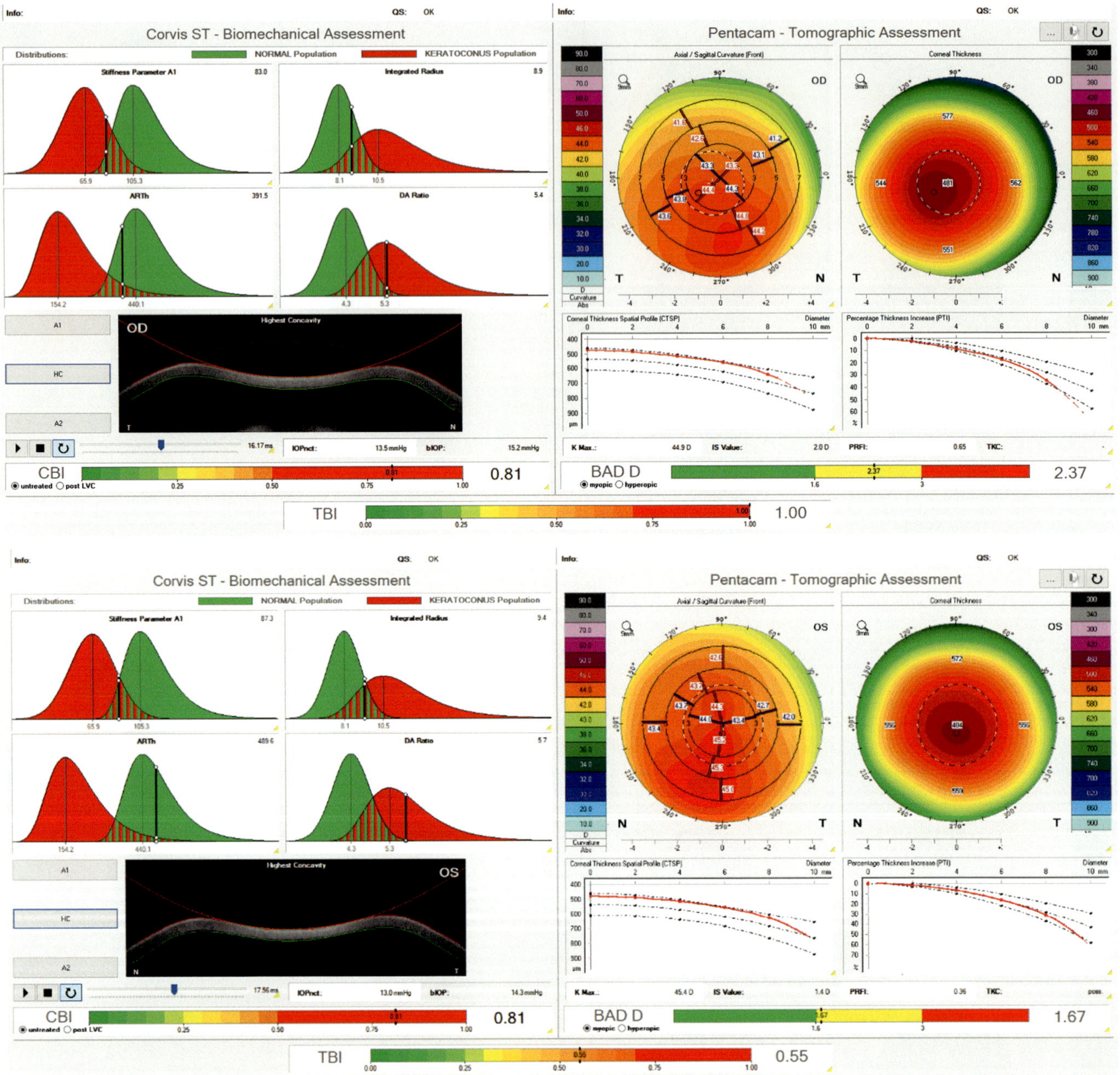

Fig. 10 Biomechanical/tomographic assessment Corvis ST® display of the same eyes as in Figs. 8 and 9. Corvis Biomechanical Index (CBI) indicating abnormal biomechanics (value 0.81, red) in both eyes. Tomographic Biomechanical Index (TBIv1) clearly indicating keratectasia in the right eye (1.00), and a suspicious value in the left eye (0.55)

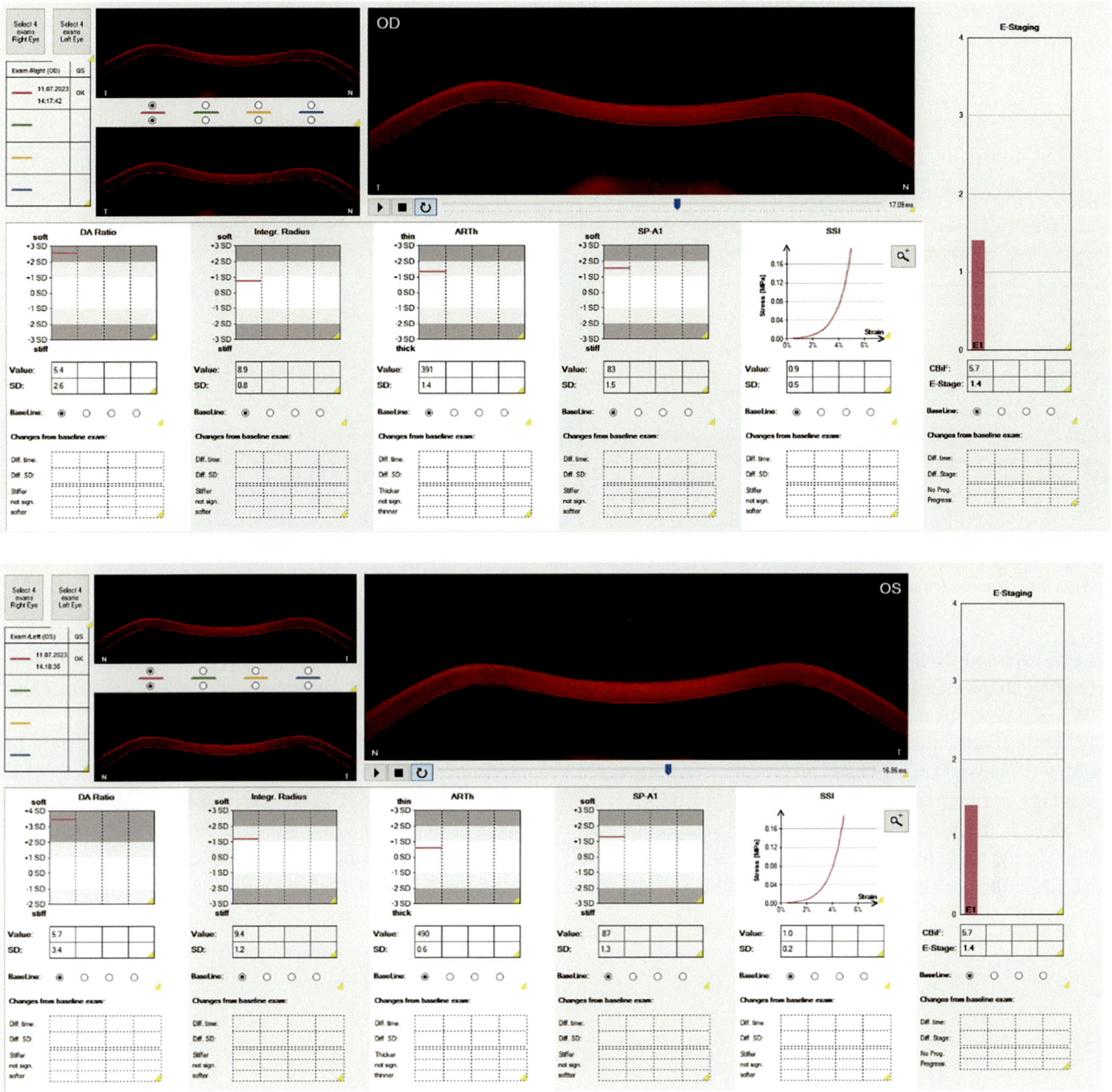

Fig. 11 Homburg Biomechanical E-staging Corvis ST® display of the same eyes as in Figs. 8–10. Biomechanical E-staging indicating abnormal corneal biomechanics in both eyes (same severity stage), thus leading to the diagnosis of subclinical keratoconus in both eyes

The Homburg Biomechanical E-Staging finally adds a severity stage of biomechanical weakening in these cases and despite different tomographic Belin/Ambrósio deviation indices (Fig. 9), it indicates comparable biomechanical E-stages for both eyes (Fig. 11).

Another example shows with-the-rule astigmatism without abnormal KC indices in both eyes (Fig. 12).

In this example, there are abnormal elevation data of posterior corneal curvature more in the right than in the

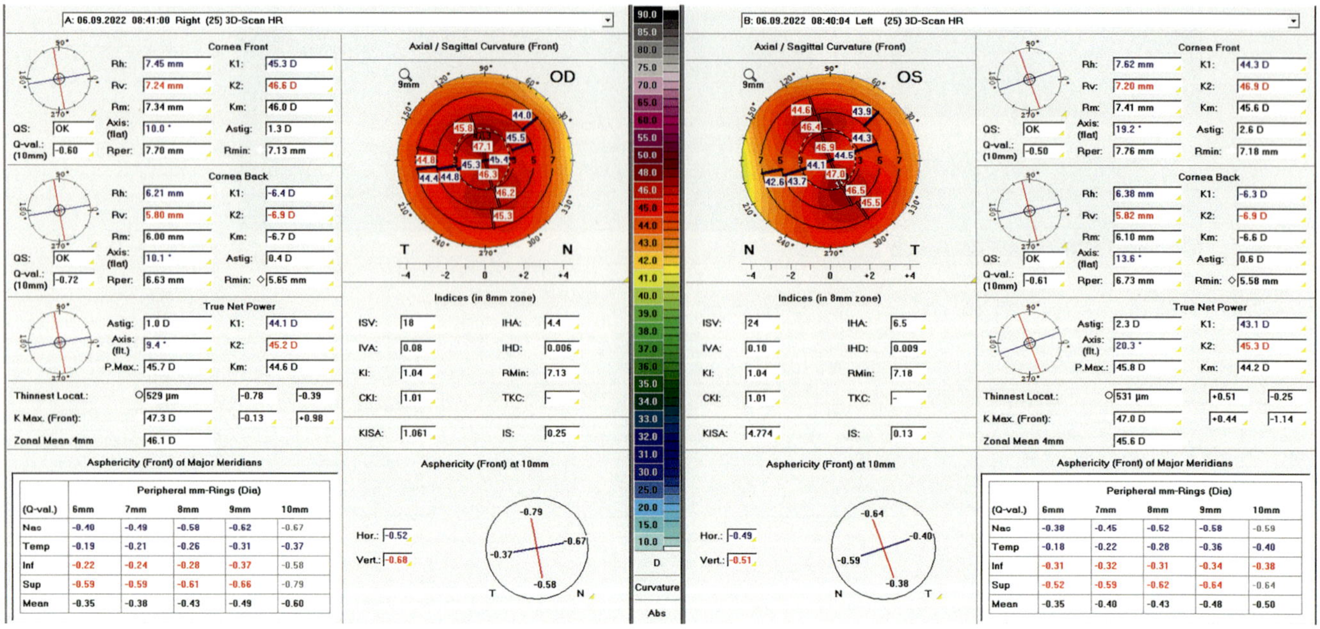

Fig. 12 Topometric Pentacam® display. Both eyes of a 36-year-old female patient with suspect of keratoconus. Slight inferior corneal steepening with unsuspicious keratoconus indices in both eyes

left eye revealed by the Belin/Ambrósio Enhanced Ectasia Screening Display (Fig. 13).

When both corneal biomechanics and tomography detect only subtle abnormalities, neither each of them can unquestionably diagnose keratectasia by itself (CBI, BAD-D, E-staging), nor their combination (TBI, Fig. 14, 15).

Although the global consensus on KC and ectatic diseases stated, that truly unilateral keratectasia does not exist [22], there exist studies about "unilateral" or very asymmetric keratectasia [23] and it is of interest to examine these eyes not only tomographically, but also biomechanically (Figs. 16–19).

In this case, the tomographically unremarkable right eye turned out to show abnormal corneal biomechanics, which may be indicative of early keratectasia. Similar findings have been reported [23], which indicates that "unilateral" keratectasia should rather be interpreted as a snapshot of very asymmetric keratectasia [19].

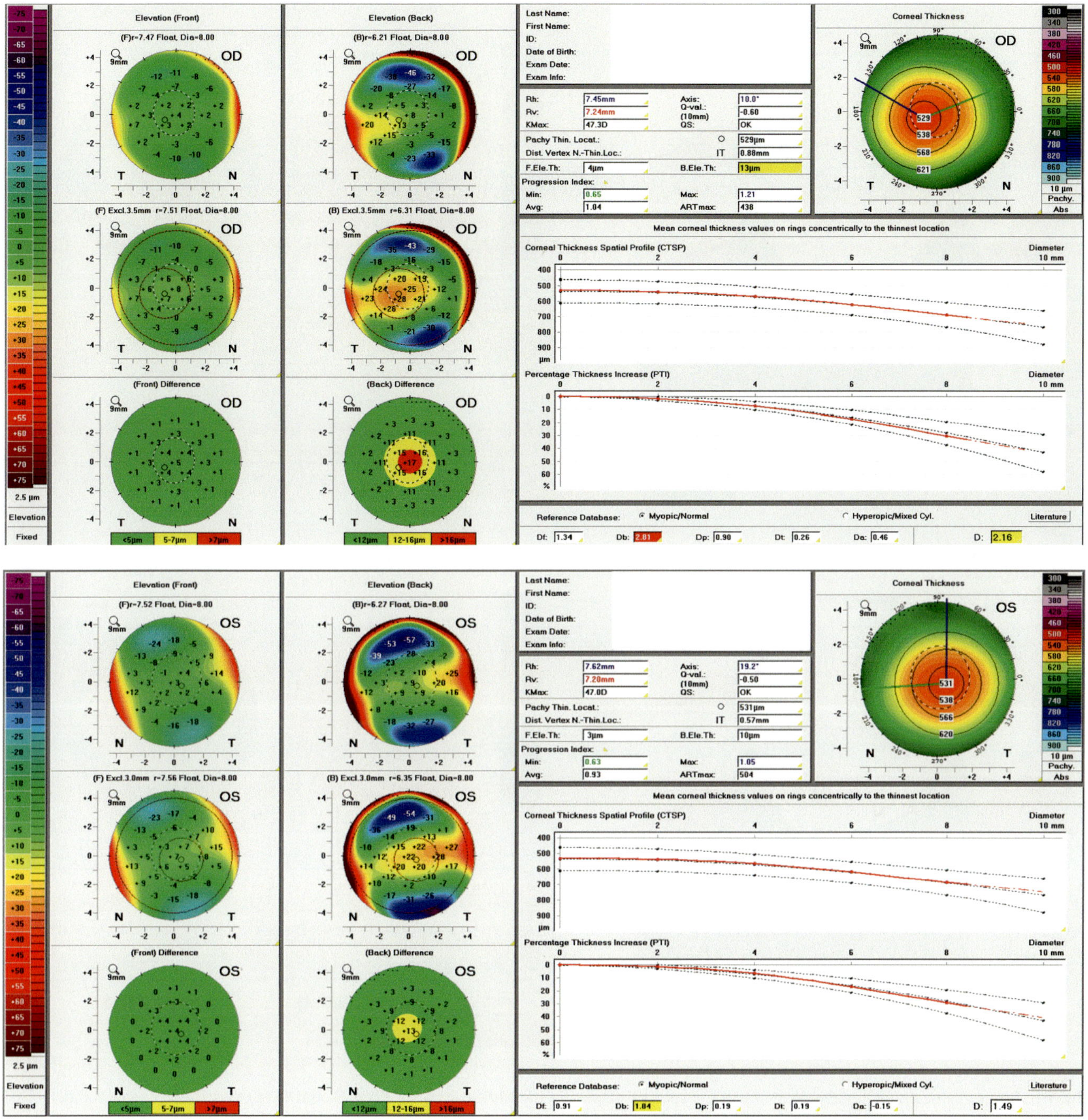

Fig. 13 Belin/Ambrósio enhanced ectasia screening Pentacam® display. Same eyes as shown in Fig. 12 with suspicious posterior elevation data shown in the difference chart. Note suspicious Belin/Ambrósio deviation indices for the right eye (OD: 2.16, OS: 1.49)

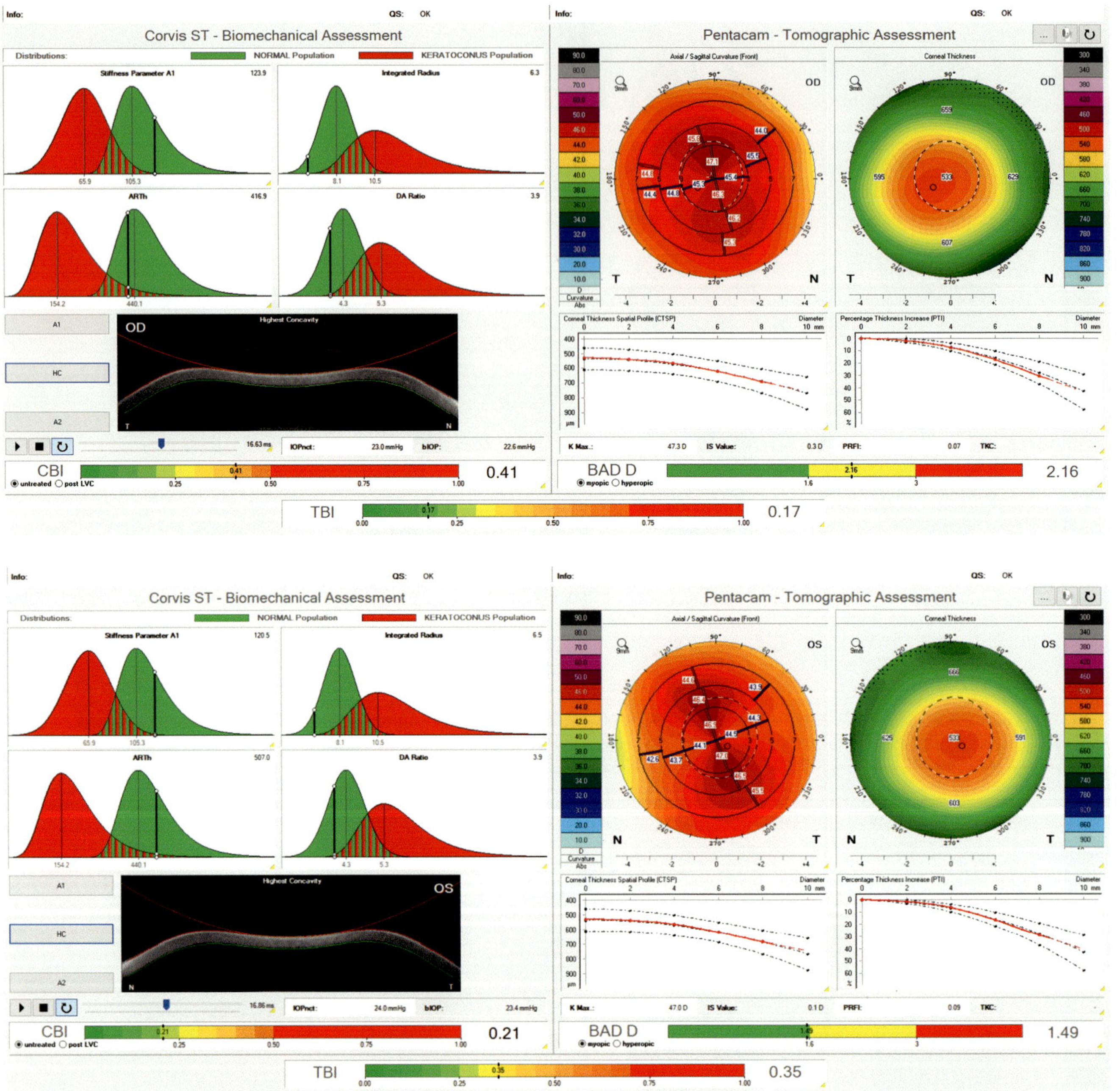

Fig. 14 Biomechanical/tomographic assessment Corvis ST® display of the same eyes as in Figs. 12 and 13. Corvis Biomechanical Index (CBI) indicating abnormal biomechanics more in the right (value 0.41, OD) than in the left eye (value 0.21, OS). Tomographic Biomechanical Index (TBIv1) with rather normal values more in the right (value 0.17, OD) than in the left eye (0.35, OS)

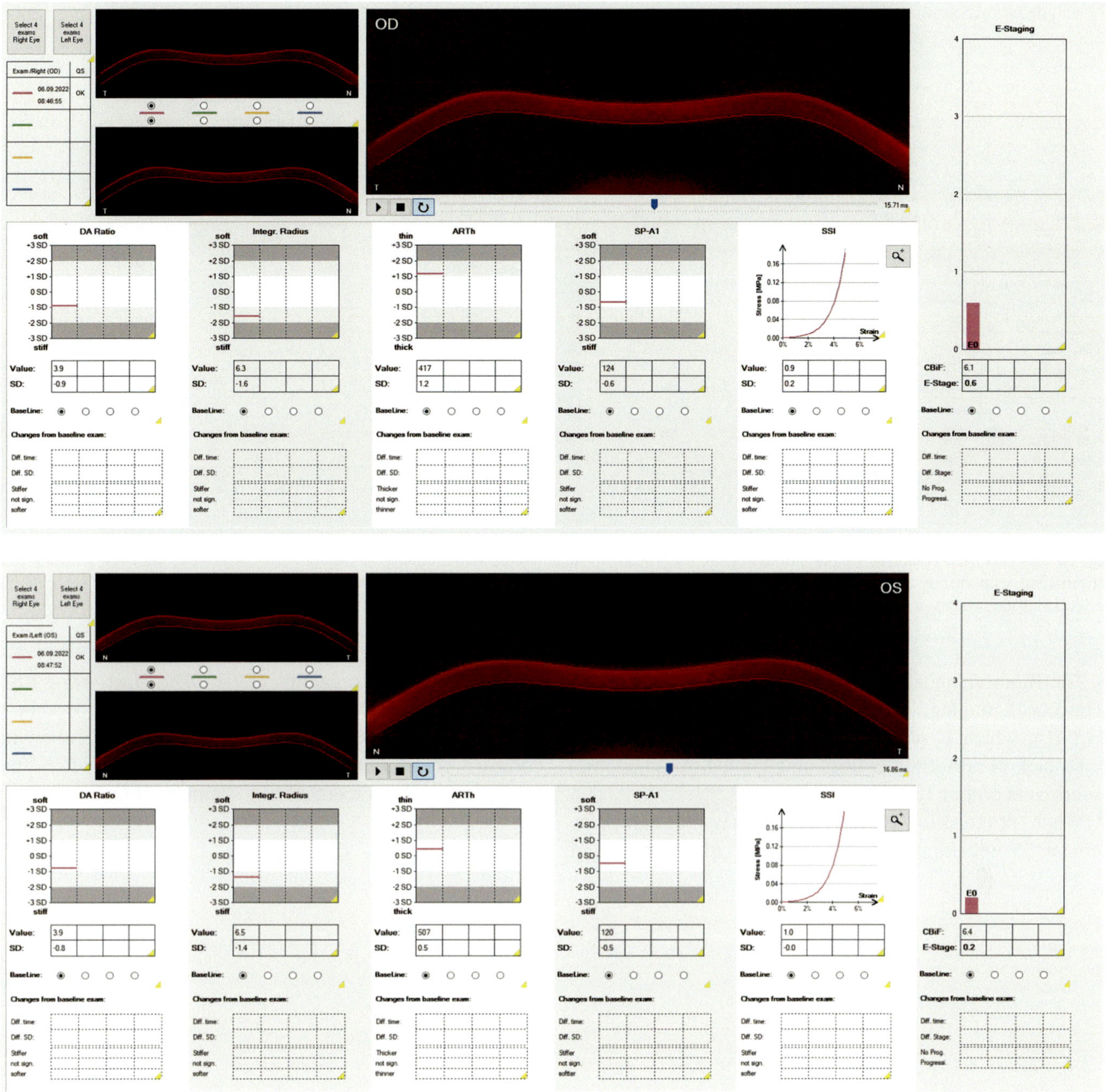

Fig. 15 Homburg Biomechanical E-Staging Corvis ST® display of the same eyes as in Figs. 12–14. E-Staging indicating only subtle abnormal corneal biomechanics more in the right than in the left eye

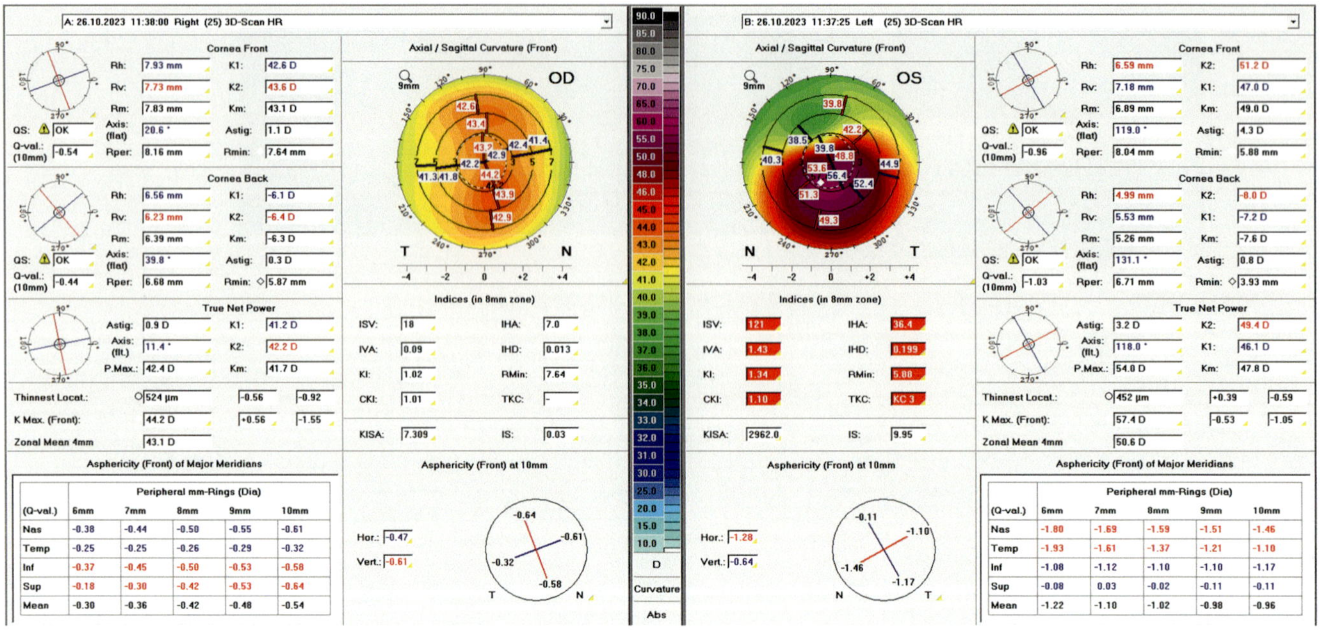

Fig. 16 Topometric Pentacam® display. Both eyes of a 27-year-old male patient with "unilateral keratoconus". Right eye showing with-the-rule astigmatism without any abnormal keratoconus indices. Left eye showing inferior thinning, abnormal keratoconus indices and a topographic keratoconus classification stage TKC3

The Biomechanical E-Staging may be used not only for keratectasia staging, but also for progression assessment (Fig. 20), which is of clinical relevance, because there is still a lack of uniformly defined and applied (tomographic) progression criteria [24–26].

When progression is detected, it may be halted by corneal crosslinking [27–29] or the implantation of intracorneal ring segments [30]. The last two CST captures show a representative course of the Homburg Biomechanical E-Staging in its current version following corneal crosslinking (Fig. 21, [26]) and after the implantation of intracorneal ring segments (Fig. 22, [31]).

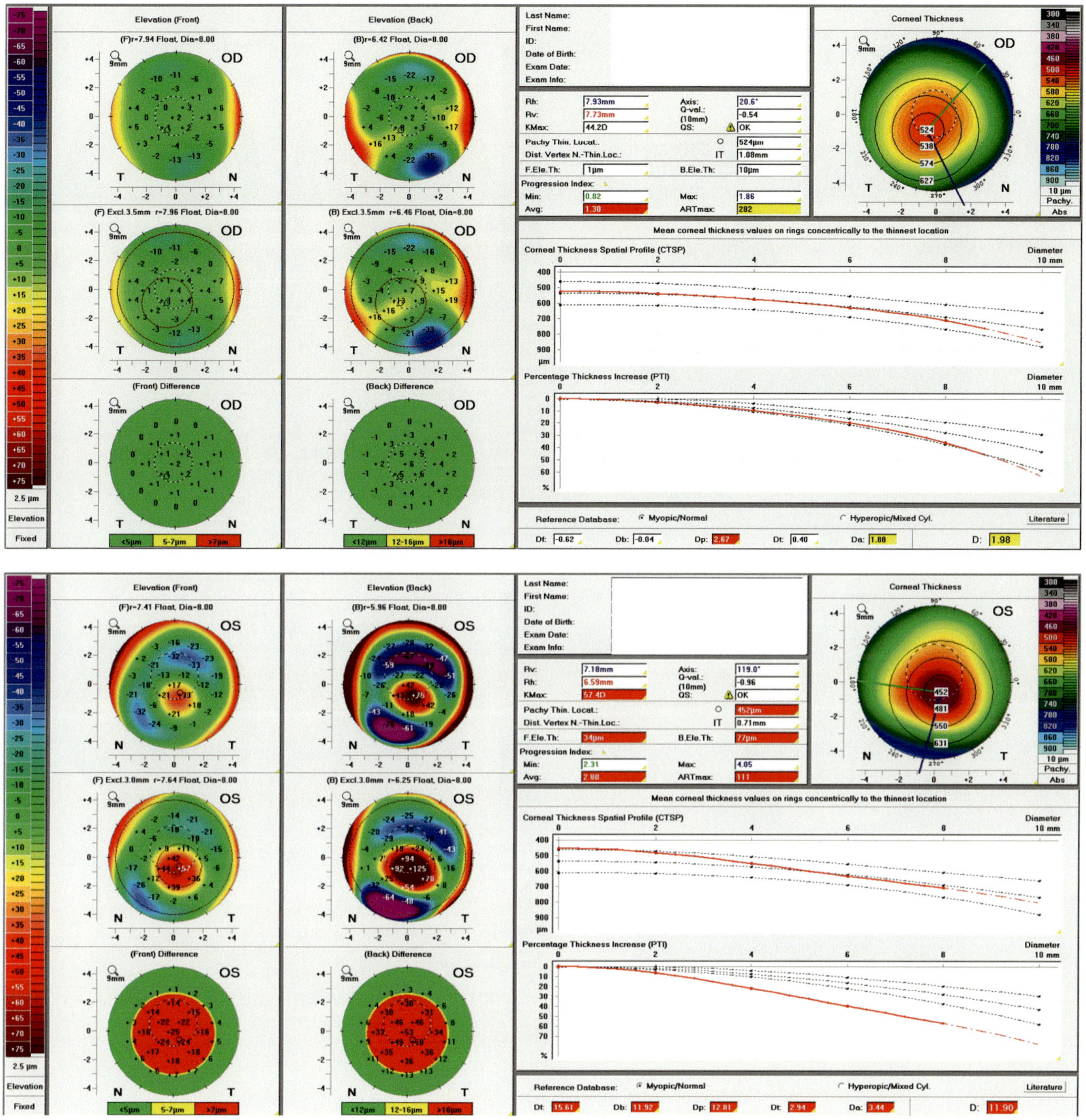

Fig. 17 Belin/Ambrósio enhanced ectasia screening Pentacam® display. Same eyes as shown in Fig. 16. Normal anterior and posterior elevation data for the right eye and suspicious Belin/Ambrósio deviation index (1.98). Abnormal anterior and posterior elevation data for the left eye with abnormal Belin/Ambrósio deviation index (11.90)

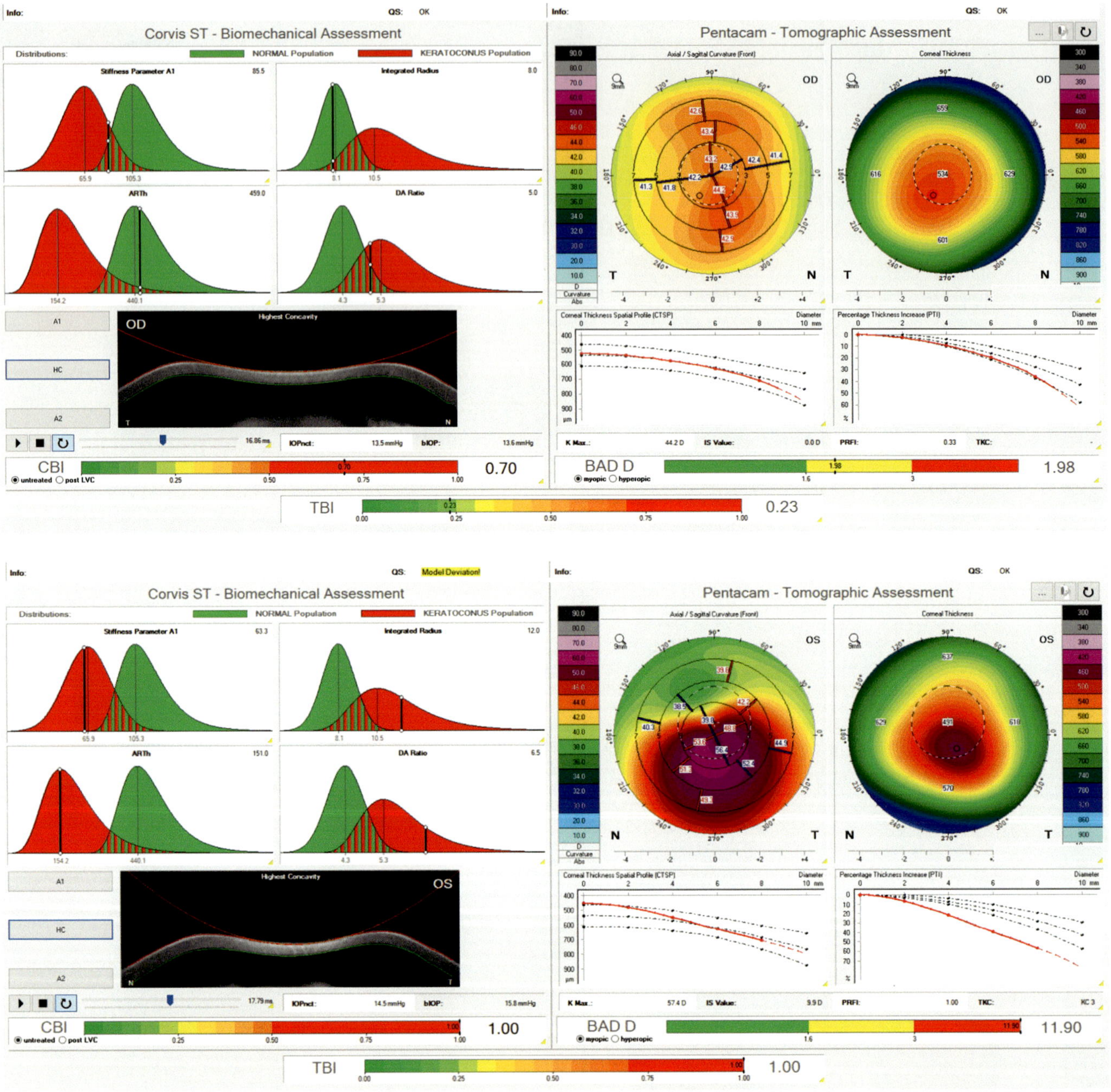

Fig. 18 Biomechanical/tomographic assessment Corvis ST® display of the same eyes as in Figs. 16 and 17. Corvis Biomechanical Index (CBI) indicating abnormal biomechanics in both the tomographically normal right eye (value 0.70, OD) and in the tomographically abnormal left eye (value 1.00, OS). Tomographic Biomechanical Index (TBIv1) with rather normal value in the right eye (value 0.23, OD) and clearly abnormal value in the left eye (1.00, OS)

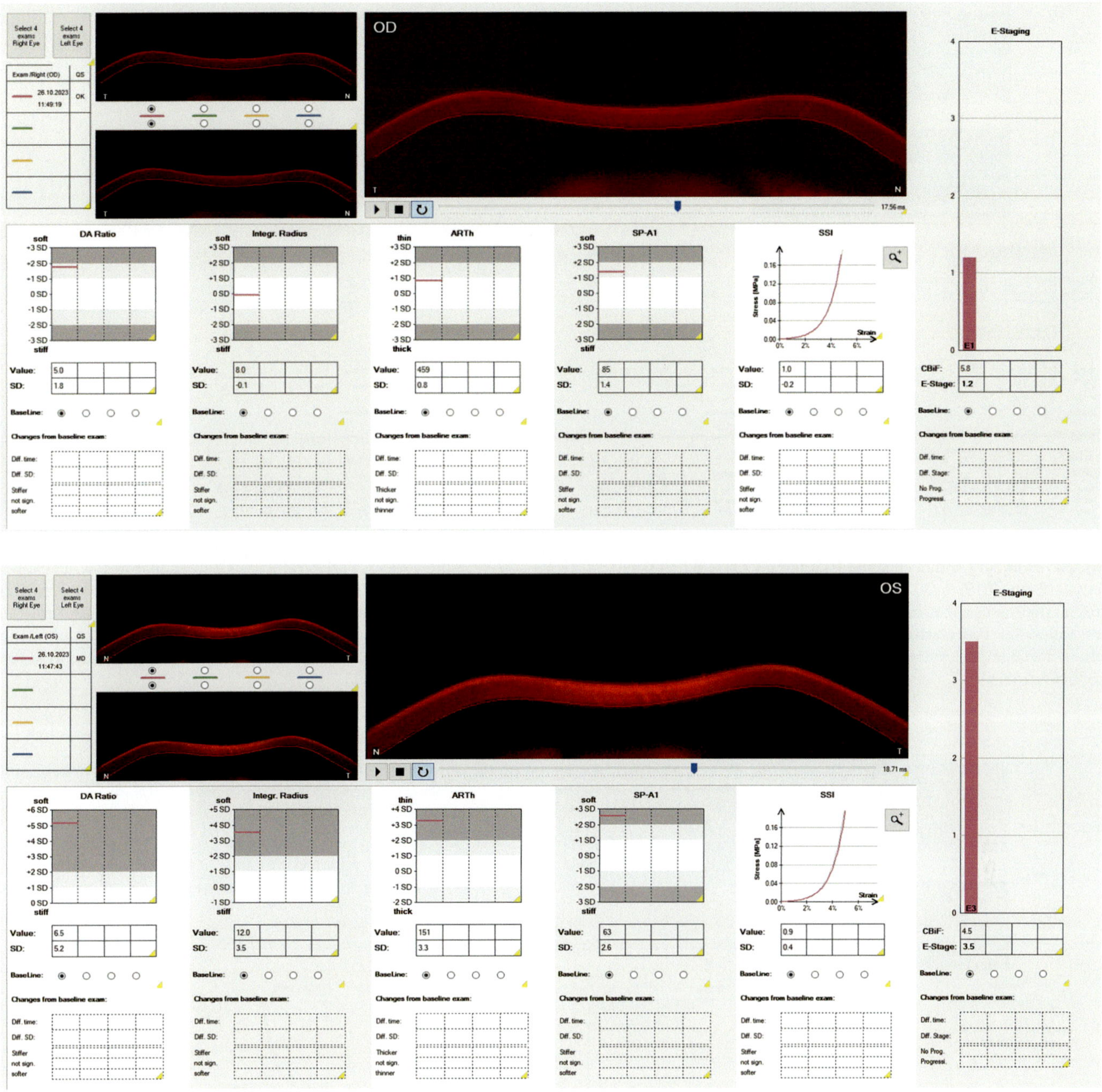

Fig. 19 Homburg Biomechanical E-Staging Corvis ST® display of the same eyes as in Figs. 16–18. Biomechanical E-Staging indicating abnormal corneal biomechanics in both the tomographically normal right eye (E1.2) and the tomographically abnormal eye (E3.5)

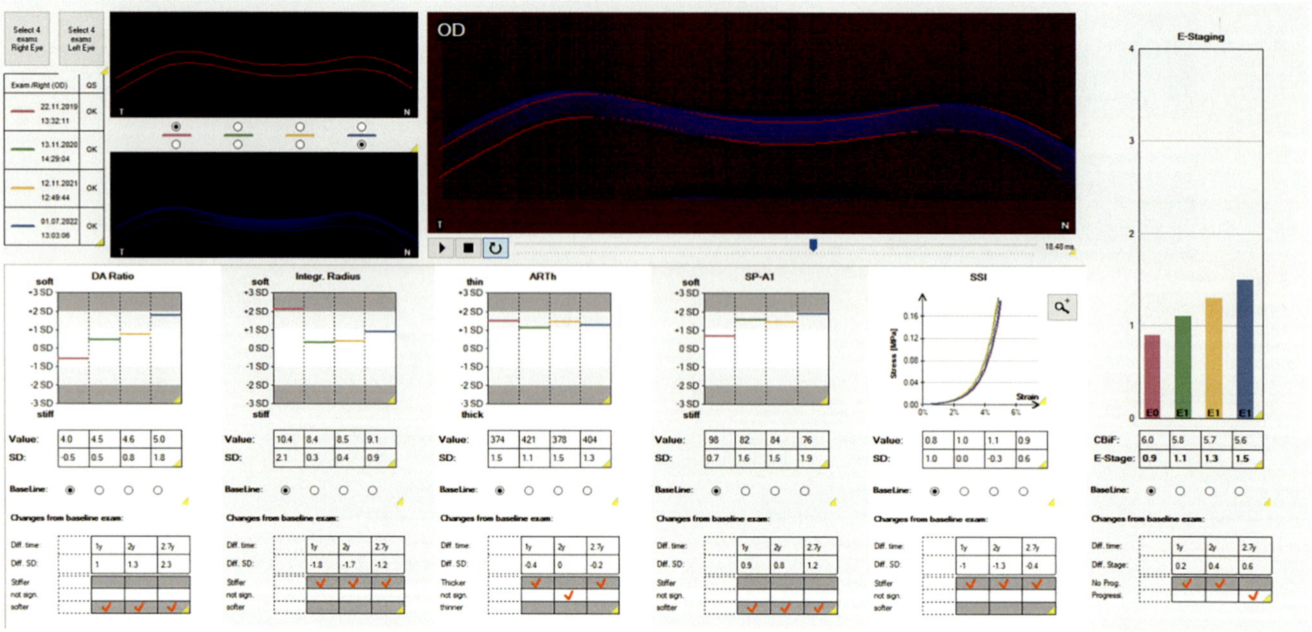

Fig. 20 Homburg Biomechanical E-Staging Corvis ST® display of a male, 27-year-old patient with keratoconus and annual follow-up examinations from 2019 to 2022. Linear progression from red (22.11.2019) to green (13.11.2020) to yellow (12.11.2021) to blue (01.07.2022). Progression assessment displayed below the individual biomechanical parameters with DA ratio and SP-A1 indicating progression from the first follow-up. Progression assessment also displayed below the Biomechanical E-Staging indicating progression at last follow-up examination (blue). Tomographic values for 2019|2020|2021|2022: K2: 44.5|44.4|44.4|44.9; Kmax: 47.6|46.8|47.1|48.4; TCT: 525|521|513|511 and BAD-D: 3.35|3.85|3.58|3.93

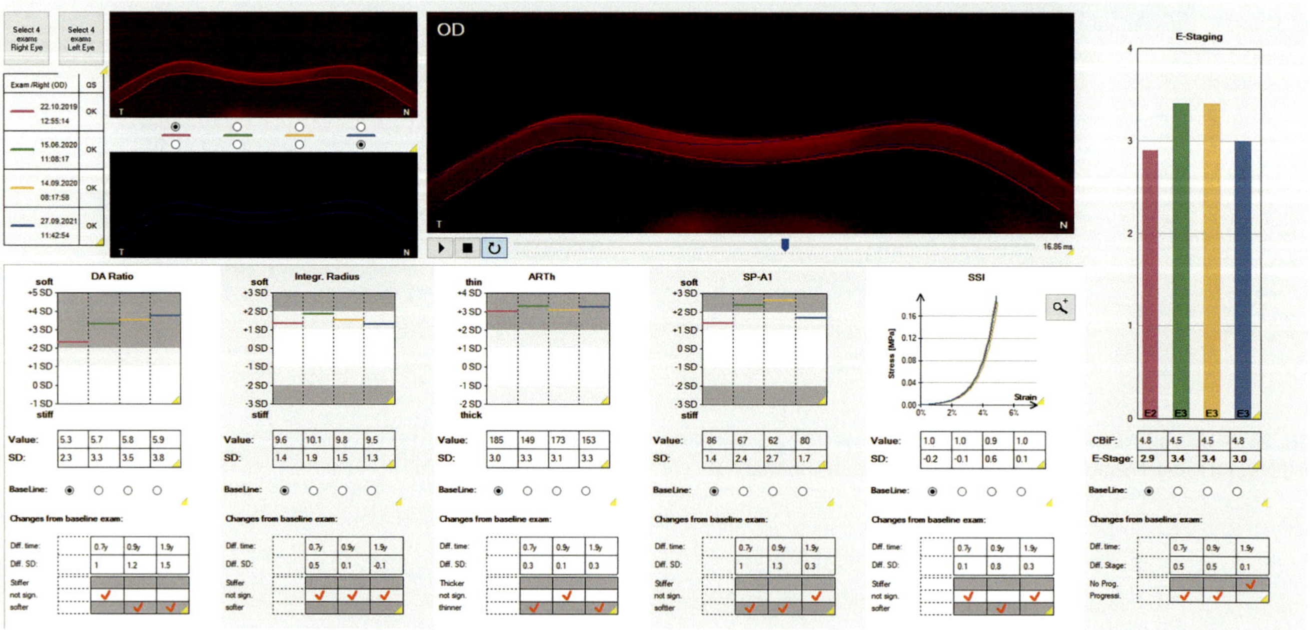

Fig. 21 Homburg Biomechanical E-Staging Corvis ST® display, representative course after accelerated corneal crosslinking. Female, 30-year-old patient with keratoconus and follow-up examinations from 2019 to 2021. Red, baseline examination (22.10.2019). Accelerated corneal crosslinking was performed one month later (18.11.2019). Green, first follow-up seven months later with biomechanical (pseudo-)progression (15.06.2020). Yellow, second follow-up with same Biomechanical E-Staging ten months after crosslinking (14.09.2020). Blue, third follow-up (27.09.2021) with biomechanical stabilization near preoperative value about two years after corneal crosslinking

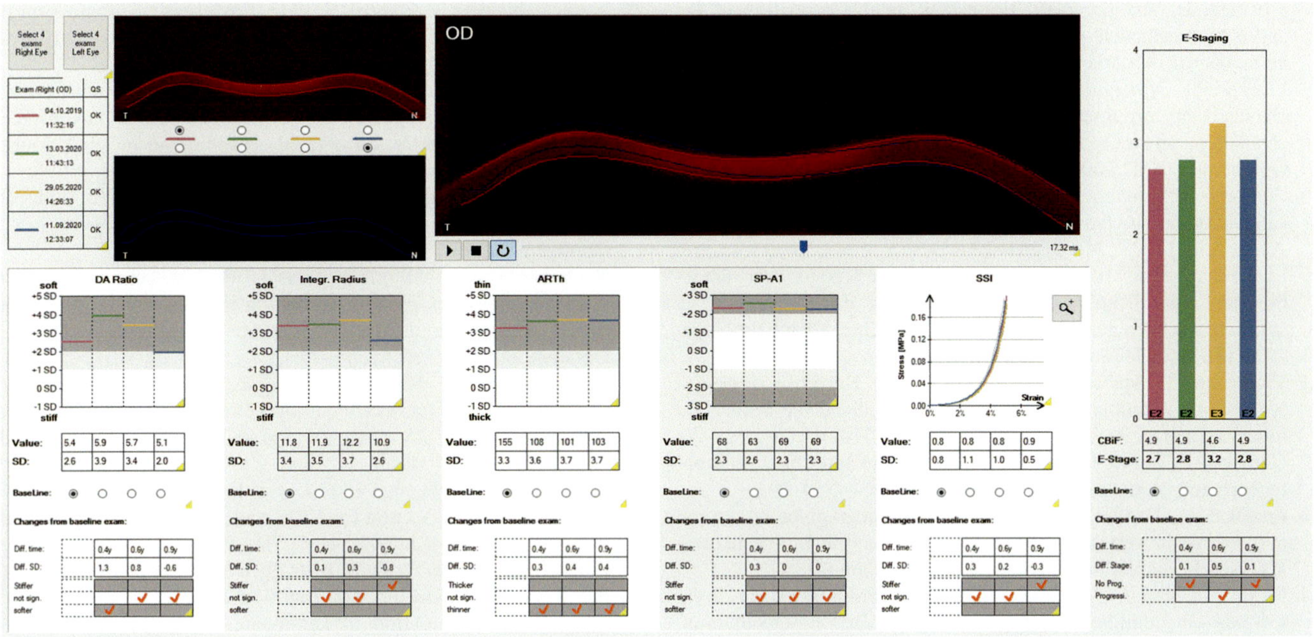

Fig. 22 Homburg Biomechanical E-Staging Corvis ST® display, representative course after implantation of intracorneal ring segments. Female, 39-year-old patient with keratoconus and follow-up examinations from 2019 to 2020. Red, baseline examination (04.10.2019). Implantation of Intacs® SK intracorneal ring segments was performed (28.11.2019). Green, first follow-up with slightly higher Biomechanical E-Staging about four months later (13.03.2020). Yellow, second follow-up with markedly higher Biomechanical E-Staging (29.05.2020). Blue, third follow-up (11.09.2020) with decreasing Biomechanical E-Staging comparable to baseline about ten months after intracorneal ring segment implantation

3 Conclusion

The measurement of corneal biomechanics and its interpretation has become an important part of the clinical diagnosis of corneal diseases. The combination of tomography and biomechanics has provided additional information that is clinically significant and can be used not only for the diagnosis, but also for the staging and progression assessment of corneal diseases and even glaucoma.

References

1. Roberts CJ, Dupps WJ. Biomechanics of corneal ectasia and biomechanical treatments. J Cataract Refract Surg. 2014;40(6):991–8.
2. Elham R, Jafarzadehpur E, Hashemi H, et al. Keratoconus diagnosis using Corvis ST measured biomechanical parameters. J Curr Ophthalmol. 2017;29(3):175–81.
3. Tian L, Ko MWL, Wang L, et al. Assessment of ocular biomechanics using dynamic ultra high-speed scheimpflug imaging in keratoconic and normal eyes. J Refract Surg. 2014;30(11):785–91.
4. Peña-García P, Peris-Martínez C, Abbouda A, et al. Detection of subclinical keratoconus through non-contact tonometry and the use of discriminant biomechanical functions. J Biomech. 2016;49(3):353–63.
5. Ambrósio R, Lopes BT, Faria-Correia F, et al. Integration of Scheimpflug-based corneal tomography and biomechanical assessments for enhancing ectasia detection. J Refract Surg. 2017;33(7):434–43.
6. Pillunat KR, Herber R, Spoerl E, et al. A new biomechanical glaucoma factor to discriminate normal eyes from normal pressure glaucoma eyes. Acta Ophthalmol. 2019;97(7):e962–7.
7. Vinciguerra R, Ambrósio R, Elsheikh A, et al. Detection of keratoconus with a new biomechanical index. J Refract Surg. 2016;32(12):803–10.
8. Vinciguerra R, Ambrósio R, Roberts CJ, et al. Biomechanical characterization of subclinical keratoconus without topographic or tomographic abnormalities. J Refract Surg. 2017;33(6):399–407.
9. Reisdorf S. Artificial intelligence for the development of screening parameters in the field of corneal biomechanics. Klin Monbl Augenheilkd. 2019;236(12):1423–7.
10. Lenk J, Haustein M, Terai N, et al. Characterization of ocular biomechanics in pellucid marginal degeneration. Cornea. 2016;35(4):506–9.
11. Mergen B, Sideroudi H, Seitz B, et al. Altered corneal biomechanics according to the biomechanical E-staging in pellucid marginal degeneration. Cornea. 2024;43(11):1361–7.
12. Goebels S, Eppig T, Wagenpfeil S, et al. Staging of keratoconus indices regarding tomography, topography, and biomechanical measurements. Am J Ophthalmol. 2015;159(4):733–8.
13. Belin MW, Duncan JK. Keratoconus: the ABCD grading system. Klin Monbl Augenheilkd. 2016;233(6):701–7.
14. Shetty R, Nuijts RMMA, Srivatsa P, et al. Understanding the correlation between tomographic and biomechanical severity of keratoconic corneas. BioMed Res Int. 2015:1–9
15. Shen Y, Han T, Jhanji V, et al. Correlation between corneal topographic, densitometry, and biomechanical parameters in keratoconus eyes. Trans Vis Sci Technol. 2019;8(3):12.
16. Koh S, Inoue R, Ambrósio R, et al. Correlation between corneal biomechanical indices and the severity of keratoconus. Cornea. 2020;39(2):215–21.

17. Flockerzi E, Vinciguerra R, Belin MW, et al. Correlation of the corvis biomechanical factor CBiF with tomographic parameters in keratoconus. J Cataract Refract Surg. 2022;48(2):215–21.
18. Flockerzi E, Vinciguerra R, Belin MW, et al. Combined biomechanical and tomographic keratoconus staging: adding a biomechanical parameter to the ABCD keratoconus staging system. Acta Ophthalmol. 2022;100(5):e1135–42.
19. Flockerzi E, Xanthopoulou K, Munteanu C, et al. The biomechanical E-staging: in vivo biomechanics in keratoconus. Klin Monbl Augenheilkd 2023; 240(6):761–73.
20. Langenbucher A, Häfner L, Eppig T, et al. Keratoconus detection and classification from parameters of the Corvis®ST: a study based on algorithms of machine learning. Ophthalmologe. 2021;118(7):697–706.
21. Vinciguerra R, Ambrósio R, Elsheikh A, et al. Detection of postlaser vision correction ectasia with a new combined biomechanical index. J Cataract Refract Surg. 2021;47(10):1314–8.
22. Gomes JAP, Tan D, Rapuano CJ, et al. Global consensus on keratoconus and ectatic diseases. Cornea. 2015;34(4):359–69.
23. Fraenkel D, Hamon L, Daas L, et al. Tomographically normal partner eye in very asymmetrical corneal ectasia: biomechanical analysis. J Cataract Refract Surg. 2021;47(3):366–72.
24. Meyer JJ, Gokul A, Vellara HR, et al. Progression of keratoconus in children and adolescents. Br J Ophthalmol. 2023;107(2):176–80.
25. Ferdi A, Nguyen V, Kandel H, et al. Predictors of progression in untreated keratoconus: a save sight keratoconus registry study. Br J Ophthalmol. 2022;106(9):1206–11.
26. Flockerzi E, Xanthopoulou K, Daas L, et al. Evaluation of dynamic corneal response parameters and the biomechanical E-staging after accelerated corneal cross-linking in keratoconus. Asia Pac J Ophthalmol (Phila). 2022;11(6):514–20.
27. Wollensak G, Spoerl E, Seiler T. Riboflavin/ultraviolet-a-induced collagen crosslinking for the treatment of keratoconus. Am J Ophthalmol. 2003;135(5):620–7.
28. Xanthopoulou K, Milioti G, Daas L, et al. Accelerated corneal crosslinking causes pseudoprogression in keratoconus within the first 6 weeks without affecting posterior corneal curvature. Eur J Ophthalmol. 2022;32(5):2565–76.
29. Xanthopoulou K, Milioti G, Daas L, et al. Accelerated corneal crosslinking for treatment of keratoconus in children and adolescents under 18 years of age. Klin Monbl Augenheilkd. 2023;240(10):1131–42.
30. Struckmeier A-K, Hamon L, Flockerzi E, et al. Femtosecond laser and mechanical dissection for ICRS and MyoRing implantation: a meta-analysis. Cornea. 2022;41(4):518–37.
31. Flockerzi E, Berger T, Seitz B, et al. Evaluation of dynamic corneal response parameters and the biomechanical E-Staging after intacs® SK implantation in keratoconus. Indian J Ophthalmol. 2024;72(Suppl 3):S495–500.

Ultrasound Biomicroscopy

Tim Berger, Zaynab Khattabi, Ursula Löw, and Berthold Seitz

Abstract

Ultrasound biomicroscopy (UBM) is a non-invasive technique that provides high-resolution images of the anterior and posterior segments of the eye, allowing for detailed analysis of the anatomy and pathology of these structures. Nowadays, UBM has become an important diagnostic modality for ophthalmologists in practice. This book chapter will provide an overview of UBM, including its principles, and clinical applications and discuss the advantages and limitations of UBM compared to other imaging modalities.

Keywords

Ultrasound biomicroscopy · Corneal opacity · Anterior segment · Diagnostic modality · Noninvasive imaging

1 Principle

Ultrasound biomicroscopy (UBM) is based on the principles of high-frequency ultrasound imaging. Ultrasound waves with high frequencies are emitted from a transducer and penetrate ocular tissues. The ultrasound waves are reflected back from different tissue interfaces, and these reflections are received by the transducer, which then converts them into electrical signals. These signals are processed and reconstructed into a high-resolution image of the anterior and posterior segment of the eye [1].

The resolution of UBM is dependent on the frequency of the ultrasound waves used. Higher frequencies provide better resolution, but penetrate less deeply into the tissue, while lower frequency waves have less resolution but penetrate deeper [2, 3].

The optimal frequency range for UBM imaging of the eye is between 35 to 50 MHz, which allows for a balance between resolution and penetration depth. UBM imaging is performed using a contact technique, in which a coupling gel is applied to the eye to ensure proper transmission of ultrasound waves between the transducer and the eye. The probe is placed in close proximity to the eye, typically with the patient in a supine position [2, 4].

2 Clinical Applications

UBM has numerous clinical applications in the diagnosis and management of various ocular diseases. The high-resolution images provided by UBM can reveal anatomical details and pathological changes in the anterior and posterior segments of the eye that are not visible with other imaging modalities.

UBM can provide information about the cornea, especially about its thickness and shape in cases of corneal edema (Fig. 1), scarring (Fig. 2) or other degenerative disorders such as corneal calcification (Figs. 3, 4 and 5) or Salzmann nodular degeneration (Fig. 6) [1, 2, 5].

UBM might be useful in evaluating the location and extent of corneal or intracameral foreign bodies. Especially the detection of secondary anterior segment changes after traumatic injuries might be important in the diagnosis and further treatment [6]. In this context, one important application is the detection and extent of corneal epithelial implantation cysts (Figs. 7, 8 and 9) [7] or similar appearing clinical findings such as an interface fluid syndrome after lamellar keratoplasty (Fig. 10) [8] or pseudocysts (Fig. 11).

T. Berger (✉) · Z. Khattabi · U. Löw · B. Seitz
Department of Ophthalmology, Saarland University Medical Center, Homburg, Germany
e-mail: tim.berger@uks.eu

B. Seitz et al. (eds.), *Atlas on Cornea*, https://doi.org/10.1007/978-3-031-65422-0_13

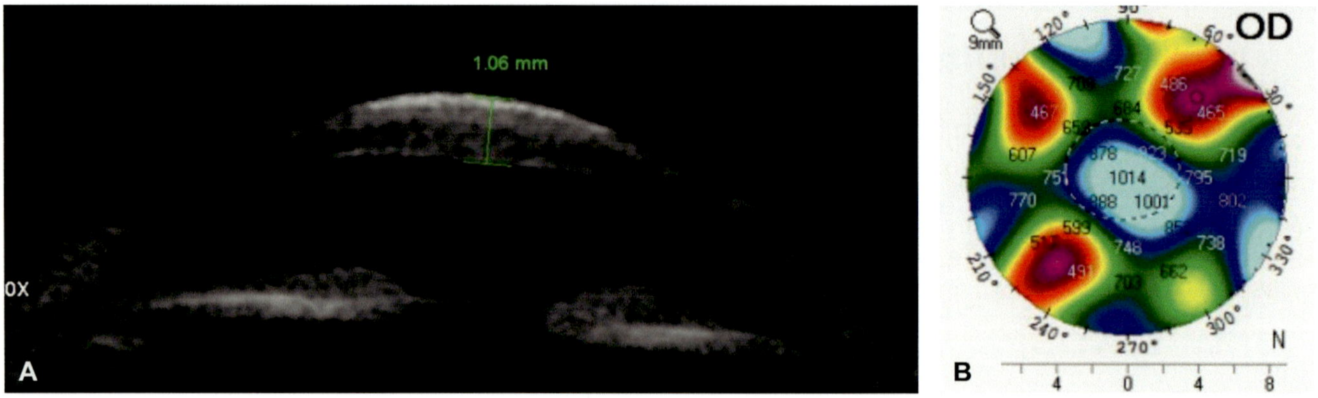

Fig. 1 Ultrasound biomicroscopy (**A**) and corresponding corneal tomography (**B**) Scheimpflug tomography, Pentacam, Oculus GmbH, Wetzlar, Germany) of a central corneal edema after Descemetorhexis without endothelial keratoplasty two weeks postoperatively. UBM enables precise measurement of the anterior segment of the eye compared to other diagnostic devices

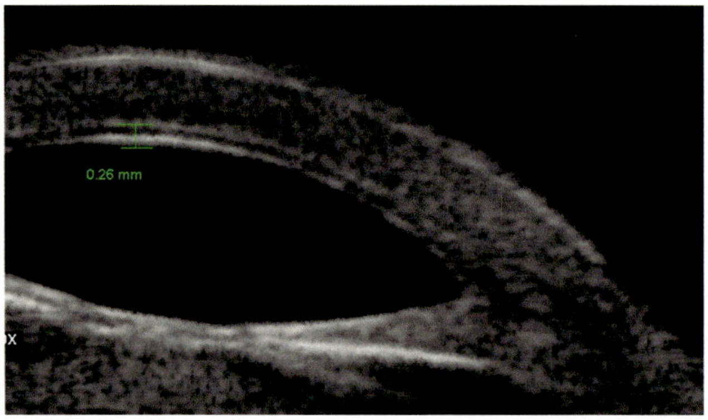

Fig. 2 Cornea after Descemet stripping automated endothelial keratoplasty (DSAEK) with sonographic identification of the interface due to fibrosis (central graft thickness: 260 µm)

It can also be used to detect other traumatic lesions such as hyphema, iridodialysis, and angle recession [6].

In cases with limited visualization of the anterior chamber, such as corneal blood staining (Figs. 12 and 13) or a subtotal or total conjunctival flap (Figs. 14 and 15), UBM may be a useful diagnostic modality [1, 3, 6, 9].

UBM is also used in the diagnosis and management of anterior segment tumours such solid dermoids of the cornea (Fig. 16) [10, 11] as well as iris (Fig. 17) and ciliary body melanomas [12]. Ocular surface tumours (Figs. 18 and 19) may also be visualized [13]. UBM is able to measure the size and extent of tumours and can help distinguish between benign and malignant lesions. Additionally, UBM can provide information on tumour invasion of surrounding structures, which is important in planning surgical intervention [10–13].

Other clinical applications of UBM include evaluation of anterior segment developmental disorders (Figs. 20, 21 and 22) that might affect the cornea, iris, and lens. UBM can provide detailed imaging of these structures, allowing for accurate diagnosis and management of these conditions [4, 14, 15].

Another important clinical application of UBM is in the diagnosis and management of glaucoma as it can provide

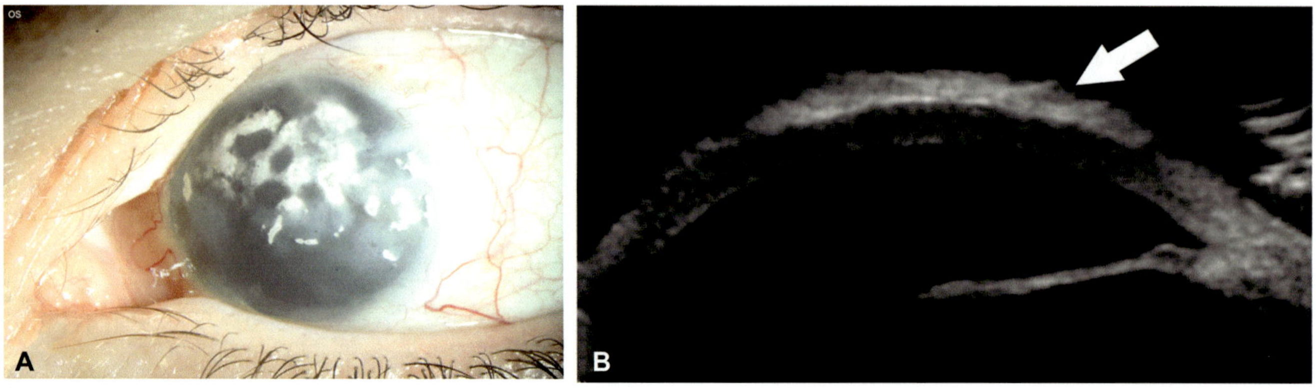

Fig. 3 Silicone oil keratopathy with pronounced corneal calcification and Salzmann nodular degeneration (**A**) The UBM image (**B**) shows hyperreflective lesion (arrow) of the cornea

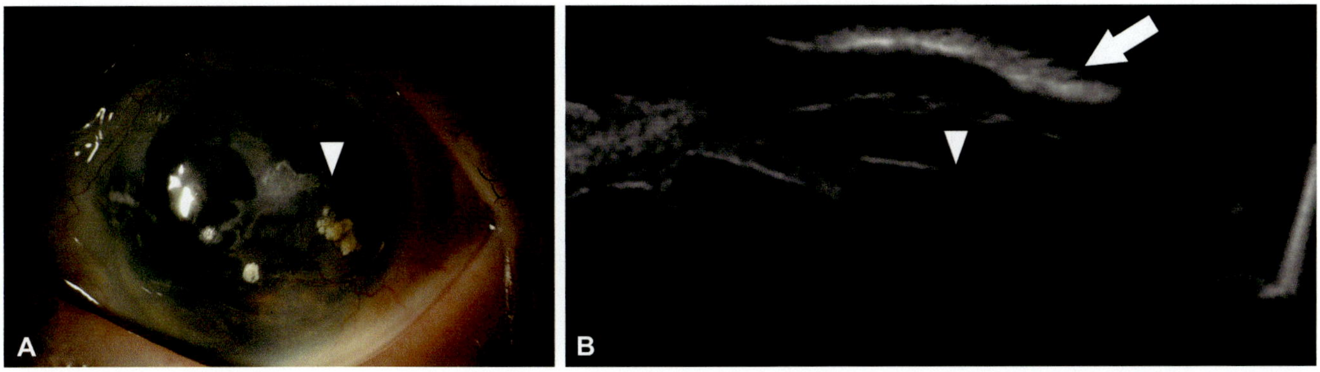

Fig. 4 Corneal calcification after ocular trauma (**A**) Sonography (**B**) reveals hyperreflective deposits (arrow) and the presence of an anterior chamber intraocular lens (arrowhead)

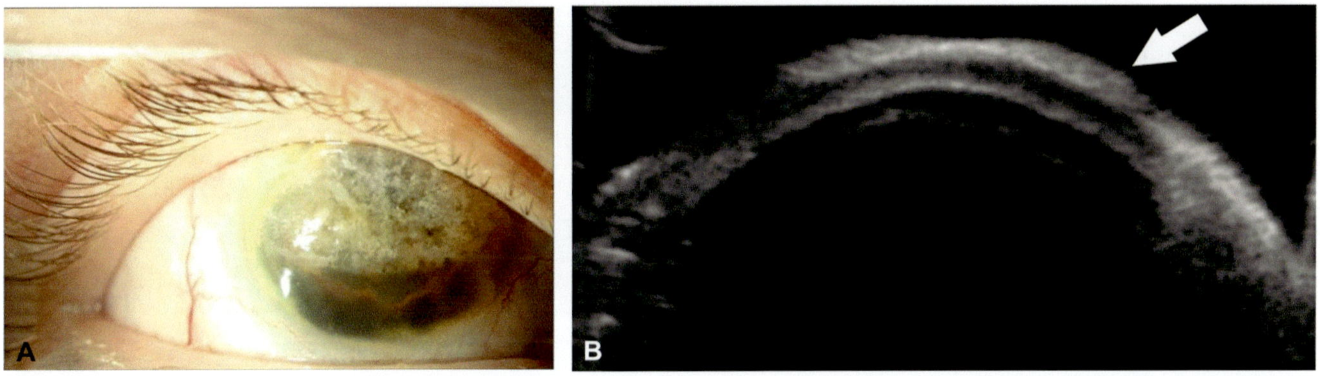

Fig. 5 Silicone oil keratopathy with corneal calcification and anterior synechiae (**A**) UBM (**B**) demonstrates hyperreflective deposits (arrow). No intraocular lens is present

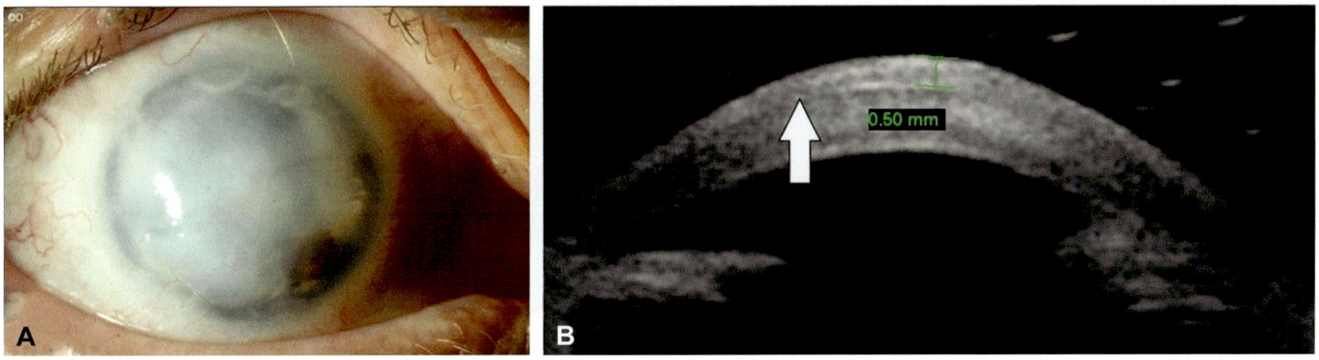

Fig. 6 Large Salzmann nodular degeneration after ocular trauma (**A**) Sonography (**B**) reveals a well demarcated Salzmann nodular degeneration (arrow, central thickness: 500 μm), anterior synechiae and aphakia

detailed images of the angle structures and trabecular meshwork [1, 16, 17]. Additionally, UBM can assess the integrity of the posterior lens capsule, diagnose ciliary body disorders, iris abnormalities, uveitis, and detect posterior segment pathologies such as retinal detachment and choroidal tumours. Measurement of lens thickness and identification of the cataract location is especially important for pediatric patients. UBM can be applied to assess the position, orientation, and stability of intraocular lenses (IOL) after cataract surgery, which can be useful in the diagnosis and management of complications such as IOL dislocation or decentration [1, 2].

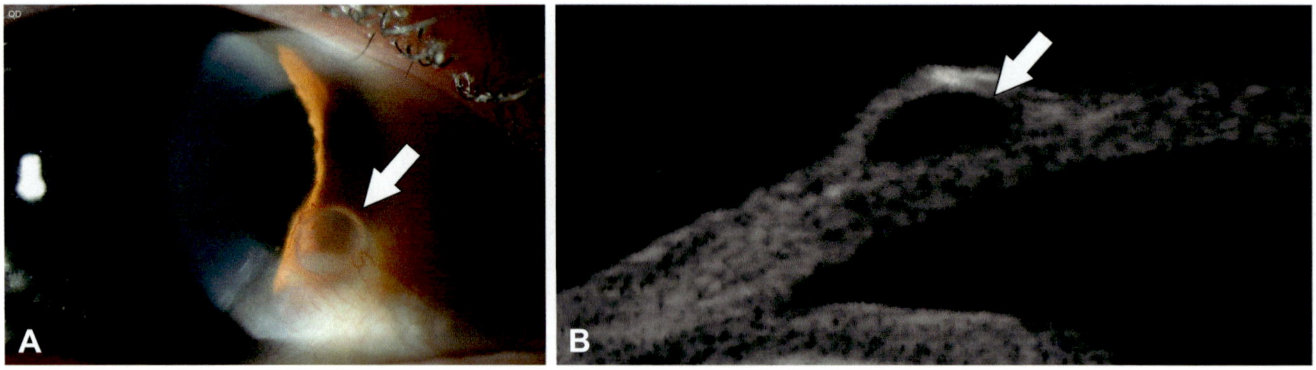

Fig. 7 Traumatic epithelial inclusion cyst (arrow) of the anterior corneal stroma after fingernail trauma (**A**) A cystic lesion with a hyporeflective cavity (arrow) is seen on sonography (**B**)

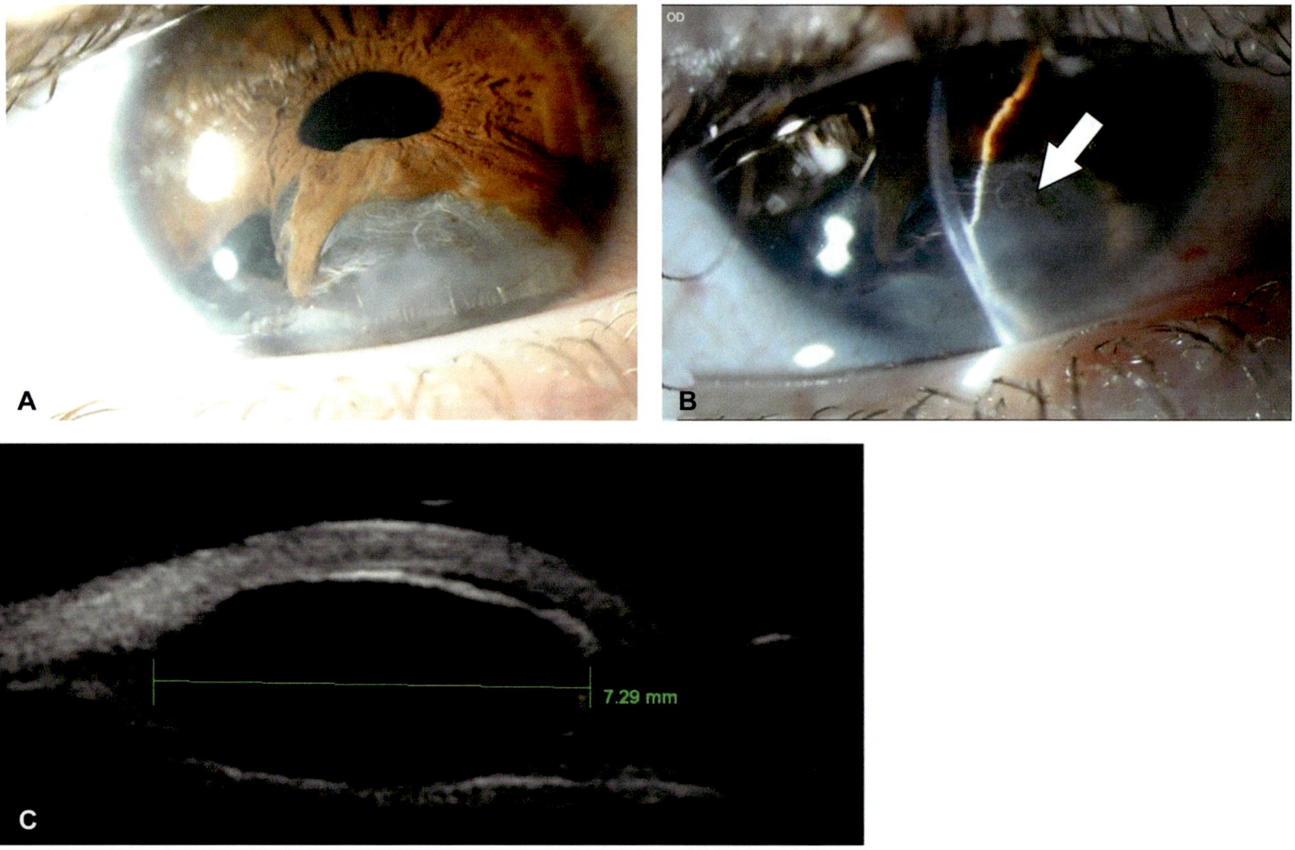

Fig. 8 Traumatic epithelial implantation cyst that occurred following ocular trauma with corneal perforation and iris prolapse ((**A**) overview, (**B**) narrow slit). Sonography is crucial to accurately determine the size (maximum longitudinal length measurement: 7.29 mm) and location of the cystic lesion (**C**)

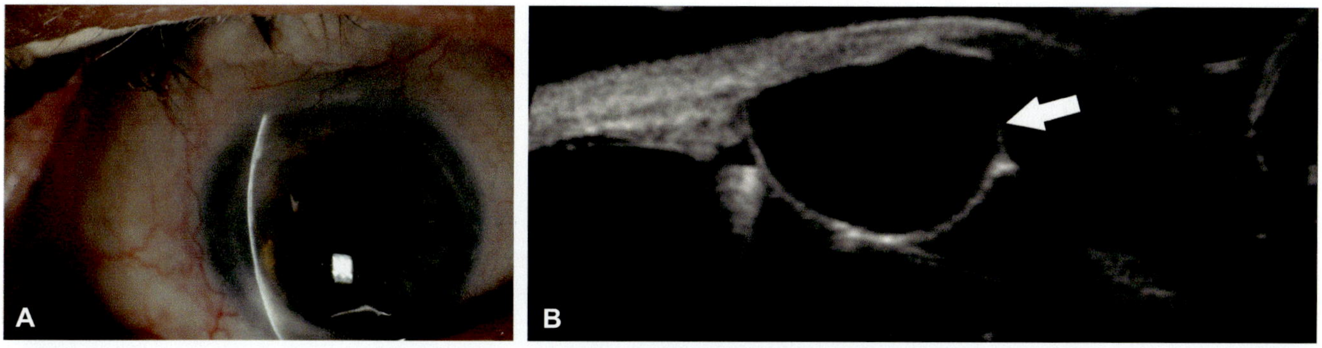

Fig. 9 Epithelial implantation cyst after emergency penetrating keratoplasty (**A**) Sonography (**B**) reveals a large cyst (arrow) at the donor-host apposition (arrowhead)

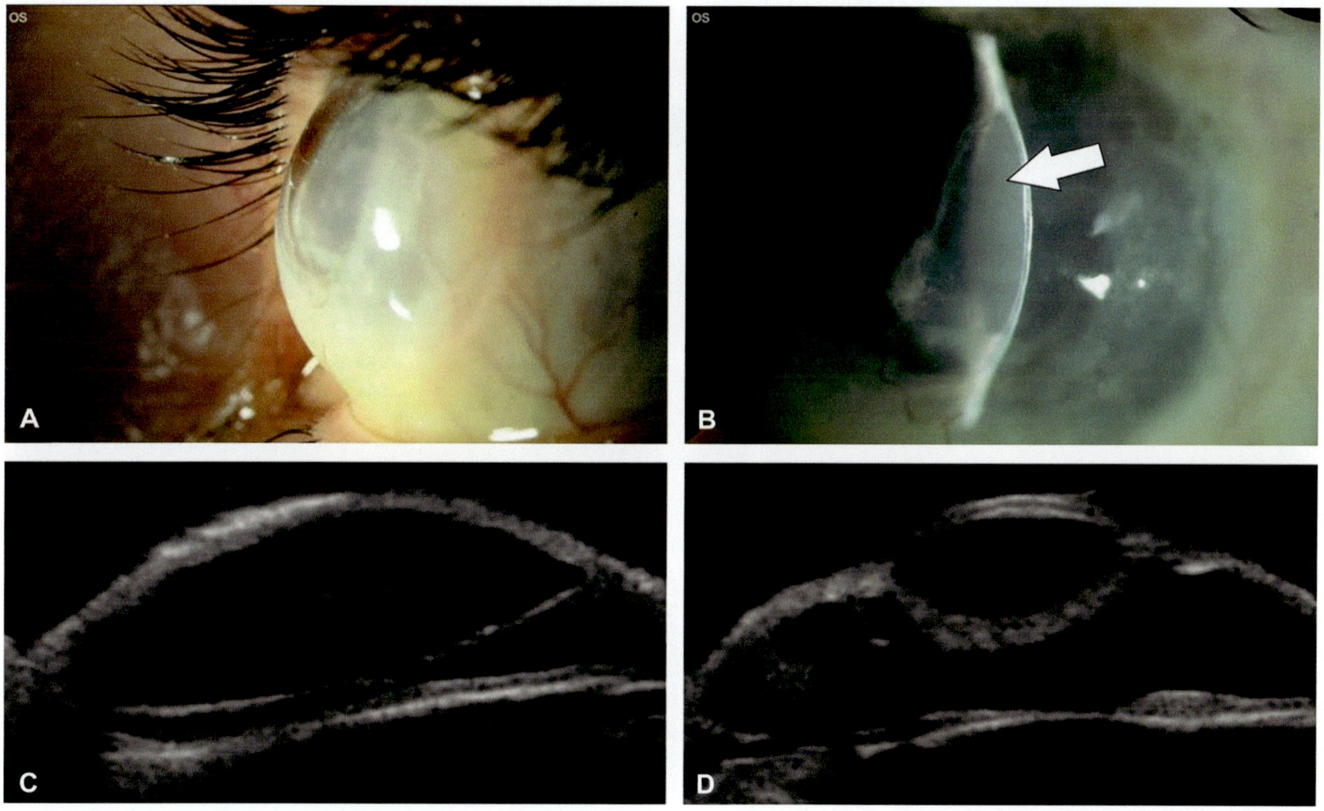

Fig. 10 Interface fluid syndrome after multiple keratoplasties (6×, most recently lamellar keratoplasty) due to keratoglobus. In side view (**A**) the cornea shows graft ectasia and the narrow slit illumination reveals interface fluid (**B**, arrow). Sonography is important to determine the size of the cavity and to differentiate between epithelial implantation cysts (thickness of the wall) (**C**,**D**)

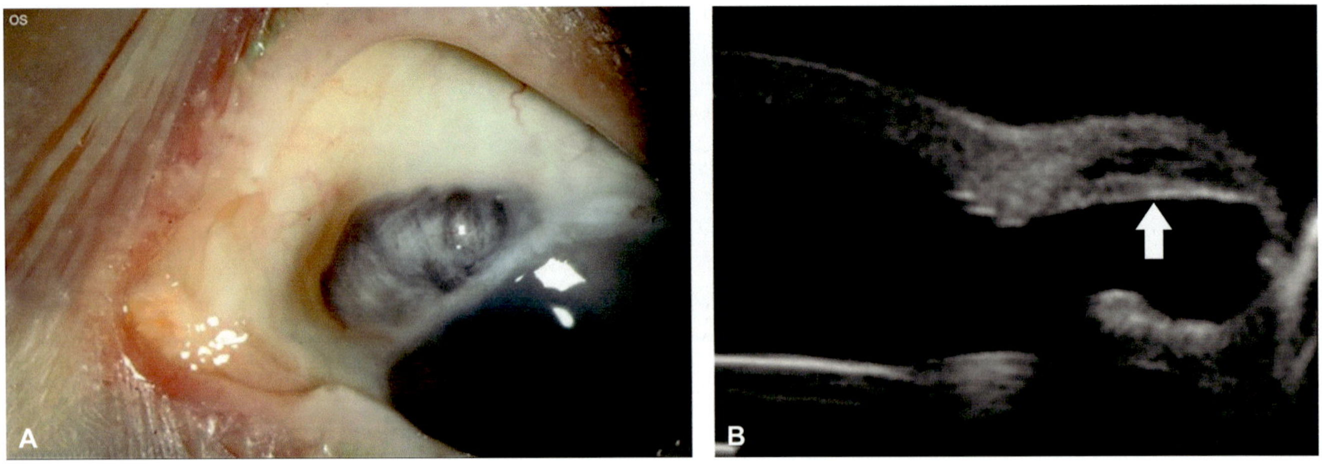

Fig. 11 Pseudocyst with iris visible under conjunctiva (**A**) following peripheral corneal perforation of unknown origin. Iris parts (arrow) are visible in pseudocyst lumen on UBM image (**B**)

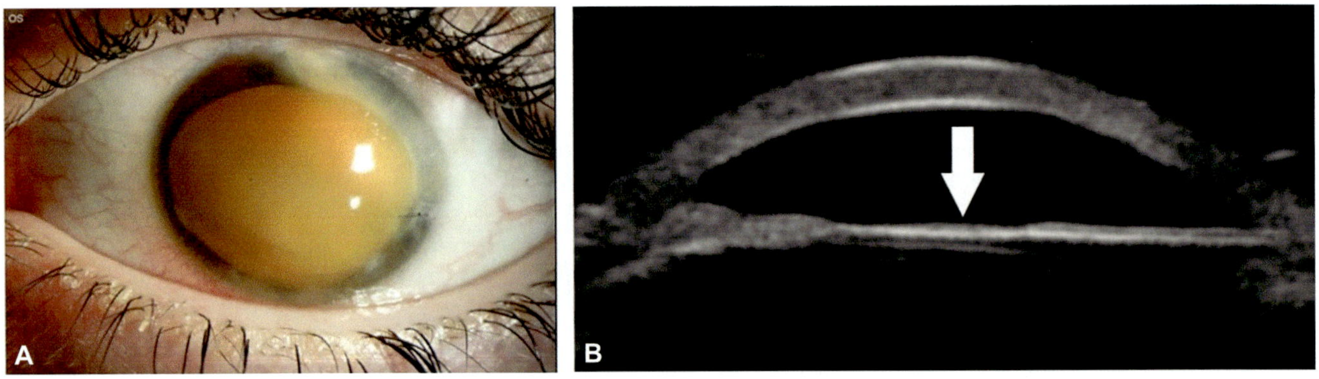

Fig. 12 Corneal blood staining with peripheral clearing of the cornea (**A**) Ultrasound (**B**) shows the presence of a fibrous occlusive membrane (arrow)

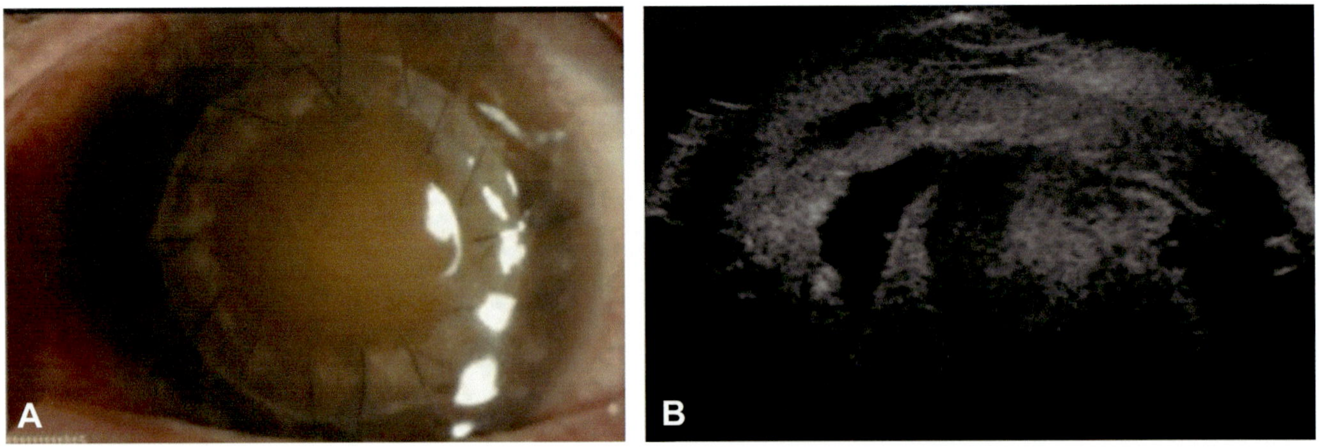

Fig. 13 Corneal blood staining observed in a graft after ocular trauma (**A**) The ultrasound image (**B**) reveals the presence of hemophthalmos, traumatic aphakia, and cyclodialysis (not shown)

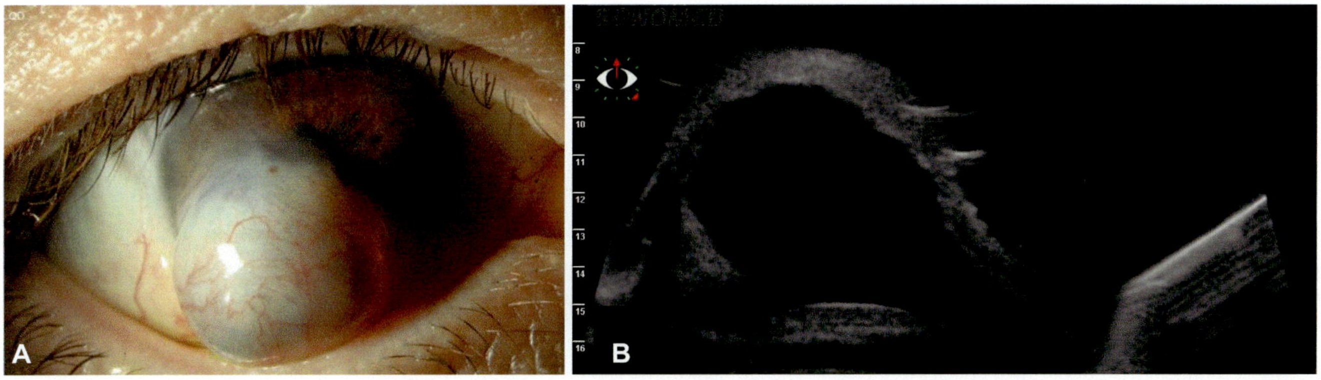

Fig. 14 Conjunctival flap following corneal perforation. The sonographic image reveals an inferior herniation of the anterior chamber, which is covered by amniotic membrane and conjunctiva

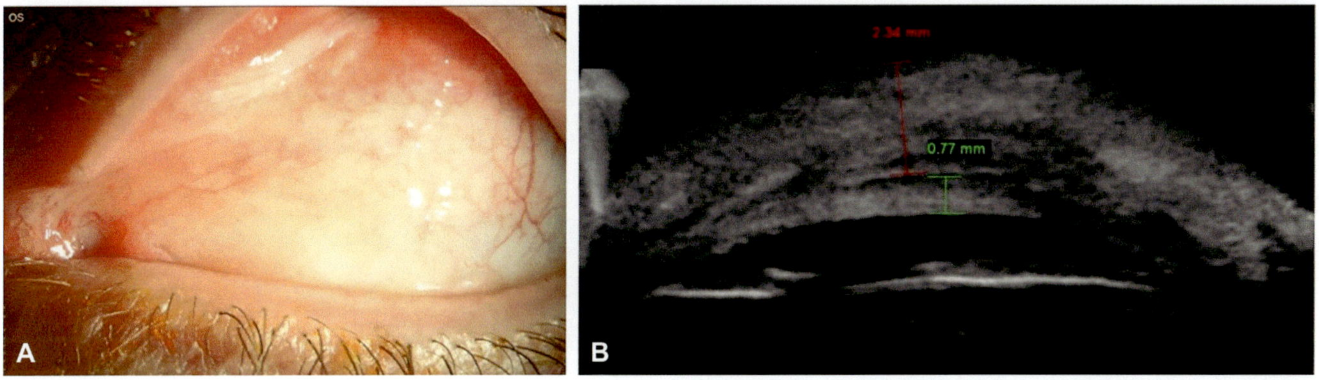

Fig. 15 Gundersen conjunctival flap (**A**) used in a patient who underwent multiple keratoplasties for infectious keratitis, following epithelial healing disorders. Ultrasound shows a conjunctival flap with a thickness of 2.3 mm (**B**)

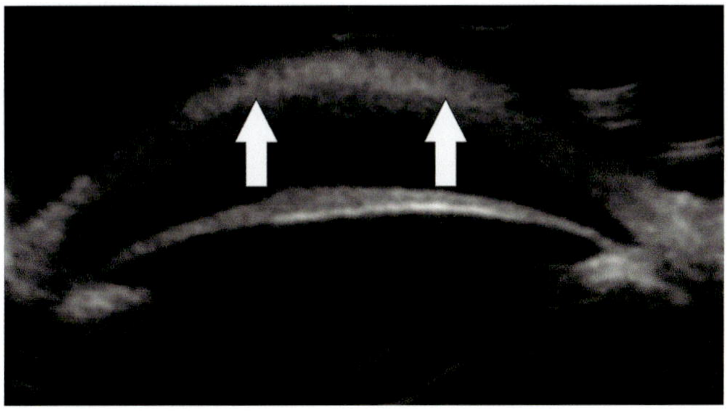

Fig. 16 Solid dermoid of the central cornea (arrows) in a 2-month-old child. UBM is important to visualize the tumour depth before surgical interventions

3 Comparison to other Imaging Modalities

UBM has several limitations that should be considered when choosing this imaging modality for clinical applications.

Disadvantages of UBM include limited penetration depth compared to other imaging modalities, which can compromise its ability to visualize deeper ocular structures.

Furthermore, UBM requires contact imaging, which might be uncomfortable for patients and may cause corneal indentation artifacts that can affect the accuracy of the measurements. The accuracy of UBM imaging is highly dependent on the operator's skill and experience in performing the examination. As it has a limited field of view and may require multiple scans to visualize the structures of interest, which might be time-consuming [17, 18].

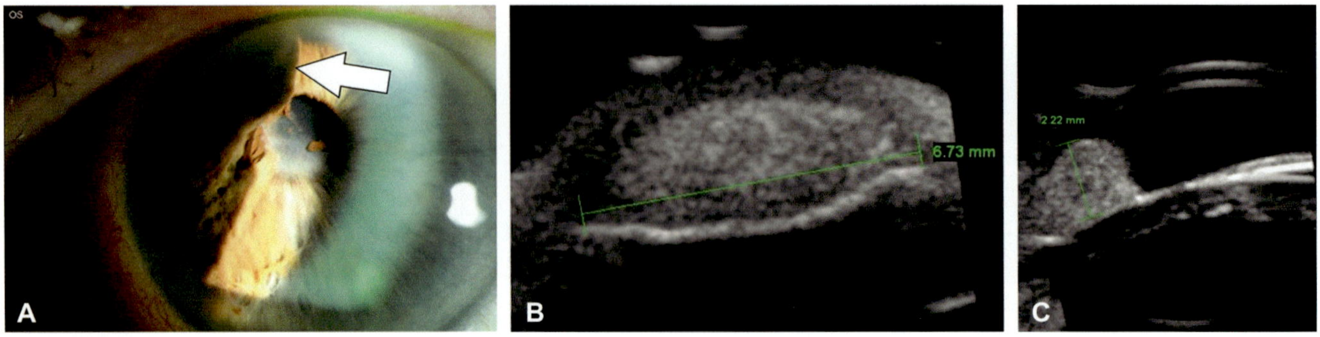

Fig. 17 Prominent iris tumour with contact to the corneal endothelium ((**A**) arrow). The ultrasound image shows a process that is indicative of an iris melanoma due to its extensive nature (**B**, **C**)

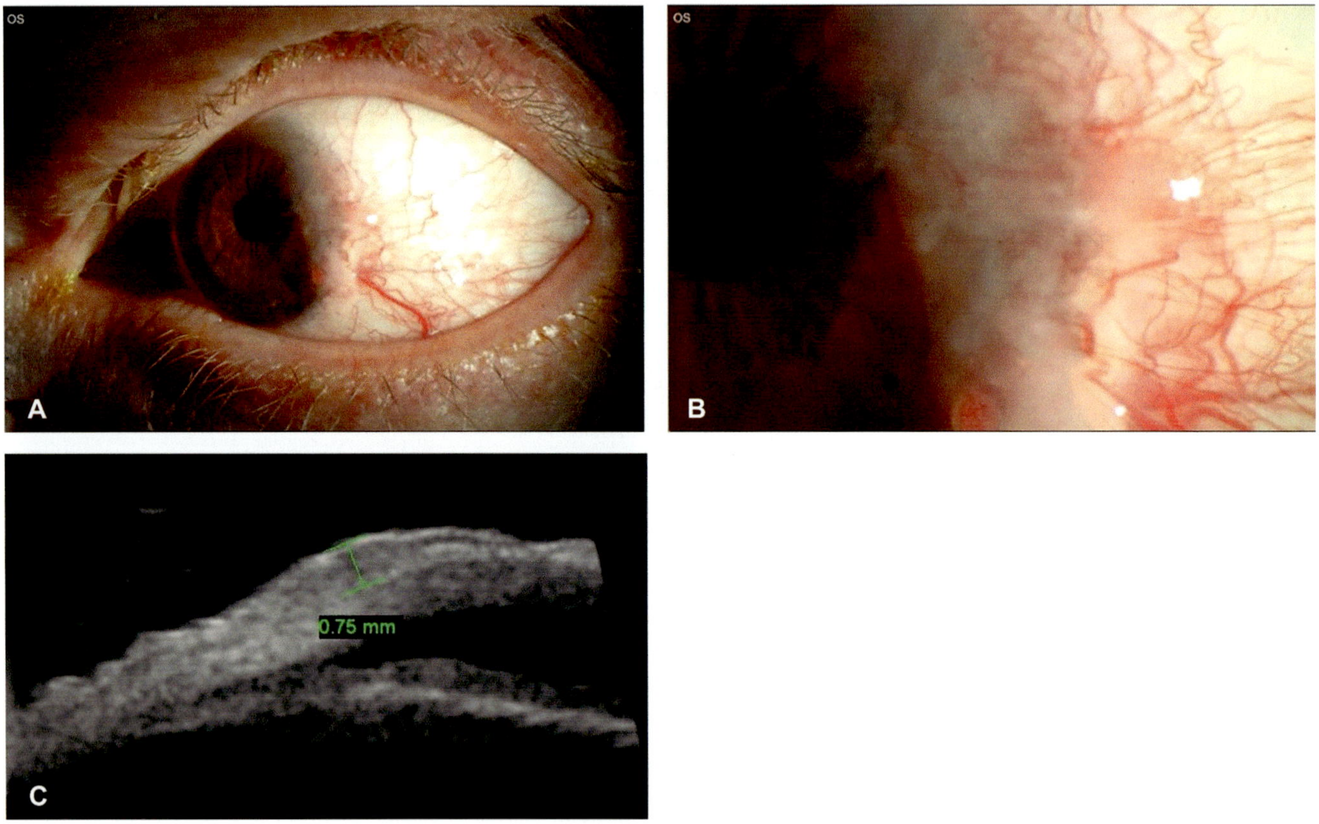

Fig. 18 Tumourous process of the conjunctiva with growth onto the cornea ((**A**) overview, (**B**) magnification). Ultrasound imaging (**C**) shows a clear demarcation between the tumourous tissue and the corneal surface

UBM and anterior segment optical coherence tomography (AS-OCT) are both imaging techniques that are used to visualize the anterior segment of the eye, but are using different technologies to produce images. AS-OCT uses low coherence interferometry to create high resolution, cross-sectional images of the anterior segment of the eye. Compared to UBM, AS-OCT may be easier to perform, as it does not require contact with the eye and can be performed quickly and with minimal discomfort to the patient. However, AS-OCT has even a more limited depth of penetration and may not be as effective at visualizing structures deep in the eye, such as the posterior segment (e.g. ciliary body) [17, 18].

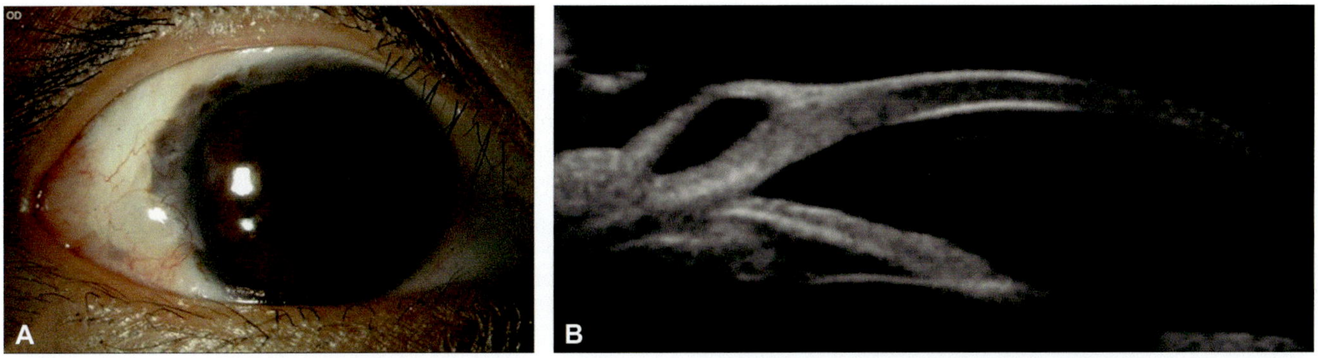

Fig. 19 Conjunctival melanosis and pterygium with a cystic formation (**A**) The ultrasound image provides a clear and detailed visualization of the cyst (**B**)

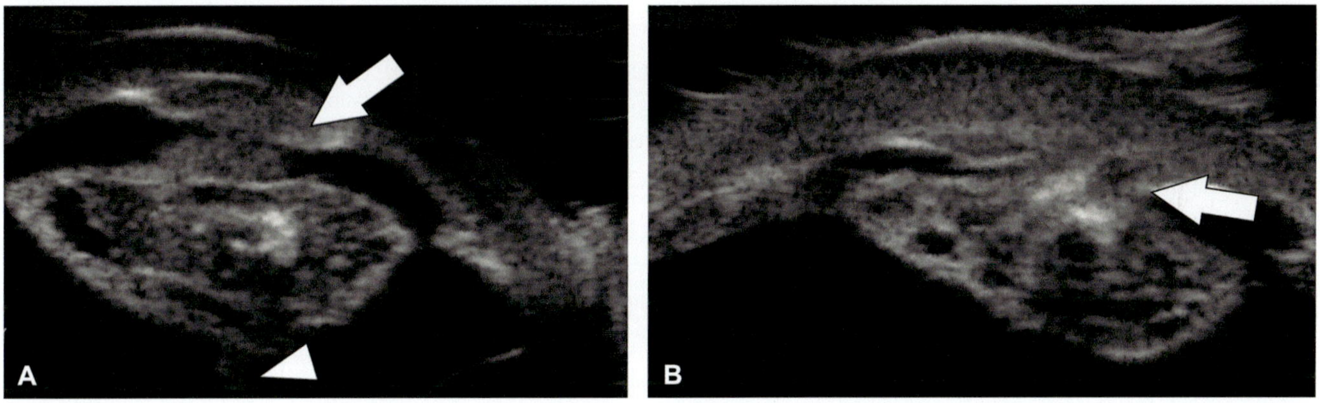

Fig. 20 Sonographic image of the anterior segment in Peters anomaly. The images of the right (**A**) and left eye (**B**) show iris and lens adjacent to the cornea (arrow), with the lens extending anteriorly and posteriorly. A persistent hyperplastic primary vitreous (a, arrowhead) is also visible on the right eye. The lens is hyper- and hyporeflective. The use of UBM imaging aids in the diagnosis and management of Peters anomaly, allowing for early intervention and improved visual outcomes

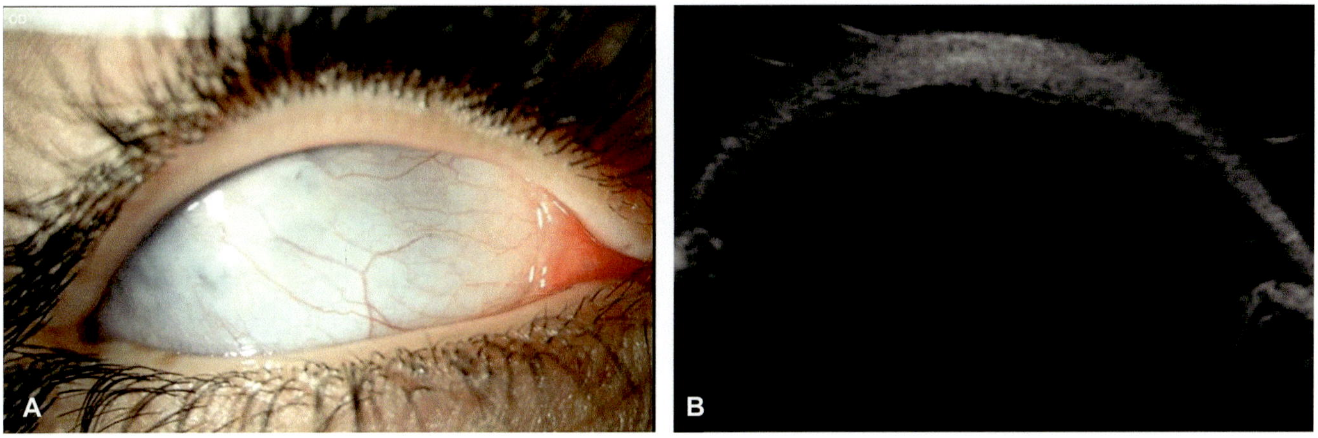

Fig. 21 Anterior segment dysgenesis with complete conjunctivalization of the cornea (**A**) Sonography demonstrates buphthalmos, aniridia, and aphakia (**B**)

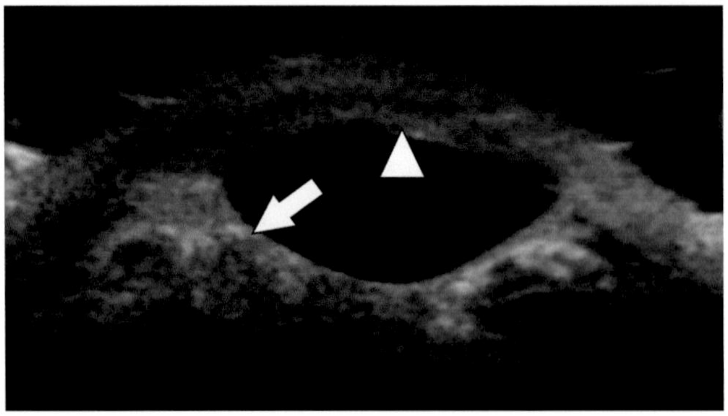

Fig. 22 Sonographic image of a patient with congenital aniridia, aphakia and progressive anterior fibrosis syndrome with fibrotic changes (arrow) and membrane formation on the corneal endothelium (arrowhead)

4 Conclusion

UBM for the diagnosis of corneal diseases is becoming less and less important in times of AS-OCT. Nowadays, there are only a few indications for UBM, such as the diagnosis of pediatric corneal diseases, which is mainly performed during an examination under anesthesia. It is important to emphasise that a high level of experience is required for a reliable diagnosis.

References

1. Pavlin CJ, Harasiewicz K, Sherar MD, Foster FS. Clinical use of ultrasound biomicroscopy. Ophthalmology. 1991;98:287–95. https://doi.org/10.1016/S0161-6420(91)32298-X.
2. He M, Wang D, Jiang Y. Overview of ultrasound biomicroscopy. J Curr Glaucoma Pract. 2012;6:25–53. https://doi.org/10.5005/jp-journals-10008-1105.
3. Foster FS, Pavlin CJ, Harasiewicz KA, Christopher DA, Turnbull DH. Advances in ultrasound biomicroscopy. Ultrasound Med Biol. 2000;26:1–27. https://doi.org/10.1016/S0301-5629(99)00096-4.
4. Alexander JL, Wei L, Palmer J, Darras A, Levin MR, Berry JL, et al. A systematic review of ultrasound biomicroscopy use in pediatric ophthalmology. Eye. 2021;35:265–76. https://doi.org/10.1038/s41433-020-01184-4.
5. Martin R. Cornea and anterior eye assessment with slit lamp biomicroscopy, specular microscopy, confocal microscopy, and ultrasound biomicroscopy. Indian J Ophthalmol. 2018;66:195. https://doi.org/10.4103/ijo.IJO_649_17.
6. Deramo VA, Shah GK, Baumal CR, Fineman MS, Correa ZM, Benson WE, et al. The role of ultrasound biomicroscopy in ocular trauma. Trans Am Ophthalmol Soc. 1998;96:355–67.
7. Marigo FA. Anterior segment implantation cysts. Arch Ophthalmol. 1998;116:1569. https://doi.org/10.1001/archopht.116.12.1569.
8. Agarwal R, Bafna R, Shakkarwal C, Sharma N. Interface fluid: A rare complication of superficial anterior lamellar keratoplasty. Indian J Ophthalmol-Case Rep. 2021;1:237–9. https://doi.org/10.4103/ijo.IJO_1275_20.
9. Abu Dail Y, Daas L, Flockerzi FA, Seitz B. Partial visual rehabilitation 5 and 6 years after a gundersen total conjunctival flap procedure. Ophthalmologie. 2022;119:203–8. https://doi.org/10.1007/s00347-021-01503-4.
10. Grant CA, Azar D. Ultrasound biomicroscopy in the diagnosis and management of limbal dermoid. Am J Ophthalmol. 1999;128:365–7. https://doi.org/10.1016/S0002-9394(99)00117-8.
11. Lanzl IM, Augsburger JJ, Hertle RW, Rapuano C, Correa-Melling Z, Cruz CS. The role of ultrasound biomicroscopy in surgical planning for limbal dermoids. Cornea. 1998;17:604. https://doi.org/10.1097/00003226-199811000-00006.
12. Conway RM, Chew T, Golchet P, Desai K, Lin S, O'Brien J. Ultrasound biomicroscopy: role in diagnosis and management in 130 consecutive patients evaluated for anterior segment tumours. Br J Ophthalmol. 2005;89:950–5. https://doi.org/10.1136/bjo.2004.059535.
13. Venkateswaran N, Sripawadkul W, Karp CL. The role of imaging technologies for ocular surface tumors. Curr Opin Ophthalmol. 2021;32:369–78. https://doi.org/10.1097/ICU.0000000000000771.
14. Chen WS, Xiang DM, Hu LX. Ultrasound biomicroscopy detects Peters' anomaly and Rieger's anomaly in infants. J Ophthalmol. 2020; 2020. https://doi.org/10.1155/2020/8346981.
15. Okamoto F, Nakano S, Okamoto C, Hommura S, Oshika T. Ultrasound biomicroscopic findings in aniridia. Am J Ophthalmol. 2004;137:858–62. https://doi.org/10.1016/j.ajo.2003.12.014.
16. Janssens R, van Rijn LJ, Eggink CA, Jansonius NM, Janssen SF. Ultrasound biomicroscopy of the anterior segment in patients with primary congenital glaucoma: a review of the literature. Acta Ophthalmol. 2022;100:605–13. https://doi.org/10.1111/aos.15082.
17. Ishikawa H. Anterior segment imaging for glaucoma: OCT or UBM? Br J Ophthalmol. 2007;91:1420–1. https://doi.org/10.1136/bjo.2007.121038.
18. Nolan W. Anterior segment imaging: ultrasound biomicroscopy and anterior segment optical coherence tomography. Curr Opin Ophthalmol. 2008;19:115–21. https://doi.org/10.1097/ICU.0b013e3282f40bba.

Diseases

Congenital Corneal Abnormalities

Barbara Käsmann-Kellner and Berthold Seitz

Abstract

Congenital corneal anomalies represent a diverse group of ocular disorders that manifest during intrauterine development or shortly after birth. Disorders of the anterior segment of the eye encompass a variety of clinical presentations including aniridia, Axenfeld and Rieger anomalies, primary congenital glaucoma, Peters anomaly, as well as syndromal associations. These conditions have a significant impact on vision due to disruption of the visual axis, and also secondary glaucoma which occurs in over 50% of patients. Ocular anterior segment disorders occur due to a complex interplay of developmental, embryological and genetic factors, and often have phenotypic overlaps and genetic heterogeneity. The reader will be presented selected causes of congenital or early emerging corneal anomalies and opacifications. There will be a categorization of the causes of corneal opacifications in infancy modified and slightly extended according to the classification of Ken Nischal et al. In addition, the aspect of Gestalt of the cornea will be described (NGP—Next Generation Phenotyping).

Keywords

Congenital · Infantile · Corneal opacification · Amblyopia · Nystagmus · Keratoplasty · Anterior segment dysplasia (ASD) · Aniridia · PAX6 · MAC

1 Introduction

1.1 Background

The anterior segment of the eye includes the cornea, iris, lens, and aqueous humor, which supplies nutrients to the avascular cornea and lens. Developmental disorders of the eye that affect this anatomical portion of the eye are collectively known as Anterior Segment Developmental Anomalies (ASDA) and are referred to as Anterior Segment Dysgenesis (ASD). These disorders exhibit a great deal of phenotypic and genetic heterogeneity and are therefore summarized here but described in detail. Some symptoms overlap, such as the tendency to develop elevated intraocular pressure (IOP). The ciliary body of the iris produces aqueous humor, which must be drained via the trabecular meshwork into Schlemm canal and the uveoscleral outflow tract. Disruption of this process is common in ASD, making secondary glaucoma a frequent complication. ASD include posterior embryotoxon, Axenfeld–Rieger syndrome, Peters anomaly/Peters Plus syndrome, primary congenital glaucoma, aniridia, congenital hereditary endothelial dystrophy, posterior polymorphous corneal dystrophy, sclerocornea, megalocornea, iridocorneal endothelial syndrome, iridogoniodysgenesis syndrome, congenital iris ectropion syndrome, and posterior keratoconus.

Although congenital or early emerging corneal opacities are rare diseases, they are the most difficult ophthalmo-pediatric diseases to treat. They usually result from genetically determined defects in the neural crest cells. They have a very high amblyogenic potential and, if occurring bilaterally, lead to severe visual impairment or even blindness. Surgery often has limited results and aims at maintaining the residual visual acuity.

B. Käsmann-Kellner (✉) · B. Seitz
Department of Ophthalmology, Saarland University Medical Center, Homburg 66424, Germany
e-mail: kaesmann@gmail.com

B. Seitz et al. (eds.), *Atlas on Cornea*, https://doi.org/10.1007/978-3-031-65422-0_14

1.2 Embryology of the Anterior Segment of the Eye and the Importance of PAX6 Gene

Embryonic development of the eye begins around the 3rd week of pregnancy and lasts until approximately the 10th week post-fertilization. Most of the diseases described in this chapter (especially common congenital corneal opacification CCO) arise during this period. Malformations of the central nervous system (CNS) occur in 14 out of 10,000 births, and these early-onset malformations often affect the ocular and orbital structures.

The development of the anterior segment of the eye occurs during embryonic development in the following stages:

1. Optic Vesicle Stage: During the third week of embryonic development, the optic vesicle invaginates to form a double-layered optic cup. The outer layer of the optic cup forms the retinal pigment epithelium (RPE), while the inner layer forms the neurosensory retina.
2. Lens Placode Stage: Around the fourth week, a thickened area of ectoderm on the surface of the optic cup forms the lens placode. The placode invaginates to form a lens pit, which eventually separates from the surface ectoderm to form the lens vesicle.
3. Hyaloid Artery and Vitreous Development: At this stage, the hyaloid artery extends into the optic cup. The hyaloid artery eventually regresses and forms the hyaloid canal, which becomes the primary vitreous.
4. Corneal Development (Fig. 1): During the fifth week, the surface ectoderm overlying the optic cup gives rise to the corneal epithelium, while the mesenchyme surrounding the optic cup gives rise to the corneal stroma and endothelium [1, 2].
5. Anterior Chamber Development (Fig. 1): The mesenchyme surrounding the optic cup also forms the iris, ciliary body, and trabecular meshwork, which together make up the anterior chamber of the eye [3–6].
6. Differentiation of Corneal Layers: By the seventh week, the corneal stroma has differentiated into five distinct layers, and the corneal endothelium has formed [7–9].

Master Gene Paired Box Gene 6 PAX6: The role of the PAX6 gene (homeobox gene) in eye and brain development is well studied and widely recognized [10, 11]. PAX6 is referred to as the "master regulator" because it controls the formation of the eye bud and the subsequent development of the various cell types within the eye (transcription factor). It is also known that mutations in the PAX6 gene lead to eye and brain developmental defects in several species [2].

However, it is also known that eye development is controlled by complex genetic regulatory networks [1]. The organogenesis of the eye is pointed out as an example of a developmental cascade of inductions. These networks include many genes and signaling pathways that interact with each other to coordinate the formation and differentiation of different cell types. PAX6 gene is part of this network and is regulated by other genes that are in turn regulated by PAX6.

PAX6 gene and the brain: PAX6 gene is also a master gene for developing the brain [2]. During embryonic development, PAX6 is active in a specific region of the developing brain called the prosencephalon or forebrain. There, PAX6 ensures the formation of specific cell types that are necessary for the formation of the various brain structures. It is also responsible for the formation of the various layers in the cortex that are important for the processing of sensory impressions and the perception of the environment.

PAX6 is in addition a gene that plays an important role in the development of organs and tissues in the body [2, 12].

Some of the organs and tissues regulated by PAX6 include:

- Nasal mucosa and formation of sensory cells
- Auditory pathways
- Pancreas: Development of the pancreas and necessary for the formation of insulin-producing cells.
- Thyroid gland: Necessary for hormone production
- Liver: Development of the liver, regulates the formation of bile ducts.
- Skin: formation of hair follicles and sweat glands
- Urinary and reproductive organs: regular development of urinary and reproductive organs, necessary for the formation of germ cells.

This list is not exhaustive, but the knowledge of the importance of the PAX6 gene is important to understand that PAX6 related anterior segment dysgenesis disease and especially PAX6 aniridia (PAX6 syndrome) are often accompanied by brain and organ development disorders and consecutive developmental, metabolic, and other diseases. This has consequences on further pediatric, genetic and therapeutic interventions.

1.3 Physiological Numbers of the Congenital and Infantile Cornea

The knowledge of the physiological measurements of the infantile cornea is essential to estimate any pathology and decide regarding possible or futile surgical intervention. Bilateral pathologies (e.g. bilateral buphthalmia without corneal opacification—mistaken for megalocornea) often are more delayed in diagnosis.

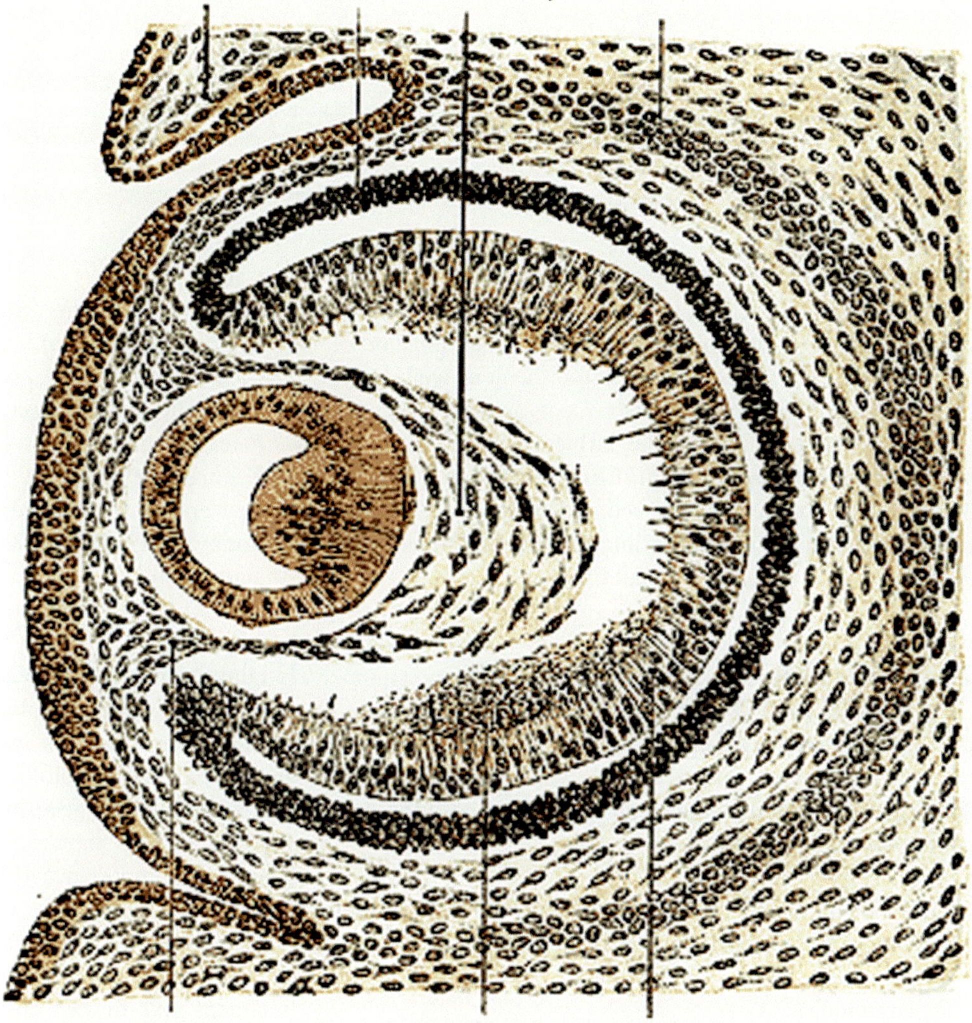

Fig. 1 Sagittal section of eye of human embryo of six weeks, showing the normal development of the eye in the middle of the organogenesis between 3rd and 10th week of pregnancy. Most conditions in this chapter arise around the 6th week. *Source* Public domain, https://commons.wikimedia.org/wiki/File:Gray867.png

Table 1 shows average physiological measurements in children aged 0–1 year and in children aged 10 years [13].

Table 1 Average physiological corneal measurements in children. As age increases, there is a significant increase in axial length (0.74 mm per doubling of age), and a non-significant trend towards lower average keratometry (−0.21 D per doubling of age) [13]

Parameter (Median)	Children aged 0–1 years	Children aged 10 years
Corneal diameter	9,5 mm	11,0 mm
Corneal thickness	0,5 mm	0,53 mm
Anterior chamber depth	3,5 mm	3,0 mm
Axial length	20,6 mm	23,1 mm
Keratometry	44,1 D	43,5 D
Intraocular pressure	12–20 mmHg	10–18 mmHg

1.4 Examination of the Infant/Toddler

Table 2 summarizes the essential features in the ophthalmological examination of children [14, 15]. It is evident that the various cooperation-related problems and the limited possibilities of examination with standard ophthalmological diagnostic equipment have a very negative and limiting significance. This is especially the case in conditions after (any) ocular surgery, especially when one depends on an accurate postoperative evaluation.

Very close collaboration with conservative pediatric ophthalmology both preoperatively and—if performed—postoperatively is an indispensable requirement for pediatric keratoplasty in the visual plasticity phase to best select occlusion therapy and timing of surgery in the face of amblyopia

Table 2 Main features of the examination of children [2, 15]

Area	Special features
Time	– Longer time during examinations – Visual acuity with Preferential Looking, LEA test takes time – Lack of compliance of the child – Longer discussions with parents – More examinations require anesthesia
Diagnostic tools	– More hand-held devices, but thus also less accurate (hand held slit lamp) – Retinoscopy essential
Documentation	– Photo documentation more difficult – Apparative corneal diagnostics not possible/only possible to a limited extent

[15]. Amblyopia treatment in congenital corneal opacification (CCO) and neonatal corneal opacification (NCO) usually is very difficult, especially in unilateral cases. Determination of refraction by retinoscopy may be very difficult as well due to CCO/NCO, and axial length measurements are necessary.

Liasis et al. [16] studied the influence of CCO on the results of the electroretinogram (ERG) and found a reduced b-wave in the absence of inner retinal dysfunction, but good ERG results can be evoked in infants with CCO post-keratoplasty in cases of normal retinal function.

2 Possible Classifications of CCO, NCO and Other Congenital Corneal Abnormalities

The following classifications can be used to describe congenital corneal abnormalities:

- The mnemonic STUMPED, which should not be used any more but which still is widely spread,
- Next Generation Phenotyping ("Gestalt") (deep phenotyping)
- Primary and secondary CCO and NCO
- Anterior segment dysgenesis (anomalies) (ASD(A)), e.g. Axenfeld–Rieger spectrum
- Aniridia as maximal variant of anterior chamber dysgenesis
- Microphthalmia-Anophthalmia-Coloboma (MAC) anomaly or spectrum
- Next Generation sequencing [17–23].

The following text will outline the different classifications and will emphasize the necessity to follow the etiological causes for inborn corneal abnormalities.

2.1 "STUMPED": Should not Be Used Any More

The mnemonic *"**STUMPED**"* was long used in older publications to remember the differential diagnoses for **c**ongenital or **n**eonatal **c**orneal **o**pacities (CCO or NCO):

- ***S***clerocornea
- ***T***ears in Descemet membrane (congenital glaucoma, rare: forceps trauma)
- ***U***lcers (infection)
- ***M***etabolic (mucopolysaccharidosis)
- ***P***eters anomaly
- ***E***dema (for example in congenitally present corneal dystrophies like congenital hereditary endothelial dystrophy (CHED), posterior polymorphous dystrophy, glaucoma)
- ***D***ermoid of limbus and/or cornea

In clinical practice, this mnemonic is still used, as it covers most of the possible etiologies of congenital corneal abnormalities. However, this mnemonic in no way respects the underlying pathophysiologic pathways of the development of the eye and the genesis of infantile corneal opacities [2, 19, 24–26]. The knowledge of the embryology of eye formation, the importance of the PAX6 gene and of possible metabolic disorders is as important as the differentiation of congenital or acquired lesions. Only a differentiated knowledge of the underlying mechanisms can lead to appropriate treatment and further clarification of possible underlying syndromes [1].

Table 3 presents a summary of possible classifications of corneal abnormalities. Each subclassification does not include all possible disease entities, and there are overlaps between the classifications. Therefore, it is useful to use a combination of the described classifications.

2.2 Gestalt: New Generation Phenotyping

Recently, New Generation Phenotyping (NGP) has become more important again, especially to avoid shotgunning requests for molecular diagnostic testing (Next generation sequencing (NGS)) [27, 28]. The NGP Gestalt Matcher is a pattern recognition algorithm used in machine learning and computer vision (examples: https://www.igsb.uni-bonn.de/en/research/gestaltmatcher, https://www.face2gene.com). Besides NGS it has several advantages, including:

Table 3 Possible classifications of congenital and neonatal corneal abnormalities

Type of classification	Definition	Examples
NGP: next generation phenotyping	AI[1] supported and Big Data guided application of advanced methods of computer vision on medical imaging data to classify rare diseases	Congenital corneal abnormalities of: – Size – Shape – Transparency
Primary CCO and NCO	CCO/NCO due to primary structural defects of the corneal tissue itself	– Corneal dystrophies – Corneal dermoids – Sclerocornea
Secondary CCO and NCO	Developmental anomalies of the anterior segment with secondary corneal involvement	– **KILD[2] (Peters)*** – ARA[3]/ARS[4] – **Aniridia*** – MAC[5] Spectrum
MAC[5]-Spectrum	Spectrum of Microphthalmia, Anophthalmia, Coloboma	– MAC[5] Anomalies – MAC[5] Spectrum with general involvement
NGS: next generation sequencing	Application of advanced genomic technologies and high-throughput sequencing methods to analyze an individual's genetic makeup with high precision and efficiency. Simultaneous analysis of multiple genetic variants	

* Described in detail in this chapter, [1]artificial intelligence, [2]kerato-irido-lenticular dysgenesis, [3]Axenfeld–Rieger Anomaly, [4]Axenfeld–Rieger Syndrome, [5]Microphthalmia-Anophthalmia-Coloboma

1. Robustness: The NGP Gestalt Matcher can recognize patterns even in the presence of noise or other forms of distortion. This applies to eye manifestations as well as to facial appearances
2. Speed: The NGP Gestalt Matcher is a fast algorithm, capable of quickly matching patterns in large datasets.
3. Accuracy: The NGP Gestalt Matcher is highly accurate, with low error rates in pattern recognition tasks.
4. Flexibility: The NGP Gestalt Matcher can be trained on a wide range of patterns and datasets

Although Gestalt matching is mainly used to analyze entire bodies and faces, we strongly advise to use the aspect of Gestalt to analyze manifestations of congenital eye diseases and use it in combination with facial appearance.

Examples for Gestalt assessments are CCO, NCO, microphthalmia, megalocornea, buphthalmia, corneal ectasia, bi- or unilaterality as well as facial stigmata like abnormal ear configuration, middle face hypoplasia, retrognathia. A recent paper [29] has shown the importance of so-called "deep phenotyping" in Peters plus syndrome.

The classification criteria for the face and the eyes are as follows:

1. **Bi- or Unilateral Involvement:** Examining whether one or both eyes are affected. Unilateral involvement more often are anomalies (changes only in the eye), while bilateral involvement more often are syndromes with extra-ocular manifestations. See Fig. 2.
2. **Atypical Axis of Lids/Lid Configuration:** Examining the orientation of eyelids, which can provide crucial diagnostic information: hyper-/hypotelorism, blepharophimosis, and upward or downward positioning. This may indicate systemic diseases like Down Syndrome, Hirschsprung Disease, Cornelia de Lange Syndrome, Apert Syndrome, WAGR Syndrome (Wilms tumor, aniridia, genitourethral abnormalities, retardation syndrome) and Stickler Syndrome (Figs. 3 and 4).
3. **Hypoplasia of Middle Face:** Identifying underdevelopment of the midface, could be hinting to Stickler and Apert syndromes (Fig. 5).
4. **Nasal Abnormalities:** Looking for anteverted nares, a broad nasal bridge, and other nasal variations (anteverted nares are typical in WAGR syndrome, Fig. 6).
5. **Lip Anomalies:** Assessing features like a harelip, narrow lip red, small oral opening, and a short philtrum. Harelip and short philtrum can occur in Peters syndrome (Figs. 7 and 8).
6. **Anomalous head position (AHP):** Evaluating head position (elevation or depression, face turn) which can vary in different syndromes (Fig. 9).
7. **Ears:** Examining the auricles for malformation, displacement, and rotation, which can hold diagnostic significance (Fig. 10) with distinct bilateral ear anomalies in Peters Plus syndrome
8. **Microphthalmia, kryptophthalmia or clinical anophthalmia:** Microphthalmia or absent eyes, sometimes associated with facial abnormalities. Often part of MAC spectrum disorders. Kryptophthalmia is a very rare disorder (Figs. 11–14).

   Microphthalmos is a congenital condition in which the affected eye is smaller than normal at birth (<9 mm in diameter). Microphthalmos is often seen in numerous chromosomal abnormalities, drug and infectious embryopathies, and quite often subsequent to a faulty closure of the embryonic fissure.

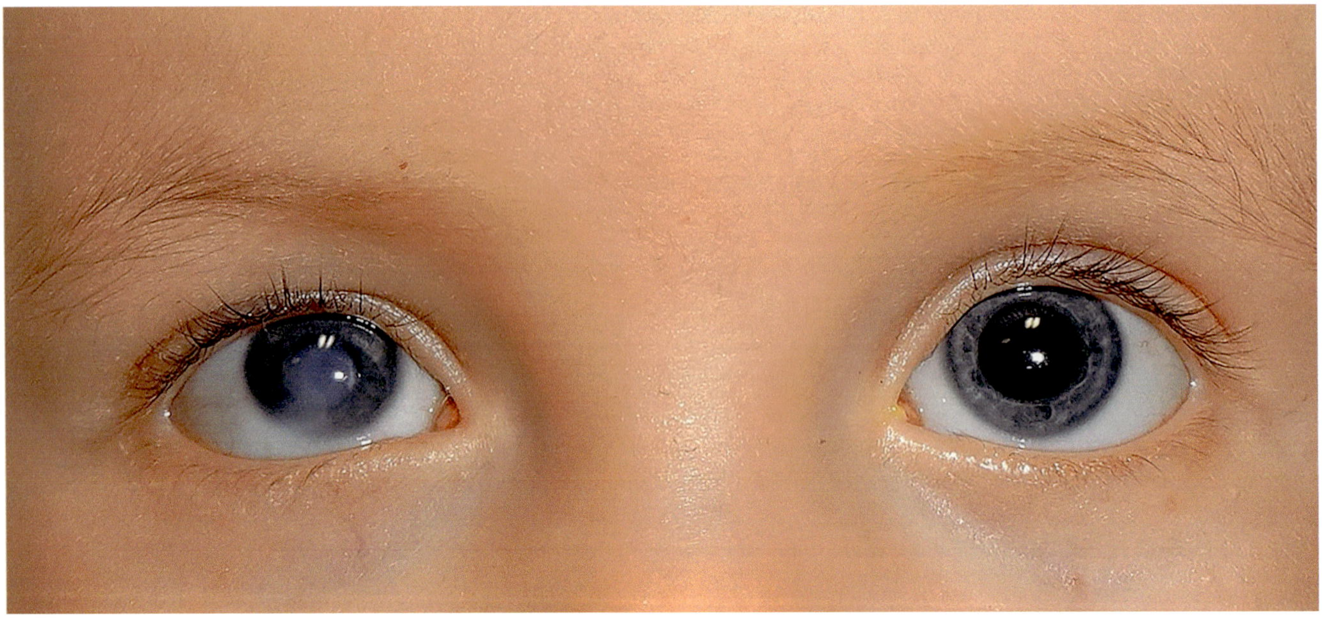

Fig. 2 Unilateral ocular abnormality: partial congenital corneal opacification, mild microphthalmia. Examination revealed Peters anomaly Type 1 (without lentocorneal adhesions), there are no systemic findings and a normal development

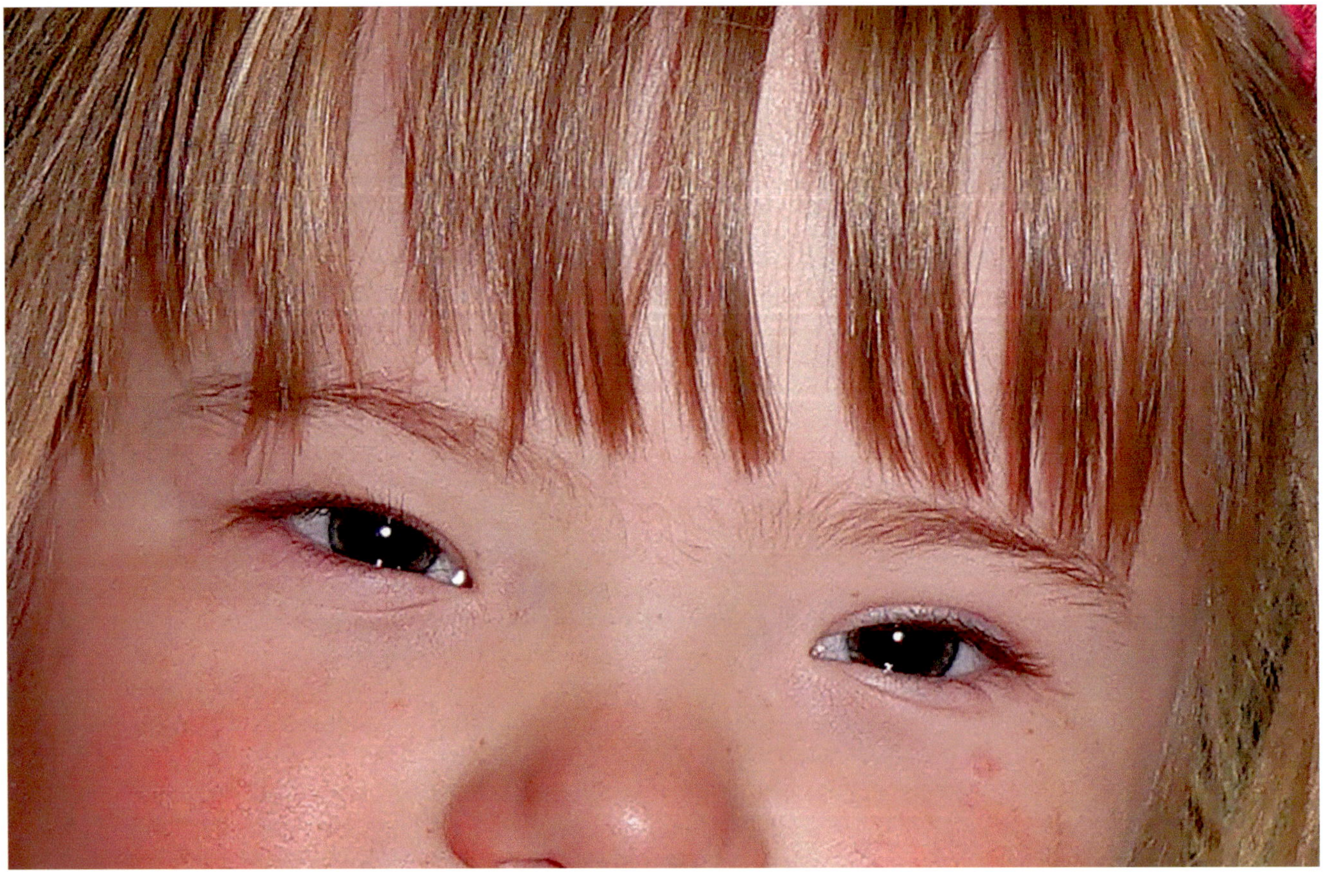

Fig. 3 Atypical lid configuration: upward slanting, can be seen in Down syndrome (as in this 4-year-old girl), Hirschsprung Disease, Cornelia de Lange Syndrome, Apert Syndrome

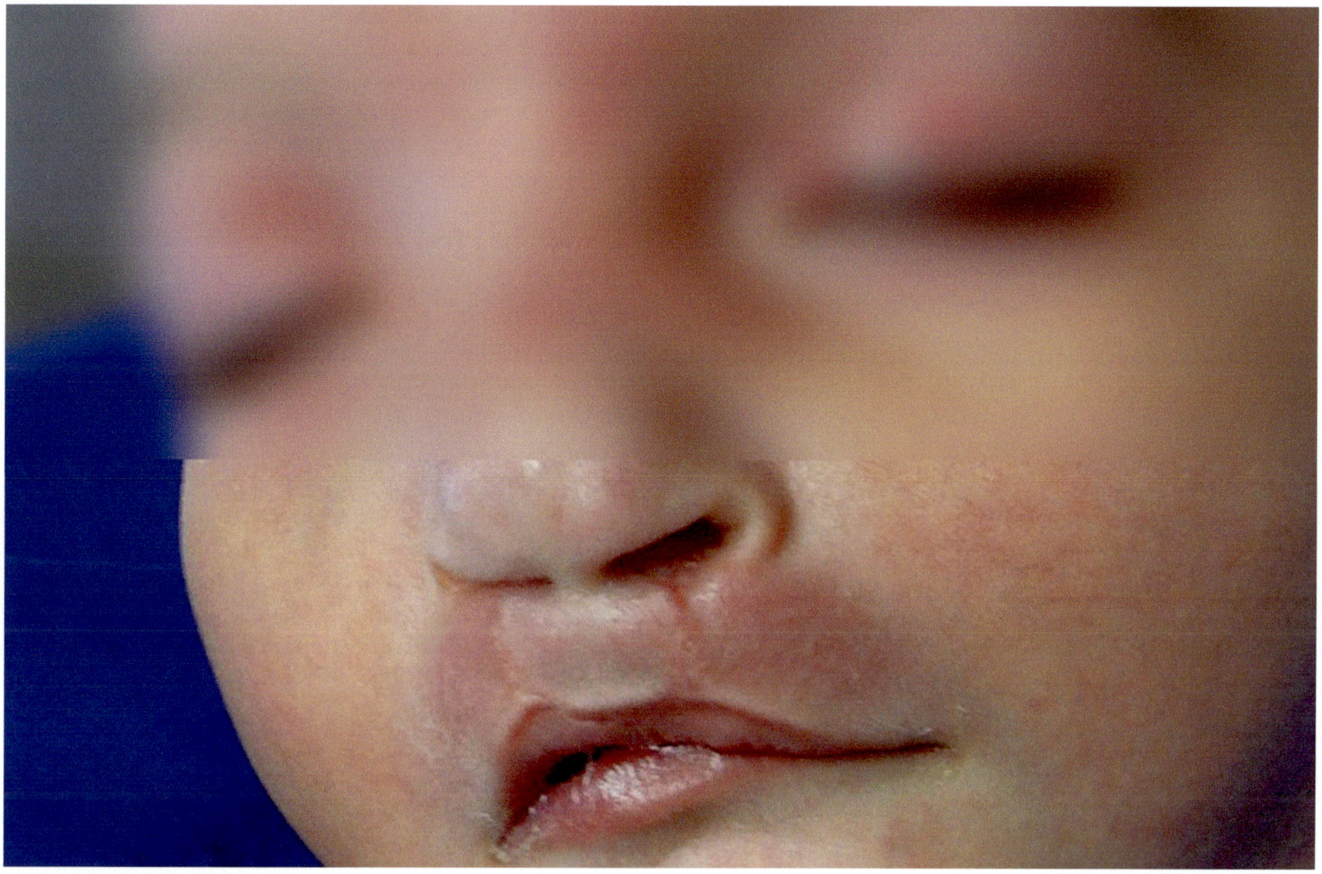

Fig. 4 Atypical lid configuration: hypertelorism, downward slanting of lids. Further facial special features: broad nose, double cleft lip and palate (post-surgery), micrognathia. Boy aged 1.5 years, has additional bilateral iris coloboma, diagnosis is Wolf–Hirschhorn syndrome

Microphthalmia with microcornea as shown in Fig. 12 is a rare anomaly. Often the orbital cyst is associated with a colobomatous defect in the microphthalmic eye. Decock et al. [30] reported that this anomaly arises between the 6th and 7th week of gestation, might be either unilateral or bilateral, and is associated with systemic anomalies. He attributes this syndrome to abnormalities in the chromosomes 3, 5, 18, and 22. Ultrasonography confirmed the presence of a chorioretinal coloboma. Histopathology revealed that the orbital cyst was made of two layers, an external layer made of dense, fibrous tissue resembling the sclera and an inner layer made of dysplastic retinal tissue. The cystic fluid resembled the cerebrospinal fluid (CSF) except for an unusual high level of beta trace protein.

Anophthalmos is a total absence of ocular tissues. True anophthalmos is rare, and its diagnosis is confirmed only after histologic examination of the orbital contents. Most instances of clinical anophthalmos are in reality cases of extremely severe microphthalmos. Genetic testing revealed no abnormalities up to now.

Sassani and Yanoff recognize three types of anophthalmos [31]:

- Primary anophthalmos, caused by suppression of the optic pits during the differentiation of the optic plate after formation of the rudiment of the forebrain. This is the case in regards to the patient in Fig. 13.
- Secondary anophthalmos, caused by the anomalous development of the anterior portion of the neural tube.
- Consecutive degenerative anophthalmos, caused by degeneration of the optic vesicle after it has been formed.

9. **Megalocornea or Classic Buphthalmia:** Assessing whether the cornea is excessively large or showing signs of classic buphthalmia, combined with tearing, pain and glare sensitivity (Fig. 15–17).
10. **Partial or Total Corneal** Opacification**:** Evaluating the extent of corneal clouding. Deep phenotyping includes the differentiation in primary and secondary opacification (see below) and might include histological characteristics (Fig. 18).

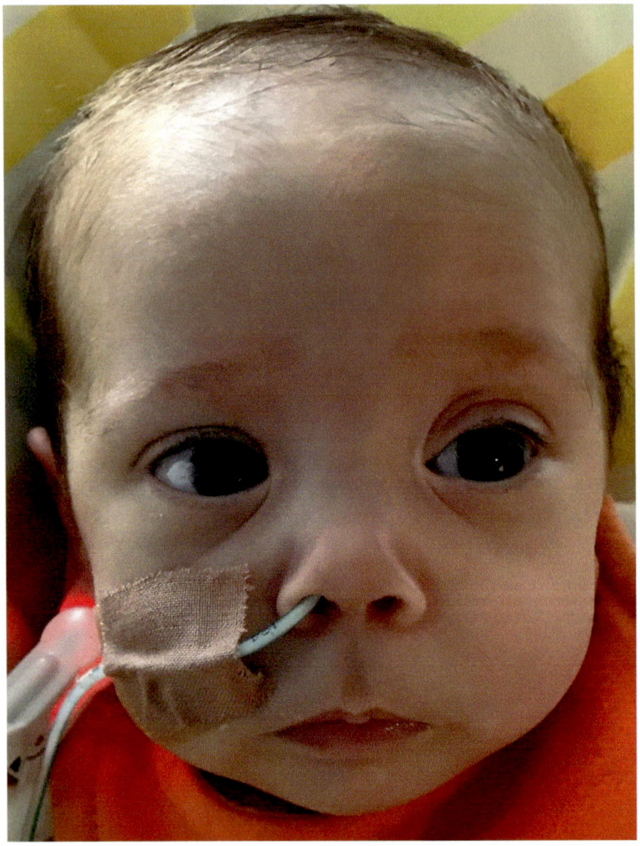

Fig. 5 Typical facial abnormalities in Stickler syndrome: a flat midface with a depressed nasal bridge, short nose, anteverted nares and a marked micrognathia, in addition exophthalmic aspect and large corneal diameter in high myopia

2.3 CCO and NCO: Epidemiology and Clinical Presentation

Primary CCO, NCO and Other Corneal Diseases (Table. 4): This section delves into developmental anomalies of the cornea itself, such as corneal dystrophies and structural defects due to dermoids. Specific conditions such as CHED, X-linked ECD, PPMD, CSCD, and CYP1B1 cytopathy are discussed.

Secondary Corneal Disease: In this category, developmental anomalies of the anterior segment (anterior segment dystrophy ASD) with secondary corneal involvement are presented. Axenfeld–Rieger Spectrum Disorders: This section focuses on a group of conditions with features overlapping with CCO and NCO, characterized by mutations in PITX2, FOXC1, and rarely PAX6. Secondary corneal diseases also include Kerato-irido-lenticular dysgenesis (KILD), irido-trabecular dysgenesis, and their correspondences with clinical entities such as Peters Anomaly, Aniridia and Sclerocornea.

Acquired Corneal Diseases: These are congenital or late-onset corneal diseases, often associated with metabolic, traumatic, infectious, and non-infectious factors. Conditions like mucopolysaccharidoses, cystinosis, keratitis, and traumatic scarring are involved. They may occur congenitally or later in life.

2.3.1 Primary CCO and NCO

Primary CCO and NCO are diseases, which are due to alterations of the corneal tissue itself. Classical examples are **corneal** dystrophies**, corneal dermoids and Microcornea/Sclerocornea**. The following images show examples of primary CCO and NCO.

Corneal Dystrophies

Congenital hereditary endothelial dystrophy (CHED) which often presents as congenital corneal edema with bilateral corneal opacifications (Fig. 18) [32], is an autosomal recessive disease (originally CHED Type 2). Former CHED Type 1 is now classified as Posterior Polymorphous Corneal Dystrophy PPCD) [32].

CHED has been mapped to chromosome 20p13 (mutation of SLC4A11 gene) and mutations in the ZEB1 gene are associated with former CHED Type 2 (=PPCD) [33].

Congenital stromal corneal dystrophy *CSCD:* Congenital Stromal Corneal Dystrophy (CSCD) is a rare, congenital, autosomal dominant corneal dystrophy characterized by non-progressive or slowly progressive clouding of the corneal stroma. It may lead to CCO (Fig. 19, right) or to NCO (Fig. 19, left [34]. The etiology of CSCD has been correlated with a deletion of the decorin gene on chromosome 12q22. Penetrating keratoplasty (PKP) is considered as treatment and there is usually no recurrence (Fig. 20) [35].

Posterior Polymorphous Corneal Dystrophy*: PPCD* Posterior Polymorphous Corneal Dystrophy (including formerly CHED Type 1) is a disorder of the corneal endothelium and Descemet membrane, producing a wide variability in clinical presentation. It appears later than CHED and therefore is a NCO. It has been mapped to four different loci on chromosomes 1, 8, 10, and 20, thus showing locus heterogeneity [36]. Although the clinical picture may be impressive (Figs. 21, 22), visual acuity often is only moderately reduced.

Structural Corneal Defects in Dermoids (Choristoma)

Corneal dermoids are congenital well-circumscribed yellow-white solid masses that involve the bulbar conjunctiva and the corneoscleral limbus (Fig. 23–28). It may occur as an isolated lesion or it can be associated with Goldenhar syndrome [19]. Hence, the patient should be evaluated for ipsilateral or bilateral preauricular skin appendages and the child should be screened for oral and skeletal abnormalities. Histopathologically, the conjunctival dermoid is a simple

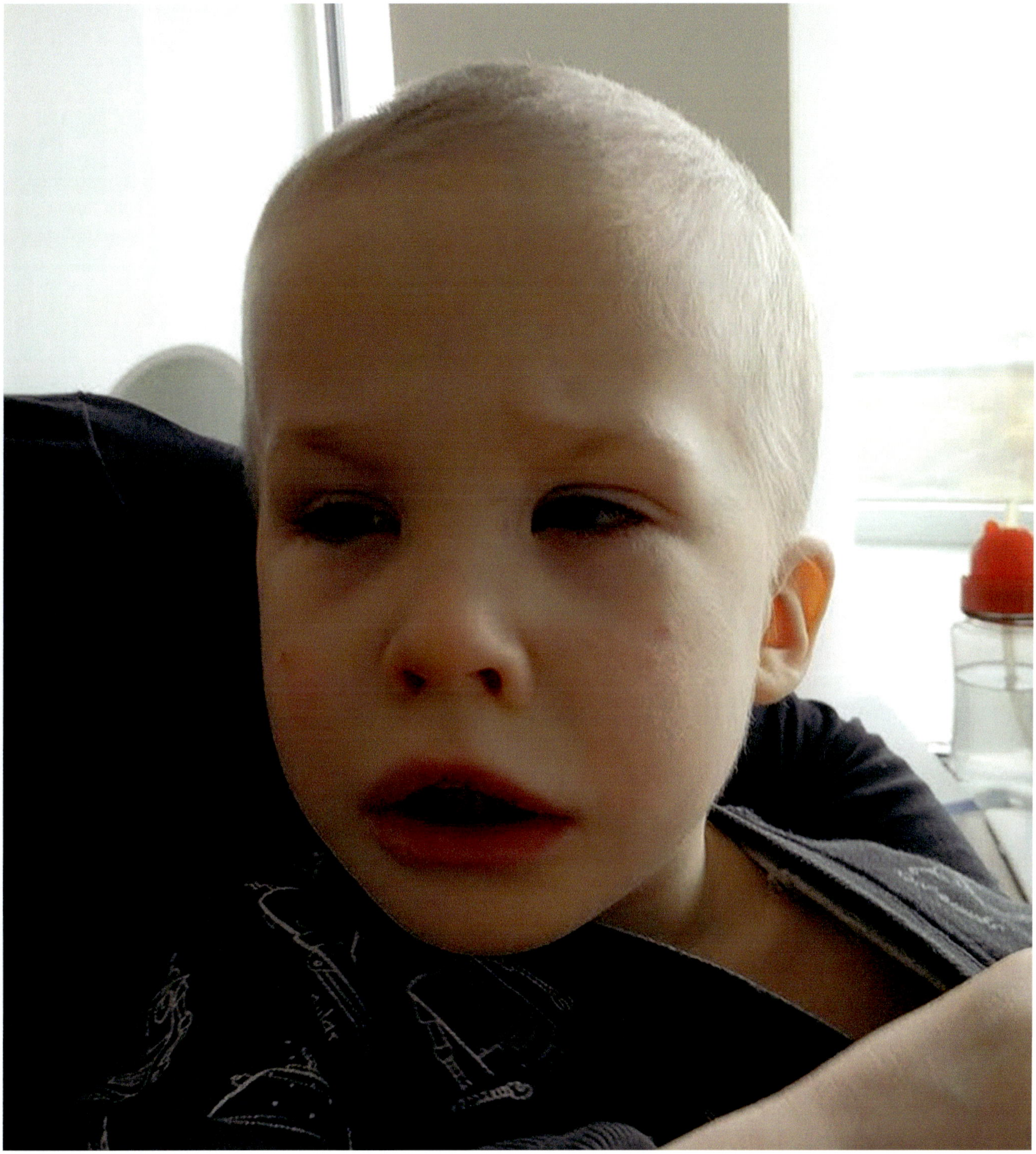

Fig. 6 Typical facial appearance of WAGR aniridia: aniridia, anteverted nares, hypotonia (open mouth), low positioned ears. This patient just undergoes chemotherapy for Wilms tumor (loss of hair)

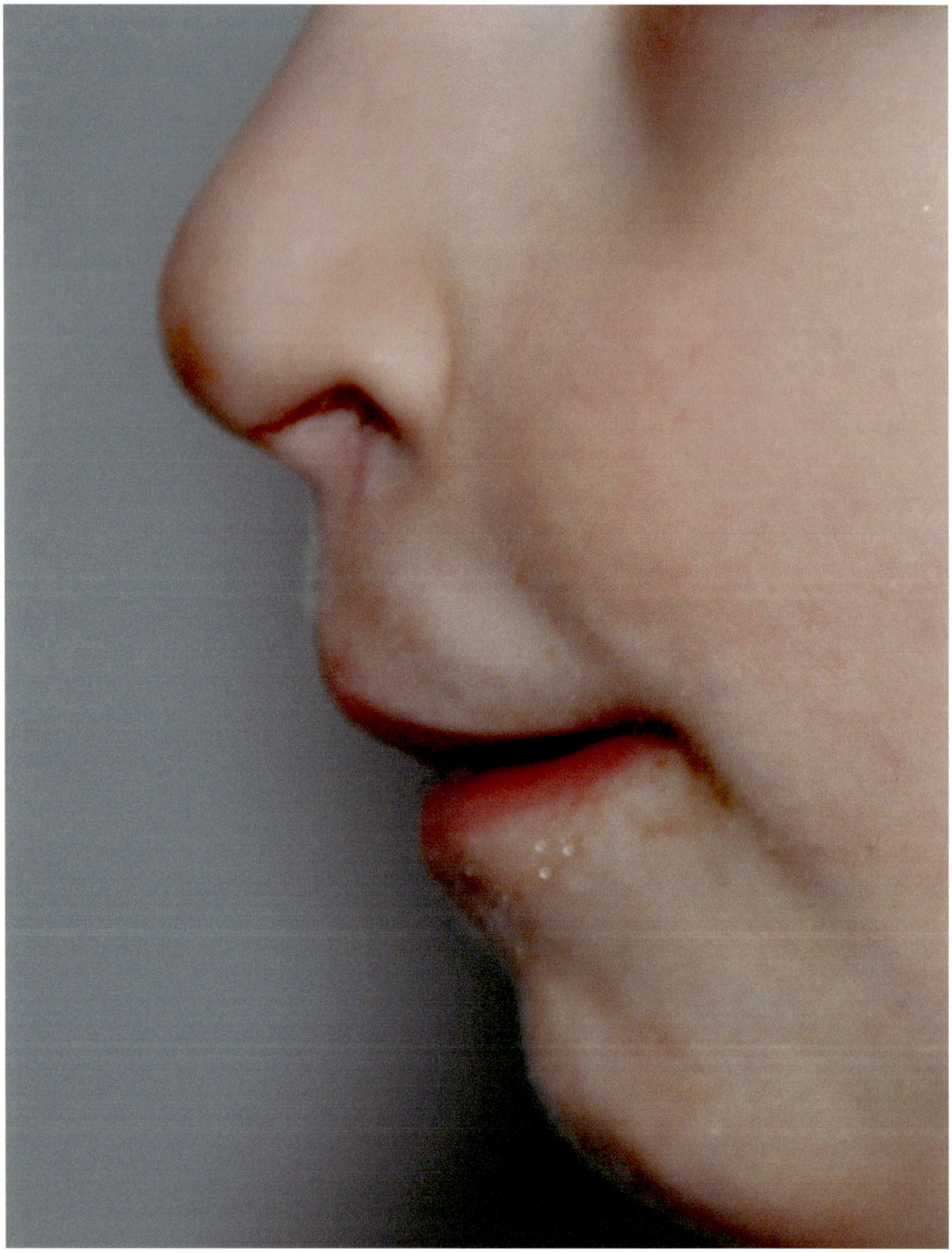

Fig. 7 Profile view of a boy with PITX2 gene associated Peters syndrome: mark short philtrum, narrow lip red, scar from surgery in harelip, micro- and retrognatia, slightly anteverted nares

choristomatous malformation that consists of dense fibrous tissue lined by conjunctival epithelium with deeper dermal elements such as hair follicles and sebaceous glands [37]. Larger or symptomatic dermoids can produce visual loss from astigmatism and from defect tear film. These are typically treated by lamellar keratosclerectomy with primary conjunctival tissue closure [38]. Neither lamellar nor penetrating keratoplasty is typically required for treatment. The ophthalmologist has to inform the parents that a grayish area in the corneal region of the former dermoid will most likely remain.

Cornea Plana, Microcornea

Cornea plana is a congenital condition where the cornea is flattened and the angle between it and the sclera is decreased [39]. This may lead to hyperopia and a hazy corneal limbus. Cornea plana has both autosomal dominant and autosomal recessive inheritance (Figs. 29–32):

1. Cornea Plana 1: AD (autosomal dominant). CNA1, Mild disease [40, 41]

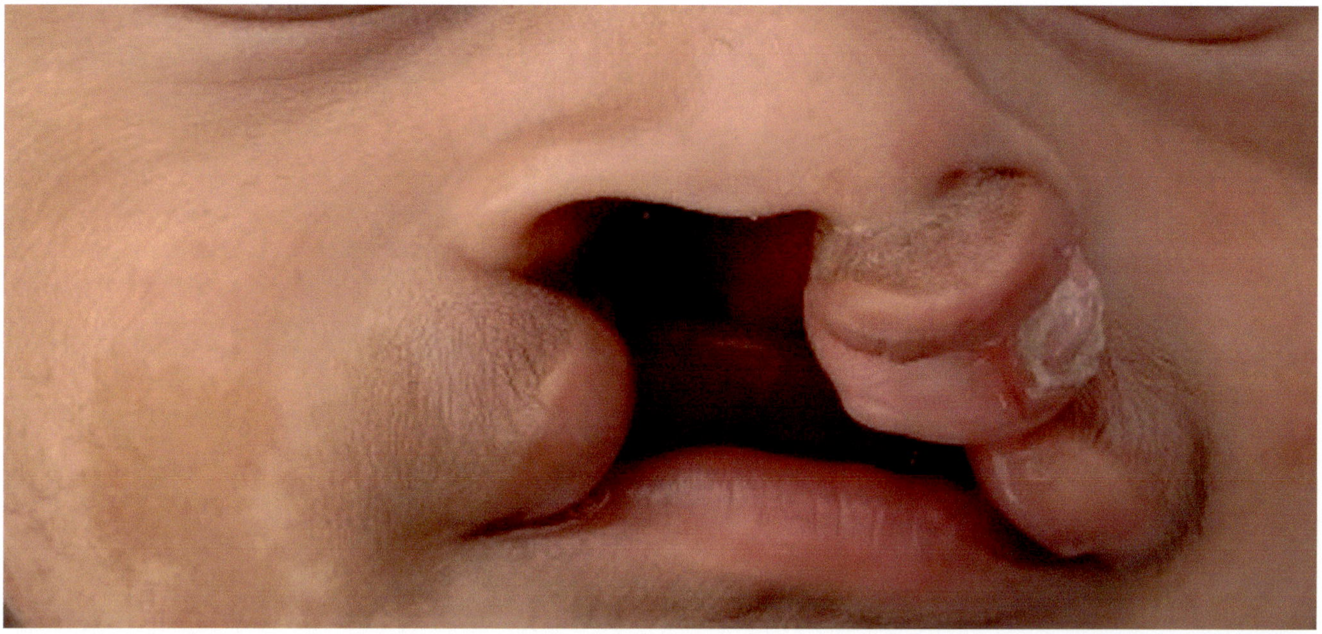

Fig. 8 Bilateral cleft lip and palate, hyperpigmented patches on the skin, ocular bilateral Peters spectrum → Peters syndrome, formerly known as Krause–Kivlin syndrome

2. Cornea Plana 2: AR (autosomal recessive). CNA2, homozygous mutation in the KERA gene. Severe disease, associated with additional ocular manifestations [42]

Cornea plana is associated with high hyperopia and especially in AD cases with secondary glaucoma.

Sclerocornea

Sclerocornea is a rare, non-progressive, bilateral, and asymmetric primary congenital disease, which has no association with inflammatory and/or infectious, causes. It is defined as diffuse (total) or peripheral opacity of the cornea, either associated or not with flat cornea and systemic changes (mental retardation, deafness, and craniofacial abnormalities) [19, 26]. Isolated sclerocornea is not associated with systemic abnormalities; there is a peripheral opacity; the central cornea is clear and sometimes flat.

Peripheral sclerocornea presents a large opacity of the peripheral cornea without a distinct limbus and is commonly associated with Rieger syndrome and Peters anomaly.

In total sclerocornea, the entire cornea is opaque and vascularized. Anterior segment ultrasonography may outline kerato-irideal and corneo-lenticular adhesions.

There is no sex predilection. The opacity of the cornea is similar to the sclera, white and vascularized, with no delimitation of the limbus, making it difficult to assess the corneal diameter correctly in cases of peripheral involvement, the central region shows up with variable transparency (Fig. 33).

In sclerocornea, there is a big overlap to other clinical entities like Peters syndrome, cornea plana type 2 and MAC spectrum disorders, which makes clinical and genetical categorization often difficult. Sometimes, even in severe sclerocornea, visual orientation is surprisingly good (see Fig. 34). Sometimes, very rare disorders can be found in sclerocornea (Fig. 35).

2.3.2 Secondary Congenital CCO and NCO

General Remarks to Anterior Segment Dysgenesis (ASD)

Anatomically, the anterior segment encompasses the cornea, anterior chamber, trabecular meshwork, iris, ciliary body, and lens. Anterior segment dysgenesis (ASD) is a group of non-acquired ocular anomalies characterized by developmental abnormalities of the anterior segment, including the cornea, iris, ciliary body, and lens. ASD is an umbrella term, which describes a spectrum of disorders originating from maldevelopment of the anterior segment and is usually associated with an increased risk of glaucoma, which might lead to blindness, if not diagnosed early. The cause is multifactorial, and many genes are involved in the development of the anterior segment (among those, PAX6 leading to the maximal form of ASD, aniridia). Part of the ASD often is Embryotoxon posterius, which is present in about 10% of the population. ASDs can be an isolated ocular anomaly or accompanied by systemic defects. In isolated cases, they are named ASD anomalies (ASDA), whereas if there are systemic comorbidities, they are named

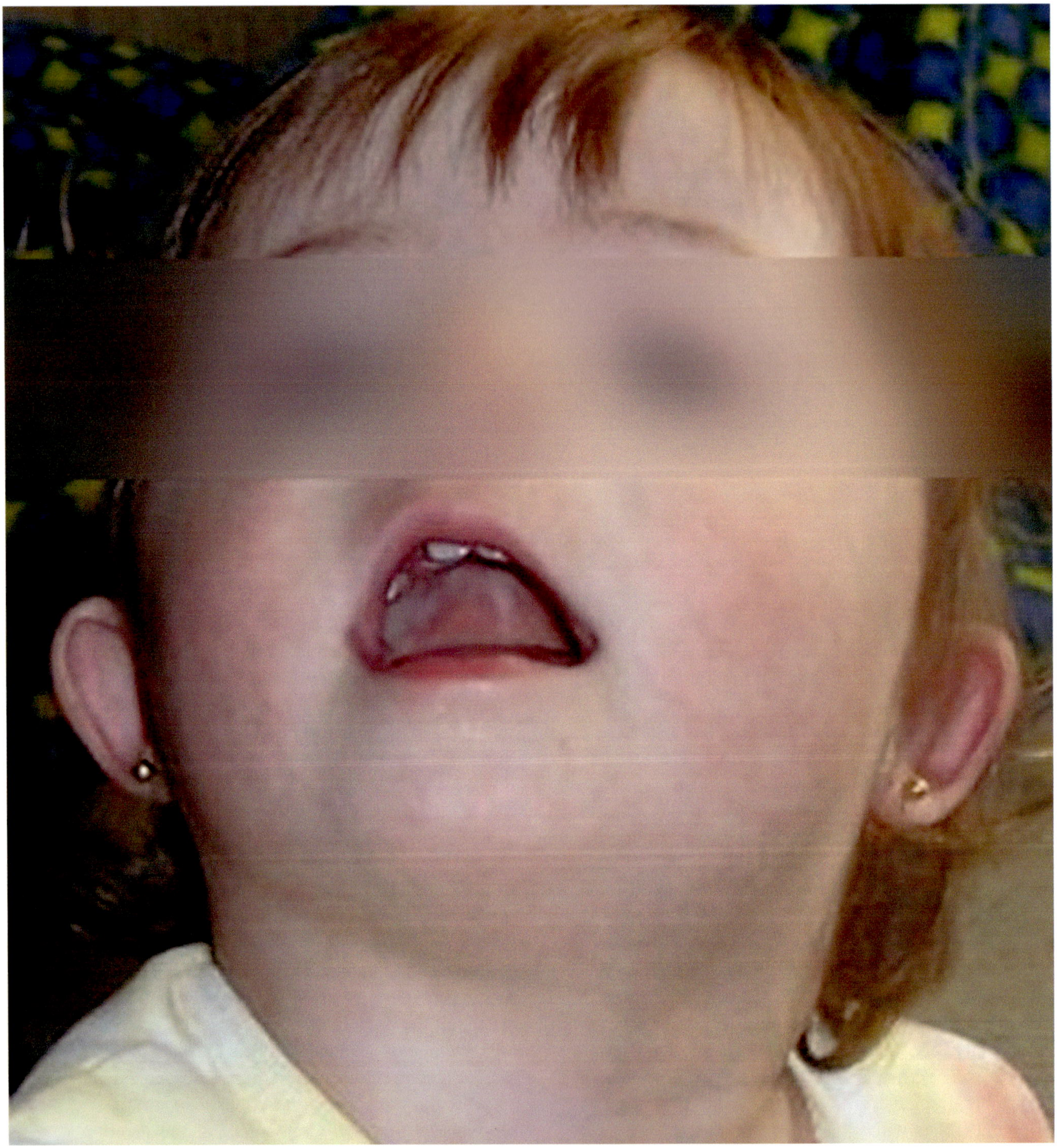

Fig. 9 Marked anomalous head position (AHP)—elevation of chin, downward gaze. In this 1.5-year-old the underlying pathology is congenital fibrosis syndrome of the extraocular muscles and ptosis

ASD syndromes (ASDS). The most common syndromes associated with ASDs are Axenfeld–Rieger syndrome (ARS), Peters Plus syndrome (PPS), Alagille syndrome, and SHORT syndrome. Glaucoma develops in approximately 60% of patients with ASD, during infancy or much later. ASDs can present as an isolated abnormality of one structure of the anterior segment, or more commonly as a combination of congenital abnormalities.

Due to the complex interplay between a number of genes during normal development of the anterior segment, pathogenic mutations in any one of these genes can consequently lead to a broad spectrum of overlapping phenotypes,

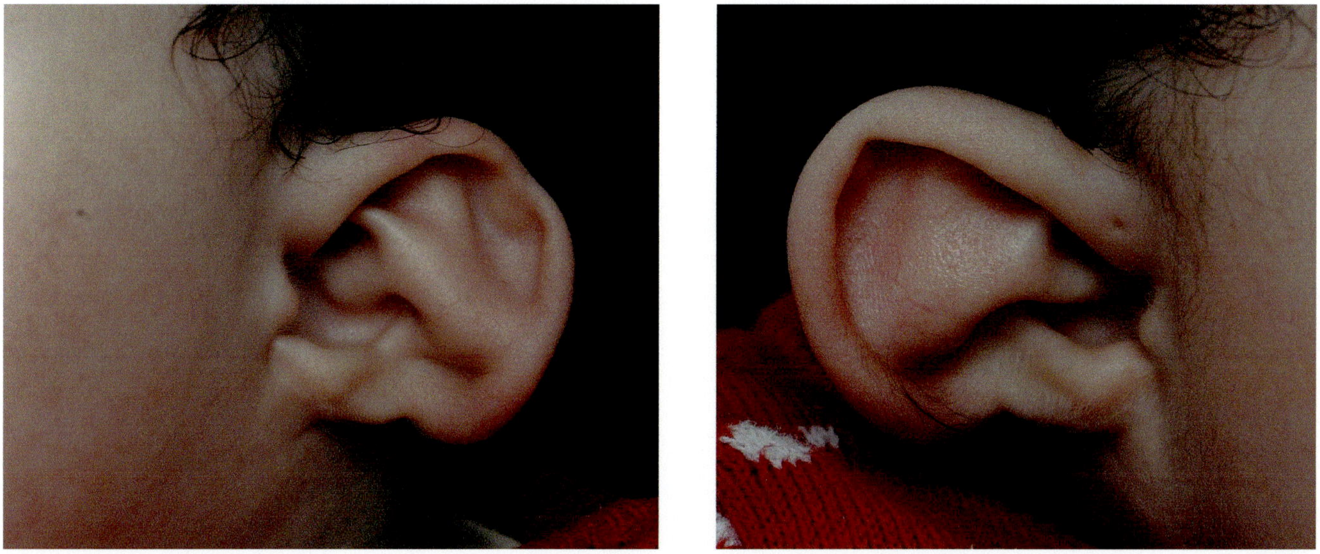

Fig. 10 Ears are especially important in Next Generation Phenotyping NGP. These are the ears of a child with ocular signs of Peters anomaly. The auricles are massively deformed. The ears indicate systemic involvement and the diagnosis therefore is Peters Syndrome. Further molecular genetic analysis revealed Oculoauricular Syndrome; OCACS: Schorderet-Munier-Franceschetti Syndrome due to mutation in the HMX1 gene

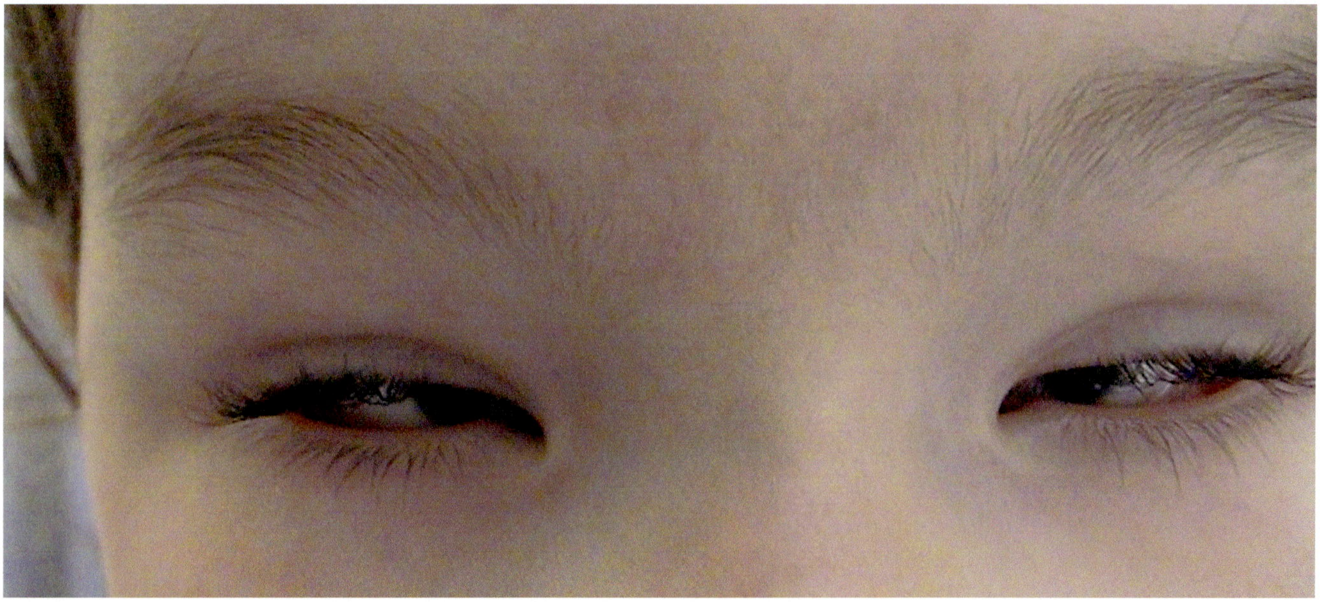

Fig. 11 Complex microphthalmia, girl aged 12 years. There was no chromosomal or molecular genetic abnormality found. In addition to microphthalmia, there was aniridia and optic nerve coloboma, normal general development (patient now visits university) consistent with Microphthalmia-Anophthalmia-Colomba (MAC) anomaly

making it challenging to assign a clinical diagnosis (see above: aniridia, sclerocornea, microcornea, microphthalmia, [43]). With an increasing understanding in genetics and genotype–phenotype correlations, a move towards a genetic diagnosis to support a clinical presentation is important to better understand ASD (Table 5).

Most patients affected by ASD have a combination of anterior segment abnormalities and in some patients, it may be associated with other congenital ocular disorders such as microphthalmia, foveal hypoplasia and optic nerve dysplasia. Figure 36 gives a schematic description of the structures of the anterior segment involved in different types of ASD.

Posterior Embryotoxon PE

Probably the mildest and most common abnormality one may consider under iridocorneal dysgenesis is simple

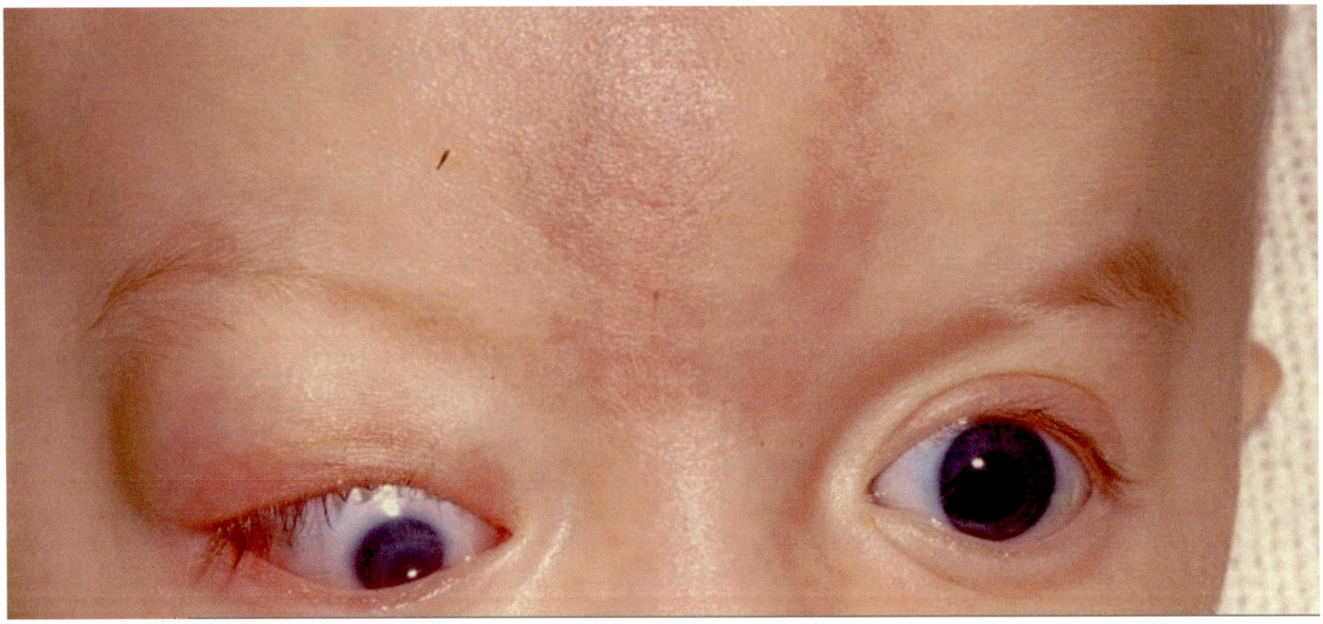

Fig. 12 Girl, 6 months. OD unilateral microphthamlia and microcornea with large orbital cyst leading to exophthalmia of the microphthalmic eye. OS atypical iris coloboma

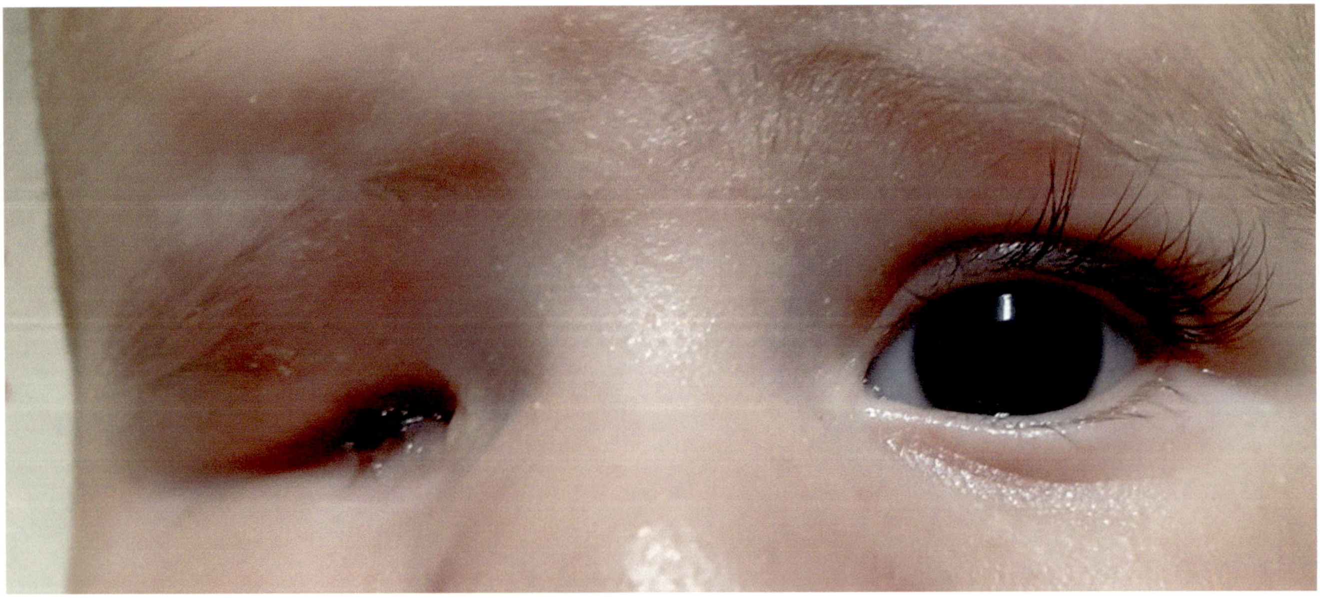

Fig. 13 Boy, 5 months. Unilateral anophthalmia, typically very short palpebral fissure width. Ultrasound did not reveal any extreme microphthalmia, nor an orbital cyst, which may be present in anophthalmia cases. Up to now, development and further pediatric and imaging examinations were within normal limits, so that we presume a MAC anomaly. Genetic testing revealed no abnormalities up to now

posterior embryotoxon, occurring normally without other evident abnormality (Figs. 37, 38).

Posterior embryotoxon (PE) refers to an anteriorly displaced and thickened Schwalbe line. Histologically, it is an iris hypoplasia with displacement of the Schwalbe line into the clear cornea. As seen on slit-lamp biomicroscopy, the grey-white Schwalbe line is concentric with and anterior to the limbus. PE can occur in 8% of the normal population, but most often occurs with Axenfeld–Rieger syndrome and arterio-hepatic dysplasia (Alagille syndrome). It is autosomal recessive.

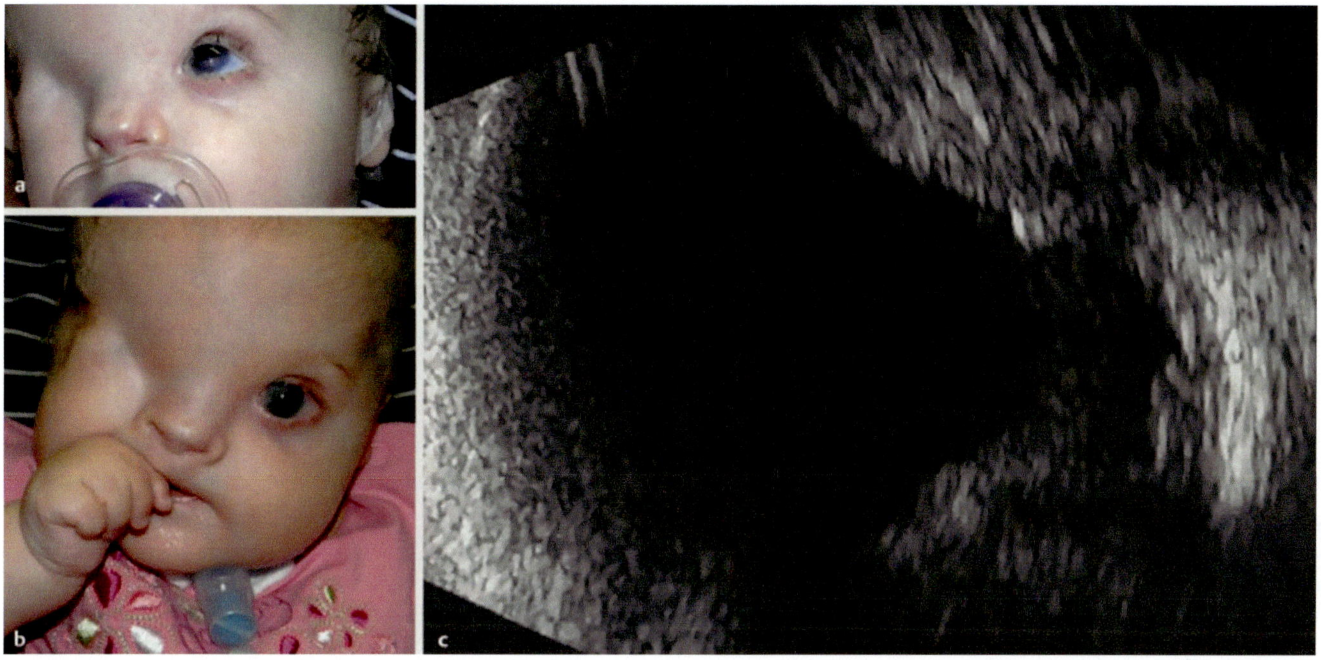

Fig. 14 Girl, 5 months at the upper left image, 12 months at the lower left image. OD true kryptophthalmia (ectodermal mesenchymal induction disorder) in Fraser Syndrome, no lid structures, no eyebrow. Ultrasound of the right side reveals kryptophthalmic colobomatous microphthalmia with a large optic nerve coloboma. VEP could evoke light perception through the skin covering the right eye. In addition, the girl had syndactylia of fingers and feet, severe laryngomalacia necessitating a tracheostomy. She now is without trachestoma, and, aged 15 years, visits high school. Fraser syndrome is caused by mutations in the FRAS1, FREM1, FREM2 or GRIP1 genes—this girl had a mutated FRAS1 gene

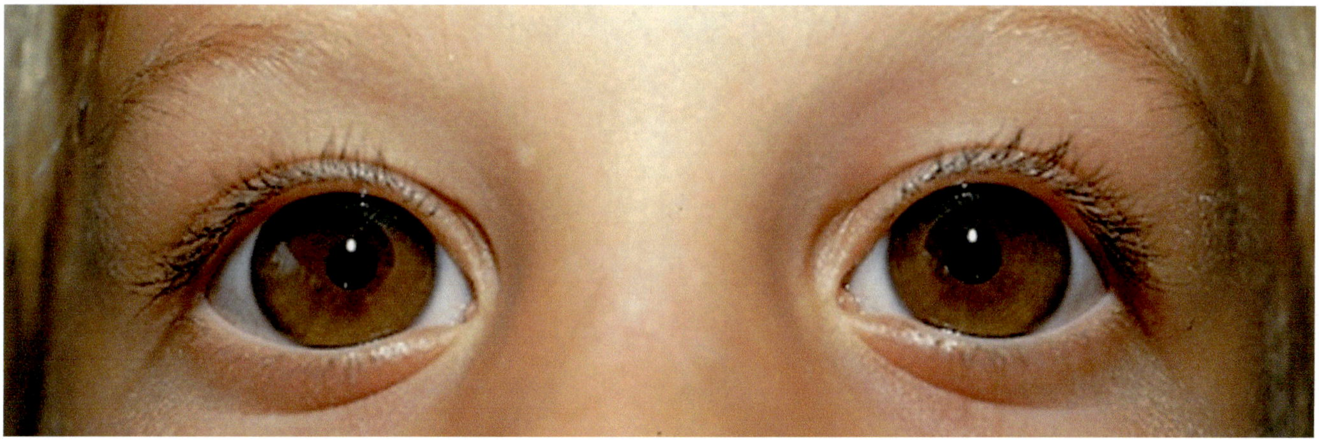

Fig. 15 Megalocornea, corneal diameter 14.5 mm, corneae clear, intraocular pressure normal

Axenfeld–Rieger Anomaly/ Syndrome (ARA/ARS)

Axenfeld anomaly is a bilateral posterior embryotoxon associated with iris strands adherent to the Schwalbe line. It occurs very rarely in isolation, but more often as part of the Axenfeld–Rieger spectrum.

Apparently, both the Axenfeld anomaly and the Rieger anomaly arise from the retention of remnants of the neural crest and the primordial endothelium at the iris and the chamber angle. Defects in the PITX2 and FOXC1 genes on chromosome 4q25 and in the FKHL7 gene on 6p25 as well as other defects have been found in various patients with Axenfeld anomaly and Rieger anomaly.

Axenfeld–Rieger anomaly (ARA) and Axenfeld–Rieger syndrome (ARS) refer to an autosomal dominant genetic condition characterized by anterior segment dysgenesis and often systemic abnormalities [2, 46]. Axenfeld anomaly is

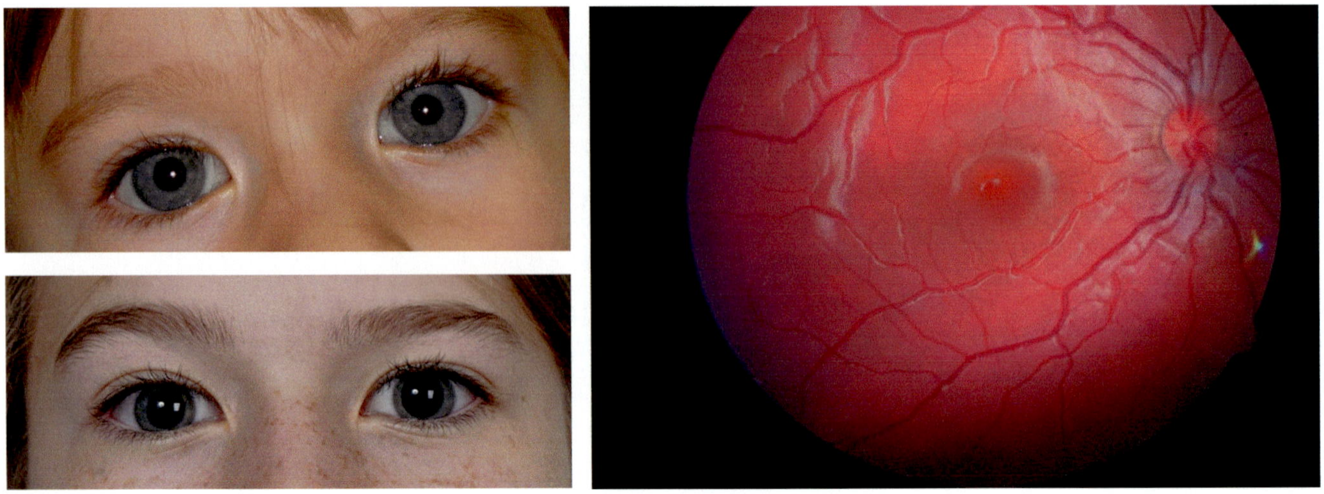

Fig. 16 Megalocornea and ocular hypertension with long follow-up. Girl, upper image: 6 years. Lower image: 16 years. Megalocornea, IOP repeatedly elevated (around 35+/5 mmHg), cornea without Haab striae, no other signs of glaucoma, refraction slightly hyperopic, axial length normal, optic nerve head OU inconspicuous. We are following the child since age 3 years, she now is 16 years, there are no changes in the findings. Visual fields normal, OCT of the optic nerve heads normal. We presume an alteration of corneal hysteresis

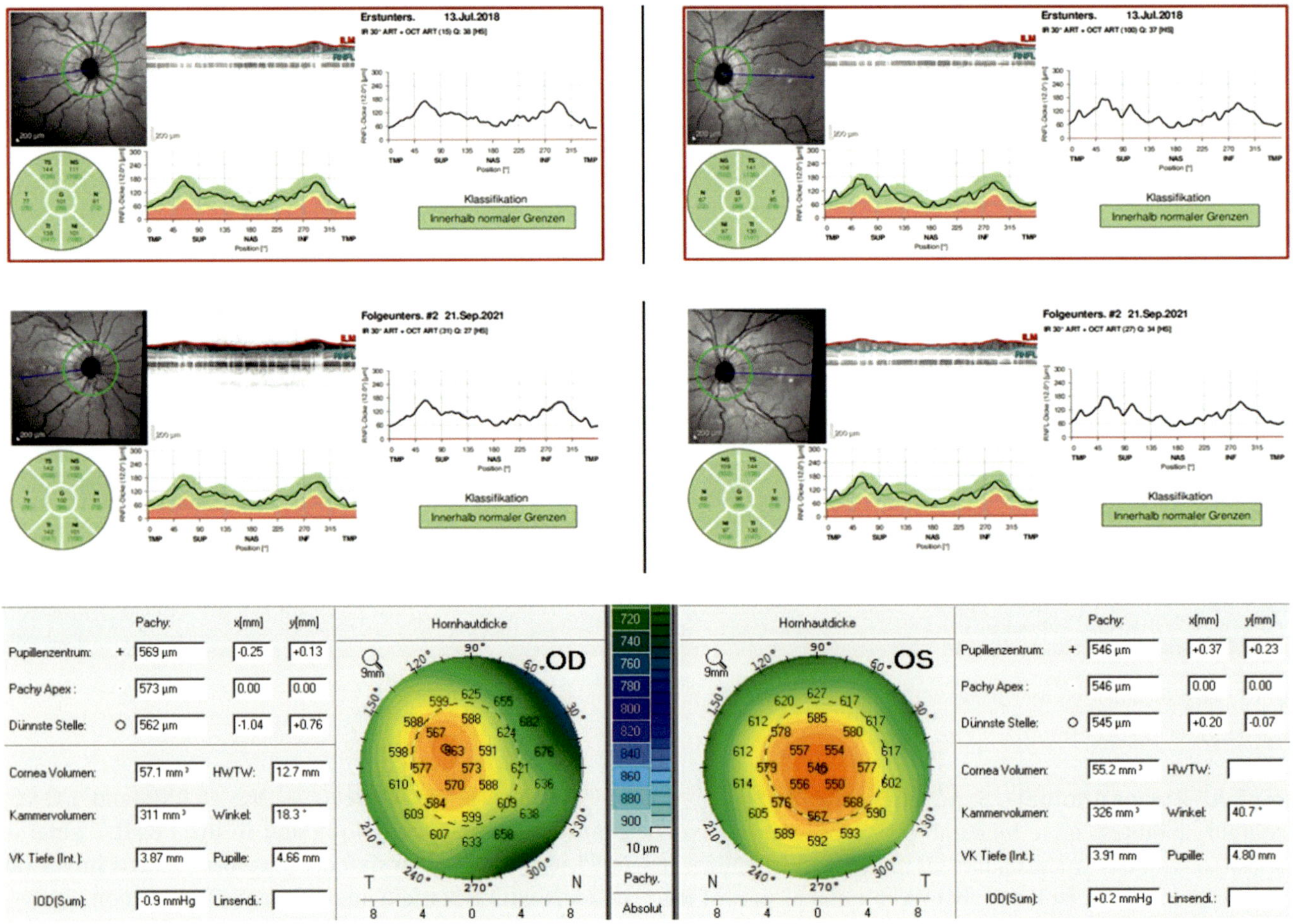

Fig. 17 Girl from Fig. 16, 16 years at the last time of examination. VA OU sc dec 1.0. IOP OD 35, OS 37. Visual fields completely normal. Optic nerve head shows no changes (see comparison between first and last exam above). Pentacam see below, normal findings without major subtraction or addition in IOP correction factor

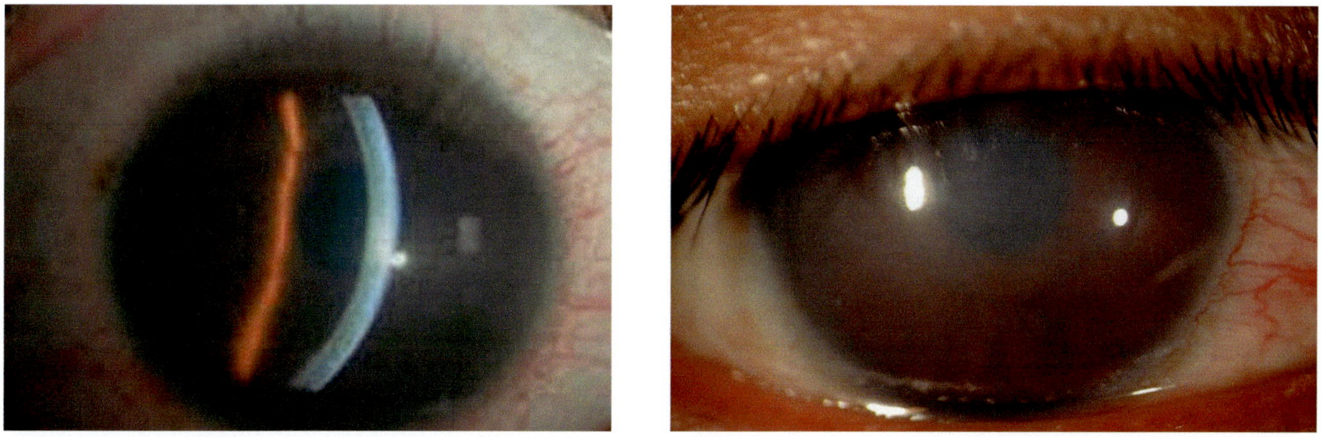

Fig. 18 Two patients with Congenital Hereditary Endothelial Dystrophy CHED, AR. CCO or NCO. Clinically diffuse, milky-glass-like corneal opacity, usually already at birth, frequently nystagmus. Poor visual acuity, high glare sensitivity, epiphora. Histology: Degeneration of endothelial cells, thickening of Descemet membrane

Table 4 Summary of the clinical entities of primary and secondary congenital corneal opacification CCO and neonatal corneal opacification NCO ([1]Microphthalmia-Anophthalmia-Coloboma, [2]Lecithin-Cholesterin-Acyltransferase)

Primary Congenital corneal abnormalities (developmental anomalies of the corneal tissue only)	Corneal dystrophies	– Posterior Polymorphic Corneal Dystrophy (PPCD) – Congenital hereditary endothelial Corneal dystrophy (CHED) – Congenital hereditary stromal dystrophy (CHSD) – X-linked hereditary endothelial dystrophy (XECD)
	Structural corneal defects in dermoids	– Isolated occurrence – Associated with syndromes (e.g. Goldenhar syndrome)
	Cornea plana	– Often associated with significant microcornea and microphthalmia
	Sclerocornea	– Partial – Total
Secondary Congenital corneal abnormalities	**KILD:** Kerato-irido-lenticular dysgenesis	– Only iridocorneal adhesions (Peters anomaly/syndrome type 1) – Lens not separated from cornea (Peters anomaly/syndrome type 2) – Lens does not form – Coloboma – Aniridia
	Irido-trabecular Dysgenesia	– Embryotoxon posterior – Infantile glaucoma – Axenfeld–Rieger anomaly/syndrome – **Aniridia**
	Primary congenital glaucoma PCG	– Common form of congenital glaucoma – May occur with non-PAX6-associated aniridia
	Microcornea, Microphthalmia (MAC[1] Spectrum)	– Isolated microphthalmia syndromes – Syndromic microphthalmia syndromes
Secondary aquired corneal diseases (often congenitally present)	Metabolic diseases/Lysosomal storage diseases	– Mucopolysaccharidoses – LCAT[2] deficiency – Tyrosinaemia – M. Fabry – Cystinosis
	Infectious keratitis	– Bacterial – Viral – Fungal – Acanthamoebae
	Traumatic	– Status after amniocentesis – Status after injury during forceps delivery

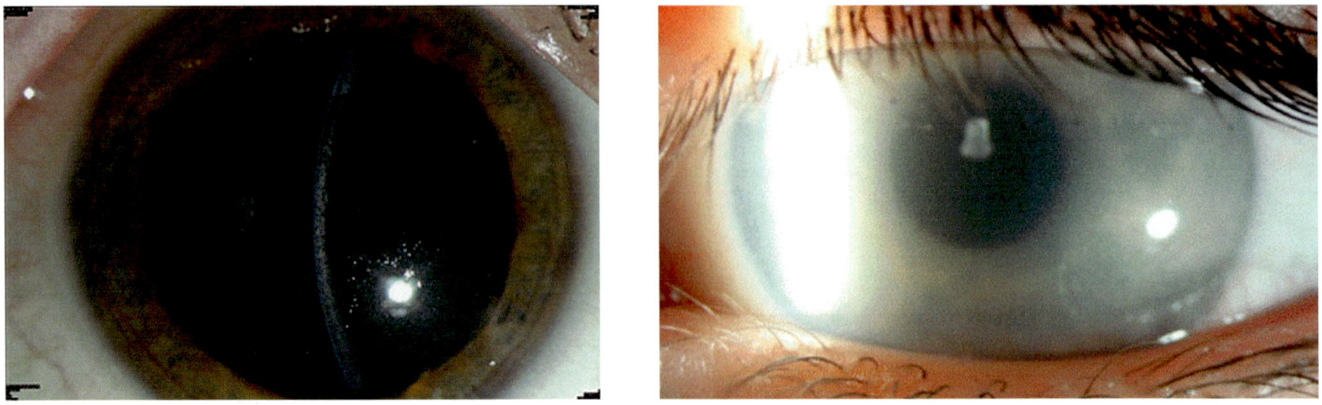

Fig. 19 Two patients with congenital stromal corneal dystrophy (CSCD)–autosomal dominant (AD). Left image: mild expression in boy aged 3 years. Corneal haze was present since birth. Right image: CCO is much more pronounced in this girl aged 2 years. Clinically, there is diffuse, pinnate opacities throughout the corneal stroma; bilateral. Histologically, there is separation of stromal lamellae and amorphous material. Visual acuity usually is severely reduced

characterized by Embryotoxon posterior (see above, Figs. 37–39), while Rieger described congenital iris abnormalities including iris hypoplasia, corectopia, and polycoria, now referred to as Rieger anomaly (Fig. 40–43). In Rieger anomaly, the anterior chamber angle is involved, as well as the cornea and iris, and glaucoma is more likely.

Axenfeld anomaly, however, can lead to congenital glaucoma as well (Fig. 39). Figures 40–43 show different manifestations of Rieger Anomaly, whereas Figs. 44–47 depict different manifestations of Axenfeld–Rieger Anomaly or Axenfeld–Rieger Syndrome.

As a rule, Axenfeld–Rieger spectrum is bilateral, but asymmetrical. Transmission in the Axenfeld–Rieger group is usually dominant (75%), but can also occur sporadically. There is evidence that a spectrum of mutations of transcription factors in chromosomal region 6p25, known as forkhead genes, are responsible for many developmental disorders of the anterior segment of the eye [2, 47]. The genes on the chromosomes 4q25 and 6p25 have been identified. The gene on chromosome 4q25 (PITX2) codes for a bicoid homeobox transcription factor. Like PAX6, this gene is expressed during eye development and is probably involved in the developmental processes of the eye [2]. The gene FOXC1 (also called FKHL7) on chromosome 6p25 belongs to a forkhead family of regulatory proteins. FOXC1 is expressed during eye development and mutations alter the dosage of the gene product. There is evidence that the FOXC1 protein and the PITX2 protein interact during eye development.

Axenfeld–Rieger syndrome is associated with systemic findings, such as dental (hypodontia, microdontia, oligodontia), facial bone defects including mid-face abnormalities (hypertelorism, maxillary hypoplasia), umbilical abnormalities (excessive peri-umbilical skin), or pituitary (empty sella syndrome, isolated growth hormone deficiency, parasellar arachnoid cyst) involvement. In addition, there may be abnormalities of the cardiovascular system (atrial septal defect) and genitalia (hypospadia, anal stenosis). The combination of Axenfeld anomaly and Rieger syndrome is known collectively as Axenfeld–Rieger syndrome (Fig. 47) [48]. Secondary glaucoma: up to 75% has been reported in those with Axenfeld–Rieger anomaly and syndrome due to FOXC1 and PITX2 mutations. Hence, regular glaucoma monitoring is mandatory.

Kerato-irido-lenticular dysplasia (KILD) [19, 26, 49]: Peters Anomaly/Peters Plus Syndrome (PA/PPS—formerly known as Krause–Kivlin Syndrome)

Peters anomaly (PA) is another disease of mesenchymal dysgenesis without systemic manifestations. Most cases occur sporadically, but there is also recessive and occasionally dominant inheritance. In 80% of cases, the disease is bilateral. The manifestations vary, with the classic type I consisting of a (para-)central stromal, eccentric or complete corneal opacity and iris strands that originate from the collarette (compare Fig. 2). It is mostly avascular, up to 75% bilateral and often asymmetrical.

Type II Peters is also referred to as KILD (kerato-iridolenticular adhesions) and is often vascularized, with the lens attached to the cornea. The AS-OCT shows no evidence of anterior lens capsule.

Initially, a central endothelial and Descemet membrane defect leads to marked corneal oedema; over time, however, the endothelium can regenerate centrally and the oedema can subside.

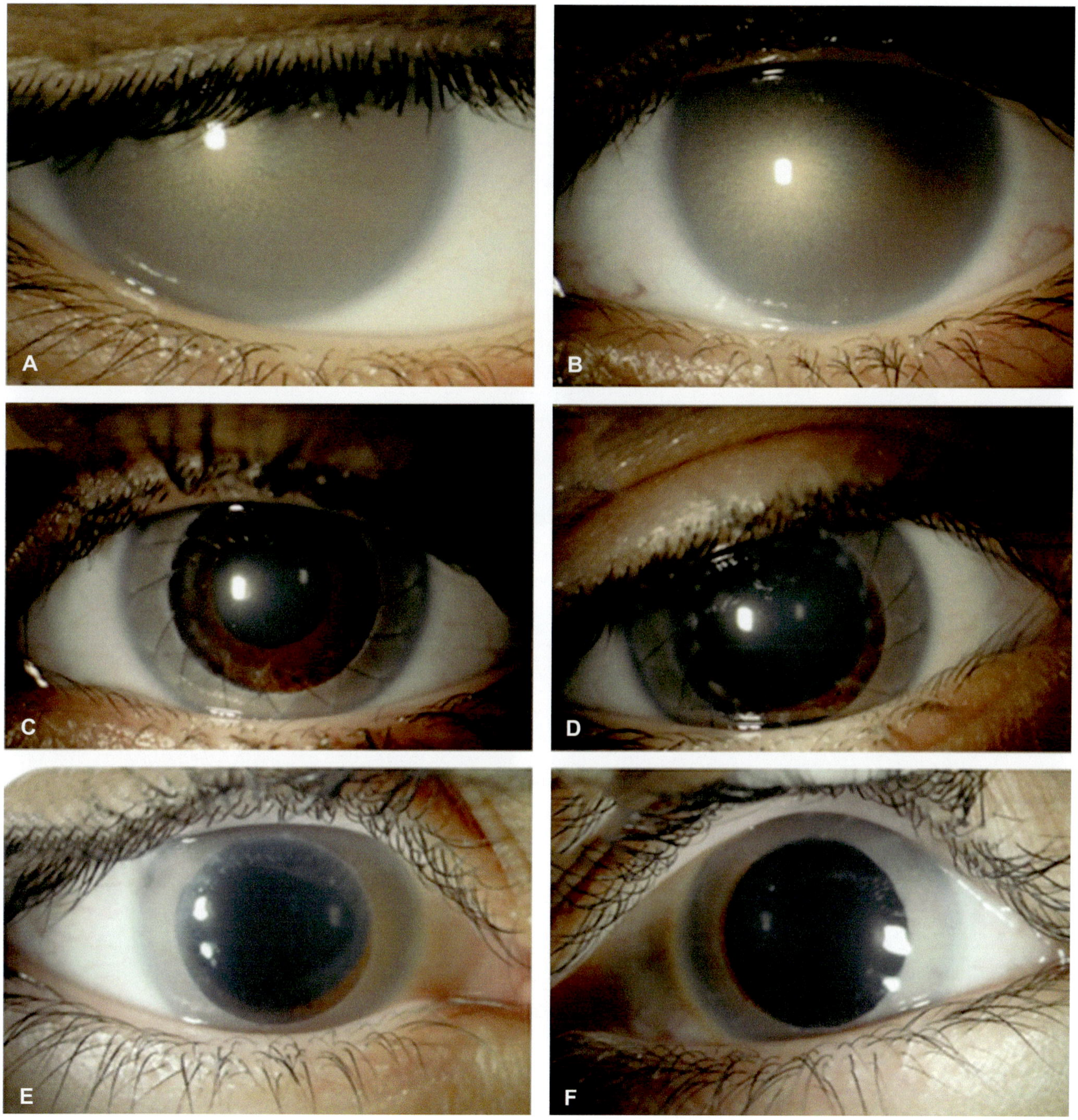

Fig. 20 Clinical findings preoperatively and after excimer laser-assisted penetrating keratoplasty for CSCD congenital stromal corneal dystrophy. (**A, B**) Age around 2 years: Diffuse greyish flake-like opacities extending to the limbus in both eyes ((**A**): right eye, (**B**): left eye). The pupil is barely visible. There are no Descemet folds, cataract, anterior synechiae or other iris abnormalities (not visible by diffuse illumination). (**C, D**) Age 2.5 and 3 years: Postoperative findings of clear grafts fixated with a double running suture according to Hoffmann of the right (**C**) and left (**D**) eye after one year. (**E, F**) Postoperative findings with clear grafts of the right (**E**) and left (**F**) eye after fourteen years. Visual acuity dec. OD 0.8, OS 0.8 [35]

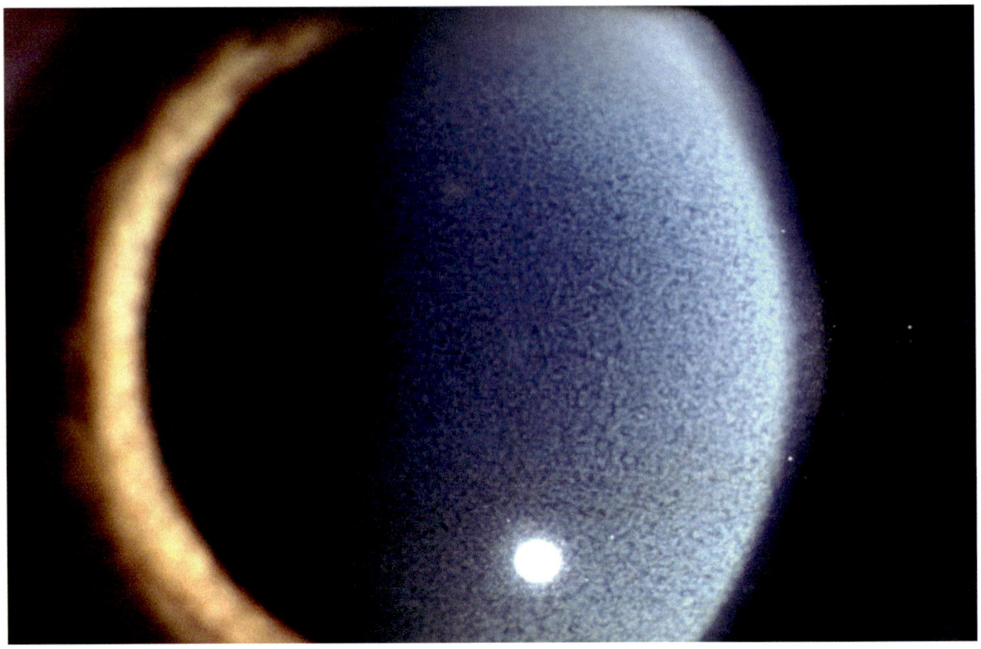

Fig. 21 PPMD: Posterior Polymorphous Corneal Dystrophy in a 3-year-old boy, autosomal dominant (AD), leading to NCO. Nodular, vesicular and ribbon-like opacities, solitary or in groups, in the posterior corneal area, rarely endothelial decompensation, often good VA

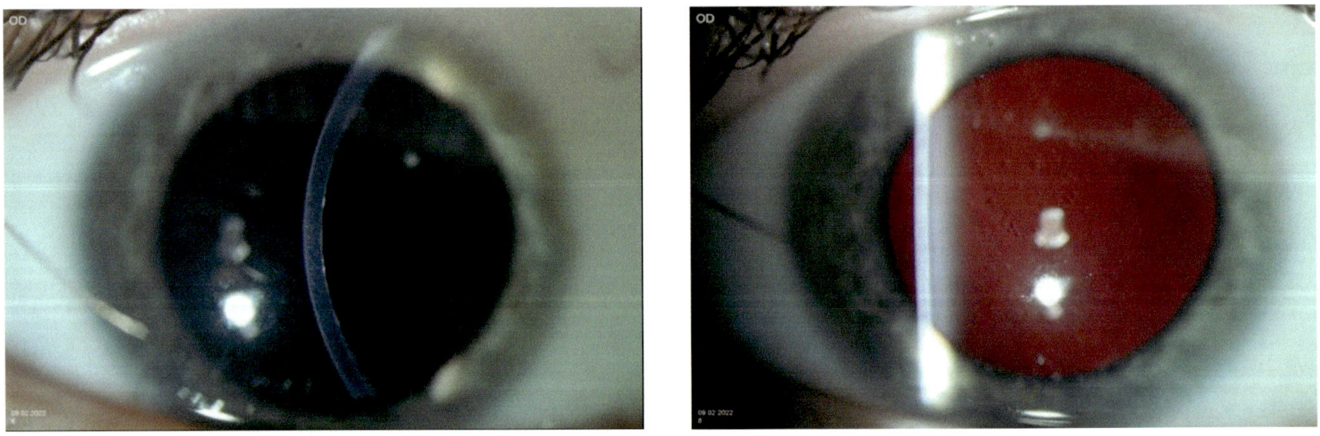

Fig. 22 PPMD: Posterior Polymorphous Corneal Dystrophy in a 14-year-old boy. VA dec OU 0.7. Histologically, there is an "epithelialization" of endothelial cells. In the rare case of irido-corneal adhesions control of IOP is necessary. Usually there is no indication for keratoplasty

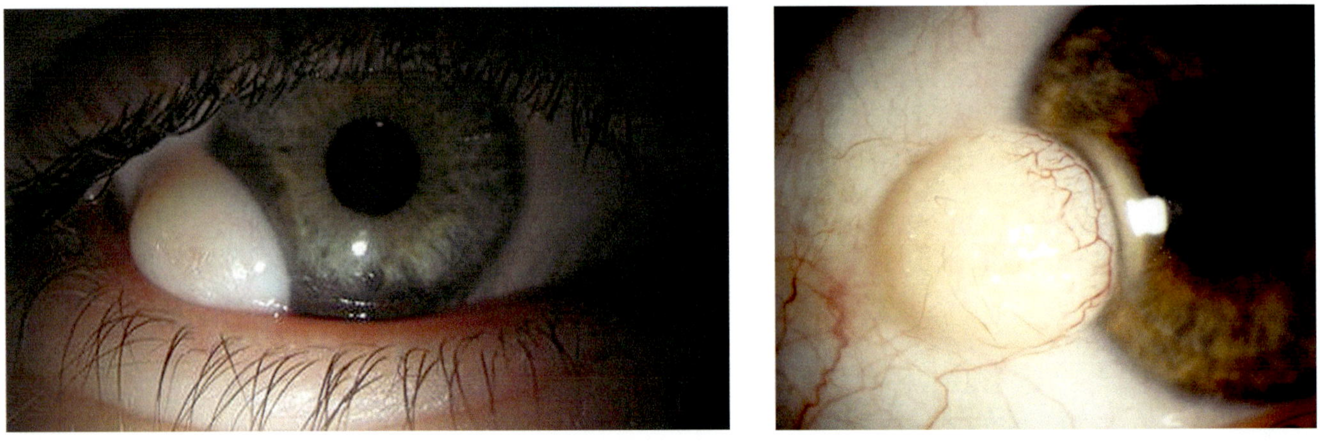

Fig. 23 Typical solid dermoids (choristomas) of the limbal region. Left image: girl, 1 year. Surgery advised due to tear film insufficiency and partial lid lag. Right image: Boy 3 years. Surgery advised due to very high astigmatism, amblyopia and deficient tear film

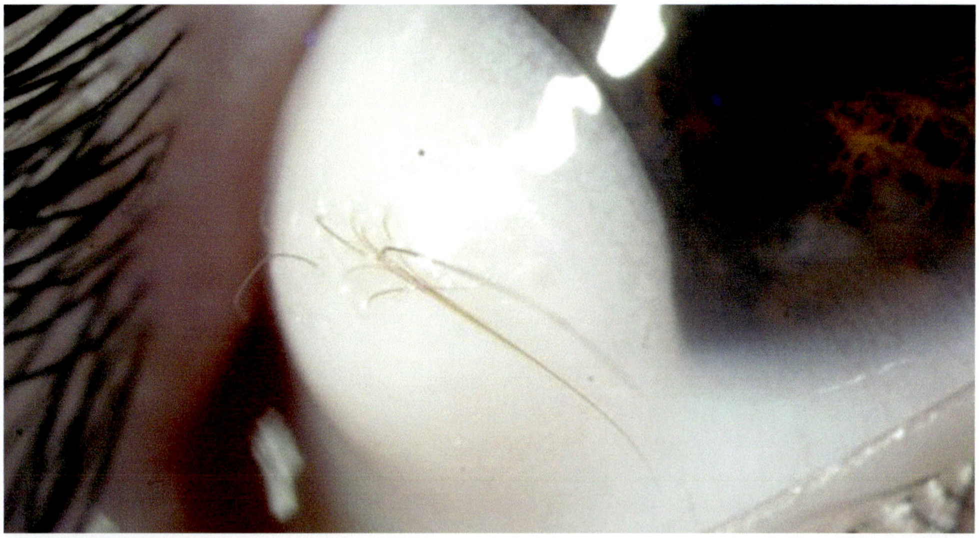

Fig. 24 Corneoscleral dermoids (choristomas) may be quite large and present with hairs, which disturb the tear film even more. In this girl, aged 1.5 years, there is lid closure insufficiency, high astigmatism and subjective discomfort, therefore a surgical excision was advised. Parents have to be informed that the involved cornea postoperatively will not be clear, but will have a grayish shade

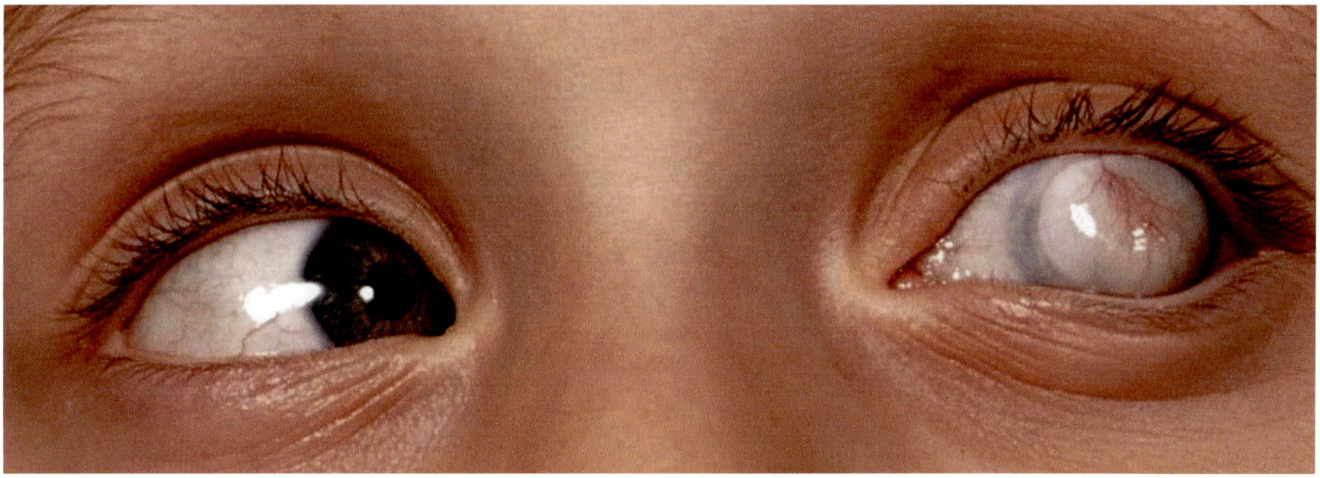

Fig. 25 OS complete corneal dermoid in a boy aged 2 years. To treat deep amblyopia a full thickness large PKP is advised, although the prognosis for improving amblyopia is small. Due to the prominent vascularization the prognosis for transparency of the transplanted cornea is reduced as well. It will, however, be a significant improvement of aesthetics

A type II variant has been characterised in which the lens adheres to the posterior cornea. Type I is usually unilateral, while type II is often bilateral [50]. Other associated ocular abnormalities often include secondary glaucoma (in more than 50% of cases), but also microcornea, cornea plana, sclerocornea, chorioretinal coloboma, iris coloboma, chamber angle and iris dysgenesis, persistent hyperplastic primary vitreous, microphthalmos, optic nerve hypoplasia and foveal hypoplasia.

The pathology of Peters anomaly shows an absence of the central Descemet membrane and endothelium, which can regenerate over time, this is sometimes used as surgical approach [51]. Other features include residual fibrosis in the opacified stroma and the central absence of Bowman layer (see Fig. 36). Changes in the TITX2, PITX3, PAX6 genes and FOXC1 gene are primarily involved in Peters anomaly, compare Table 5 (Figs. 48, 49).

Peters plus syndrome PPS (formerly known as Krause–Kivlin Syndrome

Systemic associations may include short stature, facial dysmorphia, developmental delay, syndactyly, genitourinary anomalies of the urogenital tract, brachycephaly, anomalies of the central nervous system, heart disease or deafness and delayed skeletal maturation (Fig. 50). They form the

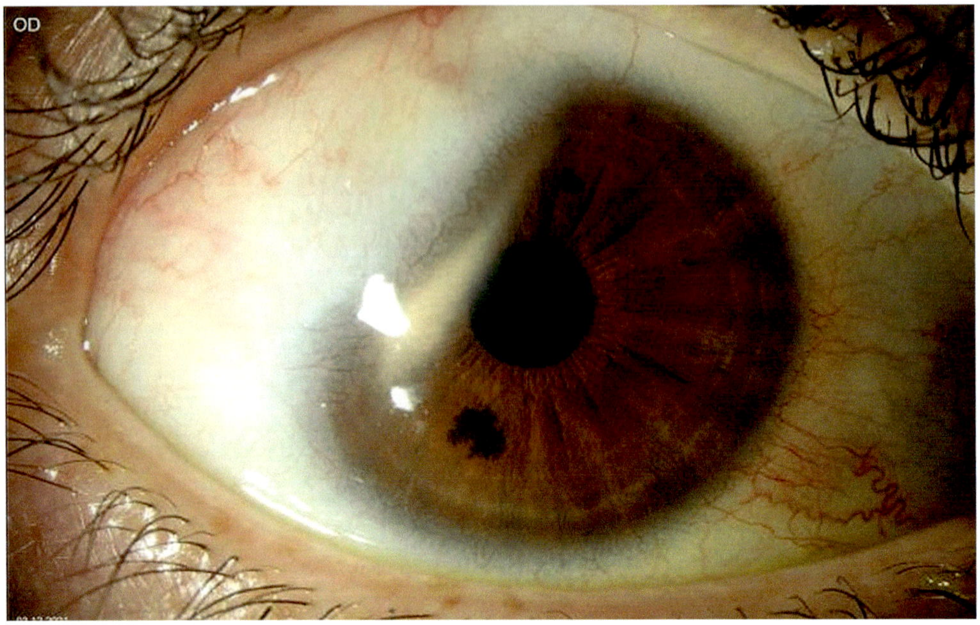

Fig. 26 Flat congenital choristoma: limbal dermoid, girl, 13 years, VA dec 0.6, no indication for surgical intervention. Compare the corneal parameters in Fig. 27

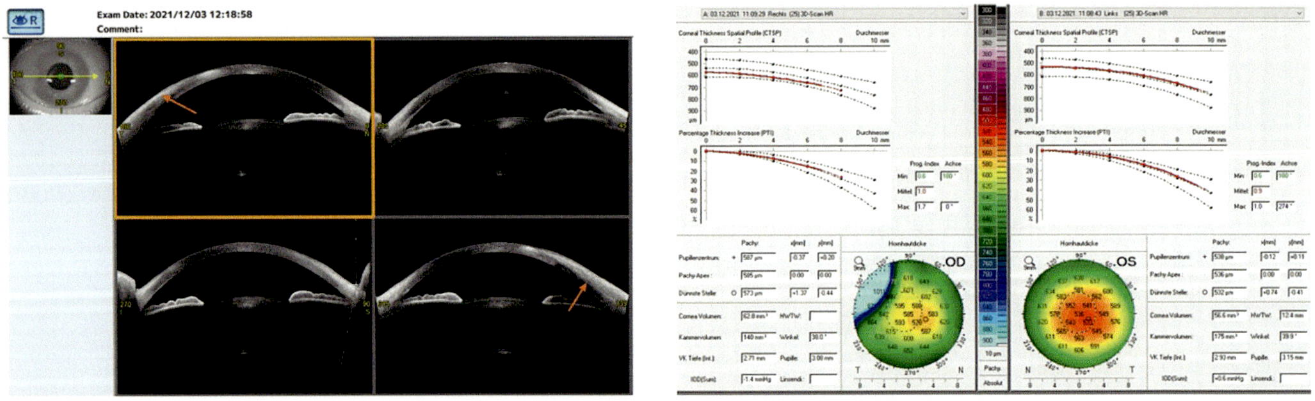

Fig. 27 Same Patient as Fig. 26. Left image: anterior segment OCT with clearly visible peripheral choristoma (arrows), right image: topography OU

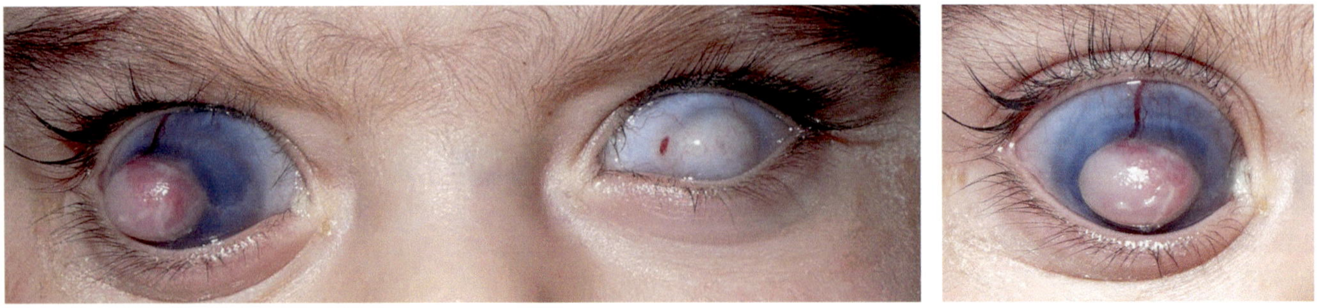

Fig. 28 Boy, 12 years. Bilateral (para-)central solid dermoid. Left image: OD: Congenital buphthalmia, (para-) central corneal dermoid with vascularization, incomplete lid closure, pain. OS: Microphthalmia, flat central dermoid. First presentation at our hospital at age 12 years

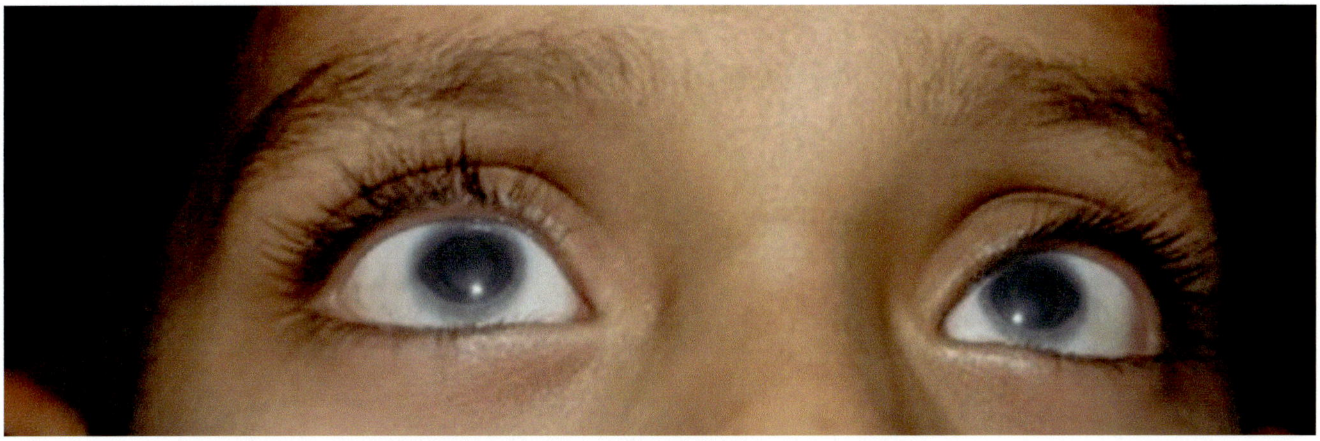

Fig. 29 Cornea plana with bluish haze, poorly demarcated corneoscleral limbus, and left sided esotropia

Fig. 30 Cornea plana sometimes is associated with sclerocornea. In this now 5 years boy, OS, a partial CCO was noticed temporally at birth, slit lamp examination showed cornea plana and limbal stem cell insufficiency temporally with corneal opacification. In addition, there was corectopia. This is type 2 Cornea plana, associated with mutations in the KERA gene, autosomal dominant (AD). Cornea plana is associated with high hyperopia and sometimes rise in IOP

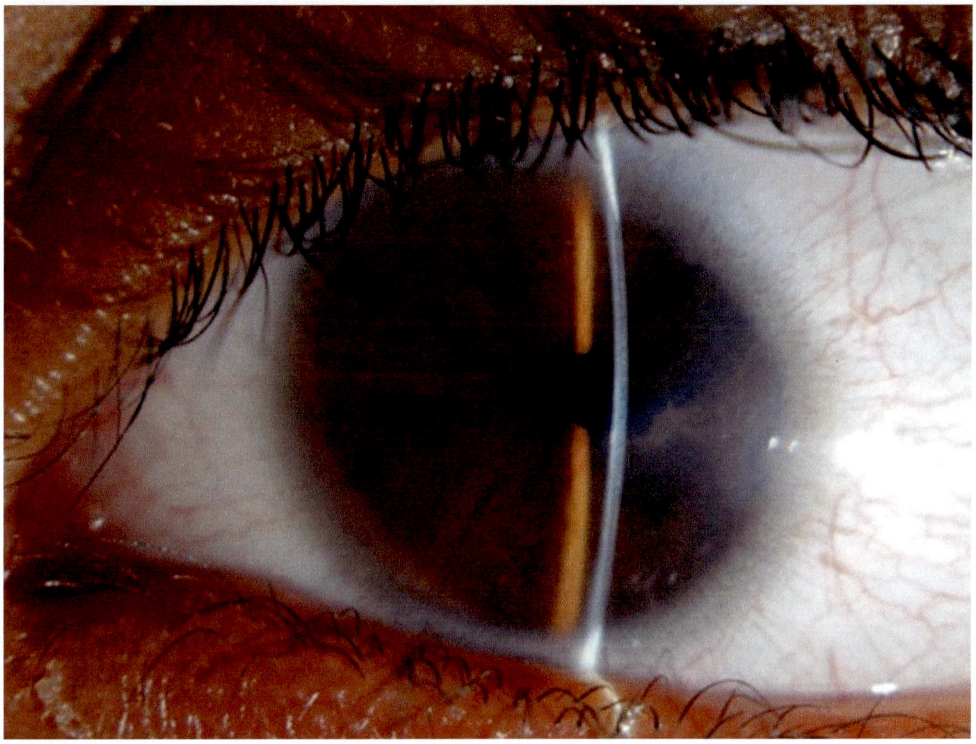

autosomal recessive Krause–Kivlin syndrome or Peters Plus syndrome (Fig. 51) [26]. Mutations in the FOXC1 gene, the PAX6 gene and the CYP1B1 gene could be the cause of PPS (see Figs. 7 and 8 for facial anomalies and Table 5).

Regarding the Treatment of Peters anomaly and Peters plus syndrome, primary therapy includes treatment of the glaucoma, which is frequently present and often difficult to treat. A penetrating keratoplasty is appropriate if the corneal opacity is bilateral. This has a poor prognosis [52]. In eyes with localised central opacity and clear mid-periphery, optical sector iridectomy can provide a simplified approach and visually effective outcome [19, 26, 53, 54].

Primary Congenital Glaucoma (CYP1B1 cytopathy) CYP1B1 cytopathy is one of the most important reasons for primary congenital glaucoma (PCG), occurring in approx. 40% of all genetically examined PCG [55, 56].

CYP1B1 cytopathy refers to a group of rare genetic disorders associated with mutations in the CYP1B1 gene (Locus GLC3A located on chromosome 2p22–p21). The GLC3A loci contains the cyctochrome P4501B1 (CYP1B1) gene, which was the first reported PCG-causing gene [57]. It codes for an enzyme that metabolizes compounds vital for the developing eye, such as fatty acids and vitamins, and is expressed in

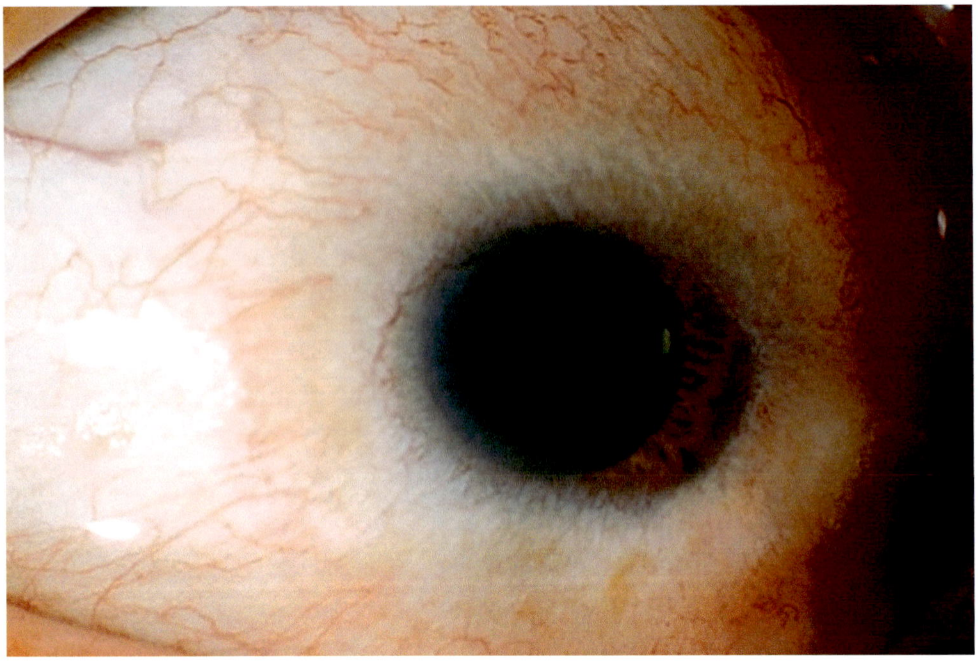

Fig. 31 Girl, 7 years. Unilateral extreme microcornea with Cornea plana OS. Limbal stem cell abnormality with partial clouding of the cornea nasally > temporally. Partial aniridia with corneal diameter 8 mm

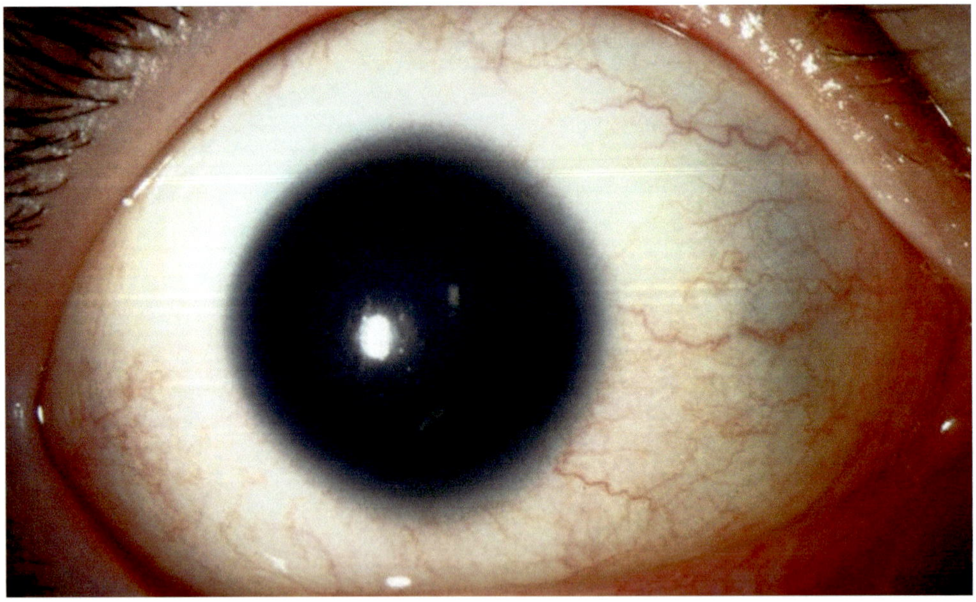

Fig. 32 Microcornea and Cornea plana can be part of anterior segment dysgenesis as well, here: complete aniridia

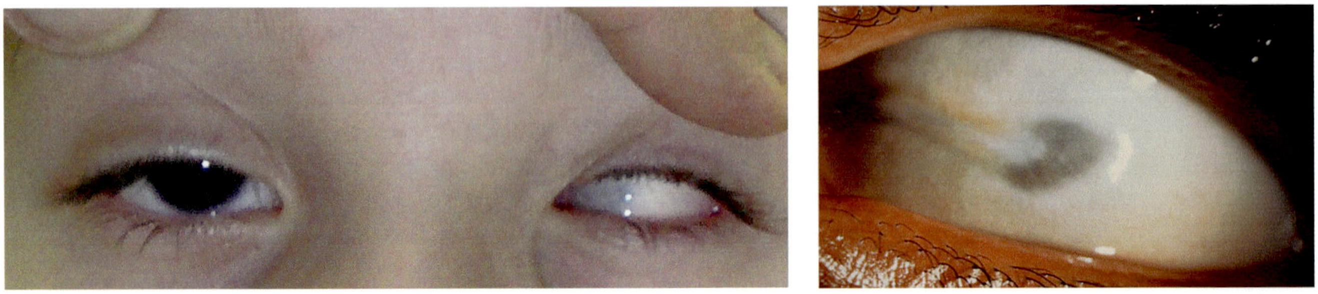

Fig. 33 Left image: Girl, 3 years. OD microphthalmia, OS more severe microphthalmia with sclerocornea. Right image: boy, OS, aged 12 years. Severe unilateral form of microphthalmia and sclerocornea

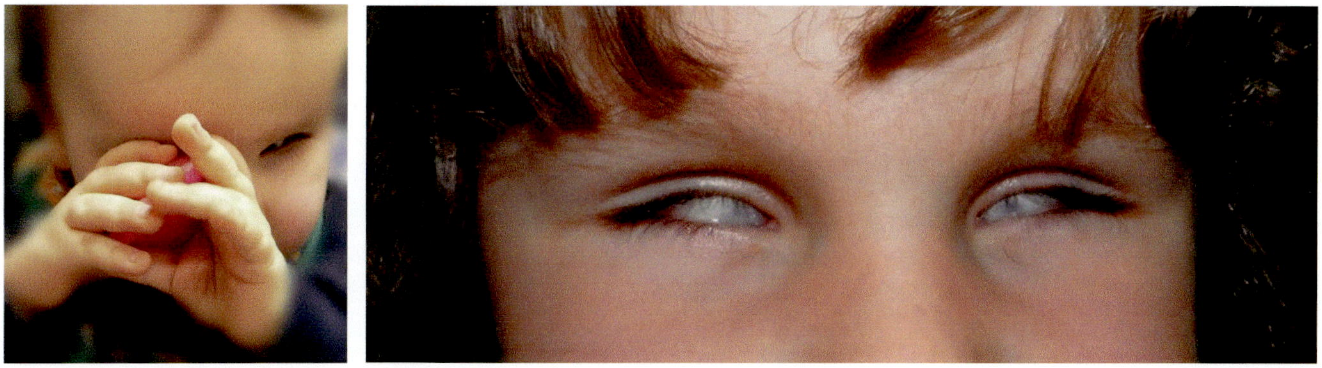

Fig. 34 Left image, Boy aged 7 months with severe microphthalmia and sclerocorneea, fixating a luminous ball. Right image: same boy as in left image, now aged 6 years. He is able to navigate within a foreign room (examination room), names colours and can pick up a spoon from the table. Genetic analysis did not reveal any anomalies

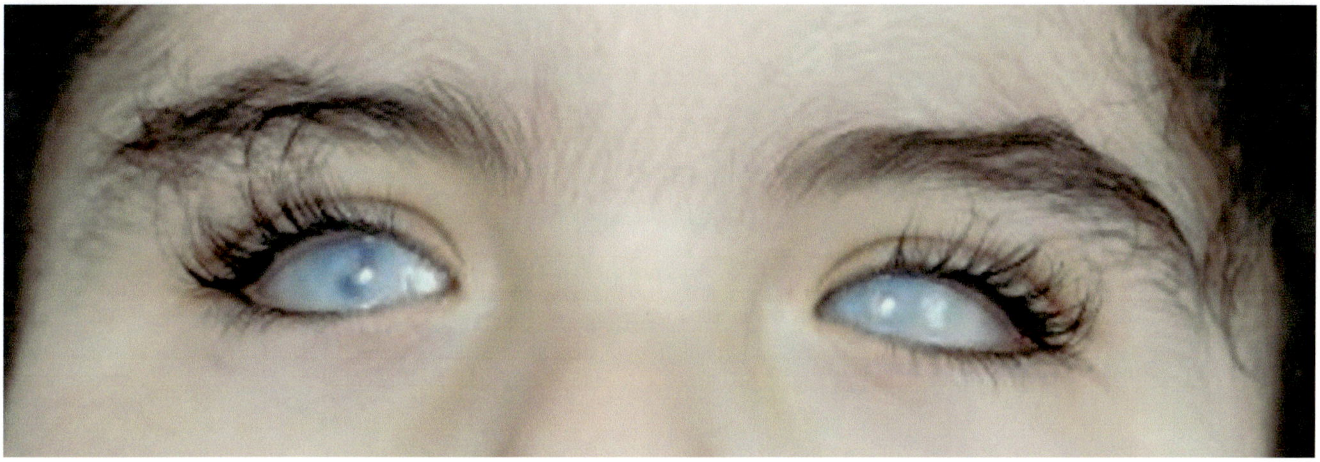

Fig. 35 OS>OD microphthalmia and sclerocornea. This boy has other facial abnormalities, compare Fig. 10: Ears are especially important in Next Generation Phenotyping NGP. The child first was diagnosed with Peters syndrome. Further molecular genetic analysis revealed Oculoauricular Syndrome (OCACS: Schorderet-Munier-Franceschetti Syndrome) due to mutation in the HMX1 gene

fetal and adult neuroepithelium and ciliary body. In zebrafish, CYP1B1 has been found to indirectly affect neural crest migration to the anterior segment and angle by playing a role in ocular fissure closure. Mutations in CYP1B1 can lead to abnormal development of the eye, causing various additional eye disorders apart from PCG (see Table 6 and Figs. 52 and 54).

The formerly described Barkan membrane could not be verified up to now. Researchers have been correlating neural crest cell (NCC) migration and differentiation with angle development and the role of CYP1B1 in ocular fissure closure, which ultimately affects NCC migration [55].

It is important to note that the features can vary among individuals with CYP1B1 cytopathy, and the severity of symptoms may differ. Table 6 gives an outlining of some relevant features of CYP1B1 cytopathy primary congenital glaucoma.

2.3.3 PAX6-Related Congenital Aniridia (Severest Form of Anterior Segment Dysgenesis), also known as PAX6 Syndrome

As mentioned in the introduction, several coordinated steps of temporally and spatially organized networked triggers (inductions) are necessary to control the development of the ocular phenotype. This is regulated at the level of transcription [2, 58–60].

The so-called master genes or DNA-binding transcription factors are crucial here PAX6, FOXC1, SOX2, FOXE3, OTX2, PITX2 and PAX2 [2, 47, 59, 61].

Aniridia is an uncommon (ca. 7000 persons in Europe) congenital bilateral disease mostly caused by mutation of the PAX6 gene. It is a pan-ocular and pro-fibrotic disorder that involves the cornea, anterior chamber, lens, retina and optic nerve [2, 14, 15, 62, 63]. Although aniridic

Table 5 Frequent genes associated with different types of anterior segment dysgenesis. Adapted from [2, 44] and from https://gene.vision/knowledge-base/anterior-segment-dysgenesis-for-doctors/ (accessed 2023-11-08); [1]autosomal recessive, [2]anterior segment dysgenesis, [3]Microphthalmia-Anophthalmia-Colomba [4]autosomal dominant

Gene (OMIM no.)	Ocular phenotypes	Inheritance
B3GALTL (#610,308)	– Peters plus syndrome	AR[1]
BMP4 (#112,262)	– ASD[2] – Microphthalmia, anophthalmia, coloboma (MAC[3]) spectrum – SHORT syndrome	AD[4]
COL4A1 (#120,130)	– Axenfeld–Rieger anomaly – Peters anomaly – MAC[3] spectrum – Congenital cataract	AD[4]
CYP1B1 (#601,771)	– Primary congenital glaucoma – Peters anomaly – Aniridia	AR[1]
FOXC1 (#601,090)	– Axenfeld–Rieger syndrome – Peters anomaly – Aniridia – Primary congenital glaucoma	AD[4]
FOXC2 (#602,402)	– Lymphoedema-distichiasis syndrome – ASD[2]	AD[4]
FOXE3 (#601,094)	– Peters anomaly – MAC[3] spectrum – ASD[2]	AD[4] or AR[1]
JAG1 (#601,920)	– Alagille syndrome – Axenfeld–Rieger Syndrome	AD[4]
LAMB2 (#150,325)	– Pierson syndrome – ASD[2]	AR[1]
NOTCH2 (#600,275)	– Alagille syndrome	AD[4]
PAX6 (#607,108)	– Aniridia – Peters anomaly – Keratitis – Isolated foveal hypoplasia – Congenital cataract – Optic nerve hypoplasia – Reduced pigmentation of the retina	AD[4]
PITX2 (#601,542)	– Axenfeld–Rieger syndrome – Peters anomaly – Iris hypoplasia	AD[4]
PITX3 (#602,669)	– ASD[2]	AD[4]

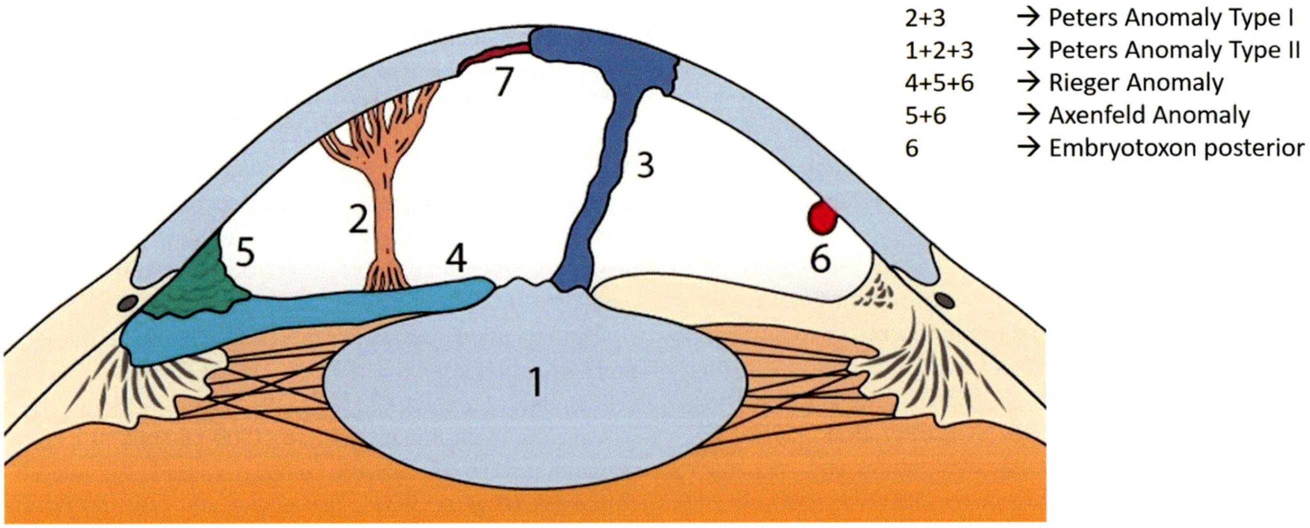

Fig. 36 Schematic description of anterior segment anomalies leading to CCO, NCO and/or glaucoma. Peters Anomaly Type I and Type II are now named KILD Syndrome: Kerato-irido-lenticular dysplasia. Adapted from: Krieglstein G, Jonescu-Cuypers C, Severin M: Atlas der Augenheilkunde. Springer Verlag Heidelberg, Berlin 1999 [45]

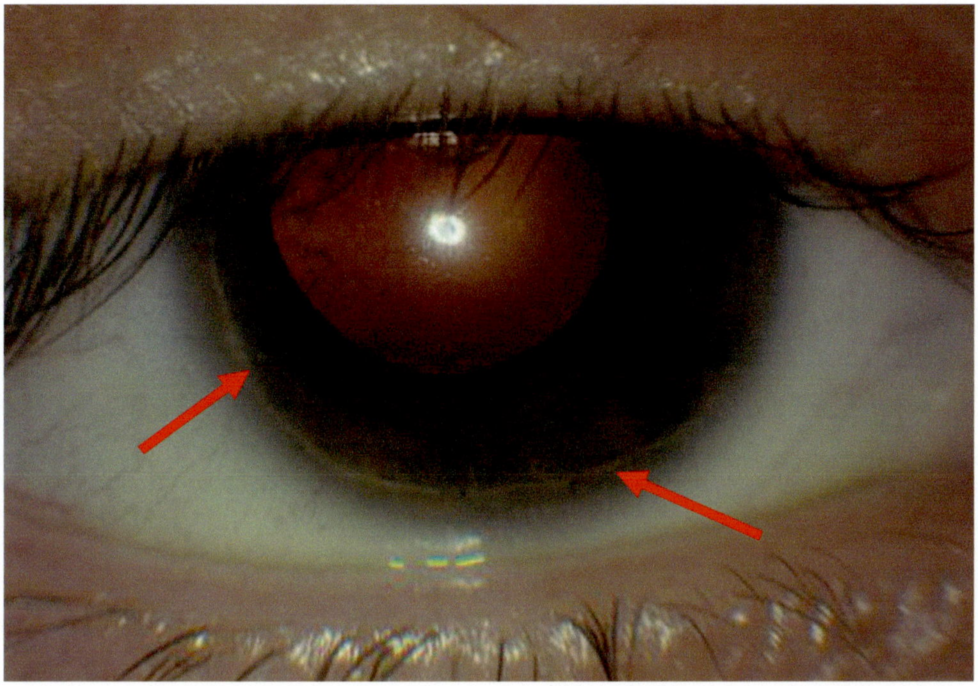

Fig. 37 Embryotoxon posterior (see arrows). Note the slightly corectopic mydriatic pupil suggestive of mild ASD

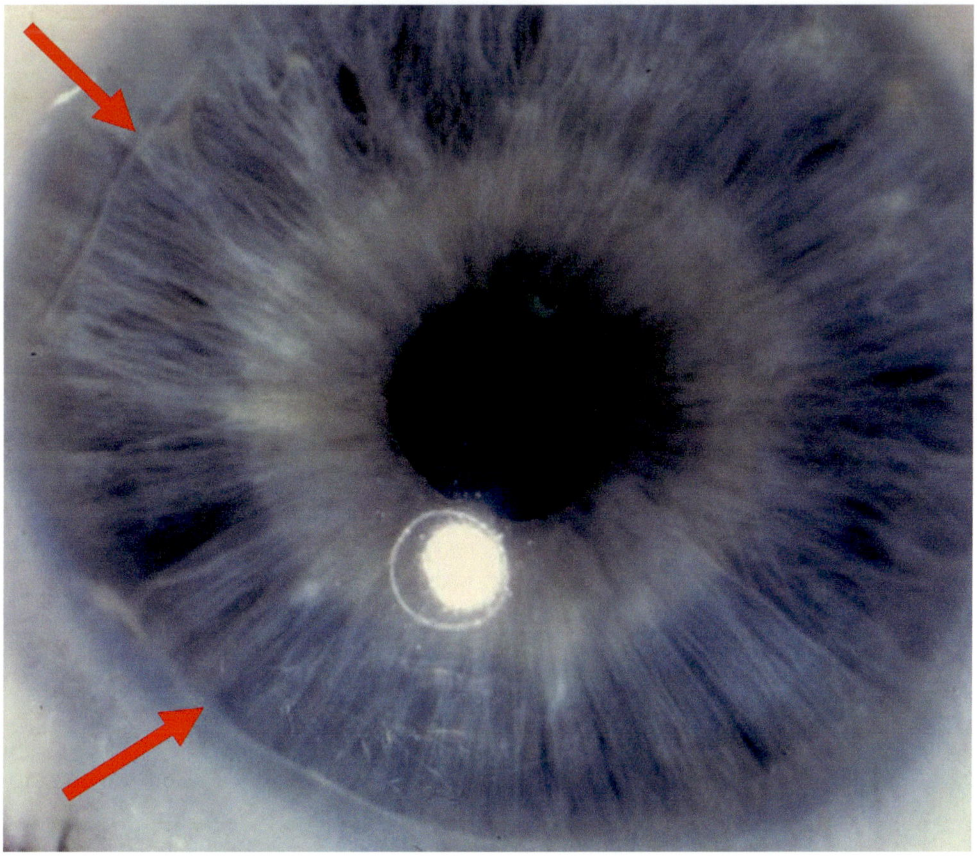

Fig. 38 Male patient with posterior embryotoxon, 12 years old, prominent Schwalbe line (arrows), full visual acuity

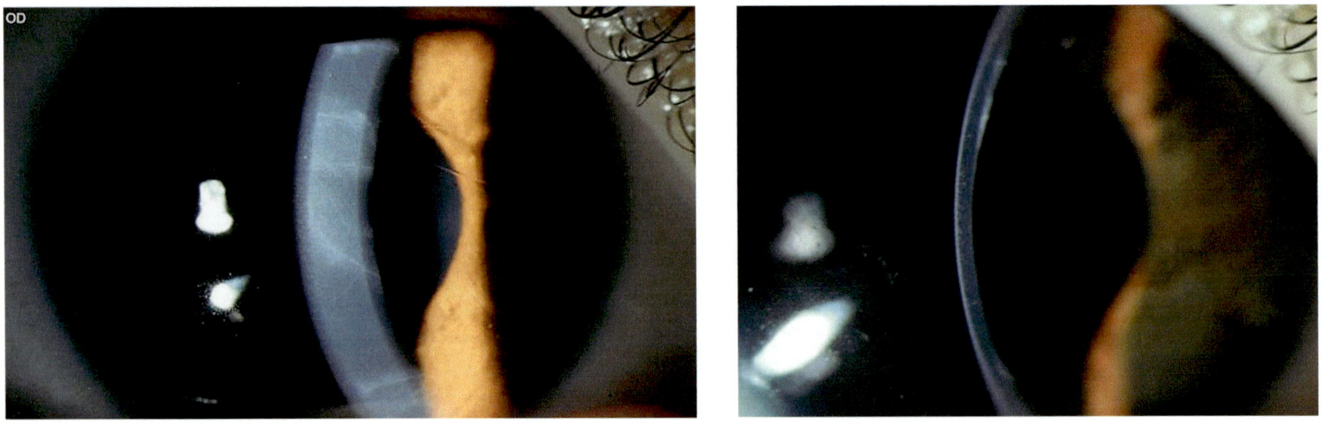

Fig. 39 3-year-old boy, OD. Since birth haze of the right cornea (CCO). Diagnosis: Axenfeld Anomaly with Haab lines. Elevated IOP. Very thin cornea due to buphthalmia. IOP could be controlled with topical antiglaucomatous drops. Deep amblyopia (dec: VA 0.02). A phakic DMEK was advised

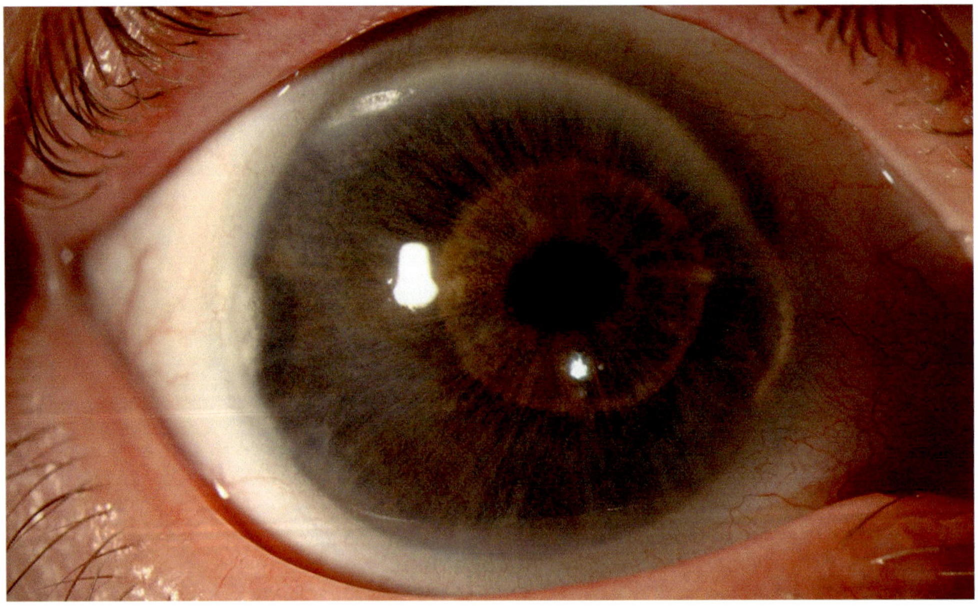

Fig. 40 Rieger Anomaly: embryotoxon posterior superior and inferior. Atypical arcus lipoides superiorly. Disrounded and corectopic pupil. Atrophic iris

keratopathy has traditionally been attributed to limbal stem cell deficiency, current evidence based on clinical observations and animal models of aniridia suggests that the proliferative potential of limbal stem cells may not initially be affected and this corneal alteration may be related to an abnormality in the limbal stem cell microenvironment, a so-called "stem cell niche" [60, 64–68]. Corneal changes in aniridic keratopathy include recurrent erosions of the corneal epithelium and ulcerations, tear film instability, dry eye, chronic pain, corneal neovascularisation, progressive corneal opacification and blindness [69–74].

PAX6 gene-associated congenital aniridia (chromosome 11) occurs in several forms: Dominant inheritance, sporadically occurring (then usually further dominant transmission), as part of WAGR or WAGRO syndrome and associated with other syndromes [75]. Furthermore, it is becoming increasingly clear that PAX6 gene-associated aniridia is associated with other systemic abnormalities (see below), which is why the term "aniridia syndrome" or "PAX6 syndrome" is increasingly being used [62, 76, 77]. For this reason, early genetic diagnosis is so essential—to rule out chromosome 11 deletion causing WAGR syndrome (with possible nephroblastoma) and to know whether PAX6 haploinsufficiency can be detected to monitor children and adults regularly for systemic associations.

PAX6 syndrome reflects the diverse embryonic influences of the master gene PAX6 on the development of various body symptoms [62, 74]. These include metabolic findings (obesity,

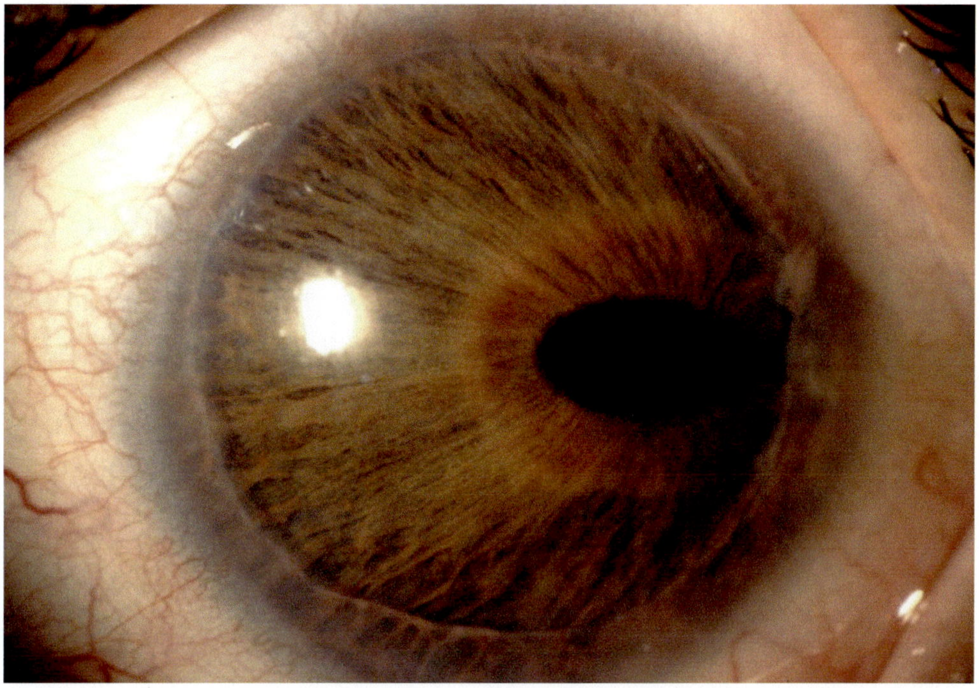

Fig. 41 Rieger Anomaly, prominent Schwalbe line and corectopia, pseudocoloboma, adherences between iris tissue and posterior cornea

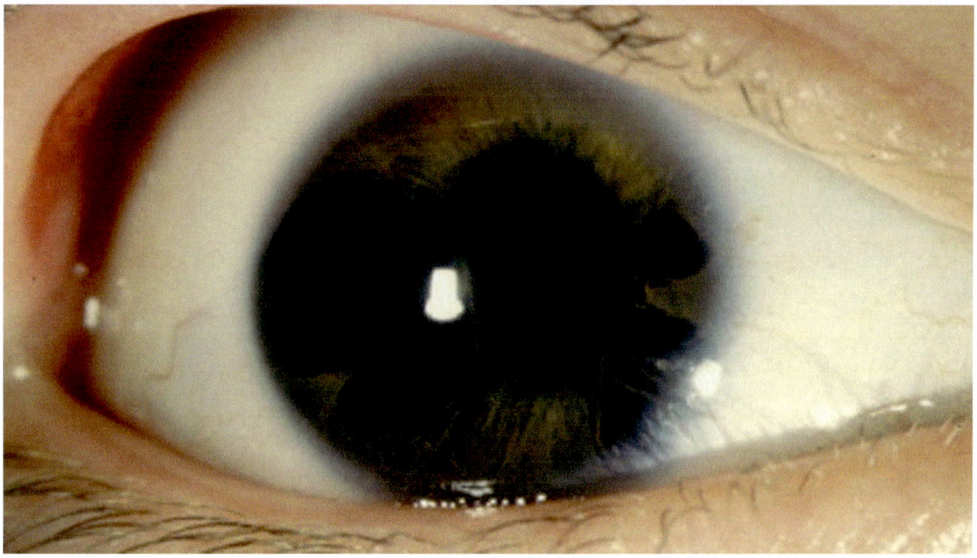

Fig. 42 Rieger Anomaly. Pseudopolycoria, disrupted iris tissue, embryotoxon posterior superiorly and temporally. High risk of developing glaucoma

impaired glucose tolerance), endocrinological findings (hypothyroidism, pituitary dysfunction, impaired melatonin secretion due to epiphyseal causes with day–night rhythm disorders) and neurological findings such as gyration disorders, corpus callosum hypoplasia, malformations of the bulbus olfactorius with hyposmia and auditory perception disorders as well as learning disabilities [12, 63, 77, 78].

Concerning corneal opacification, there may be CCO or NCO in aniridia as well. NCO, being identified as corneal clouding in infancy, is more rare than CCO and mostly due to dysregulated IOP in early infancy. It has to be differentiated from the typical PAX6 aniridia complication aniridia-associated keratopathy (AAK) which may start in early childhood, progresses slower and is not necessarily associated with elevated IOP [69, 79]. Lee et al. [72] described the prevalence of CCO in a cohort of 138 patients to be 13%, in our patients it is more rare in spite of several babies having PCG with NCO [74, 80, 81]. Figure 55 shows a girl with PAX6 haploinsufficiency and CCO, for NCO see Fig. 56.

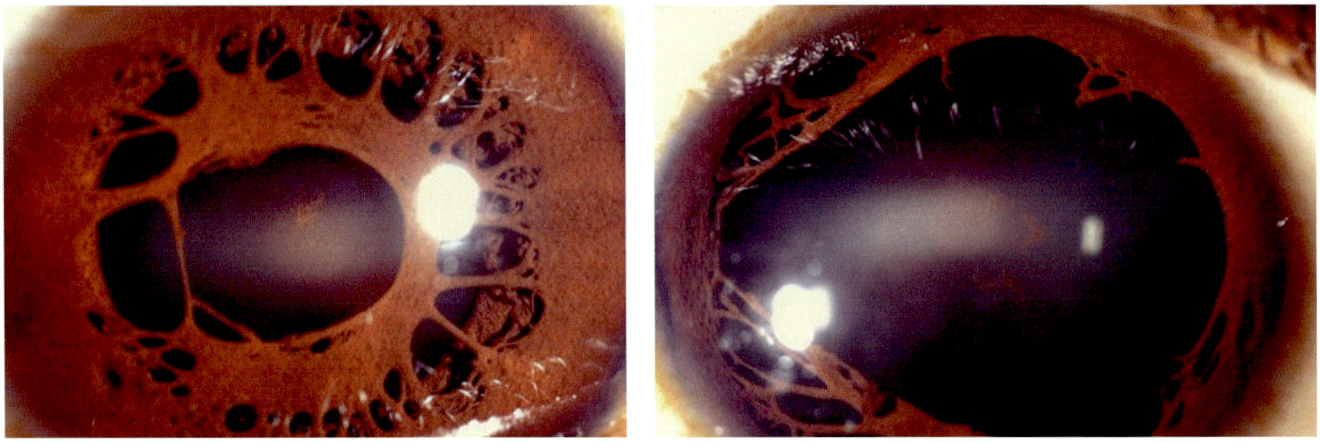

Fig. 43 Two examples of different phenotype in Rieger anomaly. Left image: boy, aged 10 years. Right image: girl, aged 8 years. Both show pseudopolycoria, both patients show pigment deposits on the anterior lens capsule. Both patients do not have glaucoma, have near to full visual acuity but are glare sensitive

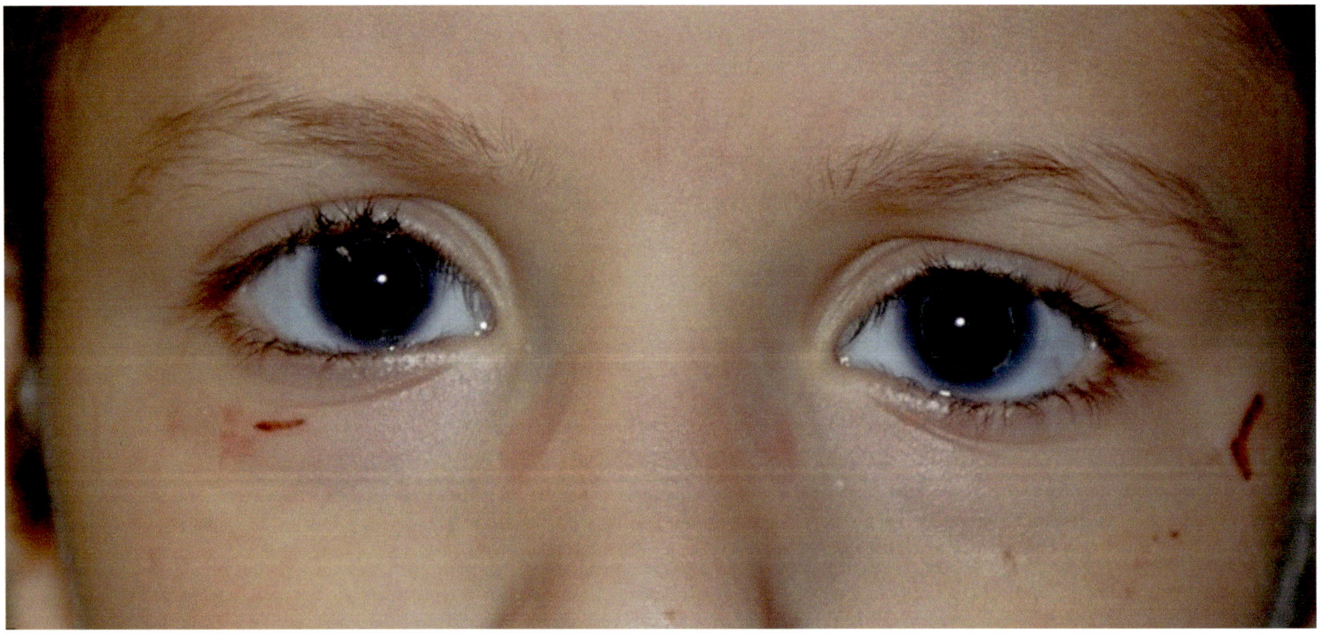

Fig. 44 Male patient, 8 years, Axenfeld–Rieger Anomaly, otherwise healthy, visual acuity dec 0.8 OU

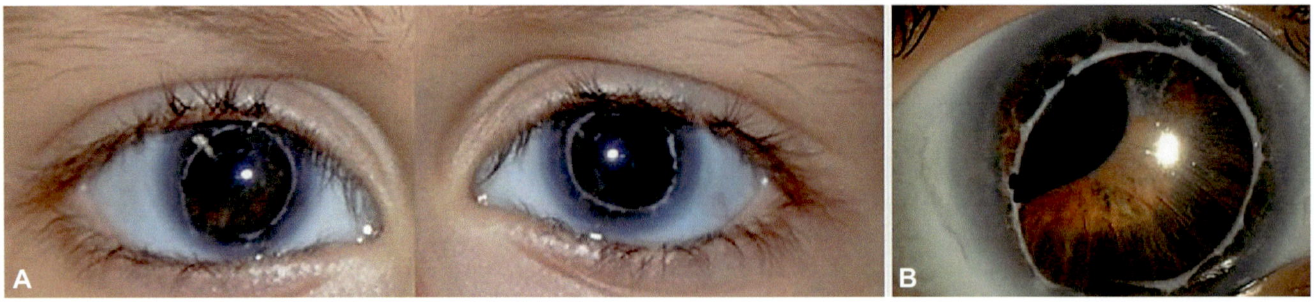

Fig. 45 Macro photos of the boy of Fig. 44: (**A**) Direct light: pair of eyes in Axenfeld–Rieger spectrum. Showed white corneal opacifications at birth. (**B**) Slit lamp: Detail of the right eye. In this case, the boy is otherwise healthy. Therefore, the correct naming is Axenfeld–Rieger Anomaly [2]

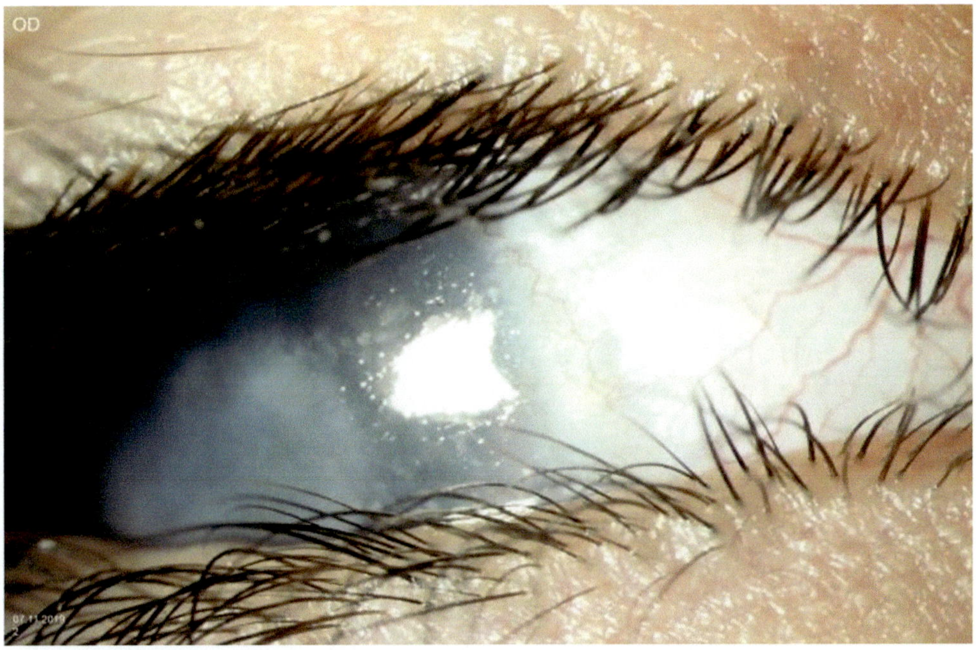

Fig. 46 1-year-old child, severely reduced cooperation, right eye with CCO, left eye not photographable due to lack of cooperation. CCO in dominant Axenfeld–Rieger Anomaly (mother affected as well)—PITX3 associated

The following Fig. 57 demonstrates a combination of CCO and rapidly progressing AAK—note especially the dense centripetal vascularization in the left image, taken under general anaesthesia.

Possible **congenital** corneal anomalies in PAX6 aniridia

- CCO (Fig. 55)
- NCO (Fig. 56)
- Rare combination of CCO/NCO and progressive AAK (Fig. 57)
- Usually at birth clear cornea (see Fig. 58)
- Mikrocornea with or without microphthalmia (Fig. 58)
- Cornea plana
- Buphthalmia (Fig. 55, 56)
- Broadened limbal area
- Delicate pannus formation as an early sign for AAK (details concerning AAK see below)
- Keratoglobus (Fig. 59)

In our registry of>350 persons with Aniridia we have not seen a vascularized CCO up to now [69, 74, 80]. Frequently the cornea in PAX6 related aniridia is clear at birth (Fig. 60).

Possible **congenital** non-corneal Anomalies in PAX6 aniridia

- Asymmetrical findings can be present! See Fig. 61
- Iris can be completely present [82]! See Figs. 61 and 62
- Microphthalmia (Fig. 61) [82]
- Ptosis (Fig. 62)
- Aniridia
  - Very variable
  - Complete iris absence apart from a small iris stump / tiny iris remnants (Fig. 60)
  - Partial aniridia (Figs. 63–65)
  - Atypical coloboma (Figs. 65, 66)
  - Corectopia in complete iris (Fig. 67)
  - Iris structure without pathological findings
  - Congenital complete or partial cataract (Fig. 68)
  - Typical: Cat. polaris anterior or (less frequently) posterior (often pyramidal shape [82]) (Figs. 64 and 69, 70)
  - persistent vascularization of the anterior lens capsule
  - Pseudofibrous hyperplasia of the anterior lens capsule (Fig. 70)
- Lens luxation or subluxation (Fig. 71)
- Lens coloboma (Fig. 71)
- Elevated IOP
- Shallow anterior chamber
- Optic nerve hypoplasia / dysplasia (Fig. 72)
- Foveal hypoplasia (Fig. 72)
- Hypopigmented fundus (Figs. 72–74)
- Colobomatous retinal defects (Fig. 73, 74)

PAX6 Aniridia Associated Complication: AAK: Aniridia Associated Keratopathy with Limbal Stem Cell Insufficiency (LSCI)

The term "limbus" comes from Latin and means "border" between two different types of tissue. In this case, it marks the border zone between the optically clear cornea and the opaque sclera. Here, the Pallisades of Vogt can be found (Fig. 75), where limbal stem cells (LSC) are located. Despite its small size, the corneoscleral limbus is a unique ocular structure that is responsible for the integrity of the cornea [83]. In general, it acts as:

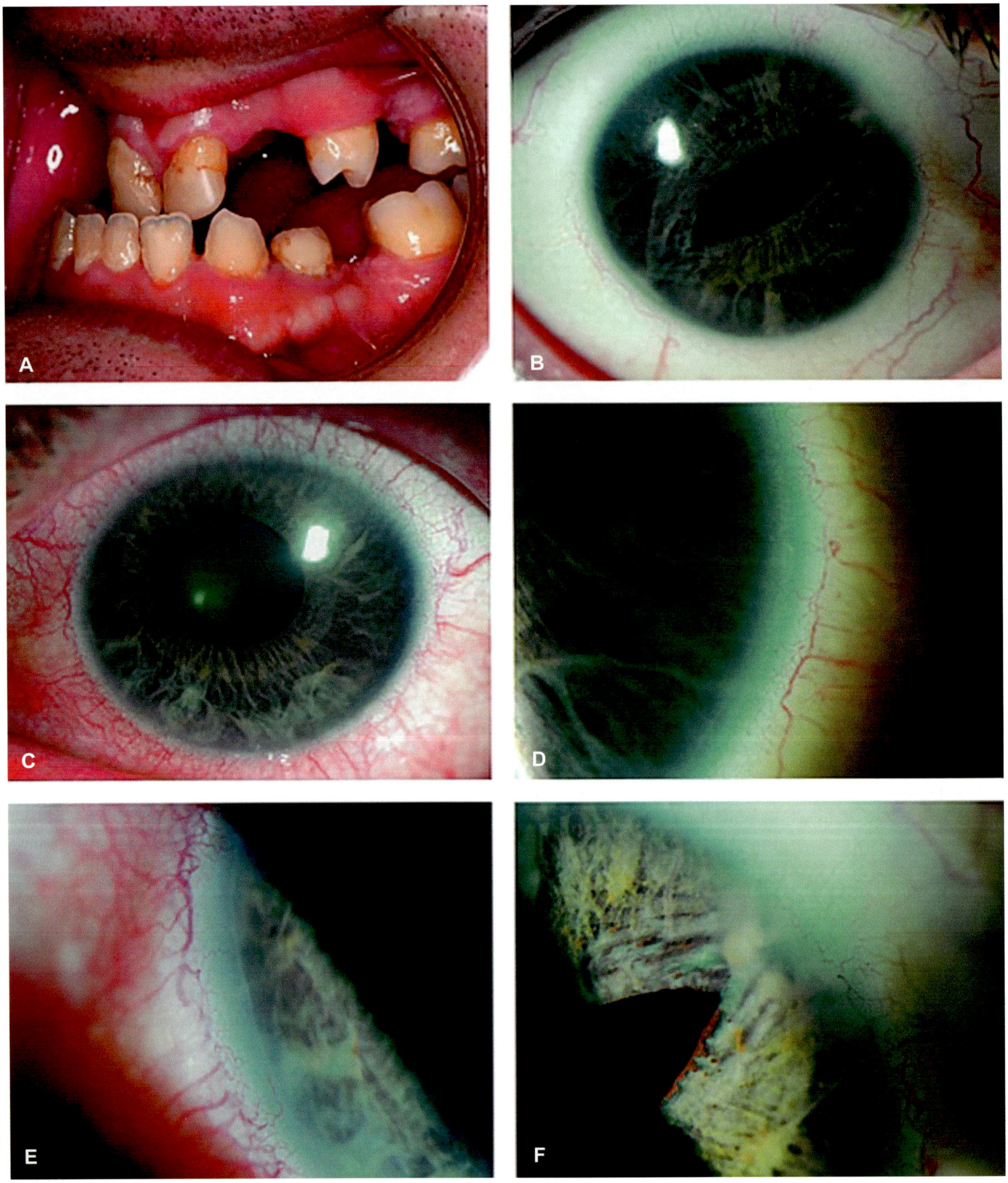

Fig. 47 Axenfeld–Rieger Syndrome: (**A**) Microdontia and hypodontia. (**B**) Abnormal pupil configuration and iris atrophy right eye. (**C**) Corectopia with iris atrophy left eye. (**D**) Posterior embryotoxon right eye. (**E**) Posterior embryotoxon left eye. (**F**) Broad peripheral anterior synechiae right eye.

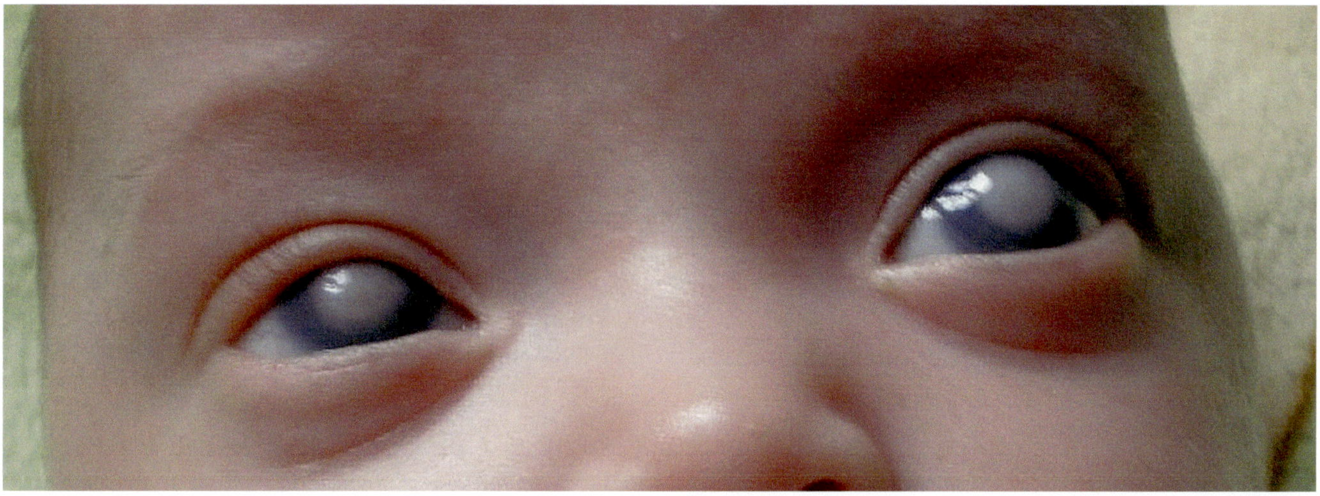

Fig. 48 Girl, 3 months. Bilateral Peters Anomaly. Up to now, the child is otherwise healthy without any systemic stigmata, therefore no Peters plus Syndrome. Ultrasound revealed Peters Anomaly Type I without lens attachment to the cornea

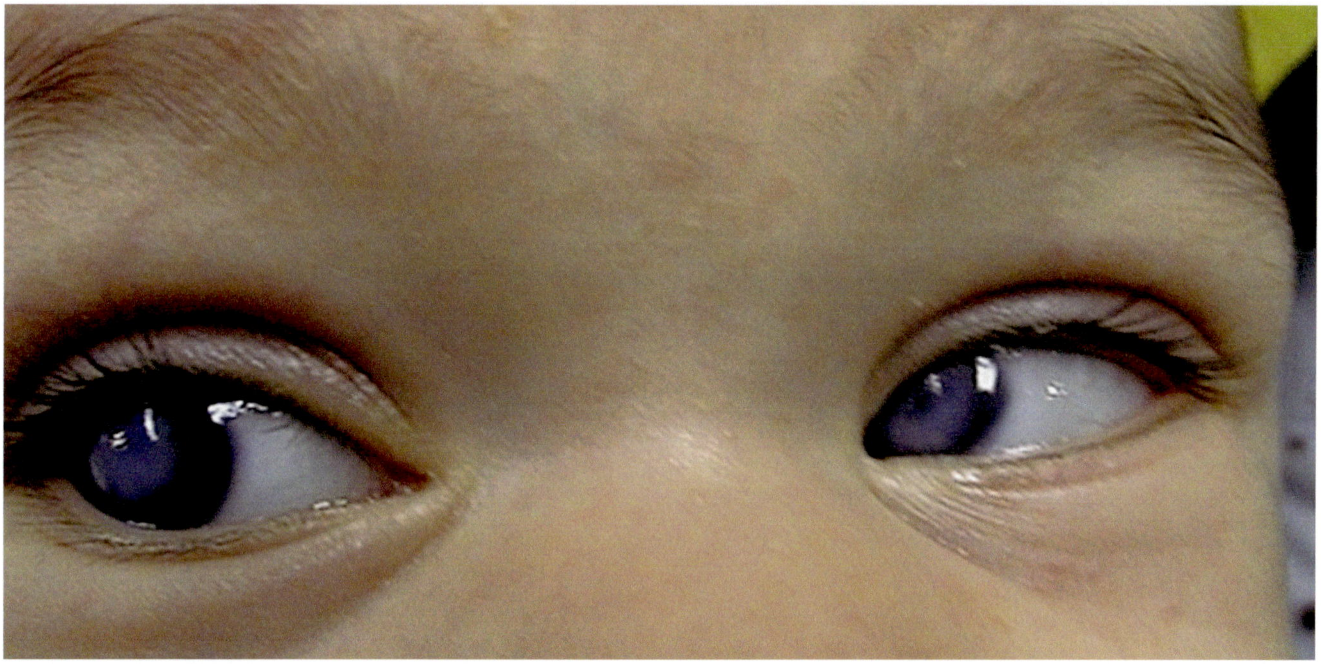

Fig. 49 Healthy girl, 18 months, Peters Anomaly, OD central corneal opacification, cornea partially clear in the periphery, OS full form of kerato-irido-lenticular dysgenesis (KILD), microphthalmia OS > OD

(1) barrier that prevents the ingrowth and migration of conjunctival cells into the corneal region,
(2) stabilizer that absorbs small pressure fluctuations to maintain corneal curvature and refractive power,
(3) site richly infiltrated with vessels and lymphatics to nourish the peripheral corneal tissue,
(4) site of aqueous humour outflow through the trabecular meshwork to maintain a regular intraocular pressure, and
(5) important niche for stem cells to regenerate corneal tissue, regulate intraocular pressure and for wound healing.

Generally, there are several etiologically different causes for limbal stem cell insufficiency [83]: genetic causes like aniridia, autosomal dominant (AD) keratitis, Ectrodactyly-ectodermal dysplasia-clefting (EEC) syndrome, but as well acquired causes like dry eye disease (DED), contact

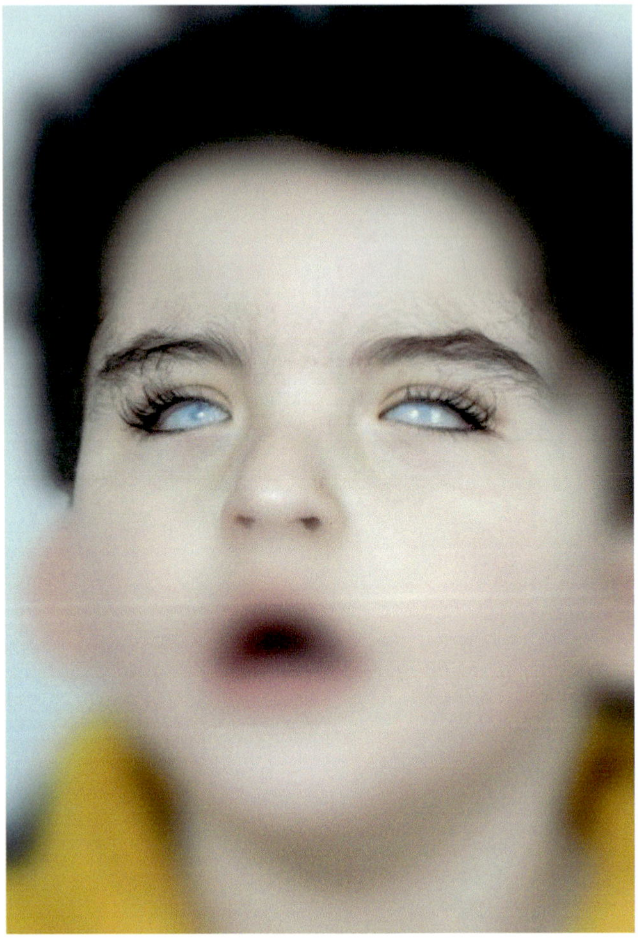

Fig. 50 10-year-old boy, multiple handicaps with Peters Plus Syndrome (PPS): severe manifestations OU (KILD), systemic signs: hypotonia, short philtrum, atypical auricles

lens wear damages, ocular burns and immunological causes such as pemphigoid-related keratopathy, medically induced LSCI, Stevens–Johnson Syndrome, post-radiation syndrome.

In aniridia, the niche function for stem cell formation is disturbed. PAX6 defects can disrupt limbal epithelial stem cell (LESC) development by first affecting the limbal niche, which in turn can affect LESC identity (Figs. 76, 77) [66, 70, 84, 85]. The PAX6 protein is a transcription factor expressed in embryonic ocular tissues and is involved in the regulation of corneal epithelial cell differentiation [83]. It has been shown that LESC are still present in young aniridia patients, but then disappear. In the course of their lives, up to 70% of those affected by aniridia develop aniridia-associated keratopathy (AAK) with an insufficiency of the limbal stem cells, impaired differentiation of the corneal epithelial cells, abnormal cell adhesion and wound healing (Fig. 78) [66, 86]. AAK is characterized by centripetal vascularisation [65], conjunctival changes and thickening of the cornea [81]. In addition to the cellular changes, a secondary inflammatory component is assumed [87, 88]. LSCI is categorized into 4 grades (Tab. 7) [66, 70]. The best prophylactic approach for LSCI-related AAK is the prophylaxis of chronic nutritional disorders of the cornea. Treatment includes preservative-free lubrication, treatment of recurrent corneal erosions by autologous serum eye drops and/ or amniotic membrane [89], bandage contact lens and/ or either penetrating keratoplasty (Homburger scheme with amniotic membrane transplantation as patch, lateral tarsorrhapy for 4 weeks [77, 79, 90] or deep anterior lamellar keratoplasty [91, 92]. Limbal stem cell transplantation is discussed, the donor however cannot be the patient himself, therefore systemic

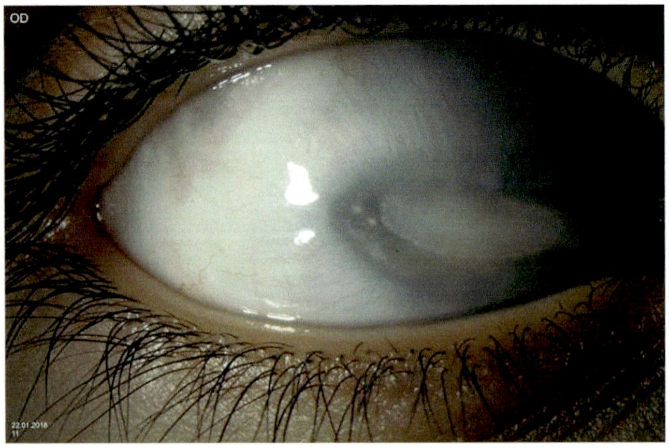

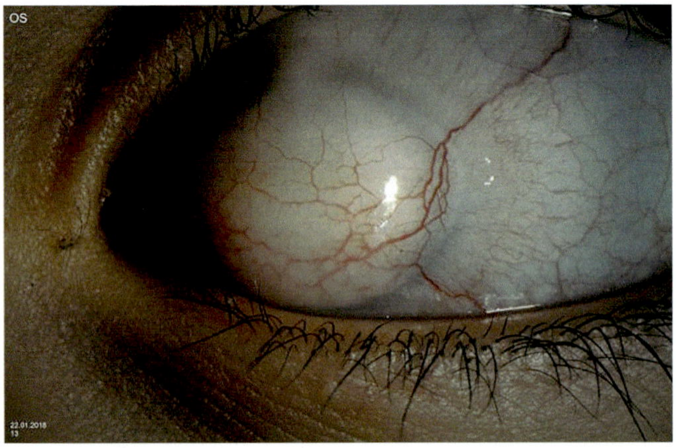

Fig. 51 13-year-old boy, PPS, multiply handicapped. First presentation at our hospital at age 13. Mixed presentation of primary CCO and secondary CCO: left image: secondary CCO in Peters Anomaly type II (KILD), right image primary CCO: large central dermoid. Ultrasound: OD microphthalmia, retina not differentiable. OS retina attached, small optic nerve diameter. Planned treatment: lamellar keratectomy for central dermoid. Visual prognosis very poor due to severe amblyopia

Table 6 Manifestations of CYP1B1-related Primary Congenital Glaucoma (PCG) [55, 57]

Features of CYP1B1 PCG	Description
Ocular abnormalities	Elevated eye pressure with pain and epiphora Increased corneal diameter Glare sensitivity
Possible additional ocular abnormalities	Iris anomalies: partial or complete aniridia Other developmental disorders of the anterior segment Opacification of the cornea Lens (sub)luxation Congenital cataract Retinal dystrophy Primary or secondary (glaucomatous) optic atrophy
Visual impairment	Low Vision to legal or absolute blindness Intense glare sensitivity
Onset	Symptoms often present at birth or early infancy
Progression	Progression varies, with many cases exhibiting gradual deterioration (difficult surgical outcomes, repeat surgeries, keratoplasty only after permanent regulation of IOP, poor prognosis post-PKP
Genetic Inheritance	Typically inherited in an autosomal recessive manner Spontaneous and dominant forms are reported Frequency: Arabic states > Europe and USA, in Arabic states the mutation of CYP1B1 for PCG is approx. 90%
Systemic Manifestations	Some cases may exhibit systemic involvement beyond the eye
Management and Treatment	Hyperosmolar eye drops Topical antiglaucomatous treatment only up until a timely surgery First: glaucoma surgery (trabeculotomy, valves) Second: keratoplasty, other procedures
Genetic Testing	Three loci for CYP1B1 mutation

Table 7 Classification of aniridia associated keratopathy (AAK) according to Lagali et al., Fries et al. [65, 66, 69, 70]

Grade of AAK	Corneal opacification	Vascularization	Conjuctivalization	Additional findings
Grade 1	Only very peripherally (pannus formation)	none	Just very peripherally	none
Grade 2	Progressive, within the outer 1/3 of the outer cornea	Often starting at 12 and 6 o´clock, progressing centripetally	Condensation of the limbo-conjunctival vessels surpassing the limbal area	DED: Dry eye disease (Sicca), occasional pain
Grade 3	Further progressive, going over the peripheral 1/3 of cornea, but center remains clear	Circularly progressive, center of cornea still free from vascularisations	Conjunctivalisation up to the middle of the cornea, corneal center still free	Recurrent corneal erosions with prolonged healing phases, pain, loss of vision, Salzmann nodules
Grade 4	Complete corneal opacification inclusive center of cornea	Limbal vessels cross the center of the cornea	Complete conjunctivalisation of the cornea	Corneal blindness, severe pain, Salzmann nodules, recurrent erosions

immune suppressive treatment is necessary. There are new research ways for treating AAK by repurposing existing FDA-approved drugs [5, 12] looking very promising.

Table 7 summarizes the classification of AAK adapted from Lagali et al. [66, 70], (see Figs. 79–92).

PAX6 Aniridia complication: Cataract

A recent publication showed that the crystalline lens in PAX6 aniridia has a smaller diameter and a smaller size than in a collective population with oculocutaneous albinism and completely translucent iris [95].

A congenital cataracta polaris anterior or posterior is frequently found, rarely a complete congenital cataract (Fig. 69). However, a premature cataract develops relatively frequently in childhood or adolescence [62, 84] (Fig. 89). There might be a dense opacification of a subluxated lens as seen in Fig. 90.

To avoid aniridia fibrosis syndrome (see below), small incision surgery with an uncoloured foldable lens should be performed. The implantation of artificial irides, large PMMA lenses and iris diaphragms for "iris replacement" are obsolete in congenital aniridia as they can lead to secondary glaucoma and aniridia fibrosis syndrome which are difficult up to impossible to control [60, 76].

PAX6 Aniridia complication: Secondary Glaucoma

Secondary glaucoma, which often occurs in early childhood or adolescence, is a complication of congenital aniridia,

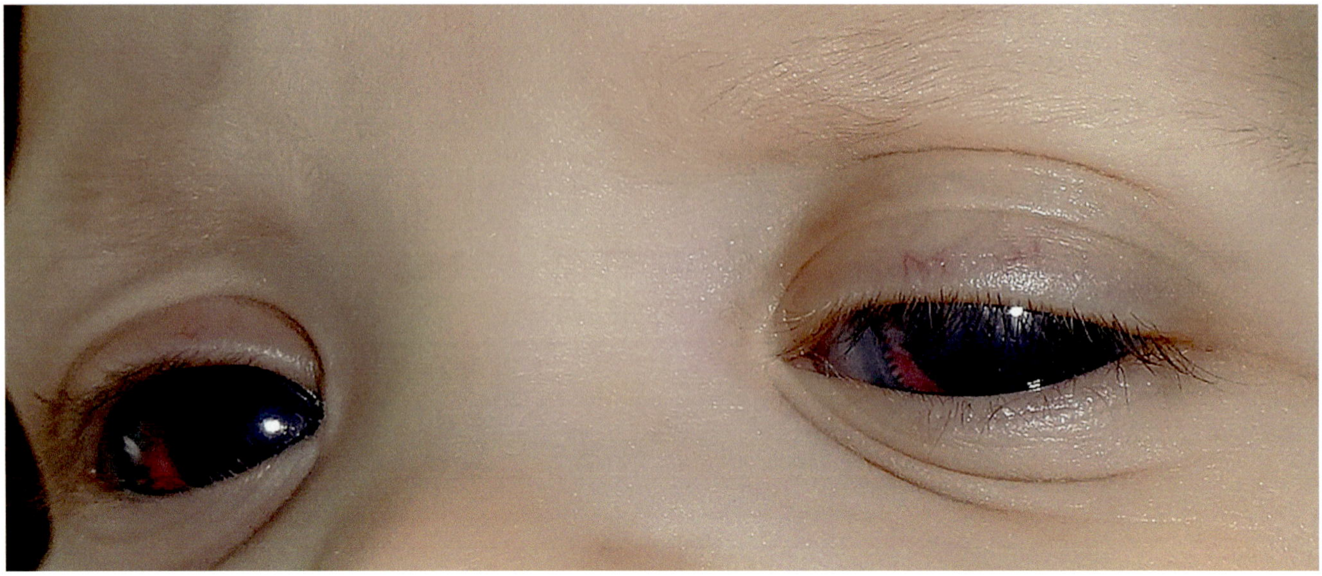

Fig. 52 NCO in 9-month-old boy, CYP1P1-related congenital glaucoma, since birth bilateral corneal opacifications, more pronounced in the left eye, progressive. Buphthalmia, elevated IOP OS > OD, in addition lens subluxation R > L, complete aniridia

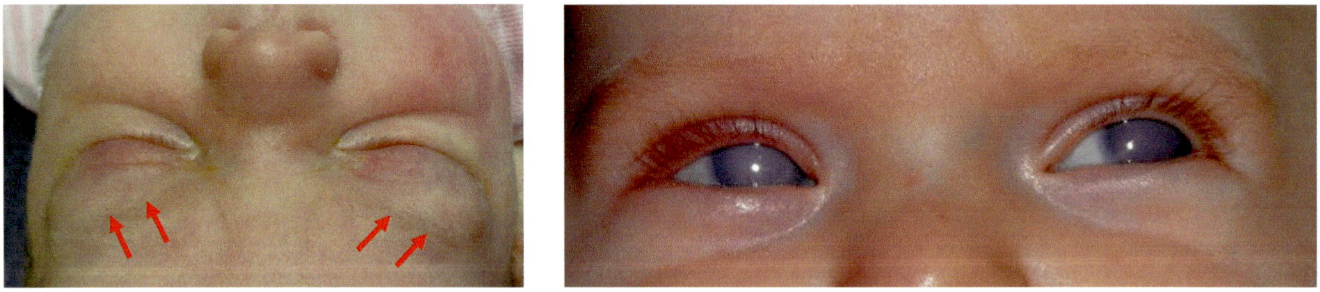

Fig. 53 Girl, 3 months, verified CYP1B1-associated anterior segment dysgenesis with complete aniridia. Type 1 PCG and severe CCO. Left image: bulging eyes. Right image: severe congenital corneal opacification, just a very tiny rim in the corneal periphery appears more clear. Complete aniridia

which can lead to irreversible blindness due to optic nerve damage [57, 62, 96–98]. The diagnosis is often made too late, as compliance with pressure measurement is reduced in children, a visual field examination is not yet possible and both the condition of the cornea and the nystagmus make optic disc OCT impossible. Ophthalmoscopic assessment of the optic disc in young patients is often made more difficult by the corneal findings; in addition, in PAX6 aniridia there are frequent abnormalities in the shape of the optic disc (e.g. dysplasia, Fig. 72), which make assessment more difficult. The corneal thickness (often increased) must also be taken into account in the IOP evaluation. Rarely, IOP is so high during pregnancy that the children are born with CCO (Fig. 91).

Years of therapeutical antiglaucomatous eye drops therapy can worsen the AAK, which is why early surgical intervention is often advised, preferably trabeculotomy as the primary intervention [57, 69, 80]

Often secondary aniridic glaucoma starts in early childhood and might be difficult to diagnose and document [99] (Fig. 92)—especially differences between both eyes are often difficult to detect in small children [77]. Frequent evaluation of IOP is necessary and can be performed by dedicated parents at home by means of the ICare® home tonometer to avoid absolute glaucoma (Fig. 93). Surgical treatment is often complicated by anatomical anomalies of the anterior chamber angle in aniridia [57, 100].

PAX6 Aniridia complication: Anterior Fibrosis Syndrome

Aniridic fibrosis syndrome (AFS) was first described by Tsai in 2005 [101] is a rare complication of invasive intraocular surgery (especially cataract extraction with intraocular lens implantation, aggravated by additional artificial lens implantation [77, 90]) that may occur in patients with congenital Aniridia (Fig. 94). It was also described

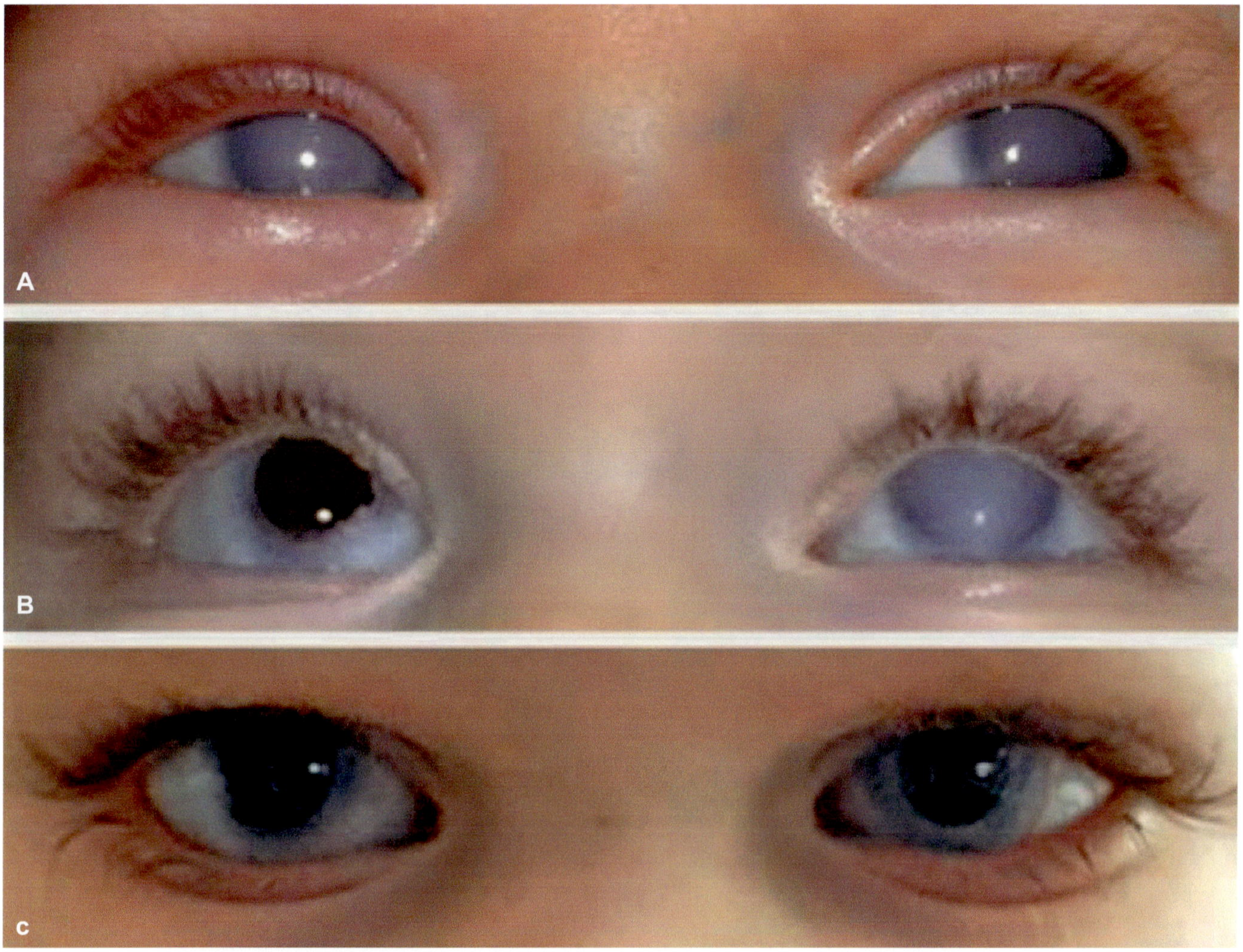

Fig. 54 CYP1B1-associated anterior segment dysgenesis [2], same girl as in Fig. 53. (**A**) CCO, congenital glaucoma, congenital corneal clouding, aniridia, findings at 3 months of age. (**B**) Findings after keratoplasty OD at 14 months of age. (**C**) Findings after keratoplasty on the contralateral eye, age 26 months

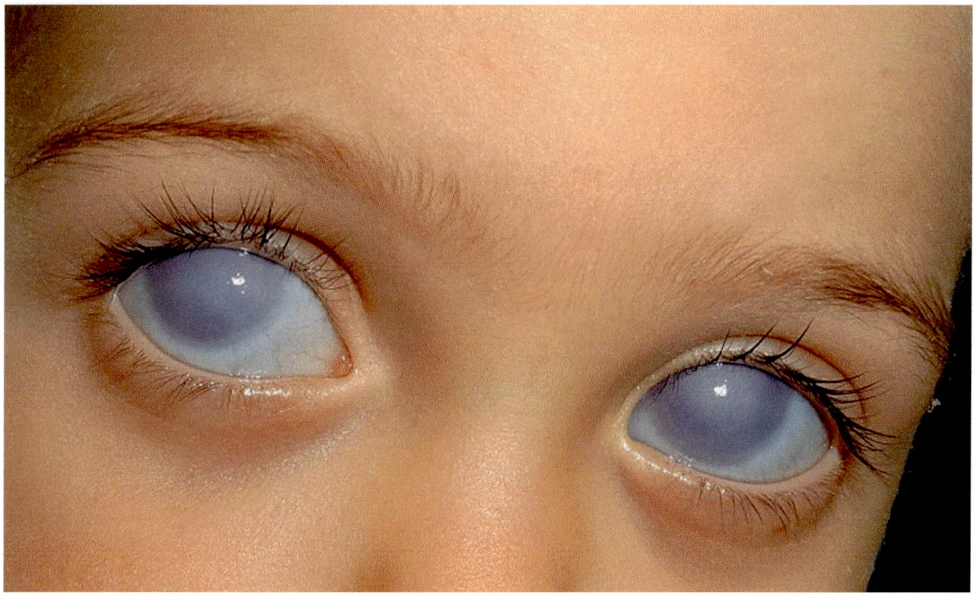

Fig. 55 6-month-old girl, CCO since birth, more pronounced in the center of the cornea, congenital glaucoma, IOP 30–40 (iCare®), buphthalmia since birth, complete aniridia (can be seen by faint red reflex peripherally), PAX6 haploinsuffiency proven

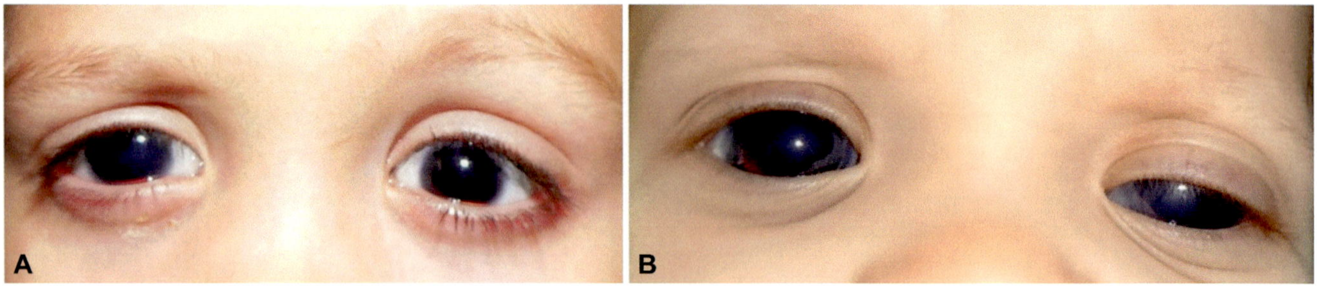

Fig. 56 NCO—neonatal progressive corneal opacification in PAX6 aniridia: (**A**) Boy, 9 months old, (**B**) Boy, aged 5 months. Since birth, the parents of both infants noted increasing haze in both eyes, in addition progressive enlargement of the eyes. Diagnosis in both boys: incomplete aniridia with buphthalmia. PAX6 haploinsufficiency proven

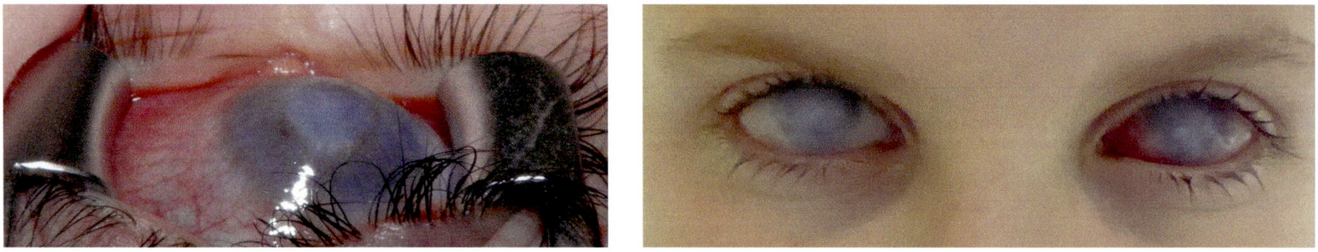

Fig. 57 CCO in combination with progressive AAK in PAX6 associated aniridia. Same boy, left image aged 2 years, right image aged 4 years. Had haze of corneas at birth plus buphthalmia with reported IOP around 50. Quickly developed severe AAK (grade 4) after having had multiple cyclophoto-lasercoagulations (CPC) of the ciliary body externally. In aniridic eyes, CPC promotes the development of AAK and should be avoided

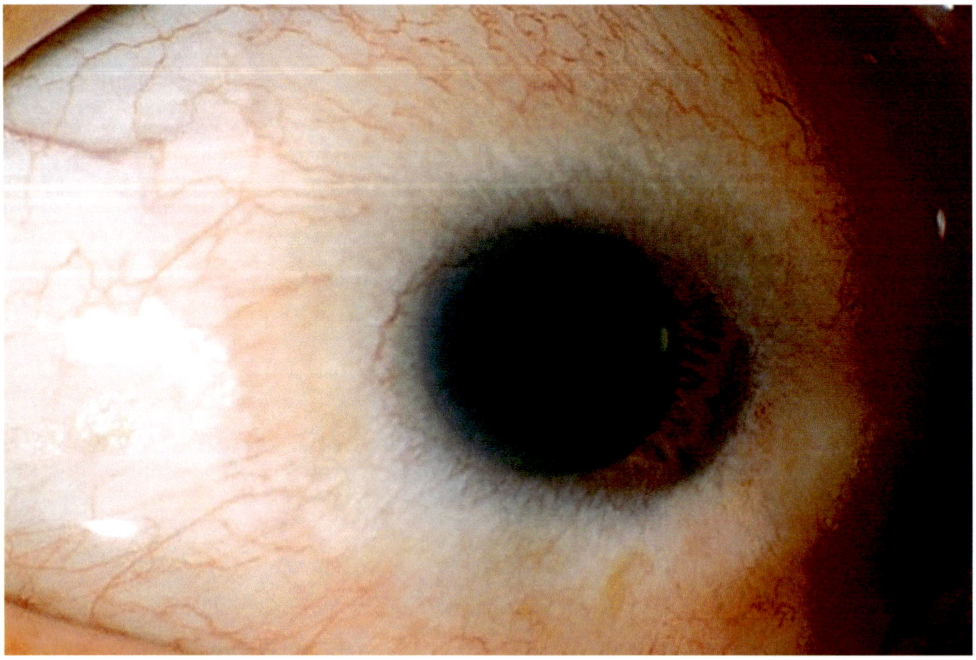

Fig. 58 Boy, now aged 7 years, bilateral microcornea without microphthalmia, beginning pannus formation circumferentially, partial aniridia, clear central and midperipheral cornea, PAX6 haploinsufficiency confirmed

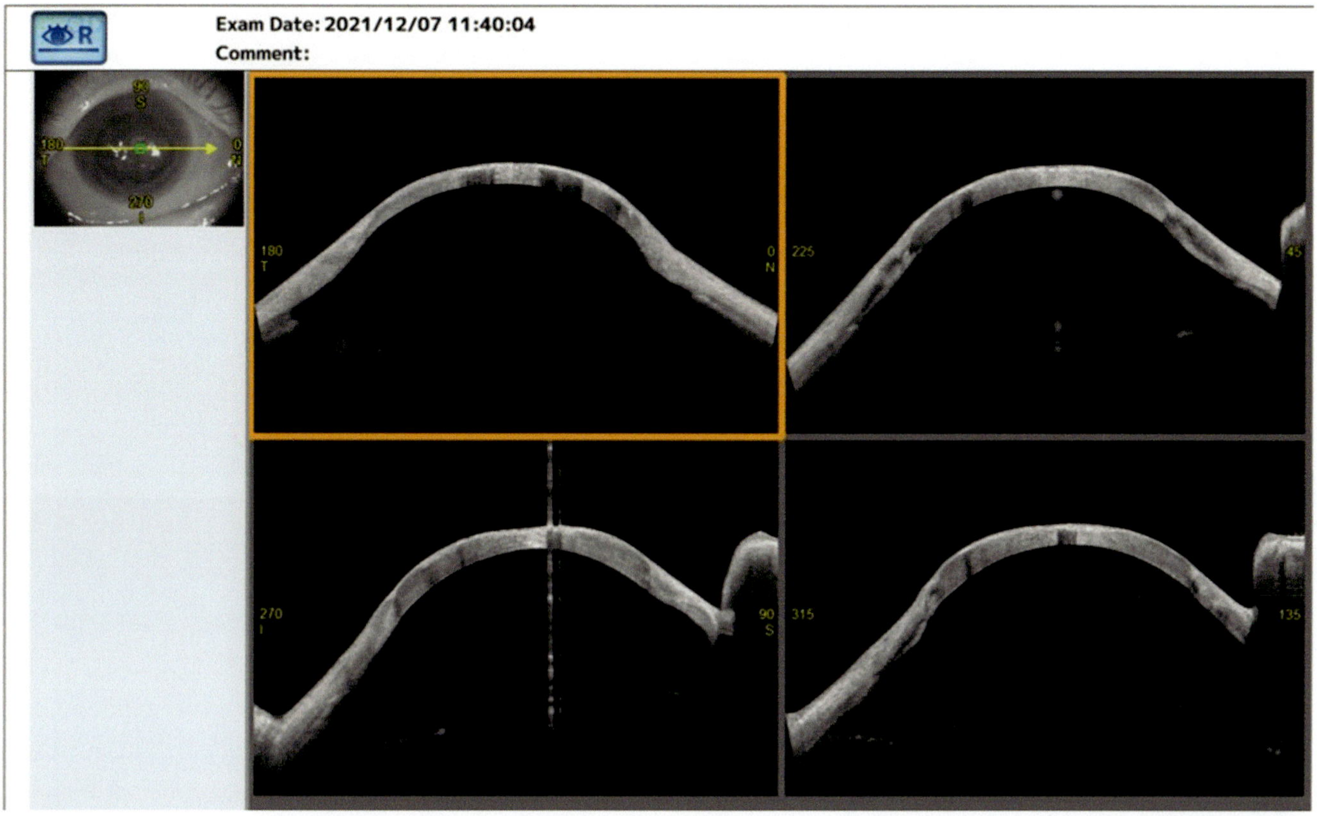

Fig. 59 12-year-old boy with aniridia and keratoglobus. PAX6 haploinsufficiency

following PKP [101]. It is characterized by a progressive fibrotic membrane overgrowth retrocorneally and within the anterior chamber after intraocular surgery. The fibrotic membrane also can involve the ciliary body and anterior retina. Histological studies showed that the extensive fibrotic tissue originated from the root of the rudimentary iris and entrapped the intraocular lens haptics. Endothelial decompensation was subsequent and very often results in phthisis bulbi with NLP. There is no preoperative test to assess the risk of developing AFS. Surgical treatment is often unsuccessful and consists of membranectomy. The basis of AFS has not yet been clarified, but in any case, the use of artificial lenses leads to a significantly increased risk. It has been recommended that only the best surgeons operate on the eyes of aniridic patients due to the potential complication of aniridic fibrosis syndrome [77, 90]. It is advisable that all implanted material goes in the capsular bag and not in the sulcus!

2.3.4 WAGR(O) Spectrum/Syndrome

WAGR(O) syndrome is a rare genetic disorder characterized by a constellation of features encompassing Wilms tumor, Aniridia, Genitourinary anomalies, and Retardation (O for Obesity). This section aims to provide a holistic understanding of the syndrome, delving into its genetic underpinnings, systemic clinical presentations, ocular abnormalities, and the prevalence of intellectual disability, obesity, and blindness.

WAGR(O) syndrome is primarily associated with deletions on chromosome 11p13 (see Fig. 95). The critical region includes the WT1 (Wilms tumor 1) and PAX6 genes. The WT1 gene plays a role in kidney and gonadal development, making individuals with WAGR syndrome susceptible to Wilms tumor and genitourinary anomalies. The lack of PAX6 due to its deletion leads to PAX6 aniridia.

Systemic Clinical Presentation

The Term WAGR(O) is an acronym for **W**ilms tumor, **a**niridia, **g**enitourethral anomalies, **r**etardation and—in selected cases—**o**besity.

Facial and general appearance: The children and adults are often hypotonic, have an open mouth, there might be saliva dripping. The nares are anteverted, the ears are low set (Fig. 96) [14].

Wilms Tumor: Approximately 50% to 60% of children with WAGR(O) syndrome develop Wilms tumor (nephroblastoma), which is a kidney cancer that usually occurs in early childhood. The risk of Wilms tumor is particularly associated with the deletion of the WT1 gene on chromosome 11p13, a key genetic factor in WAGR(O) syndrome.

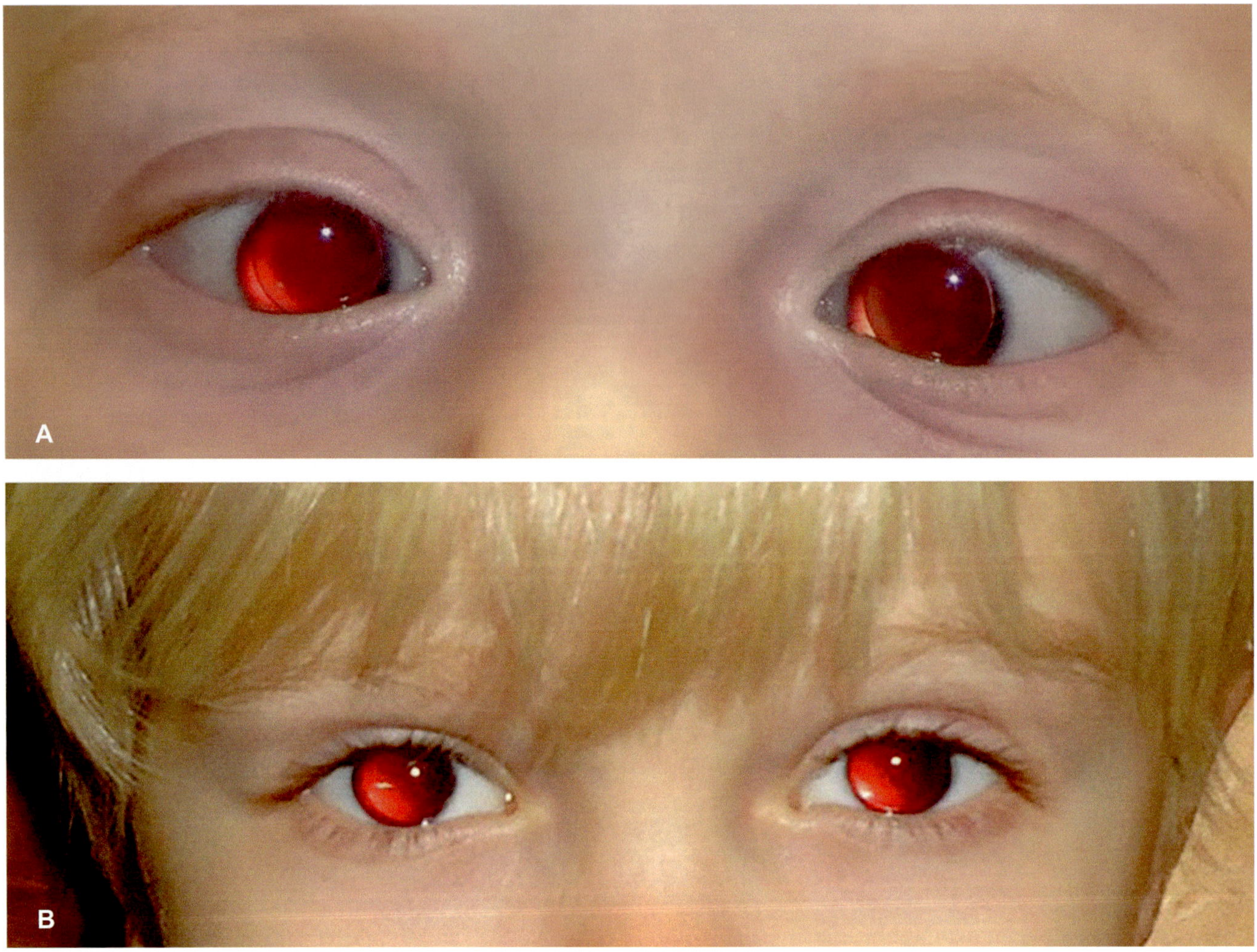

Fig. 60 Usually the cornea in aniridia is clear at birth. (**A**) Girl, 4 months. Bilateral clear cornea, no limbal pathologies. (**B**) Boy, aged 2 years, bilateral clear cornea, lens margin visible, but lens is centered, no limbal pathologies. Both children: confirmed PAX6 aniridia

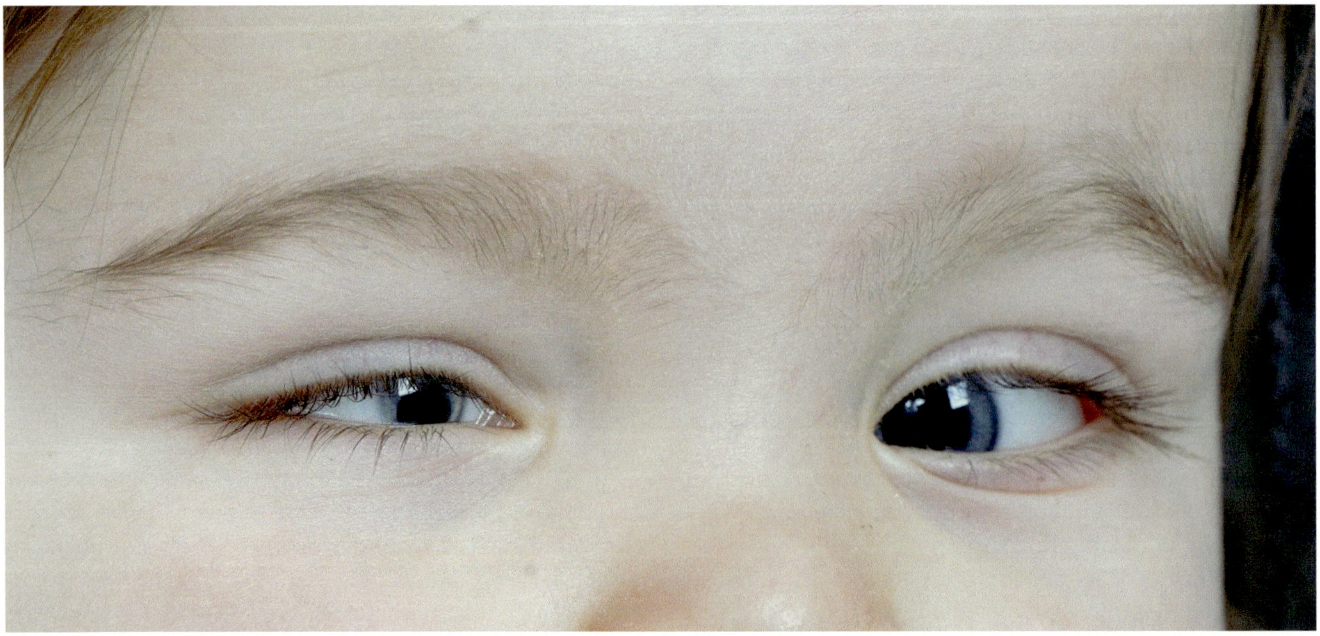

Fig. 61 Girl with PAX6 mutation, 2 years. Highly asymmetrical findings: OD microphthalmia, atypical coloboma/partial aniridia. OS with undilated pupil: slight corectopia. In the picture, the pupils are dilated. PAX6 haploinsufficiency

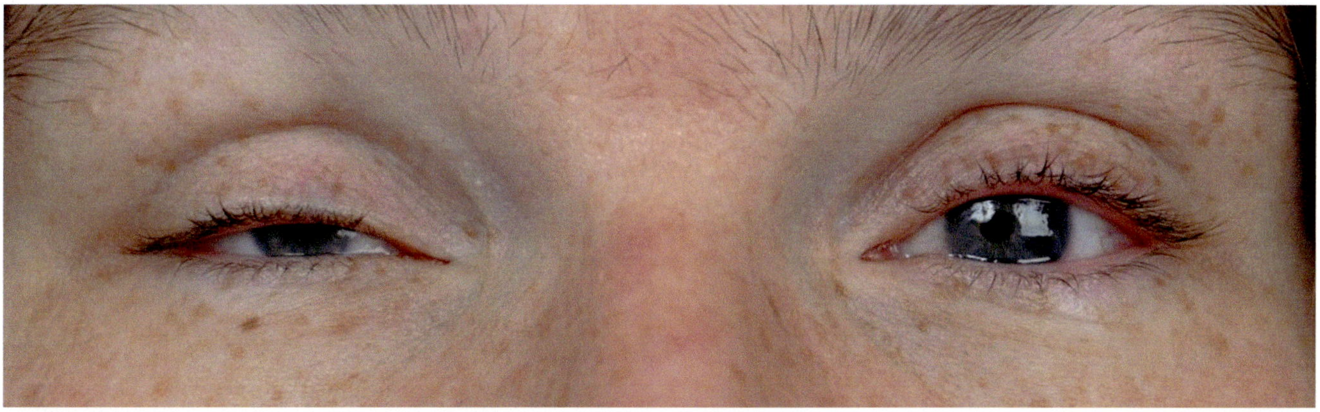

Fig. 62 Female with PAX6 mutation, now 40 years old. Congenital ptosis OD>OS, slowly progressive during adulthood

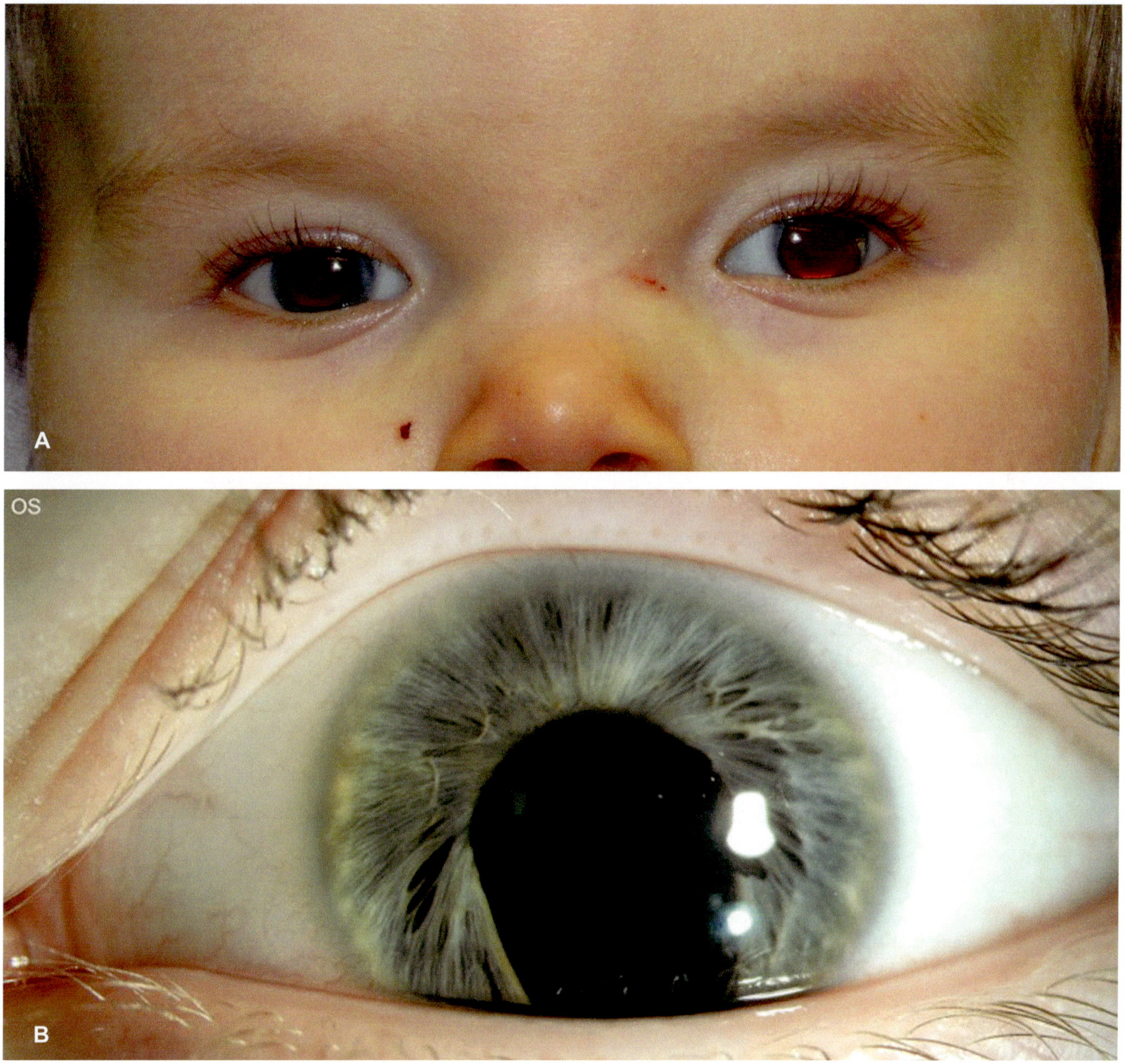

Fig. 63 (**A**) Female, aged 1.5 years. Picture taken without mydriatic eye drops. Partial aniridia both eyes, OS>OD, in OS atypical coloboma from 4 to 8 o`clock. (**B**) Male, 45 years, OS. Atypical coloboma. OD without pathological findings. Full VA OU. Son, now 12 years, has complete aniridia, VA dec 0.1. Both patients: PAX6 haploinsufficiency confirmed

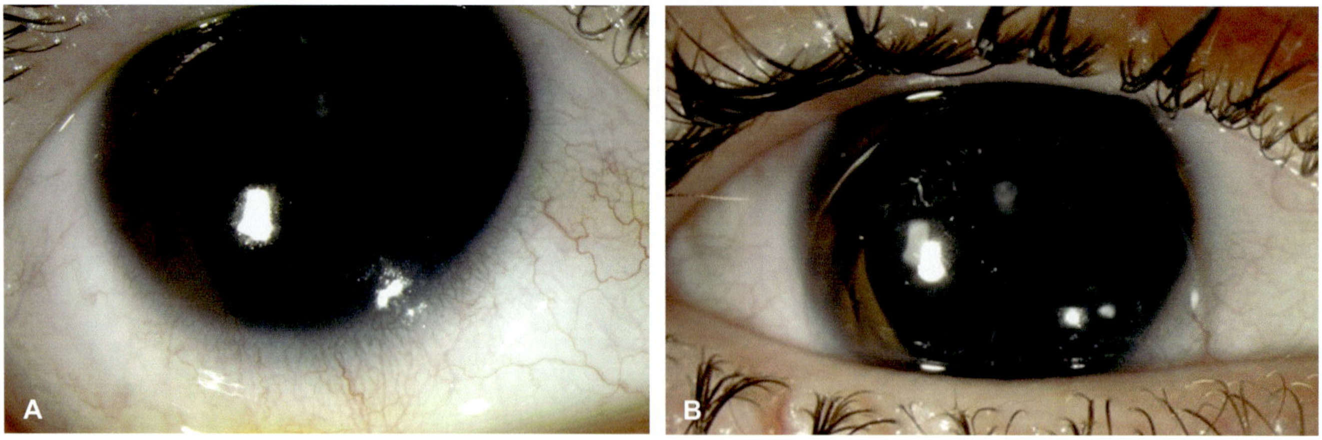

Fig. 64 (**A**) Female, now 8 years, OS. Incomplete aniridia OU, atypical coloboma. Picture taken without mydriatic medication. Cataracta polaris anterior. Beginning limbal stem cell insufficiency especially in the region where no iris is present. PAX6 haploinsuficiency confirmed. (**B**) Male, 38 years. Incomplete aniridia, clear lens apart from cataract polaris anterior, stable since birth. PAX6 mutation confirmed

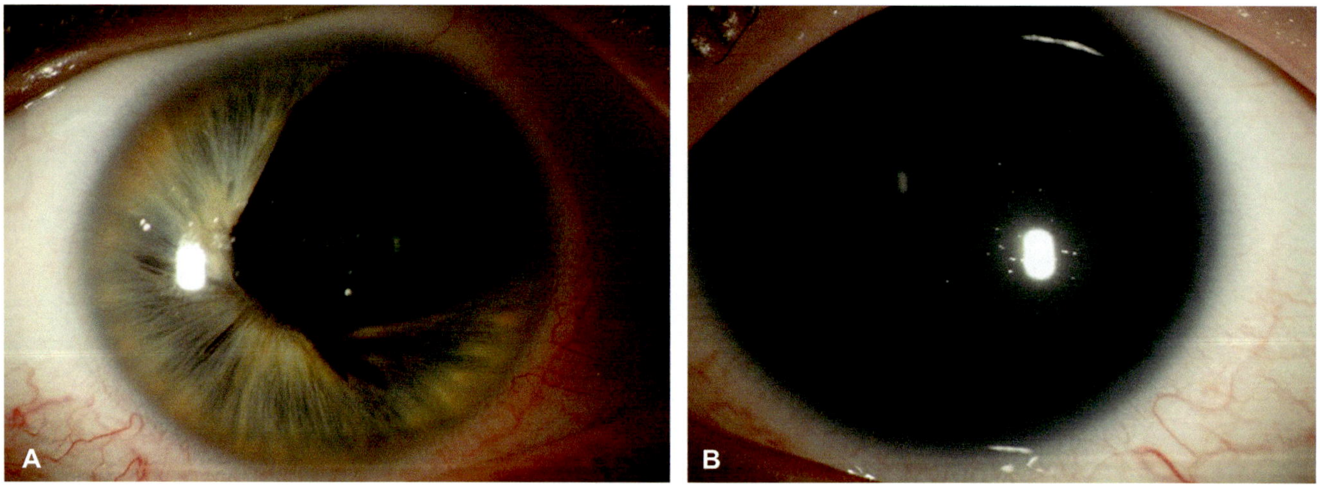

Fig. 65 Dominant PAX6 inheritance in father (**A**) and son (**B**). Father has bilateral ptosis, OU atypical coloboma, VA dec. 0.4. Son has complete aniridia, AAK Grade 1, VA dec. 0.1. They are 2 members of a family over 4 generations with 9 affected persons with aniridia

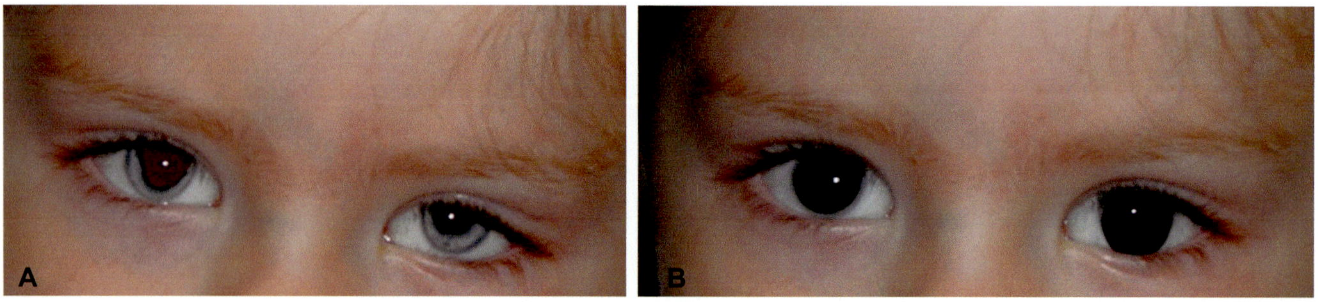

Fig. 66 (**A**) Girl, 3 years old. OD> >OS partial aniridia, OD atypical coloboma superiorly, OS corectopia. VA OD dec 0.4, OS dec 0.8. PAX6 haploinsufficiency confirmed. (**B**) Same girl as in A. Patient´s parents insisted on using darkly tinted contact lenses, in spite of warning of concerning corneal problems and in spite of the fact that on inspection the findings without contact lenses were less noticeable

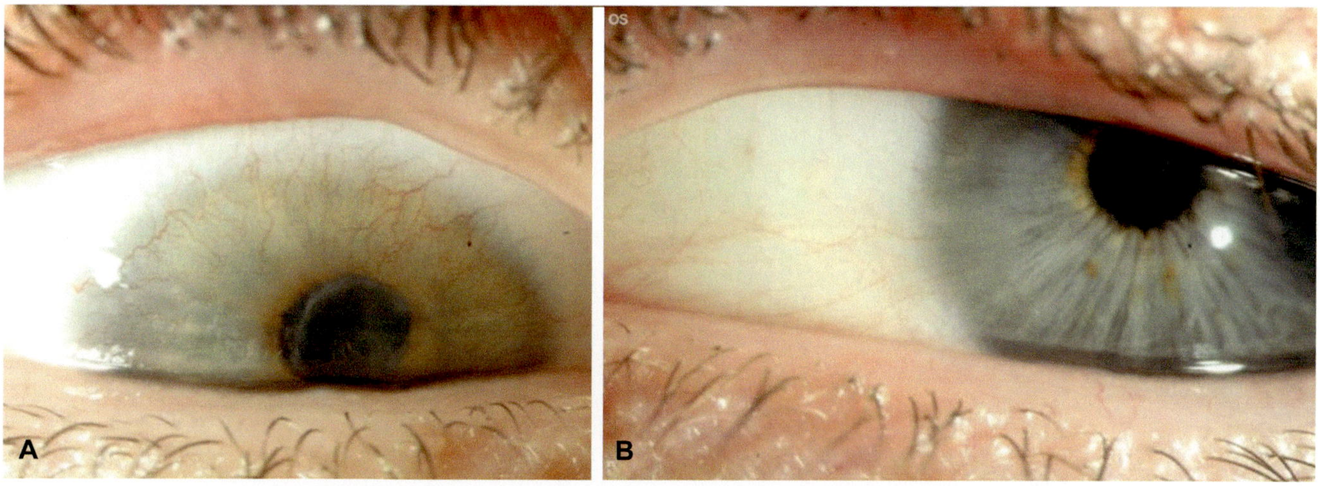

Fig. 67 Female, now 40 years. Same patient as in Fig. 63. (**A**) OD and (**B**) OS. Corectopia in completely present iris structure. Clear signs of limbal stem cell insufficiency with OD>>OS AAK. In addition, ptosis since childhood. PAX6 haploinsufficiency confirmed. Son, now 15 years, has incomplete aniridia and progressive AAK

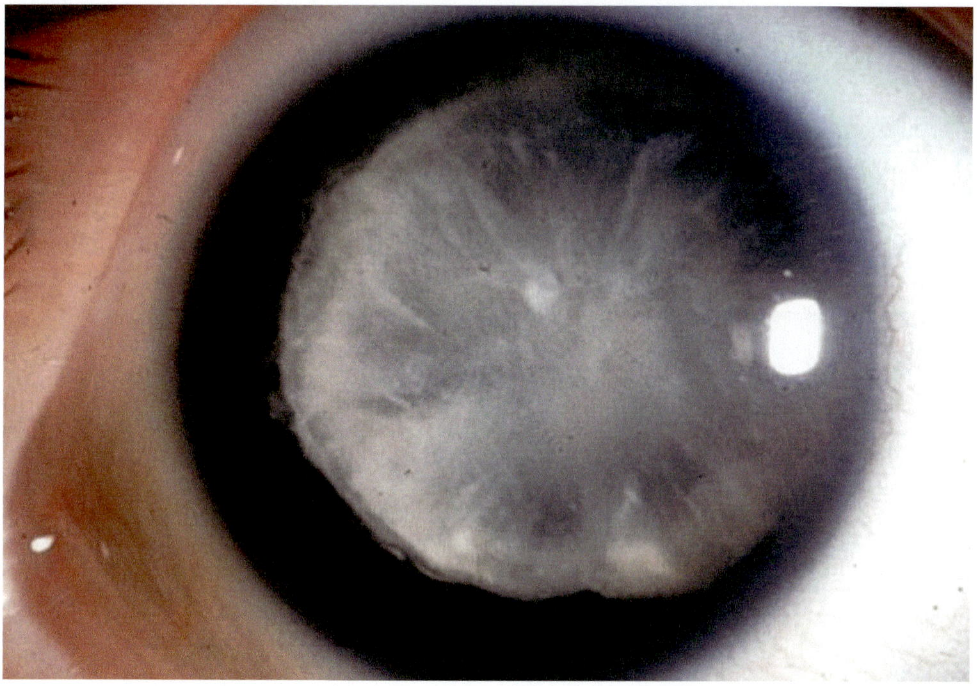

Fig. 68 Boy, aged 5 months: PAX6 related aniridia, complete aniridia, complete cataracta corticalis et nuclearis, slight pigment deposits on lens surface

This is the reason why early chromosomal examination for 11p13 deletion is mandatory. Regular and close monitoring, including imaging studies (renal ultrasound every 3 months), is crucial for early detection and effective management of Wilms tumor. It is important to note that the prevalence and risks can vary, and individual cases may exhibit differences in the expression and severity of Wilms tumor. The usual treatment consists of chemotherapy (chemotherapeutic reduction of tumor size) followed by surgery, often followed again by chemotherapy.

Ocular abnormalities

Unfortunately, the ocular sequelae of PAX6 aniridia are often especially severe: congenital cataract can be present, there is evidence of early corneal involvement and especially severe progression of AAK (Fig. 97, 98), and a high prevalence of aniridic glaucoma [10, 15, 76, 77]. In our clinical impression, even AFS occurs more often than in non-WAGR(O) PAX6 aniridic patients (Fig. 96).

All these factors contribute to a double impairment—visual and developmental. The support and promotion of

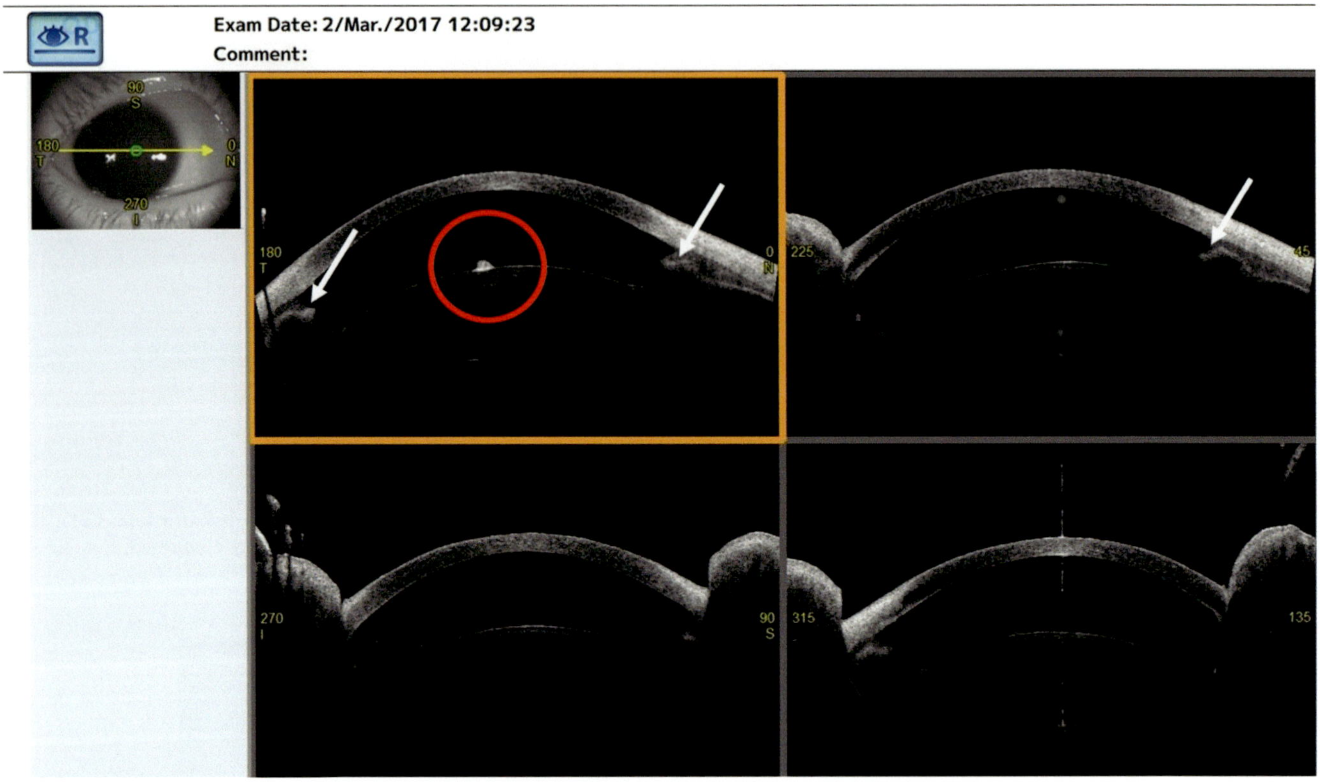

Fig. 69 5-year-old girl. OD Complete aniridia (iris stumps in anterior OCT visible, see arrows). Small anterior polar cataract OU (red circle). Usually non-progressive and visually not limitating. PAX6 haploinsufficiency

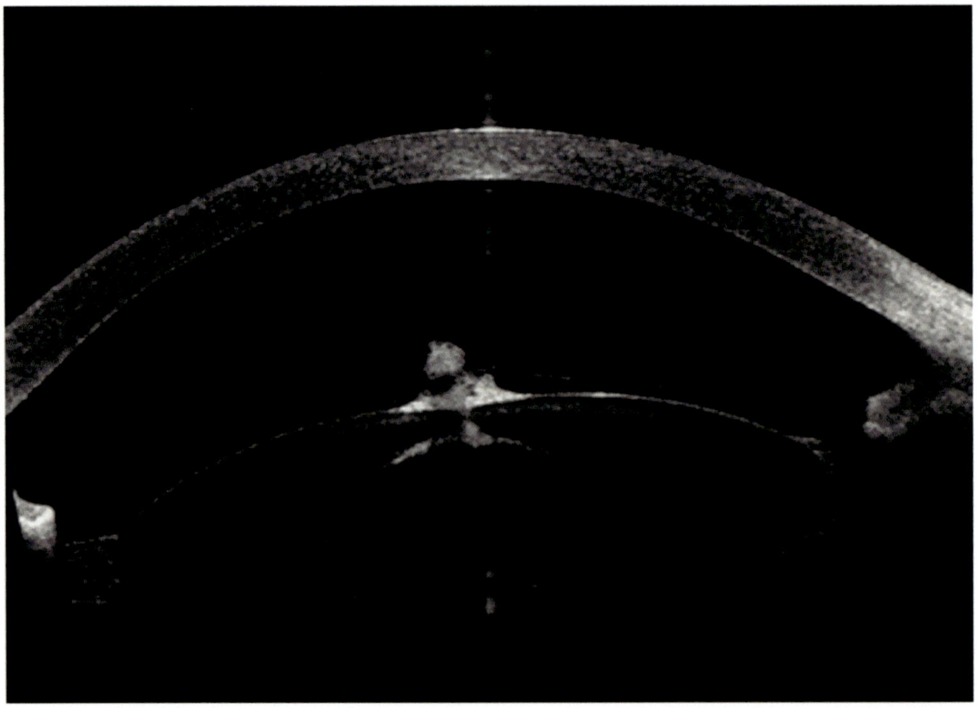

Fig. 70 Boy, now 6 years. Since birth pyramidal cataract of the anterior lens, plus pseudofibrous metaplasia of the lens capsule, PAX6 syndrome (obesity, intellectual deficits), WAGR excluded

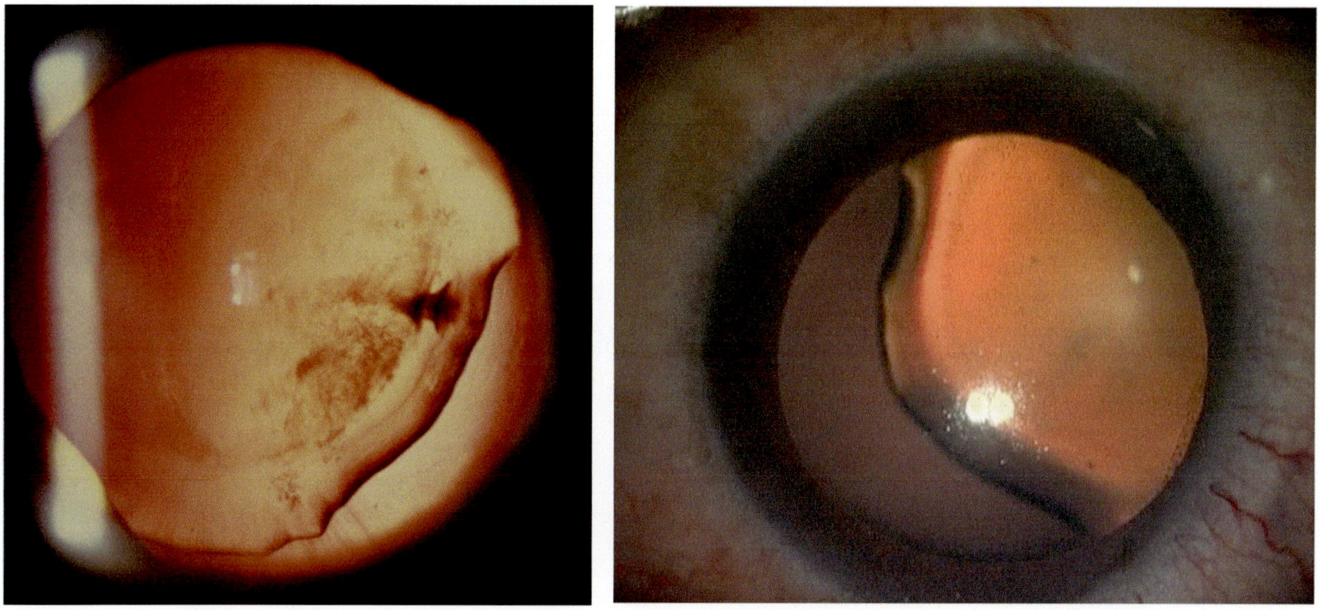

Fig. 71 Irregular fundus reflex post-partum. Examination revealed partial aniridia in both patients, incipient cortical cataract and lens coloboma in the patient on the left side, lens subluxation and visible zonula fibers. Patient on the right side shows significant lens subluxation. Both patients show PAX6 haploinsufficiency

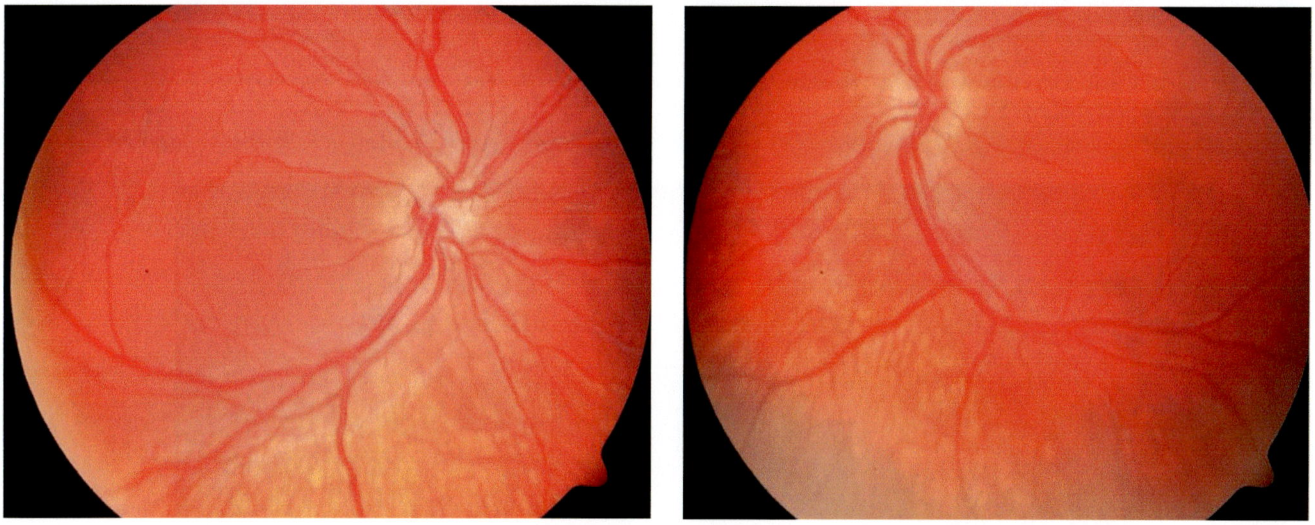

Fig. 72 7-year-old girl, OU. Partial aniridia. Fundus: Optic nerve hypoplasia, foveal hypoplasia, hypopigmented fundus aspect. PAX6 defect confirmed

developmental impairment is made much more difficult by the presence of often severe visual deficits.

The above mentioned autoaggressive behaviour aggravates ophthalmological examinations, postsurgical controls and topical treatments.

Prevalence of intellectual disability, obesity and blindness

Intellectual Disability: The prevalence of intellectual disability in individuals with WAGR(O) syndrome varies, but it is a common feature, requiring tailored educational and therapeutic interventions. In our group of 21 patients with WAGR syndrome, only three have developed intellectually normally: one girl learning Ukrainian and English Braille, one Russian student of informatics, one lawyer (the latter two have had Wilms Tumor). None of them was overweight.

Obesity: The “O” in WAGR(O) syndrome denotes an increased risk of obesity, possibly due to hormonal and genetic factors. Especially the defect of the BDNF gene

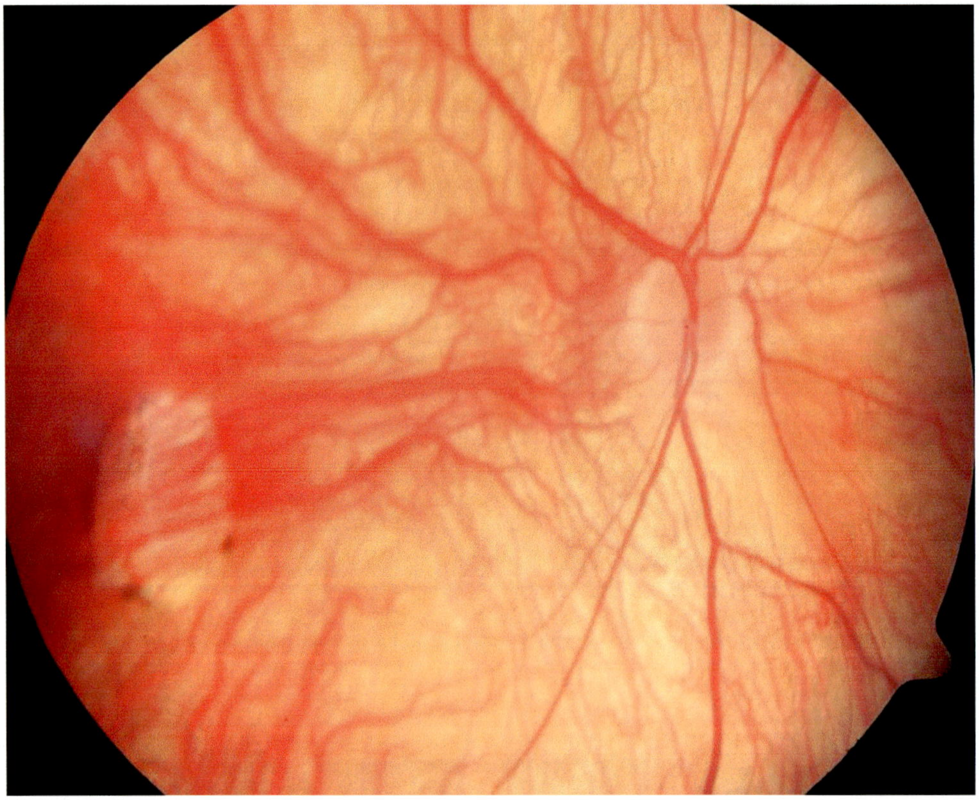

Fig. 73 12-year-old girl, OD. Partial aniridia. Fundus: Pale optic nerve head, distinctly hypopigmented fundus, paracentral coloboma temporally. PAX6 defect confirmed

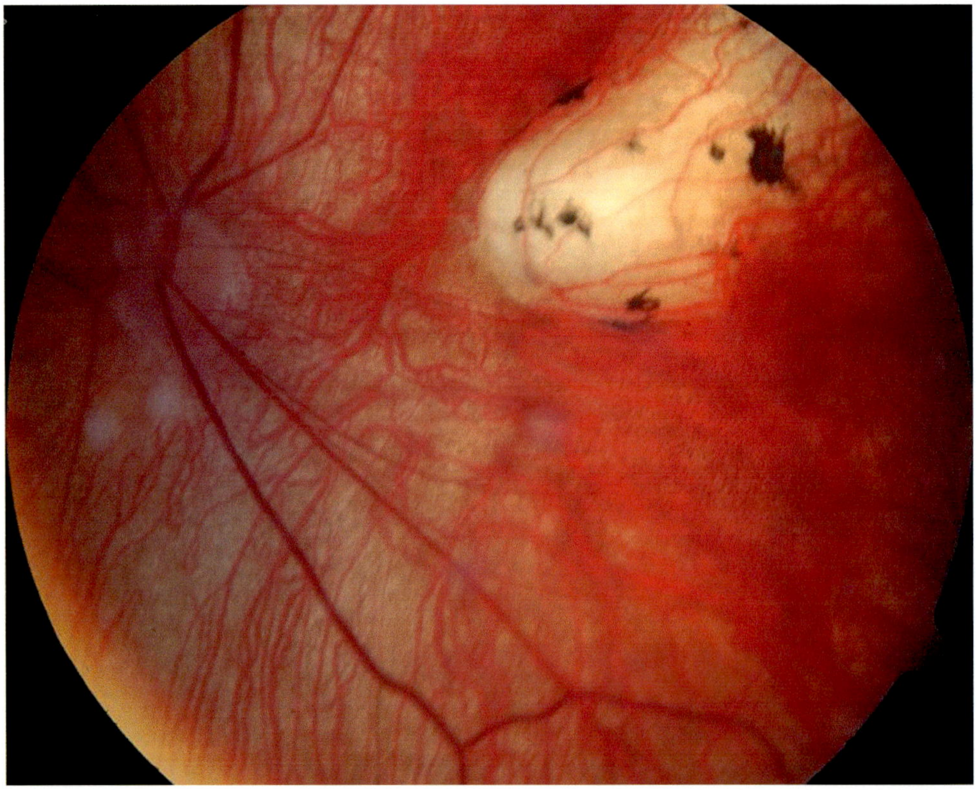

Fig. 74 Same girl as in Fig. 72, OS. Partial aniridia. Fundus: Pale optic nerve head, distinctly hypopigmented fundus, large atypical chorioretinal coloboma temporally superiorly. PAX6 defect confirmed

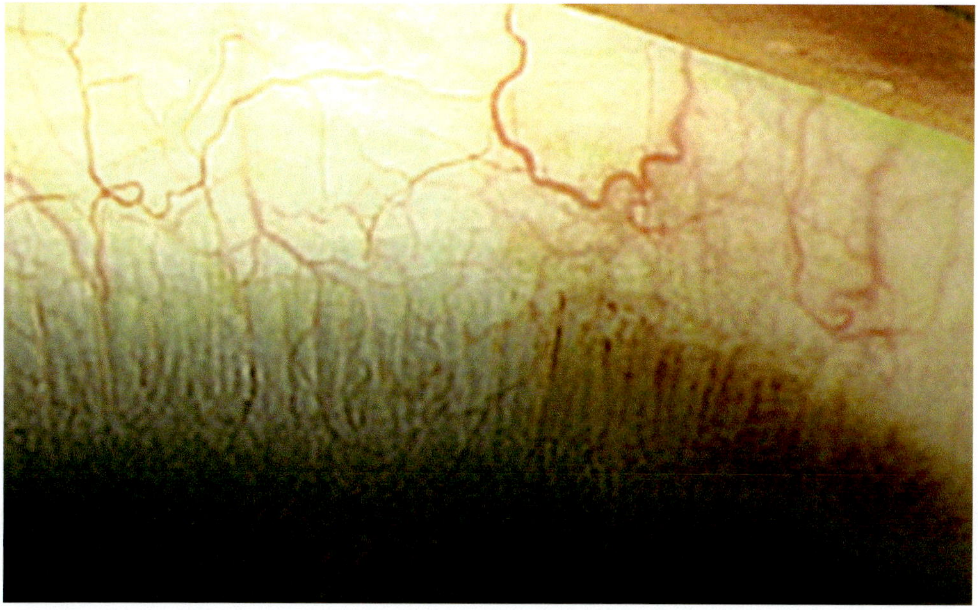

Fig. 75 Imaging of Pallisades of Vogt POV. This is the place where limbal stem cells are located [83]

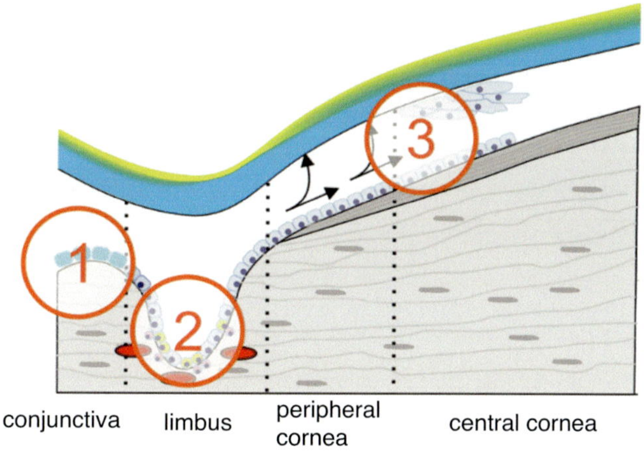

Fig. 76 Schematic illustration of limbal stem cell niche [93]. (1) Conjunctiva (overgrows the cornea in AAK) (2) Pallisades of Vogt (POV): within these are limbal stem cells (regenerate the corneal epithelium, loss or dysfunction leads to keratopathy) (3) Differentiated corneal epithelium (dysfunction favours keratopathy)

(when included in the deletion) leads to obesity and those patients are intellectually more challenged. Dietary management is crucial to prevent complications associated with obesity such as Diabetes mellitus Type II.

Blindness: Visual impairment and blindness can result from the combination of aniridia, glaucoma, and other ocular abnormalities, highlighting the importance of early intervention and regular eye examinations.

In conclusion, WAGR(O) syndrome presents a complex interplay of different defective genetic factors leading to a multifold spectrum of clinical manifestations. Early diagnosis, multidisciplinary management, and targeted systemic and ocular interventions are essential for optimizing outcomes in individuals affected by this rare and intricate syndrome.

2.4 Secondary Acquired CCO and NCO

Acquired congenital corneal opacifications and neonatal corneal opacifications are ophthalmic conditions that present unique challenges in diagnosis and management. Table 8 presents an overview of the most common secondary acquired CCO and NCO. In some children, the causes

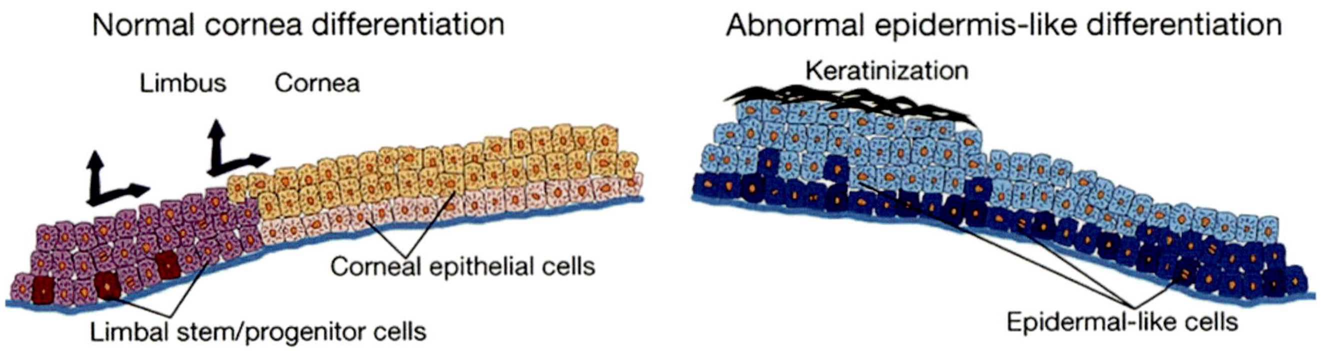

Fig. 77 Schematic drawing of limbal area in normal and in aniridic cornea. (From Ouyang et al., Nature, 2014, Vol. 511, p. 358–361, VC Macmillan Publishers Limited [94] All rights reserved (Natue Publishing Group), reproduced by permission.) [Color figure can be viewed at wileyonlinelibrary.com]. Adapted from: Käsmann-Kellner B et al (2018) Diagnostic impact of anterior segment angiography of limbal stem cell insufficiency in PAX6-related aniridia [65]

- LSC sit in Vogt Pallisades
- LSC maintain undifferentiated state
- LSC support regeneration of corneal epithelium
- LSC produce cytokines and growth factors

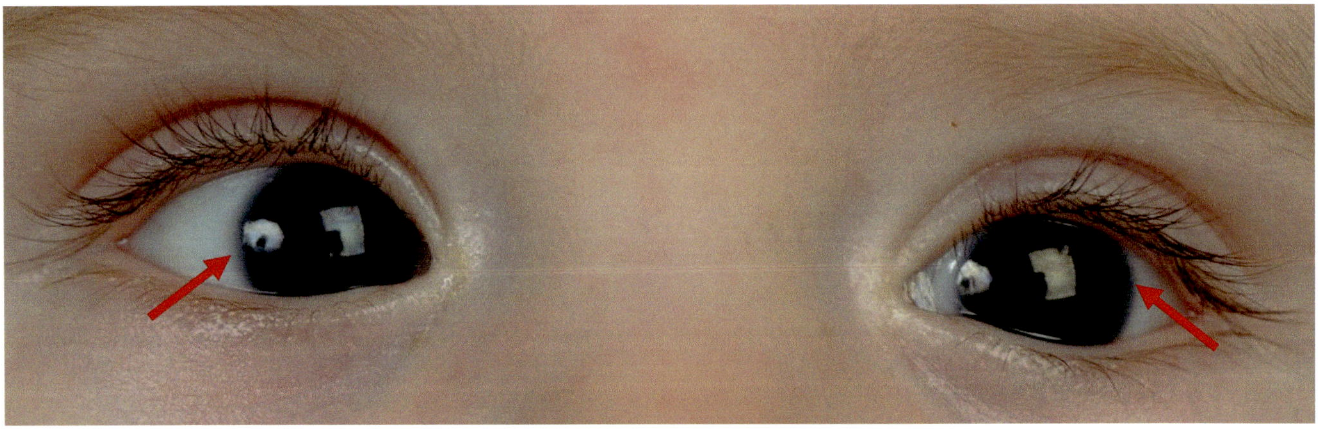

Fig. 78 Boy, aged 8 months, complete aniridia in PAX6 haploinsufficiency. **AAK grade 1**: very slight beginning avascularized pannus formation (see arrows) without any functional relevance

cannot be elucidated. The following subchapter categorizes them based on aetiological groups such as metabolic, traumatic, infectious, and others.

2.4.1 Metabolic Causes (IEM—Inborn Errors of Metabolism)

There are many possible inborn metabolic disorders, which can lead to CCO and NCO. Each of them is very rare, but in total, 1 of 800 newborns is affected by an IEM. The optical clarity of the cornea permits visualization of subtle deposition of metabolites not possible in other tissues of the body. Most metabolic diseases are inherited in an autosomal recessive manner. Generally, the metabolic disorder is a result of an enzymatic deficiency causing an accumulation of substrates, either locally or after transport into the blood stream. For few of the disorders, enzyme replacement treatment is now possible.

Most of the IEMs affect the retina (cherry red spot, secondary retinal degeneration) and the optic nerve (optic nerve atrophy), but some, especially mucopolysaccharidoses can lead to CCO and NCO (Fig. 99).

Mucopolysaccharidosis (MPS): Metabolic disorders such as mucopolysaccharidoses, a group of rare genetic conditions characterized by impaired lysosomal degradation of mucopolysaccharides, can lead to the accumulation of these substances within the cornea. Understanding the specific MPS subtype is crucial for targeted interventions and genetic counselling.

Despite systemic treatment (HSCT: Hematopoietic stem cell transplantation and ERT: Enzyme replacement therapy), no current treatment halts the progression of corneal

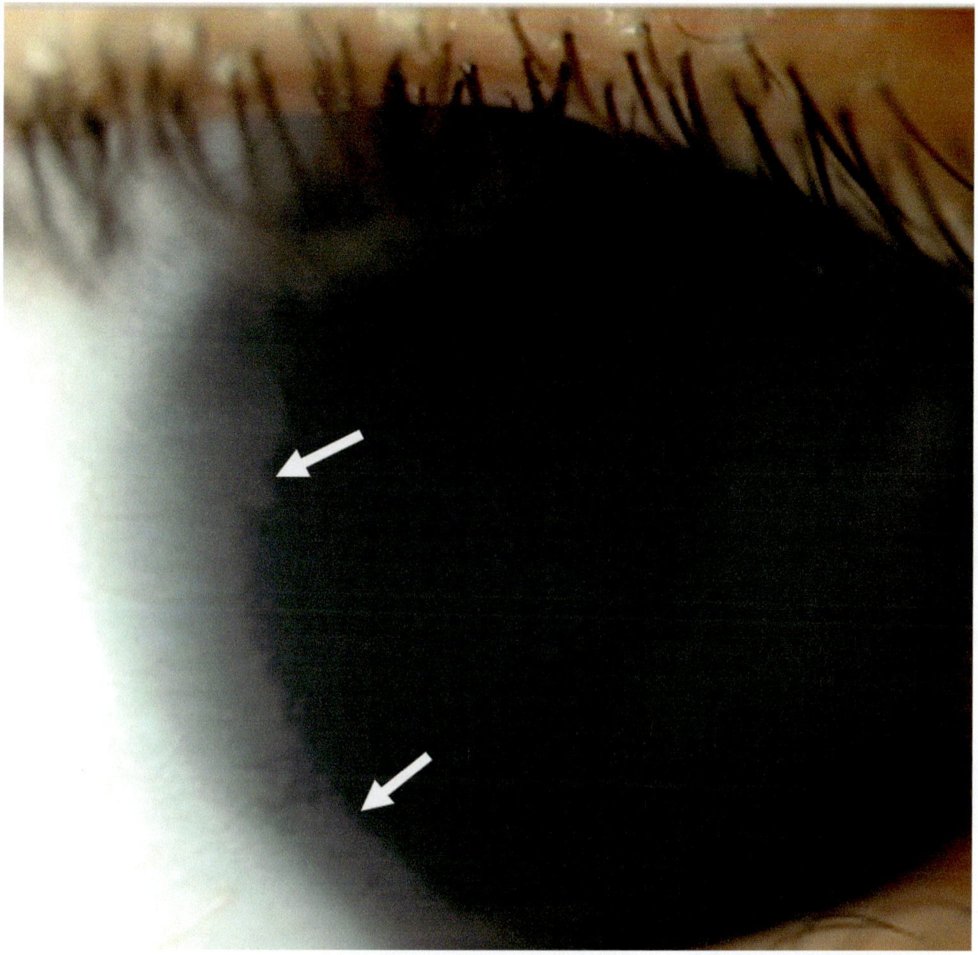

Fig. 79 8-year-old girl, OD. **AAK grade 2**: broadened pannus reaching centripetally (see arrows), but limited to outer 1/3 of cornea, beginning slight vascularization

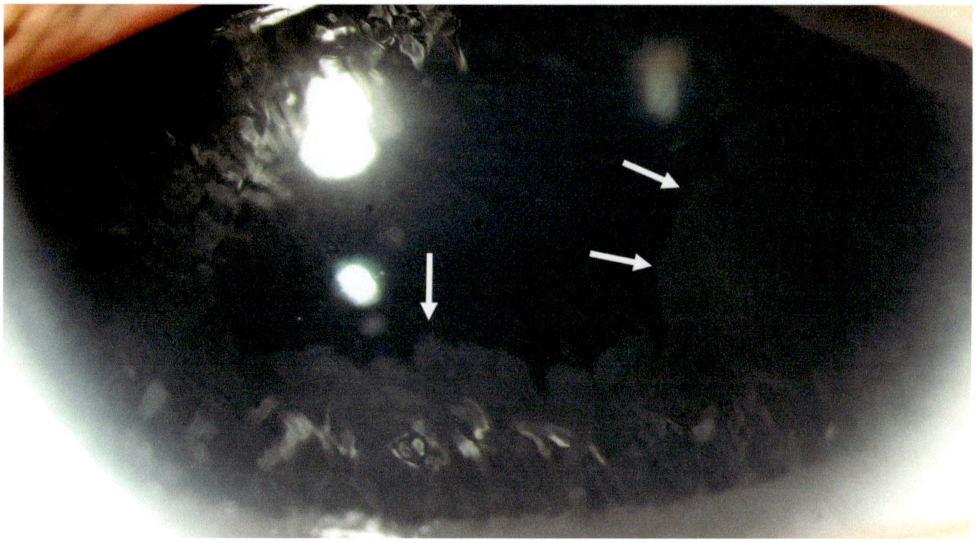

Fig. 80 9-year-old boy, OD, complete aniridia. AAK grade 2 to 3: large pannus formation, which exceeds the outer 1/3rd of the cornea especially nasally (see arrows). Still only beginning vascularization

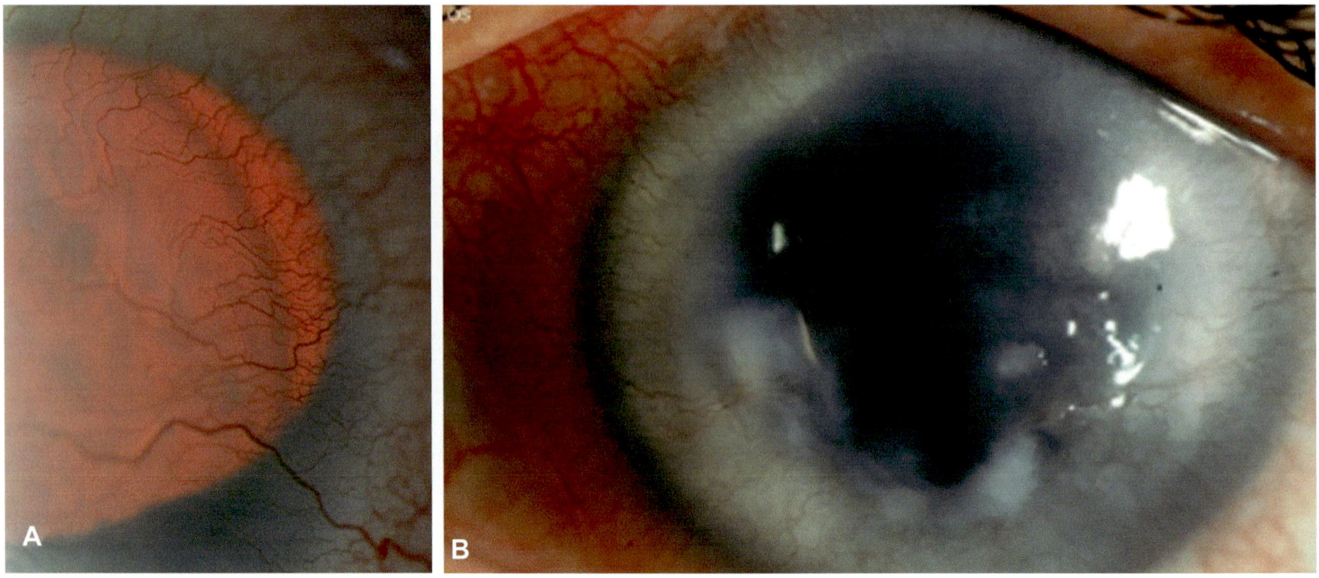

Fig. 81 2 patients with **AAK grade 3.** (**A**) 11-year-old girl, OS. Retroillumination: AAK grade 3 with distinct vascularizations, center of the cornea still clear. (**B**) 38-year-old female, OS. Grade 3 AAK with centripetally progressive vascularized pannus. In addition, typical finding in PAX6 aniridia: Salzmann nodules especially nasally and inferiorly

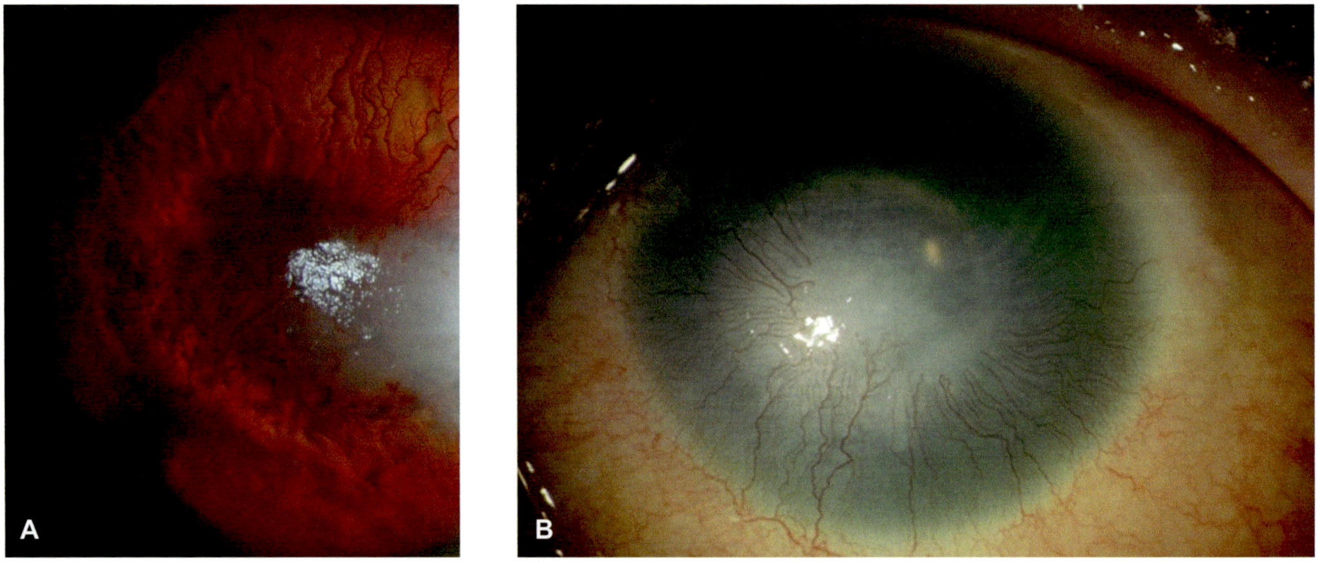

Fig. 82 2 patients with **AAK grade 4.** (**A**) 36-year-old male, OD. Retroillumination: AAK grade 4 with distinct vascularizations and central opacification of the cornea. Typical for aniridia (see center of the image): severe DED / Sicca. VA: hand motion. (**B**) 43-year-old female, OS: centripetally progressive vascularized pannus with opacification of the center of the cornea. VA: hand motion

clouding. Keratoplasty can be a beneficial intervention for patients with corneal opacification and should be considered if vision is impaired or view of the fundus precludes sufficient evaluation of the optic nerve and retina. Without systemic treatment, the graft may become opacified again, this can occur within one-year post-PKP. The efficacy of transplantation depends on the type of glycosaminoglycans (GAG) and severity of the opacification. Penetrating keratoplasty is the most performed technique, with variable success rates that can be as high as 94%.

The corneal opacification associated with MPS often is described as "matt or frosted glass". It is a diffuse, non-glare haze, which affects the entire cornea. The opacity is caused by the accumulation of GAGs in the cornea.

Lipid Metabolism Disorders: Disruptions in lipid metabolism can contribute to CCO, where abnormal

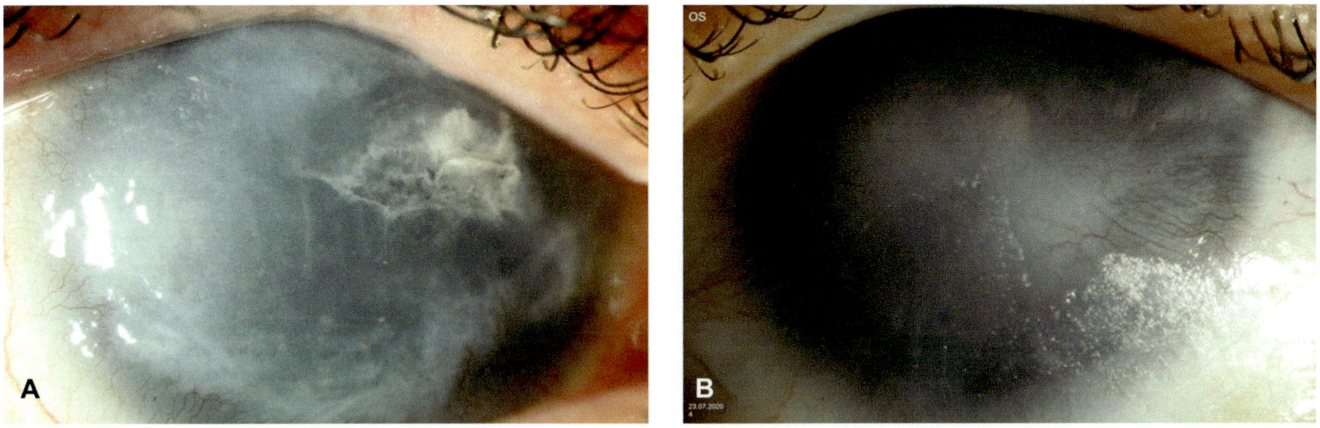

Fig. 83 2 other patients with **AAK grade 4.** (**A**) 41-year-old female, OD. AAK grade 4 with clearly less vascularizations, but deep calcifications and opaque corneal center. VA: hand motion. (**B**) 13-year-old girl, OS, WAGR(O) spectrum. Thin but overall present vascularizations, central opacification of the cornea. Typical for aniridia (see periphery of the image): severe DED / Sicca in spite of regular daily multifold treatment with autologous serum eye drops. VA: Light perception and localization

lipid deposition within the cornea leads to opacifications. Disorders such as lipid storage diseases may involve the accumulation of lipids in corneal tissues, impacting transparency. Recognition of lipid metabolism abnormalities through genetic testing and lipid analysis is essential for accurate diagnosis and appropriate management.

Corneal opacification due to lipid storage diseases can manifest as various patterns, including:

1. Ground/frosted glass opacification: This is the most common type, characterized by a diffuse, non-glare haze that affects the entire cornea. It is caused by the accumulation of abnormal lipids, such as gangliosides and globosides, in the corneal stroma.
2. Nucleated opacification: This pattern features small, round or oval opacities scattered throughout the cornea. It is associated with the accumulation of abnormal lipids in the corneal epithelium.
3. Spiculate opacification: This type presents as tiny, needle-like opacities that radiate outward from the corneal center and are confined to the epithelial layer. It is typically seen in Niemann–Pick type C disease where, however, the cherry red spot is the hallmark of the disease.
4. Cornea verticillate is the most consistent and most early disease of the lipid storage disease M. Fabry. Renal failure, peripheral neuropathy, and cardiovascular disease occur in the course of childhood.
5. Posterior corneal clouding: This type involves the accumulation of lipids in the posterior stroma or endothelium, causing a hazy appearance behind the iris.

Other Metabolic Pathways: Beyond MPS and lipid metabolism disorders, various metabolic pathways may influence corneal health. One further example is cystinosis (Fig. 100).

Cystinosis is a rare lysosomal storage disease. Cystine aggregates in all tissues and organs of the body. Usually, the infants first present with renal failure, but the ocular signs as cysteine crystals in the cornea (Fig. 100) and pigment retinopathy can aid to establish the diagnosis. The corneal deposits can be treated with cysteamine eye drops. Oral cysteamine is indicated in pigment retinopathy and all other systemic manifestations.

2.4.2 Traumatic Factors

Trauma, whether prenatal or postnatal, can contribute to corneal opacifications. In CCO, traumatic events during fetal development such as corneal perforation during amniocentesis may lead to intrauterine scar formation and corneal abnormalities (Fig. 101).

Intranatal injuries: Mechanical forces exerted on the eyes during delivery, especially in cases of difficult or prolonged labor, may cause corneal injuries. The severity of birth-related trauma can vary, ranging from mild corneal abrasions to more significant structural damage. Neonatal corneal opacifications may result from birth-related trauma (forceps damage) or external injuries (Fig. 102).

Postnatal Injuries: Postnatal trauma, such as accidental injuries or exposure to harmful substances, can contribute to corneal opacifications in both congenital and neonatal cases. The cornea's delicate structure makes it susceptible to damage from foreign bodies, chemical irritants, or mechanical trauma. Timely evaluation and appropriate treatment are essential to mitigate the impact of external injuries on corneal transparency and visual function. Figure 103 shows a Russian boy who had needed cardiothoracic surgery on his second day of life. Unfortunately, an exposition keratopathy developed during anaesthesia,

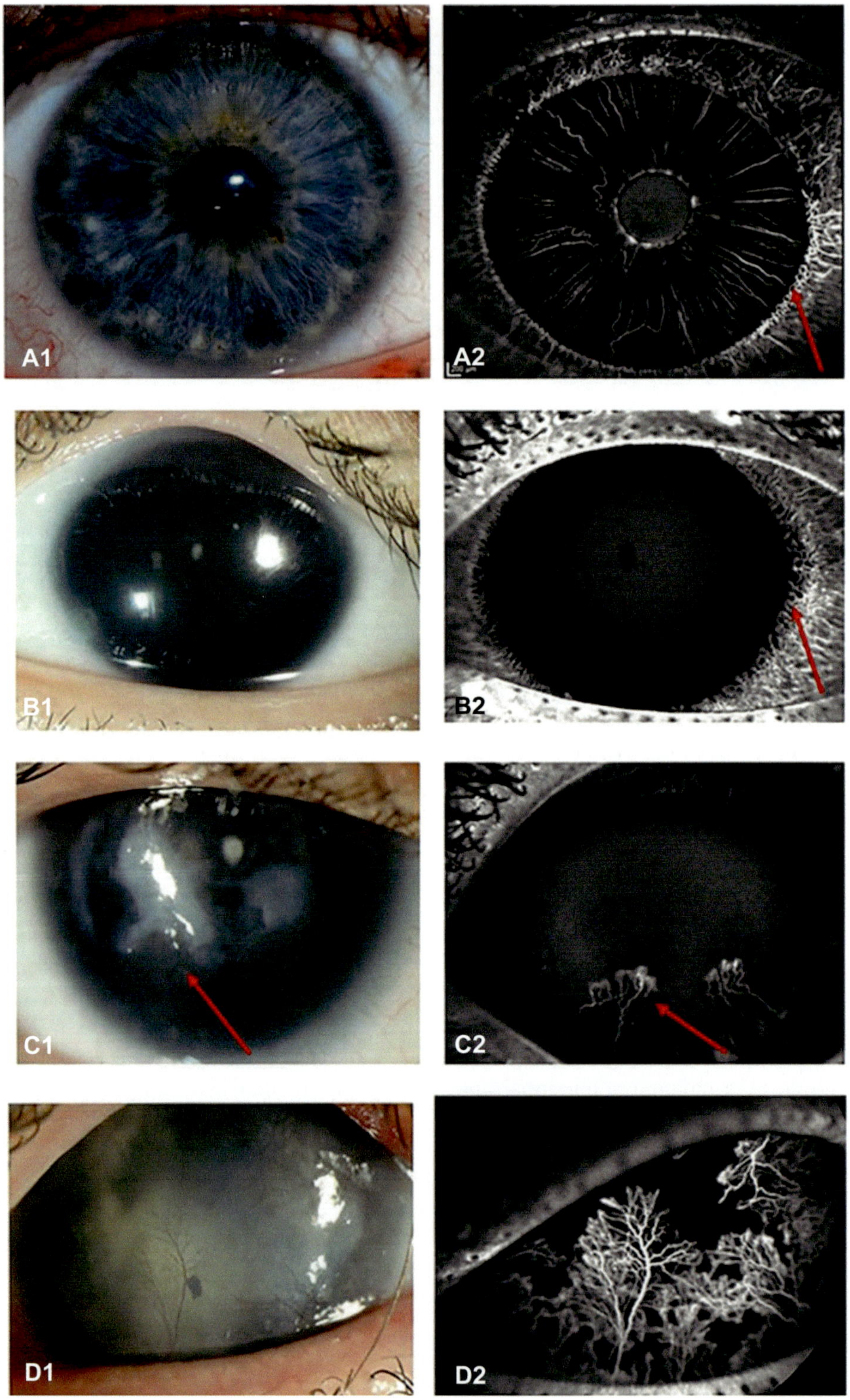

Fig. 84 Fluorescein angiographic imaging of the anterior segment in progressive AAK. (**A**) normal anterior segment angiography. (**B**) clinically very small pannus temporally at 8 o´clock. FAG: circular pannus with intense vascularizations. (**C**) AAK3 with Salzmann nodules. Not visible by biomicroscopy, distinct vessel invasion from inferior. (**D**) AAK4: The amount of dense, tree-like vascularizations only gets evident in FAG. This is a typical finding in anterior segment FAG in aniridia and AAK: the angiographic findings present the true dimension of pathological vessel invasions much more clearly than slit lamp biomicroscopy. Adapted with permission from: Käsmann-Kellner B et al. (2018) [65]

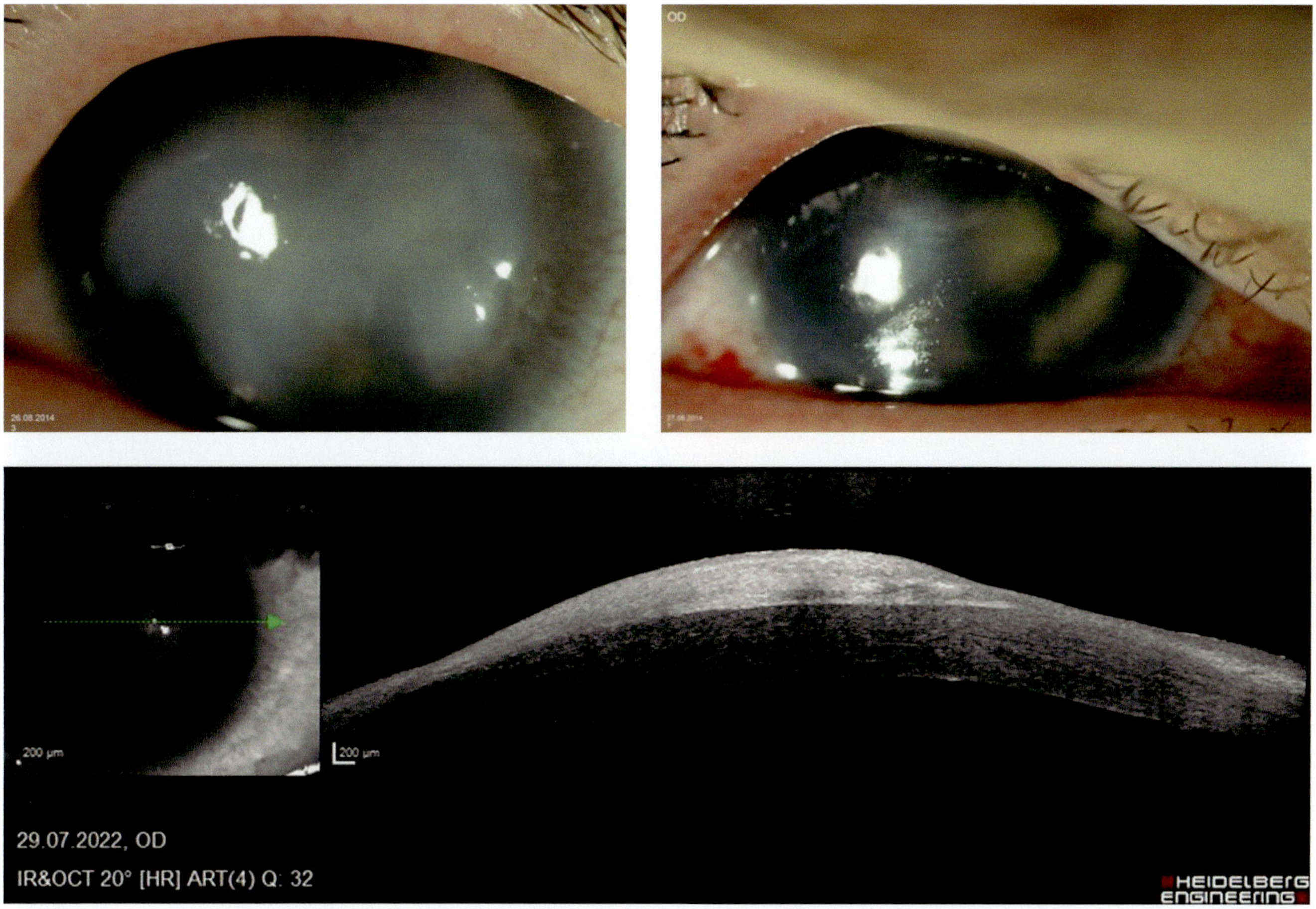

Fig. 85 Typical complication in aniridia: Salzmann nodules. Can be removed by pannectomy and PTK. Upper row: pre- and post-PTK findings. VA improved from hand motion to dec 0.1p. Lower image: preoperative anterior segment OCT showing the Salzmann nodules mounted with clear distinction from the cornea

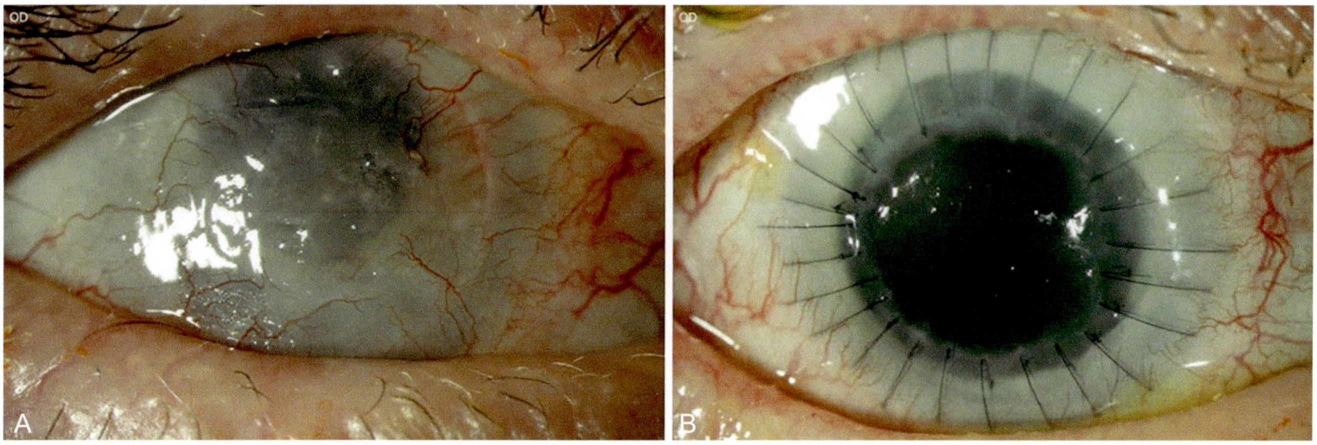

Fig. 86 Possible therapeutic approach in AAK grade 4: Homburg aniridia scheme for penetrating keratoplasty PKP [74, 84]: postoperative coverage with amniotic membrane, lateral tarsorrhaphy for 4 weeks, autologous serum eye drops 6x/daily and systemic immunosuppression. (**A**) PAX6 aniridia, female patient, aged 45 years, had previous PKP. Preoperative AAK grade 4. VA: hand motion. (**B**) Same patient, 6 months postoperatively after repeat PKP, opened lateral tarsorrhaphy. VA: dec 0.1

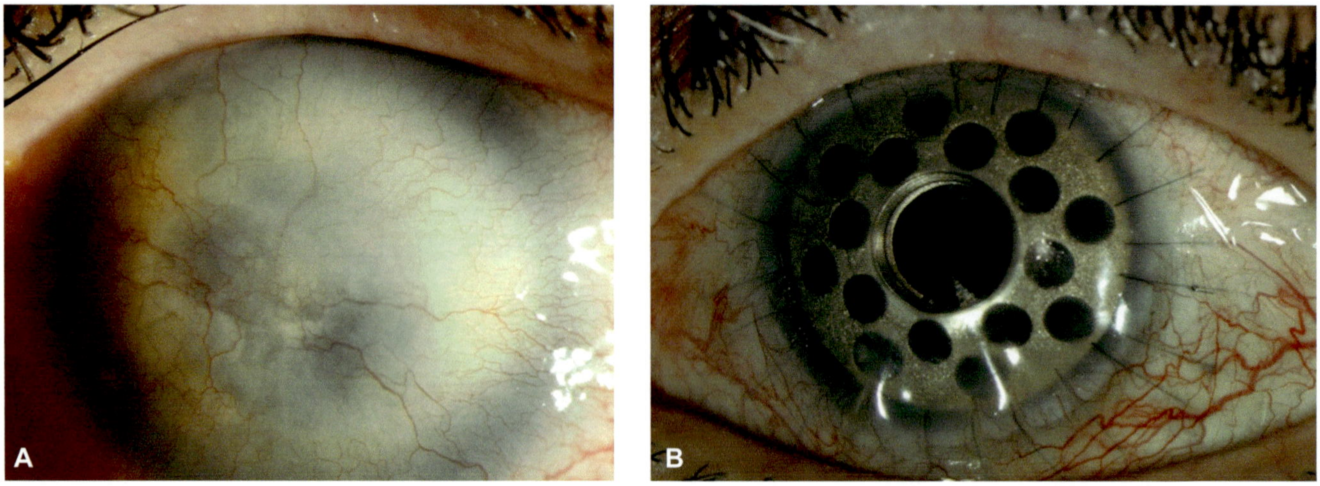

Fig. 87 Possible therapeutic approach in AAK grade 4: Boston keratoprothesis. (**A**) PAX6 aniridia, female patient from Italy. Preoperative AAK grade 4. VA: light perception (**B**) Same patient, 8 months postoperatively, VA: dec 0.1. Patient is able to read again with magnification. In Boston KPro: take care to monitor the IOP!

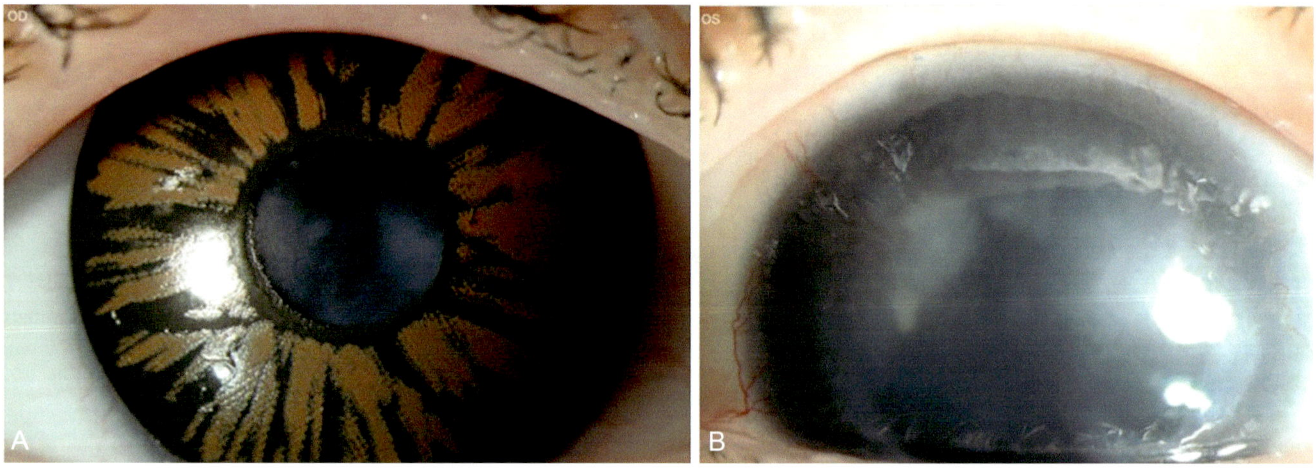

Fig. 88 Aggravation of AAK by using iris-print contact lenses. (**A**) PAX6 aniridia, male patient, aged 18. Iris print contact lens OD in situ. (**B**) Same patient, without iris print contact lens, OS. Grade 3 AAK, DED symptoms. Note the pigmented margin near the limbus, iris print contact lenses loose pigment, which will incorporate into the ocular surface and worsen AAK

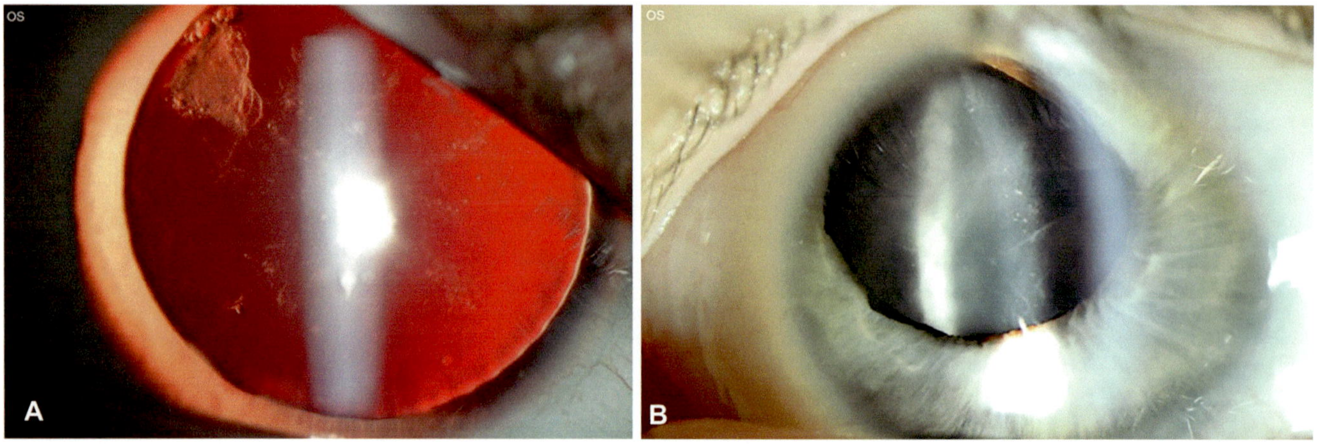

Fig. 89 Cataract formation as a complication in PAX6 aniridia. (**A**) 12-year-old boy, OS, cortical and subcapsularis posterior cataract in complete aniridia, retroillumination. (**B**) 8-year-old girl, OS, progressive cortical cataract formation in partial aniridia

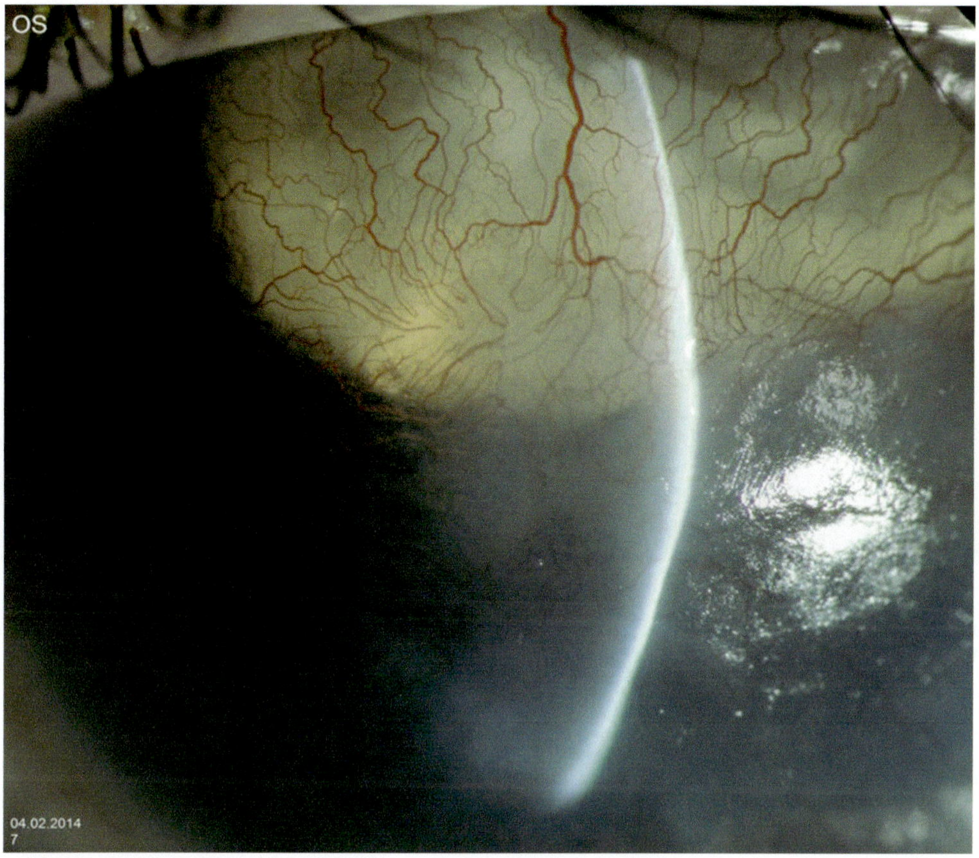

Fig. 90 15-year-old girl, OS: Subluxated cataractous lens, dense opacification of the lens, severe AAK, DED, absolute glaucoma. Due to consistent pain, the eye had to be enucleated [60]

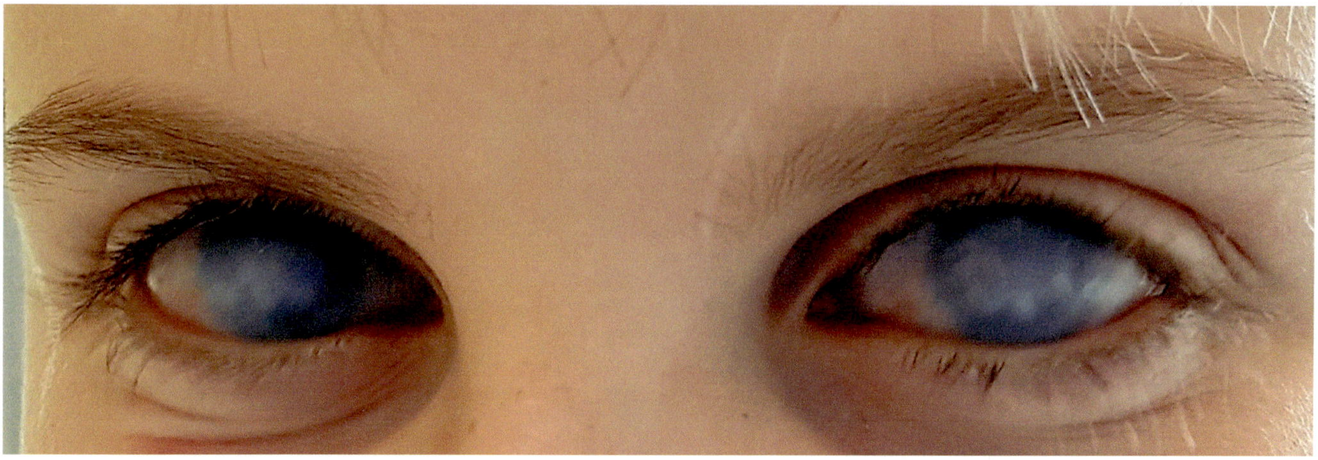

Fig. 91 2.5-year-old boy, CCO in PAX6 aniridia. The child was born with massively elevated IOP and cloudy corneas. First presentation in our hospital aged 2.5 years, externally he had already had multiple cyclophotocoagulations, which should be avoided in aniridic glaucoma

followed by the formation of a deep ulcus. In Moscow, 2 conjunctival coverages were performed, resulting in a thick vascularized corneal scar.

2.4.3 Non-Infectious Causes

A myriad of non-infectious factors can contribute to congenital corneal opacifications. This includes genetic

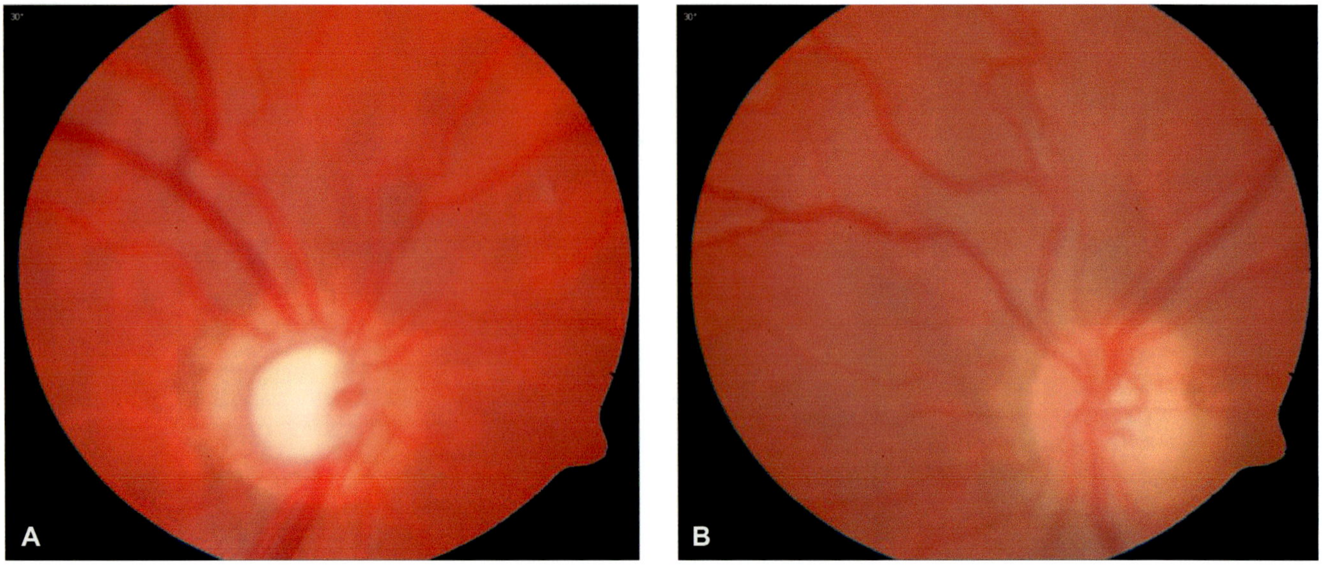

Fig. 92 Asymmetric secondary aniridia glaucoma in a 3-year-old boy with PAX6 mutation (difficult photo documentation due to age and beginning cortical cataract). (**A**) OD: progressive glaucomatous cup deepening, IOD 28–30 (Icare®). (**B**) OS: no glaucomatous changes can be seen, optic nerve head (ONH) has a normal aspect, IOP 14 (iCare®)

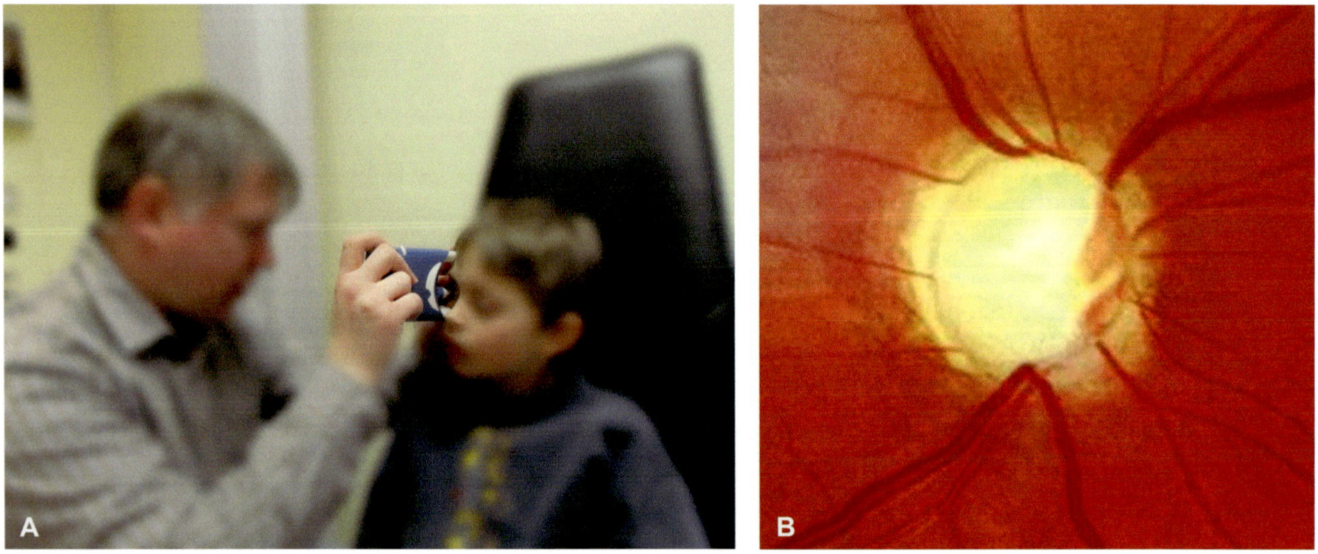

Fig. 93 9-year-old boy, bilateral secondary aniridic glaucoma in PAX6 haploinsufficiency—same problem with mother, legal blindness due to secondary glaucoma and AAK in spite of repeat PK and Boston KPro. (**A**) Father demonstrating the home care measurement of IOP by hand-held patient's Icare®. (**B**) Major secondary glaucomatous change in the optic nerve head with distinct optic atropy, legal blindness

abnormalities (see above), structural defects, and developmental anomalies.

Developmental Anomalies: Aberrations in ocular development during embryogenesis can contribute to corneal opacifications. Developmental anomalies affecting adjacent structures, such as the anterior chamber, iris or lids (Fig. 104).

One other cause of non-infectious NCO should be mentioned: radiation-induced corneal lesions (Fig. 105), which can cause persistent superficial corneal defects and has a high danger of superinfection and of the formation of ulcers.

2.4.4 Infectious Keratitis

Infections, whether congenital or acquired postnatally, pose a significant risk for corneal opacifications. This section will discuss the role of pathogens such as bacteria,

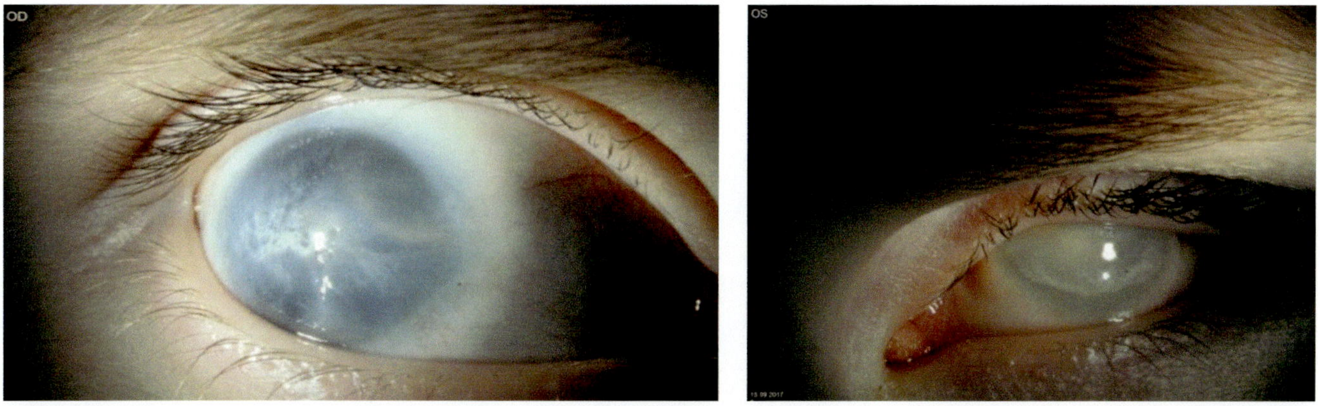

Fig. 94 10-year-old boy from Russia. In PAX6 haploinsufficiency the left image shows the OD, with AAK grade 4 (fibrotic scars, center involved, unusual: only few vascularizations), in addition elevated IOP and buphthalmia. OS shows AFS post-cataract surgery in Russia, anamnestically developed over a time of 6 months. Unfortunately, he had received systemic steroids for all the time and now presented with secondary Cushing disease and severe overweight. No surgical option for OS, NLP

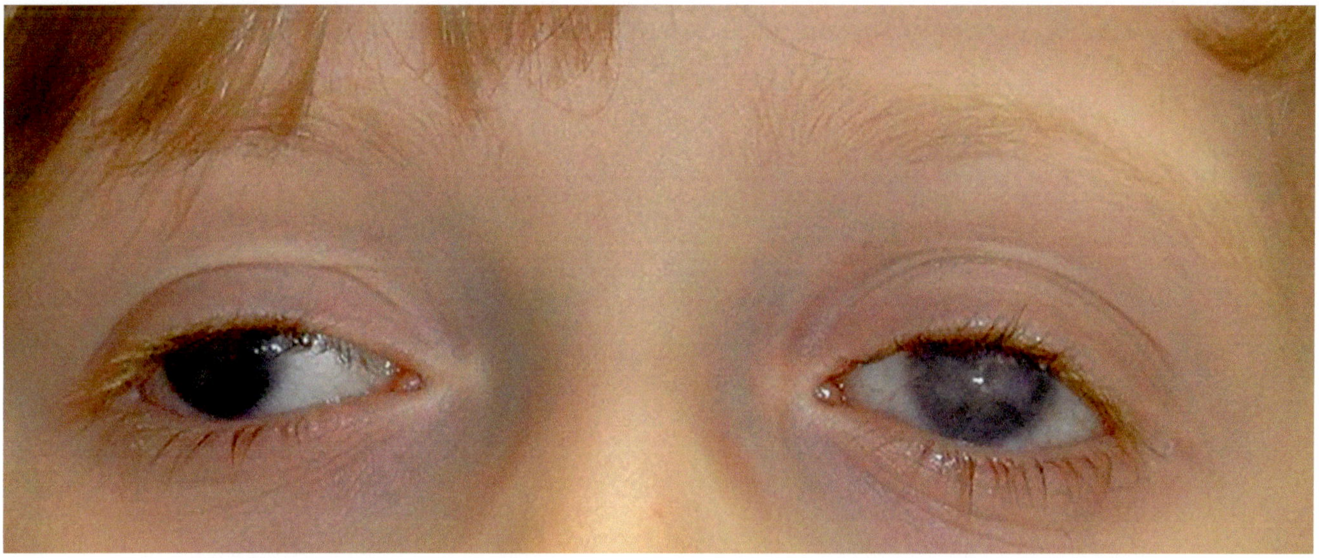

Fig. 95 6-year-old boy, WAGR Syndrome (Wilms Tumor, aniridia, genitourethral anomalies, and retardation). OD AAK grade 3, OS AAK grade 4, NCO present. Severe secondary glaucoma since age 2. The boy has had surgery and chemotherapy at age 2 due to nephroblastoma (Wilms Tumor)

viruses, and fungi in causing corneal infections in neonates. Additionally, it will explore the implications of maternal infections during pregnancy on fetal corneal development.

Infective causes contribute significantly to corneal opacifications in both congenital and neonatal cases, posing unique challenges for diagnosis and management. This summary provides a short overview of the infective factors associated with infectious corneal lesions, highlighting the specific pathogens involved and their clinical manifestations.

Bacterial Infections: Congenital corneal opacifications (CCO) and neonatal corneal opacifications (NCO) can result from bacterial infections, with pathogens such as Staphylococcus aureus, Streptococcus species, and Haemophilus influenzae being common pathogens. Bacterial keratitis may present with corneal infiltrates, ulcerations, and purulent discharge. Hyperacute conjunctivitis is primarily due to Neisseria gonorrhoeae (Fig. 106), which is a sexually transmitted disease. Gonorrhoea infection can lead to a melting of the cornea and quick perforation (Fig. 106). Neisseria meningitidis is also in the differential and is important to consider as it can lead to potentially fatal meningeal or systemic infection. It has become rare in these days, but one should especially think of this possibly in freshly migrated persons. An examination with a gynaecological smear test is obligatory.

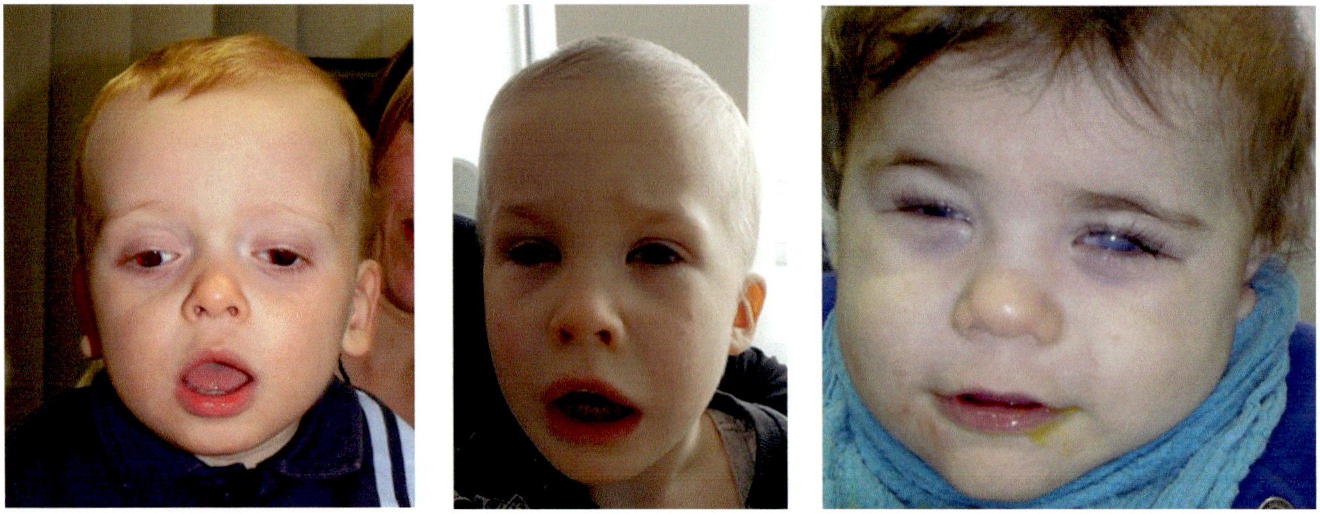

Fig. 96 Imaging with permission of all 6 parents. Typical phenotype of 3 children with WAGR syndrome. All children show hypotonia with open mouth, saliva dribbling, anteverted nares and low-set ears. Left: Boy, aged 17 months (same boy as in Fig. 100), developed nephroblastoma aged 2 years. Middle: Boy, aged 14 months, at the time of the photo under pre-surgical chemotherapy and loss of hair. Right eye: prothesis in place due to phthisis in the course of AFS following surgery to congenital cataract in Poland. Right: Boy, aged 18 months, up to now no nephroblastoma. Right eye phthisis bulbi following AFS post-surgery for glaucoma. Left eye: decompensated cornea due to secondary glaucoma

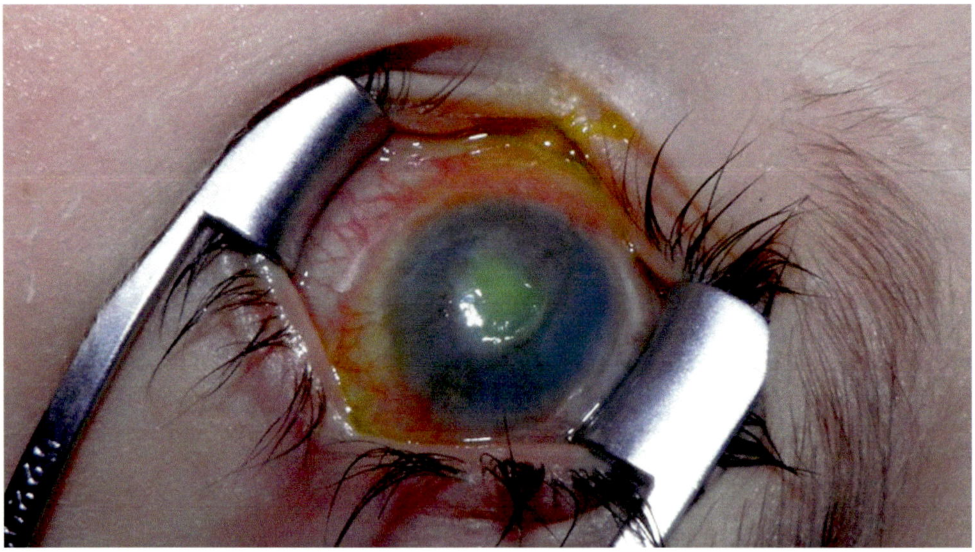

Fig. 97 3-year-old boy, WAGR syndrome. Very early onset of AAK at 8 months, now grade 4 AAK with central deep corneal ulceration

Viral Infections: Herpes simplex virus (HSV) and varicella zoster virus (VZV) are notable viral pathogens associated with corneal opacifications in neonates. Herpetic keratitis may present with deep stromal opacification (Fig. 107). Within the first year of life, a herpetic infection might manifest with dendritic or geographic corneal ulcers and vascularizations, often accompanied by photophobia and tearing (Fig. 108).

Fungal Infections: Fungal keratitis, caused by organisms like Candida and Aspergillus, can lead to corneal opacifications, particularly in neonates with compromised immune systems. Clinical manifestations may include corneal infiltrates, feathery edges, and satellite lesions. Antifungal therapy is necessary for managing fungal infections and preventing the progression of corneal damage.

Clinical Considerations: Diagnosing infective causes of corneal opacifications involves a thorough examination, including slit-lamp biomicroscopy and, when necessary, corneal cultures or polymerase chain reaction (PCR)

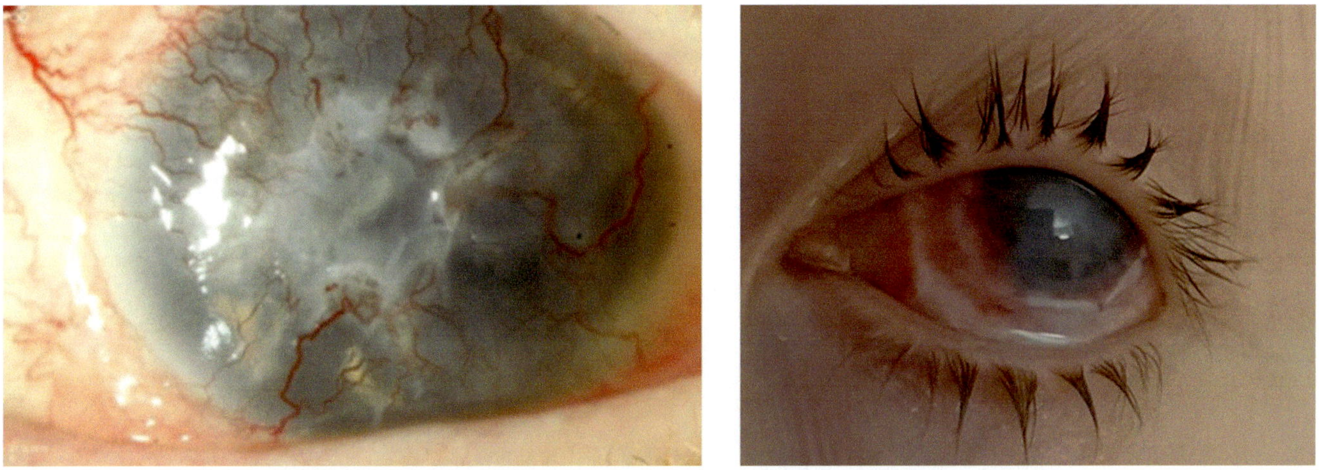

Fig. 98 12-year-old boy, WAGR(O). Left image: preoperative extensive grade 4 AAK with central fibrous scars and deep vascularization. Right image: 1 week post-allogenic limbal stem cell transplantation, lamellar keratectomy and deep anterior lamellar keratoplasty, tenon-conjunctival plastic. Amnion membrane patch and bandage contact lens in situ

Table 8 Grouped etiologies of secondarily acquired CCO and NCO

Acquired Corneal Diseases with congenital or neonatal onset	
1. Metabolic	
a. Mucopolysaccharidoses	a. Often syndromatic aspect (see NGP)
b. Cystinosis	b. Crystalline deposits, severe photophobia
c. Mucolipidoses	c. Often pediatric pathologies
2. Traumatic	
a. Forceps delivery with ocular injury	a. Striae: ruptures of Descemet membrane
3. Infectious Keratitis	
a. Bacterial (Gonococcal)	a. to c. in CCO, mostly related to natural birth. Always test the mother as well with genital smear and laboratory diagnostics
b. Viral (Herpes)	
c. Fungal	
4. Non-infectious Keratitis	
a. Lagophthalmos/exposure	a. Congenital N VII paresis, lid coloboma
b. Neurotrophic	b. Brain malformation with affection of N III
c. Steven–Johnson syndrome	c. Rare in CCO and NCO
d. Epidermolysis bullosa	d. Corneal involvement possible very early
5. Others	
a. Xeroderma pigmentosum	a. Photokeratitis, Bitot spots possible
b. Keratoglobus	b. Form anomaly (see NGP), CO later
c. Keratoconus (only > 3 years)	c. Corneal opacification rare in infancy

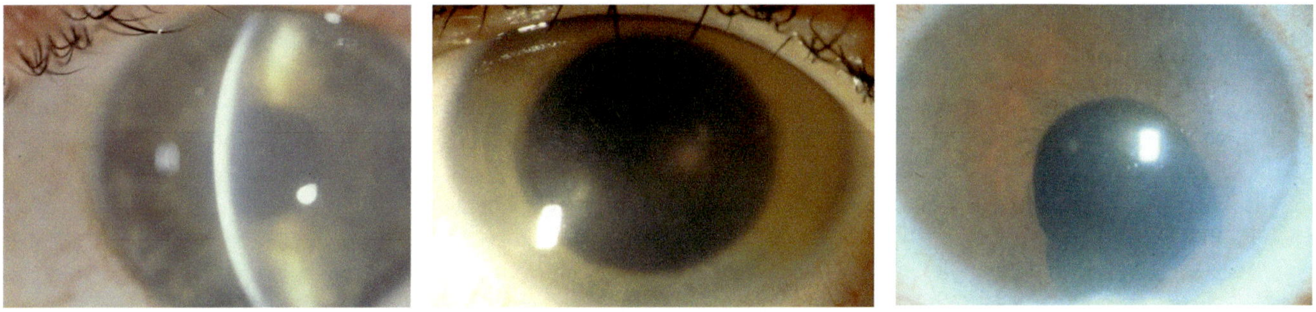

Fig. 99 Mucopolysaccharidoses (MPS) with secondary acquired CCO or NCO. Left image: MPS IS (Scheie). Middle image: MPS IH (Hunter). Right image: MPS IV (Maroteaux–Lamy), plus inferior Iris coloboma, not related to MPS IV

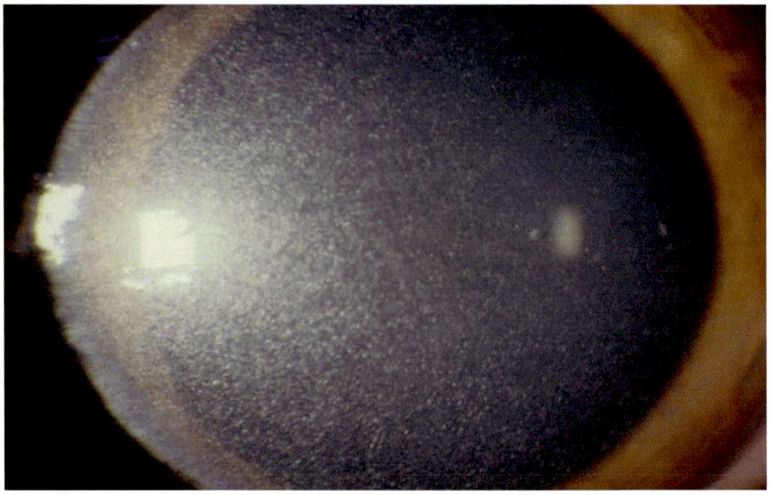

Fig. 100 Toddler, 2 years. Severe glare sensitivity. Due to early renal insufficiency cystinosis had already been diagnosed and could be confirmed by the dense crystalline corneal deposits

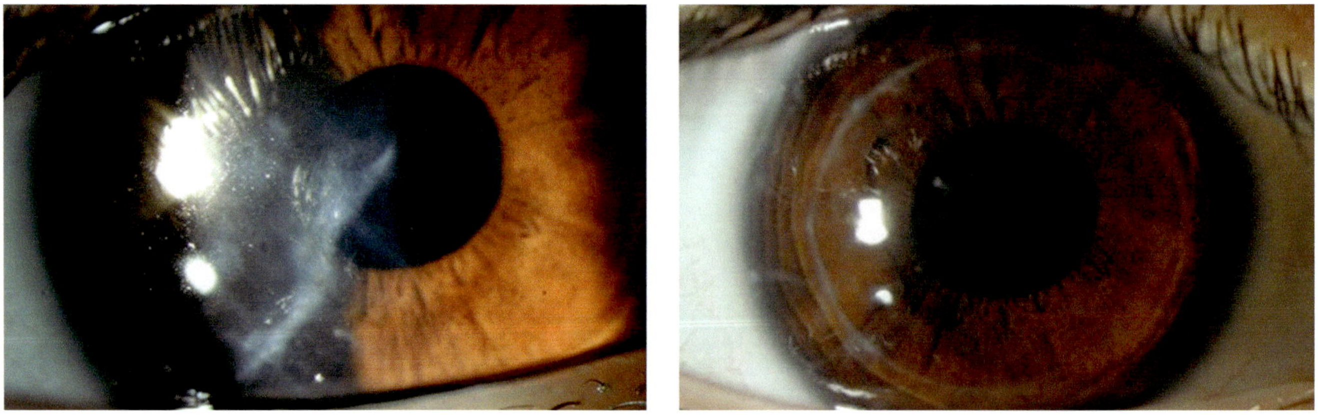

Fig. 101 Boy, first presentation in our hospital at age 8 years. Left image: CCO due to traumatic incident with perforation of the cornea during amniocentesis in utero. Right image: Clinical finding 2 years after PKP. In spite of many efforts, amblyopia treatment was not successful any more

testing. In neonates, consideration should be given to maternal history, potential exposure during birth, and systemic signs of infection. Collaboration with infectious disease specialists is valuable for comprehensive management.

In conclusion, infective causes of congenital and neonatal corneal opacifications encompass bacterial, viral, and fungal infections. Recognizing the specific pathogens involved and understanding their clinical manifestations is crucial for targeted antimicrobial or antiviral therapy. Early intervention is key to preserving corneal clarity and minimizing the impact of infective causes on visual function in affected infants.

2.4.5 Other Causes for CCO and NCO

Autoimmune Conditions: Certain autoimmune disorders may present with ocular manifestations, including corneal opacifications in neonates. Conditions such as autoimmune keratitis or immune-mediated inflammatory diseases may lead to corneal changes. Collaborating with rheumatologists and immunologists is essential for a thorough evaluation and tailored treatment strategies.

Neurological Disorders: Congenital and neonatal corneal opacifications may be associated with neurological disorders affecting the visual pathways (e.g. N. VII palsy and lagophthalmia). Neuroimaging studies and neurologic assessments are critical components of the diagnostic process in these cases.

Environmental Factors: Exposure to certain environmental factors during fetal development or early infancy may contribute to corneal opacifications. These factors can include maternal drug use, toxins, or environmental pollutants. Identification of such exposures requires a detailed history and collaboration with specialists in maternal–fetal medicine or environmental health.

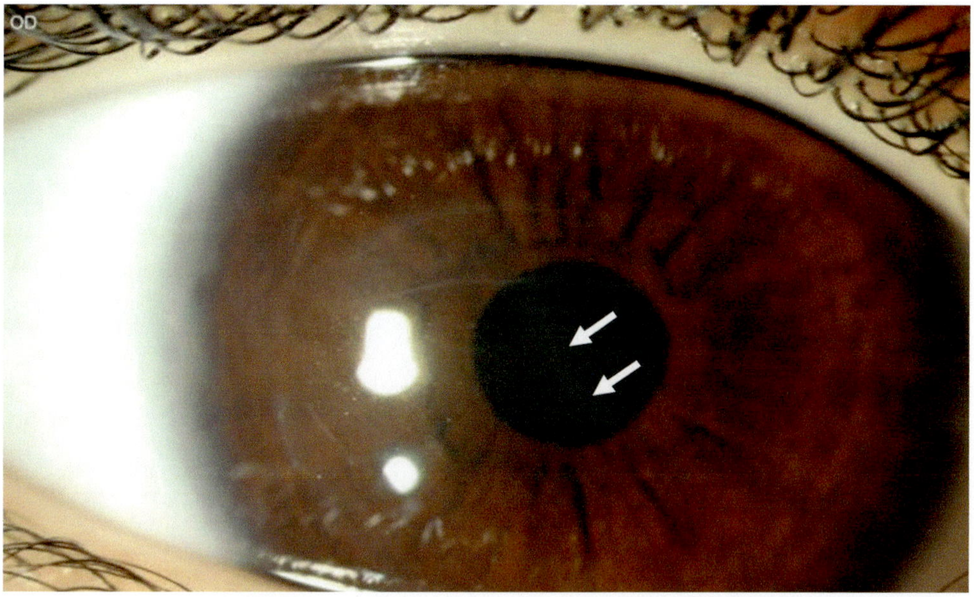

Fig. 102 2-year-old girl. NCO following prolonged birth labor and forceps delivery, resulting in atypical ruptures in Descemet membrane. In addition, the child developed secondary glaucoma

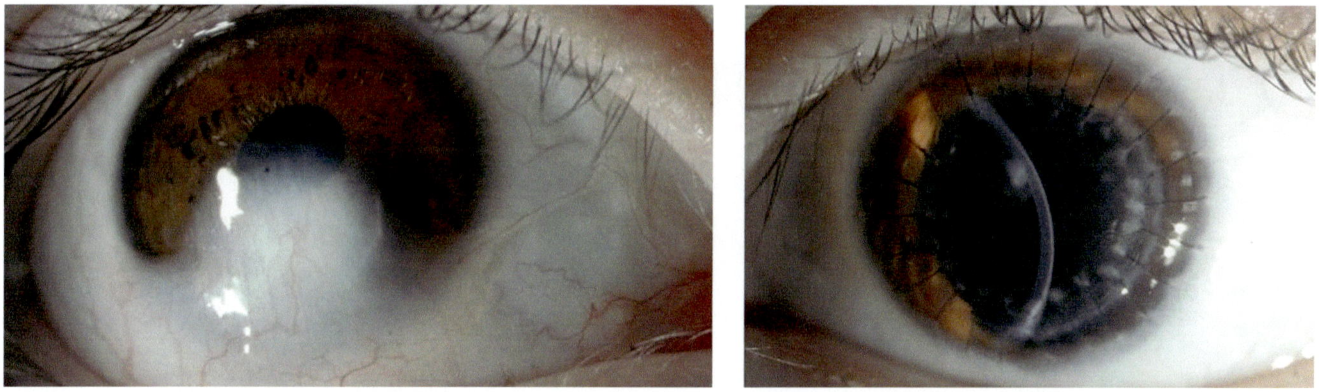

Fig. 103 1-year-old Russian boy, anamnestically had a severe congenital corneal ulcer due to lagophthalmia during anaesthesia at his 2nd day of life. Left image: Externally 2 conjunctival coverages were performed. Right image: same boy following penetrating excimer laser-assisted keratoplasty with single sutures still in place

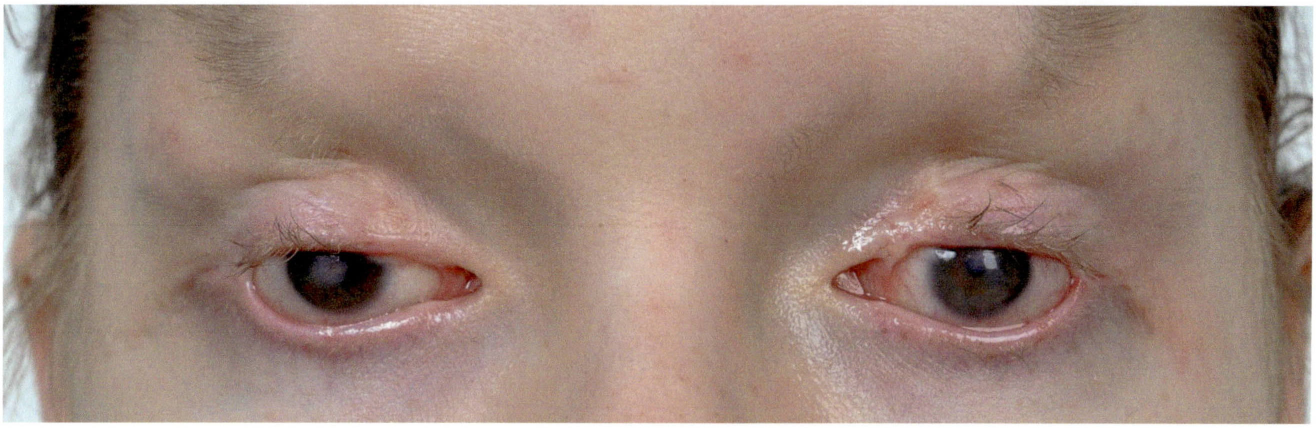

Fig. 104 Girl, now 16 years old. She was born without any upper eyelids up to and partially including the brows. On the second day of life, a bilateral Tenzel plastic was performed (mobilization of the temporal skin and trying to form a lid replacement). Already on the second day, central erosions could be observed in spite of ointment. During childhood, recurrent erosiones had to be treated frequently. Around the 6th year of life a fuctional metaplasia could be observed: she started to develop a „lid " closure and developed lashes. Due to dense corneal central scars she now is planned for keratoplasty. Symblephara nasally OS makes the surgical approach more difficult

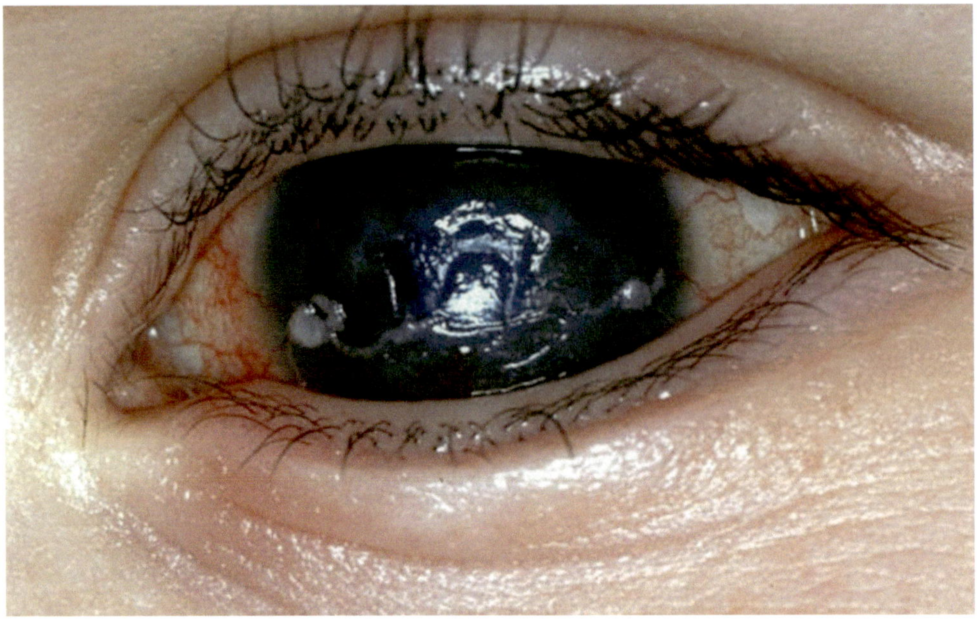

Fig. 105 1-year-old boy: OS severe epithelial lesions with beginning ulcus formation during radiation treatment due to neuroblastoma. In the further course a vascularized scar developed in the left eye, the right eye was less severely affected

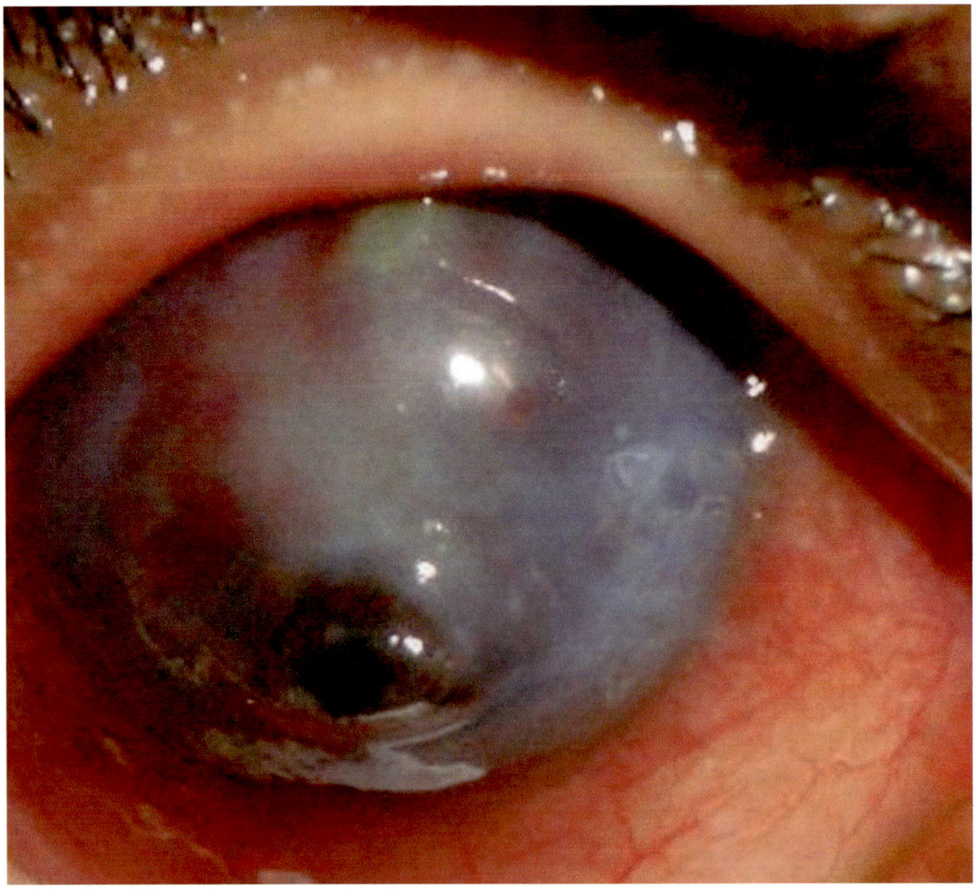

Fig. 106 Male baby, 3 days old, vaginal delivery. Hyperacute keratitis in Neisseria gonorrhoeae infection with perforation and iris prolaps at 6, immanent perforations in the periphery at 12 and in the middle periphery at 2 o'clock

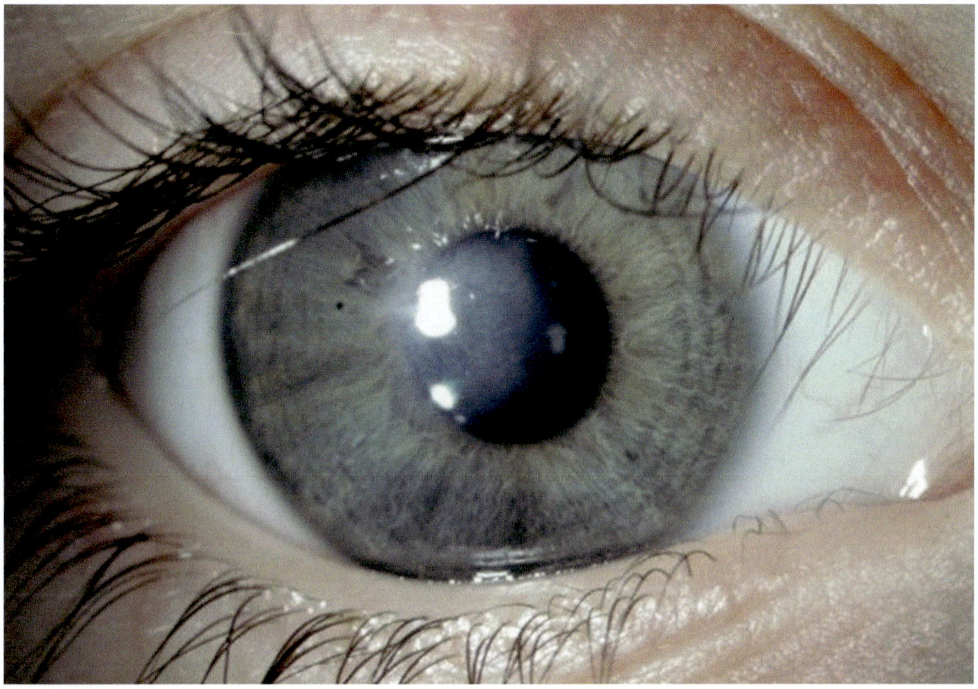

Fig. 107 Girl, now 12 months old. OD herpetic paracentral unilateral neonatal partial opacification. Opacification developed between 3rd and 4th month. Typical presentation of deep stromal herpetic keratitis. OS completely normal

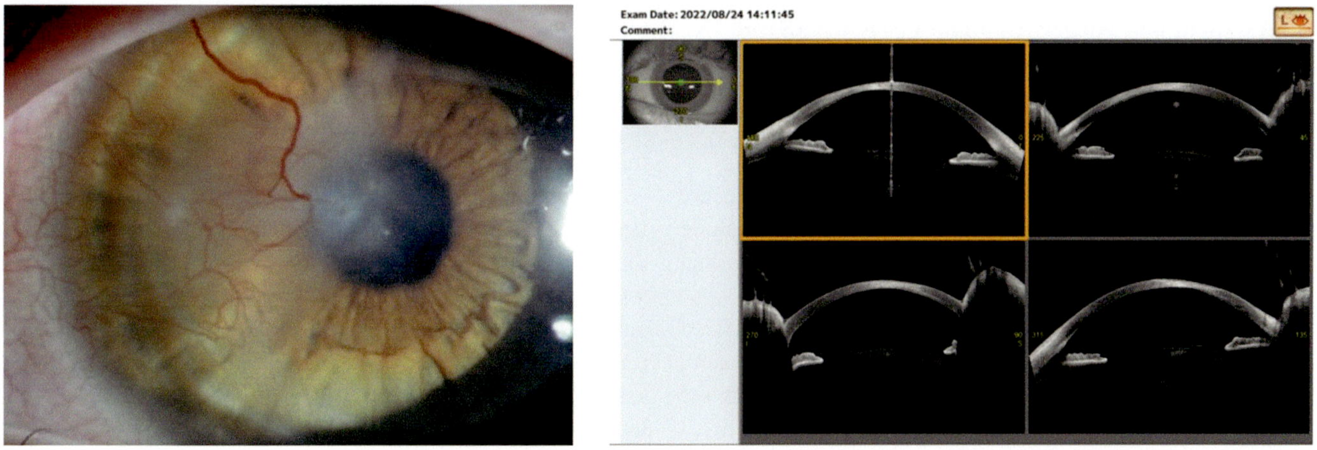

Fig. 108 NCO. Boy, aged 3 years now, developed a grayish scar of the cornea of the left eye during the first year of life. Parents presented the boy aged 2 years as they had noticed vascularizations in the opacified area. Diagnosis: herpetic corneal infection. Left image: clinical presentation, right image: anterior segment OCT with obvious thinning of the cornea in the areas of the scar

2.5 Next Generation Genotyping NGS

Although PAX6 gene is the most important gene in classical aniridia and other anterior segment dysgenesis, there are other genes, which should be evaluated if the examination of PAX6 does not yield any results.

The emphasis is on the importance of **Next Generation Sequencing (NGS)** in cases where traditional indicators do not lead to a definitive diagnosis.

The NGP classification system provides a comprehensive framework for understanding eye and facial anomalies, aiding in the identification of underlying syndromes, and guiding medical professionals towards accurate diagnoses and treatments.

The following is a list of the most important genes involved in anterior segment abnormalities [102]:

1. **PAX6 Mutations:** Mutations in the PAX6 gene can lead to aniridia, a condition characterized by the absence of the iris. These mutations can result from different mechanisms, including deletions of 11p13, disruption of the regulatory region of PAX6, or intragenic mutations. Aniridia can present with various ocular consequences such as glaucoma, cataract, macular hypoplasia, nystagmus, and limbal stem cell deficiency. Missense mutations, particularly in the DNA-binding paired domain of PAX6, can cause milder and variable phenotypes, leading to atypical forms of aniridia and related disorders.
2. **WT1 and WAGR(O) Syndrome:** Some individuals may have contiguous gene deletions of 11p13, affecting both PAX6 and the nearby WT1 gene, leading to Wilms tumor, aniridia, genitourinary abnormalities, and mental retardation (WAGR) syndrome.
3. **Other Genes Associated with Iris Abnormalities:** In addition to PAX6, other genes like PITX2, FOXC1, CYP1B1, COL4A1, and CPAMD8 have been associated with iris hypoplasia, corectopia, and polycoria.
4. **Axenfeld and Rieger Anomalies (ARA/ARS):** PITX2 and FOXC1 are the primary genes involved in ARA. Mutations in these genes can cause classic ARA and other related conditions like aniridia and primary congenital glaucoma.
5. **Alagille Syndrome:** Mutations in the JAG1 gene are associated with Alagille syndrome, which can include posterior embryotoxon, optic disc drusen, and retinal pigmentary changes.
6. **SHORT Syndrome:** SHORT syndrome is characterized by short stature, hyperextensibility, ocular depression, Rieger anomaly, and teething delay. Mutations in the PIK3R1 gene are responsible for this syndrome.
7. **Primary** Congenital **Glaucoma (PCG):** The main gene associated with PCG is CYP1B1, particularly in inbred populations. LTBP2 and FOXC1 have also been implicated in PCG, with some ethnic-specific associations. Other genes like TEK and ANGPT1 may also contribute to PCG in some cases.
8. **Peters Anomaly (PA):** PA is genetically heterogeneous and can result from mutations in genes such as PAX6, PITX2, FOXC1, PITX3, FOXE3, CYP1B1, B3GLCT (Peters Plus syndrome), and COL4A1. The lens development plays a critical role in the development of the anterior segment, and interrupted lens development can lead to various anterior segment abnormalities.
9. **FOXE3 and PITX3 Mutations:** Mutations in FOXE3 can result in a range of anterior segment abnormalities, with heterozygous mutations often associated with milder conditions, while homozygous or compound heterozygous mutations lead to more severe ocular phenotypes. FOXE3 mutations can also be linked to glaucoma.
10. **PITX3 Mutations:** Mutations in PITX3 are associated with PA, variable anterior segment abnormalities, and cataracts. A recurrent 17-bp insertion in PITX3 can cause congenital cataracts and other anterior segment abnormalities.
11. **Sclerocornea, Microphthalmia, and GJA8 Mutations:** Mutations in the GJA8 gene, usually linked to congenital cataracts, have been associated with sclerocornea, rudimentary lenses, and microphthalmia, highlighting the lens' importance in anterior segment development.

3 Conclusion

Acquired congenital corneal opacifications and neonatal corneal opacifications encompass a broad spectrum of clinical entities, each with distinct aetiological factors. By categorizing these conditions based on genetic, metabolic, traumatic, non-infectious, infectious, and other causes, this chapter aimed to enhance the understanding of ophthalmologists and researchers in the field, highlighting the progressive and highly complicated PAX6 aniridia. A comprehensive approach to diagnosis and management is essential for optimizing outcomes in patients with CCO and NCO.

Diagnosing congenital and neonatal corneal opacifications due to less conventional causes necessitates a multidisciplinary approach. Ophthalmologists should collaborate with specialists in pediatrics, rheumatology, neurology, and genetics to ensure a comprehensive evaluation. Advanced imaging techniques, genetic testing, and detailed clinical assessments are integral to identifying these diverse etiological factors.

Comprehensive management of congenital corneal anomalies involves a multidisciplinary approach, often necessitating collaboration between ophthalmologists, geneticists, and pediatric specialists. Additionally, early diagnosis through meticulous clinical evaluation, corneal imaging techniques, and genetic testing plays a crucial role in facilitating timely and effective interventions, thus optimizing visual outcomes and overall quality of life for patients with congenital corneal anomalies. Treatment options may include medical intervention, surgical correction, or, in some cases, corneal transplantation to improve visual function and ensure appropriate ocular development in affected individuals.

References

1. Herwig-Carl MC, Loeffler KU, Müller AM. Importance of investigation of fetal eyes: supplement to fetal autopsy. Pathologe. 2017;38(4):231–40.
2. Käsmann-Kellner B, Moslemani K, Seitz B. Clinical and genetic characteristics of ocular developmental disorders: MAC-spectrum, anterior segment dysgenesis. Klin Monbl Augenheilkd. 2019;236(3):269–85.
3. Amendt BA. The molecular mechanisms of Axenfeld-Rieger syndrome. Springer, New York; 2005.
4. Käsmann-Kellner B, Klemm H, Ruprecht KW. Visual acuity and refraction development in coloboma and Aniridia (author's translation) Klin Monbl Augenheilkd 2004; 221:75. https://doi.org/10.1055/s-2004-835516.
5. Moustardas P, Aberdam D, Lagali N. MAPK pathways in ocular pathophysiology: potential therapeutic drugs and challenges. Cells. 2023;12(4):617.
6. Taubenslag KJ, Scanga HL, Huey J, Lee J, Medsinge A, Sylvester CL, Cheng KP, Nischal KK. Iris anomalies and the incidence of ACTA2 mutation. Br J Ophthalmol. 2019;103(4):499–503.
7. Nischal KK, Lathrop KL. The palisades of vogt in congenital corneal opacification (an american ophthalmological society thesis). Trans Am Ophthalmol Soc. 2016;114:T8.
8. Lisch W, Weiss JS. Clinical and genetic update of corneal dystrophies. Exp Eye Res. 2019;186: 107715.
9. Mataftsi A, Islam L, Kelberman D, Sowden JC, Nischal KK. Chromosome abnormalities and the genetics of congenital corneal opacification. Mol Vis. 2011;17:1624–40.
10. Piozzi E, Allegrini D. The paediatric patient: identifying congenital aniridia as soon as possible. In: Parekh M, Poli B, Ferrari S, Teofili C, Ponzin D. Aniridia. Recent developments in scientific and clinical research. Springer Cham, Switzerland, 2015; pp. 105–118.
11. Tomqvist K. Aniridia: early diagnosis: the key roles of neonatologists, paediatrics and paediatric ophthalmologists. In: Parekh M, Poli B, Ferrari S, Teofili C, Ponzin D. Aniridia. Recent developments in scientific and clinical research. Springer Cham, Switzerland, 2015; pp. 119–122.
12. Grainger RM, Lauderdale JD, Collins JL, Trout KL, McCullen Krantz S, Wolfe SS, Netland PA. Report on the 2021 Aniridia North America symposium on PAX6, aniridia, and beyond. Ocul Surf. 2023;29:423–31.
13. Axial length and corneal curvature of normal eyes in the first decade of life. Eur J Ophthalmol. 2023; 33(6):2217–21.
14. Käsmann-Kellner B, Viestenz AR, Seitz B, Graf N, Furtwängler R. WAGR(O) syndrome—special challenges in the care of aniridia patients (author's translation)] Klin Monbl Augenheilkd. 2017; 234(10):S1–13 https://doi.org/10.1055/s-0037-1604690.
15. Käsmann-Kellner B, Moslemani K, Seitz B. Optical rehabilitation and pediatric ophthalmological care following keratoplasty for childhood corneal opacities. Ophthalmologe. 2022;119(5):462–70.
16. Liasis A, Franco E, Eldib A, Handley S, Scanga HL, Nischal KK. The influence of congenital corneal opacity on ERGs obtained using an abbreviated protocol. Ophthalmic Genet. 2023;44(1):6–10.
17. Franco E, Scanga HL, Nischal KK. Variable phenotype of secondary congenital corneal opacities associated with microphthalmia with linear skin defects syndrome. Am J Med Genet A. 2023;191(2):586–91.
18. Zhou L, Wang G, Hu B, Jiang H, Jiang F, Xu Z. Microphthalmia and anterior segment dysgenesis due to a double gene variant in GJA8 and CRYGC. Eur J Ophthalmol. 2024; 34(1):NP12–NP17.
19. Nischal KK. Recent advances in pediatric ophthalmology. In: Grzybowski (Hrsg) Current concepts in ophthalmology. Springer International Publishing, Cham. 2020; S251–74.
20. Reis LM, Amor DJ, Haddad RA, Nowak CB, Keppler-Noreuil KM, Chisholm SA, Semina EV. Alternative genetic diagnoses in Axenfeld-Rieger syndrome spectrum. Genes (Basel). 2023;14(10):1948.
21. Yousaf K, Naz S, Mushtaq A, Wohler E, Sobreira N, Ho BM, Chen LJ, Chu WK, Bashir R. Exome sequencing reveals SLC4A11 variant underlying congenital hereditary endothelial dystrophy (CHED2) misdiagnosed as congenital glaucoma. Genes (Basel). 2023;14(2):310.
22. Seitz B, Lisch W, Weiss J. The revised newest IC3D classification of corneal dystrophies. Klin Monbl Augenheilkd. 2015;232(3):283–94.
23. Riedl JC, Pfeffer N, Giers BC, Schuster AK, Vossmerbaeumer U. Postoperative results after iris reconstruction with an artificial-iris® implant with consideration of the cause of the iris defects. Eur J Ophthalmol. 2023;33(5):1946–51.
24. Boente CS, Örge FH. Anterior Segment Dysgenesis Syndromes. In: Traboulsi EI, Utz VM, editors. Practical management of pediatric ocular disorders and strabismus. New York: A case-based approach. Springer; 2016. p. 141–7.
25. Leibovitz Z, Lerman-Sagie T, Haddad L. Fetal brain development: regulating processes and related malformations. Life (Basel). 2022;12(6):809.
26. Nischal KK. Genetics of Congenital Corneal Opacification-Impact on Diagnosis and Treatment. Cornea. 2015; 34(10):S24–34.
27. Hsieh TC, Bar-Haim A, Moosa S, Ehmke N, Gripp KW, Pantel JT, Danyel M, Mensah MA, Horn D, Rosnev S, Fleischer N, Bonini G, Hustinx A, Schmid A, Knaus A, Javanmardi B, Klinkhammer H, Lesmann H, Sivalingam S, Kamphans T, Meiswinkel W, Ebstein F, Krüger E, Küry S, Bézieau S, Schmidt A, Peters S, Engels H, Mangold E, Kreiß M, Cremer K, Perne C, Betz RC, Bender T, Grundmann-Hauser K, Haack TB, Wagner M, Brunet T, Bentzen HB, Averdunk L, Coetzer KC, Lyon GJ, Spielmann M, Schaaf CP, Mundlos S, Nöthen MM, Krawitz PM. GestaltMatcher facilitates rare disease matching using facial phenotype descriptors. Nat Genet. 2022;54(3):349–57.
28. Krawitz PM. Artificial intelligence in the diagnosis of rare disorders: the development of phenotype analysis. Bundesgesundheitsblatt Gesundheitsforschung Gesundheitsschutz. 2022;65(11):1159–63.
29. Shah PR, Chauhan B, Chu CT, Kofler J, Nischal KK. Ocular phenotype of Peters-plus syndrome. Cornea. 2022;41(2):219–23.
30. Decock CE, Breusegem CM, Van Aken EH, Leroy BP, Van Den Broecke CM, Delanghe JR. High beta-trace protein concentration in the fluid of an orbital cyst associated with bilateral colobomatous microphthalmos. Br J Ophthalmol. 2007;91(6):836.
31. Sassani JW, Yanoff. Anophthalmos in an infant with multiple congenital anomalies. Am J Ophthalmol. 1977; 83(1):43–8.
32. Weiss JS, Rapuano CJ, Seitz B, Busin M, Kivelä TT, Bouheraoua N, Bredrup C, Nischal KK, Chawla H, Borderie V, Kenyon KR, Kim EK, Møller HU, Munier FL, Berger T, Lisch W. IC3D Classification of corneal dystrophies-edition 3. Cornea. 2024;43(4):466–527.
33. Lisch W, Weiss JS. Early and late clinical landmarks of corneal dystrophies. Exp Eye Res. 2020;198:108139.
34. Weiss JS, Møller HU, Aldave AJ, Seitz B, Bredrup C, Kivelä T, Munier FL, Rapuano CJ, Nischal KK, Kim EK, Sutphin J, Busin M, Labbé A, Kenyon KR, Kinoshita S, Lisch W. IC3D classification of corneal dystrophies–edition 2. Cornea. 2015;34(2):117–59.
35. Berger T, Hasenfus A, Bredrup C, Gatzioufas Z, Flockerzi F, Käsmann-Kellner B, Daas L, Flockerzi E, Knappskog PM, Stang E, Seitz B. Long-term follow-up of pediatric excimer

laser-assisted penetrating keratoplasty for congenital stromal corneal dystrophy. Cornea. 2024; 43:784–89.
36. Aldave AJ, Han J, Frausto RF. Genetics of the corneal endothelial dystrophies: an evidence-based review. Clin Genet. 2013;84(2):109–19.
37. Messmer EM. In vivo confocal microscopy–correlation to histology. Klin Monbl Augenheilkd. 2012;229(7):696–704.
38. Franco E, Gagrani M, Lalgudi VG, Shah PR, Lenhart P, Bhola R, Nischal KK. Technique for the management of extensive ocular surface lipodermoid involving the cornea of children. Cornea. 2023;42(6):770–5.
39. Khan TA, Zameer S, Janjua TA, Zahid MA, Akram A, Mallick NK. Cornea plana in a family from Pakistan: case series and literature review on the principles of management. Oman J Ophthalmol. 2023;16(2):305–9.
40. Forsius H, Damsten M, Eriksson AW, Fellman J, Lindh S, Tahvanainen E. Autosomal recessive cornea plana. A clinical and genetic study of 78 cases in Finland. Acta Ophthalmol Scand. 1998; 76(2):196–203.
41. Ramappa M, Achanta DSR, Mohamed A, Chaurasia S. Corneal endothelial alterations in recessive cornea plana: a report of 4 patients and review of literature. Ophthalmic Genet. 2020;41(6):659–62.
42. Sigler-Villanueva A, Tahvanainen E, Lindh S, Dieguez-Lucena J, Forsius H. Autosomal dominant cornea plana: clinical findings in a cuban family and a review of the literature. Ophthalmic Genet. 1997;18(2):55–62.
43. Kumar P, Hammersmith KM, Eagle R Jr. Congenital corneal opacities: diagnosis and management. In: Mannis MJ & Holland EJ, editors. Cornea. Elsevier Amsterdam; 2021. pp. 185–208.
44. Levin AV, Zanolli M, Capasso J. The wills eye handbook of ocular genetics. 1st ed. New York: Thieme; 2018.
45. Krieglstein GK, Jonescu-Cuypers CP, Severin M. Atlas der Augenheilkunde. Springer-Lehrbuch. Springer Berlin Heidelberg, Berlin, Heidelberg. 1999.
46. Colby K. Corneal diseases in children. Challenges and controversies, 1. Aufl. Essentials in Ophthalmology. Springer International Publishing, Cham. 2017.
47. Neuhann TM, Neuhann L. Human genetic diagnostics in hereditary eye diseases: what does the ophthalmologist need to know. Ophthalmologie. 2023;120(6):679–88.
48. Dhir L, Frimpong-Ansah K, Habib NE. Missed case of Axenfeld-Rieger syndrome: a case report. Cases J. 2008;1(1):299.
49. Nischal KK. A new approach to the classification of neonatal corneal opacities. Curr Opin Ophthalmol. 2012;23(5):344–54.
50. Medsinge A, Nischal KK. Cataract surgery in children with congenital keratolenticular adhesion (Peters anomaly type 2). J AAPOS. 2015;19(1):24–8.
51. Ramappa M, Chaurasia S, Mohamed A, Ramya Achanta DS, Mandal AK, Edward DP, Gokhale N, Swarup R, Nischal KK. Selective endothelialectomy in Peters anomaly: a novel surgical technique and its clinical outcomes in children. Cornea. 2022;41(12):1477–86.
52. Reichl S, Böhringer D, Richter O, Lagrèze W, Reinhard T. Long-term prognosis of Peters anomaly. Ophthalmologe. 2018;115(4):309–13.
53. Rajagopal RN, Fernandes M. Peters anomaly: novel non-invasive alternatives to penetrating keratoplasty. Semin Ophthalmol. 2023;38(3):275–82.
54. Jünemann A, Gusek GC, Naumann GO. Optical sector iridectomy: an alternative to perforating keratoplasty in Peters' anomaly. Klin Monbl Augenheilkd. 1996;209(2–3):117–24.
55. García-Antón MT, Salazar JJ, de Hoz R, Rojas B, Ramírez AI, Triviño A, Aroca-Aguilar JD, García-Feijoo J, Escribano J, Ramírez JM. Goniodysgenesis variability and activity of CYP1B1 genotypes in primary congenital glaucoma. PLoS ONE. 2017;12(4): e0176386.
56. Chouiter L, Nadifi S. Analysis of CYP1B1 gene mutations in patients with primary congenital glaucoma. J Pediatr Genet. 2017;6(4):205–14.
57. Stingl JV, Lagrèze WA, Hoffmann EM. Glaucoma in infancy and childhood. Ophthalmologie. 2023;120(3):335–44.
58. Latta L, Nordström K, Stachon T, Langenbucher A, Fries FN, Szentmáry N, Seitz B, Käsmann-Kellner B. Expression of retinoic acid signaling components ADH7 and ALDH1A1 is reduced in aniridia limbal epithelial cells and a siRNA primary cell based aniridia model. Exp Eye Res. 2019;179:8–17.
59. van Heyningen V. A journey through genetics to biology. Annu Rev Genomics Hum Genet. 2022;23:1–27.
60. Schlötzer-Schrehardt U, Latta L, Gießl A, Zenkel M, Fries FN, Käsmann-Kellner B, Kruse FE, Seitz B. Dysfunction of the limbal epithelial stem cell niche in aniridia-associated keratopathy. Ocul Surf. 2021;21:160–73.
61. Abdolkarimi D, Cunha DL, Lahne M, Moosajee M. PAX6 disease models for aniridia. Indian J Ophthalmol. 2022;70(12):4119–29.
62. Käsmann-Kellner B, Seitz B. Congenital aniridia or PAX6 syndrome. Ophthalmologe. 2014;111(12):1144.
63. Pedersen HR, Gilson SJ, Landsend ECS, Utheim ØA, Utheim TP, Baraas RC. Rod and cone dark adaptation in congenital aniridia and its association with retinal structure. Invest Ophthalmol Vis Sci. 2023;64(4):18.
64. Deng SX, Borderie V, Chan CC, Dana R, Figueiredo FC, Gomes JAP, Pellegrini G, Shimmura S, Kruse FE. The international limbal stem cell deficiency working group. Global consensus on definition, classification, diagnosis, and staging of limbal stem cell deficiency. Cornea. 2019; 38(3):364–375.
65. Käsmann-Kellner B, Latta L, Fries FN, Viestenz A, Seitz B. Diagnostic impact of anterior segment angiography of limbal stem cell insufficiency in PAX6-related aniridia. Clin Anat. 2018;31(3):392–7.
66. Lagali N, Wowra B, Fries FN, Latta L, Moslemani K, Utheim TP, Wylegala E, Seitz B, Käsmann-Kellner B. PAX6 mutational status determines aniridia-associated keratopathy phenotype. Ophthalmology. 2020;127(2):273–5.
67. López-García JS. Applications of autologous serum eye drops in aniridic keratopathy. Eur Ophthalmic Rev. 2009;3(1):51–3.
68. van Velthoven AJH, Utheim TP, Notara M, Bremond-Gignac D, Figueiredo FC, Skottman H, Aberdam D, Daniels JT, Ferrari G, Grupcheva C, Koppen C, Parekh M, Ritter T, Romano V, Ferrari S, Cursiefen C, Lagali N, LaPointe VLS, Dickman MM. Future directions in managing aniridia-associated keratopathy. Surv Ophthalmol. 2023;68(5):940–56.
69. Fries FN, Moslemani K, Utheim TP, Seitz B, Käsmann-Kellner B, Lagali NS. Early ocular surface and tear film status in congenital aniridia indicates a supportive treatment window. Br J Ophthalmol. 2023;108(1):30–6.
70. Lagali N, Wowra B, Fries FN, Latta L, Moslemani K, Utheim TP, Wylegala E, Seitz B, Käsmann-Kellner B. Early phenotypic features of aniridia-associated keratopathy and association with PAX6 coding mutations. Ocul Surf. 2020;18(1):130–40.
71. Latta L, Ludwig N, Krammes L, Stachon T, Fries FN, Mukwaya A, Szentmáry N, Seitz B, Wowra B, Kahraman M, Keller A, Meese E, Lagali N, Käsmann-Kellner B. Abnormal neovascular and proliferative conjunctival phenotype in limbal stem cell deficiency is associated with altered microRNA and gene expression modulated by PAX6 mutational status in congenital aniridia. Ocul Surf. 2021;19:115–27.
72. Lee HK, Kim MK, Oh JY. Corneal abnormalities in congenital aniridia: congenital central corneal opacity versus aniridia-associated keratopathy. Am J Ophthalmol. 2018;185:75–80.
73. Behaegel J, Tassignon MJ, Lagali N, Consejo A, Koppen C, Ní DS. Outcomes of human leukocyte antigen-matched allogeneic cultivated limbal epithelial transplantation in aniridia-associated

keratopathy-a single-center retrospective analysis. Cornea. 2022;41(1):69–77.
74. Fries FN, Náray A, Munteanu C, Stachon T, Lagali N, Seitz B, Szentmáry N, Käsmann-Kellner B. A cross-sectional analysis of 556 eyes entering the homburg aniridia centre. Klin Monbl Augenheilkd. 2024;241(3):275–82.
75. Vasilyeva TA, Marakhonov AV, Voskresenskaya AA, Kadyshev VV, Käsmann-Kellner B, Sukhanova NV, Katargina LA, Kutsev SI, Zinchenko RA. Analysis of genotype-phenotype correlations in PAX6-associated aniridia. J Med Genet. 2021;58(4):270–4.
76. Krause MA, Trout KL, Lauderdale JD, Netland PA. Visual acuity in aniridia and WAGR syndrome. Clin Ophthalmol. 2023;17:1255–61.
77. Käsmann-Kellner B, Seitz B. Aniridia syndrome: clinical findings, problematic courses and suggestions for optimization of care ("aniridia guide"). Ophthalmologe. 2014;111(12):1145–56.
78. Grant MK, Bobilev AM, Pierce JE, DeWitte J, Lauderdale JD. Structural brain abnormalities in 12 persons with aniridia. F1000Res. 2017; 6:255.
79. Farah CJ, Fries FN, Latta L, Käsmann-Kellner B, Seitz B. An attempt to optimize the outcome of penetrating keratoplasty in congenital aniridia-associated keratopathy (AAK). Int Ophthalmol. 2021;41(12):4091–8.
80. Fries FN, Náray A, Munteanu C, Stachon T, Lagali N, Seitz B, Käsmann-Kellner B, Szentmáry N. The effect of Glaucoma Treatment on Aniridia-Associated Keratopathy (AAK) - A Report from the Homburg Register for Congenital Aniridia. Klin Monbl Augenheilkd. 2025;242(5):578–83.
81. Katiyar P, Stachon T, Fries FN, Parow F, Ulrich M, Langenbucher A, Cayless A, Seitz B, Käsmann-Kellner B, Latta L, Szentmáry N. Decreased FABP5 and DSG1 protein expression following PAX6 knockdown of differentiated human limbal epithelial cells. Exp Eye Res. 2022;215:108904.
82. Chauhan BK, Medsinge A, Baumgartner MP, Scanga HL, Kamakari S, Gajdosova E, Camacho CJ, Nischal KK. Case series: Pyramidal cataracts, intact irides and nystagmus from three novel PAX6 mutations. Am J Ophthalmol Case Rep. 2018;10:172–9.
83. Moshirfar M, Masud M, Harvey DH, Payne C, Bruce E, Ronquillo YC, Hoopes PC. The multifold etiologies of limbal stem cell deficiency: a comprehensive review on the etiologies and additional treatment options for limbal stem cell deficiency. J Clin Med. 2023;12(13):4418.
84. Käsmann-Kellner B, Viestenz A, Seitz B. Aniridia guides and aniridia-syndrome (PAX6-Syndrome): do's and dont's in clinical care. In: Ponzin D (Hrsg) Aniridia. Recent developments in scientific and clinical research, 2016. Aufl. Springer, Cham. 2015; pp. 123–154.
85. Latta L, Knebel I, Bleil C, Stachon T, Katiyar P, Zussy C, Fries FN, Käsmann-Kellner B, Seitz B, Szentmáry N. Similarities in DSG1 and KRT3 downregulation through retinoic acid treatment and PAX6 knockdown related expression profiles: does PAX6 affect RA signaling in limbal epithelial cells? Biomolecules. 2021;11(11):1651.
86. Latta L, Viestenz A, Stachon T, Colanesi S, Szentmáry N, Seitz B, Käsmann-Kellner B. Human aniridia limbal epithelial cells lack expression of keratins K3 and K12. Exp Eye Res. 2018;167:100–9.
87. Altshuler A, Amitai-Lange A, Nasser W, Dimri S, Bhattacharya S, Tiosano B, Barbara R, Aberdam D, Shimmura S, Shalom-Feuerstein R. Eyes open on stem cells. Stem Cell Rep. 2023;18(12):2313–27.
88. Clahsen T, Hadrian K, Notara M, Schlereth SL, Howaldt A, Prokosch V, Volatier T, Hos D, Schroedl F, Kaser-Eichberger A, Heindl LM, Steven P, Bosch JJ, Steinkasserer A, Rokohl AC, Liu H, Mestanoglu M, Kashkar H, Schumacher B, Kiefer F, Schulte-Merker S, Matthaei M, Hou Y, Fassbender S, Jantsch J, Zhang W, Enders P, Bachmann B, Bock F, Cursiefen C. The novel role of lymphatic vessels in the pathogenesis of ocular diseases. Prog Retin Eye Res. 2023;96:101157.
89. Weischnur L, Xanthopoulou K, Munteanu C, Leonhard M, Daas L, Seitz B. Autologous serum eye drops for therapy-resistant epithelial defects of the cornea: impact of underlying disease and simultaneous amniotic transplantation in 990 applications. Ophthalmologie. 2023;120(1):43–51.
90. Seitz B, Käsmann-Kellner B, Viestenz A. Stage-related therapy of congenital aniridia. Ophthalmologe. 2014;111(12):1164–71.
91. Majo F, Muraine M. Posterior lamellar corneal graft (DSAEK) in an aphakic and congenital aniridic single eye: a case report presenting a new surgical procedure. Klin Monbl Augenheilkd. 2023;240(4):394–7.
92. Lang SJ, Böhringer D, Reinhard T. Keratoplasty in children: indications and results. Ophthalmologe. 2020;117(3):215–7.
93. Latta L, Figueiredo FC, Ashery-Padan R, Collinson JM, Daniels J, Ferrari S, Szentmáry N, Solá S, Shalom-Feuerstein R, Lako M, Xapelli S, Aberdam D, Lagali N. Pathophysiology of aniridia-associated keratopathy: developmental aspects and unanswered questions. Ocul Surf. 2021;22:245–66.
94. Ouyang H, Xue Y, Lin Y, Zhang X, Xi L, Patel S, Cai H, Luo J, Zhang M, Zhang M, Yang Y, Li G, Li H, Jiang W, Yeh E, Lin J, Pei M, Zhu J, Cao G, Zhang L, Yu B, Chen S, Fu XD, Liu Y, Zhang K. WNT7A and PAX6 define corneal epithelium homeostasis and pathogenesis. Nature. 2014;511(7509):358–61.
95. Duncan MK, Daruich A, Valleix S, Bremond-Gignac D. Reduction of lens size in PAX6-related aniridia. Exp Eye Res. 2024;238:109746.
96. Jacobson A, Mian SI, Bohnsack BL. Clinical outcomes and visual prognostic factors in congenital aniridia. BMC Ophthalmol. 2022;22(1):235.
97. Hoffmann EM. 360° trabeculotomy for pediatric glaucoma. Ophthalmologe. 2020;117(3):210–4.
98. Hsu E, Desai M. Glaucoma and systemic disease. Life. 2023;13(4):1018.
99. Arad T, Hoffmann EM, Prokosch-Willing V, Pfeiffer N, Grehn F. XEN-augmented baerveldt implantation for refractory childhood glaucoma: a retrospective case series. J Glaucoma. 2019;28(11):1015–8.
100. Viestenz A, Seitz B, Deland E, Fiorentzis M, Latta L, Viestenz A, Käsmann-Kellner B. Clinical anatomy of the anterior chamber angle in congenital aniridia and consequences for trabeculotomy/cyclophotocoagulation. Clin Anat. 2018;31(1):64–7.
101. Tsai JH, Freeman JM, Chan CC, Schwartz GS, Derby EA, Petersen MR, Holland EJ. A progressive anterior fibrosis syndrome in patients with postsurgical congenital aniridia. Am J Ophthalmol. 2005;140(6):1075–9.
102. Ma AS, Grigg JR, Jamieson RV. Phenotype-genotype correlations and emerging pathways in ocular anterior segment dysgenesis. Hum Genet. 2019;138(8–9):899–915.

Aniridia-Associated Keratopathy AAK—Genotype and Phenotype

Dina Javidjam and Neil Lagali

Abstract

Congenital aniridia is a rare genetic disorder of disrupted normal eye development. Heterozygous mutations in the *PAX6* gene are the main cause of the disease, of which over 500 distinct mutations are known to exist and lead to aniridia. Importantly, patients with aniridia are susceptible to total loss of vision from progressive aniridia-associated keratopathy (AAK), believed to be triggered by dysfunctional limbal epithelial stem cells and/or the limbal stem cell niche. In the cornea of aniridia patients, a neurotrophic deficit is also present, that is closely associated with corneal inflammation, neovascularization, and a chronic wound healing response. This chapter summarizes corneal phenotype in aniridia-associated keratopathy (AAK), including its early manifestations in relation to PAX6 mutational status (genotype). Detailed corneal imaging using slit lamp biomicroscopy, in vivo confocal microscopy (IVCM), and optical coherence tomography (OCT) are used to document phenotypic changes in the epithelial, neural, and immune cell status in relation to the genotype and the phenotypic grading of AAK, which, as a progressive pathology, is sensitive to age.

Keywords

Congenital aniridia · Genotype · Phenotype · Limbal stem cell deficiency · PAX6 gene

D. Javidjam · N. Lagali (✉)
Division of Ophthalmology, Department of Biomedical and Clinical Sciences, Linköping University, Linköping, Sweden
e-mail: neil.lagali@liu.se

1 Introduction

Congenital aniridia is a pan-ocular disease typically diagnosed and characterized by varying degrees of iris and foveal hypoplasia. In most cases, the genetic cause is a mutation in the *paired-box gene 6* (*PAX6*), resulting in haploinsufficiency of the protein product (also called PAX6) and malfunction of target genes, as *PAX6* is a transcription factor. This in turn, leads to fundamental abnormalities in the development of the eye. According to the National Organization for Rare Disorders, Aniridia is classified as a rare disease with a reported prevalence ranging from 1 in 64,000 to 1 in 96,000. However, it is important to note that the true prevalence is likely greater due to underreporting of cases. There is no data indicating that environmental exposure or drug use during pregnancy increases the probability of having a child with aniridia, and no substantial sex or racial preference has been described [1].

Aniridia has an autosomal dominant and highly penetrant hereditary pattern. Approximately two-thirds of instances are familial, with the remaining one-third occurring sporadically. The pathophysiology of congenital aniridia secondary to the genetic mutation involves multiple ocular structures, leading to keratopathy, glaucoma, cataracts, nystagmus and dry eye disease. These often arise throughout infancy or during adolescence and frequently result in significant vision impairment. Keratopathy in aniridia is called aniridic, aniridia-related, or aniridia-associated keratopathy (AAK). Even when glaucoma and cataracts are not present or adequately treated, visual acuity in aniridia patients diminishes over time, indicating that AAK is one of the most important causes of progressive vision deterioration in patients. The ocular surface alterations in AAK are attributed to a primary dysfunction and gradual breakdown of the limbal stem cell niche, driven by PAX6-related effects on both limbal melanocytes and epithelial differentiation. Therefore Limbal Stem Cell Deficiency (LSCD) is expected to have an important role in the development of keratopathy in aniridia

B. Seitz et al. (eds.), *Atlas on Cornea*, https://doi.org/10.1007/978-3-031-65422-0_15

[2]. Some of the abnormal phenotypes such as microphthalmia, optic nerve abnormalities, and Peters anomaly are more severe than conventional aniridia. The clinical manifestation of aniridia can vary substantially within some families while other families have less phenotypic diversity. The subtype of PAX6 mutation and transcription factors interacting with the gene may affect intrafamilial diversity [3].

Increasing grade of AAK is correlated with the loss of basal corneal epithelial cell phenotype and a loss of corneal subbasal nerves. A 5-point clinical AAK grading scale is typically used [4], as described in Table 1.

In this chapter, we detail that the manifestation of AAK is intricately tied to the genetic status of the patient, especially concerning mutations within the coding regions of the *PAX6* gene that lead to the protein haploinsufficiency. Additionally, we provide an in-depth examination of corneal morphology across different age groups, aiming to elucidate the observed characteristics of AAK and their potential underlying causes. The findings are grouped according to mutational status.

2 Chromosomal Mutation

Approximately one-third of sporadic and some familial aniridia cases are caused by rearrangements and whole/partial gene deletions that disrupt *PAX6*, which can also affect neighboring genes at the 11p13 chromosomal locus. In total, these mutations account for about 10% of all aniridia cases [5]. Patients with a *PAX6* gene deletion along with other flanking gene deletions (e.g., *WT1*, *FSHB*, *DCDC1*, *ELP4*, *RCN1*, *HIPK3*, *LM02*, *EHF*, and *CB44*) display a severe and aggressive AAK phenotype at a young age (4–20 years). Eighty percent of these patients also exhibit Wilms' tumor, aniridia, genitourinary anomalies, and mental retardation (WAGR) syndrome, and nearly all have poor vision, a thick opaque corneal pannus, severe corneal nerve deficit, and poor corneal sensitivity [6] (Figs. 1 and 2).

3 PTC Mutation

85% of the mutations found in aniridia are *PAX6* coding variants that cause a premature termination codon (PTC). These include nonsense variants, which account for 40% of the mutations, small insertions or deletions, which account for 30%, and splicing variants, which affect messenger RNA (mRNA) processing and are located at intron splicing sites, which account for 15% [7]. There is no obvious relationship between the position of a mutation and a particular phenotype, yet mutations involving a PTC in *PAX6* always result in aniridia or closely comparable symptoms, and yield a classical AAK phenotype. Severe and progressive vision impairment, significant iris abnormalities, and foveal hypoplasia are hallmark features of the corresponding aniridia phenotype [1] (Figs. 3, 4 and 5).

4 C-Terminal Extension Mutation

C-terminal extension mutations (CTE) (dominant negative mutations) in the *PAX6* gene originate from frameshift or point mutations that modify the C-terminus stop codon, causing run-on translation into the 3'UTR. CTE transcripts do not exhibit nonsense-mediated protein degradation, and a prolonged aberrant protein is generated. This type of mutation shows a similar classical progressive phenotype as those with PTC mutation and is frequently linked with a severe phenotype, including significant iris hypoplasia and substantial vision impairment [8] (Fig. 6).

5 Missense Mutation

A missense mutation is a non-synonymous mutation that alters an amino acid. Changes in polarity and/or protein structure result from amino acid substitutions, the majority of which occur in highly conserved residues of the paired domain of the *PAX6* gene. Disruption of the *PAX6* gene's ability to bind to DNA and transactivate target genes is a

Table 1 Clinical grading of aniridia-associated keratopathy according to a previously published scale [4]

AAK grade	Description
Grade 0	Full and undamaged limbal border that is indistinguishable from a healthy corneal limbus under the slit lamp
Grade 1	Initial collapse of the limbal boundary and early invasion of conjunctival tissue over the limbus while remaining within 1 mm of the limbal area
Grade 2	Ingrowth of conjunctival tissue into the peripheral and paracentral cornea, preserving the central 2 mm of the cornea. Can be described as vascular pannus, muddying or clouding indicating vessel ingrowth, or conjunctivalization
Grade 3	Vascularization, opacification, and corneal stromal involvement affecting the central cornea
Grade 4	End-stage advanced AAK, conjunctivalization and vascularization of the entire cornea, transformation of the anterior cornea into an opaque, thick irregular structure

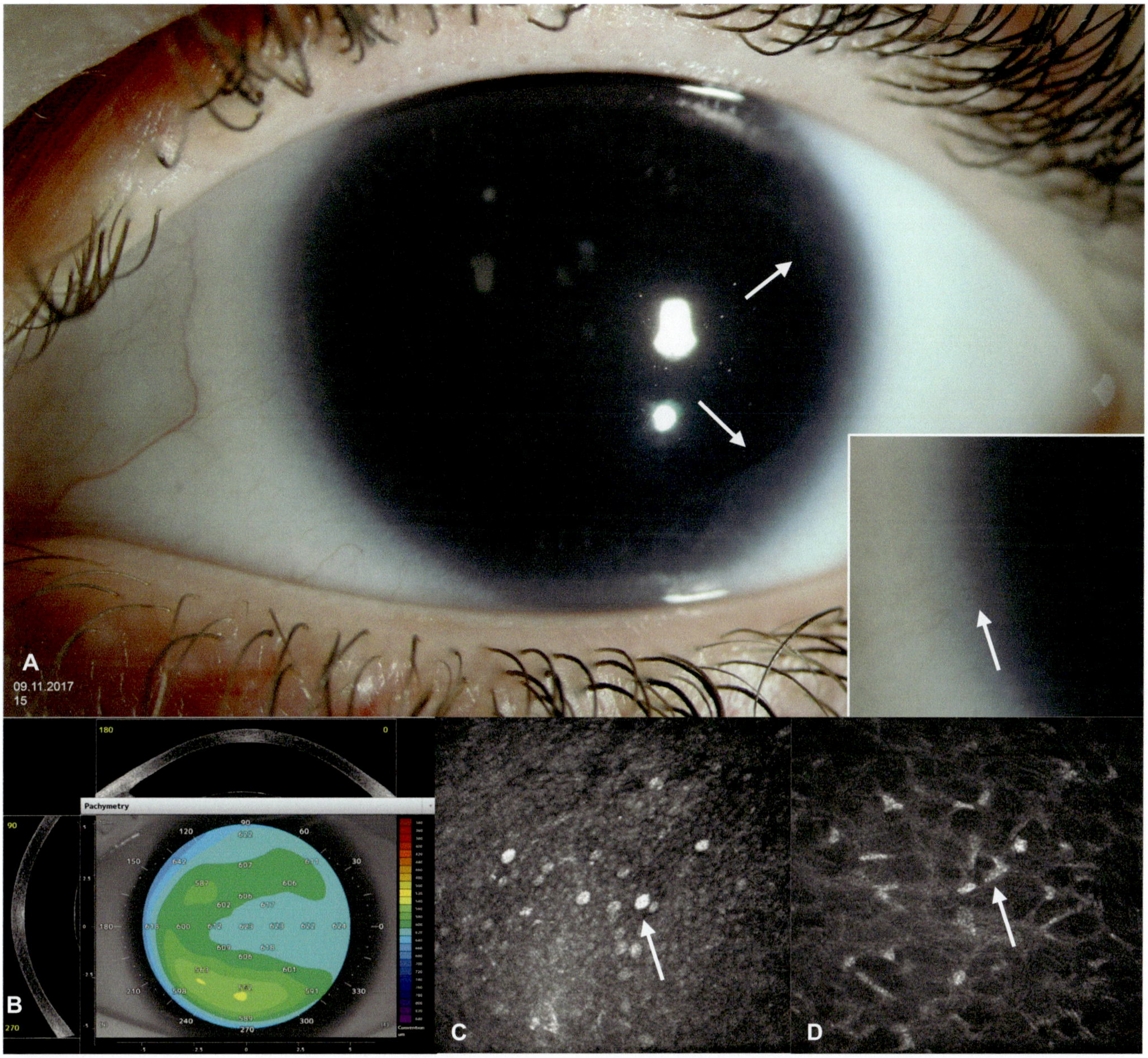

Fig. 1 A 20-year-old female patient with chromosomal mutation (PAX6, WT1, del(11) (p11.2p13)). (**A**) The cornea remains clear in the central region in this Grade 2 AAK, defined by the peripheral border of conjunctival overgrowth (arrows) (**B**) A central corneal thickness (CCT) of 623 µm is apparent on OCT, with onset of corneal thickening peripherally. (**C**) Oval-shaped goblet cells invade the peripheral cornea (arrows) with increased reflectivity relative to background basal conjunctival cells. (**D**) The corneal stroma appears normal, while peripheral vascular invasion is apparent in the limbal region (A, inset). The Snellen distance-corrected visual acuity (DCVA) for this eye was 20/400, and central corneal mechanical touch sensitivity, as measured by Cochet Bonnet esthesiometry, was 25 mm

functional consequence of non-synonymous mutations [4]. According to studies, missense mutations in the *PAX6* gene typically result in less severe aniridia symptoms. Therefore, it is anticipated that *PAX6* proteins retain some of their function due to missense mutations. However, the phenotype changes depending on the nature and location of the mutation, and predicting the missense phenotype is challenging due to the diverse activities of mutant proteins [5] (Fig. 7).

6 *PAX6* Non-Coding Region Mutation

While it was once thought that AAK was exclusive to exons of the *PAX6* gene, recent research has shown that aniridia can also result from non-coding regions of *PAX6*, such as introns, regulatory regions, and untranslated regions affecting neighboring genes such as *ELP4*, *DCDC1*, *DNAJC24*, *TRIM44*, and *IMMP1L*. Mutations in the genes *FOXC1*

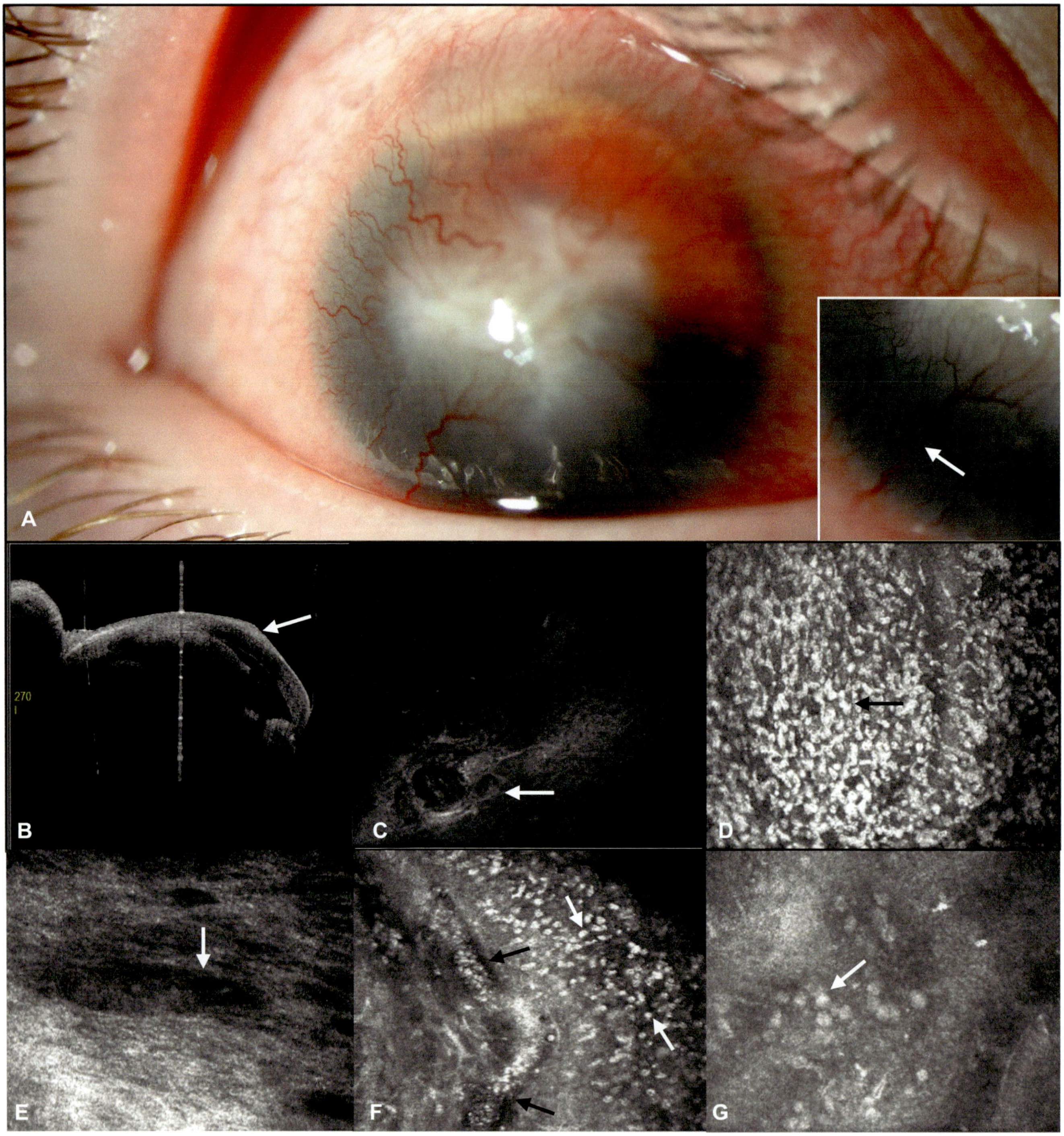

Fig. 2 Findings from a 14-year-old girl with chromosomal deletion (PAX6, WT1, del(p13-ter)) and advanced AAK. (**A**) The cornea has a Grade 4 AAK (DCVA = 20/1000, sensitivity = 10 mm), with complete conjunctivalization and vascularization, with severe vessel invasion from the limbus, followed by branching and proliferation (inset). (**B**) Uneven thickening of the cornea (arrow) is evident in the OCT image, with a central corneal thickness (CCT) measuring 1134 μm. (**C**) The point of attachment of the lens to the posterior cornea (arrow) is visible. (**D**) A substantial number of inflammatory cells (arrow) are observed in the anterior stroma. (**E**) Hyporeflective fluid-filled regions possibly representing a lymphatic vessel can be seen in the stroma (arrow). (**F**) Inflammatory cells (white arrows) accompanying a stromal blood vessel (black arrows). (**G**) Goblet cells are also apparent on the ocular surface (arrow)

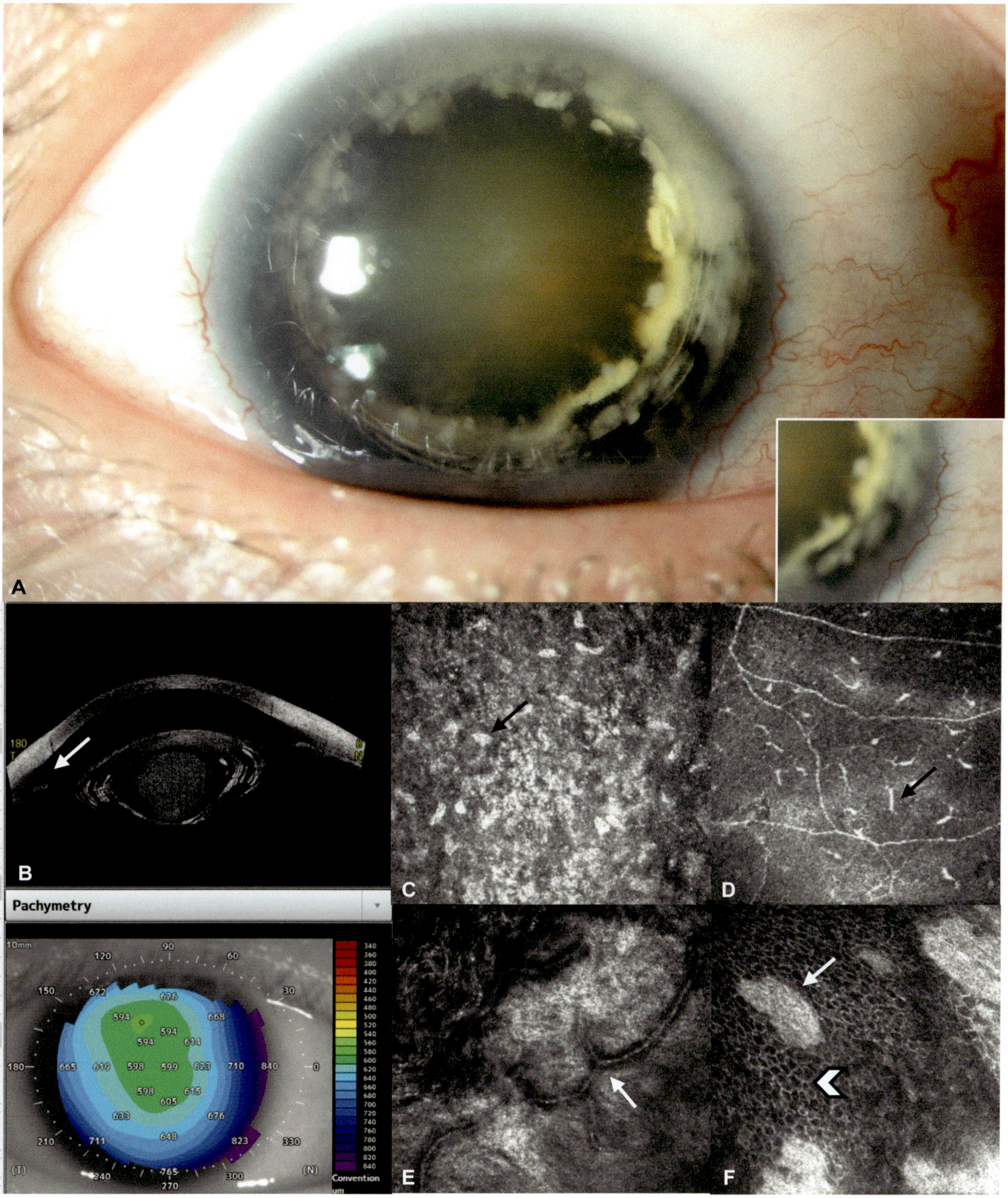

Fig. 3 AAK arising from a PTC mutation (c.130C>T) in a 46-year-old woman. (**A**) Grade 1 AAK, with vessels extending just over the limbal border (inset). Note the cataractous lens. (**B**) OCT indicates complete iris insufficiency (arrow) and a CCT of 599 μm (DCVA = 20/800, sensitivity = 30 mm). (**C**) Anterior stroma containing activated, reflective keratocytes (arrow) resulting in a corneal haze. (**D**) Reduced subbasal nerve presence with loss of normal nerve patterns. Additionally, an elevated presence of mature dendritic cells (arrow) is apparent within the central cornea. (**E**) Invasion of vessels at the limbus is visible (arrow) within an advancing fibrovascular pannus. (**F**) Mixed corneal-conjunctival phenotype is evident, with conspicuous conjunctival islands (arrow) interspersed among cornea-like wing cells displaying altered size and shape (arrowhead)

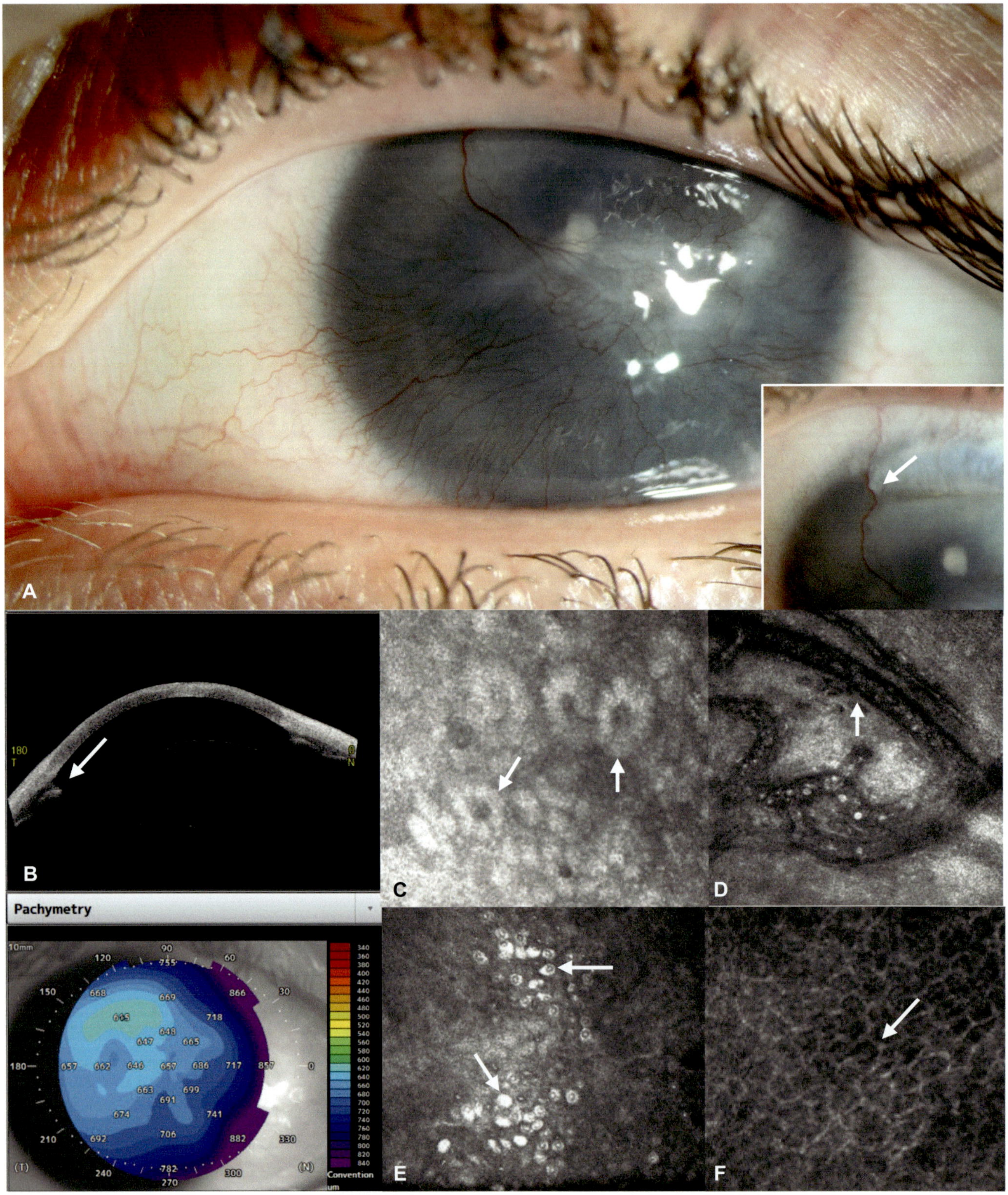

Fig. 4 A 28-year-old woman with PTK mutation (c.112_116del). (**A**) Grade 3 AAK, with fibrovascular tissue and vessel invasion from the limbus (inset). Absence of full pannus coverage with some translucent central and peripheral regions confirms a Grade 3 classification. (**B**) OCT indicates complete iris absence (DCVA = 20/750, sensitivity = 10 mm). The central corneal thickness (CCT) is 657 μm. (**C**) Goblet cells in the pannus epithelium are arranged in characteristic rosettes (arrows). (**D**) Thickened vascular trunks (arrow) are apparent in the central cornea, some with clearly visible leukocytes within the vessels. (**E**) Individual goblet cells (arrows) invading the central cornea as epithelial phenotype changes from corneal to conjunctival. (**F**) Transformation of epithelial wing cells to conjunctival-like cells, with cell borders of varying reflectivity (arrow) and large, reflective nuclei visible

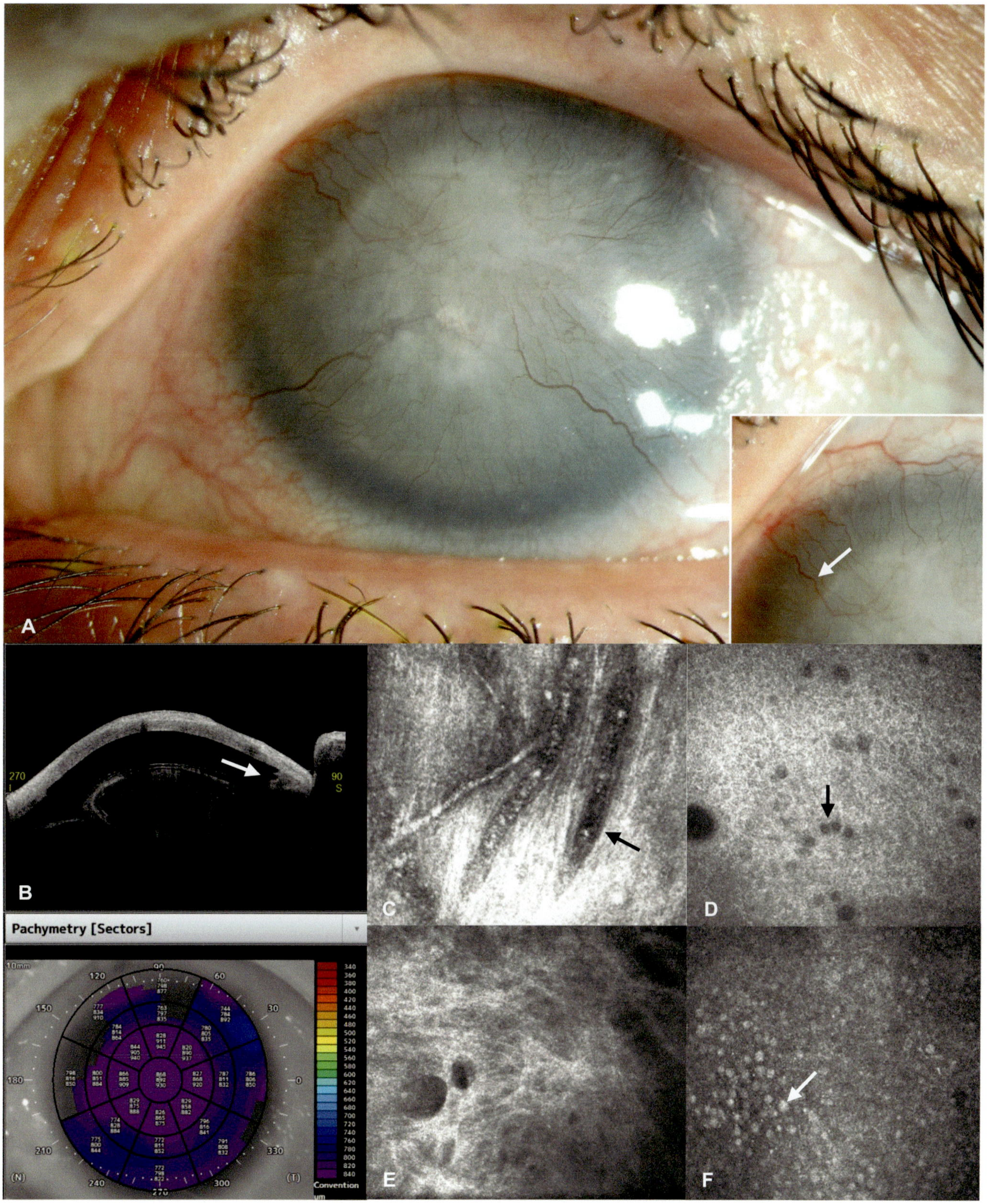

Fig. 5 46-year-old female patient with PTC mutation (c.141þ1G>A). (**A**) Grade 4 AAK, with fully vascularized and conjuntivalized cornea (DCVA = 20/2000, sensitivity = 30 mm). Extensive invasion of dilated vessels from the limbus (inset). (**B**) OCT indicates thick, opaque pannus centrally and peripherally, with complete iris absence (arrow). CCT is 891 μm. (**C**) Invasion of blood vessels (arrow) into the corneal stroma along with highly reflective, fibrous tissue. (**D**) Transformation of epithelium into a conjunctival phenotype with presence of microcysts (arrow), possibly due to disturbances in the normal fluid dynamics within the cornea. (**E**) Fibrovascular conjunctival stromal tissue present in the cornea. (**F**) Conjunctival epithelial phenotype in the cornea, with associated goblet cells (arrow)

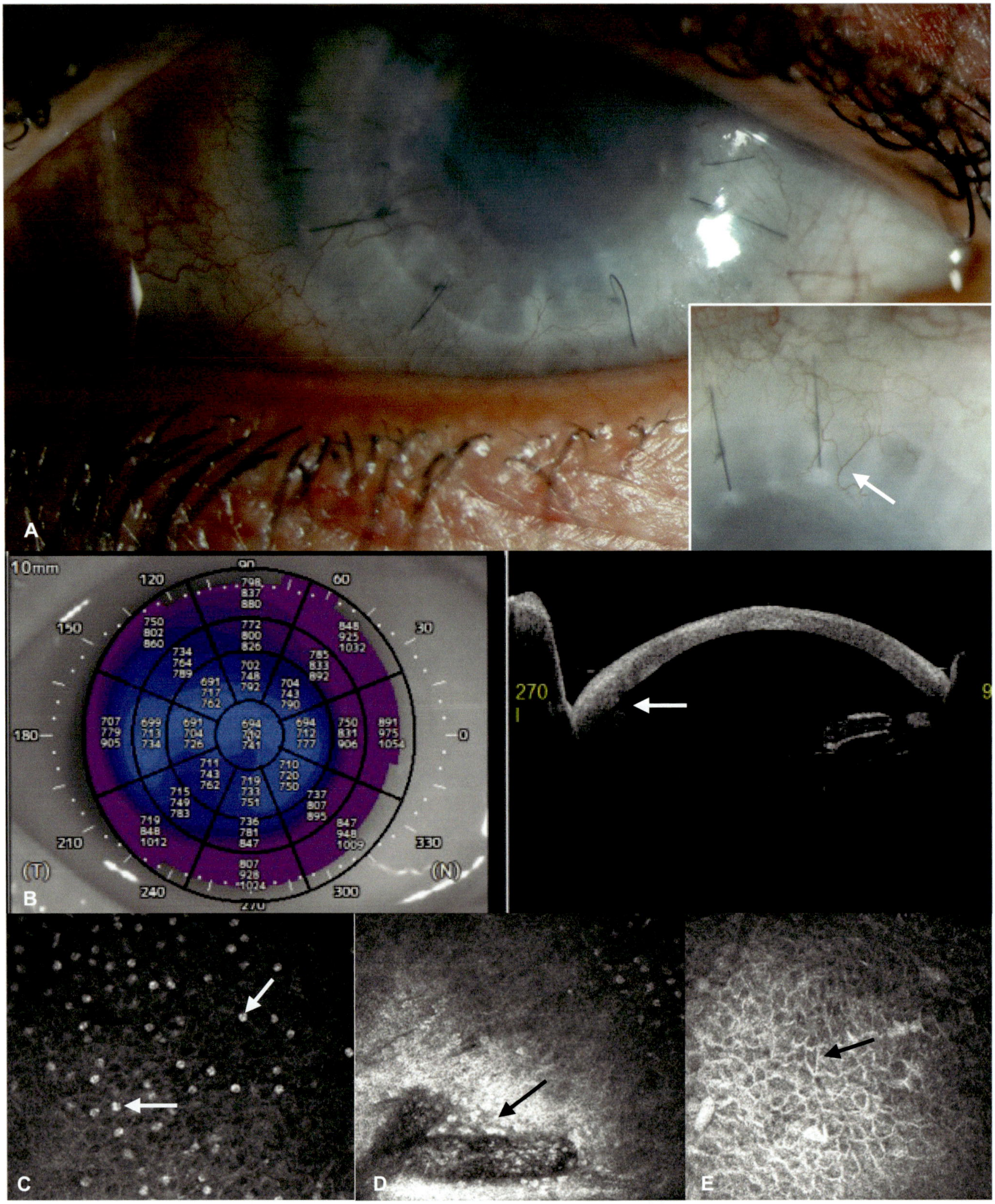

Fig. 6 A 51-year-old woman with CTE mutation in *PAX6* (c.1268A > T). (**A**) Penetrating keratoplasty (PK) surgery performed 16 months earlier in grade 3 AAK (DCVA = 20/1000, sensitivity = 10 mm). Peripheral vascularization triggered by the suture (arrow, inset). (**B**) Central corneal thickness (CCT) of 712 μm with peripheral cornea thickened to over 1000 μm. Iris hypoplasia is discernible in the OCT image (arrow). (**C**) Inflammatory cells are evident in the central corneal epithelium (arrow). (**D**) A blood vessel is observed in the corneal stroma (arrow). (**E**) Certain areas of epithelium in the central transplant region remain clear

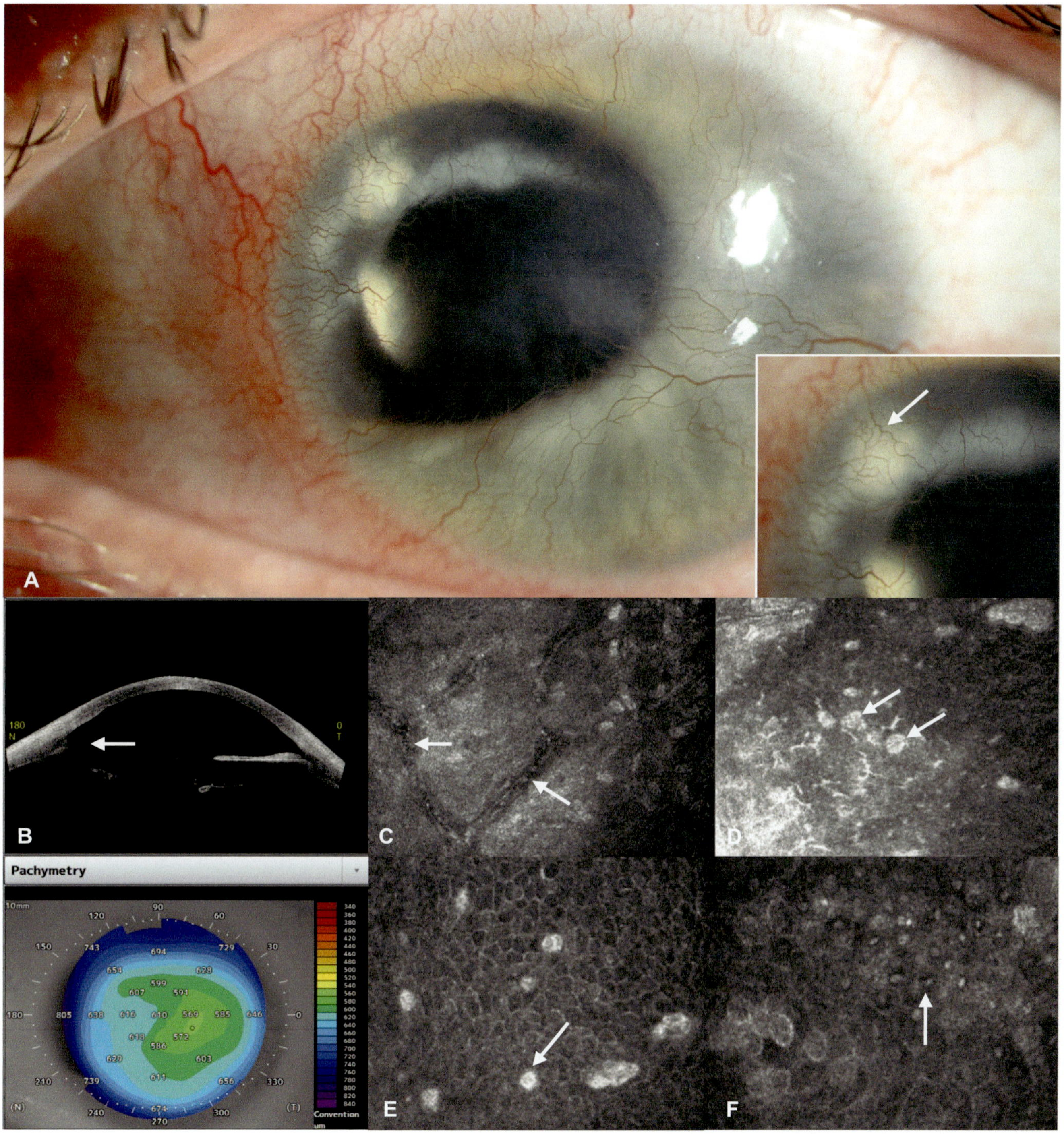

Fig. 7 Findings from a 36-year-old woman diagnosed with missense (c.266A>C). (**A**) Grade 3 AAK (DCVA = 20/200, sensitivity = 30 mm). Details of fine vessel invasion (inset, arrow). ((**B**) The OCT image reveals partial iris hypoplasia skewed to one side, and a central corneal thickness (CCT) of 610 μm. (**C**) IVCM imaging highlights the presence of vessels (arrow). (**D**) Mixed epithelial cell phenotype with 'islands' of reflective conjunctival cells (arrow) invading the peripheral cornea. (**E**) Invasion of the central corneal epithelium with conjunctival islands (arrow). (**F**) Notably, despite the significant vascularization associated with grade 3 AAK, superficial epithelial cells including nuclei and cell borders remain distinctly visible (arrow)

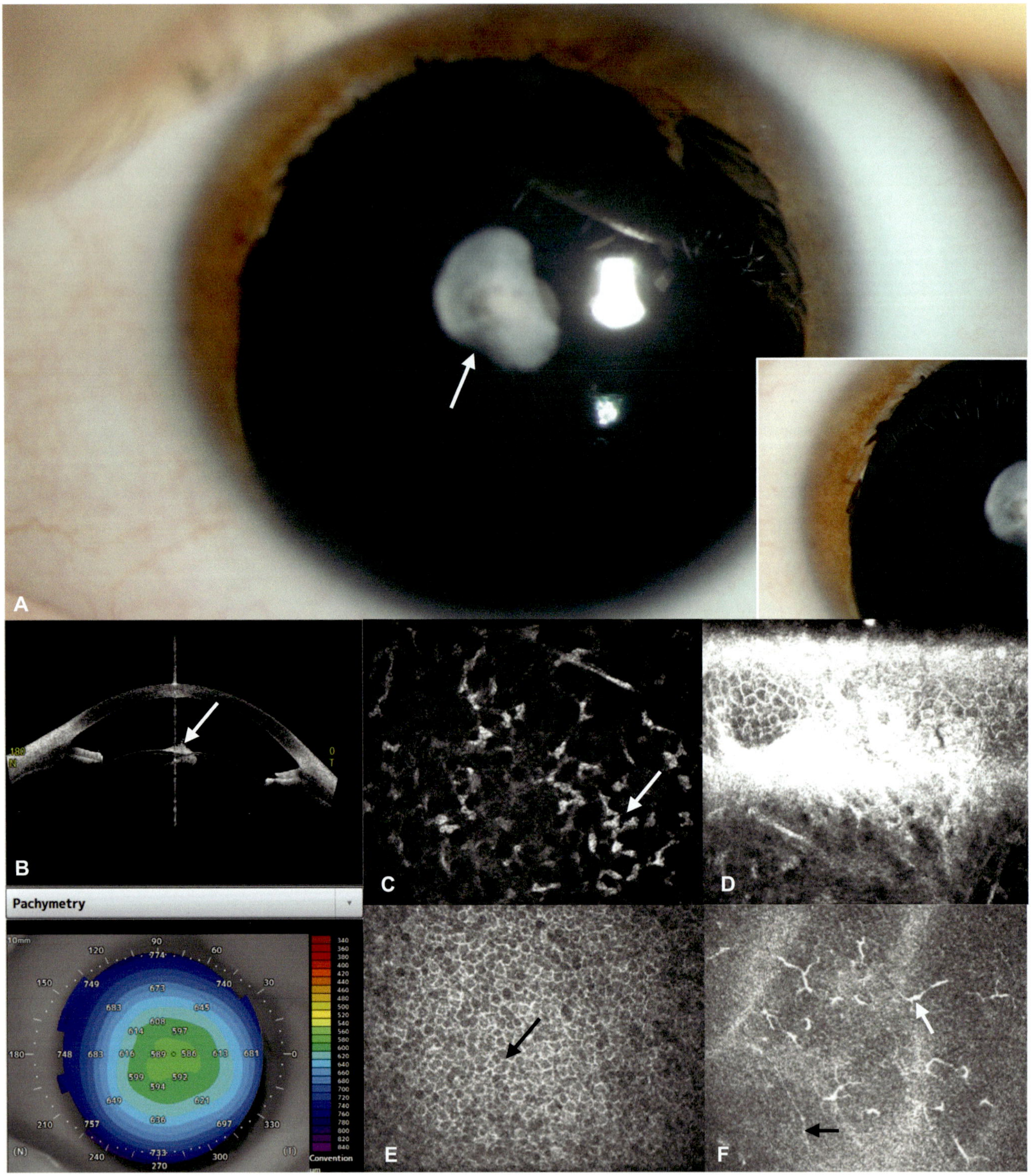

Fig. 8 A 10-year-old girl with non-coding *PAX6* (no information available). (**A**) Grade 0 AAK (DCVA = 20/80, sensitivity = 50 mm) with visible iris remnants and clear changes in the anterior lens (arrow). The limbal border (inset) remains intact. (**B**) Extensive fibrous pseudometaplasia of lens epithelial cells into the anterior chamber is visible, resulting in anterior polar cataract (arrow), with OCT revealing string-like iris remnants in the fibrous area. The CCT is 589 µm. (**C**) Some stromal keratocytes show signs of activation with brightly reflective nuclei and some cell processes visible. ((**D**) Oblique cornea section, indicating invasion of the Bowman layer and epithelium by activated stromal cells and reflective tissue. (**E**) Normal basal epithelial cell mosaic with cell borders visible (arrow). (**F**) In the central cornea, mature dendritic cells (white arrow) are present, with a very sparse presence of corneal nerves (black arrow). Note: panels A, B and F are reproduced under an open access license from [9]

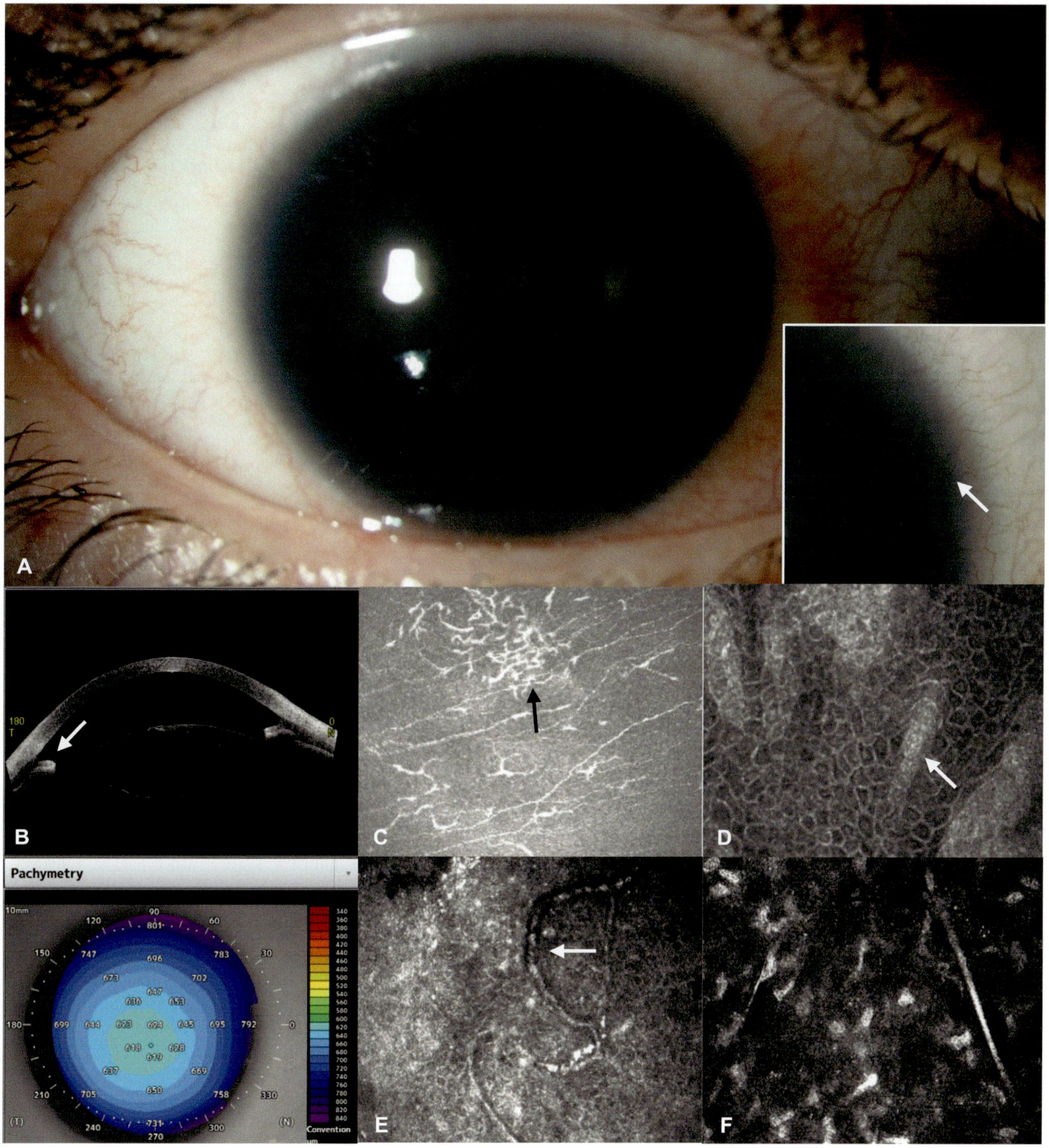

Fig. 9 Case of non-coding *PAX6* mutation in a 26-year-old woman (ELP4, DCDC1). (**A**) Grade 1 AAK is apparent (DCVA = 20/50, sensitivity = 55 mm) with breaching of the limbal border (inset, arrow). (**B**) The OCT image verifies the lack of iris, and a CCT of 624 μm. (**C**) The subbasal nerve layer contains abundant nerves, however a high density of mature dendritic cells (arrow) is present, indicating immune activation. (**D**) The corneal epithelium is transparent but, in the periphery, some epithelial cells are transformed to a conjunctival phenotype (arrow). (**E**) A vessel (arrow) invading the corneal periphery near the limbal region. (**F**) The corneal stroma appears normal

and *PITX2* mutations cause aniridia-like disorders such Axenfeld–Rieger syndrome [1]. This is known as so-called non-*PAX6* aniridia [9]. Maintaining the *PAX6* coding regions intact seems to provide enough functional *PAX6* protein to avoid the classical progressive phenotype of AAK to maintain corneal transparency. For that reason, AAK severity varies across *PAX6* cases, while patients with mutations in non-coding regions generally maintain Grade 1 AAK (Figs. 8 and 9).

7 Conclusion

The extent of ocular underdevelopment evident at birth is affected by the type and severity of *PAX6* mutation, resulting in inadequate or abnormal production of the PAX6 protein, thus influencing the spectrum of severity and progression seen in AAK. In instances of non-coding *PAX6* aniridia, the phenotype is marked by a transparent cornea, relatively satisfactory visual acuity, nearly normal density of subbasal nerves, and only moderate reduction in ocular surface sensitivity and moderate corneal thickness increase. In all instances of congenital aniridia, a mild keratopathy is evident, irrespective of the specific mutation, featuring increased corneal thickness, diminished touch sensitivity, elevated central mature dendritic cell density, increased immune activity on the ocular surface and worsened visual acuity. Both central corneal thickness (CCT) and distance-corrected visual acuity (DCVA) show strong correlations with AAK Grade across all subjects, regardless of age or mutational status. Although the sensitivity of the central cornea is typically lower in *PAX6* aniridia compared to non-coding *PAX6* mutation cases, it does not exhibit a correlation with age. In conclusion, understanding the intricate interplay between *PAX6* mutations and the resulting ocular phenotypes sheds light on the complex nature of aniridia-associated keratopathy (AAK), providing valuable insights for tailored therapeutic approaches and improved management strategies for individuals with congenital aniridia.

Acknowledgements This work was supported by the Rolf M. Schwiete Center for limbal stem cell research and congenital aniridia. With gratitude to Professor Barbara Kaesmann-Kellner, Professor Berthold Seitz, Professor Norá Szentmáry, Lorenz Latta PhD, Dr. Fabian Fries and Kayed Moslemani.

References

1. Landsend ECS, Lagali N, Utheim TP. Congenital aniridia—a comprehensive review of clinical features and therapeutic approaches. Surv Ophthalmol. 2021;66(6):1031–50.
2. Schlötzer-Schrehardt U, Latta L, Gießl A, Zenkel M, Fries FN, Käsmann-Kellner B, Kruse FE, Seitz B. Dysfunction of the limbal epithelial stem cell niche in aniridia-associated keratopathy. Ocul Surf. 2021;21:160–73.
3. Landsend ES, Utheim ØA, Pedersen HR, Lagali N, Baraas RC, Utheim TP. The genetics of congenital aniridia—a guide for the ophthalmologist. Surv Ophthalmol. 2018;63(1):105–13.
4. Lagali N, Wowra B, Fries FN, Latta L, Moslemani K, Utheim TP, Wylegala E, Seitz B, Käsmann-Kellner B. PAX6 mutational status determines aniridia-associated keratopathy phenotype. Ophthalmology. 2020;127(2):273–5.
5. Hall HN, Williamson KA, FitzPatrick DR. The genetic architecture of aniridia and gillespie syndrome. Hum Genet. 2019;138(8–9):881–98.
6. Plaisancié J, Tarilonte M, Ramos P, Jeanton-Scaramouche C, Gaston V, Dollfus H. Implication of non-coding PAX6 mutations in aniridia. Hum genet. 2018;137(10):831–46.
7. Tzoulaki I, White IM, Hanson IM. PAX6 mutations: genotype-phenotype correlations. BMC Genet. 2005 May 26;6:27.
8. Wawrocka A, Krawczynski MR. The genetics of aniridia—simple things become complicated. J Appl Genet. 2018;59(2):151–9.
9. Lagali N, Wowra B, Fries FN, Latta L, Moslemani K, Utheim TP, Wylegala E, Seitz B, Käsmann-Kellner B. Early phenotypic features of aniridia-associated keratopathy and association with PAX6 coding mutations. Ocul Surf. 2020;18(1):130–40.

Ectatic Conditions of the Cornea

Elias Flockerzi, Tim Berger, Haris Sideroudi, Loay Daas, and Berthold Seitz

Abstract

This chapter provides a short overview on the topic of ectatic conditions of the cornea. These comprise keratoconus, pellucid marginal degeneration (PMD) also known as keratotorus, keratoglobus, isolated keratoconus posticus, post-LASIK ectasia and post-keratoplasty keratectasia on the graft. Some cases of superior keratoconus or superior pellucid marginal degeneration have also been described. The diagnosis relies on slit lamp examination, epithelial mapping, corneal topography and tomography, wave front analysis and assessment of corneal biomechanics. Therapy should be adapted to the keratectasia stage and usually begins with fitting of rigid gas-permeable contact lenses, crosslinking, intracorneal ring segment implantation and ends up with deep anterior lamellar or penetrating keratoplasty.

Keywords

Keratoconus · pellucid marginal degeneration · keratoglobus · keratoconus posticus · post-LASIK keratectasia

1 Introduction

Ectatic conditions of the cornea may lead to a corneal thinning and steepening, finally resulting in high irregular astigmatism, stromal scarring and impairment of visual acuity. These corneal diseases have often similar tomographic findings and have to be differentiated from each other to make appropriate and correct treatment decisions [1].

E. Flockerzi (✉) · T. Berger · H. Sideroudi · L. Daas · B. Seitz
Department of Ophthalmology, Saarland University Medical Center, Homburg, Germany
e-mail: elias.flockerzi@uks.eu

2 Keratoconus (KC)

Keratoconus (KC) is a bilateral [2], presumably inflammatory [3] progressive ectatic condition of the human cornea [1] that leads to a paracentral corneal thinning, steepening and irregular astigmatism. The global prevalence is estimated to be about 1.38 cases per 1000 in the normal population [4] and varies geographically. Biomechanically, it is characterized by a decreased resistance to deformation when compared to healthy corneas [5]. Although chronic eye rubbing has been considered a major risk factor for developing progressive KC, the exact pathomechanism leading to KC remains still unclear. A first suspect of KC may arise if there are fluctuating refractive values and high cylinder values in general. Slit lamp examination may reveal typical clinical signs such as Vogt striae, Fleischer ring, paracentral thinning and subepithelial-stromal scarring. Vogt striae are vertical lines in the deep corneal stroma that may disappear when light pressure is applied to the eye (Fig. 1). The Fleischer ring results out of hemosiderin deposition in the basal epithelial cells because of an irregular tear film distribution around the basis of the cone (Fig. 2). Paracentral thinning, stromal scarring (Figs. 3, 4) or even a corneal hydrops with stromal oedema (Figs. 5, 6) may develop in advanced KC stages. Corneal hydrops may be treated with deep stromal compression sutures and gas injection into the anterior chamber after performing a small Nd:YAG or surgical iridotomy (Figs. 7, 8). Besides clinical slit lamp findings, KC can also be diagnosed based on retinoscopy: A scissoring reflex has been described, that safely diagnoses KC, but often underestimates its severity [6]. Corneal confocal microscopy can be used to detect subtle anomalies of the subbasal corneal nerve plexus and it has been reported that KC corneas are characterized by a significantly lower subbasal nerve plexus density and a characteristic tortuous course of the nerve fibers in comparison to healthy controls [7]—independent of whether the patients were wearing contact lenses or not.

B. Seitz et al. (eds.), *Atlas on Cornea*, https://doi.org/10.1007/978-3-031-65422-0_16

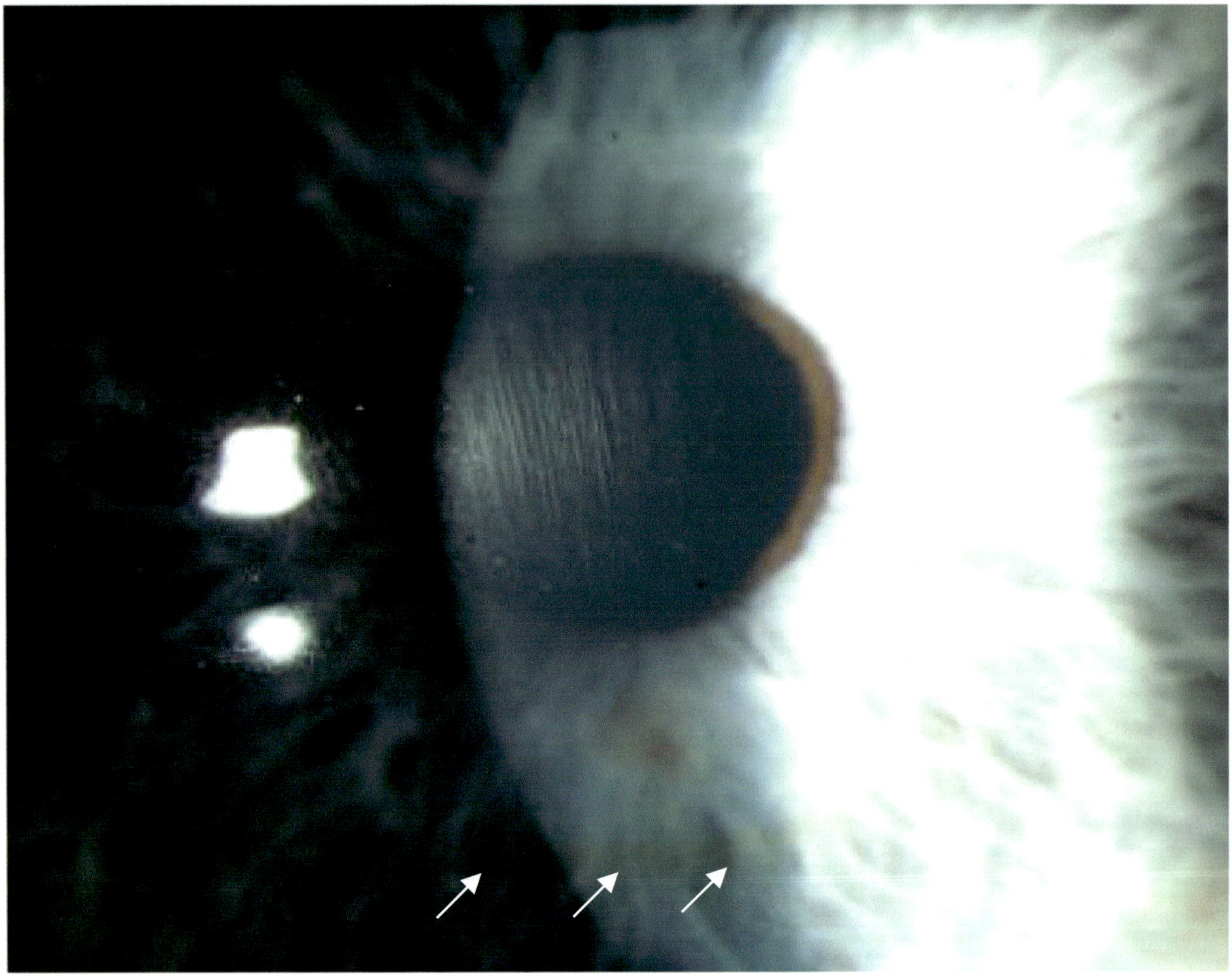

Fig. 1 Vertical Vogt striae in keratoconus. Slightly visible Fleischer ring in the lower part of the image (arrows)

Progression of KC in one eye seems to be independent of the partner eye [8] whereas inter-eye asymmetry increases with KC severity in the worse eye [9]. Different approaches to classify KC have been developed in the past. The Amsler classification was based on clinical signs and supplemented by Muckenhirn in 1984, who added corneal eccentricity. Krumeich included induced myopia, corneal radius, thickness and corneal slit-lamp findings as additional parameters [10]. One recent staging system was introduced by Belin and Duncan in 2016 [11, 12], who based it on the analyses of (1) anterior ("A") and (2) posterior ("B") corneal curvature (measured in a 3.0 mm zone centered on the thinnest corneal thickness), (3) thinnest corneal thickness itself ("C") and the distance best-corrected visual acuity ("D") including stages 0–4 for each parameter, thus enabling an individual grading of each component (see chapter "Scheimpflug-based tomography"). One monocentric study reported 8% of KC patients suffering from atopic dermatitis and 40% of KC patients from allergies [13]. The number of endothelial cells seems to decrease in advanced KC [14], and although a link with floppy eyelid syndrome has been reported, it appears that there is no interaction between dry eye syndrome and tomographic changes in KC patients [15]. Because many trisomy 21 patients are diagnosed with KC and thyroid gland dysfunction, it has been hypothesized, that hypothyroidism may be linked to KC. However, recent studies showed that KC appears to occur relatively more in euthyroid than hypothyroid patients [16] and that its severity seems to be independent of hypothyroidism [17].

The paracentral corneal thinning may also lead to an underestimation of intraocular pressure in KC patients [18]. The Corvis ST®(CST)-derived biomechanically CST-corrected intraocular pressure (bIOP) seems to be best suited for intraocular pressure measurement in KC patients [18]. The CST also provides two standard indices Corvis Biomechanical Index (CBI) and Tomographic Biomechanical Index (TBI), that cannot be used for

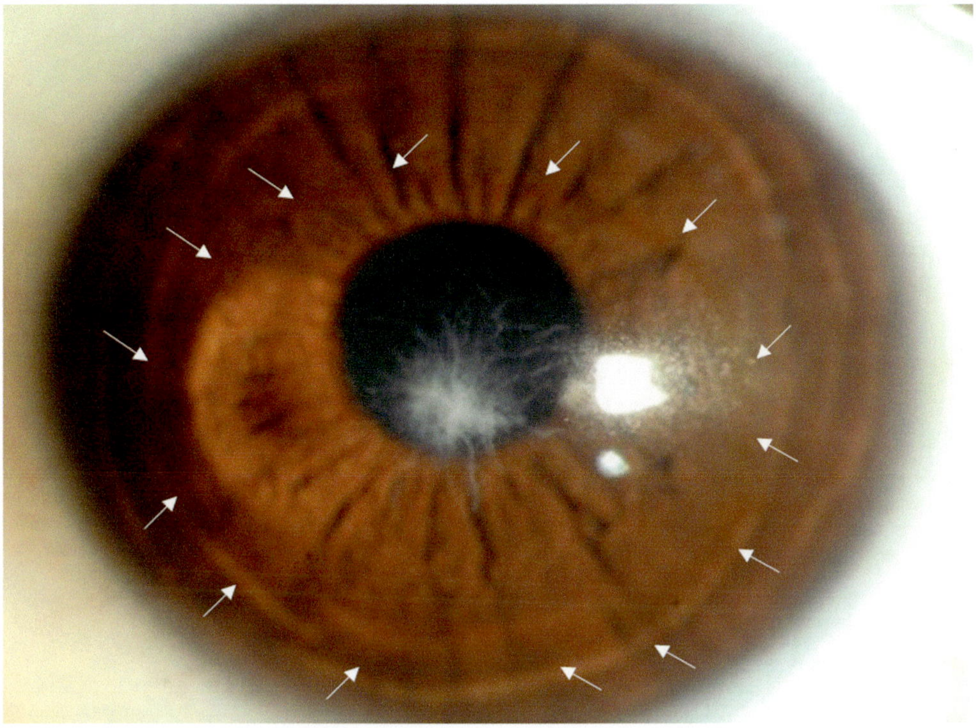

Fig. 2 Fleischer ring around the basis of the cone (arrows)

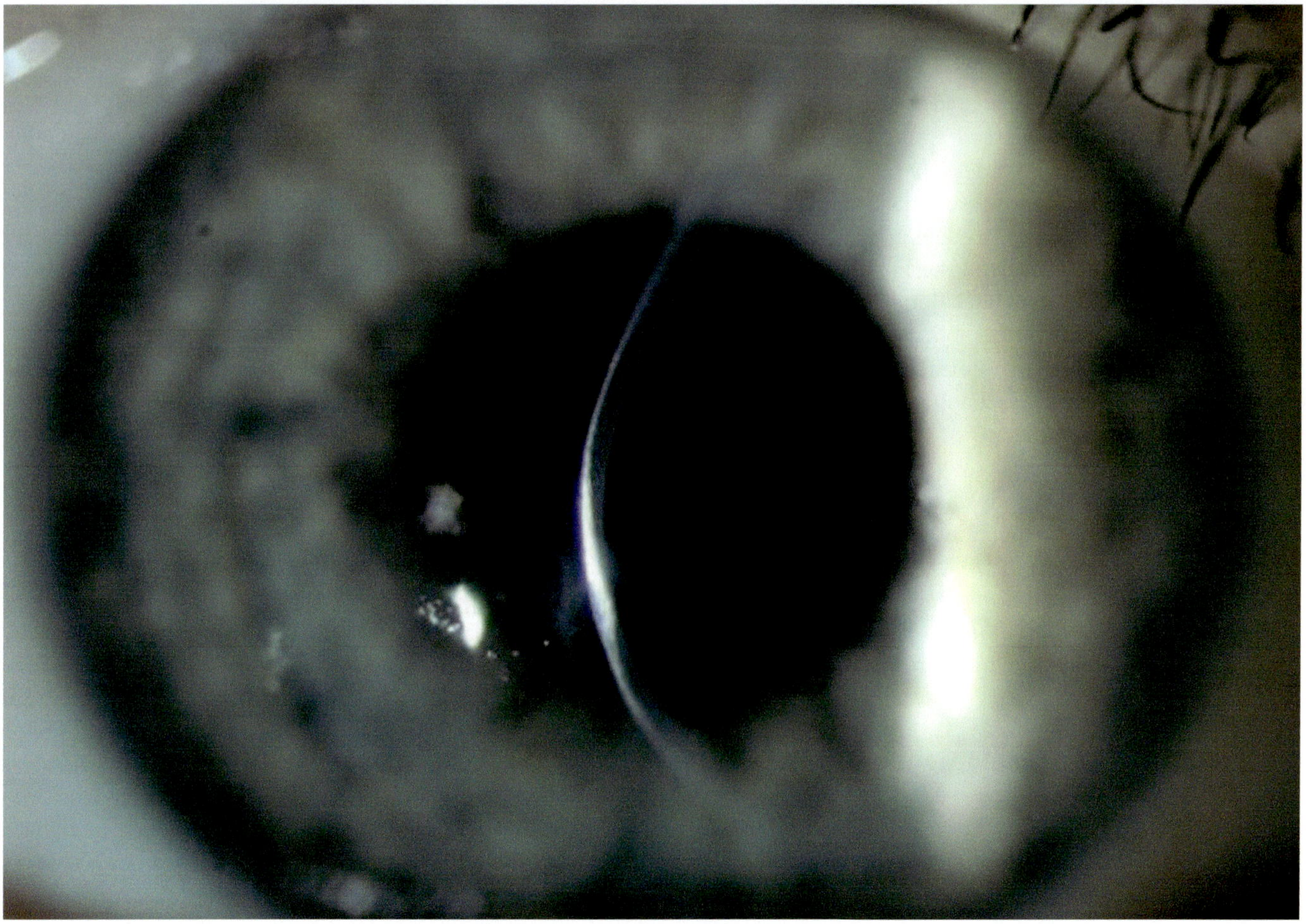

Fig. 3 Paracentral thinning and subepithelial-stromal scarring in advanced keratoconus

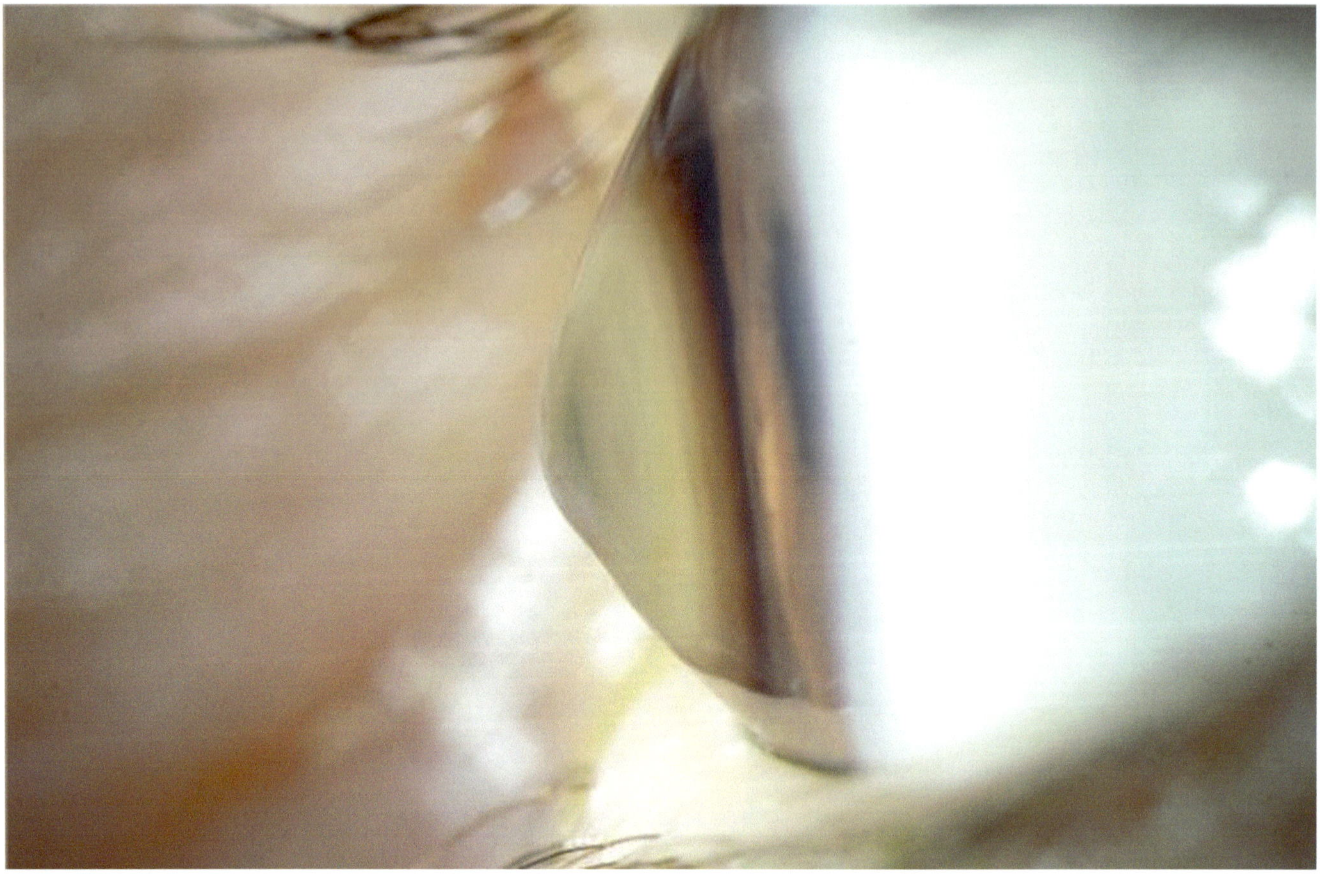

Fig. 4 Side view: paracentral thinning and steepening of the cornea in keratoconus

KC severity or progression assessment because of their nonlinear and quasi-binary behavior [19]. The Corvis Biomechanical Factor (CBiF) is the linearized term of the nonlinear CBI, and it provides biomechanical information about KC severity, thus enabling a biomechanical KC severity and progression assessment (see chapter "Corneal Visualization Scheimpflug Technology") [20].

The stage-appropriate therapy of KC includes contact lens fitting (Fig. 9) [21, 22], corneal crosslinking to stop KC progression (Fig. 10) [23, 24], implantation of intracorneal ring segments or corneal allogenic intrastromal ring segments (CAIRS; example - see also Chapter on Anterior Segment OCT) in cases of contact lens intolerance (Fig. 11) [25] and deep anterior lamellar [26] or penetrating keratoplasty (Fig. 12) in case of subepithelial or stromal scarring [27].

3 Pellucid Marginal Degeneration (PMD)

Pellucid marginal degeneration (PMD) affects the inferior periphery of the cornea and was first described in 1957 [28]. Synonymous terms are "keratotorus" or "degeneratio pellucida marginalis" [1]. "Pellucid" means "very clear" which indicates that the cornea remains generally transparent without showing the typical clinical KC signs despite advanced thinning [29]. Similar to KC, it seems to be a bilateral disease, which can lead to tears in the Descemet membrane and thus to a corneal hydrops in very advanced stages [30].

The thinning area in PMD has been described as an arcuate band of thinning in the periphery of the cornea comparable to the inferior part of a torus (doughnut form), typically reaching from the 4–8 o'clock position (Figs. 13, 14) [29, 30]. It is located in proximity about 1–2 mm away from the limbus and is separated from it by an area of normal corneal thickness [31]. The cornea above this band is characterized by (1) a normal thickness with (2) a flattening of the vertical meridian and (3) an "against-the-rule" astigmatism [29–31].

After KC, the prevalence of PMD has been reported to be higher in comparison to keratoglobus or isolated KC posticus [29, 30]. An estimation of the true PMD prevalence is difficult because it has been overdiagnosed in the past based on "crab claw", "lobster claw" or "kissing birds" patterns detected by isolated examination of corneal topography. Despite showing corneal curvature anomalies, these patterns ignore the actually proving criterion of inferior limbusparallel corneal thinning in PMD [32, 33]. This arcuate band of thinning is typically localized in a distance

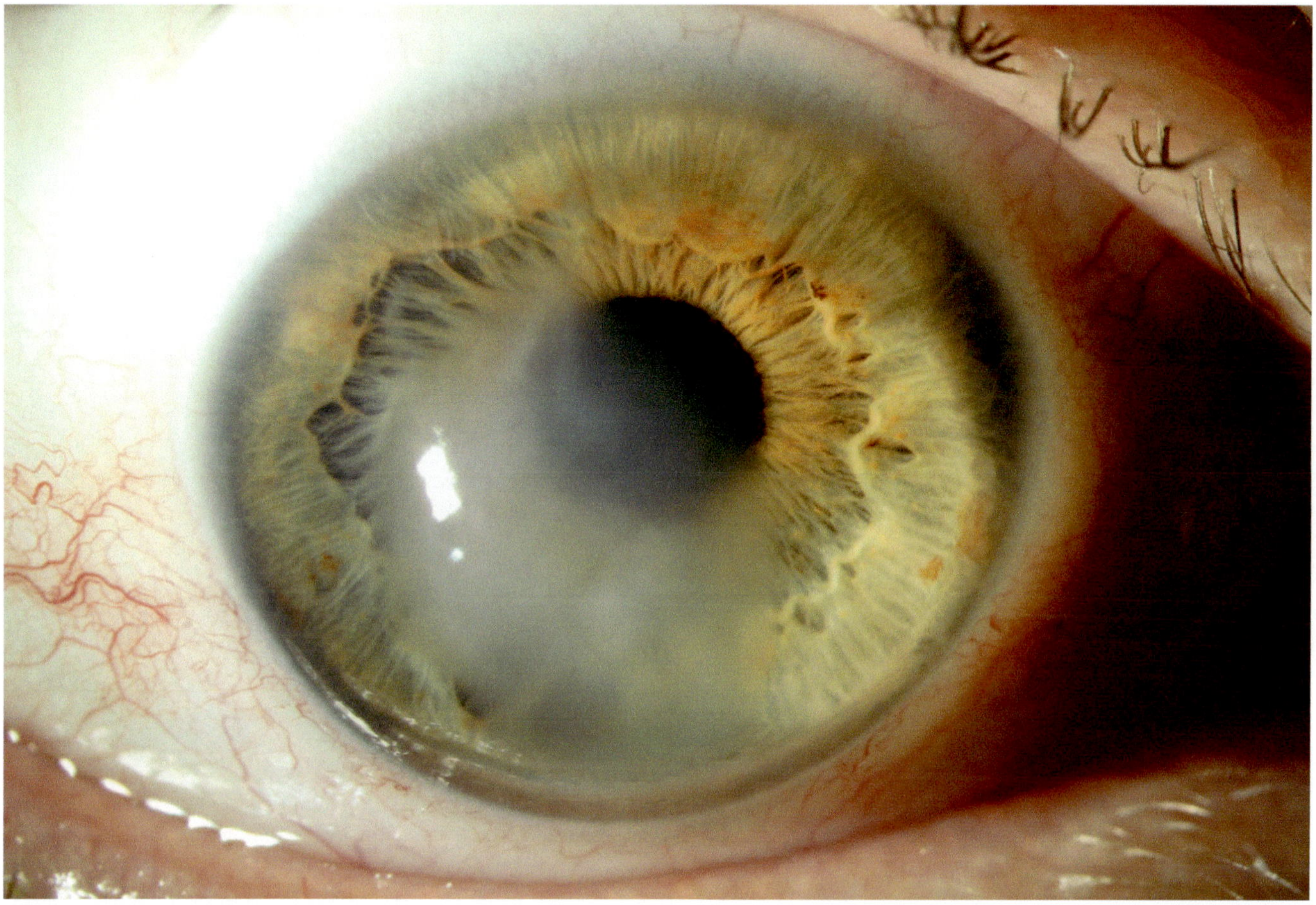

Fig. 5 Corneal hydrops with stromal edema after Descemet tear in keratoconus

of 1–2 mm from the limbus. Thus the thinned region would be located in the 10 mm zone when assuming an average corneal diameter of 12 mm [34, 35]. This area is often not covered by the topographic imaging showing anomalies as described above. Therefore, it has been recommended that PMD should nowadays be diagnosed based on a full corneal pachymetry map covering at least 12 mm in diameter [32]. For this reason, the diagnosis of PMD must be questioned when it is treated with intracorneal ring segments, since the area of maximal ectasia in PMD cases would fall outside of any currently available intracorneal ring segment [31]. Based on these criteria, some cases diagnosed as PMD based on topographic patterns as described above would rather be cases of inferior KC than PMD [36].

Corneal biomechanics were evaluated in PMD based on Ocular Response Analyzer® (ORA, Reichert Instruments, Depew, USA) and Corvis ST® (Oculus, Wetzlar, Germany) measurements. Using ORA, a lower corneal hysteresis and a lower corneal resistance factor were found in PMD compared to healthy controls [37, 38]. In view of Corvis ST® measurements, there exist controversial reports: One study did not find differences between PMD and healthy controls [37] whereas another study found a reduced corneal stiffness in PMD corneas when compared to healthy controls [39]. However, it has to be kept in mind that both devices measure mainly in the corneal center, which is less affected by the pathology in PMD.

The most common therapeutic options for true PMD are refractive correction with spectacles or contact lenses [30]. Surgically, PMD can be treated by decentered corneal crosslinking with riboflavin and ultraviolet—A light irradiation [40] or by the implantation of intracorneal ring segments [41]. Penetrating or deep anterior lamellar keratoplasty are other possible treatment options, but they have to be decentered inferiorly or with a large graft diameter and fixed with single knot sutures because of the pronounced peripheral thinning in advanced cases [42].

4 Keratoglobus

Keratoglobus is considered to be a bilateral congenital corneal disorder [1] (almost) without progression over lifetime—as opposed to KC or PMD [43]. Cases of acquired keratoglobus have also been reported [44, 45]. There exist associations with connective tissue disorders like Marfan or

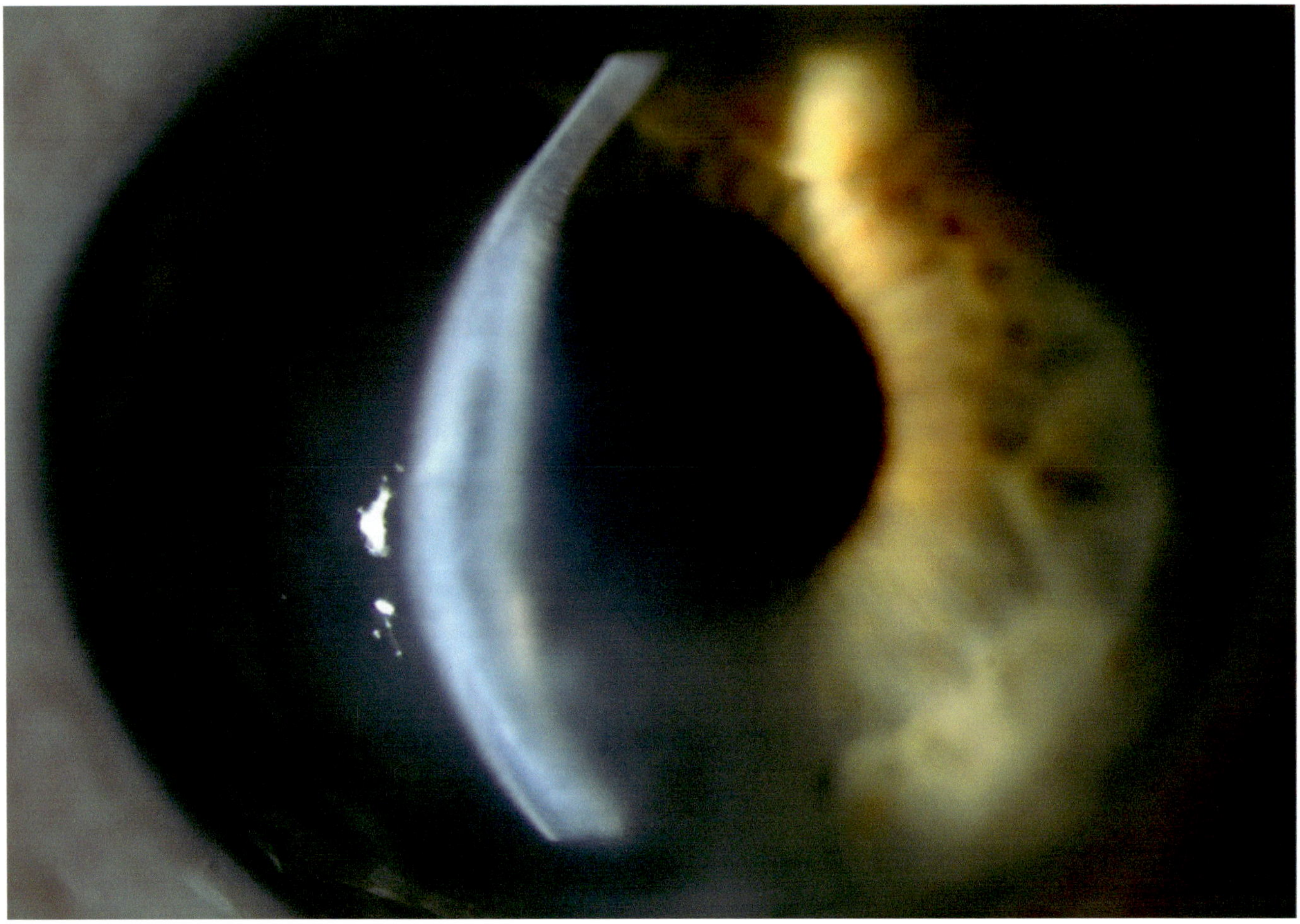

Fig. 6 Slit lamp magnification of the same eye as shown in Fig. 5. Intrastromal edema after Descemet tear in keratoconus

Ehlers–Danlos Syndrome. Characteristics include a global protrusion of the cornea with a generalized thinning from limbus to limbus and a maximal thinning in the periphery (Fig. 15) [30], whereas the typical KC signs are missing. The thinning and protrusion of the cornea induce a myopic, irregular astigmatism and make keratoglobus the most susceptible to spontaneous or trauma-induced perforation [46].

Keratoglobus has to be differentiated from megalocornea as a variant and buphthalmos in congenital glaucoma. This can be done by the analysis of glaucomatous changes that should be present in buphthalmos and by corneal thickness measurements, which are normal in megalocornea [43].

Visual rehabilitation can be achieved using spectacles or contact lenses. Contact lenses have to be handled with care, as their use may increase the risk of corneal perforation [45]. Penetrating keratoplasty may be difficult because of the circularly thinned periphery of the cornea, thus requiring very large graft diameters (e.g. 12 mm sclerocorneal transplants). A surgical alternative aiming to restore a normal corneal thickness is epikeratophakia which consisted in suturing a corneal donor lenticule on the thinned keratoglobus cornea [47]. In case of stromal scarring, a normal-thickness penetrating keratoplasty could be performed thereafter. Although good postoperative outcomes are possible, this method has been partially replaced by deep anterior lamellar keratoplasty as another treatment option for keratoglobus [42, 43].

5 Keratoconus posticus

Keratoconus posticus is characterized by a normal anterior corneal curvature [1] with mostly regular astigmatism and an abnormal posterior corneal curvature [48]. There exist two subtypes: (1) the KC posticus generalis or totalis that affects the entire posterior corneal curvature and (2) the KC posticus circumscriptus that is localized (para-) centrally and is sometimes associated with a corneal opacity [49]. Each variant is considered to be a congenital cleavage anomaly that can occur uni- or bilaterally and remains stable over lifetime [50]. Particularly unilateral cases are susceptible to develop amblyopia [51] and therefore, similar to KC, early detection and correction

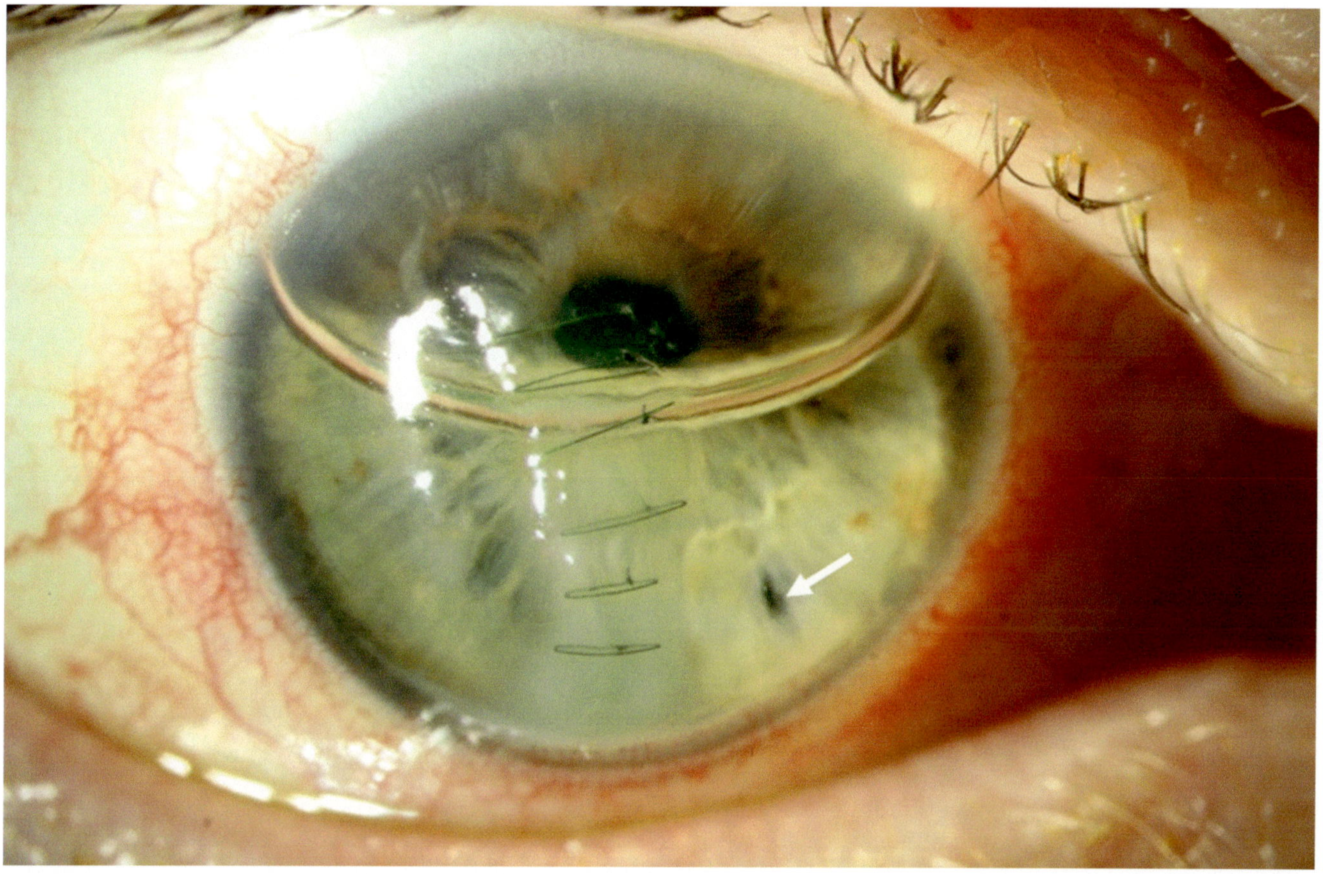

Fig. 7 Same eye as in Figs. 5, 6 one day after deep stromal compression sutures and gas injection in the anterior chamber. Resolving corneal edema. Small Nd:YAG-laser iridotomy at 05.00 o'clock to prevent an air block with subsequent rise of intraocular pressure (arrow)

with spectacles or contact lenses is crucial to prevent it. However, KC posticus is not associated with KC anterius nor has it been described to progress to it [50, 51]. Associated corneal opacities may require (rotational) keratoplasty. It has been recommended to perform an internistic workup because of associations with systemic conditions such as growth disorders, cleft formations, genitourethral malformations or musculoskeletal anomalies [52]. An overestimation of the total corneal power has to be expected even more in KC posticus than KC anterius when planning cataract surgery, thus possibly inducing a refractive surprise [51, 52].

6 Post-LASIK Keratectasia

The development of keratectasia after Laser-in-situ-keratomileusis (LASIK) defines an iatrogenic keratectasia after refractive surgery [53]. Characteristics include abnormal posterior corneal elevation [54], progressive corneal thinning and steepening similar to KC [1] (for tomographic findings, see chapter "Scheimpflug-based tomography"; for biomechanical findings, see chapter "Corneal Visualization Scheimpflug Technology") [55]. This steepening is typically located inferiorly, thus inducing myopia and astigmatism within days to years after surgery [56]. Possible risk factors include a high refractive error prior to surgery, a reduced residual stromal bed and the undetected presence of preoperative keratectasia such as KC or PMD [56, 57]. Non-surgical treatment options include contact lenses for visual rehabilitation. Surgically, corneal crosslinking may be used to halt post-LASIK keratectasia progression. The implantation of intracorneal ring segments aims to modify the anterior radius of corneal curvature and to improve visual acuity. A phakic intraocular lens can be implanted in cases of high myopia regression. Finally, advanced post-LASIK keratectasia can be treated with deep anterior lamellar or penetrating keratoplasty.

7 Superior Keratoconus and Superior Pellucid Marginal Degeneration

The differential diagnosis of superior keratectasia includes Fuchs–Terrien marginal degeneration, peripheral ulcerative keratopathy and presumably superior variants of KC and PMD [1]. There exist case reports of unilateral

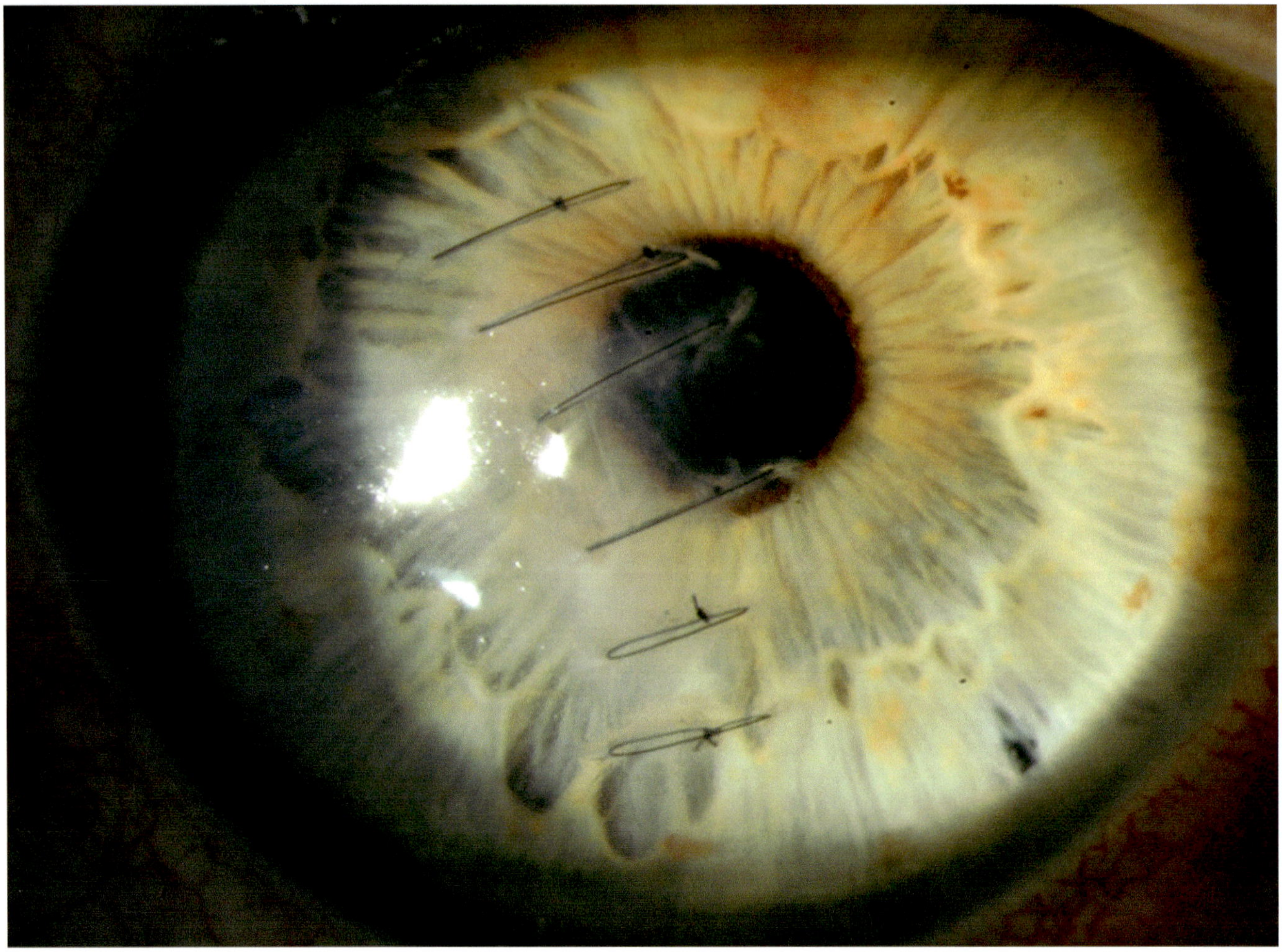

Fig. 8 Same eye as in Figs. 5, 6, 7 six weeks after deep stromal compression sutures and gas injection in the anterior chamber prior to suture removal and contact lens fitting

superior corneal steepening in children without clinical KC signs [58], superior corneal hydrops with clinical KC signs in the fellow eye [59], bilateral superior corneal protrusion with a Fleischer ring [60] and superior PMD [61]. Although these variants have been described (tomographic findings see chapter "Scheimpflug-based tomography"), the diagnosis is rare and has to be questioned critically. Sometimes, a superior corneal steepening can be found in early epithelial basement membrane dystrophy ("map-dot-fingerprint") and may also be mechanically induced, as illustrated by the case of a 62-year-old male patient with superior corneal steepening that resolved three months after surgical treatment of blepharoptosis [62].

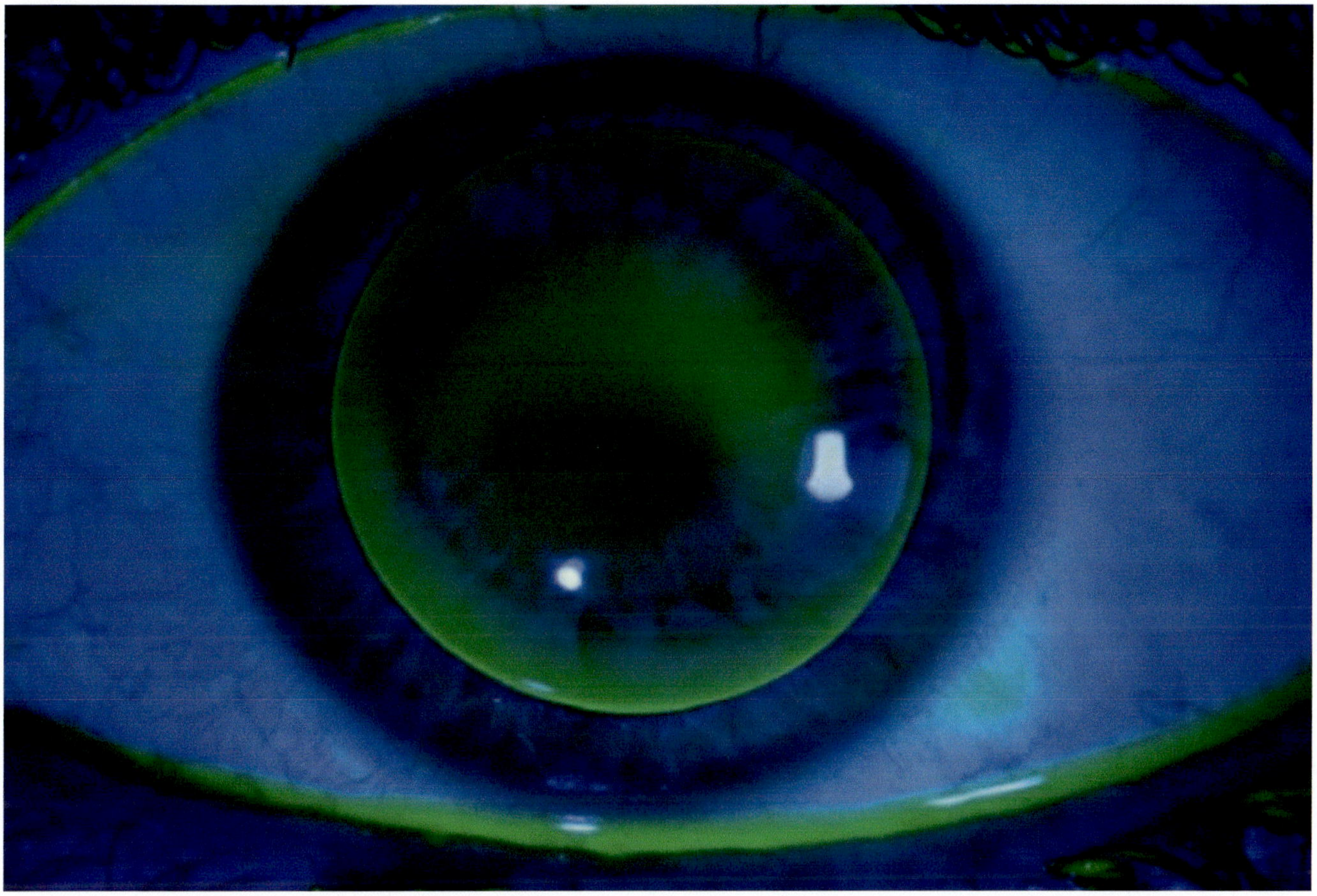

Fig. 9 Rigid gas-permeable contact lens fitting in keratoconus

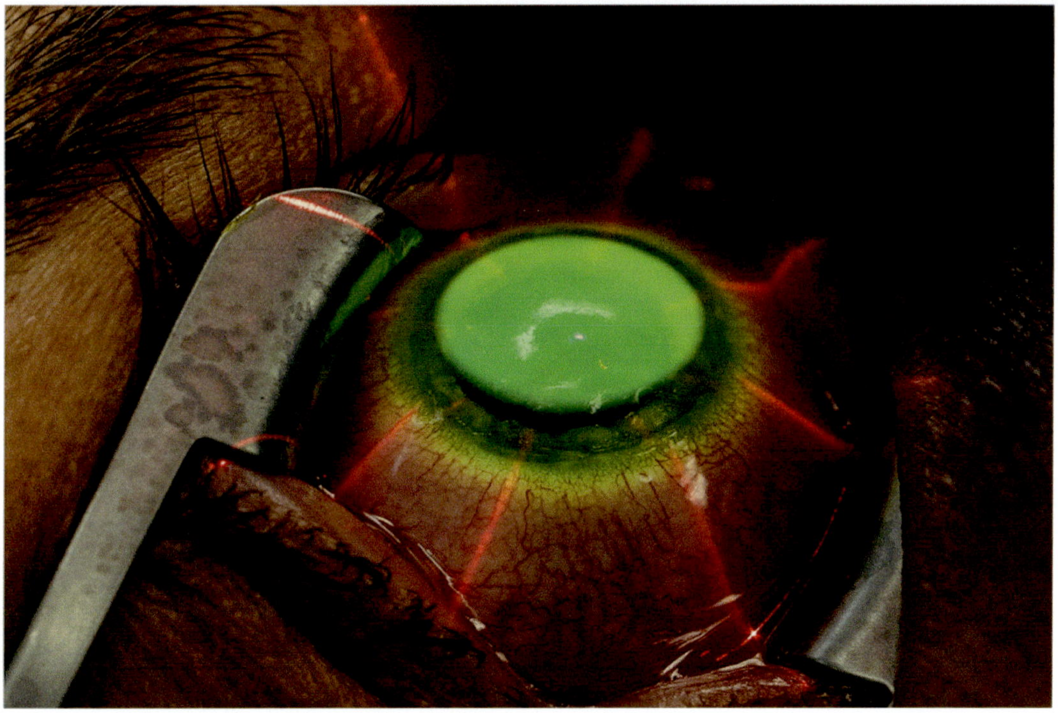

Fig. 10 Accelerated epithelium-off corneal crosslinking (9mW/cm^2, 10 min)

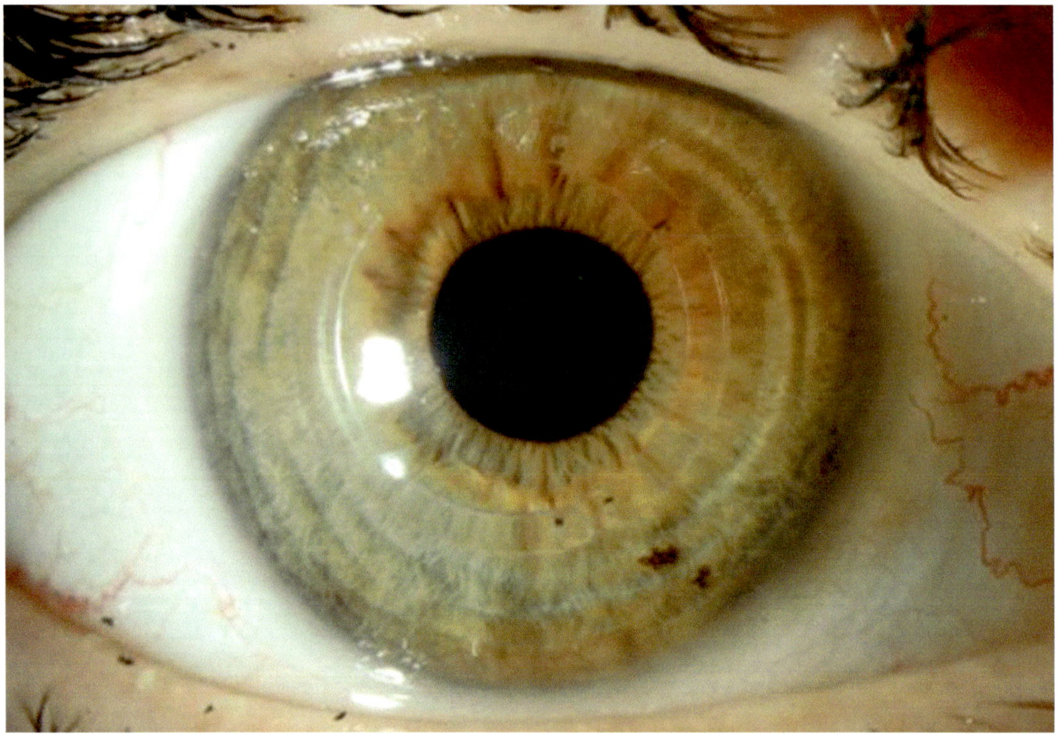

Fig. 11 Intracorneal ring segments in keratoconus (INTACS® SK, Addition Technology, Illinois, United States)

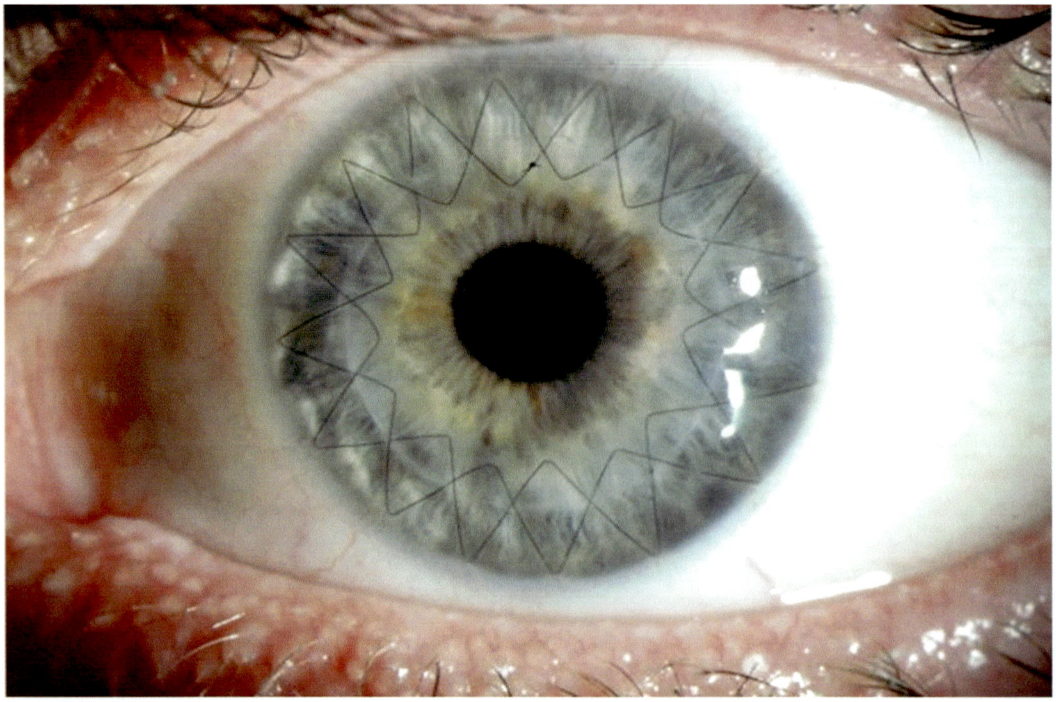

Fig. 12 Excimerlaser-assisted penetrating keratoplasty in keratoconus (8.0 mm trephination, 8.1 mm graft diameter, fixed with double-running cross-stitch suture according to Hoffmann)

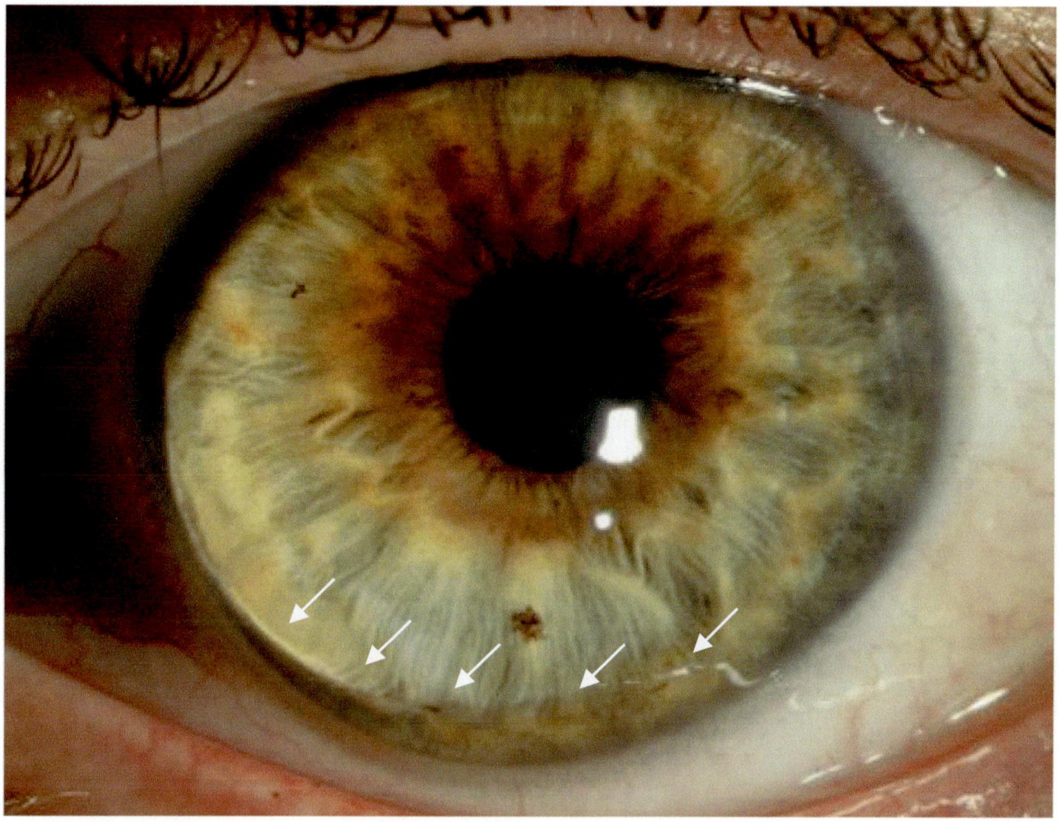

Fig. 13 Pellucid marginal degeneration with peripheral thinning and steepening of the cornea (arrows)

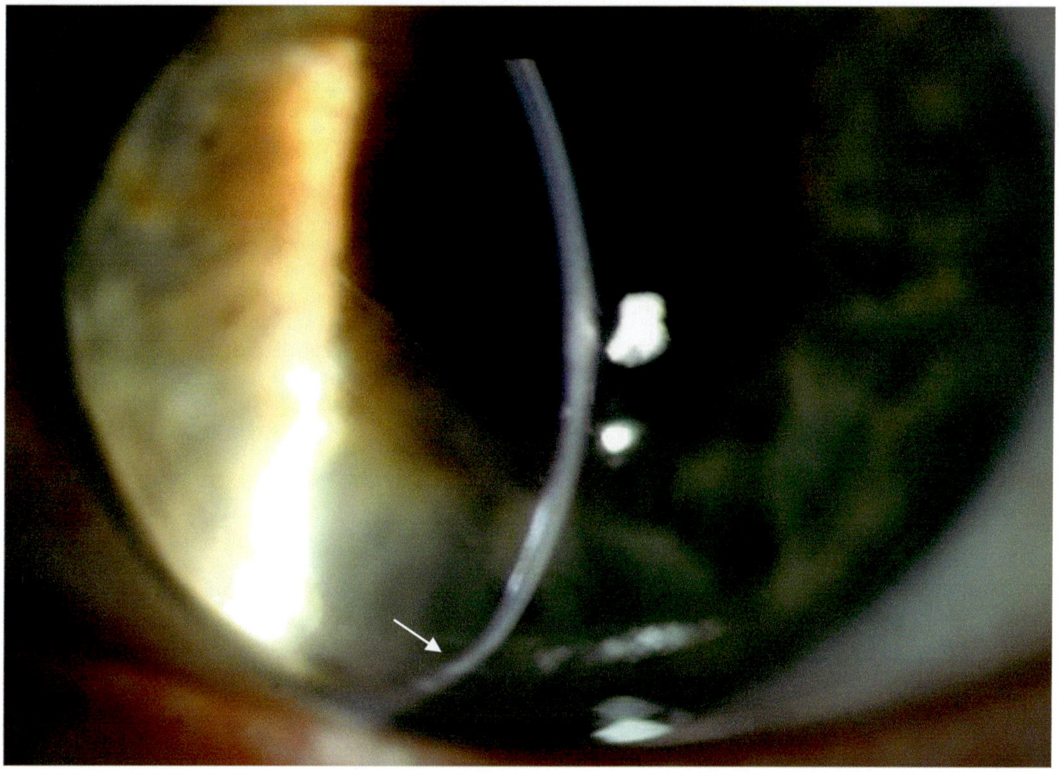

Fig. 14 Magnification of Fig. 13, pellucid marginal degeneration with peripheral thinning and steepening of the cornea (arrow)

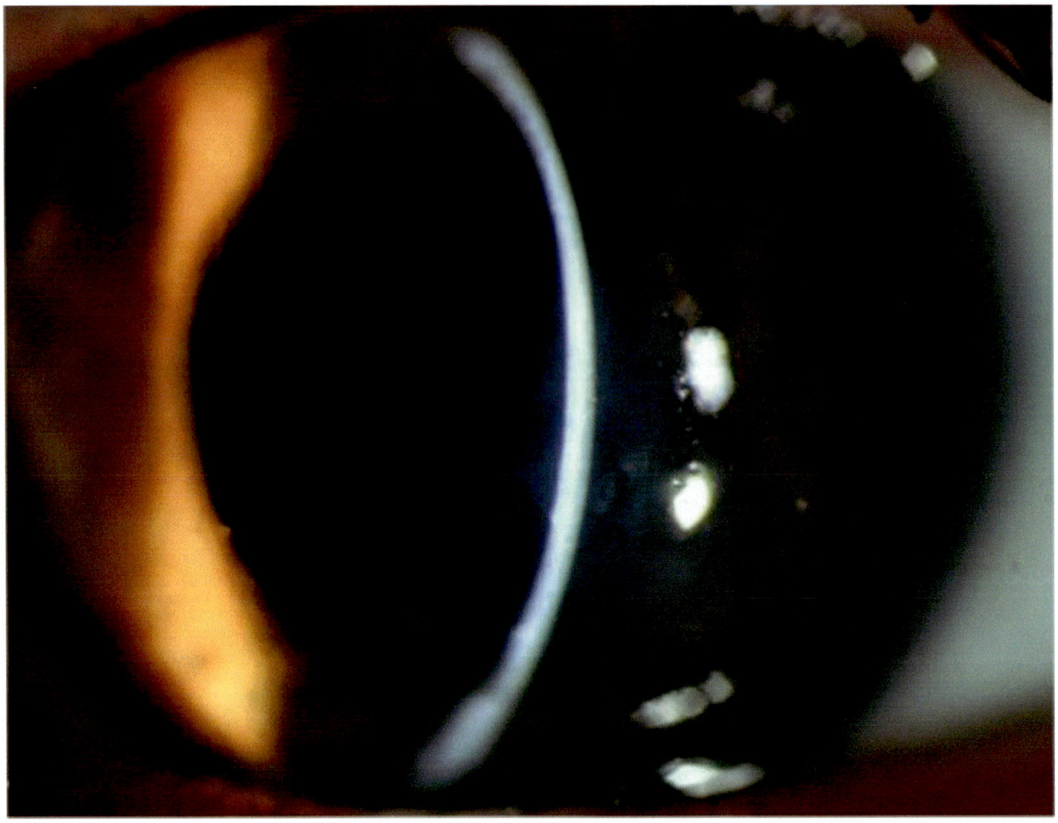

Fig. 15 Global corneal thinning in keratoglobus

8 Conclusion

Diagnostic imaging techniques enable differentiation between the different ectatic corneal diseases, which is crucial for advising patients on treatment options. The latter have been and continue to be refined to provide an individualized treatment.

References

1. Flockerzi E, Daas L, Sideroudi H, et al. Differential diagnosis of keratoconus. In: Das S, editor., et al., Keratoconus. Singapore: Springer Nature Singapore; 2022. pp. 69–88.
2. Gomes JAP, Tan D, Rapuano CJ, et al. Global consensus on keratoconus and ectatic diseases. Cornea. 2015;34(4):359–69.
3. Berger T, Szentmáry N, Chai N, et al. In vitro expression analysis of cytokines and ros-related genes in human corneal fibroblasts and keratocytes of healthy and keratoconus corneas. Ocul Immunol Inflamm. 2024;32(5):556–65.
4. Hashemi H, Heydarian S, Hooshmand E, et al. The prevalence and risk factors for keratoconus: a systematic review and meta-analysis. Cornea. 2020;39(2):263–70.
5. Ambrósio R, Lopes BT, Faria-Correia F, et al. Integration of scheimpflug-based corneal tomography and biomechanical assessments for enhancing ectasia detection. J Refract Surg. 2017;33(7):434–43.
6. Goebels S, Käsmann-Kellner B, Eppig T, et al. Can retinoscopy keep up in keratoconus diagnosis? Cont Lens Anterior Eye. 2015;38(4):234–9.
7. Flockerzi E, Daas L, Seitz B. Structural changes in the corneal subbasal nerve plexus in keratoconus. Acta Ophthalmol. 2020;98(8):e928–32.
8. Goebels S, Eppig T, Seitz B, et al. Intraindividual keratoconus progression. Klin Monbl Augenheilkd. 2017;234(8):1010–4.
9. Eppig T, Spira-Eppig C, Goebels S, et al. Asymmetry between left and right eyes in keratoconus patients increases with the severity of the worse eye. Curr Eye Res. 2018;43(7):848–55.
10. Krumeich J, Daniel J. Live-epikeratophakia and deep lamellar keratoplasty for I–III stage-specific surgical treatment of keratoconus. Klin Monbl Augenheilkd. 1997;211(2):94–100.
11. Belin MW, Duncan J, Ambrósio R, et al. A new tomographic method of staging/classifying keratoconus: the ABCD grading system. Int J Kerat Ect Cor Dis. 2015;4(3):85–93. https://doi.org/10.5005/jp-journals-10025-1105.
12. Belin MW, Duncan JK. Keratoconus: the ABCD grading system. Klin Monbl Augenheilkd. 2016;233(6):701–7.
13. Flockerzi E, Xanthopoulou K, Goebels SC, et al. Keratoconus staging by decades: a baseline ABCD classification of 1000 patients in the Homburg keratoconus center. Br J Ophthalmol. 2021;105(8):1069–75.
14. Goebels S, Eppig T, Seitz B, et al. Endothelial alterations in 712 keratoconus patients. Acta Ophthalmol. 2018;96(2):e134–9.
15. Zemova E, Eppig T, Seitz B, et al. Interaction between topographic/tomographic parameters and dry eye disease in keratoconus patients. Curr Eye Res. 2014;39(1):1–8.

16. Flaskó Z, Zemova E, Eppig T, et al. Hypothyroidism is not associated with keratoconus disease: analysis of 626 subjects. J Ophthalmol. 2019;2019:1–8.
17. Razafimino S, Flockerzi E, Zemova E, et al. Impact of hypothyroidism on tomography and biomechanics in keratoconus—cross-sectional and longitudinal assessment within the Homburg keratoconus center at the time of inclusion and after 1 year. Klin Monbl Augenheilkd. 2023;240(10):1185–91.
18. Knauf D, Seitz B, Schießl G, et al. Analysis of various modalities for intraocular pressure measurement in relation to keratoconus severity in 246 eyes of the homburg keratoconus center. Cornea. 2023;42(7):829–36.
19. Flockerzi E, Vinciguerra R, Belin MW, et al. Correlation of the corvis biomechanical factor CBiF with tomographic parameters in keratoconus. J Cataract Refract Surg. 2022;48(2):215–21.
20. Flockerzi E, Xanthopoulou K, Daas L, et al. Evaluation of dynamic corneal response parameters and the biomechanical E-staging after accelerated corneal cross-linking in keratoconus. Asia Pac J Ophthalmol (Phila). 2022;11(6):514–20.
21. Klühspies U, Grunder A, Goebels S, et al. Keratoconus lenses: the small correction miracle. Ophthalmologe. 2013;110(9):830–8.
22. Richter K, Jullien T, Klühspies U, et al. Contact lens fitting in patients with keratoconus—a retrospective assessment of 200 patients. Klin Monbl Augenheilkd. 2022;239(9):1155–63.
23. Xanthopoulou K, Milioti G, Daas L, et al. Accelerated corneal crosslinking causes pseudoprogression in keratoconus within the first 6 weeks without affecting posterior corneal curvature. Eur J Ophthalmol. 2022;32(5):2565–76.
24. Xanthopoulou K, Milioti G, Daas L, et al. Accelerated corneal crosslinking for treatment of keratoconus in children and adolescents under 18 years of age. Klin Monbl Augenheilkd. 2023;240(10):1131–42.
25. Struckmeier A-K, Hamon L, Flockerzi E, et al. Femtosecond laser and mechanical dissection for ICRS and MyoRing implantation: a meta-analysis. Cornea. 2022;41(4):518–37.
26. Daas L, Hamon L, Ardjomand N, et al. Excimer laser-assisted DALK: a case report from the Homburg keratoconus center (HKC). Ophthalmologe. 2021;118(12):1245–8.
27. Seitz B, Daas L, Hamon L, et al. Stage-appropriate treatment of keratoconus. Ophthalmologe. 2021;118(10):1069–88.
28. Schlaeppi V. The marginal inferior pelvic cortex dystrophy. Bibl Ophthalmol. 1957;12(47):672–7.
29. Moshirfar M, Edmonds JN, Behunin NL, et al. Current options in the management of pellucid marginal degeneration. J Refract Surg. 2014;30(7):474–85.
30. Jinabhai A, Radhakrishnan H, O'Donnell C. Pellucid corneal marginal degeneration: a review. Cont Lens Anterior Eye. 2011;34(2):56–63.
31. Belin MW, Asota IM, Ambrosio R, et al. What's in a name: keratoconus, pellucid marginal degeneration, and related thinning disorders. Am J Ophthalmol. 2011;152(2):157–162.e1.
32. Belin MW. Keratoconus and ectatic disease: evolving criteria for diagnosis. Klin Monbl Augenheilkd. 2020;237(6):740–4.
33. Martínez-Abad A, Piñero DP. Pellucid marginal degeneration: detection, discrimination from other corneal ectatic disorders and progression. Cont Lens Anterior Eye. 2019;42(4):341–9.
34. Rüfer F, Schröder A, Erb C. White-to-white corneal diameter: normal values in healthy humans obtained with the orbscan ii topography system. Cornea. 2005;24(3):259–61.
35. Hashemi H, Khabazkhoob M, Emamian MH, et al. White-to-white corneal diameter distribution in an adult population. J Curr Ophthalmol. 2015;27(1–2):21–4.
36. Lee BW, Jurkunas UV, Harissi-Dagher M, et al. Ectatic disorders associated with a claw-shaped pattern on corneal topography. Am J Ophthalmol. 2007;144(1):154–6.
37. Lenk J, Haustein M, Terai N, et al. Characterization of ocular biomechanics in pellucid marginal degeneration. Cornea. 2016;35(4):506–9.
38. Sedaghat MR, Ostadi-Moghadam H, Jabbarvand M, et al. Corneal hysteresis and corneal resistance factor in pellucid marginal degeneration. J Curr Ophthalmol. 2018;30(2):42–7.
39. Mergen B, Sideroudi H, Seitz B, et al. Altered corneal biomechanics according to the biomechanical E-staging in pellucid marginal degeneration. Cornea. 2024;43(11):1361–7.
40. Mamoosa B, Razmjoo H, Peyman A, et al. Short-term result of collagen crosslinking in pellucid marginal degeneration. Adv Biomed Res. 2016;5:194.
41. Ertan A, Bahadır M. Intrastromal ring segment insertion using a femtosecond laser to correct pellucid marginal corneal degeneration. J Cataract Refract Surg. 2006;32(10):1710–6.
42. Alfaro Rangel R, Szentmáry N, Lepper S, et al. 8.5/8.6-mm excimer laser–assisted penetrating keratoplasties in a tertiary corneal subspecialty referral center: indications and outcomes in 107 eyes. Cornea. 2020;39(7):806–811.
43. Wallang BS, Das S. Keratoglobus. Eye (Lond). 2013;27(9):1004–12.
44. Jacobs DS, Green WR, Maumenee AE. Acquired keratoglobus. Am J Ophthalmol. 1974;77(3):393–9.
45. Cameron JA. Keratoglobus Cornea. 1993;12(2):124–30.
46. Baillif S, Garweg JG, Grange J-D, et al. Keratoglobus: review of the literature. J Fr Ophtalmol. 2005;28(10):1145–9.
47. Kaufman HE, Werblin TP. Epikeratophakia for the treatment of keratoconus. Am J Ophthalmol. 1982;93(3):342–7.
48. Vargas V, Alió J. Posterior keratoconus—clinical aspects and anterior segment optical coherence tomography findings: a case report. Eur J Ophthalmol. 2019;29(1): NP1–5.
49. Süveges I. The histopathology of keratoconus posticus circumscriptus. Klin Monbl Augenheilkd. 1986;189(4):323–5.
50. Vajpayee RB, Sharma N. Association between anterior and posterior keratoconus. Aust N Z J Ophthalmol. 1998;26(2):181–3.
51. Silas MR, Hilkert SM, Reidy JJ, et al. Posterior keratoconus. Br J Ophthalmol. 2018;102(7):863–7.
52. Streeten BW, Karpik AG, Spitzer KH. Posterior keratoconus associated with systemic abnormalities. Arch Ophthalmol. 1983;101(4):616–22.
53. Seiler T, Koufala K, Richter G. Iatrogenic keratectasia after laser in situ keratomileusis. J Refract Surg. 1998;14(3):312–7.
54. Zhao W, Shen Y, Jian W, et al. Comparison of corneal biomechanical properties between post-LASIK ectasia and primary keratoconus. J Ophthalmol. 2020;2020:1–8.
55. Alvani A, Hashemi H, Pakravan M, et al. Post-LASIK ectasia versus keratoconus: an in vivo confocal microscopy study. Cornea. 2020;39(8):1006–12.
56. Randleman JB. Post-laser in-situ keratomileusis ectasia: current understanding and future directions. Curr Opin Ophthalmol. 2006;17(4):406–12.
57. Binder PS, Lindstrom RL, Stulting RD, et al. Keratoconus and corneal ectasia after LASIK. J Cataract Refract Surg. 2005;31(11):2035–8.
58. Weed KH, McGhee CNJ, MacEwen CJ. Atypical unilateral superior keratoconus in young males. Cont Lens Anterior Eye. 2005;28(4):177–9.
59. Tananuvat N, Leeungurasatien P, Wiriyaluppa C. Superior keratoconus with hydrops. Int Ophthalmol. 2009;29(5):419–21.
60. Prisant O, Legeais JM, Renard G. Superior keratoconus. Cornea. 1997;16(6):693–4.
61. Sridhar MS, Mahesh S, Bansal AK, et al. Superior pellucid marginal corneal degeneration. Eye (Lond). 2004;18(4):393–9.
62. Kim T, Khosla-Gupta B, Debacker C. Blepharoptosis-induced superior keratoconus. Am J Ophthalmol. 2000;130(2):232–4.

The IC3D Classification of Corneal Dystrophies—Principles, Classification and Treatment Options According to the Latest, Third IC3D Classification

Berthold Seitz, Tim Berger, Katrin Wacker and Walter Lisch

Abstract

Corneal dystrophies are a heterogeneous group of genetic diseases with a variable age of onset, clinical appearance, variable inheritance and course of progression over time. In 2005, the International Committee on Classification of Corneal Dystrophies (IC3D) was established to resolve difficulties arising from the outdated nomenclature for corneal dystrophies and to correct misconceptions in the literature. This book chapter provides an overview of the diagnostic and treatment principles of corneal dystrophies and presents the current classification of corneal dystrophies according to the revised, third IC3D classification of 2024.

Keywords

Cornea · Corneal dystrophy · International Committee for Classification of Cornea Dystrophies · IC3D

1 Introduction

Corneal dystrophies (CD) are localized opacities of the cornea in typically “white eyes”, which can be characterized by the following features [1–3]:

1. Heredity or familiarity
2. Occurrence in the 1st or 2nd decade of life
3. Typical morphology and localization within the cornea
4. Mostly bilateral, generally symmetrical occurrence
5. Mostly intrafamilial constancy of changes and progression
6. Slowly progressive course without signs of vascularization
7. No inflammatory signs
8. No exogenous causes

However, there are exceptions to some of these dystrophy definitions. Epithelial basement membrane dystrophy (EBMD) and central cloudy corneal dystrophy of François (CCDF) represent degenerative rather than hereditary disorders in the vast majority of patients [4–6]. Corneal dystrophies may be clinically unilateral, such as posterior polymorphous corneal dystrophy (PPCD). Occasionally, systemic associations are observed, as in the case of Schnyder corneal dystrophy (SCD), which might be combined with hyperlipoproteinemia [7].

2 Diagnostic Pathway for Suspected Corneal Dystrophy

The ophthalmologist is first confronted with the often difficult situation of examining a new patient with suspected CD at the slit lamp, classifying the findings correctly and following up with a conclusive consultation regarding prognosis and potential treatment options. Every ophthalmologist must be aware that a patient with finally diagnosed CD may visit his practice for at least 5 different reasons [1, 2]:

1. Visual deterioration
2. Pain (associated with red eye and epiphora)
3. Routine examination
4. Refractive problems
5. Planned family examination

B. Seitz (✉) · T. Berger
Department of Ophthalmology, Saarland University Medical Center, Homburg/Saar, Germany
e-mail: berthold.seitz@uks.eu
URL: https://www.augenklinik-saarland.de

K. Wacker
Eye Center, Albert-Ludwigs University of Freiburg, Freiburg, Germany

W. Lisch
Department of Ophthalmology, Johannes Gutenberg University Mainz, Mainz, Germany

B. Seitz et al. (eds.), *Atlas on Cornea*, https://doi.org/10.1007/978-3-031-65422-0_17

A detailed anamnesis (current anamnesis, ocular anamnesis, family anamnesis) is obligatory. Patients with CD may show the aspect of acute corneal inflammation. However, this so-called inflammation is often caused by corneal epithelial defects, particularly in anterior CD, and does not represent a primary inflammatory condition. Especially epithelial, but also endothelial CD, can imitate bacterial or viral keratitis due to secondary epithelial defects [8]. In case of corneal changes and consecutive subjective complaints, the contralateral eye should always be examined for corneal opacities. A bilateral corneal opacity is suspicious for an existing CD even if there is a difference in severity between both eyes. However, before a diagnosis of CD can be made, skin diseases in combination with eyelid changes (meibomian gland dysfunction) and dysfunctional tear syndrome (such as in rosacea and atopy) must be excluded [8].

In order to detect key findings (so-called "landmarks") for the correct classification of CD, both opacity patterns and opacity units must be determined during slit lamp examination [1, 8–10]. Opacity patterns are determined by (1) horizontal extent, (2) vertical extent ("depth"), and (3) the clarity/opacity of the cornea in between. The horizontal extension is assessed in the wide slit, the depth extension in the blade-thin, very bright slit. The examination with retroillumination after drug-induced mydriasis, is indispensable, not only for the exact classification of the opacity units [1]. Both eyes should always be examined in mydriasis with retroillumination and compared. Overall, this results in clinical key findings that can be different for each CD and, therefore, represents an important differential diagnostic characteristic. An examination of the anterior chamber angle, the lens and the posterior segment of the eye is also essential for differential diagnostic considerations. The clinical examination should be supplemented with further diagnostics of the anterior (e.g. anterior segment optical coherence tomography—AS-OCT, endothelial cell specular microscopy, in-vivo confocal microscopy) and posterior segment of the eye [11].

Hereditary corneal diseases may be a phenomenon limited to the cornea or may be accompanied by abnormalities in other parts of the eye (examination of the entire eye) or the body (e.g. symptoms or signs of systemic diseases). In any case, hereditary metabolic diseases with corneal manifestations must be differentiated from CD. The ophthalmologist can make a significant contribution to the diagnosis of a systemic disease through atypical corneal findings.

Familial amyloidosis (known as Meretoja syndrome or hereditary gelsolin amyloidosis) is a systemic disease caused by pathogenic variants of the gelsolin gene [12]. Affected individuals exhibit neuropathy of the facial nerves and a flabby, mask-like face (so-called "cutis laxa"). The corneal findings in familial amyloidosis are similar to those of lattice CD, but the lattice lines are less numerous, begin peripherally and spread centrally. Therefore, this clinical picture is no longer referred to as lattice corneal dystrophy type 2 [12]. In advanced stages, corneal epithelial erosions and neurotrophic keratopathy may occur, which is why keratoplasty is associated with a high rate of graft failure in contrast to lattice CD [13]. The correct differentiation of clinically similar findings is, therefore, also of prognostic importance.

With the introduction and development of genotypic analyses (e.g. blood sample or oral mucosal swab with subsequent DNA extraction), knowledge of CD has steadily increased, allowing inaccuracies in the nomenclature to be clarified [14]. Although the medical history and clinical examination are usually the mainstays of diagnosis, only genetic testing leads to the clinical confirmation. Genotyping revealed both genotypic heterogeneity, i.e. a single CD such as Meesmann corneal dystrophy (MECD) could be assigned to different genes (*KRT3* and *KRT12*), and phenotypic heterogeneity, i.e. the *TGFBI* gene was assigned to different allelic dystrophy phenotypes, such as Reis–Bücklers corneal dystrophy (RBCD), Thiel–Behnke corneal dystrophy (TBCD), granular corneal dystrophy type 1 (GCD1), granular corneal dystrophy type 2 (GCD2) and lattice corneal dystrophy (LCD) [15, 16].

The diagnosis of CD in pediatric patients remains challenging, largely because most publications contain photographs of CD with the classic findings in adulthood. There is a relatively small number of well-documented early findings, often showing only very subtle corneal changes in childhood. Early findings are sometimes very distinct from the classic manifestations of CD in adulthood. Children with CD often present to the ophthalmologist not because of visual impairment, but because of eye pain caused by dystrophy-related corneal erosions. The family examination as well as a genetic examination are often of decisive importance in making a diagnosis in such cases.

3 Treatment of Corneal Dystrophies

The following section explains the basic principles of conservative and surgical treatment of CD [17]. A detailed description of the treatment options for individual CD is provided in the revised third edition of the IC3D [18].

In general, conservative or surgical treatment of CD is indicated for symptomatic and/or functional complaints. CD affecting the epithelial/subepithelial area or the anterior corneal stroma can lead to foreign body sensation or pain (e.g. recurrent corneal erosions, dry eye), as well as an irregular corneal surface with reduced visual acuity and quality. However, some CD are usually asymptomatic and require no treatment. Conservative treatment of CD mainly involves the application of tear substitutes and, in severe cases, the insertion of a therapeutic bandage contact lens. The choice of the surgical procedure depends on the symptoms, the clinical findings and the assessment of the device-based diagnostics. In addition, the patient should have realistic expectations and be informed about potential complications (residual opacities, recurrences). The risk of recurrence depends on the underlying CD.

Excimer laser-assisted phototherapeutic keratectomy (excimer PTK) has a promising prognosis for prominent and superficial changes. In contrast, localized lesions with stromal thinning or deeper manifestation show an unfavorable prognosis. Superficial CD such as EBMD or GCD2 (GCD1 with typically deeper manifestation) can be treated very well with excimer PTK. In SCD, 50% of all affected patients have crystalline deposits, which are always located subepithelially and might affect the optical center. These superficial crystalline deposits can be treated well with the excimer PTK, whereas the diffuse opacities in SCD may affect the entire corneal stroma. The amyloid deposits in LCD, which are typically located in the deep stroma, are also difficult to access with the excimer laser. Macular corneal dystrophy (MCD) has acid mucopolysaccharides that can affect all structures from epithelium to endothelium (development of endothelial decompensation is possible) and extend from limbus to limbus. Since the superficial deposits in MCD can lead to an irregular topography (so-called "pseudokeratoconus" profile), excimer PTK can contribute to surface regularization, even if deep deposits remain (CAVE: corneas in MCD are typically thinned) [19]. Determination of ablation depth should be performed with the AS-OCT, as Scheimpflug-based systems do not provide reliable thickness measurements in opacified corneas (CAVE: increased hyperopia with increasing ablation depth). To minimize the recurrence of CD and avoid the risk of stromal scarring (large ablation depth, repeat excimer PTK, excimer PTK after keratoplasty), mitomycin C 0.02% should be used intraoperatively for 60–90 s [20].

Penetrating keratoplasty (PKP) or deep anterior lamellar keratoplasty (DALK, no endothelial graft rejection) may be indicated for diffuse or deep stromal involvement [21, 22]. Preparation of the recipient bed in anterior lamellar keratoplasty should always be performed up to the "crystal clear" Descemet membrane, as residual stroma of the recipient (e.g. superficial ALK) might lead to dense opacities in the interface area. The individual risk of recurrence must be taken into account in the decision-making process for each surgical procedure [23]. While MCD after PKP rarely causes recurrences, GCD2 (in contrast to GCD1) and LCD are characterized by a postoperative course with early recurrences [24, 23]. In addition, epithelial healing disorders can occur postoperatively (especially in LCD), which is why subsequent treatment with autologous serum eye drops should be considered after surgery [25]. Descemet Membrane Endothelial Keratoplasty (DMEK) is the method of choice for endothelial CD [26].

4 The International Committee for the Classification of Corneal Dystrophies (IC3D)

In July 2005, the "International Committee on Classification of Corneal Dystrophies" (IC3D) was established with the support of the American Cornea Society. This working group consisted of 17 cornea experts from the USA, Asia and Europe. The task of the working group was to develop a new, internationally accepted classification of CD and to correct the deficiencies of the centuries-old phenotype-based method of classifying CD. The aim was to avoid misinterpretations and misnomers for the different CD in the future.

In 2008 and 2011, the first IC3D publications attempted to develop a "new system for the classification of CD" by integrating the then current information on phenotype, pathology, and especially genetics [15, 16]. In addition, templates for each CD were provided including name, abbreviation, MIM (Mendelian Inheritance in Men), eponym, inheritance, gene locus, mutation, onset, clinical signs, course, symptoms, light microscopy, electron microscopy, confocal microscopy, as well as characteristic slit lamp photographs in color, essential literature information and category classification.

The different CDs were divided into 4 categories (Table 1) according to clinical and genetic knowledge [15, 16]. The second edition of IC3D was published in 2015 [27, 28], followed by a revised third edition in 2024 [18]. This book chapter presents the various CD according to the current IC3D classification [18].

Table 1 IC3D categories of corneal dystrophies

Category	Description
1	Well-defined disease entity with known gene
2	Well-defined disease entity with unknown gene but known gene locus
3	Well-defined disease entity with unknown gene locus
4	Poorly defined disease entity with unknown gene locus

5 The Revised Third IC3D Classification of Corneal Dystrophies

The revised third edition of the IC3D classification (Table 2) divides CDs into 4 different groups:

1. Epithelial and subepithelial dystrophies
2. Epithelial–stromal TGFBI dystrophies
3. Stromal dystrophies
4. Endothelial dystrophies

5.1 Epithelial and Subepithelial Dystrophies

5.1.1 Epithelial Basement Membrane Dystrophy

Epithelial basement membrane dystrophy (EBMD, so-called map dot fingerprint dystrophy) is a very common corneal dystrophy [29]. Because most cases are not inherited, it must be assumed that it is more likely to be a degenerative disease (Category 4). The symptoms can vary and range from asymptomatic courses, pain by recurrent

Table 2 Classification of corneal dystrophies (3rd edition of the IC3D classification) [18]

Group	Name of the corneal dystrophy	IC3D abbreviation	Category (C)	Figures
Epithelial and subepithelial dystrophies	Epithelial basement membrane dystrophy	EBMD	C3	1–6
	Epithelial recurrent erosion dystrophies: – Epithelial recurrent erosion dystrophy – Franceschetti corneal dystrophy – Dystrophia Smolandiensis – Dystrophia Helsinglandica	EREDs ERED FRCD DS DH	 C1 C4 C4 C4	–
	Subepithelial mucinous corneal dystrophy	SMCD	C4	–
	Meesmann corneal dystrophy	MECD	C1	7–10
	Lisch epithelial corneal dystrophy	LECD	C1	11–12
	Gelatinous drop-like corneal dystrophy	GDLD	C1	13–14
Epithelial–stromal TGFBI dystrophies	Reis–Bücklers corneal dystrophy	RBCD	C1	15–17
	Thiel–Behnke corneal dystrophy	TBCD	C1	18–21
	Lattice corneal dystrophies: – Classic LCD – LCD variants	LCD	 C1 C1	22–28
	Granular corneal dystrophy, type 1	GCD1	C1	29–41
	Granular corneal dystrophy, type 2	GCD2	C1	42–52
Stromal dystrophies	Macular corneal dystrophy	MCD	C1	53–60
	Schnyder corneal dystrophy	SCD	C1	61–70
	Congenital stromal corneal dystrophy	CSCD	C1	71–72
	Fleck corneal dystrophy	FCD	C1	73
	Posterior amorphous corneal dystrophy	PACD	C1	–
	Central cloudy dystrophy of François	CCDF	C4	74–75
	Pre-Descemet corneal dystrophies: – Pre-Descemet corneal dystrophy (Cornea farinata) – Punctiform and polychromatic pre-Descemet corneal dystrophy	PDCDs: PDCD PPPCD	 C4 C1	– 76
Endothelial dystrophies	Fuchs endothelial corneal dystrophy	FECD	C1, C2, or C3	–
	Posterior polymorphous corneal dystrophy	PPCD	C1	77–87
	Congenital hereditary endothelial dystrophy	CHED	C1 or C3	88–91
	X-linked endothelial corneal dystrophy	XECD	C2	92–93

erosions or visual impairment by secondary induced irregular corneal astigmatism. Clinical key findings include "maps", "Cogan dots", "fingerprint lines" and a "bleb" pattern. The maps are irregular islands of thickened, gray, hazy epithelium with circumscribed borders, which are mainly found in the central or paracentral cornea (Figs. 1 and 2). Cogan dots are irregular round, oval or comma-shaped putty-gray intraepithelial opacities in the central or paracentral cornea (Fig. 3). "Fingerprints" (Figs. 4 and 5) are parallel, curved lines that typically occur paracentrally and are best visualized by using retroillumination. Cogan dots are always combined with subtle maps (Fig. 6A). The surgical treatment of choice is an excimer PTK to remove the corneal opacities and to increase the number of hemidesmosomes (Fig. 6B).

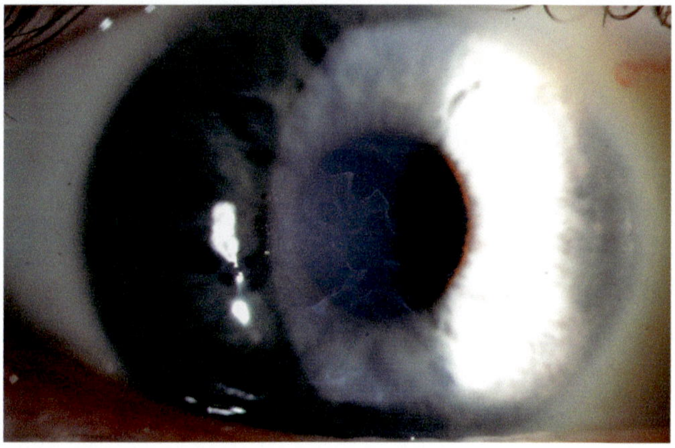

Fig. 1 Epithelial basement membrane dystrophy showing irregular islands of thickened, greyish epithelium with circumscribed borders ("maps")

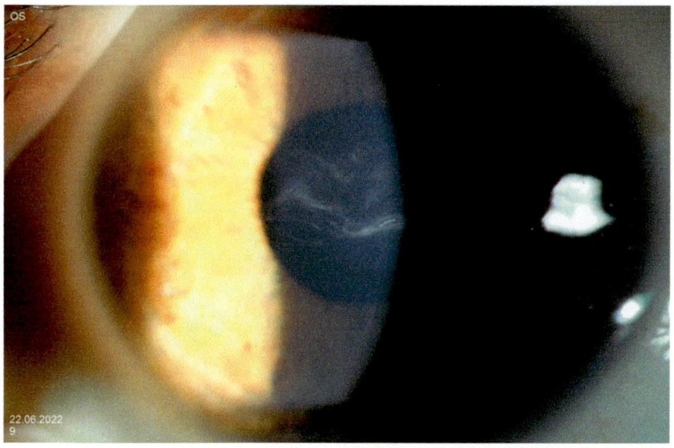

Fig. 2 Severe epithelial basement membrane dystrophy with maps in the optical center

5.1.2 Epithelial Recurrent Erosion Dystrophies

The epithelial recurrent erosion dystrophies (EREDs) include the following dystrophies:

1. Epithelial recurrent erosion dystrophy (ERED) [30]
2. Franceschetti corneal dystrophy (FRCD) [31]
3. Dystrophia Smolandiensis (DS) [32]
4. Dystrophia Helsinglandica (DH) [33]

In 2015, mutations in the collagen 17 alpha 1 gene (*COL17A1*) were described for the autosomal dominant inherited ERED (category 1) [30]. No genetic locus or gene could be identified for the other three category 4 CDs (FRCD, DS, and DH).

In the first decade of life, recurrent corneal erosions occur that last up to 7 days. During the pain-free intervals, no corneal changes are clinically visible. In middle age, with increasing frequency of recurrences, subepithelial or raised, keloid-like corneal scars might develop, leading to visual impairment in up to 50% of patients in their late thirties. However, the frequency and severity of recurrent corneal erosions decreases in the fourth decade of life.

5.1.3 Subepithelial Mucinous Corneal Dystrophy

Subepithelial mucinous corneal dystrophy (SMCD) has been described in one family (no inheritance pattern known) and is characterized by diffuse bilateral subepithelial corneal opacities that are most dense in the central cornea [34]. The symptoms and clinical findings of SMCD are similar to those of ERED.

5.1.4 Meesmann Corneal Dystrophy

Meesmann corneal dystrophy (MECD) is inherited in an autosomal dominant manner and represents an example of phenotypic heterogeneity as one phenotype is caused by two different genes (12q13, keratin 3—*KRT3* and 17q12 keratin 12—*KRT12*) [35]. In most cases, the dystrophy is asymptomatic. However, increased light sensitivity, foreign body sensation and recurrent epithelial erosions have been described. It is characterized by tiny intraepithelial cysts that extend to the limbus of the cornea. These diffuse white–gray opacities of MECD observed by direct illumination might have a distinct border and vary in pattern (Figs. 7 and 8). Using indirect illumination, the gray opacities appear as single clear microcysts, which is a clinical landmark of MECD (Figs. 9 and 10). Multiple coalescing cysts might lead to linear opacities.

5.1.5 Lisch Epithelial Corneal Dystrophy

In 1992, Walter Lisch et al. first described the distinctive bilateral clinical and histologic signs in a large family of six generations and one singular unilateral male from Germany and two singular unilateral and bilateral

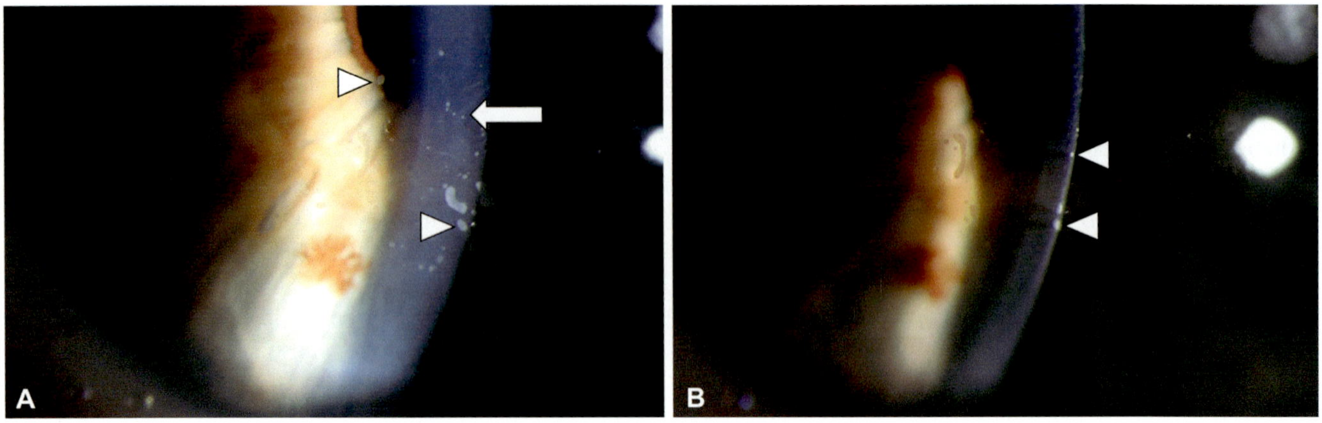

Fig. 3 Epithelial basement membrane dystrophy with oval and comma-shaped, grey, intraepithelial opacities (Cogan dots, arrowheads). Cogan dots are always combined with subtle maps (arrow) (**A** broad slit illumination, **B** thin slit illumination)

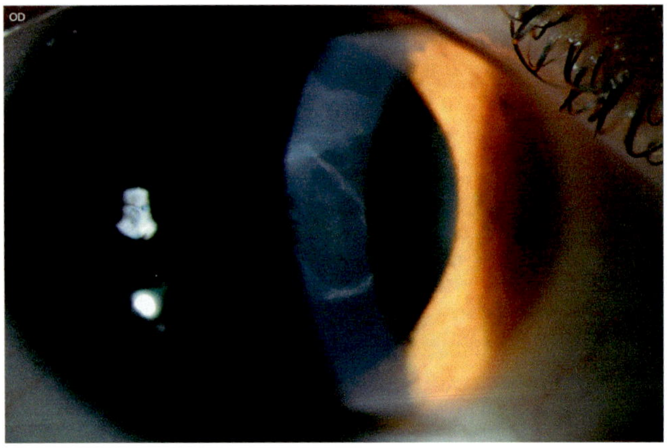

Fig. 4 Epithelial basement membrane dystrophy demonstrating advanced "Maps"

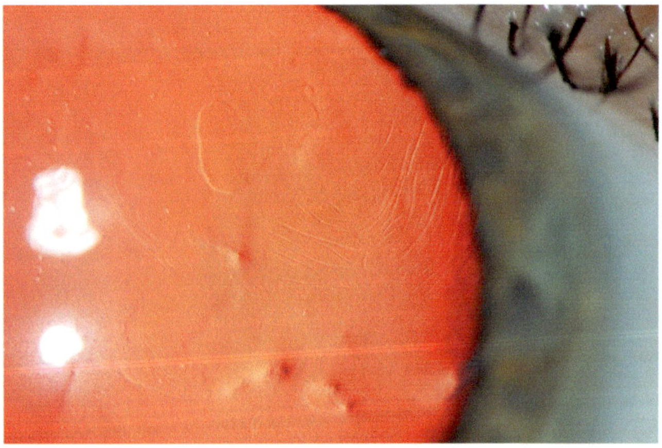

Fig. 5 Epithelial basement membrane dystrophy with fingerprint lines that can be observed by retroillumination

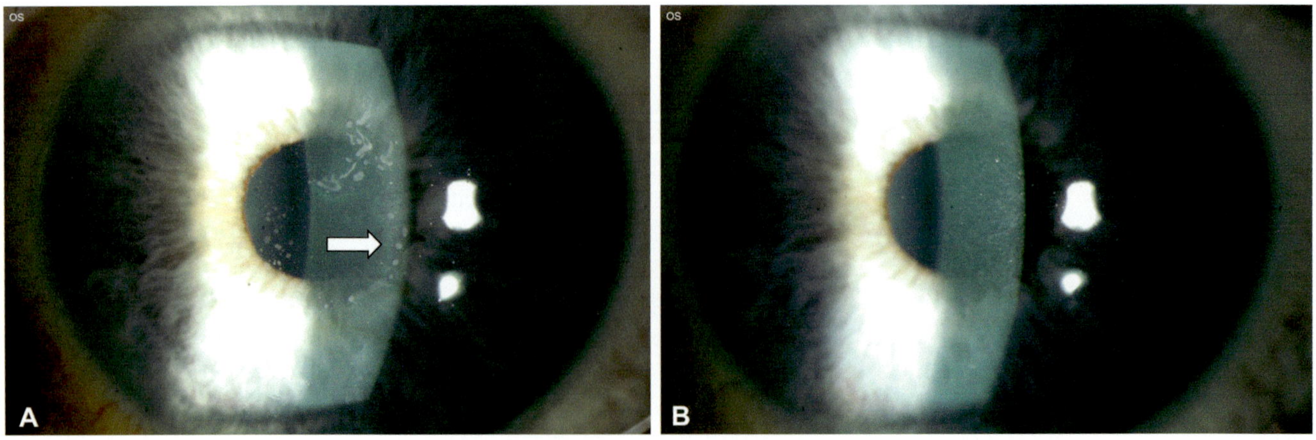

Fig. 6 Epithelial basement membrane with pronounced Cogan dots, which are always combined with subtle maps (**A**) margin of the maps marked by arrow). Postoperative results showing complete removal of the opacities six weeks after excimer laser-assisted phototherapeutic keratectomy (**B**)

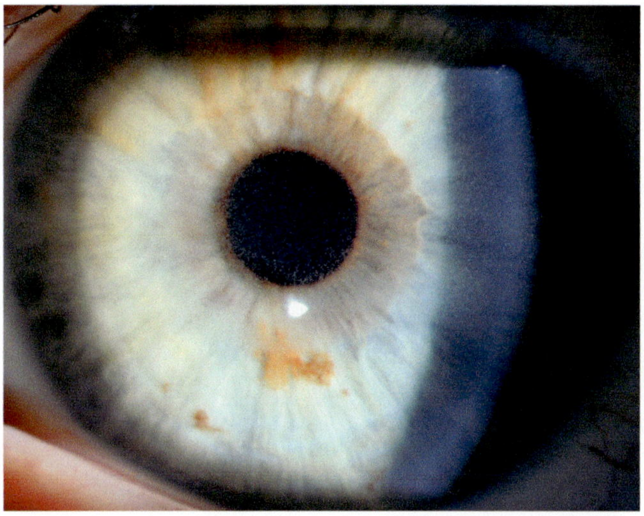

Fig. 7 Meesmann corneal dystrophy with multiple intraepithelial cysts

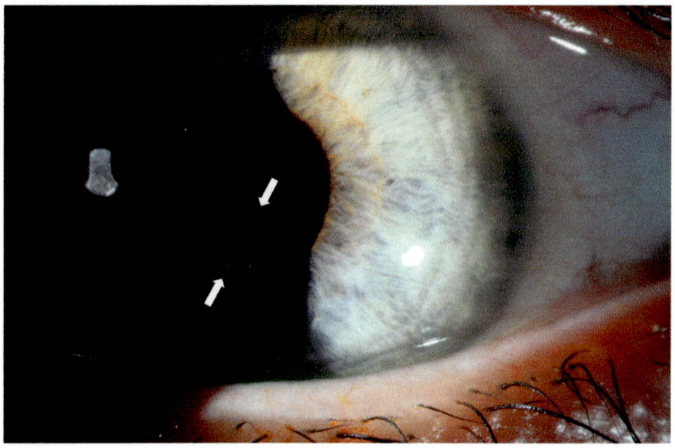

Fig. 8 Meesmann corneal dystrophy with a vortex-shaped pattern (arrows). Superficial cysts can be visualized after fluorescein vital staining

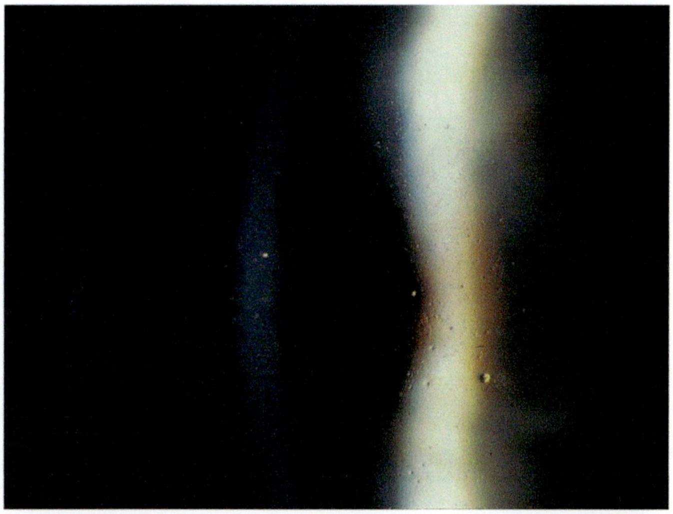

Fig. 9 Meesmann corneal dystrophy with clear intraepithelial microcysts demonstrated by indirect illumination

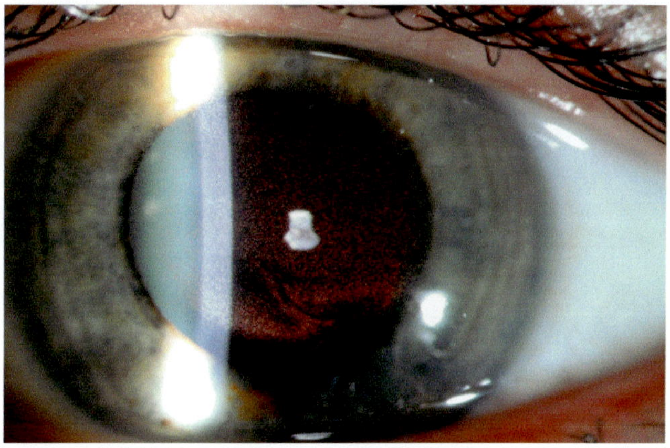

Fig. 10 Meesmann corneal dystrophy with isolated, clear intraepithelial microcysts visualized by retroillumination

females of the USA [36]. Lisch epithelial corneal dystrophy (LECD, autosomal dominant, 19p13.2, Mucolipin 1—*MOLN1*) is characterized by localized grayish opacities (Fig. 11) associated with a whorled, radial or flame/feathery-like shape that relatively often extend to the corneal limbus in a club-shaped pattern [36, 37]. Typically, crowded tiny clear microcysts can be observed in both eyes by indirect illumination with dilated pupils. The examination under pharmacologically dilated pupils is therefore very important for the diagnosis, as the indirect appearance is a characteristic clinical landmark of LECD (Fig. 12). All hereditary forms are bilateral. The clinical course is mostly asymptomatic and slowly progressive. However, these opacities might cause visual deterioration when affecting the central cornea.

5.1.6 Gelatinous Drop-Like Corneal Dystrophy

Gelatinous drop-like corneal dystrophy (GDLD) has an autosomal recessive inheritance pattern (1p32, Tumor-associated calcium signal transducer 2—*TACSTD2*) with onset in the first to second decade of life. GDLD is rare in the USA and Europe and occurs mainly in Japan [38]. Typical clinical findings are subepithelial amyloid deposits that are initially observed in the central cornea, which can later develop into a group of small multiple nodules (so-called mulberry configuration). Recurrent corneal epithelial erosions or superficial vascularization is common. Later in life, patients may also show progression of stromal opacities or develop larger nodular kumquat-like lesions [38].

GDLD has four phenotypic varieties: 1. Typical mulberry, 2. Band keratopathy, 3. Stromal opacity, 4. Kumquat-like. One of the most striking clinical features of GDLD is

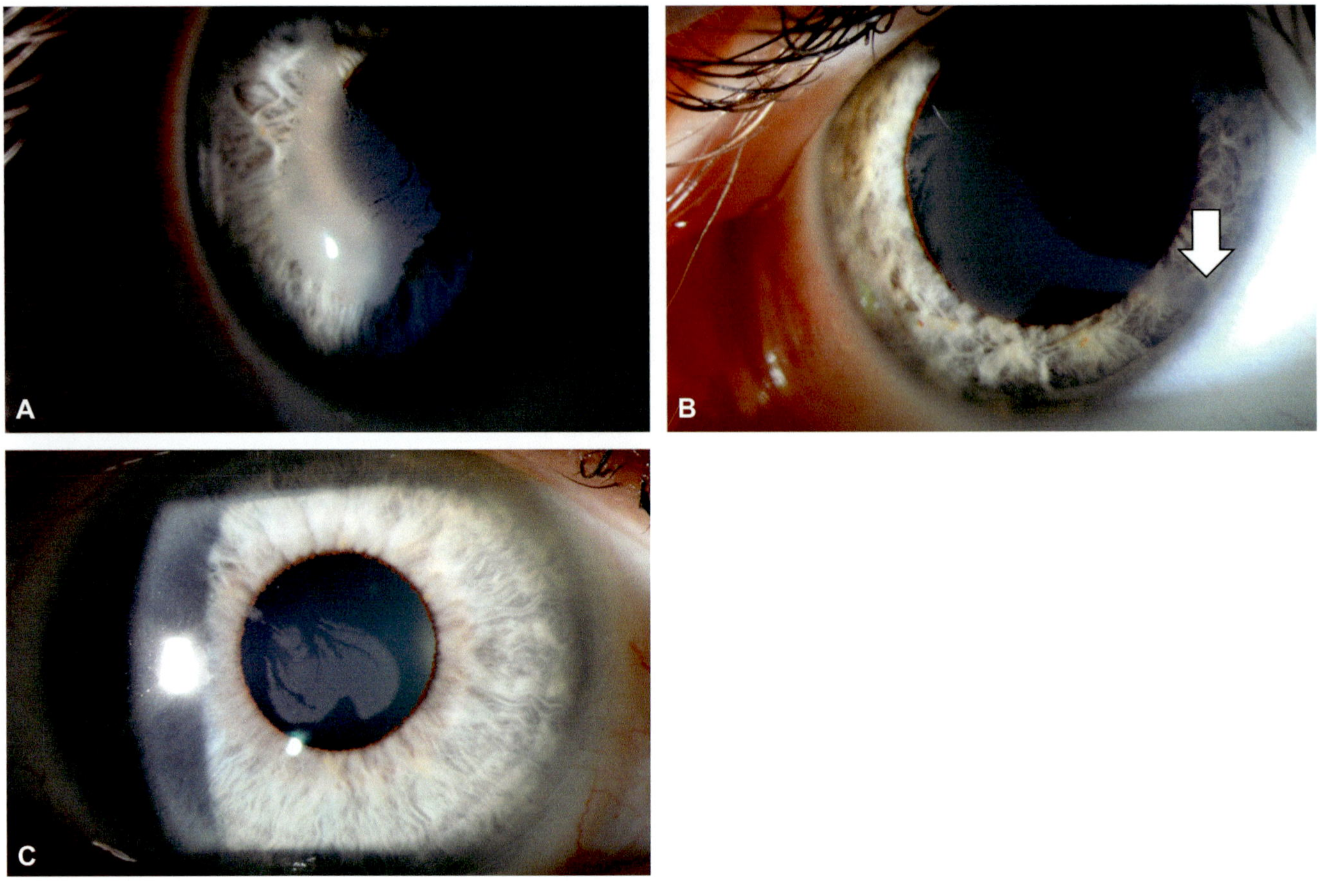

Fig. 11 Lisch epithelial corneal dystrophy (**A**–**C**) demonstrating diffuse grayish epithelial opacities of different patterns (radial, feathery or flame-shaped). The opacity might extend to the corneal limbus (best visible in figure (**B**), arrow)

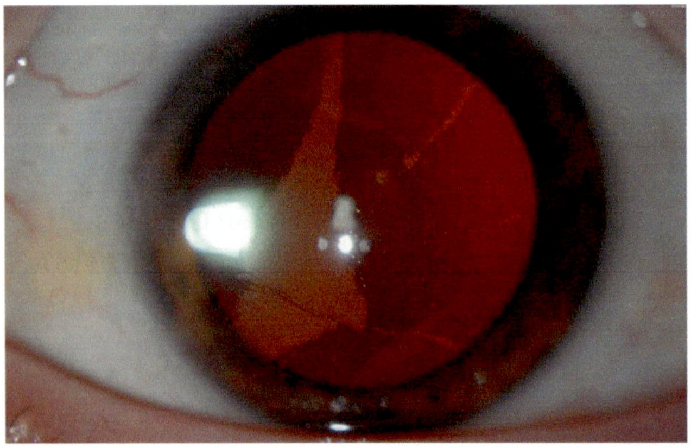

Fig. 12 Lisch epithelial corneal dystrophy demonstrates multiple crowded and clear microcysts in indirect illumination

the increased fluorescein permeability of the corneal epithelium [39].

The risk of recurrence after surgical procedures such as excimer PTK or penetrating keratoplasty (Figs. 13 and 14) is very high (up to 70%) [38].

5.2 Epithelial–Stromal *TGFBI* Dystrophies

The second edition of the IC3D, published in 2015, introduced the epithelial–stromal *TGFBI* CD (TGFBI: Transforming Growth Factor Beta Induced) as a new anatomical category in the classification of CD [28]. Mutations in the *TGFBI* gene on chromosome 5q31 were detected in several cases of anterior CD as early as 1994 and 1997 [40, 41].

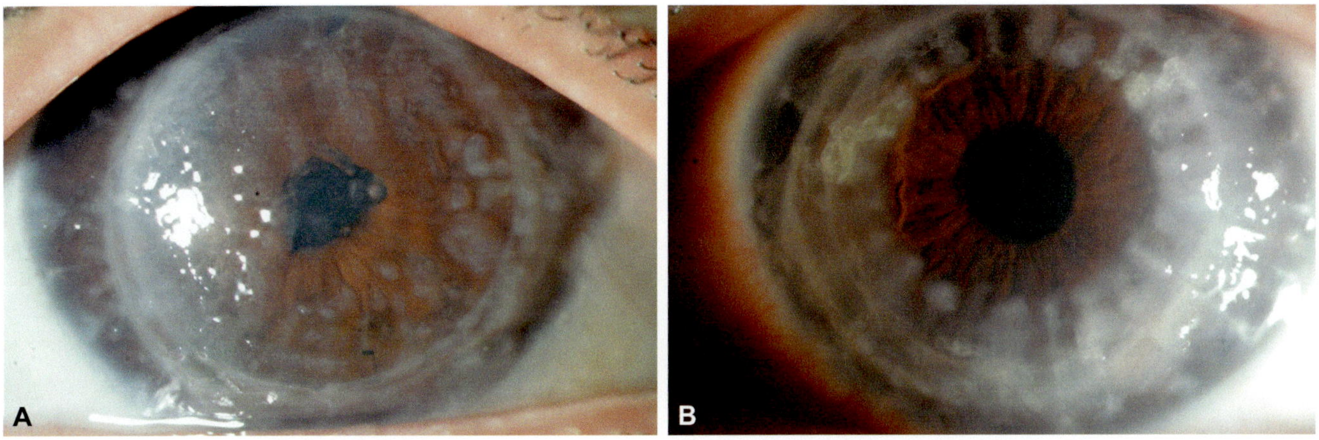

Fig. 13 Gelatinous drop-like corneal dystrophy in a 28-year-old man with recurrence after penetrating keratoplasty (OD: 5 years ago/OS: 2 years ago) demonstrating multiple amyloid nodules in the right (**A**) and left (**B**) eye. Amyloid deposits are clearly visible in the left eye along the suture tracks (**B**)

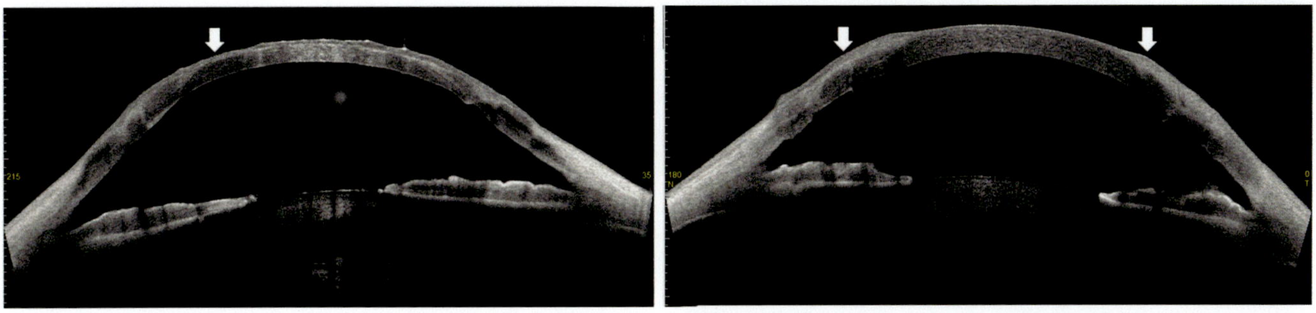

Fig. 14 Anterior segment optical coherence tomography in recurrent gelatinous drop-like corneal dystrophy after penetrating keratoplasty (OD: (**A**)/OS: (**B**)). The amyloid deposits appear as hyperreflective lesions (arrows) on the corneal graft. The clinical findings are provided in Fig. 13

The group of epithelial–stromal *TGFBI* CD (autosomal dominant) demonstrate phenotypic heterogeneity with a single gene causing different allelic dystrophy phenotypes (RBCD, TBCD, GCD1, GCD2 and LCD).

5.2.1 Reis–Bücklers Corneal Dystrophy

Reis–Bücklers corneal dystrophy (RBCD) is characterized by confluent irregular and coarse geographic-like opacities (landmark of RBCD, Figs. 15, 16 and 17) of varying density at the level of Bowman layer and the superficial stroma (rapid progression). The opacities are initially more pronounced in the central cornea, while in advanced stages the deeper stroma and the limbus are usually affected as well. The distinction between RBCD and TBCD is particularly difficult in early stages. While RBCD tends to

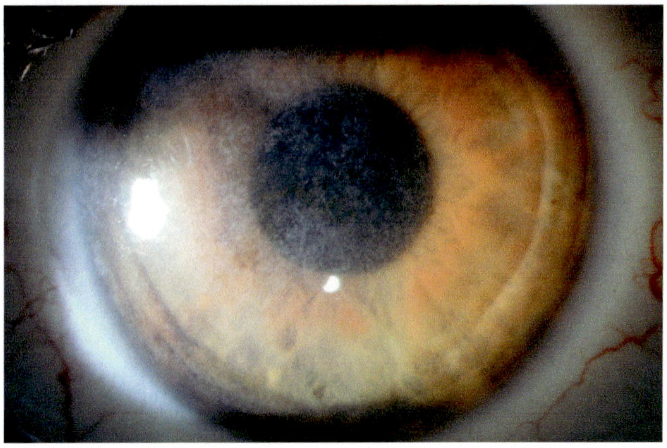

Fig. 15 Reis–Bücklers corneal dystrophy with irregular and coarse geographic corneal opacities

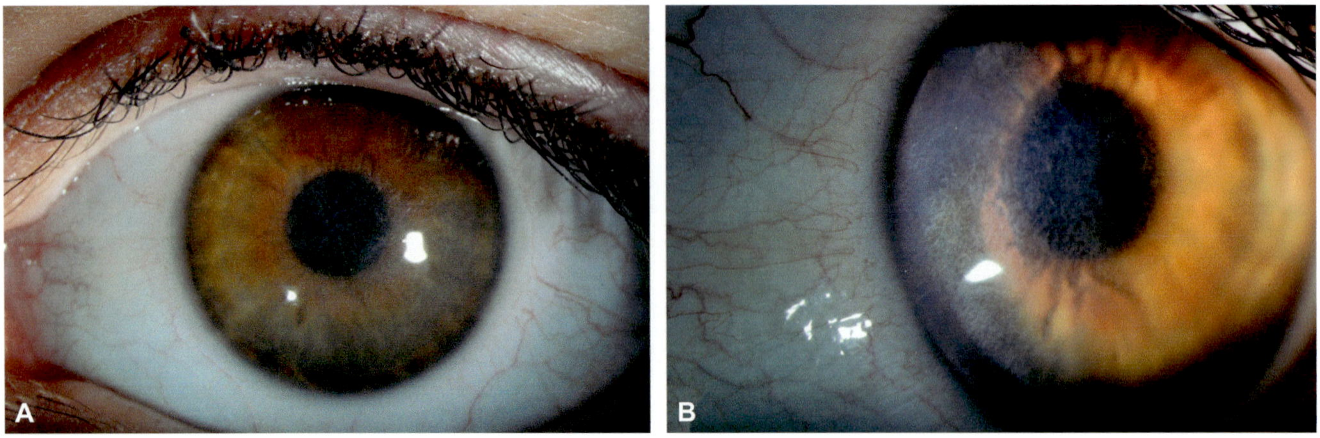

Fig. 16 Reis–Bücklers corneal dystrophy showing corneal opacities extending to the corneal limbus (**A**: overview, **B**: broad slit illumination)

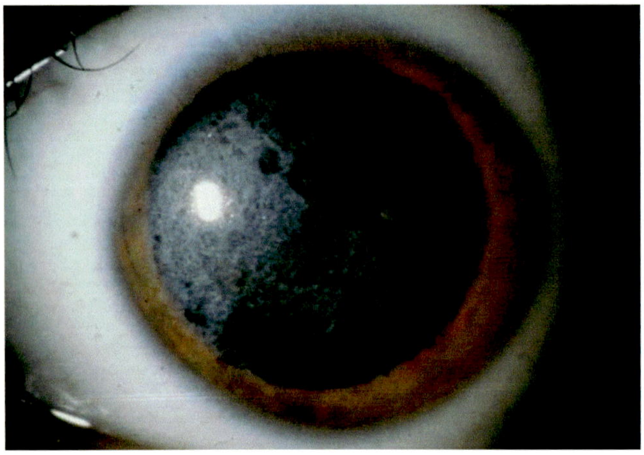

Fig. 17 Advanced stage of Reis–Bücklers corneal dystrophy with geographic opacities. In contrast to Thiel–Behnke corneal dystrophy, the margins of the opacity are sharply defined

exhibit irregular diffuse corneal opacities with clear interruptions, TBCD shows a reticular formation, particularly in the center of the cornea. Symptoms include painful, recurrent corneal erosions even before corneal opacities are visible. Significant visual impairment develops as the disease progresses.

5.2.2 Thiel–Behnke Corneal Dystrophy

In early stages of Thiel–Behnke corneal dystrophy (TBCD), irregularly shaped and scattered opacities may appear at the level of Bowman layer (Figs. 18, 19 and 20). As the disease progresses, the typical symmetrical, honeycomb-shaped subepithelial opacities (landmark of TBCD) are present. The peripheral cornea is usually not affected in the beginning. However, the opacities may extend to deeper stromal layers and the corneal periphery up to a distance of 1–2 mm from the corneal limbus. In the first and second decade of life,

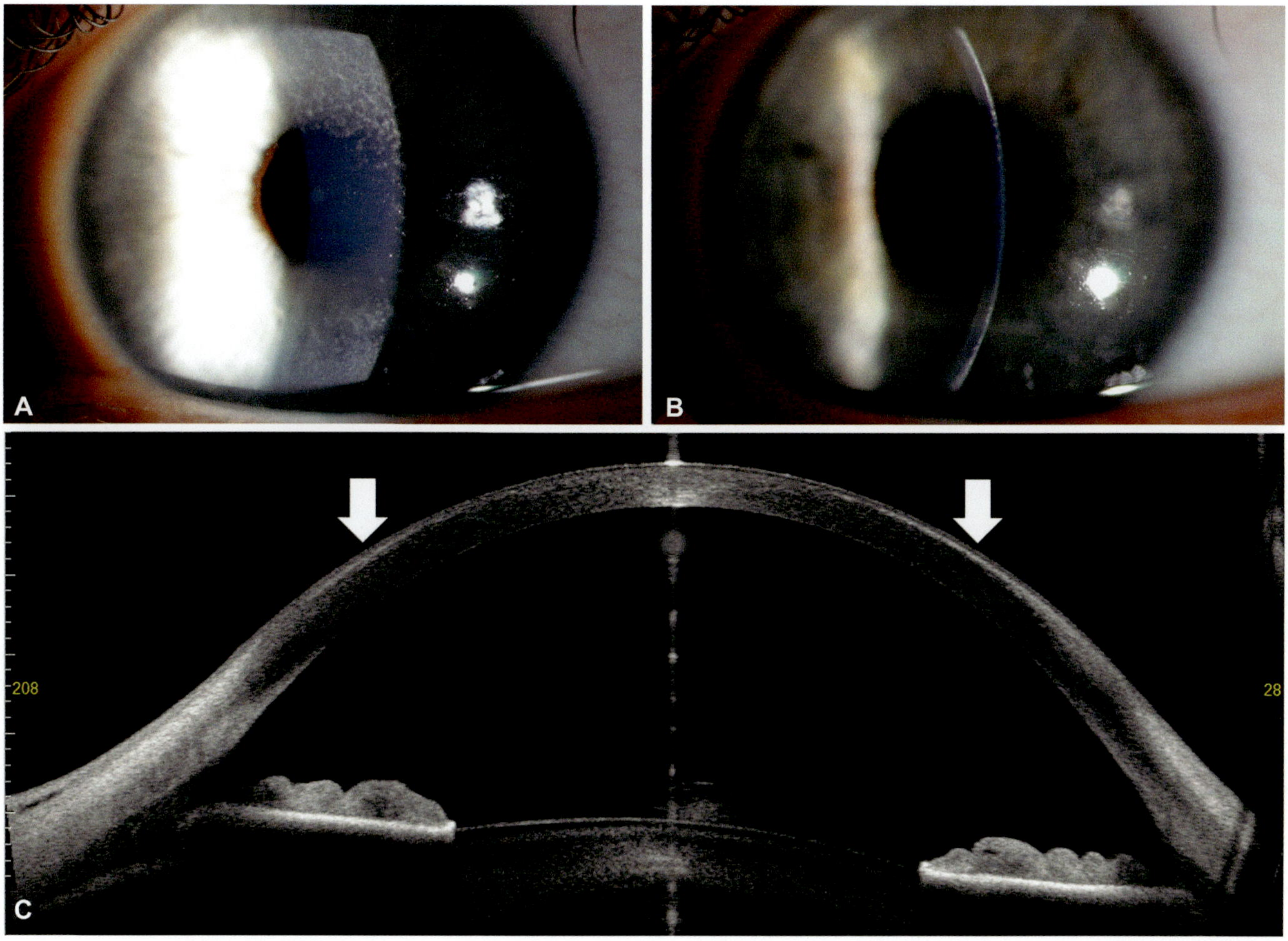

Fig. 18 Early findings of Thiel–Behnke corneal dystrophy in a 10-year-old male child. The corneal opacities extend to the midperiphery, sparing the central cornea and are limited to the superficial corneal layers ((**A**) broad slit illumination, (**B**) thin slit illumination). Anterior segment optical coherence tomography (**C**) demonstrating midperipheral/peripheral subepithelial hyperreflective lesions (arrows)

painful episodes can occur due to recurrent corneal epithelial erosions, which decrease in frequency over time. Advanced corneal opacities result in visual deterioration in later stages. The course is similar but often less aggressive and frequent than RBCD. However it is difficult to distinguish TBCD from RBCD in individual cases, especially in early stages.

Anterior segment optical coherence tomography may be an important tool in assessing the disease because, unlike RBCD, TBCD shows an extensive sawtooth pattern (Fig. 21) of hyperreflective material on the surface of Bowman layer [42].

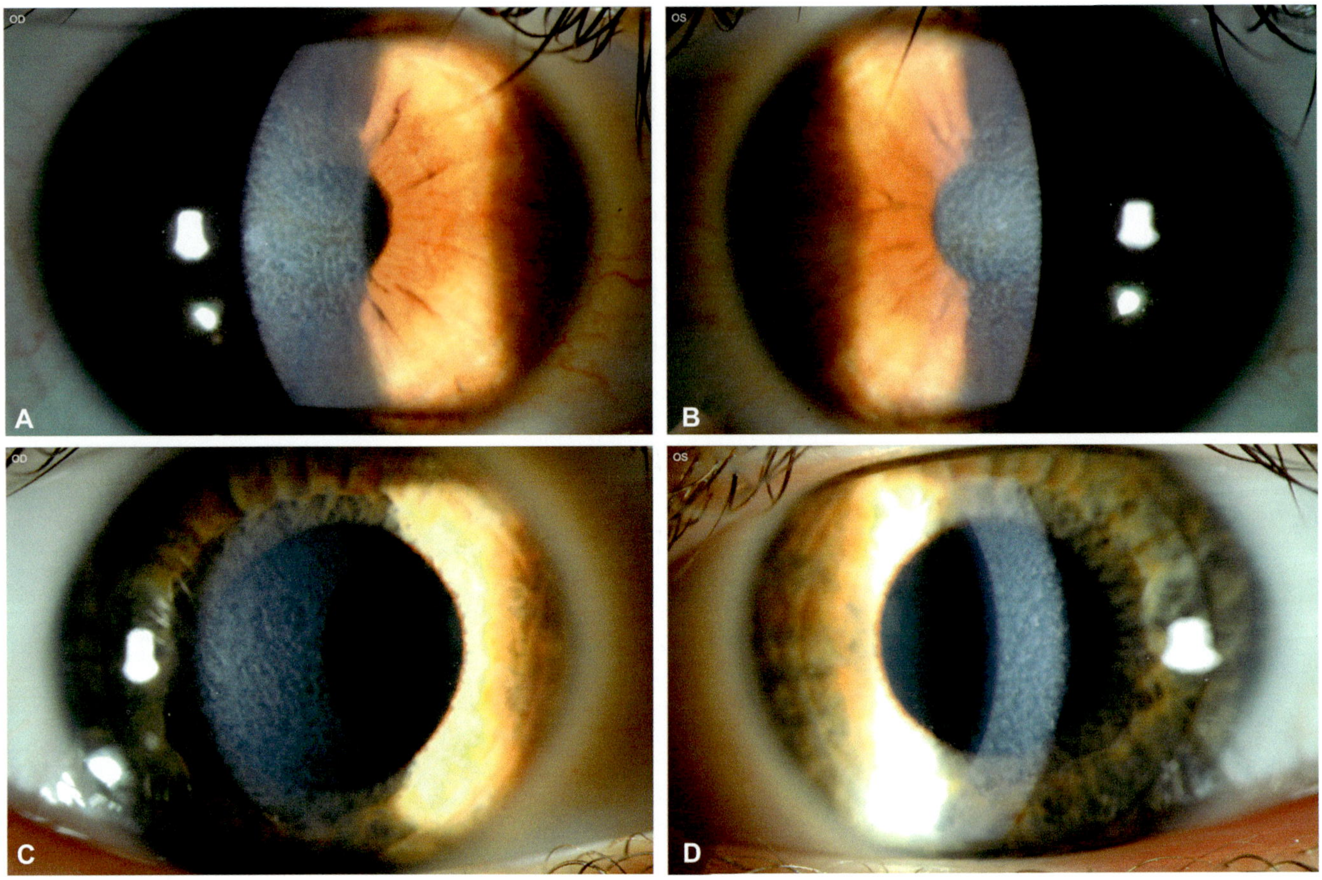

Fig. 19 Thiel–Behnke corneal dystrophy in a 35-year-old man (OD: **A**/OS: **B**) and in a 21-year-old man (OD: **C**/OS: **D**), shown with broad slit illumination. The clinical findings (honeycomb-shaped subepithelial opacities) are mostly symmetrical and equally pronounced compared to the fellow eye

5.2.3 Lattice Corneal Dystrophies

Lattice corneal dystrophies (LCDs) are divided into classic LCD and the LCD variants. While classic LCD is associated with an R124C mutation in the *TGFBI* gene, the growing group of LCD variants are due to other *TGFBI* mutations [43]. The third edition of the IC3D classification proposes a nomenclature system for LCD variants in which the actual names are based primarily on genotype rather than phenotype [18]. The first clinical signs of classic LCD (Figs. 22 and 23) are central, superficial, patchy opacities that usually appear by the end of the first decade. Simultaneously, thin branching refractile lines and/or subepithelial, whitish, ovoid dots might occur. These lines initially develop in the superficial central cornea, subsequently spreading centrifugally and into the deeper stroma (Fig. 24). However, the peripheral stroma remains clear. In later stages of the disease, subepithelial opacities of the central and paracentral cornea occur simultaneously with central and paracentral lattice lines causing diffuse central haze by the second to third decade of life. The

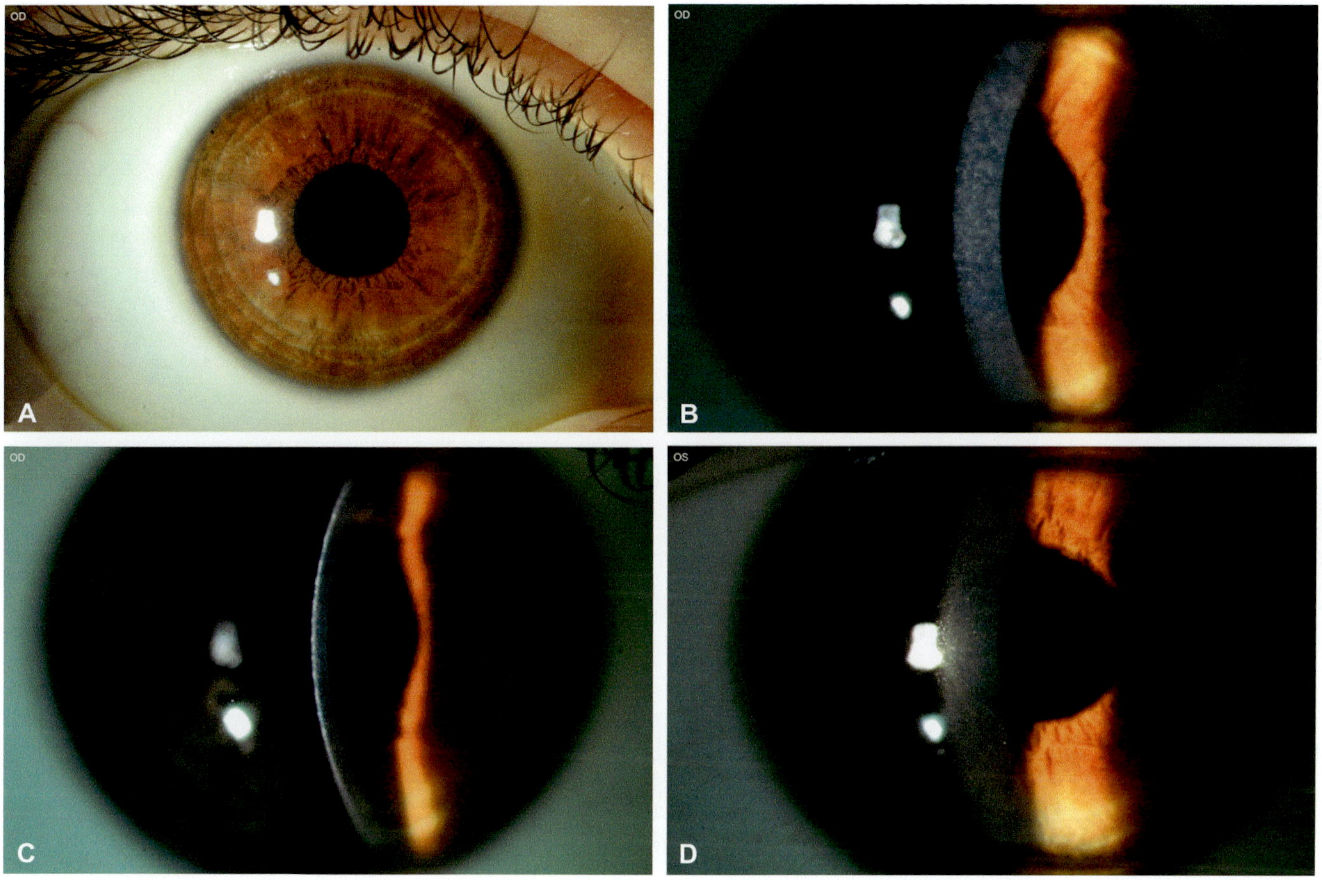

Fig. 20 Thiel–Behnke corneal dystrophy in a 14-year-old female child (**A**). The honeycomb-like subepithelial opacities are best visualized using a broad (**B**) and very thin slit illumination (**C**). As the deposits are usually localized in the superficial corneal layers, they can be completely removed after excimer laser-assisted phototherapeutic keratectomy (**D**)

clinical findings are usually asymmetrical and can also only appear unilaterally. Symptoms include painful episodes due to recurrent erosions (Fig. 25) and visual impairment. Although the phenotype of LCD variants is typically similar, it is not identical to that of classic LCD [18]. For example, some variants lack the distinct lattice lines (Fig. 26), which can make the clinical diagnosis of LCD more difficult. Nevertheless, all variants show histopathologically corneal amyloid deposits as the primary diagnostic feature.

In comparison to the variants, which are geographically limited, classic LCD is widespread and has been described in five continents. The literature now includes more than 80 different variants of LCD [18]. The age of onset and the depth of the deposits differ from variant to variant, and some variants occasionally show a very heterogeneous opacity pattern. These variants may initially be misdiagnosed as other CD such as EBMD, RBCD, TBCD or GCD until genotyping provides clarity. Similar to classic LCD,

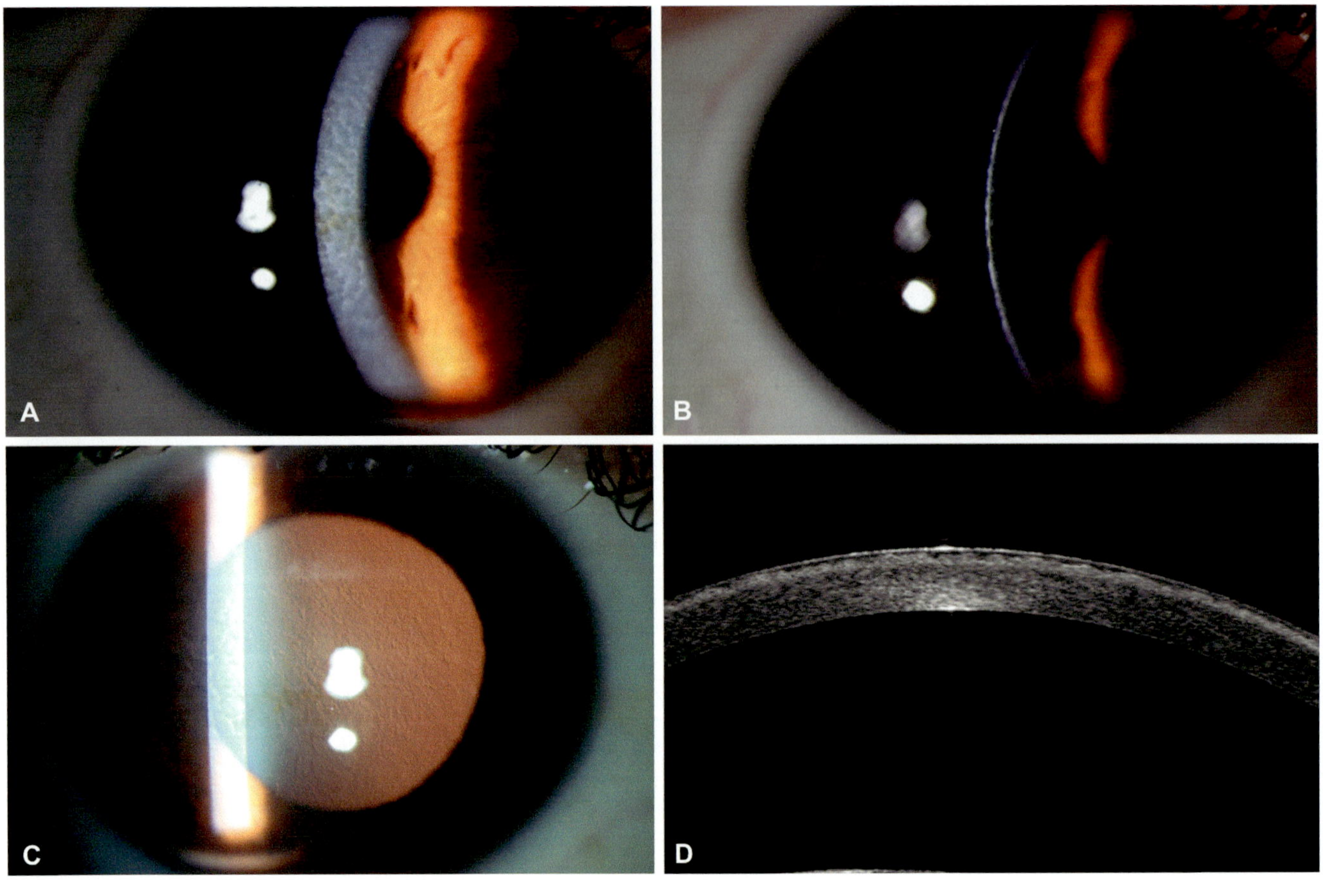

Fig. 21 Thiel–Behnke corneal dystrophy showing the characteristic appearance with broad slit illumination (**A**), thin slit illumination (**B**) and with retroillumination (**C**). The corresponding optical coherence tomography (**D**) demonstrates a typical sawtooth pattern of hyperreflective material in Bowman layer

there are phenotypic differences between both eyes and also between individual patients with the same variant [18]. Superficial lattice lines can be successfully removed after excimer PTK (Fig. 27). However, the recurrence of lattice lines often affects deeper stromal layers, making them inaccessible to excimer PTK (Fig. 28).

5.2.4 Granular Corneal Dystrophy, Type 1

The early findings in childhood may be non-specific and manifest as a vortex pattern of very small brownish granules (Figs. 29 and 30) in the form of lines above Bowman layer (clinical landmark in children). With further disease progression, well-defined, discrete granules appear grayish-white under direct illumination with a clear stroma in between (Figs. 31 and 32). These crumb-like granules increase in size (0.1–0.3 mm) and number, are more irregular in shape, unsystematically distributed, and may coalesce resulting in a snowflake appearance (clinical landmark in adults, Figs. 33, 34 and 35). The granules consist of extremely small, transparent dots with the appearance of vacuoles, glassy splinters or crushed

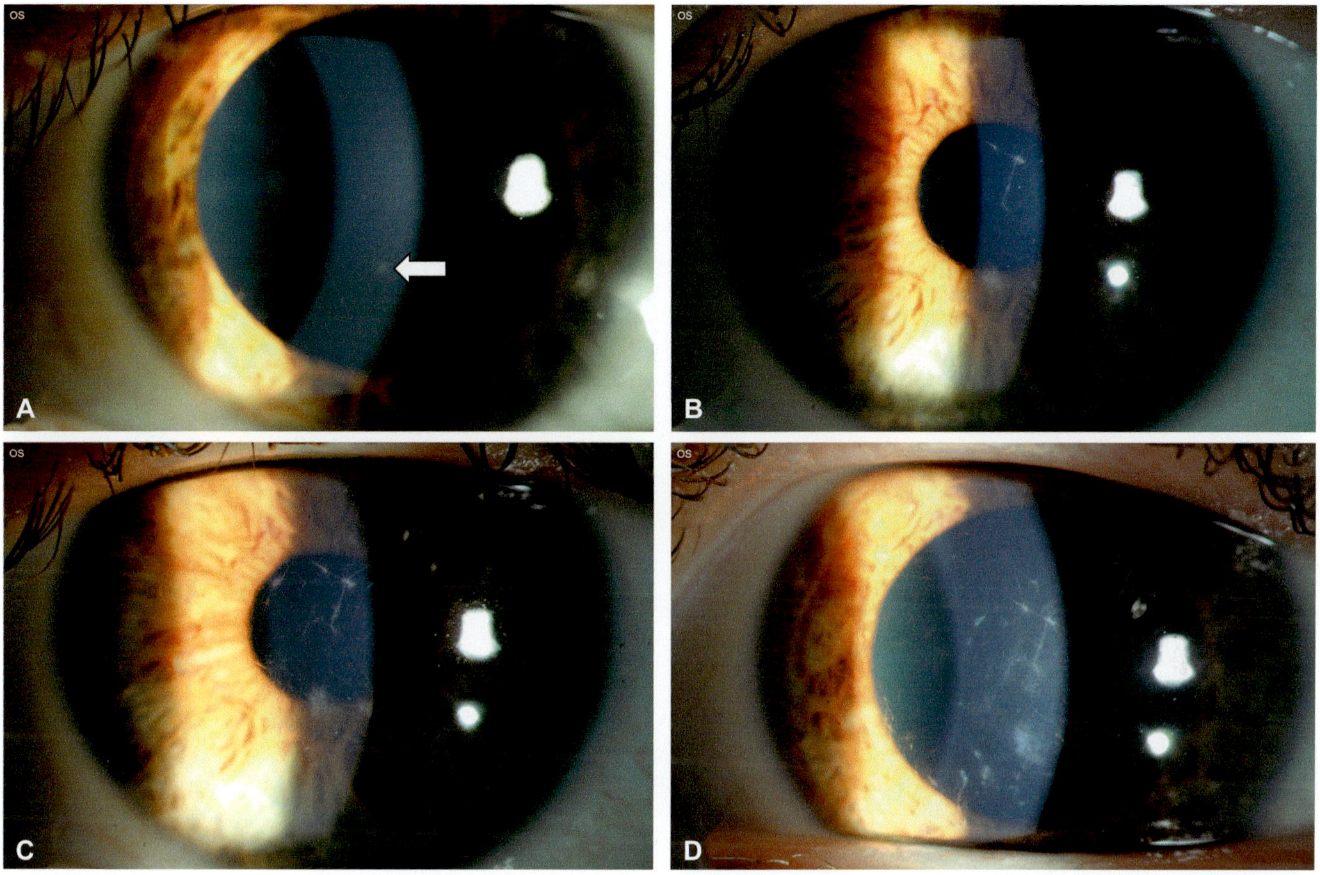

Fig. 22 Progression of lattice corneal dystrophy. At the age of 10 years, only single patchy opacities (white arrow) are visible (**A**). The first thin lattice lines appear in the central cornea at the age of 13 years (**B**) and increase in density by the age of 15 years (**C**). The subepithelial corneal opacities between the lattice lines increase at the age of 17 years (**D**)

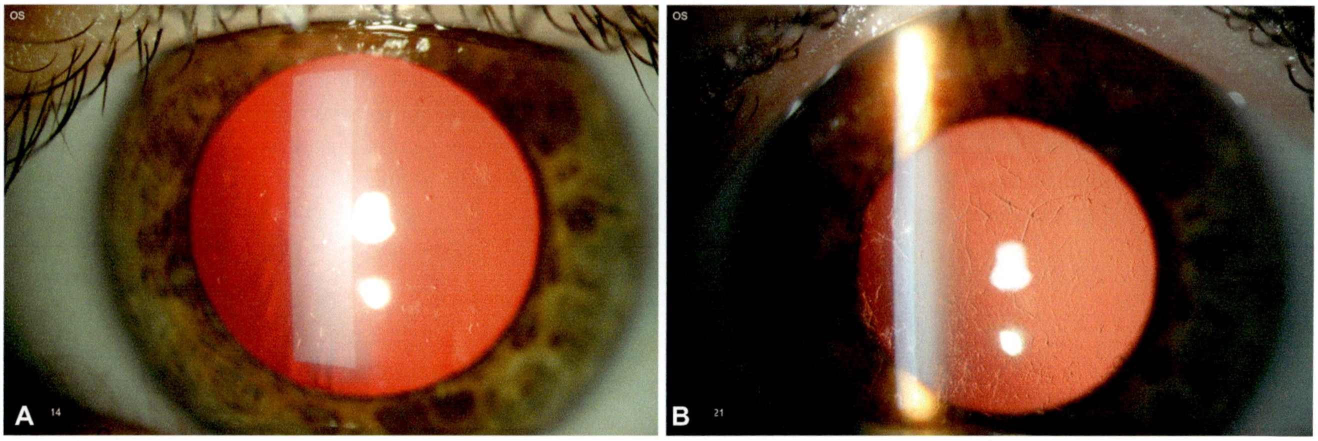

Fig. 23 Progressive lattice corneal dystrophy at the age of 10 (**A**) and 17 (**B**) years, visualized by retroillumination. There is a pronounced increase in lattice lines seven years later. The photographs using direct illumination are displayed in Fig. 22

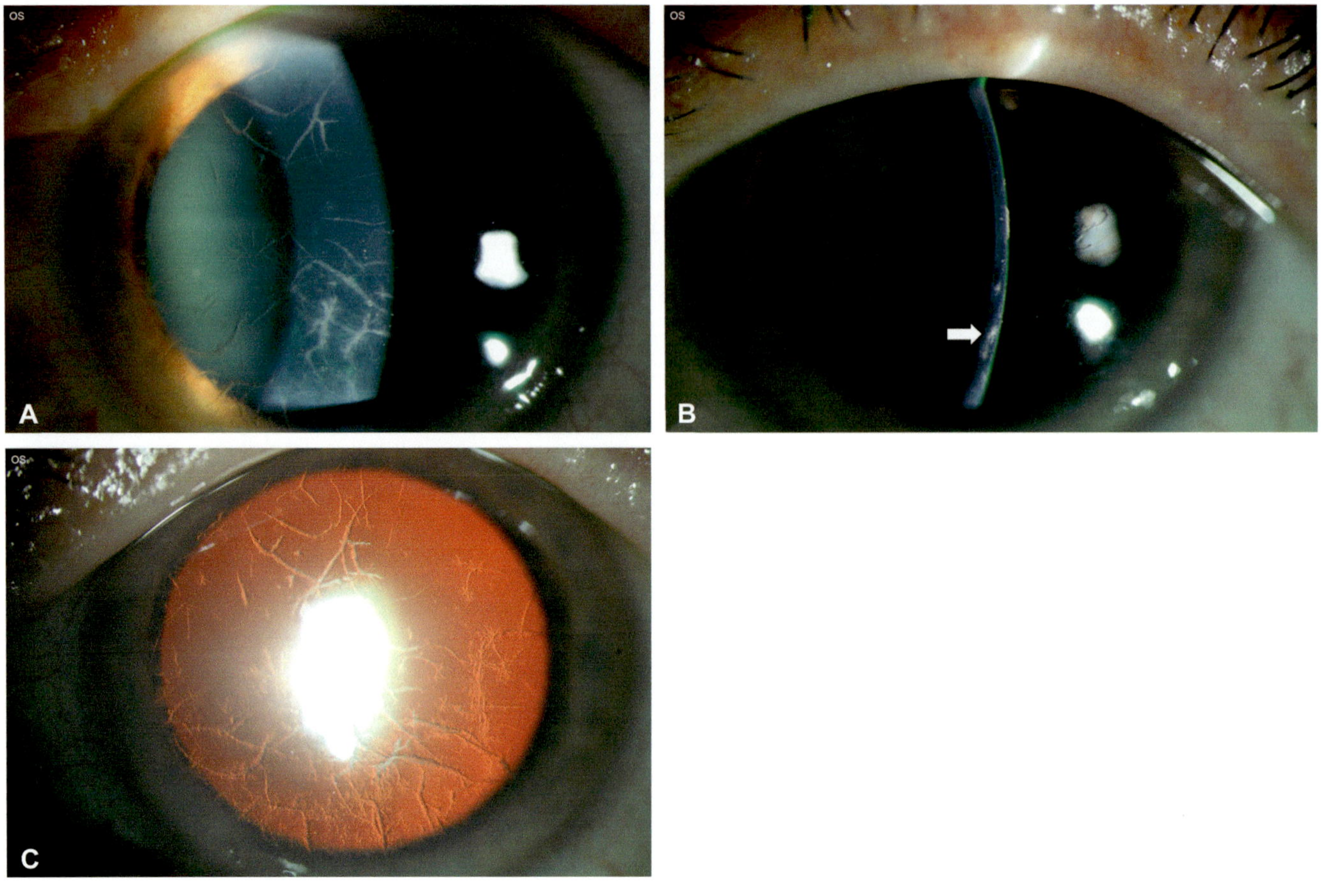

Fig. 24 Advanced lattice corneal dystrophy with direct illumination (**A**, **B**) and retroillumination (**C**). The thin slit image (**B**, arrow) demonstrates amyloid deposits down to the deeper stromal layers

breadcrumbs and can be visualized very well with retroillumination. The cornea between the deposits is clear. The peripheral stroma is affected, but the limbus is generally free of deposits. In advanced stages, the granules affect the deeper corneal stroma down to the Descemet membrane. Furthermore, the granules become increasingly confluent (Fig. 36), especially in the superficial cornea, which leads to deterioration in visual acuity by the fifth decade of life. Early symptoms include glare and photophobia, while visual acuity decreases with age as the opacity progresses. Homozygotes have more severe manifestations and symptoms. Recurrence patterns vary widely, with recurrences occurring as early as one year after surgery. Laser procedures such as excimer PTK may cause exacerbation with

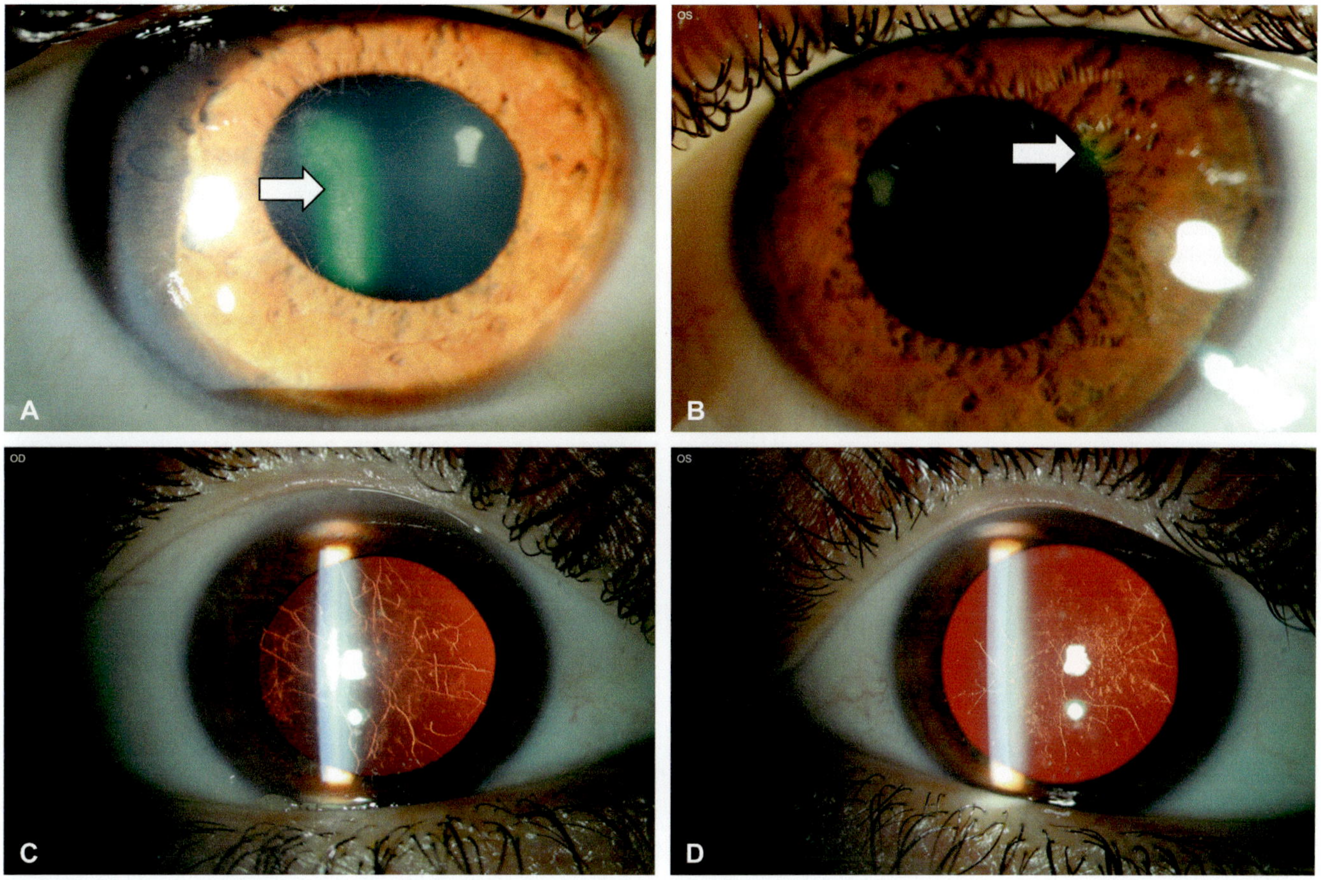

Fig. 25 Lattice corneal dystrophy with recurrent erosions (arrows) in both eyes displayed by direct illumination and retroillumination (OD: **A**, **C**/OS: **B**, **D**)

increased deposition of granular material (Figs. 37 and 38). After keratoplasty, deposits in the graft initially occur centrally and superficially (Fig. 39) and occasionally take on a vortex pattern suggestive of epithelial involvement [44]. Furthermore, deposits are also found at the graft–host junction or along suture tracks (Figs. 40 and 41).

5.2.5 Granular Corneal Dystrophy, Type 2

In heterozygotes, the initial clinical signs are subtle and characterized by small white stromal dots that may develop small spokes or thorns. However, GCD1 and GCD2 are not easy to distinguish in the early stages. As the disease progresses (more by individual growth than by an increase in the number of opacities), all eyes develop superficial, whitish, round patches with moth-eaten centers that may

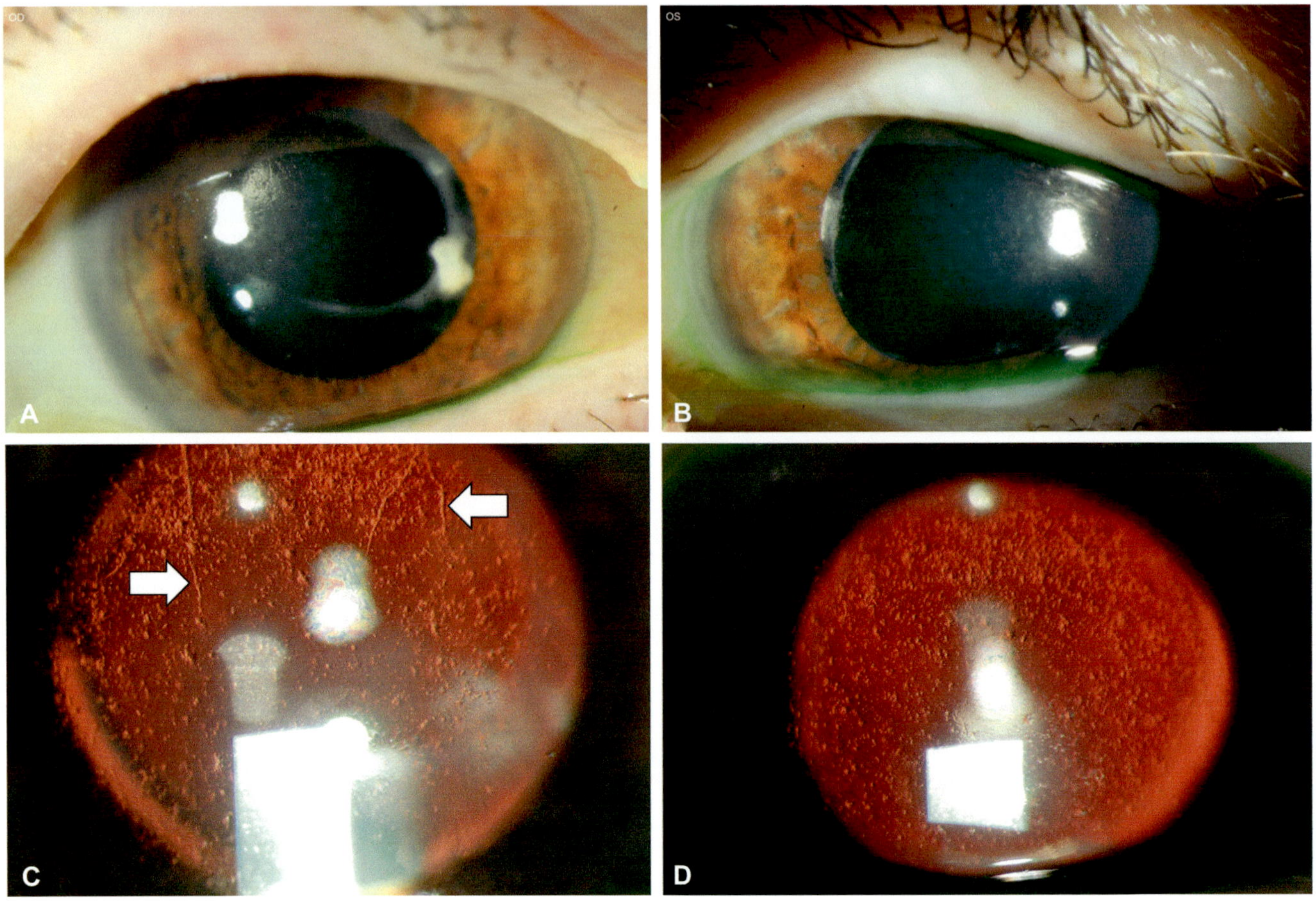

Fig. 26 Seventy-five-year-old woman with lattice corneal dystrophy in both eyes (OD: **A**/OS: **B**). In the right eye, retroillumination revealed punctate changes with multiple lattice lines (**C**, arrows), while the latter were absent in the fellow eye (**D**)

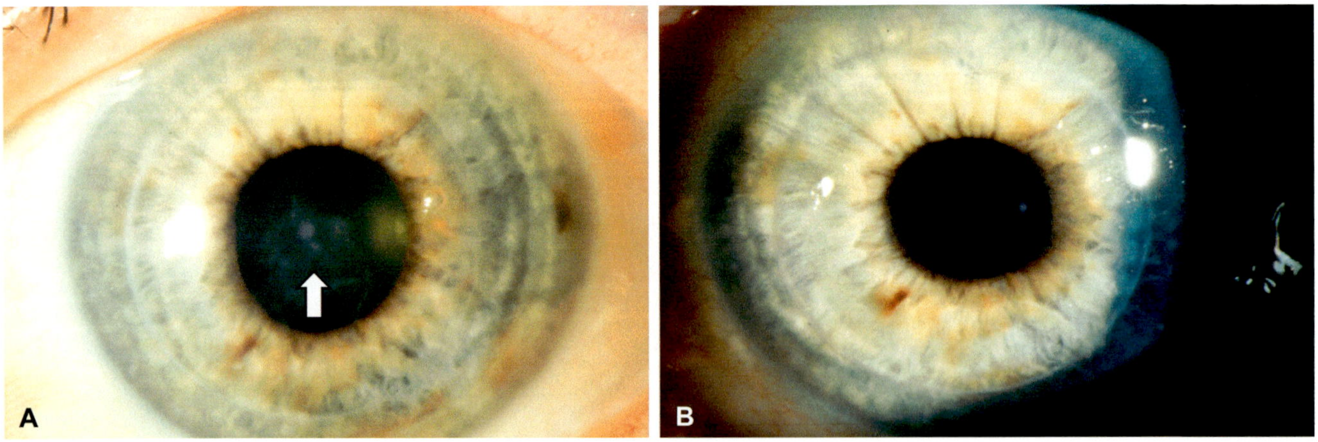

Fig. 27 Recurrence of lattice corneal dystrophy in the graft after penetrating keratoplasty (**A**, arrow). The superficial amyloid deposits can be completely removed by excimer laser-assisted phototherapeutic keratectomy (**B**)

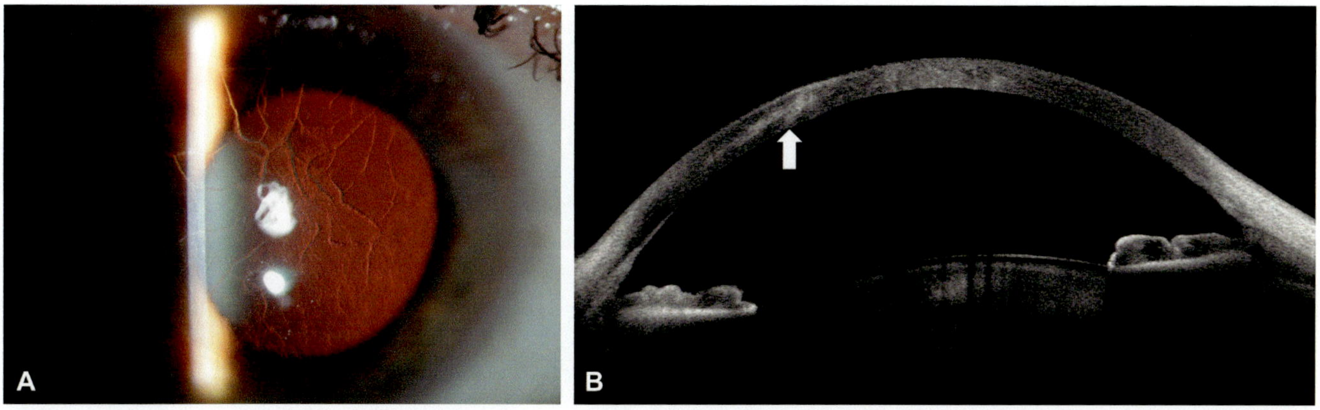

Fig. 28 Lattice corneal dystrophy with pronounced, thick lattice lines (**A** retroillumination). Anterior segment optical coherence tomography (**B**) demonstrates that the hyperreflective amyloid deposits are located in the deep stromal layer (arrows)

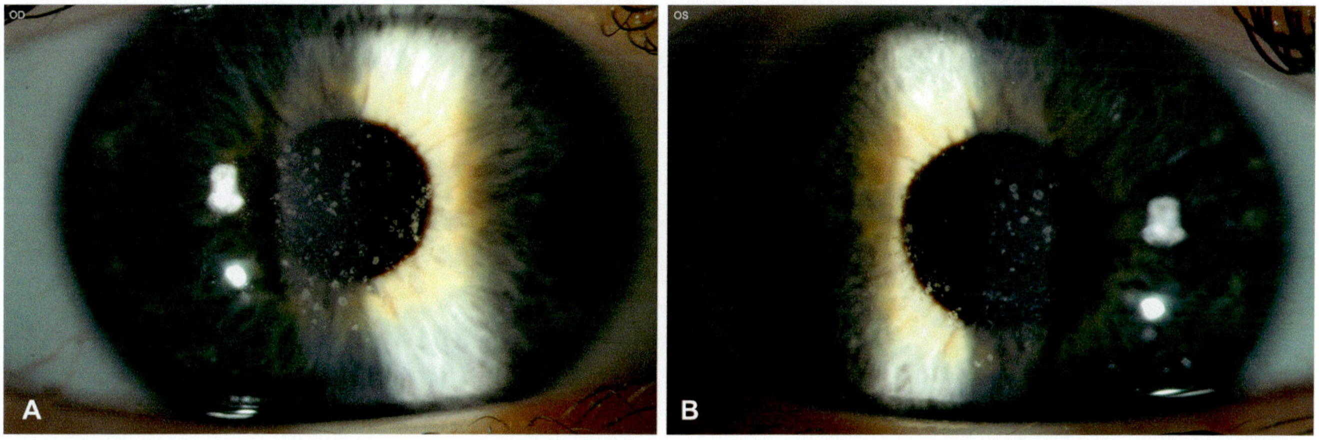

Fig. 29 Granular corneal dystrophy type 1 in a 13-year-old child with small granular deposits in both eyes (OD: **A**/OS: **B**)

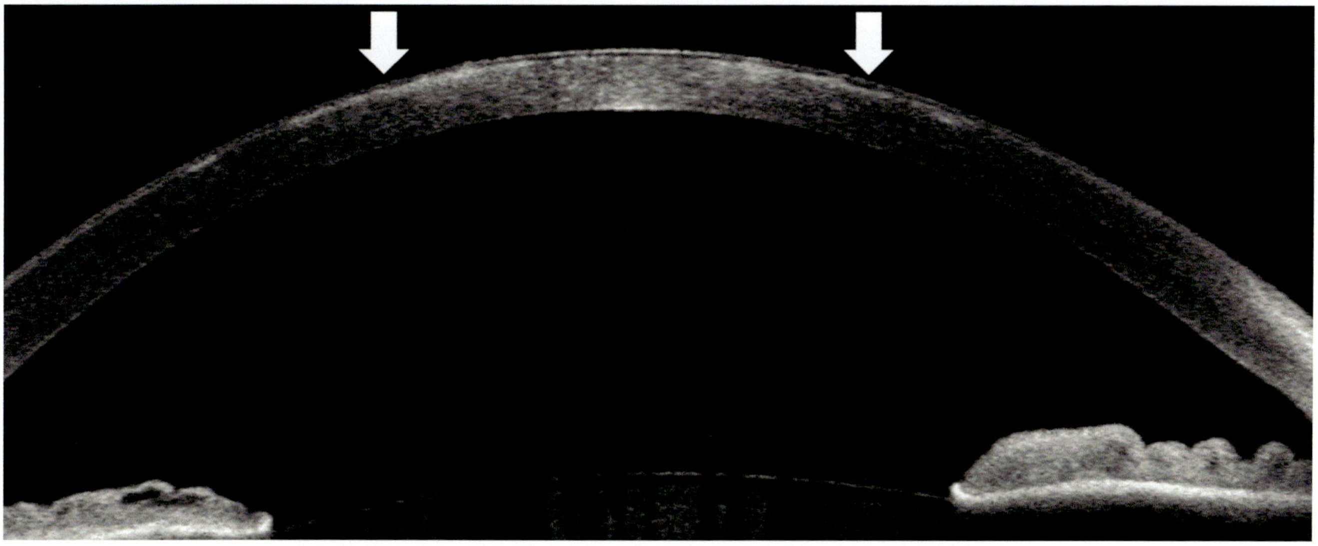

Fig. 30 Anterior segment optical coherence tomography in granular corneal dystrophy type 1 demonstrating hyperreflective subepithelial deposits (arrows) in a 13-year-old child (see Fig. 29 for clinical presentation)

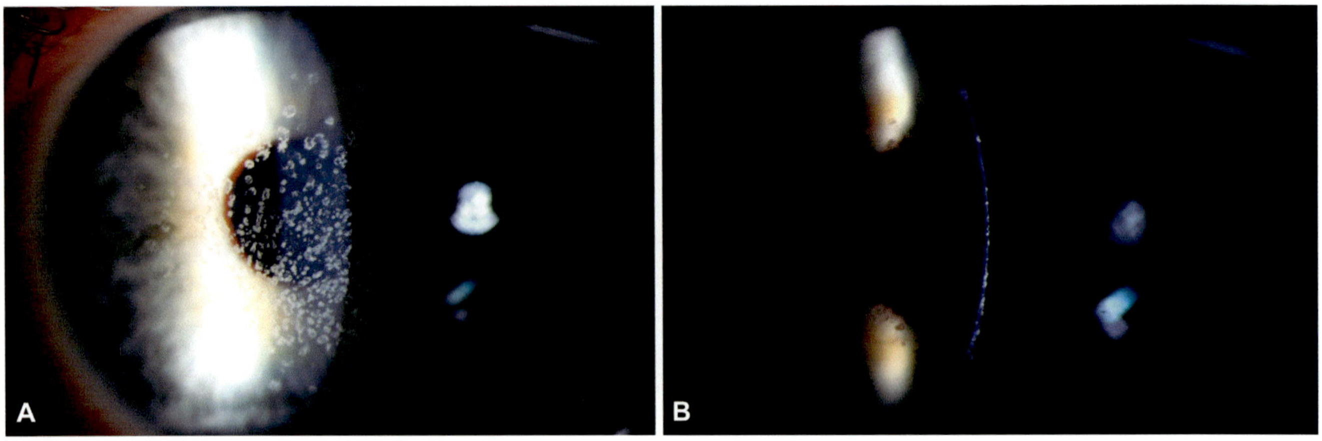

Fig. 31 Granular corneal dystrophy type 1 in a 16-year-old child, demonstrated by broad (**A**) and thin slit illumination (**B**). The granular changes are small, irregular in shape and are limited to the anterior stroma

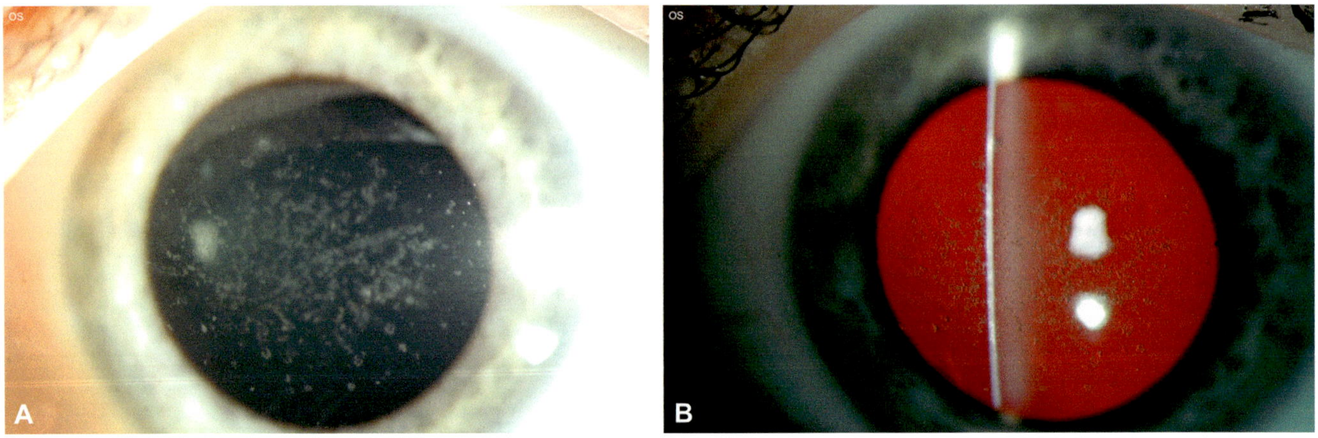

Fig. 32 Granular corneal dystrophy type 1 in a 22-year-old woman. The granular changes become increasingly confluent ((**A**) overview, (**B**) retroillumination)

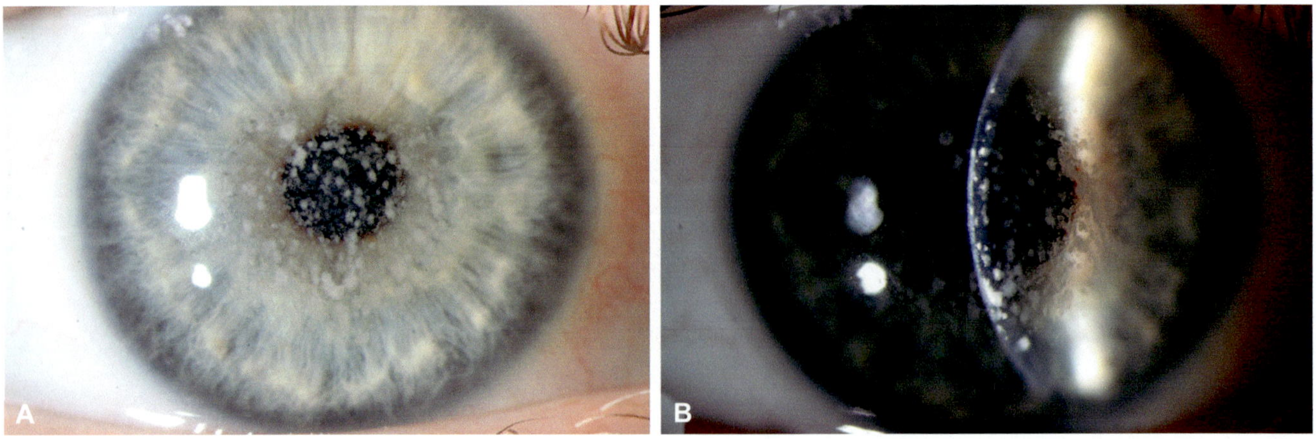

Fig. 33 Granular dystrophy type 1 in a 34-year-old woman (**A**). The thin slit illumination (**B**) shows granular deposits in the deep corneal stroma just in front of Descemet membrane

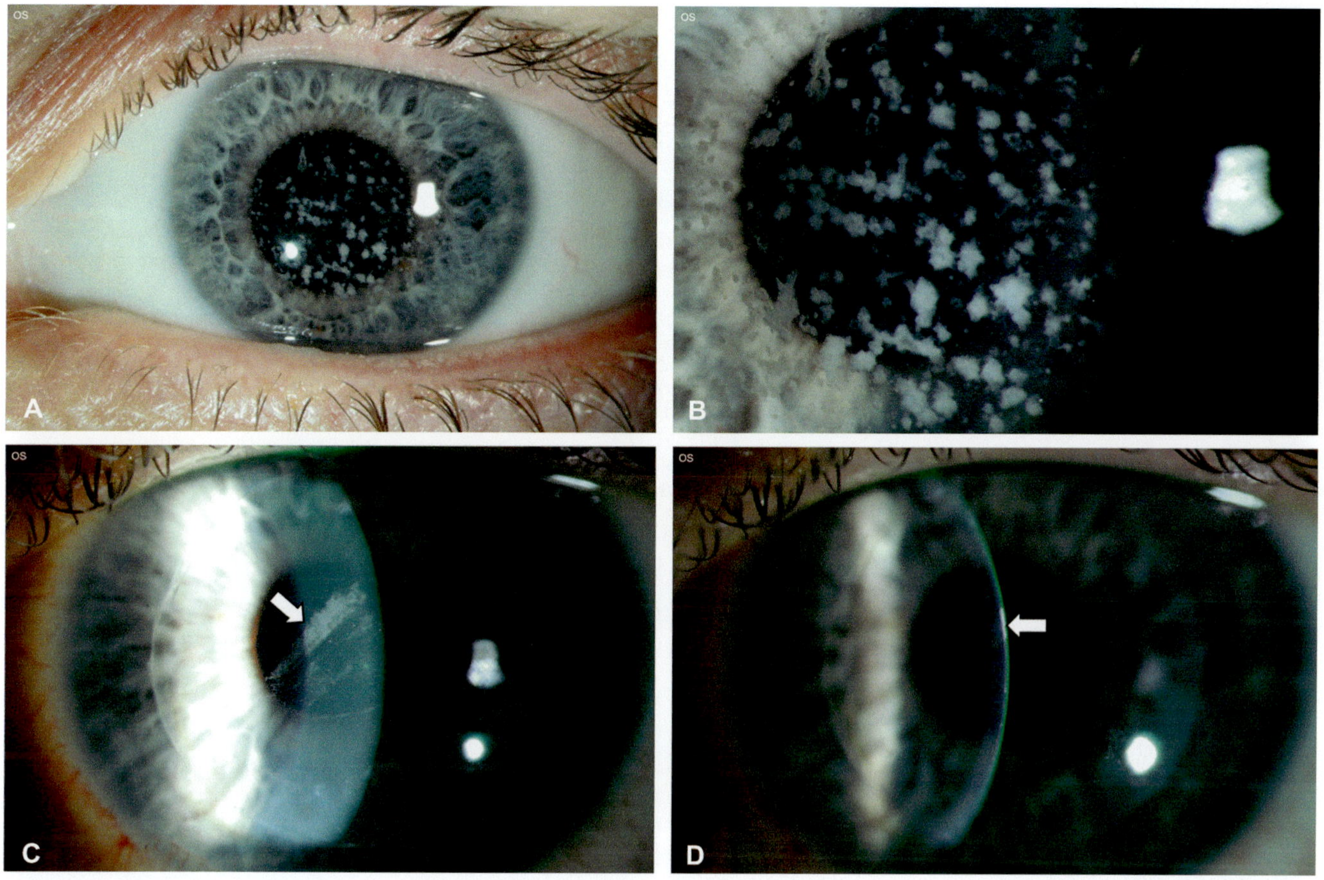

Fig. 34 Advanced granular corneal dystrophy type 1 (snowflake appearance) in a 36-year-old man ((**A**) overview, (**B**) magnification). A superficial, band-like recurrence of the dystrophy (arrows) occurred in the central cornea within 4 years after penetrating keratoplasty ((**C**) broad slit illumination, (**D**) thin slit illumination)

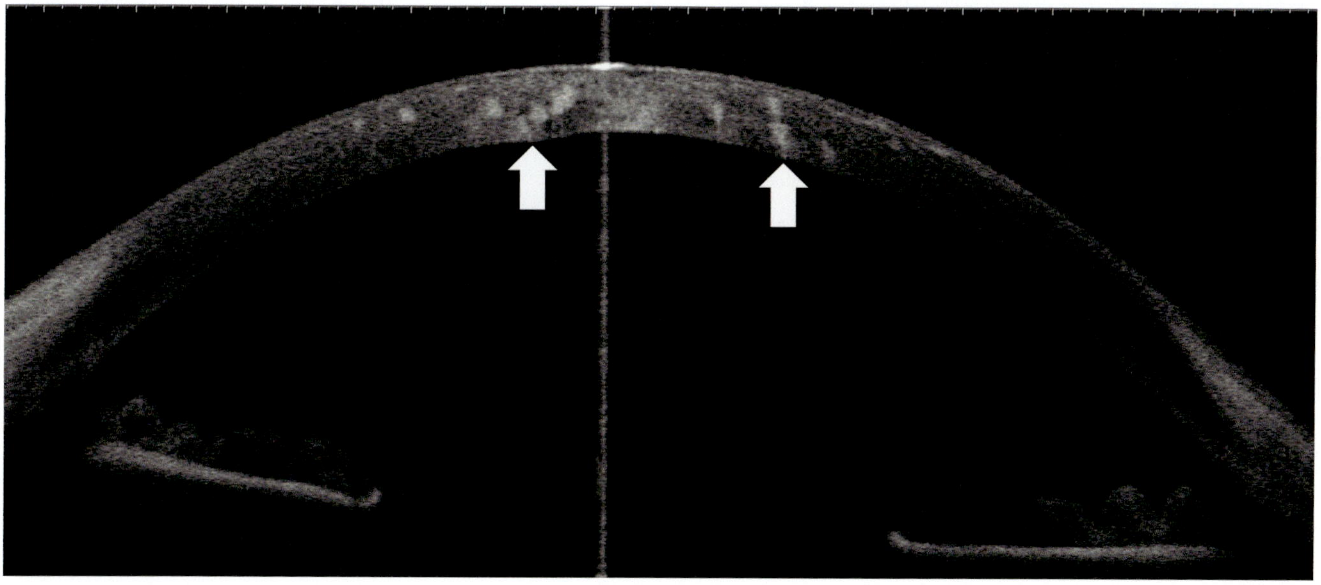

Fig. 35 In classic granular corneal dystrophy type 1, the hyperreflective deposits (arrows) are also found in deeper stromal layers. The clinical findings are shown in Fig. 34 (**A, B**)

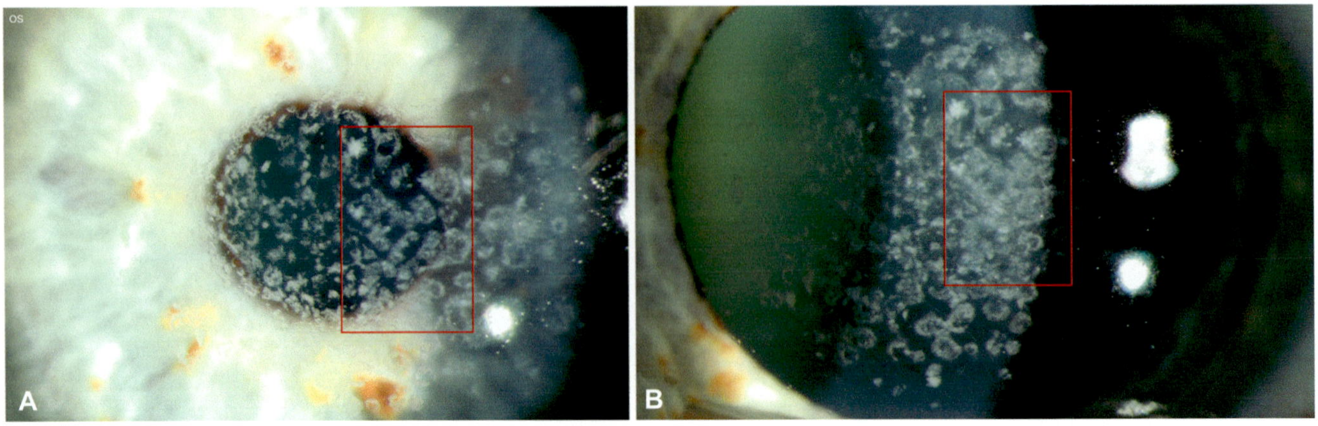

Fig. 36 Granular corneal dystrophy type 1 in a 57-year-old woman (**A**). Within 4 years there is a pronounced increase in granular opacities (**B**). The red box represents the identical areas between the two periods of time

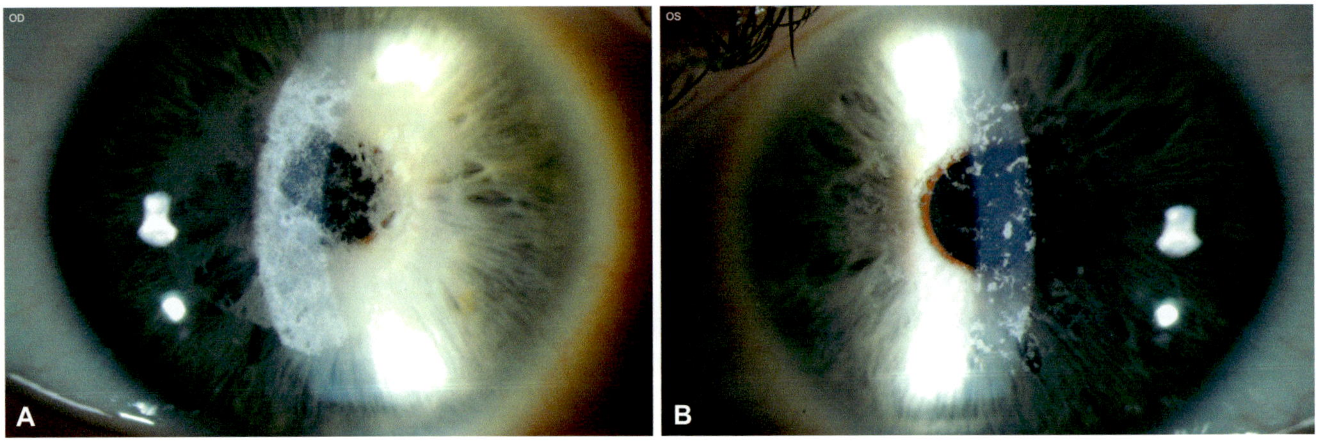

Fig. 37 Granular corneal dystrophy type 1 in a 35-year-old man. Previously, excimer laser-assisted phototherapeutic keratectomy was performed on the right (**A**) and left (**B**) eye 12 years ago. While the left eye shows multiple, deep deposits, the right eye demonstrates more severe findings with a dense geographic corneal opacity

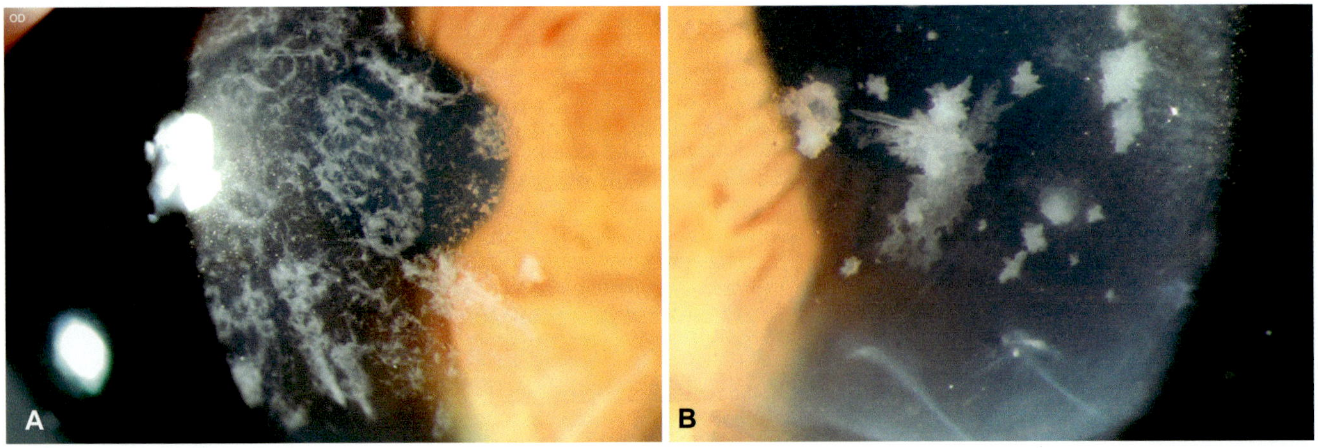

Fig. 38 Granular corneal dystrophy, type 1 in a 61-year-old woman. Two phototherapeutic keratectomies were performed on the right eye, resulting in dense deposits of granular material (reticular appearance). The left eye showed granular deposits in various forms, some with glassy splinters, 14 years after a penetrating keratoplasty

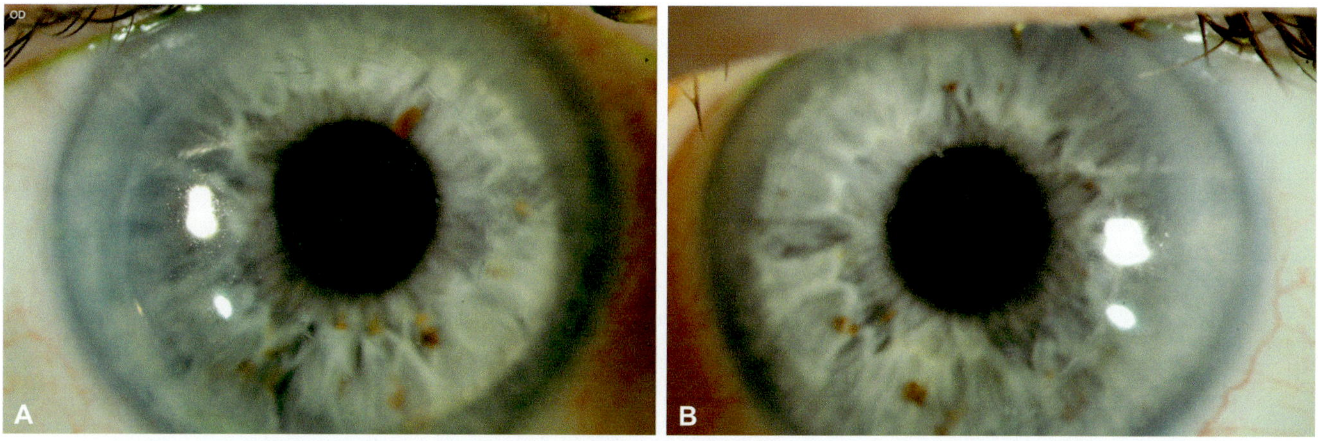

Fig. 39 Recurrence of granular corneal dystrophy type 1 after penetrating keratoplasty in a 66-year-old man. Superficial granular deposits in the central cornea are seen in the right (**A**) and left (**B**) eye after 9 (OD) and 6 (OS) years

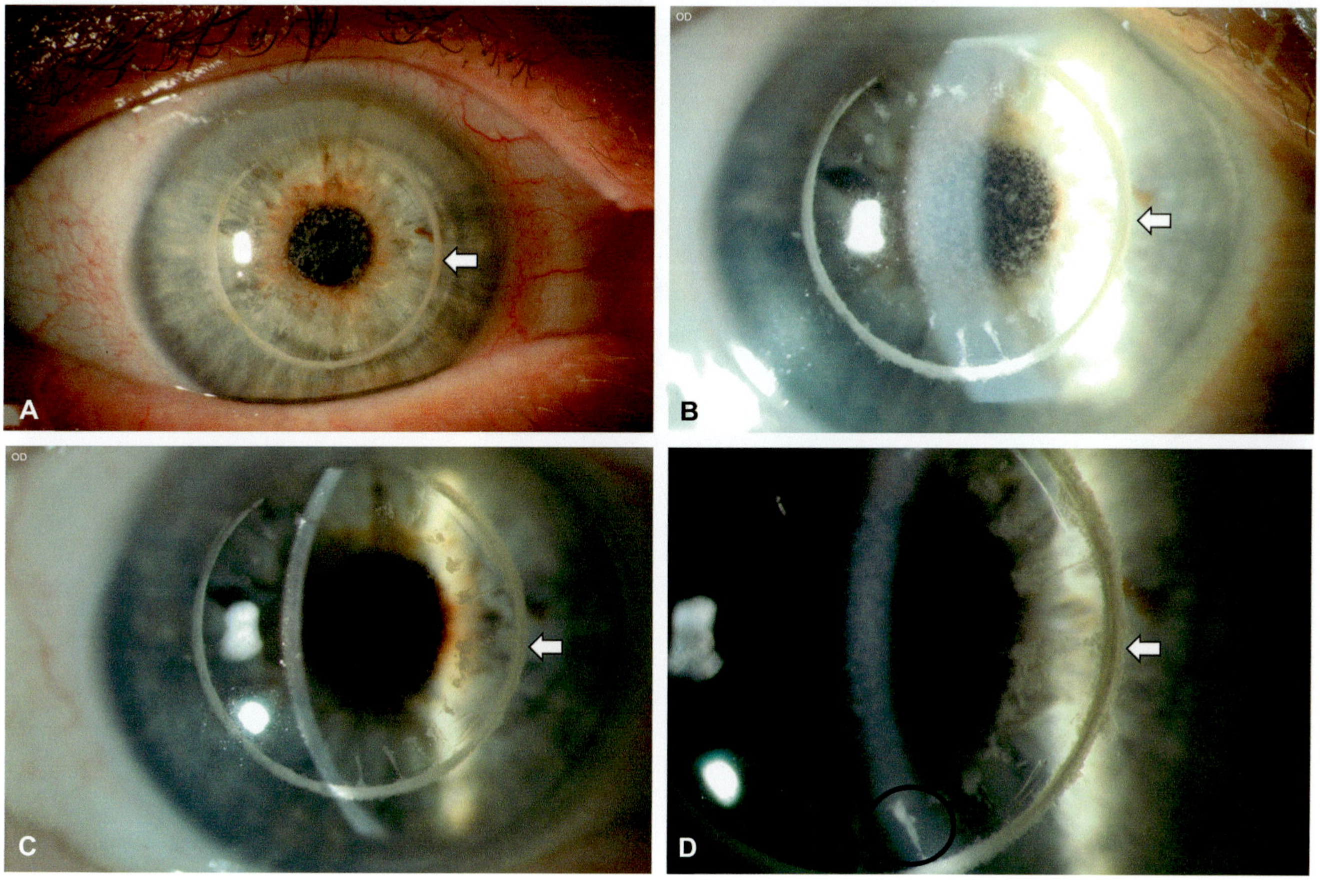

Fig. 40 Penetrating keratoplasty (15 years ago) in granular corneal dystrophy type 1 with pronounced granular deposits at the graft–host junction (arrows) and along the suture tracks (**D** circle) ((**A**) overview, (**B**) broad slit illumination, (**C**) thin slit illumination, (**D**) indirect illumination)

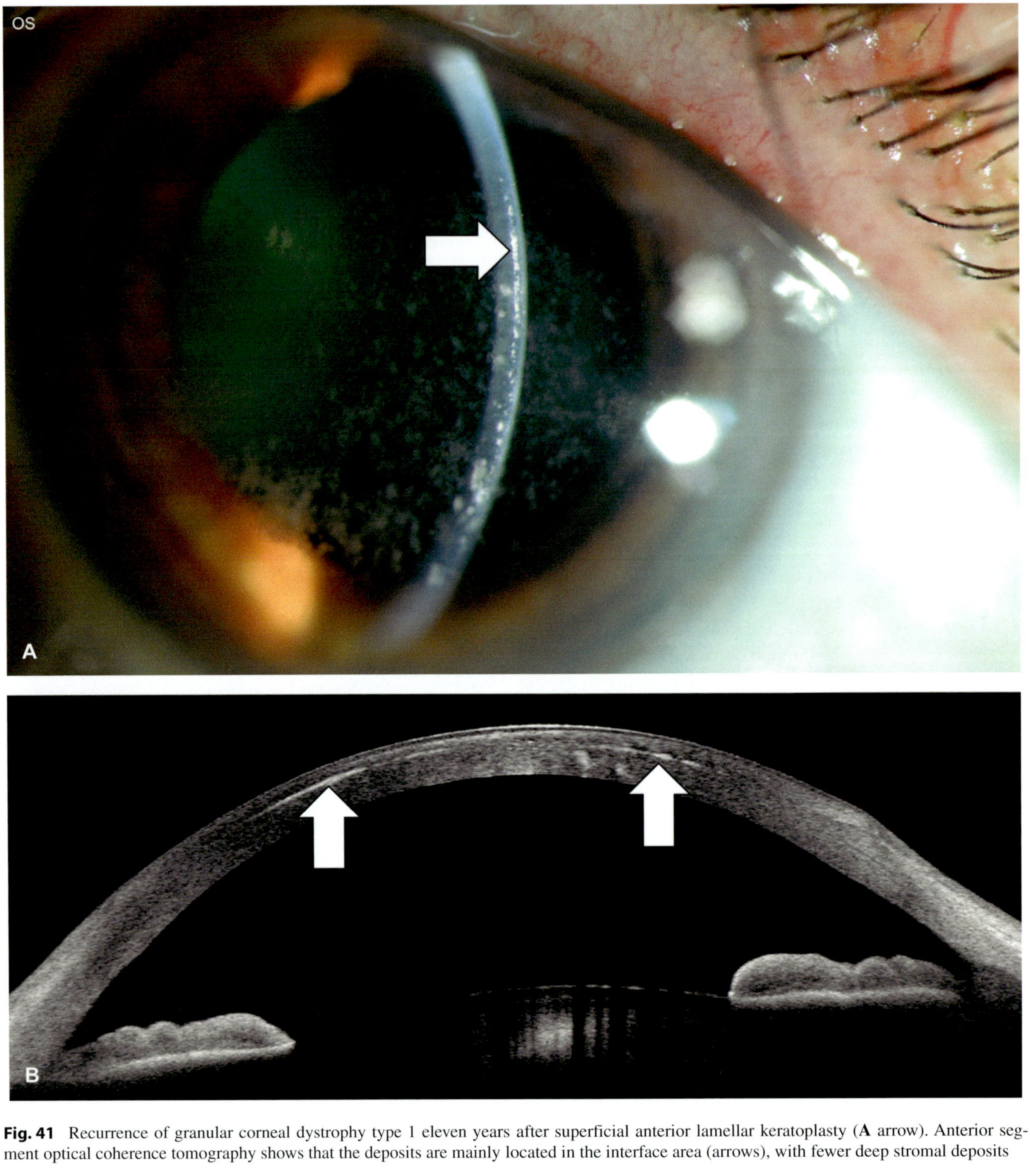

Fig. 41 Recurrence of granular corneal dystrophy type 1 eleven years after superficial anterior lamellar keratoplasty (**A** arrow). Anterior segment optical coherence tomography shows that the deposits are mainly located in the interface area (arrows), with fewer deep stromal deposits

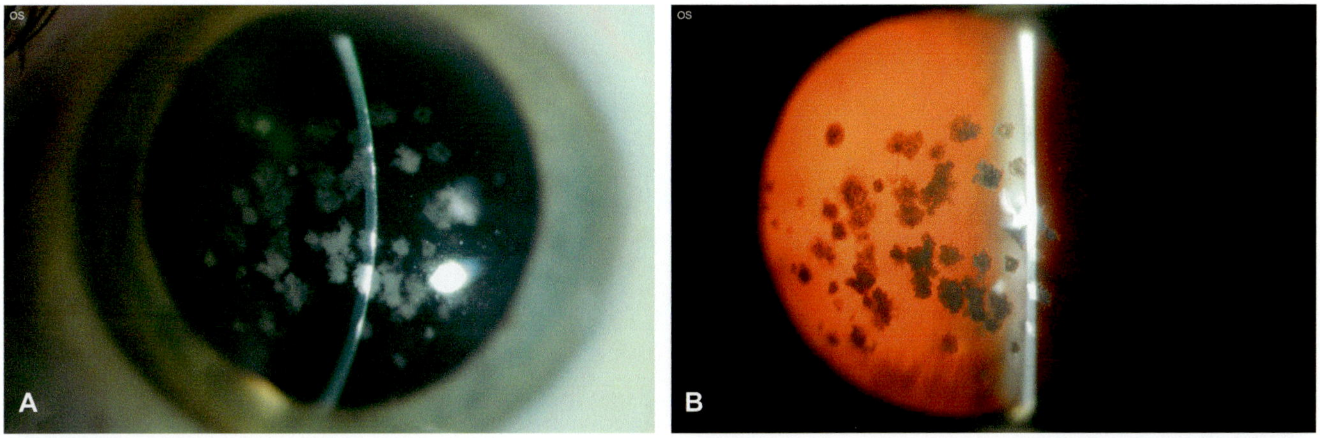

Fig. 42 Granular corneal dystrophy type 2 with multiple superficial granular deposits (discs) in a 76-year-old man ((**A**) thin slit illumination, (**B**) retroillumination)

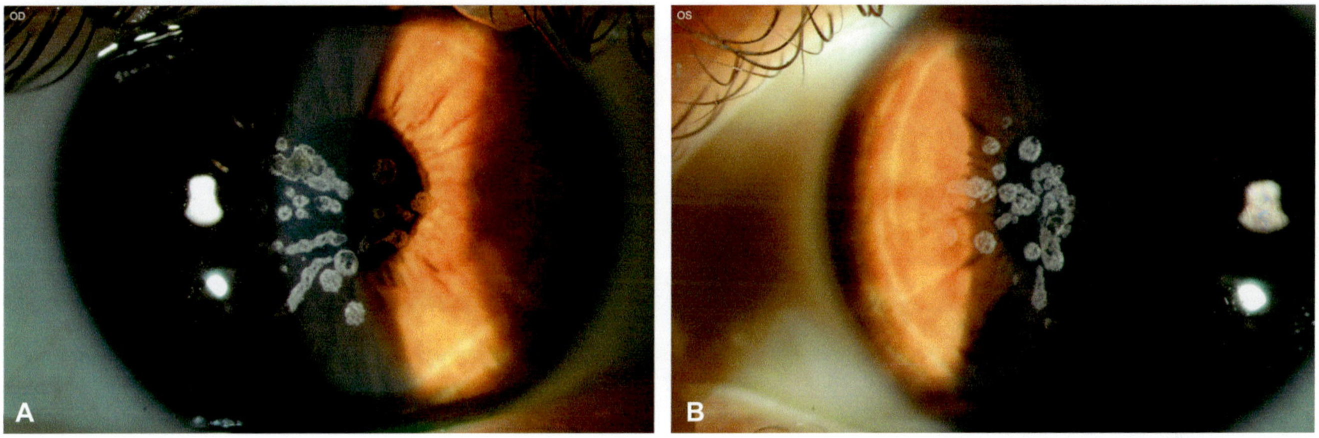

Fig. 43 Granular corneal dystrophy type 2 in a 46-year-old woman. The granular deposits show a ring-like appearance in both eyes (OD: (**A**)/ OS: (**B**)). In contrast to type 1, the deposits are not as numerous and are located in the superficial corneal layers

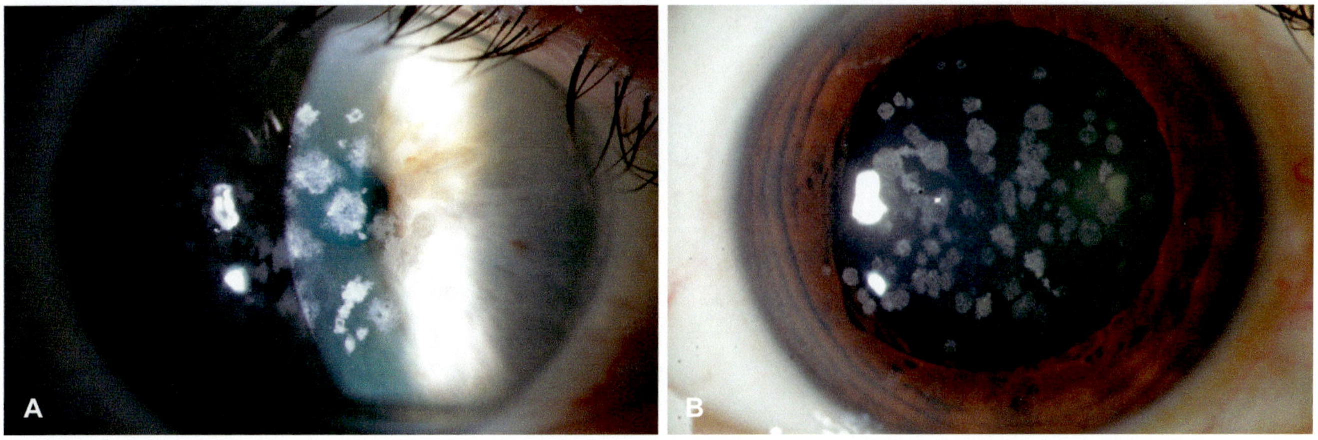

Fig. 44 Granular corneal dystrophy type 2 in two different individuals. Typically, the deposits are superficial, round patches with moth-eaten centers (ring-shaped)

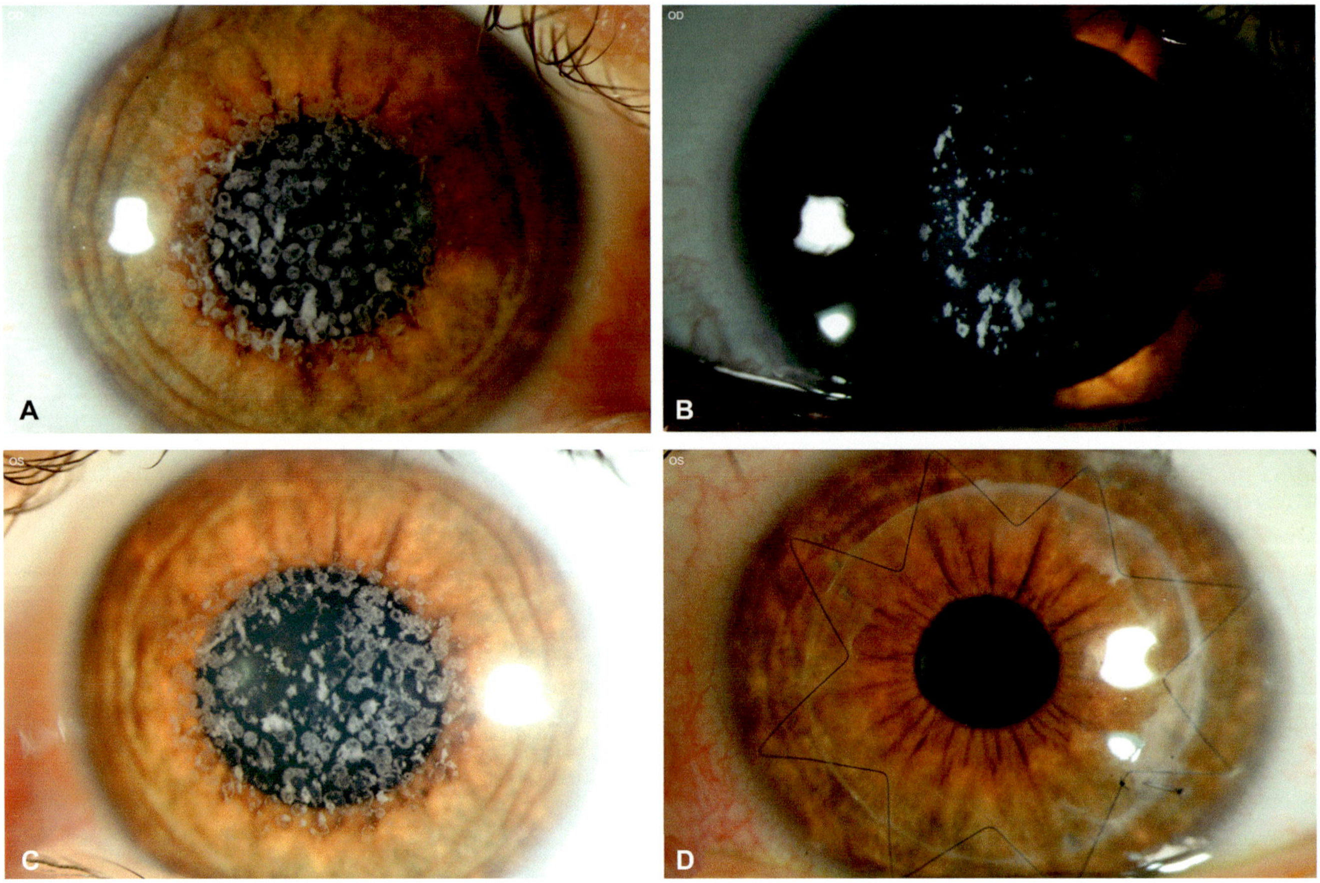

Fig. 45 Granular corneal dystrophy type 2 with multiple ring-shaped granular opacities in both eyes (OD: (**A**)/OS: (**C**)). Excimer laser-assisted phototherapeutic keratectomy was performed on the right eye (**B**), which removed most of the superficial opacities. In contrast, penetrating keratoplasty was performed on the left eye (**D**)

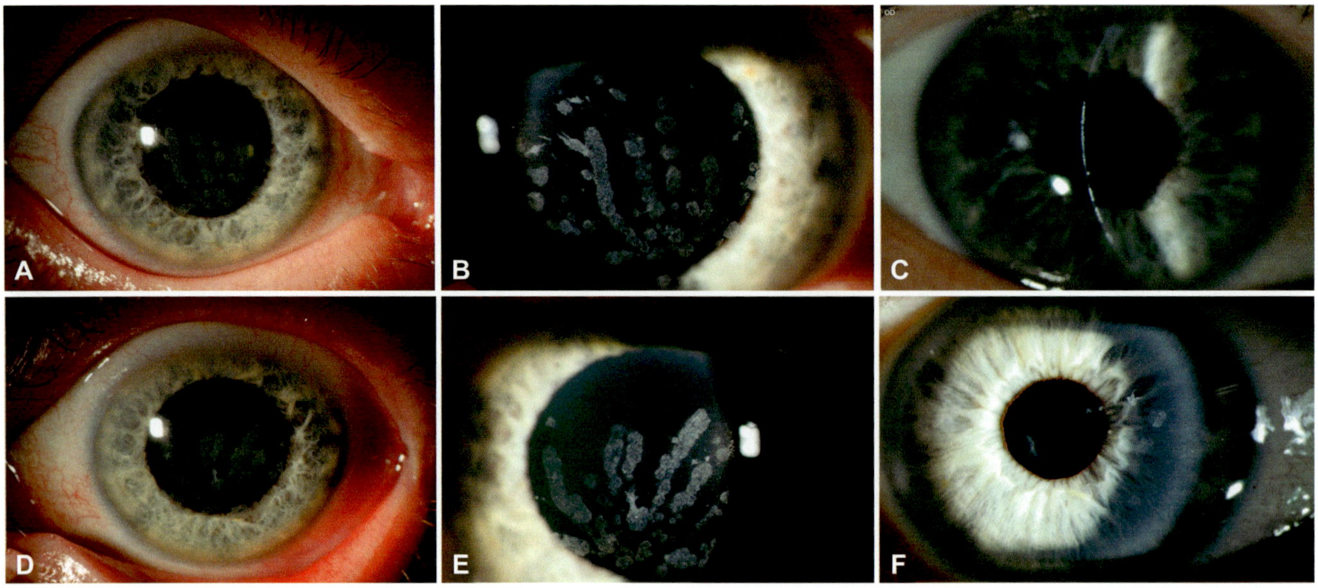

Fig. 46 Granular corneal dystrophy type 2 with finger-like deposits in both eyes (OD: **A**–**C**/OS: **D**–**E**) in a 53-year-old woman. Excimer laser-assisted phototherapeutic keratectomy was performed on the left eye (**F**), which removed most of the superficial deposits

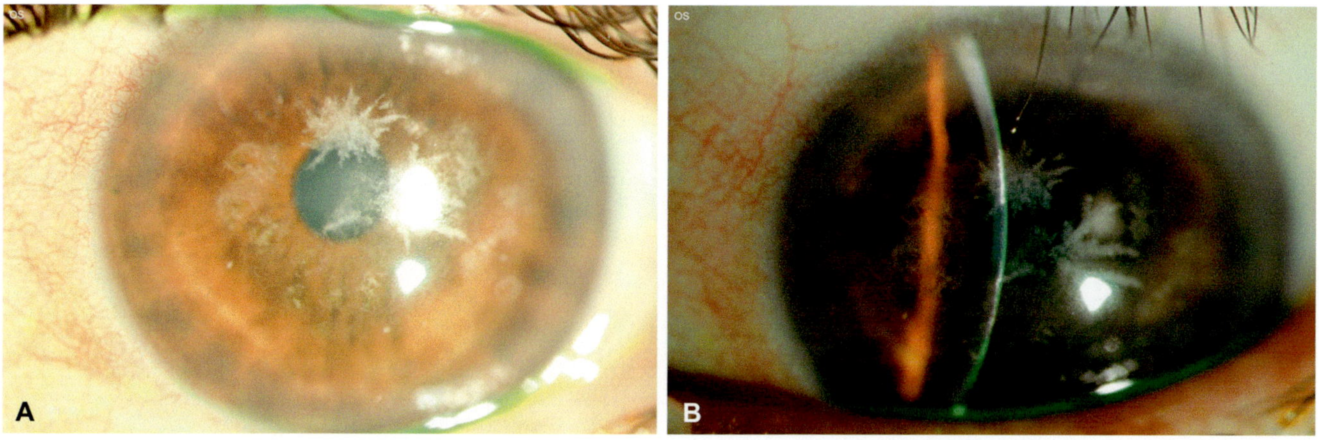

Fig. 47 Granular corneal dystrophy type 2 in a 60-year-old man. Compared to granular corneal dystrophy type 1, there are fewer deposits. These superficial deposits might have a star/spider-like appearance ((**A**) overview, (**B**) thin slit illumination)

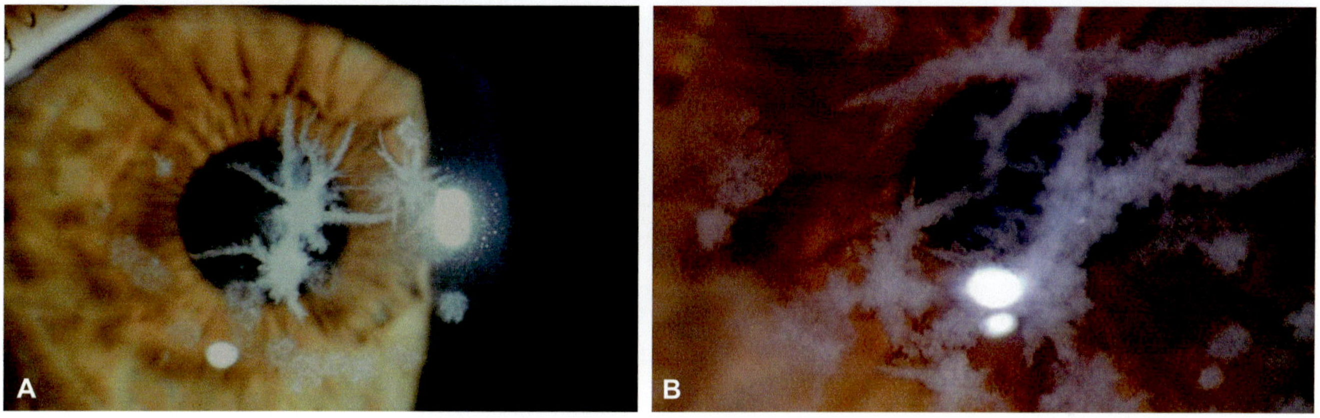

Fig. 48 Granular corneal dystrophy type 2 with star-shaped deposits in two individuals (**A**, **B**)

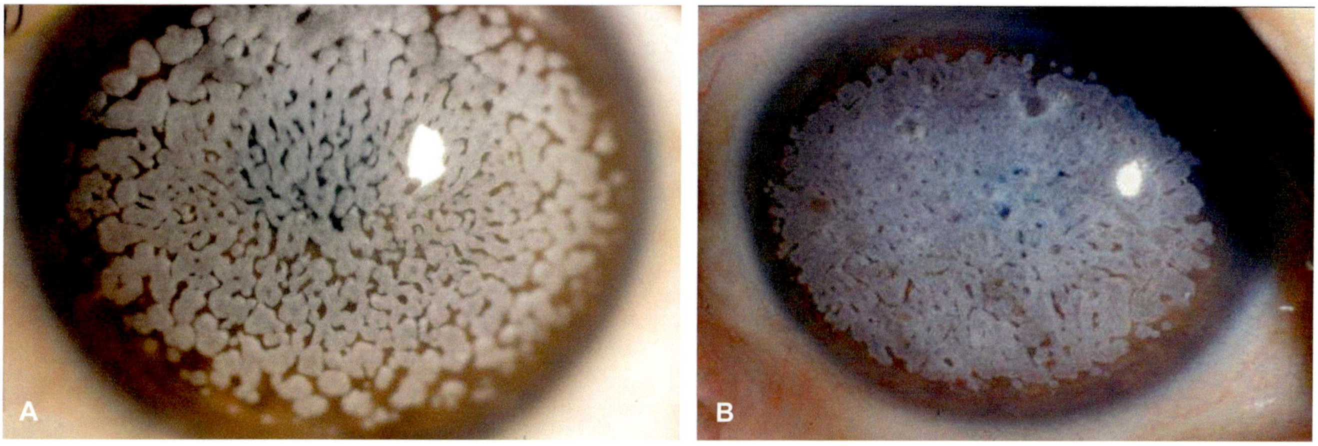

Fig. 49 Homozygote granular corneal dystrophy type 2 with denser and confluent opacities in two individuals (**A**, **B**)

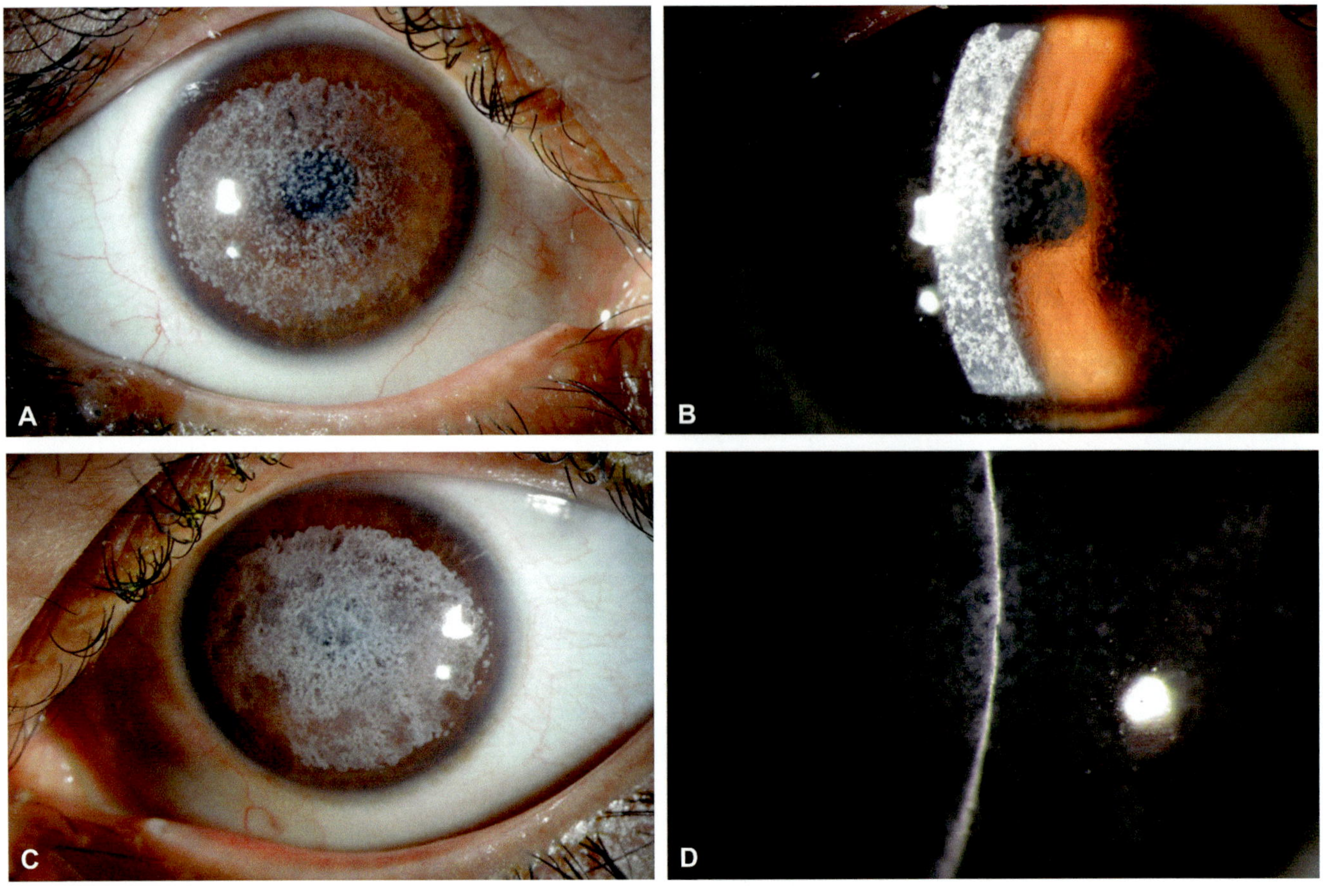

Fig. 50 Homozygous granular corneal dystrophy type 2 in a 38-year-old woman (OD: **A**, **B**/OS: **C**, **D**). The superficial granular deposits are dense and confluent. The corneal limbus is free of deposits

resemble discs (Fig. 42) or rings (Figs. 43, 44 and 45), often in finger-like arrangement (Fig. 46). Other commonly found clinical signs include spiky anterior to midstromal deposits that are star-, icicle-, or spider-shaped (Figs. 47 and 48). Sometimes short lines can be recognized, which must be distinguished from lattice lines in LCD. The lines in GCD2 are thicker, whiter, may have bulbs or spikes and cross less frequently than the thinner lattice lines in classic LCD. Heterozygous GCD2 is characteristically associated with less stromal opacities than GCD1. In contrast, homozygous patients (Figs. 49, 50 and 51) may exhibit very dense, large, irregular opacities with increasing depth as the disease progresses. In case of central involvement, visual acuity may

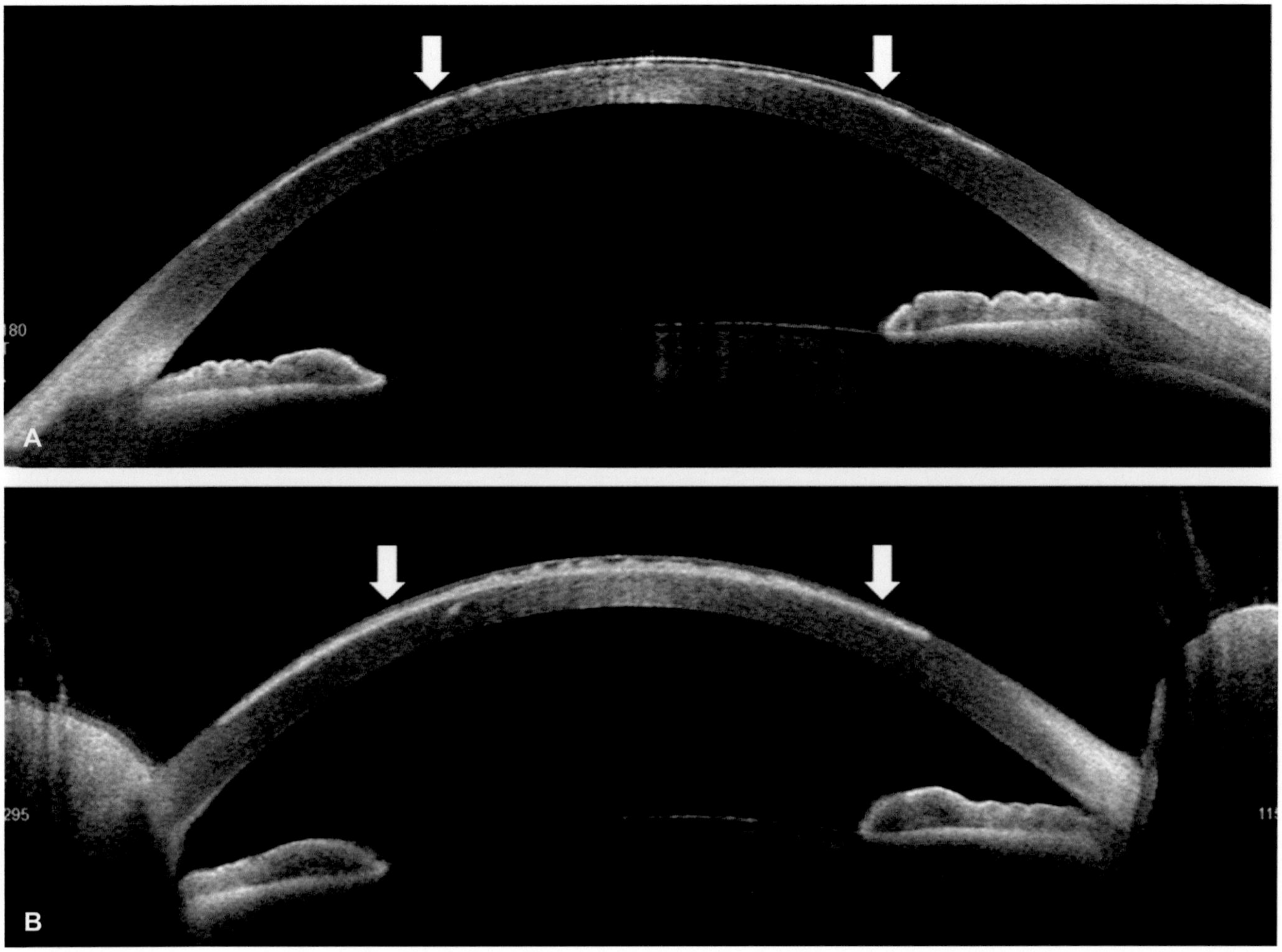

Fig. 51 Anterior segment optical coherence tomography in homozygous granular corneal dystrophy type 2 showing a superficial, dense, hyperreflective lesion (arrow) in the right (**A**) and left (**B**) eye

be noticeably reduced. In contrast to GCD1, recurrent erosions are less frequent.

In GCD2, laser-in-situ-keratomileusis can lead to an accelerated accumulation of granular deposits in the interface (Fig. 52), resulting in massive protein accumulation several years after the procedure [45, 46].

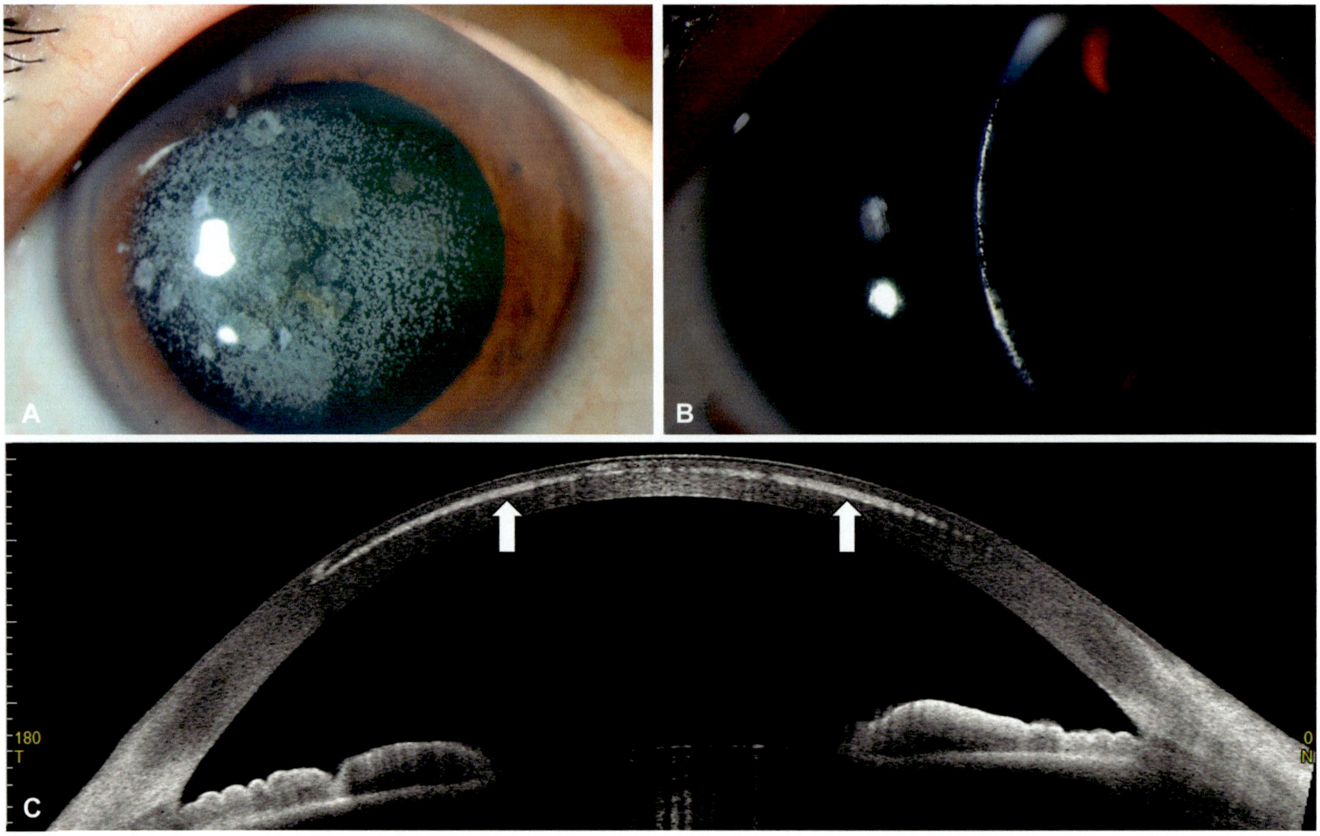

Fig. 52 Granular corneal dystrophy type 2 in a 59-year-old patient. Laser-in-situ-keratomileusis was previously performed 10 years ago, which resulted in a pronounced formation of hyalin deposits in the interface area (**A**, **B**). The anterior segment optical coherence tomography is showing the hyperreflective granular deposits along the interface (arrows), (**C**)

5.3 Stromal Dystrophies

5.3.1 Macular Corneal Dystrophy

In early stages of macular corneal dystrophy (MCD, autosomal recessive, 16q22.1, Carbohydrate sulfotransferase 6—*CHST6*), central, superficial, irregular whitish fleck-like opacities (macules) develop, which can later involve the limbus and the deep stroma down to Descemet membrane and the endothelium (Figs. 53, 54, 55 and 56). Progressive diffuse opacification ("haze") develops at the same time, involving the entire stroma of the cornea in later stages, causing severe vision loss by the third decade of life ("large snowflakes and fog"). Unlike granular corneal dystrophy, MCD is characterized by progressive diffuse haze formation between the fleck-like opacities. While the larger central fleck-like opacities are found in the superficial stroma, the smaller and more discrete peripheral opacities are located in the deep corneal stroma. Anterior stromal and subepithelial deposits (Figs. 57 and 58) may result in significant refractive error by affecting the anterior corneal surface leading to irregular astigmatism. Another important

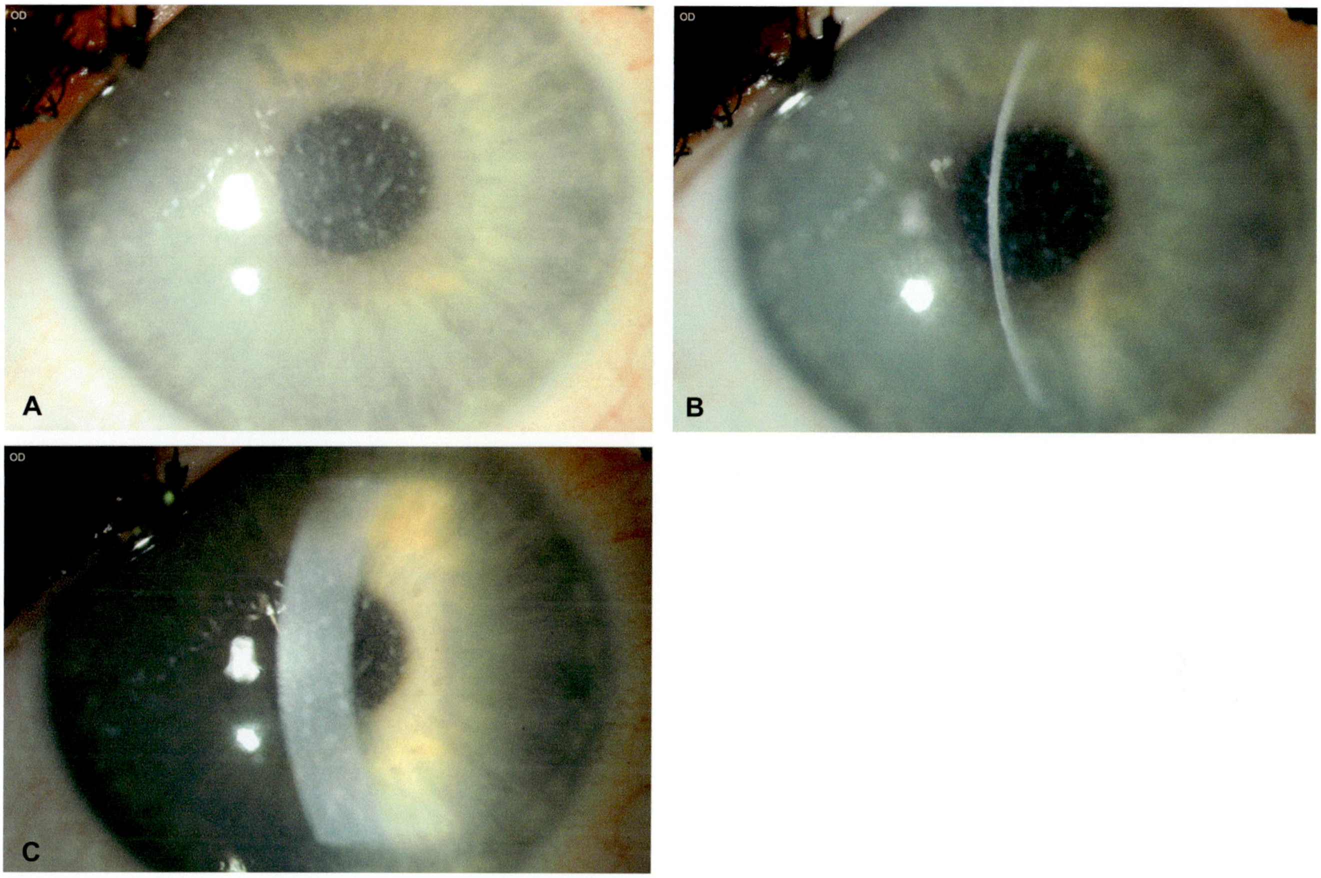

Fig. 53 Macular corneal dystrophy in a 24-year-old woman ((**A**) overview). The fleck-like lesions are small. The cornea is diffusely thinned with dense haze ((**B**) thin slit illumination, (**C**) broad slit illumination)

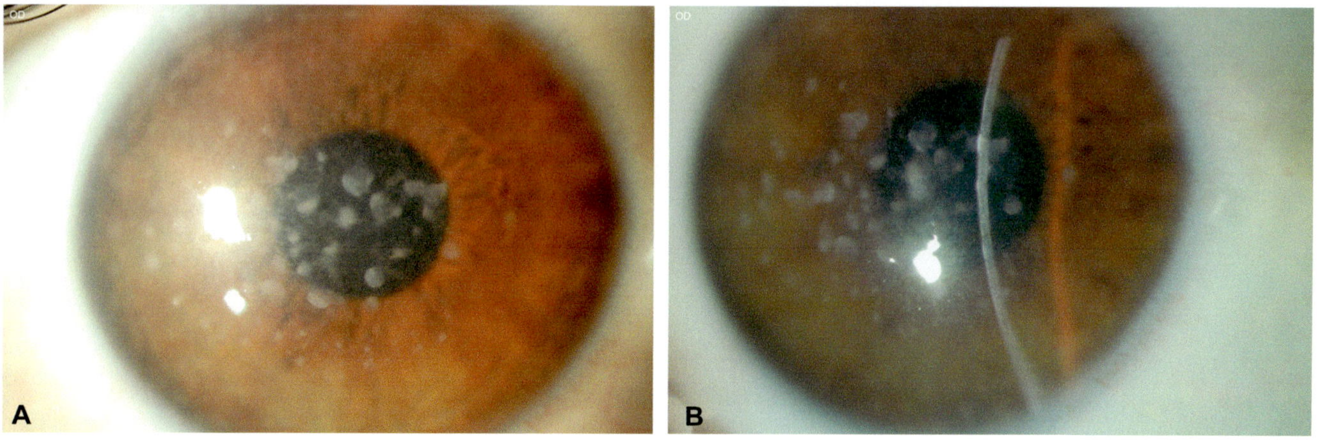

Fig. 54 Macular corneal dystrophy with multiple fleck-like deposits (**A**) and corneal thinning (best visible with thin slit illumination, **B**) in a 33-year-old woman

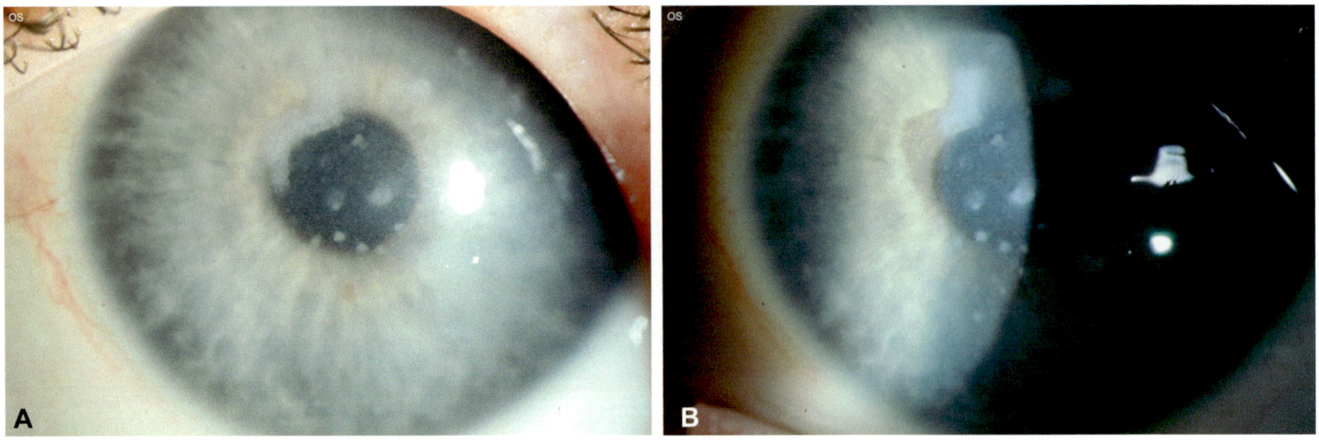

Fig. 55 Macular corneal dystrophy in a 24-year-old woman with larger fleck-like opacities and haze ((**A**) overview, (**B**) broad slit illumination)

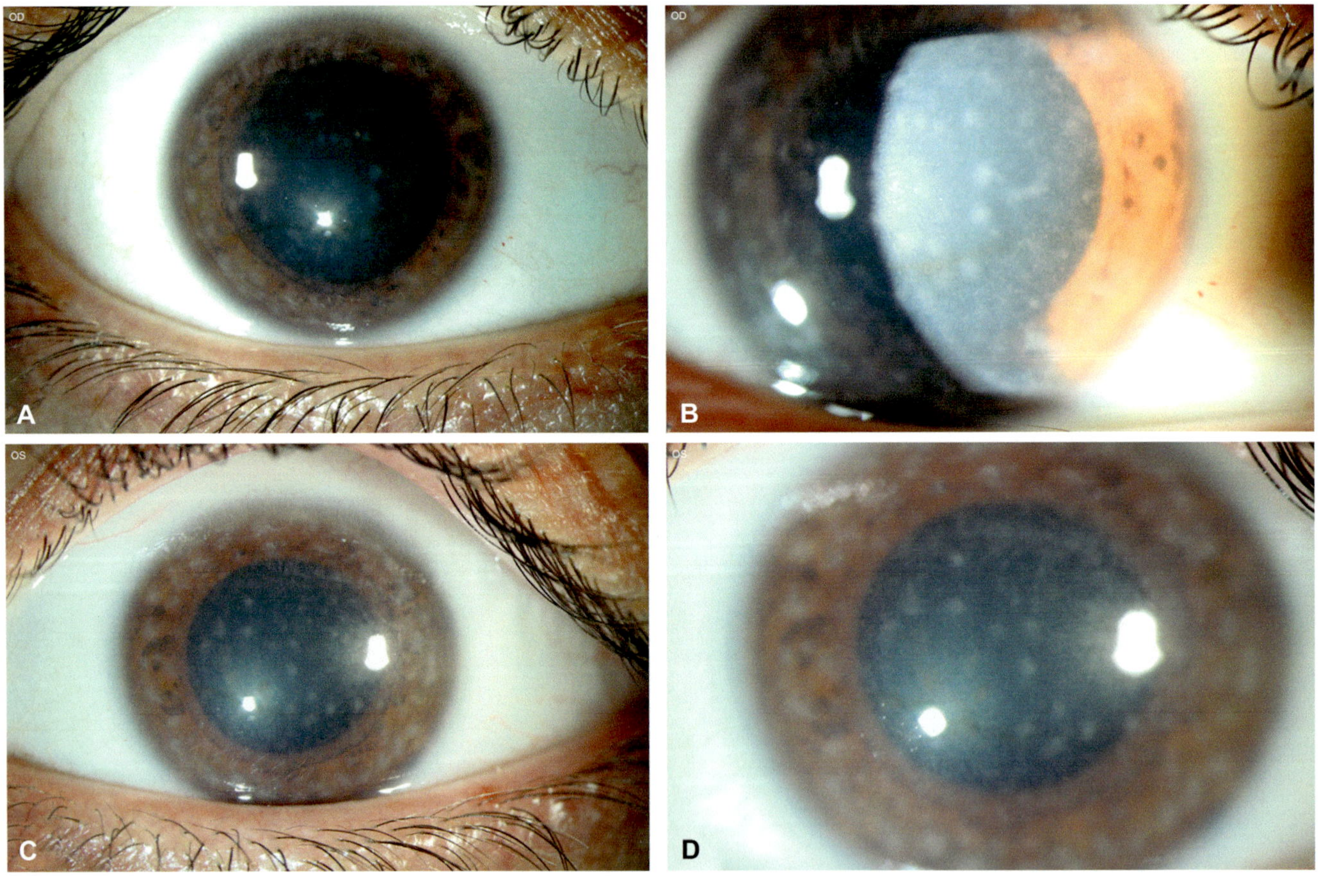

Fig. 56 Macular corneal dystrophy in a 27-year-old man. There are multiple small patchy opacities (leopard fur-like appearance) with corneal haze in both eyes (OD: **A**, **B**/OS: **C**, **D**) which extend to the limbus

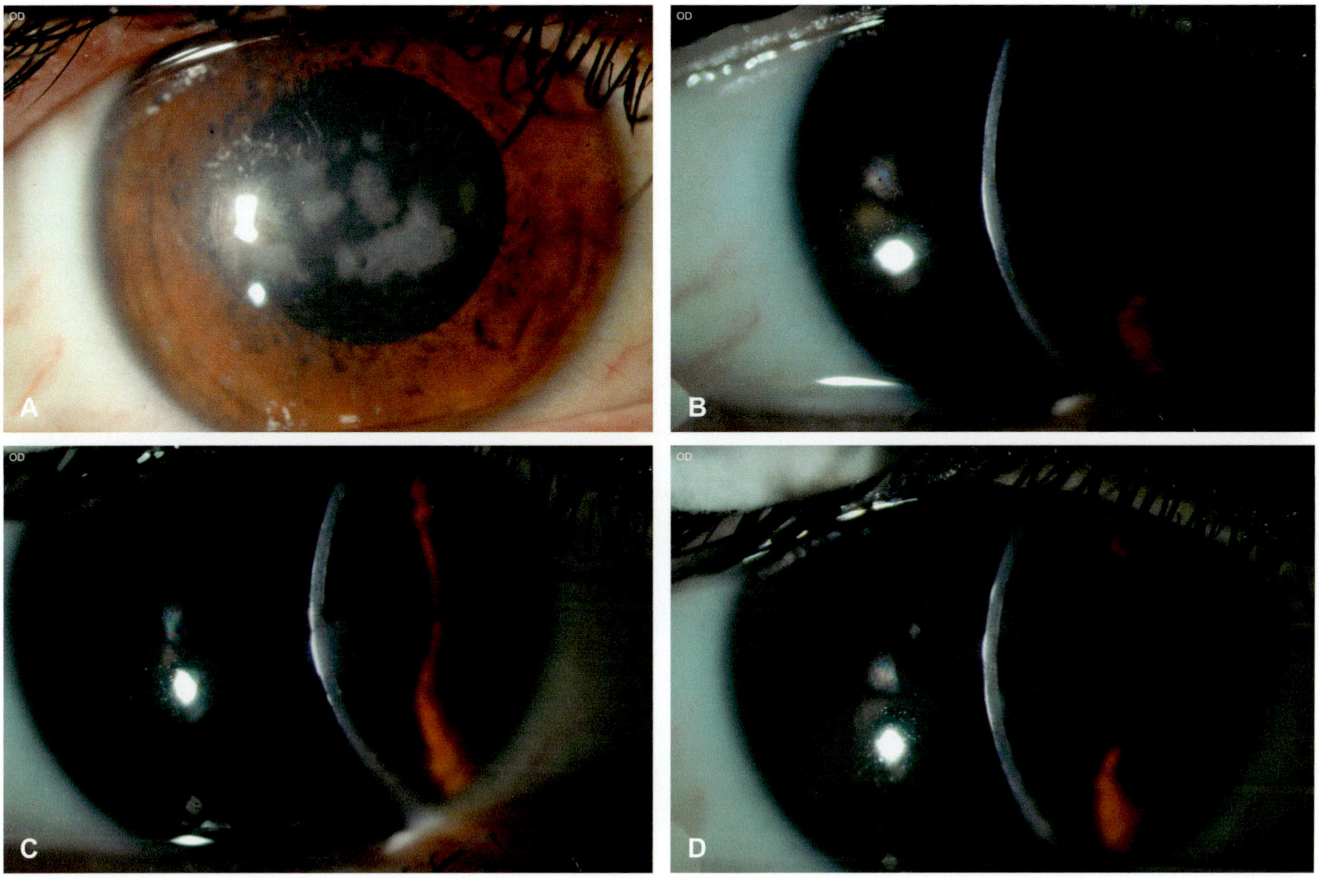

Fig. 57 Macular corneal dystrophy in a 29-year-old man (**A**). There are dense and large patchy deposits that are elevated and cause an irregular surface (**B–D** thin slit illumination of different areas)

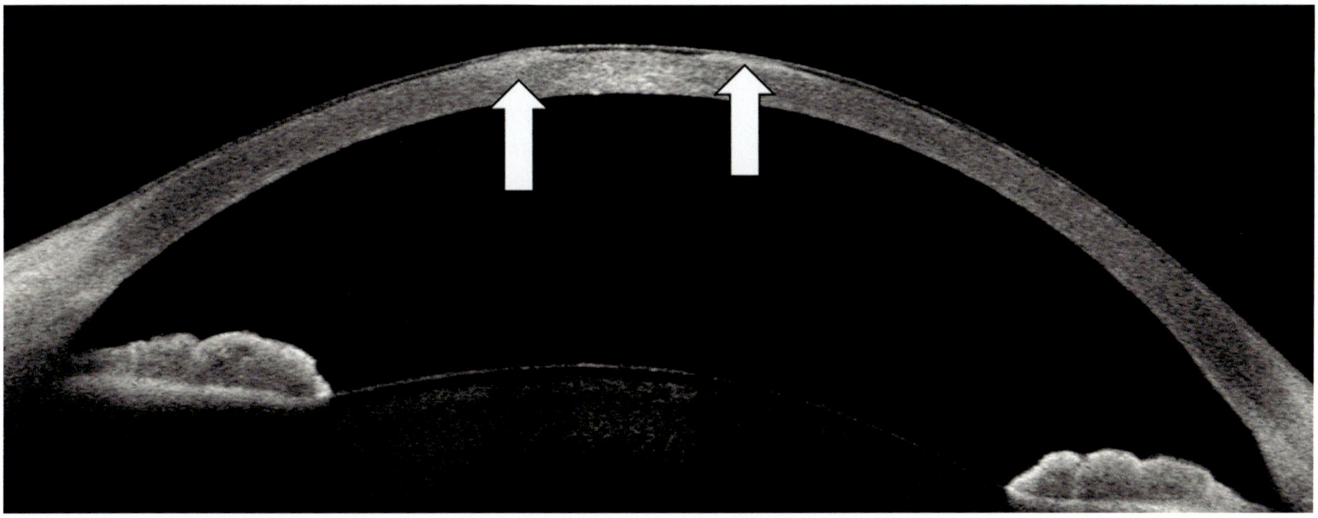

Fig. 58 Anterior segment optical coherence tomography in macular corneal dystrophy. Note the superficial hyperreflective deposits (arrows), which represent the fleck-like opacities. However, fine deposits reach down to Descemet membrane

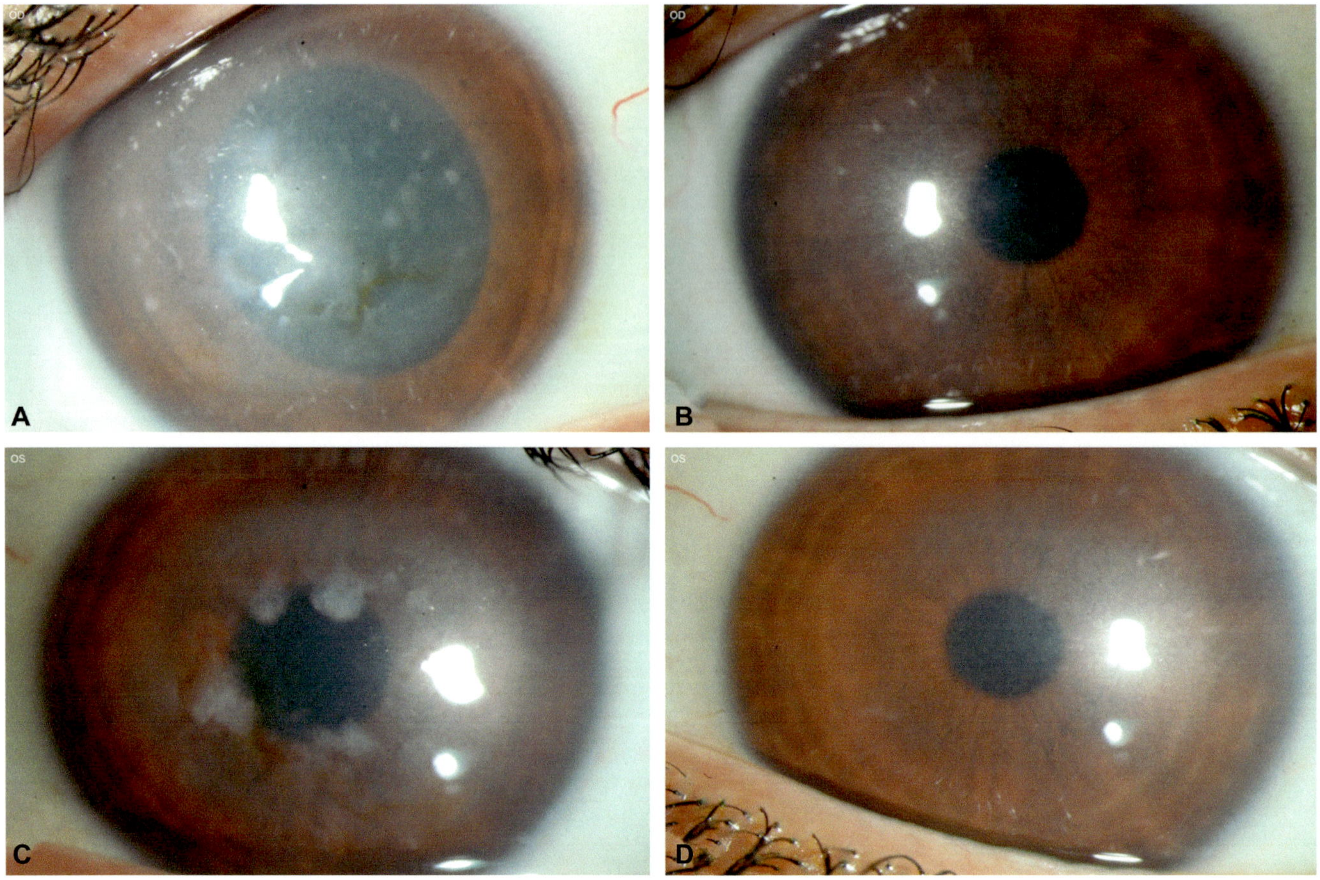

Fig. 59 Macular corneal dystrophy with fleck-like opacities and diffuse haze in both eyes of a 35-year-old woman (**A** OD/**C** OS). After excimer laser-assisted phototherapeutic keratectomy, the superficial white flecks were removed completely, whereas the diffuse pan-stromal haze remained (**B** OD/**D** OS)

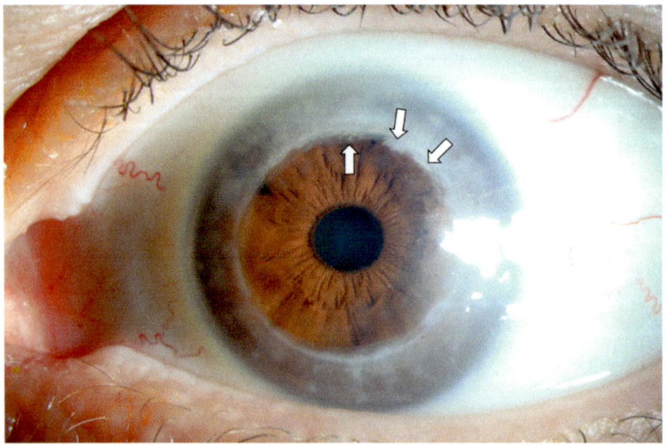

Fig. 60 Penetrating keratoplasty for macular corneal dystrophy 40 years ago. The central graft is totally clear. Stromal deposits at the graft–host junction indicate a dystrophy recurrence in the graft (arrows). The remaining host cornea is diffusely opacified up to the limbus

characteristic feature of MCD is a progressive corneal thinning, which is caused by a reduction in interfibrillar spacing [47, 48]. Endothelial decompensation is not common but may appear in later stages. Excimer PTK is a suitable option for removing the large, central fleck-like opacities, which are generally localized in the anterior stroma [49] (Fig. 59). Clinically relevant recurrences after keratoplasty are very rare, most grafts are still clear decades later [24] (Fig. 60).

5.3.2 Schnyder Corneal Dystrophy

Schnyder corneal dystrophy (SCD) is an autosomal dominant corneal disorder (1p36, UbiA prenyltransferase domain-containing protein 1—*UBIAD1*) [50, 51–55].

The disease can manifest in childhood (Figs. 61 and 62), however, the diagnosis is mostly made in the second or third decade of life. The clinical findings usually depend

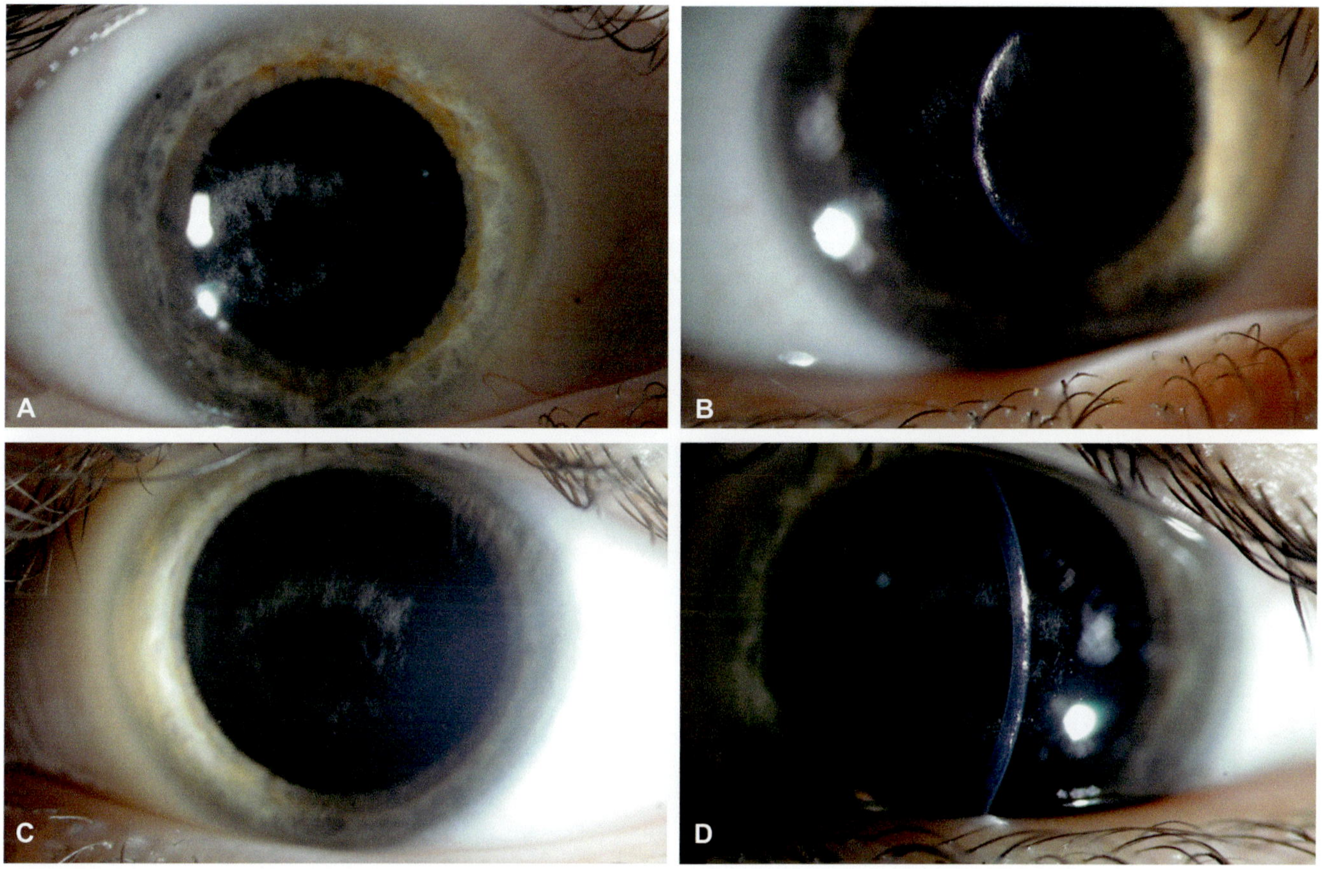

Fig. 61 Early findings of Schnyder corneal dystrophy in an 8-year-old male child. There are superficial, ring-shaped crystalline deposits in the right (**A**, **B**) and left (**C**, **D**) eye. The characteristic midperipheral opacity and the arcus lipoides are absent. Diagnosis may be more difficult in early findings as the typical morphological changes are not yet present

on the patient's age. In early stages, patients of 23 years and younger might present a ring-like or disc-like central corneal opacity and/or central crowded comma-shaped subepithelial crystals (Figs. 63 and 64). Arcus lipoides might be present between age 23 and 38 years (Fig. 65). Mid-peripheral panstromal opacities also develop after the age of 38 years, making the entire cornea appear opaque (Figs. 66 and 67). It is important to note that corneal crystals are only found in 50% of patients with SCD. Furthermore, crystals may be unilateral and can occur late in the disease. Corneal crystals in SCD have a comma-shaped look, which is important in the differential diagnosis of punctiform crystals that occur in cystinosis or paraproteinemic keratopathy associated with monoclonal gammopathy of undetermined significance (MGUS). The crystalline deposits are localized subepithelially and can be removed effectively with an excimer

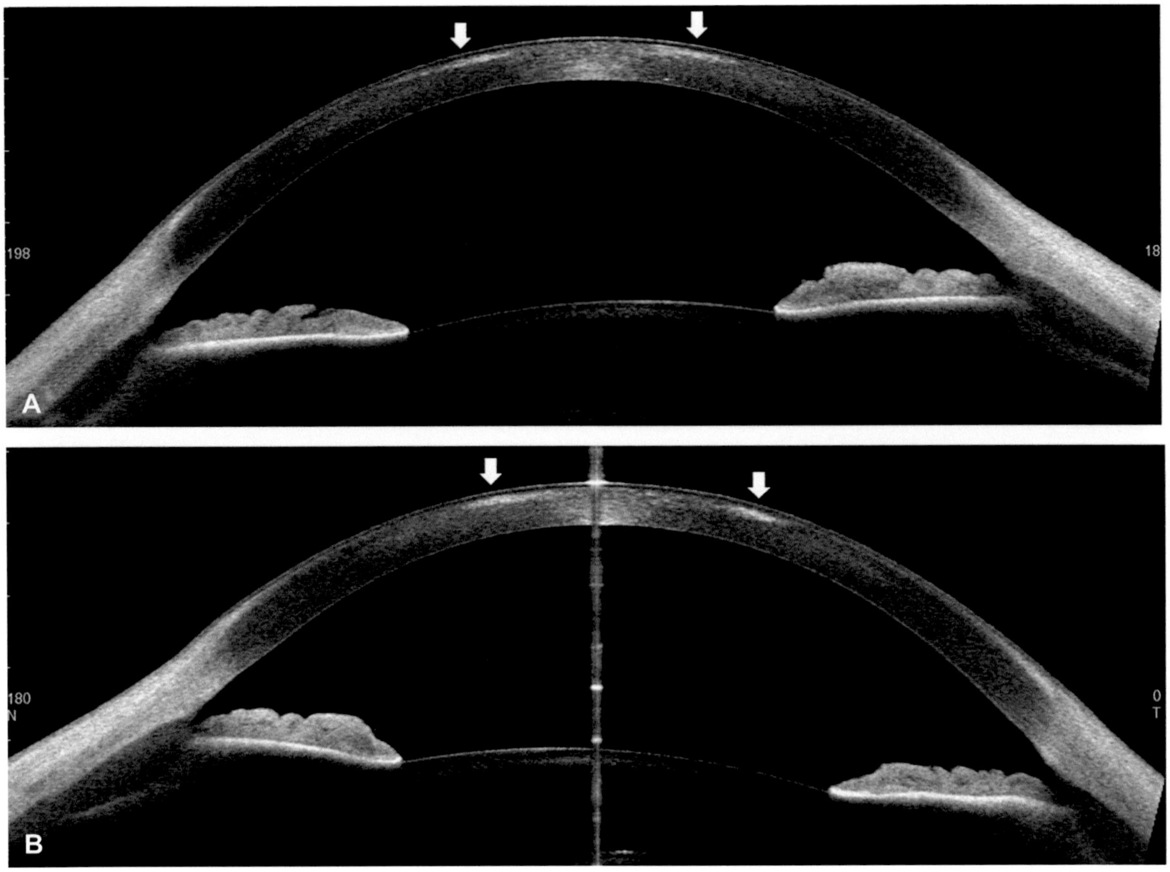

Fig. 62 In early Schnyder dystrophy at the age of 8 years, only subepithelial-anterior stromal crystalline deposits are seen by anterior segment optical coherence tomography (hyperreflective changes: arrows). The clinical findings are shown in Fig. 61

laser-assisted phototherapeutic keratectomy (Fig. 68), however the pan-stromal opacities remain and may lead to severe visual impairment. In such cases, penetrating keratoplasty might help to improve vision (Fig. 69). The prognosis after keratoplasty is generally good, but small subepithelial crystalline opacities may appear on the graft over time (Fig. 70).

Congenital Stromal Corneal Dystrophy

Congenital stromal corneal dystrophy (CSCD) is inherited in an autosomal dominant manner (12q21.33, Decorin—*DCN*) [56, 57]. This stromal dystrophy is characterized by diffuse, bilateral corneal clouding (clinical landmark) with flake-like whitish opacities throughout the stroma of the entire cornea that occur at

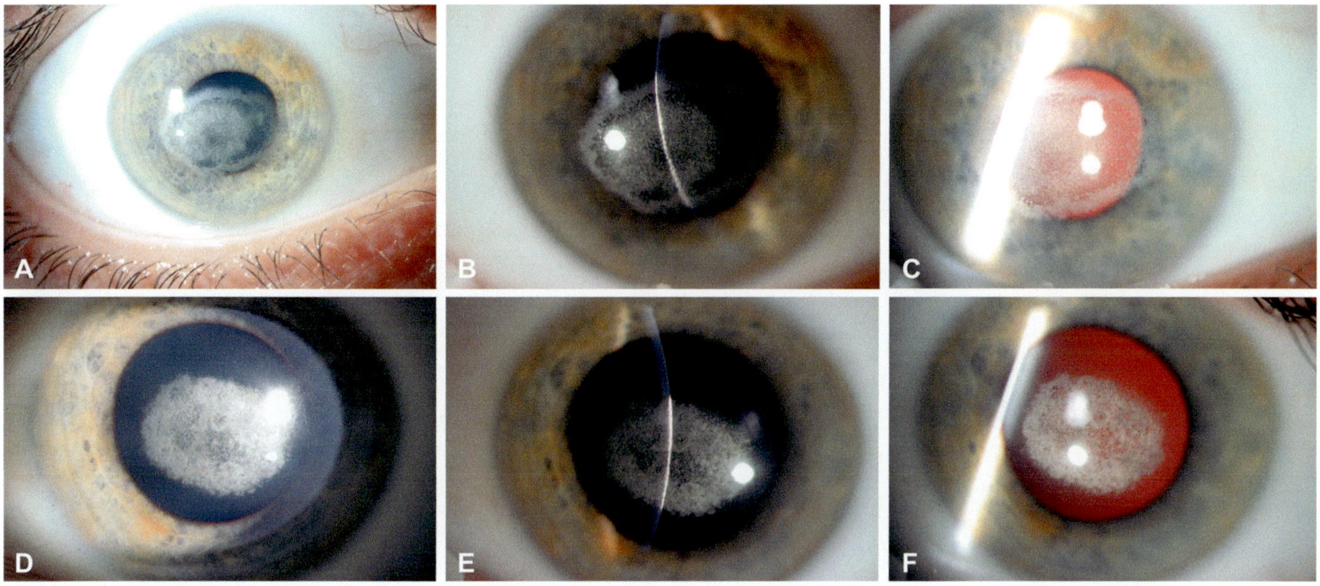

Fig. 63 Schnyder corneal dystrophy in a 28-year-old man (OD: **A**–**C**/OS: **D**–**F**). There are dense, island-shaped crystalline deposits that are superficially localized (**B**, **E**). There is no arcus lipoides

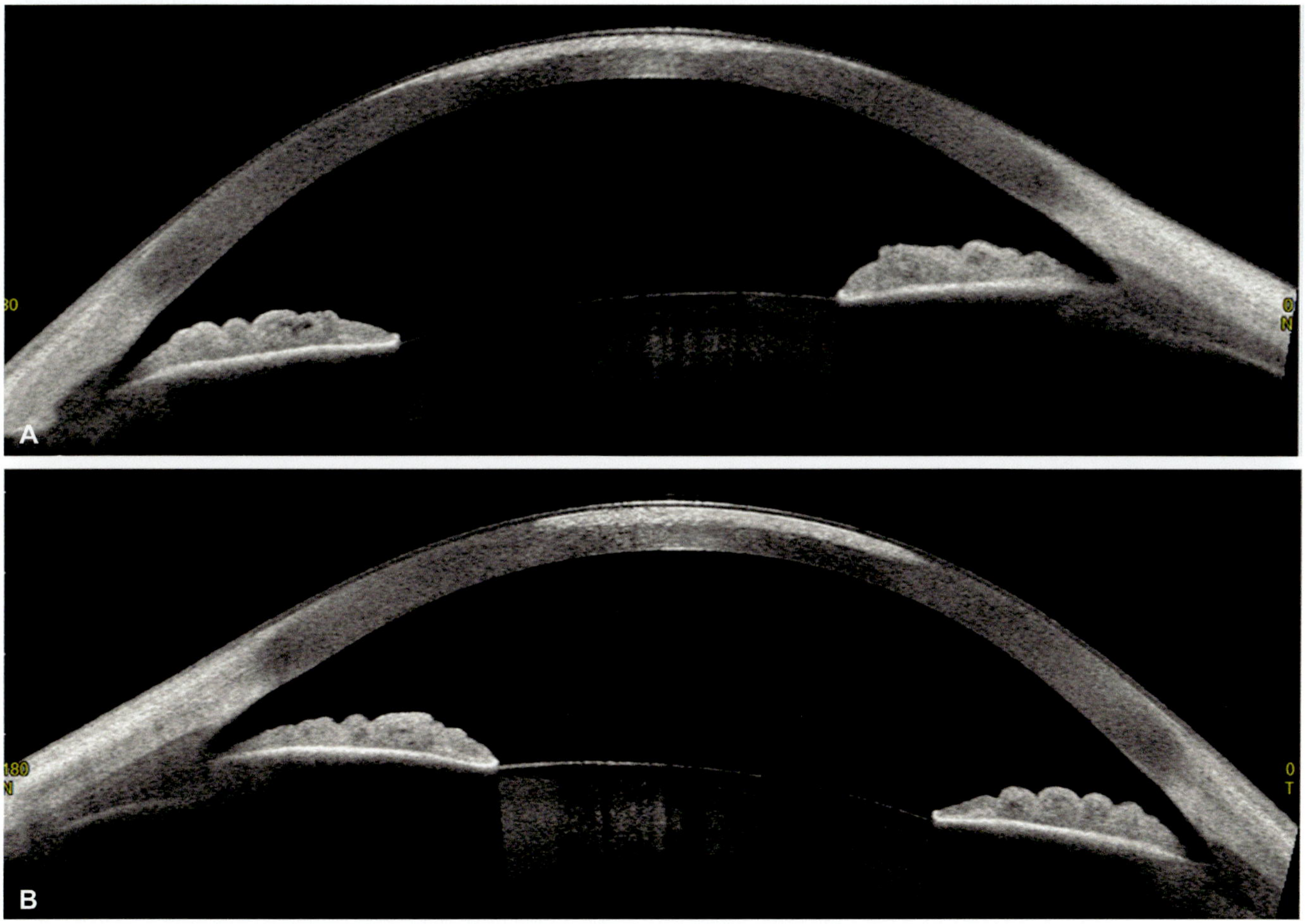

Fig. 64 Anterior segment optical coherence tomography in Schnyder corneal dystrophy with dense crystalline deposits demonstrated by a hyperreflective lesion extending into the anterior corneal stroma in the right (**A**) and left eye (**B**). The clinical findings are provided in Fig. 63

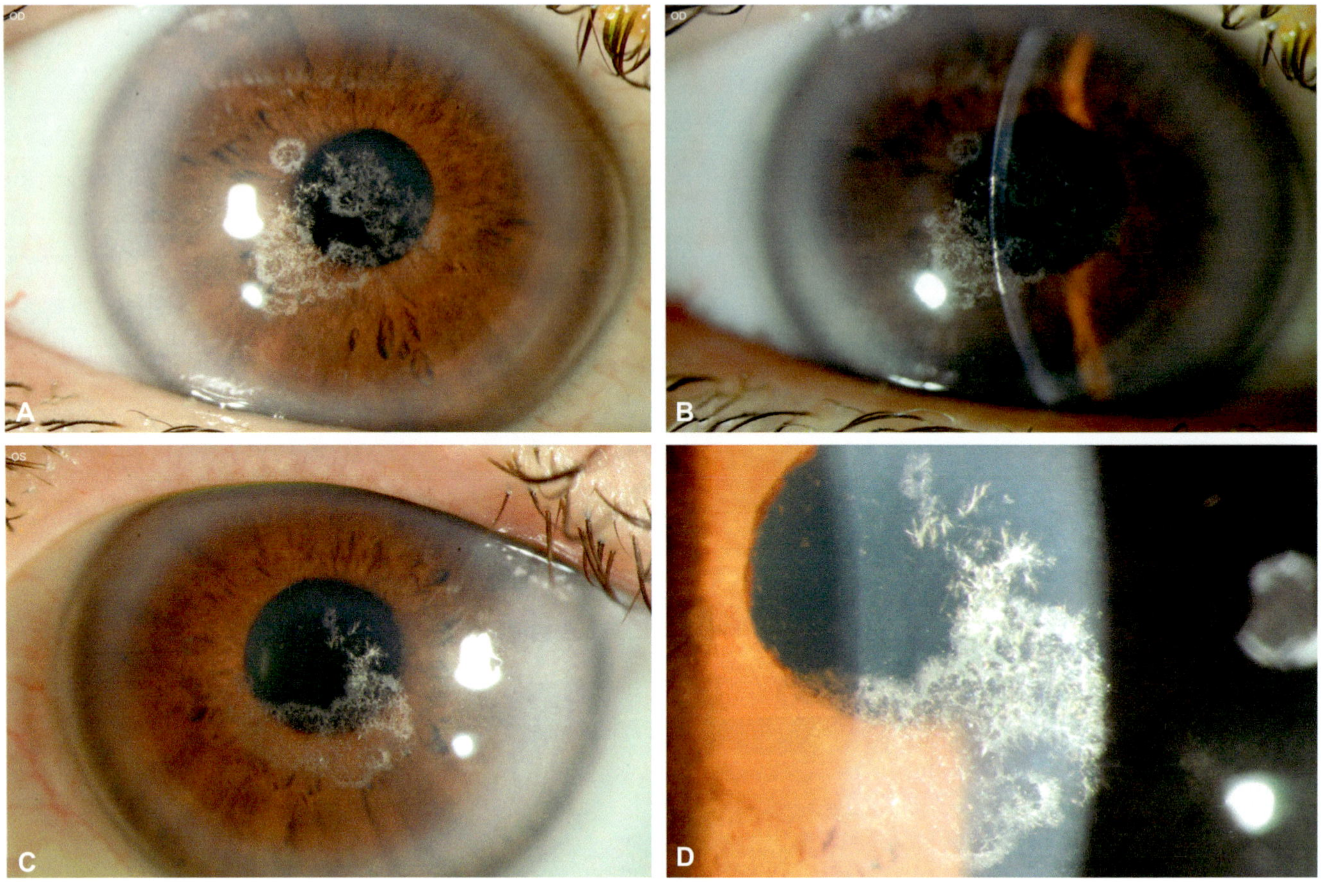

Fig. 65 Schnyder corneal dystrophy in a 41-year-old woman (OD: **A**, **B**/OS: **C**, **D**). Both eyes demonstrate an arcus lipoides and subepithelial crystalline deposits (best visible in (**B**))

or shortly after birth and are thought to increase in number with age as patients describe progressive visual deterioration over time (Figs. 71 and 72) [58]. Due to the severe pan-stromal stromal opacity, there is a high risk of amblyopia.

5.3.3 Fleck Corneal Dystrophy

The autosomal dominant inherited Fleck corneal dystrophy (FCD; 2q34, phosphoinositide kinase, FYVE finger—*PIK-FYVE*) is characterized by subtle, small discoid opacities or discrete, flat, gray–white, dandruff-like, and occasionally

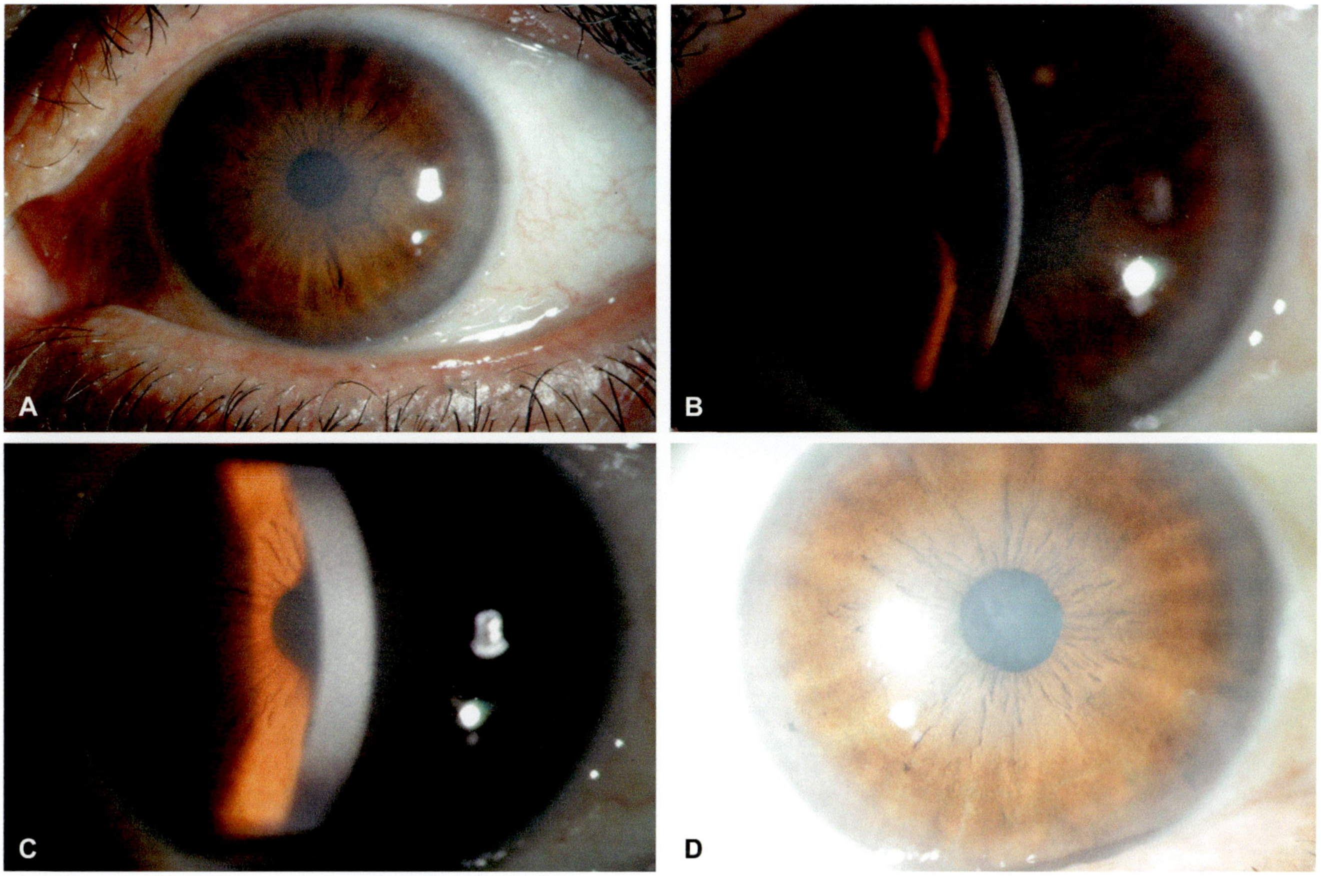

Fig. 66 Schnyder corneal dystrophy with arcus lipoides and a central opacity extending to the midperiphery of the cornea in the left ((**A**) overview, (**B**) thin slit illumination, (**C**) broad slit illumination) and right eye ((**D**) overview). No crystals are present

ring-shaped opacities scattered sparsely throughout any level of the otherwise clear stroma (Fig. 73). Most cases are asymptomatic (sometimes photophobia) and do not need conservative or surgical treatment [59, 60, 61].

5.3.4 Posterior Amorphous Corneal Dystrophy

Posterior amorphous corneal dystrophy (PACD) is an autosomal inherited corneal dystrophy caused by haploinsufficiency of small leucine-rich proteoglycans

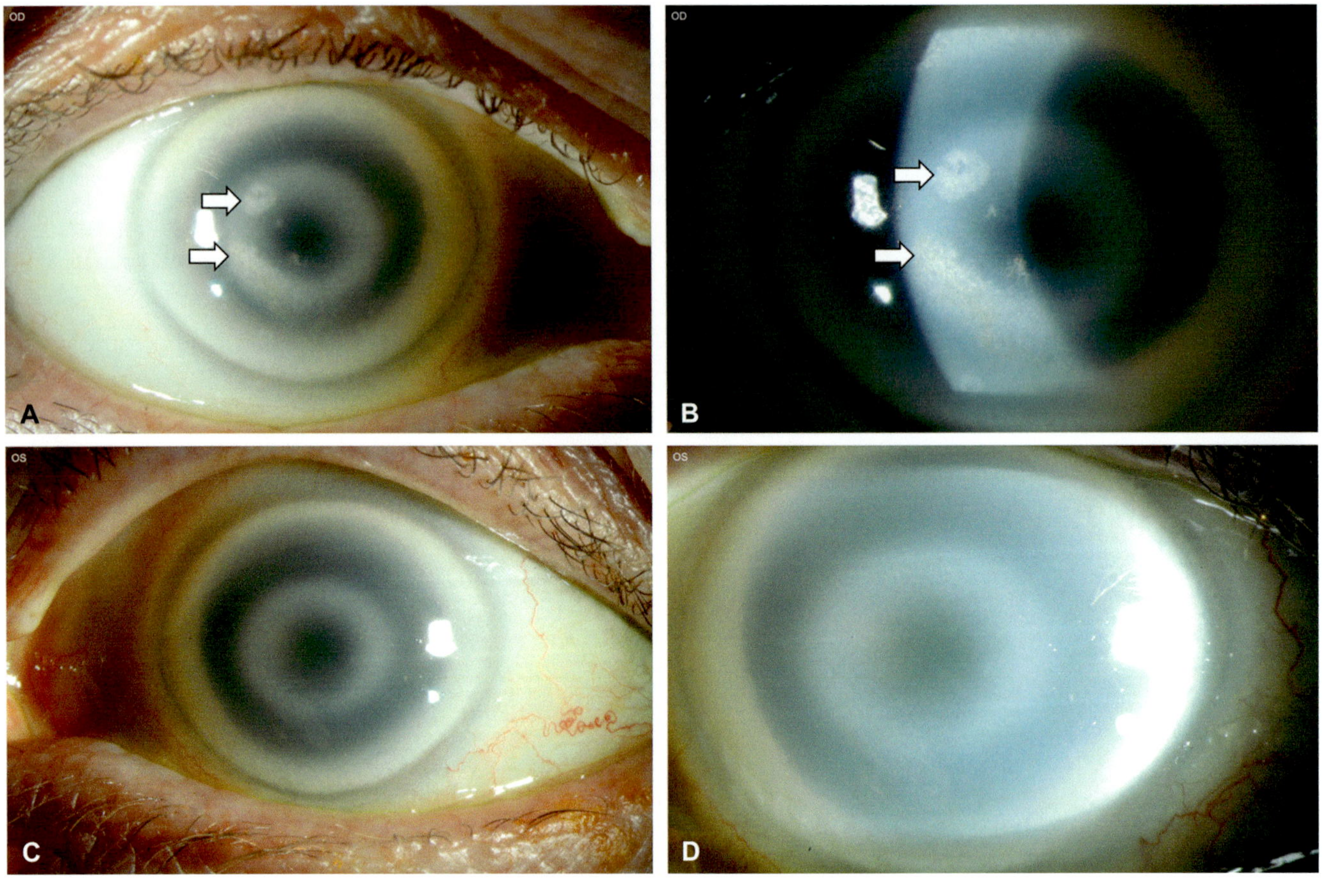

Fig. 67 Schnyder corneal dystrophy with an advanced arcus lipoides, a dense midperipheral opacity ring, and pan-stromal opacities (OD: **A**, **B**/ OS: **C**, **D**). Crystalline deposits are only present in the right eye (**A**, **B** arrows)

(12q21.33, keratocan—*KERA*, lumican—*LUM*, decorin—*DCN*, epiphycan—*EPYC*) [62]. It is characterized by diffuse grey, sheet-like opacities, which can be found in any layer of the corneal stroma, but mainly posteriorly. The diffuse opacities may be interrupted by transparent stromal areas.

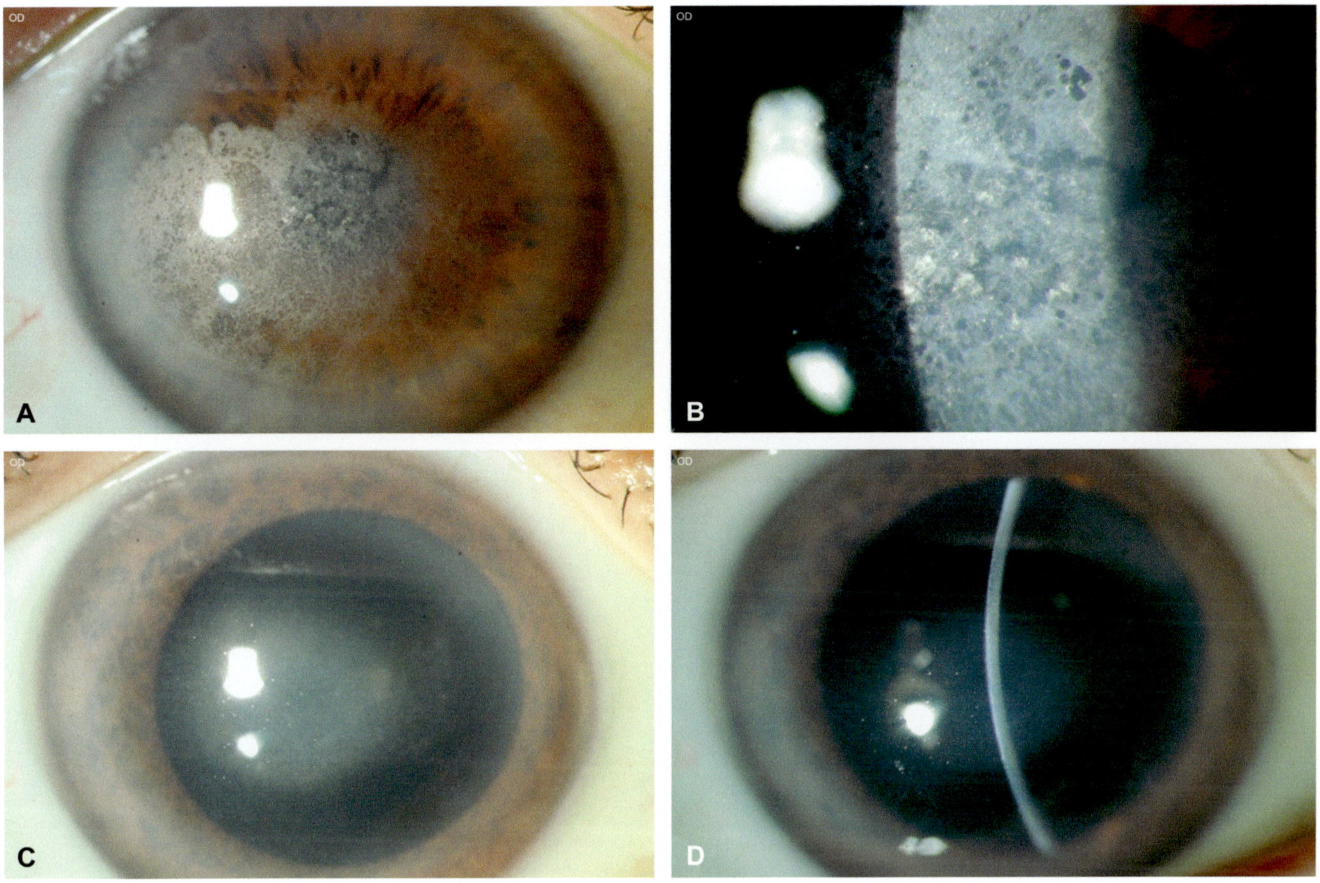

Fig. 68 Severe Schnyder corneal dystrophy with dense crystalline deposits (**A**, **B**) in a 41-year-old man. The subepithelial crystalline deposits could be removed completely after excimer laser-assisted phototherapeutic keratectomy. However, the pan-stromal opacities remain (**C**, **D**)

5.3.5 Central Cloudy Dystrophy of François

Central cloudy dystrophy of François (CCDF) is probably more a degenerative disease than a real corneal dystrophy (Category 4). The clinical findings include a polygonal central cloudy grey-white stromal opacity (Figs. 74 and 75), which is separated by linear areas of clear cornea (leather-like crocodile appearance).

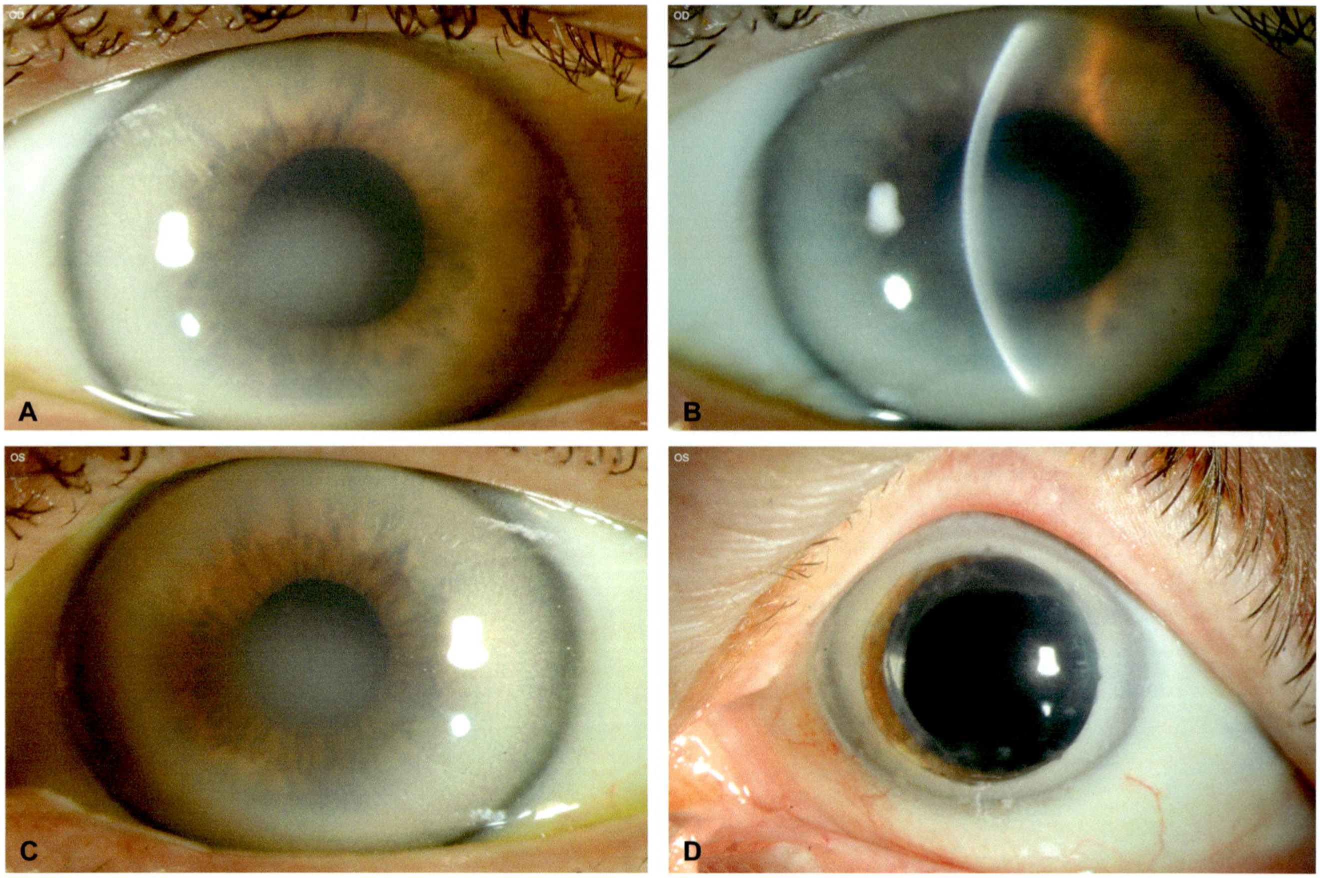

Fig. 69 Schnyder corneal dystrophy in a 71-year-old woman. There is a dense arcus lipoides, a central discoid opacity and pan-stromal opacities in both eyes (OD: **A**, **B**/OS: **C**). Penetrating keratoplasty was performed on the left eye (**D**) with a completely clear graft three years later

5.3.6 Pre-Descemet Corneal Dystrophies

The Pre-Descemet corneal dystrophies (PDCDs) include the Pre-Descemet corneal dystrophy (PDCD, Cornea farinata) and the punctiform and polychromatic pre-Descemet corneal dystrophy (PPPCD). While cornea farinata represents more a degenerative disease, PPPCD is caused by a mutation of the Peroxiredoxin 3 gene (*PRDX3*) on chromosome 10q26.11 [63]. Cornea farinata is characterized by fine and focal, polymorphic, gray opacities, which are located in the posterior corneal

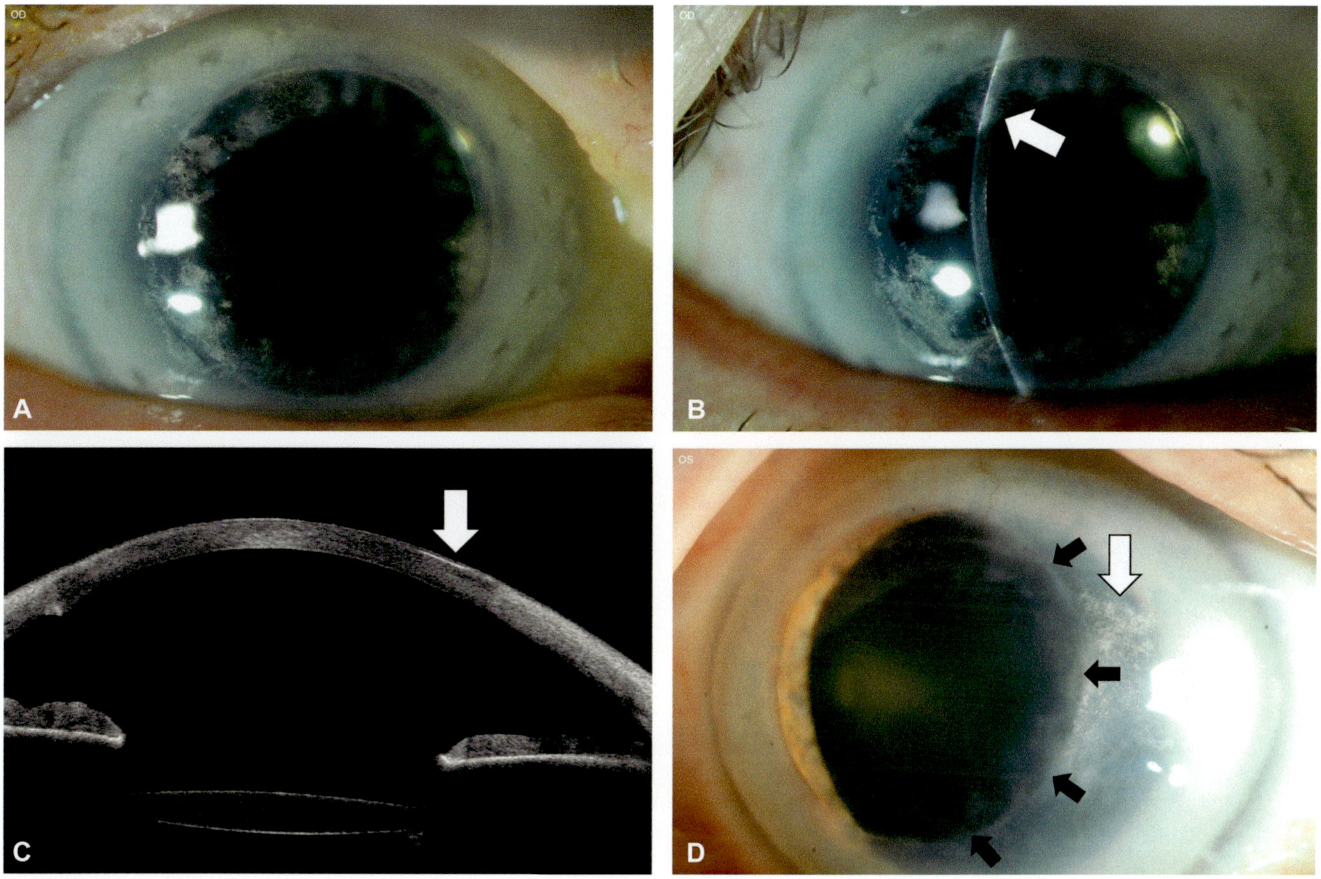

Fig. 70 Superficial recurrence with subepithelial crystalline deposits (arrows) at the graft periphery eight years after penetrating keratoplasty for Schnyder dystrophy ((**A**) overview, (**B**) thin slit illumination, (**C**) anterior segment optical coherence tomography). Another case (**D**) of subepithelial crystalline deposits (white arrow) at the graft–host junction (black arrows) 15 years after penetrating keratoplasty (small graft diameter and nasally decentered)

stroma immediately anterior to Descemet membrane. In contrast, the opacities in PPPCD (Fig. 76) are larger, polychromatic and more punctate than in cornea farinata. These changes not only emphasize the importance of genomic analysis today, but also highlight the

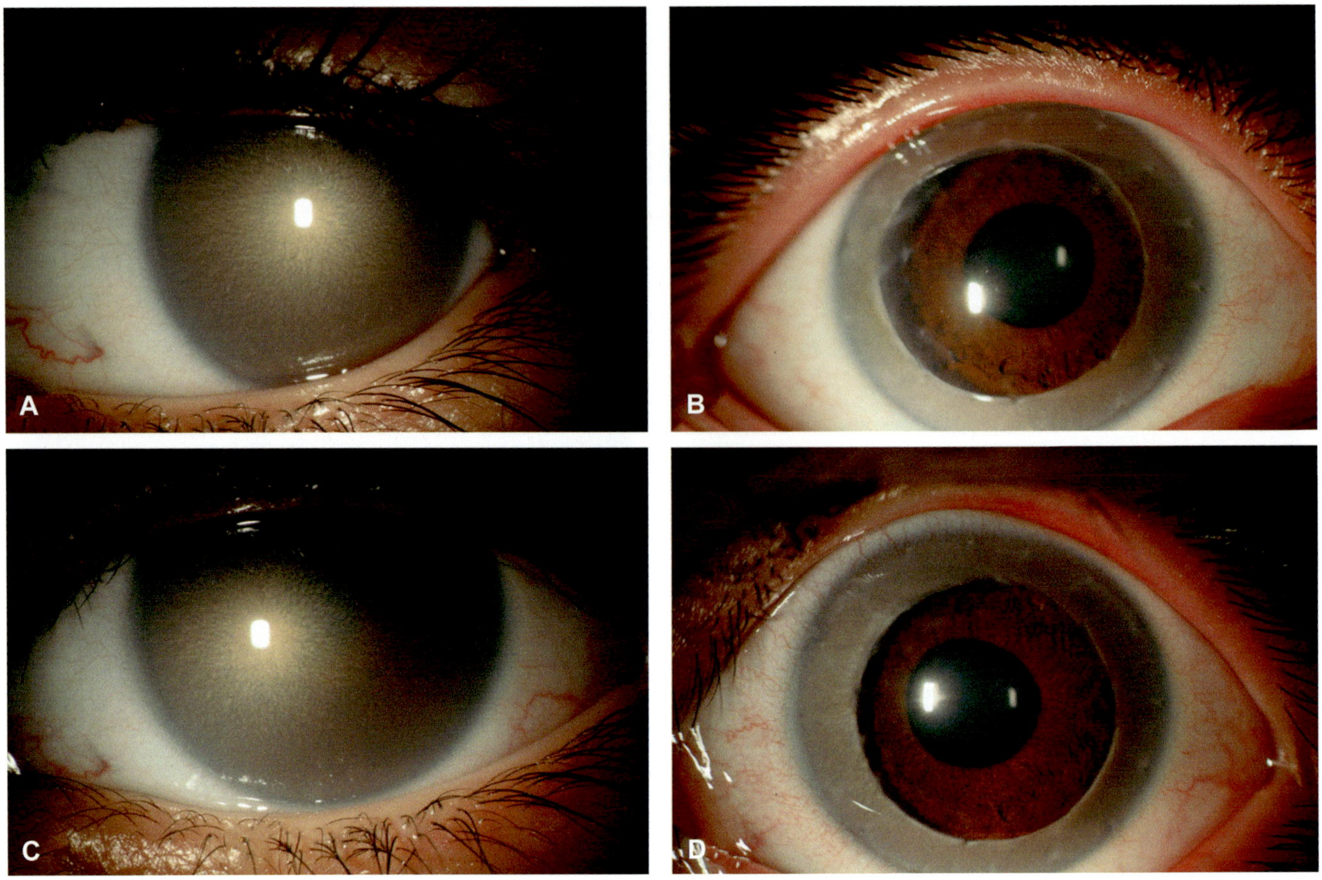

Fig. 71 Congenital stromal corneal dystrophy in a male child (OD: **A**/OS: **C**) with diffuse, grayish, snowflake-like opacity affecting the entire stroma and extending to the limbus. Following penetrating keratoplasty (OD: **B**/OS: **D**) at the age of 2½ and 3 years, the corneal graft is totally clear until 14 years postoperatively with a completely opacified host cornea

importance of updating the classification of CD at regular intervals [18].

5.4 Endothelial Dystrophies

5.4.1 Fuchs Endothelial Corneal Dystrophy

A detailed description of Fuchs endothelial corneal dystrophy (FECD) can be found in Chap. 18.

5.4.2 Posterior Polymorphous Corneal Dystrophy

Posterior polymorphous corneal dystrophy (PPCD) is divided into 3 subtypes (category 1). These include PPCD1 (20p11.2, Ovo-like zinc finger 2—*OVOL2*), PPCD3 (10p11.22, Zinc finger E-box-binding homeobox 1—*ZEB1*), and PPCD4 (8q22.3, Grainyhead-like transcription factor 2—*GRHL2*). In contrast to most dystrophies, PPCD is often asymmetric. Clinical findings vary widely in terms of Descemet membrane and endothelial

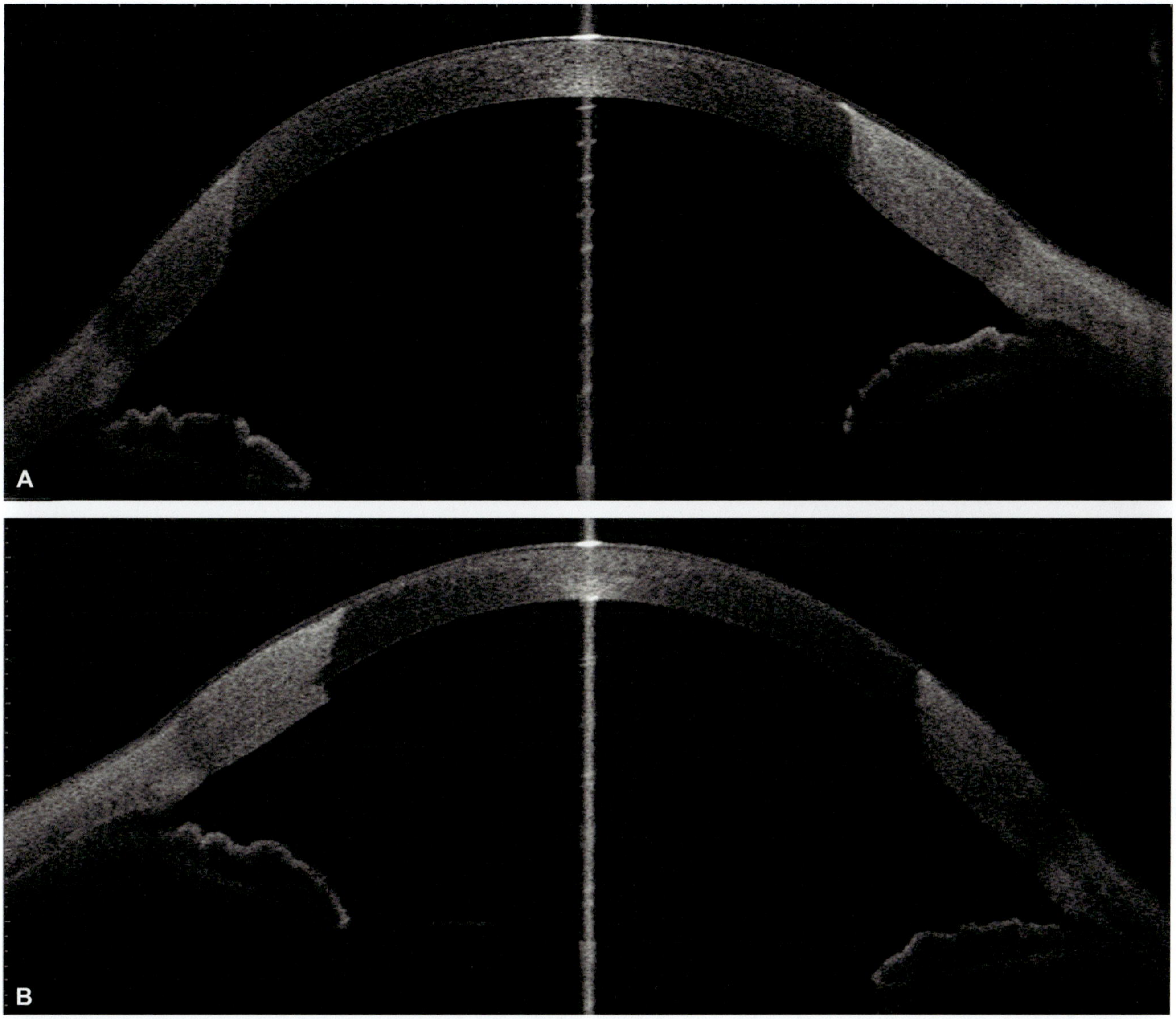

Fig. 72 Anterior segment optical coherence tomography in a 4-year-old male child after excimerlaser-assisted penetrating keratoplasty for congenital stromal corneal dystrophy (OD: **A**/OS: **B**). The host cornea demonstrates a pronounced hyperreflectivity affecting the entire cornea, while the corneal graft is completely normal. Note the straight laser incision edges of the graft–host junction. The clinical findings are provided in Fig. 71 (**B, D**)

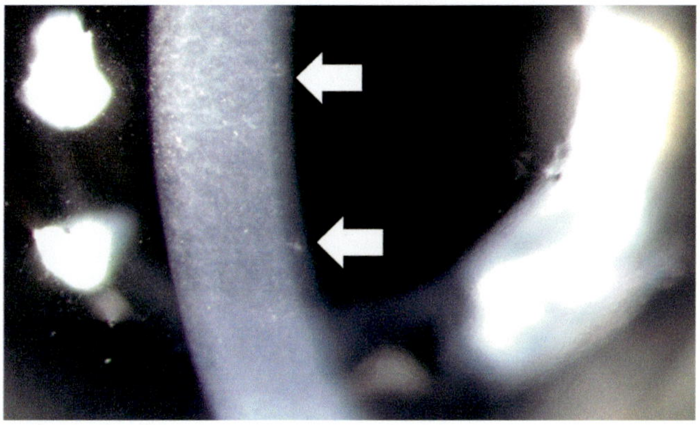

Fig. 73 Fleck corneal dystrophy in a 71-year-old woman. There are small, scattered opacities (arrows) in the otherwise clear corneal stroma

opacities, ranging from plaque-like lesions (Figs. 77, 78 and 79) to geographic gray opacities or vesicular changes (mostly in PPCD3, Figs. 80, 81, 82 and 83).

The vesicular lesions (Fig. 77) might be single or grouped and are often surrounded by gray circular opacities. Another characteristic sign are "railroad tracks" (Figs. 84, 85 and 86), which appear as parallel gray-white endothelial bands with white flaky material along the bands that may extend over the entire cornea. In advanced stages, especially in PPCD1, severe verrucous lesions of the posterior corneal surface may develop [64]. PPCD is usually asymptomatic, however, in case of endothelial

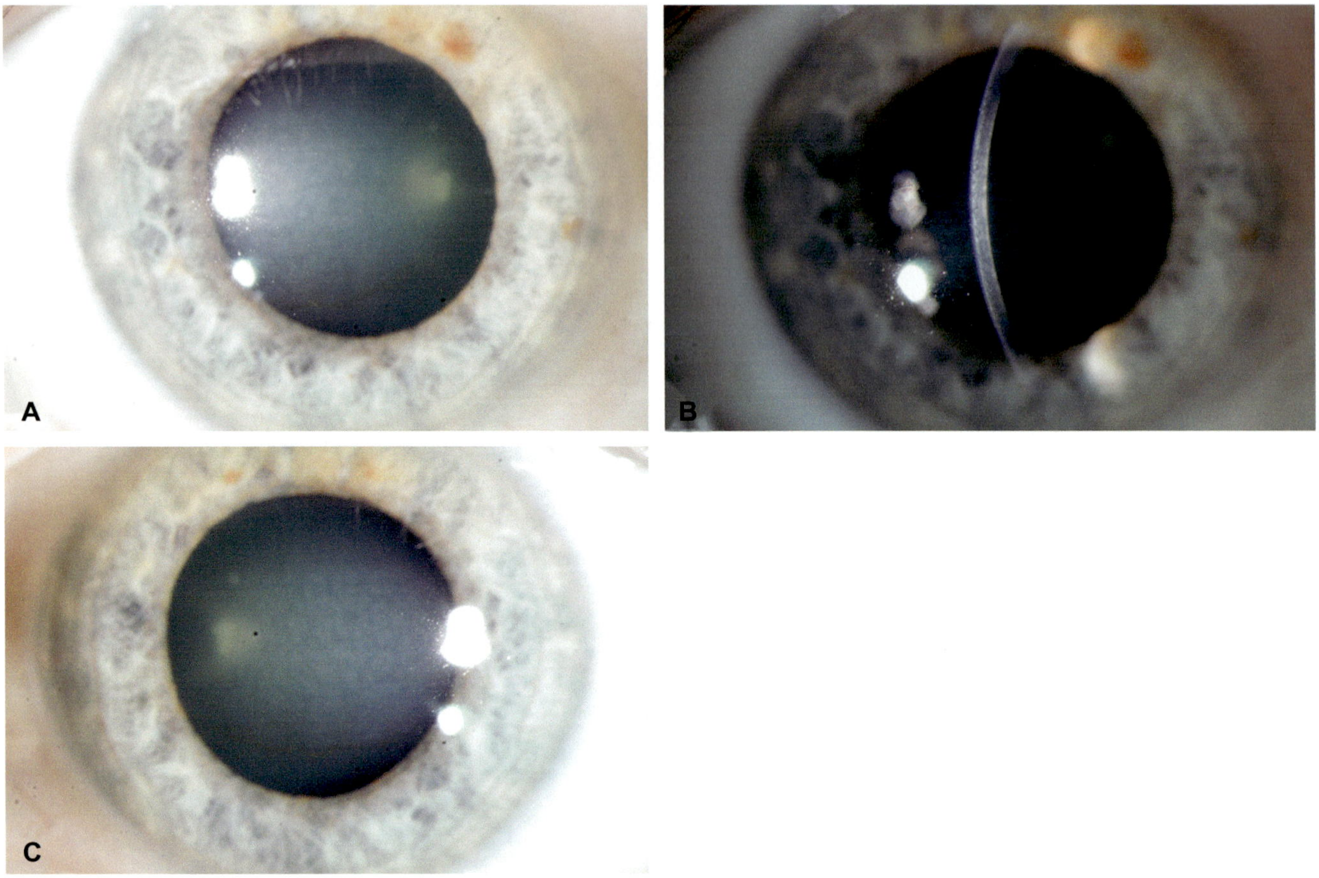

Fig. 74 Central cloudy dystrophy of François in a 71-year-old man demonstrating a polygonal cloudy gray-white stromal opacity, which is separated by linear areas of clear cornea (OD: **A**, **B**/OS: **C**)

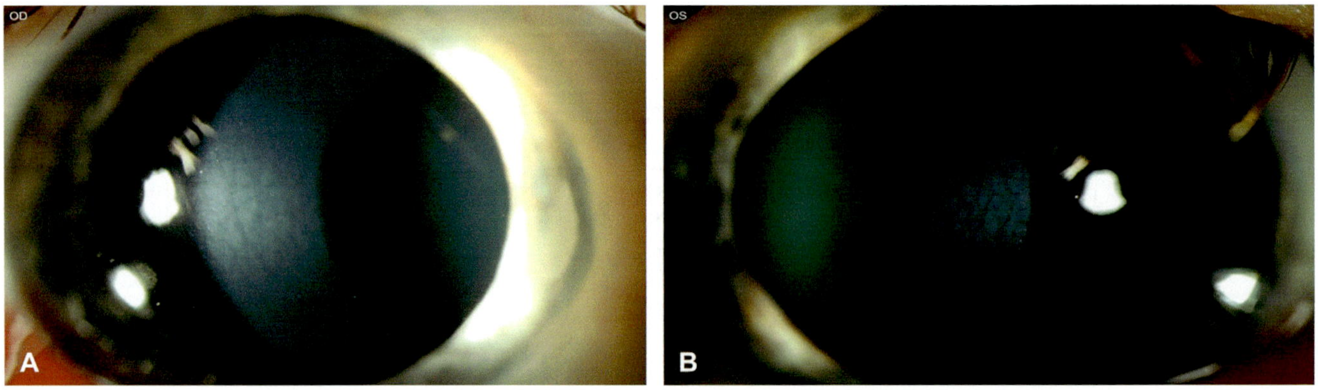

Fig. 75 Central cloudy dystrophy of François demonstrated by broad slit illumination (OD: **A**/OS: **B**)

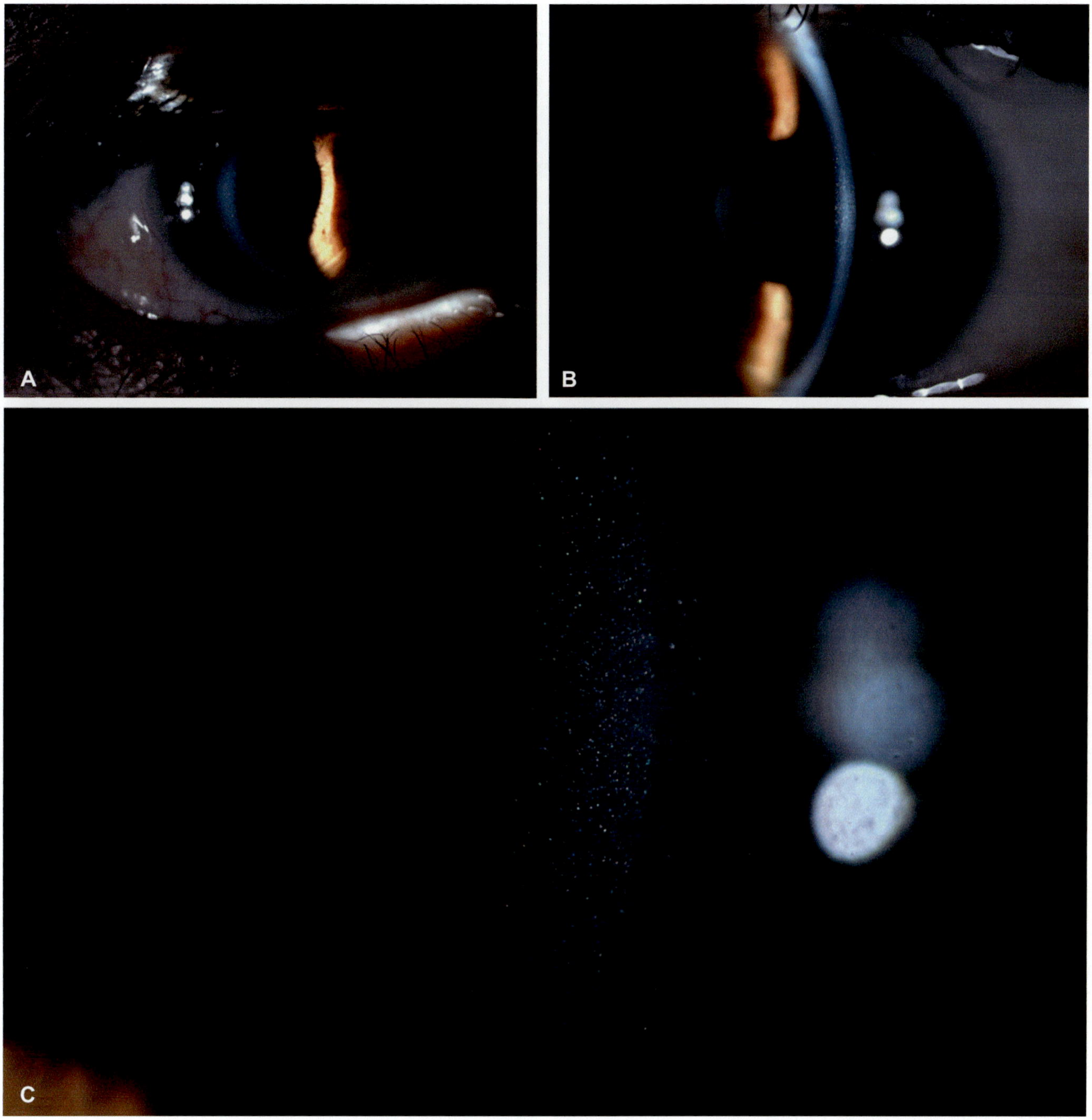

Fig. 76 Punctiform and polychromatic pre-Descemet corneal dystrophy with polychromatic crystalline deposits at the posterior corneal stroma, which are denser centrally (**A** overview, **B** thin slit, **C** magnification) (with permission of Dr. Pablo Martí Rodrigo, Barcelona)

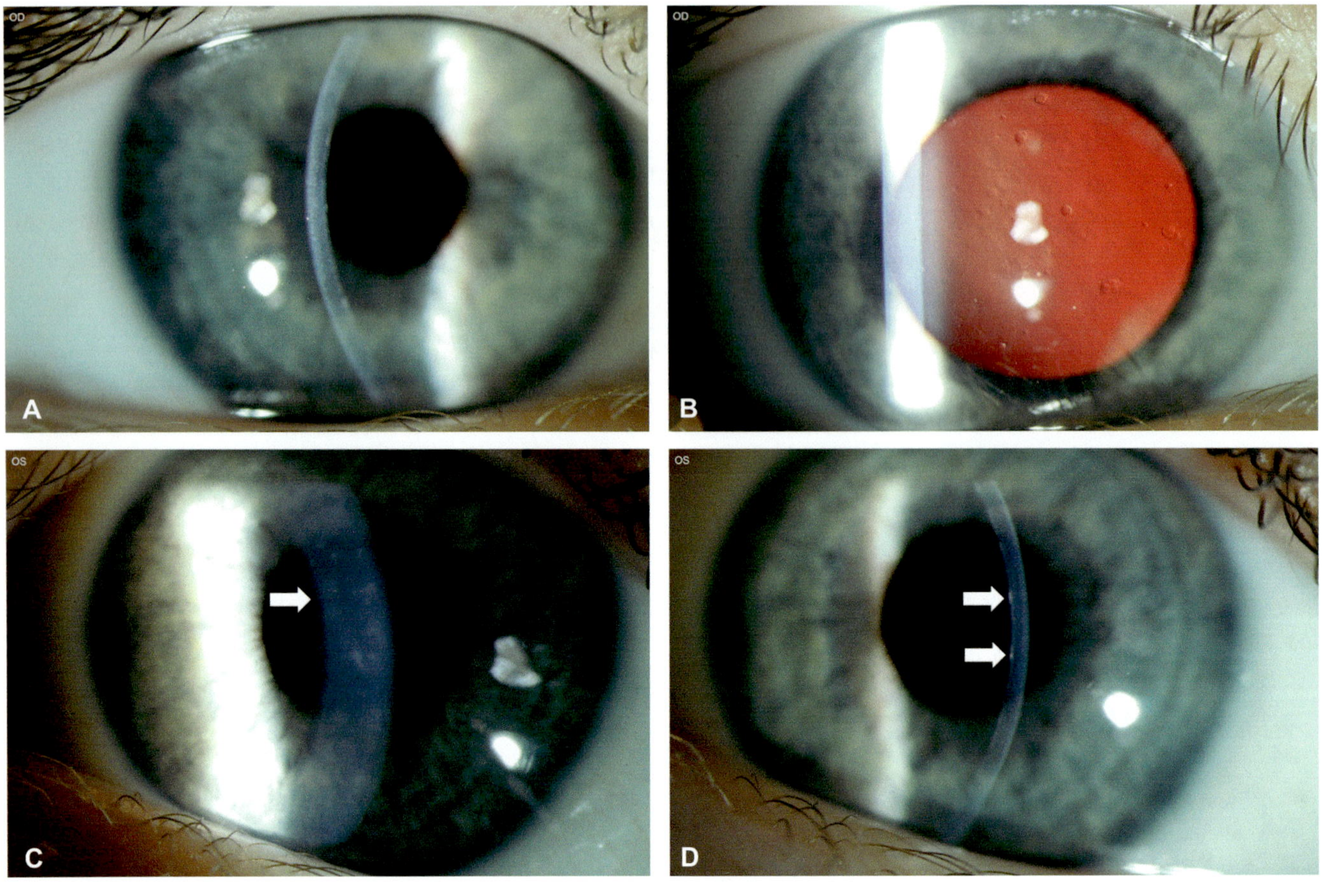

Fig. 77 Posterior polymorphous corneal dystrophy in a 4-year-old female child. The right eye (**A**, **B**) shows several vesicular lesions that are best recognized by retroillumination (**B**). The findings are more pronounced in the left eye (**C**, **D**, arrows) with multiple grayish opacities. Asymmetrical findings are frequently found in posterior polymorphous corneal dystrophy

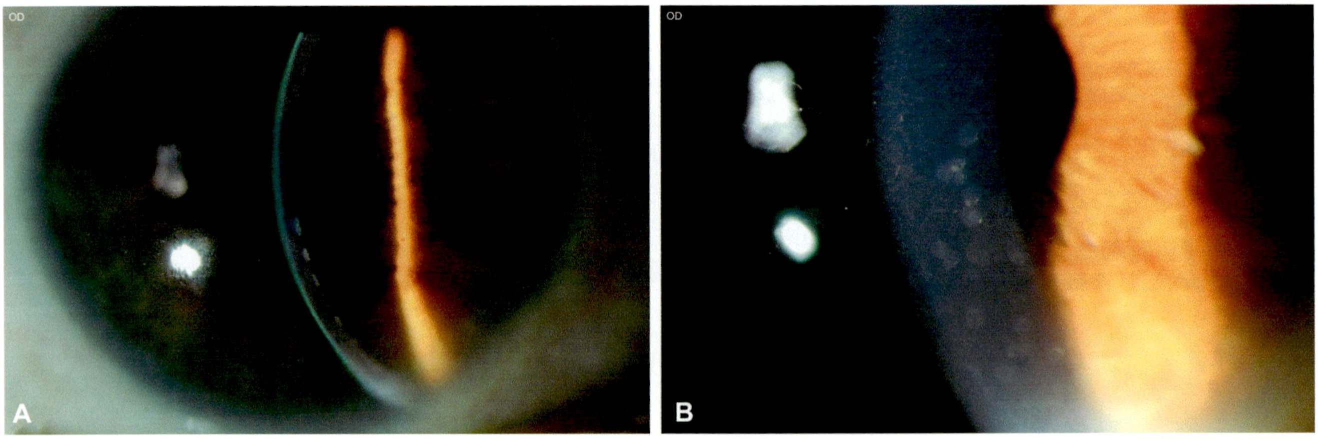

Fig. 78 Posterior polymorphous corneal dystrophy in a 31-year-old man with coin-like, barely prominent lesions of the posterior corneal surface ((**A**) thin slit illumination, (**B**) broad slit illumination)

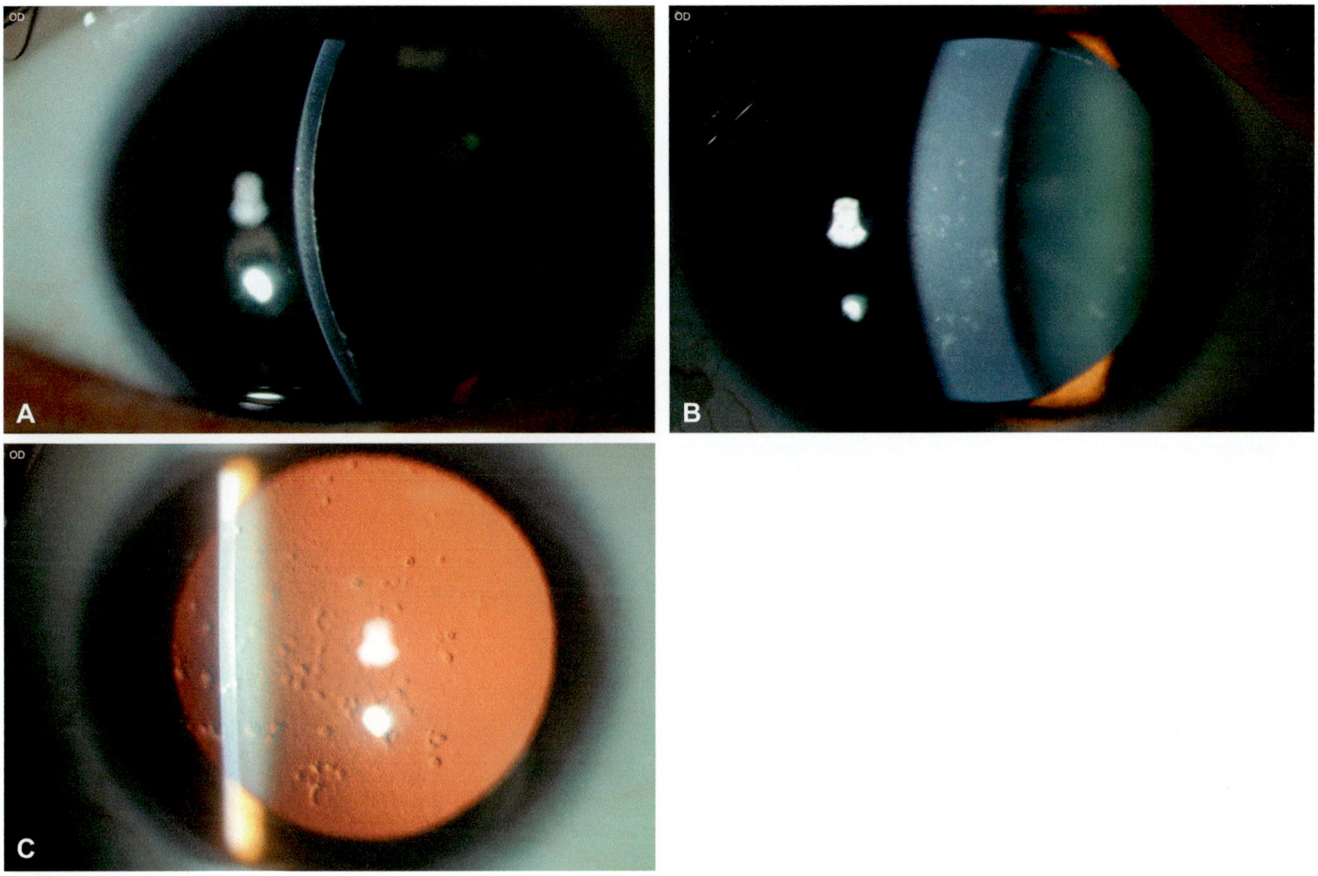

Fig. 79 Posterior polymorphous corneal dystrophy in a 41-year-old man. There are multiple flaky, gray opacities on the posterior corneal surface, which are slightly prominent (**A**, **B**). Retroillumination (**C**) demonstrates a diffuse distribution

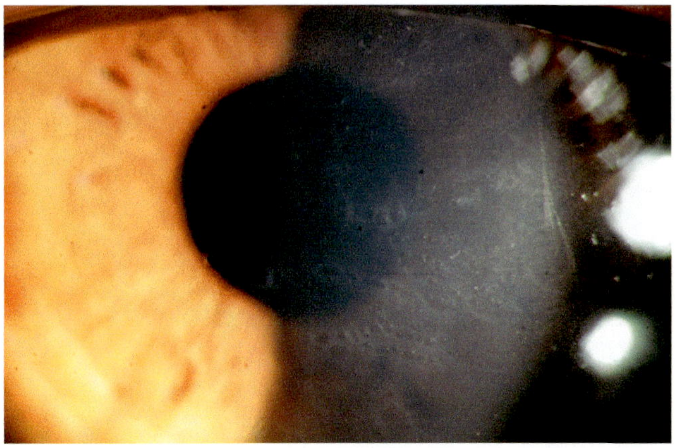

Fig. 80 Posterior polymorphous corneal dystrophy in a 24-year-old woman with vesicular lesions arranged in a pearl-chain pattern

decompensation (20–25%, Fig. 87) it is associated with vision loss and pain. One third of all eyes may develop secondary glaucoma.

5.4.3 Congenital Hereditary Endothelial Dystrophy

Congenital hereditary endothelial dystrophy (CHED) is an autosomal recessive (20p13, Solute carrier family 4, sodium borate transporter, member 11—*SLC4A11*) endothelial dystrophy (category 1).

It is mostly bilateral, but often asymmetric. The cornea is characterized by corneal clouding ranging from diffuse haze to ground-glass, milky appearance resulting from a primary endothelial dysfunction (Figs. 88, 89, 90 and 91). The corneal stroma is severely thickened (2–3 times thicker

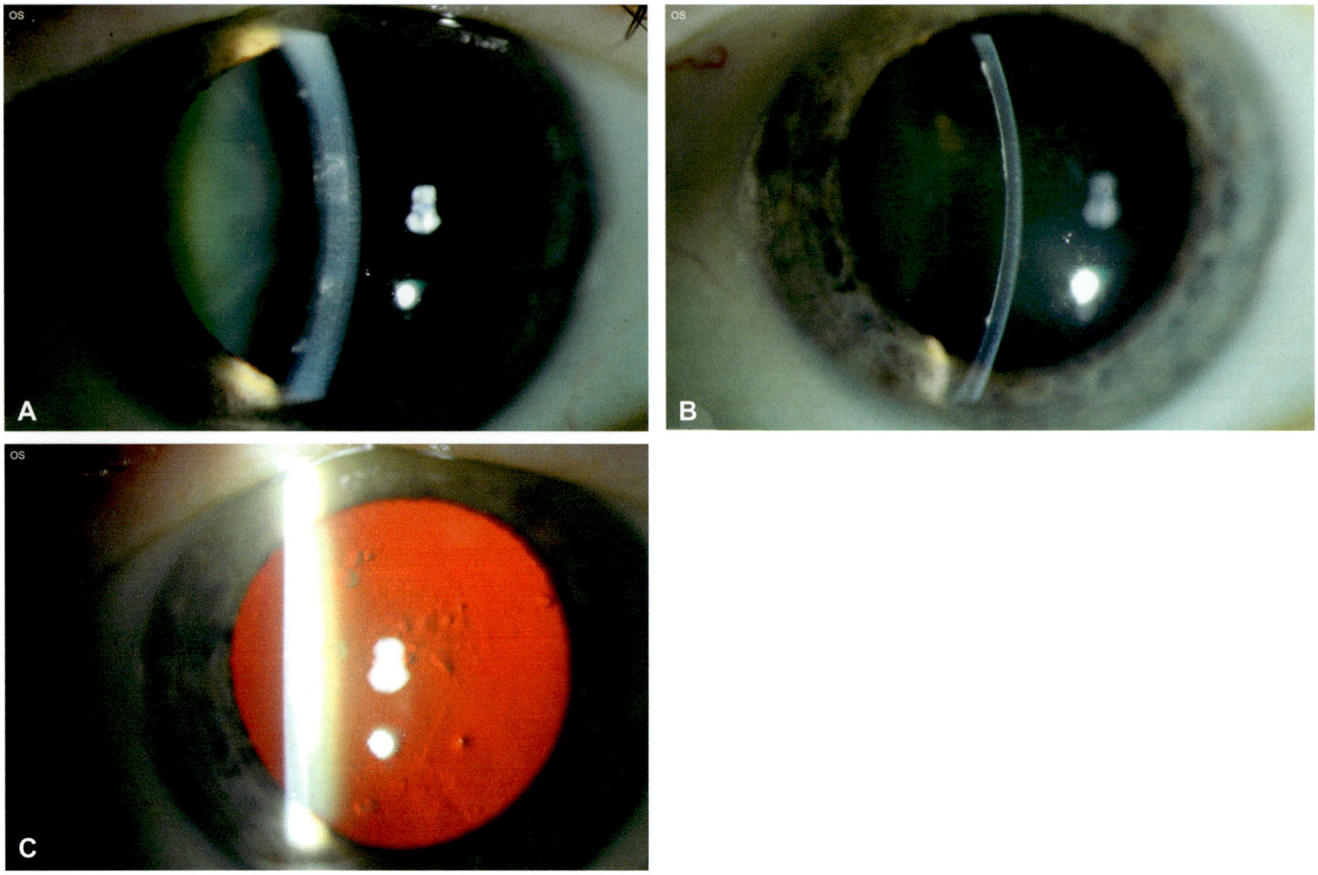

Fig. 81 Posterior polymorphous corneal dystrophy with grayish opacities and verrucous lesions at the level of Descemet membrane and endothelium in a 69-year-old woman

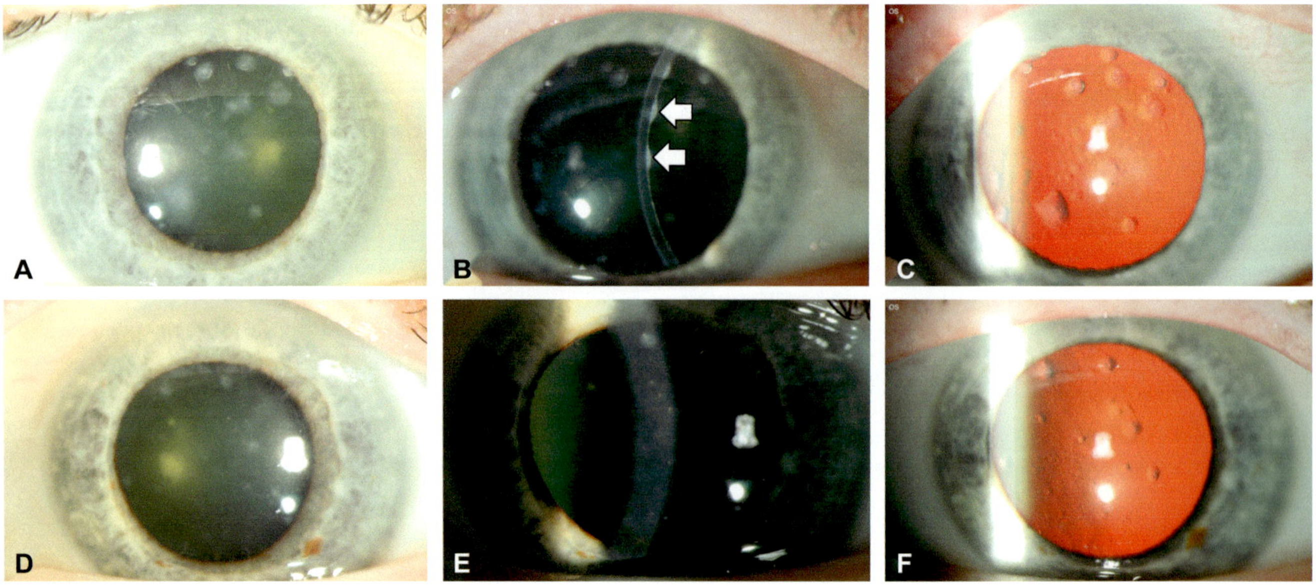

Fig. 82 Posterior polymorphous corneal dystrophy (type 1) in a 62-year-old woman with severe verrucous lesions (arrows) in both eyes (OD: **A**–**C**/OS: **D**–**F**). The thin slit image (**B**) demonstrates the prominent verrucous lesions of the posterior corneal surface

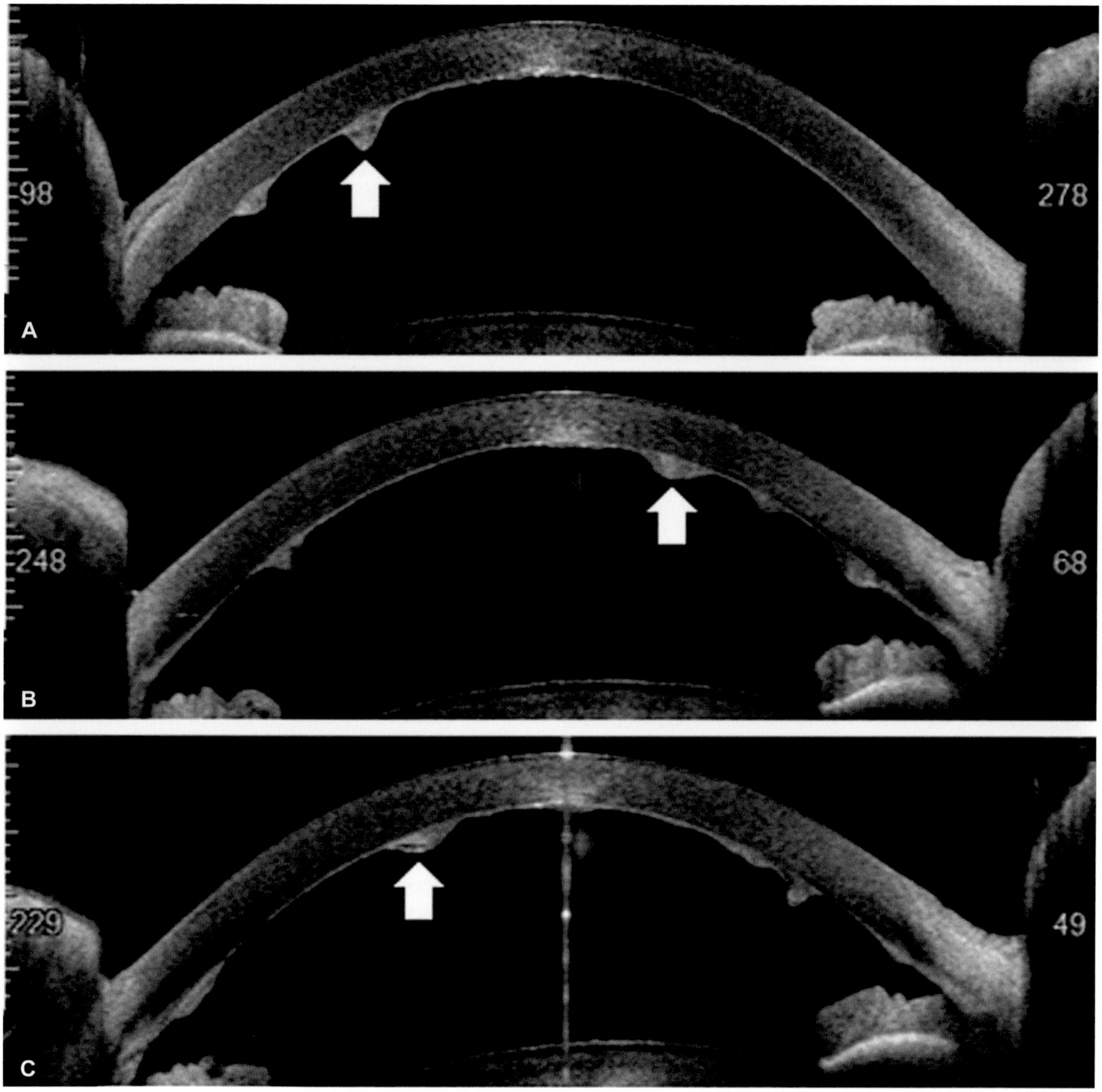

Fig. 83 Anterior segment optical coherence tomography in posterior polymorphous corneal dystrophy with prominent vesicular lesions of the posterior corneal surface (arrows) in different sections. The clinical findings are provided in Fig. 81

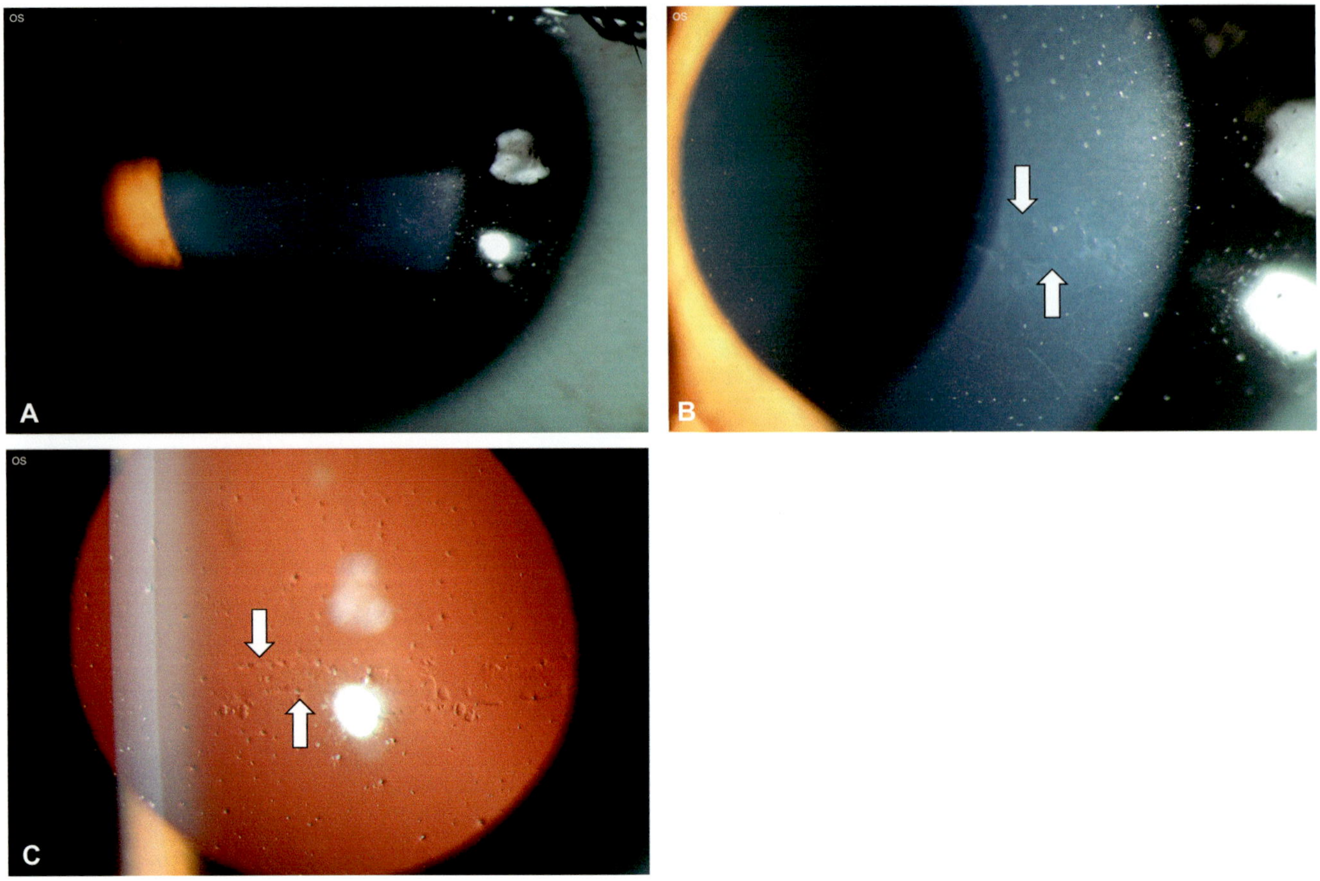

Fig. 84 Posterior polymorphous corneal dystrophy with railroad tracks (arrows) in a 13-year-old female child ((**A**) overview, (**B**) broad slit illumination, (**C**) retroillumination)

than a normal cornea) but with minimal epithelial edema. Corneal edema leads to blurred vision, whereas tearing or photophobia are rare.

5.4.4 X-linked Endothelial Corneal Dystrophy

X-linked endothelial corneal dystrophy (XECD) is a rare endothelial CD inherited in an X-linked dominant manner (Xq25, category 2). To date, this CD has only been described in one large Austrian family in 2006 (Figs. 92 and 93) [65]. Since then, no further families have been described worldwide.

The clinical signs of XECD differ between male and female carriers:

Male Carriers

1. Diffuse corneal opacities (ranging from corneal haze to milky appearance) because of severe moon crater endothelial changes of the cornea
2. Secondary band-shaped corneal degeneration combined with moon crater endothelial changes

Female Carriers

1. Only moon crater endothelial changes with variable presentation. To date, no decompensation of the cornea has been observed

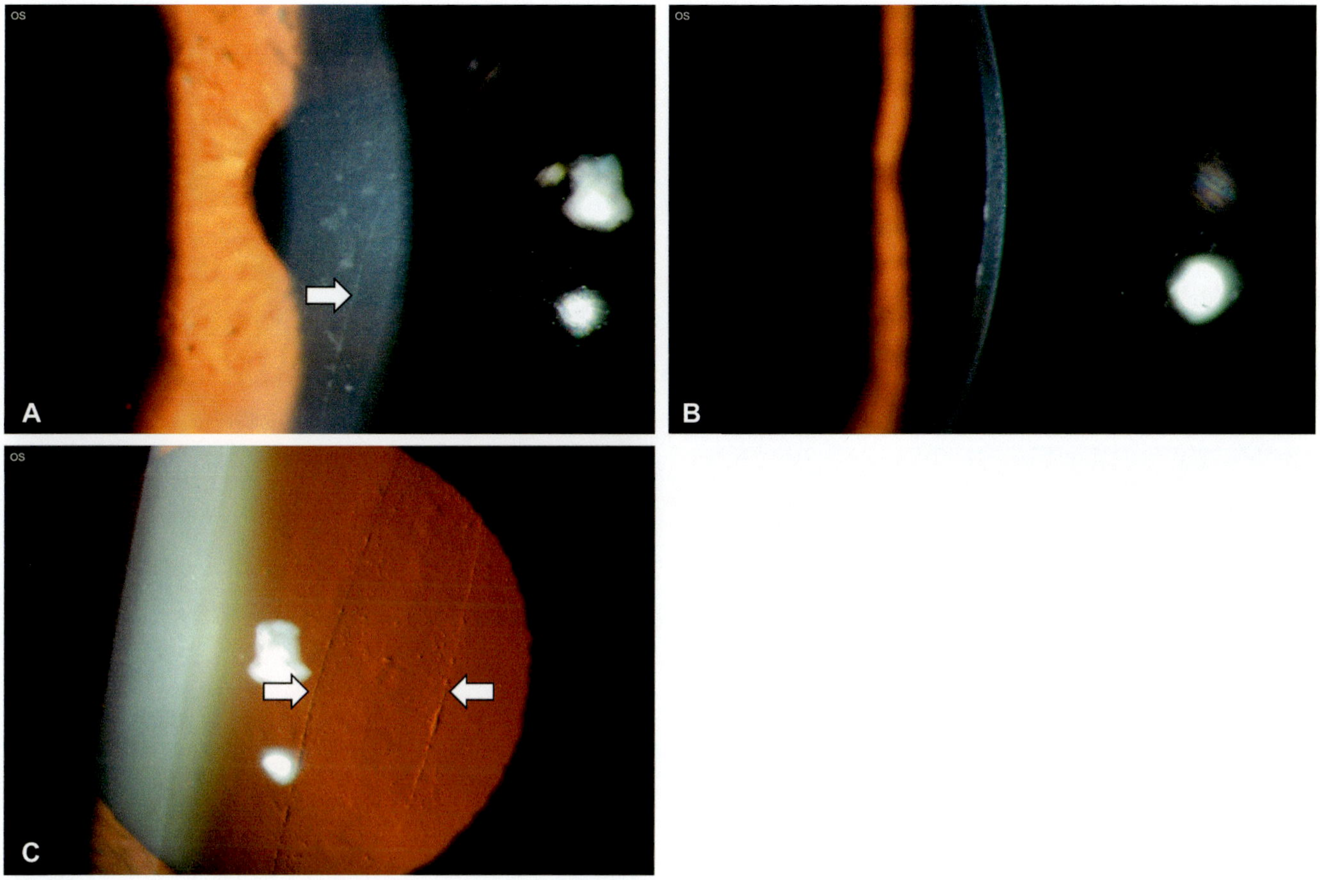

Fig. 85 Posterior polymorphous corneal dystrophy demonstrating vertical railroad tracks (arrows) with flake-like material along the bands in a 63-year-old man ((**A**) broad slit illumination, (**B**) thin slit illumination, (**C**) retroillumination)

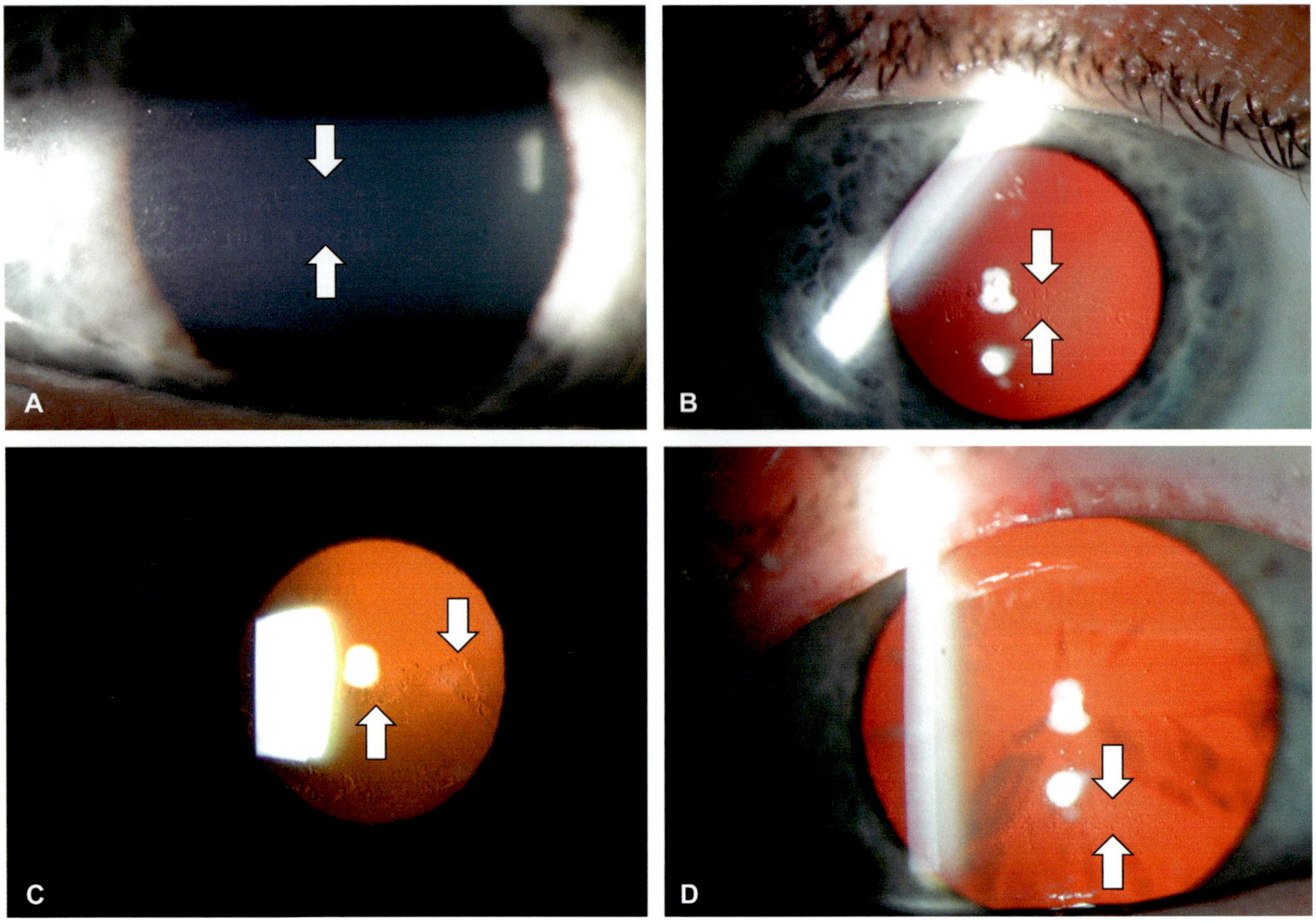

Fig. 86 Posterior polymorphous corneal dystrophy demonstrating parallel gray-white endothelial bands (so called "railroad tracks") in three individuals ((**A**), (**B**) direct illumination with corresponding retroillumation, (**C**) two horizonal railroad tracks, (**D**) railroad tracks in the lower part of the cornea)

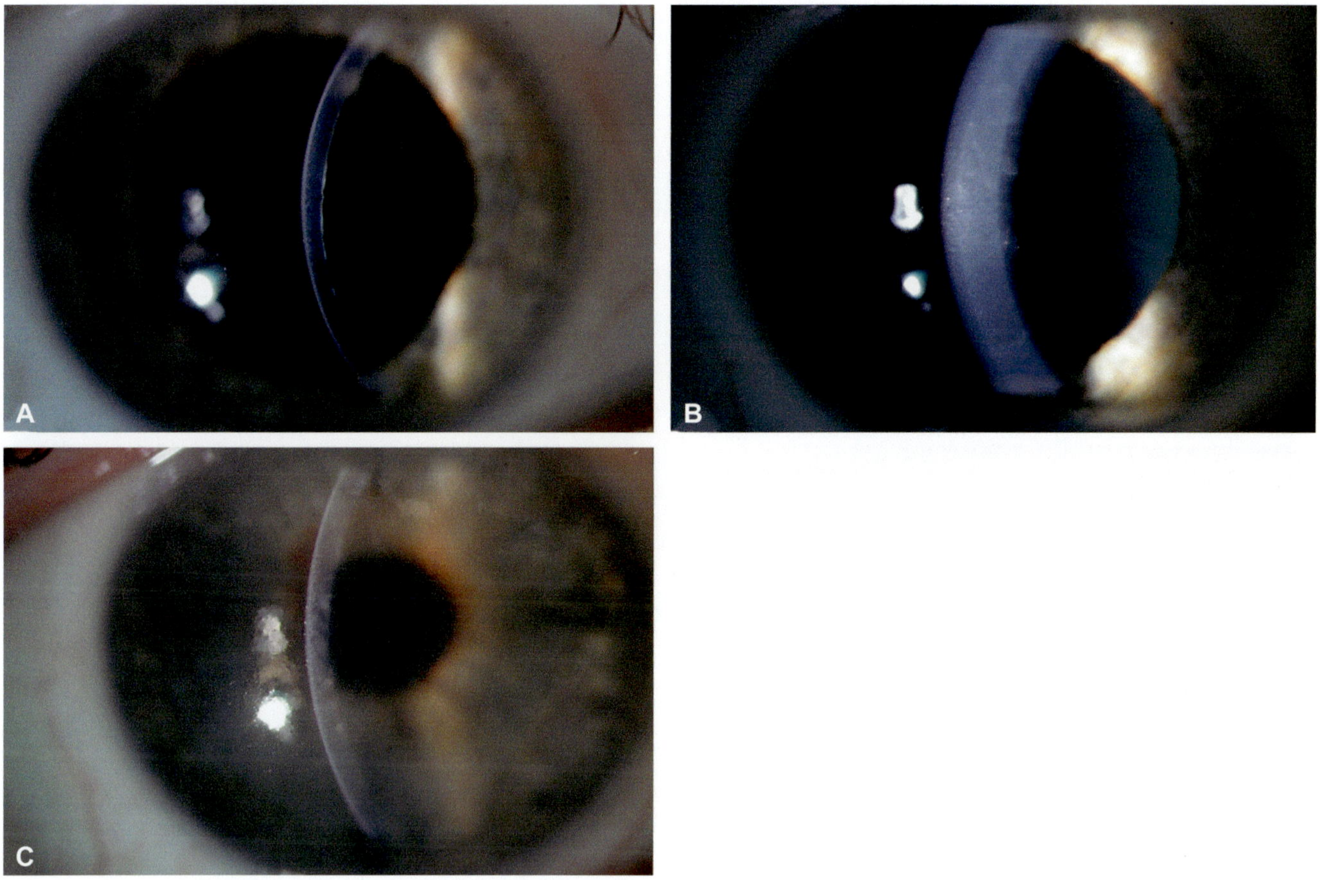

Fig. 87 Posterior polymorphous corneal dystrophy with development of endothelial decompensation. Shown are the findings of a 42-year-old man with posterior grayish changes and few Descemet folds ((**A**) thin slit illumination, (**B**) broad slit illumination). Two months later ((**C**) thin slit illumination), there is progressive endothelial decompensation with epithelial edema and increasing Descemet folds (details of the iris become blurred), requiring Descemet membrane endothelial keratoplasty (DMEK)

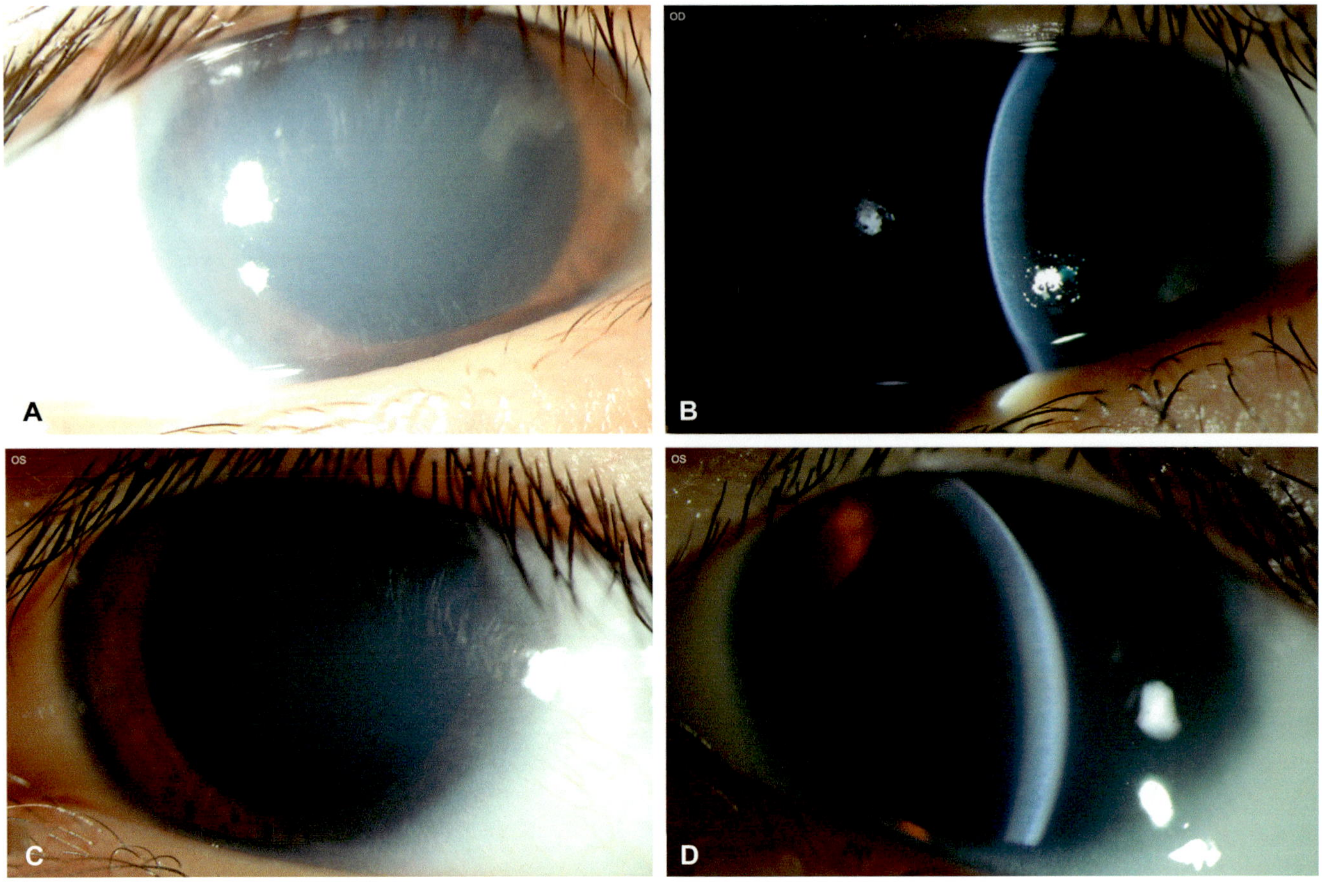

Fig. 88 Congenital hereditary endothelial dystrophy demonstrating thickened, hazy corneas in a 4-year-old male child (OD: **A**, **B**/OS: **C**, **D**)

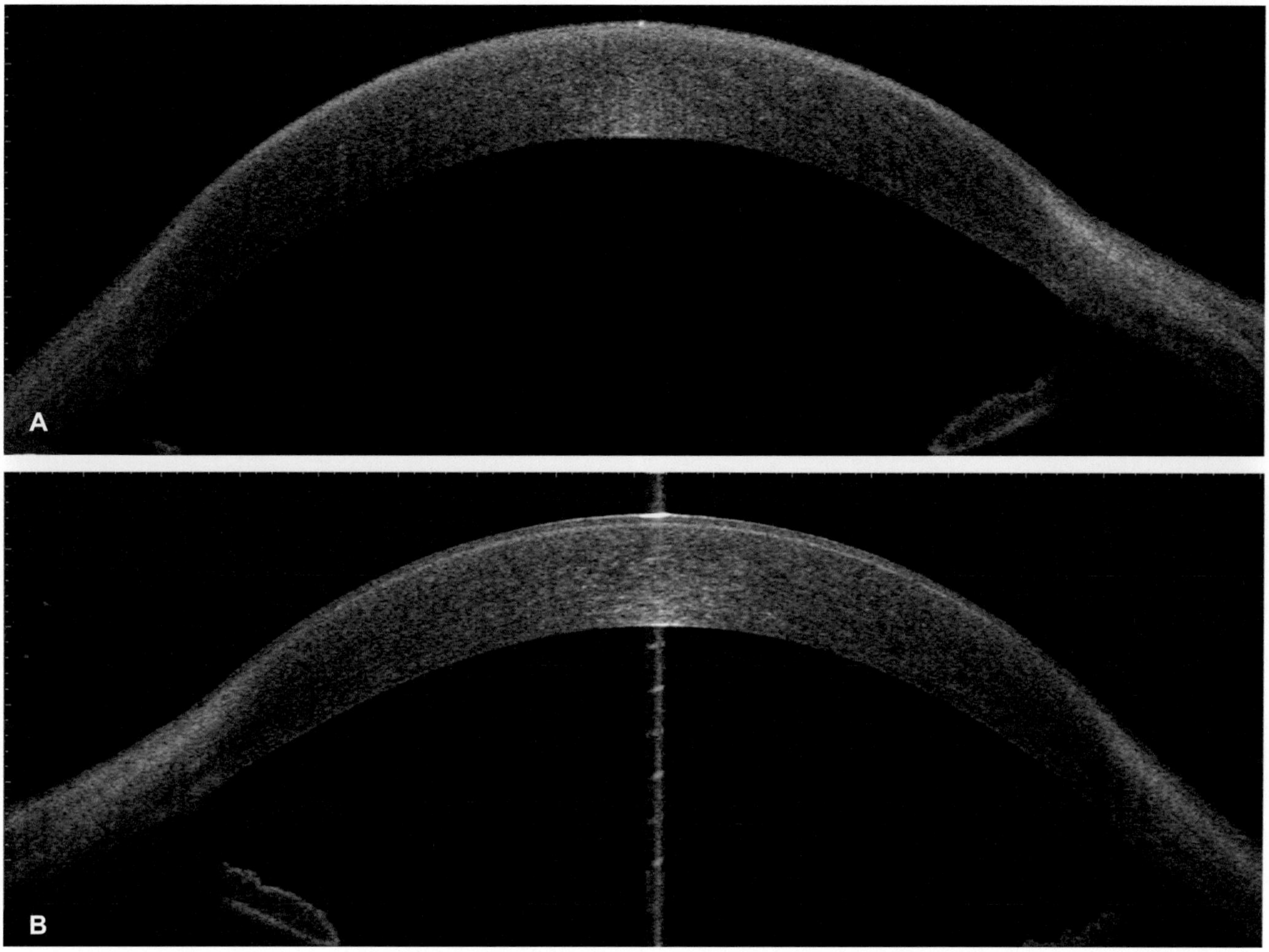

Fig. 89 Anterior segment optical coherence tomography in congenital hereditary endothelial dystrophy showing diffuse thickened corneas in a 4-year-old male child (OD: **A**/OS: **B**). The clinical findings are provided in Fig. 88

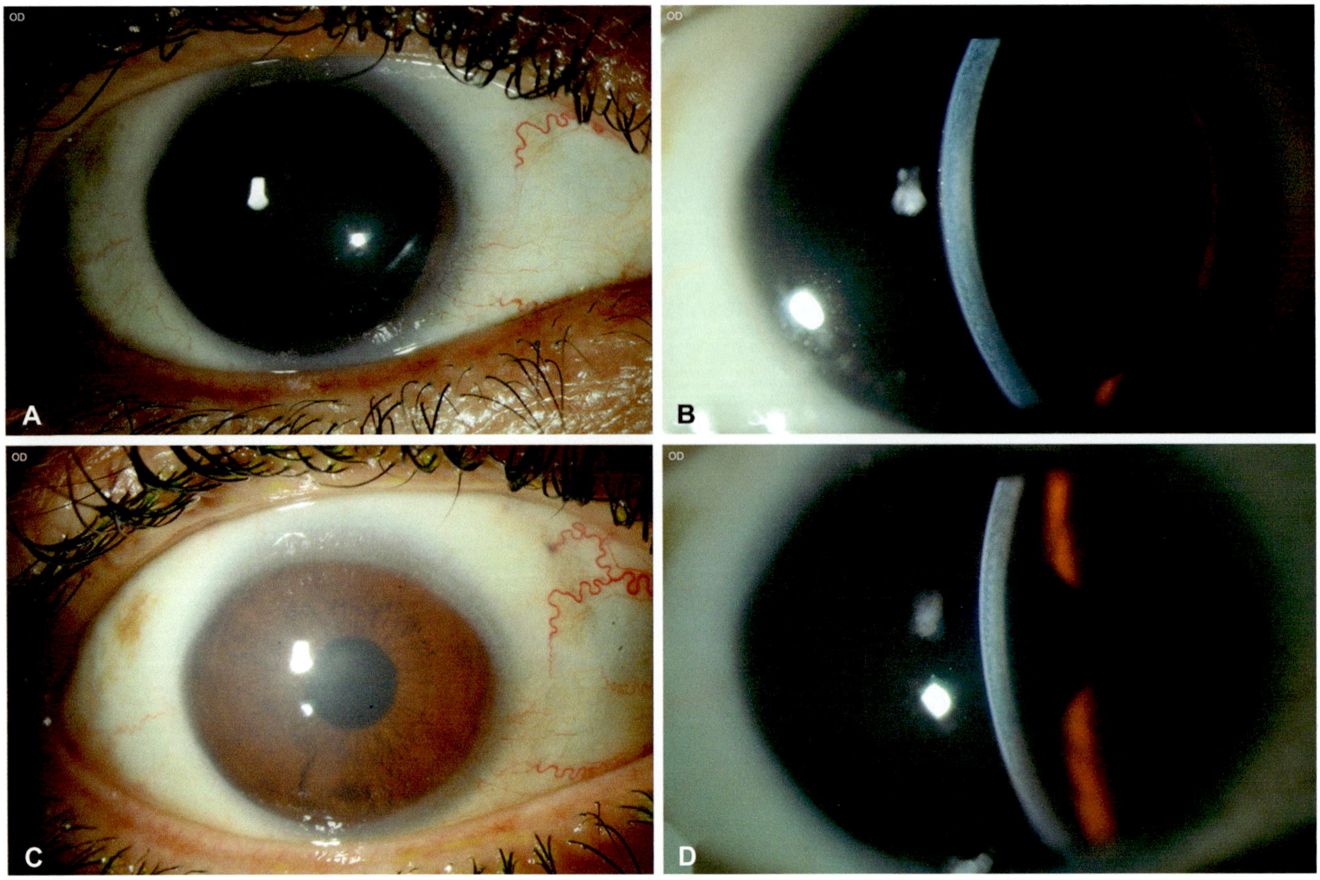

Fig. 90 Congenital hereditary endothelial dystrophy demonstrating a thickened, hazy cornea of the right eye in a 38-year-old man ((**A**) overview, (**B**) thin slit illumination). (**C, D**) The bottom row shows relatively stable clinical findings after 7 years without surgical intervention

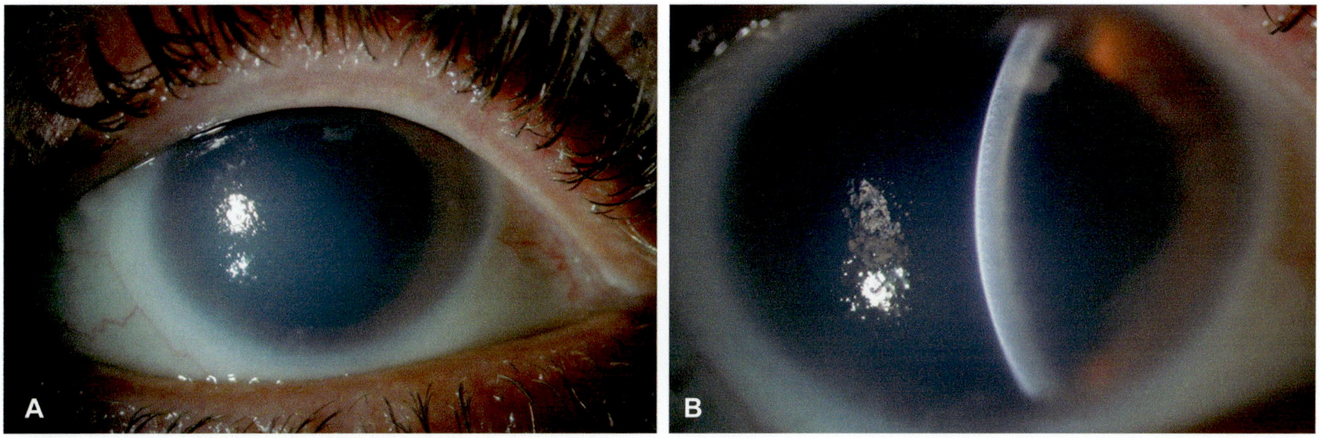

Fig. 91 Congenital hereditary endothelial dystrophy demonstrating a severely thickened, milky cornea in a 40-year-old man ((**A**) overview, (**B**) thin slit illumination)

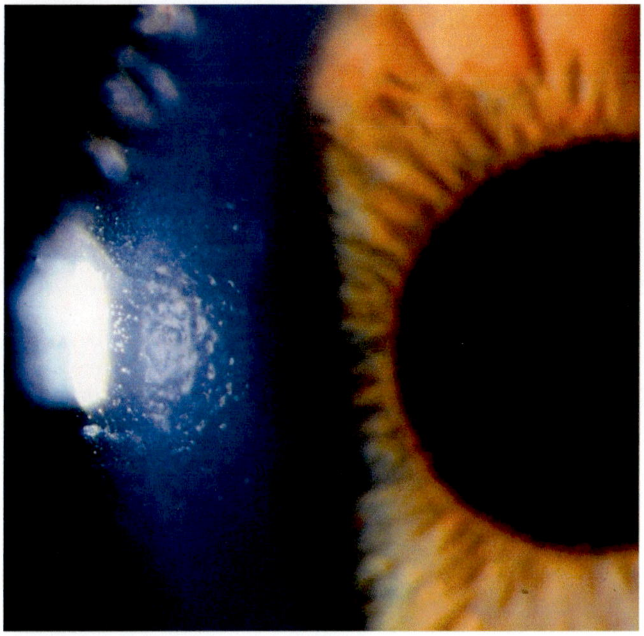

Fig. 92 X-linked endothelial corneal dystrophy with moon crater-like endothelial changes visualized by direct illumination

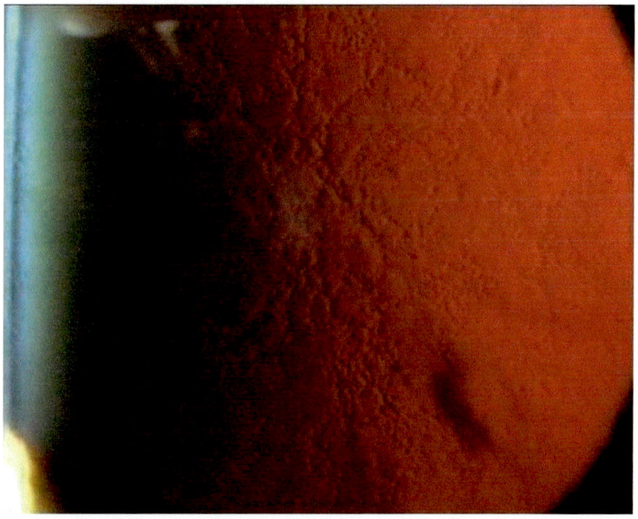

Fig. 93 X-linked endothelial corneal dystrophy with moon crater-like endothelial changes visualized by indirect illumination

6 Conclusion

CDs are inherited deposits of various materials restricted to the cornea with a typical morphology. These diseases are mostly bilateral, sometimes asymmetrical, progress slowly without primary signs of inflammation or exogenous causes. In their third edition, the International Committee on the Classification of Corneal Dystrophies (IC3D) lists 22 entities which are updated on a regular basis. These entities are characterized by 4 categories (from 1 = well defined disease entity with known gene to 4 = poorly defined disease entity with unknown gene locus). If necessary, corneal dystrophies can be very well treated with excimer PTK, anterior lamellar, posterior lamellar or penetrating keratoplasty. Recurrences are to be expected after treatment.

References

1. Lisch W, Seitz B. New international classification of corneal dystrophies and clinical landmarks. Klin Monbl Augenheilkd. 2008;225:616–22. https://doi.org/10.1055/s-2008-1027552.
2. Lisch W, Seitz B. New international classification of corneal dystrophies. Ophthalmologie. 2011;108:883–97. https://doi.org/10.1007/s00347-011-2388-8.
3. Lisch W, Weiss JS. Clinical and genetic update of corneal dystrophies. Exp Eye Res. 2019;186:107715. https://doi.org/10.1016/j.exer.2019.107715.
4. Bramsen T, Ehlers N, Baggesen LH. Central cloudy corneal dystrophy of François. Acta Ophthalmol. 1976;54:221–6. https://doi.org/10.1111/j.1755-3768.1976.tb00435.x.
5. François J. A new heredofamilial dystrophy of the cornea. J Genet Hum. 1956;5:189–96.
6. Strachan IM. Cloudy central corneal dystrophy of Francois. Five cases in the same family. Br J Ophthalmol. 1969;53:192–4. https://doi.org/10.1136/bjo.53.3.192.
7. Brownstein S, Jackson WB, Onerheim RM. Schnyder's crystalline corneal dystrophy in association with hyperlipoproteinemia: histopathological and ultrastructural findings. Can J Ophthalmol. 1991;26:273–9.
8. Lisch W, Seitz B. Masquerade keratitis due to hereditary corneal disorders. Klin Monbl Augenheilkd. 2011;228:504–8. https://doi.org/10.1055/s-0031-1273344.
9. Lisch W, Seitz B. The clinical landmarks of corneal dystrophies. Dev Ophthalmol. 2011;48:9–23. https://doi.org/10.1159/000324075.
10. Lisch W, Weiss JS. Early and late clinical landmarks of corneal dystrophies. Exp Eye Res. 2020;198:108139. https://doi.org/10.1016/j.exer.2020.108139.
11. Berger T, Flockerzi E, Daas L, Hamon L, Khattabi Z, Berger M, Seitz B. Modern corneal diagnostics as the key for the correct classification of the disease and optimal treatment decisions. Ophthalmologie. 2023;120:1238–50. https://doi.org/10.1007/s00347-023-01919-0.
12. Carrwik C, Stenevi U. Lattice corneal dystrophy, gelsolin type (Meretoja's syndrome). Acta Ophthalmol. 2009;87:813–9. https://doi.org/10.1111/j.1755-3768.2009.01686.x.
13. Mattila JS, Krootila K, Kivelä T, Holopainen JM. Penetrating keratoplasty for corneal amyloidosis in familial amyloidosis, finnish type. Ophthalmology. 2015;122:457–63. https://doi.org/10.1016/j.ophtha.2014.09.035.
14. Weiss JS, Willoughby CE, Abad-Morales V, Turunen JA, Lisch W. Update on the corneal dystrophies—genetic testing and therapy. Cornea. 2022;41:1337–44. https://doi.org/10.1097/ICO.0000000000002857.
15. Weiss J, Møller H, Lisch W, Kinoshita S, Aldave AJ, Belin MW, Kivelä T, Busin M, Munier FL, Seitz B, Sutphin J, Bredrup C, Mannis MJ, Rapuano C, Van Rij G, Kim EK, Klintworth GK. The IC3D classification of the corneal dystrophies. Klin Monbl Augenheilkd. 2011;228:S1–39. https://doi.org/10.1055/s-0029-1245895.
16. Weiss JS, Møller HU, Lisch W, Kinoshita S, Aldave AJ, Belin MW, Kivelä T, Busin M, Munier FL, Seitz B, Sutphin J, Bredrup C, Mannis MJ, Rapuano CJ, Van Rij G, Kim EK, Klintworth GK. The IC3D classification of the corneal dystrophies. Cornea. 2008;27:S1–42. https://doi.org/10.1097/ico.0b013e31817780fb.
17. Seitz B, Lisch W. Stage-related therapy of corneal dystrophies. Dev Ophthalmol. 2011;48:116–53. https://doi.org/10.1159/000324081.
18. Weiss JS, Rapuano CJ, Seitz B, Busin M, Kivelä TT, Bouheraoua N, Bredrup C, Nischal KK, Chawla H, Borderie V, Kenyon KR, Kim EK, Møller HU, Munier FL, Berger T, Lisch W. IC3D classification of corneal dystrophies-edition 3. Cornea. 2024;43:466–527. https://doi.org/10.1097/ICO.0000000000003420.
19. Szentmáry N, Seitz B, Langenbucher A, Schlötzer-Schrehardt U, Hofmann-Rummelt C, Naumann GO. Histologic and ultrastructural changes in corneas with granular and macular dystrophy after excimer laser phototherapeutic keratectomy. Cornea. 2006;25:257–63. https://doi.org/10.1097/01.ico.0000176603.87376.d8.
20. Kim TI, Pak JH, Chae JB, Kim EK, Tchah H. Mitomycin C inhibits recurrent Avellino dystrophy after phototherapeutic keratectomy. Cornea. 2006;25:220–3. https://doi.org/10.1097/01.ico.0000164830.79970.71.
21. Daas L, Hamon L, Ardjomand N, Safi T, Seitz B. Excimer laser-assisted DALK: a case report from the Homburg Keratoconus Center (HKC). Ophthalmologe. 2021;118:1245–48. https://doi.org/10.1007/s00347-021-01342-3.
22. Seitz B, Langenbucher A, Kus MM, Küchle M, Naumann GOH. Nonmechanical corneal trephination with the excimer laser improves outcome after penetrating keratoplasty. Ophthalmology. 1999;106:1156–65. https://doi.org/10.1016/S0161-6420(99)90265-8.
23. Marcon AS, Cohen EJ, Rapuano CJ, Laibson PR. Recurrence of corneal stromal dystrophies after penetrating keratoplasty. Cornea. 2003;22:19–21. https://doi.org/10.1097/00003226-200301000-00005.
24. Bischoff-Jung M, Flockerzi E, Hasenfus A, Viestenz A, Matoula P, Schlötzer-Schrehardt U, Seitz B. Recurrence of macular corneal dystrophy on the graft 50 years after penetrating keratoplasty. GMS Ophthalmol Cases. 2020;10:Doc34. https://doi.org/10.3205/oc000161.
25. Das S, Langenbucher A, Seitz B. Delayed healing of corneal epithelium after phototherapeutic keratectomy for lattice dystrophy. Cornea. 2005;24:283–7. https://doi.org/10.1097/01.ico.0000138853.26332.55.
26. Flockerzi E, Turner C, Seitz B, Collaborators GSG, GeKeR Study Group. Descemet's membrane endothelial keratoplasty is the predominant keratoplasty procedure in Germany since 2016: a report of the DOG-section cornea and its keratoplasty registry. Br J Ophthalmol. 2024;108:646–53 https://doi.org/10.1136/bjo-2022-323162.
27. Seitz B, Lisch W, Weiss J. The revised newest IC3D classification of corneal dystrophies. Klin Monbl Augenheilkd. 2015;232:283–94. https://doi.org/10.1055/s-0041-100774.

28. Weiss JS, Møller HU, Aldave AJ, Seitz B, Bredrup C, Kivelä T, Munier FL, Rapuano CJ, Nischal KK, Kim EK, Sutphin J, Busin M, Labbé A, Kenyon KR, Kinoshita S, Lisch W. IC3D classification of corneal dystrophies-edition 2. Cornea. 2015;34:117–59. https://doi.org/10.1097/ICO.0000000000000307.
29. Laibson PR. Microcystic corneal dystrophy. Trans Am Ophthalmol Soc. 1977;74:488–531.
30. Jonsson F, Byström B, Davidson AE, Backman LJ, Kellgren TG, Tuft SJ, Koskela T, Rydén P, Sandgren O, Danielson P, Hardcastle AJ, Golovleva I. Mutations in collagen, type XVII, alpha 1 (COL17A1) cause epithelial recurrent erosion dystrophy (ERED). Hum Mutat. 2015;36:463–73. https://doi.org/10.1002/humu.22764.
31. Lisch W, Bron AJ, Munier FL, Schorderet DF, Tiab L, Lange C, Saikia P, Reinhard T, Weiss JS, Gundlach E, Pleyer U, Lisch C, Auw-Haedrich C. Franceschetti hereditary recurrent corneal erosion. Am J Ophthalmol. 2012;153:1073–81.e4. https://doi.org/10.1016/j.ajo.2011.12.011.
32. Hammar B, Björck E, Lagerstedt K, Dellby A, Fagerholm P. A new corneal disease with recurrent erosive episodes and autosomal-dominant inheritance. Acta Ophthalmol. 2008;86:758–63. https://doi.org/10.1111/j.1600-0420.2007.01123.x.
33. Hammar B, Björck E, Lind H, Lagerstedt K, Dellby A, Fagerholm P. Dystrophia Helsinglandica: a new type of hereditary corneal recurrent erosions with late subepithelial fibrosis. Acta Ophthalmol. 2009;87:659–65. https://doi.org/10.1111/j.1755-3768.2008.01308.x.
34. Feder RS. Subepithelial mucinous corneal dystrophy. Arch Ophthalmol. 1993;111:1106. https://doi.org/10.1001/archopht.1993.01090080102025.
35. Irvine AD, Corden LD, Swensson O, Swensson B, Moore JE, Frazer DG, Smith FJ, Knowlton RG, Christophers E, Rochels R, Uitto J, McLean WH. Mutations in cornea-specific keratin K3 or K12 genes cause Meesmann's corneal dystrophy. Nat Genet. 1997;16:184–7. https://doi.org/10.1038/ng0697-184.
36. Lisch W, Steuhl KP, Lisch C, Weidle EG, Emmig CT, Cohen KL, Perry HD. A new, band-shaped and whorled microcystic dystrophy of the corneal epithelium. Am J Ophthalmol. 1992;114:35–44. https://doi.org/10.1016/S0002-9394(14)77410-0.
37. Patterson K, Chong JX, Chung DD, Lisch W, Karp CL, Dreisler E, Lockington D, Rohrbach JM, Garczarczyk-Asim D, Müller T, Tuft SJ, Skalicka P, Wilnai Y, Samra NN, Ibrahim A, Mandel H, Davidson AE, Liskova P, Aldave AJ, Bamshad MJ, Janecke AR. Lisch epithelial corneal dystrophy is caused by heterozygous loss-of-function variants in MCOLN1. Am J Ophthalmol. 2024;258:183–95. https://doi.org/10.1016/j.ajo.2023.10.011.
38. Kaza H, Barik MR, Reddy MM, Mittal R, Das S. Gelatinous drop-like corneal dystrophy: a review. Br J Ophthalmol. 2017;101:10–5. https://doi.org/10.1136/bjophthalmol-2016-309555.
39. Kinoshita S, Nishida K, Dota A, Inatomi T, Koizumi N, Elliott A, Lewis D, Quantock A, Fullwood N. Epithelial barrier function and ultrastructure of gelatinous drop-like corneal dystrophy. Cornea. 2000;19:551–5. https://doi.org/10.1097/00003226-200007000-00029.
40. Munier FL, Korvatska E, Djemaï A, Le Paslier D, Zografos L, Pescia G, Schorderet DF. Kerato-epithelin mutations in four 5q31-linked corneal dystrophies. Nat Genet. 1997;15:247–51. https://doi.org/10.1038/ng0397-247.
41. Stone EM, Mathers WD, Rosenwasser GOD, Holland EJ, Folberg R, Krachmer JH, Nichols BE, Gorevic PD, Taylor CM, Streb LM, et al. Three autosomal dominant corneal dystrophies map to chromosome 5q. Nat Genet. 1994;6:47–51. https://doi.org/10.1038/ng0194-47.
42. Vajzovic LM, Karp CL, Haft P, Shousha MA, Dubovy SR, Hurmeric V, Yoo SH, Wang J. Ultra high-resolution anterior segment optical coherence tomography in the evaluation of anterior corneal dystrophies and degenerations. Ophthalmology. 2011;118:1291–6. https://doi.org/10.1016/j.ophtha.2010.12.015.
43. Milovanova E, Gomon S, Rocha G. Classic lattice corneal dystrophy: a brief review and summary of treatment modalities. Graefe's Arch Clin Exp Ophthalmol. 2024;262:1667–81. https://doi.org/10.1007/s00417-023-06297-6.
44. Lyons CJ, McCartney AC, Kirkness CM, Ficker LA, Steele AD, Rice NS. Granular corneal dystrophy. Visual results and pattern of recurrence after lamellar or penetrating keratoplasty. Ophthalmology. 1994;101:1812–7. https://doi.org/10.1016/s0161-6420(94)31096-7.
45. Chao-Shern C, Me R, DeDionisio LA, Ke BL, Nesbit MA, Marshall J, Moore CBT. Post-LASIK exacerbation of granular corneal dystrophy type 2 in members of a chinese family. Eye. 2018;32:39–43. https://doi.org/10.1038/eye.2017.265.
46. Poulsen ET, Nielsen NS, Jensen MM, Nielsen E, Hjortdal J, Kim EK, Enghild JJ. LASIK surgery of granular corneal dystrophy type 2 patients leads to accumulation and differential proteolytic processing of transforming growth factor beta-induced protein (TGFBIp). Proteomics. 2016;16:539–43. https://doi.org/10.1002/pmic.201500287.
47. Dudakova L, Palos M, Svobodova M, et al. Macular corneal dystrophy and associated corneal thinning. Eye. 2014;28:1201–5. https://doi.org/10.1038/eye.2014.164.
48. Quantock AJ, Meek KM, Ridgway AEA, Bron AJ, Thonar EJ. Macular corneal dystrophy: reduction in both corneal thickness and collagen interfibrillar spacing. Curr Eye Res. 1990;9:393–8. https://doi.org/10.3109/02713689008999628.
49. Hafner A, Langenbucher A, Seitz B. Long-term results of phototherapeutic keratectomy with 193-nm excimer laser for macular corneal dystrophy. Am J Ophthalmol. 2005;140:392.e1–392.e. https://doi.org/10.1016/j.ajo.2005.03.052.
50. Nickerson ML, Kostiha BN, Brandt W, Fredericks W, Xu KP, Yu FS, Gold B, Chodosh J, Goldberg M, Lu DW, Yamada M, Tervo TM, Grutzmacher R, Croasdale C, Hoeltzenbein M, Sutphin J, Malkowicz SB, Wessjohann L, Kruth HS, Dean M, Weiss JS. UBIAD1 mutation alters a mitochondrial prenyltransferase to cause schnyder corneal dystrophy. PLoS ONE. 2010;5:e10760. https://doi.org/10.1371/journal.pone.0010760.
51. Weiss JS. Visual morbidity in thirty-four families with Schnyder crystalline corneal dystrophy (an American Ophthalmological Society thesis). Trans Am Ophthalmol Soc. 2007;105:616–48.
52. Weiss JS. Schnyder corneal dystrophy. Curr Opin Ophthalmol. 2009;20:292–8. https://doi.org/10.1097/ICU.0b013e32832b753e.
53. Weiss JS. More on Schnyder corneal dystrophy. Ophthalmology. 2009;116:2260. https://doi.org/10.1016/j.ophtha.2009.07.022.
54. Weiss JS, Khemichian AJ. Differential diagnosis of Schnyder corneal dystrophy. Dev Ophthalmol. 2011;48:67–96. https://doi.org/10.1159/000324078.
55. Weiss JS, Kruth HS, Kuivaniemi H, Tromp G, White PS, Winters RS, Lisch W, Henn W, Denninger E, Krause M, Wasson P, Ebenezer N, Mahurkar S, Nickerson ML. Mutations in the UBIAD1 gene on chromosome short arm 1, region 36, cause Schnyder crystalline corneal dystrophy. Invest Ophthalmol Vis Sci. 2007;48:5007–12. https://doi.org/10.1167/iovs.07-0845.
56. Bredrup C, Knappskog PM, Majewski J, Rødahl E, Boman H. Congenital stromal dystrophy of the cornea caused by a mutation in the decorin gene. Invest Opthalmol Vis Sci. 2005;46:420–6. https://doi.org/10.1167/iovs.04-0804.
57. Bredrup C, Stang E, Bruland O, Palka BP, Young RD, Haavik J, Knappskog PM, Rødahl E. Decorin accumulation contributes to the stromal opacities found in congenital stromal corneal dystrophy. Invest Ophthalmol Vis Sci. 2010;51:5578–82. https://doi.org/10.1167/iovs.09-4933.
58. Berger T, Hasenfus A, Bredrup C, et al. Long-term follow-up of pediatric excimer laser-assisted penetrating keratoplasty for

congenital stromal corneal dystrophy. Cornea. 2024;43:784–9 https://doi.org/10.1097/ICO.0000000000003519.
59. Can E, Kan E, Akgün Hİ. Clinical features and in-vivo confocal microscopic imaging of fleck corneal dystrophy. Semin Ophthalmol. 2013;28:239–41. https://doi.org/10.3109/08820538.2012.760629.
60. Li S, Tiab L, Jiao X, Munier FL, Zografos L, Frueh BE, Sergeev Y, Smith J, Rubin B, Meallet MA, Forster RK, Hejtmancik JF, Schorderet DF. Mutations in PIP5K3 are associated with François-Neetens Mouchetée Fleck corneal dystrophy. Am J Hum Genet. 2005;77:54–63. https://doi.org/10.1086/431346.
61. Nicholson DH, Green WR, Cross HE, Kenyon KR, Massof D. A clinical and histopathological study of François-Neetens speckled corneal dystrophy. Am J Ophthalmol. 1977;83:554–60. https://doi.org/10.1016/0002-9394(77)90566-9.
62. Kim MJ, Frausto RF, Rosenwasser GOD, Bui T, Le DJ, Stone EM, Aldave AJ. Posterior amorphous corneal dystrophy is associated with a deletion of small leucine-rich proteoglycans on chromosome 12. PLoS ONE. 2014;9: e95037. https://doi.org/10.1371/journal.pone.0095037.
63. Choo CH, De Los Bueis AB, Chung DD, Aldave AJ. Confirmation of PRDX3 c.568G>C as the genetic basis of punctiform and polychromatic pre-descemet corneal dystrophy. Cornea. 2022;41:779–81. https://doi.org/10.1097/ICO.0000000000002828.
64. Berger T, Seitz B, Löw U, Flockerzi F, Schlötzer-Schrehardt U, Daas L. Descemet membrane endothelial keratoplasty (DMEK) for severe verrucous posterior polymorphous corneal dystrophy with uncommon clinical and ultrastructural findings. Klin Monbl Augenheilkd. 2024;241:1081–90. https://doi.org/10.1055/a-1862-8403.
65. Schmid E, Lisch W, Philipp W, Lechner S, Göttinger W, Schlötzer-Schrehardt U, Müller T, Utermann G, Janecke AR. A new, X-linked endothelial corneal dystrophy. Am J Ophthalmol. 2006;141:478–87. https://doi.org/10.1016/j.ajo.2005.10.020.

Fuchs Endothelial Corneal Dystrophy FECD

Katrin Wacker and Thomas Reinhard

Abstract

Fuchs endothelial corneal dystrophy (FECD) manifests typically in the fifth or sixth decade of life. Focal posterior collagenous excrescences in the central cornea, so-called guttae, are the diagnostic hallmark on slit-lamp exam. In FECD, progressive endothelial dysfunction leads to corneal edema. Chronic edema results in characteristic morphological and anatomical changes in all corneal layers that impair corneal transparency and optics. Endothelial keratoplasty promises near complete visual rehabilitation by replacing the abnormal Descemet membrane and corneal endothelium if remodeling in the host cornea is not too advanced.

Keywords

Corneal edema · Guttae · Corneal fibrosis · Corneal tomography · Disease severity · Staging

1 Introduction

Fuchs endothelial corneal dystrophy (FECD) is characterized by posterior collagenous excrescences in the central cornea, so-called guttae, and progressive corneal edema resulting in reduced corneal transparency and impaired vision [1].

Since the first description of the disease in 1910 [2], our understanding of morphology and therapy has improved tremendously. Pathognomonic changes in morphology are present in all corneal layers early in the course of the disease as a result of subclinical corneal edema. With the advent of endothelial keratoplasty, in particular Descemet membrane endothelial keratoplasty (DMEK), complete visual rehabilitation is possible if not prevented by progressive and irreversible scar formation in the remaining host cornea and other eye diseases [3–5]. This chapter will review and display morphological changes characteristic for FECD relevant for staging disease severity and indication for surgical therapy.

2 Corneal Endothelial Cells

In FECD, dysfunction of the endothelial barrier and pump results in impaired hydration control [6–9]. As disease progresses, guttae disrupt the regular hexagonal array of the corneal endothelial cell layer (Fig. 1) [10, 11]. Corneal endothelial cells get lost, presumably through apoptosis induced by guttae microenvironment, or show adaptive responses such as enlargement, migration, and redistribution [12–18].

3 Descemet Membrane and Guttae

Descemet membrane becomes abnormal and thickens with FECD progression. The Descemet membrane of eyes with FECD can appear grey with a focal, island-shaped fibrillary layer (Fig. 2). The posterior layer of Descemet membrane thickens with multiple layers of basement membrane-like material [19, 20].

Guttae are the diagnostic hallmark of FECD on slit-lamp exam (Fig. 3). Guttae develop as focal collagenous excrescences adjacent to a thickened and ultrastructurally modified Descemet membrane [20, 22, 23]. In FECD, guttae are located in the center of the cornea with an oval distribution pattern that becomes confluent over time [24–26]. To grade disease severity, the number and confluence of guttae can

K. Wacker (✉) · T. Reinhard
Eye Center, Albert-Ludwigs University of Freiburg, Freiburg, Germany
e-mail: katrin.wacker@uniklinik-freiburg.de; wacker@dr-wacker.de

K. Wacker
Herbolzheim, Germany

B. Seitz et al. (eds.), *Atlas on Cornea*, https://doi.org/10.1007/978-3-031-65422-0_18

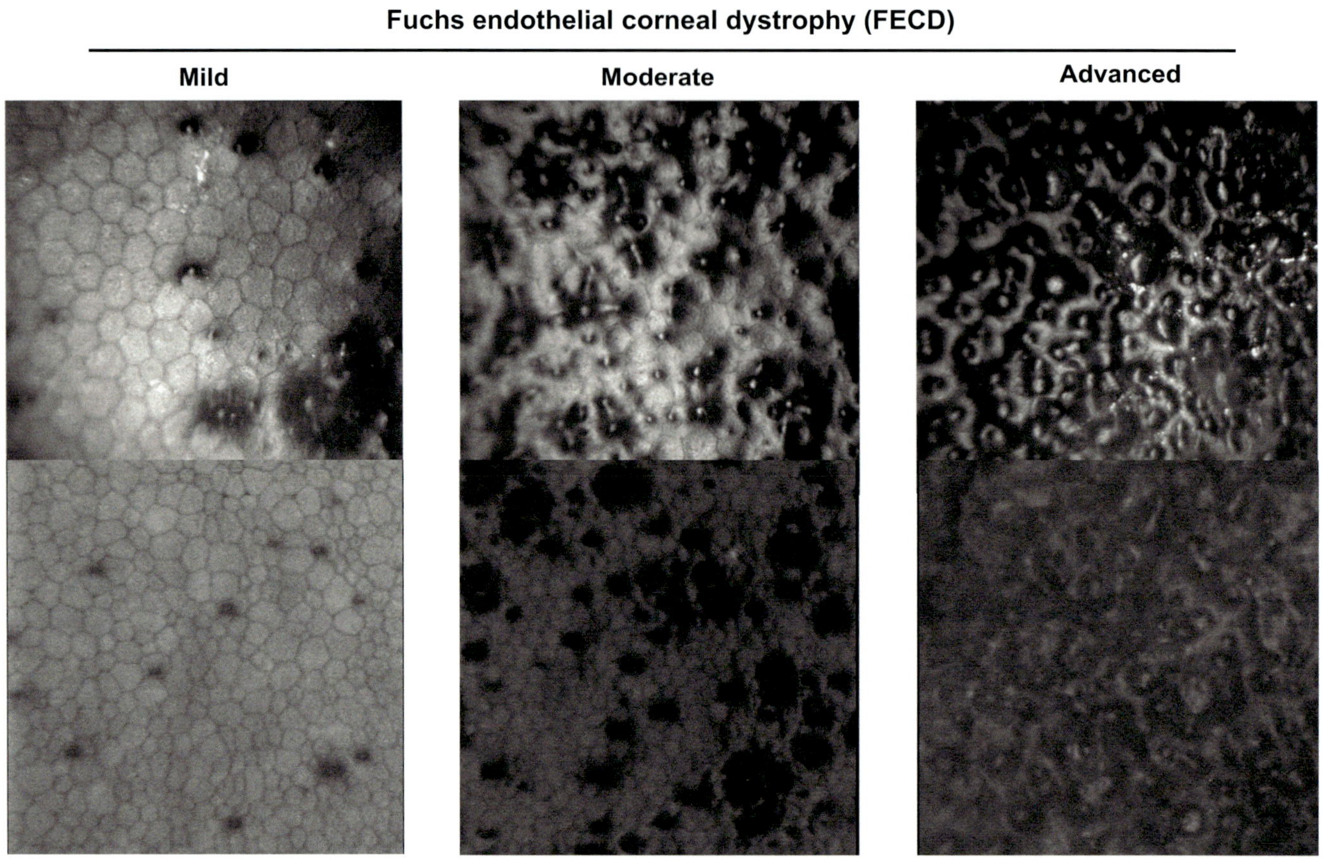

Fig. 1 **Corneal endothelial cells in Fuchs dystrophy (FECD).** Confocal microscopy (*upper row*) and specular microscopy (*lower row*) images of corneal endothelial cells in FECD. Guttae appear as dark spots and become confluent with disease progression

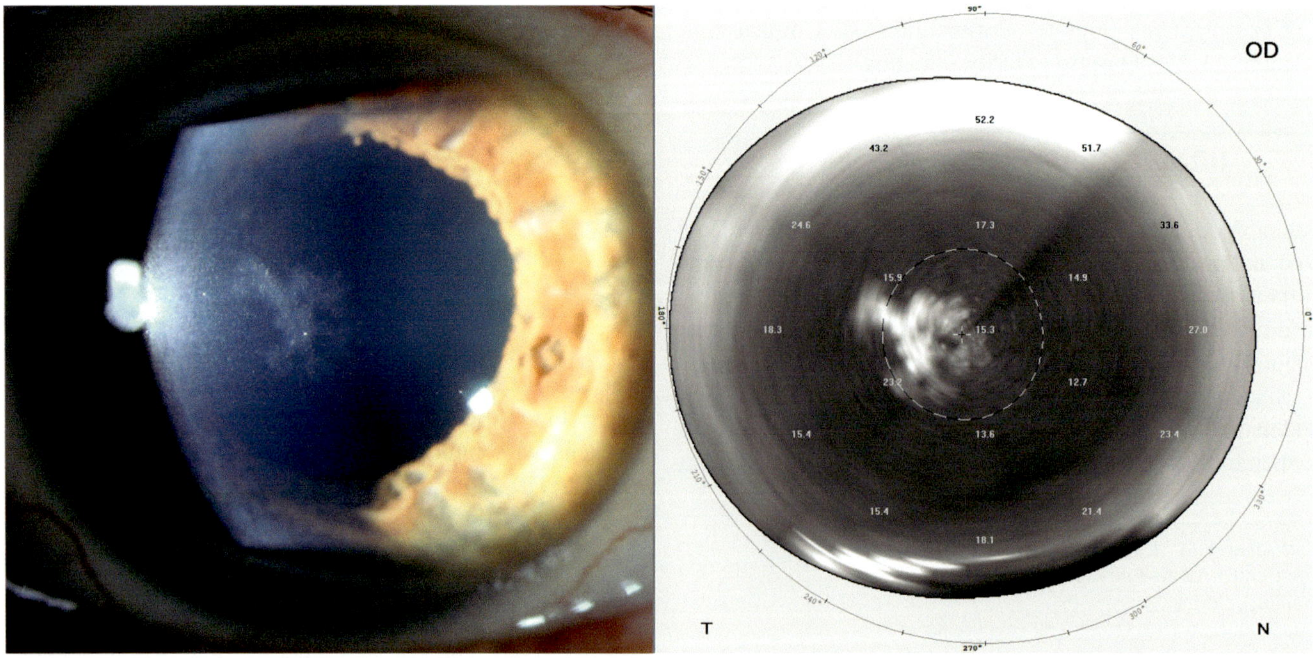

Fig. 2 **Descemet membrane in Fuchs dystrophy (FECD).** Fibrillary layer visible on slit-lamp exam with broad tangential illumination and in Scheimpflug imaging. Thieme license 5390390845977 for reprint from Zander, Jiang [21]

be determined on slit-lamp exam or using computer-based analysis of retroillumination photographs [26–28].

4 Corneal Edema

Progressive endothelial dysfunction results in corneal edema. In clinically advanced FECD, an area of stromal edema becomes visible on slit-lamp exam (Fig. 4). The focal, central localization and the bilateral nature of edema accompanied by guttae may help in differentiating FECD from other etiologies of corneal edema such as pseudophakic bullous keratopathy [21].

Identifying corneal edema early in the course of the disease is key, given the risk of progressive and irreversible remodeling in all corneal layers, including those that are not restored by endothelial keratoplasty [3–5]. While Ernst Fuchs initially described the disease as *dystrophia epithelialia corneae* without slit-lamp's biomicroscopy, even on slit-lamp exam, more subtle features of edema may be easily missed by cornea specialists [31]. Scheimpflug tomography and anterior segment optical coherence tomography

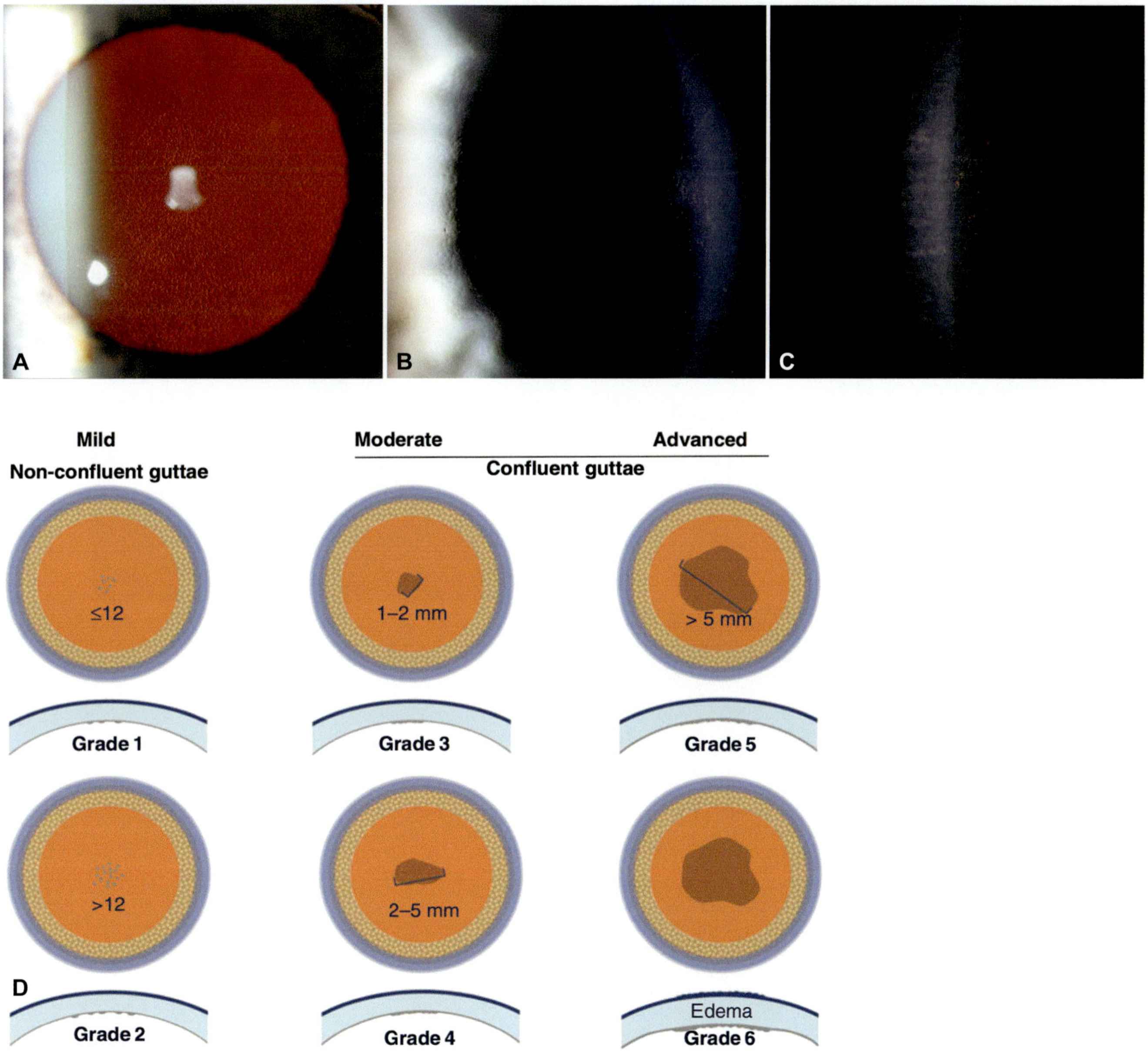

Fig. 3 Guttae in Fuchs dystrophy (FECD). (**A**) Retroillumination photos of distribution and confluence of guttae. Guttae are predominantly localized in the interpalpebral zone with a more horizontal than vertical distribution pattern. (**B**) "Beaten metal" appearance of the cornea with blurred iris details. (**C**) Pigment deposits may accompany guttae. (**D**) Modified Krachmer grading based on presence and confluence of guttae and the presence of edema. Springer license 5336380980122 for reprint from Wacker, McLaren [29].

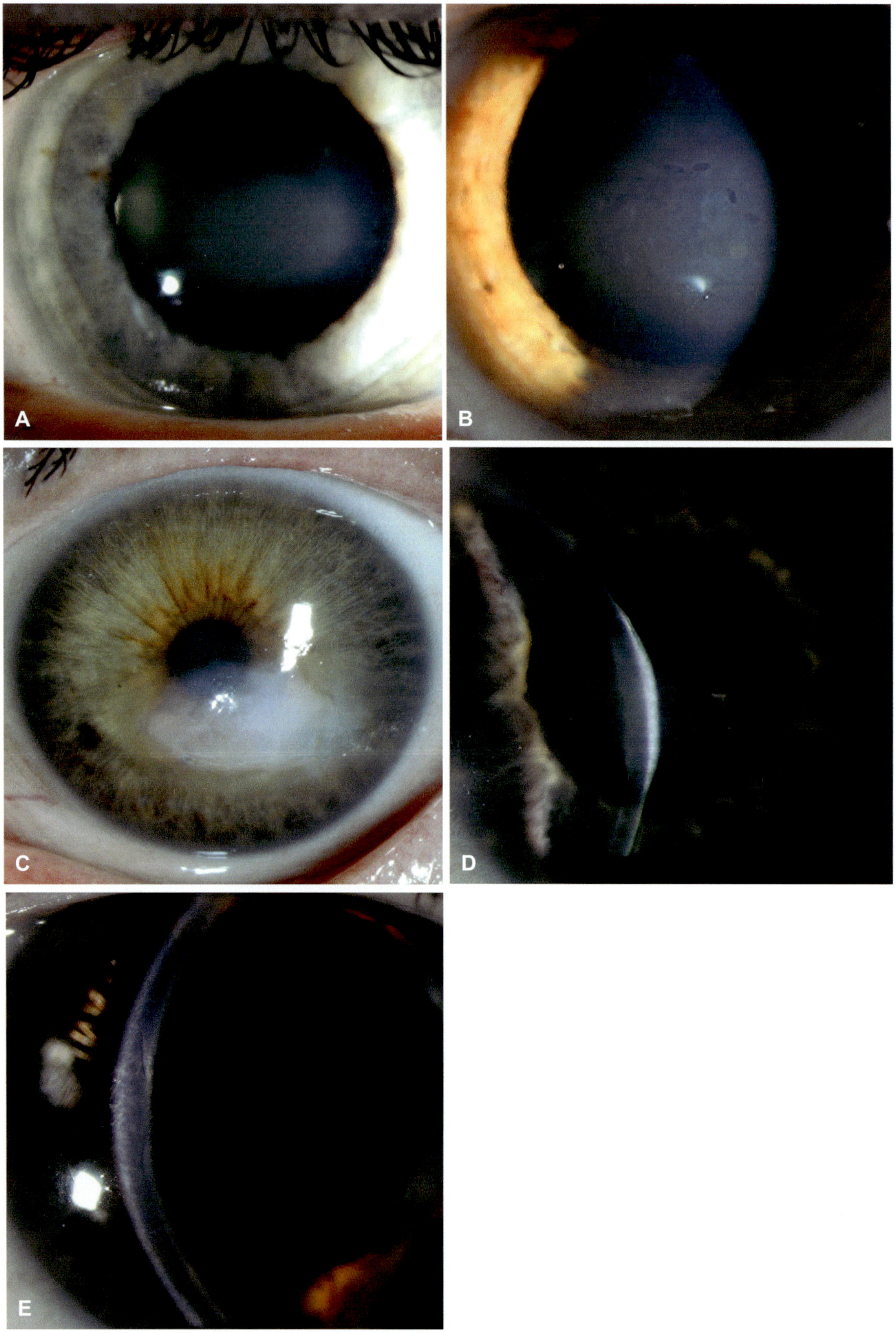

Fig. 4 **Corneal edema on slit-lamp exam in Fuchs dystrophy (FECD)**. Characteristic signs of edema include (**A**) focal ground glass haze and microcystic epithelial edema, (**B**) subepithelial bullae, (**C**) pannus formation, (**D**) changes to the corneal curvature, and (**E**) Descemet or deep stromal folds. Springer licenses 50141831 for reprint from Wacker, Reinhard [30]

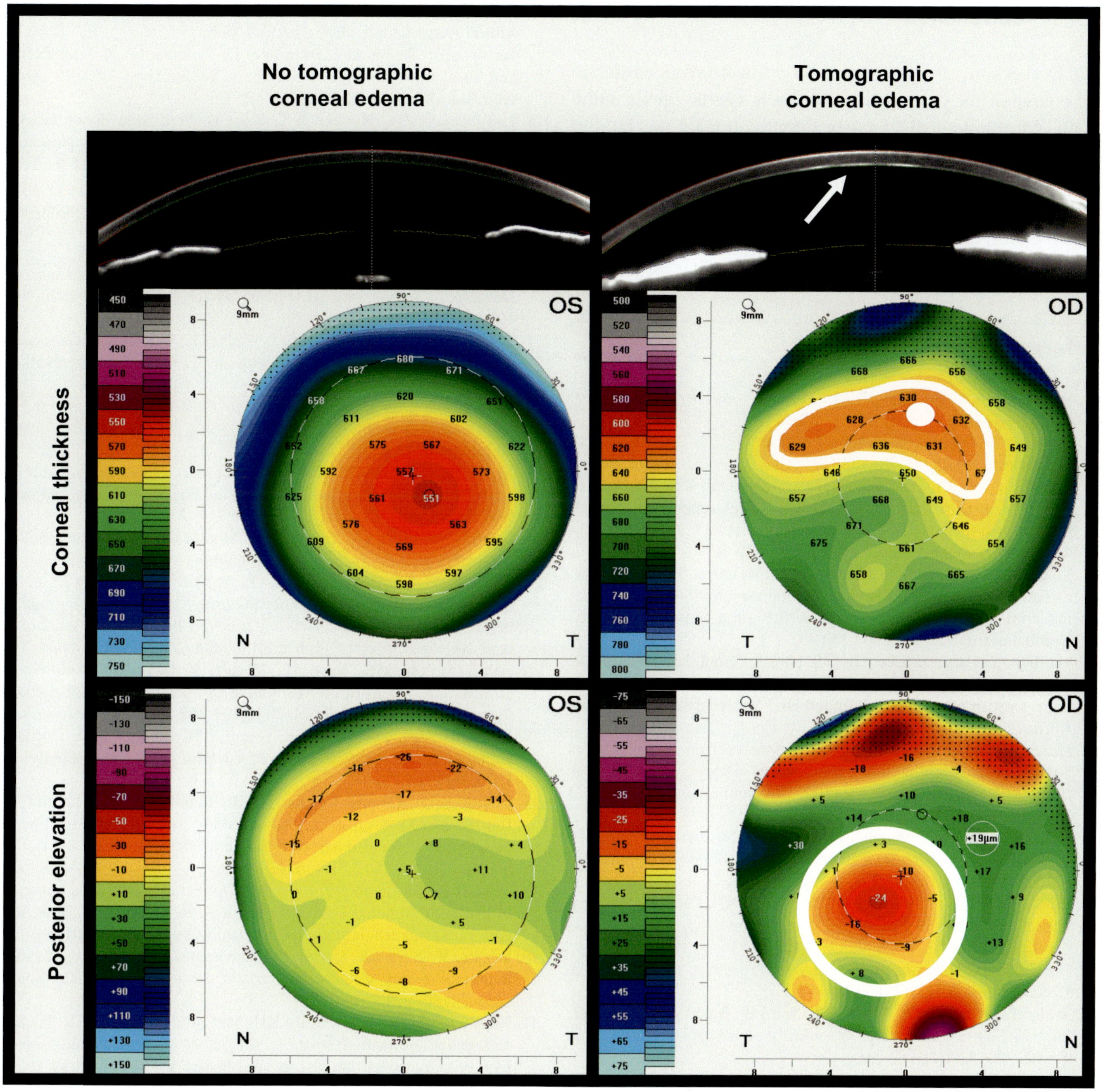

Fig. 5 **Corneal edema on Scheimpflug tomography in Fuchs dystrophy (FECD)**. Characteristic features of tomographic edema include irregular lines of equal corneal thickness (isopachs), displacement of the point of thinnest corneal thickness from its inferior-temporal location (*white dot*), and an area of focal posterior corneal depression [35, 37]. Thieme license \\ for reprint from Zander, Jiang [21]

have improved the assessment of corneal curvatures, structure, and thickness profile [32–34]. Tomographic features of focal corneal edema are visible earlier in the course of the disease before they become visible on slit-lamp exam (Fig. 5) [35, 36].

Chronic corneal edema changes the regularity of the anterior cornea. Longstanding edema with poorly adherent epithelium may result in a folded basement membrane, scarring, pannus formation, or vascularization [24, 38–40]. Even when guttae are not confluent and edema is not visible on slit-lamp exam, anterior corneal changes already result in keratocyte depletion and an increase of corneal backscatter and high-order aberrations, which may persist even five years after restoration of endothelial function [4, 36, 41–43].

5 Conclusion

FECD alters the architecture of all corneal layers earlier in the course of the disease than edema is visible on slit-lamp exam. Morphological changes directly impair the quality of the retinal image by inducing high-order aberrations and disability glare. To prevent irreversible changes to the cornea that limit complete visual rehabilitation after restoration of the endothelial function, early detection and staging of disease severity is desirable.

References

1. Wilson SE, Bourne WM. Fuchs' dystrophy. Cornea. 1988;7(1):2–18.
2. Fuchs E. Dystrophia epithelialis corneae. Graefes Arch Klin Exp Ophthalmol. 1910;76:478–508.
3. Dapena I, Yeh RY, Baydoun L, Cabrerizo J, van Dijk K, Ham L, et al. Potential causes of incomplete visual rehabilitation at 6 months postoperative after Descemet membrane endothelial keratoplasty. Am J Ophthalmol. 2013;156(4):780–8.
4. Wacker K, Baratz KH, Maguire LJ, McLaren JW, Patel SV. Descemet stripping endothelial keratoplasty for Fuchs' endothelial corneal dystrophy: five-year results of a prospective study. Ophthalmology. 2016;123(1):154–60.
5. van Dijk K, Parker J, Liarakos VS, Ham L, Frank LE, Melles GR. Incidence of irregular astigmatism eligible for contact lens fitting after Descemet membrane endothelial keratoplasty. J Cataract Refract Surg. 2013;39(7):1036–46.
6. Leber T. Studien über den Flüssigkeitswechsel im Auge. Graefes Arch Klin Exp Ophthalmol. 1873;19(2):87–185.
7. Maurice DM. The location of the fluid pump in the cornea. J Physiol. 1972;221(1):43–54.
8. Polse KA, Brand R, Mandell R, Vastine D, Demartini D, Flom R. Age differences in corneal hydration control. Invest Ophthalmol Vis Sci. 1989;30(3):392–9.
9. Wacker K, McLaren JW, Kane KM, Baratz KH, Patel SV. Corneal hydration control in Fuchs' endothelial corneal dystrophy. Invest Ophthalmol Vis Sci. 2016;57(11):5060–5.
10. Bourne WM. Corneal endothelium—past, present, and future. Eye Contact Lens. 2010;36(5):310–4.
11. Weiss JS, Møller HU, Aldave AJ, Seitz B, Bredrup C, Kivelä T, et al. IC3D classification of corneal dystrophies—edition 2. Cornea. 2015;34(2):117–59.
12. Borderie VM, Baudrimont M, Vallee A, Ereau TL, Gray F, Laroche L. Corneal endothelial cell apoptosis in patients with Fuchs' dystrophy. Invest Ophthalmol Vis Sci. 2000;41(9):2501–5.
13. Kocaba V, Katikireddy KR, Gipson I, Price MO, Price FW, Jurkunas UV. Association of the Gutta-induced microenvironment with corneal endothelial cell behavior and demise in Fuchs endothelial corneal dystrophy. JAMA Ophthalmol. 2018;136(8):886–92.
14. Ong Tone S, Kocaba V, Bohm M, Wylegala A, White TL, Jurkunas UV. Fuchs endothelial corneal dystrophy: the vicious cycle of Fuchs pathogenesis. Prog Retin Eye Res. 2021;80:100863.
15. Böhringer D, Böhringer S, Poxleitner K, Birnbaum F, Schwartzkopff J, Maier P, et al. Long-term graft survival in penetrating keratoplasty: the biexponential model of chronic endothelial cell loss revisited. Cornea. 2010;29(10):1113–7.
16. Reinhard T, Böhringer D, Huschen D, Sundmacher R. Chronic endothelial cell loss of the graft after penetrating keratoplasty: influence of endothelial cell migration from graft to host. Klin Monbl Augenheilkd. 2002;219(6):410–6.
17. Birnbaum F, Reinhard T, Böhringer D, Sundmacher R. Endothelial cell loss after autologous rotational keratoplasty. Graefes Arch Clin Exp Ophthalmol. 2005;243(1):57–9.
18. Langenbucher A, Nguyen NX, Seitz B. Predictive donor factors for chronic endothelial cell loss after nonmechanical penetrating keratoplasty in a regression model. Graefes Arch Clin Exp Ophthalmol. 2003;241(12):975–81.
19. Johnson DH, Bourne WM, Campbell RJ. The ultrastructure of Descemet's membrane. I. Changes with age in normal corneas. Arch Ophthalmol. 1982;100(12):1942–7.
20. Bourne WM, Johnson DH, Campbell RJ. The ultrastructure of Descemet's membrane. III. Fuchs' dystrophy. Arch Ophthalmol. 1982;100(12):1952–5.
21. Zander DB, Jiang J, Reinhard T, Wacker K. Corneal oedema: aetiology, diagnostic testing, and treatment. Klin Monbl Augenheilkd. 2022;239(6):752–9.
22. Iwamoto T, DeVoe AG. Electron microscopic studies on Fuchs' combined dystrophy. I. Posterior portion of the cornea. Invest Ophthalmol. 1971;10(1):9–28.
23. Yuen HK, Rassier CE, Jardeleza MS, Green WR, de la Cruz Z, Stark WJ, et al. A morphologic study of Fuchs dystrophy and bullous keratopathy. Cornea. 2005;24(3):319–27.
24. Adamis AP, Filatov V, Tripathi BJ, Tripathi RC. Fuchs' endothelial dystrophy of the cornea. Surv Ophthalmol. 1993;38(2):149–68.
25. Fujimoto H, Maeda N, Soma T, Oie Y, Koh S, Tsujikawa M, et al. Quantitative regional differences in corneal endothelial abnormalities in the central and peripheral zones in Fuchs' endothelial corneal dystrophy. Invest Ophthalmol Vis Sci. 2014;55(8):5090–8.
26. Soh YQ, Peh GSL, Naso SL, Kocaba V, Mehta JS. Automated clinical assessment of corneal guttae in Fuchs endothelial corneal dystrophy. Am J Ophthalmol. 2021;221:260–72.
27. Krachmer JH, Purcell JJ Jr, Young CW, Bucher KD. Corneal endothelial dystrophy. A study of 64 families. Arch Ophthalmol. 1978;96(11):2036–9.
28. Louttit MD, Kopplin LJ, Igo RP Jr, Fondran JR, Tagliaferri A, Bardenstein D, et al. A multicenter study to map genes for Fuchs endothelial corneal dystrophy: baseline characteristics and heritability. Cornea. 2012;31(1):26–35.
29. Wacker K, McLaren JW, Patel SV. Optical and anatomic changes in Fuchs Endothelial Dystrophy corneas. In: Cursiefen C, Jun AS, editors. Springer International Publishing Switzerland; 2017.
30. Wacker K, Reinhard T, Maier P. Pathogenesis and diagnostic evaluation of Fuchs' endothelial corneal dystrophy. Ophthalmologe. 2019;116(3):221–7.
31. Repp DJ, Hodge DO, Baratz KH, McLaren JW, Patel SV. Fuchs' endothelial corneal dystrophy: subjective grading versus objective grading based on the central-to-peripheral thickness ratio. Ophthalmology. 2013;120(4):687–94.
32. Kwon RO, Price MO, Price FW Jr, Ambrosio R Jr, Belin MW. Pentacam characterization of corneas with Fuchs dystrophy treated with Descemet membrane endothelial keratoplasty. J Refract Surg. 2010;26(12):972–9.
33. Brunette I, Sherknies D, Terry MA, Chagnon M, Bourges JL, Meunier J. 3-D characterization of the corneal shape in Fuchs dystrophy and pseudophakic keratopathy. Invest Ophthalmol Vis Sci. 2011;52(1):206–14.
34. Wacker K, McLaren JW, Patel SV. Directional posterior corneal profile changes in Fuchs' endothelial corneal dystrophy. Invest Ophthalmol Vis Sci. 2015;56(10):5904–11.
35. Sun SY, Wacker K, Baratz KH, Patel SV. Determining subclinical edema in Fuchs endothelial corneal dystrophy. Revised classification using Scheimpflug tomography for preoperative assessment. Ophthalmology. 2019;126(2):195–205.

36. Wacker K, McLaren JW, Amin SR, Baratz KH, Patel SV. Corneal high-order aberrations and backscatter in Fuchs' endothelial corneal dystrophy. Ophthalmology. 2015;122(8):1645–52.
37. Zander D, Grewing V, Glatz A, Lapp T, Maier PC, Reinhard T, et al. Predicting edema resolution after Descemet membrane endothelial keratoplasty for Fuchs dystrophy using Scheimpflug tomography. JAMA Ophthalmol. 2021;139(4):423–30.
38. Eagle RC Jr, Laibson PR, Arentsen JJ. Epithelial abnormalities in chronic corneal edema: a histopathological study. Trans Am Ophthalmol Soc. 1989;87:107–19; discussion 19–24.
39. Morishige N, Yamada N, Teranishi S, Chikama T, Nishida T, Takahara A. Detection of subepithelial fibrosis associated with corneal stromal edema by second harmonic generation imaging microscopy. Invest Ophthalmol Vis Sci. 2009;50(7):3145–50.
40. Chaurasia S, Price MO, McKee Y, Price FW Jr. Descemet membrane endothelial keratoplasty combined with epithelial debridement and mitomycin-C application for Fuchs dystrophy with preoperative subepithelial fibrosis or anterior basement membrane dystrophy. Cornea. 2014;33(4):335–9.
41. Amin SR, Baratz KH, McLaren JW, Patel SV. Corneal abnormalities early in the course of Fuchs' endothelial dystrophy. Ophthalmology. 2014;121(12):2325–33.
42. Hecker LA, McLaren JW, Bachman LA, Patel SV. Anterior keratocyte depletion in Fuchs endothelial dystrophy. Arch Ophthalmol. 2011;129(5):555–61.
43. Patel SV, McLaren JW. In vivo confocal microscopy of Fuchs endothelial dystrophy before and after endothelial keratoplasty. JAMA Ophthalmol. 2013;131(5):611–8.

PEX Keratopathy and its Differentiation from Fuchs Dystrophy

Ursula Schlötzer-Schrehardt

Abstract

Pseudoexfoliation (PEX) has long been known to compromise all anterior segment structures including the cornea, particularly the corneal endothelium. Based on clinical and histopathological evidence, a specific endotheliopathy has been described in PEX eyes, leading to early loss of endothelial cells and early diffuse corneal endothelial decompensation. It results from a diseased corneal endothelium and its active involvement in the fibrotic PEX process. Clinically and histopathologically, PEX keratopathy is characterized by (1) decrease in endothelial cell density associated with marked variations in cell size and shape; (2) pronounced pigment dispersion and phagocytosis of melanin granules by endothelial cells; (3) fibroblastic transformation of endothelial cells; (4) active production of PEX fibrils by degenerative endothelial cells, which may appear as hyperreflective deposits on clinical examination; and (5) irregular diffuse thickening of the Descemet membrane with foci of incorporated PEX aggregates, but without guttae formations. Elevated intraocular pressure may aggravate endothelial changes but appears not to be their primary cause. PEX and Fuchs endotheliopathies can be mainly differentiated by presence or lack of typical PEX fibrils or typical guttae. PEX keratopathy plays a significant role in the clinical management of PEX patients, representing a rather common risk factor for corneal edema following ocular surgery but a relatively rare indication for endothelial keratoplasty.

U. Schlötzer-Schrehardt (✉)
Department of Ophthalmology, Friedrich-Alexander University of Erlangen-Nürnberg, Erlangen, Germany
e-mail: ursula.schloetzer-schrehardt@uk-erlangen.de

Keywords

Pseudoexfoliation syndrome · PEX keratopathy · Fuchs dystrophy · Corneal endothelium · Descemet membrane

1 Introduction

Pseudoexfoliation (PEX) syndrome represents an age-related, generalized metabolic disorder of the extracellular matrix, that leads to progressive accumulation of an abnormal fibrillar extracellular material, termed PEX material, in various intra- and extraocular tissues [1]. PEX syndrome occurs in all geographic regions worldwide with reported prevalence rates averaging about 10–15% of the general population over the age of 60 [2]. It affects all tissues of the anterior eye segment, skin, blood vessels and visceral organs including heart, lungs and meninges. It is clinically diagnosed by observation of dandruff-like white flakes of PEX material on ocular structures, particularly the anterior lens surface and the pupillary border of the iris. The terms exfoliation or pseudoexfoliation syndrome have been alternatively used for this entity, although the process does not represent a true exfoliation of the lens capsule. It can be rather described as a fibrotic process, which is characterized by an excessive production and disordered aggregation of elastic microfibrils into highly cross-linked fibrillar aggregates, which progressively accumulate in affected tissues. This fibrotic process appears to result from the effects of multiple genes, with *LOXL1* (*lysyl oxidase-like 1*) representing the strongest genetic risk factor, in combination with environmental, stress and dietary factors [3]. The characteristic PEX fibrils appear to be multifocally produced by various cell types lining the aqueous-bathed ocular surfaces, e.g. the nonpigmented ciliary epithelium, iris pigment epithelium, and trabecular endothelium. This abnormal matrix process results in a broad spectrum of ocular complications associated with PEX syndrome.

B. Seitz et al. (eds.), *Atlas on Cornea*, https://doi.org/10.1007/978-3-031-65422-0_19

PEX syndrome is typically associated with an increased risk for development of open-angle glaucoma and subluxation of the crystalline or intraocular lens. In addition, the PEX-associated tissue alterations also predispose to angle-closure glaucoma, cataract, pigment dispersion from the iris, poor mydriasis, blood-aqueous barrier dysfunction, posterior synechiae, dry eye disease, retinal vein occlusion as well as serious complications in cataract surgery [4]. Systemic associations are primarily related to vasculopathy, including transient ischemic attacks, stroke, myocardial infarction, aortic aneurysms, cerebrovascular insufficiency, Alzheimer's disease, and hearing loss as well as to elastic tissue abnormalities, including inguinal hernias, pelvic organ prolapse, chronic obstructive pulmonary disease and obstructive sleep apnea [5].

The involvement of the cornea in the PEX process, which may lead to early corneal endothelial decompensation, is less aware in clinical practice, because the subtle clinical signs may be easily overlooked or misinterpreted as "atypical Fuchs endothelial corneal dystrophy" (FECD) [6]. However, there is a clear association between corneal endothelial alterations and PEX syndrome, which tend to be amplified in PEX glaucoma. Based on characteristic clinical and histopathological alterations of the posterior cornea, Naumann and Schlötzer-Schrehardt [7] defined a PEX-associated corneal endotheliopathy or "PEX keratopathy" as a distinct clinical entity and cause of corneal endothelial decompensation. The overall concept of this chapter is to describe the clinical and histopathological features of PEX keratopathy, its clinical relevance and its differentiation from classical FECD.

2 PEX Keratopathy

2.1 Clinical Signs

PEX keratopathy represents a bilateral asymmetric, slowly progressing disease of the corneal endothelium and its basement membrane, i.e. Descemet membrane (DM). Changes at the corneal endothelial layer may be seen clinically by slit-lamp biomicroscopy as mild corneal edema, diffusely involving the entire cornea, in association with a diffusely thickened DM without formation of guttae and diffuse pigment deposition on the corneal endothelium [7] (Fig. 1). In addition, one or more undulating pigmented lines can be observed in the peripheral cornea anterior to or on Schwalbe line (Sampaolesi line). Occasionally, focal retrocorneal flakes of whitish PEX material can be clinically observed adhering to the corneal endothelium, which may be erroneously interpreted as inflammatory precipitates [8] (Fig. 2). Although not all patients with PEX will present with a clinically manifest keratopathy, involving the retrocorneal accumulation of PEX material, PEX patients show consistent alterations of the corneal endothelium.

Specular microscopy reveals a significantly reduced corneal endothelial cell density (ECD) and pronounced changes in cell size (polymegethism) and shape (pleomorphism) in eyes with PEX compared to controls, with an average reduction of ECD by 10–15% [7, 9–13]. Alterations were observed in both clinically affected and unaffected contralateral eyes and have been confirmed by confocal scanning biomicroscopy, which also shows hyperreflective endothelial deposits in the majority of PEX eyes [14–17] (Fig. 3A, B). These observations suggest that the corneal endothelium may be one of the earliest intraocular structures with observable (and measurable) damage before the presence of PEX material on the lens or iris. The progressive cell loss induces compensatory changes in remaining endothelial cells, which migrate, enlarge and become more heterogenous with loss of hexagonality. However, these processes appear to be independent of the presence of glaucoma, with no significant differences in ECD between PEX syndrome and PEX glaucoma in most studies [13, 14, 18–20]. Some studies found a statistically significant lower ECD in PEX glaucoma eyes compared to primary open-angle glaucoma (POAG) eyes, suggesting that elevated IOP and PEX are independent factors damaging the endothelium [20, 21]. Consistently, there is only a weak correlation between IOP and ECD, showing that IOP is not the main causative factor for endothelial cell loss. Rather, PEX-specific pathogenetic factors in the anterior segment or aqueous humor, such as anterior chamber hypoxia with increased oxidative stress or blood-aqueous barrier defects with influx of serum proteins, have been suggested to cause endothelial cell degeneration [7]. Nevertheless, endothelial cell counts appear to decrease with severity of disease: When PEX patients were classified into mild, moderate and severe disease stages (based on the quantity of PEX material deposits on the iris or lens and the presence of glaucoma), the disease stage was found to correlate with decreasing ECD [20, 22] (Fig. 3C). Thus, ECD may have potential as clinical biomarker for PEX to assess severity of disease [17].

Aside from endothelial alterations, PEX keratopathy seems to affect all layers of the cornea, justifying the term "PEX keratopathy". Using in vivo confocal scanning laser microscopy, other degenerative alterations have been observed in both PEX and contralateral eyes, including significantly reduced cell densities in the basal epithelial layer and corneal stroma as well as significantly reduced subbasal nerve densities, which correlated with decreased corneal sensitivity [16, 23–26]. No consistent trends were found when analyzing differences in central corneal thickness (CCT) among control, PEX syndrome and PEX glaucoma groups [17].

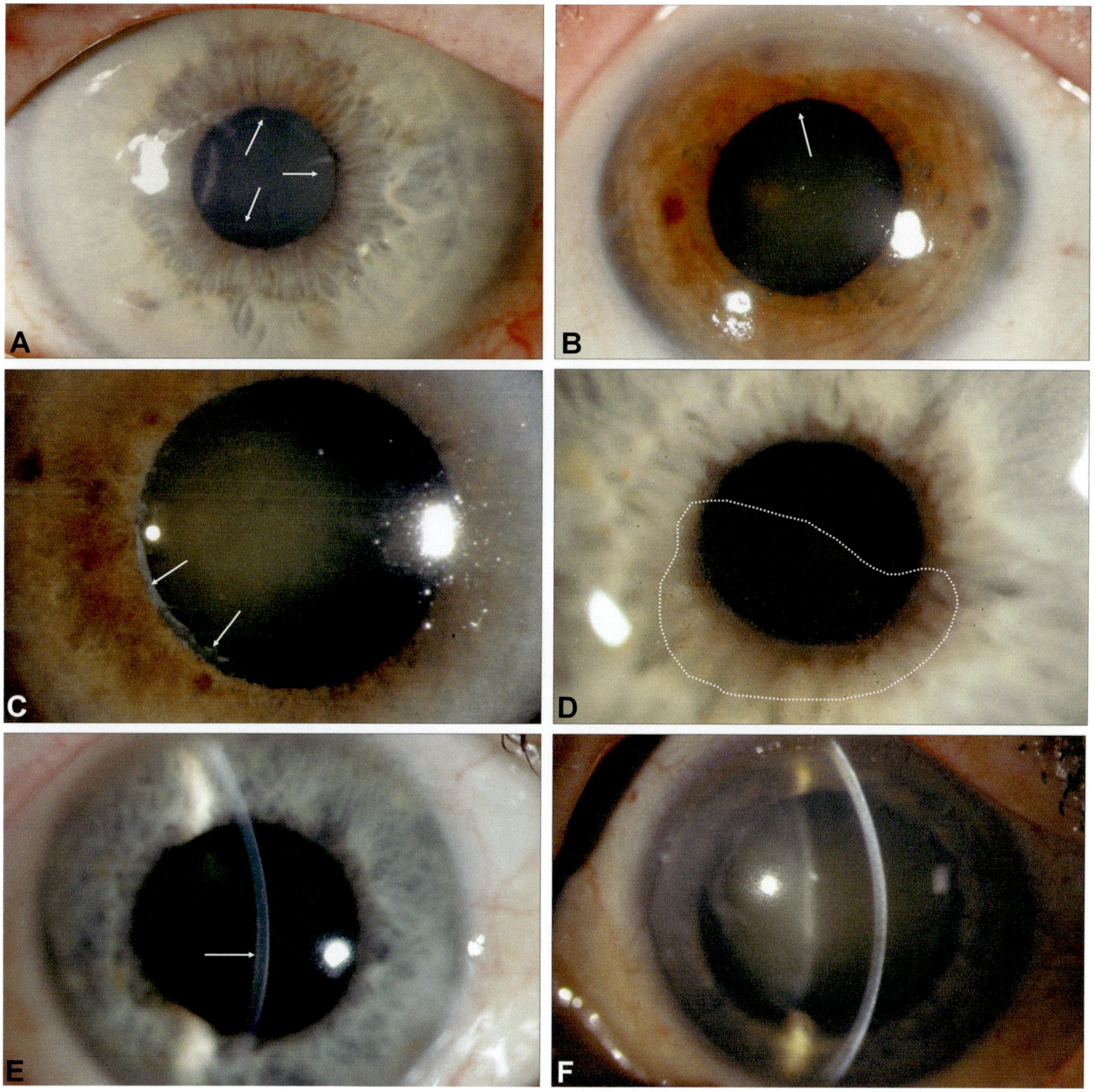

Fig. 1 Clinical features of PEX keratopathy. (**A–C**) Diffuse corneal edema in three patients with PEX syndrome after moderate rise in intraocular pressure; arrows indicate PEX material deposits on the peripheral lens surface. (**D**) Pronounced pigment dispersion (dashed area) on the posterior surface of the cornea. (**E, F**) Slit-lamp examination showing subtle hyperreflective endothelial deposits (**E**, arrow) and diffuse corneal thickening (**F**) (Figure (**C**) from Naumann and Schlötzer-Schrehardt [7]; with permission)

2.2 Histopathological Features

The active involvement of the corneal endothelium in the PEX process has been first described by Schlötzer-Schrehardt and Naumann [27]. By analyzing three corneas from PEX patients, they demonstrated focal retrocorneal aggregates that either adhered loosely to the endothelium or were incorporated into DM thereby forming large posterior protrusions or warts (Fig. 4A–C). These aggregates consisted of PEX material intermingled with pigment granules and detached, pigmented endothelial cells. They obviously corresponded to the hyperreflective deposits seen clinically by confocal microscopy (Fig. 3A). In the affected areas, the endothelial layer appeared irregular and discontinuous with

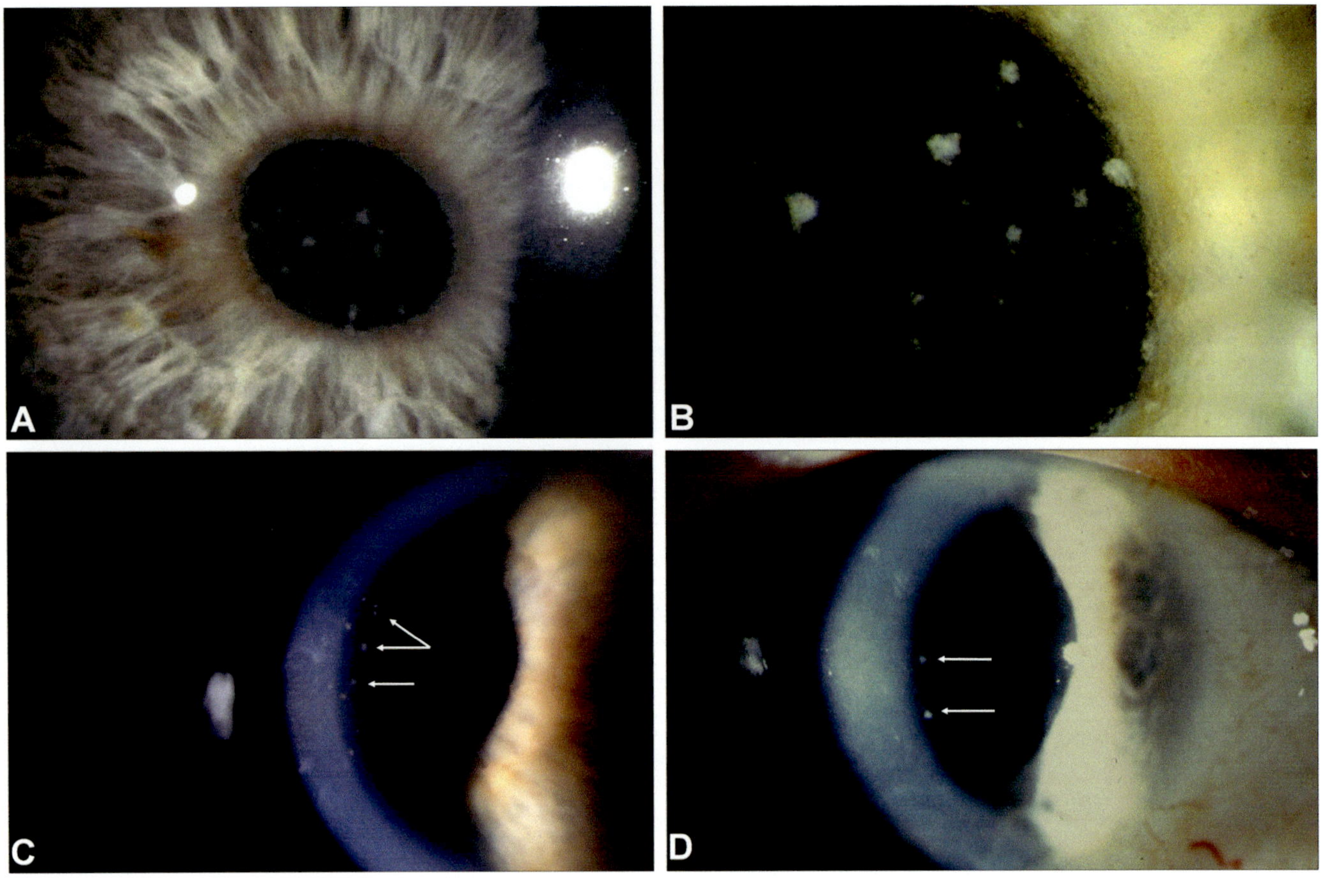

Fig. 2 Clinical features of PEX keratopathy. (**A**–**D**) Retrocorneal deposits (arrows) of PEX material in four patients with PEX syndrome

detaching, degenerating, heavily pigmented endothelial cells. As a result of corneal endothelial dysfunction, DM was abnormally thickened.

Electron microscopy confirmed the presence of typical PEX fibrils, which represent the gold standard for diagnosis, within these deposits and provided evidence for a focal production of PEX fibrils by corneal endothelial cells in situ (Fig. 4D, E). Ultrastructural evidence included the origin of PEX fibrils from surface pits and invaginations of the endothelial cell membrane, and well-developed secretory organelles, indicating increased metabolic activity. PEX fiber production occurred along apical endothelial cell surfaces facing the aqueous humor and was accompanied by a loss of cell polarity and partial or complete detachment from DM. Thus, accumulations of PEX material always concurred with defects in the endothelial layer. Subsequent reendothelialization of denuded areas of DM by neighbouring fibroblastic endothelial cells, undergoing endothelial-to-mesenchymal transition, led to overgrowth and incorporation of PEX aggregates, cellular debris, and pigment granules into DM (Fig. 4F, G). Following incorporation, the PEX deposits are no longer clinically/biomicroscopically visible, providing a possible explanation, why only a small percentage of PEX eyes shows retrocorneal flaky deposits on clinical examination. Associated with these specific changes, the corneal endothelium showed also non-specific ultrastructural alterations, including pronounced phagocytosis of pigment granules and abnormal basement membrane production resulting in an irregular thickening of DM.

These initial observations were subsequently corroborated in 22 corneal buttons obtained from PEX patients who underwent penetrating keratoplasty for irreversible corneal decompensation [7]. In this consecutive series, the morphological alterations of the posterior cornea, which were independent of the presence of glaucoma, included the following features:

- Discontinuous endothelial layer including degenerative endothelial cells with large amounts of phagocytosed pigment granules.
- Abnormal irregular thickening of DM (range 12–41 μm; normal 10–12 μm) and formation of irregular protrusions or warts, but no typical guttae.
- Fibrillar PEX aggregates adhering to or incorporated into DM in part of specimens.

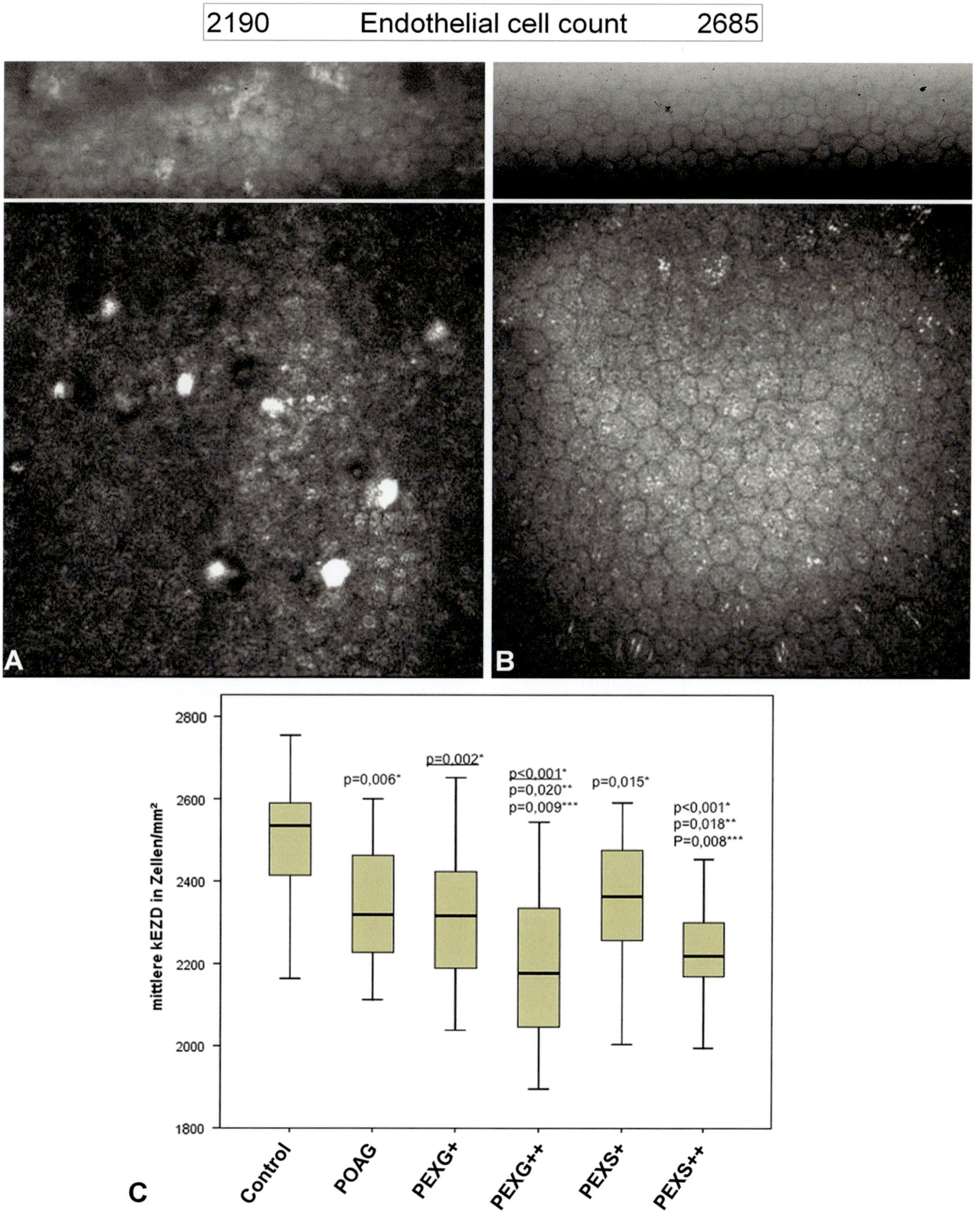

Fig. 3 Corneal endothelial cell count and morphology in a patient with clinically unilateral PEX syndrome by specular microscopy and confocal microscopy. (**A**) Polymorphous and attenuated endothelial cells together with whitish hyperreflective deposits in the affected eye. (**B**) Corneal endothelial cells with mild pleomorphism in the contralateral eye. (**C**) Mean corneal endothelial cell density (cells/mm^2) in healthy controls (n = 19), patients with primary open-angle glaucoma (POAG, n = 19), patients with secondary glaucoma due to mild (PEXG+, n = 18) or pronounced PEX (PEXG++, n = 17), and patients with mild (PEXS+, n = 17) or pronounced (PEXS++, n = 17) PEX syndrome. Statistically significant differences were assessed by Mann–Whitney U-test after Bonferroni correction (* relative to control; ** relative to POAG; *** relative to PEXG+ and PEXS+) (Figure (**C**) from Zimmermann et al. [20]; with permission)

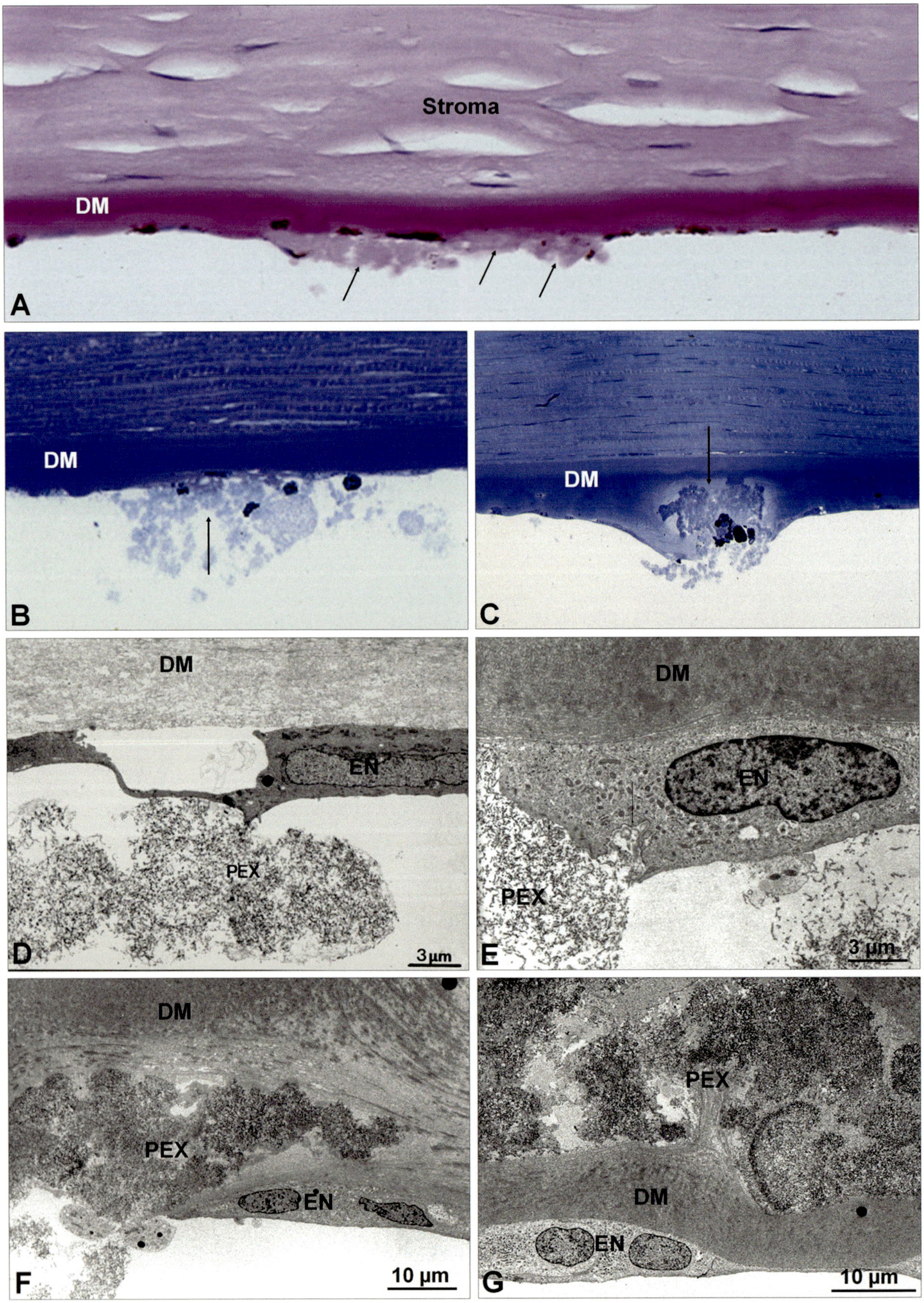

Fig. 4 Histopathologic features of PEX keratopathy. (**A**) Light microscopic appearance (PAS staining) of the posterior cornea in a patient with PEX keratopathy showing irregular thickening of Descemet membrane (DM), hyperpigmented fibroblastic endothelial cells, and focal PEX material accumulations (arrows). (**B**), (**C**) Focal PEX material aggregates (arrows) adhering to and incorporated into DM in association with hyperpigmented detached endothelial cells (semithin section, toluidine blue; magnification ×350). (**D**), (**E**) Transmission electron micrographs showing PEX material in association with a corneal endothelial cell (EN) detaching from DM (**D**) and in association with an apical surface invagination (arrow) of an endothelial cell (**E**). (**F**), (**G**) Transmission electron micrographs showing incorporation of PEX material aggregates into DM by overgrowing fibroblastic endothelial cells (EN)

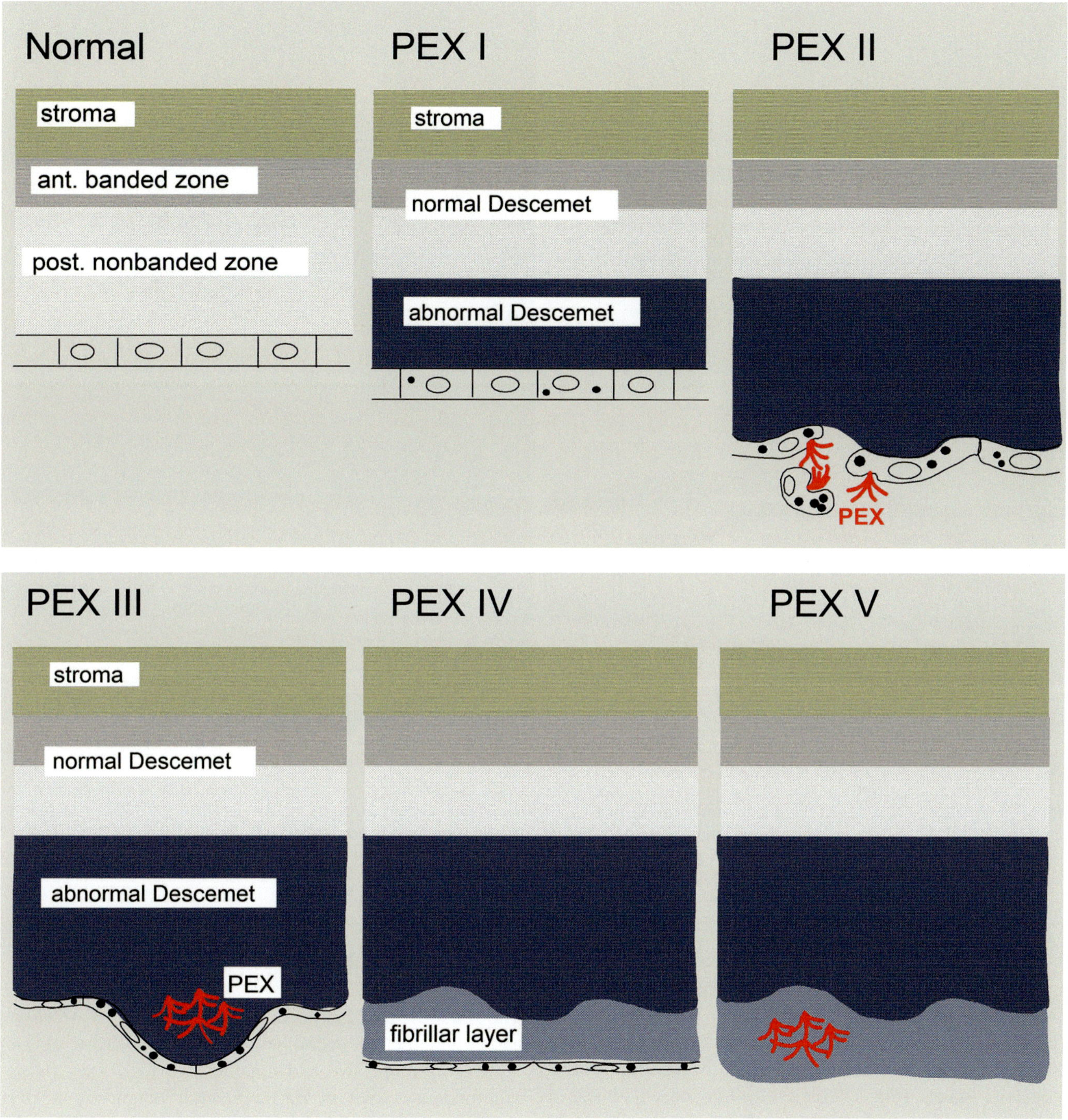

Fig. 5 Schematic representation of gradual alterations of the corneal endothelium and Descemet membrane (DM) in PEX keratopathy proceeding from stage 1 to 5 compared with the normal structure. (I) Production of an abnormal posterior banded layer of DM by diseased endothelial cells, accompanied by phagocytosis of pigment granules; (II) thickening of the abnormal posterior banded zone and production of PEX fibrils by detaching, melanin-containing endothelial cells along their apical surface; (III) incorporation of PEX material into Descemet membrane by overgrowing fibroblast-like endothelial cells; (IV) additional production of a posterior fibrillar layer by fibroblast-like endothelial cells; (V) degeneration and loss of endothelial cells leaving a denuded, thickened Descemet membrane containing focal PEX aggregates

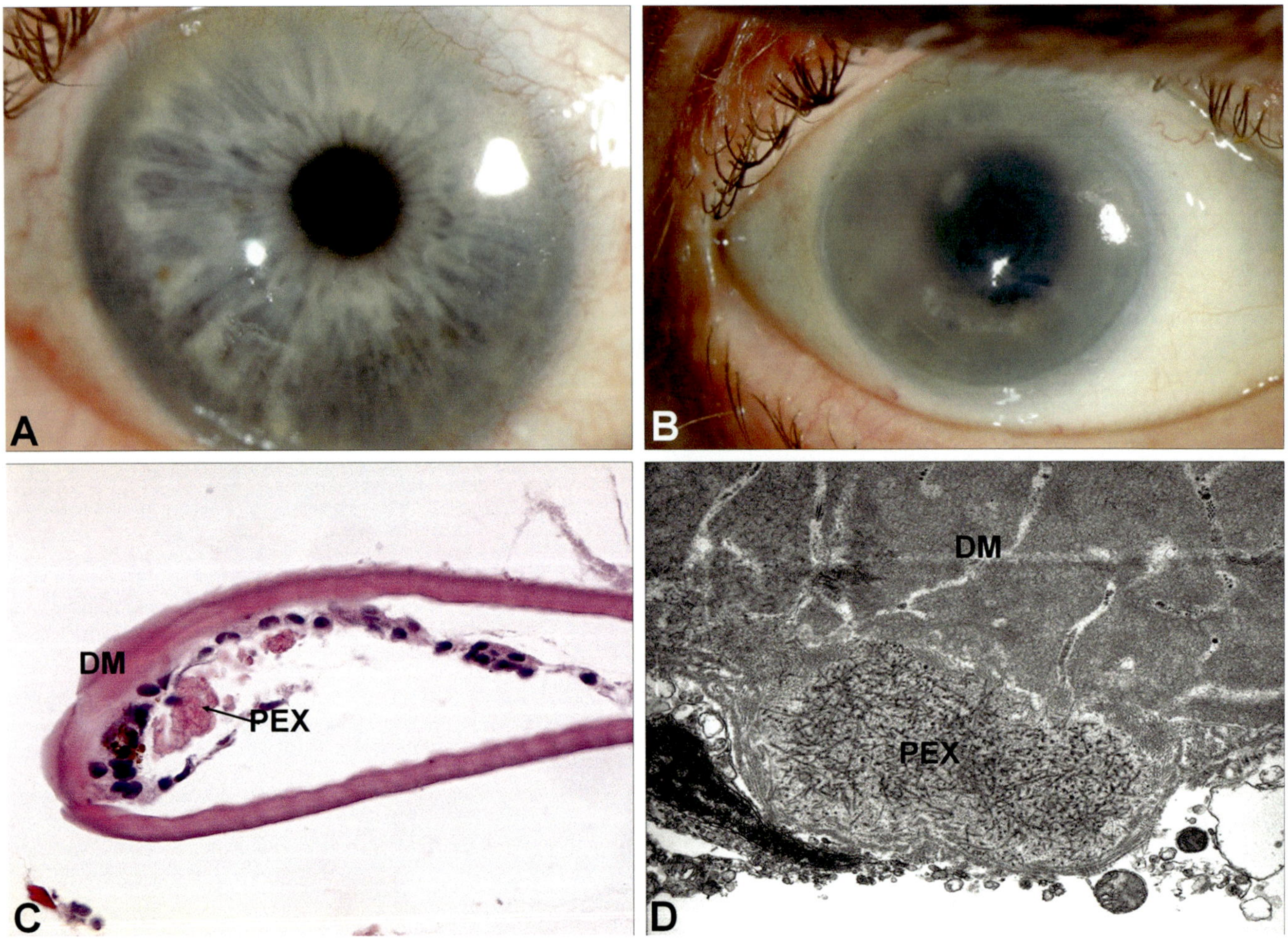

Fig. 6 Preexisting PEX syndrome in donor corneas used for Descemet membrane endothelial keratoplasty (DMEK). (**A**), (**B**) A 74-year-old patient with Fuchs dystrophy before (**A**) and 3 months after DMEK (**B**) with primary graft failure. (**C**), (**D**) Light microscopic (**C**) and electron microscopic (**D**) appearance of explanted DMEK graft showing retrocorneal deposits of PEX material, in association with pigmented endothelial cells, indicating the presence of PEX keratopathy in the donor

– Fibroblastic transformation of attenuated endothelial cells depositing an additional posterior fibrillar layer onto DM.

The slowly progressing morphological alterations of endothelium and DM in PEX keratopathy could be graded into five sequential stages (Fig. 5): (I) Production of an abnormal posterior banded layer of DM by diseased and attenuated endothelial cells; (II) further thickening of the abnormal posterior banded zone and focal production of PEX fibrils by detaching, melanin-containing endothelial cells along their apical surface; (III) incorporation of PEX fiber aggregates into DM by overgrowth of neighboring fibroblast-like endothelial cells; (IV) additional deposition of a posterior fibrillar layer by fibroblast-like endothelial cells; and (V) progressive loss of endothelial cells leaving a denuded, thickened Descemet membrane containing focal PEX aggregates.

2.3 Clinical Relevance

The endothelial dysfunction may explain a relatively early endothelial decompensation, which can develop both in normotensive and hypertensive PEX eyes following moderate rises in IOP, e.g. after diagnostic mydriasis [7]. Lowering of IOP may lead to corneal clearing, but additional damage to the compromised endothelium, e.g. by minor intraoperative trauma, may lead to endothelial decompensation. Since the threshold for an intraoperative endothelial trauma is much lower and the probability of a postoperative endothelial decompensation is much higher in PEX eyes than in non-PEX eyes, an accurate diagnosis is important to avoid intra- and post-operative complications. The percentage of endothelial cell loss was significantly greater in PEX eyes (9.0%) than in controls (3.4%) 1 and

Table 1 Clinical and histopathological differential diagnosis of Fuchs endothelial corneal dystrophy and pseudoexfoliation (PEX) keratopathy

	PEX keratopathy	Fuchs dystrophy
Clinical signs		
Manifestation	Bilateral asymmetric	Bilateral asymmetric
Age of onset	60–70 years	50–60 years
Female: male ratio	2: 1	3–4: 1
Posterior corneal surface	Hyperreflective deposits	Guttae
Pigment dispersion	+++	+
Endothelial cell loss	+++	++
Pleomorphism, polymegethism	+++	++
Decompensation pattern	Diffuse	Central
Histopathological features		
Descemet membrane	Diffusely thickened with focal irregular protrusions	Thickened with free or buried guttae
Thickness of Descemet membrane	16–45 μm	14–30 μm
Posterior fibrillar layer	(++)	(++)
PEX fibrils	+++	–
Melanin phagocytosis	+++	+
Fibroblastic transformation	+++	++

+ = mild; ++ = moderate; +++ = marked; – = absent

3 months postoperatively and was associated with a greater increase in CCT [28–30]. However, 6–7 years after cataract surgery, no statistically significant differences in ECD and CCT between eyes with and without PEX were observed [31]. In a 10-year single-center, retrospective cohort study, eyes with PEX had significantly higher rates of corneal edema following cataract surgery [32]. Corneal decompensation following filtering surgery with the ExPRESS mini glaucoma shunt device has been also described in PEX eyes [33]. Thus, the corneal endotheliopathy may potentiate the known complications of anterior segment surgery in PEX eyes, and preoperative assessment of endothelial status and close postoperative follow-up is recommended.

In advanced stages of disease, irreversible corneal endothelial decompensation may occur and present an indication for corneal transplantation, either full-thickness keratoplasty or posterior lamellar keratoplasty [34, 35]. However, the proportion of patients requiring corneal endothelial transplantation is low (in our Department 2.3% in 2010–2011) compared to patients with FECD. Still, DMEK has been reported effective for the treatment of endothelial dysfunction in PEX patients [35]. In 6 eyes with PEX undergoing DMEK, there was no primary graft failure, and none of the patients required re-bubbling. When outcomes were compared with FECD (n = 8), no statistical difference was observed in CCT. However, postoperative visual acuity was significantly worse, as was ECD, in the PEX than in the FECD group at 1, 3 and 4 months postoperatively. Differences remained statistically significant even after adjustment for age. These differences may be related to an increased breakdown of the blood-aqueous barrier in PEX eyes. Elevated cytokine levels, including pro-inflammatory cytokines and pro-fibrotic growth factors, in the aqueous humor may facilitate enhanced degeneration and apoptosis of endothelial cells.

Another issue of clinical relevance is the suitability of cornea donor tissue from PEX eyes for corneal transplantation. Because of a pre-damaged corneal endothelium the transplants may more frequently lead to graft failure. In one study, 1/7 cases of primary graft failure was due to preexisting PEX in the donor cornea [36] (Fig. 6). Moreover, in more than 10 patients suffering from keratoconus requiring penetrating keratoplasty at less than 40 years of age, who had received donor tissues beyond 75 years of age, we and others observed postoperative development of intraocular PEX manifestations in the operated eye [37, 38]. This may be a peculiar coincidence or a reaction to surgery, but may also indicate that PEX is a transmissible disease. As a practical consequence, corneas from donors suffering from advanced PEX syndrome may be less suitable for corneal transplantation.

3 PEX Keratopathy Versus Fuchs Dystrophy

In a consecutive series of 2238 penetrating corneal grafts from 1995 to 2003 in our Department, 72 (3.2%) were diagnosed with histopathologically confirmed PEX keratopathy (unpublished data). PEX keratopathy may have been previously misdiagnosed as "atypical non-guttate Fuchs dystrophy". Abbott et al. [6] described 6 patients with unilateral endothelial dysfunction, reduced endothelial cell counts and corneal edema, differing histologically from FECD, and suggested that they represent either a variant of FECD or a form of endothelial disease of unknown etiology. More recently, non-guttate FECD was also suggested to cause progressive unilateral corneal endothelial failure of unknown etiology in 11 patients [39]. However, a case report on two patients with bullous keratopathy of unknown etiology showed that PEX keratopathy was the underlying cause [40]. A subsequent small-scale survey in Japan reported that the number of diagnosed PEX keratopathy among all cases with bullous keratopathy of unknown etiology increased from 36.4 to 58.8% within 3 years [16]. In view of the increased life expectancy of populations, the prevalence of PEX keratopathy is expected to continue to further increase.

FECD, in contrast, is the most common form of corneal endothelial dystrophy. This bilateral asymmetric disease typically occurs around the age of 50–60 years and with a greater incidence in women than men at a ratio of 3–4:1 [41]. It is characterized by a progressive loss of corneal endothelial cells, which is associated with increased variations in size and shape as well as transition of endothelial cells into a fibroblast-like phenotype (endothelial-to-mesenchymal transition), causing corneal edema. The diseased endothelial cells produce an abnormally thickened DM with circumscribed drop-like excrescences, termed guttae, which represent the clinical and histopathologic hallmark of FECD. In advanced stages, the guttae can be buried by a posterior fibrillar layer deposited onto DM by fibroblast-like endothelial cells.

Although FECD and PEX keratopathy share certain features, both endotheliopathies can be differentiated clinically and histopathologically, mainly by the presence or lack of typical guttae or typical PEX fibrils (Table 1). Clinical examination of FECD patients using slit-lamp biomicroscopy, specular microscopy or confocal microscopy shows the presence of individual and/or confluent guttae, variable amounts of pigmentation of the posterior cornea, and alterations in endothelial cell morphology and density, predominantly in the corneal centre causing a predominantly central corneal edema (Fig. 7A). This pattern of corneal edema can be distinguished from the diffuse corneal edema in PEX eyes, which is often associated with the presence of hyperreflective deposits and pronounced pigment dispersion on the posterior surface (Fig. 7B). ECD reduction is less progressive in FECD, and cell counts were reported to be 16% less than in age-matched controls, but 21% less in PEX eyes and even 35% less in PEX glaucoma eyes [10].

Histopathologically, FECD is characterized by abnormal thickening of DM and formation of guttae as well as a less pronounced endothelial cell loss, fibroblastic transformation, and pigment phagocytosis of endothelial cells (Fig. 7C, E). Diffuse, irregular thickening of DM is more pronounced in PEX keratopathy with focal irregular protrusions but no typical guttae formations. In particular, foci of typical PEX fibrils can be occasionally found in association with heavily pigmented, detaching endothelial cells on and/or within DM (Fig. 7D, F). Additional formation of a posterior fibrillar layer by fibroblast-like endothelial cells can occur in advanced stages of both PEX keratopathy and FECD, as it represents an unspecific sign of endothelial-to-mesenchymal transition in response to stress and progressive cell loss.

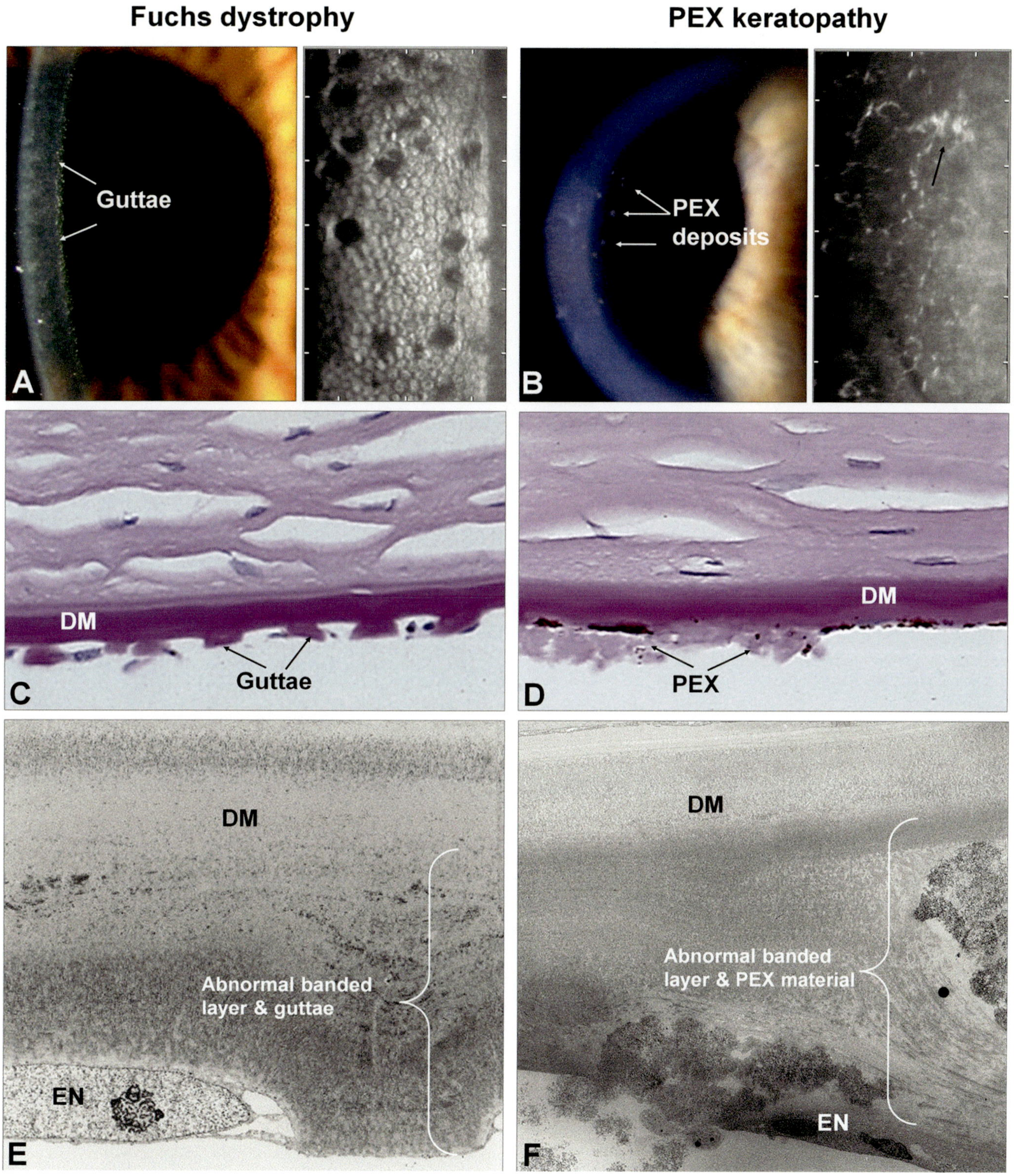

Fig. 7 Clinical and histopathological differential diagnosis between Fuchs corneal dystrophy and PEX keratopathy. (**A**) Typical guttae of Descemet membrane in Fuchs dystrophy shown by slit-lamp biomicroscopy and confocal microscopy. (**B**) Retrocorneal PEX deposits in PEX keratopathy shown by slit-lamp biomicroscopy and confocal microscopy. (**C**) Light micrograph showing abnormal Descemet membrane (DM) with typical guttae in Fuchs dystrophy. (**D**) Light micrograph showing focal PEX material accumulations and hyperpigmented fibroblastic endothelial cells in PEX keratopathy. (**E**, **F**) Transmission electron micrographs showing abnormal posterior banded layer of DM with typical guttae in Fuchs dystrophy (**E**) and inclusions of PEX material in PEX keratopathy (**F**) (EN, endothelium)

4 Conclusion

PEX keratopathy should be taken into consideration as one possible cause for corneal edema of unknown etiology. Compared to FECD, it represents a relatively rare indication for corneal endothelial transplantation, but a rather frequent risk factor for cataract and glaucoma surgery in PEX patients. The implications of PEX on the corneal endothelium are clinically relevant, predisposing to early corneal decompensation after intraocular surgery and highlighting the importance of preoperative assessment of the corneal endothelial status in PEX patients. Intraoperatively, the use of a dispersive viscoelastic material that coats and protects the corneal endothelial surface may be considered. In vivo confocal microscopy, showing reduced ECD and hyperreflective deposits, is a useful tool to assist in proper diagnosis even at early stages of disease. The use of corneal buttons from donors with PEX syndrome may be questioned.

References

1. Schlötzer-Schrehardt U, Naumann GOH. Perspective—ocular and systemic pseudoexfoliation syndrome. Am J Ophthalmol. 2006;141:921–37.
2. Ritch R, Schlötzer-Schrehardt U. Exfoliation syndrome. Surv Ophthalmol. 2001;45(4):265–315.
3. Schlötzer-Schrehardt U. Molecular biology of exfoliation syndrome. J Glaucoma. 2018;27(Suppl 1):S32–7.
4. Conway RM, Schlötzer-Schrehardt U, Küchle M, Naumann GO. Pseudoexfoliation syndrome: pathological manifestations of relevance to intraocular surgery. Clin Exp Ophthalmol. 2004;32(2):199–210.
5. Chung H, Arora S, Damji KF, Weis E. Association of pseudoexfoliation syndrome with cardiovascular and cerebrovascular disease: a systematic review and meta-analysis. Can J Ophthalmol. 2018;53(4):365–72.
6. Abbott RL, Fine BS, Webster RG Jr, Paglen PG, Spencer WH. Specular microscopic and histologic observations in nonguttate corneal endothelial degeneration. Ophthalmology. 1981;88(8):788–800.
7. Naumann GOH, Schlötzer-Schrehardt U. Keratopathy in pseudoexfoliation syndrome as a cause of corneal endothelial decompensation. Ophthalmology. 2000;107:1111–24.
8. Chern KC, Meisler DM, Rockwood EJ, Lowder CY. Pseudoexfoliation syndrome masquerading as uveitis. Am J Ophthalmol. 1994;118:392–3.
9. Miyake K, Matsuda M, Inaba M. Corneal endothelial changes in pseudoexfoliation syndrome. Am J Ophthalmol. 1989;108:49–52.
10. Knorr HLJ, Jünemann A, Händel A, Naumann GOH. Morphometrische und qualitative Veränderungen des Hornhautendothels bei Pseudoexfoliations-syndrom. Fortschr Ophthalmol. 1991;88:786–9.
11. Seitz B, Müller EE, Langenbucher A, Kus MM, Naumann GO. Endothelial keratopathy in pseudoexfoliation syndrome: quantitative and qualitative morphometry using automated video image analysis. Klin Monbl Augenheilkd. 1995;207:167–75.
12. Wang L, Yamasita R, Hommura S. Corneal endothelial changes and aqueous flare intensity in pseudoexfoliation syndrome. Ophthalmologica. 1999;213(6):387–91.
13. Inoue K, Okugawa K, Oshika T, Amano S. Morphological study of corneal endothelium and corneal thickness in pseudoexfoliation syndrome. Jpn J Ophthalmol. 2003;47(3):235–9.
14. Wali UK, Bialasiewicz AA, Rizvi SG, Al-Belushi H. In vivo morphometry of corneal endothelial cells in pseudoexfoliation keratopathy with glaucoma and cataract. Ophthalmic Res. 2009;41(3):175–9.
15. Sbeity Z, Palmiero PM, Tello C, Liebmann JM, Ritch R. Non-contact in vivo confocal scanning laser microscopy in exfoliation syndrome, exfoliation syndrome suspect and normal eyes. Acta Ophthalmol. 2011;89(3):241–7.
16. Zheng X. New findings for an old disease: morphological studies on pseudoexfoliation syndrome-related keratopathy and binocular asymmetry. Cornea. 2013;32(Suppl 1):S84–90.
17. Palko JR, Qi O, Sheybani A. Corneal alterations associated with pseudoexfoliation syndrome and glaucoma: a literature review. J Ophthalmic Vis Res. 2017;12(3):312–24.
18. Wang M, Sun W, Ying L, Dong XG. Corneal endothelial cell density and morphology in Chinese patients with pseudoexfoliation syndrome. Int J Ophthalmol. 2012;5(2):186–9.
19. Tomaszewski BT, Zalewska R, Mariak Z. Evaluation of the endothelial cell density and the central corneal thickness in pseudoexfoliation syndrome and pseudoexfoliation glaucoma. J Ophthalmol. 2014;2014:123683.
20. Zimmermann N, Wünscher M, Schlötzer-Schrehardt U, Erb C. Corneal endothelial cell density and its correlation with the severity of pseudoexfoliation. Klin Monbl Augenheilkd. 2014;231(2):158–63.
21. Sarowa S, Manoher JM, Jain K, Singhal Y, Devathia D. Qualitative and quantitative changes of corneal endothelial cells and central corneal thickness in pseudoexfoliation syndrome and pseudoexfoliation glaucoma. Int J Med Sci Public Health. 2016;5:2526–30.
22. Aoki T, Kitazawa K, Inatomi T, Kusada N, Horiuchi N, Takeda K, Yokoi N, Kinoshita S, Sotozono C. Risk factors for corneal endothelial cell loss in patients with pseudoexfoliation syndrome. Sci Rep. 2020;10(1):7260.
23. Zheng X, Shiraishi A, Okuma S, Mizoue S, Goto T, Kawasaki S, Uno T, Miyoshi T, Ruggeri A, Ohashi Y. In vivo confocal microscopic evidence of keratopathy in patients with pseudoexfoliation syndrome. Invest Ophthalmol Vis Sci. 2011;52(3):1755–61.
24. Kocabeyoglu S, Mocan MC, Irkec M, Karakaya J. In vivo confocal microscopic evaluation of corneas in patients with exfoliation syndrome. J Glaucoma. 2016;25(2):193–7.
25. Yüksel N, Emre E, Pirhan D. Evaluation of corneal microstructure in pseudoexfoliation syndrome and glaucoma: in vivo scanning laser confocal microscopic study. Curr Eye Res. 2016;41(1):34–40.
26. Terracciano L, Cennamo M, Favuzza E, Julia L, Caporossi O, Mencucci R. An in vivo confocal microscopy study of corneal changes in pseudoexfoliation syndrome. Eur J Ophthalmol. 2019;29(5):555–60.
27. Schlötzer-Schrehardt U, Dörfler S, Naumann GOH. Corneal endothelial involvement in pseudoexfoliation syndrome. Arch Ophthalmol. 1993;111:666–74.
28. Kaljurand K, Teesalu P. Exfoliation syndrome as a risk factor for corneal endothelial cell loss in cataract surgery. Ann Ophthalmol (Skokie). 2007 Winter;39(4):327–33.
29. Hayashi K, Manabe S, Yoshimura K, Kondo H. Corneal endothelial damage after cataract surgery in eyes with pseudoexfoliation syndrome. J Cataract Refract Surg. 2013;39(6):881–7.

30. Hasegawa Y, Nejima R, Mori Y, Sakisaka T, Minami K, Miyata K, Oshika T. Risk factors for corneal endothelial cell loss by cataract surgery in eyes with pseudoexfoliation syndrome. Clin Ophthalmol. 2016;30(10):1685–9.
31. Ostern AE, Drolsum L. Corneal endothelial cells 6–7 years following cataract surgery in patients with pseudoexfoliation syndrome. Acta Ophthalmol. 2012;90(5):408–11.
32. Ong AY, Shalchi Z. Outcomes of cataract surgery in pseudoexfoliation syndrome in England: 10-year retrospective cohort study. J Cataract Refract Surg. 2021;47(2):165–71.
33. Tojo N, Hayashi A, Miyakoshi A. Corneal decompensation following filtering surgery with the Ex-PRESS(®) mini glaucoma shunt device. Clin Ophthalmol. 2015;17(9):499–502.
34. Nguyen NX, Lattermann V, Schlötzer-Schrehardt U, Seitz B. Functional outcomes after penetrating keratoplasty in pseudoexfoliation syndrome (PEX)-keratopathy. Klin Monbl Augenheilkd. 2004;221:819–24.
35. Tase S, Shimizu T, Hayashi T, Tabuchi H, Niimi K, Mizuki N, Kato N. Descemet's membrane endothelial keratoplasty for pseudoexfoliation syndrome: a case series. BMC Ophthalmol. 2019;19(1):119.
36. Ćirković A, Schlötzer-Schrehardt U, Weller JM, Kruse FE, Tourtas T. Clinical and ultrastructural characteristics of graft failure in DMEK: 1-year results after repeat DMEK. Cornea. 2015;34(1):11–7.
37. Küchle M, Naumann GOH. Occurrence of pseudoexfoliation following penetrating keratoplasty for Keratoconus. Br J Ophthalmol. 1992;76:98–100.
38. Milioti G, Löw U, Gatzioufas Z, Ninios K, Schirra F, Seitz B. Early manifestation of a pseudoexfoliation syndrom after a cornea transplantation. Klin Monbl Augenheilkd. 2011;228(3):249–51.
39. Lee WH, Tey A, Gales K, Mudhar HS, Figueiredo FC. Progressive idiopathic unilateral corneal endothelial failure of unknown aetiology in phakic eyes. Br J Ophthalmol. 2018;102(12):1634–9.
40. Zheng X, Inoue Y, Shiraishi A, Hara Y, Goto T, Ohashi Y. In vivo confocal microscopic and histological findings of unknown bullous keratopathy probably associated with pseudoexfoliation syndrome. BMC Ophthalmol. 2012;22(12):17.
41. Ong Tone S, Kocaba V, Böhm M, Wylegala A, White TL, Jurkunas UV. Fuchs endothelial corneal dystrophy: the vicious cycle of Fuchs pathogenesis. Prog Retin Eye Res. 2021;80:100863.

Monoclonal Gammopathies of Undetermined Significance (MGUS)—The Role of the Cornea Specialist

Walter Lisch

Abstract

The appearance of chameleon-like corneal opacities in monoclonal gammopathies (MG) is not well known in Ophthalmology. Today, the hematologists distinguish between three forms of MG: Multiple Myeloma (MM); Smoldering Multiple Meloma (SMM) and Monoclonal Gammopathy of Undetermined Significance (MGUS). MGUS and SMM are percursors of MM and are asymptomatic disorders from the hematological view. MGUS is a hidden disorder and one of the most common premalignant disorders in Western countries, with a prevalence of 3.2% in the white general population 50 years of age or older. However, in MGUS there are many corneal opacities from the ophthalmological view, which can also reduce the visual acuity. The purpose of this chapter was to show four patients with distinct corneal opacities that enabled the hematological diagnosis of MGUS.

Keywords

Monoclonal gammopathies · MGUS · Distinct corneal opacities · Lattice corneal dystrophy · Occurrence

1 Introduction

According to a 1984 study by Kyle et al. [1], monoclonal gammopathies can be divided into systemic monoclonal gammopathy, such as multiple myeloma (MM) and similar diseases, and MGUS formerly known as benign monoclonal gammopathy. The International Myeloma Working Group defined three criteria for the diagnosis of MGUS: (1) M protein concentration in serum of 3 g/dL or less, (2) a proportion of plasma cells in the bone marrow of 10% or less, and (3) absence of lytic bone lesions, anemia, hypercalcemia, and renal insufficiency (so-called CRAB lesions) related to the proliferation of monoclonal plasma cells [2].

Smoldering (asymptomatic) multiple myeloma (SMM) needs to be distinguished from MGUS because of a higher risk of progression to MM. Among 21,463 residents of Olmsted County, Minnesota, MGUS was found in 694 (3.2%) [1]. The isotype of the monoclonal immunoglobulin was IgG in 68.9% of the 694 patients with MGUS, IgM in 17.2%, IgA in 10.8%, and biclonal in 3.0%. Regrettably, however, no slit lamp examination of the cornea was performed. At the end of their article Kyle et al. [1] wrote that the presented study is "generally representative of the white population of the United States." Bourne examined with the group of Kyle et al. 100 random patients with MM at the slit lamp and saw only in one patient corneal crystals [3]. They concluded that the examination on the slit lamp is not useful in screening of monoclonal gammopathies. This statement may be not correct in view of the following case reports.

2 Corneal Involvement in Monoclonal Gammopathies

The initial description of corneal noncrystalline deposits in association with paraproteinemia was by Meesmann in 1934 in the setting of MM [4]. Blobner was the first to describe crystalline deposits in the whole cornea associated with a paraproteinemia [5]. In 1958, Bürki reported a patient with MM and bilateral corneal crystals [6]. The definitive evidence that corneal crystals in gammopathies are immunoglobulins was demonstrated by Klintworth et al. in 1978 using immunofluorescence and immunoperoxidase techniques [7]. The earlier ophthalmological opinion was that the classic corneal involvement consists only of bilateral crystals in

W. Lisch (✉)
Hanau, Germany
e-mail: prof.dr.lisch@augenklinik-hanau.de

B. Seitz et al. (eds.), *Atlas on Cornea*, https://doi.org/10.1007/978-3-031-65422-0_20

Table 1 There are 51, mostly singular cases of MGUS- or SMM-induced PPK in the literature from 1934 to 2015

Patients	First and wrong diagnosis		MGUS- or SMM-induced PPK
29	Schnyder CD or cystinosis	+	Crystalline-like PPK
9	Lattice CD	+	Lattice-like PPK
4	Granular CD	+	Granular-like PPK
15	Keratitis/Scleritis	+	Peripheral band-like PPK
9	Brown discoloration of Descemet membrane	+ and Hypercupremia	Lewis syndrome [9]
4	Stromal CD	+	Stromal-flake-like PPK
1	Reis–Bücklers CD	+	Geographic-like PPK
4	Cornea verticillata (Fabry disease or drug-induced)	+	Verticillata-like PPK

SPE Serum-Protein-Electrophoresis; *MGUS* Monoclonal Gammopathy of Undetermined Significance; *SMM* Smoldering Multiple Myeloma; *CD* Corneal Dystrophy; *PPK* Paraproteinemic Keratopathy

MM or rarely in the so-called benign monoclonal gammopathies, often combined with diffuse stromal opacities. In 1991, Steuhl et al. reported about such connections [8].

3 Paraproteinemic Keratopathy (PPK) in Form of Distinct Corneal Opacities in MGUS and SMM

From 1934 to 2015, there have been 51 different publications in the world literature, mostly isolated cases of MGUS or SMM-induced PPK. The first diagnosis was either a different form of corneal dystrophy or an inflammatory disorder but not the correct diagnosis in the sense of a distinct paraproteinemic keratopathy (Table 1).

We will provide four examples of corneal involvement in elderly patients that the ophthalmologist submitted the patient with suspicious corneal diagnosis to the hematology to perform a Serum-Protein-Electrophoresis (SPE) to confirm or exclude a paraproteinemic keratopathy (PPK).

4 Suspicious Corneal Opacities May Lead to the Hematological Diagnosis of MGUS or SMM

4.1 Case 1

82-year-old female patient showing the aspect of Lattice corneal dystrophy (LCD) (Fig. 1). LCD is an autosomal dominant inherited disorder. Therefore, our question to the patient was if other affected members of the cornea exist in her family. There were no other family members. Our first diagnosis was either a new mutation of LCD or PPK. The costs of Serum-Protein-Electrophoresis (SPE) are much cheaper than the DNA analysis. That is why we submitted the patient to the clinic of Hematology to perform a SPE. The result was positive and we could diagnose MGUS-induced Lattice-like PPK. The consequence of our diagnosis is a regular check once a year hematologically and ophthalmologically. There are some publications with regard to Lattice-like PPK [10, 11].

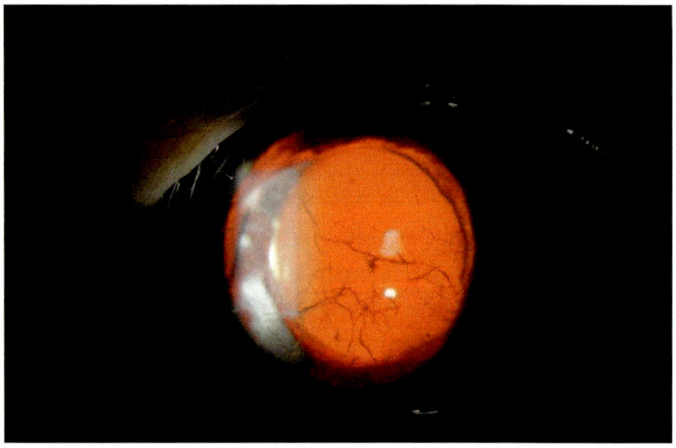

Fig. 1 82-year-old female patient with Lattice-like paraproteinemic keratopathy in indirect illumination. MGUS after Serum-Protein-Electrophoresis (SPE). After posterior phakoemulsification and artificial posterior lens implantation

4.2 Case 2

62-year-old male patient (from Tero Kivelä, Helsinki) showing the aspect of anterior reticulated corneal opacification (Fig. 2A, B). The slit lamp examination could exclude a Lattice corneal dystrophy (LCD). There were no affected family members of the cornea in his family. The patient was submitted to the clinic of Hematology to perform a SPE to confirm or exclude a monoclonal gammopathy. The hematological result was MGUS and the Finish ophthalmologists could diagnose MGUS-induced reticulated-like PPK. It is a new type with regard to the new classification of MGUS-induced PPK [12]. Duke-Elder presented in his System of Ophthalmology 1977 in Vol VIII, Part 2 on page 926 an own chapter about "Superficial Reticular Dystrophy of Koby [13]. This disorder is probably equal with Reticular-like PPK.

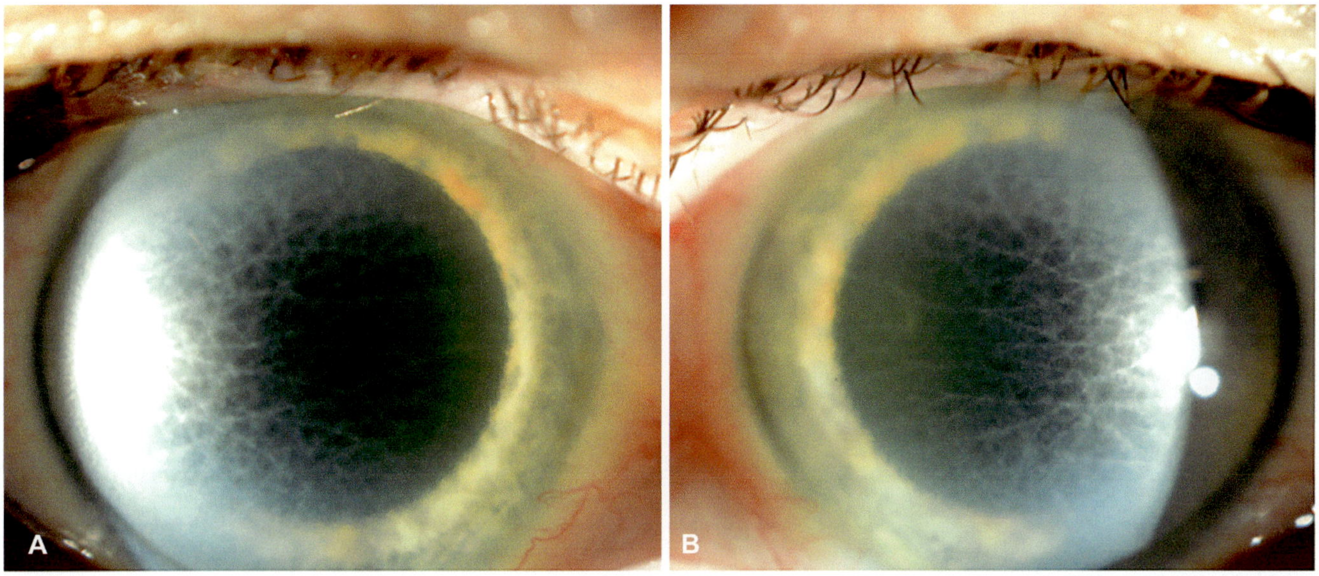

Fig. 2 (**A**) (Photograph courtesy of Tero Kivelä, MD). 62-year-old male patient. Right eye: Reticular-like paraproteinemic keratopathy (SPE-MGUS). (**B**) (Photograph courtesy of Tero Kivelä, MD). 62-year-old male patient. Left eye: Reticular-like paraproteinemic keratopathy (SPE-MGUS)

4.3 Case 3

63-year-old female patient came to the ophthalmologist because she suffered from constant bilateral red eye. My early diagnosis would be: peripheral lipid keratopathy. The patient was very scared. After much hesitation, she agreed to undergo a hematological examination. The hematological result was SMM and we could diagnose SMM-induced mild elevated peripheral band-like PPK (Fig. 3A, B) [12]. The hematologists discussed a probable systemic chemotherapy. There was an improvement of the bilateral red eye during the systemic therapy, but not of the peripheral corneal involvement. The red eye was interpreted as foreign body irritation as a result of the elevated peripheral corneal band.

4.4 Case 4

64-year-old female who suffered from a mild deterioration of her right visual acuity. The BCVA right was 0.8. The BCVA left was 1.0. The first Ophthalmologist interpreted that as an unspecific age-related deterioration. The slit lamp examination disclosed a mild and diffuse opacification of the corneal stroma (Fig. 4). We suggested to perform a hematological examination. The hematological result was MGUS and we could diagnose MGUS-induced mild, stromal-like PPK. Six monthly ophthalmological and hematological check-ups were suggested.

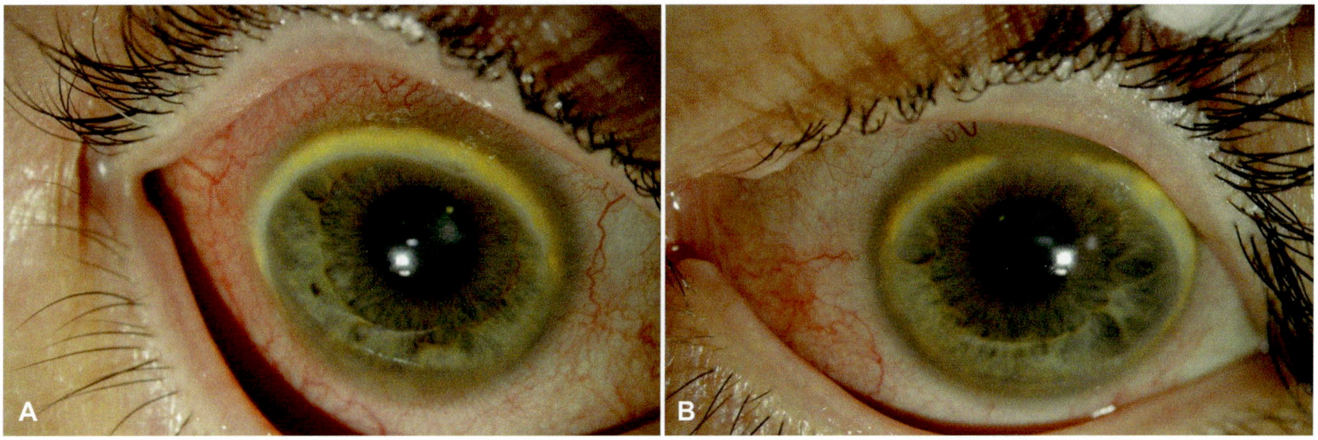

Fig. 3 (**A**) 63-year-old female patient. Right eye: red conjunctiva and peripheral band-like (particularly above) paraproteinemic keratopathy (SPE-SMM). Constant red eye. (**B**) 63-year-old female patient. Left eye: red conjunctiva and peripheral band-like paraproteinemic keratopathy (SPE-SMM). Constant red eye

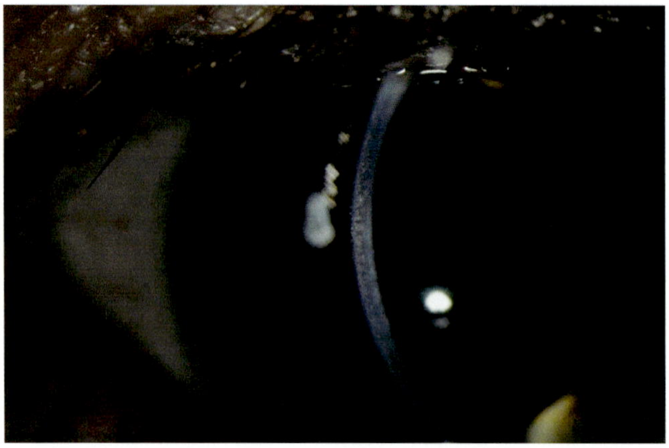

Fig. 4 64-year-old female patient. Right eye: very mild diffuse opacities of corneal stroma disclosing diffuse stromal-like paraproteinemic keratopathy (SPE-MGUS)

5 Occurrence of MGUS and PPK-Induced Patient Opacites

In my opinion, the hemo-epidemiologiocal studies on MGUS and MGUS-induced PPK are very vague. For example, the Southern California hematologists were unable to provide me with any relevant information about the incidence of MGUS and MGUS-induced PPK. To report uncertain numbers, I refer to the epidemiological study by Kyle et al. [1].

I try to calculate:

For Germany	81.6 million inhabitants
	36.5 million inhabitants older than 50 years
	1.2 (3%) million MGUS
	12,000 (1%) inhabitants with MGUS-induced PPK?
For USA	46,000 (1%) inhabitants with MGUS-induced PPK?

There are authors who suggest the new term "Monoclonal gammopathy of ocular significance" [14].

6 Conclusion

Today, MGUS-induced PPK is diagnosed much more frequently than previously. Every MGUS patients should be submitted from the hematologist to the ophthalmologist for slit lamp examination to find out a normal cornea or a specific corneal involvement in the sense of MGUS-induced PPK. The ophthalmologist should submit any older patient with unclear corneal changes to a hematologist with the question of a monoclonal gammopathy. However, it should be avoided as far as possible to diagnose a corneal finding as a degenerative, age-related change without having previously performed an SPE with the hematologist to rule out a MGUS-induced PPK. It is known today, that the MGUS-performed corneal changes can be very subtle!

Close collaboration between Hematology and Ophthalmology seems necessary to better assess the incidence of MGUS and MGUS-induced PPK [15].

References

1. Kyle RA, Therneau TM, Rajkumar SV, et al. Prevalence of monoclonal gammopathy of undetermined significance. N Engl J Med. 2006;345:1362–9.
2. International Myeloma Working Group. Criteria for the classification of monoclonal gammopathies, multiple myeloma and related disorders: a report of the International Myeloma Working Group. Br J Ophthalmol. 2003;121:749–57.
3. Bourne WM, Kyle RA, Brubacker RF, Greip PR. Incidence of corneal crystals in the monoclonal gammopathies. Am J Ophthalmol. 1989;107:192–3.
4. Meesmann A. Über eine eigenartige Hornhautdegeneration (?) (Ablagerung des Bence-Jones-schen Eiweisskörpers in der Hornhaut). Ber Dtsch Ophthalmol Ges. 1934;50:311–5.
5. Blobner F. Kristallinische Degeneration der Bindehaut und Hornhaut. Klin Monbl Augenheilkd. 1938;100:588–93.
6. Bürki E. Über Hornhautveränderungen bei einem Fall von multiplem Myelom (Plasmacytom). Ophthalmologica. 1958;135:566–72.
7. Klintworth GK, Bredehoeft SJ, Reed JW. Analysis of corneal crystalline deposits in multiple myeloma. Am J Ophthalmol. 1978;86:303–13.
8. Steuhl K-P, Knorr M, Rohrbach JM, et al. Paraproteinemic corneal deposits in plasma cell myeloma. Am J Ophthalmol. 1991;111:312–8.
9. Lisch W, Vossmerbäumer U. Corneal opacity and copper levels of the Lewis syndrome after systemic chemotherapy. Am J Ophthalmol Case Rep. 2020;20:100926.
10. Spiegel P, Grossniklaus HE, Reinhart WJ, Thomas RH. Unusual presentation of paraproteinemic corneal infiltrates. Cornea. 1990;9:81–5.
11. Lisch W, Saikia P, Pitz S, et al. Chameleon-like appearance of immunotactoid keratopathy. Cornea. 2012;31:55–8.
12. Lisch W, Wasielica-Poslednik J, Kivelä T, et al. The hematological definition of monoclonal gammopathy of undetermined significance in relation to paraproteinemic keratopathy (An American Ophthalmological Society Thesis). Trans Am Ophthalmol Soc. 2016;114:T7(1–21).
13. Duke-Elder S. Superficial reticular dystrophy of Koby. Syst Ophthalmol. 1977; VIII(Part 2):926.
14. Karakus S, Gottsch JD, Caturegjh P, Eghrari AO. Monoclonal gammopathy of ocular significance. Am J Ophthalmol Case Rep. 2019;15:100471.
15. Szentmáry N, Kormányos K, Gábor T, et al. Szewèszeti tümetek és szemészeti társbetegségek monoklonális gammopathiával járó kórbépehben. Hematològia - Transfeeziológia. 2021;54:82–8.

Limbal Stem Cell Deficiency

Ursula Schlötzer-Schrehardt and Friedrich E. Kruse

Abstract

Regeneration and repair of the corneal epithelium rely on a population of stem cells residing in the basal epithelial layer at the corneoscleral limbus within a specialized niche microenvironment. Damage to or dysfunction of this population lead to limbal stem cell deficiency (LSCD), a rare but debilitating and potentially blinding ocular surface disease, that can be caused by many hereditary and acquired conditions, most frequently ocular burns. Management of LSCD requires an accurate diagnosis including staging of LSCD severity using clinical, laboratory and in vivo-imaging techniques. A variety of medical and surgical procedures, which transfer autologous or allogeneic stem cells onto the diseased eyes of LSCD patients, have been developed and clinically validated to reconstitute the corneal epithelium. Given some limitations of established procedures, novel therapeutic approaches are needed. In this chapter, we will discuss the etiology, demographics, clinical manifestation, classification, diagnosis as well as current and future treatment modalities of LSCD.

Keywords

Limbal stem cells · Limbal stem cell deficiency · Limbal stem cell transplantation · CLET · COMET · Corneal epithelium

U. Schlötzer-Schrehardt (✉) · F. E. Kruse
Department of Ophthalmology, Friedrich-Alexander University of Erlangen-Nürnberg, Erlangen, Germany
e-mail: ursula.schloetzer-schrehardt@uk-erlangen.de

F. E. Kruse
e-mail: friedrich.kruse@uk-erlangen.de

1 Limbal Stem Cells and Their Niche

The corneal epithelium is a rapidly regenerating stratified squamous epithelium. Stable homeostasis of corneal epithelial cells is an important prerequisite for the integrity of the ocular surface and thus for corneal transparency and visual function. Under both normal conditions as well as following injury, epithelial homeostasis is achieved by a distinct population of unipotent stem cells located in the basal epithelium at the corneoscleral limbus [1]. Limbal epithelial stem cells (LESCs) are quiescent, slow-cycling cells, which can divide throughout life both symmetrically to self-renew and asymmetrically to produce daughter or progenitor cells, which migrate centripetally into the basal layer of the corneal epithelium and eventually differentiate into corneal epithelial cells [2].

LESCs and their progeny reside within small clusters in an anatomically protected region, at the bottom of limbal epithelial crypts, which are clinically identified as palisades of Vogt (Fig. 1A–C) [3]. LESCs can be localized by positive expression of putative stem/progenitor cell markers, such as ABCG2, ΔNp63α, ABCB5, keratin (K)15, and N-cadherin, and the absence of corneal epithelial differentiation markers, such as K3 and K12 [4, 5]. LESC quiescence and proliferation are maintained in balance through complex interactions with niche cells, extracellular matrix components, blood vessels, and nerves within a specialized and highly regulated environment, known as the limbal stem cell niche (Fig. 1D–F) [6, 7]. The limbal niche contains several types of supporting cells, including limbal melanocytes, limbal mesenchymal stromal cells, and transmigrating immune cells, secreting soluble growth and survival factors. Niche-specific extracellular matrix constituents convey biophysical and biochemical signals via specific cell–matrix interactions [8, 9]. Whereas interactions of LESCs with niche-specific matrix components, such as laminin-511, have been well characterized and utilized for corneal epithelial tissue engineering [10], the cross-talk of LESCs with different niche cell populations is subject of

B. Seitz et al. (eds.), *Atlas on Cornea*, https://doi.org/10.1007/978-3-031-65422-0_21

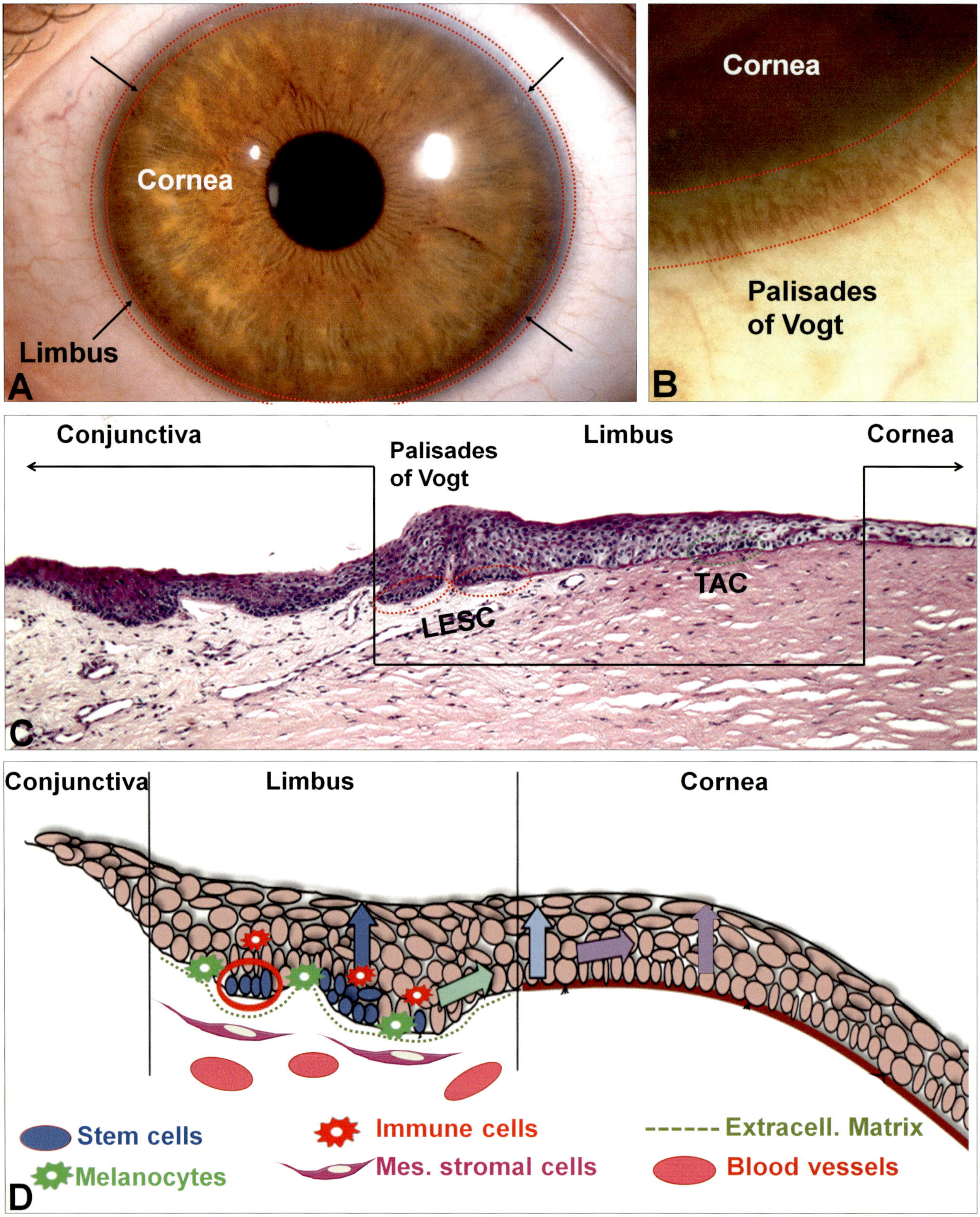

Fig. 1 Limbal stem cells and their niche. (**A**) Clinical appearance of a normal eye. (**B**) Clinical appearance of the limbal region forming the palisades of Vogt. (**C**) Light micrograph showing the limbal region and clusters of limbal epithelial stem cells (LESC, red circles) at the bottom of the palisades of Vogt as well as their progenitor or transient amplifying cells (TAC, green circle) (PAS staining). (**D**) Schematic of the limbal niche

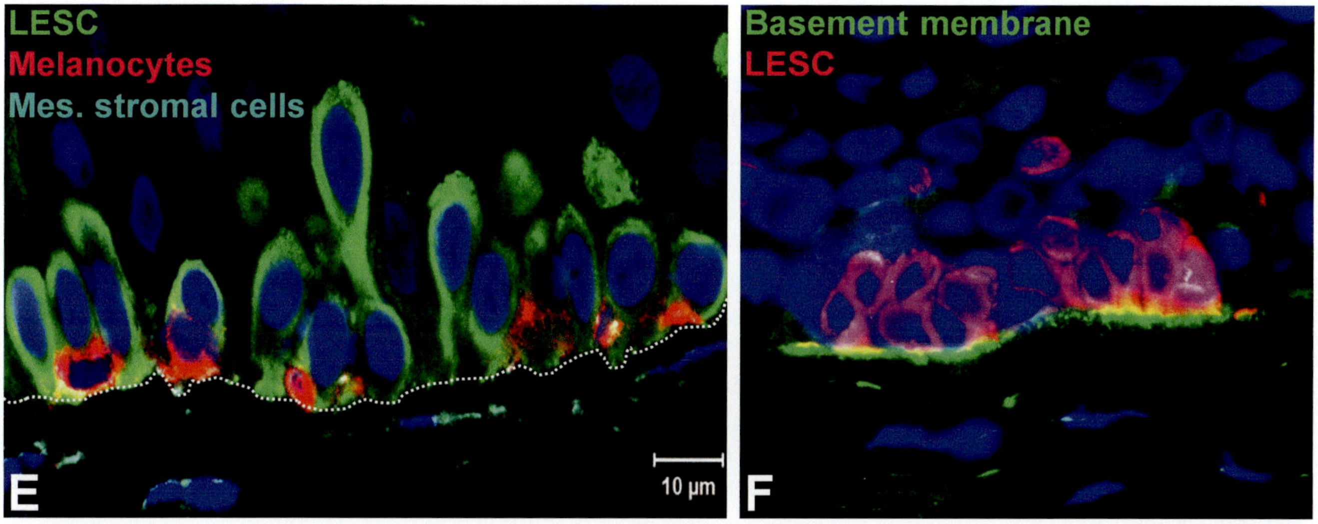

Fig. 1 (**E**) Immunohistochemistry of corneoscleral tissue section showing LESC cluster comprising keratin 15 (K15)-positive epithelial stem cells (green), Melan-A-positive melanocytes (red), vimentin-positive mesenchymal stromal cells (cyan). The basement membrane is indicated by a dashed line; nuclei are counterstained with 4′,6-diamidino-2-phenylindole (blue). (**F**) Immunohistochemistry showing limbus-specific basement membrane staining for laminin-511 (green) in association with K15-positive LESC (red)

active research. Both limbal mesenchymal stromal cells and melanocytes have been shown to physically interact with LESCs to prevent their differentiation and maintain their self-renewal capability [11]. Both niche cell populations have been also acknowledged for their potent immunomodulatory, anti-inflammatory and anti-angiogenic properties making them attractive tools for clinical applications and future regenerative cell therapies [12, 13]. In animal models of limbal stem cell disease, limbal mesenchymal stromal cells have been shown to reduce corneal neovascularization, stromal opacification, inflammation, and edema. Furthermore, immune cells have been recently shown to act as niche cells for LESCs and to regulate maintenance of an undifferentiated stem cell phenotype [14].

Normal function of LESCs is a prerequisite for maintenance and regeneration of the corneal epithelium and acts as a barrier against the invasion of conjunctival epithelium onto the corneal surface [15]. In vivo experimental evidence suggested that a certain number of LESCs, covering approximately 25–35% of the limbus, is necessary to sustain corneal epithelial homeostasis and an intact limbal barrier [16]. Any extensive dysfunction or depletion of LESCs in combination with the destruction of their niche results in limbal barrier breakdown and may lead to partial or total LSCD. Although LSCD is a rare disease with an estimated prevalence of up to 1–5/10,000 (www.orphanet.net), it leads to decreased vision and ocular discomfort in affected patients resulting in a significant impairment of their quality of life.

2 Definition of LSCD

LSCD is an ocular surface disease caused by a decrease in the population and/or function of LESCs, which leads to the inability to sustain the normal homeostasis of the corneal epithelium [17]. The disease is characterized by conjunctivalization (i.e. replacement of the normal corneal by conjunctival epithelium), and other signs of epithelial dysfunction including persistent or recurrent epithelial defects, corneal neovascularization, chronic inflammation, scarring, and pannus formation. Functional consequences are ocular discomfort, pain and decreased vision up to functional blindness. Partial LSCD is characterized by sectoral conjunctivalization of the corneal surface and the presence of residual LESCs. Total LSCD is characterized by conjunctivalization of the entire corneal surface due to complete loss of LESCs. LSCD may present as an isolated entity or in association with other ocular surface abnormalities including severe dry eye disease, chronic inflammation and neurotrophic keratopathy.

3 Classification of LSCD

Whereas idiopathic LSCD is a rare and poorly characterized condition [18], both acquired and inherited conditions more commonly result in partial or total LSCD.

3.1 Acquired LSCD

Chemical and thermal trauma appears to be the leading cause of LSCD [17, 19]. Chemical injuries seem to be far more common than thermal injuries, and result in both LESC and niche destruction. Alkali burns seem to be more common than acid burns, and occur more frequent in males than in females. Thermal injuries can result from exposure to extreme heat or cold.

Iatrogenic causes, such as prolonged contact lens wear, can induce LSCD [17]. The pathophysiology of contact lens-induced LSCD is supposed to be multifactorial involving mechanical, hypoxic and toxic insults [20]. Ocular surgery with limbal involvement, e.g. extensive pterygium surgery, tumor excision, and glaucoma surgery with use of antimetabolites, can induce LSCD. Topical drugs, in particular antimetabolites, and preservatives in eye drops have been also reported as potential causes.

Other potential causes of LSCD include long-standing bullous keratopathy, chronic inflammatory eye conditions and infectious diseases such as trachoma and herpes keratitis [17]. Immunologic disorders, particularly Stevens–Johnson syndrome and toxic epidermal necrolysis, are commonly associated with chronic ocular surface inflammation and LSCD. Mucous membrane pemphigoid is also associated with chronic inflammation and LSCD. Vernal and atopic keratoconjunctivitis as well as graft-versus-host disease after allogeneic hematopoietic stem cell transplantation may lead to LSCD as well.

3.2 Hereditary LSCD

Genetic disorders that have been associated with LSCD include congenital aniridia, Peter's anomaly, dyskeratosis congenita, dominantly inherited keratitis, Turner syndrome, xeroderma pigmentosum, epidermolysis bullosa, and others [17]. Congenital aniridia, caused by haploinsufficiency of the PAX6 transcription factor, may frequently lead to aniridia-associated keratopathy (AAK), which is characterized by a slowly progressing LSCD eventually leading to corneal conjunctivalization and loss of vision [21]. Development of AAK has been initially attributed to a primary deficiency or gradual depletion of LESC. However, a recent single-case study demonstrated marked alterations of the limbal niche and suggested that ocular surface alterations in AAK are caused by a primary dysfunction and gradual breakdown of the limbal stem cell niche [22].

4 Demographics of LSCD

Whereas precise epidemiologic data are not available, it is acknowledged that the leading cause of LSCD is ocular burn which represents at least 2/3 of reported cases [17, 19]. A comprehensive epidemiologic analysis involving almost 2000 eyes from two ophthalmological centers in India reported that the majority of patients presented with total unilateral LSCD, and the most frequent causes were ocular burn (84%) followed by Stevens–Johnson syndrome (4%), atopic keratoconjunctivitis (3%) and mucous membrane pemphigoid (2%). In cases of bilateral LSCD, the major causes were atopic keratoconjunctivitis and ocular burn (30% each) followed by Stevens–Johnson syndrome (23%), congenital aniridia (9%) and mucous membrane pemphigoid (4%) [23]. In a large retrospective series of patients with LSCD referred to a specialized center in the United States, LSCD was mostly bilateral (70%) [24]. The most common etiologies were congenital aniridia (30.9%), chemical or thermal injuries (20.6%), contact lens (16.8%), Stevens–Johnson syndrome (SJS, 10.4%), and iatrogenic (7.3%). Out of 100 consecutive patients with LSCD referred to a specialized center in the UK, the main cause of LSCD was ocular burn (61%), especially chemical burn, which primarily affected young men [19]. Most patients presented with total unilateral LSCD. Notably, assault with ammonia has recently emerged as an important mechanism of LSCD. Other causes included congenital aniridia, mitomycin C toxicity, and chronic use of topical medication with preservatives.

5 Diagnosis of LSCD

The diagnosis of LSCD is based on medical history, clinical presentation and diagnostic tests (Fig. 2) [17, 25, 26]. The clinical manifestation of LSCD can vary depending on the severity and duration of the disease. Recurrent erosions are typically the first sign of LSCD and lead to sudden pain in the eye. Other frequent symptoms include decreased vision, recurrent episodes of pain, foreign body sensation, tearing, dryness, blepharospasm, photophobia, conjunctival hyperemia, and ocular discomfort. The International LSCD Working Group's Global Consensus has recently published their comprehensive guidelines on the clinical presentation, classification, diagnosis, and staging of LSCD [17].

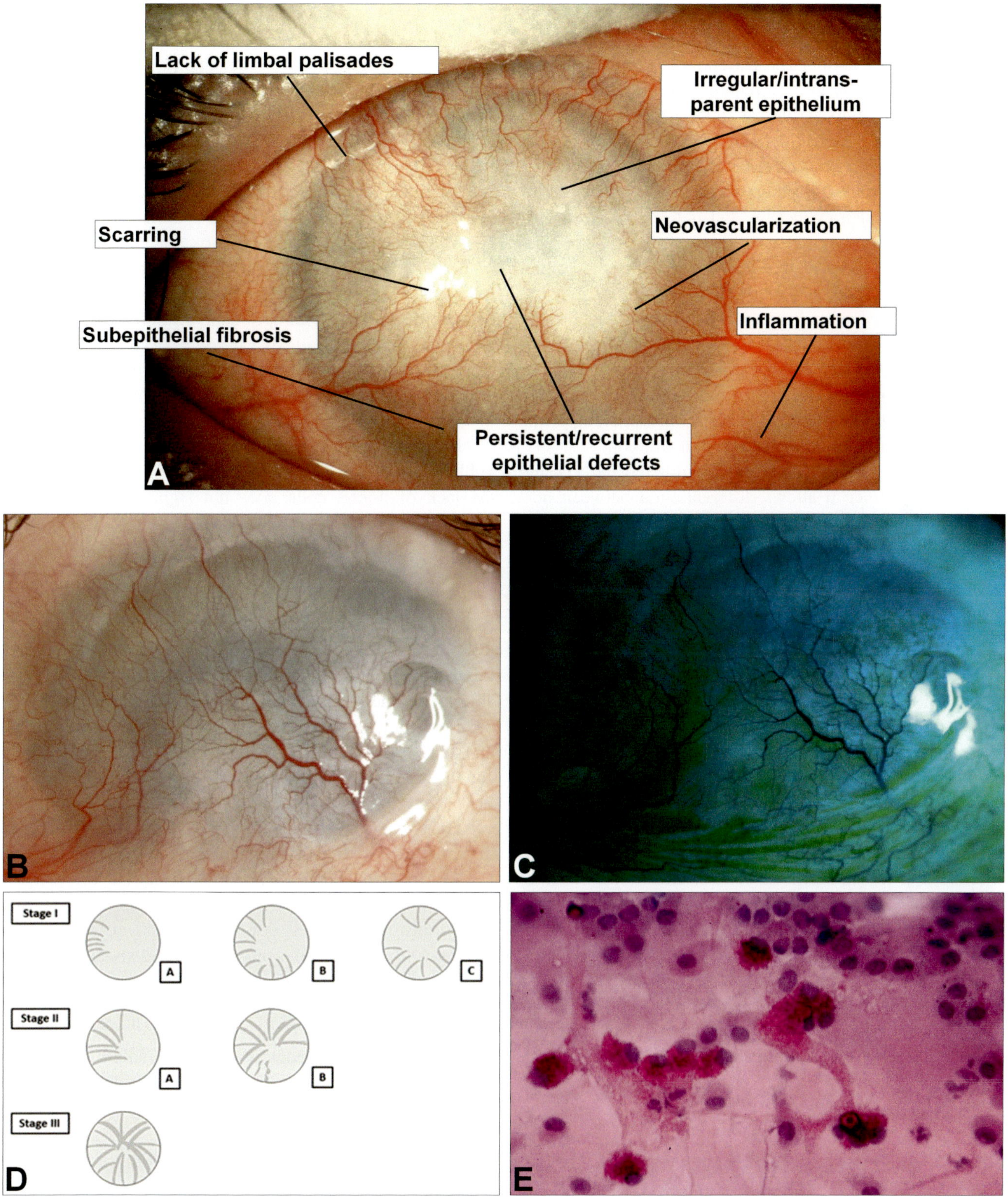

Fig. 2 Diagnosis of limbal stem cell deficiency (LSCD). (**A**) Clinical appearance of an eye with total LSCD, corneal opacification and neovascularization showing typical signs. ((**B**), (**C**) Eye of a 23-year-old male patient with severe stage of LSCD (visual acuity: light perception) after alkali burn under bright light (**B**) and fluorescein staining under cobalt blue light (**C**) showing pronounced neovascularization and fluorescein pooling in areas of abnormal epithelium and conjunctivalization. (**D**) Staging system of LSCD as previously established by the LSCD International Working Group [17]. (**E**) Detection of conjunctival goblet cells on the corneal surface using impression cytology and PAS staining

5.1 Clinical Examination

The absence of a normal corneal epithelial phenotype and the gradual transition into a conjunctival epithelial phenotype generate the typical clinical signs of LSCD. Thus, the epithelium on the corneal surface may show either a conjunctival phenotype or a mixture of corneal and conjunctival epithelial cells. Slit-lamp biomicroscopy can reveal signs of epithelial irregularities and defects, neovascularization, peripheral pannus formation, and corneal opacities [17, 25]. In early or moderate LSCD, the abnormal epithelium spreads in a spiral pattern from the limbus and has been described as vortex keratopathy or whorl-like epitheliopathy. In more advanced stages of LSCD, persistent and/or recurrent epithelial defects, neovascularization, sub-epithelial fibrosis, fibrovascular pannus, and corneal stromal scarring can be observed (Fig. 2A). Absence or flattening of the limbal palisades of Vogt may be noted in addition.

Fluorescein staining can confirm epithelial defects and abnormalities, since it allows differentiation between normal corneal and abnormal conjunctival epithelium on the surface. Under normal conditions corneal epithelial surface cells are firmly connected by tight junctions, which are impermeable to fluorescein molecules. In contrast, the conjunctival epithelium lacks tight junctions, allowing diffusion of fluorescein into the paracellular spaces and revealing abnormal staining after several minutes of fluorescein instillation ("late fluorescein staining") [17]. The intensity of the staining varies according to the state of the diease: In mild or early stages of LSCD, only a punctate fluorescein staining pattern may be seen. As the disease becomes more severe, a clear demarcation line may sometimes be visible between the area covered by the corneal and conjunctival epithelial cells in sectoral LSCD (Fig. 2B, C).

According to the extent of corneal and limbal involvement, LSCD can be classified into 3 stages (Table 1, Fig. 2D) [17]. The stages are correlated with a gradual decrease in basal epithelial cell density of the central cornea.

However, clinical examination alone is often not sufficient for an accurate diagnosis and staging, because clinal signs can be very subtle. Additional diagnostic tests should, therefore, be performed to confirm the diagnosis of LSCD.

5.2 Impression Cytology

LSCD is often diagnosed by detection of conjunctival goblet cells on the corneal surface using impression cytology, which used to be considered as the diagnostic "gold standard" for conjunctivalization in LSCD [17, 25]. The technique is simple, cheap and marginally invasive. Cellulose acetate filters are often used to collect superficial epithelial cells, which are then subjected to cytological examination. Histological staining with hematoxylin and eosin (H&E) or periodic acid-Schiff stain (PAS) is often used to identify goblet cells (Fig. 2E). Immunohistochemistry allows detection of conjunctival epithelial, e.g. K7, K13, K19, and goblet cell markers, e.g. MUC1 and MUC5AC, in collected cells [27, 28]. The lack of corneal epithelial differentiation (i.e. K12) and progenitor makers (i.e. K15) can also be used to support the diagnosis of LCSD.

However, studies have confirmed that the detection of goblet cells has a high specificity but low sensitivity, and the lack of goblet cells does not signify the absence of LSCD. Therefore, additional tests are required for a definite diagnosis.

5.3 In Vivo-Imaging Techniques

In vivo laser scanning confocal microscopy (IVCM) and anterior segment optical coherence tomography (AS-OCT) have emerged as valuable non-invasive diagnostic tools for LSCD [17, 25]. IVCM findings of the central cornea indicating LSCD include the presence of a conjunctival epithelial phenotype and goblet cells, reduction of basal epithelial cell density, increased basal epithelial cell size, epithelial thinning, and reduction of sub-basal nerve density [26]. IVCM findings in the limbal area comprise the absence or flattening of limbal palisades and crypts, absence of a clear transition between conjunctival and corneal epithelia, reduction of basal epithelial cell density, increased basal epithelial cell size, epithelial thinning, and occasional presence of inflammatory cells. These signs correlate with severity of LSCD.

AS-OCT with a spectral domain resolution of 3 μm of both the central cornea and limbus has emerged as an

Table 1 Staging of LSCD based on clinical presentation

Stage I: normal corneal epithelium within the 5 mm central cornea	A. Limbal involvement < 50%
	B. Limbal involvement ≥ 50% < 100%
	C. Limbal involvement 100%
Stage II: central 5 mm of the cornea affected	A. Limbal involvement < 50%
	B. Limbal involvement ≥ 50% < 100%
Stage III: entire corneal surface involved	

alternative imaging technique for LSCD, allowing for a larger field of view compared to IVCM. While it does not offer the same degree of optical resolution at the cellular level, it may prove useful in measuring corneal epithelial thickness, pannus depth and the presence of corneal vessels [29]. Presence of the palisades of Vogt and limbal crypts, epithelial thickness, and transition between the hyporeflective corneal epithelium and the hyperreflective conjunctival epithelium can be assessed semi-quantitatively in the limbal region. Consistent with IVCM, the central and limbal epithelial thickness decreased in eyes with LSCD and correlated with disease severity [30].

Deng and colleagues developed a comprehensive staging system by multimodal in vivo imaging to quantitate basal epithelial cell density, basal cell morphology, epithelial thickness, and corneal nerve fiber density [31]. They showed that basal epithelial cell density, central corneal epithelial thickness, and corneal nerve fiber length were the best parameters to differentiate LSCD from healthy eyes.

6 Therapy of LSCD

The treatment of LSCD is aimed at reconstruction of the corneal epithelium and stabilization of the ocular surface. Therapeutic options depend on the etiology, severity, extent, and laterality of the disease. The International LSCD Working Group's Global Consensus has recently published their comprehensive guidelines on the medical and surgical management of LSCD as a stepwise flowchart (Fig. 3A) [32]. Briefly, stages I and IIA can often be managed by medical treatment, whereas stages IIB and III require surgical treatment, eventually by transplantation of LESCs. Advanced LSCD represents a contraindication for conventional corneal transplantation, i.e. penetrating keratoplasty, because the ocular surface will not re-epithelialize properly without replenishment of the depleted stem cell pool.

Mild cases or partial LSCD may be medically treated with lubricating eye drops, ointments, anti-inflammatory drugs, topical antibiotics, and therapeutic contact lenses to protect the cornea. Moderate to severe cases or total LSCD may require surgical intervention, such as sectoral conjunctival epitheliectomy, amniotic membrane transplantation, or LESC transplantation to promote re-epithelialization [32]. However, ocular surface comorbidities, such as chronic inflammation, infections, and severe dry eye disease, which compromise the function of residual LESCs and threaten the survival of transplanted LESCs, should be treated in advance [26]. Stem cell-based transplantation options include keratolimbal or conjunctival limbal grafts, simple limbal epithelial grafts, and ex vivo expanded limbal and oral mucosal epithelial cells [33, 34]. In general, autologous procedures should be preferred over allogeneic approaches, because they offer better success rates and avoid the risks of immunosuppression [35].

6.1 Limbal Tissue Transplantation

In LSCD patients a variety of procedures which transfer healthy stem cells onto diseased eyes have been described (Fig. 3B) [32–34]. Initially, large conjunctival limbal tissue biopsies, taken from either the patient's contralateral healthy eye in unilateral cases (conjunctival limbal autograft, CLAU) or from the eye of an allogeneic living donor in bilateral cases (conjunctival limbal allograft, CLAL), were used to reconstitute the corneal epithelium [36, 37]. A modified approach uses post-mortem donor eyes as allogeneic tissue source (keratolimbal allograft, KLAL) [38]. From 1989 to 2006, CLAU transplantation was the most commonly performed procedure for unilateral severe LSCD with excellent outcomes. Up to 88% of eyes had good long-term results showing an improvement of the ocular surface and visual acuity with only few complications (Fig. 4A) [39, 40]. The limitation of this approach is that it requires removal of 40–50% of the donor limbus, which poses the risk of iatrogenic LSCD in the healthy contralateral or living-related donor eye. CLAL or KLAL transplantation showed much lower success rates, primarily because of immunologic rejection despite of immunosuppression [38, 41].

6.2 Cultivated Limbal Epithelial Transplantation (CLET)

To reduce the risk of iatrogenic LSCD in a healthy donor eye, ex vivo-expansion and transplantation of LESCs isolated from a small limbal biopsy (1–2 mm^2) has been established. Since the pioneering work by Pellegrini et al. [42] using mouse embryonic fibroblasts as feeder cells for LESCs, many protocols have been developed to isolate and cultivate LESCs from either the patient's healthy contralateral eye (autologous CLET) or a donor eye (allogeneic CLET) [43]. Following direct outgrowth from limbal explants or prior enrichment by clonal growth on a feeder layer, LESCs are expanded on transplantable carriers to generate multilayered epithelial sheets for transplantation (Fig. 3C). The carrier materials most frequently used for LESC transplantation are human amniotic membrane and fibrin gels. In 2015, Holoclar (Chiesi Farmaceutici) was conditionally approved as the first stem cell-based

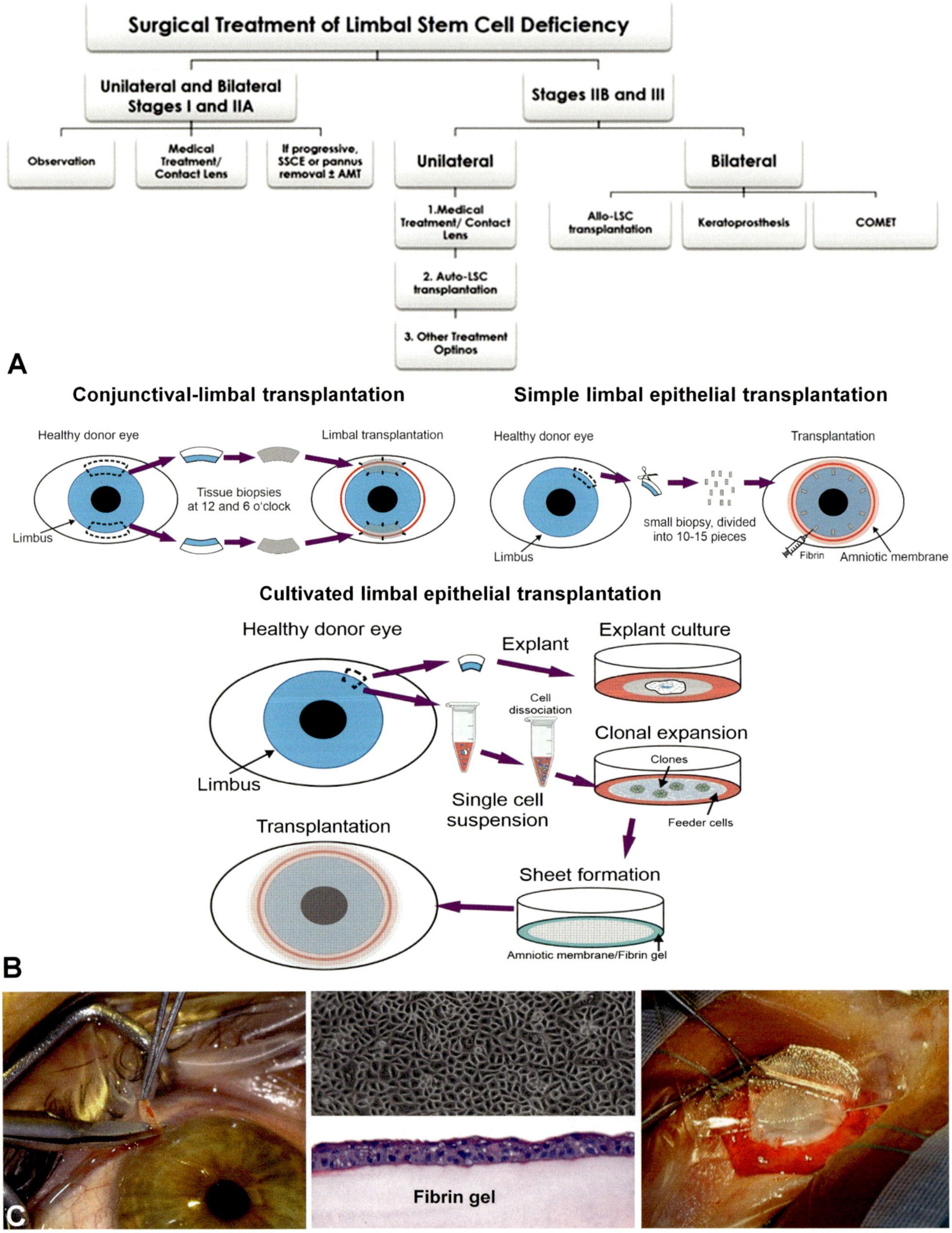

Fig. 3 Therapy of limbal stem cell deficiency (LSCD). (**A**) Flowchart of management strategies of different stages of LSCD as previously established by the LSCD International Working Group [32]. (**B**) Schematics of stem cell-based transplantation options, including conjunctival limbal transplantation, simple limbal epithelial transplantation and cultivated limbal epithelial transplantation. (**C**) Cultivated limbal epithelial transplantation procedure showing surgical harvesting of a limbal biopsy from the donor eye (left), ex vivo expansion of limbal epithelial cells on fibrin gel and formation of a multilayered epithelial sheet (center), and transplantation of the epithelial sheet on the recipient eye (right)

medicinal product by the European Medicines Agency (EMA) for clinical use [44]. Holoclar is a commercially available CLET therapy, which consists of autologous LESC-derived corneal epithelial cells, including about 3.5% stem cells, cultivated on a 2.2 cm diameter fibrin gel as a carrier. Its efficacy and safety has been assessed in a multinational, multicentre, prospective, open-label, uncontrolled clinical phase IV trial. However, the application for Holoclar is limited to patients suffering from unilateral LSCD as a result of ocular burns. Nevertheless, CLET procedure currently represents the only widely applied stem cell-based therapy in clinical ophthalmology [45].

CLET has become the standard treatment of choice for LSCD in various clinical centers. Overall, CLET has proven as a successful technique to treat LSCD by supporting corneal re-epithelialization while causing rare donor complications, with similar outcomes than that of CLAU (Fig. 4B, C). Despite many variables between clinical studies, long-term success rates, defined as a fully epithelialized and avascular corneal surface, in autologous procedures have been reported to average about 70% [35, 43, 46, 47]. For bilateral disease, allograft transplantation had been reported with much lower success rates primarily due to immunological problems [35]. An essential prerequisite of epithelial grafts for long-term restoration of the ocular surface is the presence of an adequate number of stem cells, which can be preoperatively determined by the presence of ΔNp63α-positive cells within the graft [43, 45] (Fig. 5).

However, CLET is an expensive procedure that requires GMP-concordant cell culture facilities. Recently, allogeneic LESCs have been isolated from cadaveric donor eyes based on their positive expression of the surface marker ABCB5, expanded in vitro and manufactured as an advanced therapy medicinal product. Suspended in fibrin gel, the enriched ABCB5+ cells are engrafted onto the diseased ocular surface and covered with a bandage contact lens. Currently, this product is being tested in a multicenter phase I/IIa clinical trials for the treatment of LSCD [48].

6.3 Simple Limbal Epithelial Transplantation (SLET)

For the treatment of unilateral LSCD, SLET offers a more cost-effective and easier-to-perform alternative approach, which avoids the need for GMP-compliant LESC cultivation ex vivo [49]. In order to expand the LESCs directly on the patient's affected eye in vivo, multiple tiny pieces of limbal tissue, taken from the healthy contralateral eye, are uniformly placed on amniotic membrane and grafted onto the patient's diseased eye. Cell outgrowth from the limbal explants leads to corneal re-epithelialization typically within 2 weeks. Reported success rates are similar to those of CLAU and CLET and average about 70–80% [50, 51].

6.4 Cultivated Oral Mucosal Epithelial Transplantation (COMET)

For treatment of patients with bilateral ocular surface disease, COMET has been developed as an autologous surgical procedure for restoration of the corneal surface [52, 53]. In this approach, oral mucosal epithelial cells are isolated from a biopsy (3–10 mm^2) of the patient's own buccal mucosal epithelium and expanded on human amniotic membrane or on temperature-responsive polymer surfaces to generate carrier-free cell sheets. Several clinical studies supported the safety and efficacy of this approach, with long-term success rates between 50 and 65% [54]. However, peripheral neovascularization following transplantation has been reported to occur in more than 90% of patients and has been considered a drawback of this procedure [55]. It has also been reported that oral mucosal epithelial cell grafts rarely transdifferentiate to a corneal epithelial phenotype, as indicated by lacking expression of cornea-specific cytokeratin K12 [56]. Still, COMET is currently the only clinically approved transplantation technique using non-ocular cell types.

6.5 Keratoprostheses

Finally, various types of keratoprostheses (KPros) have been used for visual rehabilitation in patients with severe bilateral LSCD, who are not amenable to transplantation and keratoplasty [57, 58]. The most commonly used types are the Boston type I- and type II-Kpro and the osteo-odonto-KPro. Despite early success of visual recovery, complications, such as melting, fungal keratitis, endophthalmitis and glaucoma development, increase with follow-up time [32, 59].

6.6 Future Strategies

By stabilization of the corneal surface epithelium, current transplantation procedures are of great benefit for patients suffering from LSCD. However, they also have their limitations, such as recurrent corneal neovascularization, underlining the need for further improvements

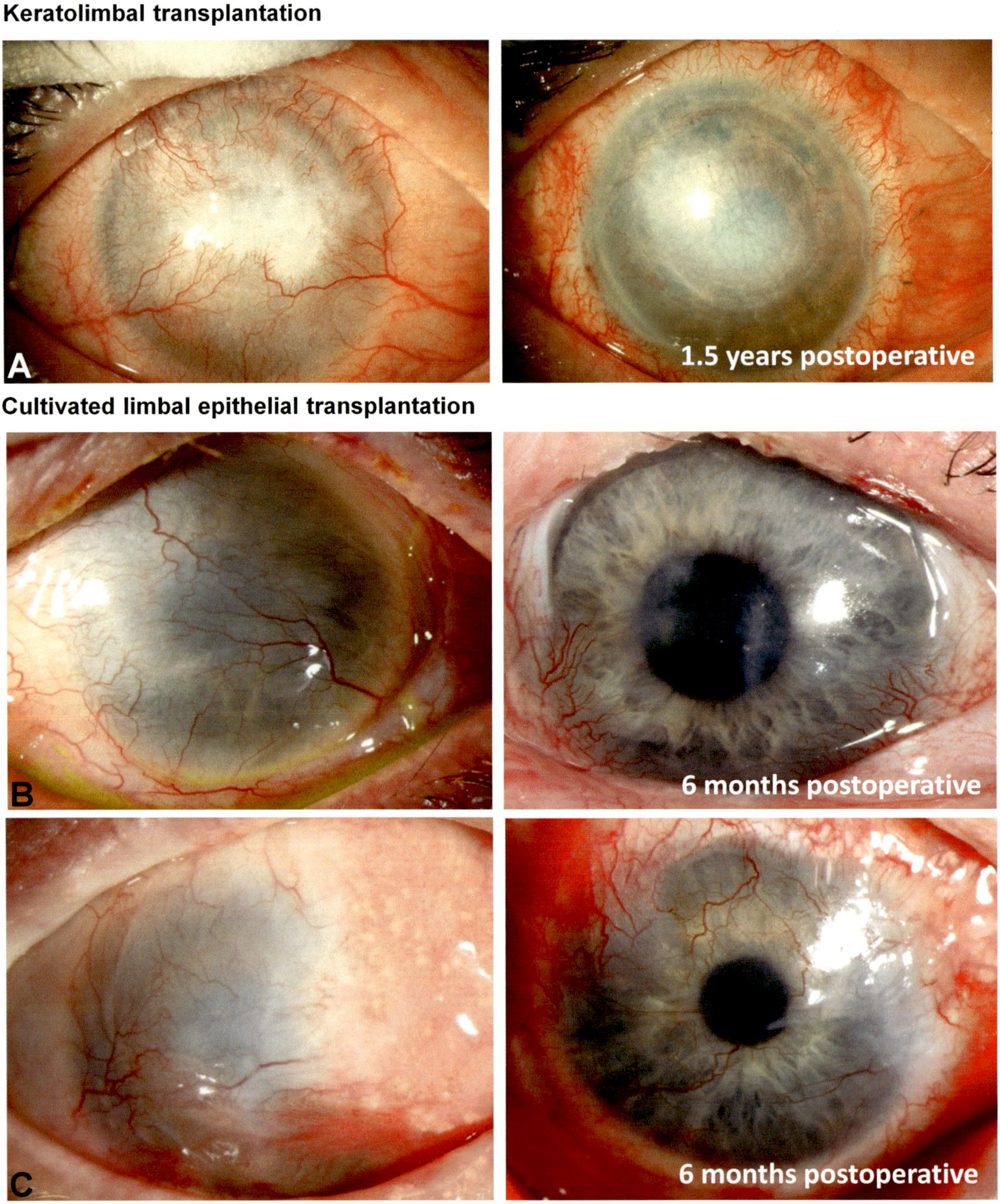

Fig. 4 Therapy of limbal stem cell deficiency (LSCD). (**A**) Pre- and postoperative clinical images of a patient with unilateral total LSCD after chemical burn, who had received a large keratolimbal autograft; 1.5 years post-transplantation there was persistent stromal opacification and preservation of the limbal barrier [37]. (**B**, **C**) Pre- and postoperative clinical images of two 27-year-old males patient with unilateral total LSCD after fireworks injury (visual acuity; hand movements); 6 months post-transplantation, visual acuity has been improved (0.15) through re-epithelialization, but recurrent peripheral corneal neovascularization was also observed

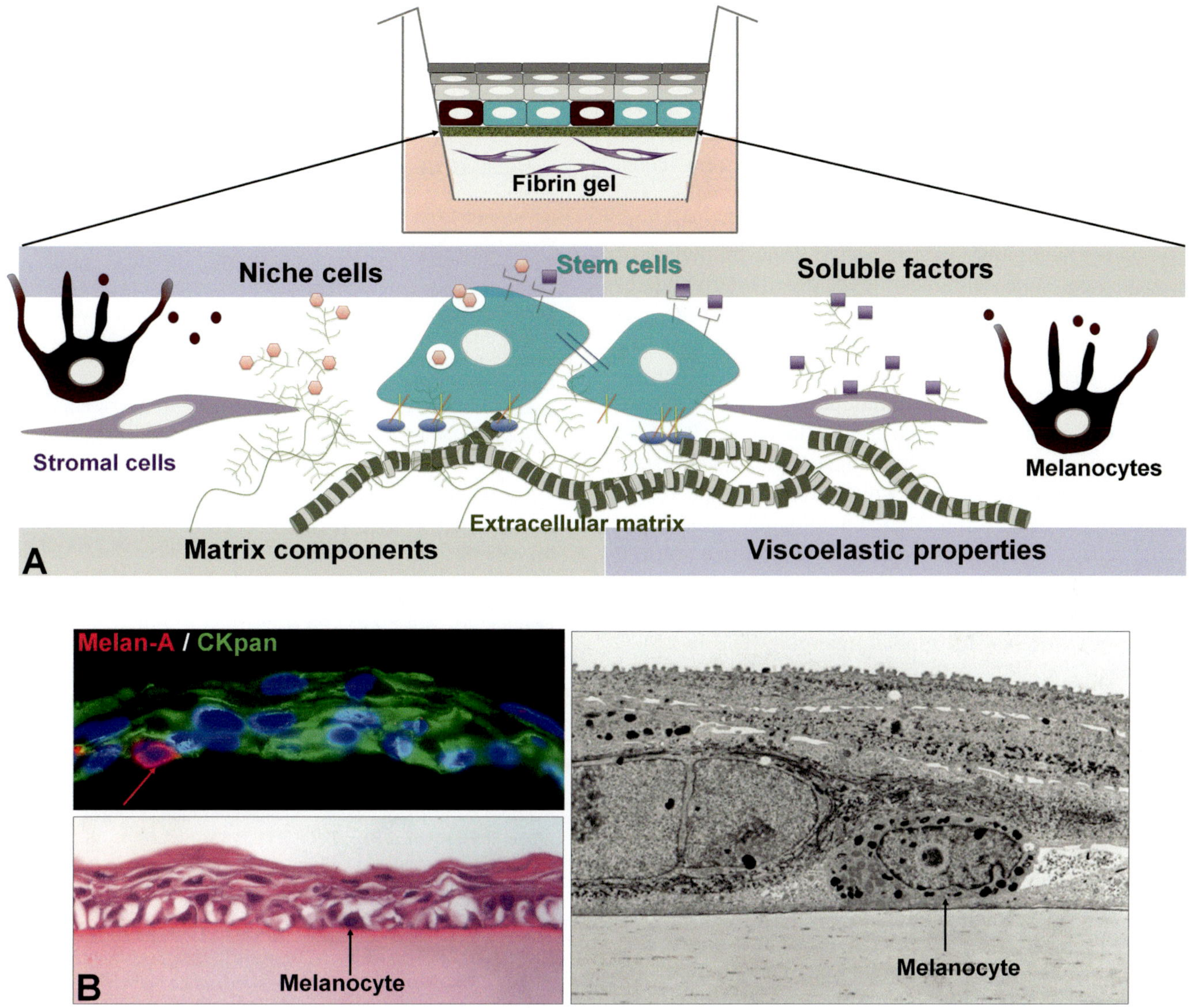

Fig. 5 Future therapeutic strategies for limbal stem cell deficiency (LSCD): focus on the limbal stem cell niche. (**A**) Schematic of future approaches for ex vivo expansion of limbal stem cells by incorporating various cellular and non-cellular niche factors into the culture system [63]. (**B**) Corneal epithelial tissue engineering using limbal melanocytes for co-culture with limbal stem cells. Epithelial constructs on fibrin gel containing cytokeratin-positive epithelial cells and Melan A-positive melanocytes (arrows) are shown by immunohistochemistry (top right), light microscopy (bottom right) and transmission electron microscopy (left)

and advancements [59]. The overarching goal of novel approaches is the maintenance of a stem cell phenotype in culture and after transplantation. One limitation of current cultivation/transplantation procedures is, that they do not appear to support the survival of stem cells in the grafts, because these lack essential components of the niche microenvironment [60]. It has been reported that as early as one month after transplantation, no donor cells can be observed in the recipient's ocular surface epithelium. Thus, current research activities aim at incorporating key components of the limbal niche, e.g. specific matrix components or niche cells, into the culture systems, to improve stem cell survival during cultivation and following transplantation (Fig. 4) [61–63]. Nevertheless, full success in transplantation of limbal epithelium is currently hampered by our limited understanding of the niche-specific factors that govern self-renewal, maintenance and proliferation of LESCs.

Moreover, most of the available culture protocols still utilize xenogeneic, allogeneic and/or undefined culture components including murine feeder cells, bovine serum, amniotic membrane, and a number of animal-derived growth additives. In order to further improve and standardize this therapeutic approach, researchers have focused on the introduction of safer and xenofree culture procedures to avoid the use of xenobiotics [64].

Alternative approaches have emerged that make use of epithelial stem cells that have been isolated from the conjunctiva, epidermis or hair follicle and that can be directed towards a corneal epithelial cell lineage by appropriate extrinsic cues. Non-epithelial cells used for ocular surface reconstruction include mesenchymal stem cells, dental pulp stem cells, umbilical cord stem cells, and embryonic stem cells [65]. The potent immunomodulatory, anti-inflammatory and anti-angiogenic properties of mesenchymal stem cells make them excellent candidates for tissue engineering or treatment of injuries to the cornea and limbus. In a proof-of-concept clinical trial, the transplantation of allogeneic bone marrow-derived mesenchymal stem cells using amniotic membrane as carrier proved as equally efficient as allogeneic CLET in LSCD patients [66]. Finally, induced pluripotent stem cells (iPSC)-derived LESCs, which offer potential for an unlimited source of differentiated autologous corneal epithelial cells, are currently under investigation in a phase I/IIa clinical trial in Japan [67, 68]. Non-cellular therapies including amniotic membrane derivatives, soluble growth factors, or exosomes are another emerging field in LSCD therapy [61].

7 Conclusion

In recent years, there have been significant developments in diagnostic tools and treatment modalities of LSCD by using stem cell-based transplantation approaches in combination with corneal epithelial tissue engineering. Currently, CLET, SLET and COMET procedures are the only widely applied stem cell-based therapies in ophthalmology, which have been clinically validated. In general, autologous procedures have a higher success rate in restoring a stable ocular surface than allogeneic procedures, but in terms of safety and efficacy the transplantation modalities seem to be comparable [34, 69]. Successful LESC transplantation also requires co-treatment of ocular surface comorbidities, such as ocular inflammation, dry eye, eyelid abnormalities, and neurotrophic keratopathy. However, to ensure long-term functionality of transplants and long-term regeneration of the ocular surface, further improvements, such as standardization of culture conditions, preservation of stem cell phenotype during cultivation, and development of biomimetic and xenobiotic-free culture systems, are required to advance this therapeutic strategy. Restoration of the limbal niche, both in vitro and in vivo, is crucial in maintaining the function of patient's residual LESCs and ensuring the survival of transplanted LESCs.

References

1. Bonnet C, González S, Roberts JS, Robertson SYT, Ruiz M, Zheng J, Deng SX. Human limbal epithelial stem cell regulation, bioengineering and function. Prog Retin Eye Res. 2021;85:100956.
2. Cotsarelis G, Cheng SZ, Dong G, Sun TT, Lavker RM. Existence of slow-cycling limbal epithelial basal cells that can be preferentially stimulated to proliferate: implications on epithelial stem cells. Cell. 1989;57(2):201–9.
3. Townsend WM. The limbal palisades of Vogt. Trans Am Ophthalmol Soc. 1991;89:721–56.
4. Schlötzer-Schrehardt U, Kruse FE. Identification and characterization of limbal stem cells. Exp Eye Res. 2005;81(3):247–64.
5. Gonzalez G, Sasamoto Y, Ksander BR, Frank MH, Frank NY. Limbal stem cells: identity, developmental origin, and therapeutic potential. Wiley Interdiscip Rev Dev Biol. 2018;7(2). https://doi.org/10.1002/wdev.303
6. Li W, Hayashida Y, Chen YT, Tseng SC. Niche regulation of corneal epithelial stem cells at the limbus. Cell Res. 2007;17(1):26–36.
7. Robertson SYT, Roberts JS, Deng SX. Regulation of limbal epithelial stem cells: importance of the niche. Int J Mol Sci. 2021;22(21):11975.
8. Schlötzer-Schrehardt U, Dietrich T, Saito K, Sorokin L, Sasaki T, Paulsson M, Kruse FE. Characterization of extracellular matrix components in the limbal epithelial stem cell compartment. Exp Eye Res. 2007;85(6):845–60.
9. Polisetti N, Zenkel M, Menzel-Severing J, Kruse FE, Schlötzer-Schrehardt U. Cell adhesion molecules and stem cell-niche-interactions in the limbal stem cell niche. Stem Cells. 2016;34(1):203–19.
10. Polisetti N, Sorokin L, Okumura N, Koizumi N, Kinoshita S, Kruse FE, Schlötzer-Schrehardt U. Laminin-511 and -521-based matrices for efficient ex vivo-expansion of human limbal epithelial progenitor cells. Sci Rep. 2017;7(1):5152.
11. Dziasko MA, Daniels JT. Anatomical features and cell-cell interactions in the human limbal epithelial stem cell niche. Ocul Surf. 2016;14(3):322–30.
12. Polisetti N, Gießl A, Zenkel M, Heger L, Dudziak D, Naschberger E, Stich L, Steinkasserer A, Kruse FE, Schlötzer-Schrehardt U. Melanocytes as emerging key players in niche regulation of limbal epithelial stem cells. Ocul Surf. 2021;22:172–89.
13. Al-Jaibaji O, Swioklo S, Connon CJ. Mesenchymal stromal cells for ocular surface repair. Expert Opin Biol Ther. 2019;19(7):643–53.
14. Collin J, Queen R, Zerti D, Bojic S, Dorgau B, Moyse N, Molina MM, Yang C, Dey S, Reynolds G, Hussain R, Coxhead JM, Lisgo S, Henderson D, Joseph A, Rooney P, Ghosh S, Clarke L, Connon C, Haniffa M, Figueiredo F, Armstrong L, Lako M. A single cell atlas of human cornea that defines its development, limbal progenitor cells and their interactions with the immune cells. Ocul Surf. 2021;21:279–98.
15. Tseng SC. Concept and application of limbal stem cells. Eye (Lond). 1989;3(Pt 2):141–57.
16. Huang AJ, Tseng SC. Corneal epithelial wound healing in the absence of limbal epithelium. Invest Ophthalmol Vis Sci. 1991;32(1):96–105.
17. Deng SX, Borderie V, Chan CC, Dana R, Figueiredo FC, Gomes JAP, Pellegrini G, Shimmura S, Kruse FE; and The International Limbal Stem Cell Deficiency Working Group. Global consensus on definition, classification, diagnosis, and staging of limbal stem cell deficiency. Cornea. 2019;38(3):364–75.

18. Espana EM, Grueterich M, Romano AC, Touhami A, Tseng SC. Idiopathic limbal stem cell deficiency. Ophthalmology. 2002;109(11):2004–10.
19. Cartes C, Lako M, Figueiredo FC. Referral patterns of patients with limbal stem cell deficiency to a specialized tertiary center in the United Kingdom. Ophthalmol Ther. 2021;10(3):535–45.
20. Rossen J, Amram A, Milani B, Park D, Harthan J, Joslin C, McMahon T, Djalilian A. Contact lens-induced limbal stem cell deficiency. Ocul Surf. 2016;14(4):419–34.
21. Landsend ECS, Lagali N, Utheim TP. Congenital aniridia—a comprehensive review of clinical features and therapeutic approaches. Surv Ophthalmol. 2021;66(6):1031–50.
22. Schlötzer-Schrehardt U, Latta L, Gießl A, Zenkel M, Fries FN, Käsmann-Kellner B, Kruse FE, Seitz B. Dysfunction of the limbal epithelial stem cell niche in aniridia-associated keratopathy. Ocul Surf. 2021;21:160–73.
23. Vazirani J, Nair D, Shanbhag S, Wurity S, Ranjan A, Sangwan V. Limbal stem cell deficiency-demography and underlying causes. Am J Ophthalmol. 2018;188:99–103.
24. Cheung AY, Sarnicola E, Denny MR, Sepsakos L, Auteri NJ, Holland EJ. Limbal stem cell deficiency: demographics and clinical characteristics of a large retrospective series at a single tertiary referral center. Cornea. 2021;40(12):1525–31.
25. Le Q, Xu J, Deng SX. The diagnosis of limbal stem cell deficiency. Ocul Surf. 2018;16(1):58–69.
26. Bonnet C, Roberts JS, Deng SX. Limbal stem cell diseases. Exp Eye Res. 2021;205:108437.
27. Poli M, Burillon C, Auxenfans C, Rovere MR, Damour O. Immunocytochemical diagnosis of limbal stem cell deficiency: comparative analysis of current corneal and conjunctival biomarkers. Cornea. 2015;34(7):817–23.
28. Liang Q, Le Q, Wang L, Cordova D, Baclagon E, Garrido SG, Levin M, Jin Y, Tseng CH, Rao J, Deng SX. Cytokeratin 13 is a new biomarker for the diagnosis of limbal stem cell deficiency. Cornea. 2022;41(7):867–73.
29. Lee WD, Devarajan K, Chua J, Schmetterer L, Mehta JS, Ang M. Optical coherence tomography angiography for the anterior segment. Eye Vis (Lond). 2019;6:4.
30. Liang Q, Le Q, Cordova DW, Tseng CH, Deng SX. Corneal epithelial thickness measured using anterior segment optical coherence tomography as a diagnostic parameter for limbal stem cell deficiency. Am J Ophthalmol. 2020;216:132–9.
31. Le Q, Chauhan T, Cordova D, Tseng CH, Deng SX. Biomarkers of in vivo limbal stem cell function. Ocul Surf. 2022;23:123–30.
32. Deng SX, Kruse F, Gomes JAP, Chan CC, Daya S, Dana R, Figueiredo FC, Kinoshita S, Rama P, Sangwan V, Slomovic AR, Tan D; and the International Limbal Stem Cell Deficiency Working Group. Global consensus on the management of limbal stem cell deficiency. Cornea. 2020;39(10):1291–302.
33. Holland EJ. Management of limbal stem cell deficiency: a historical perspective, past, present, and future. Cornea. 2015;34(Suppl 10):S9–15.
34. Figueiredo FC, Glanville JM, Arber M, Carr E, Rydevik G, Hogg J, Okonkwo A, Figueiredo G, Lako M, Whiter F, Wilson K. A systematic review of cellular therapies for the treatment of limbal stem cell deficiency affecting one or both eyes. Ocul Surf. 2021;20:48–61.
35. Le Q, Chauhan T, Yung M, Tseng CH, Deng SX. Outcomes of limbal stem cell transplant: a meta-analysis. JAMA Ophthalmol. 2020;138(6):660–70.
36. Kenyon KR, Tseng SC. Limbal autograft transplantation for ocular surface disorders. Ophthalmology. 1989;96(5):709–22; discussion 722–3.
37. Kruse FE, Reinhard T. Die Limbustransplantation zur Rekonstruktion der Augenoberfläche [Limbus transplantation for reconstruction of the ocular surface]. Ophthalmologe. 2001;98(9):818–31.
38. Cheung AY, Eslani M, Kurji KH, Wright E, Sarnicola E, Govil A, Holland EJ. Long-term outcomes of living-related conjunctival limbal allograft compared with keratolimbal allograft in patients with limbal stem cell deficiency. Cornea. 2020;39(8):980–5.
39. Daya SM. Conjunctival-limbal autograft. Curr Opin Ophthalmol. 2017;28(4):370–6.
40. Borderie VM, Ghoubay D, Georgeon C, Borderie M, de Sousa C, Legendre A, Rouard H. Long-term results of cultured limbal stem cell versus limbal tissue transplantation in stage III limbal deficiency. Stem Cells Transl Med. 2019;8(12):1230–41.
41. Eslani M, Cheung AY, Kurji K, Pierson K, Sarnicola E, Holland EJ. Long-term outcomes of conjunctival limbal autograft in patients with unilateral total limbal stem cell deficiency. Ocul Surf. 2019;17(4):670–4.
42. Pellegrini G, Traverso CE, Franzi AT, Zingirian M, Cancedda R, De Luca M. Long-term restoration of damaged corneal surfaces with autologous cultivated corneal epithelium. Lancet. 1997;349(9057):990–3.
43. Rama P, Ferrari G, Pellegrini G. Cultivated limbal epithelial transplantation. Curr Opin Ophthalmol. 2017;28(4):387–9.
44. Pellegrini G, Ardigò D, Milazzo G, Iotti G, Guatelli P, Pelosi D, De Luca M. Navigating market authorization: the path holoclar took to become the first stem cell product approved in the European Union. Stem Cells Transl Med. 2018;7(1):146–54.
45. Pellegrini G, Rama P, Di Rocco A, Panaras A, De Luca M. Concise review: hurdles in a successful example of limbal stem cell-based regenerative medicine. Stem Cells. 2014;32(1):26–34.
46. Sangwan VS, Basu S, Vemuganti GK, Sejpal K, Subramaniam SV, Bandyopadhyay S, Krishnaiah S, Gaddipati S, Tiwari S, Balasubramanian D. Clinical outcomes of xeno-free autologous cultivated limbal epithelial transplantation: a 10-year study. Br J Ophthalmol. 2011;95(11):1525–9.
47. Baylis O, Figueiredo F, Henein C, Lako M, Ahmad S. 13 years of cultured limbal epithelial cell therapy: a review of the outcomes. J Cell Biochem. 2011;112(4):993–1002.
48. Norrick A, Esterlechner J, Niebergall-Roth E, Dehio U, Sadeghi S, Schröder HM, Ballikaya S, Stemler N, Ganss C, Dieter K, Dachtler AK, Merz P, Sel S, Chodosh J, Cursiefen C, Frank NY, Auffarth GU, Ksander B, Frank MH, Kluth MA. Process development and safety evaluation of $ABCB5^+$ limbal stem cells as advanced-therapy medicinal product to treat limbal stem cell deficiency. Stem Cell Res Ther. 2021;12(1):194.
49. Sangwan VS, Basu S, MacNeil S, Balasubramanian D. Simple limbal epithelial transplantation (SLET): a novel surgical technique for the treatment of unilateral limbal stem cell deficiency. Br J Ophthalmol. 2012;96(7):931–4.
50. Shanbhag SS, Patel CN, Goyal R, Donthineni PR, Singh V, Basu S. Simple limbal epithelial transplantation (SLET): review of indications, surgical technique, mechanism, outcomes, limitations, and impact. Indian J Ophthalmol. 2019;67(8):1265–77.
51. Vazirani J, Ali MH, Sharma N, Gupta N, Mittal V, Atallah M, Amescua G, Chowdhury T, Abdala-Figuerola A, Ramirez-Miranda A, Navas A, Graue-Hernández EO, Chodosh J. Autologous simple limbal epithelial transplantation for unilateral limbal stem cell deficiency: multicentre results. Br J Ophthalmol. 2016;100(10):1416–20.
52. Inatomi T, Nakamura T, Koizumi N, Sotozono C, Kinoshita S. Current concepts and challenges in ocular surface reconstruction using cultivated mucosal epithelial transplantation. Cornea. 2005;24(8 Suppl):S32–8.
53. Cabral JV, Jackson CJ, Utheim TP, Jirsova K. Ex vivo cultivated oral mucosal epithelial cell transplantation for limbal stem cell deficiency: a review. Stem Cell Res Ther. 2020;11(1):301.

54. Nakamura T, Kinoshita S. New hopes and strategies for the treatment of severe ocular surface disease. Curr Opin Ophthalmol. 2011;22(4):274–8.
55. Kiritoshi S, Oie Y, Nampei K, Sato S, Morota M, Nishida K. Anterior segment optical coherence tomography angiography in patients following cultivated oral mucosal epithelial transplantation. Am J Ophthalmol. 2019;208:242–50.
56. Nishida K, Yamato M, Hayashida Y, Watanabe K, Yamamoto K, Adachi E, Nagai S, Kikuchi A, Maeda N, Watanabe H, Okano T, Tano Y. Corneal reconstruction with tissue-engineered cell sheets composed of autologous oral mucosal epithelium. N Engl J Med. 2004;351(12):1187–96.
57. Avadhanam VS, Smith HE, Liu C. Keratoprostheses for corneal blindness: a review of contemporary devices. Clin Ophthalmol. 2015;9:697–720.
58. Aravena C, Bozkurt TK, Yu F, Aldave AJ. Long-term outcomes of the Boston type I keratoprosthesis in the management of corneal limbal stem cell deficiency. Cornea. 2016;35(9):1156–64.
59. Lee WB, Shtein RM, Kaufman SC, Deng SX, Rosenblatt MI. Boston keratoprosthesis: outcomes and complications: a report by the American Academy of Ophthalmology. Ophthalmology. 2015;122(7):1504–11.
60. Nakamura T, Inatomi T, Sotozono C, Koizumi N, Kinoshita S. Ocular surface reconstruction using stem cell and tissue engineering. Prog Retin Eye Res. 2016;51:187–207.
61. Ghareeb AE, Lako M, Figueiredo FC. Recent advances in stem cell therapy for limbal stem cell deficiency: a narrative review. Ophthalmol Ther. 2020;9(4):809–31.
62. Yazdanpanah G, Haq Z, Kang K, Jabbehdari S, Rosenblatt ML, Djalilian AR. Strategies for reconstructing the limbal stem cell niche. Ocul Surf. 2019;17(2):230–40.
63. Soleimani M, Cheraqpour K, Koganti R, Baharnoori SM, Djalilian AR. Concise review: bioengineering of limbal stem cell niche. Bioengineering (Basel). 2023;10(1):111.
64. Schlötzer-Schrehardt U, Freudenberg U, Kruse FE. Zukunftstechnologie Tissue-Engineering: Fokus auf die Stammzellnische [The emerging technology of tissue engineering: focus on stem cell niche]. Ophthalmologe. 2017;114(4):327–40.
65. Nieto-Nicolau N, Martínez-Conesa EM, Velasco-García AM, Aloy-Reverté C, Vilarrodona A, Casaroli-Marano RP. Xenofree generation of limbal stem cells for ocular surface advanced cell therapy. Stem Cell Res Ther. 2019;10(1):374.
66. Masood F, Chang JH, Akbar A, Song A, Hu WY, Azar DT, Rosenblatt MI. Therapeutic strategies for restoring perturbed corneal epithelial homeostasis in limbal stem cell deficiency: current trends and future directions. Cells. 2022;11(20):3247.
67. Calonge M, Pérez I, Galindo S, Nieto-Miguel T, López-Paniagua M, Fernández I, Alberca M, García-Sancho J, Sánchez A, Herreras JM. A proof-of-concept clinical trial using mesenchymal stem cells for the treatment of corneal epithelial stem cell deficiency. Transl Res. 2019;206:18–40.
68. Hayashi R, Ishikawa Y, Katori R, Sasamoto Y, Taniwaki Y, Takayanagi H, Tsujikawa M, Sekiguchi K, Quantock AJ, Nishida K. Coordinated generation of multiple ocular-like cell lineages and fabrication of functional corneal epithelial cell sheets from human iPS cells. Nat Protoc. 2017;12(4):683–96.
69. Mahmood N, Suh TC, Ali KM, Sefat E, Jahan UM, Huang Y, Gilger BC, Gluck JM. Induced pluripotent stem cell-derived corneal cells: current status and application. Stem Cell Rev Rep. 2022;18(8):2817–32.

Bacterial Keratitis

Loïc Hamon, Sören L. Becker, and Berthold Seitz

Abstract

Bacterial infections are by far the most common cause of infectious keratitis in high-income countries. The clinical appearance can vary widely depending on the type and species of bacteria, ranging from small superficial infiltrates to necrotizing forms. The multiple classes of available antibiotics render the therapeutic scope varied and complex, especially before pathogen specification and antibiotic sensitivity testing. This chapter focuses on the clinical, diagnostic and therapeutic approaches to bacterial keratitis.

Keywords

Keratitis · Bacteria · Bacillus · Coccus · Polymerase chain reaction · Culture · Antibiotics · Antibiotic sensitivity testing · Crosslinking · Keratoplasty

1 Introduction

Bacteria have the lead in term of infectious keratitis in United States of America (USA) and Europe, representing more than 90% of all diagnosed microbial keratitis [1, 2]. On the contrary, they represent a minor part of microbial keratitis compared to fungal keratitis in pacific Asia and India, with only 34% [3]. The prevalence of bacterial keratitis varies with age, job, socio-economic status and other predisposing conditions or risk factors. Concerning the pathophysiology, most bacteria need a break of the epithelial layer to penetrate into the cornea, thus inducing a **bacterial keratitis** (Fig. 1). Nevertheless, some bacteria such as *Neisseria* sp. or *Corynebacterium* sp. are able to penetrate intact epithelium. The severity of the infection greatly depends on the pathogen agent and the therapeutic response to local antibiotics and could extend in endophthalmitis with potential blindness.

The following chapter focuses on differential diagnosis between bacterial pathogens and on stage-appropriate therapy.

2 Risk Factors

Risk factors are in principle all localized or systemic conditions that could alternate the integrity of the epithelial layer and thus let bacteria penetrate into the stroma, or reduce the patient's local or systemic immune response against microbial agents. Major risk factors are summarized in Table 1.

A major risk factor for severe bacterial keratitis, principally for young patients without underlying diseases, is the (mis)use of **contact lenses** (CL) (Fig. 2). Contact lens-associated keratitis can present with pathogens such as *Pseudomonas aeruginosa*, or, less frequently, other Gram-negative species such as *Serratia* species (sp.), and show not rarely mixed infections with fungus or the parasite *Acanthamoeba* sp. Therefore, contact lens-associated keratitis needs particularly attention in order to target pathogens as fast as possible and thus optimize the therapy.

L. Hamon (✉) · B. Seitz
Department of Ophthalmology, Saarland University Medical Center, Homburg/Saar, Germany
e-mail: hamon.loic@outlook.com

B. Seitz
e-mail: berthold.seitz@uks.eu

L. Hamon
Department of Ophthalmology, Clinique Notre-Dame de Grâce, Charleroi, Belgium

S. L. Becker
Institute of Medical Microbiology and Hygiene, Saarland University Medical Center, Homburg/Saar, Germany
e-mail: becker.soeren@uks.eu

B. Seitz et al. (eds.), *Atlas on Cornea*, https://doi.org/10.1007/978-3-031-65422-0_22

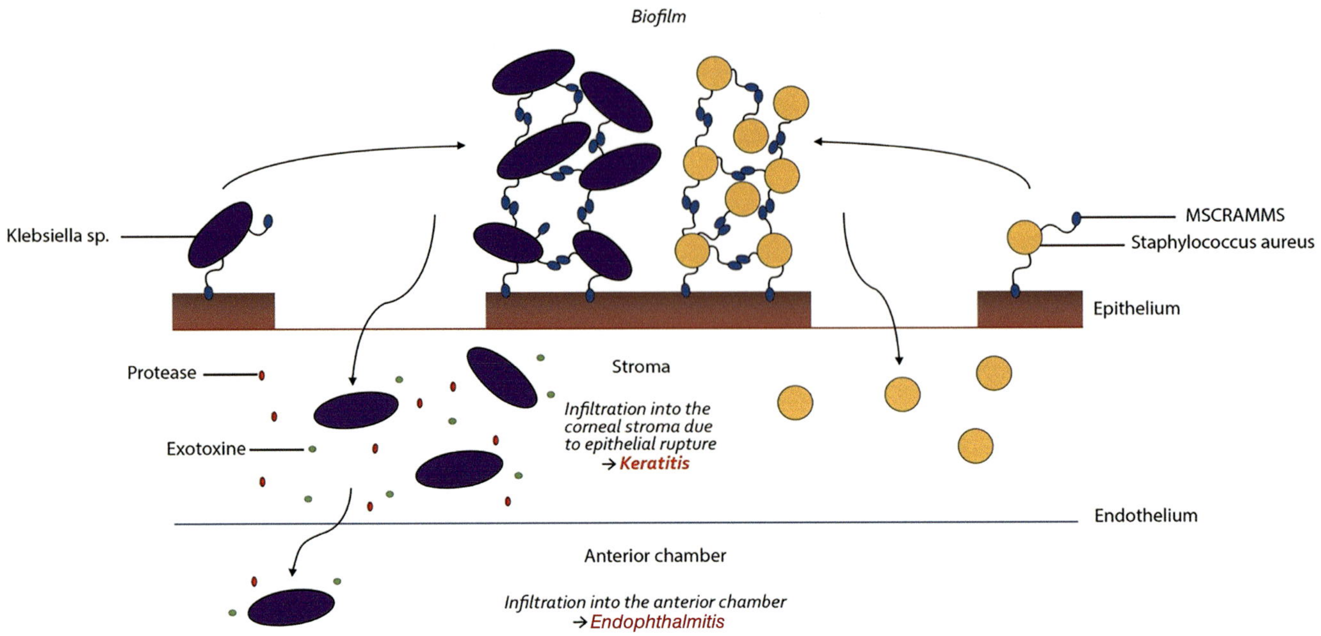

Fig. 1 **Pathophysiology of bacterial keratitis**. In case of disruption of the epithelial barrier, bacteria can adhere to the margin of damaged epithelium surface using epithelial glycoproteins and bacterial surface adhesins (so-called microbial surface components recognizing adhesive matrix molecules—*MSCRAMMS*) to create a protective film for bacteria (biofilm), favorizing bacterial resistance against immune response [4]. A microbiological infiltration into the cornea is called **keratitis**. Gram-negative bacteria are generally not very virulent and rarely penetrate deep into the stroma. In contrast, gram-positive bacteria can produce proteases, exotoxins and lipopolysaccharides (LPS) in order to degrade stromal basement membrane and extracellular matrix. In case of melting of the deep stromal tissue, bacterial infiltration into the anterior chamber is possible, thus causing **endophthalmitis**

Table 1 Risk factors for bacterial keratitis

Ocular		Systemic	
Contact lenses		Diabetes mellitus	
Acute trauma	Corneal injury	Atopic dermatitis (rosacea, neurodermitis)	
	Corneal foreign body	Collagenosis, vasculitis	Sjögren syndrome
	Corneal perforation		Rheumatoid arthritis
Eyelid pathologies	Eyelid malposition	Vitamin A deficiency	
	Trichiasis	Immune deficiency	AIDS
	Lagophthalmos		Systemic immunosuppressive therapy
	Blepharitis	Graves' disease	
Chronic alteration of ocular surface	Dry eye syndrome		
	Expositional keratopathy		
	Corneal hypoesthesia (e.g. after herpes virus infection)		
Chronic use of local immunosuppressive therapy			

3 Symptoms and Clinical Aspect

Patients with bacterial keratitis present typically in general or ophthalmologic emergency with unspecific symptoms such as (peri-)ocular pain, foreign body sensation, photophobia, epiphora, secretions, decrease on visual acuity or acute contact lens intolerance. The diagnosis can be realized clinically using a slit lamp, with the typical presence of an epithelial defect associated with stromal white-grayish or -yellowish infiltrates (Figs. 3, 4, 5 and 6). Atypical infiltrates such as ring infiltrates can also be observed in bacterial keratitis (Fig. 7) [9], particularly for patients presenting immunodeficiency [10]. The clinical aspect gives a good indication of the severity of the keratitis but is never sufficient to specify the pathogen(s) involved.

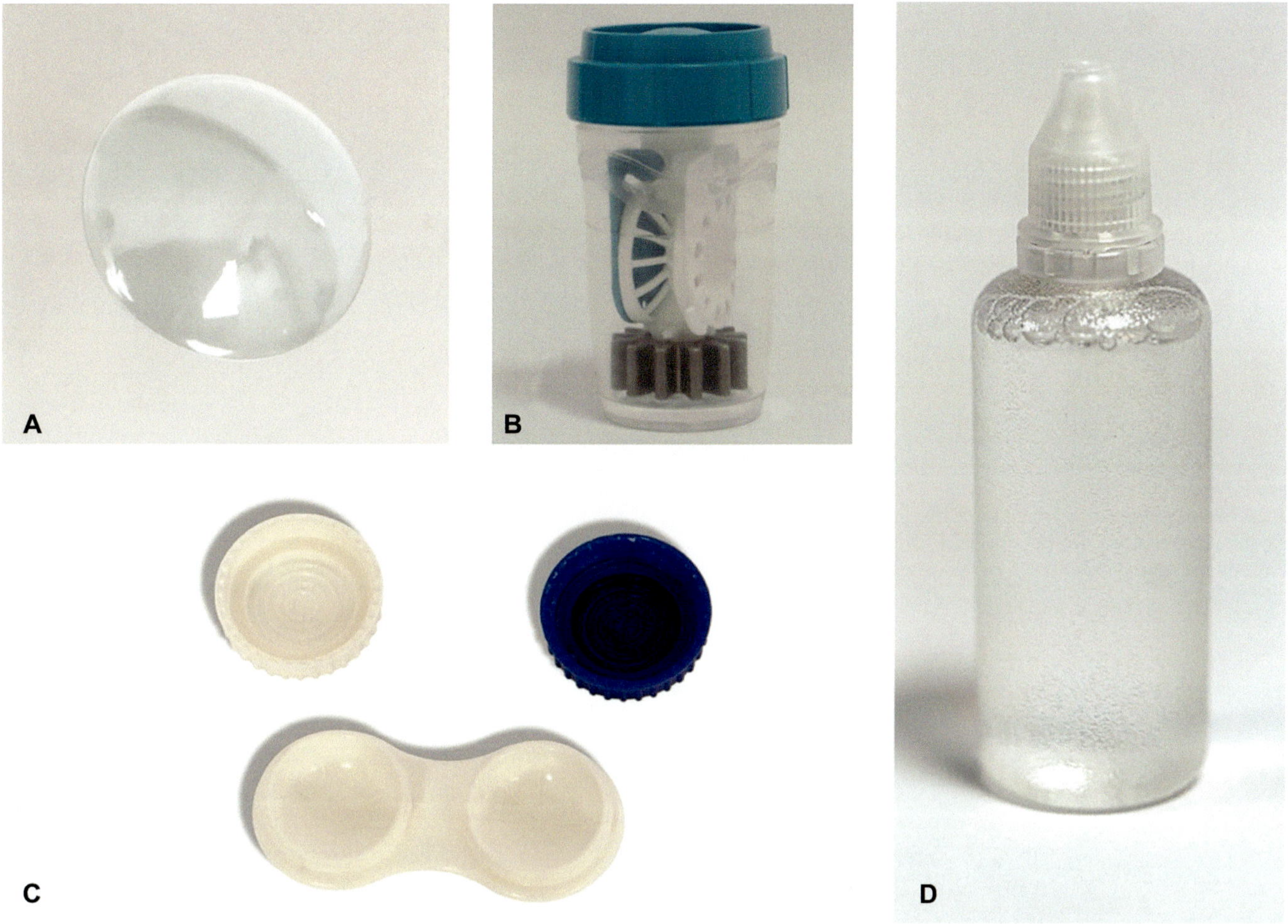

Fig. 2 **Contact lens-associated keratitis**. (**A**) Soft contact lens (CL). (**B, C**) CL cases. (**D**) CL cleaning solution. CL and all elements involved in contact lens hygiene can contain or retain germs and are a high provider of keratitis, especially in young healthy population. Keratitis incidence varies with the CL wearing duration, with reported incidences of 3–5 per 10,000 for daily CL and 20 per 10,000 for monthly CL [5, 6]. Also, CL stiffness and material are important criteria, with higher risk using soft CL compared to rigid CL or silicon hydrogel lenses compared to hydroxyethylmethacrylate CL [7]. Finally, wearing CL during night increases the risk of keratitis by 6.5 [8]. In case of CL-associated keratitis, it is recommended to send not only the CL but also the case and a sample of cleaning solution for microbiological analysis

4 Pathogen Identification

Pathogen identification is performed by analyses of tissue or liquid samples (scratches, swabs, punctions or biopsies), preferably prior to initiation of antibiotic therapy. Potential bacterial agents can be preliminarily identified based on their microscopic morphology (cocci or rods/bacilli) and their characteristics on Gram stain (Gram-positive: blue-darkish; Gram-negative: reddish color), using light microscopy (Fig. 8), which allows to guide first therapeutic decisions (Table 2).

Culture from corneal scratch, corneal or conjunctival swab or anterior chamber punction (in case of hypopyon) remains currently the gold standard for pathogen identification [13]. The culture is performed in laboratory in liquid nutrient medium (broth culture) or on agar plates by microbiologists and usually takes 24–72 h for common pathogens; however, prolonged incubation of up to several weeks might be required for fastidious pathogens and mycobacteria (Fig. 9).

Most culture-grown isolates can be unambiguously identified using matrix-assisted laser desorption/ionization time-of-flight (MALDI-TOF) mass spectrometry. In addition to identification, this technique can also be employed for further characterizations, e.g. proteomic fingerprinting of an organism (Fig. 10).

As additional tests, pan-bacterial and/or pan-fungal polymerase chain reaction (PCR) assays might be useful to detect pathogens that could be missed by culture alone. However, PCR is also prone to false-negative results, especially in the case of oligobacterial infections. A limitation

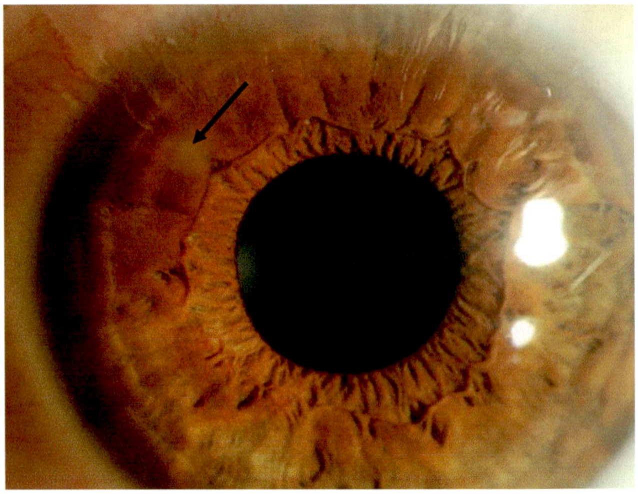

Fig. 3 ***Staphylococcus aureus*** **keratitis** presenting a small white–gray-cream, cloudy, well-demarcated stromal infiltrate (*arrow*). Keratitis presenting this aspect have a mostly good prognosis under topical therapy

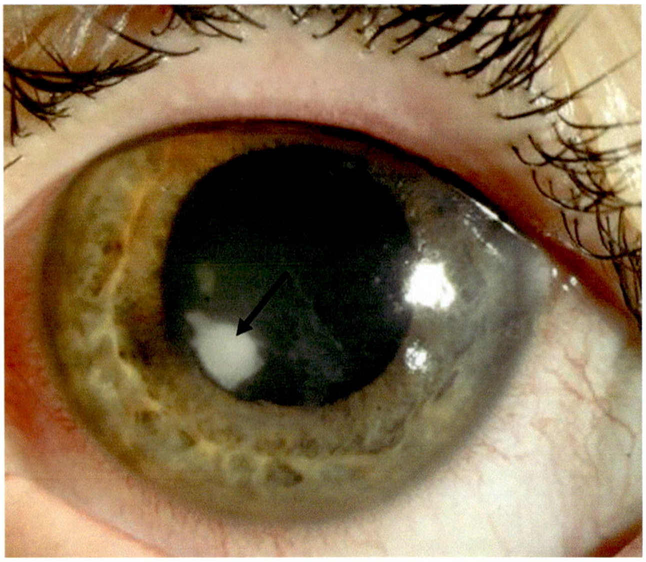

Fig. 5 ***Klebsiella*** **sp. keratitis** presenting a medium-sized, white-creamy, completely opaque and well demarcated infiltrate (*arrow*). Such infiltrates require high frequency local therapy and daily controls as long as no significant improvement is visible

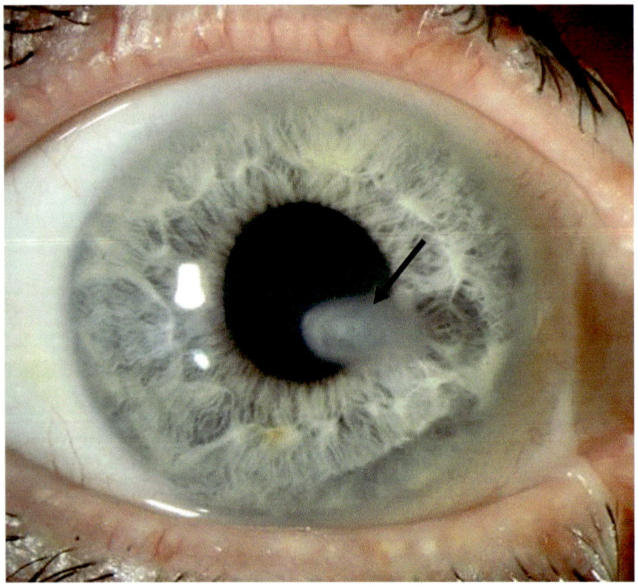

Fig. 4 ***Pseudomonas*** **sp. keratitis** presenting a medium-sized, more opaque, well-demarcated infiltrate (*arrow*) with central ulceration. Despite a relatively reassuring clinical aspect, it is important to be vigilant regarding a potentially rapid deterioration

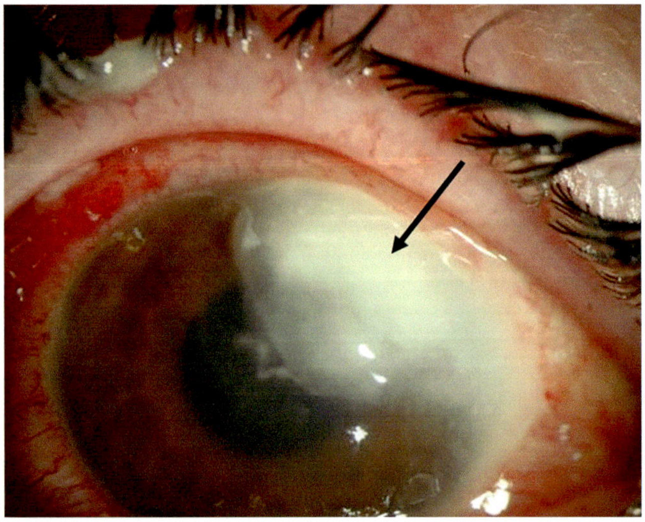

Fig. 6 ***Pseudomonas aeruginosa*** **keratitis** presenting a large, creamy and purulent infiltrate (*arrow*) with dirty aspect. Pseudomonas keratitis frequently presents with rapid progression into the deep stroma, which may lead to corneal perforation

of PCR is its inability to differentiate between vital and non-vital pathogens, which does not allow the assessment of the activity of the infection.

In vivo confocal microscopy has shown an important role in the diagnosis of microbial keratitis, particularly for the early detection of fungi [14] and acanthamoeba [15]. On the contrary, in vivo confocal microscopy appeared mostly valueless in bacterial keratitis, showing very atypical pictures [16] (Fig. 11).

5 Therapy

The therapeutical approach in case of keratitis is often limited to a topical antibiotic treatment. Since systemic therapy has (almost) no role in bacterial keratitis, the following recommendations concern only topical therapy (eye drops or ointments). The conservative therapeutical approach for bacterial keratitis is divided into two crucial steps:

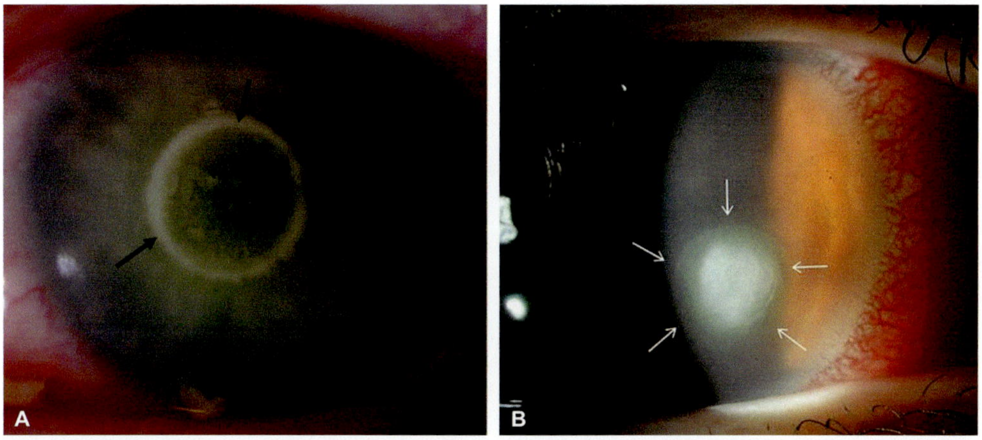

Fig. 7 **Ring infiltrate**. (**A**) ***Moraxella atlantae* keratitis** presenting an atypical **ring infiltrate** (arrows). Reprinted with permission of Elsevier. Am J Ophthalmol Case Reports, Vol. 7, A. Barash, T.Y. Chou, Moraxella atlantae keratitis presenting with an infectious ring ulcer, pp. 62–65. Copyright (2017). (**B**) Discrete immune ring around a dense bacterial infiltrate (arrows). Ring infiltrates are an unusual finding in gram-negative bacterial keratitis due to focal immune reaction involving bacterial exotoxins, damaged host cells, complement and immune complexes with chemotactically attraction of polymorphonuclear leukocytes [9, 11]. Ring infiltrates, also known as *Wessely immune ring*, are more typically seen in acanthamoeba keratitis but are not pathognomonic [12]. Reprinted with permission of Springer Nature. Ophthalmologe, Issue 118, Weinstein I, Fries FN, Szentmáry N, Seitz B, Daas L. [Distinctive Wessely immune ring in keratitis—a chameleon], pp. 53–55. Copyright (2021)

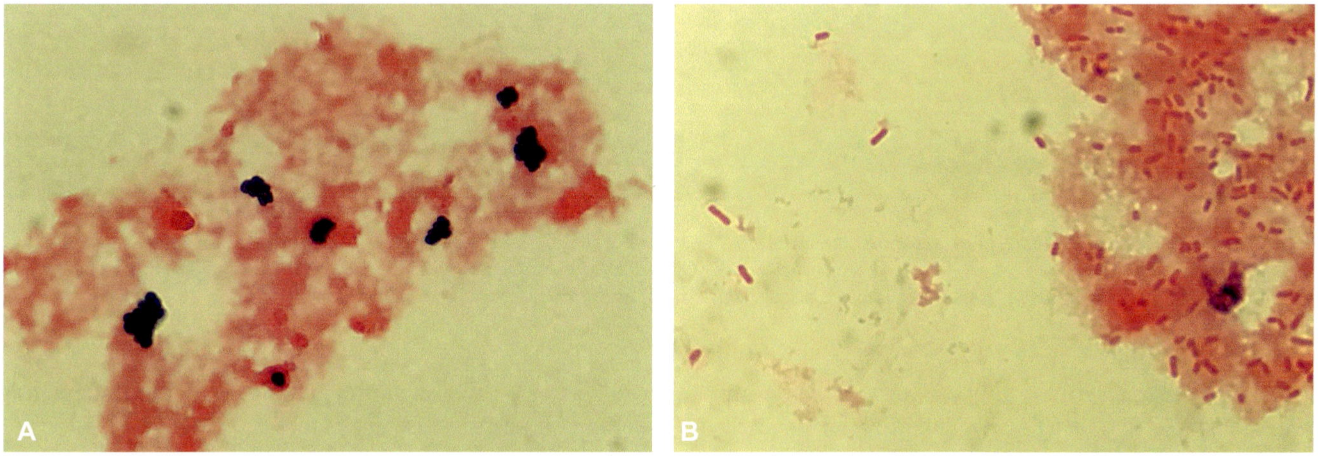

Fig. 8 **Direct examination of Gram-stained bacteria using light microscopy**. (**A**) Typical appearance of Gram-positive (=dark-blueish color) cocci (e.g. *Staphylococcus epidermidis*). (**B**) Typical appearance of Gram-negative (=red-colored) rods (e.g. *Klebsiella pneumoniae*)

(1) **Empirical therapy**, before identification of the pathogen, based on severity and pathogen probability [18]. Topical therapy should be started as soon as possible, before pathogen identification. A too moderate therapy could be contraproductive. Therapy should begin with sufficient posology [6]. Topical application of quinolones can be a reasonable first choice in cases of isolated superficial infiltrate, e.g. moxifloxacin 8x/d. In more alarming cases, multiple or large infiltrates, combination therapy might be beneficial, e.g. moxifloxacin + cefuroxime or moxifloxacin + polyspectran® (polymyxin B + Neomycin + Gramicidin) every half an hour alternatively for a few days. The frequency can be rapidly reduced in case of improvement. In case of intraocular involvement or stromal necrosis, topical steroid therapy should be slowly initiated after improvement under antibiotics [19].

(2) **Therapy adjustment**, after pathogen identification. Topical gyrase inhibitors (e.g. ciprofloxacin, ofloxacin, moxifloxacin, …) are usually efficient against staphylococci, streptococci, *Pseudomonas* spp. and other Gram-negative bacteria. Aminoglycosides (e.g. gentamycin, tobramycin, …) are also efficient against staphylococci and *Pseudomonas* spp. For anaerobic bacteria, lincosamides (e.g. clindamycin) are commonly used.

Table 2 Frequent pathogen agents for bacterial keratitis

Coccus		Bacillus		
Gram +	Gram −	Gram +	Gram −	Acid-fast bacilli
Staphylococcus aureus	*Moraxella* spp.	*Corynebacterium diphtheriae*	*Escherichia coli*	*Mycobacterium* spp.
Coagulase-negative staphylococci	*Neisseria gonorrhoeae*	*Bacillus* spp.	*Klebsiella pneumoniae*	*Nocardia* spp.
Streptococcus pneumoniae	*Neisseria meningitidis*		*Morganella morganii*	
Streptococcus pyogenes			*Pseudomonas* spp.	
Viridans streptococci			*Serratia marcescens*	
Anaerobic cocci			*Acinetobacter* spp.	
			Proteus spp.	

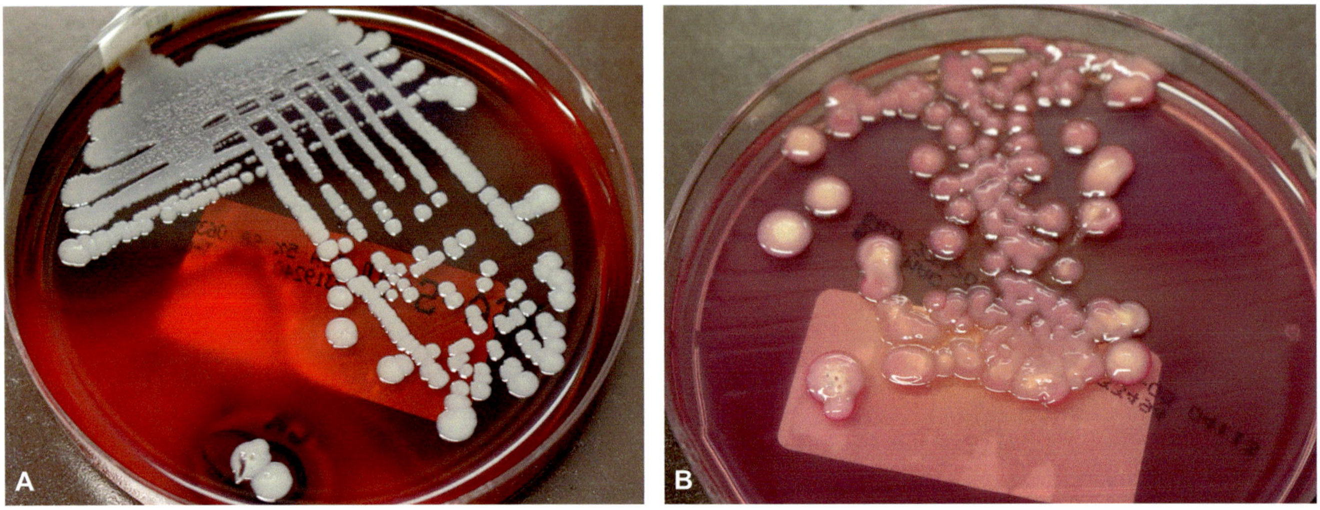

Fig. 9 **Bacterial growth on agar plate cultures**. Bacteria are streaked on petri dishes containing specific agar media. These agar plates are then incubated at 35–37 °C for several days to detect bacteria. (**A**) Growth of a beta-haemolytic *Staphylococcus aureus* on a blood agar plate. (**B**) Growth of *Klebsiella pneumoniae* on MacConkey agar, a specific medium for Gram-negative bacteria

If antibiotic sensitivity testing was performed during the culture (Fig. 12), the therapy should be adapted to specific resistances and sensitivities (Fig. 13) [20].

In case of deterioration under topical therapy, the addition of systemic antibiotics could be beneficial and a complementary surgical approach should be considered. In this context, photoactivated chromophore for infectious keratitis crosslinking (PACK-CXL) seems to be a useful adjuvant therapy in (therapy-resistant) bacterial keratitis, with up to 85.7% therapeutical success and faster epithelial healing [22, 23]. Alternatively, steam cautery procedure [24] or argon cold plasma therapy (ionization of plasma at "low" temperature in the infected corneal tissue) also showed promising results, reducing broad spectrum of pathogens without damaging the ocular surface [25].

For more severe cases with fulminant evolution, hypopyon or corneal perforation, a penetrating keratoplasty (PKP) is indicated [26]. The PKP should be performed without delay (not before assessment of conservative therapeutic effect but also **not too late**!), in order to reduce the risk of endophthalmitis and maximize the success of surgery. The PKP can also be combined with lens extraction or cataract surgery [27]. In such cases, the addition of systemic broad-spectrum antibiotics might be beneficial. A large diameter transplant (e.g. 10.0/10.5 mm) may be necessary with 32 single sutures, allowing the removal of loose or infected sutures postoperatively [28, 29] (Fig. 14).

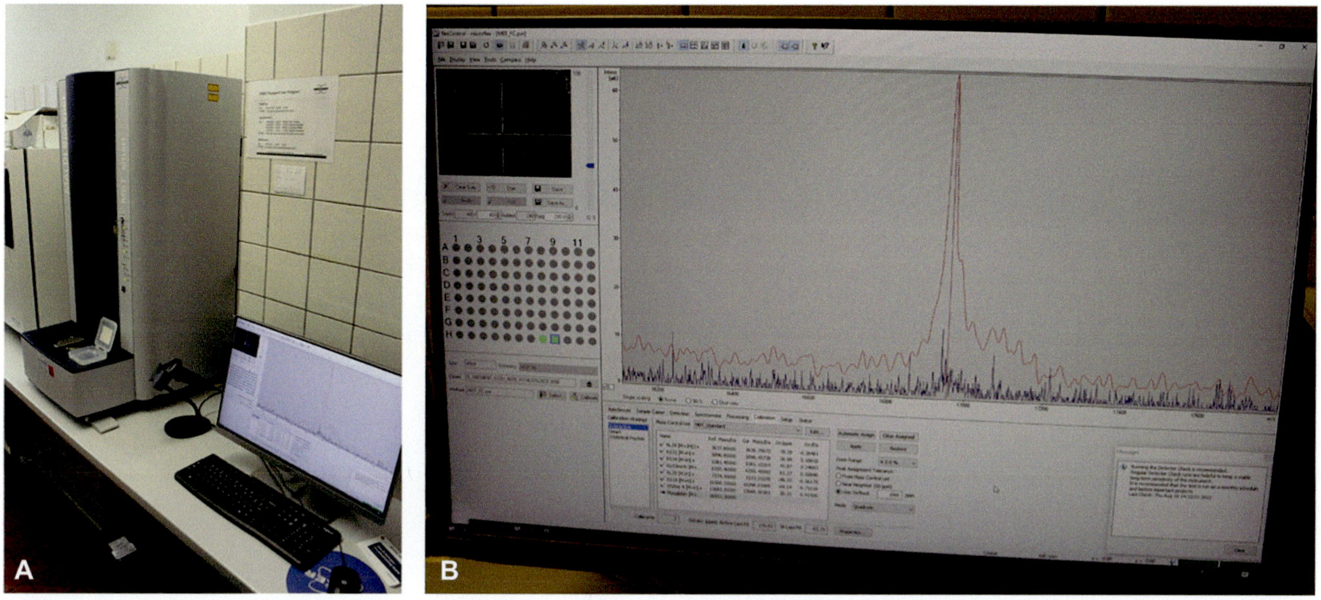

Fig. 10 **Matrix-assisted laser desorption/ionization time-of-flight (MALDI-TOF) mass spectrometry** is nowadays a standard technique for a rapid identification of culture-grown bacteria to the species level. (**A**) MALDI-TOF mass spectrometer. (**B**) Overview of the accompanying software, displaying specific measurement results. Reprinted with permission of Springer Nature Journal of Ophthalmic Inflammation and Infection, Issue 1, Vol. 10, Soleimani M, Masoumi A, Khodavaisy A, Heidari M, Haydar AA, Izadi A. Current diagnostic tools and management modalities of Nocardia keratitis, p. 36. Copyright (2011)

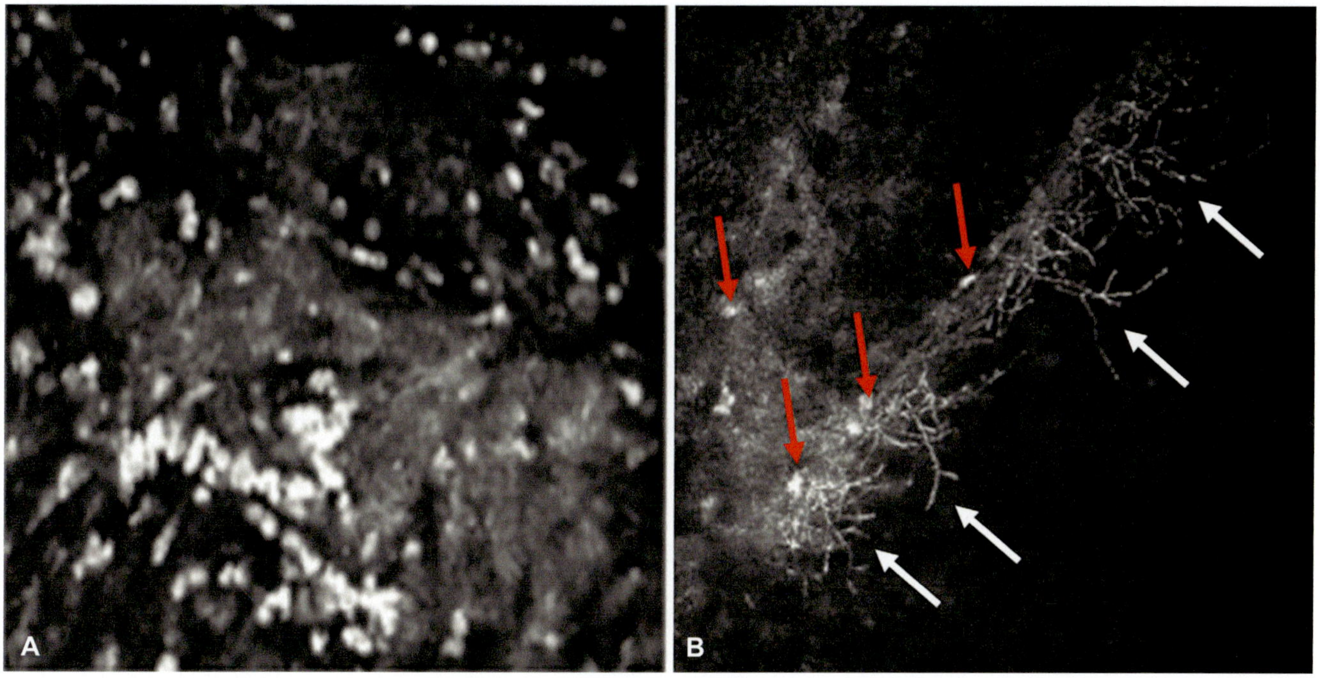

Fig. 11 **In vivo confocal microscopy**. (**A**) **Staphylococcus keratitis**. No typical aspect in in vivo confocal microscopy. The numerous round hyperreflective structures correspond to inflammatory cells (neutrophils and macrophages) and are particularly evident at infiltrate margins. (**B**) **Nocardia keratitis**. Thin hyperreflective interlocking filaments at infiltrate margin (*white arrows*), corresponding to *Nocardia* sp., with surrounding round hyperreflective structures (*red arrows*), corresponding to inflammatory cells [17]. Nocardia filaments are thinner than fungal hyphae but could be easily misinterpreted as fungal structures. Reprinted with permission of Springer Nature Journal of Ophthalmic Inflammation and Infection, Issue 1, Vol. 10, Soleimani M, Masoumi A, Khodavaisy A, Heidari M, Haydar AA, Izadi A. Current diagnostic tools and management modalities of Nocardia keratitis, p. 36. Copyright (2011)

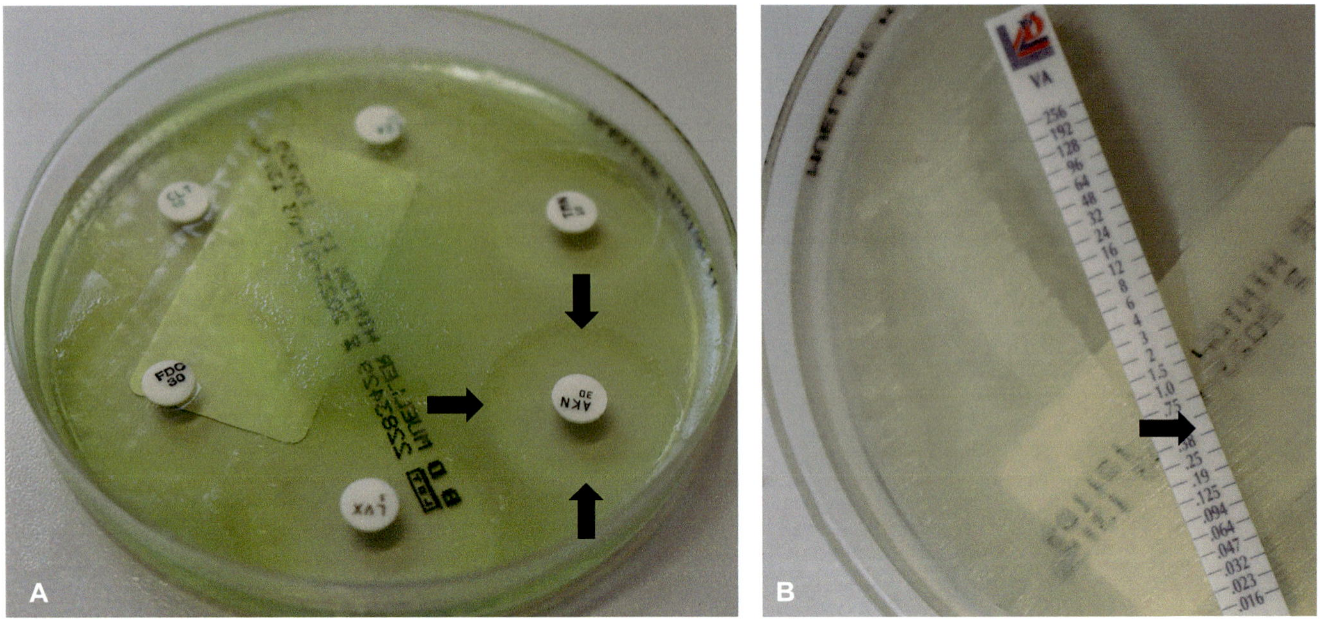

Fig. 12 **Antibiotic susceptibility testing**. The bacterium is streaked on a nutrient agar plate and is then exposed to antibiotic-containing disks or strips. If bacterial growth is inhibited, a clear inhibition zone becomes visible around the antibiotic (*black arrows*). (**A**) Disc diffusion method. (**B**) Epsilometry. The strip contains an ascending concentration of the antibiotic, which allows to identify the exact minimal inhibitory concentration (MIC) of the antibiotic

Culture

[1] Staphylococcus epidermidis **isolated**

Antibiogram	**[1]**		**[1]**
Flucloxacillin	S	Daptomycin	S
Cefazolin	S	Vancomycin	S
Gentamicin	**R**	Doxycyclin	**R**
Ciprofloxacin	S	Tigecyclin	S
Moxifloxacin	S	Fosfomycin	S
Erythromycin	**R**	Fusidinsäure	**R**
Clindamycin	S	Co-trimoxazol	S
Linezolid	S		

A

Culture

[1] Pseudomonas aeruginosa **after enrichment**

Antibiogram	**[1]**		**[1]**
Piperacillin/Tazobactam	I	Tobramycin	I
Ceftazidim	I	Amikacin	S
Cefepim	I	Ciprofloxacin	I
Imipenem	I	Levofloxacin	I
Meropenem	S		

B

Fig. 13 **Typical reports of culture with antibiotic sensitivity testing**. (**A**) Corneal scratch positive for *staphylococcus epidermidis*, showing multi-sensitivity to antibiotics but resistance against gentamycin, erythromycin, doxycycline and fusidic acid. In such cases, a local monotherapy with commercially available antibiotics (e.g. moxifloxacin eye drops) is generally sufficient. (**B**) Corneal scratch positive for *pseudomonas aeruginosa*, showing mostly intermediate sensitivity, except for meropenem and amikacin. In case of intermediate sensitivity, **fortified eye drops** with (classically 10×) higher concentration can be used, ideally as polytherapy with 2 or more antibiotic classes [21]

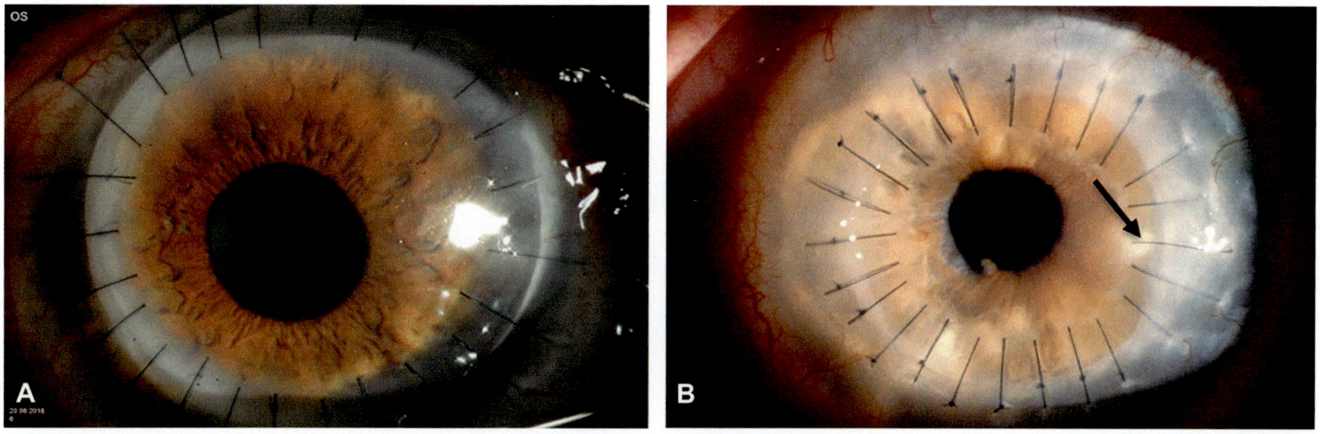

Fig. 14 **Penetrating keratoplasty**. (**A**) **Cornea after emergency penetrating keratoplasty ("à chaud") for fulminant pseudomonas spp. keratitis**. In case of acute keratitis, it is essential to use a large dimension graft (e.g. 10.0/10.5 mm or even more) to avoid recurrence as well as (24–32) single sutures to allow their removal in case of localized infection [26]. (**B**) Patient after emergency penetrating keratoplasty "à chaud" presenting a focal **infiltrate with loosening suture** (*arrow*)

6 Conclusion

Bacterial keratitis can present clinically in various forms. Appropriate therapy requires rapid treatment initiation and possibly identification of the pathogen and determination of its antimicrobial susceptibility pattern. Although the gold standard remains culture, the diagnostic yield might be improved by adjunctive PCR analyses. Topical antibiotic therapy should be started before pathogen identification and then further adapted after diagnosis. A surgical approach can be considered in case of deterioration despite appropriate therapy.

References

1. Ting DSJ, Settle C, Morgan SJ, Baylis O, Ghosh S. A 10-year analysis of microbiological profiles of microbial keratitis: the North East England Study. Eye. 2018;32:1416–7. https://doi.org/10.1038/s41433-018-0085-4.
2. Alexandrakis G, Alfonso EC, Miller D. Shifting trends in bacterial keratitis in South Florida and emerging resistance to fluoroquinolones. Ophthalmology. 2000;107:1497–502. https://doi.org/10.1016/s0161-6420(00)00179-2.
3. Lalitha P, Manoharan G, Karpagam R, Prajna NV, Srinivasan M, Mascarenhas J, Das M, Porco TC, Lietman TM, Cevallos V, Keenan JD. Trends in antibiotic resistance in bacterial keratitis isolates from South India. Br J Ophthalmol. 2016;101:108–13. https://doi.org/10.1136/bjophthalmol-2016-308487.
4. Lakhundi S, Siddiqui R, Khan NA. Pathogenesis of microbial keratitis. Microb Pathog. 2017;104:97–109. https://doi.org/10.1016/j.micpath.2016.12.013.
5. Cheng KH, Leung SL, Hoekman HW, Beekhuis WH, Mulder PG, Geerards AJ, Kijlstra A. Incidence of contact-lens-associated microbial keratitis and its related morbidity. Lancet. 1999;354:181–5. https://doi.org/10.1016/S0140-6736(98)09385-4.
6. Rachwalik D, Pleyer U. Bacterial keratitis. Klin Monbl Augenheilkd. 2015;232:738–44.
7. Stapleton F, Keay L, Edwards K, Naduvilath T, Dart JK, Brian G, Holden BA. The incidence of contact lens-related microbial keratitis in Australia. Ophthalmology. 2008;115:1655–62. https://doi.org/10.1016/j.ophtha.2008.04.002.
8. Stapleton F, Edwards K, Keay L, Naduvilath T, Dart JK, Brian G, Holden B. Risk factors for moderate and severe microbial keratitis in daily wear contact lens users. Ophthalmology. 2012;119:1516–21. https://doi.org/10.1016/j.ophtha.2012.01.052.
9. Barash A, Chou TY. Moraxella atlantae keratitis presenting with an infectious ring ulcer. Am J Ophthalmol Case Rep. 2017;7:62–5. https://doi.org/10.1016/j.ajoc.2017.06.003.
10. Chaidaroon W, Supalaset S. Corneal ring infiltrates caused by serratia marcescens in a patient with human immunodeficiency virus. Case Rep Ophthalmol. 2016;7:359–63. https://doi.org/10.1159/000448023.
11. Ijiri Y, Yamamoto T, Kamata R. The role of Pseudomonas aeruginosa elastase in corneal ring abscess formation in pseudomonal keratitis. Graefes Arch Clin Exp Ophthalmol. 1993;231:521–8. https://doi.org/10.1007/BF00921117.
12. Weinstein I, Fries FN, Szentmáry N, Seitz B, Daas L. Distinctive Wessely immune ring in keratitis—a chameleon. Ophthalmologe. 2021;118:53–5. https://doi.org/10.1007/s00347-020-01084-8.
13. Pleyer U, Behrens-Baumann W. Bacterial keratitis. Current diagnostic aspects. Ophthalmologe. 2007;104:9–14. https://doi.org/10.1007/s00347-006-1466-9.
14. Sourlis C, Seitz B, Roth M, Hamon L, Daas L. Outcomes of severe fungal keratitis using in vivo confocal microscopy and early therapeutic penetrating keratoplasty. Clin Ophthalmol. 2022;16:2245–54. https://doi.org/10.2147/OPTH.S358709.
15. Daas L, Viestenz A, Schnabel PA, Fries FN, Hager T, Szentmáry N, Seitz B. Confocal microscopy as an early relapse marker for acanthamoeba keratitis. Clin Anat. 2018;31:60–3. https://doi.org/10.1002/ca.22925.
16. Kumar RL, Cruzat A, Hamrah P. Current state of in vivo confocal microscopy in management of microbial keratitis. Semin Ophthalmol. 2010;25:166–70. https://doi.org/10.3109/08820538.2010.518516.
17. Soleimani M, Masoumi A, Khodavaisy S, Heidari M, Haydar AA, Izadi A. Current diagnostic tools and management modalities of Nocardia keratitis. J Ophthalmic Inflamm Infect. 2020;10:36. https://doi.org/10.1186/s12348-020-00228-w.

18. Austin A, Lietman T, Rose-Nussbaumer J. Update on the management of infectious keratitis. Ophthalmology. 2017;124:1678–89. https://doi.org/10.1016/j.ophtha.2017.05.012.
19. Ni N, Srinivasan M, McLeod SD, Acharya NR, Lietman TM, Rose-Nussbaumer J. Use of adjunctive topical corticosteroids in bacterial keratitis. Curr Opin Ophthalmol. 2016;27:353–7. https://doi.org/10.1097/ICU.0000000000000273.
20. Jorgensen JH, Ferraro MJ. Antimicrobial susceptibility testing: a review of general principles and contemporary practices. Clin Infect Dis. 2009;49:1749–55. https://doi.org/10.1086/647952.
21. Chiquet C, Romanet JP. Prescribing fortified eye drops. J Fr Ophtalmol. 2007;30:423–30. https://doi.org/10.1016/s0181-5512(07)89618-5.
22. Papaioannou L, Miligkos M, Papathanassiou M. Corneal collagen cross-linking for infectious keratitis: a systematic review and meta-analysis. Cornea. 2016;35:62–71. https://doi.org/10.1097/ICO.0000000000000644.
23. Ting DSJ, Henein C, Said DG, Dua HS. Photoactivated chromophore for infectious keratitis Corneal cross-linking (PACK-CXL): a systematic review and meta-analysis. Ocul Surf. 2019;17:624–34. https://doi.org/10.1016/j.jtos.2019.08.006.
24. Maier P, Birnbaum F, Reinhard T. Steam cautery of the cornea in microbial keratitis. Ophthalmologe. 2008;105:79–80. https://doi.org/10.1007/s00347-007-1652-4.
25. Reitberger HH, Czugala M, Chow C, Mohr A, Burkovski A, Gruenert AK, Schoenebeck R, Fuchsluger TA. Argon cold plasma—a novel tool to treat therapy-resistant corneal infections. Am J Ophthalmol. 2018;190:150–63. https://doi.org/10.1016/j.ajo.2018.03.025.
26. Seitz B, Szentmáry N, El-Husseiny M, Viestenz A, Langenbucher A, Naumann GO. The penetrating keratoplasty (PKP): a century of success. In: Hjortdal J, ed. Corneal transplantation. Cham: Springer; 2016. p. 67–92.
27. Berger T, Seitz B, Flockerzi E, Suffo S, Daas L. Indications and results of emergency penetrating keratoplasty with simultaneous cataract surgery ("triple-PKP à chaud"). Cornea. 2023;42:272–9. https://doi.org/10.1097/ICO.0000000000003035.
28. Jonas JB, Budde WM. Loosening of single versus double running sutures in penetrating keratoplasty for keratoconus. Graefes Arch Clin Exp Ophthalmol. 1999;237:522–3. https://doi.org/10.1007/s004170050273.
29. Alfaro Rangel R, Szentmáry N, Lepper S, Milioti G, Daas L, Langenbucher A, Seitz B. Large-diameter penetrating keratoplasties are mostly due to very severe infectious keratitis and cannot always prevent secondary enucleation. Klin Monbl Augenheilkd. 2022;239:1361–8. https://doi.org/10.1055/a-1396-4787.

The Chameleon of "Herpetic Keratitis"—Different Manifestations Require Different Therapeutic Approaches

Berthold Seitz and Arnd Heiligenhaus

Abstract

Keratitis of herpetic origin, which is common in Europe, is mostly caused by herpes simplex virus type I (HSV) and its appearance is like a chameleon. It can usually be treated successfully if the different, typically unilateral forms of this disease are known: 1. epithelial keratitis (dendritica/geographica), 2. stromal keratitis (necrotizing vs. non-necrotizing = "interstitial"), 3. endotheliitis (="disciform keratitis"), 4. so-called "metaherpetic keratitis" (=neurotrophic keratopathy), 5. (vascularized) corneal scars. The therapeutic regimen is deliberately adapted to the form of appearance. Concomitant ocular hypertension should be treated primarily with medication in the acute stage (avoid prostaglandin analogues!). After keratoplasty and in case of frequent severe keratitis episodes, systemic acyclovir application (2×400 mg/day) for at least 1 year is the current standard!

Keywords

Herpetic keratitis · Keratitis dendritica · Disciform keratitis · Interstitial keratitis · Ulcerative necrotizing stromal keratitis · Metaherpetic keratitis · Chameleon · Therapeutic regimen

B. Seitz (✉)
Department of Ophthalmology, Saarland University Medical Center, Homburg/Saar, Germany
e-mail: berthold.seitz@uks.eu
URL: https://www.augenklinik-saarland.de

A. Heiligenhaus
Eye Department at St. Franziskus Hospital, Münster, Germany

1 Introduction

Up until about 30 years ago, an uncontrollable keratitis geographica (Fig. 1) often represented the "beginning of the end" (suture loosening, infiltrate, melting, immune reaction, bacterial superinfection, endophthalmitis …) of the graft after repeated corneal transplantation for keratitis of herpetic origin. Today, the herpes simplex virus type I (HSV) has largely lost its terror as a frequent causative agent of keratitis in Europe. However, in order to do justice to the individual clinical picture, it is imperative that the term "herpetic keratitis" is not used undifferentiated in everyday clinical practice.

2 Primary Infection, Latency and Recurrence

HSV type 1 is isolated in over 95% of cases of herpetic infection of the upper half of the body, while type 2 is predominant in the genital area. 50–90% of all people experience an HSV infection during their lifetime. Primary infection with HSV type 1 usually occurs in early childhood, while type 2 is acquired either at birth or more commonly between 16 and 30 years of age through sexual contact with an infected person.

The primary infection often causes viremia. This in turn causes the formation of humoral antibodies, which remain detectable throughout life, and cell-mediated immune responses. Often, such an infection is subclinical. Subsequent HSV infections in individuals who have already undergone primary infection are almost always recurrent, although de novo infection, i.e., infection by a different strain of HSV, is possible [1, 2].

After primary ocular or—much more frequently—oral or facial HSV infection, the virus establishes a latent infection (latency) in the neurons of the trigeminal nerve, especially the ganglion Gasseri [3, 4]. Based on current data,

B. Seitz et al. (eds.), *Atlas on Cornea*, https://doi.org/10.1007/978-3-031-65422-0_23

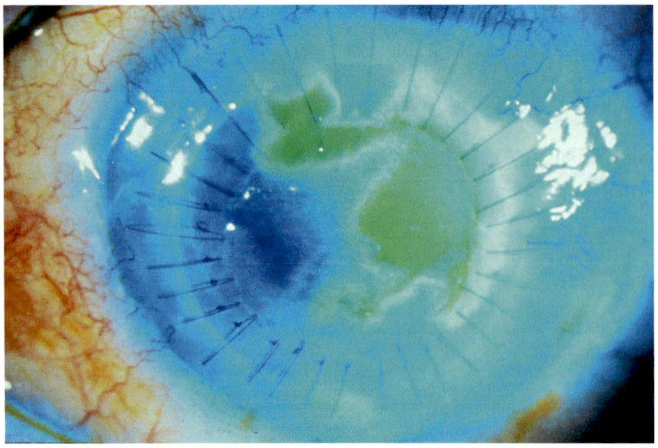

Fig. 1 Keratitis herpetica geographica—recurrence on the graft (vital staining with fluorescein and blue light)

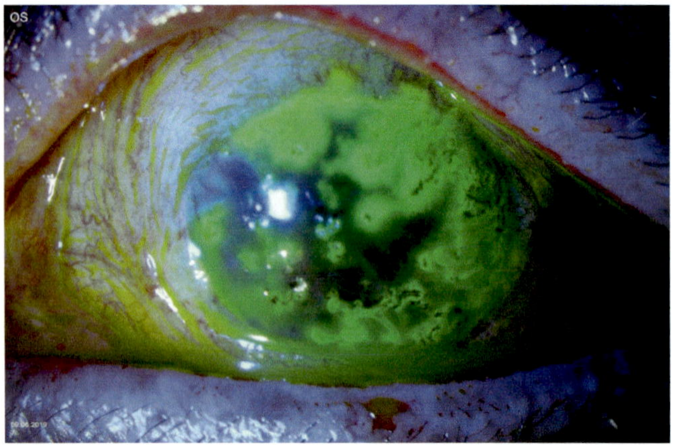

Fig. 2 Severe epithelial herpes simplex virus keratitis in a patient with HIV

it is likely that HSV may also remain latent in the cornea [3, 5, 6]. Viruses are in a dynamic state of perpetual, slow replication of a portion of their genome (latency-associated transcription, LAT). During latency, the expression of lytic genes is largely suppressed. LAT inhibits apoptosis and productive infection, thereby allowing survival of infected neurons and promoting the cycle of latency and reactivation of HSV in the sensory ganglion [7].

The host immune system is responsible for preventing disseminated infection and controlling HSV latency [8]. Due to the relative absence of viral gene expression and HSV latency confined to the cell, the virus can escape elimination by the immune system. When the host–virus balance is disrupted, local recurrence occurs. Numerous factors are known to trigger recurrences—e.g. trauma such as excimer laser keratectomy, sunlight (especially UV component), menstruation, fever, physical and emotional stress, corticosteroids, immunosuppression, and adrenaline [9]. Unfortunately, it is still uncertain as to what causes the disturbance of the balance in detail.

During reactivation, the latent virus re-enters the lytic replication phase, after which the virus returns to the site of primary infection or to the peripheral part of the innervating nerve branch by retrograde axonal transport. Occasionally, the virus infects neurons in adjacent regions of the same ganglion or even other ganglia to infect new sites in the body. The frequency of HSV reactivation correlates with the severity of the primary infection, the viral strain, and the immune status of the infected person.

The recurrence rate increases with the number of previous recurrences. The frequency of recurrences is about 10% after one year, 50% after 10 years and over 60% after 20 years. Recurrence after primary ocular herpetic infection occurs in at least 1/3 of cases, of which 50% develop the disease more than once [10, 11]. Recurrences are particularly frequent in HIV-infected individuals and other immunodeficiencies, such as atopy, or under immunosuppressive therapy (Fig. 2). Earlier corneal stromal involvement increases the likelihood of subsequent stromal inflammation. The incidence of stromal keratitis is 2–5% at initial manifestation and increases to 20–40% at further recurrences [12, 13].

3 Diagnosis of Keratitis of Herpetic Origin

In Europe, HSV is a very common cause of keratitis. **This should always be kept in mind!** Typically, the disease is unilateral (exceptions more often in childhood, Fig. 3 [14]). Regarding anamnesis, a past ocular inflammation (i.e. recurrence) can often be inquired about. A reduction in corneal sensitivity is indicative but need not be present in endotheliitis. Similarly, there is often a discrepancy between the severity of the objective findings and the subjective pain. There are typically no conjunctival follicles. **Vital stains** (e.g., Rose Bengal or fluorescein/blue light or Lissamine Green) are very helpful for biomicroscopic diagnosis at the slit lamp (Fig. 4).

Only in case of atypical symptoms laboratory diagnostics are useful. While serological tests are irrelevant, real-time PCR from corneal tissue or tear film is able to confirm suspicion and determine the amount of viral genome in the tissue. A large number of HSV gene copies are detectable in patients with steroid therapy, frequent relapses, severe disease, corneal neovascularization and graft failure [15].

Recent studies indicate that even the clinically inconspicuous contralateral cornea may show subclinical changes in sensitivity, nerve fiber density, and endothelial density in the presence of HSV or Zoster keratitis [16–19].

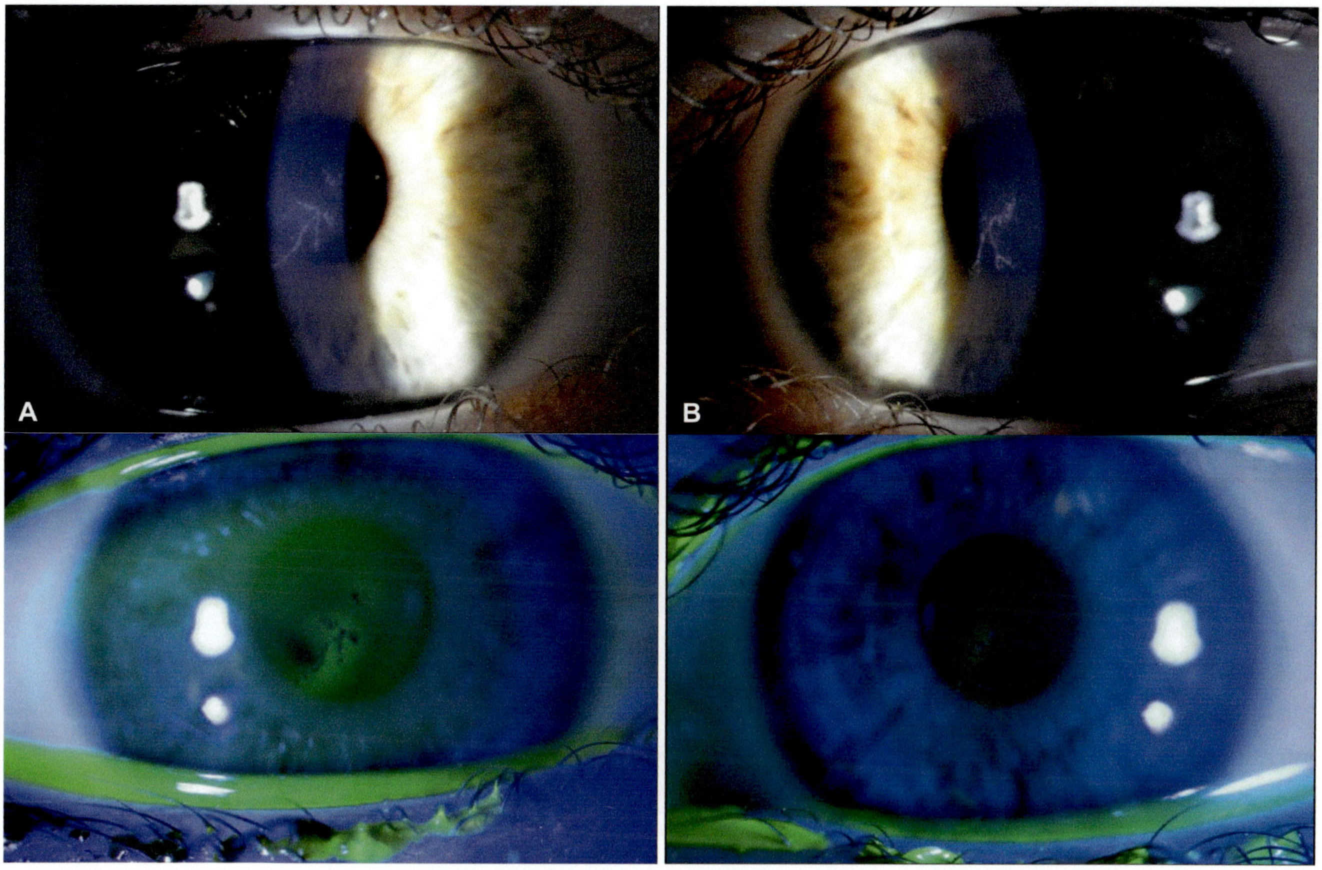

Fig. 3 Bilateral keratits dendritica in a 12-year-old girl. (**A**) OD, (**B**) OS

4 Classification of Keratitis of Herpetic Origin

Keratitis of herpetic origin is always a recurrence, except for the rare primary corneal infection.

Keratitis of herpetic origin can be present as (Table 1):

1. Infectious epithelial keratitis (Keratitis dendritica/ geographica).
2. Stromal immunological keratitis either necrotizing (so-called "ulcerative necrotizing stromal keratitis") or non-necrotizing (so-called "interstitial keratitis").
3. Endotheliitis (so-called "disciform keratitis").
4. Neurotrophic keratopathy (so-called "metaherpetic keratitis").
5. It is not uncommon that it ends as more or less dense disciform or multifocal corneal scars with stromal thinning and with more or less severe stromal neovascularization (typically one or few vascular strains).

However, the aforementioned clinical pictures can also emerge from each other and coexist. Uveitis with/without acute ocular hypertension may be present simultaneously.

This classification is modified from Holland and Schwartz [20], which the authors consider clearer for practical use than that of Liesegang [21] and that of Sundmacher [1].

4.1 Epithelial Herpetic Keratitis

Keratitis dendritica is common (Fig. 5). In the early stages, dot or star-shaped opaque plaques of swollen epithelial cells can be observed. This develops into keratitis dendritica or, if these lesions are confluent, keratitis geographica (especially after corticosteroid therapy). Epithelial infiltrates with bulbous extensions containing replicating virus are typical of the dendritic lesions. Within a few days, a light subepithelial infiltrate develops, which often remains after corneal abrasion [22].

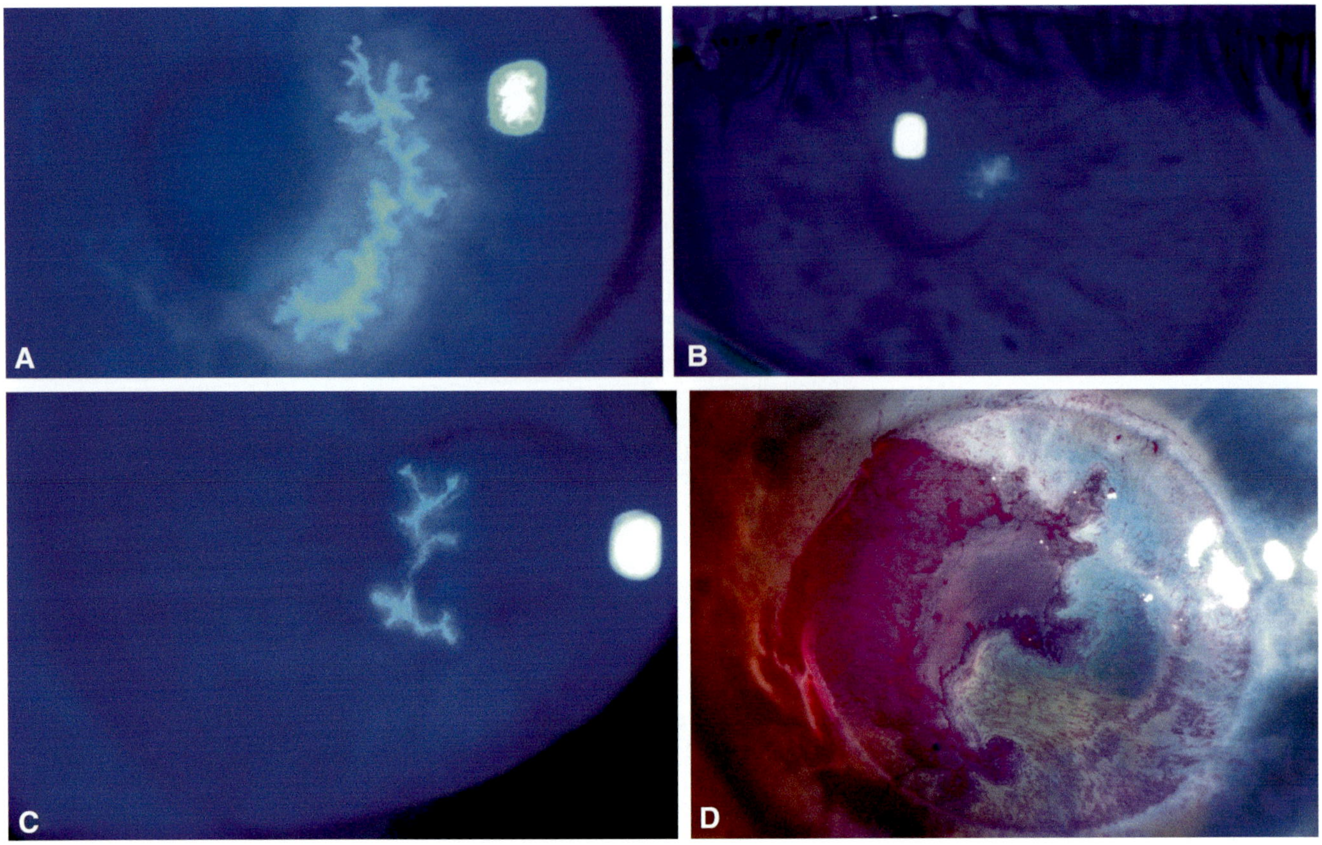

Fig. 4 (**A, C**) Classical keratitis dendritica (vital staining with fluorescein and blue light), (**D**) Keratitis herpetica geographica—recurrence on the graft (vital staining with Rose Bengal)

Table 1 Classification of herpetic keratitis (modified after Holland and Schwartz 1999 [20])

• Infectious epithelial keratitis (Keratitis dendritica/geographica)
• Stromal immune-mediated keratitis → necrotizing ("ulcerative necrotizing stromal keratitis" = "ulcer"); infectious and immunological → non-necrotizing ("interstitial keratitis"); immunological
• Endotheliitis ("disciform keratitis"); immunological
• Neurotrophic keratopathy (so-called "metaherpetic keratitis")
• (Vascularized) disciform corneal scars
• Keratouveitis

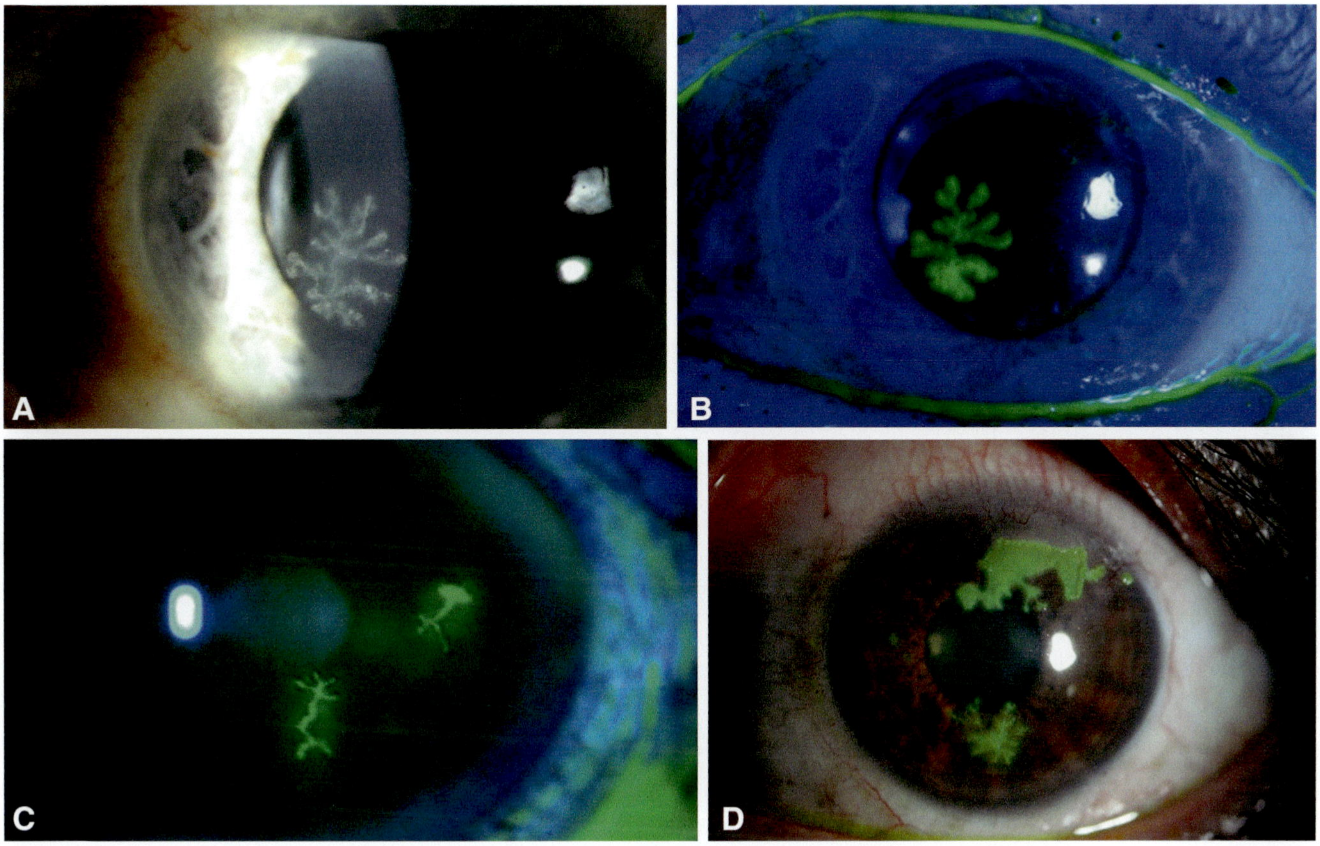

Fig. 5 (**A**) Artful keratitis dendritica (slit lamp overview). (**B**) Artful keratitis dendritica (vital staining with fluorescein and blue light), (**C, D**) Bifocal keratitis dendritica (vital staining with Lissamine Green)

4.2 Stromal Immune-Mediated Herpetic Keratitis

In this case, a distinction has to be made between 1. ulcerative necrotizing stromal keratitis (so-called "herpetic ulcer") and 2. "interstitial keratitis".

4.2.1 Ulcerative Necrotizing Stromal Keratitis (So-Called "Herpetic Ulcer"): Abundant Replicating Virus Plus Immune Response

In the ulcer, abundant active (replicating) virus is found in the stroma (Fig. 6). The ulcer base and margins exhibit a dense, whitish inflammatory infiltrate and edema. Delayed healing and recurrence result in dense scarring, tissue loss, and neovascularization. If left untreated, the risk of perforation is very high. Typically, the disease progresses initially without hypopyon, but it is not uncommon for the ulcer to be superinfected with bacteria. Usually, the finding is unilateral and corneal sensitivity is more or less markedly decreased. Virus genome and antigen can be detected in the affected corneal tissue [23].

4.2.2 Interstitial Keratitis: Immune Reaction Without Replicating Virus

In interstitial keratitis, the inflammatory reaction in the stroma dominates without thickening (Fig. 7). A combination of a T-cell mediated and antigen–antibody complement cascade due to viral antigen remaining in the stroma is thought to be involved [1, 6]. Recurrent interstitial keratitis can lead to keratoconus-like morphologic findings [24].

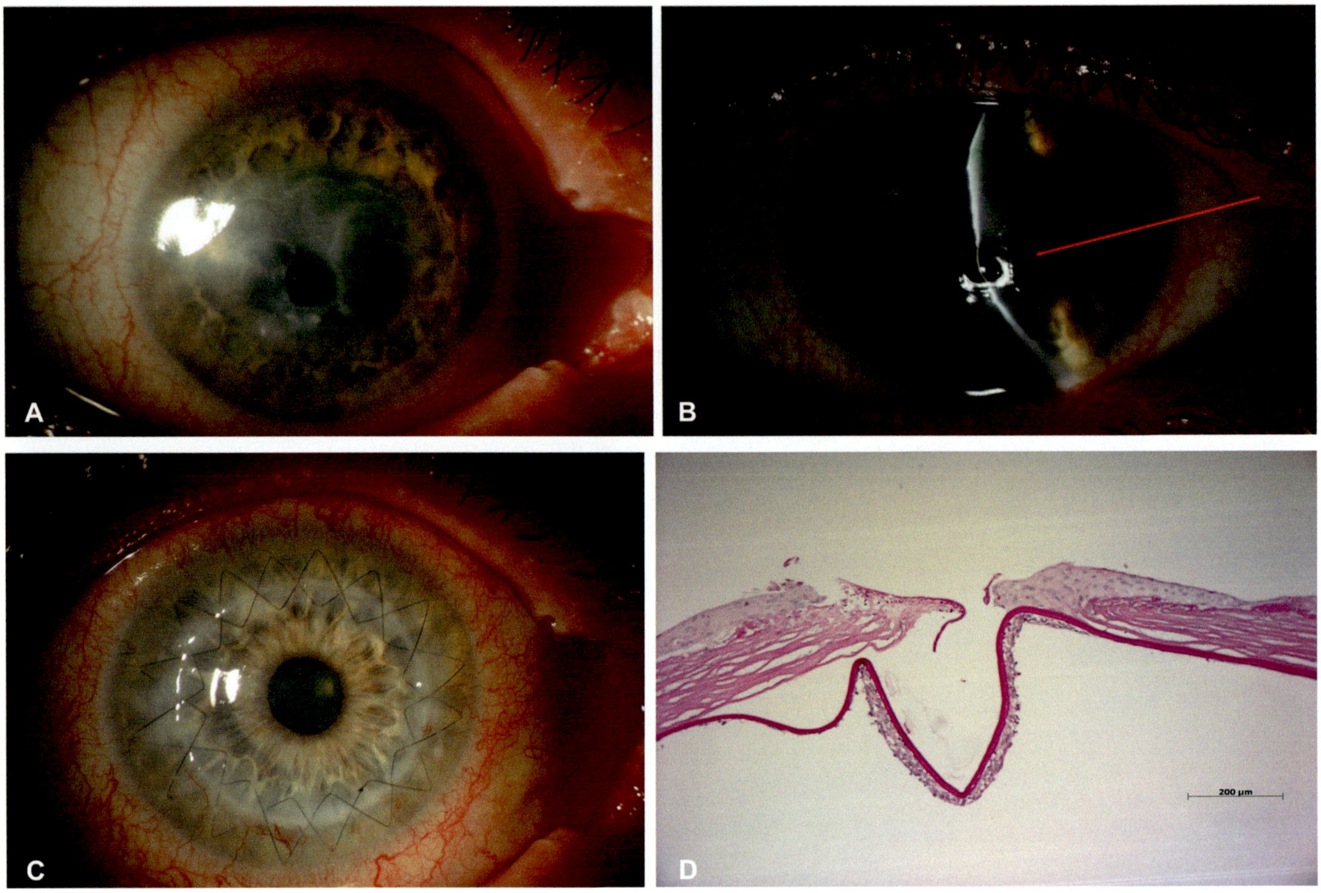

Fig. 6 Ulcerative necrotising stromal keratitis ("herpetic ulcer") with descemetocele. (**A**) Overview, (**B**) slit (arrow points to descemetocele), (**C**) 3 days after penetrating excimer laser keratoplasty à chaud (7.5/7.6 mm) with double continuous cross-stich suture according to Hoffmann, (**D**) histology: descemetocele with granulomatous reaction along Descemet membrane (thanks to Prof. Bohle, Pathological Institute of the UKS)

4.3 Keratitis Disciformis ("Endotheliitis"): Stromal Edema and Retrocorneal Precipitates

Approximately every 6th patient with epithelial herpes later develops keratitis disciformis. Clinically, a focal (Fig. 8A), sometimes also diffuse (Fig. 8B) stromal edema (without infiltrate!) with microcystic epithelial edema, Descemet folds and more or less fine (dendritic) retrocorneal precipitates are found. Besides the direct viral infection of the endothelium **(HSV-Ag persists in the corneal endothelium!)** [5], immunological processes (T-cell mediated immune reaction) are probably predominant [6, 20].

As a differential diagnosis (DD), the retinal, intracameral, floating foreign body after a windshield injury must always be excluded. Sometimes patients remember such an incident only after "forced anamnesis". Further DD include poorly executed phacoemulsification, acute glaucoma, and advanced Fuchs endothelial dystrophy, which, however, can already be ruled out by a skilled slit-lamp examination of the contralateral side.

In "**concomitant uveitis**", slit lamp examination also reveals cells in the anterior chamber and a positive Tyndall effect. Uveitis is triggered by cytolytic viral replication in uveal tissue and trabecular meshwork. This is followed by an antiviral immune response. The HSV and its genome can be detected in the aqueous humor [25, 26]. Histologically, a cellular infiltrate in the iris stroma and perineuritis as well as perivasculitis can be detected. Underlying the sectorial iris atrophies and hemorrhages is an inflammation-related occlusive vasculitis. Cytolytic viral replication in the trabecular endothelium can often lead to ocular hypertension. Persistent ocular hypotony may result in ischemia-induced necrosis of the ciliary body [27–29].

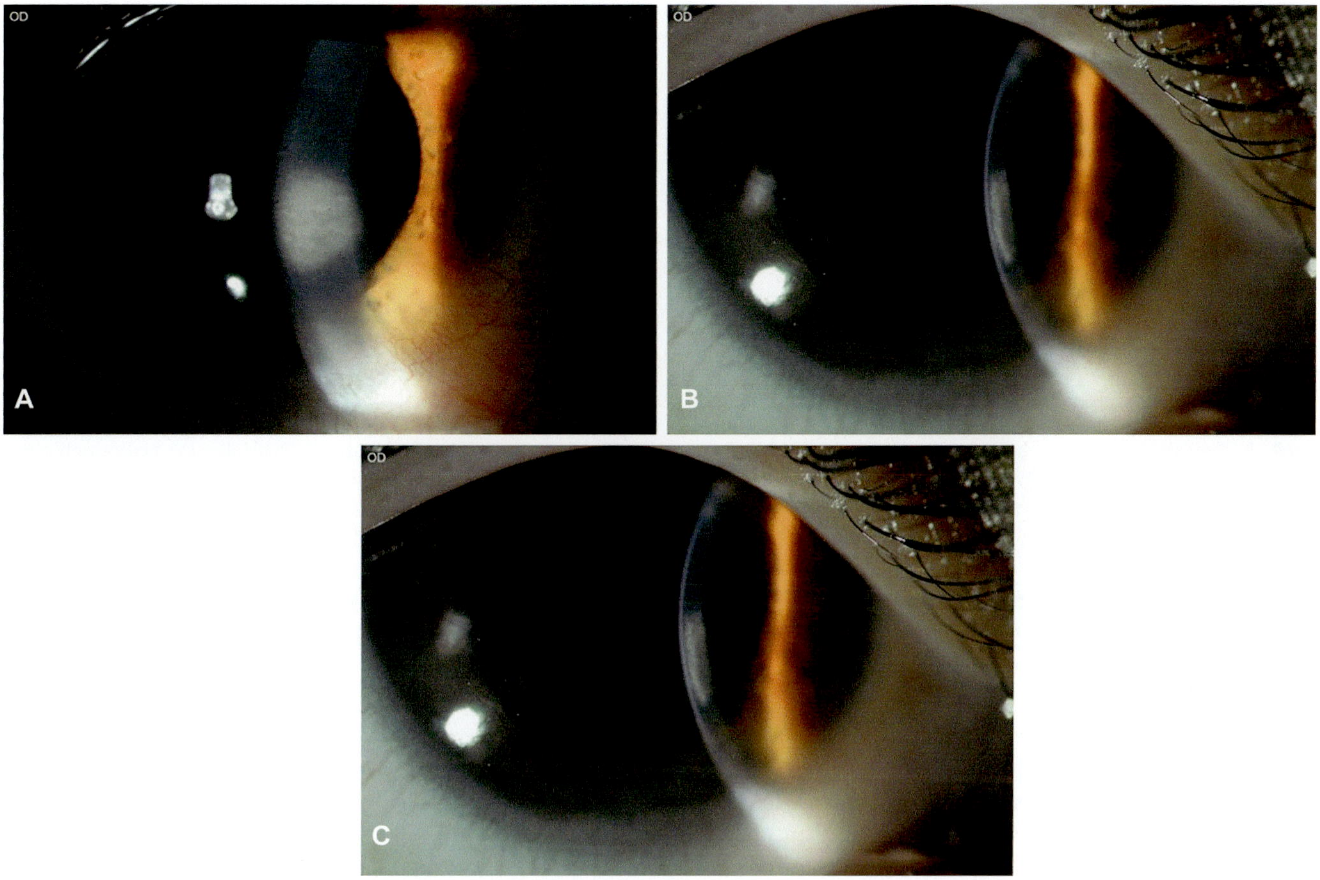

Fig. 7 "Interstitial keratitis" without necrosis, without ulceration, without stromal thickening: (**A**) overview, (**B**) central slit, (**C**) midperipheral slit

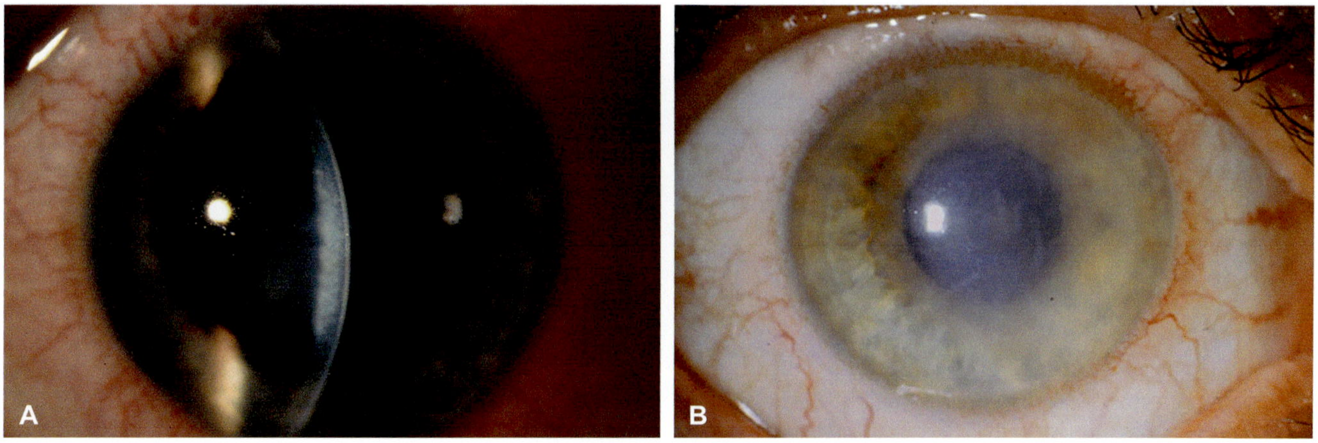

Fig. 8 So-called "disciform keratitis" can present either as (**A**) focal or (**B**) diffuse (DD: free floating foreign body in the anterior chamber) herpetic endotheliitis

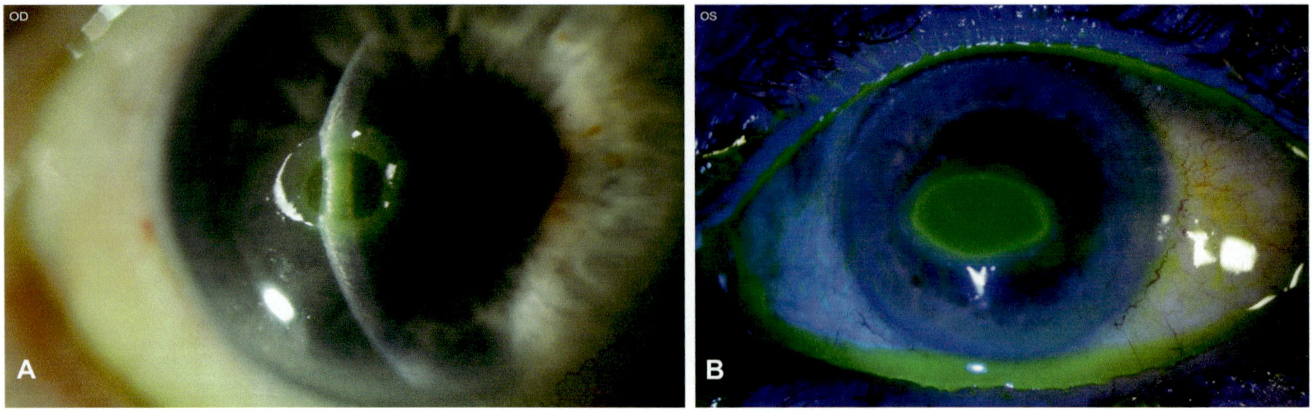

Fig. 9 Ulcerative neurotrophic keratopathy in sense of a therapy-resistant so-called "metaherpetic keratitis". Typically, the neurotrophic epithelial defects do not show a polygonal, but a round (Fig. 9A) or oval (Fig. 9B) border: the defect takes the smallest circumference of the given area!

Typical of **herpetic keratouveitis** are:

- Focal iris pigment leaf defects (DD: condition after acute angle-closure glaucoma)
- Secondary ocular hypertension in "trabeculitis"
- Fast posterior synechia formation
- Spontaneous anterior chamber bleeding possible (due to formation of bridging vessels or vasculitis/necrosis in iris and chamber angle)
- Also possible as isolated anterior uveitis without keratitis [1, 30]

4.4 So-Called "Metaherpetic Keratitis": Mainly Surface Disturbances

The so-called "metaherpetic keratitis" is typically a late stage ("burnt-out herpes") with impaired corneal innervation and persistent loss of corneal sensitivity and reduced tear secretion in the sense of a **neurotrophic keratopathy**. The cause, in addition to the infection itself, is often drug damage ("overtreated ulcer"). Typically, there is no immune reaction and no viral replication any more [2, 20]!

Surface disorders analogous to those of a neurotrophic keratopathy of other origin are predominant [31]. Following the usual classification, the disorders according to Mackie [32] can range from **(1) keratopathia superficialis punctata to (2) corneal erosion to (3) metaherpetic ulcer** with defect of Bowman layer (Fig. 9). Typically, the neurotrophic epithelial defects do not show a polygonal but a round (Fig. 9A) or oval (Fig. 9B) boundary: the defect occupies the smallest circumference for the given area!

4.5 (Vascularized) Stromal Corneal Scars with Stromal Thinning

A more or less vascularized, disciform or multifocal stromal corneal scar with stromal thinning represents the typical late stage after frequently recurrent (ulcerating) herpetic keratitis, which is typically accompanied by irreversible visual loss of various degrees (Fig. 10).

5 Therapy of the Different Manifestations of Keratitis of Herpetic Origin (Table 2)

5.1 Epithelial Herpetic Keratitis

Topical therapy consists of either gancyclovir gel 5x, acyclovir ointment 5x, trifluorothymidine (TFT) eye drops 5x (available through international pharmacies), or bromovinyldeoxyuride (BVDU) ointment 5x gradually tapering over a few (usually 2–3) weeks. Although these drugs have similar efficacy, the more modern agents are better tolerated [33–36].

Toxic or allergic reactions are not uncommon in long-term therapy. According to recent publications, resistance to viral drugs is increasing, even in patients with intact immune systems [37–39].

Topical vidarabine and foscarnet have been suggested in the case of acyclovir resistance [38]. Cidofovir has not gained acceptance at effective doses because of severe local toxicity.

Systemic acyclovir therapy is not primarily necessary. However, the 2nd Herpetic Eye Disease Study (HEDS)

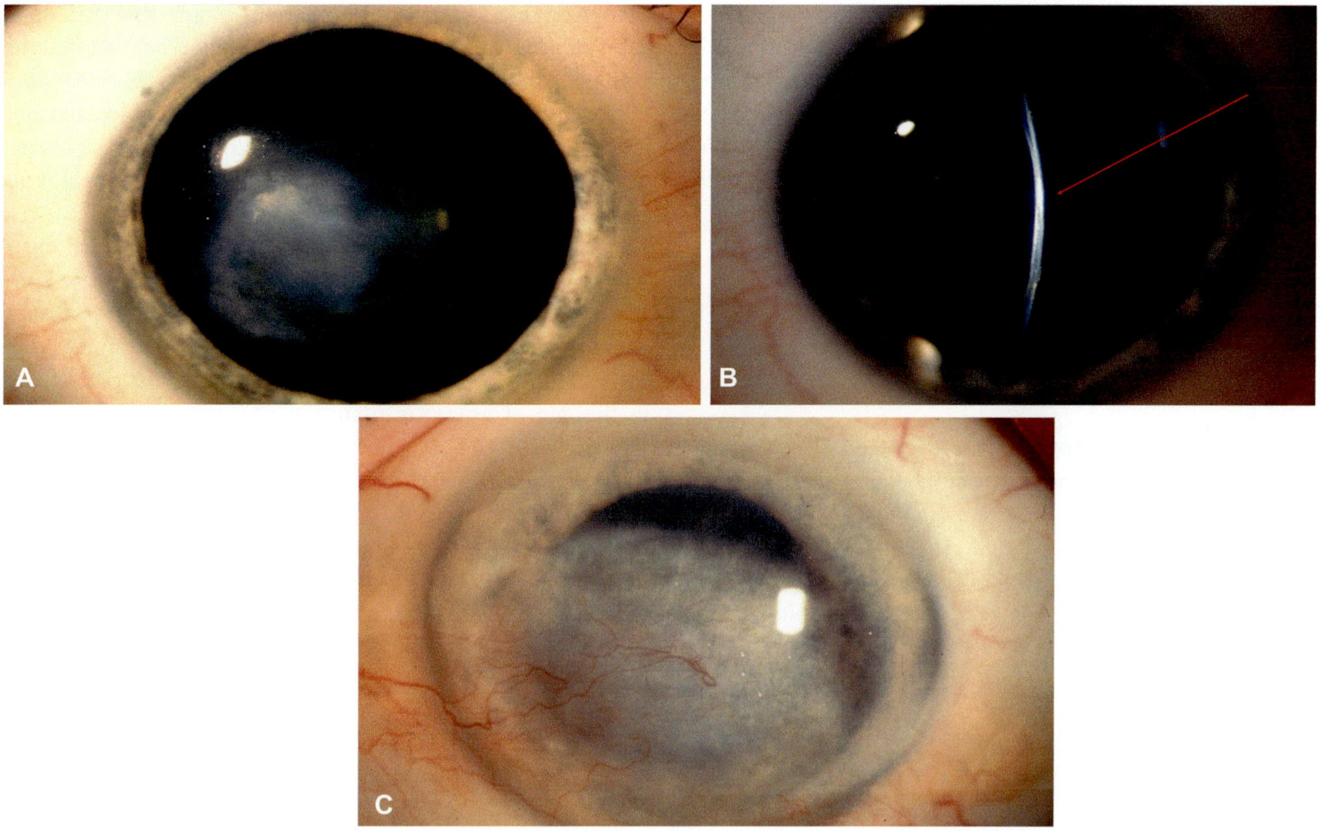

Fig. 10 (**A**) Avascularized central disciform scar with stromal thinning, (**B**) slit, (**C**) moderately vascularized disciform central scar. This is not high-risk for keratoplasty!

Table 2 Overview of drug therapy for "herpetic keratitis" (according to Seitz et al. 2011 [2])

Type of disease	Virustatics		Corticosteroids	Antibiotics	Cycloplegics	Care
	Topical	Systemic	Topical/systemic			
Epithelial keratitis	+	–	*CI/CI*	(+)	–	(+)
Stromal keratitis						
Infectious	+	+	(+)/(+)	+	+	–
Interstitial	+	(+)	+/(+)	–	(+)	–
Disciform keratitis	+	(+)	+/(+)	–	(+)	–
So-called "Metaherpetic Keratitis"	((+))	–	((+))/–	–	–	++

+ = recommended; (+) = recommended under special circumstances; ((+)) rather not —sometimes low doses as a precaution; CI = contraindicated

showed that acyclovir 2 × 400 mg times daily p.o. for one year significantly reduced the recurrence rate and progression to stromal keratitis [11]. This treatment strategy is indicated only in patients with a high recurrence rate, severe epithelial progression (e.g. geographic or multiple lesions), transition to the stromal form, and after keratoplasty. Short-term oral acyclovir treatment (for 3 weeks) did **not** reduce (in contrast to long-term administration) the likelihood of transition to stromal herpetic keratitis when observed for one year [10].

CAVE: Local corticosteroids are contraindicated in epithelial HSV keratitis!

Since spontaneous healing usually occurs after 2–3 weeks and the recurrence rate as well as the frequency of secondary stromal involvement are similar with and without therapy, the value of therapy is to shorten the duration of the disease. Gentle partial swab abrasion of the corneal epithelium with a cotton swab can remove nearly 100% of the viruses along with the epithelium [1]. Nowadays, abrasion followed by local antibiotic treatment (!) seems to be recommended only in patients with extensive lesions, delayed healing or possible development of resistance due to the availability of well effective antiviral drugs.

5.2 Stromal Immune-Mediated Herpetic Keratitis

5.2.1 Ulcerative Necrotizing Stromal Keratitis (So-Called "Herpetic Ulcer")

Local: Gancyclovir gel 5x or Acyclovir ointment 5x and antibiotics (e.g. moxifloxacin eye drops 5x), cycloplegics (e.g. atropine EDO eye drops 2x). **Initially, steroids should not be given!** However, since clinically and experimentally accompanying inflammation plays a major role [6], topical steroids should be added cautiously a few days after sufficient antiviral and antibiotic treatment [22, 33]. Since cyclosporine A achieves effective T-lymphocyte blockage and anti-inflammation, but does not increase the risk of ulceration and perforation, it is a potentially helpful additional drug, especially in the acute ulcerative phase [33, 40].

Systemic: Acyclovir 5×400/800 mg orally for about 4 weeks, then reduce to 2×400 mg. In eyes with necrotizing HSV keratitis, additional treatment with a systemic antiviral agent improves the final outcome.

Keratoplasty à chaud should be limited to perforation in the age of amniotic membrane transplantation (AMT). Otherwise, AMT (typically as a "multigraft sandwich" [41]) allows to postpone keratoplasty from the acute stage into the irritation-free, and thus prognostically much more favorable interval [41–46]. If keratoplasty à chaud becomes necessary in case of a perforation risk, it can also be combined with simultaneous amniotic membrane transplantation as a patch (Fig. 11) [47]. In case of focal

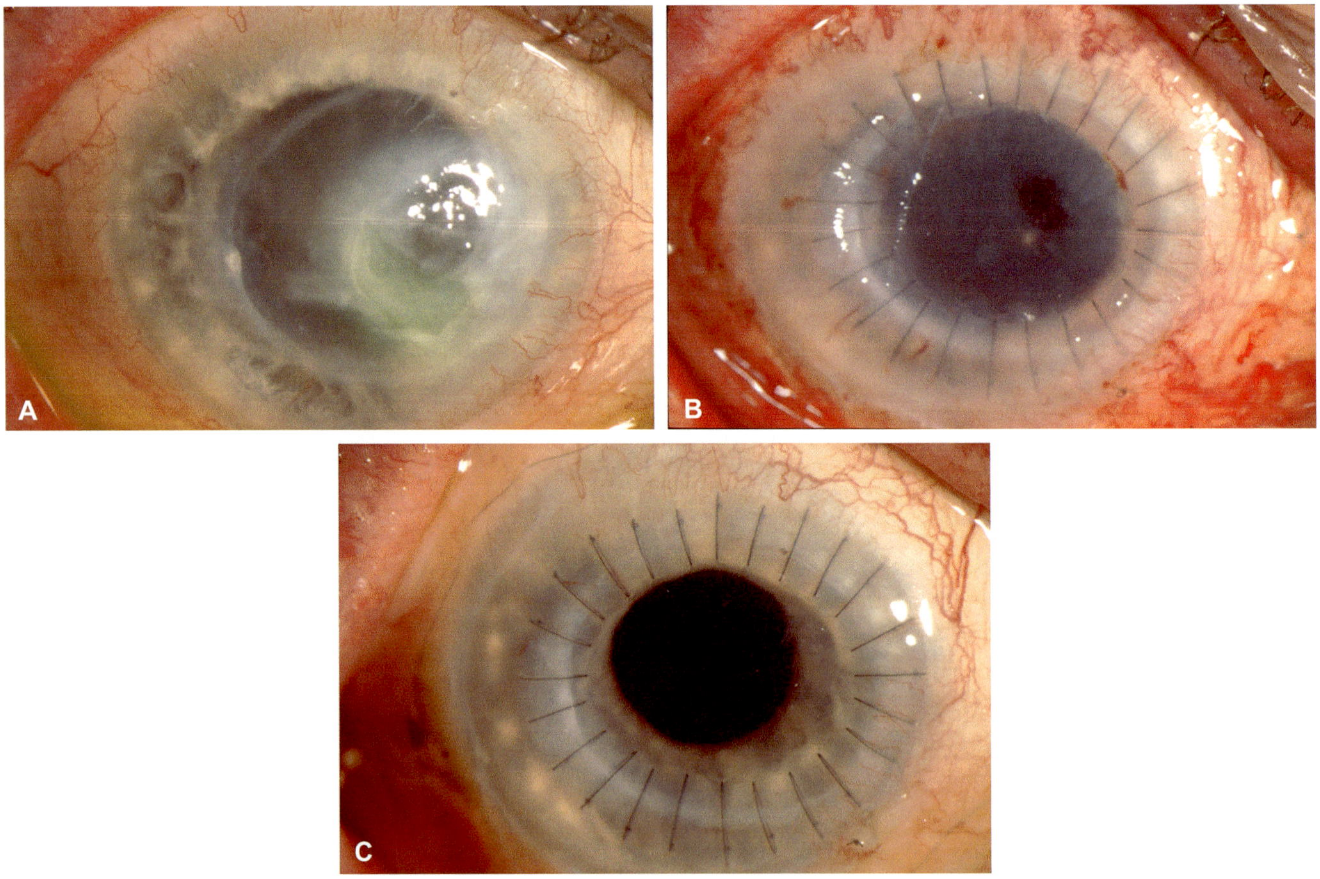

Fig. 11 (**A**) Descemetocele after ipsilateral autologous rotational keratoplasty for herpetic corneal scars + cataracta nuclearis brunescens, (**B**) first day after eccentric elliptical triple procedure à chaud (excimer laser trephination 7.0×8.0/7.1/8.1 mm) + simultaneous amnion membrane transplantation AMT as patch, (**C**) 10 days postoperatively the patch is no longer present, the episcleral 10–0 nylon threads still need to be removed

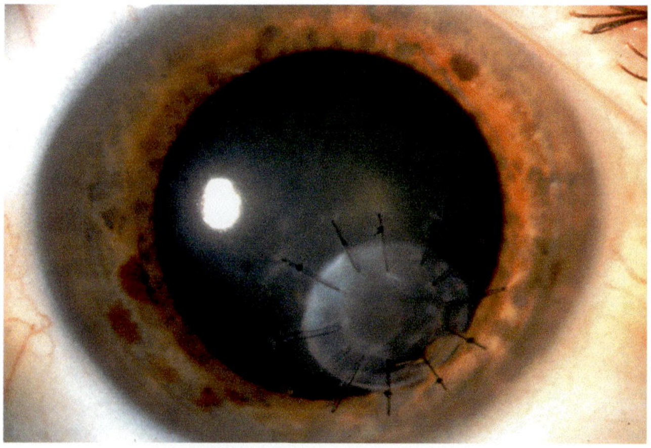

Fig. 12 Eccentric mini-keratoplasty à chaud (3.5/3.8 mm) for focally perforated ulcerative necrotizing stromal keratitis of herpetic origin

perforation, an eccentric tectonic mini-keratoplasty may be indicated (Fig. 12) [48, 49]. Phototherapeutic keratectomy (PTK) with the excimer laser is contraindicated [50]!

CAVE: Non-steroidal anti-inflammatory drugs are contraindicated in view of a possible corneal perforation!

5.2.2 Interstitial Keratitis

To date, the majority of authors recommend **combined therapy with topical corticosteroids and viral drugs** [1, 22, 33]. Primarily, topical therapy with gancyclovir gel 5x or acyclovir ointment (5x) and prednisolone acetate eye drops 5–8x is recommended. Both drugs are slowly tapered off in parallel with reduction of the application every 2 weeks. A reduction of the dose should only be done if there is no irritation clinically (no inflammatory infiltration and edema in the stroma, no active keratoprecipitates). If the effect is insufficient and in case of pronounced keratouveitis or secondary glaucoma, it is recommended to add acyclovir 5×400 mg for 6 weeks systemically, with subsequent reduction to 2×400 mg over several months (alternatively valaciclovir 3×1 g, later 2×500 mg). Long-term prophylaxis with 400 mg acyclovir twice daily reduced the stromal recurrence rate from 28 to 14% [11].

In case of resistance to therapy, systemic steroids should also be considered in the short term—always tapering off. **Surgical therapy is not indicated**. In cases of chronic course, topical cyclosporine A eye drops 3x should be considered for steroid sparing [40, 51].

5.3 Keratitis Disciformis ("Endotheliitis")

Topical corticosteroids are therapeutically indispensable because of the immunological processes [1, 2, 22, 33]. To prevent epithelial recurrence (reactivation of cytolytic viral replication), virustatics (topical and/or systemic) become necessary simultaneously.

The individual recommendation for therapy depends on the severity of keratouveitis or herpetic trabeculitis: Prednisolone acetate (or Loteprednol) eye drops 5x, Gancyclovir gel or Acyclovir ointment 5x: reduce both every 2 weeks—but only if there is no irritation—by 1 application per day, leave with 1x steroid early and 1x Gancyclovir gel or Acyclovir ointment at night for several months. If no improvement, reactivation under dose reduction and anterior uveitis, systemic administration of acyclovir, 5×400 mg 6 weeks, then reduction to 2×400 mg for 3–6 months. Alternatively, valaciclovir 3×1 g for 6 weeks, then 2×500 mg over 3–6 months. Systemic corticosteroids (e.g., 100 mg Urbason rapidly tapered) are administered in refractory disease, severe anterior uveitis, and/or trabeculitis (Fig. 13).

In corneal endothelial decompensation, DMEK can be performed today with very good success but under systemic acyclovir protection [42, 52, 53]. In case of recurrent DMEK or PKP failure, a herpetic [54, 55] or cytomegaloviral [56, 57] origin should always be considered and excluded ex juvantibus and/or by aqueous humor analysis [58, 59].

CAVE: Prostaglandin analogues are relatively contraindicated for pressure reduction in secondary ocular hypertension because they may maintain or increase the inflammatory state!

CAVE: Non-steroidal anti-inflammatory drugs have no role in the therapy of disciform keratitis.

5.4 So-Called "Metaherpetic Keratitis": Mainly Surface Disturbances

All toxic eye drops (virustatics, corticosteroids and all eye drops with preservatives) are discontinued and preservative-free and phosphate-free tear substitutes (preferably with hyaluronic acid), nourishing gels and eye ointments containing vitamin A or dexpanthenol are applied instead. A pressure patch at night may be temporarily beneficial. Very helpful today is the option of **autologous serum eye drops**, which we apply 100% 5–10x per day [60]. In case of resistance to therapy, **therapeutic contact lenses** may be useful, in case of ulcerative processes, **collagenase inhibitors** may be useful [61, 62].

In persistent cases, we perform **amniotic membrane transplantation** (AMT—usually as a patch), **botulinum toxin injection** to induce temporary iatrogenic ptosis, or (temporary) lateral tarsorrhaphy. Today, a **Gundersen flap** must be considered **ultima ratio** [62, 63].

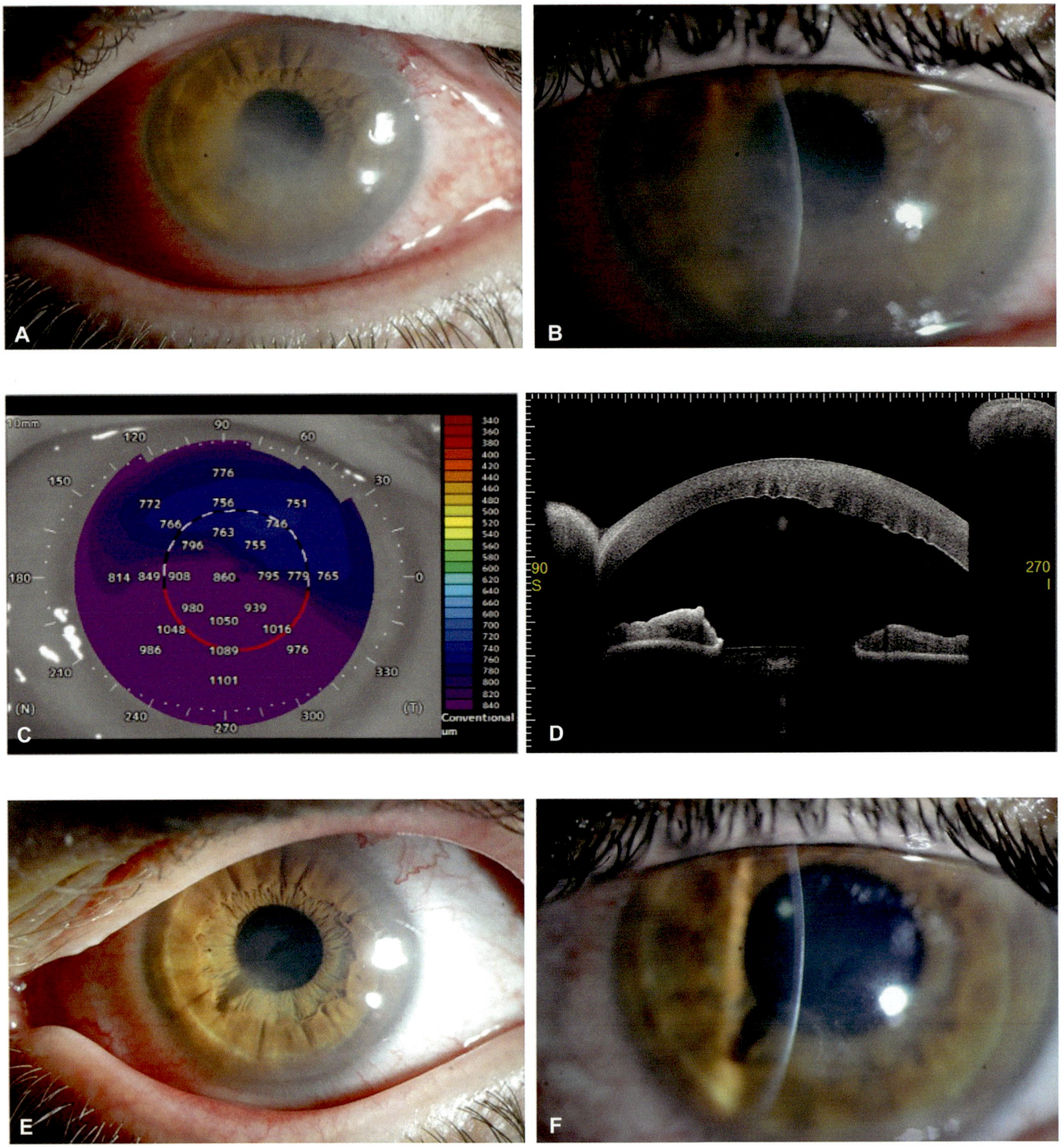

Fig. 13 Disciform keratitis since 2 weeks treated only with Acyclovir ointment, VA 20/200, corneal thickness paracentral-inferiorly 1050 µm, (**A**) slit lamp—Overview, (**B**) thin slit, (**C**) thickness map, (**D**) AS-OCT vertical section. 6 days after addition of systemic Acyclovir and topical and systemic corticosteroids rapid increase of VA to 20/25, corneal thickness paracentral-inferiorly decreases to 653 µm, (**E**) slit lamp overview. (**F**) thin slit

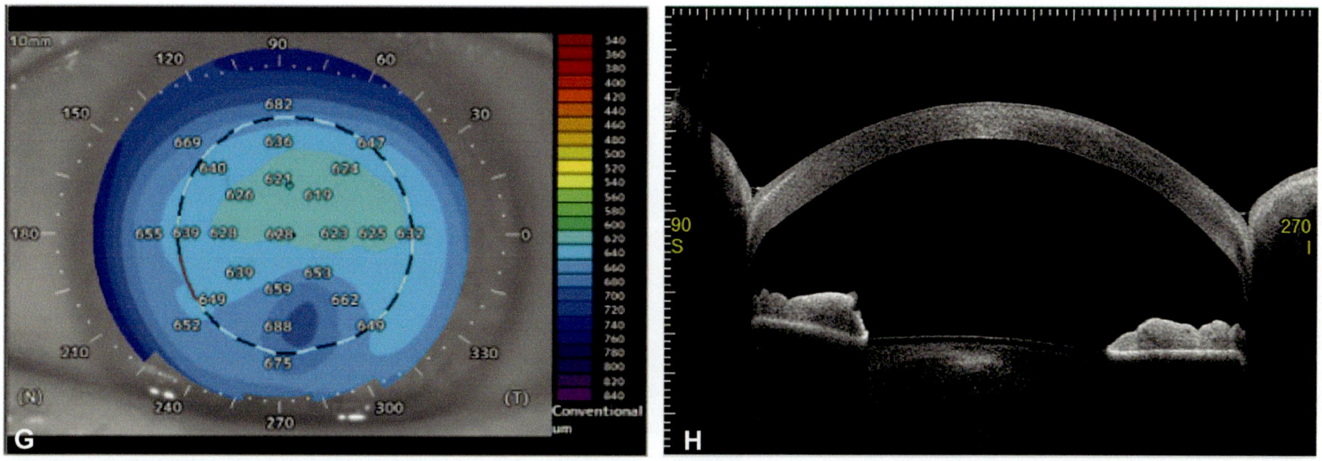

Fig. 13 (**G**) thickness map, (**H**) AS-OCT vertical section

5.5 (Vascularized) Stromal Corneal Scars with Stromal Thinning

Due to the depth of the scar and stromal thinning, excimer laser PTK is rarely useful—if at all, only under systemic acyclovir protection [50]. We tend to refrain from lamellar keratoplasty because of the viral persistence in the endothelium demonstrated by Holbach, Asano and Naumann [5]. For the same reason, ipsilateral autorotation keratoplasty is generally not recommended [64].

In principle and if possible, penetrating keratoplasty should not be carried out until the eye has been free of inflammation for six months (Fig. 14). In case of persistent interstitial keratitis/endotheliitis, we postpone corneal transplantation and apply topical corticosteroids and gancyclovir gel or acyclovir ointment (Fig. 15).

Initial experience shows that a reduction of neovascularization can be achieved with the application of anti-VEGF eye drops [65]. This seems to be particularly useful in cases of vision-reducing central neovascularization with lipid keratopathy or in preparation for elective keratoplasty. However, in recurrent inflammation, this therapy has no convincing long-term effect [22].

CAVE: *Persistent corneal edema is an indication of a still active process and therefore surgical intervention should be delayed.*

CAVE: *After keratoplasty, steroids should not be applied without acyclovir protection!*

Postoperatively, acyclovir in a dosage of 2×400 mg daily p.o. for 1 year [66] helps to avoid a flare-up of the viral infection in the graft with/without subsequent rejection reaction, if necessary together with long-term therapy with topical gancyclovir gel or acyclovir application as an ointment directly before going to bed. Occasional dendritiform epitheliopathies on the PKP graft (Fig. 16) may be resistant to therapy for weeks [67].

NOTE: In principle, transplant reactions should always be treated in combination with gancylovir/acyclovir and steroids, because a herpes recurrence can never be practically excluded according to the textbook (immune reaction: precipitates limited to the graft!).

6 Transmission of HSV from Donor to Recipient in the Context of Corneal Transplantation

There is an association between HSV and donor endothelial loss in organ culture ("severe endothelial necrosis") [68]. Primary graft failure after uncomplicated PKP due to keratoconus/PMD in young patients is very rare, but the cause often remains unclear [69, 70]. Organ cultured donor tissue

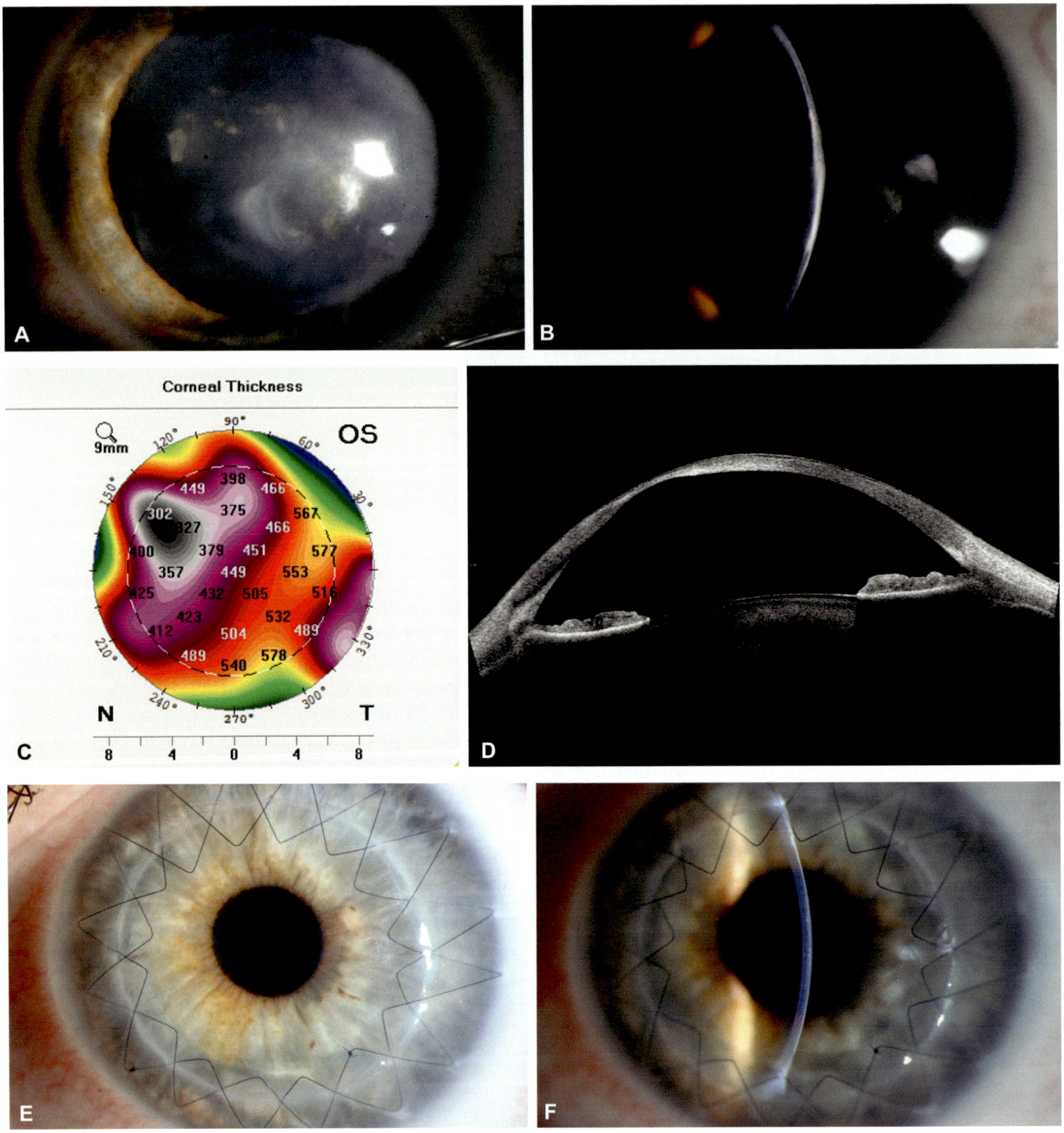

Fig. 14 30-year-old lady with full-thickness corneal scars, major corneal thinning and minor peripheral corneal neovascularization after multiple recurrences of ulcerative necrotizing stromal keratitis. VA: 20/200. Last recurrence of inflammation more than 1 year ago. Three university eye departments argued against corneal transplantation ("too thin, too high risk of recurrence on the graft, too high risk of immunological graft rejection"). (**A–D**) Before penetrating keratoplasty (**A**) overview, (**B**) thin slit, (**C**) thickness map: thinnest point 302 µm in the midperiphery, AS-OCT: midperipheral thinning of the cornea), (**E–H**) 5 weeks after excimer laser assisted penetrating keratoplasty with double running cross-stitch suture according to Hoffmann, VA20/30 (**E**) overview, (**F**) thin slit

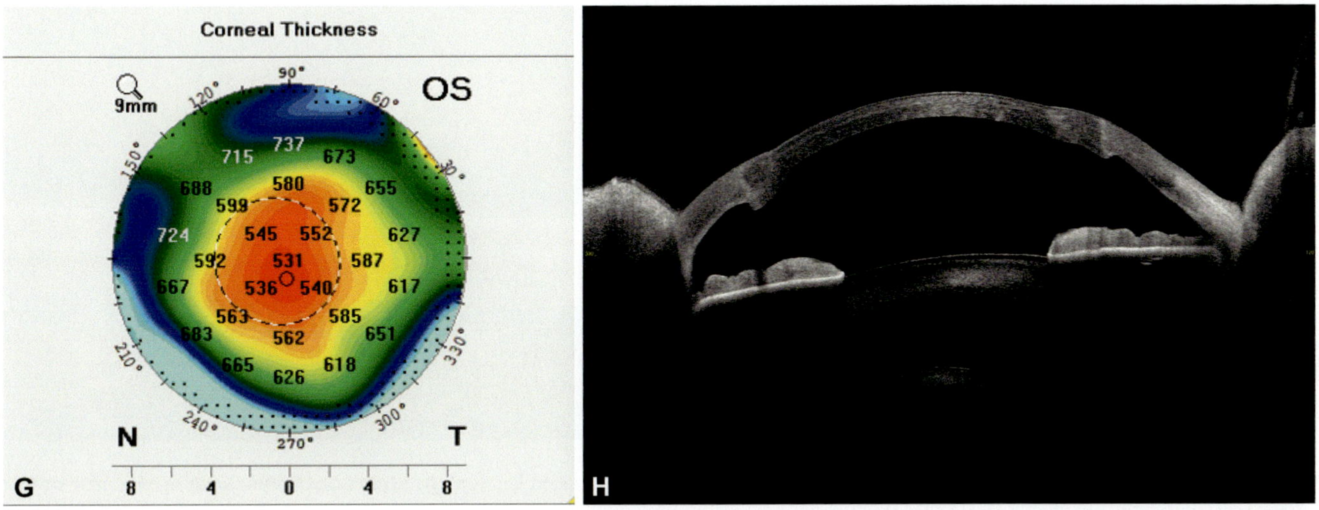

Fig. 14 (**G**) thickness map: homogeneous thickness distribution, (**H**) AS-OCT: favorable apposition at the graft-host junction

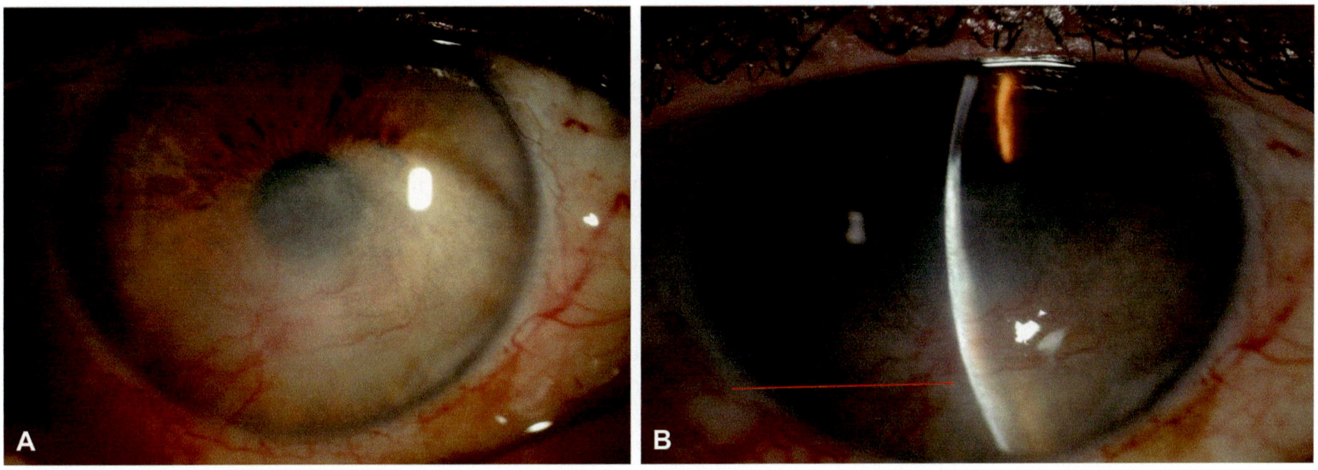

Fig. 15 (**A**) Long existing interstitial keratitis and endotheliitis of herpetic origin with pronounced stromal vascularization and clear inflammatory activity, (**B**) slit lamp image: focally thickened cornea due to endothelial decompensation

can very rarely transmit HSV to the patient in the setting of corneal transplantation [71]. Ping-pong infection from the infected graft to the host and back to the new graft may be responsible for delayed failure of further grafts—if adequate antiviral therapy is not administered [72].

On the other hand, a positive HSV-Ag finding in clinically inconspicuous corneas may exacerbate after keratoplasty. Therefore, it has been recommended to routinely submit a portion of the excised pathologic cornea—but not the corneoscleral remnant ring after graft harvest—to virology for HSV PCR [15]. In a study of 2230 consecutive corneal excisates, 29 (1.5%) excisates without a history of herpes (e.g. keratectasia) were HSV PCR positive. This percentage increased to 5% with a clinical picture of fungal keratitis [73].

In any primary graft failure, the possibility of herpetic endotheliitis of the graft should be considered and the patient treated accordingly (see above) [59, 74, 75].

7 Prophylaxis of Herpetic Recurrences

Safe prophylaxis of herpes recurrences without side effects, as often demanded by concerned patients and parents of children involved, is not possible. However, the following approaches have proven effective in practice:

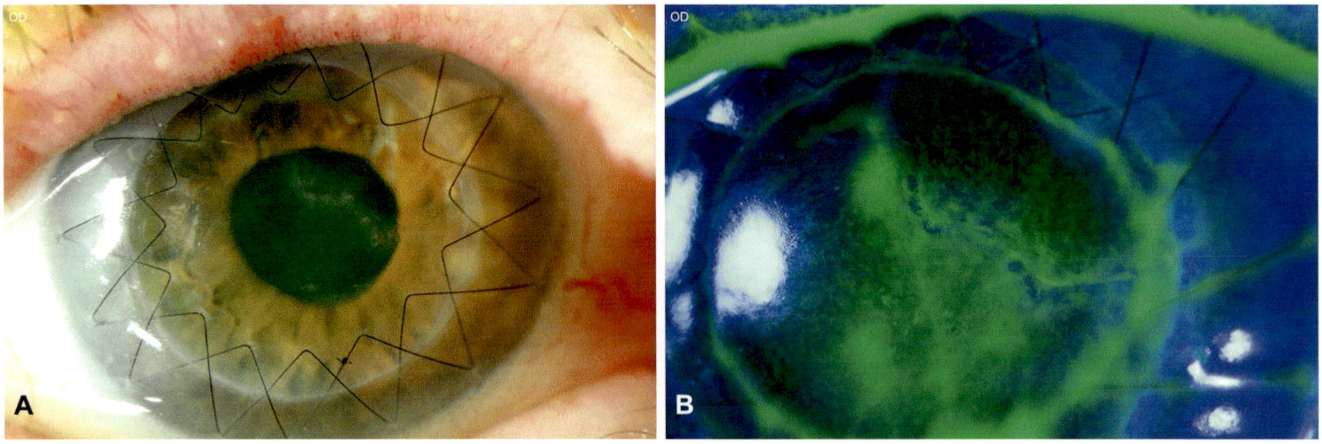

Fig. 16 (**A**) Recurrence of keratitis dendritica after penetrating excimer laser-assisted keratoplasty with 8 orientation teeth in avascular stromal corneal scar after recurring ulcerative stromal keratitis herpetic origin with double continuous cross-stich suture, (**B**) vital staining with fluorescein and blue light

- Gancylovir gel or Acyclovir ointment 1x directly before bedtime
- Artificial tears consistently!!
- 2×400 mg Acyclovir orally for months [76]
- In case of endotheliitis or interstitial keratitis: 1x prednisolone acetate eye drop 1x

A multicenter study confirmed the prophylactic benefit of low-dose acyclovir (400 mg orally 2 times daily) [11], especially for stromal keratitis. In epithelial HSV recurrences under long-term acyclovir administration, it should be considered that viral resistance may be present. The clinical relevance of the observation that acyclovir resistance is more frequently detected under long-term acyclovir therapy needs further investigation [77, 78].

NOTE: Gancylovir gel or Acyclovir ointment administered at night is applied just before closing the eyes when going to sleep.

8 Conclusion

Herpetic keratitis is a chameleon and various clinical pictures can also emerge from each other and coexist. Uveitis with/without acute ocular hypertension may be present simultaneously. Different manifestations of the disease require different therapeutic approaches. **Topical corticosteroids are contraindicated in epithelial HSV keratitis!** In ulcerative necrotizing stromal keratitis, AMT (typically as a "multigraft sandwich") in the acute stage allows to postpone keratoplasty into the irritation-free, and thus prognostically much more favorable, interval. In interstitial keratitis, the inflammatory reaction in the stroma dominates. In endothelial keratitis disciformis, same as in interstitial keratitis, topical corticosteroids are therapeutically indispensable because of the immunologic processes involved. Prostaglandin analogues are relatively contraindicated for pressure reduction in ocular hypertension in the context of keratouveitis herpetica, because they may maintain or increase the inflammatory state. The so-called "metaherpetic keratitis" is typically a late stage ("burnt out herpes") with impaired corneal innervation and persistent loss of corneal sensitivity and reduced tear secretion in the sense of a neurotrophic keratopathy.

After keratoplasty, acyclovir in a dosage of 2×400 mg daily p.o. for 1 year helps to avoid a recurrence of the viral infection in the graft with/without subsequent rejection. In 1.5% of PKP excisates without herpes anamnesis (e.g., in keratectasias), the HSV PCR is positive (5% in clinical picture of fungal keratitis) [73]. In principle, suspected transplant reactions should always be treated in combination with gancylovir/acyclovir and steroids, because a simultaneous herpes recurrence can never be excluded in practice according to the textbook (immune reaction: precipitates limited to the graft!).

References

1. Sundmacher R. Color atlas of herpetic eye disease. Berlin/Heidelberg: Springer; 2009.
2. Seitz B, Heiligenhaus A. "Herpetic keratitis". Various expressions require different therapeutic approaches. Ophthalmologe. 2011;108:385–95.
3. Cook SD, Hill JH. Herpes simplex virus: molecular biology and the possibility of corneal latency. Surv Ophthalmol. 1991;36:140–8.

4. Gordon YJ, Romanowski E, Araullo T, Cruz McKnight JLC. HSV-1 corneal latency. Invest Ophthalmol Vis Sci. 1991;32:663–5.
5. Holbach LM, Asano N, Naumann GOH. Infection of the corneal endothelium in herpes simplex keratitis. Am J Ophthalmol. 1998;126:592–4.
6. Remeijer L, Osterhaus ADME, Verjans GMGM. Human herpes simplex virus keratitis: the pathogenesis revisited. Ocul Immunol Inflamm. 2004;12:255–85.
7. Roizman B, Knipe DM, Whitley RJ. Herpes simplex virus. In: Knipe DM, Howley PM, editors. Fields virology. 5th ed. Lippincott Williams & Wilkins; 2007. p. 2502–7.
8. Sheridan BS, Knickelbein JE, Hendricks RL. CD8 T cells and latent herpes simplex virus type 1: keeping the peace in sensory ganglia. Expert Opin Biol Ther. 2007;7:1323–31.
9. HEDS The Herpetic Eye Disease Study Group. Psychological stress and other potential triggers for recurrence of herpes simplex virus eye infections. Arch Ophthalmol. 2000;118:1617–25.
10. HEDS The Herpetic Eye Disease Study Group. A controlled trial of oral acyclovir for the prevention of stromal keratitis or iritis in patients with herpes simplex virus epithelial keratitis. The epithelial keratitis trial. Arch Ophthalmol. 1997;115:703–12.
11. HEDS The Herpetic Eye Disease Study Group. Acyclovir for the prevention of recurrent herpes simplex virus eye disease. N Engl J Med. 1998;339:300–6.
12. Liesegang TJ. Epidemiology of ocular herpes simplex: natural history in Rochester, Minn, 1950 through 1982. Arch Ophthalmol. 1989;107:1160–5.
13. HEDS The Herpetic Eye Disease Study Group. Predictors of recurrent herpes simplex virus keratitis. Cornea. 2001;20:123–8.
14. Fiorentzis M, Szentmáry N, Seitz B. Bilateral vascularized disciform corneal scar of herpetic origin in a child. Ophthalmologe. 2015;112:162–5.
15. Remeijer L, Duan R, van Dun JM, Wefers Bettink MA, Osterhaus ADME, Verjans GMG. Prevalence and clinical consequences of herpes simplex virus type 1 DNA in human cornea tissues. J Infect Dis. 2009;200:11–9.
16. Cavalcanti BM, Cruzat A, Sahin A, Pavan-Langston, Samayoa E, Hamrah P. In Vivo confocal microscopy detects bilateral changes of corneal immune cells and nerves in unilateral herpes zoster ophthalmicus. Ocul Surf. 2018;16:101–11.
17. Hamrah P, Cruzat A, Dastjerdi MH, Zheng L, Shahatit BM, Bayhan HA, Dana R, Pavan-Langston D. Corneal sensation and subbasal nerve alterations in patients with herpes simplex keratitis: an in vivo confocal microscopy study. Ophthalmology. 2010;117:1930–6.
18. Liu X, Xu S, Wang Y, Jin X, Shi Y, Zhang H. Bilateral limbal stem cell alterations in patients with unilateral herpes simplex keratitis and herpes zoster ophthalmicus as shown by in vivo confocal microscopy. Invest Ophthalmol Vis Sci. 2021;62:12.
19. Müller RT, Pourmirzaie R, Pavan-Langston D, Cavalcanti BM, Aggarwal S, Colón C, Jamali A, Cruzat A, Hamrah P. In vivo confocal microscopy demonstrates bilateral loss of endothelial cells in unilateral herpes simplex keratitis. Invest Ophthalmol Vis Sci. 2015;56:4899–906.
20. Holland EJ, Schwartz GS. Classification of herpes simplex virus keratitis. Cornea. 1999;18:144–54.
21. Liesegang TJ. Classification of herpes simplex virus keratitis and anterior uveitis. Cornea. 1999;18:127–43.
22. Seitz B, Heiligenhaus A. The chameleon of herpetic keratitis—diagnosis and therapy. Klin Monbl Augenheilkd. 2015;232:745–53.
23. Holbach LM, Font RL, Naumann GOH. Herpes simplex stromal and endothelial keratitis. Ophthalmology. 1990;97:722–8.
24. Hanet MS, Zimpfer A, Lepper S, Seitz B. Keratoconus-like tomographic changes in a case of recurrent interstitial keratitis. J Ophthalmic Inflamm Infect. 2018;8:4.
25. De Groot-Mijnes JD, Rothova A, Van Loon AM, Schuller M, Ten Dam-Van Loon NH, De Boer JH, Schuurman R, Weersink AJ. Polymerase chain reaction and Goldmann-Witmer coefficient analysis are complimentary for the diagnosis of infectious uveitis. Am J Ophthalmol. 2006;141:313–8.
26. Schacher S, Garweg JG, Russ C, Böhnke M. Diagnosis of herpetic uveitis and keratouveitis. Klin Monbl Augenheilkd 1998;212:359–62.
27. Naumann GOH, Gass J, Font R. Histopathology of herpes zoster ophthalmicus. Am J Ophthalmol. 1968;65:533–41.
28. Ozan-Yueksel T, Heinz C, Heiligenhaus A, Hammer CM, Luetjen-Drecoll E. Morphological changes in trabeculectomy specimens in different kinds of uveitis glaucoma. Curr Eye Res. 2011;36:442–8.
29. Bustos DE, Atherton SS. Detection of herpes simplex virus type 1 in human ciliary ganglia. Invest Ophthalmol Vis Sci. 2002;43:2244–9.
30. van der Lelij A, Ooijman FM, Kijlstra A, Rothova A. Anterior uveitis with sectoral iris atrophy in the absence of keratitis: a distinct clinical entity among herpetic eye diseases. Ophthalmology. 2000;107:1164–70.
31. Cursiefen C, Seitz B, Kruse FE. Neurotrophic keratitis. Ophthalmologe. 2005;102:7–14.
32. Mackie IA. Role of the corneal nerves in destructive disease of the cornea. Trans Ophthalmol Soc UK. 1978;98:343–7.
33. Behrens-Baumann W. Herpes simplex keratitis. A short overview of the current therapy. Klin Monbl Augenheilkd 2010;227:388–92.
34. Hoh HB, Goldschmidt P, Easty DL. Comparative efficacy of ganciclovir and acyclovir ointment in the treatment of herpes simplex dendritic keratitis. Curr Eye Res. 1992;101:68–72.
35. Power WJ, Benedict-Smith A, Hillery M, Brady K, Collum LMT. Randomized double-blind trial of bromovinyldeoxyuridine (BVDU) and trifluorothymidine (TFT) in dendritic corneal ulceration. Br J Ophthalmol. 1991;75:649–51.
36. Sundmacher R. Therapy of herpetic diseases of the anterior eye segment. Klin Monbl Augenheilkd. 1985;186:421–3.
37. Bacon TH, Levin MJ, Leary JJ, Sarisky RT, Sutton D. Herpes simplex virus resistance to acyclovir and penciclovir after two decades of antiviral therapy. Clin Microbiol Rev. 2003;16:114–28.
38. Duan R, de Vries RD, van Dun JM, van Loenen FB, Osterhaus AD, Remeijer L, Verjans GM. Acyclovir susceptibility and genetic characteristics of sequential herpes simplex virus type 1 corneal isolates from patients with recurrent herpetic keratitis. J Infect Dis. 2009;200:1402–14.
39. Spira C, Szentmáry N, Hasenfus A, Sauter M, Smola S, Seitz B. Therapy refractory stromal Herpes keratitis under aciclovir. Ophthalmologe. 2014;111:654–9.
40. Heiligenhaus A, Steuhl KP. Topical cyclosporin A in patients with herpes simplex stromal keratitis Graefe's. Arch Clin Exp Ophthalmol 1999;237:435–8.
41. Seitz B, Resch M, Schlötzer-Schrehardt U, Hofmann-Rummelt C, Sauer R, Kruse FE. Histopathology and ultrastructure of human corneas after amniotic membrane transplantation. Arch Ophthalmol. 2006;124:1487–90.
42. Alfaro Rangel R, Lepper S, Szentmáry N, Langenbucher A, Seitz B. Herpes simplex virus keratitis in a University Tertiary Referral Centre—clinical features and surgical approaches. Klin Monbl Augenheilkd. 2021;238:989–95.
43. Heiligenhaus A, Bauer D, Meller D, Steuhl KP, Tseng SC. Improvement of HSV-1 necrotizing keratitis with amniotic membrane transplantation. Invest Ophthalmol Vis Sci. 2001;42:1969–74.
44. Heiligenhaus A, Li H, Hernandez Galindo EE, Koch J, Steuhl KP, Meller D. Management of acute ulcerative and necrotizing herpes simplex and zoster keratitis with amniotic membrane transplantation. Br J Ophthalmol. 2003;87:1215–9.

45. Hoffmann S, Szentmáry N, Seitz B. Amniotic membrane transplantation for the treatment of infectious ulcerative keratitis before elective penetrating keratoplasty. Cornea. 2013;32:1321–5.
46. Resch MD, Schlötzer-Schrehardt U, Hofmann-Rummelt C, Sauer R, Kruse FE, Beckmann MW, Seitz B. Integration patterns of cryopreserved amniotic membranes into the human cornea. Ophthalmology. 2006;113:1927–35.
47. Seitz B, Das S, Sauer R, Hofmann-Rummelt C, Beckmann MW, Kruse F. Simultaneous amniotic membrane patch in high-risk keratoplasty. Cornea. 2011;30:269–72.
48. Riedel T, Seitz B, Langenbucher A, Naumann GO. Morphological results after eccentric perforating keratoplasty. Ophthalmologe. 2001;98:639–46.
49. Riedel T, Seitz B, Langenbucher A, Naumann GOH. Visual acuity and astigmatism after eccentric penetrating keratoplasty—a retrospective study on 117 patients. Klin Monbl Augenheilkd. 2002;219:40–5.
50. Seitz B, Langenbucher A. Phototherapeutic keratectomy in corneal dystrophies. In: Reinhard T, Larkin F, editors. Essentials in ophthalmology—corneal and external eye disease. Berlin: Springer; 2008. p. 55–82.
51. Rao SN. Treatment of herpes simplex virus stromal keratitis unresponsive to topical prednisolone 1% with topical cyclosporine 0.05%. Am J Ophthalmol. 2006;141:771–2.
52. Asi F, Milioti G, Seitz B. Descemet membrane endothelial keratoplasty for corneal decompensation caused by herpes simplex virus endotheliitis. J Cataract Refract Surg. 2018;44:106–8.
53. Seitz B, Daas L, Flockerzi E, Suffo S. Descemet membrane endothelial keratoplasty DMEK—donor and recipient step by step. Ophthalmologe. 2020;117:811–28.
54. Matar C, Seitz B, Daas L. Recurrent DMEK failure. Ophthalmologe. 2021;118:719–23.
55. Zarei-Ghanavati S, Alizadeh R, Yoo S. Herpes simplex virus endotheliitis following Descemet's membrane endothelial keratoplasty. J Ophthalmic Vis Res. 2015;10:184–6.
56. Anshu A, Chee SP, Mehta JS, Tan DT. Cytomegalovirus endotheliitis in Descemet's stripping endothelial keratoplasty. Ophthalmology. 2009;116:624–30.
57. Basilious A, Chew HF. Topical ganciclovir for prophylaxis of cytomegalovirus endotheliitis in endothelial keratoplasty. Cornea. 2019;38:120–2.
58. Seitz B, El-Husseiny M, Langenbucher A, Szentmáry N. Prophylaxis and management of complications in penetrating keratoplasty. Ophthalmologe. 2013;110:605–13.
59. Seitz B, Daas L, Wykrota AA, Flockerzi E, Suffo S. Graft failure after PKP and DMEK: what is the best option? Klin Monbl Augenheilkd. 2022;239:775–85.
60. Weischnur L, Xanthopoulou K, Munteanu C, Daas L, Leonhard M, Seitz B. Autologous serum eye drops for therapy-resistant epithelial defects of the cornea: impact of underlying disease and simultaneous amniotic transplantation in 990 applications. Ophthalmologie. 2023;120:43–51.
61. Dua HS, Said DG, Messmer EM, Rolando M, Benitez-Del-Castillo JM, Hossain PN, Shortt AJ, Geerling G, Nubile M, Figueiredo FC, Rauz S, Mastropasqua L, Rama P, Baudouin C. Neurotrophic keratopathy. Prog Retin Eye Res. 2018;66:107–31.
62. Seitz B, Grütereich M, Cursiefen C, Kruse FE. Conservative and surgical treatment of neurotrophic keratopathy. Ophthalmologe. 2005;102:15–26.
63. Abu Dail Y, Daas L, Flockerzi FA, Seitz B. Partial visual rehabilitation 5 and 6 years after a Gundersen total conjunctival flap procedure. Ophthalmologe. 2022;119:203–8.
64. Quintin A, Serfözö A, Daas L, Suffo S, Seitz B. Autologous contralateral and ipsilateral rotational penetrating keratoplasty— a case series and mini-review. Klin Monbl Augenheilkd. 2025;242:52–61
65. Saravia M, Zapata G, Ferraiolo P, Racca L, Berra A. Anti-VEGF monoclonal antibody-induced regression of corneal neovascularisation and inflammation in a rabbit model of herpetic stromal keratitis. Graefes Arch Clin Exp Ophthalmol. 2009;247:1409–16.
66. van Rooij J, Rijneveld WJ, Remeijer L, Völker-Dieben HJM, Eggink CA, Geerards AJM, Mulder PGH, Doornenbal P, Beekhuis WH. Effect of oral acyclovir after penetrating keratoplasty for herpetic keratitis. A placebo-controlled multicenter trial. Ophthalmology. 2003;110:1916–9.
67. Rezende RA, Uchoa UB, Raber IM, Rapuano CJ, Laibson PR, Cohen EJ. New onset of herpes simplex virus epithelial keratitis after penetrating keratoplasty. Am J Ophthalmol. 2004;137:415–9.
68. Sengler U, Reinhard T, Adams O, Krempe C, Sundmacher R. Herpes simplex virus infection in the media of donor corneas during organ culture: frequency and consequences. Eye. 2001;15:644–7.
69. Cockerham GC, Krafft AE, McLean IW. Herpes simpex virus in primary graft failure. Arch Ophthalmol. 1997;115:586–9.
70. Biswas S, Suaresh P, Bonshek RE, Corbitt G, Tullo AB, Ridgway AE. Graft failure in human donor corneas due to transmission of herpes simplex virus. Br J Ophthalmol. 2000;84:701–5.
71. Nche EN, Katzir A, Solomon A, Wolf D, Panet A, Lavy I. Occurrence of herpes viruses in morphologically normal corneas. Cornea. 2023;42:412–5.
72. Stavridis E, Gatzioufas Z, Hasenfus A, Sauter M, Smola S. Seitz B Ping-pong transmission of herpes simplex virus 1 following corneal transplantation. Ophthalmologe. 2012;109:1017–21.
73. Tóth G, Berkó-Göttel B, Seitz B, Langenbucher A, Stachon T, Pluzsik MT, Nagy ZZ, Smola S, Szentmáry N. Herpes simplex virus PCR in 2230 explanted corneal buttons. Acta Ophthalmol. 2022;100:e77–82.
74. Abu Dail Y, Daas L, Flockerzi E, Munteanu C, Kahlert J, Smola S, Seitz B. PCR testing for herpesviruses in aqueous humor samples from patients with and without clinical corneal endothelial graft rejection. J Med Virol. 2024;96(3):e29538.
75. Gatzioufas Z, Hasenfus A, Gyöngyössy B, Stavridis E, Sauter M, Smola S, Seitz B. Repeat corneal graft failure due to graft-to-host herpetic infection. J Ophthalmic Inflamm Infect. 2013;28:24.
76. Luccarelli SV, Lucentini S, Martellucci CA, Marelli L, Sacchi M, Nucci P. Impact of adherence (compliance) to oral acyclovir prophylaxis in the recurrence of herpetic keratitis: long-term results from a pediatric cohort. Cornea. 2021;40:1126–31.
77. van Velzen M, van de Vijver D, van Loenen FB, Osterhaus ADME, Remeijer L, Verjans GMGM. Acyclovir prophylaxis predisposes to antiviral-resistant recurrent herpetic keratitis. J Infect Dis. 2013;208:1359–65.
78. Verjans GMGM, Heiligenhaus A. Herpes simplex virus-induced ocular diseases: detrimental interaction between virus and host. Curr Immunol Rev. 2011;7:310–27.

Acanthamoeba Keratitis

Nóra Szentmáry, Alan Cayless, Fabian N. Fries, Loay Daas, Lei Shi, and Berthold Seitz

Abstract

The typical clinical appearance of acanthamoeba keratitis includes pseudodendritiformic epitheliopathy, multifocal stromal infiltrates, ring infiltrate, perineural infiltrate, broad-based anterior synechiae, secondary glaucoma, iris atrophy and mature cataract. Rare complications are sterile anterior uveitis, scleritis, chorioretinitis and retinal vasculitis. In 83–93% of cases, acanthamoeba keratitis patients are contact lens wearers. Acanthamoeba keratitis is diagnosed by polymerase chain reaction (PCR), confocal microscopy, in vitro culture and histopathological examination. There are currently only case series on the safety and effectivity of medical and surgical treatment of acanthamoeba keratitis and to date there have been no randomised controlled clinical studies. After early diagnosis, acanthamoeba keratitis can often be successfully treated using triple topical therapy with polyhexamide, propamidine isethionate and neomycin. Topical therapy should be continued for up to 1 year. In therapy-resistant cases corneal cryotherapy, amniotic membrane transplantation, crosslinking therapy and therapeutic keratoplasty can be performed.

Keywords

Acanthamoeba keratitis · Clinical signs · Diamidine · Biguanide · Treatment

N. Szentmáry (✉) · F. N. Fries · L. Shi
Dr. Rolf M. Schwiete Center for Limbal Stem Cell and Congenital Aniridia Research, Saarland University, Homburg/Saar, Germany
e-mail: nora.szentmary@uks.eu

A. Cayless
School of Physical Sciences, The Open University, Milton Keynes, UK

F. N. Fries · L. Daas · B. Seitz
Department of Ophthalmology, Saarland University Medical Center, UKS, Homburg/Saar, Germany

1 Introduction

Acanthamoeba keratitis (AK) is a rare but potentially devastating ocular infection, occuring mostly in contact lens wearers. *Acanthamoeba* are ubiquitous, free-living protozoa, present in air, soil, dust, drinking water and also in sea water. There is a dormant resilient cyst and an infective trophozoite form.

AK is often misdiagnosed and treated as herpetic, bacterial or mycotic keratitis, since many signs and symptoms may look similar to other kinds of keratitis. It is challenging for an ophthalmologist to find the right diagnosis [1, 2], and consequently, diagnosis is often delayed and ophthalmologists tend to observe a heterogeneous and protracted clinical course.

1.1 *Acanthamoeba* Physiology and Life Cycle

Acanthamoeba is present in two forms: trophozoites and cysts.

The so called vegetative form or trophozoite has a size of 25–40 μm and is fed from bacteria, algae and yeasts. Enterobacteria are especially preferred through *Acanthamoebae* but some *Acanthamoeba* species house bacteria as endosymbionts [3].

The double-walled cysts have a 13–20 μm size and survive antibiotics, low temperatures (for example 15 months at −15 °C), high doses of UV-light and γ-radiation. In adverse conditions, *Acanthamoeba* trophozoites form cysts which may survive for more than 24 years.

*Acanthamoeb*a are classified through their rDNA-sequence-types (T1–T12) (Stothard). AK is most often caused by the T4 genotype [4–10].

B. Seitz et al. (eds.), *Atlas on Cornea*, https://doi.org/10.1007/978-3-031-65422-0_24

1.2 Acanthamoeba Keratitis Pathophysiology

In cases of corneal infection, as a first step *Acanthamoeba* are attached to the corneal epithelial cells through the Mannose-binding protein. This binding supports secretion of metalloproteinase, serin- and cysteinproteinase by *Acanthamoeba,* resulting in cytotoxic effects on human corneal epithelial cells and keratocytes and supporting deeper corneal penetration of *Acanthamoebae* [11–13].

Acanthamoeba may also migrate along corneal nerves and damage these [14, 15].

1.3 Epidemiology, Risk Factors and Prevention

The first reports on AK were published in the seventies [16, 17]. With increasing use of contact lenses, its incidence increased in the 1980s [18–20], reaching an incidence of 1 in 30,000 contact lens wearers in the 1990s (Great Britain, Hong Kong) [21]. Nowadays about 5% of contact-lens-associated keratitis is caused by *Acanthamoebae* [22, 23].

The main risk factors are: extended use of contact lenses (daily lenses have a lower risk) [24–26], wearing contact lenses in the bath, and cleaning lenses with tap water or saliva instead of a dedicated lens cleaning solution [27]. Additional risk factors are corneal surface damage, exposure to contaminated water and low socioeconomic status [28, 29].

A study of contact lens cleaning solutions has proven that only those containing hydrogen peroxide are effective against all Acanthamoeba strains [30].

2 Acanthamoeba Keratitis Diagnostics

In cases showing clinical signs of AK, diagnostics must always be performed. We use in vivo confocal microscopy and in vitro diagnostics such as polymerase-chain-reaction (PCR), histopathological examination, or microbiological culture [31–35]. All diagnostic methods, including the analysed material and the sensitivity of the method are summarised in Table 1.

As a first step, having recognised clinical signs of AK, it is important to use appropriate diagnostic methods. These are summarised as follows:

In vivo *confocal microscopy* has more than 90% sensitivity in experienced hands, however only Acanthamoeba cysts are well recognised using this method [33–35]. *Polymerase-chain-reaction (PCR)* of corneal scrapings showed the highest sensitivity at 84–100%, and may give a result within 60 min [36–39]. However, PCR has the potential disadvantage that non-living *Acanthamoeba* genetic material may also give a positive result [3].

In vitro *culture* may have between 0 and 70% sensitivity. This technique uses the fact the *Acanthamoeba* grows well on *Escherichia coli (E. coli)* and *Acanthamoeba* forms lines in an *E. coli* covered plate. This method has the disadvantage of being fairly slow, typically giving results within 3 weeks [40–42].

Presence of *Acanthamoeba* may also be verified through *histopathological analysis*, with 31–65% sensitivity. Corneal scrapings or excised or explanted tissue from keratoplasty may be analysed using periodic acid Schiff, Masson, Gram, Giemsa, Grocott-methamine-silver or calcofluor-white stainings [36, 43, 44].

Table 1 We use in vivo confocal microscopy and in vitro diagnostics such as polymerase-chain-reaction (PCR), histopathological examination, or microbiological culture in acanthamoeba keratitis [2, 31–34]

Diagnostic method	Analyzed material	Sensitivity
In-vivo confocal microscopy	In vivo corneal examination	Above 90% with experienced examiner
Polymerase-chain reaction (PCR)	Corneal scrapings (epithelium) or corneal biopsy + contact lens case and cleaning solution	84–100%
In-vitro culture	Corneal scrapings (epithelium) or corneal biopsy + contact lens case and cleaning solution	0–77%
Histopathological analysis	Corneal scrapings or excision or explanted tissue from keratoplasty	31–65%

Table 2 Clinical symptoms and their time of presentation in acanthamoeba keratitis

Clinical symptom	Time	Special properties
Chameleon-like epithelial changes ("dirty epithelium") (Fig. 1A)	Within the first 2 weeks in 50% of the patients	Grey epithelial opacities, pseudodendritiformic epitheliopathy, epithelial microerosions or microcysts
Multifocal stromal infiltrates (Fig. 2A)	Within the first 2 weeks	Mostly central and paracentral
Ringinfiltrate/Wessely immune ring (Figs. 1B and 2A)	In the first month in 20% of the patients incidence increases with time	From polymorphonuclear leukocytes, antigen–antibody complex and complement
Perineural infiltrate (Fig. 3)	In the first month of the disease in 2.5–63% of the patients	Radial, from limbus to middle stroma, results in loss of corneal nerve fibres
Sterile anterior uveitis, scleritis, broad-based anterior synechiae, secondary glaucoma, iris atrophy, mature cataract (Fig. 4), chorioretinitis, retinal vasculitis	Late symptoms, following months	Rare! Reason unknown (treatment or disease?) [79, 80]

3 Clinical Symptoms

In early stages of the disease, about 75–90% of all patients are misdiagnosed, as typical AK symptoms are difficult to associate [5, 9]. Analysis of the *German Acanthamoeba Keratitis Registry* has shown that Acanthamoeba keratitis patients have been incorrectly diagnosed as having either herpetic (47.6% of cases), mycotic (25.2%) or bacterial (3.9%) keratitis [33]. Typically, in Germany, the correct AK diagnosis was not arrived at before 2.8 ± 4.0 months (range 0–23 months) after the appearance of the first clinical symptoms [33].

In about 23% of cases [2, 31, 44–46] a mixed infection involving co-infection with virus, bacteria or fungi is present.

Clinical signs of AK are the following [44–55] **(Table 2)**:

- Chameleon-like epithelial changes ("dirty epithelium", pseudodentritiformic epitheliopathy, epithelial microerosions and microcysts) (Figs. 1A and 2A)
- Multifocal stromal infiltrates (Fig. 2A)
- Ring infiltrate ("Wessely immune ring") (Fig. 2A)
- Peripheral perineural infiltrate (Fig. 3)
- Common complications: broad-based anterior synechiae, secondary glaucoma, iris atrophy, mature cataract (Fig. 4), persistent epithelial defect
- Rare complications: sterile anterior uveitis, scleritis (Fig. 4)
- Very rare complications: chorioretinitis and retinal vasculitis

4 Differential Diagnosis

"Dirty epithelium" and pseudodendritiformic epitheliopathy have to be differentiated from an epithelial *herpetic* keratitis (dendritic or geographic). These do not have round spot-like widenings at the endings of the epithelial erosions, unlike herpetic epithelial keratitis.

In the absence of bacterial or mycotic superinfection of an AK, the stromal infiltrates in AK in the early stages of the disease are multifocal, dot-like (resembling unsharp-edged stromal stars) and partly transparent. In contrast, *bacterial* or *mycotic* stromal infiltrates are thicker and typically monofocal. Nevertheless, satellite infiltrates in fungal keratitis may imitate multifocal stromal infiltrates of AK.

The Wessely immune ring may be present in bacterial, mycotic or acanthamoeba keratitis. The clinical image of the stromal infiltrates at the same time differentiates these clinical entities.

5 Acanthamoeba Keratitis Treatment

There are currently only case series on the safety and effectivity of medical and surgical treatment of AK and to date there have been no randomised controlled clinical studies.

5.1 Conservative Treatment

5.1.1 Diamidine and Biguanide

Diamidines, such as propamidin-isoethionat (Brolene), hexamidin-diisoethionat (Hexacyl) and dibromopropamidin (Golden Eye) are used in 0.1% concentration [56–58]. *Biguanides,* such as polyhexamethilen-biguanide (polyhexanid) (Lavasept) and chlorhexidin (Curasept) are applied in 0.02% concentration [2].

The concentration dependent effect of diamidines and biguanides on human epithelial cells, keratocytes and endothelial cells have already been described, and propamidin-isoethionate as diamidine and chlorhexidin as biguanide seem to be the least cytotoxic. However, these may reduce

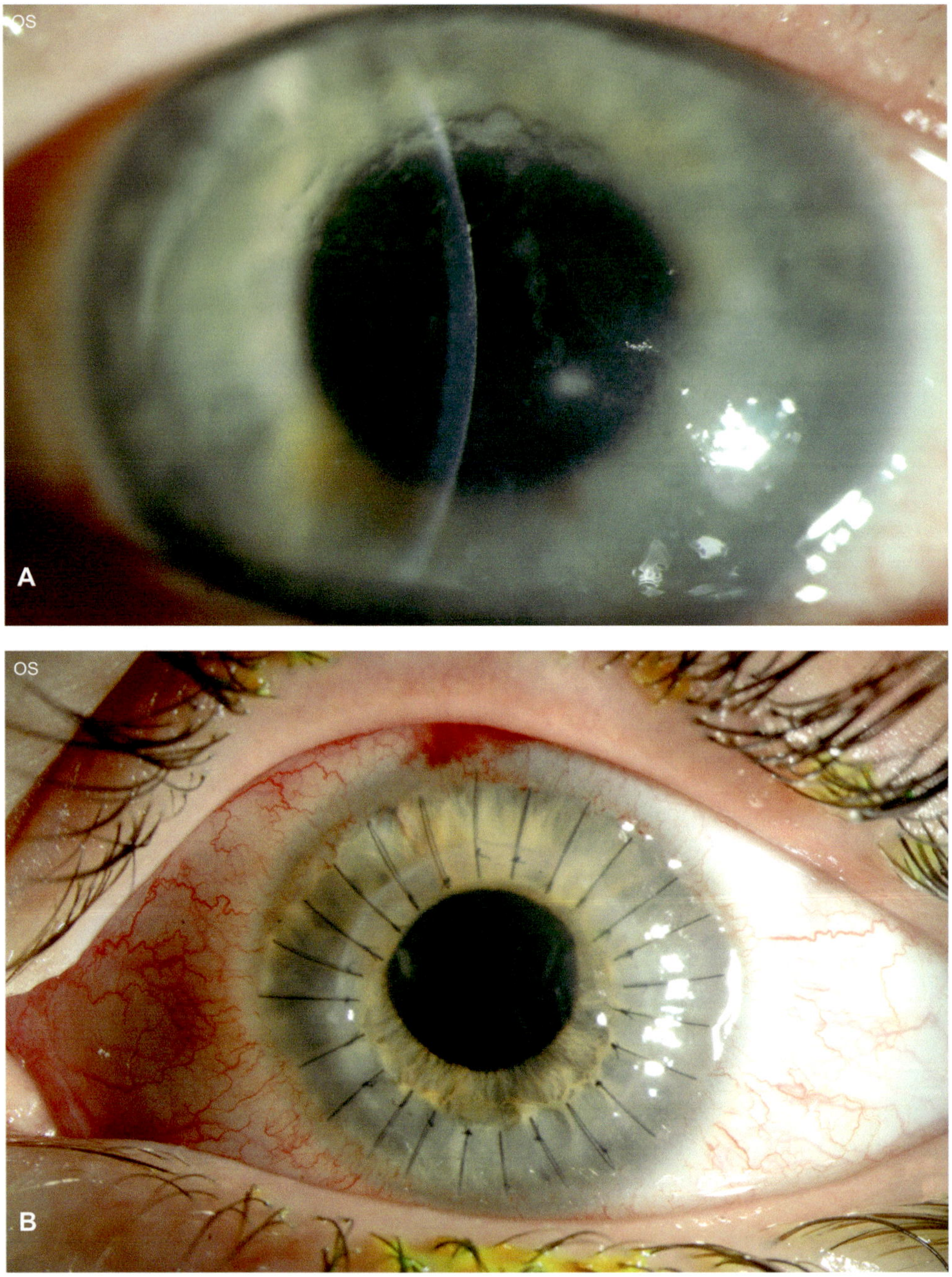

Fig. 1 "Dirty epithelium" (**A**) and six months later excimer laser penetrating keratoplasty with interrupted sutures (**B**), in acanthamoeba keratitis

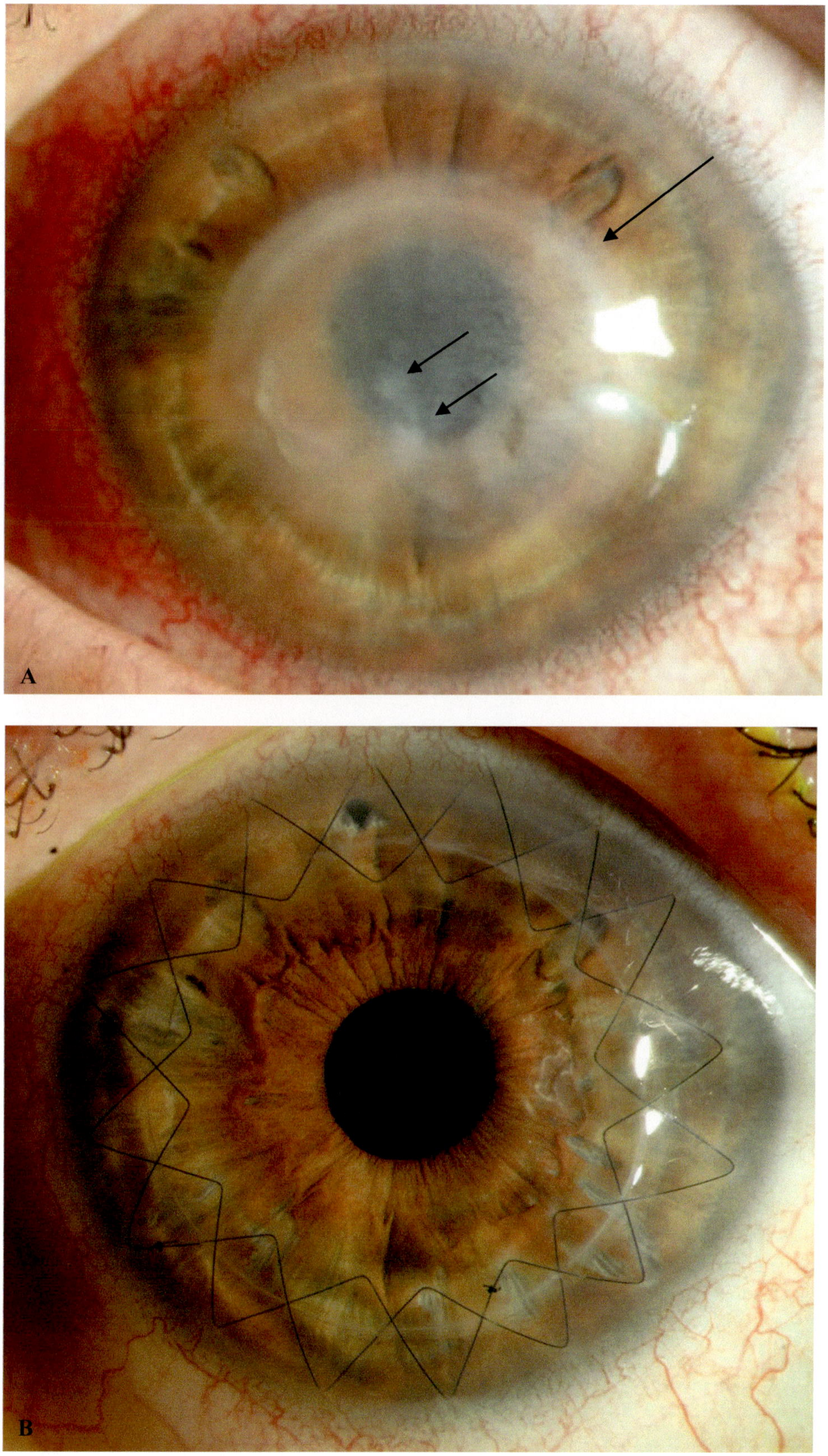

Fig. 2 Dirty epithelium, incomplete ring infiltrate (long arrow) and multifocal stromal infiltrates (small arrows) in acanthamoeba keratitis (**A**). One week later after excimer laser penetrating keratoplasty with double-running sutures (**B**)

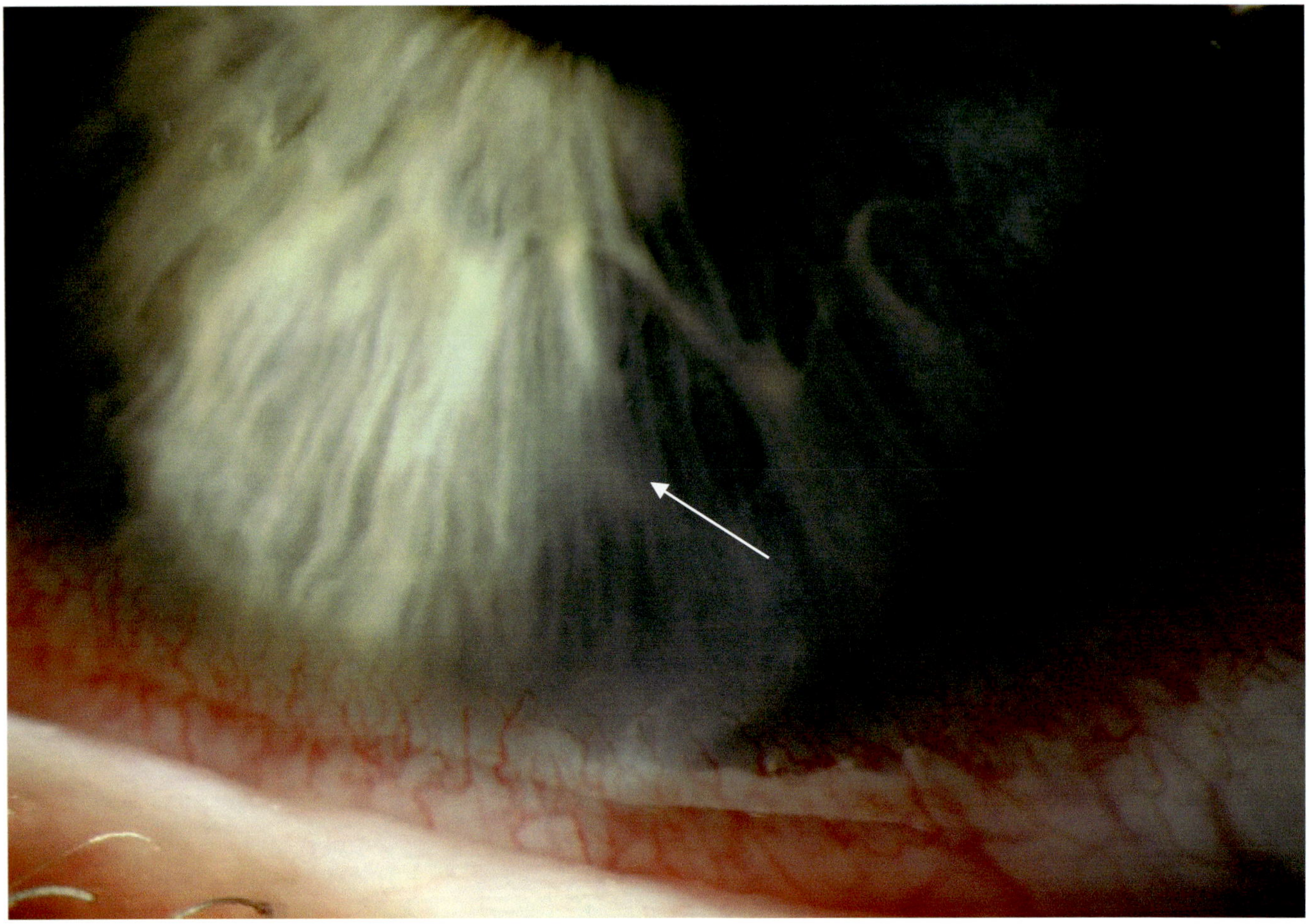

Fig. 3 Perineuritis in acanthamoeba keratitis (arrow) (contact lens wearer)

proliferation and migration of human corneal cells more than other diamidines and biguanides [59].

5.1.2 Antibiotics

Neomycin kills trophozoites, prevents bacterial superinfection [60] and reduces bacterial load, as a food source for *Acanthamoeba* [2].

5.1.3 Povidone-Iodine and Miltefosine

An in vitro experiment reported on a better anticystic effect of 1% povidon-iodine than propamidin-isoethionat or polyhexanid. However, these results have not been verified in clinical studies [61].

Miltefosine has been shown to be effective against *Acanthamoeba* in vitro [62].

5.1.4 Steroids

Topical use of steroids may suppress the clinical signs of AK, for as long as they are used. Their disadvantage is that they support excystment and an increase in the number of throphozoites. However, a patient with AK and severe inflammation may also benefit from their use. Steroids should never be used without additional topical antiseptics and should never be applied at early stage of AK treatment (never in the first week even after appropriate diagnosis) [63, 64]. When stopping topical steroids, a Wessely immune ring may develop within 2 days in patients with AK.

5.1.5 Antifungals

Miconazole and Clotrimazole have been previously used as topical treatment of AK [65, 66]. In addition, there are reports on topical and systemic voriconazole use in these patients [65–67]. An in vitro study described better anticystic effect using natamycin in contrast to propamidin-isoethionat or polyhexamethilen-biguanid [61]. However, data on clinical use of natamycin in AK patients is not available.

In Germany, we suggest topical application of polyhexamethilen-biguanid, propamidin-isoethionat and Neomycin as triple-therapy in case of AK [2]. To date there have been no randomised controlled clinical trials on the safety and effectivity of conservative treatment in AK.

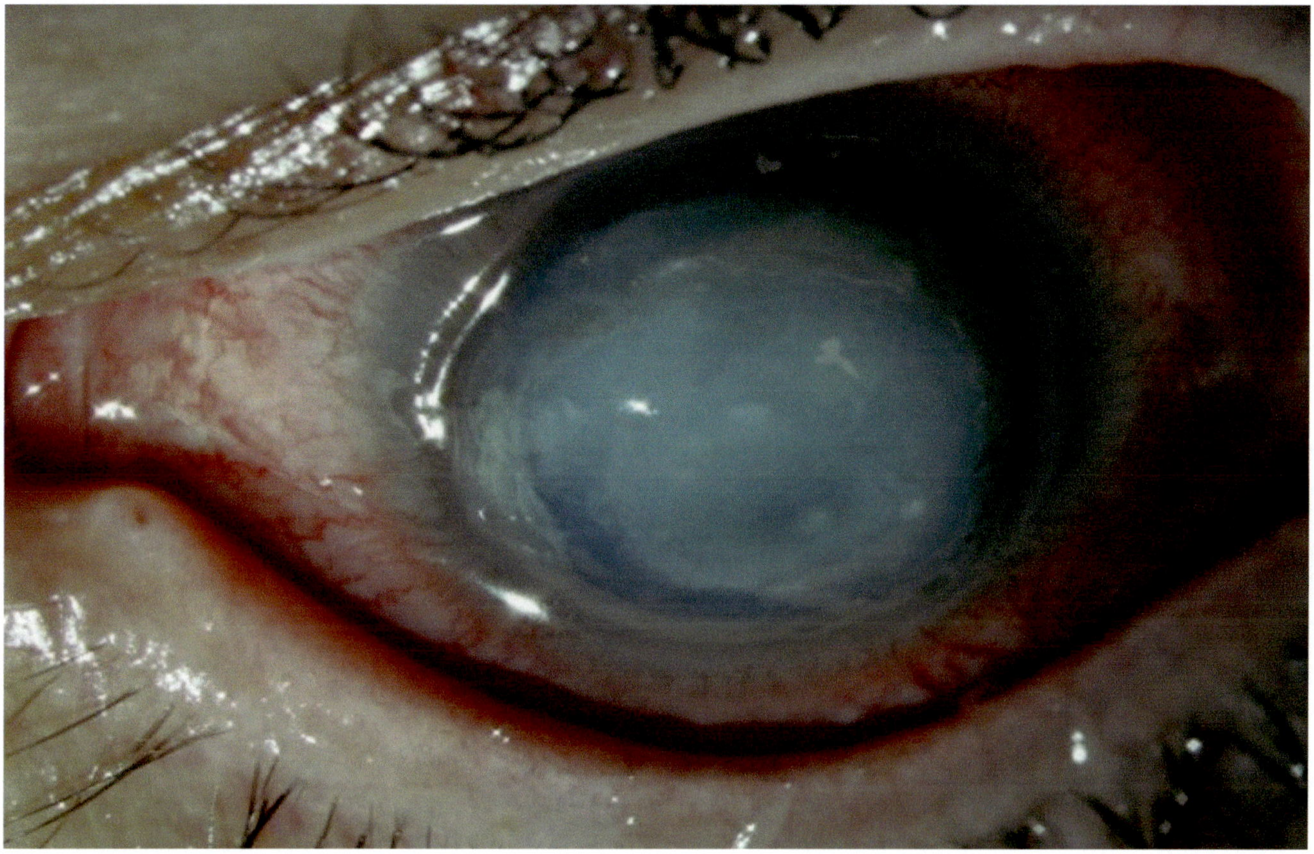

Fig. 4 Scleritis, corneal ulcer, iris atrophy, persistent mydriasis and mature cataract in severe acanthamoeba keratitis

During the first two days a "surprise attack" can be initiated with polyhexamethilen-biguanide and propamidin-isoethionat every quarter to half an hour during day and night. Then, until the sixth day, polyhexamethilen-biguanide and propamidin-isoethionat are applied every hour and only during the day (06:00–24:00). Over the following 4 weeks, eyedrop use is reduced to every 2 h. Additionally, neomycin is also applied five times a day [60]. In therapy resistant cases, we may change polyhexamethilen-biguanide to chlorhexidin, or increase the concentration (for polyhexamethilen-biguanide to 0.08%, for chlorhexidin to 0.2%).

To the best of our current knowledge, combination therapy using diamidine, biguanide and antibiotics should be continued in descending doses for up to 1 year.

5.1.6 Surgical Treatment

Diagnostic and therapeutic epithelial abrasion aims to remove microorganisms resulting in a better penetration of topical medication [68]. If topical conservative treatment does not improve clinical signs and symptoms, a corneal cryotherapy, amniotic membrane transplantation, or penetrating keratoplasty may be performed. In therapy resistant cases, a crosslinking treatment as a photodynamic therapy may be used, in some cases repeatedly.

Corneal cryotherapy is an adjuvant treatment of topical therapy. The infected corneal areas, or the recipient area before penetrating keratoplasty will be treated using a cold cryoprobe 2–3 times ("freeze–thaw–freeze") until ice crystals are formed in the corneal stroma [69]. As part of a penetrating keratoplasty, cryotherapy is circularly used (about 2 s at −80 °C to the recipient bed) before recipient trephination. The effect of this type of cryotherapy on limbal epithelial stem cells has currently not been clarified.

An *Amniotic Membrane Transplantation* (AMT) may be used, especially for persistent epithelial defects or ulcers as a "Patch", "Graft" or "Sandwich" and may help to reach a quiet state of the eye [70]. In many cases, AMT has to be repeated several times in order to reach epithelial closure.

Photodynamic Therapy (PDT) may be an alternative treatment option in therapy resistant infectious keratitis [71]. The successful use of Riboflavin-UVA Crosslinking in AK has been summarised in a case series in 2011 [72]. Nevertheless, in cases of stromal infiltrates, UVA-light penetration to the corneal stroma may be reduced. An accelerated crosslinking in AK is not suggested.

In cases of AK expansion in direction of the corneoscleral limbus, an early penetrating keratoplasty has to be done, in order to perform the excision in uninfected corneal tissue. In cases of progressive, therapy resistant ulceration over weeks and months, with peripheral reparative neovascularisation, we suggest an early (<5 months disease course) à chaud penetrating keratoplasty [73] (Figs. 1B and 2B). The origin of frequent therapy resistant epithelial defects in the transplanted tissue after PKP, has not yet been clarified. Potential treatment options of these epithelial defects are (1) autologous serum, (2) AMT, (3) Cacicol20® or (4) Neurotrophic Growth Factor (NGF).

Following penetrating keratoplasty, we continue the use of the above described topical treatment for up to 1 year [2, 74]. However, there have also been no controlled clinical trials related to this topic. Perhaps local therapy may be stopped earlier, in order to avoid persistent epithelial defects, peripheral anterior synechiae and mature cataract. Confocal microscopy may be useful in diagnosis of AK recurrences [32].

In cases of perforated corneal ulcers, a nonmechanical, excimer laser-assisted keratoplasty is best performed [75]. Using an elliptical excimer laser trephination with metal masks, the infected corneal area can be removed with a more homogeneous distance from the limbal vessels, especially in typically elliptical shaped AK [76].

Some authors suggest at least a 3 months-long observation period without inflammatory signs, following discontinuation of conservative therapy before planning an elective penetrating keratoplasty, following AK. In such elective PKPs, graft survival may be up to 100% after 5 years and 67% after 10 years [73, 77–80].

Today, the novel concept of early "low load keratoplasty" may avoid disastrous long-standing keratitis cases without healing over more than 12 months [81, 82].

6 Conclusion

AK presents in early stages with grey-dirty epithelium, pseudodendritiformic epitheliopathy, perineuritis, multifocal stromal infiltrates, ring infiltrates and in later stages with scleritis, iris atrophy, anterior synechiae, secondary glaucoma, mature cataract and chorioretinitis. As a conservative treatment, triple-topical therapy (polyhexamethilen-biguanide, propamidin-isoethionat, neomycin) can be used for up to one year. In therapy resistant cases, surgical treatment options such as corneal cryotherapy, amniotic membrane transplantation, riboflavin-UVA crosslinking and penetrating keratoplasty may be applied.

References

1. Meltendorf C, Duncker G. Acanthamoeba keratitis. Klin Monbl Augenheilkd. 2011;228:R29–R43.
2. Szentmáry N, Goebels S, Matoula P, et al. Acanthamoeba keratitis—a rare and often late diagnosed disease. Klin Monbl Augenheilkd. 2012;229:521–8.
3. Weekers PH, Bodelier PL, Wijen JP, et al. Effects of grazing by the free-living soil amobae Acanthamoeba castellanii, Acanthamoeba polyphaga, and Hartmannella vermiformis on various bacteria. Appl Environ Microbiol. 1993;59:2317–9.
4. Gupta S, Das SR. Stock cultures of free-living amebas: effect of temperature on viability and pathogenicity. J Parasitol. 1999;85:137–9.
5. De Jonckheere J, van de Voorde H. Differences in destruction of cysts of pathogenic and nonpathogenic Naegleria and Acanthamoeba by chlorine. Appl Environ Microbiol. 1976;31:294–7.
6. Khunkitti W, Lloyd D, Furr JR, et al. Acanthamoeba castellanii: growth, encystment, excystment and biocide susceptibility. J Infect Dis. 1998;36:43–8.
7. Brown TJ, Cursons RT. Pathogenic free-living amebae (PFLA) from frozen swimming areas in Oslo, Norway. Scan J Infect Dis. 1977;9:237–40.
8. Aksozek A, McClellan K, Howard K, et al. Resistance of Acanthamoeba castellanii cysts to physical, chemical, and radiological conditions. J Parasitol. 2002;88:621–3.
9. Mazur T, Hadas E, Iwanicka I. The duration of the cyst stage and the viability and virulence of Acanthamoeba isolates. Trop Med Parasitol. 1995;46:106–8.
10. Stothard DR, Hay J, Schroeder-Deidrich JM, et al. Fluorescent oligonucleotide probes for clinical and environmental detection of Acanthamoeba and the T4 18S rRNA gebe sequence type. J Clin Microbiol. 1999;37:2687–93.
11. Panjwani N. Pathogenesis of acanthamoeba keratitis. Ocul Surf. 2010;8:70–9.
12. Clarke DW, Niederkorn JY. The pathophysiology of acanthamoeba keratitis. Trends Parasitol. 2006;22:175–80.
13. Hadas E, Mazur T. Proteolytic enzymes of pathogenic and nonpathogenic strains of Acanthamoeba spp. Trop Med Parasitol. 1993;44:197–200.
14. Moore MB, McCulley JP, Kaufman HE, et al. Radial keratoneuritis as a presenting sign in acanthamoeba keratitis. Ophthalmology. 1986;93:1310–5.
15. Alfawaz A. Radial keratoneuritis as a presenting sign in acanthamoeba keratitis. Middle East Afr J Ophthalmol. 2011;18:252–5.
16. Naginton J, Watson PG, Payfair TJ, et al. Amoebic infection of the eye. Lancet. 1974;2:1537–40.
17. Jones DB, Visvesvara GS, Robinson NM. Acanthamoeba polyphaga keratitis and Acanthamoeba uveitis associated with fatal meningoencephalitis. Trans Ophthalmol Soc UK. 1975;95:221–32.
18. Ku JY, Chan FM, Beckingsale P. Acanthamoeba keratitis cluster: and increase in acanthamoeba keratitis in Australia. Clin Exp Ophthalmol. 2009;37:181–90.
19. Moore MB, McCulley JP, Newton C, et al. Acanthamoeba keratitis. A growing problem in soft and hard contact lens wearers. Ophthalmology 1987;94:1654–61.
20. Schaumberg DA, Snow KK, Dana MR. The epidemic of acanthamoeba keratitis: where do we stand? Cornea. 1998;17:3–10.
21. Seal DV. Acanthamoeba keratitis update—incidence, molecular epidemiology and new drugs for treatment. Eye (Lond). 2003;17:893–905.

22. Butler TK, Males JJ, Robinson LP, et al. Six-year review of acanthamoeba keratitis in New South Wales, Australia: 1997–2002. Clin Exp Ophthalmol. 2005;33:41–6.
23. Acharya NR, Lietman TM, Margolis TP. Parasites on the rise: a new epidemic of acanthamoeba keratitis. Am J Ophthalmol. 2007;144:292–3.
24. McAllum P, Bahar I, Kaiserman I, et al. Temporal and seasonal trends in acanthamoeba keratitis. Cornea. 2009;28:7–10.
25. Radford CF, Lehmann OJ, Dart JK, et al. National acanthamoeba keratitis study group. Acanthamoeba keratitis: multicentre survey in England 1992–1996. Br J Ophthalmol. 1998;82:1387–92.
26. Chew HF, Yildiz EH, Hammersmith KM, et al. Clinical outcomes and prognostic factors associated with acanthamoeba keratitis. Cornea. 2011;30:435–41.
27. Hammersmith KM. Diagnosis and management of acanthamoeba keratitis. Curr Opin Ophthalmol. 2006;17:327–31.
28. Stehr-Green JK, Bailey TM, Visvesvara GS. The epidemiology of acanthamoeba keratitis in the United States. Am J Ophthalmol. 1989;107:331–6.
29. Sharma S, Garg P, Rao GN. Patient characteristics, diagnosis, and treatment of non-contact lens related acanthamoeba keratitis. Br J Ophthalmol. 2000;84:1103–8.
30. Johnston SP, Sriram R, Qvarnstrom Y, et al. Resistance of Acanthamoeba cysts to disinfection in multiple contact lens solutions. J Clin Microbiol. 2009;47:2040–5.
31. Dart JK, Saw VP, Kilvington S. Acanthamoeba keratitis: diagnosis and treatment update 2009. Am J Ophthalmol. 2009;148:487–99.
32. Daas L, Viestenz A, Schnabel P, et al. Confocal microscopy in acanthamoeba keratitis as an early relapse-marker. Clin Anat. 2018;31:60–3.
33. Daas L, Szentmáry N, Eppig T, et al. The German acanthamoeba keratitis register: initial results of a multicenter study. Ophthalmologe. 2015;112:752–63.
34. Pfister DR, Cameron JD, Krachmer JH, et al. Confocal microscopy findings of acanthamoeba keratitis. Am J Ophthalmol. 1996;121:119–28.
35. Duguid IG, Dart JK, Morlet N, et al. Acanthamoeba keratitis treated with polyhexamethyl biguanide and propamidine. Ophthalmology. 1997;104:1587–92.
36. Lehmann OJ, Green SM, Morlet N, et al. Polymerase chain reaction analysis of corneal epithelial and tear samples in the diagnosis of acanthamoeba keratitis. Invest Ophthalmol Vis Sci. 1998;39:1261–5.
37. Qvarnstrom Y, Visvesvara GS, Sriram R, et al. Multiplex real-time PCR assay for simultaneous detection of Acanthamoeba spp., Balamuthia mandrillaris, and Naegleria fowleri. J Clin Microbiol. 2006;44:3589–95.
38. Thompson PP, Kowalski RP, Shanks RM, et al. Validation of real-time PCR for laboratory diagnosis of acanthamoeba keratitis. J Clin Microbiol. 2008;46:3232–6.
39. Mathers WD, Sutphin JE, Folberg R, et al. Outbreak of keratitis presumed to be caused by Acanthamoeba. Am J Ophthalmol. 1996;121:129–42.
40. Reinhard T, Behrens-Baumann W. Anti-infective drug therapy in ophthalmology—Part 4: Acanthamoeba keratitis. Klin Monbl Augenheilkd. 2006;223:485–91.
41. Aspöck H. Grundzüge der Diagnostik. In: Hiepe T, Lucius R, Gottstein B, editors. Allgemeine Parasitologie mit den Grundzügen der Immunologie, Diagnostik und Bekämpfung. Stuttgart: Parey in MVS Medizinverlage; 2006. p. 339–457.
42. Bacon AS, Frazer DG, Dart JK, et al. A review of 72 consecutive cases of acanthamoeba keratitis, 1984–1992. Eye (Lond). 1993;7:719–25.
43. Sharma S, Athmanathan S, Atha-Ur-Rasheed M, et al. Evaluation of immunoperoxidase staining technique in the diagnosis of acanthamoeba keratitis. Indian J Ophthalmol. 2001;49:181–6.
44. Claerhout I, Goegebuer A, Van Den Broecke C, et al. Delay in diagnosis and outcome of acanthamoeba keratitis. Graefes Arch Clin Exp Ophthalmol. 2004;242:648–53.
45. Awwad ST, Petroll WM, McCulley JP, et al. Updates in acanthamoeba keratitis. Eye Contact Lens. 2007;33:1–8.
46. Perry HD, Donnenfeld ED, Foulks GN, et al. Decreased corneal sensation as an initial feature of acanthamoeba keratitis. Ophthalmology. 1995;102:1565–8.
47. Patel DV, McGhee CN. Acanthamoeba keratitis: a comprehensive photographic reference of common and uncommon signs. Clin Experiment Ophthalmol. 2009;37:232–8.
48. Papathanassiou M, Gartry D. Steril corneal ulcer with ring infiltrate and hypopyon after recurrent erosions. Eye. 2007;21:124–6.
49. Thomas KE, Purcell TL, Tanzer DJ et al. Delayed diagnosis of microsporidial stromal keratitis: unusual Wessely ring presentation and partial treatment with medications against Acanthamoeba. BMJ Case Rep. 2011. pii: bcr0820103233. https://doi.org/10.1136/bcr.08.2010.3233.
50. Kremer I, Cohen EJ, Eagle RC Jr, et al. Histopathologic evaluation of stromal inflammation in acanthamoeba keratitis. CLAO J. 1994;20:45–8.
51. Clarke DW, Alizadeh H, Niederkorn JY. Failure of Acanthamoeba castellanii to produce intraocular infections. Invest Ophthalmol Vis Sci. 2005;46:2472–8.
52. Shigeyasu C, Shimazaki J. Ocular surface reconstruction after exposure to high concentrations of antiseptic solutions. Cornea. 2012;31:59–65.
53. Awwad ST, Heilman M, Hogan RN, et al. Severe reactive ischemic posterior segment inflammation in acanthamoeba keratitis: a new potentially blinding syndrome. Ophthalmology. 2007;114:313–20.
54. Herz NL, Matoba AY, Wilhelmus KR. Rapidly progressive cataract and iris atrophy during treatment of acanthamoeba keratitis. Ophthalmology. 2008;115:866–9.
55. Kelley PS, Dossey AP, Patel D, et al. Secondary glaucoma associated with advanced acanthamoeba keratitis. Eye Contact Lens. 2006;32:178–82.
56. Larkin DF, Kilvington S, Dart JK. Treatment of acanthamoeba keratitis with polyhexamethylene biguanide. Ophthalmology. 1992;99:185–91.
57. Ficker L, Seal D, Warhurst D, et al. Acanthamoeba keratitis—resistance to medical therapy. Eye (Lond). 1990;4(Pt 6):835–8.
58. Wright P, Warhurst D, Jones BR. Acanthamoeba keratitis successfully treated medically. Br J Ophthalmol. 1985;69:778–82.
59. Shi L, Stachon T, Seitz B, Wagenpfeil S, Langenbucher A, Szentmáry N. The effect of antiamoebic agents on viability, proliferation and migration of human epithelial cells, keratocytes and endothelial cells, in vitro. Curr Eye Res. 2018;43:725–33.
60. Elder MJ, Kilvington S, Dart JK. A clinicopathologic study of in vitro sensitivity testing and acanthamoeba keratitis. Invest Ophthalmol Vis Sci. 1994;35:1059–64.
61. Sunada A, Kimura K, Nishi K, et al. In vitro evaluations of topical agents to treat acanthamoeba keratitis. Ophthalmology. 2014;121:2059–65.
62. Polat ZA, Walochnik J, Obwaller A, et al. Miltefosine and polyhexamethylene biguanide: a new drug combination for the treatment of acanthamoeba keratitis. Clin Exp Ophthalmol. 2014;42:151–8.
63. McClellan K, Howard K, Niederkorn JY, et al. Effect of steroids on Acanthamoeba cysts and trophozoites. Invest Ophthalmol Vis Sci. 2001;42:2885–93.

64. Carnt N, Optom B, Robaei D, et al. The impact of topical corticosteroids used in conjunction with antiamoebic therapy on the outcome of acanthamoeba keratitis. Ophthalmology. 2016;123:984–90.
65. D'Aversa G, Stern GA, Driebe Jr WT. Diagnosis and successful medical treatment of Acanthamoeba keratitis. Arch Ophthalmol. 1995;113:1120–3.
66. Amoils SP, Heney C. Acanthamoeba keratitis with live isolates treated with cryosurgery and fluconazole. Am J Ophthalmol. 1999;127:718–20.
67. Oldenburg CE, Acharya NR, Tu EZ, et al. Practice patterns and opinions in the treatment of acanthamoeba keratitis. Cornea. 2011;30:1363–8.
68. Brooks Jr. JG, Coster DJ, Badenoch PR. Acanthamoeba keratitis. Resolution after epithelial debridement. Cornea. 1994;13:186–9.
69. Klüppel M, Reinhard T, Sundmacher R, et al. Therapy of advanced amoeba keratitis with keratoplasty à chaud and adjuvant cryotherapy. Ophthalmologe. 1997;94:99–103.
70. Seitz B, Resch MD, Schlötzer-Schrehardt U, et al. Histopathology and ultrastructure of human corneas after amniotic membrane transplantation. Arch Ophthalmol. 2006;124:1487–90.
71. Szentmáry N, Goebels S, Bischoff M, et al. Photodynamic therapy (PDT) for infectious keratitis. Ophthalmologe. 2012;109:165–70.
72. Khan YA, Kashiwabuchi RT, Martins SA, et al. Riboflavin and ultraviolet light a therapy as an adjuvant treatment for medically refractive acanthamoeben keratitis: report of 3 cases. Ophthalmology. 2011;118:324–31.
73. Laurik KL, Szentmáry N, Daas L, Langenbucher A, Seitz B. Early penetrating keratoplasty à chaud may improve outcome in therapy-resistant acanthamoeba keratitis. Adv Ther. 2019;36:2528–40.
74. Hager T, Hasenfus A, Stachon T, et al. Crosslinking and corneal cryotherapy in acanthamoeba keratitis—a histological study. Graefes Arch Clin Exp Ophthalmol. 2016;254:149–53.
75. Seitz B, Langenbucher A, Kus MM, et al. Nonmechanical corneal trephination with the excimer laser improves outcome after penetrating keratoplasty. Ophthalmology. 1999;106:1556–64.
76. Szentmáry N, Langenbucher A, Kus MM, et al. Elliptical nonmechanical corneal trephination—intraoperative complications and long-term outcome of 42 consecutive penetrating keratoplasties. Cornea. 2007;26:414–20.
77. Robaei D, Carnt N, Minassian DC, et al. Therapeutic and optical keratoplasty in the management of acanthamoeba keratitis: risk factors, outcomes, and summary of the literature. Ophthalmology. 2015;122:17–24.
78. Ehlers N, Hjordtal J. Are cataract and iris atrophy toxic complications of medical treatment of acanthamoeba keratitis? Acta Ophthalmol Scand. 2004;82:228–31.
79. Iovieno A, Gore DM, Carnt N, et al. Acanthamoeba sclerokeratitis: epidemiology, clinical features and treatment outcomes. Ophthalmology. 2014;121:2340–7.
80. Shi L, Hager T, Fries FN, Daas L, Holbach L, Hofmann-Rummelt C, Zemova E, Seitz B, Szentmáry N. Reactive uveitis, retinal vasculitis and scleritis as ocular end-stage of acanthamoeba keratitis: a histological study. Int J Ophthalmol. 2019;12:1966–71.
81. Abu Dail Y, Flockerzi E, Szentmáry N, Seitz B, Daas L. Acanthamoeba keratitis: what is the best time for keratoplasty in patients with resistance to conservative therapy? Klin Monbl Augenheilkd. 2025;242:629–635.
82. Abu Dail Y, Flockerzi E, Munteanu C, Szentmáry N, Seitz B, Daas L. Rethinking keratoplasty for patients with acanthamoeba keratitis: early "Low Load Keratoplasty" in contrast to late optical and therapeutic keratoplasty. Microorganisms. 2024;12:1801.

Mycotic Keratitis

Loay Daas, Yaser Abu Dail, and Berthold Seitz

Abstract

Fungal keratitis is a serious eye disease. Its incidence increased significantly in industrial countries such as Germany in recent years, largely due to the increased wearing of soft contact lenses (CL). The clinical presentation of fungal keratitis is variable and cannot be clearly distinguished from other types of CL-associated keratitis at early stages. The time required to identify the correct organism and the delay in administering the correct therapy (including early penetrating keratoplasty) often result in a poor long-term outcome and a higher enucleation rate in mycotic keratitis than in other cases of microbial keratitis. Fungal keratitis cannot be excluded by the absence of typical clinical symptoms. Therefore, further diagnostics, including same-day in vivo confocal microscopy, are required to determine the causative agent and the resistance spectrum.

Keywords

Mycotic keratitis · Candida · Fusarium · Aspergillus · Mycotic co-infection · Confocal microscopy

1 Introduction

Fungi can be broadly divided into filamentous fungi and yeast fungi (Fig. 1) [1–3]:

- **The filamentous group** includes Fusarium and Aspergillus. They are found mainly after trauma and in contact lenses (CL) users (Fig. 1A).
- **The group of yeasts** includes Candida species and is more common in immunocompromised patients (Fig. 1B).

The global incidence of mycotic keratitis is estimated to be at least 1 million cases per year, and probably about 100 000 eyes are enucleated annually due to delayed diagnosis and poor therapeutic outcomes [4]. Although the most common cases of infection are male agricultural workers in developing countries secondary to ocular trauma with organic material [5], fungal keratitis has also increased significantly in Western countries such as Germany in recent years, largely due to the increased wearing of soft CL [1, 6].

The large international outbreak of contact lens-associated fungal keratitis in 2005–2006 in developed countries and recent results from the German Fungal Keratitis Registry showed how certain filamentous fungal species, such as Fusarium sp., can lead to devastating disease, up to eye loss in otherwise young and healthy patients [1, 7–9].

2 Clinical Presentation of Mycotic Keratitis

The clinical presentation of fungal keratitis is variable and cannot be clearly distinguished from other types of CL-associated keratitis at early stages [10] (Fig. 2). The existence of co-infection may also obscure the characteristic symptoms of mycotic keratitis. This often leads to a delay in diagnosis and therapy as well as a worse prognosis [1, 10, 11]. The most common initial misdiagnosis in mycotic keratitis is bacterial keratitis [11].

Signs in early stages are often ambiguous. These include foreign body sensation, redness, decrease in visual acuity, epiphora, purulent discharges, pain, and sensitivity to light. Common clinical findings include Satellite lesions,

L. Daas (✉) · Y. Abu Dail · B. Seitz
Department of Ophthalmology, Saarland University Medical Center, Homburg, Germany
e-mail: loay.daas@uks.eu

B. Seitz et al. (eds.), *Atlas on Cornea*, https://doi.org/10.1007/978-3-031-65422-0_25

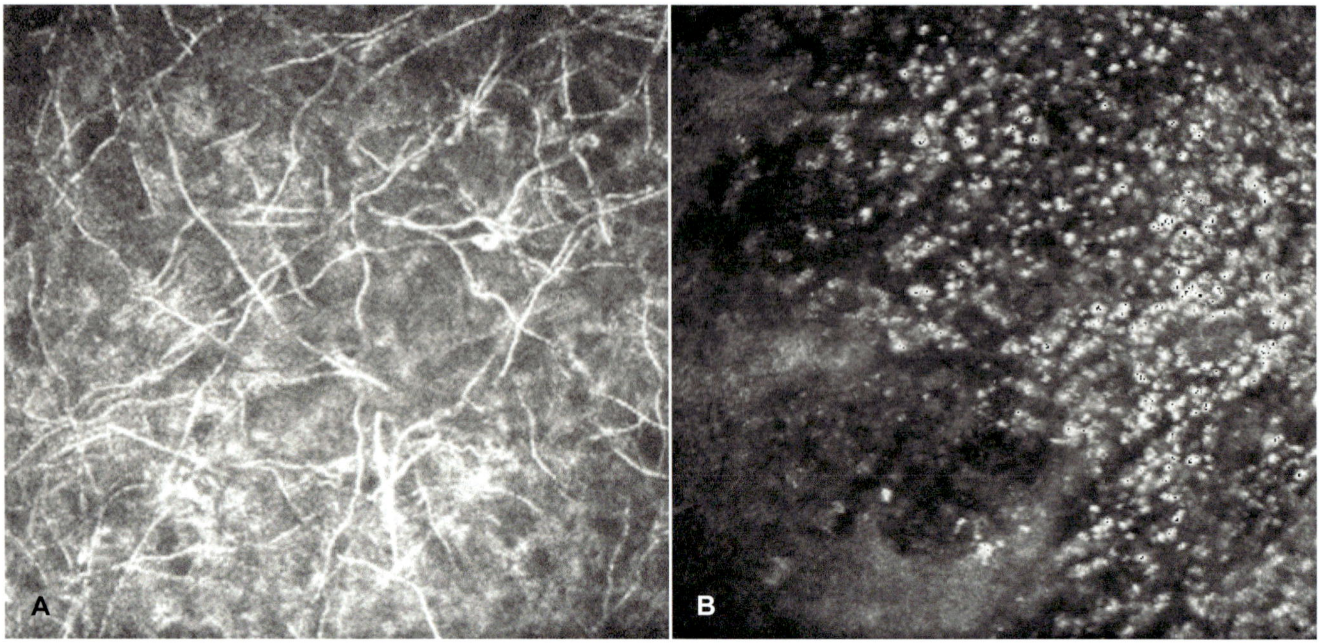

Fig. 1 (**A**) Filamentous mycotic keratitis with Aspergillus under Confocal microscopy. (**B**) Mycotic keratitis with Candida yeasts under confocal microscopy

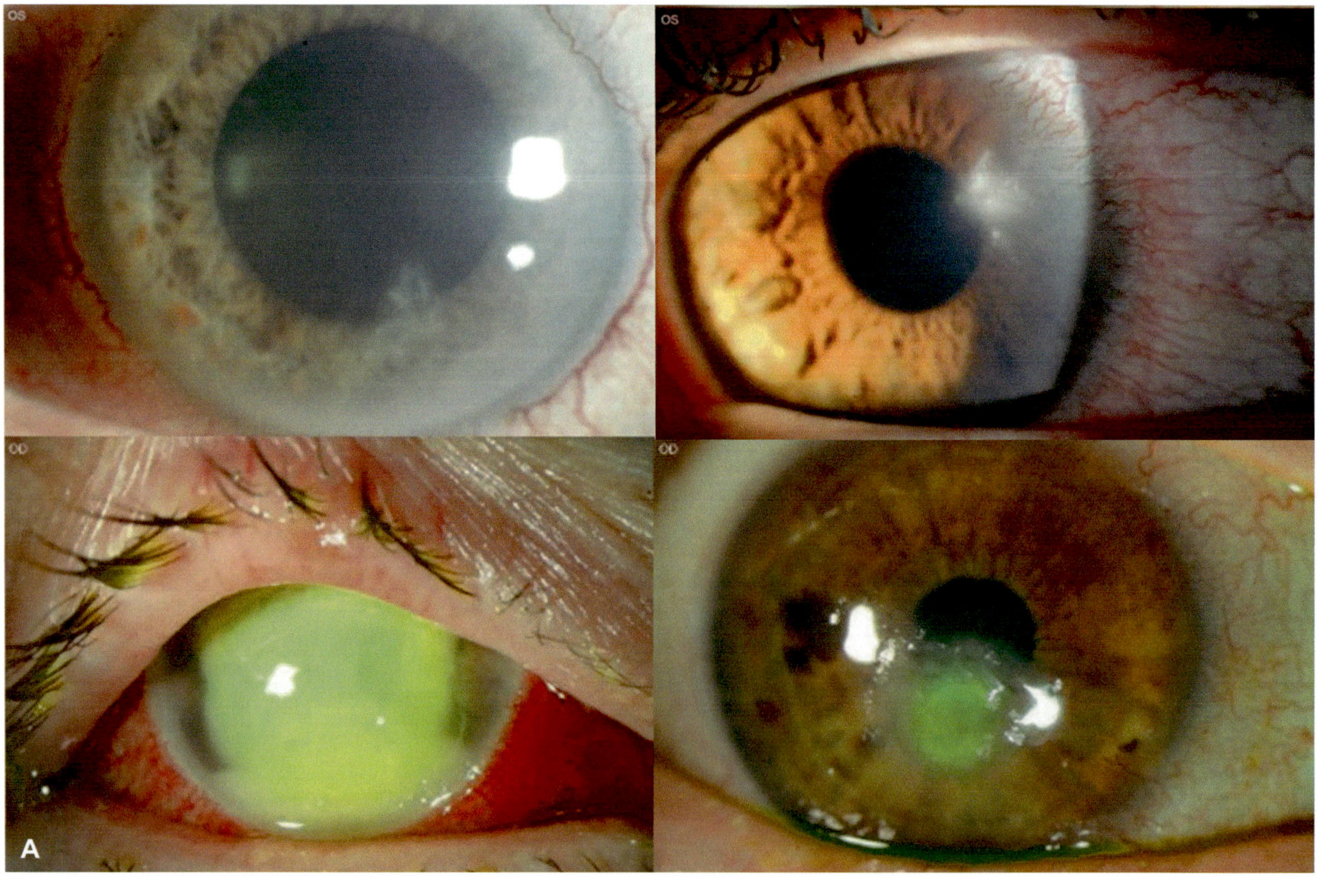

Fig. 2 Various and atypical clinical presentations of fungal keratitis caused by different species should be noted. It is important to recognize the diversity in clinical findings and severity of keratitis caused by the same species, as well as the potential similarities in clinical presentation among different species. (**A**) Fusaria

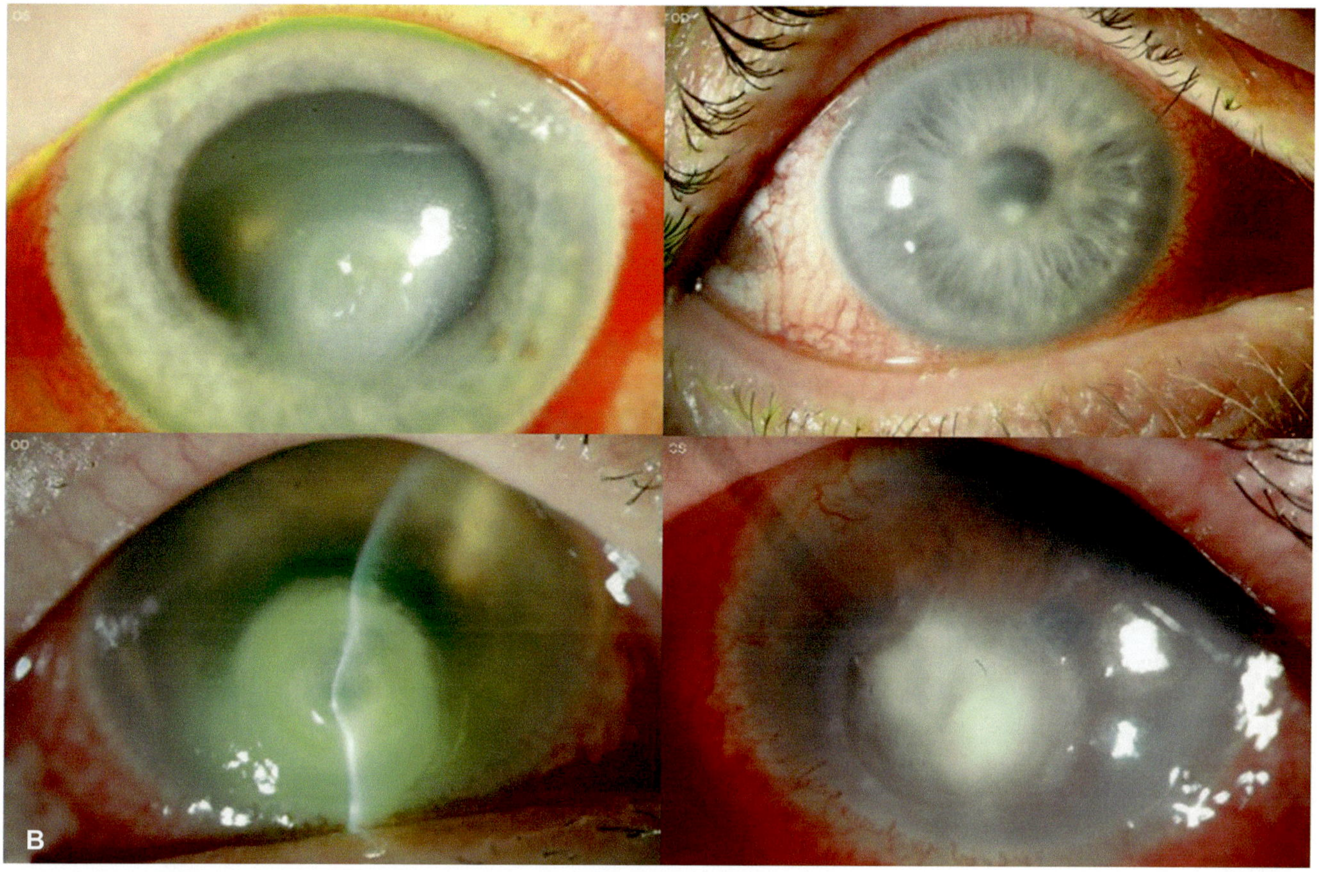

Fig. 2 (**B**) Candida

endothelial plaques, rough greyish surface, raised intact epithelium, as well as irregular marginal area (map-like, fider-like or washed out) [12, 13]. Other symptoms include the pyramid-shaped hypopyon (Behrens-Baumann sign 1) and the prominent stromal infiltration with intact epithelium (Behrens-Baumann sign 2) [14] (Fig. 3).

3 Diagnosis of Mycotic Keratitis

According to the German fungal keratitis register, the accurate diagnosis of mycotic keratitis took an average of 17 days in contact lens users and 12 days in non-contact lens users [1]. This indicates that the diagnosis of mycotic keratitis is still being delayed. By employing a combination of diagnostic methods such as in-vivo confocal microscopy, polymerase chain reaction (PCR), culture growth, and histopathology, it is possible to attain a precise and timely diagnosis (Fig. 4). Depending on the experience of the investigator, confocal microscopy shows the best sensitivity with 94% followed by PCR, in vitro cultivation and histopathological examination. In vivo confocal microscopy can also be used for early diagnosis in cases of recurrent mycotic keratitis [15]. It is strongly recommended that all diagnostic procedures are performed simultaneously in all cases [11, 16]. In case of reduced intraocular visualisation, an ultrasound examination should be performed to exclude intraocular involvement.

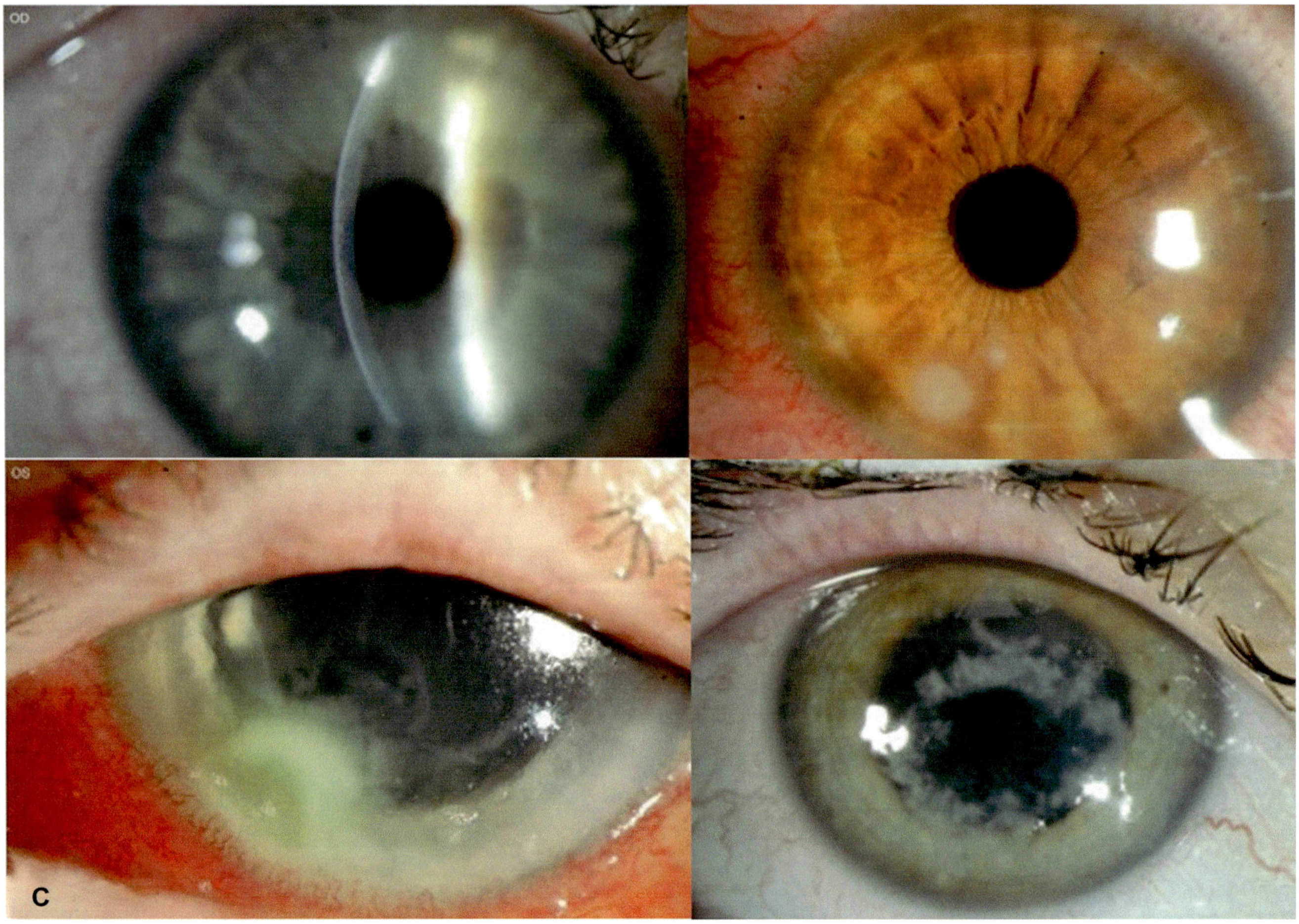

Fig. 2 (**C**) Aspergillus. Co-infections could further obscure the characteristic findings of mycotic keratitis

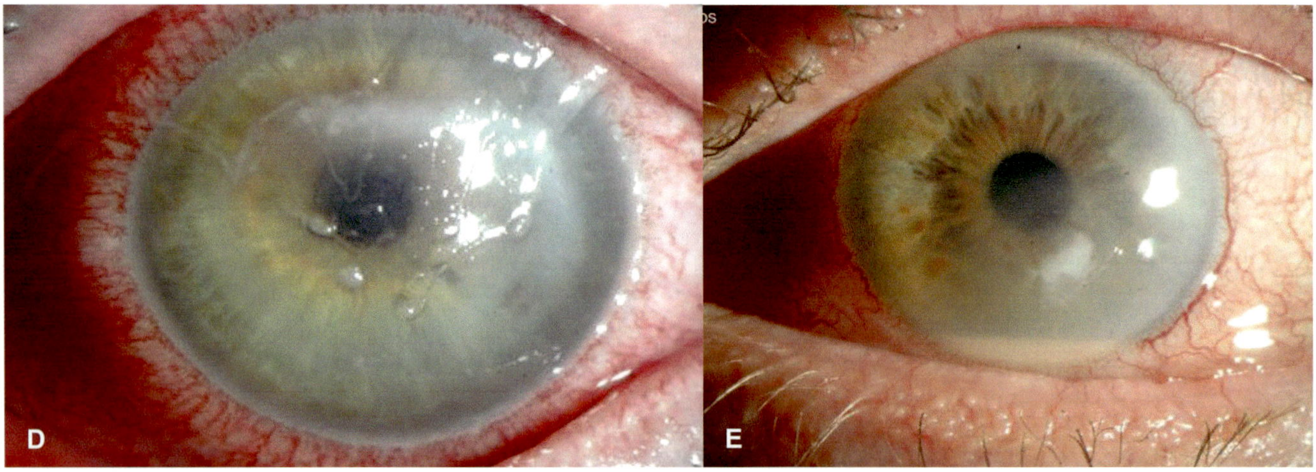

Fig. 2 (**D**) Mycotic keratitis with co-infection of Acanthamoeba. Note the ring infiltrate typical of Acanthamoeba keratitis. (**E**) Mycotic keratitis with co-infection of Staphylococcus aureus. Note the non-pyramidal hypopyon typical of a bacterial infection

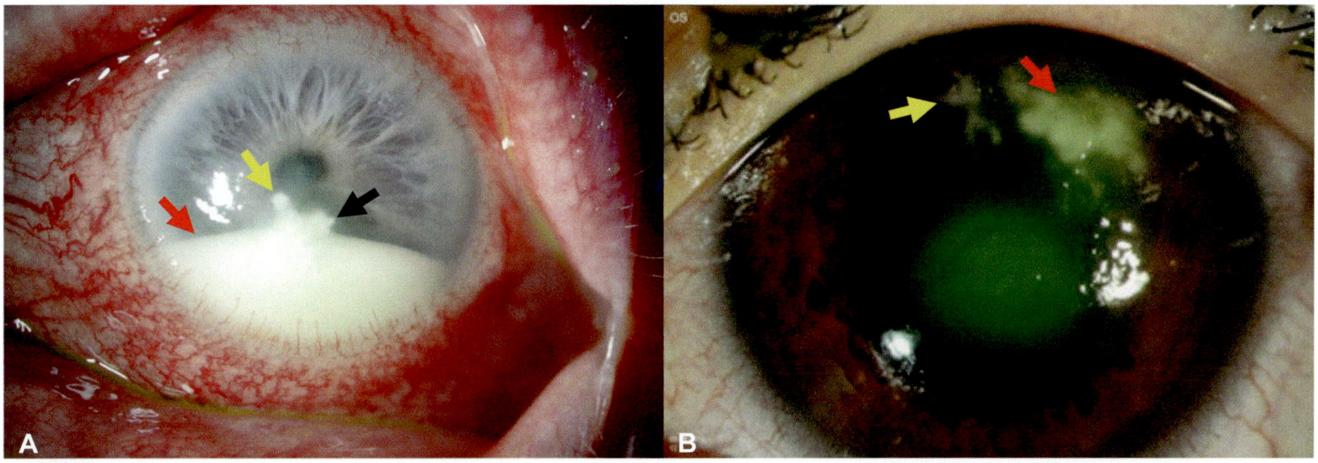

Fig. 3 (**A**) Behrens-Baumann sign 1: Cone- or pyramid-shaped hypopyon (red arrow). Incorporation of leukocytes into the fungal scaffold in the anterior chamber of the eye. Main lesion (black arrow) and satellite lesions (yellow arrow) (**B**) Behrens-Baumann sign 2: Infiltrate under largely intact epithelium. Fungal elements that have passed through corneal epithelium proliferate to such an extent that the cornea appears thickened. Note the geographical prominent infiltration with irregular marginal area (red arrow) as well as the satellite infiltrate (yellow arrow)

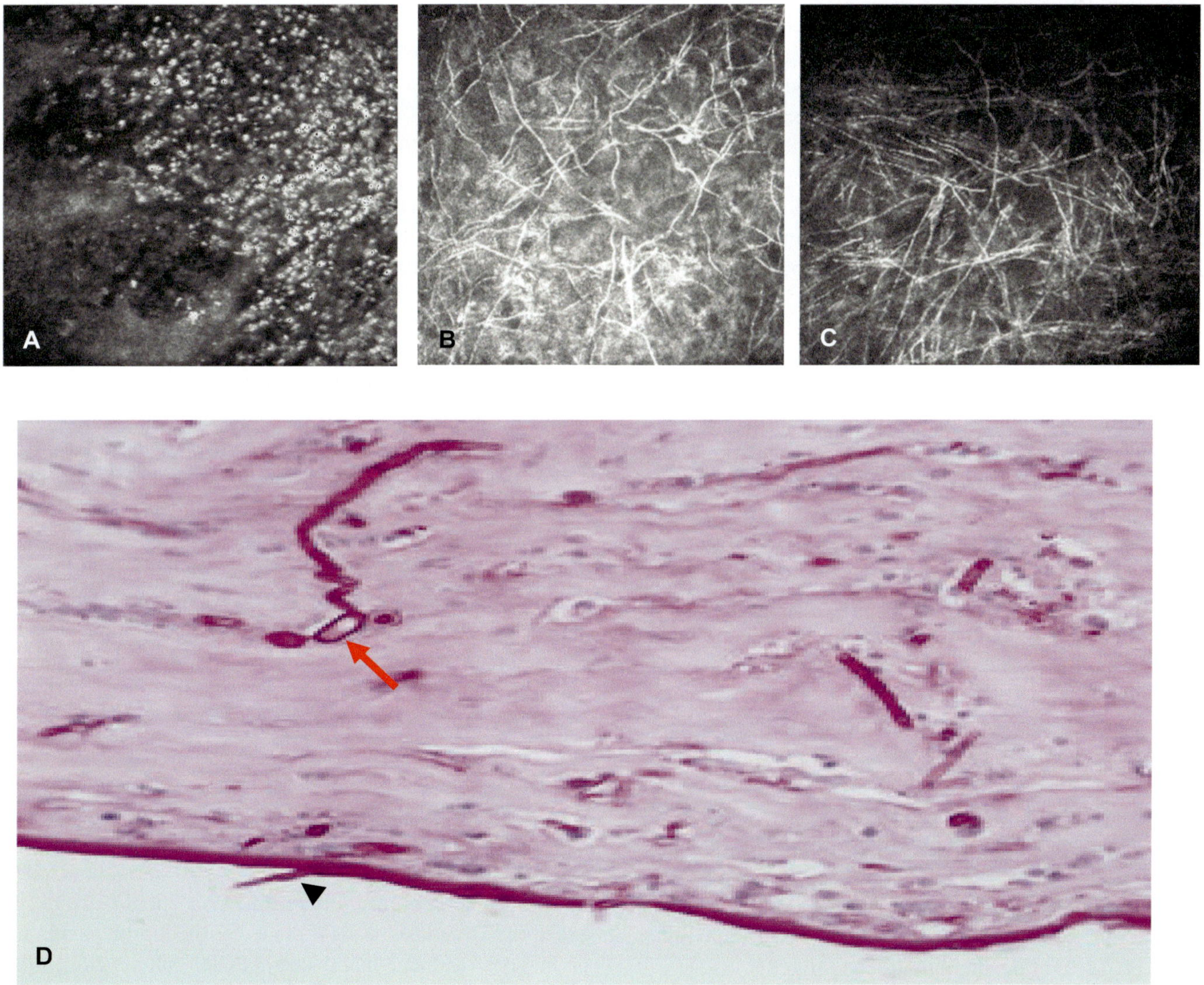

Fig. 4 In-vivo confocal microscopy in mycotic keratitis (**A**) Candida: note the yeasts (**B**) Aspergillus (**C**) Fusaria (**D**) Mycotic hyphae within the posterior corneal stroma (red arrow) with penetration of the Descemet membrane (black arrow)

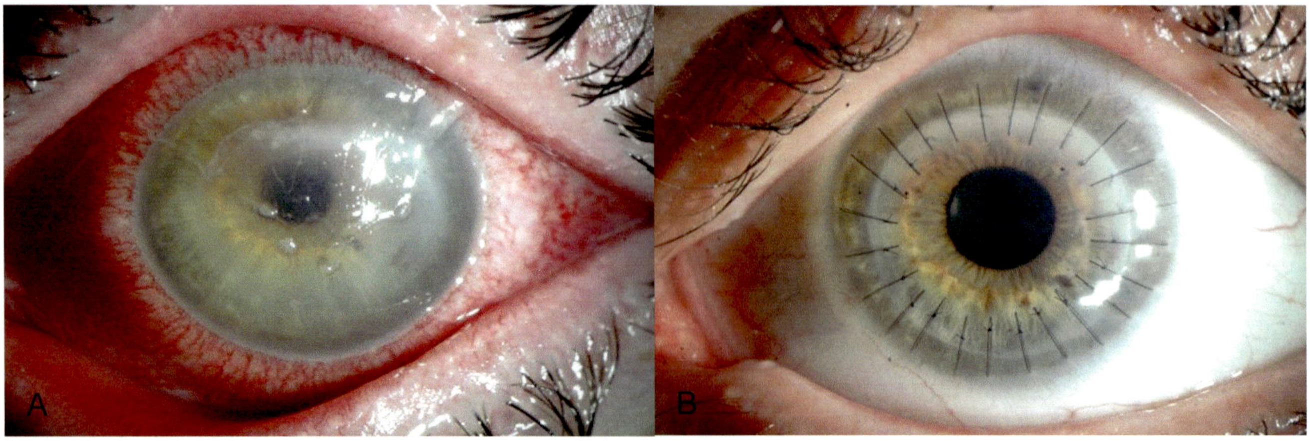

Fig. 5 (**A**) a 30-year-old patient with contact lens-associated mycotic keratitis with co-infection with Acanthamoeba. (**B**) Same eye 6 months after a 8.5/8.6 mm penetrating excimer laser-assisted keratoplasty

4 Conservative Therapy of Mycotic Keratitis

Voriconazole 2% eyedrops is the drug of choice if pathogen is unknown. In case of fusarium and aspergillus, Natamycin 5% eyedrops and systemic therapy with voriconazole should be immediately added [13]. Systemic voriconazole should also be administered as 6 mg/kg i.v. twice in the first 24 h and then 4 mg/kg i.v. twice a day as maintenance dose, or 400 mg twice in the first 24 h and then 300 mg p.o. twice a day as maintenance dose [3, 13]. In the case of candida, amphotericin B 0.5% eyedrops should be added. In persistent candida infections, natamycin 5% eyedrops and systemic voriconazole can also be added [13]. Eyedrops should initially be administered every 30–60 min until the clinical regression of infection is reached. Afterwords, eyedrops should be continued five times daily for 2–3 months and then stopped without tapering. Antimycotic therapy should always be optimized according to the antibiogram results as soon as possible. Terbinafine 0.25% eyedrops and 250 mg p.o. once daily could also be considered in cases with sensitive fungi unresponsive to other antimycotics [17]. Other, less frequently used, antimycotics are summarized in a review by Behrens-Baumann et al. [3]. Considering the substantial molecular weight of Natamycin and Amphotericin B, it is highly advisable to perform corneal abrasion before commencing topical therapy and to repeat it every other day when using these agents.

5 Surgical Therapy of Mycotic Keratitis

The severity of mycotic keratitis is reflected in the high percentage of consequent keratoplasties (29–67%) and enucleations (7–12%) in the literature [2, 11, 16, 18].

We recommend performing a penetrating keratoplasty (PKP) before the anterior chamber gets affected (Fig. 5). Because fungal hyphae can penetrate Descemet membrane (Fig. 4D), we do not recommend performing deep anterior lamellar keratoplasty (DALK).

The first step is washing the anterior chamber with antimycotic drugs and removing all membranes from the chamber angle via irrigation/aspiration. The next step is performing a PKP with a large diameter to achieve a safety distance and minimize the recurrence risk [19]. A circular intrastromal voriconazole injection with a 30-gauge needle at the excision site of the host stroma after completion of suture placement may also be performed to increase the safety of the procedure in terms of preventing recurrence of infection [20–23]. Repeated intracameral injection of voriconazole, e.g. every two days, also helps reducing the recurrence rate. Surgery should always be performed with a preparedness to perform a pars plana vitrectomy in case of intravitreal involvement.

Postoperatively, repeated anterior chamber lavage with irrigation/aspiration and intracameral injection of antimycotic agents should be performed every two days. Topical antimycotics should be applied at least for 2 months. The initiation of topical steroids should be delayed for a minimum of 7–10 days after penetrating keratoplasty (PKP), commencing with a low dosage [24]. More details about microsurgical treatment of fungal keratitis can be reviewed from our recent open access overview [25].

6 Conclusion

Mycotic keratitis shows atypical and variable corneal findings. The presence of co-infection should always be expected. Diagnosis is best made by the simultaneous use of in vivo confocal microscopy, PCR, culture cultivation, and histopathology. In cases of unknown pathogens, voriconazole 2% eyedrops should be empirically used. In case of fusaria, natamycin 5% eyedrops should also be added. A surgical therapy using a PKP with a large diameter as well as circular, intrastromal injection of voriconazole into the host cornea and preparedness for pars plana vitrectomy should be performed before involvement of the anterior chamber. Postoperatively, repeated anterior chamber lavage with irrigation/aspiration and intracameral injection of antimycotic agents should be performed every two days. Topical antimycotics should be applied at least for 2 months and not be tapered. Topical steroids are to be first applied at least 7–10 days after PKP starting with a low dose. Early diagnosis, therapy and surgical intervention (within days to few weeks) are essential for a good visual prognosis and to avoid enucleation.

References

1. Roth M, Holtmann C, Daas L, Kakkassery V, Kurzai O, Geerling G, and German Fungal Keratitis Registry Study Group. Results from the German fungal keratitis registry: significant differences between cases with and without a history of contact lens use. Cornea. 2021 Nov 1;40(11):1453–61.
2. Nielsen SE, Nielsen E, Julian HO, Lindegaard J, Højgaard K, Ivarsen A, et al. Incidence and clinical characteristics of fungal keratitis in a Danish population from 2000 to 2013. Acta Ophthalmol. 2015;93(1):54–8.
3. Behrens-Baumann W, Finis D, Mackenzie C, Roth M, Geerling G. Keratomycosis–therapy standards and new developments. Klin Monbl Augenheilkd. 2015;232(6):754–64.
4. Brown L, Leck AK, Gichangi M, Burton MJ, Denning DW. The global incidence and diagnosis of fungal keratitis. Lancet Infect Dis. 2021;21(3):49–57.
5. Gopinathan U, Sharma S, Garg P, Rao G. Review of epidemiological features, microbiological diagnosis and treatment outcome of microbial keratitis: experience of over a decade. Indian J Ophthalmol. 2009;57(4):273–9.
6. Khor WB, Aung T, Saw SM, Wong TY, Tambyah PA, Tan AL, et al. An outbreak of Fusarium keratitis associated with contact lens wear in Singapore. JAMA. 2006;295(24):2867–73.
7. Morgan PB, Efron N. A decade of contact lens prescribing trends in the United Kingdom (1996–2005). Cont Lens Anterior Eye. 2006;29(2):59–68.
8. Gaujoux T, Chatel MA, Chaumeil C, Laroche L, Borderie VM. Outbreak of contact lens-related Fusarium keratitis in France. Cornea. 2008;27(9):1018–21.
9. Chang DC, Grant GB, O'Donnell K, Wannemuehler KA, Noble-Wang J, Rao CY, et al. Multistate outbreak of Fusarium keratitis associated with use of a contact lens solution. JAMA. 2006;296(8):953–63.
10. Alfaro Rangel R, Szentmáry N, Lepper S, Milioti G, Daas L, Langenbucher A, et al. Large-diameter penetrating keratoplasties are mostly due to very severe infectious keratitis and cannot always prevent secondary enucleation. Klin Monbl Augenheilkd. 2022;239(11):1361–8.
11. Sourlis C, Seitz B, Roth M, Hamon L, Daas L. Outcomes of severe fungal keratitis using in vivo confocal microscopy and early therapeutic penetrating keratoplasty. Clin Ophthalmol. 2022;16:2245–54.
12. Thomas PA, Kaliamurthy J. Mycotic keratitis: epidemiology, diagnosis and management. Clin Microbiol Infect. 2013;19(3):210–20.
13. Roth M, Steindor F, Kurzai O, Behrens-Baumann W, Mackenzie CR, Geerling G. Mycotic keratitis: clinical signs, diagnosis, therapy. Augenheilkunde up2date. 2020;10:8–16.
14. Behrens-Baumann W. Keratomycosis: diagnosis and therapy. Ophthalmologe. 2009;106(5):471–80.
15. Daas L, Bischoff-Jung M, Viestenz A, Seitz B, Viestenz A. Confocal microscopy as an early relapse marker after keratoplasty due to Fusarium solani keratitis. Ophthalmologe. 2017;114(1):66–9.
16. Roth M, Daas L, Renner-Wilde A, Cvetkova-Fischer N, Saeger M, Herwig-Carl M, et al. The German keratomycosis registry: Initial results of a multicenter survey. Ophthalmologe. 2019;116(10):957–66.
17. Tayel SA, El-Nabarawi MA, Tadros MI, Abd-Elsalam WH. Positively charged polymeric nanoparticle reservoirs of terbinafine hydrochloride: preclinical implications for controlled drug delivery in the aqueous humor of rabbits. AAPS PharmSciTech. 2013;14(2):782–93.
18. Tuft SJ, Tullo AB. Fungal keratitis in the United Kingdom 2003–2005. Eye (Lond). 2009;23(6):1308–13.
19. Berger T, Seitz B, Flockerzi F, Daas L. Recurrent filamentous fungal keratitis caused when the primarily selected graft diameter was too small. Klin Monbl Augenheilkd. 2022.
20. Kalaiselvi G, Narayana S, Krishnan T, Sengupta S. Intrastromal voriconazole for deep recalcitrant fungal keratitis: a case series. Br J Ophthalmol. 2015;99(2):195–8.
21. Nejabat M, Yaqubi N, Khosravi A, Zomorodian K, Ashraf MJ, Salouti R. Therapeutic effect of intrastromal voriconazole, topical voriconazole, and topical natamycin on fusarium keratitis in rabbit. J Ophthalmol. 2016.
22. Prakash G, Sharma N, Goel M, Titiyal JS, Vajpayee RB. Evaluation of intrastromal injection of voriconazole as a therapeutic adjunctive for the management of deep recalcitrant fungal keratitis. Am J Ophthalmol. 2008;146(1).
23. Sharma N, Agarwal P, Sinha R, Titiyal JS, Velpandian T, Vajpayee RB. Evaluation of intrastromal voriconazole injection in recalcitrant deep fungal keratitis: case series. Br J Ophthalmol. 2011;95(12):1735–7.
24. Wang T, Li S, Gao H, Shi W. Therapeutic dilemma in fungal keratitis: administration of steroids for immune rejection early after keratoplasty. Graefes Arch Clin Exp Ophthalmol. 2016;254(8):1585–9.
25. Seitz B, Abu Dail Y, Berger T, Suffo S, Flockerzi E, Flockerzi F, Daas L. Fungal keratitis in Germany: Diagnostics, conservative and microsurgical treatment. Ophthalmologie. 2025;122:652–69.

Autoimmune Keratitis

Elisabeth M. Messmer

Abstract

Autoimmune keratitis may occur idiopathic, postinfectious, or postoperatively. It may present as an ocular disease only or may manifest as part of a general disease such as allergy as well as potentially lethal collagen vascular disease or franc vasculitis. Correct diagnosis and management are of utmost importance to prevent sequelae, preserve vision, and may be lifesaving for the patient.

Keywords

Peripheral ulcerative keratitis · Cogan syndrome · Diffuse lamellar keratitis · Vernal keratoconjunctivitis · Thygeson's keratitis · Superior limbic keratoconjunctivitis

1 Staphylococcal Peripheral Corneal Infiltrates

Small, round to oval subepithelial peripheral corneal infiltrates are the hallmark of staphylococcal associated peripheral keratitis indicating an immune reaction to staphylococcal antigen (Fig. 1). They are typically localized in the corneal periphery with predilection at 10–11, 1–2, 4–5 and 7–8 clock hours. These infiltrates typically leave a small **clear margin** to the limbus and are accompanied by a triangular-shaped conjunctival hyperemia (Fig. 2). They are often associated and caused by blepharitis/meibomitis/meibomian gland dysfunction (MGD). Formerly, this disease has been referred to as "infect-allergic marginal keratitis".

E. M. Messmer (✉)
Department of Ophthalmology, LMU University Hospital, LMU Munich, Mathildenstrasse 8, Munich 80336, Germany
e-mail: emessmer@med.uni-muenchen.de

B. Seitz et al. (eds.), *Atlas on Cornea*, https://doi.org/10.1007/978-3-031-65422-0_26

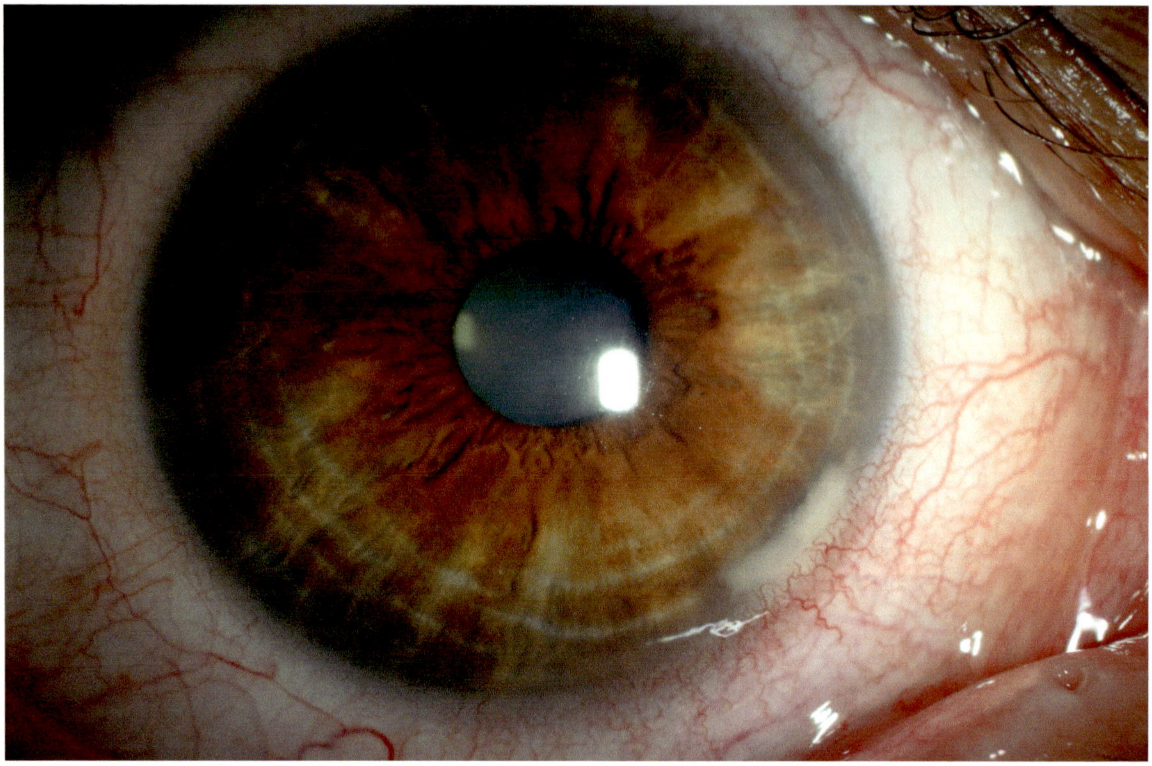

Fig. 1 Staphylococcal peripheral corneal infiltrate

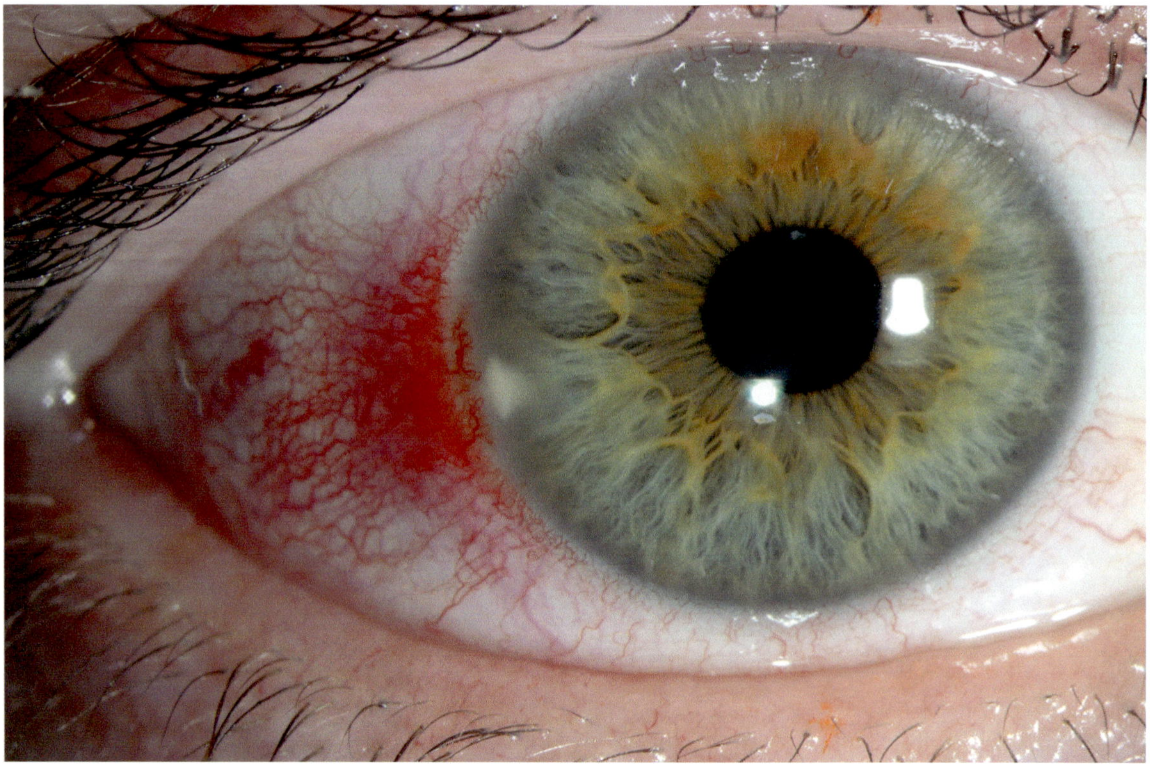

Fig. 2 Staphylococcal peripheral corneal infiltrate with triangular shaped conjunctival hyperemia

2 Corneal Phlyctenule

Phlyctenular keratoconjunctivitis is a nonspecific autoimmune response (allergic hypersensitivity reaction to an endogenous toxin) in the cornea (Fig. 3) and/or conjunctiva to a variety of distinct conditions. In developed countries it is mostly due to staphylococcal infection. Worm infections and tuberculosis must be considered in developing countries.

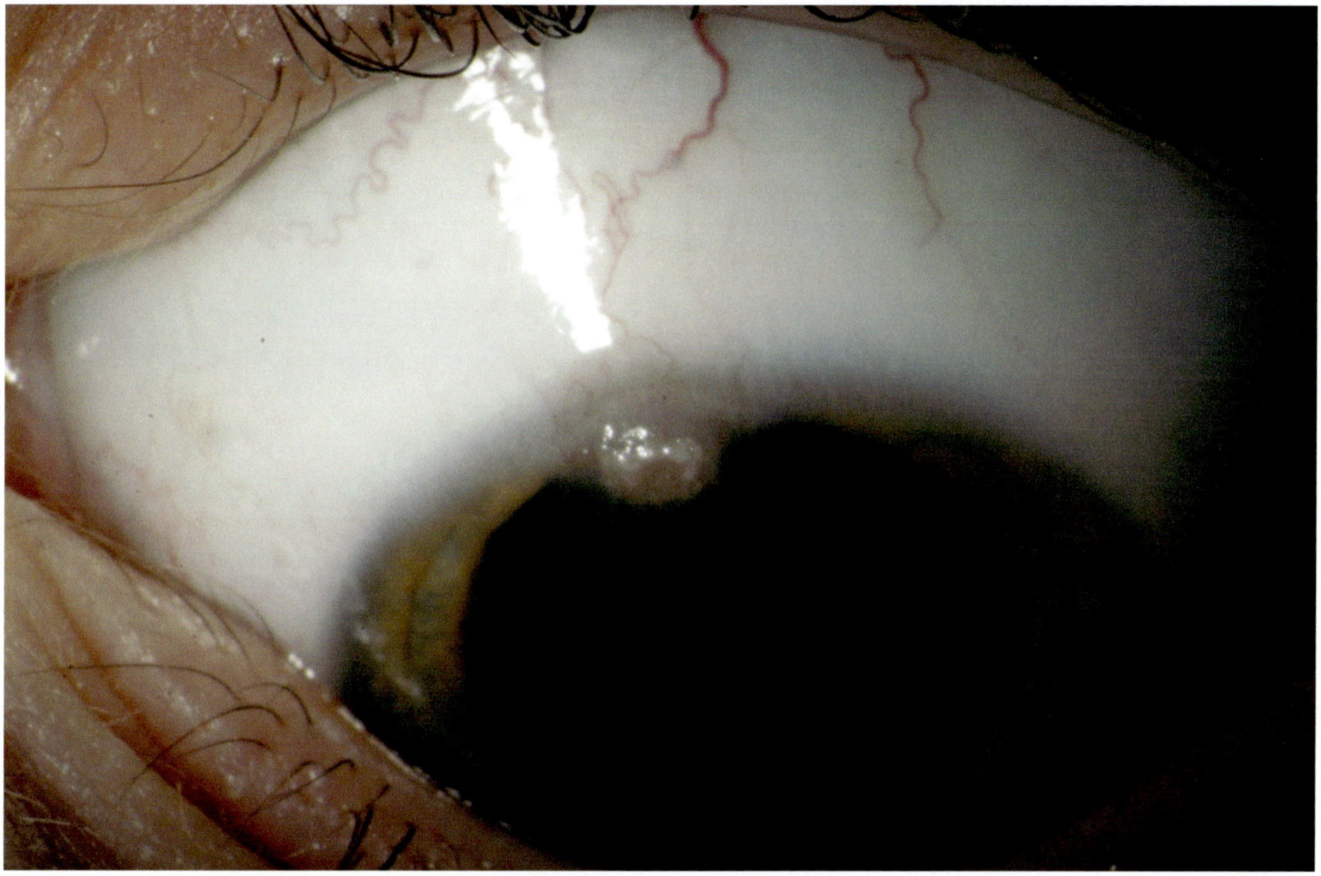

Fig. 3 Corneal phlyctenule in a child with meibomian gland dysfunction most probably due to staphylococcal infection

3 Peripheral Ulcerative Keratitis (PUK)

Peripheral ulcerative keratitis (PUK) is defined as a crescent-shaped stromal inflammation of the juxtalimbal cornea with epithelial defect and progressive stromal ulceration. PUK can be bacterial, viral, mycotic and/or caused by acanthamoeba. Most frequently it is, however, the (primary) manifestation of collagen vascular disease and/or systemic vasculitis.

3.1 PUK Associated with Collagen Vascular Disease and Systemic Vasculitis

PUK can develop in the course of rheumatoid arthritis (Figs. 4 and 5A, B, C), psoriasis arthritis (Fig. 6), granulomatosis with polyangiitis, recurrent polychondritis, systemic lupus erythematodes (Fig. 7), classic polyarteriitis nodosa, microscopic polyangiitis, and Churg-Strauss syndrome. The sclera is typically involved and may develop necrotizing scleritis. Untreated, the systemic condition may be lethal. Therefore, immediate diagnosis and treatment of the ocular condition may be lifesaving.

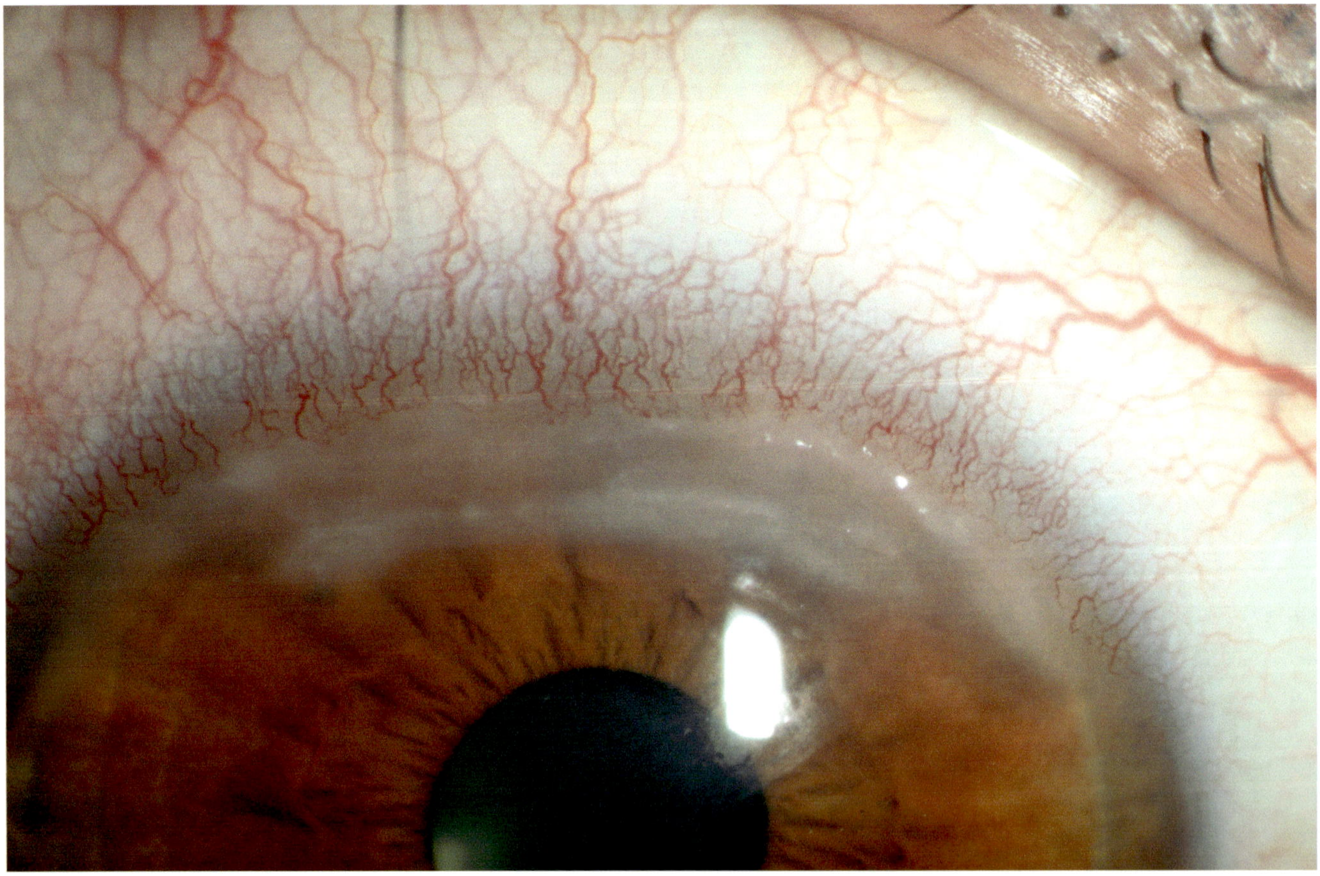

Fig. 4 Peripheral ulcerative keratitis associated with rheumatoid arthritis

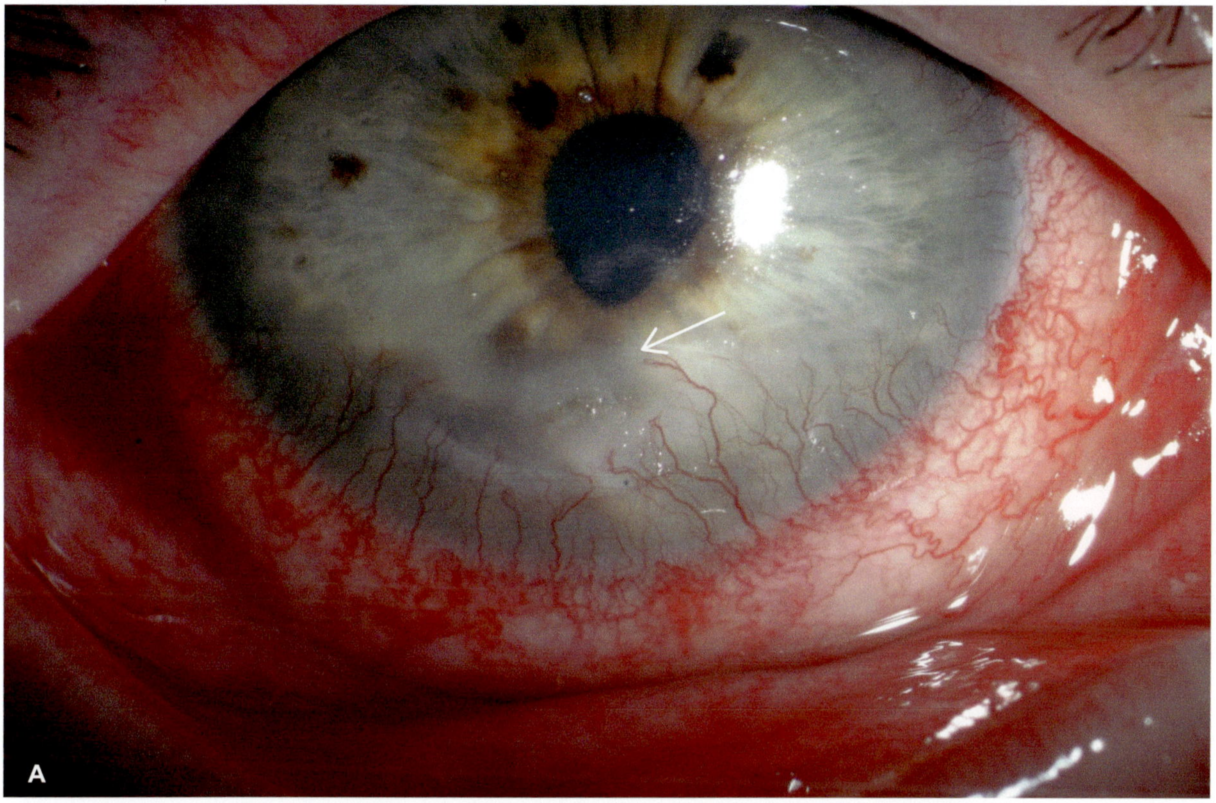

Fig. 5A Peripheral ulcerative keratitis with small corneal perforation (arrow) associated with rheumatoid arthritis.

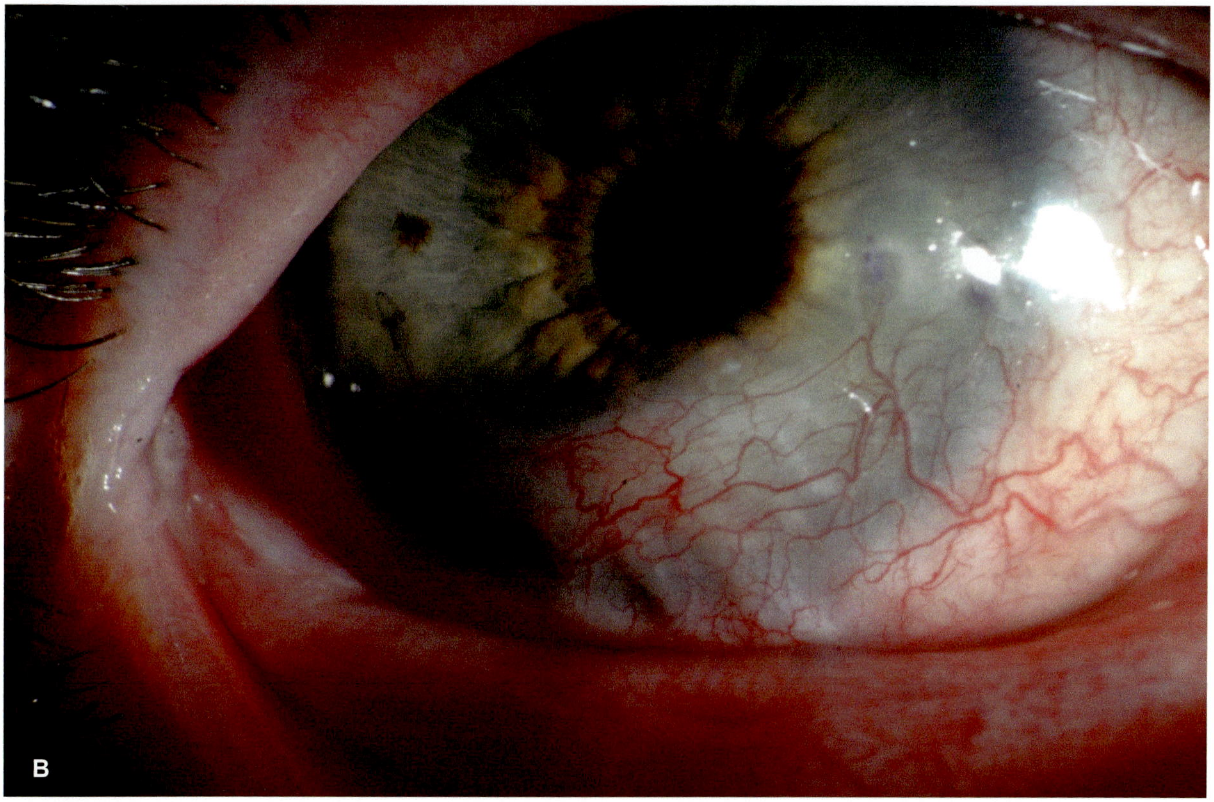

Fig. 5B Peripheral ulcerative keratitis after conjunctival flap surgery performed under immunosuppressive treatment with oral corticosteroids and methotrexate

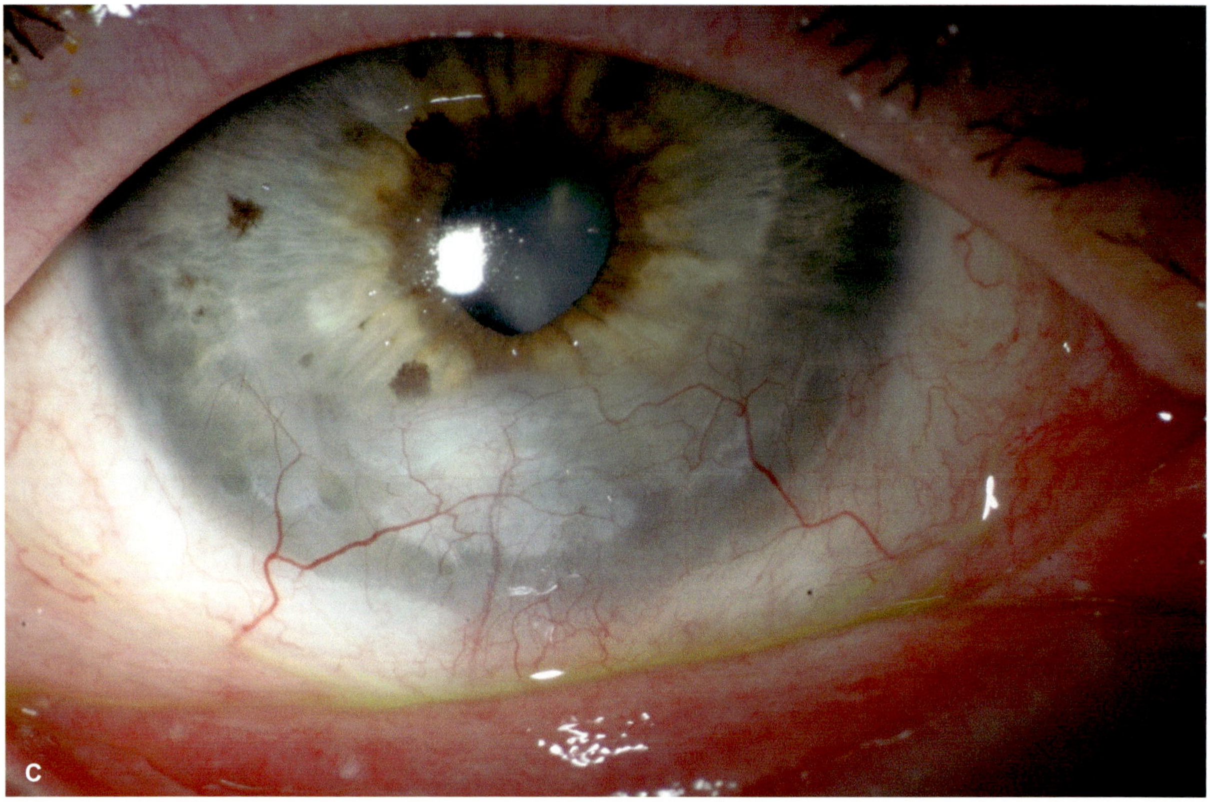

Fig. 5C 1 year following conjunctival flap surgery with satisfying visual acuity

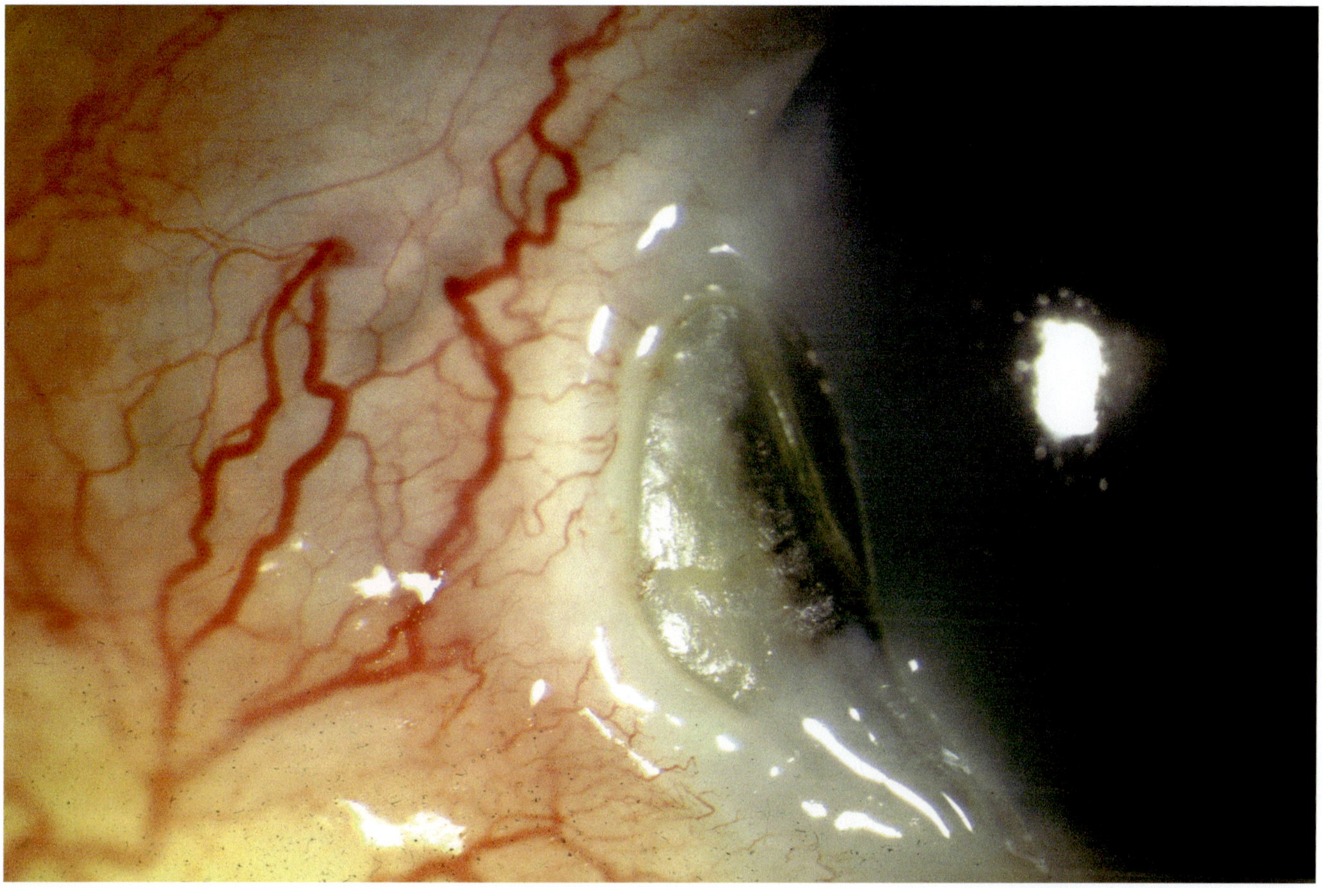

Fig. 6 Peripheral ulcerative keratitis associated with psoriasis arthritis

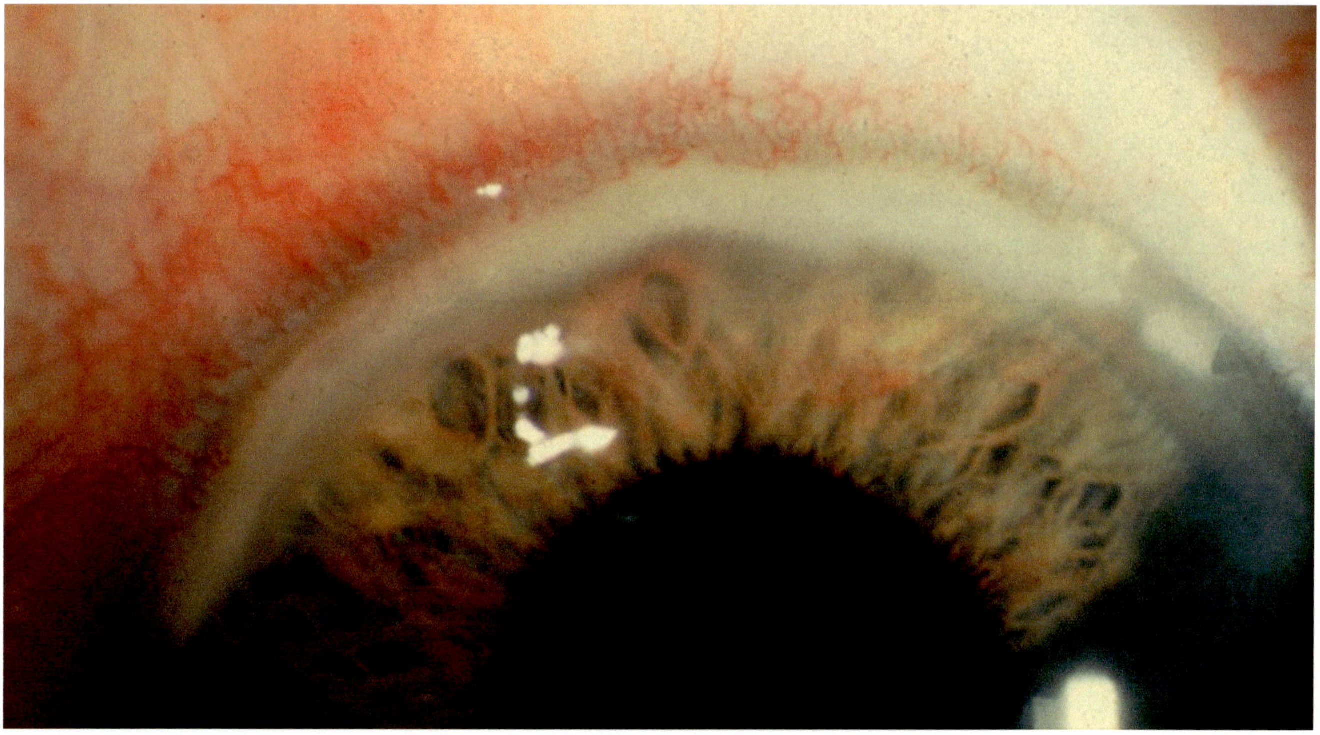

Fig. 7 Peripheral ulcerative keratitis associated with systemic lupus erythematodes

4 Mooren Ulcer

The pathogenesis of Mooren ulcer is not completely understood. Associations with worm infections, chronic hepatitis C, herpes simplex virus and varicella zoster virus infections, syphilis and tuberculosis have been described. It may occur after ocular trauma and eye surgery. Mooren's ulcer is a diagnosis of exclusion. Small peripheral stromal infiltrates develop rapidly epithelial defects and ulcerations that—in contrast to staphylococcal infiltrates—reach the limbus. The ulcerations typically progress circumferentially and from the limbus to the center (Fig. 8). A typical finding is an abrupt transition from involved to non-involved cornea with an **overhanging edge** of the ulcer (Fig. 9). Scleral involvement is rare in contrast to PUK associated with collagen vascular disease and systemic vasculitis.

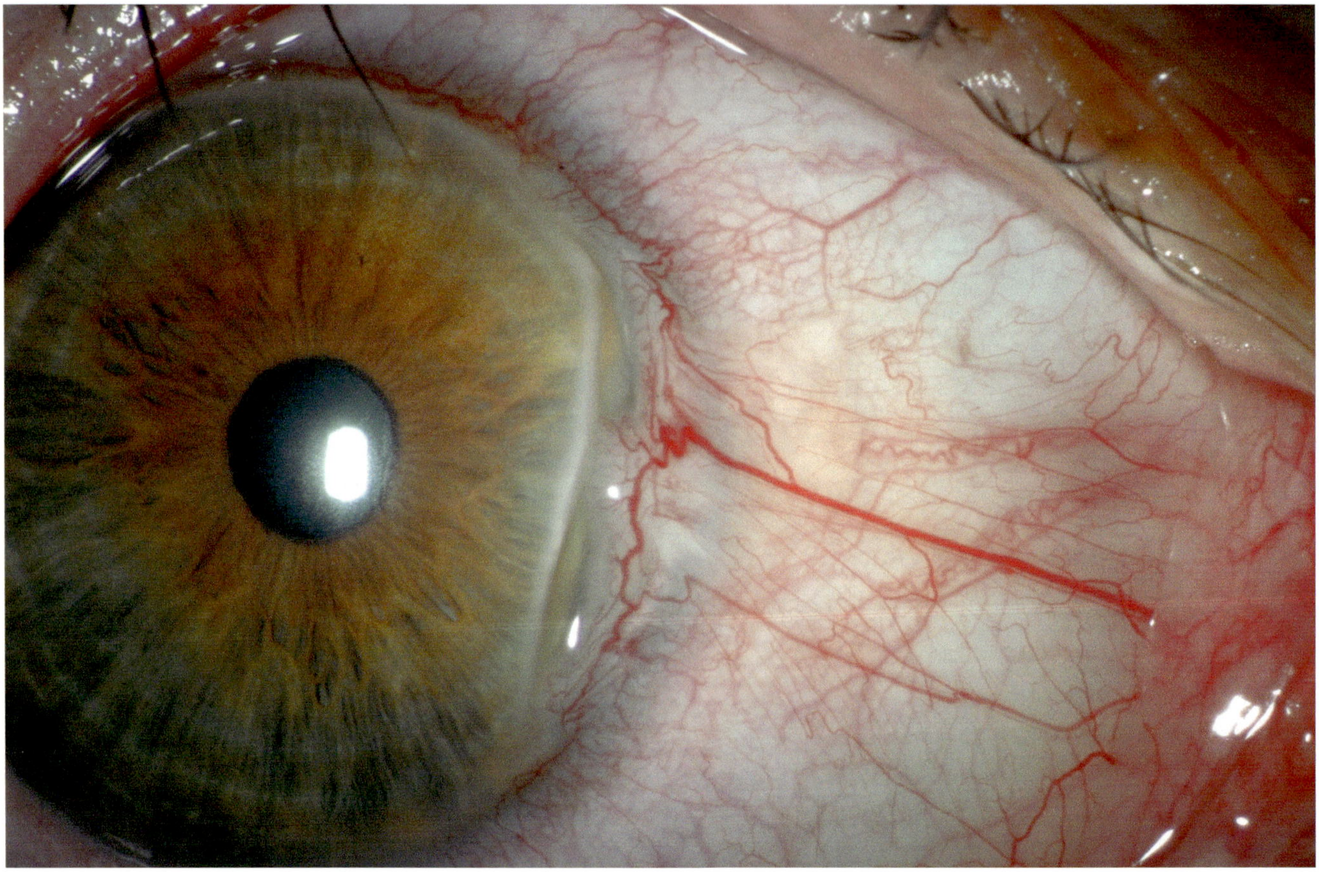

Fig. 8 Mooren ulcer with circumferential ulceration including the limbus. No scleral involvement

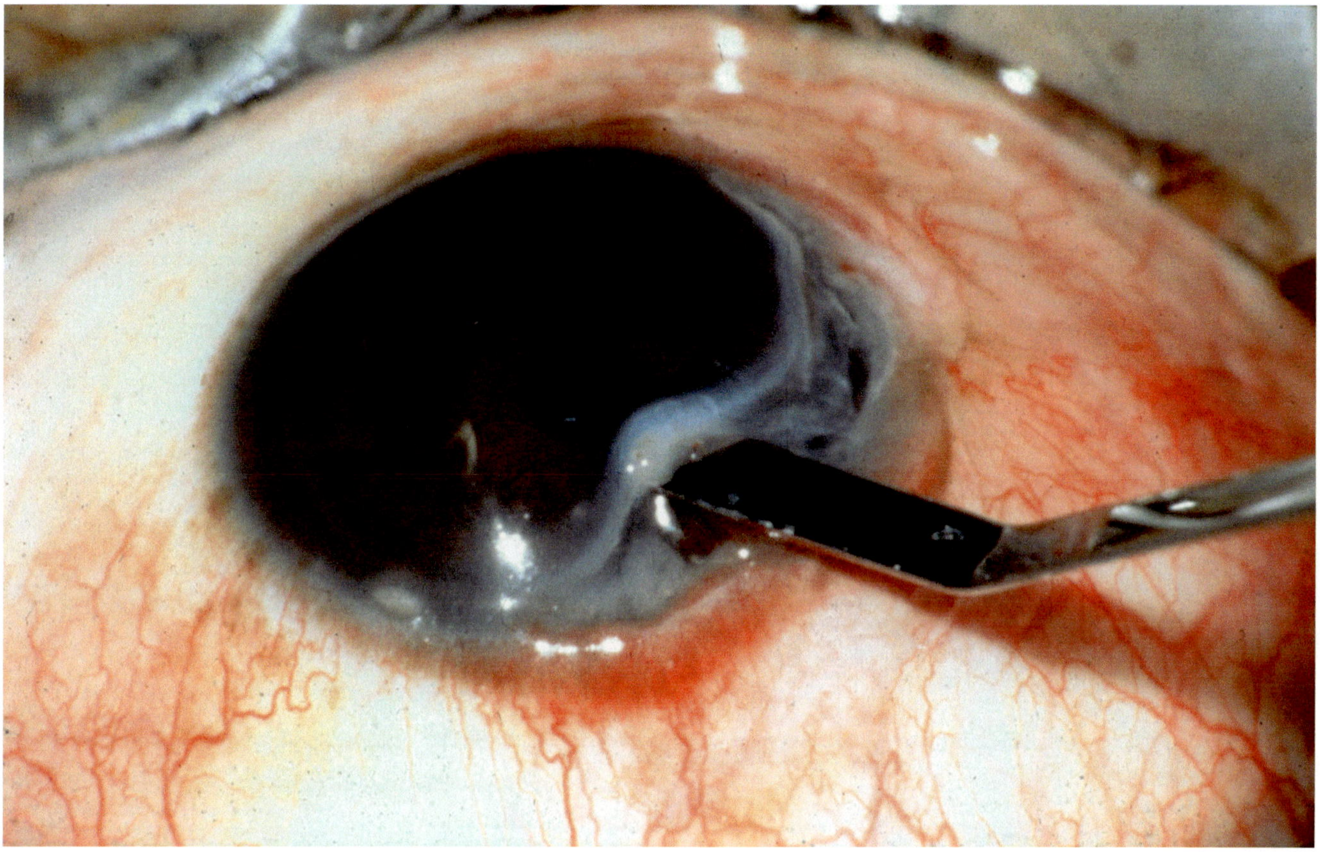

Fig. 9 Undermining edge of Mooren ulcer

5 Interstitial keratitis (Cogan Syndrome)

Cogan syndrome is an autoimmune disease characterized by inflammation of the inner ears and the eyes, presenting with vestibulo-auditory dysfunction and interstitial keratitis. It may be associated with life-threatening systemic vasculitis in 10% of cases. It typically affects young adults. Humoral and cellular immune responses to a common antigen in cornea and inner ear are suggested pathomechanisms. It acutely manifests with diffuse or sectoral subepithelial infiltrates and progresses to classical interstitial keratitis (Fig. 10 and 11). (Epi-) scleritis and panuveitis may complicate the disease. It usually responds to steroid treatment and immunomodulatory therapy but may end up in vascularized corneal scarring with irregular astigmatism.

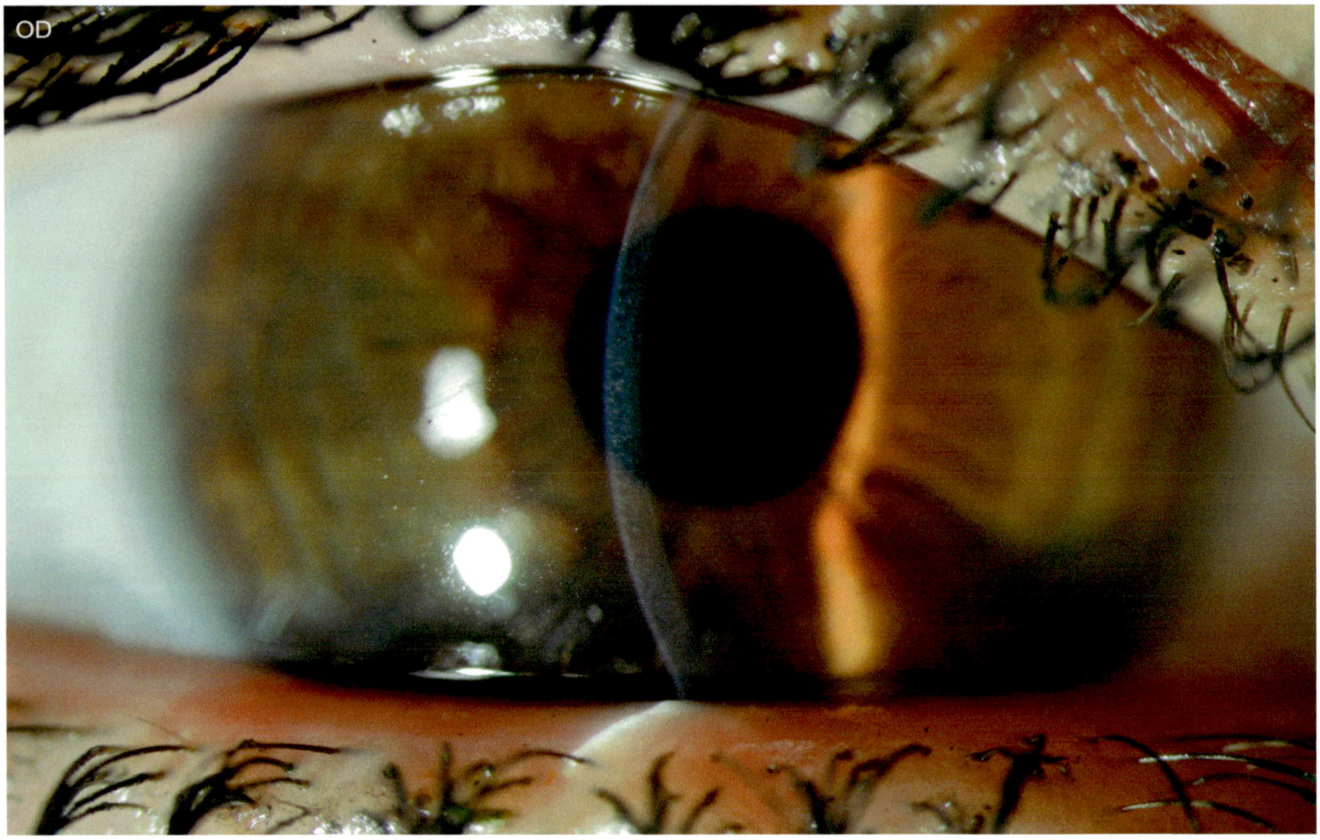

Fig. 10 Interstitial keratitis with multiple fine diffuse infiltrates subepithelially and in the mid-corneal stroma (right eye). Courtesy of: Springer

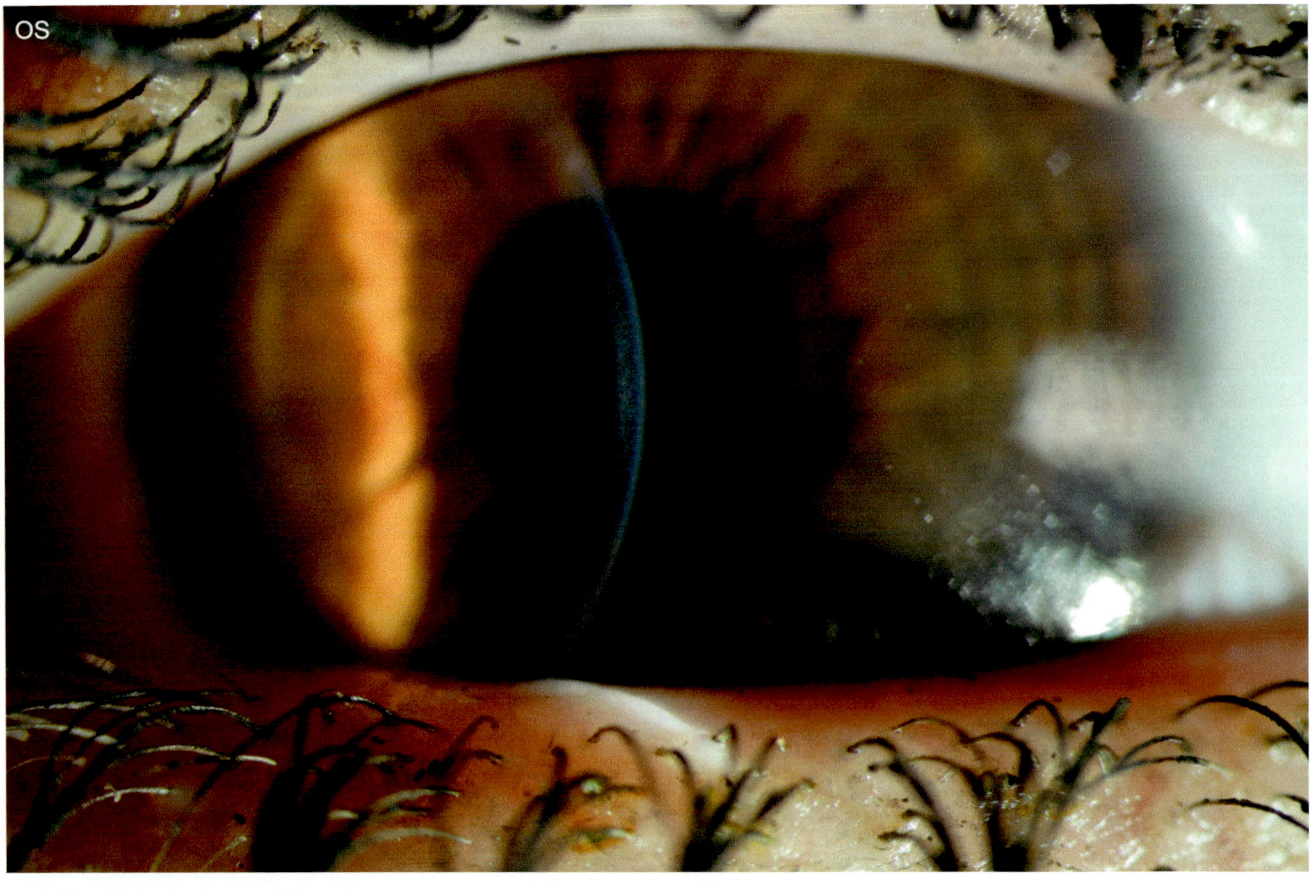

Fig. 11 Interstitial keratitis with fine infiltrates in the mid-corneal stroma in otherwise inconspicuous and non-irritant findings (left eye). Courtesy of: Springer

6 Diffuse Lamellar Keratitis Following LASIK

The most frequent non-infectious corneal complication after LASIK is a diffuse lamellar keratitis (DLK or SOS (sands of sahara)), an inflammatory reaction along the stromal interface (Fig. 12). Microkeratome oil, metallic debris of the microkeratome, meibomian secretions and bacterial endotoxins are discussed as pathogenetic factors. Risk factor for the development of DLK is a postoperative epithelial defect. Severe DLK with central involvement can lead to stomal melt and induction of irregular astigmatism caused by large striae due to localized tissue loss.

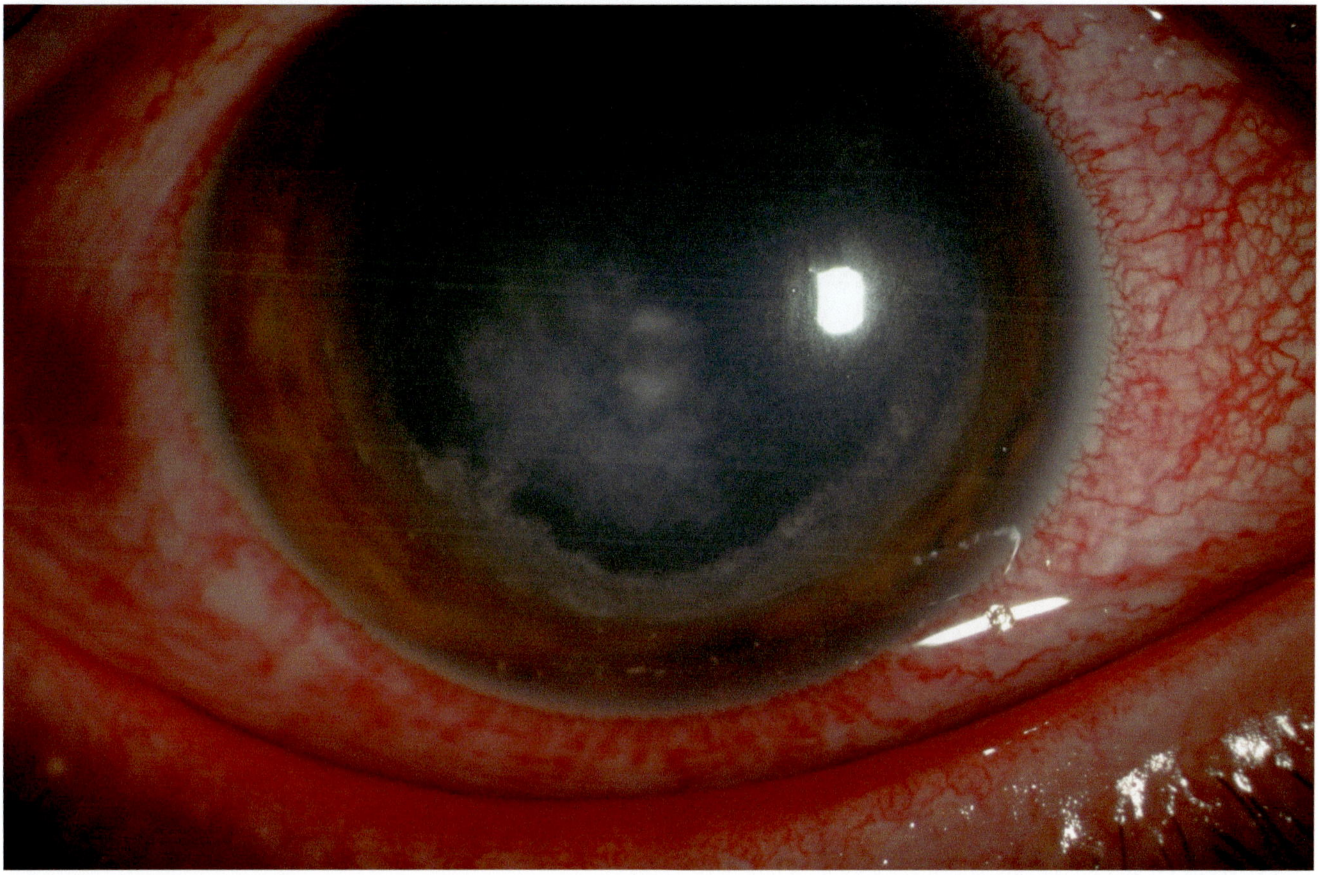

Fig. 12 Diffuse lamellar keratitis following LASIK

7 Vernal Keratoconjunctivitis (VKC)

Vernal keratoconjunctivitis is characterized by tarsal (giant) papillae and/or limbal papillae/gelatinous limbal infiltrates (Figs. 13 and 14). Corneal shield ulcers and plaques are rare complications of VKC (Fig. 15). They are maintained by the mechanical action of conjunctival papillae and toxic mediators released by eosinophils and mast cells. Major basic protein and eosinophil cationic protein accumulate in the ulcer and thus disturb epithelial migration and healing of the shield ulceration.

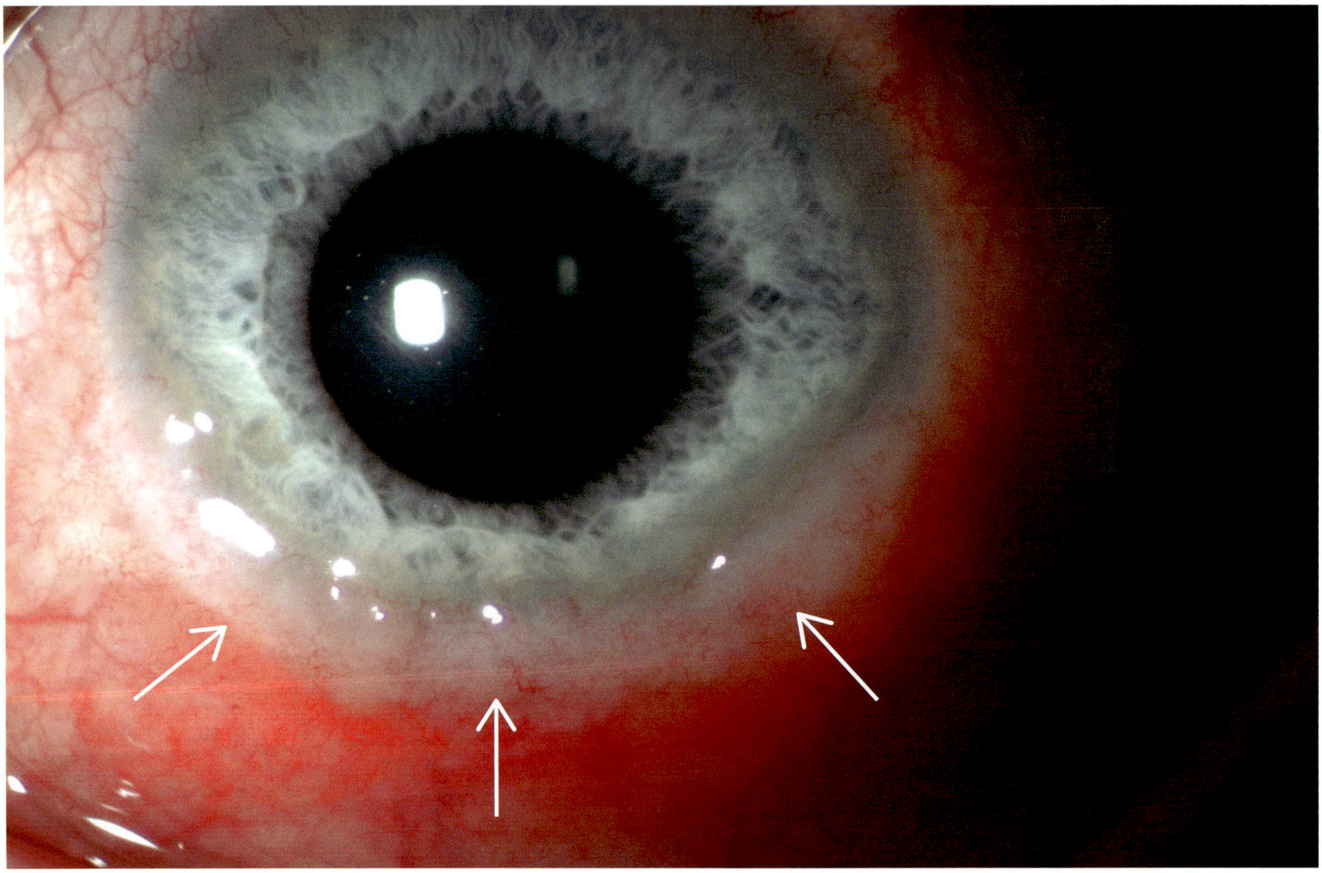

Fig. 13 Vernal keratoconjunctivitis with limbal gelatinous infiltrates (arrows)

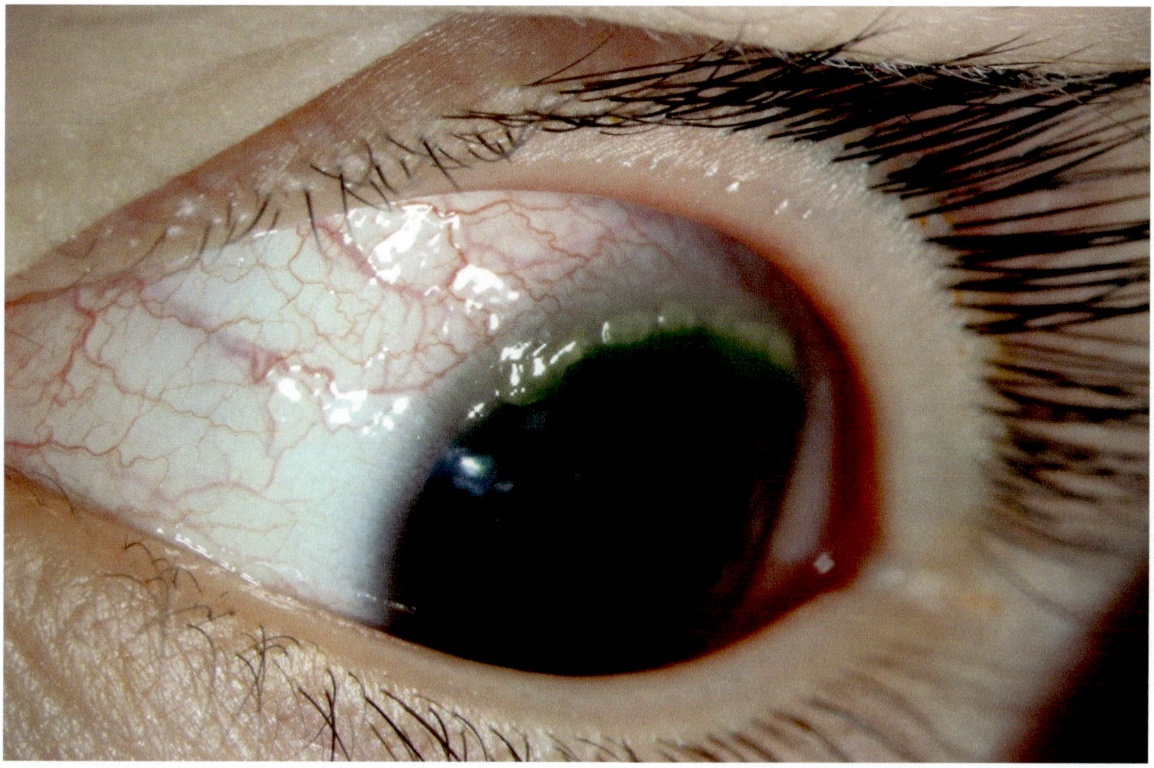

Fig. 14 Vernal keratoconjunctivitis with limbal papillae

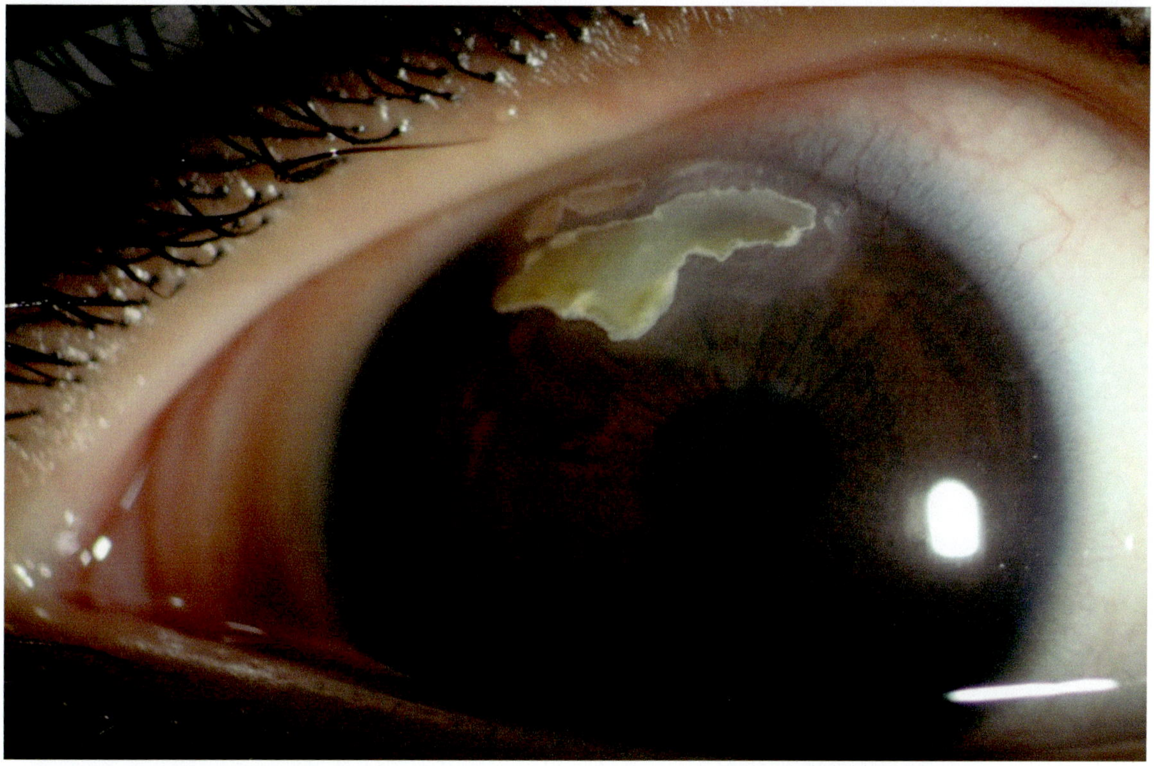

Fig. 15 Vernal keratoconjunctivitis with Shield ulceration

8 Thygeson Keratitis

Thygeson superficial punctate keratitis is a chronic and recurrent corneal epitheliopathy mainly of children and young adults characterized by small, elevated, round (sometimes star-shaped), white–gray intraepithelial lesions (Fig. 16) that typically present bilaterally and stain with fluorescein (Fig. 17). Pathogenetic mechanisms proposed include viral infection, autoimmune-mediated, and immune response to viral infection.

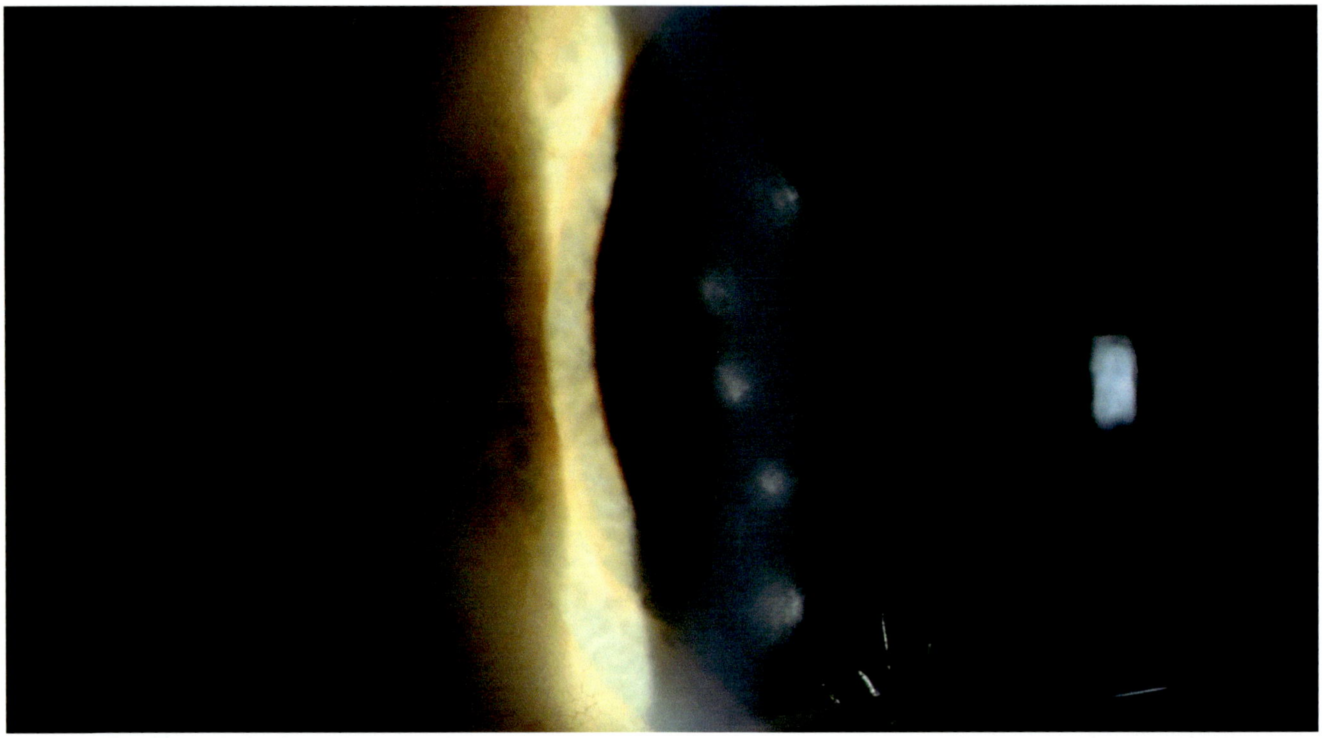

Fig. 16 Thygeson keratitis

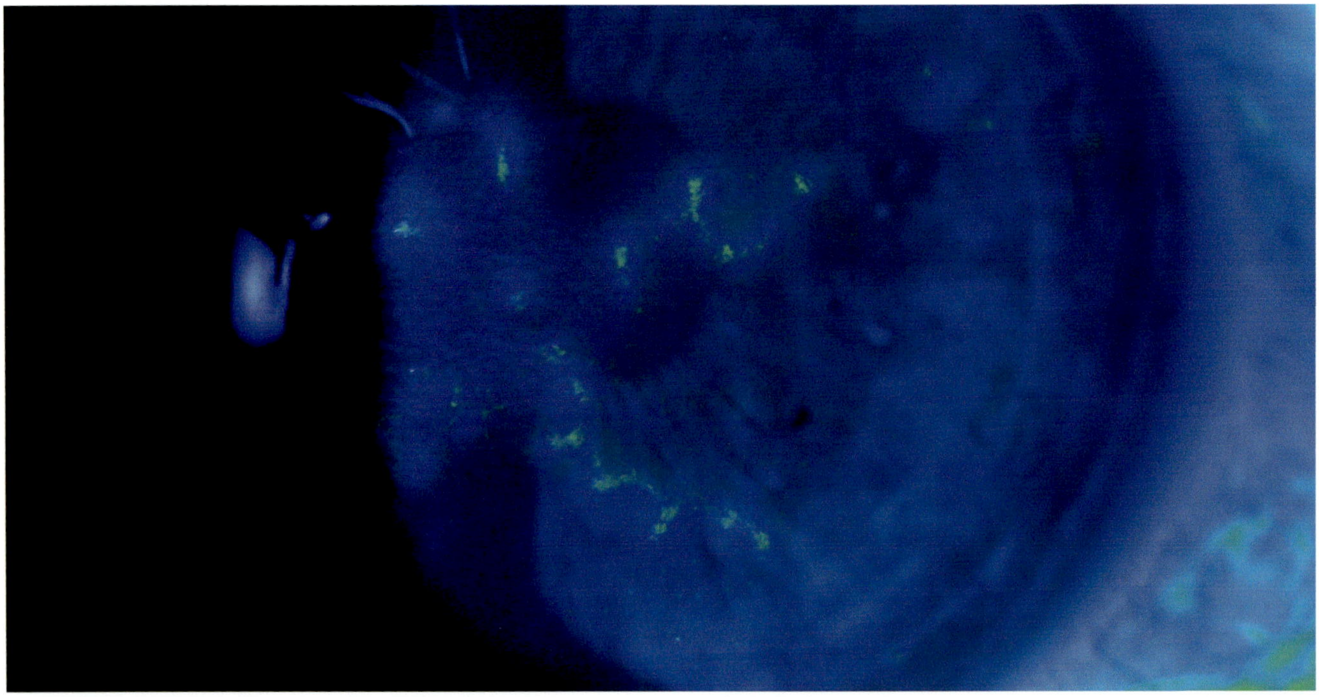

Fig. 17 Thygeson keratitis. Epithelial lesions stain with fluorescein

9 Epidemic Keratoconjunctivitis

Epidemic keratoconjunctivitis (EKC) is a highly contagious adenoviral infection (serotypes 8 and 19). It occurs mostly bilateral with the second eye following 3–7 days later. Superficial punctate keratopathy may develop during the acute phase of disease. Pseudomembranes may develop acutely resulting in symblepharon formation. Visual impairment can persist for months because of autoimmune subepithelial nummular corneal infiltrates (Figs. 18 and 19) and irregular astigmatism.

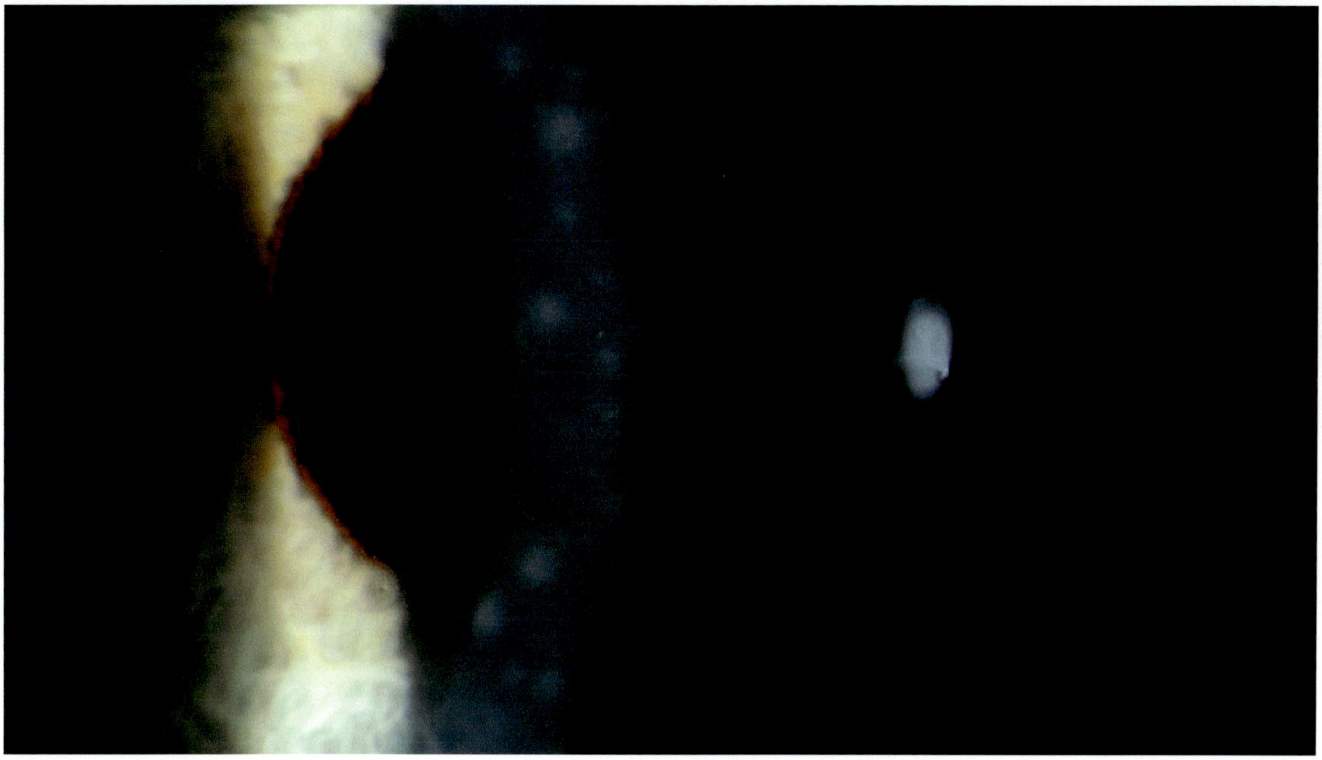

Fig. 18 Autoimmune subepithelial nummular corneal infiltrates in epidemic keratoconjunctivitis

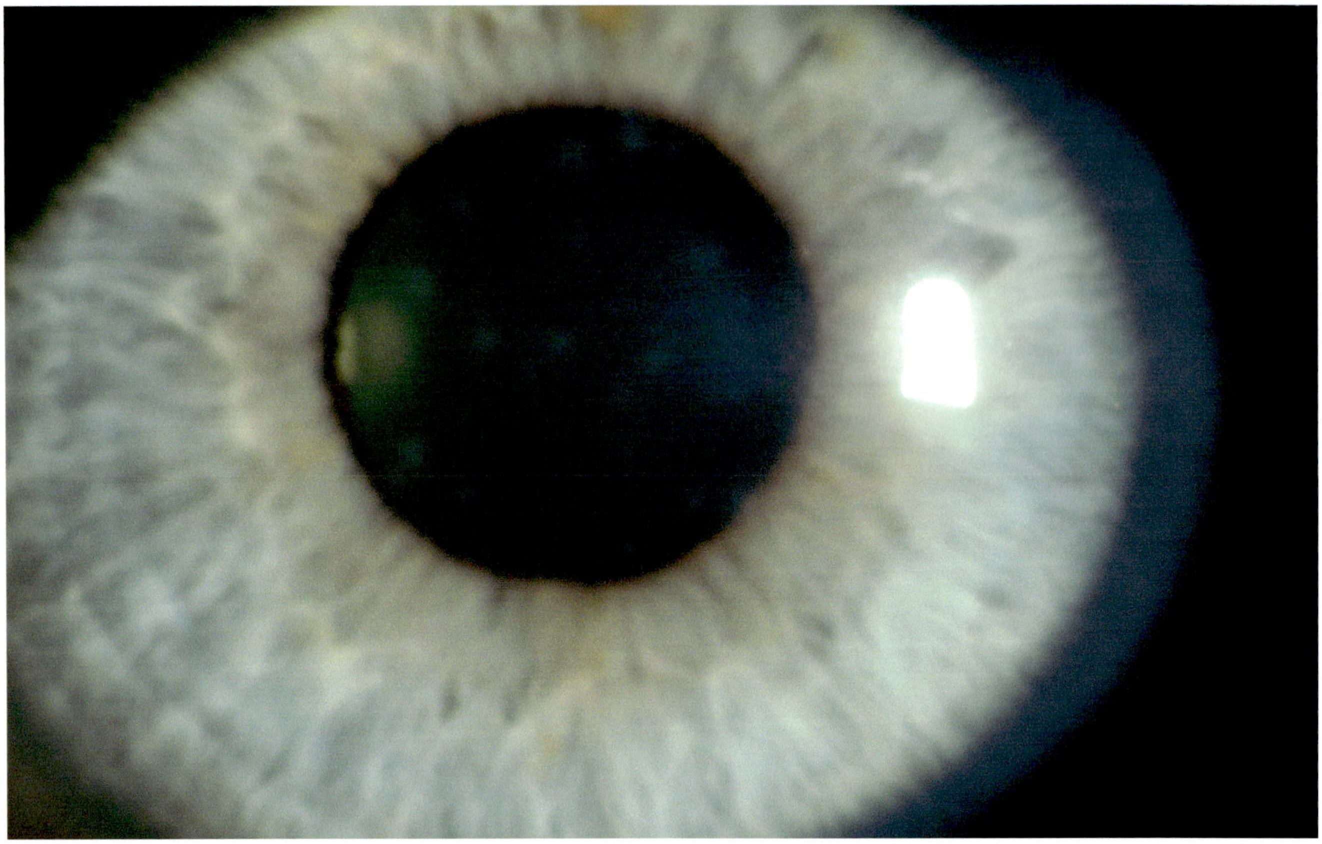

Fig. 19 Autoimmune subepithelial nummular corneal infiltrates in epidemic keratoconjunctivitis

10 Superior Limbic Keratoconjunctivitis

Superior limbic keratoconjunctivitis (SLK) is characterized by a bilateral chronic inflammation of the superior limbus and superior bulbar and tarsal conjunctiva (Fig. 20). Patients often show fine punctate staining of the limbus and the adjacent area (Fig. 21), sometimes associated with the development of filaments. SLK can be associated with non-ocular conditions such as **thyroid disease**. It is thought to be related to mechanical friction, tear film instability, or an autoimmune/inflammatory etiology.

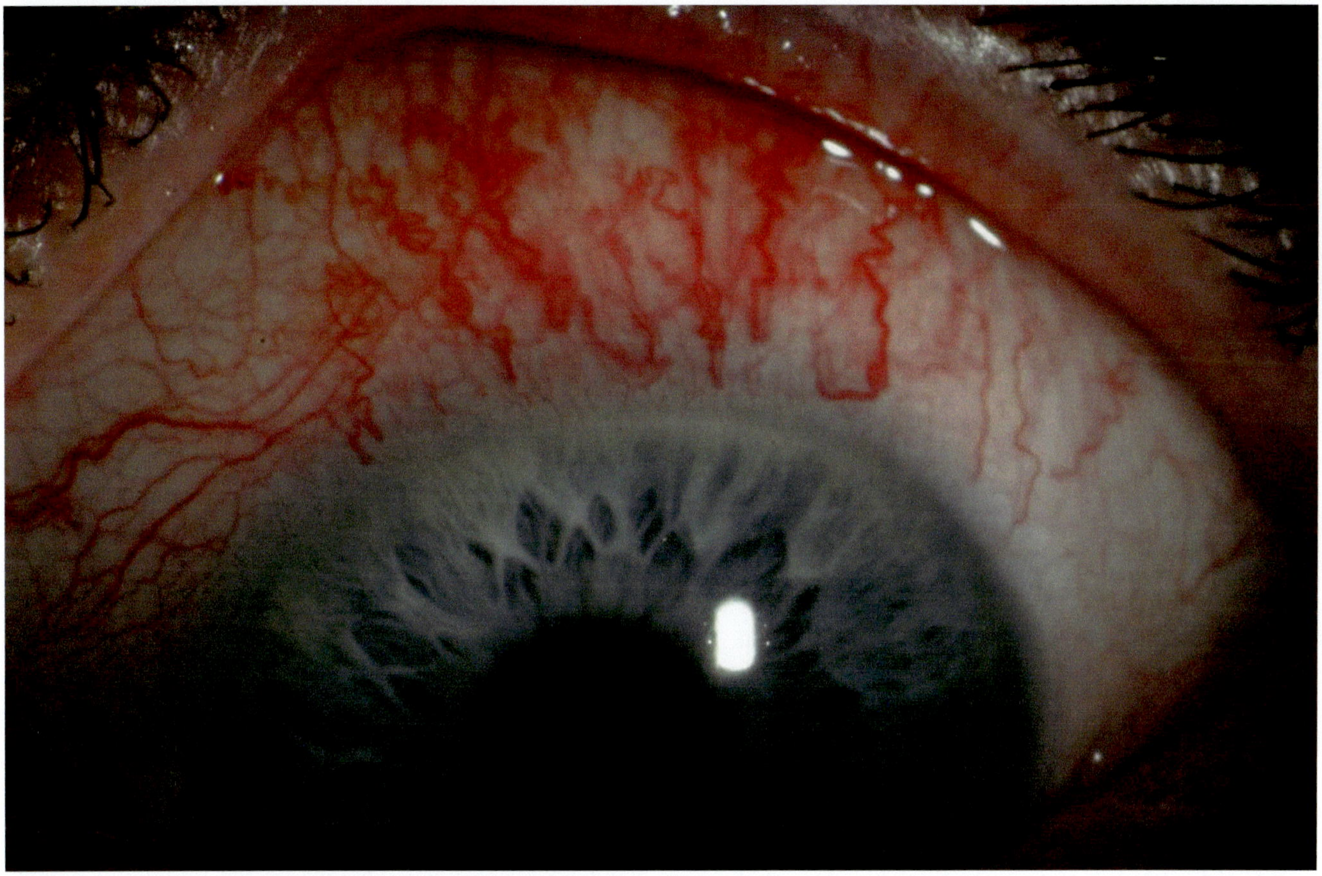

Fig. 20 Superior limbic keratoconjunctivitis

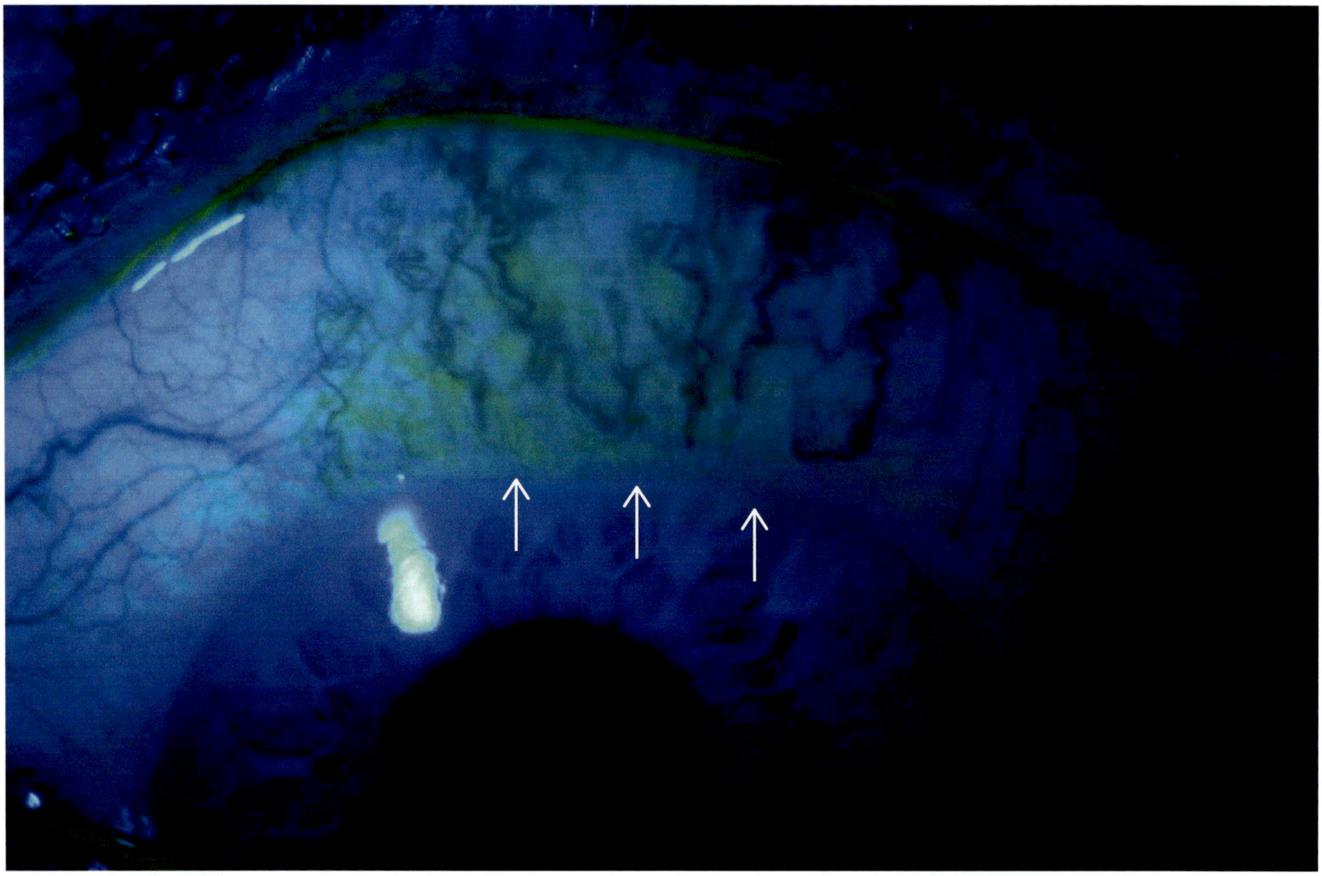

Fig. 21 Superior limbic keratoconjunctivitis with punctate fluorescein staining (arrows) of the limbus and the adjacent area

11 Conclusion

The differential diagnosis of autoimmune keratitis may be a challenge for the ophthalmologist. A profound ocular and systemic patient history together with the knowledge of specific clinical features allows the correct diagnosis in most cases. Microbiological swabs may exclude an infectious cause. Further laboratory investigations are sometimes needed to exclude or proof systemic disease. In most instances, topical and/or anti-inflammatory treatments together with specific measurements indicated by the distinct disease process are mandatory. Prognosis depends on the individual diagnosis and may reach from complete healing up to corneal scarring with cloudy corneas, induced astigmatism, and/or vision loss.

References

1. Alhassan MB, Rabiu M, Agbabiaka IO. Interventions for Mooren's ulcer. Cochrane Database Syst Rev 2014; 22: CD006131.
2. Cao Y, Zhang W, Wu J et al. Peripheral ulcerative keratitis associated with autoimmune disease. Pathogenesis and treatment. J Ophthalmol 2017: https://doi.org/10.1155/2017/7298026.
3. Durtette C, Hachulla E, Resche-Rigon M, et al. Cogan syndrome: characteristics, outcome and treatment in a French nationwide retrospective study and literature review. Autoimmunity Rev. 2017;16:1219–23.
4. Gupta Y, Kishore A, Kumari P, et al. Peripheral ulcerative keratitis. Surv Ophthalmol. 2021;66:977–98.
5. Johnson JD, Harissi-Dagher M, Pineda R, et al. Diffuse lamellar keratitis: incidence, associations, outcomes, and a new classification. J Cataract Refract Surg. 2001;27:1560–6.
6. Lahoti S, Weiss M, Johnson DA, Kheirkhah A. Superior limbic keratoconjunctivitis: a comprehensive review. Surv Ophthalmol. 2022;67:331–41.
7. Mandal N, Yeung SN, Tadrous C, Iovieno A. Thygeson's superficial punctate keratitis. Graefe's Arch Clin Exp Ophthalmol. 2022;260:1837–41.
8. Marjanovic I, Löw U, Seitz B. Unilateral photophobia as initial symptom of severe systemic disease. Ophthalmologe. 2016;113:1078–81.
9. Messmer EM. Sterile Keratitis. Klin Monatsbl Augenheilkd. 2019;236:1235–50.
10. Mondino BJ. Inflammatory diseases of the peripheral cornea. Ophthalmology. 1988;95:463–72.
11. Reddy JC, Basu S, Saboo US, et al. Management, clinical outcomes, and complications of shield ulcers in vernal keratoconjunctivitis. Am J Ophthalmol. 2013;155:550–9.
12. Reinstein CZ, Stuart AJ, Vida RS, et al. Incidence and outcomes of sterile multifocal inflammatory keratitis and diffuse lamellar keratitis after SMILE. J Refract Surg. 2018;155:550–9.
13. Sangwan VS, Zafirakis P, Foster CS. Mooren's ulcer: current concepts in management. Indian J Ophthalmol. 1997;45:7–17.

Dry Eye Disease DED (Including Blepharitis/Meibomitis/Meibomian Gland Dysfunction)

Elisabeth M. Messmer

Abstract

Dry Eye Disease Dry eye disease (DED) is common with a worldwide prevalence between 5 to 34%. It is defined as a "multifactorial disease of the tears and ocular surface that results in symptoms of discomfort, visual disturbance, and tear film instability with potential damage to the ocular surface. It is accompanied by increased osmolarity of the tear film and inflammation of the ocular surface". Classification into "dry eye with reduced tear production (aqueous-deficient)" and "dry eye with increased evaporation of the tear film mainly caused by blepharitis and meibomian gland dysfunction (MGD) (hyperevaporative)" has proved useful on practical grounds.

Keywords

Dry eye disease · Blepharitis · Meibomian gland dysfunction · Filamentary keratitis · Rosacea · Blepharokeratoconjunctivitis

1 Clinical Signs of Dry Eye Disease

Clinical signs are short tear film break up time (Fig. 1), conjunctival staining (Fig. 2), and corneal staining (Figs. 3 and 4). In severe aqueous deficient DED painful filamentary keratitis may develop composed of degenerated epithelial cells and mucus (Fig. 5). Severe aqueous deficient DED may be complicated by corneal perforation (Fig. 6).

E. M. Messmer (✉)
Department of Ophthalmology, University Hospital, LMU Munich, Mathildenstrasse 8, Munich 80366, Germany
e-mail: emessmer@med.uni-muenchen.de

B. Seitz et al. (eds.), *Atlas on Cornea*, https://doi.org/10.1007/978-3-031-65422-0_27

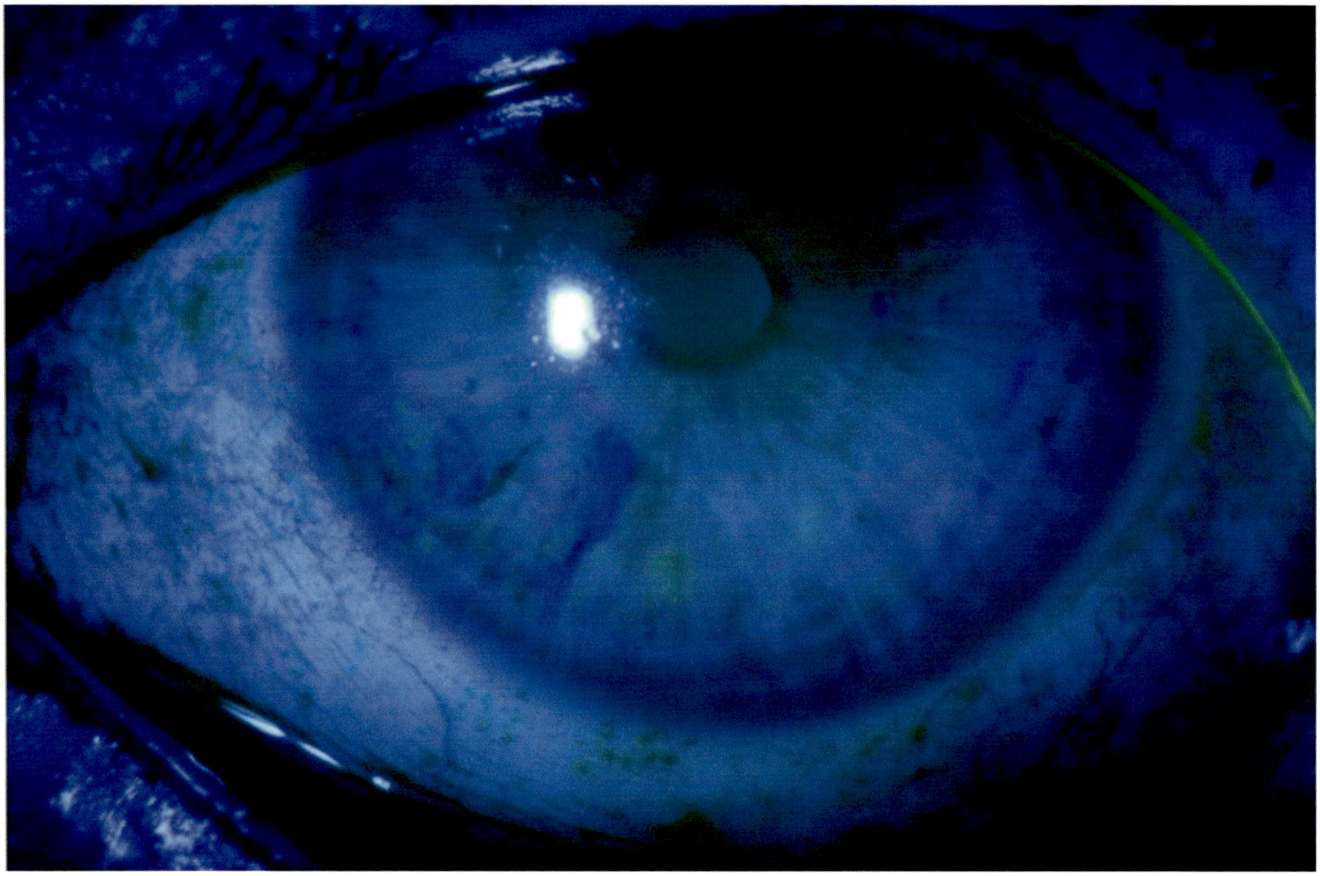

Fig. 1 Short tear film break up time of 5 s (normal > 10 s) in patient with DED

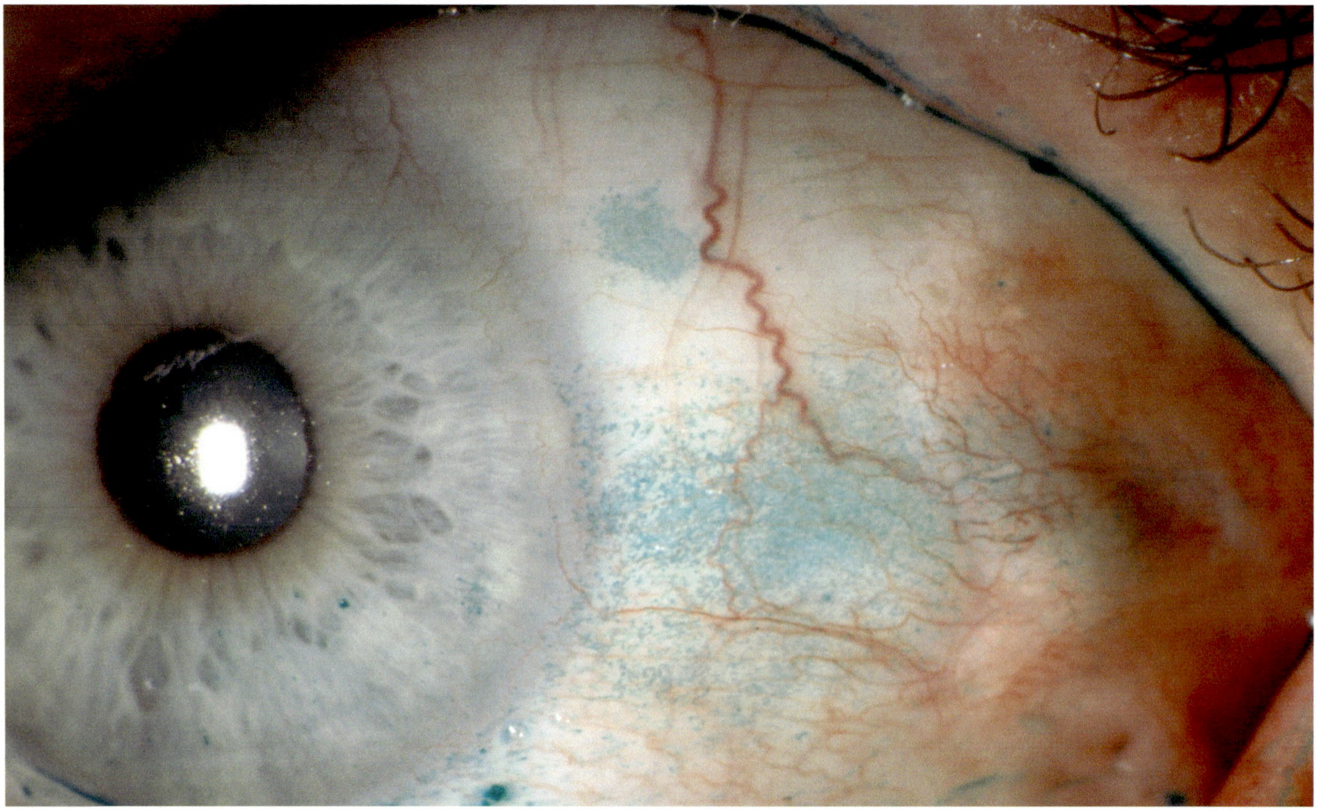

Fig. 2 Conjunctival staining with lissamine green in patient with DED

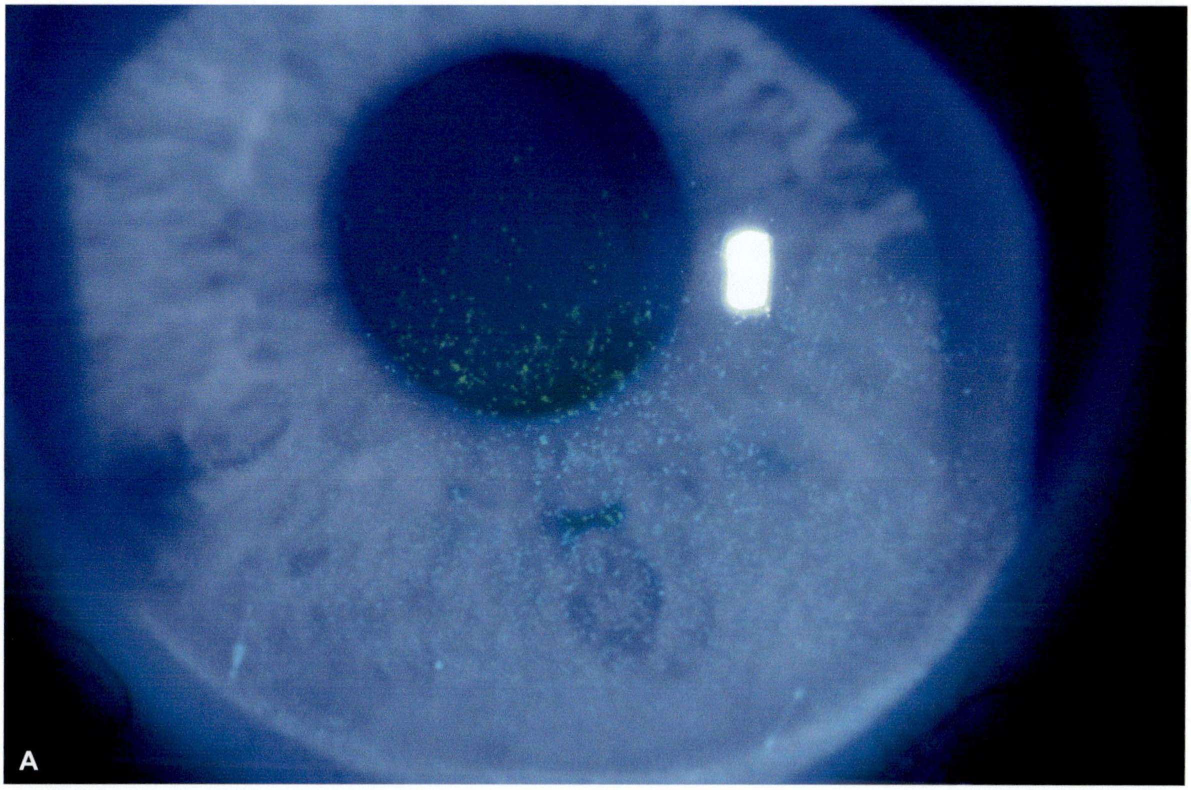

Fig. 3 (**A**) Moderate corneal fluorescein staining (superficial punctate keratopathy)

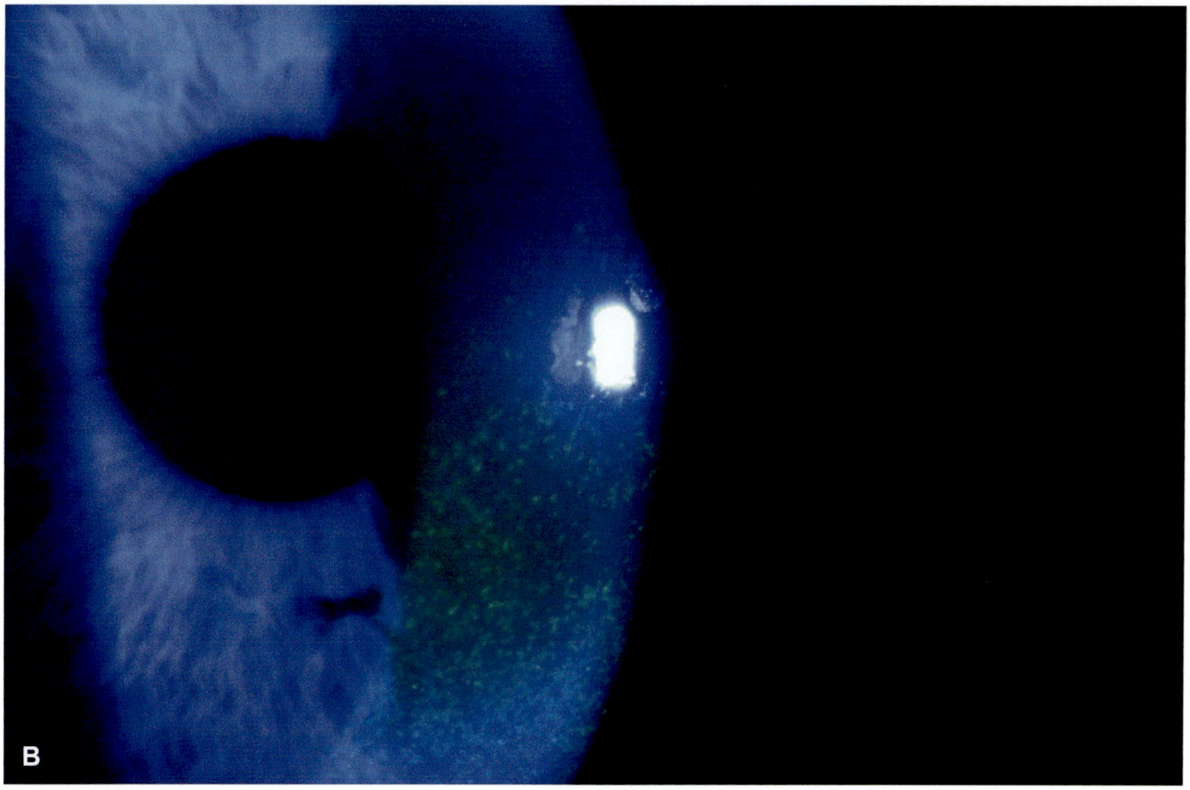

Fig. 3 (**B**) Moderate corneal fluorescein staining (superficial punctate keratopathy)

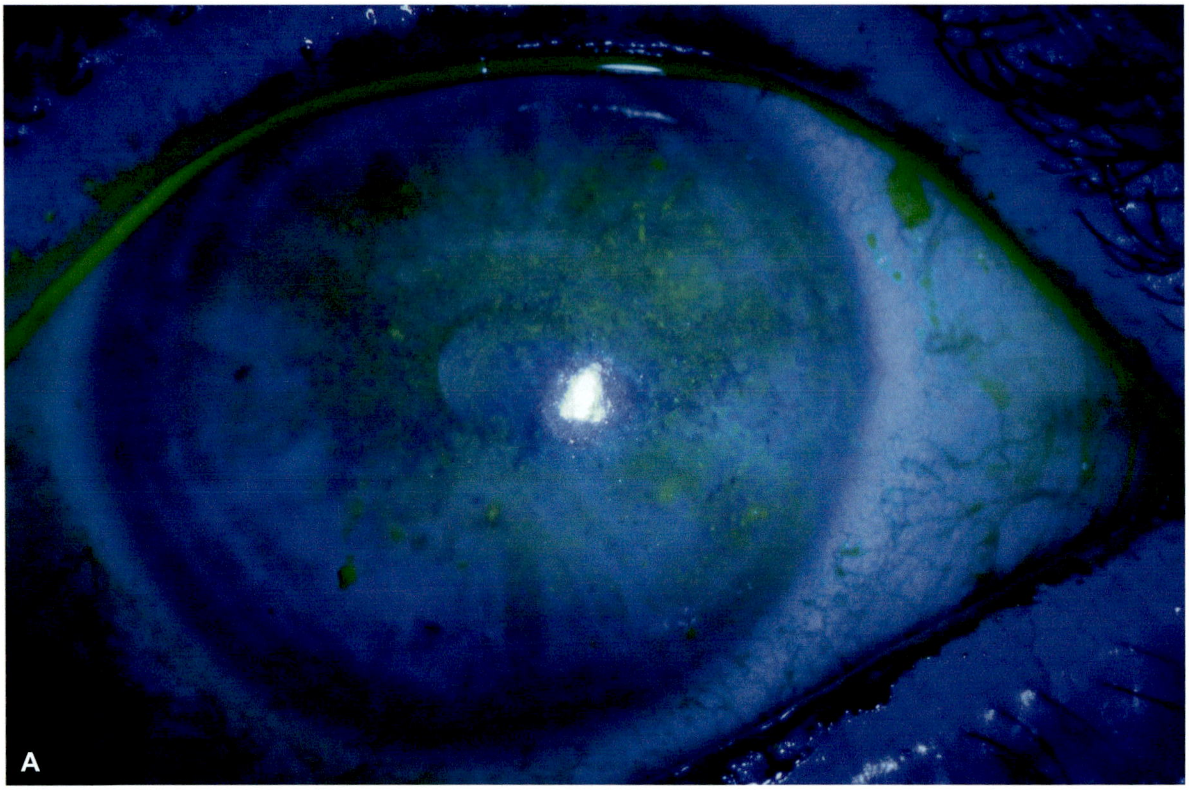

Fig. 4 (**A**) Severe corneal fluorescein staining (superficial punctate keratopathy) in a patient with DED associated with Sjögren syndrome

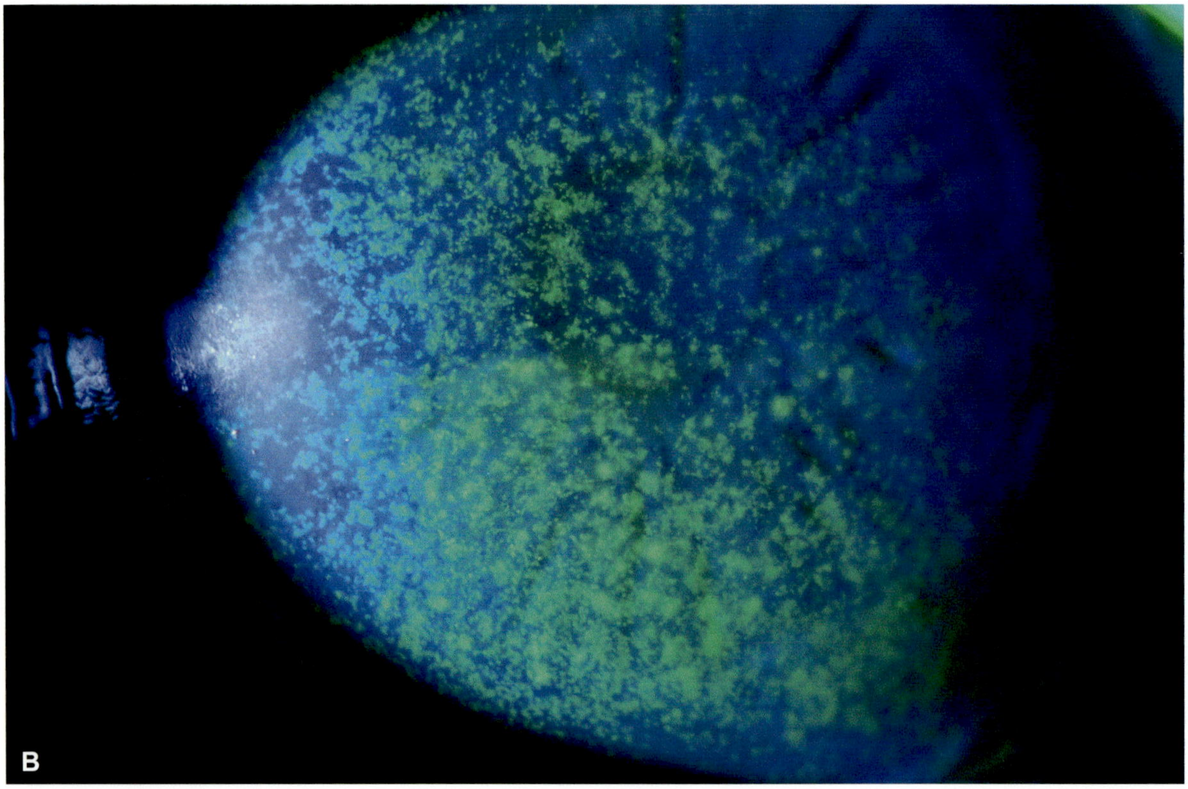

Fig. 4 (**B**) Severe corneal fluorescein staining (superficial punctate keratopathy) in another patient with DED associated with Sjögren syndrome

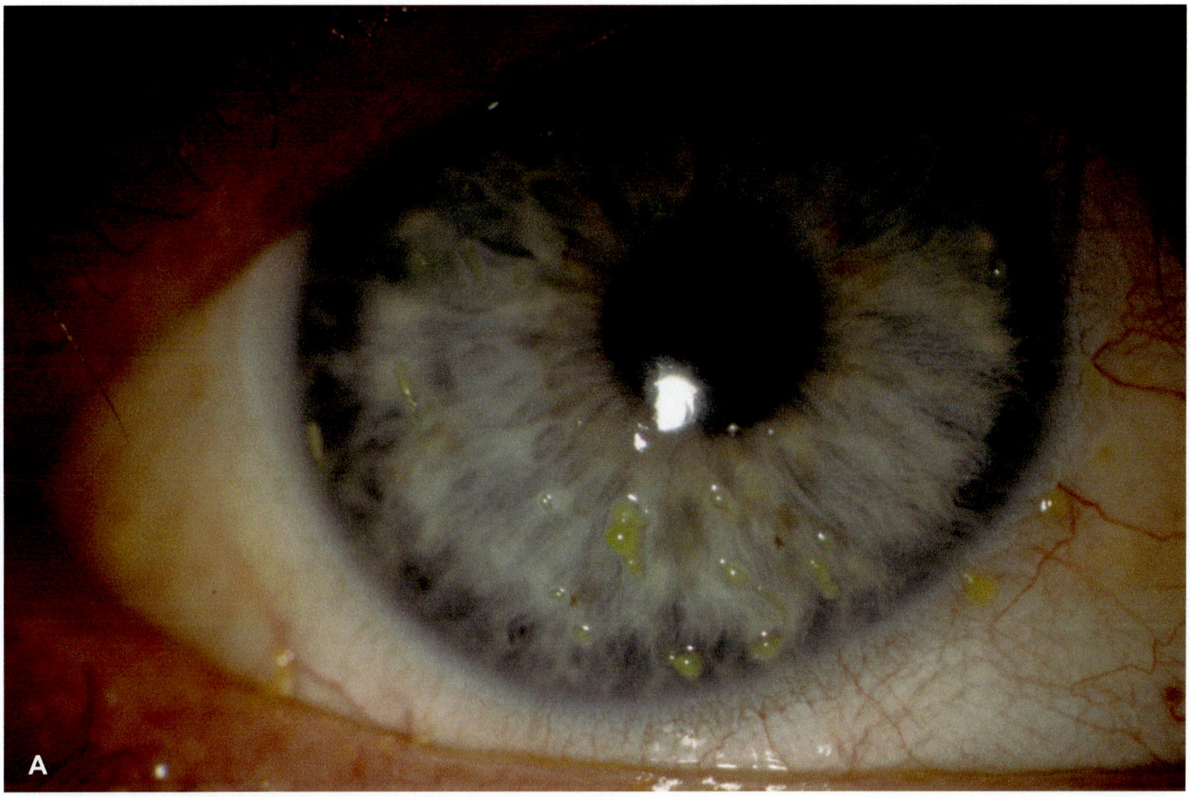

Fig. 5 (**A**) Filamentary keratitis in severe DED

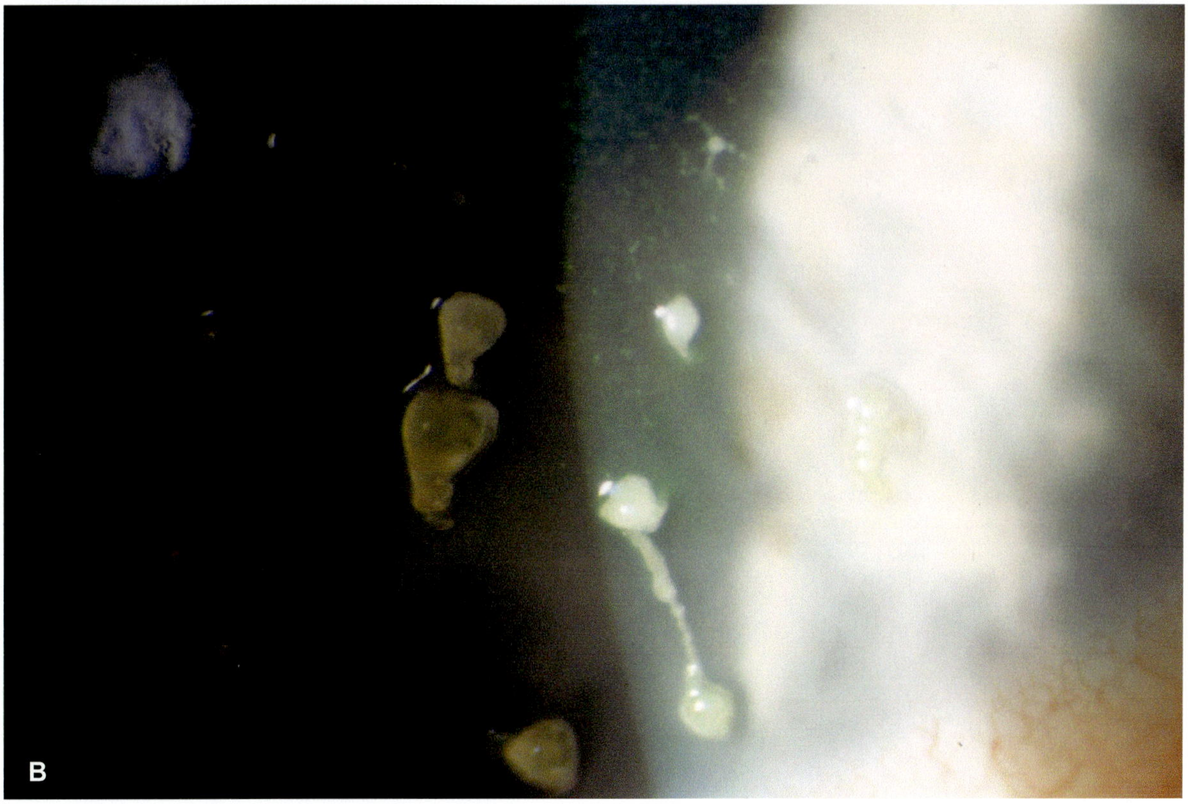

Fig. 5 (**B**) Filamentary keratitis in severe DED (large magnification)

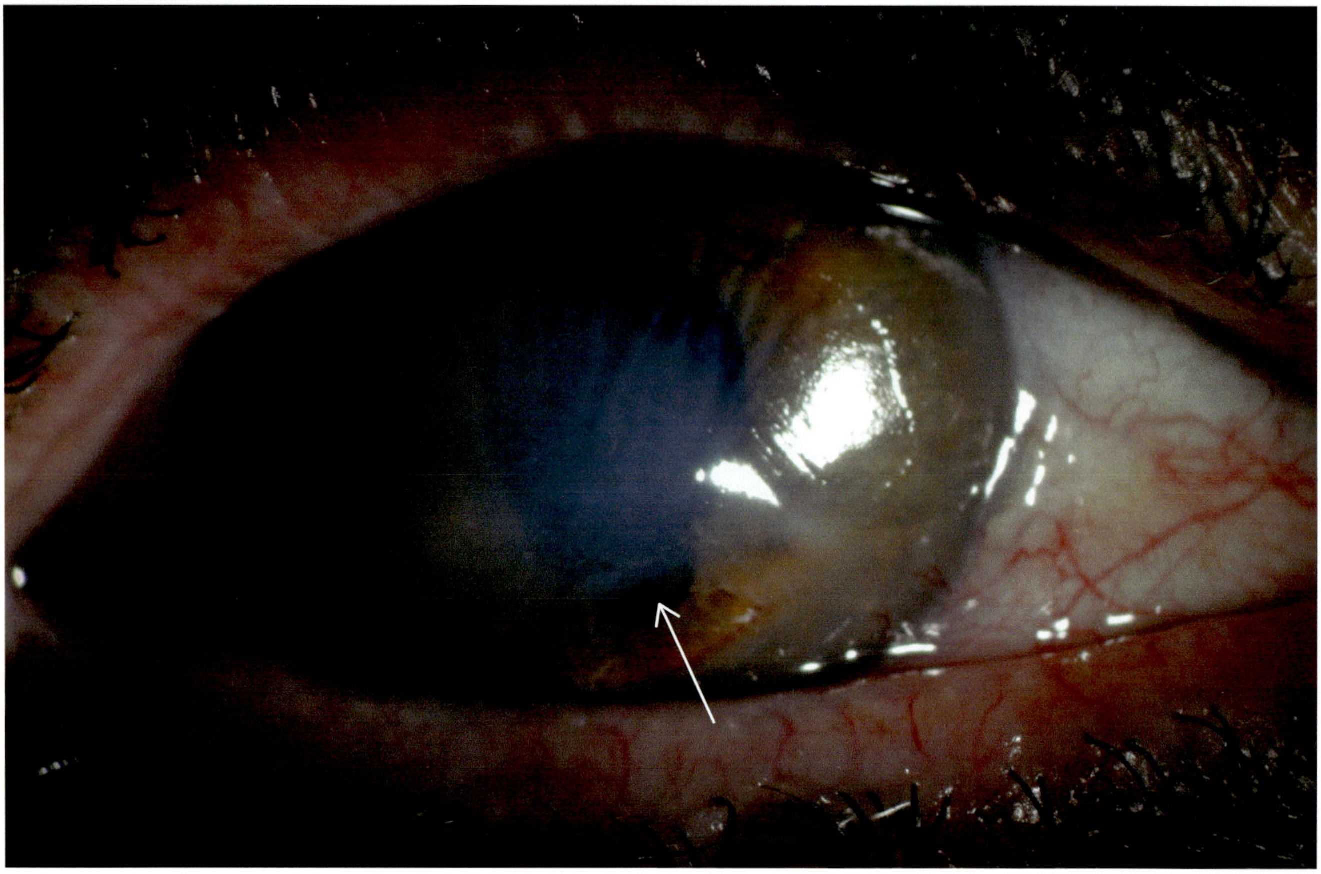

Fig. 6 Corneal perforation (arrow) in patient with severe DED associated with secondary Sjögren syndrome in rheumatoid arthritis

2 Meibomian Gland Dysfunction

Meibomian gland dysfunction (MGD) is common and may be seen in up to 80% of patients with DED. It is characterized by a foamy tear film caused by changes in the fatty acid composition of the meibum (Fig. 7) and changes at the lid margin including telangiectasias (Fig. 8), and conjunctivalization as well as keratinization of the lid margin (Fig. 9). Meibomian glands are typically obstructed. A thickened, yellowish, sometimes tooth-paste-like meibum can be expressed (Fig. 10A–D).

MGD can be associated with skin diseases such as seborrheic dermatitis (Fig. 11A, B) and rosacea. Staphylococcal infiltrates, limbal insufficiency with pannus formation and phlyctenules may complicate MGD in these patients (Figs. 12A, B and 13).

MGD/Meibomitis/blepharitis may be complicated by the development of (recurrent) hordeola, obstructed/infected glands of Zeis or Moll (external) or meibomian glands (internal) (Fig. 14). Moreover, lipogranulomatous inflammation of obstructed meibomian glands may cause (recurrent) chalazion in MGD.

An hyperinfestation with Demodex mites is considered a pathogenetic event in MGD. Rarified and broken lashes as well as collarette formation around lash bases (Fig. 15) are typically seen clinically.

Anterior blepharitis typically refers to inflammation around the lid skin, eye lashes and lash follicles. It can be subdivided into staphylococcal and seborrheic variants. Staphylococcal blepharitis is characterized by hyperemia and edema of the anterior lid margin with sticky eyelids and loss of lashes (Fig. 16). Seborrheic blepharitis is associated with scale-like oily flakes around the lash base.

Blepharokeratoconjunctivitis in childhood is one of the most common reasons for pediatric consultations in ophthalmology. It is a chronic inflammatory condition of the lid margin (Figs. 17 and 18) with secondary conjunctival and corneal involvement (Fig. 19). The pathogenesis of this disorder is unclear, but it has been proposed to be associated with early skin and mucous membrane colonization with Staphylococcus spp., the immune-genetic susceptibility of the affected patients, hypersensitivity responses against bacterial antigens as well as staphylococcal exotoxins. It is believed that children are more susceptible to corneal

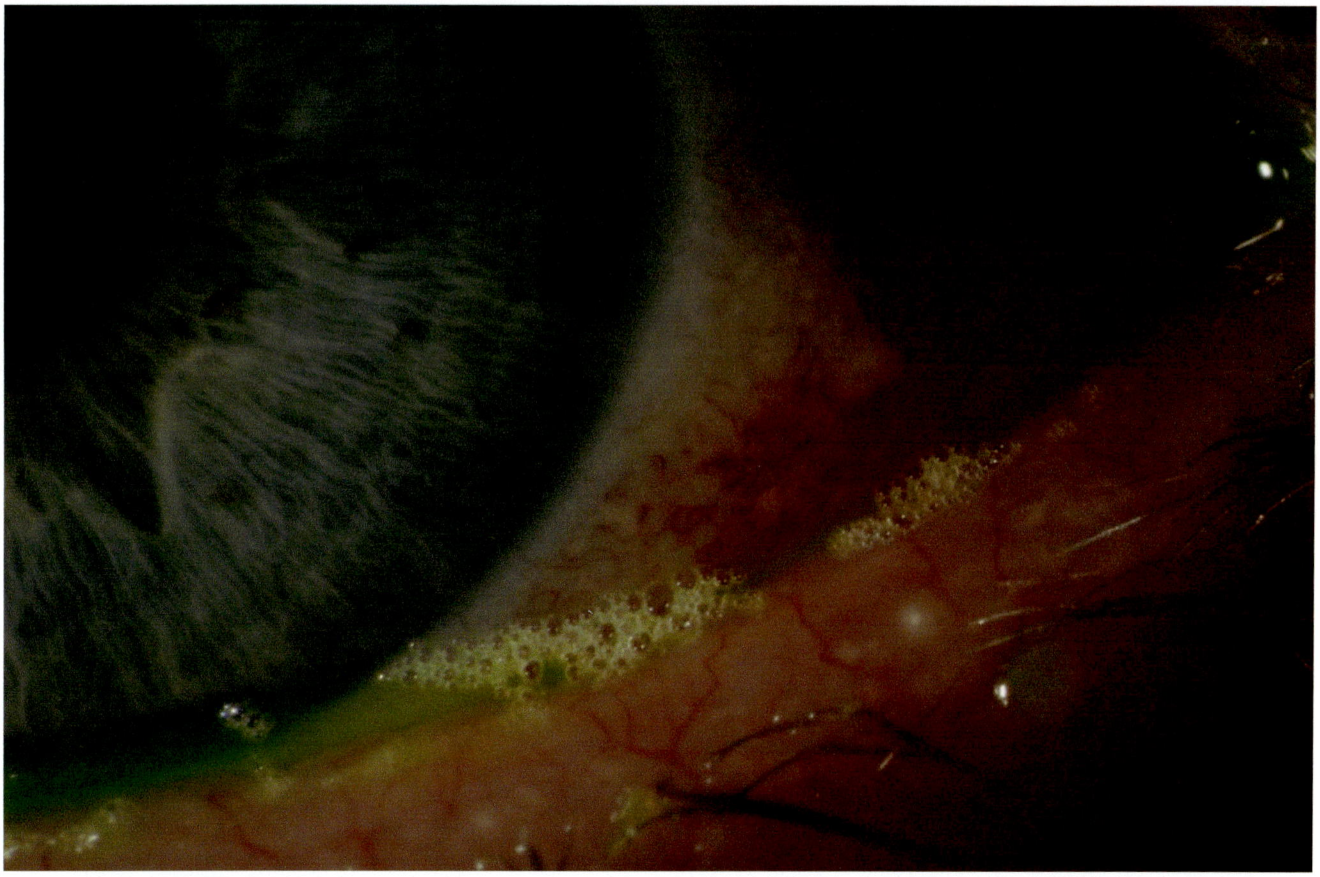

Fig. 7 Foamy tear film in MGD

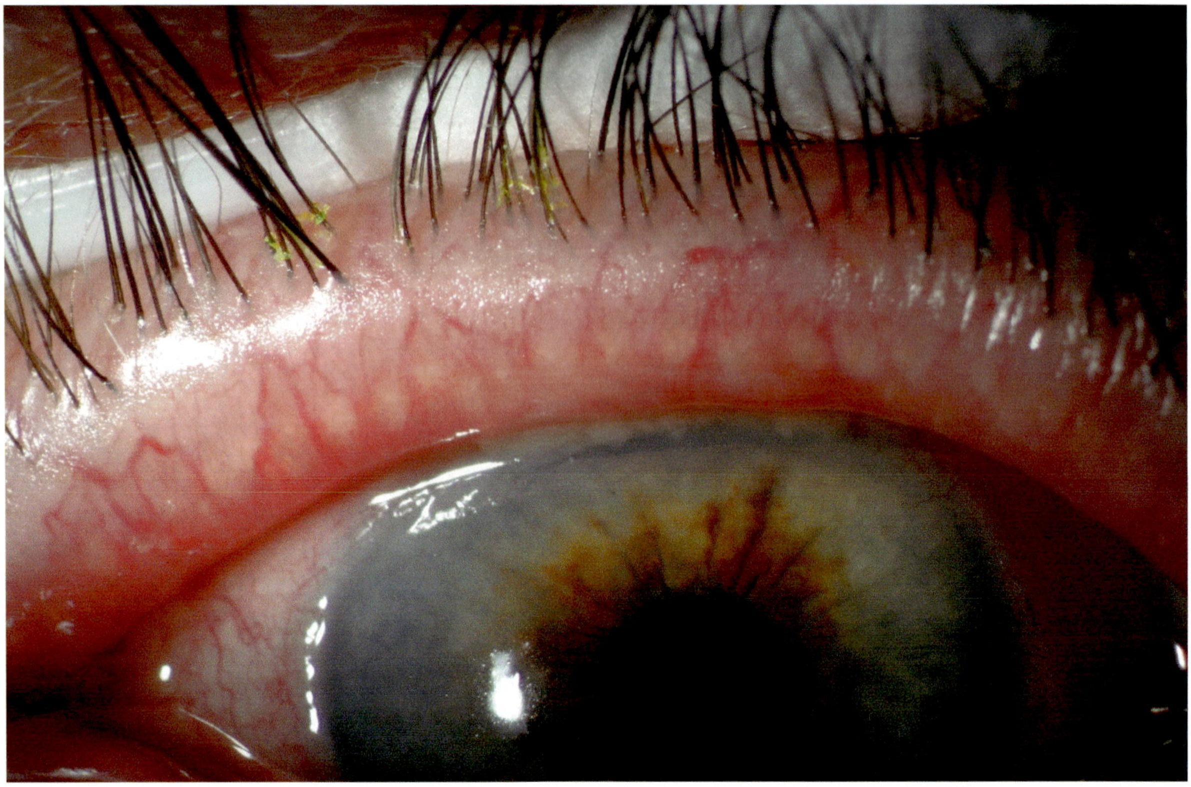

Fig. 8 Teleangiectasias of the lid margin in MGD

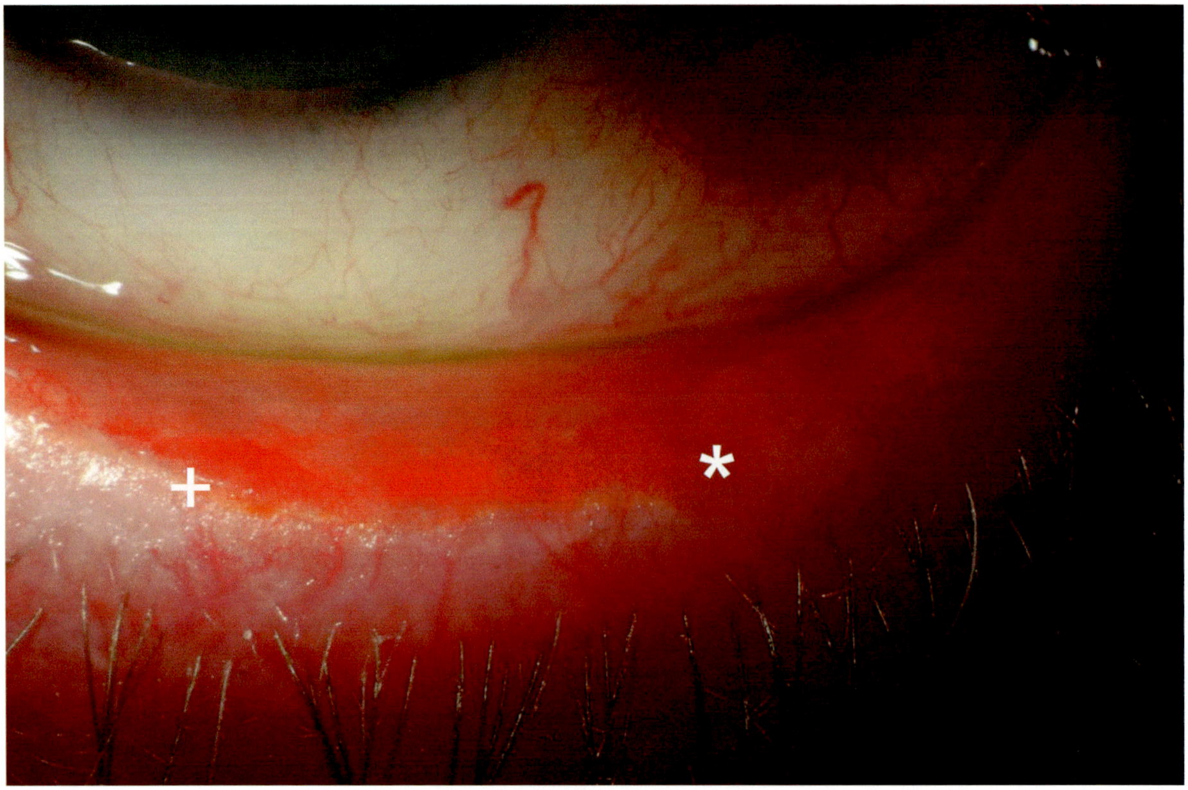

Fig. 9 Conjunctivalization (*) and keratinization (+) of the lid margin in MGD

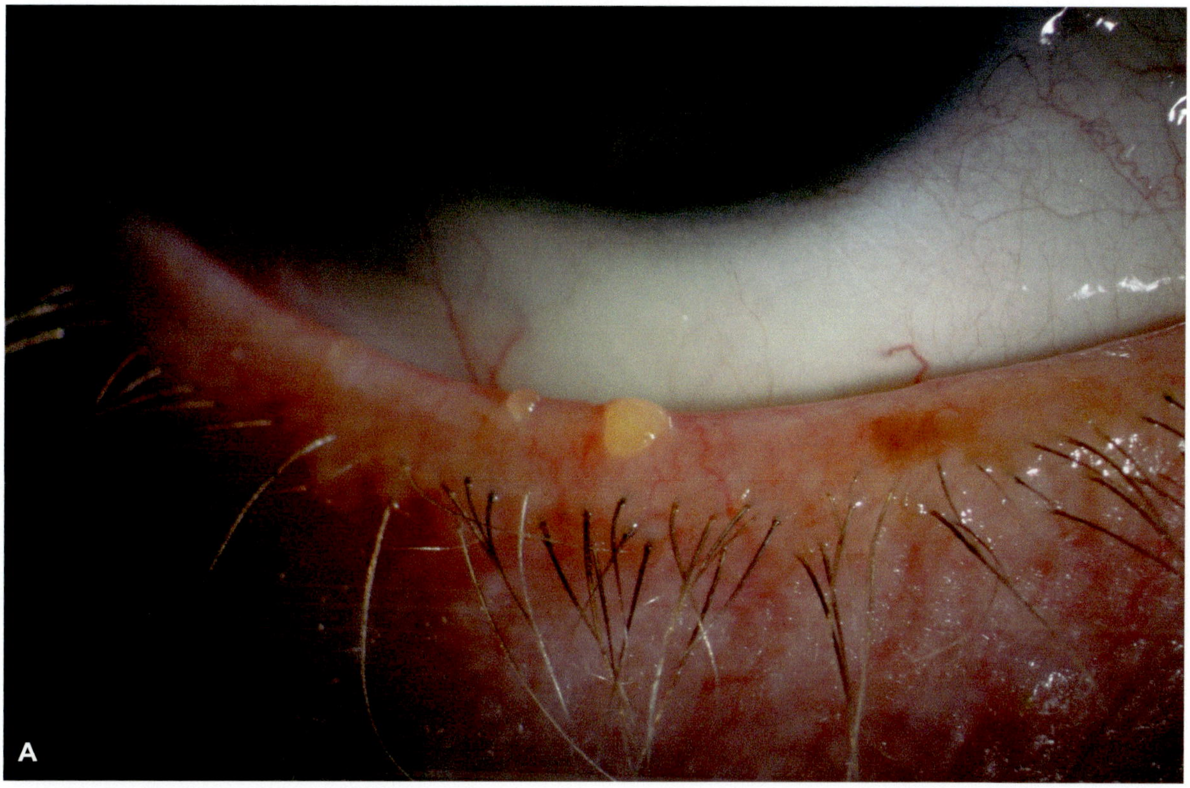

Fig. 10 (**A**) Obstructed Meibomian glands in MGD

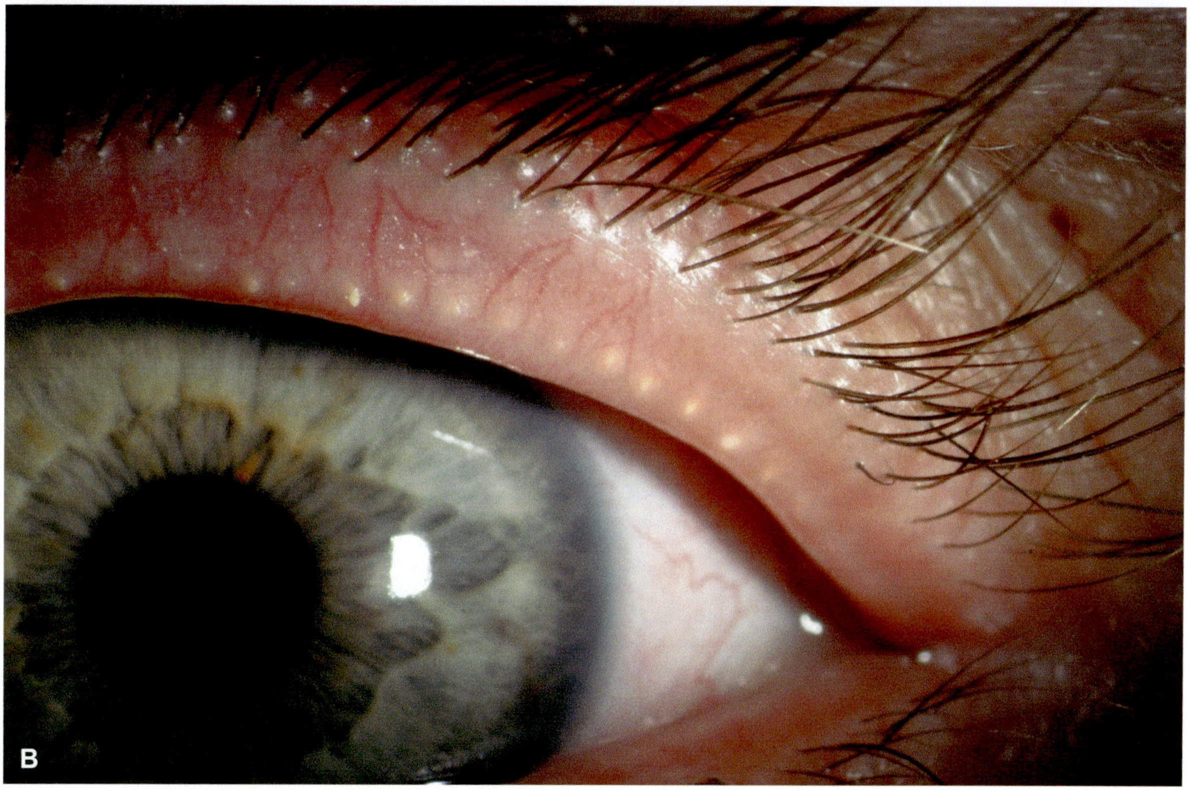

Fig. 10 (**B**) Lidmargins with telangiectasias. Obstructed meibomian glands in MGD

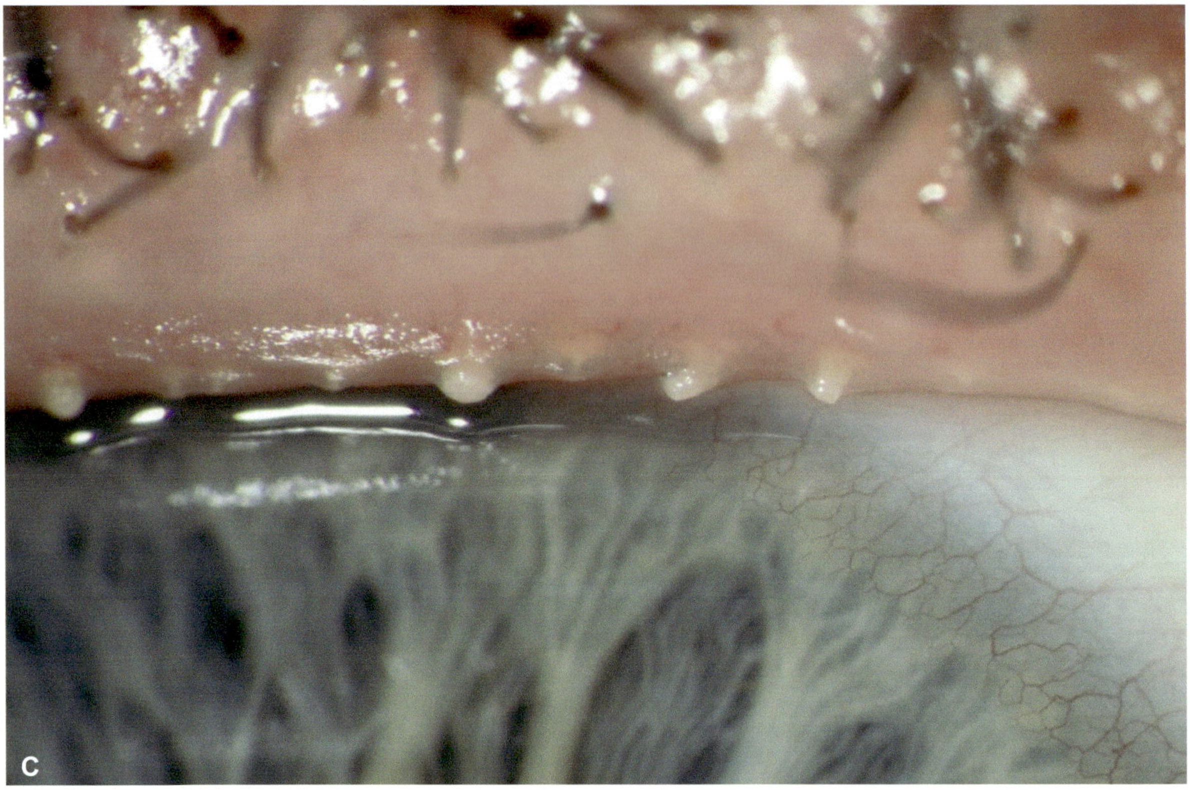

Fig. 10 (**C**) Severely obstructed meibomian gland exhibiting white, thickened meibom secretions

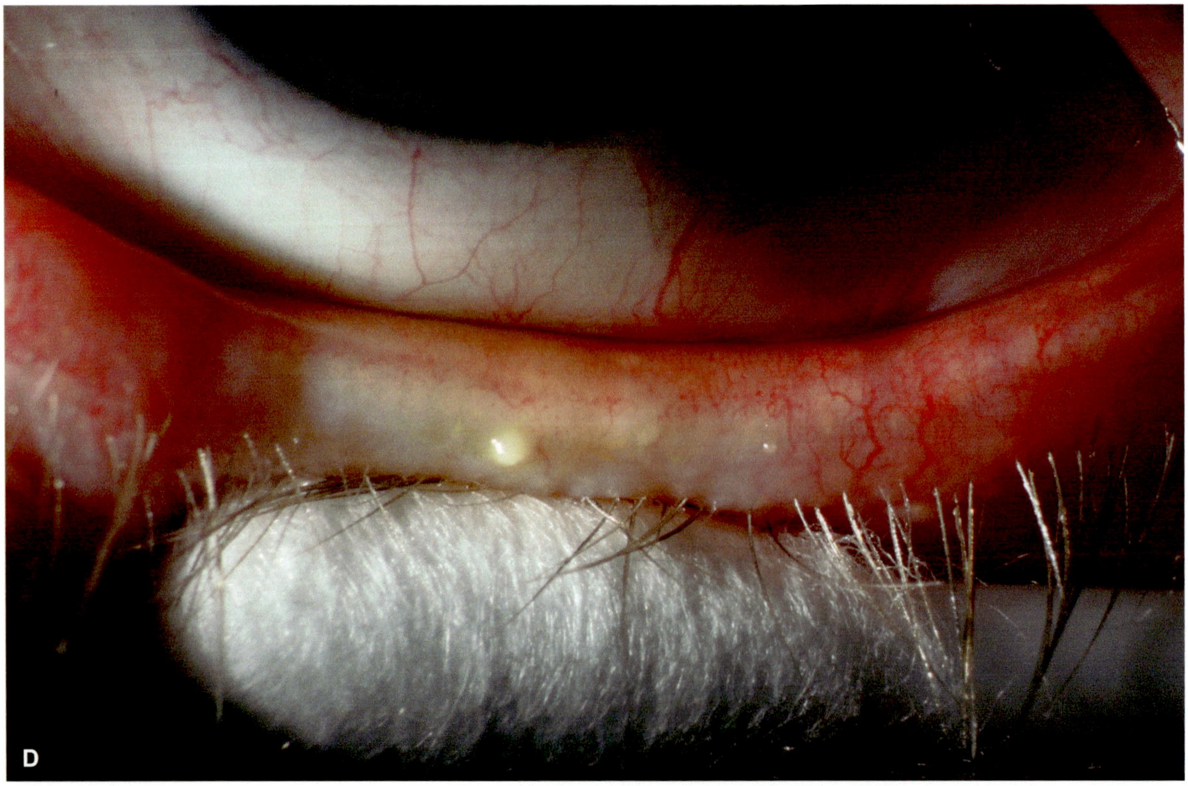

Fig. 10 (**D**) Only small amounts of thickened opaque meibum can be expressed with considerate pressure onto the meibomian glands

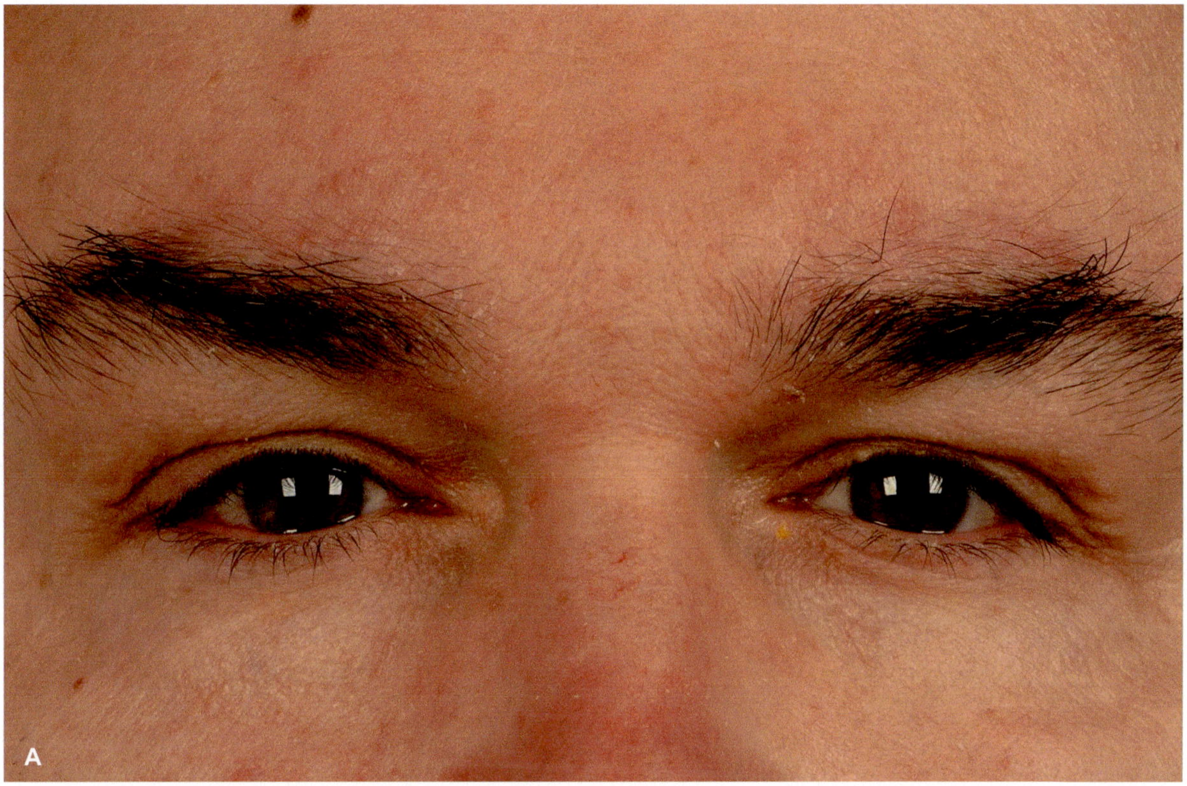

Fig. 11 (**A**) MGD in patient with seborrheic dermatitis. Skin changes in seborrheic dermatitis at forehead and in between eyebrows

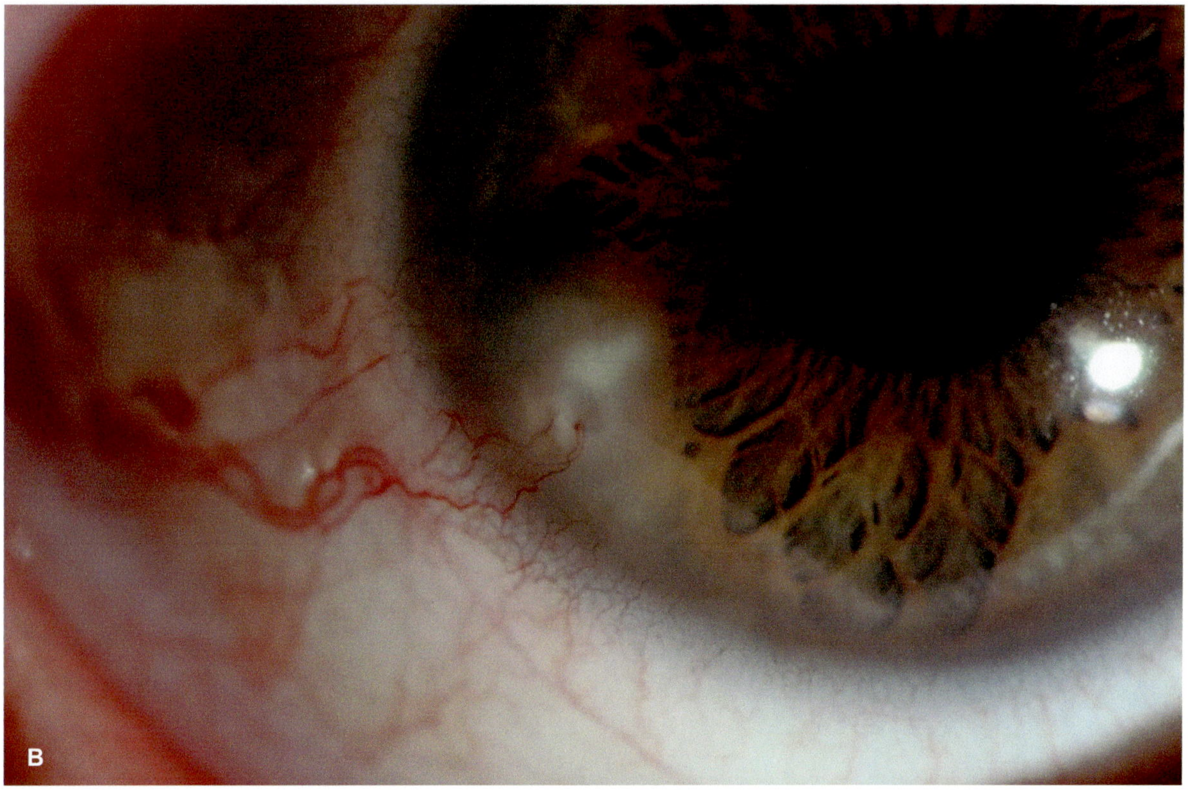

Fig. 11 (**B**) MGD in patient with seborrheic dermatitis. Staphylococcal infiltrate associated with MGD in seborrheic dermatitis

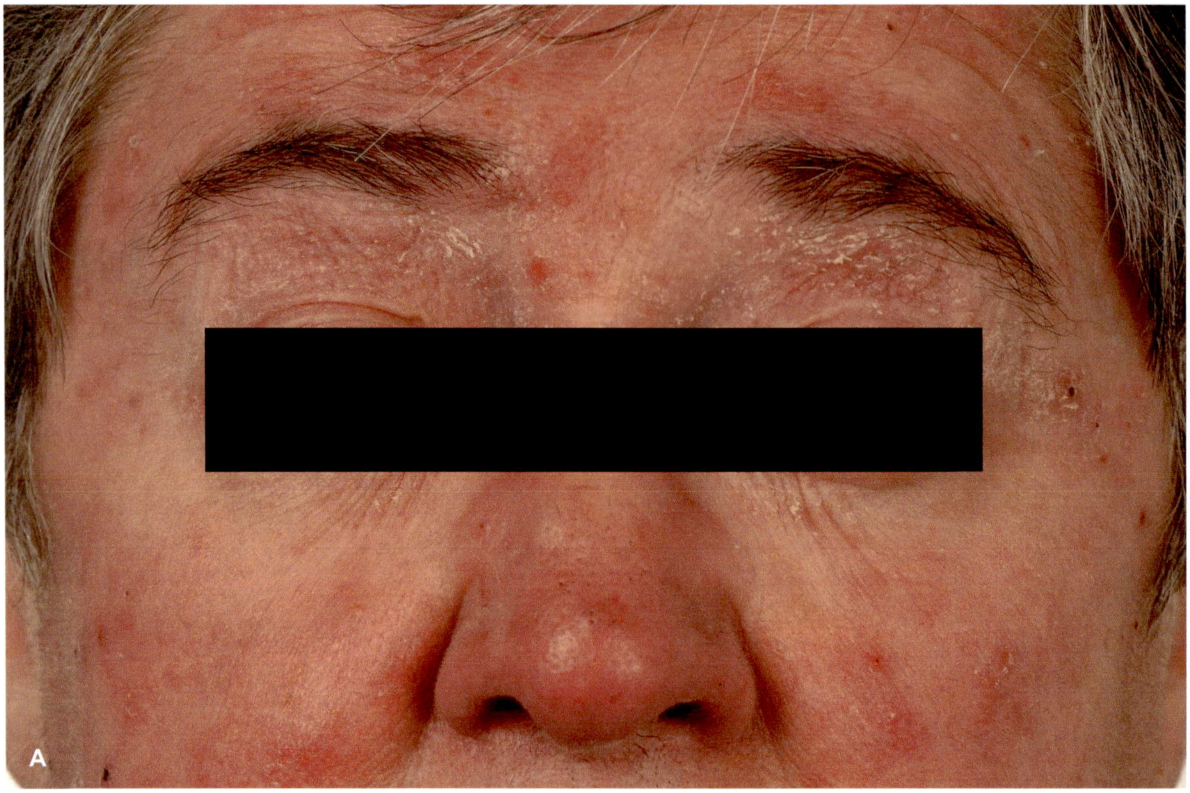

Fig. 12 (**A**) Complicated MGD in patient with rosacea. Dermal papule and pustule formation in patient with rosacea

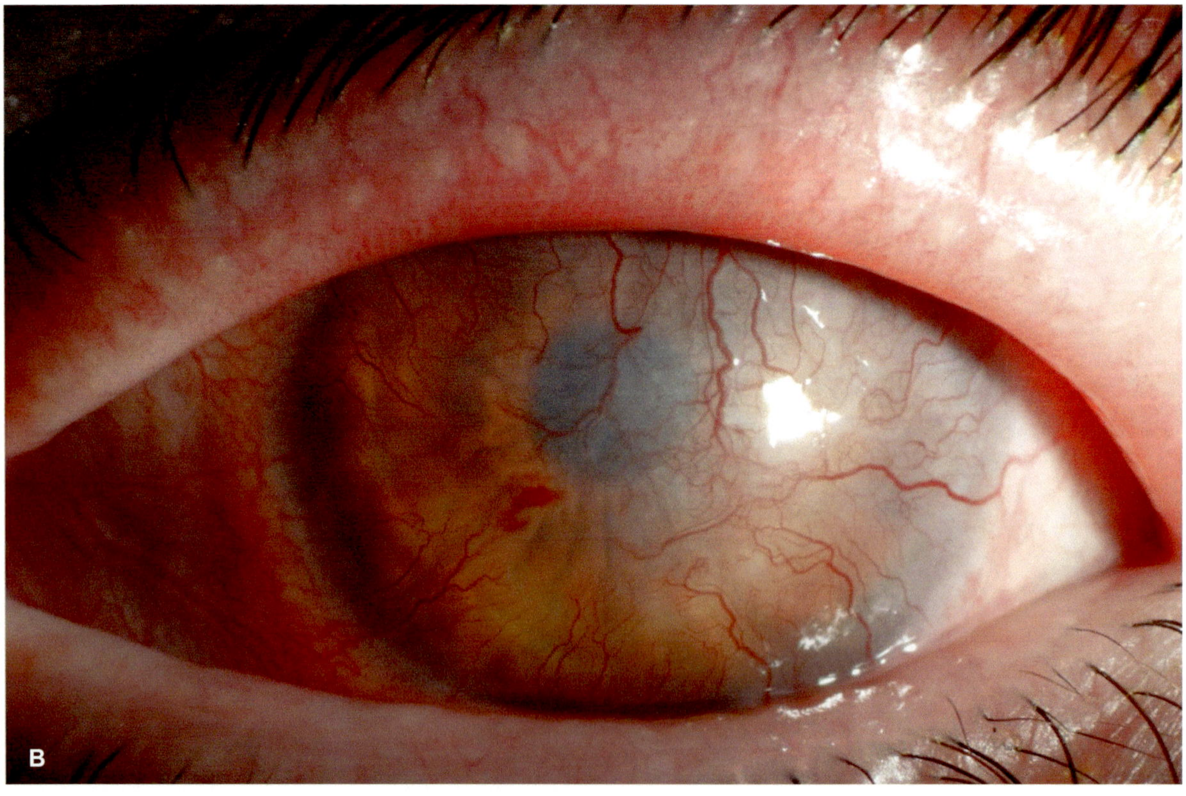

Fig. 12 (**B**) Complicated MGD in patient with rosacea. Limbal insufficiency in patient with MGD associated with rosacea

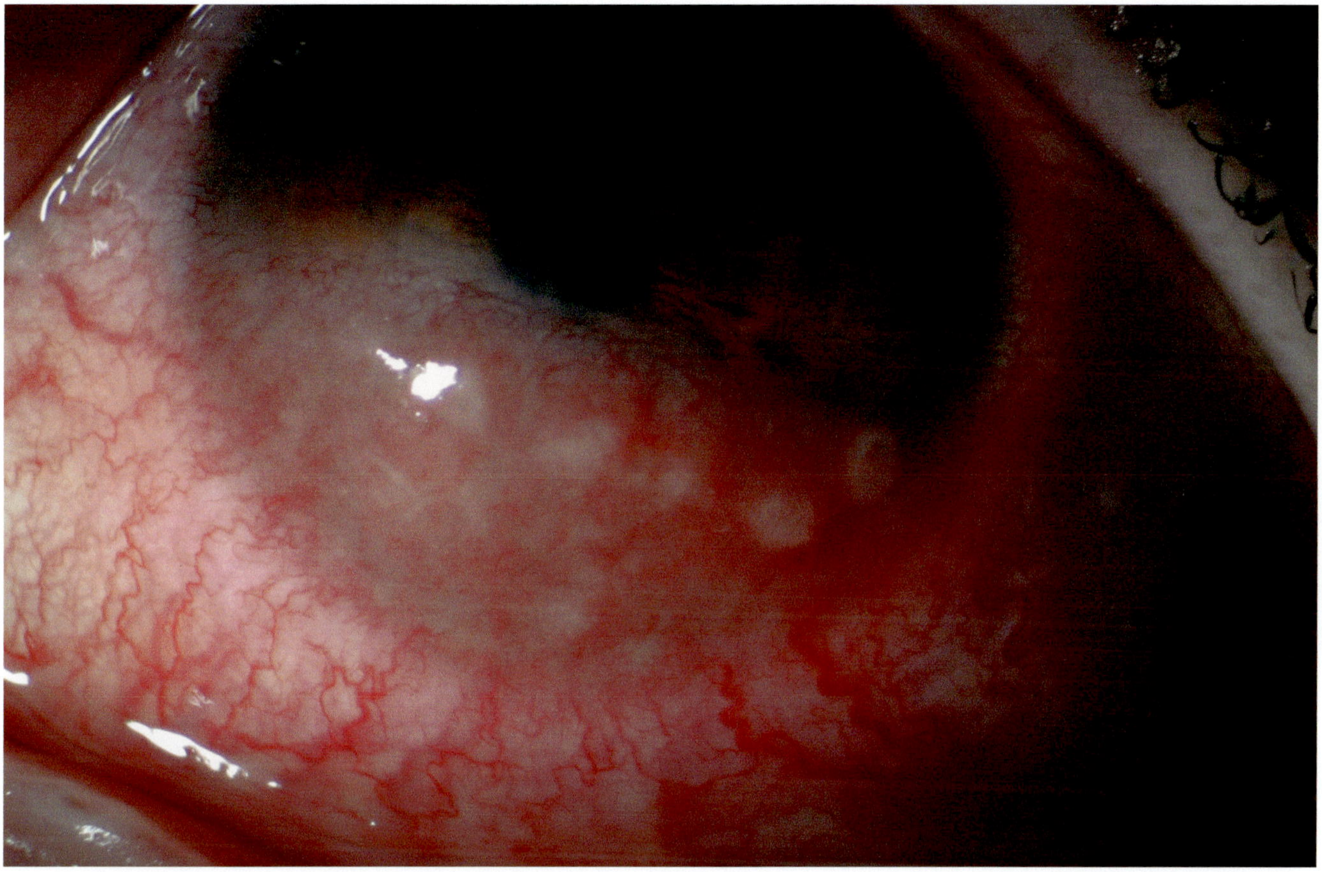

Fig. 13 Pannus and Phlyctenule formation in patient with MGD associated with rosacea

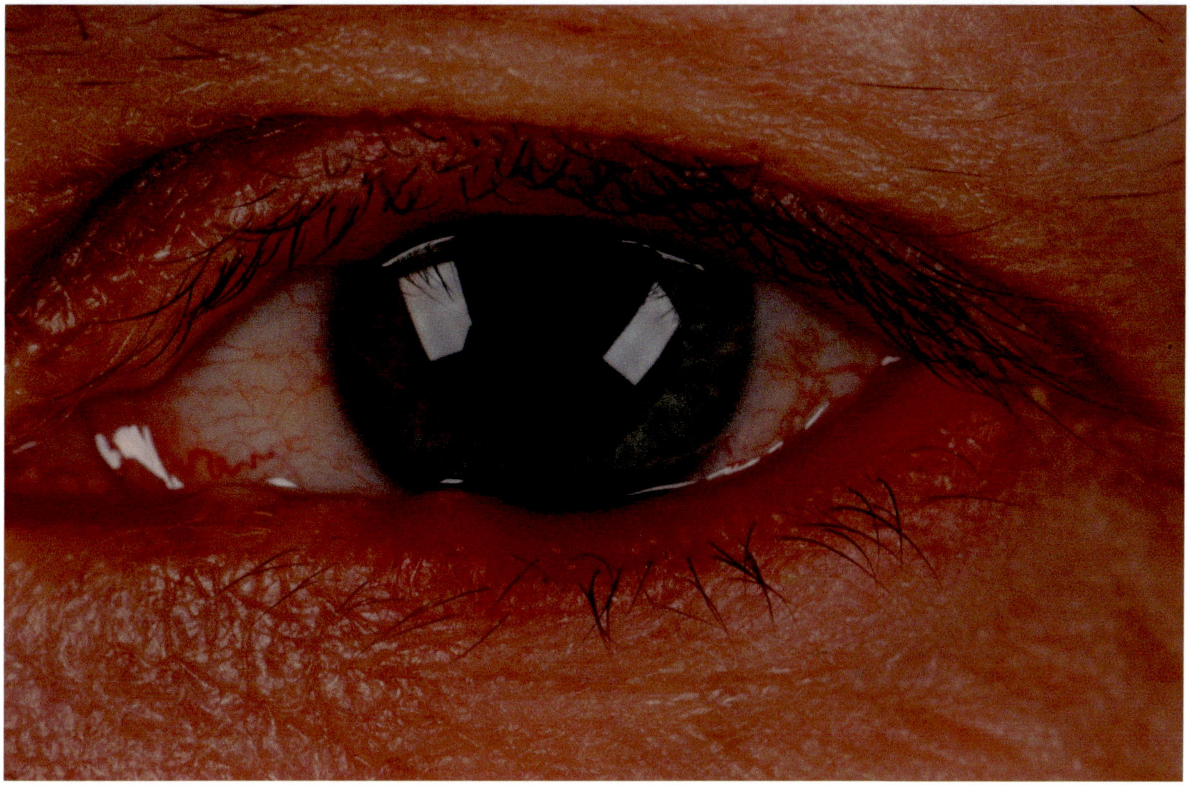

Fig. 14 Multiple hordeola in patient with MGD

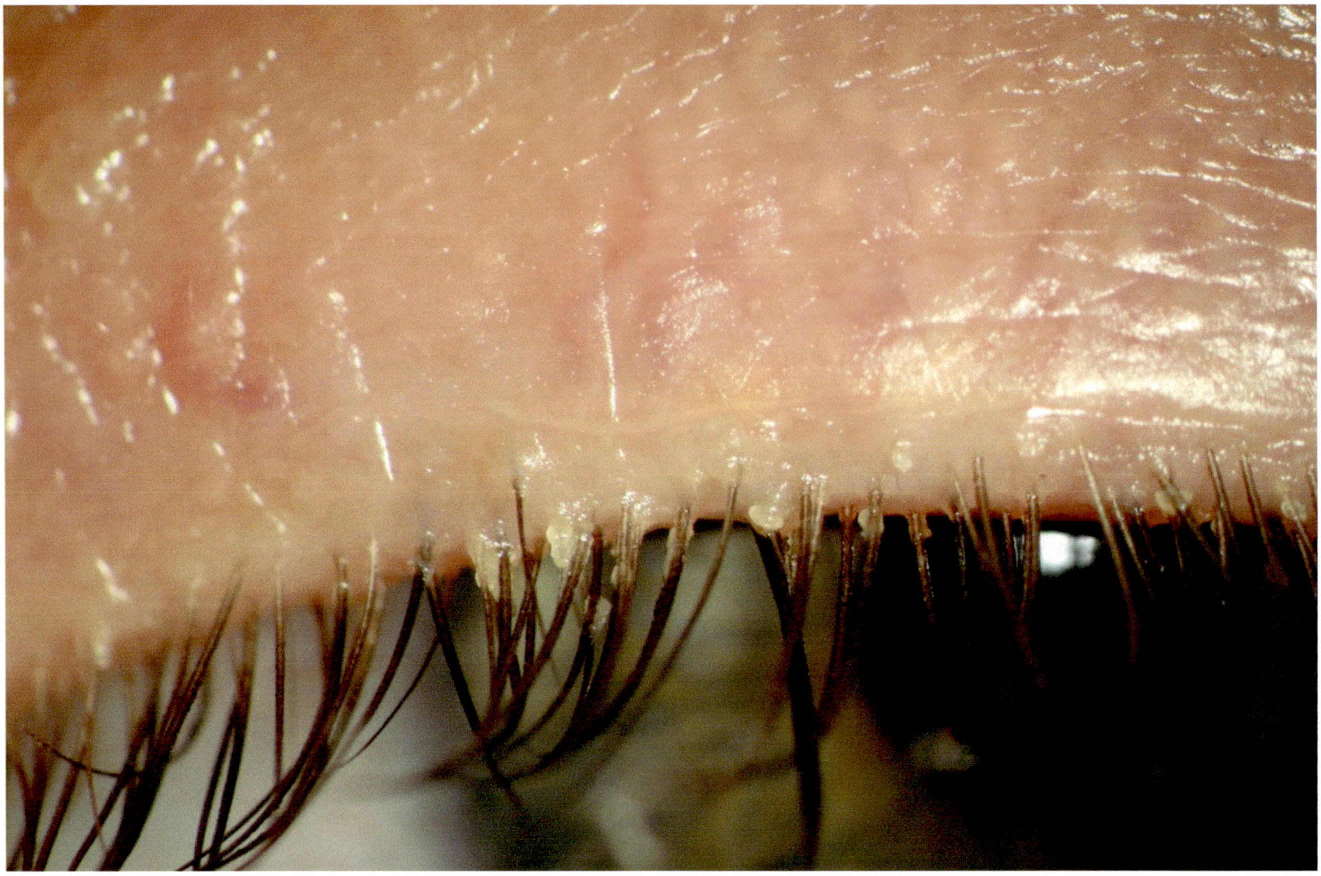

Fig. 15 Collarette formation around lash bases in MGD associated with Demodex hyperinfestation

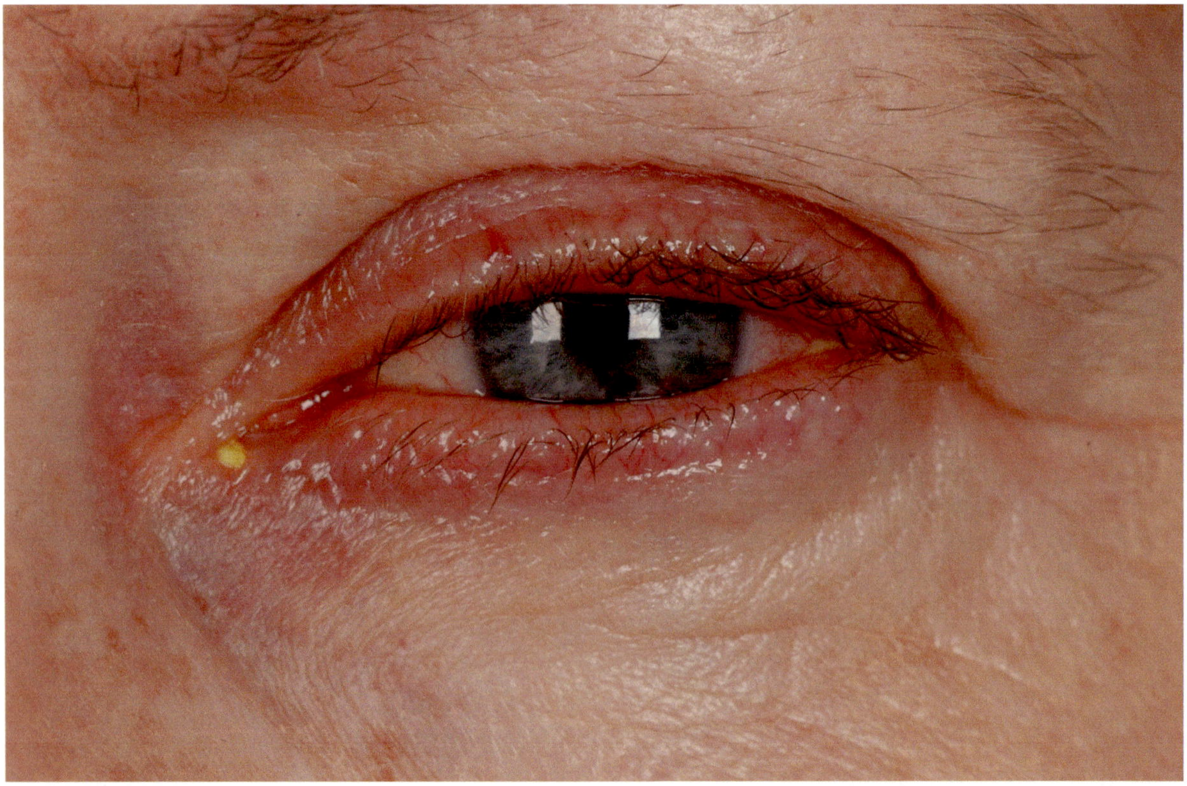

Fig. 16 Anterior blepharitis

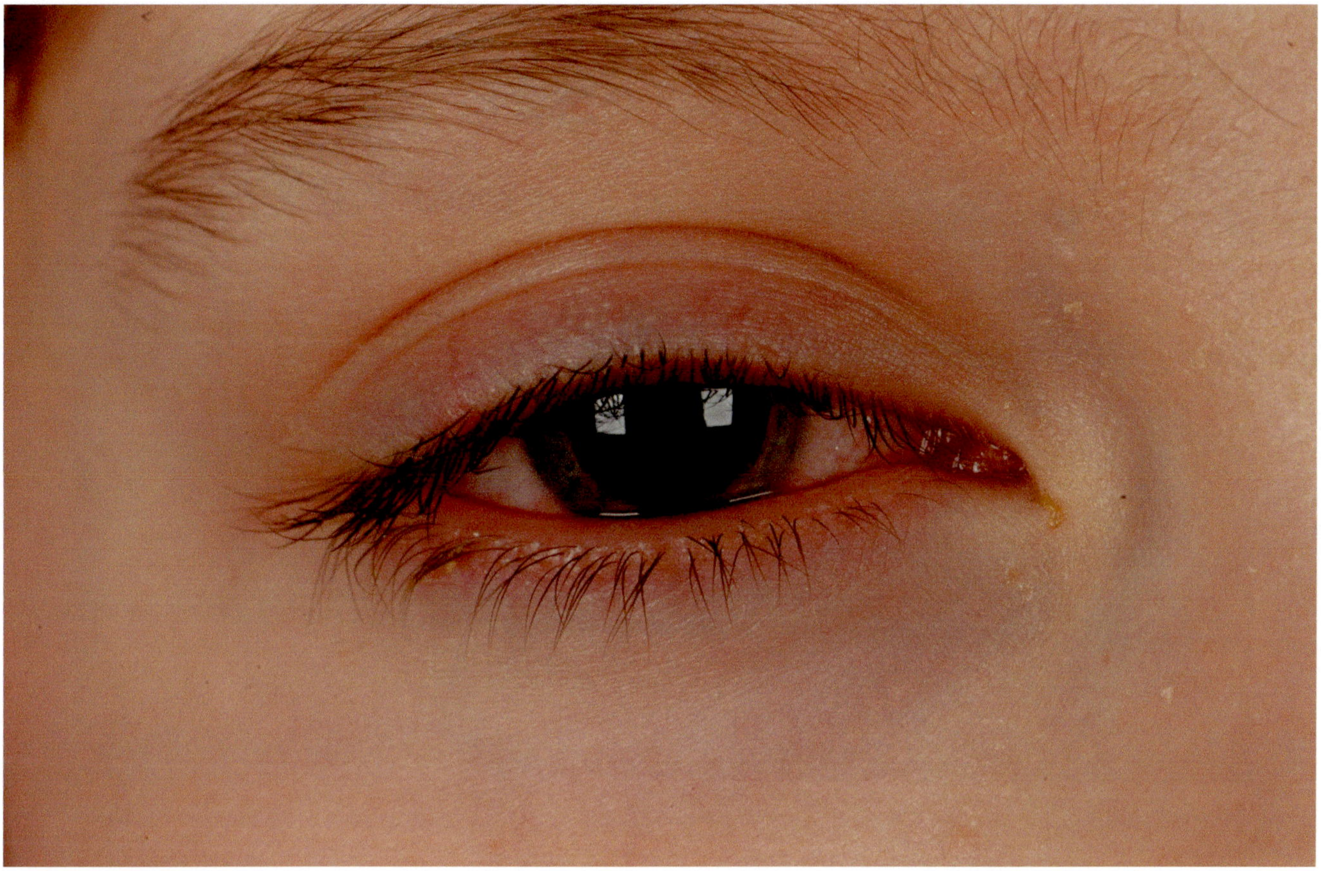

Fig. 17 Blepharokeratoconjunctivitis in 8-year-old child

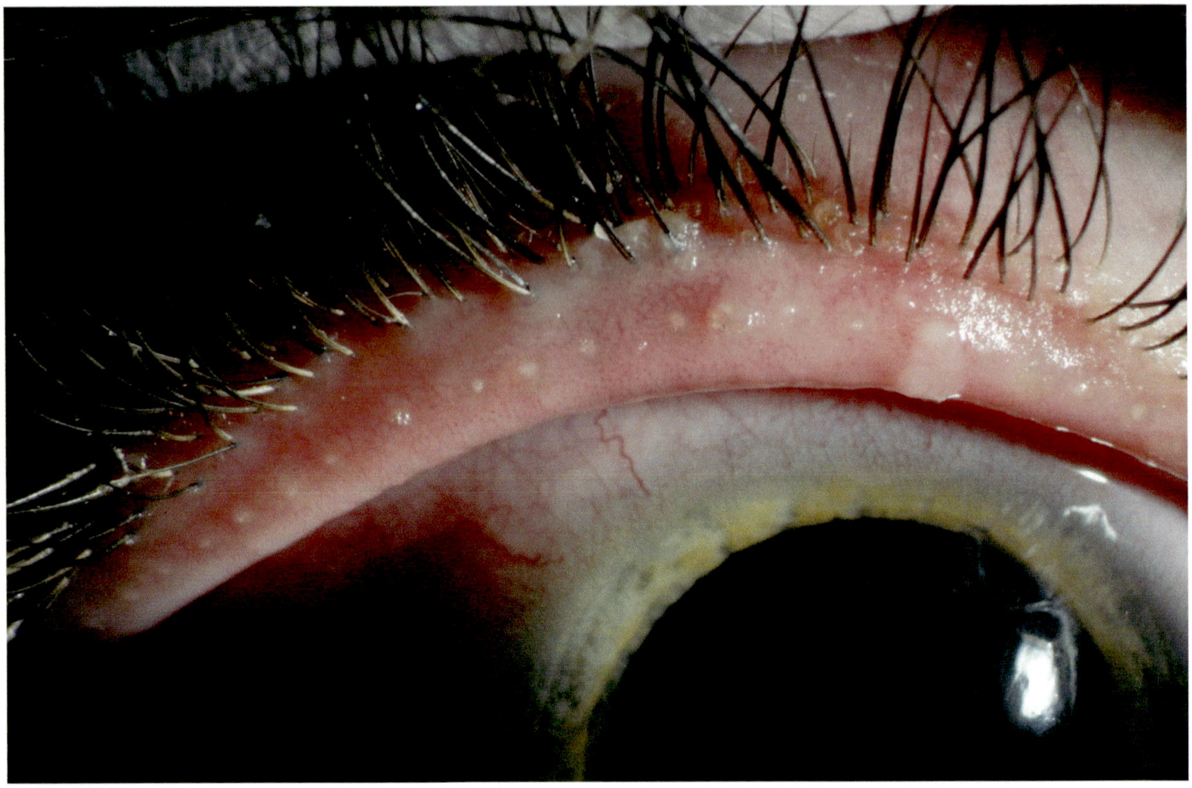

Fig. 18 (A) Blepharokeratoconjunctivitis in 8-year-old child. Massive blepharitis with obstructed meibomian glands and collarette formation around lash bases

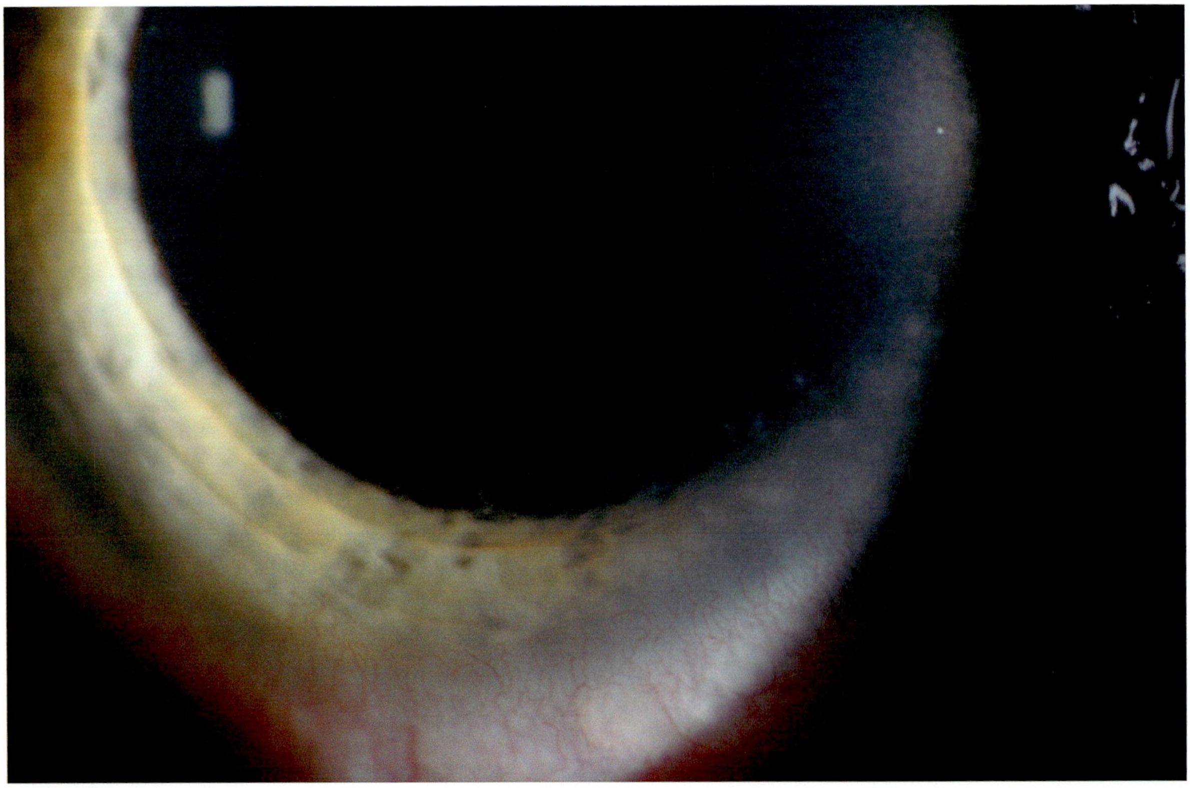

Fig. 18 (B) Blepharokeratoconjunctivitis in 8-year-old child. Corneal epithelial and subepithelial corneal infiltrates inferiorly

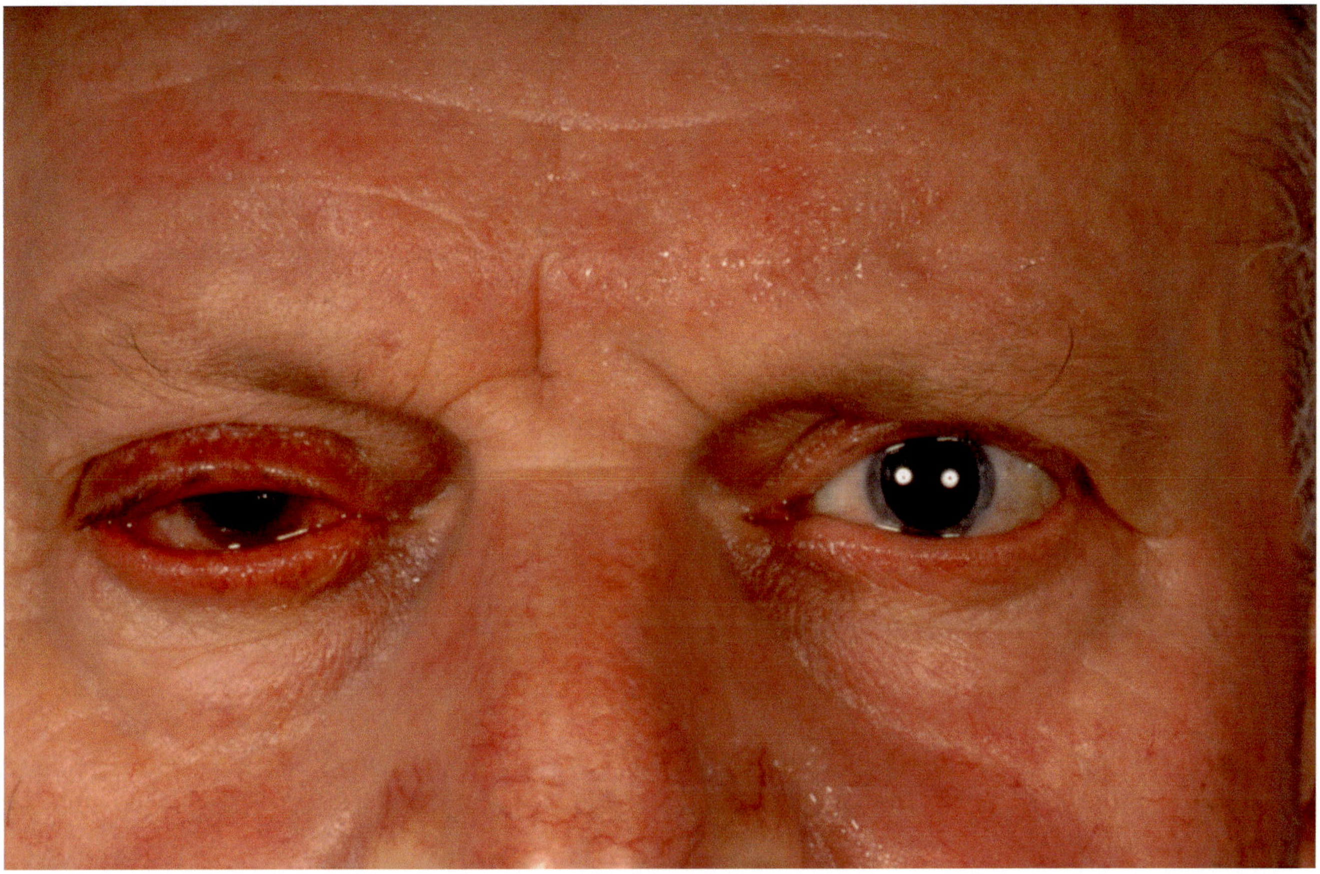

Fig. 19 Meibomian gland carcinoma OD imitating unilateral blepharitis

damage from an exaggerated and immature immune adaptive response against these bacterial components.

Unilateral blepharitis is uncommon. Meibomian gland carcinoma must be ruled out (Fig. 19).

3 Conclusion

Dry Eye Disease (DED) is common with a worldwide prevalence of 5 to 34%. Aqueous deficient DED is characterized by reduced tear production as well as ocular surface corneal staining and may be associated with autoimmune disease such as Sjögren disease. It may progress to filamentary keratitis, corneal ulceration, and perforation. Hyperevaporative DED due to MGD presents with typical pathology in lid margins, meibomian gland secretions, and with a reduced tear film quality. MGD may be associated with dermatological disease such as rosacea and seborrheic dermatitis and may be complicated by corneal infiltrates, ulceration, and neovascularization. Hordeola and chalazia may form. MGD or frank blepharitis may be induced or worsened by Demodex hyperinfestation. Blepharokeratoconjunctivitis is also a childhood disease and may be quite treatment refractory. Unilateral blepharitis is rare and may be caused by underlying meibomian gland carcinoma.

References

1. Bron AJ, de Paiva CS, Chauhan SK, et al. TFOS DEWS II pathophysiology report. Ocul Surf. 2017;15:438–510.
2. Craig JP, Nichols KK, Akpek EK, et al. TFOS DEWS II definition and classification report. Ocul Surf. 2017;15:276–83.
3. Fromstein SR, Harthan JS, Patel J, Opitz DL. Demodex blepharitis: clinical perspectives. Clin Optom (Auckl) 2018;10:57–63
4. Geerling G, Tauber J, Baudouin C, et al. The international workshop on meibomian gland dysfunction: report of the subcommittee on management and treatment of meibomian gland dysfunction. Invest Ophthalmol Vis Sci. 2011;52:2050–64.
5. Gupta N, Dhawan A, Beri S, D'souza P. Clinical spectrum of pediatric blepharokeratoconjunctivitis. J AAPOS. 2010;14:527–9.
6. Jones L, Downie LE, Korb D, et al. TFOS DEWS II management and therapy report. Ocul Surf. 2017;15:575–628.
7. Knop E, Knop N, Millar T, et al. The international workshop on meibomian gland dysfunction: report of the subcommittee on anatomy, physiology, and pathophysiology of the meibomian gland. Invest Ophthalmol Vis Sci. 2011;52:1938–78.
8. Messmer EM. The pathophysiology, diagnosis, and treatment of dry eye disease. Dtsch Arztebl Int. 2015;112:71–81.

9. Nelson JD, Shimazaki J, Benitez-del-Castillo JM, et al. The international workshop on meibomian gland dysfunction: report of the definition and classification subcommittee. Invest Ophthalmol Vis Sci. 2011;52:1930–7.
10. Rodriguez-Garcia A, Gonzalez-Godinez S, Lopez-Rubio S. Blepharokeratoconjunctivitis in childhood: corneal involvement and visual outcome. Eye. 2016;30:438–46.
11. Shah PP, Stein RL, Perry HD. Update on the management of Demodex Blepharitis. Cornea. 2022;41:934–9.
12. Schaumberg DA, Nichols JJ, Papas EB, et al. The international workshop on meibomian gland dysfunction: report of the subcommittee on the epidemiology of, and associated risk factors for. MGD Invest Ophthalmol Vis Sci. 2011;52:1994–2005.
13. Shields JA, Saktanasate J, Lally SE, Carrasco JR, Shields CL. Sebaceous carcinoma of the ocular region: the 2014 professor Winifred Mao lecture. Asia Pac J Ophthalmol (Phila). 2015;4:221–7.
14. Sobolewska B, Schaller M, Zierhut M. Rosacea and dry eye disease. Ocul Immunol Inflamm. 2022;30:570–9.
15. Tavassoli S, Wong N, Chan E. Ocular manifestations of rosacea: a clinical review. Clin Exp Ophthalmol. 2021;49:104–17.
16. Tomlinson A, Bron AJ, Korb DR, et al. The international workshop on Meibomian gland dysfunction: report of the diagnosis subcommittee. Invest Ophthalmol Vis Sci. 2011;52:2006–49.
17. Wolffsohn JS, Arita R, Chalmers R, et al. TFOS DEWS II diagnostic methodology report. Ocul Surf. 2017;15:539–74.

Ocular Graft-versus-Host Disease GvHD

Philipp Steven, Volkan Tahmaz, and Leonie Menghesha

Abstract

This chapter describes a very common, severe complication after allogeneic hematopoetic stem cell transplantation (aHSCT). Ocular graft-versus-host disease (oGVHD) is an autoimmunological entity that occurs in up to 60% of patients after aHSCT. Due to its fast onset and rapid progression, oGVHD may lead to severe tissue damage, consecutive loss of visual function and pain and therefore significant reduction of quality-of-life. Examples of different forms and stages of oGVHD are presented and supplemented with therapeutic suggestions.

Keywords

Ocular graft-versus-host disease · Bone marrow transplantation · Allogeneic hematopoetic stem cell transplantation · Complications · Dry eye

1 Introduction

Ocular graft-versus-host disease (oGVHD) is one of the most common complications following allogeneic hematopoetic stem cell transplantation (aHSCT) for treatment of hemato-oncological malignancies. Patients develop oGVHD in up to 60% of the cases.

P. Steven (✉) · V. Tahmaz · L. Menghesha
Department of Internal Medicine I and Department of Ophthalmology, Medical Faculty, University Hospital of Cologne, Cologne, Germany
e-mail: philipp.steven@uk-koeln.de

2 Acute oGVHD

As early as several weeks to 2–3 months after aHSCT acute oGVHD develops in presumably 10% of the patients [1, 2]. Acute oGVHD is characterized by unspecific chemosis, mimicking allergic conjunctivitis, which is often unresponsive to topical anti-allergic medication. More severe cases demonstrate (pseudo-) membranous conjunctivitis, which responds to high-frequency topical steroids [3] (Figs. 1, 2, 3 and 4).

3 Chronic oGVHD

Far more common, chronic oGVHD develops mainly between 5–25 months after aHSCT [4, 5]. The current understanding of chronic GVHD consists of 3 pathologically distinct phases of disease: 1: Tissue damage and acute inflammatory response due to chemotherapy, irradiation and conditioning regimen, 2. Chronic inflammation with immune cell proliferation and loss of peripheral immunological tolerance and 3. Fibrosis and deposition of immunoglobulins [6]. Clinically, chronic oGVHD may onset with mild blepharitis, keratitis, conjunctivitis and reduced tearfilm stability and volume, appearing as generic dry eye disease [7, 8]. However, typically disease progresses rapidly towards severe blepharitis, meibomian gland loss [9], severe conjunctivitis and keratitis, superior limbal keratoconjunctivitis and complete failure of tear production. Conjunctival scarring and fornix shortening occurs in some patients (Figs. 5, 6, 7, and 8).

Diagnosis of chronic oGVHD is often delayed, as symptoms may start slightly and remain undetected or unnoticed due to other more pressing topics following aHSCT such as skin GVHD, adjustment of systemic medications and low frequency ophthalmic consultations [10]. Therefore, it is recommended to perform eye examinations before and after aHSCT at defined timepoints to detect pathological changes as early as possible and to start aggressive

B. Seitz et al. (eds.), *Atlas on Cornea*, https://doi.org/10.1007/978-3-031-65422-0_28

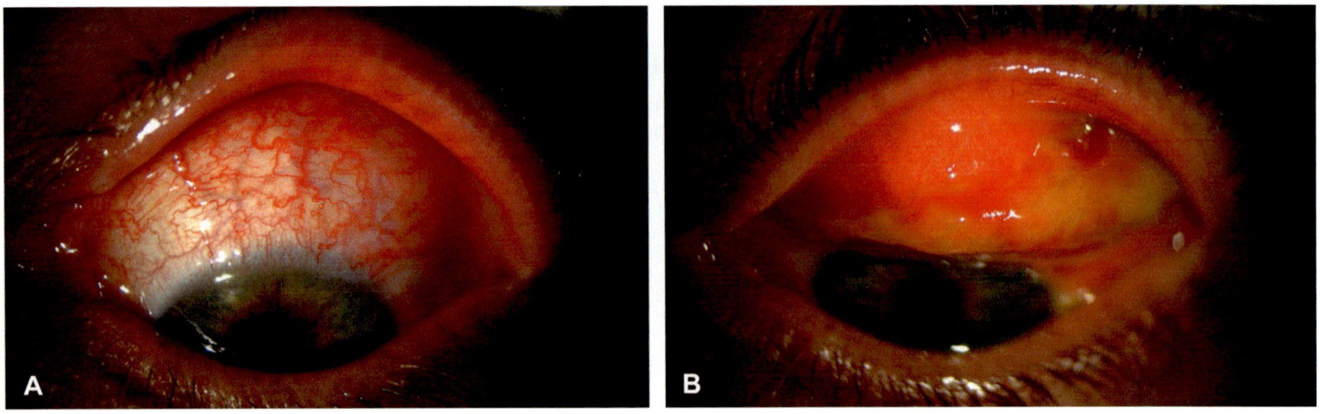

Fig. 1 Acute oGVHD in a 36-year-old patient, 3 months after aHSCT due to acute myeloid leukemia. (**A**) Severe conjunctivitis with increased blood flow and tortuous vessels, (**B**) Membranes of the upper tarsal conjunctiva. Improvement with residual scarring was achieved with topical treatment using high dose corticosteroids over 4 weeks, short term antibiotics for 5 days and lubrication using artificial tears and ointments

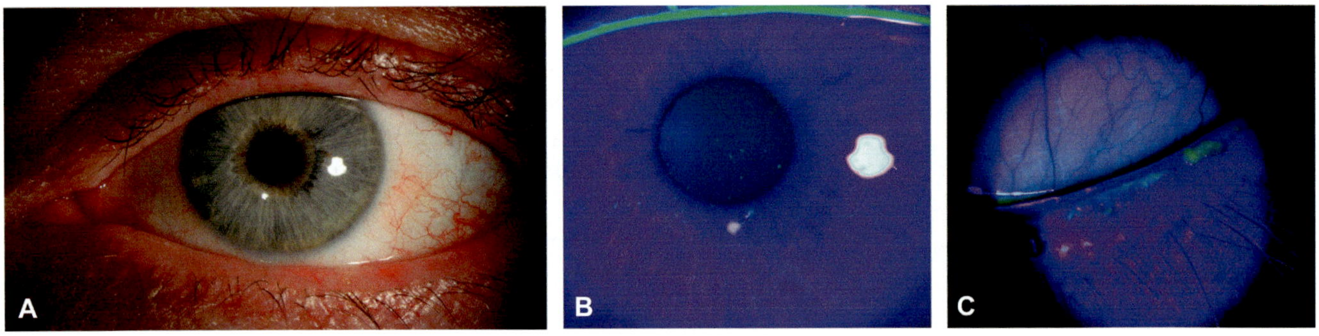

Fig. 2 Mild chronic oGVHD (**A**) unobtrusive anterior segment in slit lamp microscopy. (**B**) mild corneal fluoresceine staining. (**C**) anterior dislocation of Marx line with mild signs of blepharitis. Despite limited signs of ocular surface inflammation, immediate therapy using local anti-inflammatory medication in addition to artificial tears is mandatory and should be closely monitored. Male patient, 47 years, 2 years after aHSCT due to acute lymphatic leukemia

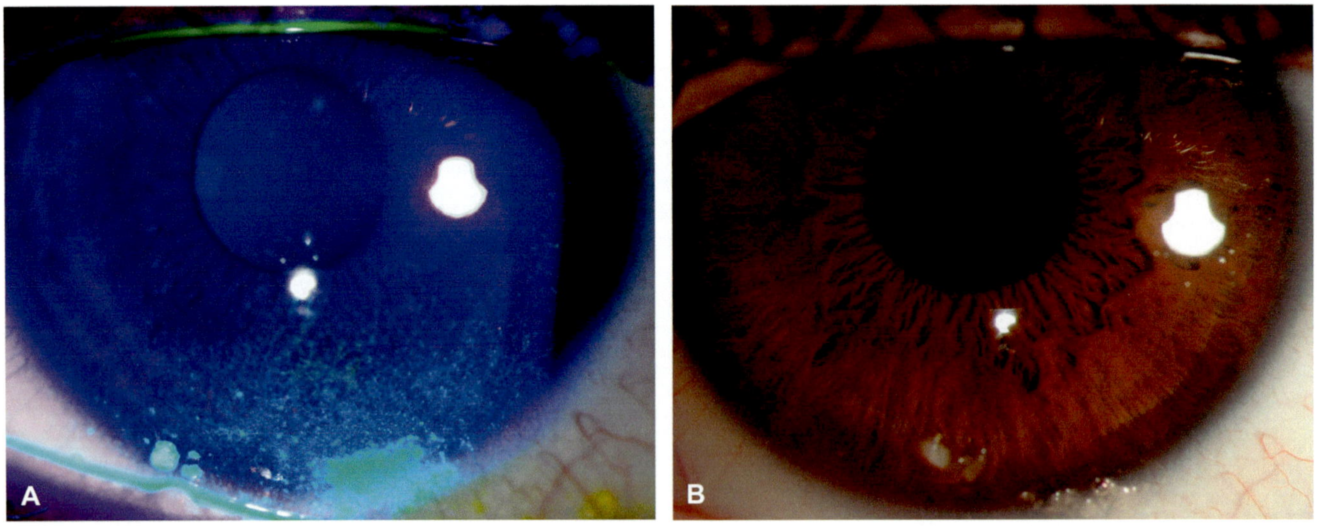

Fig. 3 Corneal epitheliopathy is a key finding in chronic oGVHD. Grading should always performed using intravital staining, e.g. with fluoresceine dye (**A**) as slitlamp biomicroscopy (**B**) may lead to underestimation of epithelial barrier impairment. Male patient, 25 years, 3 years after aHSCT due to Hodgkin Lymphoma

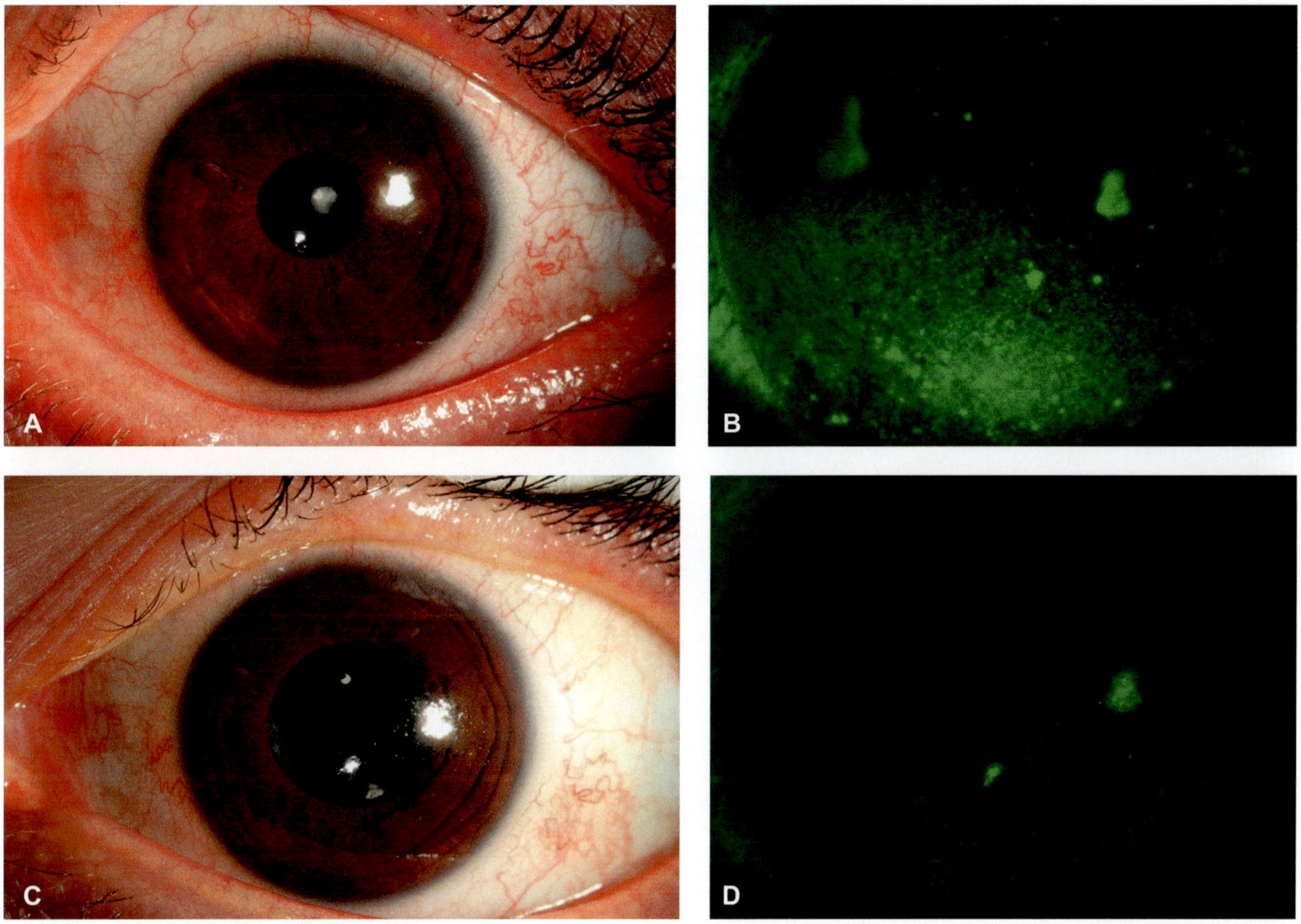

Fig. 4 (**A+B**) Severe corneal epitheliopathy (grade 5, Oxford grading scheme) in a 36-year-old female patient, 9 years after aHSCT due to acute myeloid leukemia. (**C+D**) Topical cyclosporine 3x/day for 3 months, additional topical corticosteroids 2x/day and intensive application of artificial tears lead to significant improvement with reduced redness and corneal staining

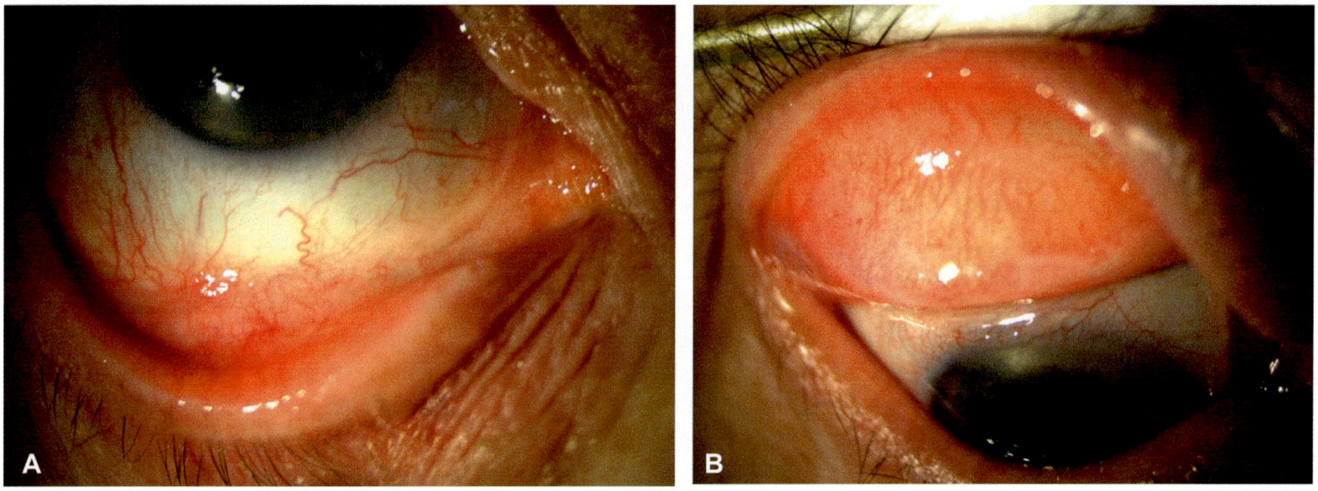

Fig. 5 Female patient, 75 years, 6 years after aHSCT due to myelodysplastic syndrome. Cicatrization and shortening of inferior fornix (**A**) and scarring of tarsal conjunctiva (**B**)

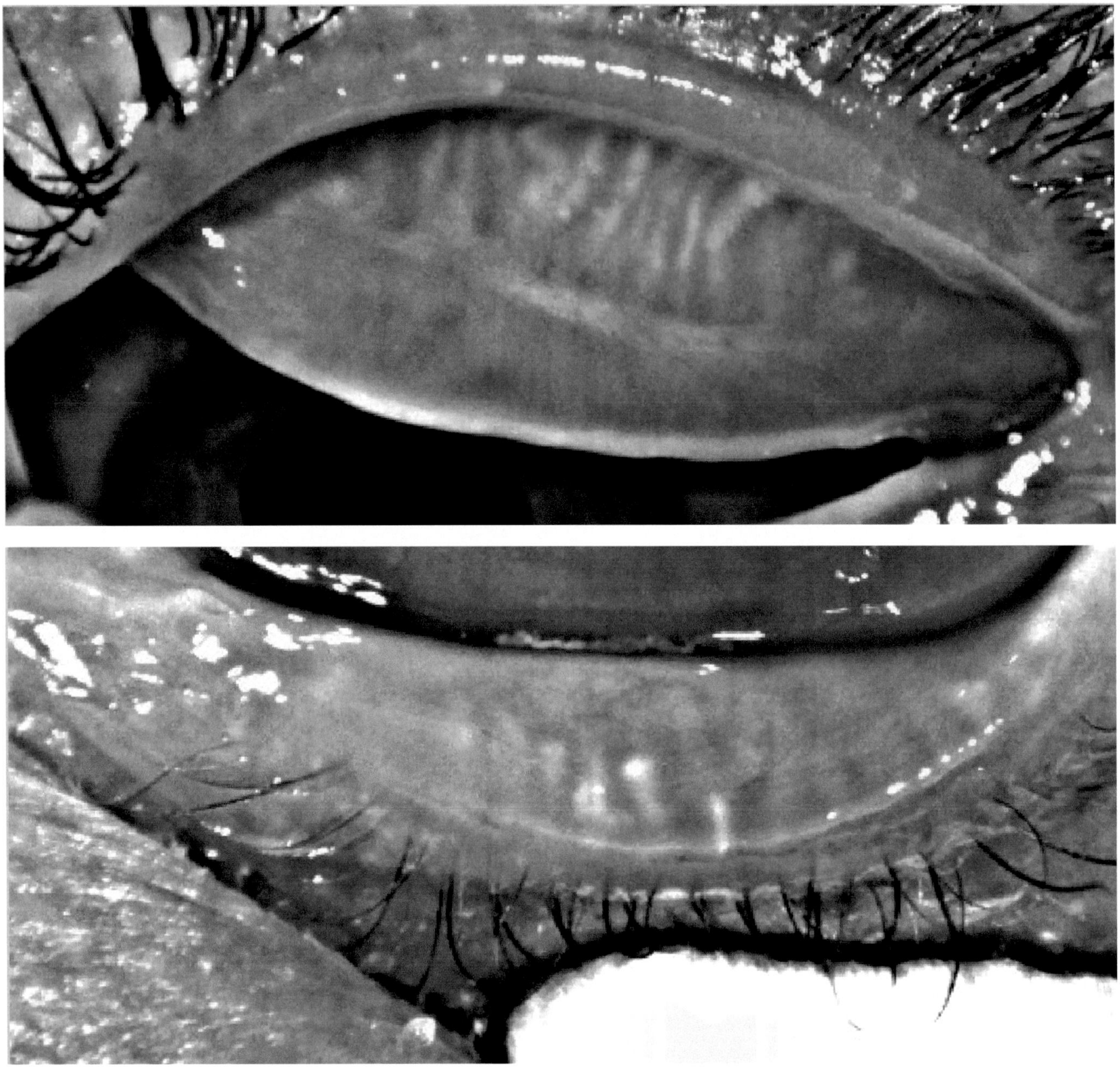

Fig. 6 Significant loss of meibomian glands of upper and lower eye lid in a 51-year-old female patient, 1 year after aHSCT due to acute myeloid leukemia

treatment within the "window-of-opportunity" [11]. This regimen enhances the chance to slow-down, delay or even prevent severe disease progress. Treatments include lubrication with eye drops and/or ointments [12], topical immunosuppressive drugs such as corticosteroids and cyclosporine and in more severe cases regenerative treatment approaches using blood-derived eye drops (serum or plasma eye drops) [13] or most recently Insulin eye drops. Other therapeutic options include scleral contact lenses [14] and some centers use punctual plugs [15] (Figs. 9, 10, 11 and 12).

Untreated, chronic oGVHD often progresses very fast into severe disease states with high inflammatory activity leading to increased and irreversible tissue damage. Severe epithelial barrier dysfunction increases the risk for infections, corneal scarring and neovascularization and consecutive loss of vision. The vastly impaired function of the main lacrimal gland together with loss of meibomian glands and destruction of the lid margin structure causes a severe aqueous-deficient and evaporative dry eye phenotype and consecutive discomfort, burning, dryness up to

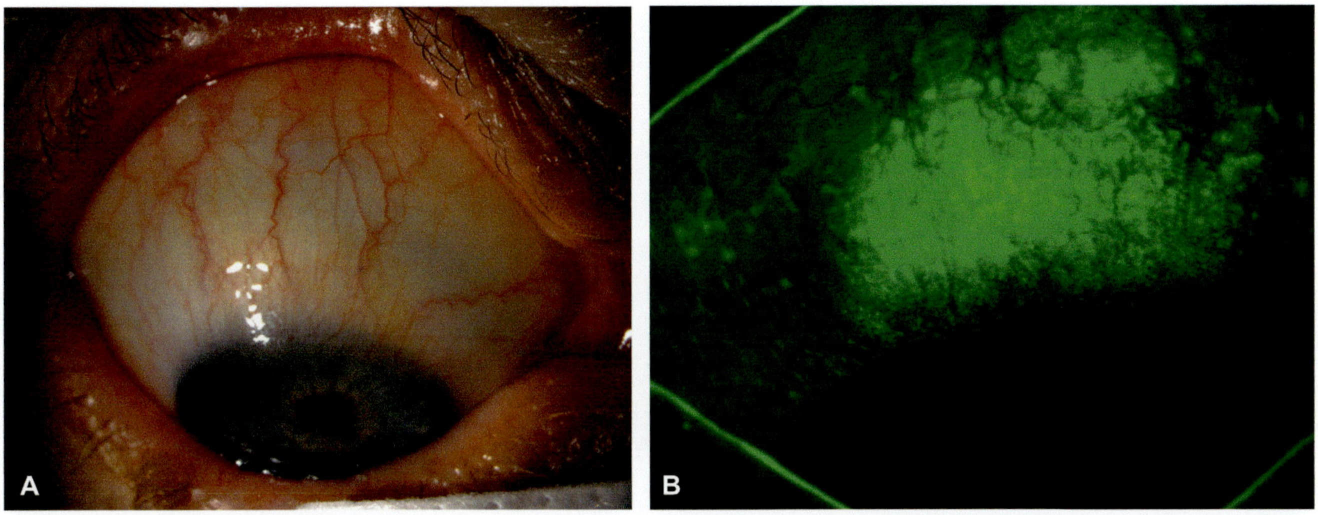

Fig. 7 Superior limbal keratokonjunctivitis is a very frequent finding in chronic oGVHD, but is often overlooked in slit lamp examination. 66-year-old male patient, 20 years after aHSCT due to osteomyelofibrosis. (**A**) Right eye in downward gaze with slightly increased conjunctival blood vessels. (**B**) Fluoresceine staining reveals severe superior limbal keratokonjunctivitis

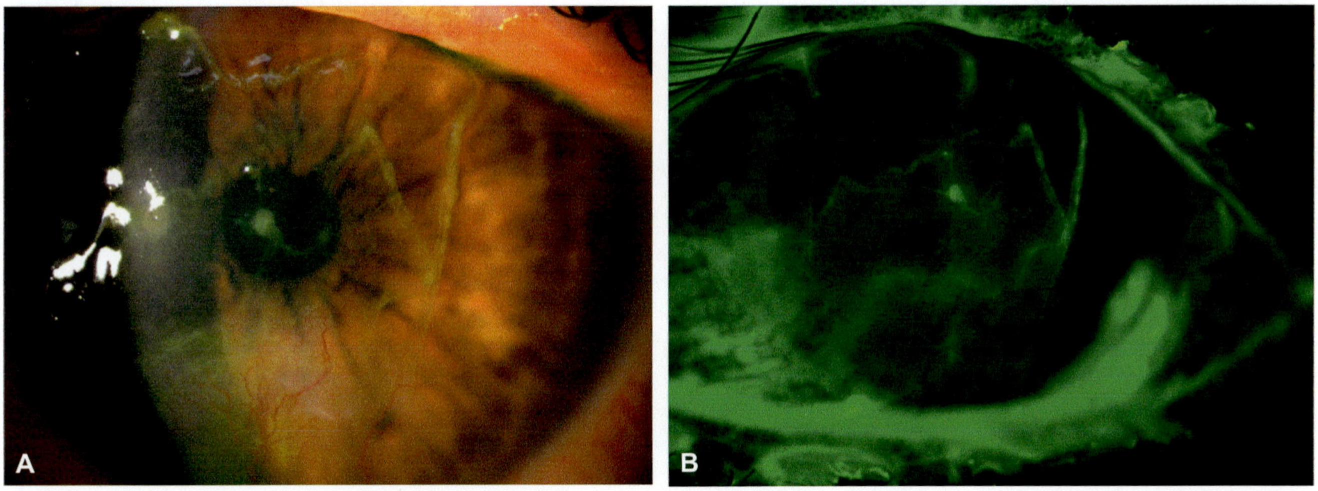

Fig. 8 Activation of the innate immune system is part of oGVHD pathogenesis. Nuclear extracellular traps (NETs) are extracellular DNA strands, that are excessively secreted by neutrophils and visible as sticky webs on the ocular surface (**A+B**) [21]. Microbiology revealed very sporadic S. aureus in conjunctival swabs. Therapy in this 28-year-old female patient, 4 years after aHSCT due to pro-B-acute lymphatic leukemia included topical corticosteroids, antibiotics, heparin and acetylcysteine eye drops

pain sensation. Severe chronic oGVHD leads to disabilities to read, drive, perform daily life tasks and may lead to immobilization and repeated phases of hospitalization [16].

Complications such as corneal perforation [17] should be avoided at all costs, as penetrating keratoplasty often fails due to impaired epithelial wound healing and increased risk of graft rejection.

It has to be noted, that oGVHD may also affect the posterior segment [18]. Furthermore, the requirement of high dose systemical steroids enhance the risk of secondary glaucoma and cataract development [19]. Cataract surgery has a higher risk of complications and extended peri-operative care should be applied [20].

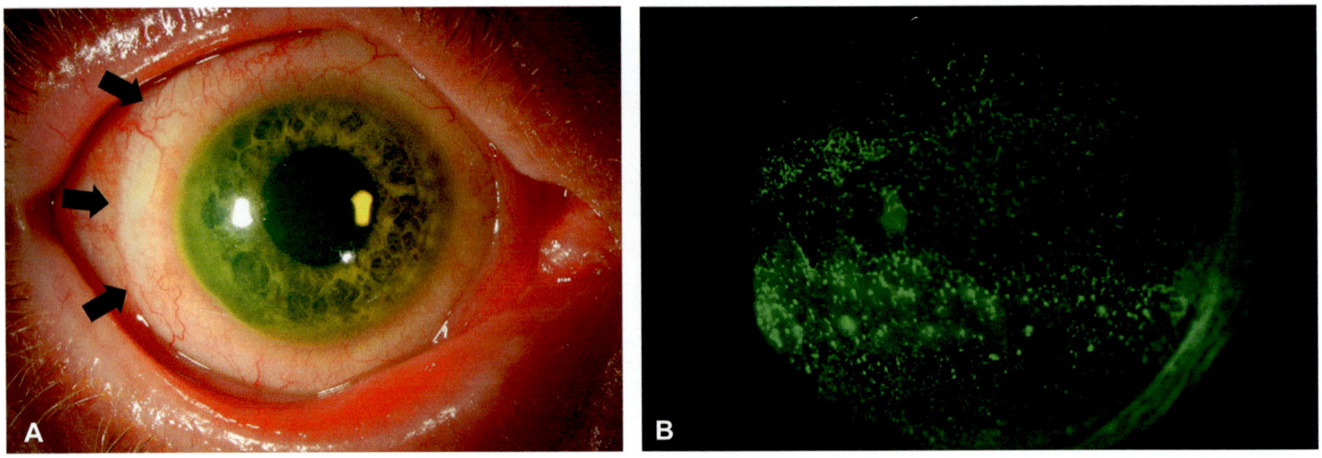

Fig. 9 Fitting of scleral contact lenses (arrows) is a feasible therapeutic option. Scleral lenses are large rigid lenses, in which the haptic is located on the conjunctiva/sclera (**A**) arrows and a reservoir between cornea and lens is filled with saline or artificial tears. Scleral lenses may be used in patients with severe corneal epitheliopathy (**B**) to improve vision as they cover the cornea without contact

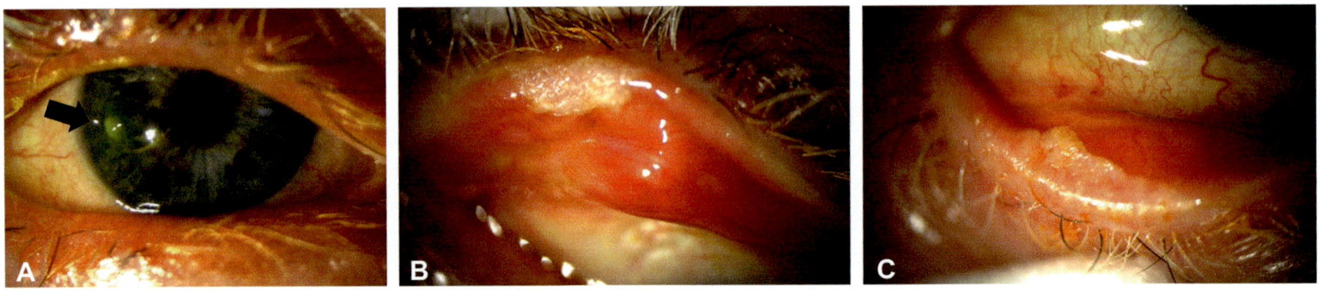

Fig. 10 Corneal perforation (**A**) (arrow) and metaplastic transformation (**B, C**) of upper and lower lid margins of the right eye. 51-year-old female patient, 2 years after aHSCT due to acute myeloid leukemia

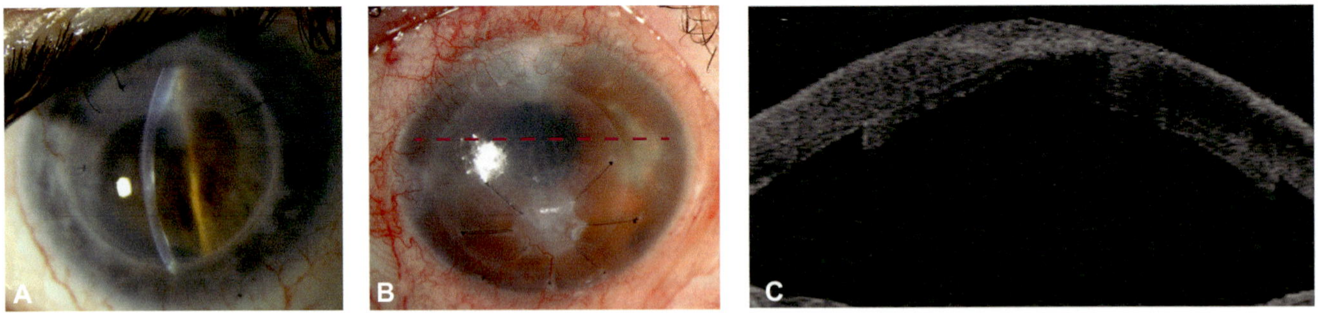

Fig. 11 High-risk corneal surgery in chronic oGVHD. (**A**) Penetrating keratoplasty was performed 3 times after previous 4x amniotic membrane transplantation and crosslinking after autologous transplantation of the submandibular gland and development of non-healing corneal ulcerations. After endothelial failure, the 60-year-old male patient (aHSCT 2011 due to plasmocytoma) was lost to follow-up. (**B**) 70-year-old male patient, 5 years after aHSCT due to acute myeloid leukemia, developed corneal decompensation, a non-healing epithelial defect and stromal melting after cataract surgery. Treatment included amniotic membrane transplantation and DSAEK (red dotted line: section plane for (**C**). (**C**) OCT image of B demonstrating DSAEK lamella attached to the posterior surface of the cornea

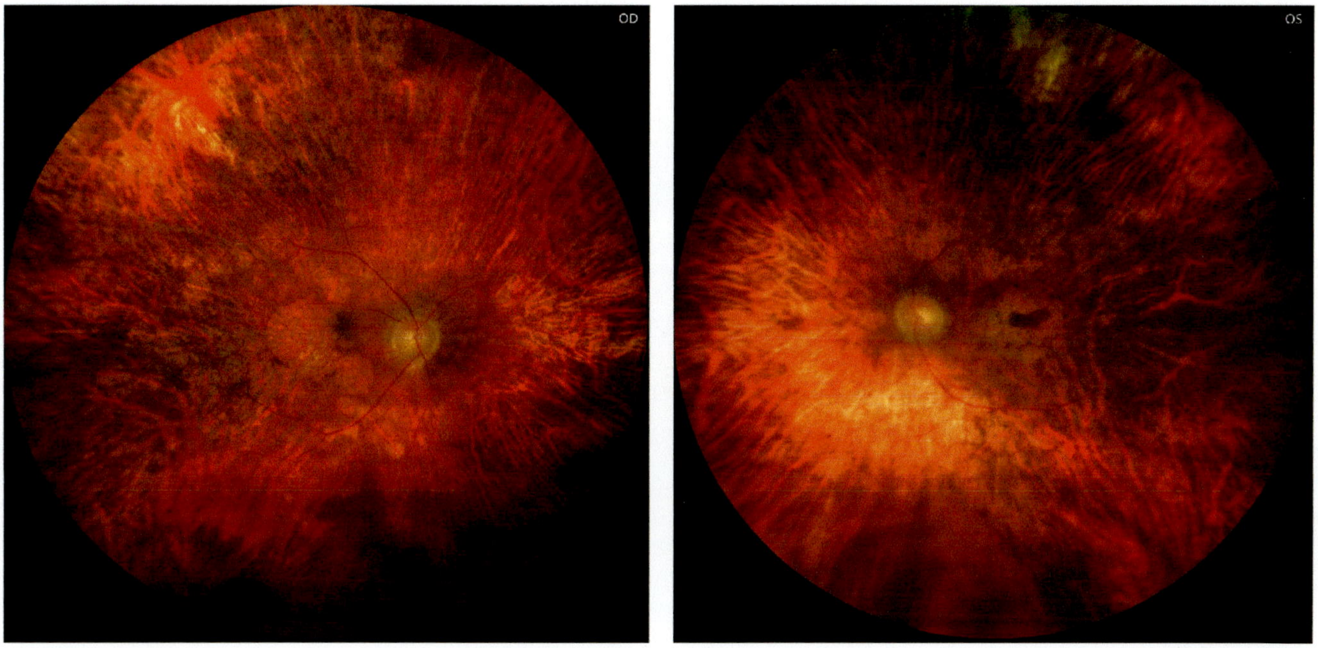

Fig. 12 Ocular GVHD is not restricted to the ocular surface, but may also affect the retina. Right and left eye of a 74-year-old male patient, 18 years after aHSCT due to osteomyelofibrosis who developed a non-infectious, panuveitis, treated with repeated intravitreal injections of corticosteroids

4 Conclusion

The entire eye needs to be examined at each appointment following aHSCT and ocular GVHD should not be treated as generic forms of dry eye but aggressively under increased awareness.

References

1. Kitko CL, Pidala J, Schoemans HM, Lawitschka A, Flowers ME, Cowen EW, et al. National institutes of health consensus development project on criteria for clinical trials in chronic graft-versus-host disease: IIa. The 2020 clinical implementation and early diagnosis working group report. Transplant Cell Ther. 2021;27(7):545–57.
2. Wolff D, Radojcic V, Lafyatis R, Cinar R, Rosenstein RK, Cowen EW, et al. national institutes of health consensus development project on criteria for clinical trials in chronic graft-versus-host disease: IV. The 2020 highly morbid forms report. Transplant Cell Ther. 2021;27(10):817–35.
3. Liu YC, Gau JP, Lin PY, Liu CJ, Liu CJ, Liu JH, et al. Conjunctival acute graft-versus-host disease in adult patients receiving allogeneic hematopoietic stem cell transplantation: a cohort study. PLoS ONE. 2016;11(11): e0167129.
4. Filipovich AH. Diagnosis and manifestations of chronic graft-versus-host disease. Best Pract Res Clin Haematol. 2008;21(2):251–7.
5. Kim SK, Smith JA, Dunn JP. Chronic Ocular Graft versus Host Disease. In: Vogelsang GB, Pavletic SZ, editors. Chronic graft versus host disease: interdisciplinary management. New York: Cambridge University Press; 2009. p. 199–206.
6. Zeiser R, Blazar BR. Pathophysiology of chronic graft-versus-host disease and therapeutic targets. N Engl J Med. 2017;377(26):2565–79.
7. Siebelmann S, Jing B, Cursiefen C, Steven P. Non-invasive diagnosis of ocular graft-versus-host disease. Klin Monbl Augenheilk. 2015;232(5):652–7.
8. Dietrich-Ntoukas T, Cursiefen C, Westekemper H, Eberwein P, Reinhard T, Bertz H, et al. Diagnosis and treatment of ocular chronic graft-versus-host disease: report from the German-Austrian-Swiss consensus conference on clinical practice in chronic GVHD. Cornea. 2012;31(3):299–310.
9. Engel LA, Wittig S, Bock F, Sauerbier L, Scheid C, Holtick U, et al. Meibography and meibomian gland measurements in ocular graft-versus-host disease. Bone Marrow Transplant. 2015;50(7):961–7.
10. Rapoport Y, Freeman T, Koyama T, Engelhardt BG, Jagasia M, Savani BN, et al. Validation of international chronic ocular graft-versus-host disease (GVHD) group diagnostic criteria as a chronic ocular GVHD-specific metric. Cornea. 2017;36(2):258–63.
11. S1-Leitlinie Okuläre graft-versus-host-Erkrankung. S1-guideline DOG BVA. 1.1 ed: AWMF; 2020.
12. Steven P, Augustin AJ, Geerling G, Kaercher T, Kretz F, Kunert K, et al. Semifluorinated alkane eye drops for treatment of dry eye disease due to Meibomian gland disease. J Ocul Pharmacol Ther. 2017.
13. Tahmaz V, Gehlsen U, Sauerbier L, Holtick U, Engel L, Radojska S, et al. Treatment of severe chronic ocular graft-versus-host disease using 100% autologous serum eye drops from a sealed manufacturing system: a retrospective cohort study. Br J Ophthalmol. 2016.
14. Jacobs DS, Rosenthal P. Boston scleral lens prosthetic device for treatment of severe dry eye in chronic graft-versus-host disease. Cornea. 2007;26(10):1195–9.
15. Sabti S, Halter JP, Braun Frankl BC, Goldblum D. Punctal occlusion is safe and efficient for the treatment of keratoconjunctivitis

sicca in patients with ocular GvHD. Bone Marrow Transplant. 2012;47(7):981–4.
16. Sun YC, Chai X, Inamoto Y, Pidala J, Martin PJ, Flowers ME, et al. Impact of Ocular Chronic Graft-versus-Host Disease on Quality of Life. Biol Blood Marrow Transplant. 2015;21(9):1687–91.
17. Inagaki E, Ogawa Y, Matsumoto Y, Kawakita T, Shimmura S, Tsubota K. Four cases of corneal perforation in patients with chronic graft-versus-host disease. Mol Vis. 2011;17:598–606.
18. Mirza N, Zierhut M, Korn A, Bornemann A, Vogel W, Schmid-Horch B, et al. Graft versus self (GvS) against T-cell autoantigens is a mechanism of graft-host interaction. Proc Natl Acad Sci U S A. 2016;113(48):13827–32.
19. Tichelli A, Gratwohl A, Egger T, Roth J, Prunte A, Nissen C, et al. Cataract formation after bone marrow transplantation. Ann Intern Med. 1993;119(12):1175–80.
20. Gehlsen U, Faust C, Blecha C, Dietrich-Ntoukas T, Eberwein P, Issleib S, et al. Outcomes and complications of cataract surgery in patients with chronic ocular graft-versus-host-disease-a multicenter, retrospective analysis. Graefes Arch Clin Exp Ophthalmol. 2022;260(8):2613–22.
21. Arafat SN, Robert MC, Abud T, Spurr-Michaud S, Amparo F, Dohlman CH, et al. Elevated neutrophil elastase in tears of ocular graft-versus-host disease patients. Am J Ophthalmol. 2017;176:46–52.

Vernal KeratoConjunctivitis VKC and Atopic KeratoConjunctivitis AKC

Uwe Pleyer

Abstract

Keratoconjunctivitis vernalis (VKC) and Atopic keratoconjunctivitis (AKC) are bilateral, recurrent disorders of the ocular surface that can lead to severe cornea alterations. Clinical characteristics are the formation of giant papillae in the tarsus region (diameter > 1 mm) and/or changes near the limbus ("trantas dots"). The etiology and pathophysiology remain unclear. Clinical findings and immunohistological examinations suggest that complex (both IgE-dependent and IgE-independent immunopathological) changes are involved. Predisposing factors include endocrine, genetic, neurogenic as well as environmental and socioeconomic influences. Whereas VKC affects mostly children and often has a self-limiting course, onset of AKC is commonly later and runs a prolonged clinical course. Clinically VKC and AKC are very similar and there is controversy regarding classification of both disorders. It has been proposed that VKC is a childhood form of AKC that evolves into AKC in adulthood.

Antihistamines, mast cell stabilizers and, if necessary, topical steroids have proven effective as acute therapy. However, this treatment approach is insufficient in severe cases and cannot completely avoid recurrence. Immunomodulators such as Ciclosporin A and tacrolimus are alternative agents, especially for long-term therapy. In AKC patients, vision-threatening complications occur including transformation to malignancies.

Keywords

Allergy · Corticosteroids · Cyclosporine A · Ocular allergy · Ocular surface · Vernal keratoconjunctivitis

1 Introduction

Vernal keratoconjunctivitis (VKC) and atopic keratoconjunctivitis (AKC) are recurrent bilateral inflammatory diseases of the ocular surface [1–3]. Clinically, these disorders share some similarities but there is controversy regarding classification of both entities. More recent concepts on the pathogenesis of these disorders indicate an impaired epithelial barrier that enhances allergen uptake, leading to activation of an overreacting immune response and chronic inflammation [4]. Epithelial barrier dysfunction has been recently implicated in the development of allergic diseases such as eczema and asthma [5]. In line with this background, further atopic diseases are often present in the history of affected individuals. This is especially true for AKC, where atopic dermatitis is a *conditio sine qua non*. The main criteria and differences between both entities are shown in Table 1 [2, 6].

2 VKC Clinical Findings and Diagnosis

The clinical presentation is characterized by three manifestations, which can be seen as:

1. Limbal
2. Tarsal or
3. Mixed type.

All three manifestations are associated with intense itching, redness, lacrimation, photophobia and a mucinous, viscous

U. Pleyer (✉)
Department of Ophthalmology, Charité—Universitätsmedizin Berlin, Corporate Member of Freie Universitaet Berlin, Humboldt Universitaet zu Berlin and Berlin Institute of Health, Campus Virchow Klinikum, Berlin, Germany
e-mail: uwe.pleyer@charite.de

B. Seitz et al. (eds.), *Atlas on Cornea*, https://doi.org/10.1007/978-3-031-65422-0_29

Table 1 Main clinical criteria and differences between Keratoconjunctivitis vernalis (VKC) and Atopic keratoconjunctivitis (AKC)

Feature	VKC	AKC
Age at beginning	**Predominantly in childhood**	**Teenagers, young adults**
Gender	**Boys > Girls**	**No gender dominance**
Seasonal	**Increased in spring**	**Perennial**
Lid findings consistence of secretion	**Viscous discharge**	**Often eczema, blepharitis rather "watery"**
Conjunctival scarring	–	**Conjunctival scarring Symblepharon possible**
"Horner-Trantas dots"	**Horner-Trantas dots as a typical finding may occur**	**Rare**
Corneal neovascularization	**Rare Vernalis Plaque**	**Stromal neovascularization in the late course**
Conjunctival smear	**Typical: Eosinophilic granulocytes**	**Rare: Eosinophilic granulocytes**
Prognosis	**Favorable often regression after puberty**	**Often chronically progressive often associated with Keratoconus, Cataract**

discharge [1–3]. Blepharospasm and blurring of vision often impair quality of life substantially and the term "morning misery" is perfectly well choosen.

2.1 Limbal VKC

Limbal VKC presents with small gelatinous, yellow-white deposits that occur at the limbal region, which are called "Horner-Trantas dots" (Fig. 1). They are initially found predominantly in the upper circumference and can subsequently affect the entire limbus. Morphologically, these are eosinophilic granulocytes and epithelial cell deposits. With adequate treatment, the lesions completely recede; in some patients a somewhat pale and scarred limbus remains (Fig. 2). It is still unclear whether the milder limbal VKC represents an early stage of the other two forms.

2.2 Tarsal VKC

In Europe, the tarsal form predominates, while limbal VKC is more common in Asia and Africa [1]. Giant papillae are the pathognomonic finding of the usually more severe tarsal VKC; therefore, the upper eyelid should always be "everted" (Fig. 3).

These "cobble stone-like changes" can range in size from 1 to 8 mm and correlate with persistence and severity of symptoms. Not infrequently, clinically a pseudoptosis may occur. In the acute stage, the giant papillae are covered by viscous discharge. During active exacerbations, giant papillae increase in size and shrink only slowly, even with adequate therapy. It is interesting to observe that after years, however, the papillae can also completely regress. Based on the clinical findings, Bonini et al. suggested a grading scale on the severity of VKC.

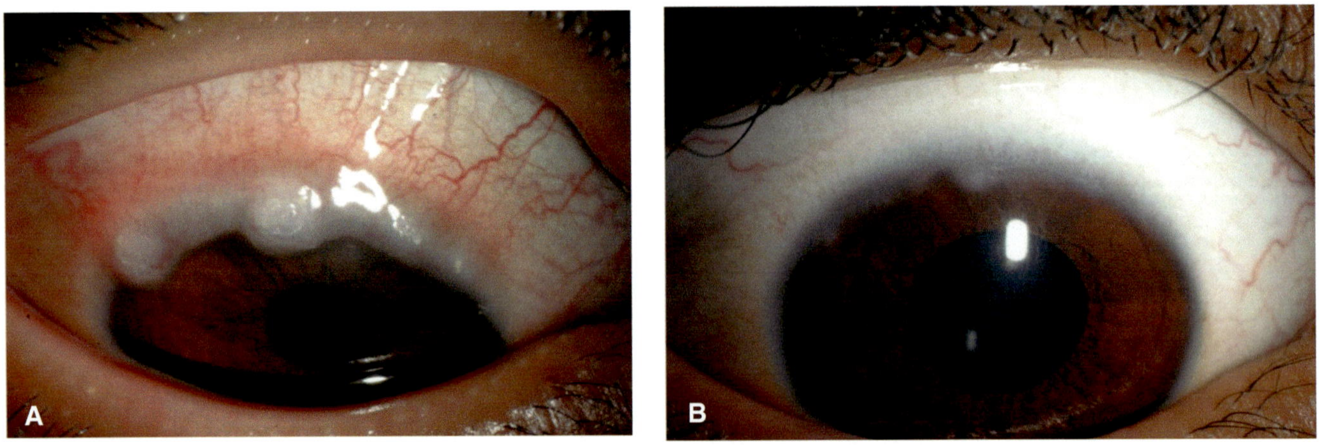

Fig. 1 (**A**) Horner-Trantas dots in a six-year girl with limbal vernal keratoconjunctivitis. (**B**) Following treatment with topical Loteprednol 1x/d combined with Cyclosporine A eye drops 1% 2x/d figure. From: Pleyer U, Leonardi A [3]

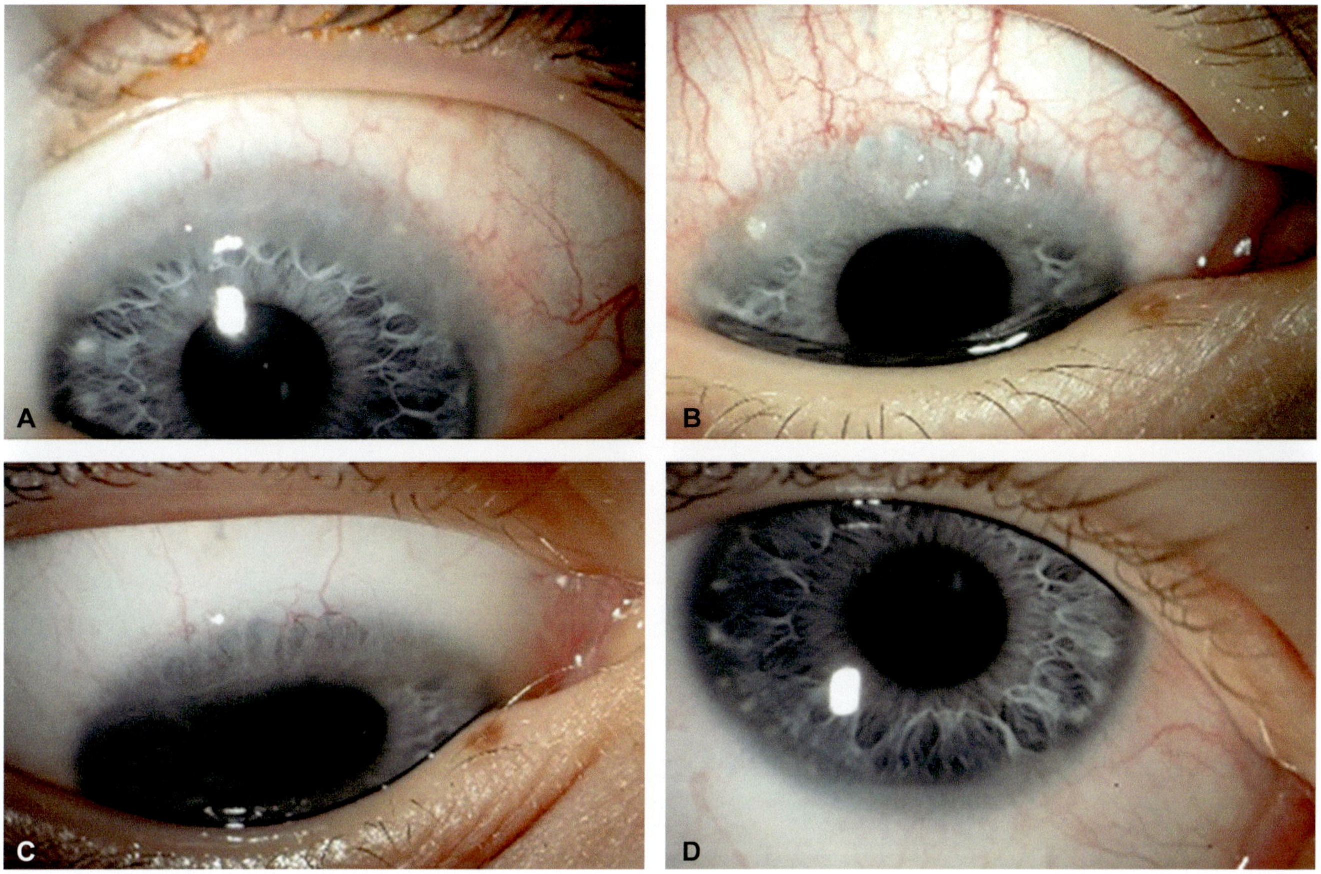

Fig. 2 (**A**, **B**) Bilateral Horner-Trantas dots in a 7-year-old-boy. (**C**, **D**) Following treatment with systemic Omalizumab (for concomitant allergic asthma). From: Rossberg S, Pleyer U, Lau S [13]

2.3 Corneal Involvement

Corneal findings vary due to the severity of the disease and are more frequent in tarsal VKC. Inflammatory changes of the entire ocular surface may lead to keratitis, punctate epithelial erosions and eventually to macro-erosions [3, 8]. Metalloproteinases and eosinophilic cationic protein are presumably involved in corneal damage and lead to persistence of the epithelial defect. In case of impaired wound healing, plaque-like lesions may result. Further progression leads to persistent Bowman layer erosion and a "shield ulcer" may develop (Fig. 4). These often oval-shaped defects are predominantly localized in the upper half of the cornea and sharply demarked. Shield ulcers are seen in about 5–10% of VKC cases [1, 3]. Long term healing often occurs with scarring and irregular astigmatism and leads to permanent visual impairment.

3 Diagnosis

The diagnosis of VKC is based on history, symptoms and findings. Not uncommon, the family history discloses that parents or siblings are (30–50%) also affected by atopy. Children often present already with further allergic diseases such as skin eczema (about 10%), rhinitis (20%) and asthma (up to about 30%) [3]. In some children, VKC precedes the remaining allergic manifestations. This association is more common in tarsal versus limbal VKC.

Further investigations are rarely indicated. Cytology or biopsy of the conjunctiva may reveal eosinophils and neutrophils. As a less invasive procedure tear fluid can be collected, with highly elevated IgE concentrations. Commercial kits are available for semi-quantitative testing.

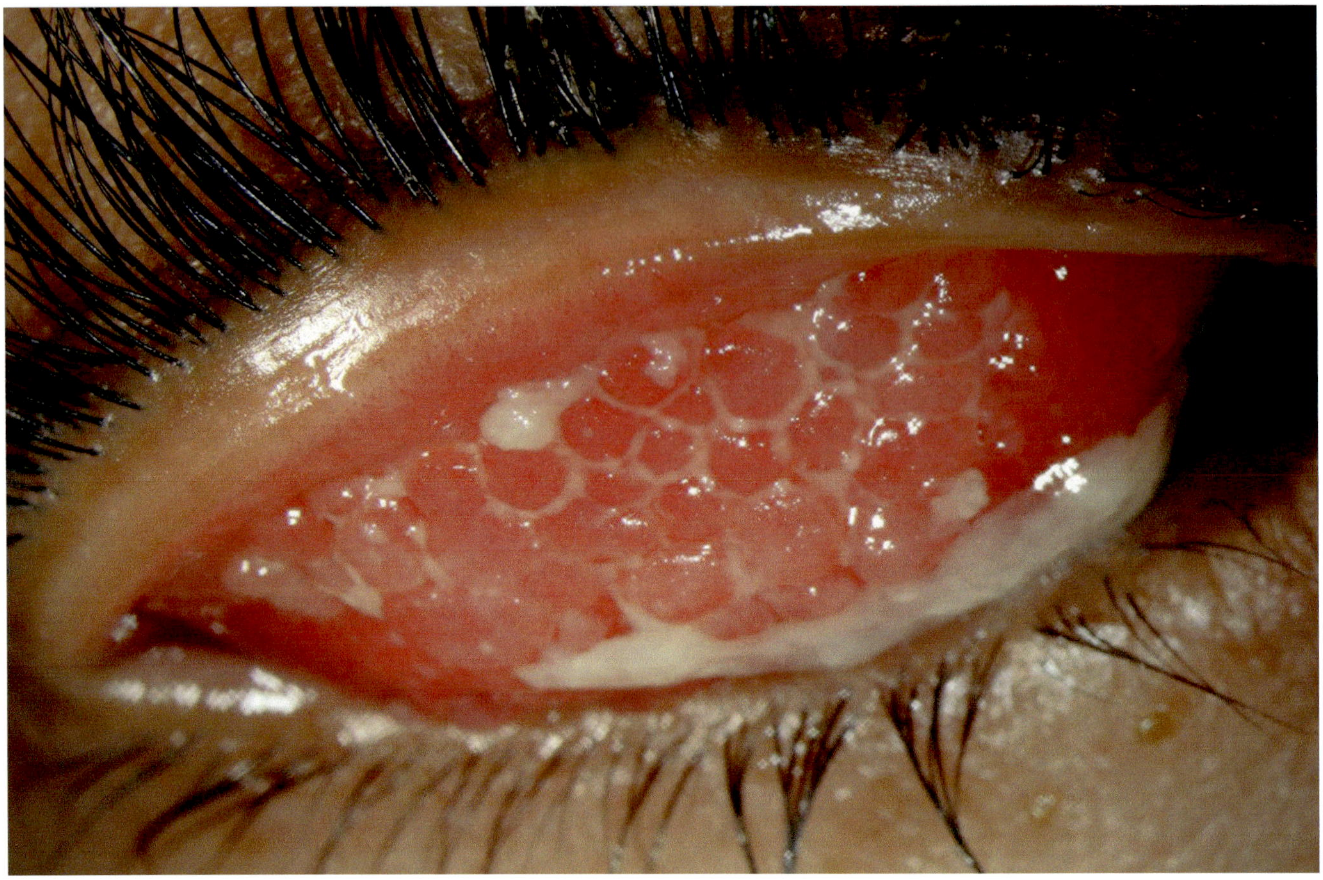

Fig. 3 Giant papillae in a 12-year-old boy suffering from tarsal vernal keratoconjunctivitis, following everted upper eye lid

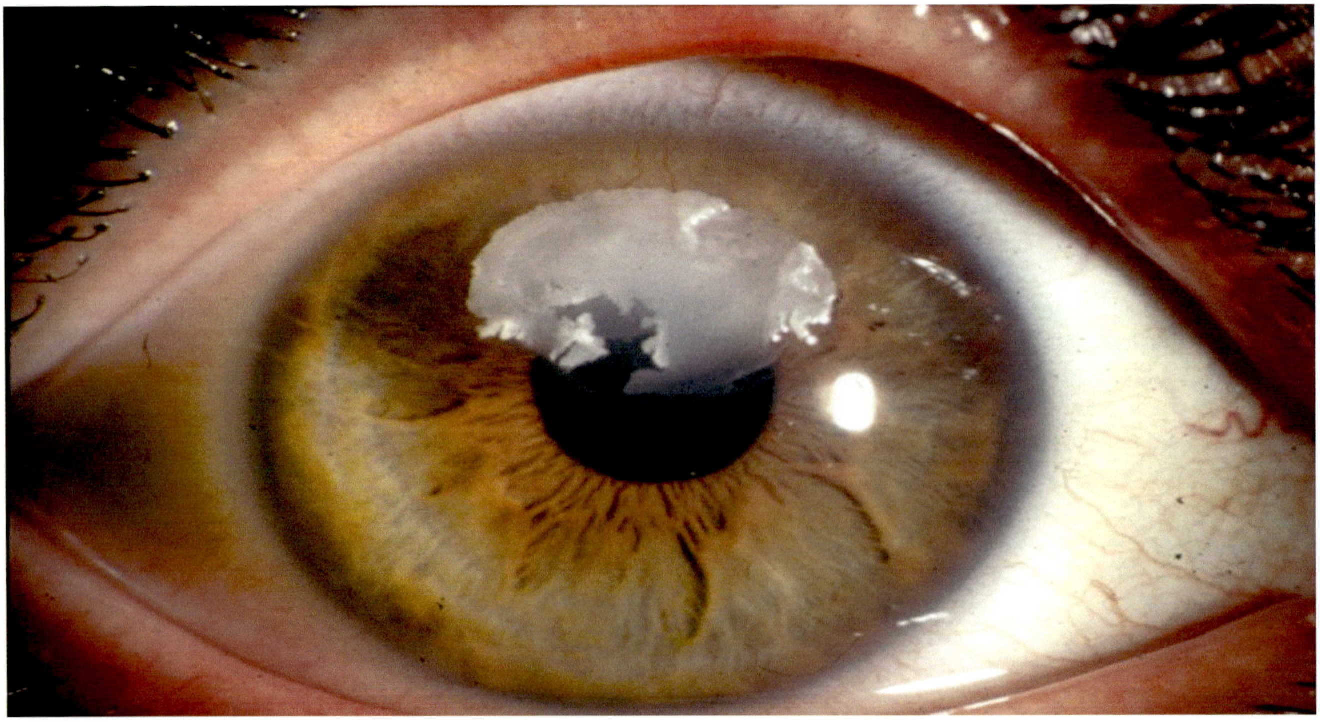

Fig. 4 "Shield ulcer" in a 7-year-old boy with tarsal vernal keratoconjunctivitis

4 Allergic Diagnostics

Conjunctival provocation test

About 15–20% of children react to topically applied (test) allergens at the conjunctiva. This diagnostic procedure is probably the most sensitive to support a specific sensitization and, if it may initiate specific immunotherapy. The test needs to be carried out in the non-irritant season [9].

Specific serum IgE

Examination of total and specific serum IgE may be diagnostically meaningful in VKC or AKC patients. Notable only about half of the patients have elevated, specific IgE values and the clinical course of IgE-positive and -negative children does not differ.

Differential diagnosis

Main differential diagnosis that have to be considered, are other allergic conditions, mainly AKC and giant papillary conjunctivitis, e.g. in contact lens wearers.

5 Conservative Therapy

Avoidance of any possible trigger (allergens) as well as conservative management such as cool compresses, lubricants and artificial tears are first line options [10].

A brief outline of a step latter treatment approach based on topical applied agents is provided in Fig. 5. Notable long-term immunomodulation with the calcineurin inhibitor cyclosporine A has been tested in RCTs and is FDA/EMA approved [11]. In severe affected children systemic therapy might be needed [12–14].

6 Surgical Treatment

In treatment-refractory courses, excision of giant papillae has occasionally been practiced and combined with mitomycin C or steroid injections into the tarsus [15]. CO_2 laser application has also be used to remove giant papillae. Cryocoagulation of the giant papillae is not recommended, since it often leads to pronounced scarring and fibrosis.

7 Shield Ulcer

If epithelial defects persist despite topical measures (lubricants, therapeutic contact lens), amniotic membrane transplants have proven successful. After debridement of plaque-like changes, re-epithelialization is usually achieved within a week. Limbus stem cell transplantation has also been used successfully [8, 16].

Local: Antihistamines, mast cell stabilizers.

Systemic: Antihistamines.

From grade 3: Topical cyclosporine A, tacrolimus, steroids, systemic specific immunotherapy.

8 Atopic Keratoconjunctivitis Clinical Findings and Diagnosis

Atopic keratoconjunctivitis (AKC) is a chronic ocular surface inflammatory disorder that, by definition is associated with atopic dermatitis [6]. Commonly there is a family

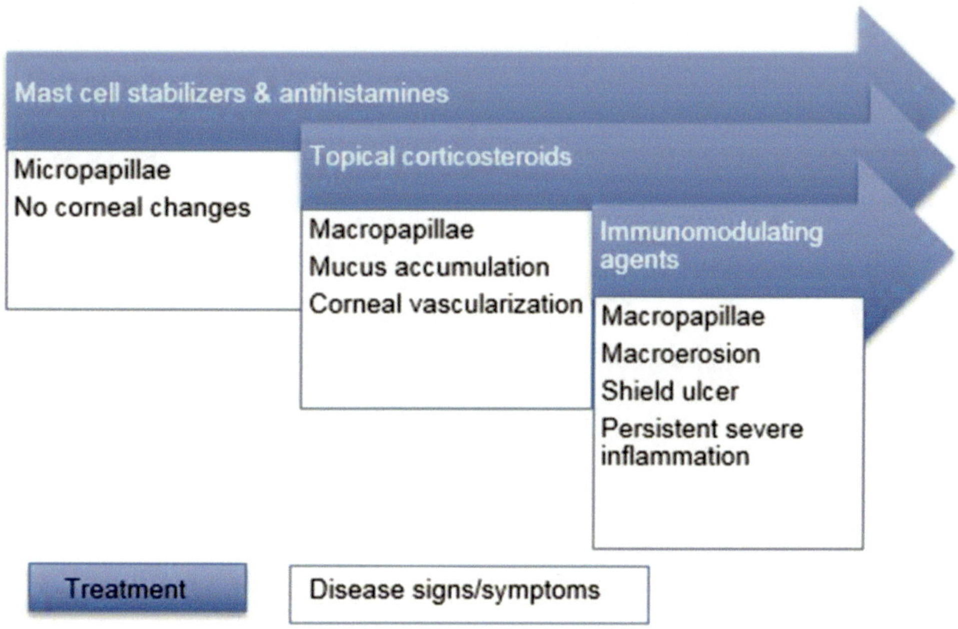

Fig. 5 "Step ladder" for conservative treatment approach in VKC patients

history with other allergic disorders e.g. asthma or urticaria. Interestingly AKC patients already are often affected by atopic dermatitis since childhood, whereas ocular involvement appears often decades later in life. Other associated disorders include asthma, allergic rhinitis and allergic response to environmental allergens.

Cardinal symptoms of AKC are similar to VKC patients including bilateral itching, tearing, photophobia and impaired vision [2, 17]. Important clinical findings are already visible in the periorbital (skin) region. Eczematous skin lesions, madarosis and chronic blepharitis are common (Fig. 6). Just like patients with VKC, there is often a viscous mucous secretion that can be interpreted as an activity sign of inflammation. Giant papillae can also occur with AKC but are more rare and smaller. Due to chronic conjunctivitis, symblephara are possible, which must be differentiated e.g. from ocular pemphigoid (Fig. 7).

Corneal involvement is common in AKC and may be sight-threatening. Alterations of the ocular surface initially often present with punctate epitheliopathy that may progress to plaque formation and corneal subepithelial scarring. If left untreated neovascularization may develop with subsequent pannus formation and corneal thinning eventually leading to corneal ectasia (keratoconus) or perforation [18]. Other clinical findings include early (anterior or posterior polar) cataracts. Due to immunological dysregulation, patients with AKC are predisposed to (bilateral!) Herpes simplex keratitis and even neoplasia [2] (Fig. 8).

9 Diagnosis

The diagnosis of AKC is mainly clinical, based on (dermatological) history, symptoms and clinical findings [17]. Due to the association with dermatitis, cooperation with dermatologists is recommended to secure the diagnosis and to support the therapeutic management. Among other investigations, skin prick testing may establish atopic disease. Serum IgE levels may also indicate the severity of systemic atopy. Also, tear IgE levels correlate with the clinical severity of AKC. Impression cytology or conjunctival biopsy may clarify potential neoplastic changes.

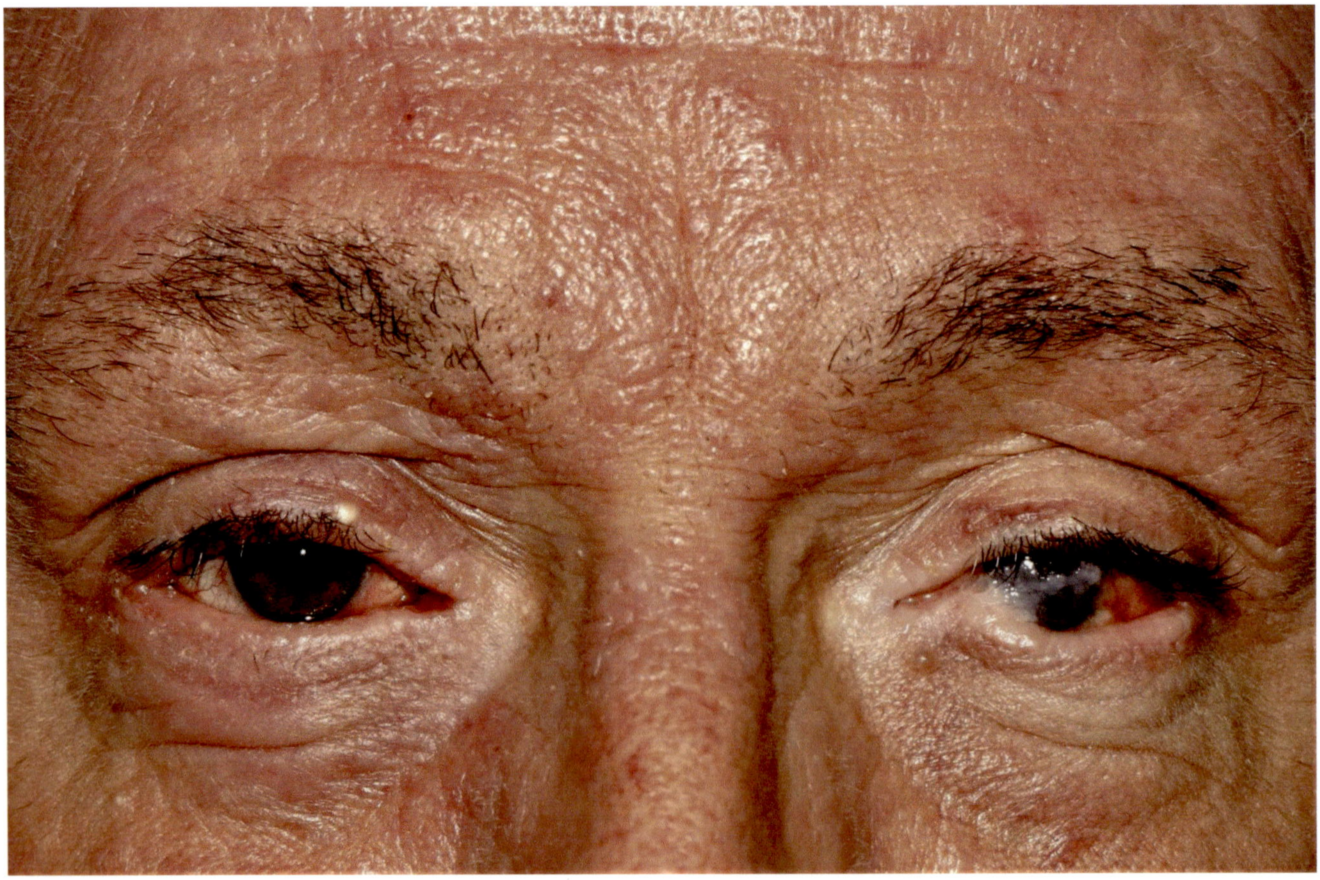

Fig. 6 Clinical findings in 53-year-old male with atopic keratoconjunctivitis. Notice: Periocular eczema, madarosis, symblephara (left eye) and corneal haze

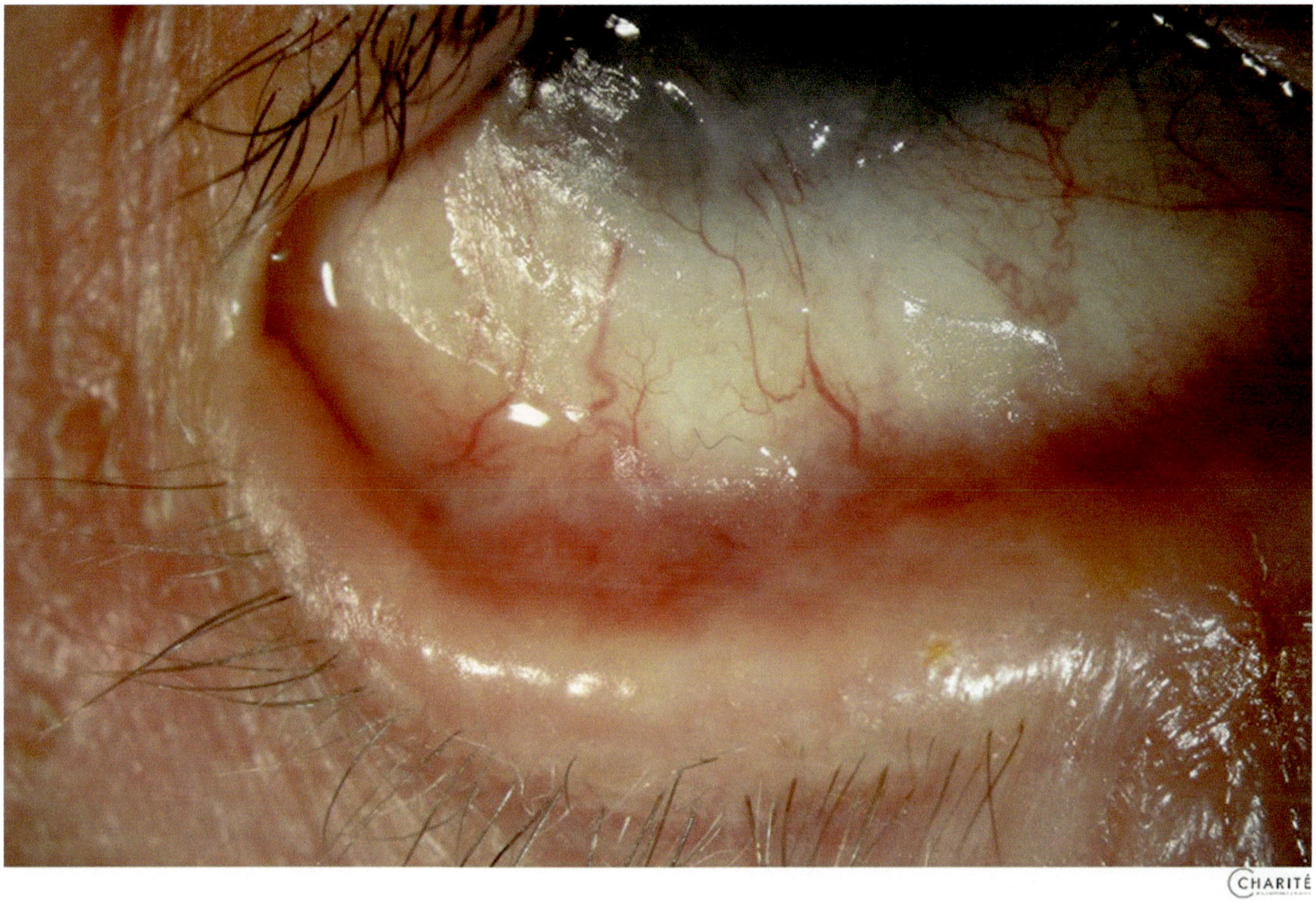

Fig. 7 Clinical findings in atopic keratoconjunctivitis. Notice: Symblephara and conjunctival and corneal keratinization

10 Therapy

Atopic keratoconjunctivitis needs long-term treatment to prevent complications such as scarring or thinning of the cornea. In the early stages of the disease, treatment of AKC is based on allergen avoidance and a step latter approach of pharmacotherapeutic agents similar to those used in the VKC [10, 19, 20]. The treatment of atopic eczema has improved significantly in recent years. In severely affected patients presenting with progressive cicatrization, neovascularisation or peripheral ulcerative keratopathy, systemic therapy may be indicated. A close cooperation with dermatologists often is helpful. Systemically applied agents, immunomodulatory agents such as cyclosporine or tacrolimus have been successfully used, but need drug monitoring [21]. More recently biologic DMARDs have been introduced in atopic dermatitis. These agents are targeting e.g. IgE, IL-5, IL-5 receptor α, IL-4 receptor α, and IL-13 and have significantly improved recent treatment results [22].

Especially using systemic therapy, many patients also have favorable effects with regard to eye involvement. Of particular interest is the treatment with dupilumab [23]. This agent blocks interleukin (IL)-4 and IL-13 and is approved for patients aged ≥ 12 years with moderate-to-severe atopic dermatitis. Even when conjunctivitis is a known comorbidity of atopic dermatitis it is of interest that Dupilumab led in clinical trials to a higher conjunctivitis incidence than placebo-treated patients. Therefore, close monitoring of these patients is necessary [24].

Corneal alterations are not uncommon in AKC. Amniotic membrane transplantation has proven to be effective for persistent corneal epithelial defects. Penetrating keratoplasty may be indicated in patients with keratoconus and AKC. Here, attention should be paid to intensive postoperative follow-up care (systemic immunosuppressive therapy, cyclosporine A, if necessary). Although rare, ocular surface neoplasia in association with AKC occur but no consensus exists on treatment. Most commonly topical interferon-alpha-2b or topical 5-fluorouracil have been used [25].

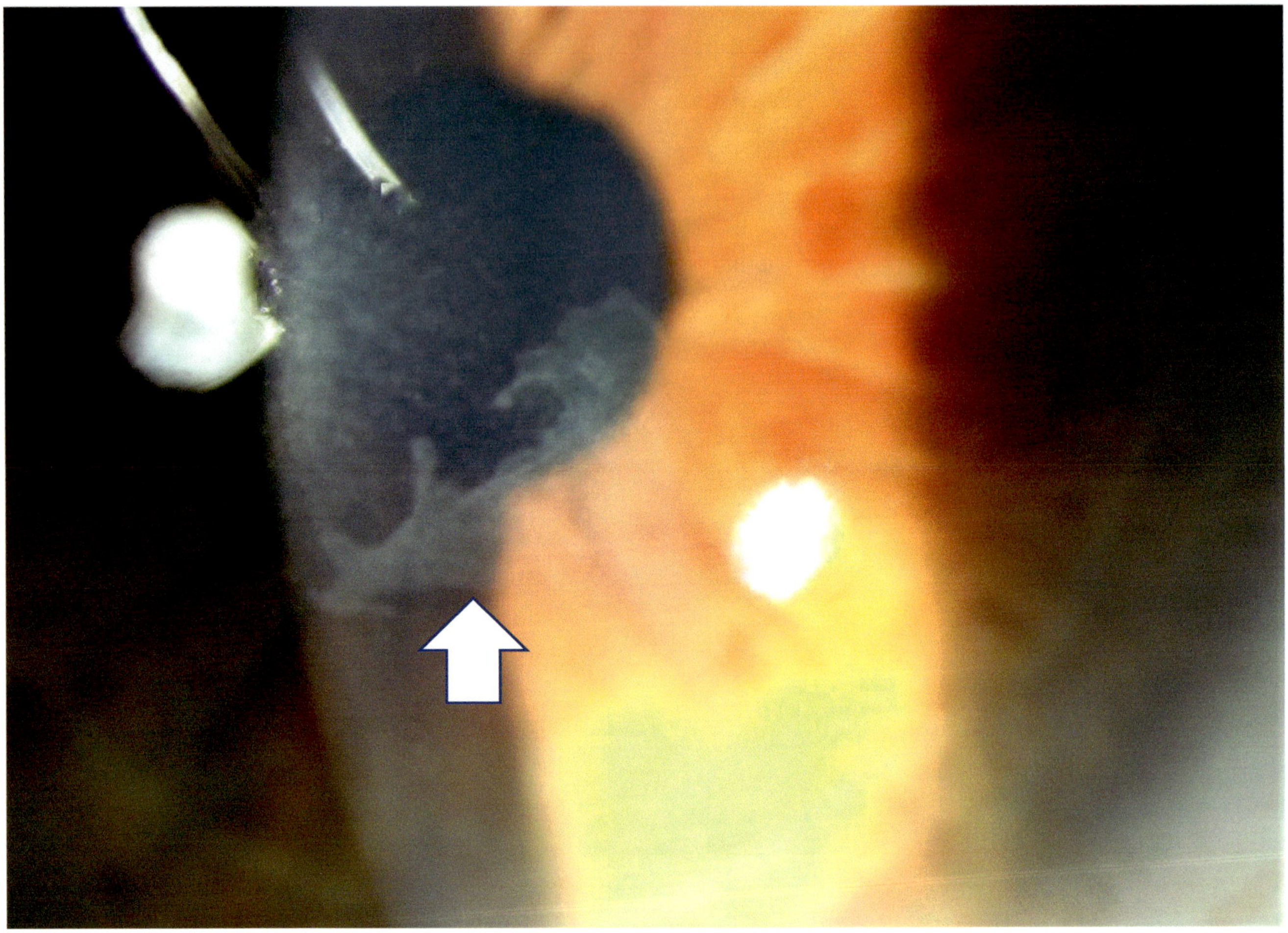

Fig. 8 Clinical findings in atopic keratoconjunctivitis (same patient as Fig. 6). Right eye: Notice cornea with suspected Corneal Intraepithelial Neoplasia (CIN)

11 Conclusion

VKC and AKC are chronic, immune-mediated (allergic) diseases of the ocular surface. It can be assumed that due to the general increase in prevalence of allergic disorders, these patients will be seen more frequently. Not uncommonly, the diagnosis is delayed and yet not adequately treated. Symptoms and clinical findings are highly variable and may severely affect the cornea. Treatment options have expanded in recent years. The prognosis is considered favorable under adequate therapy, but more than 30% of patients suffer from lifelong residuals and complications.

References

1. Vichyanond P, Pacharn P, Pleyer U, Leonardi. A Vernal keratoconjunctivitis: a severe allergic eye disease with remodeling changes. Pediatr Allergy Immunol 2014;25(4):314–22. https://doi.org/10.1111/pai.12197.
2. Heinz C et al. In: Pleyer U. Entzündliche Augenerkrankungen; Seite 129, Springer Verlag Berlin, Heidelberg. 2021;S 215–227.
3. Pleyer U, Leonardi A. Vernal keratoconjunctivitis. Ophthalmologe. 2015;112(2):177–89. https://doi.org/10.1007/s00347-014-3184-z.
4. Singh N, Diebold Y, Sahu SK, Leonardi A. Epithelial barrier dysfunction in ocular allergy. Allergy. 2022;77(5):1360–72. https://doi.org/10.1111/all.15174.
5. Fukuda K, Ishida W, Kishimoto T, Nakajima I, Miura Y, Sumi T, Yamashiro K. Role of damage-associated molecular patterns (DAMPs/Alarmins) in severe ocular allergic diseases. Cells. 2022;11(6):1051. https://doi.org/10.3390/cells11061051.
6. Patel N, Venkateswaran N, Wang Z, Galor A. Ocular involvement in atopic disease: a review. Curr Opin Ophthalmol. 2018;29(6):576–81.
7. Bonini S, Sacchetti M, Mantelli F, Lambiase A. Clinical grading of vernal keratoconjunctivitis. Curr Opin Allergy Clin Immunol. 2007;7(5):436–41. https://doi.org/10.1097/ACI.0b013e3282efb726.
8. Feizi S, Javadi MA, Alemzadeh-Ansari M, Arabi A, Shahraki T, Kheirkhah A. Management of corneal complications in vernal keratoconjunctivitis: a review. Ocul Surf. 2021;19:282–9.
9. Fauquert JL, Jedrzejczak-Czechowicz M, Rondon C et al. Interest group on ocular allergy (IGOA) from the European academy of allergy and clinical immunology. Conjunctival allergen provocation test: guidelines for daily practice. Allergy 2017;72(1):43–54 https://doi.org/10.1111/all.12986.

10. Roumeau I, Coutu A, Navel V. Efficacy of medical treatments for vernal keratoconjunctivitis: a systematic review and meta-analysis. J Allergy Clin Immunol. 2021;148(3):822–34. https://doi.org/10.1016/j.jaci.2021.03.026.
11. Leonardi A, Doan S, Aragona P, et al. Topical cyclosporine a cationic ophthalmic emulsion in paediatric vernal keratoconjunctivitis: pooled analysis of randomised novative and vektis trials. Eye (Lond). 2023;37(11):2320–6. https://doi.org/10.1038/s41433-022-02342-6.
12. Kim SE, Nowak V, Quartilho A, Larkin F, Hingorani M, Tuft S, Dahlmann-Noor A. Systemic interventions for severe atopic and vernal keratoconjunctivitis in children and young people up to the age of 16 years. Cochrane Database Syst Rev 2020;10(10): CD013298. https://doi.org/10.1002/14651858.CD013298.
13. Rossberg S, Pleyer U, Lau S. Omalizumab in three children with severe vernal keratoconjunctivitis. Allergo J. 2020;29:28–35. https://doi.org/10.1007/s15007-020-2581-7.
14. Yu L, Zhang H, Pan J, Ye L. Pediatric usage of Omalizumab: a promising one. World Allergy Organ J. 2021;14(12): 100614. https://doi.org/10.1016/j.waojou.100614.
15. Jain AK, Sukhija J. Low dose mitomycin-C in severe vernal keratoconjunctivitis: a randomized prospective double blind study. Indian J Ophthalmol. 2006;54(2):111–6. https://doi.org/10.4103/0301-4738.25832.PMID:16770028.doi:10.1016/j.jtos.2020.10.005.
16. Singh V, Shukla S, Ramachandran C, et al. Science and art of cell-based ocular surface regeneration. Int Rev Cell Mol Biol. 2015;319:45–106. https://doi.org/10.1016/bs.ircmb.2015.07.001.
17. Brémond-Gignac D, Nischal KK, Mortemousque B, Gajdosova E, Granet DB, Chiambaretta F. Atopic keratoconjunctivitis in children: clinical features and diagnosis. Ophthalmology. 2016;123(2):435–7.
18. Nivenius E, Montan P. Spontaneous corneal perforation associated with atopic keratoconjunctivitis: a case series and literature review. Acta Ophthalmol. 2015;93(4):383–7.
19. Yazu H, Fukagawa K, Shimizu E, Sato Y, Fujishima H. Long-term outcomes of 0.1% tacrolimus eye drops in eyes with severe allergic conjunctival diseases. Allergy Asthma Clin Immunol. 2021;17(1):11. https://doi.org/10.1186/s13223-021-00513-w.
20. González-López JJ, López-Alcalde J, Morcillo Laiz R, Fernández Buenaga R, Rebolleda Fernández G. Topical cyclosporine for atopic keratoconjunctivitis. Cochrane Database Syst Rev 2012;9:CD009078.
21. Salek MS, Finlay AY, Luscombe DK et al. Cyclosporin greatly improves the quality of life of adults with severe atopic dermatitis. A randomized, double-blind, placebo-controlled trial. Br J Dermatol 1993;129(4):422–430.
22. Fukuda K, Kishimoto T, Sumi T, Yamashiro K, Ebihara N. Biologics for allergy: therapeutic potential for ocular allergic diseases and adverse effects on the eye. Allergol Int. 2023;72(2):234–44. https://doi.org/10.1016/j.alit.2022.09.005.
23. Bansal A, Simpson EL, Paller AS, Siegfried EC, et al. Conjunctivitis in Dupilumab clinical trials for adolescents with atopic dermatitis or asthma. Am J Clin Dermatol. 2021;22:101–15. https://doi.org/10.1007/s40257-020-00577-1.
24. Wohlrab J, Wollenberg A, Reimann H, Pleyer U, Werfel T. Interdisziplinäre Handlungsempfehlung bei Dupilumab-assoziierten entzündlichen Augenerkrankungen Hautarzt. 2019;70(1):64–67 https://doi.org/10.1007/s00105-018-4316-1.
25. Zhang L, Mercado C, Galor A, Holland EJ, Wang G, Karp CL. Challenging treatment of ocular surface squamous neoplasia in patients with atopic disease. Ocul Immunol Inflamm. 2019;27(2):288–93. https://doi.org/10.1080/09273948.2017.1394470.

Ocular Rosacea

Uwe Pleyer

Abstract

Rosacea is a chronic inflammatory skin condition of unknown etiology. Four distinct subtypes have been classified with type IV being ocular rosacea. Ocular rosacea is a chronic, inflammatory condition that may occur even in the absence of skin changes. It is characterized by bilateral blepharitis and meibomitis, which may subsequently alter the entire ocular surface including the cornea. Corneal involvement has been reported in up to 50% of rosacea patients and ranges from punctate epithelial keratopathy to corneal neovascularization, infiltrates, epithelial ulceration and even perforation. The diagnosis is largely based on clinical findings, although it is often delayed in the absence of cutaneous changes, particularly in children.

Keywords

Cornea · Dry eye · Keratitis · Meibomian gland dysfunction · Treatment

1 Introduction

Rosacea is classified as a chronic inflammatory skin disease of unknown aetiology. There are indications that dysregulation of the innate immune system and changes in the microbiome (skin and gut) are pathogenic factors. Often, triggering factors such as sun exposure, emotional distress, spicy foods, alcohol or coffee consumption as well as certain medications can be identified in patient's medical history [1, 2].

Rosacea may occur in children, but most frequently affects individuals in their 3rd–6th decade of life with a female predominance (3:1) (Fig. 1A–C). Paediatric rosacea is considered to be rare, but seems underreported since typical skin changes are often absent or difficult to diagnose.

2 Diagnosis

Based on clinical findings rosacea is classified into four subtypes (Rosacea Society Expert Committee) [3]:

- Erythematotelangiectatic
- Papulopustular
- Phymatous
- Ocular rosacea

General skin changes in rosacea present as chronic inflammatory skin changes with facial redness, especially in the area of the nose and periorbital region (Fig. 2). Another clinical hallmark are telangiectasias. Further changes may present as papululopustular skin manifestations. Rhinophyma of the nose is most commonly seen in men over 40 years of age and may occur as a late finding in more advanced stages of the disease (Fig. 3).

As own entity and with pronounced changes similar to rosacea, Morbihan's disease presents with insidious swelling of the forehead, cheeks and periorbital region [4].

2.1 Ocular Rosacea

Ocular rosacea is likely to be underdiagnosed. This is mainly related to its rather unspecific signs and symptoms. Common symptoms of ocular rosacea result from

U. Pleyer (✉)
Department of Ophthalmology, Charité–Universitätsmedizin Berlin, Corporate Member of Freie Universitaet Berlin, Humboldt Universitaet zu Berlin and Berlin Institute of Health, Campus Virchow Klinikum, Berlin, Germany
e-mail: uwe.pleyer@charite.de

B. Seitz et al. (eds.), *Atlas on Cornea*, https://doi.org/10.1007/978-3-031-65422-0_30

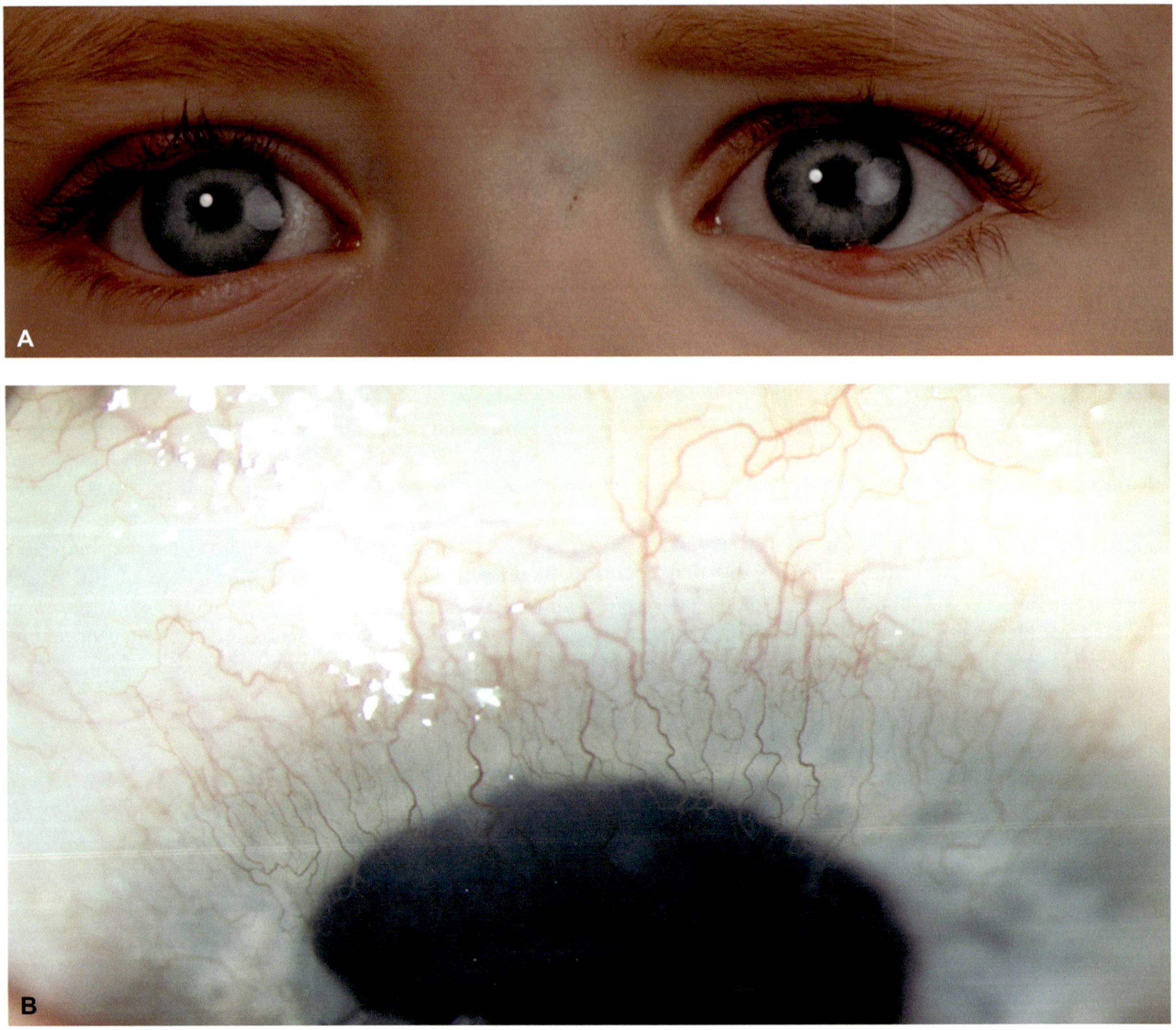

Fig. 1 (**A**) Four-year-old girl with ocular rosacea, presenting with a 6-month history of epiphora and recurrent bilateral hordeola. (**B**) Left eye—upper limbal region (same girl)

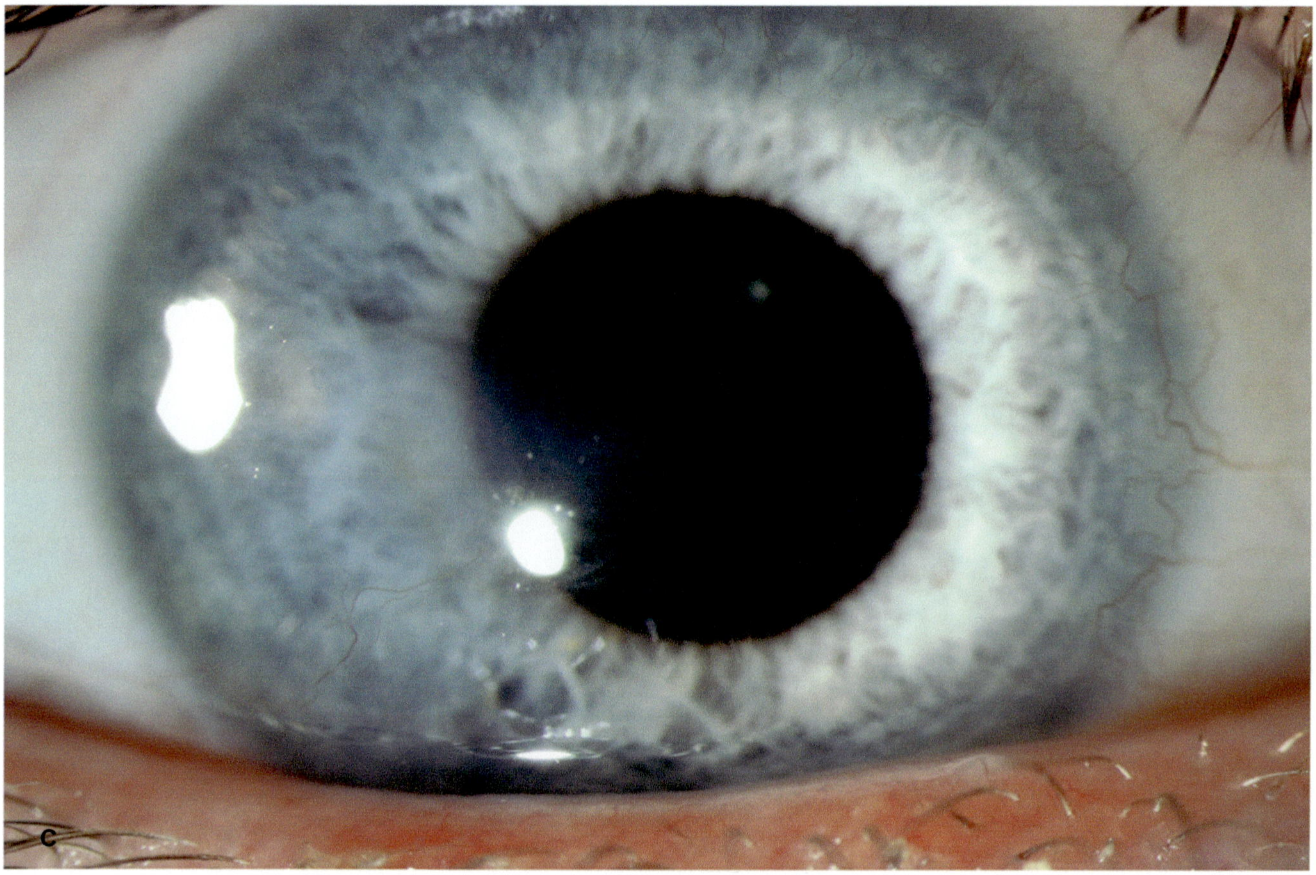

Fig. 1 (C) Left eye—notice: circular neovascularization at the limbal region (same girl)

meibomian gland dysfunction resulting in an "evaporative dry eye". Complaints frequently start already in the morning and hence may offer a hint regarding the differential diagnosis of a hypovolemic dry eye, which often show increased symptoms at later hours [1].

In more severely affected patients, visual impairment with blurred vision and light sensitivity may occur resulting in impaired quality of life. Still, early diagnosis of ocular rosacea is important since ocular signs may even precede skin changes and early treatment may prevent disease progression. The hallmarks of ocular rosacea include bilateral chronic blepharitis and meibomian gland dysfunction. At the slit lamp, typical findings present as telangiectasia (Fig. 4) of the eyelid margin and dysfunction of the meibomian glands in more than 90% of patients. Several studies have reported an association between the severity and extent of skin teleangiectasia and ocular findings [5, 6]. Due to meibomian gland dysfunction, almost all patients develop an evaporative dry eye [5–7].

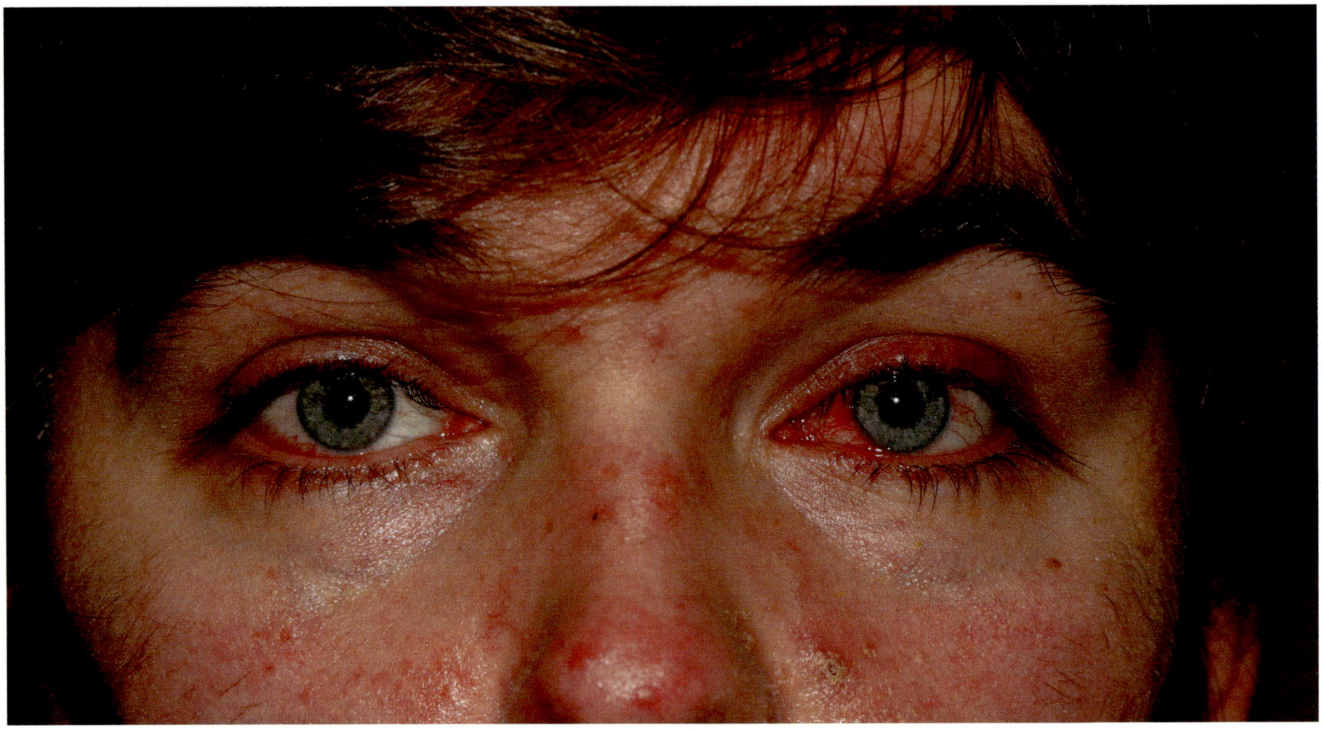

Fig. 2 Clinical presentation of oculocutaneous and ocular rosacea. A patient with nasal and facial erythema, with telangiectasia, blepharophyma, meibomitis and phlyctenules

2.2 Cornea Involvement

The cornea is affected in up to 30% of patients with any type of rosacea and up to 50% in ocular rosacea. Initially corneal involvement presents as superficial punctate keratitis, typically affecting the lower third of the peripheral cornea. These superficial changes may progress to recurrent corneal epithelial erosions. Secondary superinfection in these patients is reported. Persistent epithelial alterations and chronic inflammation of the ocular surface are considered as the driving force leading to peripheral corneal neovascularization. In more severely affected patients, it may present with subepithelial marginal triangular infiltrates (phlyctenules) (Fig. 5). If left untreated, these infiltrates may progress further centrally and may result in stromal ulceration and even perforation [2] (Table 1).

3 Management

Due to its unspecific and multifactorial aetiology no standard therapy is established. General measures concern lifestyle changes (avoidance of triggers, change in diet) [1, 3]. In mild forms of ocular rosacea, topical ophthalmological treatment can be sufficient. In ocular rosacea physical measures such as eyelid care are usually recommended to

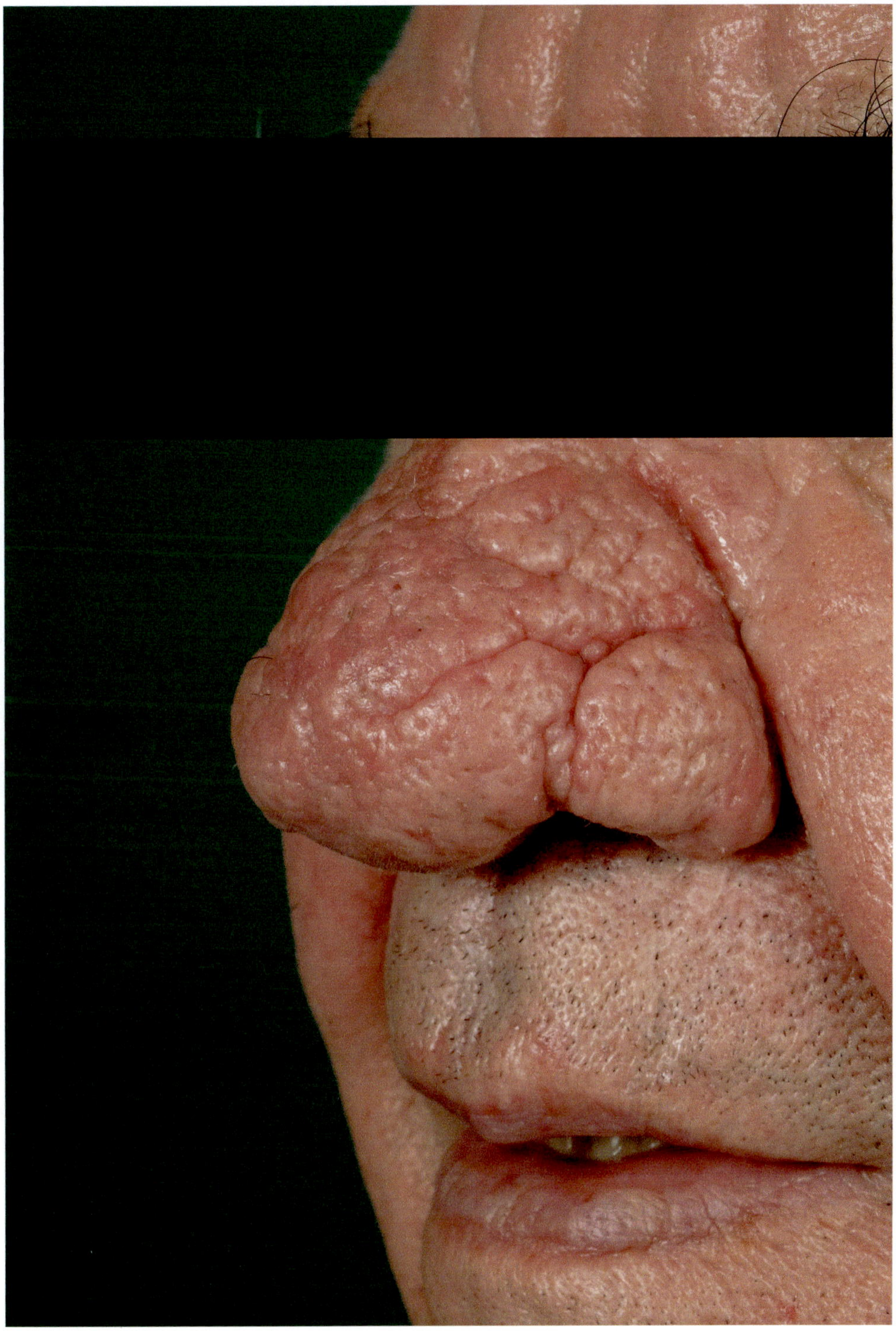

Fig. 3 Rhinophyma—nodular swelling and congestion of the nose in an advanced stage of rosacea. (Courtesy of: Department for Otorhinolaryngology, Head and Neck Surgery, Saarland University Medical Center)

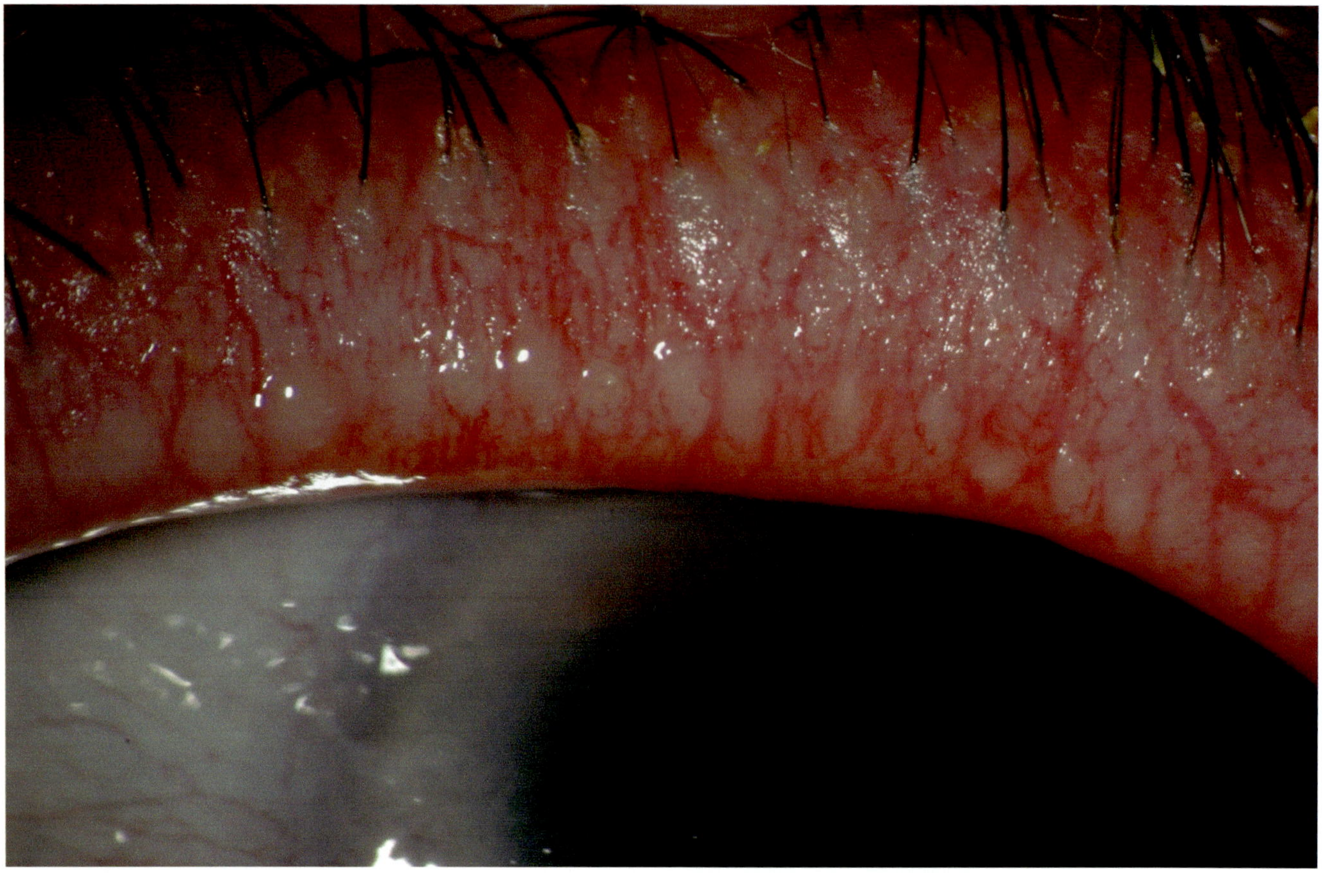

Fig. 4 Blepharitis with telangiectasia, blepharophyma, and meibomitis

improve meibomian gland function. This can be supported by warm compresses. Secondary changes of the tear film may benefit symptomatically from (lipid-containing) tear substitution [9, 10].

A broad spectrum of topical anti-inflammatory agents has been used to treat ocular rosacea.

This includes topical unpreserved soft steroids, Ciclosporin A and azithromycin.

Notable, as in systemic treatments all medications have to be used for prolonged times [1, 8, 10, 11].

Systemic antimicrobial agents such as doxycycline and minocycline play a significant role in therapy due to their anti-inflammatory effect in rosacea and often have a favourable influence in patients with moderate type of ocular disease [1, 3]. It is important that a long-term application takes place, as therapeutic effects may only occur after weeks. It is believed, that anti-inflammatory effects are due to downregulation of metalloproteinases and other proinflammatory mediators. Long-term treatment benefits of biophysical treatment measures such as "Lipiflow" and "Intense Puls Light Therapy" are still inconclusive and are currently not reimbursed (in Germany) [1, 12]. An overview of the therapeutic measures for the different forms of rosacea is provided in Flowchart 1.

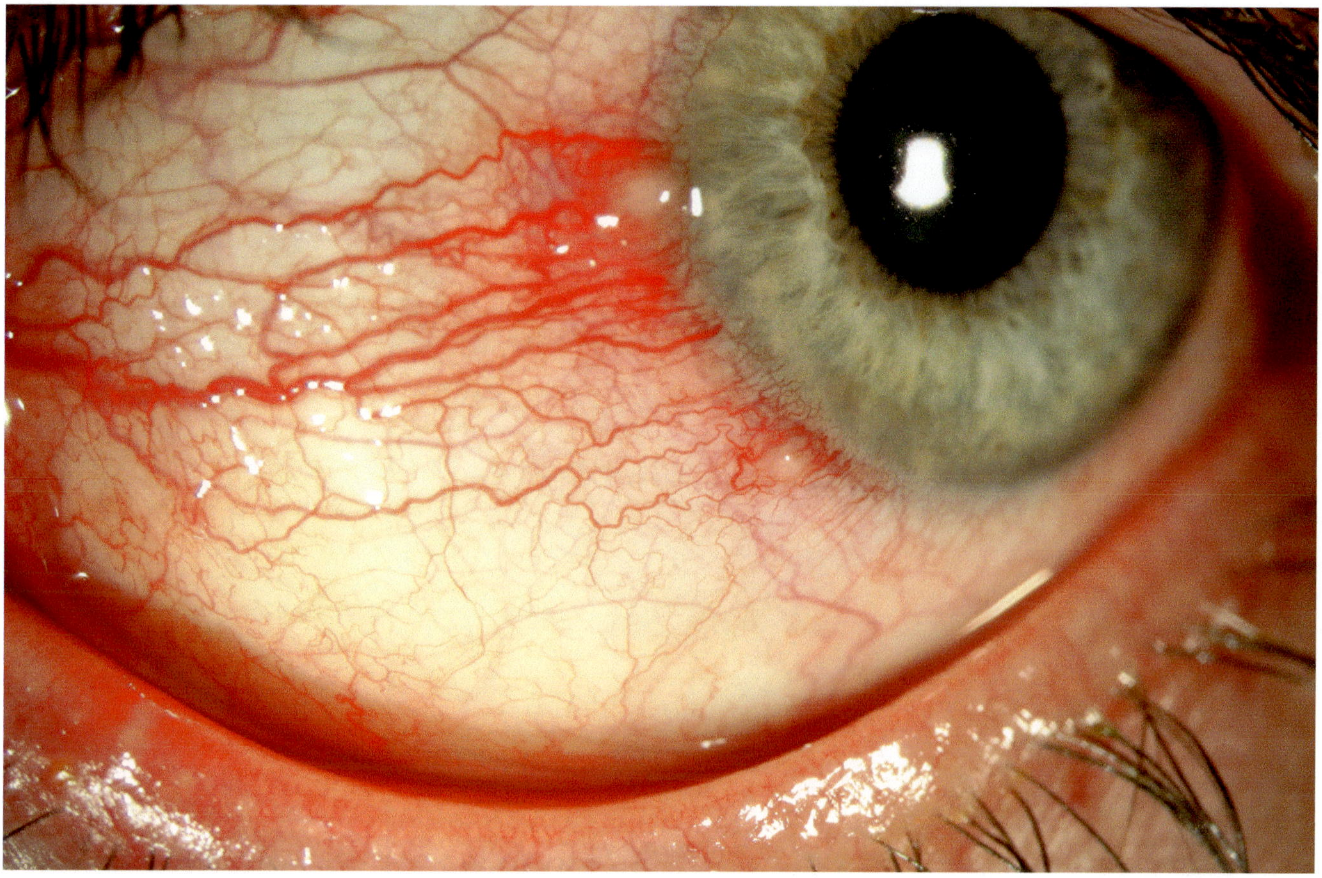

Fig. 5 Left eye of the same patient (Fig. 1) with telangiectasia, blepharophyma, meibomitis and phlyctenules

Table 1 Primary and secondary features of rosacea. Adapted from the national rosacea society expert committee (3)

Diagnostic features	Major features	Minor features
Persistent centrofacial erythema associated with periodic intensification by potential trigger factors	Flushing/transient centrofacial erythema	Burning sensation of the skin
	Inflammatory papules and pustules	Burning sensation of the skin
	Telangiectasia Ocular Lid margin telangiectasia	Oedema
	Blepharitis/Keratitis/conjunctivitis/sclerokeratitis	Dry sensation of the skin

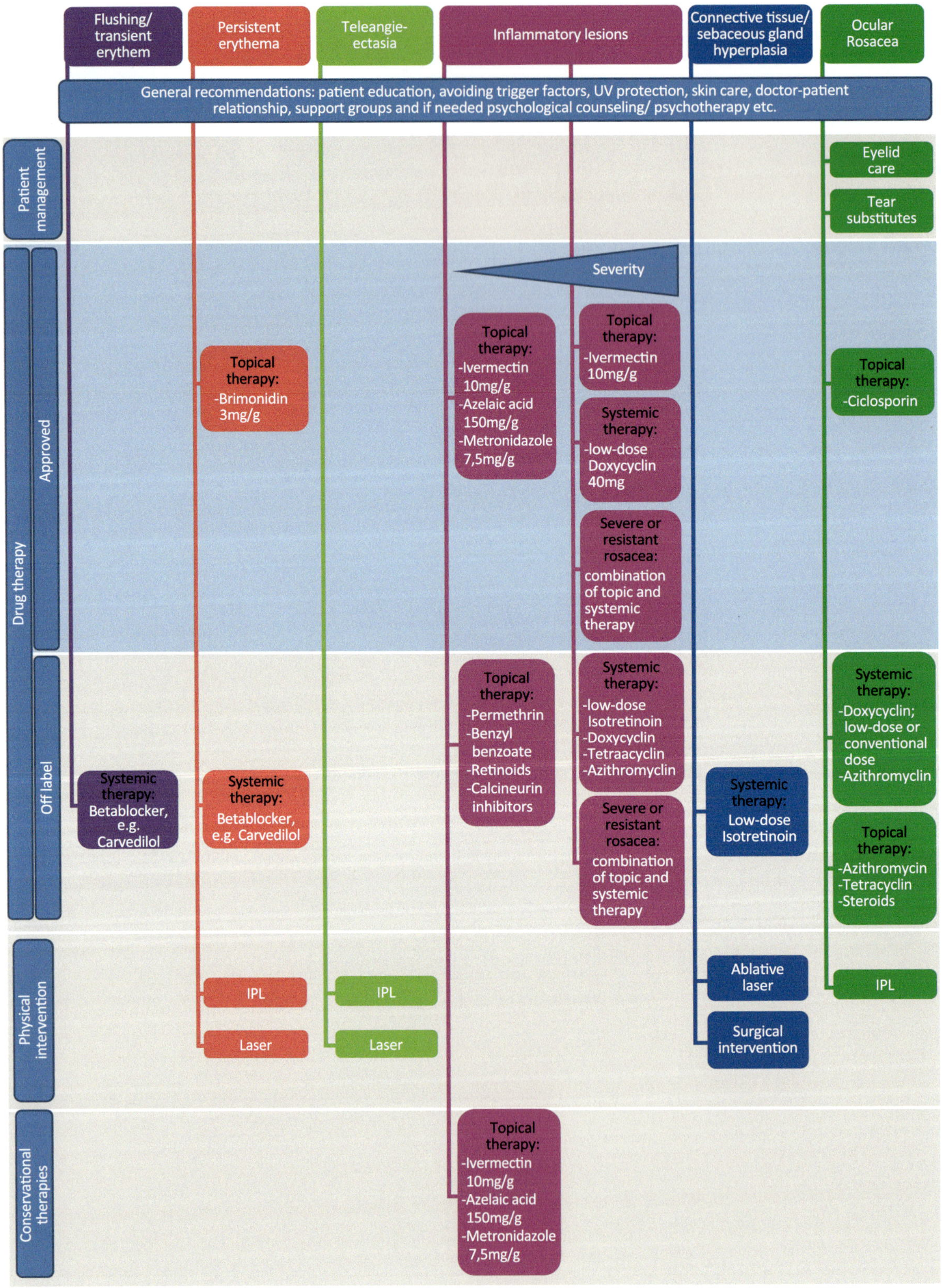

Flowchart 1 Indicating treatment options in rosacea [1]

4 Conclusion

Rosacea is a common chronic skin disorder with a wide range of clinical findings. Ocular involvement is frequent and may present as an isolated type of the disease spectrum. Ocular findings are characterized by bilateral inflammatory changes, which may include the cornea. If left untreated, ocular rosacea may cause varying degrees of ocular morbidity and significant impaired quality of life.

References

1. Clanner-Engelshofen BM, Bernhard D, Dargatz S, et al. S2k guideline: rosacea. J Dtsch Dermatol Ges. 2022;20(8):1147–65. https://doi.org/10.1111/ddg.14849.
2. Tavassoli S, Wong N, Chan E. Ocular manifestations of rosacea: a clinical review. Clin Exp Ophthalmol. 2021;49(2):104–17. https://doi.org/10.1111/ceo.13900.
3. Thiboutot D, Anderson R, Cook-Bolden F. Standard management options for rosacea: the 2019 update by the national rosacea society expert committee. J Am Acad Dermatol. 2020;82(6):1501–10. https://doi.org/10.1016/j.jaad.2020.01.077.
4. Carruth BP, Meyer DR, Wladis EJ, et al. Extreme eyelid lymphedema associated with rosacea (Morbihan disease): case series, literature review, and therapeutic considerations. Ophthalmic Plast Reconstr Surg. 2017;33:S34–8.
5. Palamar M, Degirmenci C, Ertam I, Yagci A. Evaluation of dry eye and Meibomian gland dysfunction with meibography in patients with rosacea. Cornea. 2015;34:497–9.
6. Woo YR, Cho M, Ju HJ et al. Ocular comorbidities in rosacea: a case-control study based on seven institutions. J Clin Med. 2021;10(13):2897. https://doi.org/10.3390/jcm10132897.
7. Qian L, Wei W. Identified risk factors for dry eye syndrome: a systematic review and meta-analysis. PLoS One. 2022;17(8):e0271267. https://doi.org/10.1371/journal.pone.0271267.
8. Geerling G, Baudouin C, Aragona P et al. Emerging strategies for the diagnosis and treatment of meibomian gland dysfunction. In: Proceedings of the OCEAN group meeting. Ocul Surf. 2017;15:179–92.
9. Jones L, Downie LE, Korb D, et al. TFOS DEWS II management and therapy report. Ocul Surf. 2017;15:575–628.
10. van Zuuren EJ, Fedorowicz Z, Tan J, et al. Interventions for rosacea based on the phenotype approach: an updated systematic review including GRADE assessments. Br J Dermatol. 2019;181(1):65–79. https://doi.org/10.1111/bjd.17590.
11. Schechter BA, Katz RS, Friedman LS. Efficacy of topical cyclosporine for the treatment of ocular rosacea. Adv Ther. 2009;26:651–9.
12. Vergés C, March de Ribot F, Salgado-Borges J, Gonzalez J. Prospective evaluation of intense pulsed light treatment for Meibomian gland dysfunction and blepharitis due to ocular rosacea. Eur J Dermatol. 2022;32(4):505–515. https://doi.org/10.1684/ejd.2022.4301.

Mucous Membrane Pemphigoid with Ocular Involvement

Mathias Roth, Rémi Yaïci, Maria Borrelli, and Gerd Geerling

Abstract

Mucous membrane pemphigoid (MMP) refers to a heterogeneous group of autoimmune bullous disorders. The disease is characterized by recurrent inflammation and progressive scarring that can affect all mucous membranes with varying frequencies. Ocular involvement presents the clinician with a diagnostic challenge as cicatricial conjunctivitis includes over 30 differential diagnoses, and specific diagnostic tests are negative in up to half of the cases. Fibrosis begins with minor changes such as subepithelial fibrosis, e.g. on the upper tarsal plate or next to the plica semilunaris. In the further course, fornix shortening or symblephara may develop. This can lead to entropion and trichiasis, possibly leading to chronic keratopathy with recurrent corneal erosions and vascularization. In the final stage, an ankyloblepharon develops, possibly limiting all eye movement ("frozen globe"). MMP is also a therapeutic challenge, as only very few randomized clinical trials have so far been performed due to the rarity of the disease. Patient management requires good collaboration with other specialties, the use of immunosuppressants and, only when inflammatory activity is under control, surgical rehabilitation. However, it is important to remember that seemingly trivial surgical procedures can trigger exacerbation of the disease and progression of fibrosis.

Keywords

Cicatrizing conjunctivitis · Symblepharon · Ankyloblepharon · Mucous membrane pemphigoid · Autoimmune disease · Ocular manifestation

1 Introduction

Mucous membrane pemphigoid (MMP) is a chronic blistering autoimmune disease and belongs to the group of pemphigoid diseases [1, 2]. It is a rare condition without geographic or ethnic predilection. In Germany, the incidence is estimated at 2 new cases per million population annually [3, 4]. The prevalence is about 24.6 per million population, which corresponds to about 2,000 cases in Germany (5). Women seem to be affected slightly more often than men [4, 5]. The average age at onset is between 60 and 68 years of age [6–15]. In children, MMP is extremely rare but can occur [16–18]. The disease most frequently manifests itself on the mucous membranes close to the skin, especially the oral mucosa (Fig. 1) followed by the conjunctiva—without blister formation—, nasal or nasopharynx and the anogenital mucous membranes. However, the mucous membranes of the larynx, esophagus, urethra, and rectum may also be affected. Approximately 70% of MMP patients will develop ocular manifestations [19–21]. Therefore, patients with MMP without ocular involvement should have regular ophthalmologic examinations and ophthalmologists need to be aware of the typical clinical signs. Vice versa, in case of ocular involvement, appropriate examinations by dermatologists, ENT and gynecology specialists should be requested and repeated once the diagnosis has been confirmed [10]. A well-targeted medical history regarding possible extraocular involvement can already be indicative of a possible multisite disease (Table 1).

The investigation of a suspected case can be challenging, as cicatricial conjunctivitis includes over 30 differential

Supplementary Information The online version contains supplementary material available at https://doi.org/10.1007/978-3-031-65422-0_31.

M. Roth (✉) · R. Yaïci · M. Borrelli · G. Geerling
Department of Ophthalmology, University Hospital Dusseldorf, Dusseldorf, Germany
e-mail: mathias.roth@med.uni-duesseldorf.de

B. Seitz et al. (eds.), *Atlas on Cornea*, https://doi.org/10.1007/978-3-031-65422-0_31

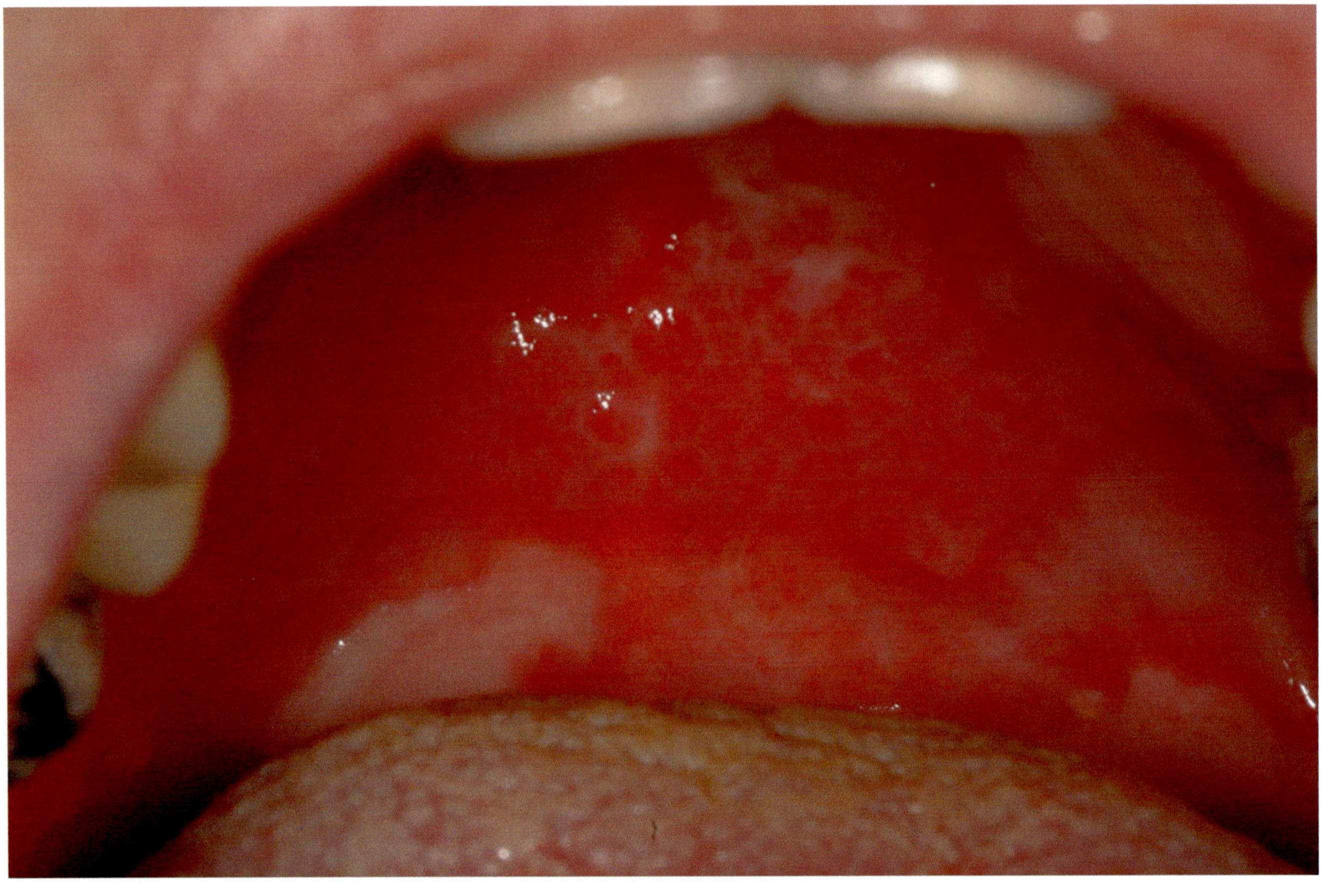

Fig. 1 **Extraocular findings of ophthalmological patients**. Besides the ocular findings, this patient also showed an oral involvement, which typically appears as red or ulcerated whitish patches. Blisters may occur but tend to easily burst and leave ulcers. This patient presented with numerous mouth ulcers on the hard palate. Overall, 80% of the patients with mucous membrane pemphigoid show multisite involvement. It is therefore essential to ask about symptoms that may refer to an extraocular location. An exhaustive targeted history is summarized in Table 1

Table 1 Medical history. The key role of the ophthalmic or other clinician is to systematically inquire about other possible organic damage. With the help of a well-targeted history, an ophthalmologist can already point to a possible multisite disease

	Medical history
For all sites:	Time of first onset of symptoms and lesions on mucous membranes
Mouth	Stomatitis, gingival bleeding, painful feeding
Skin	Occurrence of skin changes (erosions/blisters)
Nasal cavity	Painful lesions in nasal cavities, frequent nosebleeds
Esophagus	Dysphagia,
Trachea	Dysphonia, dyspnea
Genitals	Dysuria, vaginal synechiae, increasing foreskin tightness, dyspareunia, genital erosions
General	Weight loss

diagnoses, and specific tests can be negative in up to 50% of cases [10, 22]. Direct immunofluorescence (IF) microscopy from perilesional tissue to detect basement membrane associated bound IgG, IgA and/or complement C3, combined with serological testing for circulating autoantibodies are recommended. In most patients, the serum antibodies titers are low and depending upon which antibodies are tested, the proportions of positivity vary. Circulating autoantibodies are determined by indirect IF assays, ELISA or immunoblotting [23]. The major target antigen in MMP is BP180, followed by BP230 [1]. An important target antigen is laminin 332, which has been associated with the simultaneous presence of malignancies, i.e. paraneoplastic pemphigoid [24–31].

Table 2 Staging of Mucous membrane pemphigoid according to Foster

	Findings for staging according to Foster [21]
Stage I	Chronic conjunctivitis with subepithelial fibrosis (Fig. 2)
Stage II	Shortening of the inferior fornix (see Fig. 3)
Stage III	Symblepharon formation (see Fig. 4)
Stage IV	Ankyloblepharon and keratinization of the ocular surface, "Frozen globe" (see Fig. 8)

In most cases, patients with MMP need a long-term treatment with steroid-sparing immunosuppressive agents according to a stepladder approach [32]. Thus, interdisciplinary collaboration is not only essential in diagnosis of mucous membrane pemphigoid, but also in its therapy, especially when it comes to biologicals and i. v. immunoglobulin application.

2 Clinical Findings

There are different systems for staging of the ocular manifestation of the disease. The frequently used Foster staging system is based on clinical findings (see Table 1) and thus will be used to depict the course of the disease in this chapter [21] (Table 2).

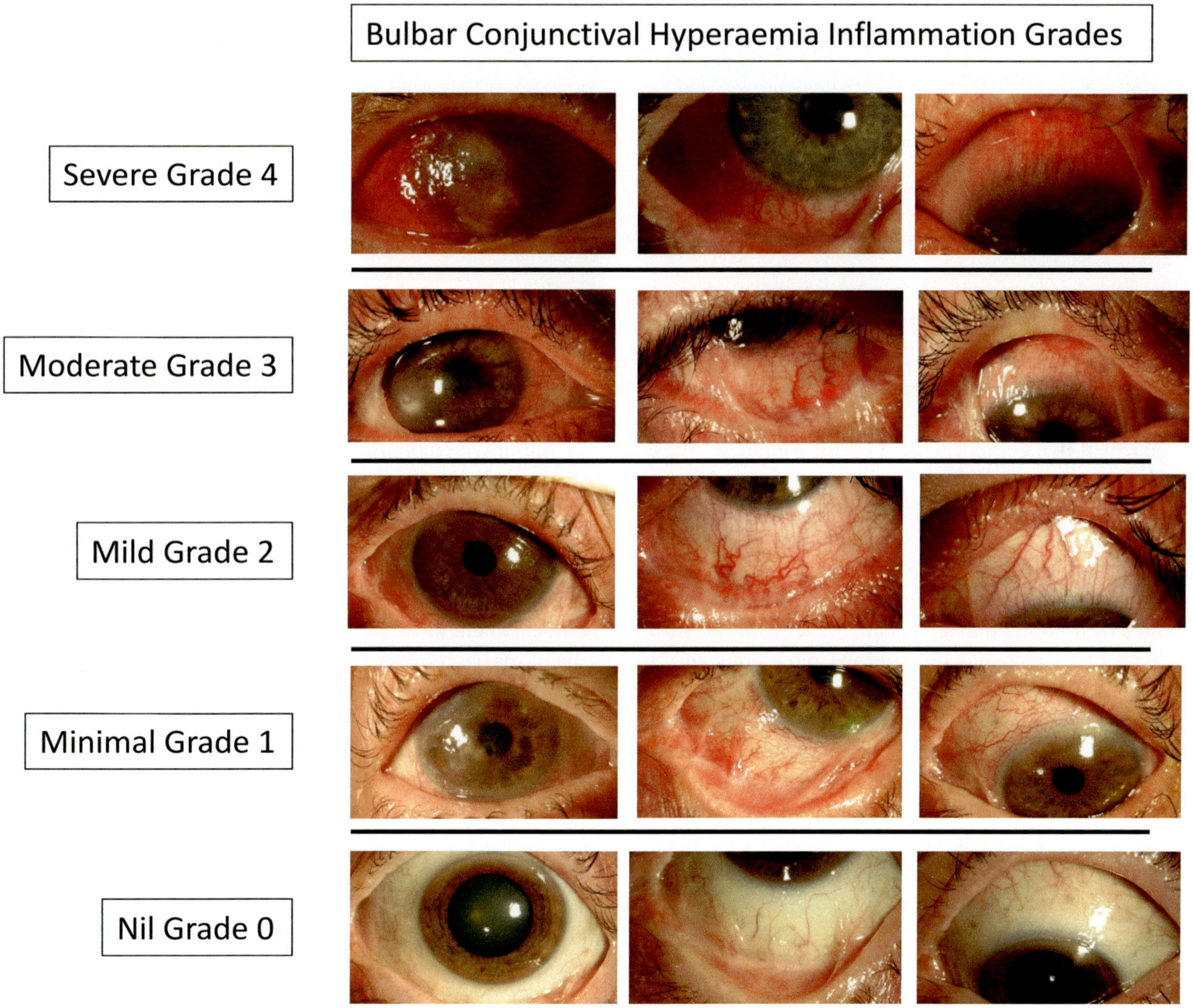

Fig. 2 **Grading of Hyperemia (modified according to Ong et al.** [10]). The most suitable parameter to determine the disease activity (corresponding to inflammatory activity) in ocular involvement of MMP is conjunctival hyperemia. To standardize and classify conjunctival hyperemia into nil, minimal, mild, moderate and severe disease activity of ocular involvement, a visual analogue scale is recommended [10]

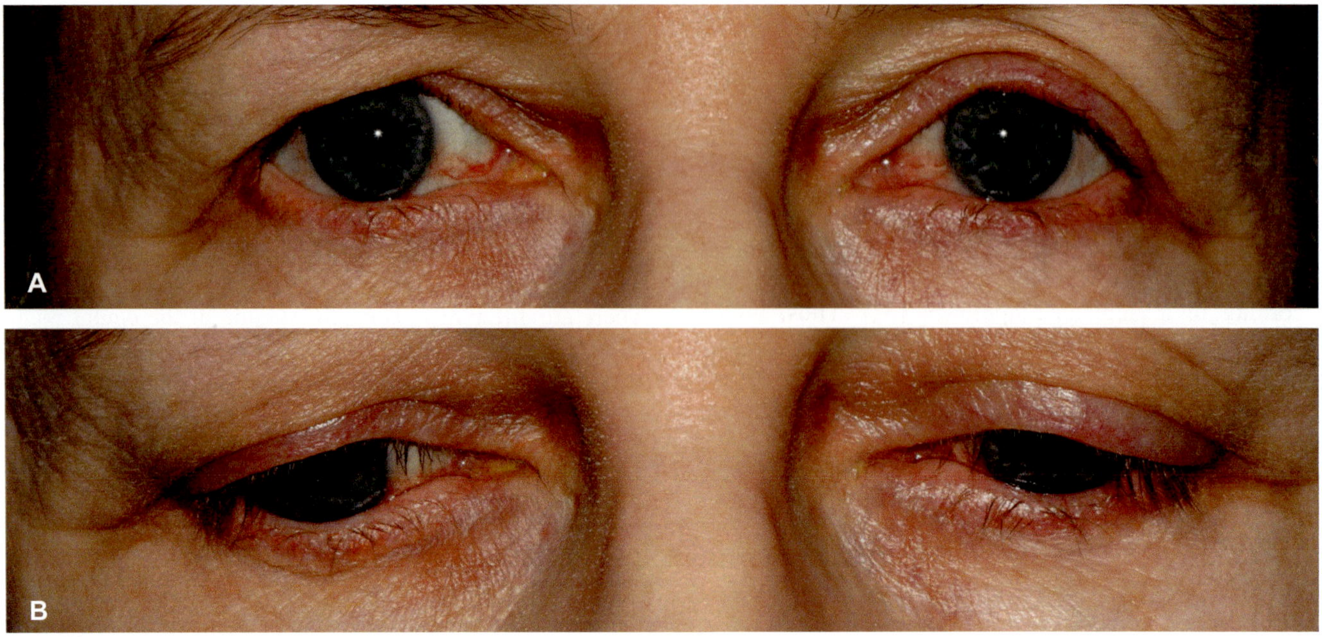

Fig. 3 **Unspecific initial signs and symptoms**. This 56-year-old female patient had been treated for severe dry eye due to Rosacea for 9 years. She presented because of increasing redness, tearing, burning and foreign body sensation. The clinical examination revealed an unspecific presentation with a mild, medially pronounced conjunctival hyperemia (**A**) meibomian gland dysfunction, and blepharitis (**B**) Slit lamp examination revealed subtle signs of cicatricial conjunctivitis (see Fig. 2) and diagnostics specific for mucous membrane pemphigoid were initiated, confirming the diagnosis of mucous membrane pemphigoid by biopsy and direct immunofluorescence

It is important to note, that, due to a lack of correlation of disease stage with disease activity, none of the currently available staging systems can be used for indication or guidance of immunosuppressive therapy [33]. However, conjunctival hyperemia can be a useful parameter to assess the inflammatory activity. Ong et al. developed a visual analog scale to differentiate between minimal, mild, moderate and severe disease activity (Fig. 2) [34].

Ocular involvement is usually bilateral, although asymmetric involvement of either eye is possible [35, 36]. Conjunctival inflammation occurs in temporally variable episodes of spontaneous relapses and remissions and leads to progressive scarring and subsequent shrinkage of the conjunctiva. But even in clinically apparently calm phases, this irreversible, subepithelial fibrosing process can progress insidiously [37, 38]. This may lead to obstruction of the lacrimal gland excretory ducts and accessory lacrimal glands with decreased production of aqueous tear film [39]. Increasing demise of conjunctival goblet cells may reduce the mucin phase of the tear film, and occlusion of the meibomian gland orifices may reduce the lipid phase. This influence on all three phases of the tear film results in both a quantitative and qualitative tear deficiency with instability of the tear film.

Initially, symptoms are indistinguishable from those of dry eye. The patients complain of redness, tearing, burning and foreign body sensation [40]. Also, clinically the findings with meibomian gland dysfunction, blepharitis and conjunctival injection may resemble chronic (blepharo)-conjunctivitis sicca (Fig. 3). Due to this initially unspecific clinical picture, it takes on average about 2 years until a diagnosis is confirmed by biopsy [41]. For this reason, a thorough slit lamp examination and awareness of possible early signs of the disease are particularly important in cases of unclear recurrent and refractory conjunctivitis. At the beginning of the disease, changes mostly in the medial canthus with flattening of the plica semilunaris and caruncle, but also a shortening of the lateral canthus can be indicative [10, 14, 42] (Foster I; Fig. 4). Subepithelial fibrosis may initially be very subtle and visible as fine white striae

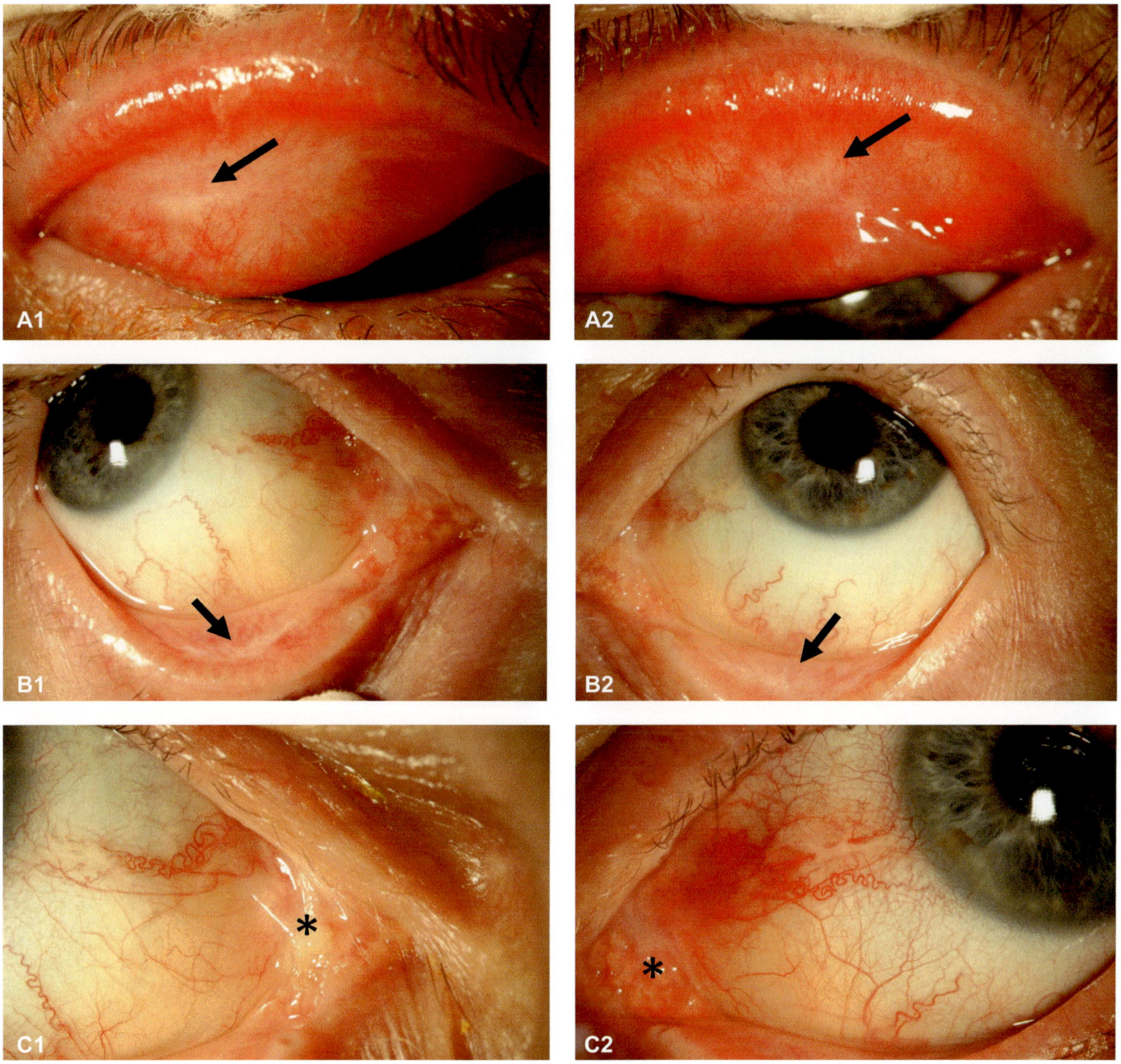

Fig. 4 **Foster Stage I**. In the same patient as in Fig. 1, slit lamp examination revealed fine white linear scarring in the upper tarsus (**A**, black arrows) and the lower fornices (**B**, black arrows). Initially these changes due to subepithelial fibrosis may only be very subtle as in (**A1**) and (**B2**). For this reason, all patients with a chronic conjunctival inflammation, possibly also with spontaneous remissions and relapses, need to undergo a thorough slit lamp examination including ectropionizing. (**C**) The medial canthus shows progressive scarring with loss of the plica semilunaris and caruncle (asterisks). Usually, as in this case, both eyes are affected. It is important to be aware, that even in clinically apparently calm eyes, subepithelial fibrosis can progress and lead to further shrinkage of the conjunctiva [37, 38]. (Figs. 4/(**A1**) and 4/(**C2**) from Geerling et al. Clinical aspects of ocular mucosal pemphigoid. Ophthalmologie. 2023;120:472–477)

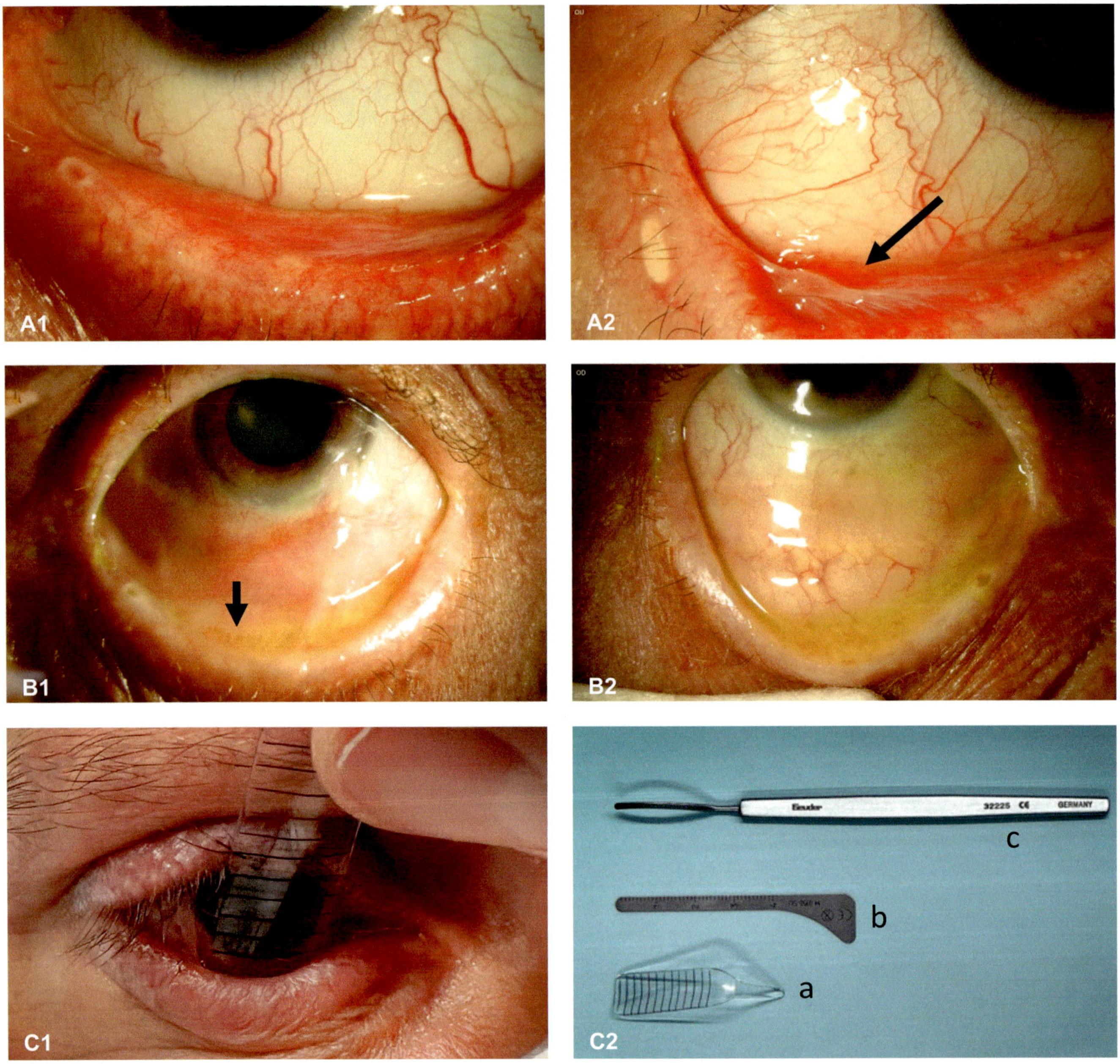

Fig. 5 **Foster Stage II**. Progressive conjunctival shrinkage results in shortening of the fornices (Normal fornix depth [45–48]: lower fornix ca. 10–11 mm; upper fornix: ca. 14–15 mm). In (**A2**), the traction in the conjunctiva in the lower fornix due to the progressive scarring can be seen (black arrow). In (**B1**) and (**B2**), an advanced shortening of the fornix can be observed, the traction in the conjunctiva can be seen again (**B1**, black arrow). Due to progressive fibrosis even in apparently quiet phases, fornix depth can gradually decrease over time and thus is an important parameter to measure progression. As shown in (**C1**), depth of the fornices should regularly be measured. **C2** shows specific devices. Wiliams et al. developed a transparent and atraumatic device made of PMMA that is not commercially (**C2**, **a**) [47]. The flexible measurement device by Steven et al. is commercially available in Germany (**C2**, **b**), but also a curved Vogt scleral ruler can be used (**C2**, **c**)

in the lower fornix or subtarsally (Fig. 4). The progressive conjunctival shrinkage results in a shortening of the fornices (Foster II; Fig. 5) and the formation of symblephara (Foster III; Fig. 6). Increasing qualitative and quantitative tear deficiency causes severe dry eye, possibly leading to corneal and conjunctival keratinization. Eyelid malposition and trichiasis (Figs. 7 and 8) exacerbate the keratopathy and may lead to the formation of corneal epithelial

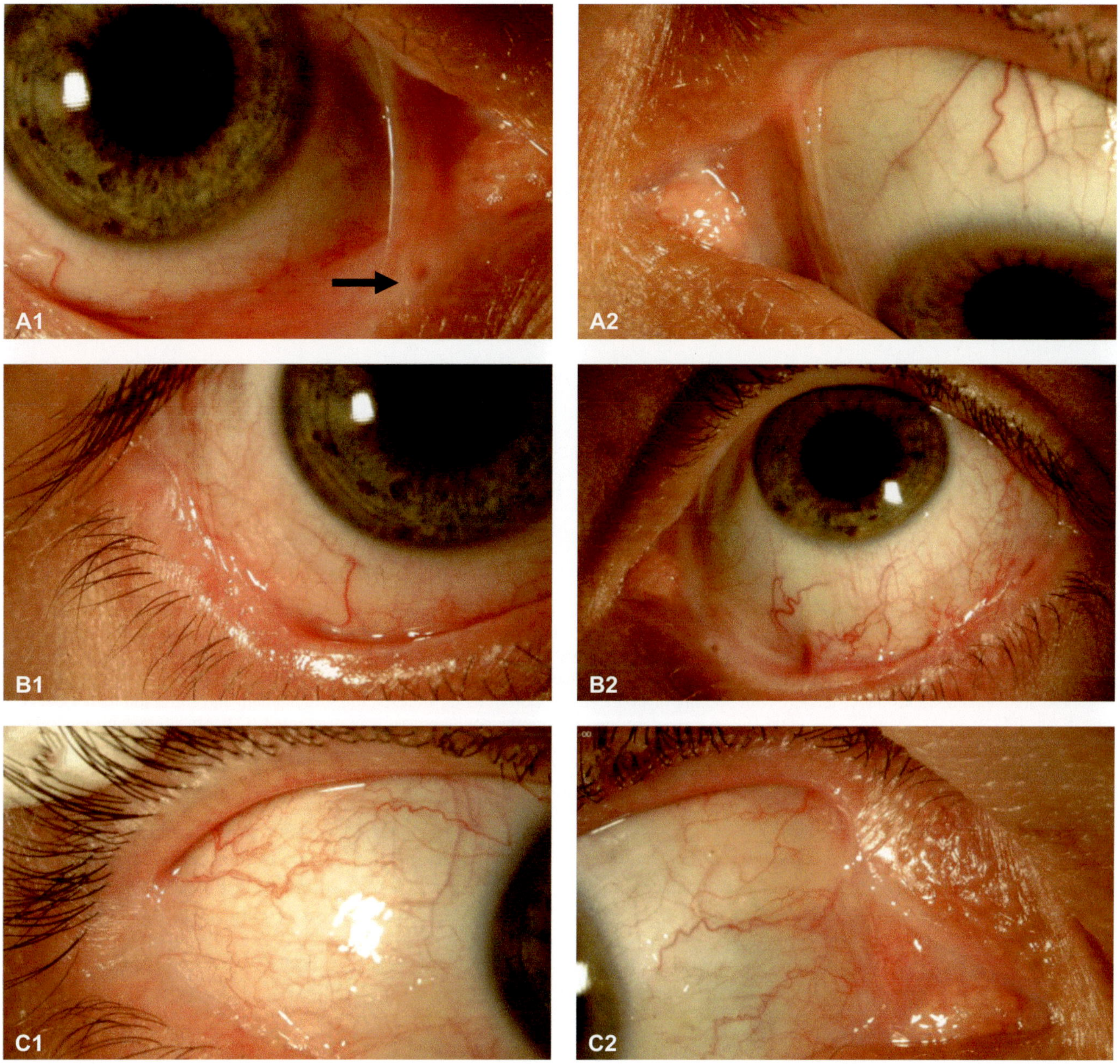

Fig. 6 **Foster Stage III**. This 37-year-old male patient presented for the first time in 2015. Apart from increasing dry eye symptoms, he was complaining of inflammatory changes on the palate and recurrent mouth ulcers throughout the last two years. Examination revealed bilateral, advanced symblephara in the upper (**A**) and lower (**B**) fornix, as well as in canthal area (**C**). The punctum of the right eye showed early signs of fibrotic obstruction (**A1**, arrow). A mucosal biopsy from nose and mouth were negative. Biopsy of the conjunctiva and blood tests were repeated and confirmed an anti-laminin 332 positive mucous membrane pemphigoid. Due to his young age, this patient has a higher risk for more severe and rapidly progressive disease [7, 10, 49]. Due to the possible association of laminin 332 with malignancies, a screening was initiated but remained without a result

defects, neovascularization, or even perforations with corresponding visual loss (Fig. 9) [10, 14, 40, 43]. If surgery is necessary to correct eyelid malposition (Figs. 7 and 8), opening of the conjunctiva needs to be avoided strictly to prevent exacerbation of the disease. In a part of the patients an inflammatory involvement of the peripheral cornea occurs. This so-called “limbitis” leads to damage of limbal stem cells and is associated with a more severe course of

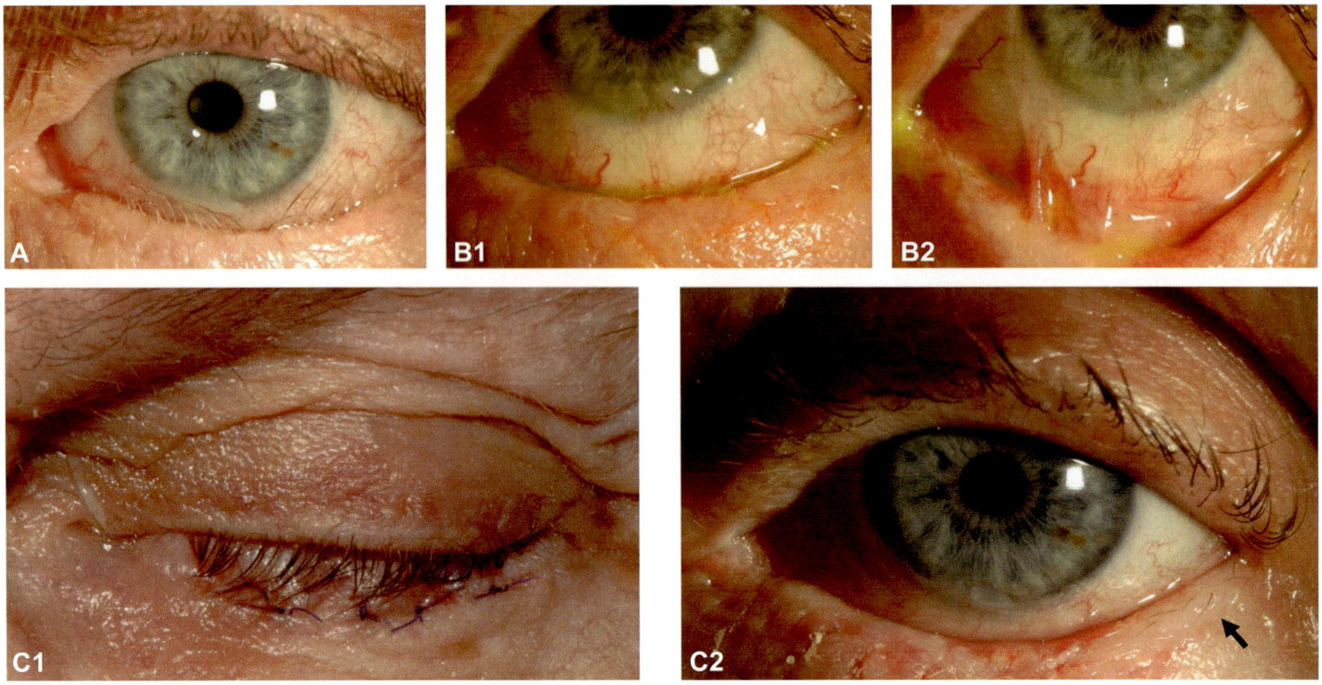

Fig. 7 **Eyelid malposition and trichiasis**. Eyelid malposition, trichiasis and possibly limbal stem cell deficiency exacerbate keratopathy and may lead to the formation of corneal epithelial defects, neovascularization or even perforation with corresponding visual loss. (**A**) Shows a patient with severe trichiasis due to an entropion of the lower lid in 2009. (**B1**) During the next 5 years, the patient underwent electrolysis treatment of aberrant lashes every year (note reduction of eyelashes), nevertheless some trichiasis remained. (**B2**) Although both eyes appeared clinically calm at all examinations under therapy with 500 mg mycophenolate mofetil b.i.d., fibrosis, the symblephara and entropion increased. (**C1**) Thus, lower lid retractor tightening procedure (Jones procedure; no opening the conjunctiva!) was performed (**C2**) After removal of sutures an outward turn of the remaining eyelashes can be recognized (black arrow)

the disease [22, 33, 44] (Fig. 10). Further progression may result in ankyloblepharon (Foster IV) possibly limiting ocular motility (Fig. 11). The final stage of the disease is often associated with severe loss of visual acuity. As keratoplasty of any type tends to have a poor prognosis due to the increased risk of graft failure in those cases, keratoprothesis with biological haptics may be a better choice in patients with terminal bilateral disease (Fig. 11).

Fig. 8 **Anterior lamella repositioning**: Thirty-nine-years-old patient presented with trichiasis, conjunctival hyperemia, foreign body sensation ▶ and reduced vision. Clinical examination revealed upper lid entropium with lash ptosis, scarred upper tarsal conjunctiva, lower fornix symblepharon, conjunctival hyperemia and corneal pannus suspected of a mucous membrane pemphigoid. We planned a conjunctival biopsy and upper lid anterior lamella repositioning to reduce corneal exposure to ptotic eyelashes (**A1**, **B1**). Surgery was performed in local anesthesia. The amount of skin to be excided safely to lift the anterior lamella is marked (**B2**, **B3**); The anterior lamella is prepared down to the lash line (**B4**), a grey-line split is performed to obtain extra eversion of the lashes (**B5**). Three double-armed absorbable sutures are anchored in a "U-fashion" in the tarsal plate and are tied just above the lashes (**B6**). The skin incision is closed with interrupted absorbable sutures (**B7**), which are removed after 10 days. The patient discomfort and vision improved

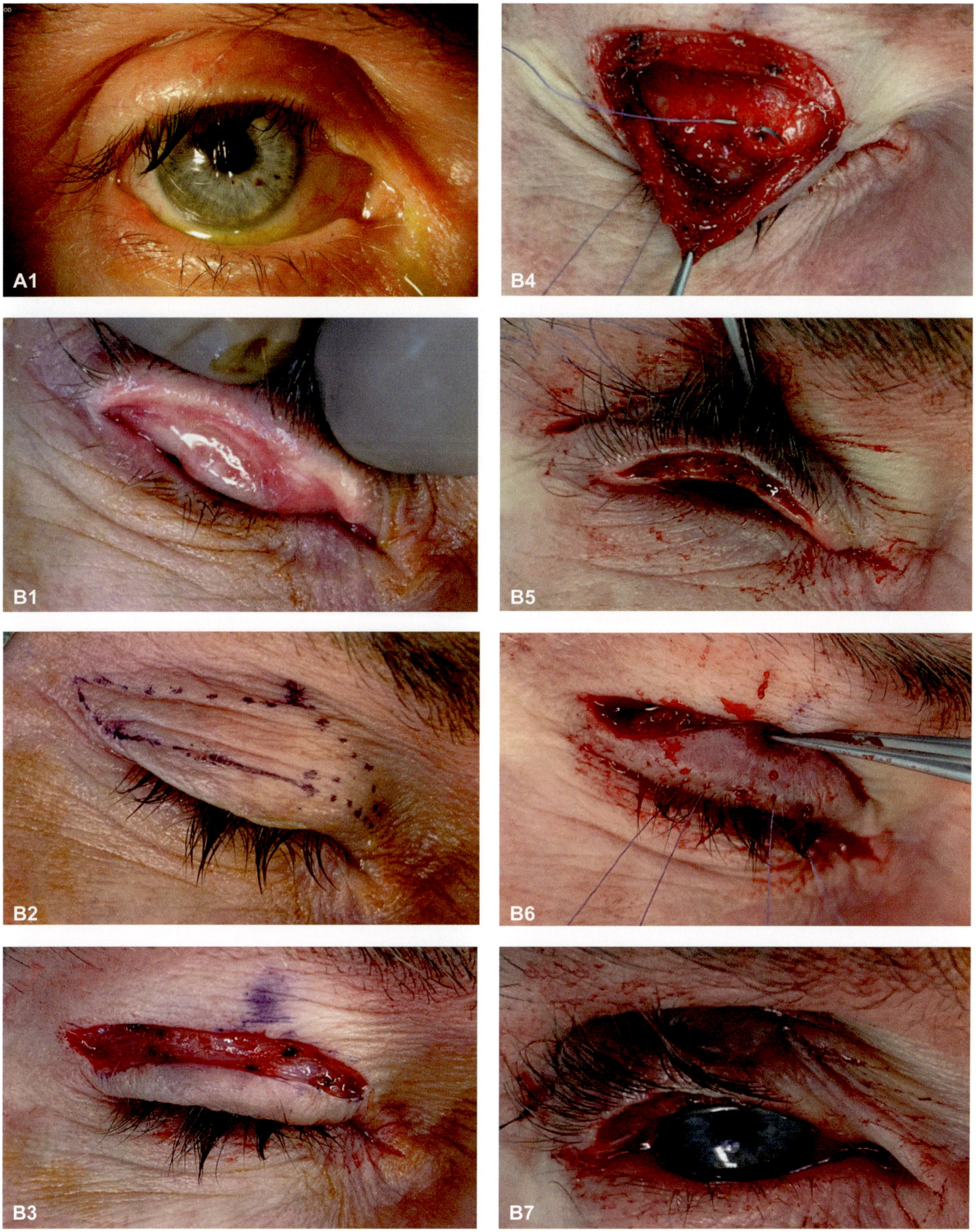
A1
B4
B1
B5
B2
B6
B3
B7

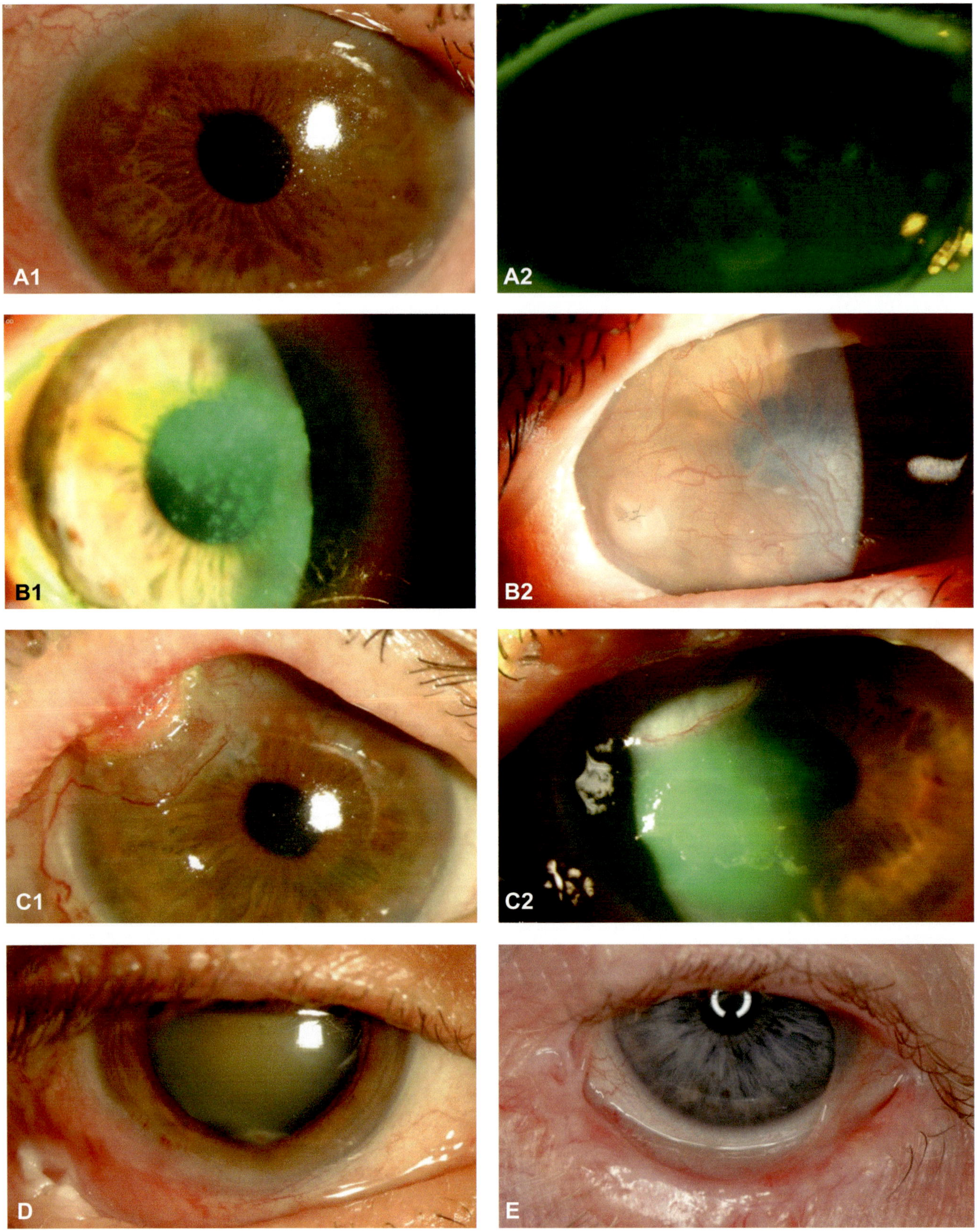
A1
A2
B1
B2
C1
C2
D
E

◀ **Fig. 9** **Ocular surface findings**. (**A1**) On slit lamp examination the tear film appeared to be more viscous. (**A2**) In the same patient, a pronounced irregularity of the tear film and ocular surface can be visualized with fluorescein staining. (**B**) 5 years after first presentation, the patient from Fig. 4 developed severe punctate keratopathy with microerosions due to trichiasis (**B1**). Another 3 years later, the same patient presented again with further progression including peripheral corneal neovascularization and ankyloblepharon (**B2**). (**C**) A 76-year-old female patient developed a symblepharon encroaching the upper limbus (**C1**) and 3 months later an adjacent corneal ulcer (**C2**). (**D**) Age, as well as the often long-term inflammatory reaction and the need for steroid therapy are risk factors for the development of lens opacities, as shown in this patient. Cataract surgery should only be performed in an inflammation-free state or under maximum control of inflammation [50]. (**E**) This 81-year-old male patient showed advanced symblephara and a beginning ankyloblepharon. Such findings, as well as the symblepharon in (**C1**), can lead but not necessarily limit ocular motility. (Video available as online supplement: QR code)

Please scan to access video content

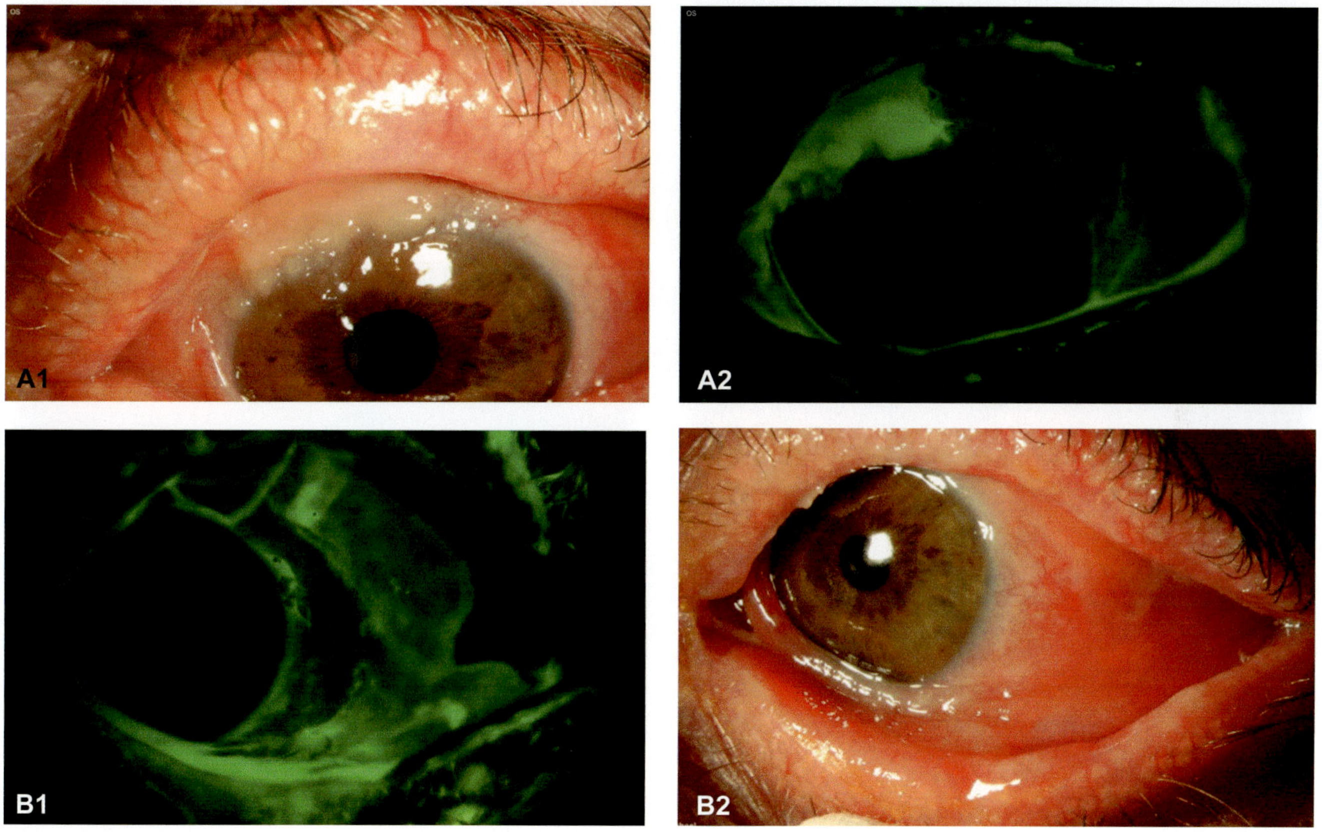

Fig. 10 **Limbal stem cell deficiency.** Increasing qualitative and quantitative tear deficiency lead to severe dry eye with chronic conjunctivitis. In some patients limbitis develops, that may lead to stem cell failure. Limbitis is an important prognostic sign, as it is associated with a more severe course of the disease [22, 33, 44]. (**A1**) shows limbitis in a 59-year-old patient, including peripheral infiltrates similar to Horner-Trantas dots in vernal keratoconjunctivitis. (**A2**) Fluoresceine staining shows the conjunctival erosion in the inflamed area of the limbus. Although treated with intravenous cyclophosphamide and prednisolone, the same patient developed extensive conjunctival erosions (**B1**) which are easily missed without dye use (**B2**). Six months later the patient passed away due to a severe uro-sepsis

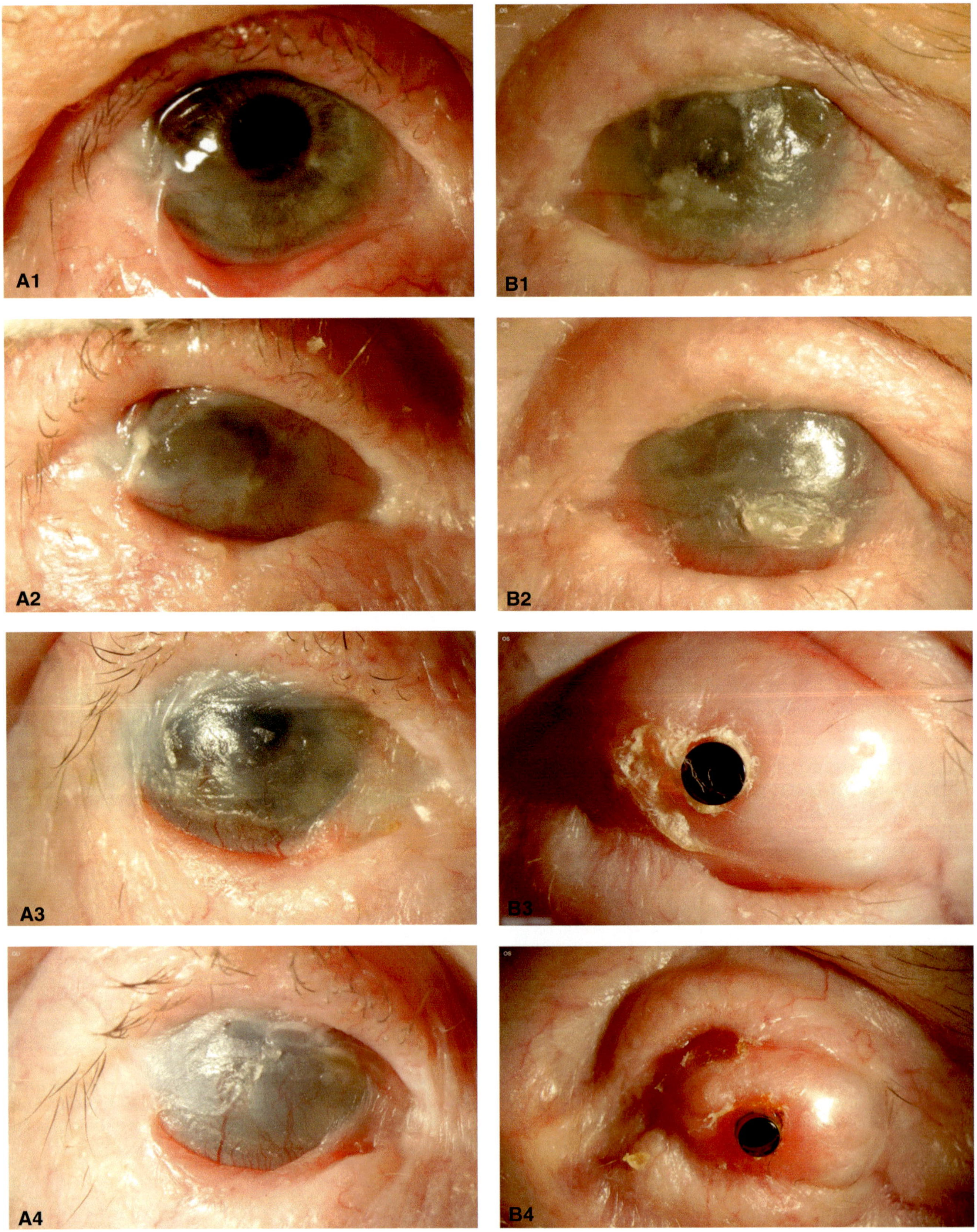

Fig. 11 **Foster Stage IV**. Further progression may result in keratinization of the entire ocular surface and ankyloblepharon. This figure shows the evolution of the right (**A**) and left eye (**B**) of one patient over 33 months. In this period, the right eye (**A**) progressed from stage III to stage IV and a so called "Frozen globe" (**A4**). A morph video of this progress is available as online supplement: QR code. The left eye (**B**) underwent an osteo-odonto-keratoprothesis surgery for visual rehabilitation achieving a best corrected visual acuity of 0.4 (52). (Fig. 11/(**A3**) from Geerling et al. Clinical aspects of ocular mucosal pemphigoid. Ophthalmologie, 2023;120:472–477 and Fig. 11/(**B4**) from Geerling et al. Treatment of ocular mucous membrane pemphigoid. Ophthalmologie, 2023; 120:496–501)

Please scan to access video content

3 Conclusion

Mucous membrane pemphigoid is a therapeutic challenge that can be addressed surgically when inflammatory activity is under control. In order to achieve this, interdisciplinary cooperation for this complex condition is helpful and necessary.

References

1. Beek N van, Zillikens D, Schmidt E. Bullous autoimmune dermatoses: clinical features, diagnostic evaluation, and treatment options. Dtsch Arztebl Int. 2021;118:413–20.
2. Amber KT, Murrell DF, Schmidt E, Joly P, Borradori L. Autoimmune Subepidermal Bullous Diseases of the Skin and Mucosae: Clinical Features, Diagnosis, and Management. Clin Rev Allerg Immu. 2018;54(1):26–51.
3. Bertram F, Bröcker E, Zillikens D, Schmidt E. Prospective analysis of the incidence of autoimmune bullous disorders in Lower Franconia, Germany. J Dtsch Dermatol Ges. 2009;7(5):434–40.
4. Beek N, Weidinger A, Schneider SW, Kleinheinz A, Gläser R, Holtsche MM, et al. Incidence of pemphigoid diseases in Northern Germany in 2016—first data from the Schleswig-Holstein registry of autoimmune bullous diseases. J Eur Acad Dermatol. 2021;35(5):1197–202.
5. Hübner F, Recke A, Zillikens D, Linder R, Schmidt E. Prevalence and age distribution of pemphigus and pemphigoid diseases in Germany. J Invest Dermatol. 2016;136(12):2495–8.
6. Radford CF, Rauz S, Williams GP, Saw VPJ, Dart JKG. Eye (Lond). 2012;26(9):1199–208.
7. Hong GH, Khan IR, Shifera AS, Okeagu C, Thorne JE. Incidence and clinical characteristics of ocular involvement in mucous membrane pemphigoid. Ocul Immunol Inflamm. 2018;27(5):1–5.
8. Higgins GT, Allan RB, Hall R, Field EA, Kaye SB. Development of ocular disease in patients with mucous membrane pemphigoid involving the oral mucosa. Br J Ophthalmol. 2006; 90(8):964–7.
9. Long Q, Zuo YG, Yang X, Gao TT, Liu J, Li Y. Clinical features and in vivo confocal microscopy assessment in 12 patients with ocular cicatricial pemphigoid. Int J Ophthalmol. 2016;9(5):730–7
10. Ong HS, Setterfield JF, Minassian DC, Dart JK. Mucous membrane pemphigoid study group 2009–2014. Mucous membrane pemphigoid with ccular involvement: the clinical phenotype and its relationship to direct immunofluorescence findings. Ophthalmology. 2018;125(4):496–504.
11. Labowsky MT, Stinnett SS, Liss J, Daluvoy M, Hall RP, Shieh C. Clinical implications of direct immunofluorescence findings in patients with ocular mucous membrane Pemphigoid. Am J Ophthalmol. 2017;183:48–55.
12. Chiganer EH, Albera P. Ocular cicatricial pemphigoid: Conjunctival biopsy findings and its relationship to ocular's inflammation and scarring. Rev Mex Oftalmol. 2017;91(3):134–41.
13. Hui X, Zhang H. Analysis of clinical characteristics of cicatricial pemphigoid in 35 cases. Int J Ophthalmol [Internet]. 2010;10(9):1829–31.
14. Foster CS, Neumann R, Tauber J. Long term results of systemic chemotherapy for ocular cicatricial pemphigoid. Doc Ophthalmol. 1992;82(3):223–9.
15. Thorne JE, Anhalt GJ, Jabs DA. Mucous membrane pemphigoid and pseudopemphigoid. Ophthalmology. 2004;111(1):45–52.
16. Hübner F, König IR, Holtsche MM, Zillikens D, Linder R, Schmidt E. Prevalence and age distribution of pemphigus and pemphigoid diseases among paediatric patients in Germany. J Eur Acad Dermatol. 2020;34(11):2600–5.
17. Kharfi M, Khaled A, Anane R, Fazaa B, Kamoun MR. Early onset childhood cicatricial pemphigoid: a case report and review of the literature. Pediatr Dermatol. 2010;27(2):119-–24.
18. Flores-Climente V, Rozas-Muñoz E, Martínez-Grau A, Aucouturier F, Luna S, Baselga E. Childhood ocular mucous membrane pemphigoid successfully treated with rituximab. Pediatr Dermatol. 2019;36(6):984–5.
19. Chan LS. Mucous membrane pemphigoid. Clin Dermatol. 2001;19(6):703–11.
20. Fleming TE, Korman NJ. Cicatricial pemphigoid. J Am Acad Dermatol. 2000;43(4):571–94.
21. Foster CS. Cicatricial pemphigoid. T Am Ophthal Soc. 1986;84:527–663.
22. Hofmann SC, Günther C, Böckle BC, Didona D, Ehrchen J, Gaskins M, et al. S2k-Leitlinie zur Diagnostik und Therapie des Schleimhautpemphigoids. Jddg J Der Deutschen Dermatologischen Gesellschaft. 2022;20(11):1530–52.
23. Leverkus M, Schmidt E, Lazarova Z, Bröcker EB, Yancey KB, Zillikens D. Antiepiligrin Cicatricial pemphigoid: an underdiagnosed entity within the spectrum of scarring autoimmune subepidermal bullous diseases? Arch Dermatol. 1999;135(9):1091–8.
24. Egan CA, Lazarova Z, Darling TN, Yee C, Cote T, Yancey KB. Anti-epiligrin cicatricial pemphigoid and relative risk for cancer. Lancet. 2001;357(9271):1850-1.
25. Terra JB, Pas HH, Hertl M, Dikkers FG, Kamminga N, Jonkman MF. Immunofluorescence serration pattern analysis as a diagnostic criterion in antilaminin-332 mucous membrane pemphigoid: immunopathological findings and clinical experience in 10 Dutch patients. Brit J Dermatol. 2011;165(4):815–22.
26. Hayakawa T, Furumura M, Fukano H, Li X, Ishii N, Hamada T, et al. Diagnosis of oral mucous membrane pemphigoid by means of combined serologic testing. Oral Surg Oral Medicine Oral Pathology Oral Radiology. 2014;117(4):483–96.
27. Matsushima S, Horiguchi Y, Honda T, Fujii S, Okano T, Tanabe M, et al. A case of anti-epiligrin cicatricial pemphigoid associated with lung carcinoma and severe laryngeal stenosis: review of Japanese cases and evaluation of risk for internal malignancy. J Dermatology. 2004;31(1):10–5.
28. Goletz S, Probst C, Komorowski L, Schlumberger W, Fechner K, van Beek N, et al. A sensitive and specific assay for the serological diagnosis of antilaminin 332 mucous membrane pemphigoid. Brit J Dermatol. 2019;180(1):149–56.
29. Gasparini G, Cozzani E, Zenzo GD, Salemme A, Dematté E, Vassallo C, et al. Anti-laminin 332 antibody detection using biochip immunofluorescence microscopy in a real-life cohort of Italian patients with mucous membrane pemphigoid. European J Dermatology Ejd. 2021.
30. Li X, Qian H, Natsuaki Y, Koga H, Kawakami T, Tateishi C, et al. Clinical and immunological findings in 55 patients with

anti-laminin 332-type mucous membrane pemphigoid. Brit J Dermatol. 2021;185(2):449–51.
31. Schmidt E, Rashid H, Marzano AV, Lamberts A, Zenzo GD, Diercks GFH, et al. European Guidelines (S3) on diagnosis and management of mucous membrane pemphigoid, initiated by the European academy of Dermatology and Venereology—part II. J Eur Acad Dermatol. 2021.
32. Elder MJ, Bernauer W, Leonard J, Dart JK. Progression of disease in ocular cicatricial pemphigoid. Br J Ophthalmol. 1996;80(4):292--6.
33. Ong HS, Minassian D, Rauz S, Mehta JS, Dart JK. Validation of a clinical assessment tool for cicatrising conjunctivitis. Ocular Surf. 2020;18(1):121–9.
34. Miserocchi E, Baltatzis S, Roque MR, Ahmed AR, Foster CS. The effect of treatment and its related side effects in patients with severe ocular cicatricial pemphigoid. Ophthalmology. 2002;109(1):111–8.
35. Saw VPJ, Dart JKG, Rauz S, Ramsay A, Bunce C, Xing W, et al. Immunosuppressive therapy for ocular mucous membrane pemphigoid strategies and outcomes. Ophthalmology. 2007;115(2):253-261.e1.
36. Williams GP, Radford C, Nightingale P, Dart JKG, Rauz S. Evaluation of early and late presentation of patients with ocular mucous membrane pemphigoid to two major tertiary referral hospitals in the United Kingdom. Eye (Lond). 2011;25(9):1207–18.
37. Saw VP, Schmidt E, Offiah I, Galatowicz G, Zillikens D, Dart JK, Calder VL, Daniels JT. Profibrotic phenotype of conjunctival fibroblasts from mucous membrane pemphigoid. Am J Pathol. 2011;178(1):187–97.
38. Mondino BJ, Brown SI. Ocular cicatricial pemphigoid. Ophthalmology. 1981;88(2):95–100.
39. Mameletzi E, Hamedani M, Majo F, Guex-Crosier Y. Clinical Manifestations of Mucous Membrane Pemphigoid in a Tertiary Center. Klin Monbl Augenheilkd. 2012;229(4):416–9.
40. Mehra T, Guenova E, Dechent F, Würth F, Zierhut M, Röcken M, et al. Diagnostic relevance of direct immunofluorescence in ocular mucous membrane pemphigoid. Jddg J Der Deutschen Dermatologischen Gesellschaft. 2015;13(12):1268Trans Ophthalmol Soc U K (1962). 1979;99(1):141–574.
41. Wright P. Enigma of ocular cicatricial pemphigoid. A comparative study of clinical and immunological findings. Transactions of the Ophthalmological Societies of the United Kingdom [Internet]. 1979;99(1):141–5. Trans Ophthalmol Soc U K (1962). 1979;99(1):141–5.
42. Cheung AY, Sarnicola E, Denny MR, Sepsakos L, Auteri NJ, Holland EJ. Limbal stem cell deficiency: demographics and clinical characteristics of a large retrospective series at a single tertiary referral center. Cornea. 2021;40(12):1525–31.
43. Dart JK. The 2016 Bowman Lecture Conjunctival curses: scarring conjunctivitis 30 years on. Eye (Lond). 2017;31(2):301–332.
44. Bobba S, Devlin C, Girolamo ND, Wakefield D, McCluskey P, Chan E, et al. Incidence, clinical features and diagnosis of cicatrising conjunctivitis in Australia and New Zealand. Eye. 2018;32(10):1636–43.
45. Khan IJ, Ghauri AJ, Hodson J, Edmunds MR, Cottrell P, Evans S, et al. Defining the limits of normal conjunctival fornix anatomy in a healthy South Asian population. Ophthalmology. 2014;121(2):492–7.
46. Jutley G, Carpenter D, Hau S, Booth D, Jasim HA, Tay E, et al. Upper and lower conjunctival fornix depth in healthy white caucasian eyes: a method of objective assessment. Eye. 2016;30(10):1351–8.
47. Williams GP, Saw VPJ, Saeed T, Evans ST, Cottrell P, Curnow SJ, et al. Validation of a fornix depth measurer: a putative tool for the assessment of progressive cicatrising conjunctivitis. Brit J Ophthalmol. 2011;95(6):842.
48. Kawakita T, Kawashima M, Murat D, Tsubota K, Shimazaki J. Measurement of fornix depth and area: a novel method of determining the severity of fornix shortening. Eye. 2009; 23(5):1115–9.
49. Rauz S, Maddison PG, Dart JK. Evaluation of Mucous Membrane Pemphigoid with Ocular Involvement in Young Patients. Ophthalmology. 2005;112(7):1268–74.
50. Geerling G, Dart JKG. Management and outcome of cataract surgery in ocular cicatricial pemphigoid. Graefe's Archive Clin Exp Ophthalmol. 2000;238(2):112–8.
51. Schmidt E, Benoit S, Kampik D, Hille K, Geerling G. Tibial bone keratoprosthesis: reversing blindness in mucous membrane pemphigoid. J Dtsch Dermatol Ges. 2017;15(10):1024–1026.

Stevens–Johnson Syndrome SJS/Toxic Epidermal Necrolysis TEN

Arnd Heiligenhaus and Jan Ehrchen

Abstract

Stevens–Johnson syndrome (SJS)/toxic epidermal necrolysis (TEN) is defined as a rare and serious, widespread, vesiculobullous rash with epidermal sloughing and necrosis of the skin and mucous membrane involvement, usually of eyes, oral cavity, and genitals. Drugs are the most common cause of SJS/TEN. Ocular involvement in SJS/TEN occurs in 20% to 90% of cases, being almost 100% in more severe TEN. Acute-stage severe ocular complications are defined as severe conjunctivitis with pseudomembranes and epithelial defects of the conjunctiva and cornea. Consequences such as persistent corneal epithelial defects, which present a risk of infection and tissue destruction of the stroma, represent severe ocular complications of chronic disease. Long-term visual impairment constitutes a major burden of disease, occurring in about 25–50% of patients. Histological confirmation from skin biopsy at disease onset with the hallmark finding of subepidermal split formation is obligatory to exclude potential differential diagnoses. Early transfer to specialized units, such as dermatological centers, intensive care, or burn units should be initiated to improve survival. Early diagnosis, early withdrawal of the suspected initiating drug, immediate and appropriate care in the acute phase, and appropriate follow-up by cornea specialists are important to prevent vision impairment.

A. Heiligenhaus (✉)
Uveitis Zentrum, Augenzentrum Am St. Franziskus Hospital, Münster, Deutschland
e-mail: arnd.heiligenhaus@uveitis-zentrum.de
URL: http://www.uveitis-zentrum.de

J. Ehrchen
Leitung Autoimmunerkrankungen; Klinik Für Dermatologie, Universitätsklinikum Münster (UKM), Münster, Deutschland
e-mail: jan.ehrchen@ukmuenster.de

Keywords

Stevens–Johnson syndrome · Toxic epidermal necrolysis · Eye · Complications · Diagnosis · Therapy

1 Clinical Characteristics in Stevens–Johnson Syndrome and Toxic Epidermal Necrolysis

Stevens and Johnson in 1922 first described a life-threatening disease-causing blistering of the skin and mucous membranes, named Stevens–Johnson syndrome (SJS) [1]. In 1956, Lyell established the term toxic epidermal necrolysis (TEN) to describe the extensive detachment of the epidermis that resembled scaled skin [2]. Fuchs' syndrome is considered to be a pure mucosal variant of SJS. SJS/TEN is defined as an acute, widespread vesiculobullous rash with epidermal sloughing and necrosis of the skin and mucous membrane involvement, usually of eyes, oral cavity, and genitals. SJS/TEN are rare and serious diseases, putting patients' lives in danger during the acute phase and commonly leaving them with a severe burden of illness in the long term. SJS and TEN likely describe the same disease, but with differences in severity [3]. Hence, SJS involves < 10% of the total body surface area (BSA), whereas SJS-TEN affects 10–30%, and TEN > 30% of BSA, respectively.

Epidemiology

With incidence rates of 0.4–7/1 Mio residents [4, 5], SJS and TEN are rare diseases. Indeed, within the PubMed literature between 1980 and 2017, only about 850 cases with probable or definite SJS/TEN have been reported. Although SJS/TEN can occur at any age, two peaks of disease onset have been described, one in childhood and another one between the second and third decade of life [6]. Reported disease occurrence in children accounts for about 1/3 of patients [6, 7].

B. Seitz et al. (eds.), *Atlas on Cornea*, https://doi.org/10.1007/978-3-031-65422-0_32

Burden of illness

Worldwide burden of illness is substantial, as prolonged hospitalization, high mortality (up to 50% in elderly), and diverse long-term consequences impairing quality of life may develop [8]. Owing to the extensive skin involvement and secondary complications, the mortality of TEN can be up to three times higher than that of SJS.

Risk factors

Risk factors for SJS/TEN development include immunocompromised states, e.g., HIV, malignancy, and generalized immune-mediated disease. Racial and genetic predisposition for SJS has been suspected. Certain ethnicities, particularly patients of Asian descent, are at increased risk for drug-induced SJS/TEN.

The underlying hypersensitivity reaction to particular triggers may be linked to certain HLA alleles [9–11]. In addition to microbial infection and medicines (see below), a combination of multiple gene polymorphisms and their interactions have been suggested to contribute strongly to the onset of SJS/TEM [12]. Certain HLA subtypes were identified as biomarkers for severe ocular complications in SJS patients [13]. Significant associations between certain HLA genotypes and cold medicine-induced SJS/TEN with severe ocular complications were distinguished. However, as these drugs are commonly freely available worldwide, genetic screening prior to their use might not be feasible.

Drugs are the most common cause of SJS/TEN. Drugs such as antibiotics, anti-infective sulfonamides, sulfasalazine, oxicam-type nonsteroidal anti-inflammatory drugs (NSAIDS), allopurinol, and aromatic anticonvulsants are known risk factors for the disease (Table 1) [14]. In a nationwide study, culprit drugs included anticonvulsants (most frequent), allopurinol, amoxicillin, dorzolamide, and acetaminophen [15]. In FDA regulatory actions, seventeen hematology/oncology products (e.g., checkpoint inhibitors), eight antimicrobials, six radiocontrast agents, deflazacort, and febuxostat were labeled for SJS/TEN. A 20-year database review of children with SJS/TEN disclosed morbilliform rash (83%) and blisters (39%) as the predominant presentation, with common oral (97%) and eye (84%) involvement, mostly induced by drugs (72%; antiepileptics 36%) [16]. Within a large dataset from a major tertiary eye hospital in the UK, oral antibiotics (penicillins, sulfa drugs, and tetracyclines) were causative in half of the chronic SJS patients and nonsteroidal drugs and anticonvulsants in 7–8% of them [6].

Among nondrug infectious causes, herpesvirus, mycoplasma pneumonia, tuberculosis, and human immunodeficiency virus (HIV) are known risk factors for SJS/TEN. Lastly, vaccinations are also implicated as triggering factors (e.g., human papillomavirus, mumps, measles, rubella, hepatitis B, influenza, anthrax, and tetanus [14]).

Clinical phases

SJS/TEN patients may present with a prodromal phase of fever, malaise, cough, stinging eyes, and sore throat, preceding mucocutaneous disease. The acute phase of mucocutaneous disease is characterized by diffuse erythema typically located at the trunk, face, feet, and hands. Then, bullae may develop and large sheets of epidermis may separate from the dermis, resulting in widespread erosions (Fig. 1) as well as desquamation of mucosa (primarily oral (Fig. 2) and ocular). Cutaneous lesions also include target-like lesions. "Target lesions" are less than 3 cm in diameter, round, and involve 2–3 concentric zones of color change, usually a central area of dusky erythema and often blister formation, sometimes a middle paler zone of edema, and an outer ring of erythema with a defined edge (Fig. 3). Target lesions plus involvement of at least two mucous membranes comprise SJS, while widespread epidermal necrolysis > 30% body surface area defines TEN. The condition can be associated with multi-organ failure, sepsis, gastrointestinal hemorrhage, and pulmonary embolism.

Table 1 Drugs associated with a high risk for developing Stevens–Johnson syndrome/toxic epidermal necrolysis

Carbamazepin
Lamotrigene
Nevirapine
Phenobarbital
Phenytoin
Allopurinol
Antibiotics, especially beta lactams
Anti-infective sulfonamides, like cotrimoxazole
Sulfasalazine
Oxicame non-steroidal anti-inflammatory drug
Dorzolamide and Methazolamide

NSAID = non-steroidal anti-inflammatory drugs

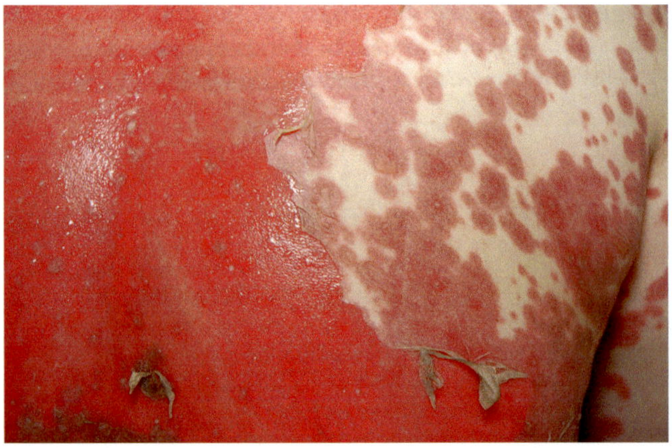

Fig. 1 SJS/TEN target lesions and extensive erosive areas at the trunk

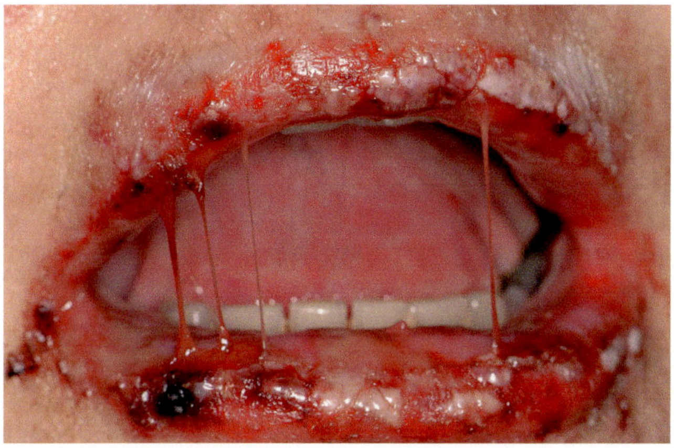

Fig. 2 SJS/TEN extensive erosive lesions on the lips

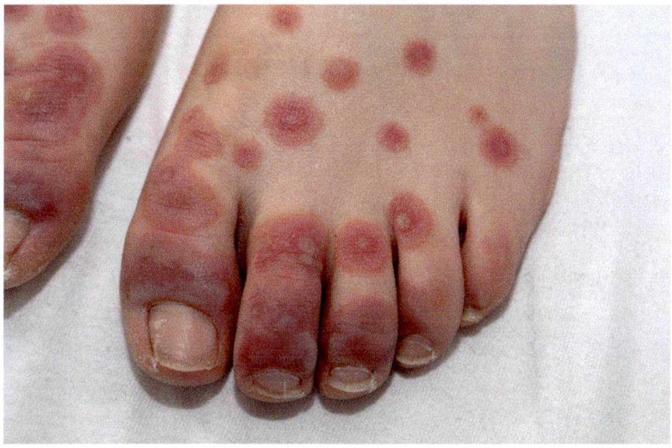

Fig. 3 Target lesions, round lesions with concentric zones of color change, a central area of dusky erythema and blister formation, a middle paler zone of edema, and an outer ring of erythema with defined edge

While SJS/TEN typically are self-limiting, lasting 6–8 weeks after onset, the acute stage may be followed by a relentless chronic course characterized by multi-organ sequelae with increased morbidity and reduced quality of life. Remitting inflammation and chronic ocular surface disease are observed in 30–50% of patients, and particularly in TEN [17–19].

2 Eye Involvement in SJS/TEN

Ocular involvement in SJS/TEN occurs in 20% and up to 90% of cases, being almost 100% in the more severe TEN [5, 20, 21]. Eye involvement might not be appreciated during the initial disease stage. However, acute conjunctivitis can develop even before or within several hours to days after the initial mucocutaneous lesions have become apparent [22].

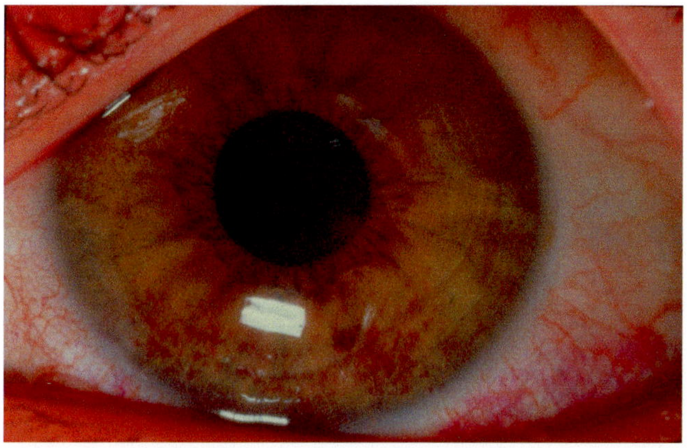

Fig. 4 Stevens–Johnson syndrome. Chronic phase. Punctate keratitis. Bengal rose staining of cornea and conjunctiva

Ocular sequelae vary from mild dry eyes, mucopurulent conjunctivitis, punctate keratitis (Fig. 4) to pseudomembranous/membranous conjunctivitis, with or without early corneal involvement. Subsequently, entropion with severe corneal scarring and ulceration and perforation may follow [23]. While no clear correlation between skin and eye disease has previously been found, recent studies suggest that disease severity, older age, and higher S100A8/A9 and granulysin levels help to predict acute severe ocular complications [24].

No standardized distinction between "acute" and "chronic" SJS/TEN has been found. While this distinction may be between 3 and 6 months after disease onset [25], some studies have used an arbitrary cut-off of 12 months to define chronic disease [26].

Acute-stage severe ocular complications are defined as severe conjunctivitis with pseudomembranes and epithelial defects of the conjunctiva and cornea. Consequences such as persistent corneal epithelial defects, constituting a risk of infection and tissue destruction of the stroma, represent severe ocular complications of chronic disease. Severe ocular surface complications may persist long after the systemic condition has subsided. In addition, chronic ocular disease in SJS/TEN tends to be progressive and unpredictable, with poor correlation with the severity of acute ocular complications [21, 27]. Persistent ocular surface inflammation can result in a multitude of long-standing sequelae. These include dry eye disease, eyelid malposition (ectropion, entropion, lagophthalmos), misdirected lashes (trichiasis, distichiasis; Fig. 5), posterior eyelid keratinization, conjunctival disease (keratinization, symblepharon, and ankyloblepharon; Fig. 6), and corneal disease (epithelial defects, thinning, scarring, neovascularization, and limbal stem cell deficiency) (Fig. 7) [25]. Corneal complications (neovascularization and opacification) are correlated with the worst long-term visual prognosis [26].

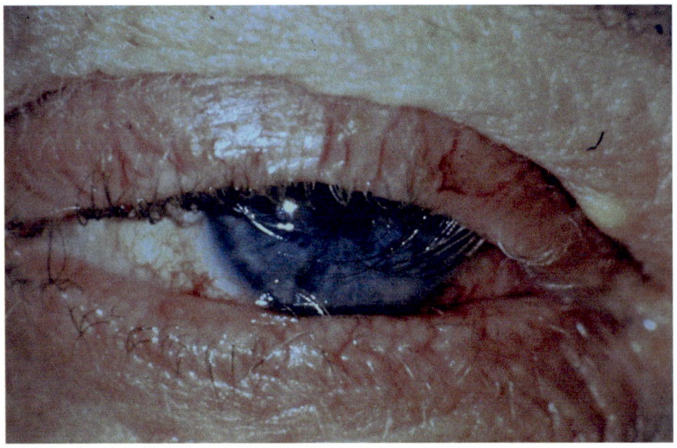

Fig. 5 Stevens–Johnson syndrome. Entropion, trichiasis

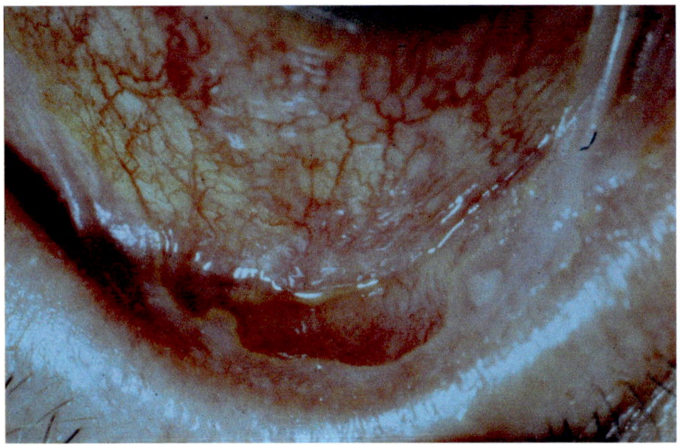

Fig. 6 Stevens–Johnson syndrome. Chronic stage. Symblepharon, lid margin keratinization

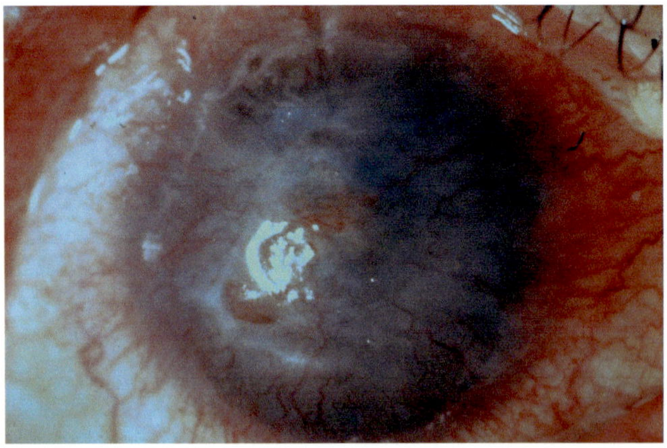

Fig. 7 Toxic epidermal necrolysis. Chronic stage. Corneal scarring, neovascularization, limbal stem cell deficiency

Fibrosis of the superotemporal conjunctiva around the ducts of the lacrimal gland—which drain tears onto the ocular surface—represents the main etiology for aqueous deficiency dry eye in the patients [28]. Severe dry eye, however, not only results from aqueous tear deficiency, but also from decreased wettability (by corneal surface change via squamous metaplasia/keratinization) of the corneal surface and increased evaporation (due to Meibomian gland dysfunction) [29].

Prevalence of visual disturbances and eye dryness correlated with acute ocular severity [22]. Proinflammatory cytokines in tears were increased in chronic SJS patients [30]. Attempts have been made to categorize the different phenotypes of acute ocular surface disease in SJS/TEN patients [22, 31, 32]. These categories are not mutually exclusive and can occur either simultaneously or sequentially (Table 2).

3 Long-Term Prognosis in SJS/TEN

Eye disease

Long-term sequelae from SJS/TEN are serious and not rare. The severity of the underlying disease during the acute phase and initial ocular lesions constitutes the main risk of severe long-term eye damage [33, 34].

Data from the RegiSCAR study demonstrate that at 8 weeks, most survivors suffer from skin (88%) and eye symptoms (70%), and these symptoms were present at 5 years in about two-thirds of patients [8]. Many of the patients suffered from psychological sequelae and did not return to premorbid activities or to gainful employment. Notably, poor initial vision, disease duration, and limbal stem cell deficiency are predictors for poor final outcome [6].

In 30–50% of SJS/TEN patients, long-term complications may develop, including symblepharon, lid margin keratinization, trichiasis, entropium, dry eye syndrome, corneal neovascularization, and persistent epithelial defects [17, 35]. Long-term visual impairment is a major burden of SJS that developed in about 25–50% of patients reported previously [6, 26, 36]. Symblepharon, keratinization, limbal stem cell deficiency, and corneal neovascularization and opacification (Fig. 8) are major contributors to severe visual outcome. Almost 2/3 of SJS/TEN children not receiving appropriate therapy were eventually blind [37].

Mucocutaneous disease

Since necrolysis is limited to the epidermis, scar formation at the skin is not a frequent complication of SJS/TEN. However, it can occur if large areas of the skin are involved

Table 2 Grading systems for acute phase Stevens–Johnson syndrome/toxic epidermal necrolysis

Sotozono et al. 2015 [22]			
Ocular surface grading system (each, grade 0–3):			
Corneal complications		Superficial punctate keratopathy	
		Epithelial defect	
		Loss of the palisades of Vogt	
		Conjunctivalization	
		Neovascularization	
		Opacification	
		Keratinization	
Conjunctival complications		Hyperemia	
		Symblepharon formation	
Eyelid complications		Trichiasis	
		Mucocutaneous junction involvement	
		Meibomian gland involvement	
		Punctal damage	
Grade 1: Conjunctival hyperemia; no corneal, conjunctival, or eyelid margin defects			
Grade 2: Corneal, conjunctival, or eyelid margin defects without membranes			
Grade 3: Corneal, conjunctival, or eyelid margin defects with membranes			
Gregory 2016 [31]			
	Lid margin	Cornea	Conjunctiva (bulbar and palpebral)
Mild	No staining	No staining	hyperemia, without stain
Severe	Staining > 1/3 of lid margin length on at least 1 lid	Any epithelial defect more than punctate staining	(+) staining > 1 cm
Extremely severe	Staining > 1/3 of lid margin length on more than 1 lid	Any epithelial defect more than punctate staining	multiple areas of stain > 1 cm
Thorel et al. 2020 [32]			
Stage 0		No ocular involvement	
Stage 1		Conjunctival hyperemia	
Stage 2		Pseudomembranous conjunctivitis	
		Reversible conjunctival adhesion	
		Slight fornix foreshortening	
		Superficial punctate keratitis	
Stage 3		Corneal ulceration	
		Symblepharon/irreversible conjunctivalization	

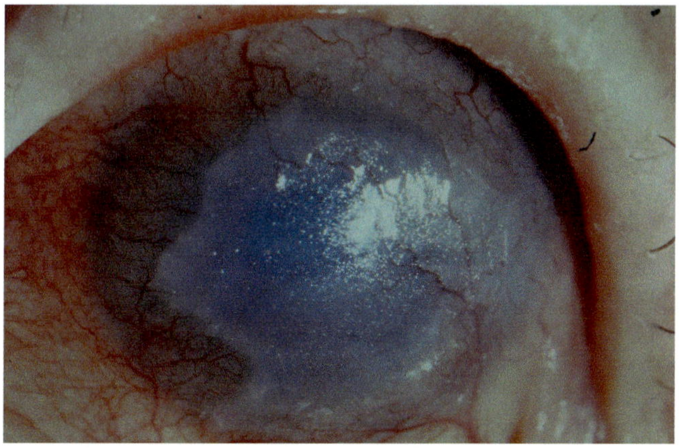

Fig. 8 Stevens–Johnson syndrome. Chronic stage. Dry eye, limbal stem cell deficiency, corneal neovascularization and scar formation

and if secondary complications such as infections arise. Moreover, long-lasting dyspigmentation of the skin is a common finding. Post-inflammatory scarring and strictures can develop at mucosal surfaces, for example, the esophagus or the genital mucosa, but the oral cavity and the lips are usually spared. Nail dystrophy and alopecia are also observed as cutaneous complications of disease.

SJS/TEN may also be complicated by obliterative bronchitis or bronchiolitis, bronchiectasis, esophageal stricture, recurrent cystitis, lingual ulcerations, and recurrent oral aphthae. Keloid variants with chronic pain and pruritus of the involved areas may develop. The presence of extensive necrolysis, idiopathic nature of disease, old age, elevated urea, creatinine and glucose levels, neutropenia, lymphopenia, and thrombocytopenia are linked to a poor prognosis.

Table 3 SCORTEN ("Severity-of-Illness Score for Toxic Epidermial Necrolysis") scale

Risk factor	0	1
Age	<40 years	>40 years
Associated malignancy	No	Yes
Heart rate (beats/min)	<120	>120
Serum BUN (Blood Urea Nitrogen) (mg/dL)	<27	>27
Detached or compromised body surface	<10%	>10%
Serum bicarbonate (mEq/L)	>20	<20
Serum glucose (mg/dL)	<250	>250

* Adapted from Guegan et al. 2006 [38]

Table 4 Mortality

No of risk factors	Mortality rate (%)
0–1	3.2
2	12.1
3	35.3
4	58.3
5 or more	>90

* Adapted from Guegan et al. 2006 [38]

The score of toxic epidermal necrolysis (SCORTEN) scale [38] (Table 3) has been validated to determine the mortality (Table 4) and is considered to be the gold standard for prognosis.

4 Immunopathogenesis in SJS/TEN

Current evidence demonstrates that specific HLA alleles predispose to developing SJS/TEN after exposure to particular drugs. The mutations or polymorphisms of drug metabolic enzymes, transporters, receptors, immune system genes, and T cell-mediated apoptosis signaling pathways that contribute to SJS/TEN are important prerequisites to disease development.

T cells appear as important mediators in disease, interacting with particular HLA/peptide/T cell receptor complexes on keratinocytes, thereby inducing adaptive immune responses and adverse reactions. Infiltrating CD8+cytotoxic T cells and NK cells via secreting cytolytic proteins, chemokines (e.g., granulysin, perforin/granzyme) and intracellular enzymes (caspases), and Fas-FasL then cause profound apoptotic keratinocyte death. Hence, tumor necrosis factor-α (TNF-α) and interleukin-6 (IL-6) as well as cytotoxic T cells and their secretory products are found in blister fluid [39–41].

5 Diagnostic Approaches in SJS/TEN

Differential diagnosis

As about one third of cases may be misdiagnosed, histological confirmation from skin biopsy at disease onset with the hallmark finding of subepidermal split formation is obligatory [42] to exclude potential differential diagnoses. Other cutaneous diseases resulting in widespread blister formation can be distinguished by intraepidermal split formation (pemphigus disease, including paraneoplastic pemphigus and staphylococcal split skin syndrome), or the absence of immunoglobulin depositions (pemphigoid group of diseases, including linear IgA dermatosis) in direct immunofluorescence. The latter is especially important as linear IgA dermatosis can be associated with drug intake (especially vancomycin) and may clinically mimic SJS/TEN. Lupus erythematodes can sometimes mimic SJS/TEN (Rowell Syndrome) but can usually be distinguished by paraffin-embedded histology.

Skin biopsy

Histopathologic examination remains the gold standard for diagnosis of blistering disorders, including SJS/TEN. The typical histological finding is an interface dermatitis with a sparse infiltration of mainly CD4+and CD8-positive T cells in the papillary dermis and extensive epidermal necrosis, resulting in widespread separation of the epidermis from the dermis or focal subepidermal blister formation. If SJS/TEN is clinically suspected, several skin biopsies should be taken. Frozen sections are suitable both for rapid diagnosis confirming subepidermal spilt formation and for direct immunofluorescence staining of respective immunoglobulins to exclude autoimmune blistering disease. A paraffin-embedded specimen is required for routine histology.

Importantly, SJS/TEN is a clinical diagnosis, requiring immediate therapeutic action, even before the results from skin biopsies are available. Rapid onset of widespread skin lesions after a prodromal phase, induction of skin blisters by shear forces (rubbing the skin horizontally with slight pressure, Nikolski sign), and history of intake of drugs typically associated with SJS/TEN implies the diagnosis of SJS/TEN until proven otherwise. Identifying the disease-inducing cause is of utmost importance. With every day of continuing the causal drug the outcome worsens. Novel validated biomarkers, immunoassays, and genetic studies for prompt identification of the initiating drug are highly desired as it is currently not possible to identify the causal drug by routine allergological testing in the initial phase of the disease. Therefore, every drug that is being administered should be evaluated according to the possibility that it is a causal agent for SJS/TEN and also according to the acute medical indication for drug intake. Usually, SJS/TEN develops during the first 2 months after initiating drug therapy. Moreover, some drugs are more likely to induce SJS/TEN than others, and these drugs (see Table 1) must be stopped immediately. Generally, it is advisable in the current therapeutic setting to discontinue any drugs for which there is no vital indication.

6 Treatment and General Considerations

Hospital setting and care team

SJS/TEN behave like a superficial dermal burn with fluid shifts, hypermetabolism, and high nutritional requirements. Therefore, an interdisciplinary approach to SJS/TEN management is needed, involving in particular dermatologists, ophthalmologists, burn surgeons, gynecologists, immunologists, and pharmacologists. Early transfer to specialized units, such as dermatological centers, intensive care, or burn units should be initiated to improve survival. Early diagnosis, early withdrawal of the suspected initiating drug, immediate and appropriate care in the acute phase, and appropriate follow-up by cornea specialists are important to prevent vision impairment.

Anti-inflammatory treatment

Due to the lack of effective immunomodulatory treatment, some experts advise that treatment in the acute phase of disease should primarily involve cessation of potential causative drugs, symptomatic treatment, and best supportive care [32].

Previous observations clearly indicate that ongoing inflammation in SJS/TEN commonly causes fibrosis, and that this is independent of exogenous factors. While inflammation commonly does not respond properly to topical anti-inflammatory treatment, systemic disease-modifying anti-rheumatic drugs (DMARDs) are potentially useful. However, as DMARDs have previously been found to induce disease, they should be used with particular caution. Despite the lack of high-quality evidence regarding the therapeutic effects, many specialized centers use anti-inflammatory treatment during the initial phase of disease.

Although systemic corticosteroids are of particular importance and are commonly used during the acute phase of disease, there is controversy regarding their efficacy since increased morbidity and mortality have been occasionally reported in retrospective analyses. However, both dosage and length of treatment with corticosteroids varied considerably in these studies, hindering a high-quality evaluation. Especially the use of moderate oral dosages up to 1 mg/kg body weight may be inferior to other treatment options, such as TNF inhibitors [41]. However, if high doses of corticosteroids are used for short periods of time (e.g., administered intravenously for 3–5 days), patients improved rapidly and no increased mortality was found in several case series [43, 44]. Accordingly, registry studies (RegiSCAR group) do not support an increase in mortality associated with systemic corticosteroids [45]. However, as there are no data from controlled studies, the controversy regarding corticosteroids remains. There is agreement that the well-known adverse effects of corticosteroids limit their use during the chronic phase. Recent data on the use of DMARDs (e.g., cyclosporine and TNF-α Inhibitors) suggest that these drugs may reduce recurrence rates and disease progression in the chronic phase.

Supportive care

In addition to pain control, an important initial goal is prevention of secondary infection primarily by non-adhesive wound dressings and topical treatment with antiseptics. Systemic antibiotics should only be used when there is clear evidence of bacterial infection. Surgical debridement of the skin must be avoided whenever possible. Tense blisters should be punctured, but the epidermal roof should be left in place whenever possible. Shear force must be avoided when handling the patient.

Oral feeding is encouraged to prevent GIT restriction. The target for caloric intake is 20–30 kcal/kg body weight per day. Blood glucose should be monitored daily and hyperglycemia > 180 mg/dl should be corrected with insulin [46]. The use of proton pump inhibitors can be considered if corticosteroids are given at high doses. Careful monitoring of fluid balance is important and strict input/output charts maintained to prevent renal impairment. As temperature control is impaired in these patients due to loss of the integument, an ambient room temperature between 25 and 32°C is required. Pulmonary hygiene including postural drainage to prevent secondary lung complications is advisable. Prophylactic anticoagulation is necessary in bedridden patients. Low-molecular-weight heparins are preferred if kidney parameters are within normal ranges.

Treatment of the skin

Modern non-adhesive wound dressings and topical antiseptics in gel formations and paraffin-based ointments are used to aid reepithelization and to prevent secondary skin infections. Systemic antibiotics should only be administered when there is clear evidence of bacterial infection. Surgical debridement of the skin must be avoided. Tense blisters should be punctured, but the epidermal roof should be left in place whenever possible. Shear force must be avoided.

In the case of scar formation as a consequence of extensive skin involvement and complications, further treatment options include scar massage, silicon sheeting, and the use of pressure garments. Scarring may also be treated with medical laser devices. Regular mouthwashes with antiseptic and analgesic preparations are warranted. Paraffin-based ointments should be applied to the lips regularly. Severe urogenital involvement may require urethral catheterization. In men, regular foreskin mobilization is warranted.

Daily clinical examination and patient history as well as routine testing for inflammatory parameters are warranted to detect infections. While routine microbial testing is advised by some authorities, it cannot distinguish between colonization and infection. Systemic antibiotics should only be used when there is credible evidence of bacterial infection.

Systemic anti-inflammatory medication, rationale and agents

Activated T cells, especially cytotoxic T cells, are critically involved in mediating epidermal necrolysis; therefore, attempts to improve the course of disease have been made by administering anti-inflammatory or immunosuppressive drugs. As the disease is rare, prospective high-quality studies addressing this question are lacking (for a review, see [47]). DMARDs are used as early treatment, aiming to arrest epidermal necrosis, particularly in cases of recurrent and SJS/TEN and when complications have developed [35, 48–50]. As potential treatment options, corticosteroids, TNF inhibitors, cyclosporine, and intravenous immunoglobulin (IVIG) are currently the treatments most widely used in Europe [51].

Several studies have suggested that cyclosporine has beneficial effects in patients with SJS/TEN, including an open-label trial using an initial dose of 3 mg/kg body weight/day and with subsequent tapering [52]. Survival was better than predicted by SCORTEN in this analysis. While some studies suggest that the effects of cyclosporine are superior to those of other agents, this may in part be due to selection of patients with a better prognosis [53].

Recent studies, including a randomized trial comparing etanercept with moderate doses of oral steroids, suggest beneficial effects (e.g., faster reepithelization) of TNF-alpha inhibitors in patients with SJS/TEN [41]. The effect of TNF inhibition on survival is less clear. No difference in mortality was noted in the randomized clinical trial by Wang et al. [41], while a better survival than predicted by SCORTEN was described after using TNF inhibitors in a recent open case series [54]. Currently, the value of TNF-alpha inhibitors in disease management is still uncertain.

The data on IVIG are particularly controversial as an increased mortality was observed in a previous prospective study [55] using an IVIG dose of 2 g/kg body weight given over 2 days. It has been argued that higher doses may be required in SJS/TEN patients [56]. Moreover, a combination of IVIG with systemic corticosteroids compared to IVIG alone was associated with a better survival in another cohort study [45]. Thus, the role of IVIG in SJS/TEN remains uncertain. However, the fact that IVIGs are not associated with an increased risk of infection is a compelling reason to consider this therapy in patients with TEN and life-threatening comorbidities, e.g., in patients with cancer under treatment with immune checkpoint inhibitors [57].

Given the sparse high-quality data from controlled clinical trials and the heterogeneity of treatment protocols, it is currently not possible to evaluate the hierarchy or even the general role of anti-inflammatory treatments for managing patients with SJS/TEN. However, bearing these limitations in mind, beneficial effects are possible and a recent systematic meta-analysis did show better survival for some treatment options, e.g., cyclosporine, and no worse survival for any anti-inflammatory treatment analyzed [47].

7 Management of Eye Disease and Ocular Sequelae in SJS/TEN

Acute, early phase

As the primary goal in the acute phase is saving patients´ lives, ocular involvement may often be missed, thereby obscuring vision. Hence, immediate care (preferably 24–48 h after disease onset) by an ophthalmologist is mandatory, even before diagnosis is confirmed by skin biopsy [39]. Then, 1–2 daily reevaluations are required, as disease may progress rapidly [25].

For clinical management, grading systems to assess the severity of acute surface disease in SJS/TEN have been established [22]. Here, periocular skin, eyelid position and margin, patency of the lacrimal puncta, direction of the eyelashes, status of the Meibomian gland orifices, height of the tear meniscus, quality of the tear film, ocular surface keratinization, conjunctiva, and cornea (with use of fluorescein to assess breakdown) should be examined carefully and eyelids everted with the use of lid retractors (Table 5). Pain medication or sedatives may be required for

Table 5 Windows of opportunity for ophthalmic intervention in Stevens–Johnson syndrome/toxic epidermal necrolysis

SJS/TEN: phase of disease	Ocular findings
Acute	Ocular surface/eyelid margin epithelial defect
	Pseudomembrane formation
Chronic	Posterior eyelid margin keratinization
	Trichiasis/distichiasis
	Tear deficiency
	Persistent epithelial defect

Each finding should trigger an intervention to mitigate likely further vision loss. (*Kohanim et al. 2016; [62])

proper examinations. Saline rinses remove mucous and tear film debris and may aid in providing better visibility of the ocular surface. Presence of membranes should be assessed. Repeated measurement of depth and area of the fornix and determining whether symblepharon is present have been suggested for proper disease monitoring [58].

Management protocols for patients with severe ocular surface disease (e.g., SJS/TEN) follow a stepladder approach, including management of dryness, epithelial defects, limbal stem cell deficiency, lid disease (trichiasis, lid malposition, and Meibomian gland dysfunction), and inflammation. Lid surgery (excision of lash follicles, lid split and anterior lamellar repositioning, and mucous membrane grafts), the use of scleral contact lenses, amniotic membrane transplantation and surface reconstructive surgery, and systemic immunosuppression might be considered [6, 32].

Frequent lubrication (every 1–2 h and ointment at bedtime) should be ensured and non-preserved hyaluronate preparations preferred. Punctal occlusion and retinoid acid drops may be considered. Serum eye drops—containing a variety of anti-inflammatory molecules [59]—may be used for severe dry eye and epithelial disintegration. Tegaderm™ or plastic wrap may be applied in severe sloughing, and soft therapeutic contact lens and moisture chambers in exposure keratopathy. Topical antibiotics are recommended for patients with ocular epithelial defects to prevent secondary infection [60, 61].

Topical corticosteroid eyedrops (prednisolone acetate 1%), and probably cyclosporine/tacrolimus, and corticosteroid ointment to the eyelid margins should be given as required individually. Generally, unpreserved eyedrop formulations should be preferred. High-dose pulsed corticosteroids administered within the first few days after disease onset have been beneficial in improving disease outcome in some studies [43]. However, as the use of systemic steroids for acute SJS/TEN is controversial, it may be preferentially given in patients with severe eye disease.

Membranes/pseudomembranes should be lysed and removed frequently. As mechanical synechiolysis may induce mechanical trauma, their benefits must be weighed against the intervention-induced inflammation.

For nonhealing erosions or superficial ulcers, tarsorraphy, punctal occlusion (cautery), bandage contact lenses (e.g., high oxygen-transmissible silicone hydrogel CL with medium water content), and/or amniotic membrane transplantation (AMT) might be considered. Initially, misdirected eyelashes can be epilated. The beneficial effect of amnion supposedly relies on its antimicrobial and immunomodulatory properties, and it promotes epithelization. A randomized control trial showed that AMT is a useful adjunct to medical treatment in maintaining vision and a stable ocular surface [62]. Indeed, early AMT (within 5–10 days after symptom onset) is promising to prevent poor outcome and severe shortening of the fornix [28, 63, 64]. Indications for AMT include any corneal defect, staining of the eyelid margin > 1/3 of its length, any conjunctival staining > 1 cm at its greatest diameter, and/or pseudomembrane formation [31, 62]. Disorders of the eyelid margin anatomy are key risk factors for chronic progression, thus indicating AMT. A beneficial effect of AMT on visual outcome and severe ocular complications has been shown [65] (Table 6).

The possible sources of keratinized epithelium at the posterior lid margin could be associated with adjacent anterior eyelid epidermis, hyperkeratinized epithelium from the Meibomian gland ductal orifices, or de novo metaplasia of the conjunctival epithelium [66]. For keratopathy related to lid margin keratinization, prosthetic replacement of ocular surface ecosystem (PROSE) lenses might be helpful or excision combined with AMT or mucous membrane grafting (MMG) could be considered.

The use of systemic immunosuppression in SJS/TEN in the acute phase of disease is still controversial. While systemic corticosteroid treatment did not significantly improve

Table 6 Suggested initial management of acute ocular Stevens–Johnson syndrome/toxic epidermal necrolysis based on a simple clinical grading system

Grade	Grade defined	Management
0	No ocular involvement	AT 4x/day
1	Conjunctival hyperemia	Moxi 3x/day
		Pred 6x/day
		FML 6x/day
		AT hourly, as feasible
2	Ocular surface/eyelid margin epithelial defect or pseudomembrane formation	Use above therapies, plus consider AMT
3	Ocular surface/eyelid margin epithelial defect and pseudomembrane formation	Use above therapies, plus consider AMT

AT: artificial tears. Moxi: moxifloxacine 0.5% ophthalmic solution. Pred: prednisolone acetate 1% ophthalmic suspension.
FML: fluorometholone 0.1% ophthalmic ointment. AMT: amniotic membrane transplantation.
*Adapted from Yip et al. 2005 [67]

ocular outcomes in some studies, improved ocular outcome was reported by others. IVIG, either given alone or in combination with corticosteroids, did not improve outcome [27, 67]. Furthermore, there is limited evidence for the use of plasmapheresis, cyclosporine, TNF alpha antibodies, or thalidomide (TNF-α inhibitor), IL-6 antibodies, or cyclophosphamide in the acute phase of disease, as the data in previous publications were controversial [60, 61].

Late/chronic phase

Re-evaluation intervals should be guided by disease severity [61], in general beginning 1 month after the acute phase and continued at 2–4 monthly intervals thereafter. Schirmer´s test should be performed and vital dye staining (e.g., fluorescein) carried out to assess corneal and conjunctival integrity. Superficial punctate keratopathy should be addressed, too, as it may progress to corneal opacification.

The primary goal of management is to preserve/restore vision and reduce inflammation and persistent discomfort. In the chronic phase of disease, the complex ocular sequelae need to be managed, including symblepharon, lid malformation, trichiasis, conjunctival keratinization, limbal stem cell deficiency, corneal pannus, and dry eye.

Chronic ocular complications in SJS/TEN can persist despite topical treatment. Poor understanding of the underlying pathophysiology and lack of a standardized approach have resulted in a paucity of data regarding suitable treatment options. Mostly, late surface failure is the consequence of limbal stem cell destruction during the acute phase of disease. Thereafter, chronic cicatricial sequelae, such as trichiasis, entropion, and exposure, contribute to progressive alteration of the surface.

Medical treatment

Severe and chronic inflammation in SJS/TEN patients may result in lacrimal duct atrophy, goblet cell and lipid component loss, squamous metaplasia, Meibomian gland atrophy, and complex tear film disorders, involving aqueous, mucin, and lipid layers. Conversely, severe dry eye may increase ocular surface inflammation. Thereby, in addition to frequently applying preservative-free artificial tears, cyclosporin A eye drops may be helpful to improve signs and symptoms. Although lacrimal puncta are commonly scarred during the acute inflammatory phase of disease, punctal cautery may be applied in the others. Topical antibiotics reduce the risk of secondary infection (Fig. 9).

The primary goal of managing chronic SJS/TEN is to control inflammation. Nonprogressive cicatrization does not require systemic DMARDs treatment. For controlling recurrent or chronic inflammation, which develops in a minority of patients [35, 48], topical steroids and also serum eye drops are primarily used. Ongoing surface inflammation and progressive conjunctival fibrosis in the absence of exogenous aggravating factors suggest a possible role for DMARDs in the chronic phase of disease in selected patients. Within a large set of patients with chronic SJS, a third of patients received DMARDs [6]. Hence, cyclosporin A, azathioprine, methotrexate, mycophenolate, cyclophosphamide, and infliximab have been administered for persistent and remitting inflammatory courses of disease.

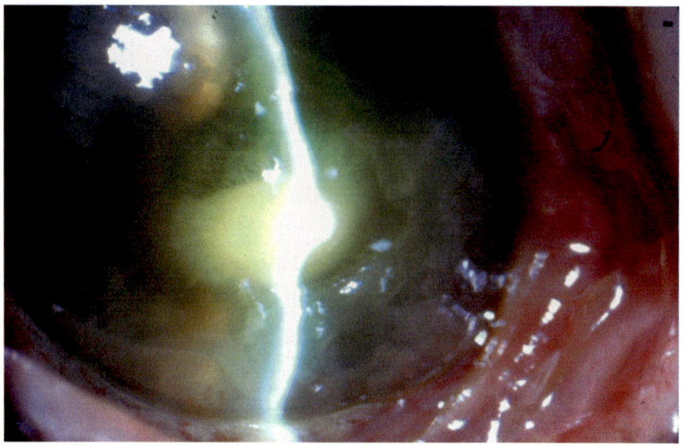

Fig. 9 Toxic epidermal necrolysis. Chronic stage. Limbal stem cell deficiency, persistent epithelial defect, secondary corneal ulceration, and fungal keratitis

Surgical interventions

Surgical treatment may be required, with techniques adapted to an individual's needs. Systemic corticosteroids and DMARDs may be considered to control inflammation prior to and after ocular surgery. Insufficient control of inflammation may eventually result in entropion, lid margin keratinization, and trichiasis and in subsequent ocular surface irritation (corneal staining and neovascularization), corneal opacification or melting, and blindness. Therefore, epilation and contact lens use may be indicated and thereafter AMT and fornix reconstruction (probably also with MMG).

Destruction of the mucocutaneous junction during the acute stage of disease may result in the overgrowth of keratinized skin epithelium onto the tarsal conjunctiva, predisposing the patient to subsequent conjunctival and corneal deterioration. Topical vitamin A, rigid contact lens, or scleral lens use may then be beneficial. Surgical removal of keratinization, probably with the use of autologous MMG may be indicated in severe posterior margin keratinization associated with corneal epitheliopathy, neovascularization, and discomfort. However, proper technique and timing are still controversial [6, 17, 61, 62].

To release scars in the skin and treat lagophthalmus, tarsorrhaphy may be indicated. For the management of entropion or ectropion, lateral canthoplasty, tarsal anterior lamellar repositioning, tarsal fracture, anterior lamellar repositioning, posterior lamellar tightening, or tarsoconjunctival advancement may be performed as required individually.

Allogeneic limbal or keratolimbal allografts have been used in advanced corneal opacification and stem cell deficiency. However, the procedures have been associated with high rejection rates although they were performed under systemic DMARDs. Photodynamic therapy with verteporfin, probably combined with additional topical bevacizumab, could be applied in patients with advanced corneal neovascularization. Gundersen flap might be considered for corneal covering, but fornix foreshortening and symblepharon may preclude the procedure.

Tectonic procedures (lamellar of full-thickness grafts) are performed in patients with severe, persistent epithelial defects, corneal melting, or perforation. However, the long-term prognosis after surgery in SJS/TEN patients is poor due to the high risk of failure, corneal melting, and perforation. Possible alternative options include cyanacrylate glue with bandage contact lens (in perforations < 2 mm), AMT, or keratoprosthesis.

While fornix shortening often can be left untreated, reconstruction may be warranted for patients with severe lid margin keratinization, trichiasis, and surface epithelial damage and to enable contact lens fitting.

With cultivated oral mucosal epithelial cell sheets transplantation (COMET), complete reepithelization of the cornea was achieved at about 1 year postoperatively in a small patient series [68]. AMT (Figs.10A and B) or MMG might also represent good options to reconstruct eyelid margin and fornix and to improve punctate keratopathy, haze, and corneal vascularization [69].

For the end-stage of disease and as the last resort, Boston-type keratoprosthesis (Fig. 11) or modified osteo-odonto-keratoprosthesis may be considered for visual rehabilitation in patients with bilateral end-stage ocular surface disease. However, these treatments have been associated with high complication rates (e.g., infection, retinal detachment, and glaucoma) [69, 70]. Due to the complexity of keratoprosthesis procedures and intensive follow-up, this procedure should only be performed by well-trained surgeons in tertiary centers [61].

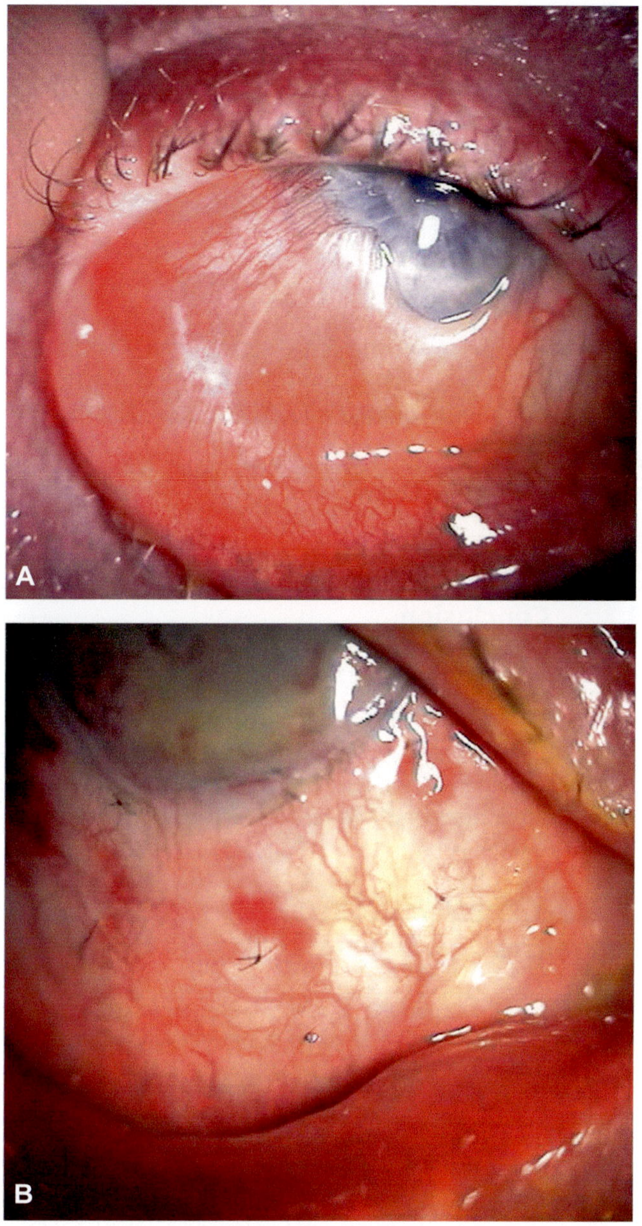

Fig. 10 (**A**) Stevens–Johnson syndrome. Late stage. Advanced scar formation with motility limitations and dry eye disorder. Before amniotic membrane transplantation. (**B**) Stevens–Johnson syndrome. Late stage. 4 weeks after amniotic membrane transplantation

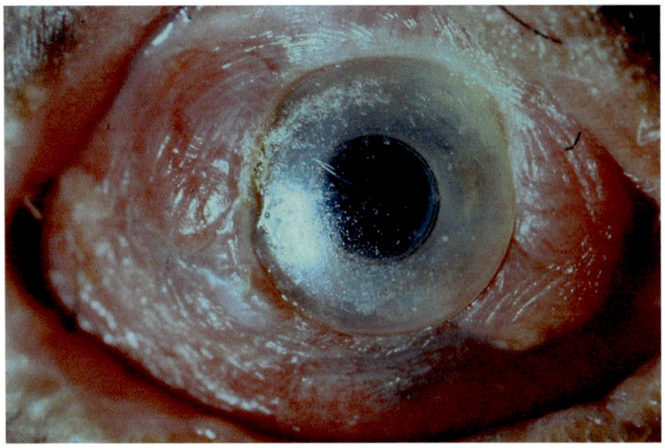

Fig. 11 Stevens–Johnson syndrome. Boston-type keratoprosthesis. Courtesy of C.S. Foster, Boston

8 Conclusion

Stevens–Johnson syndrome (SJS)/toxic epidermal necrolysis (TEN) is a rare and serious widespread, vesiculobullous rash, often with ocular involvement. Severe ocular complications probably leading to long-term visual impairment commonly occur. Prompt diagnosis and transfer to specialized interdisciplinary care may improve survival and visual outcome.

References

1. Stevens AM, Johnson FC. A new eruptive fever associated with stomatitis and ophthalmia: a report of two cases in children. Am J Child. 1922;24:526–33.
2. Lyell A. Toxic epidermal necrolysis: an eruption resembling scaling of the skin. Br J Dermatol. 1956;68:355–61. https://doi.org/10.1111/j.1365-2133.1956.tb12766.x.
3. Kelly JP, Auquier A, Rzany B, Naldi L, Bastuji-Garin S, Correia O, et al. An international collaborative case-control study of severe cutaneous adverse reactions (SCAR): design and methods. J Clin Epidemiol. 1995;48:1099–108. https://doi.org/10.1016/0895-4356(95)00004-n.
4. Rzany R, Mockenhaupt M, Baur S, Schröder W, Stocker U, Mueller J, et al. Epidemiology or erythema exsudativum multiforme majus, Stevens-Johnson syndrome, and toxic epidermal necrolysis in Germany (1990–1992): structure and results of a population-bases registry. J Clin Epidemiol. 1996;49:769–73. https://doi.org/10.1016/0895-4356(96)00035-2.
5. Yang MS, Lee JY, Kim J, Kim GW, Kim BK, Kim JY, et al. Incidence of Stevens-Johnson syndrome and toxic epidermal necrolysis: a nationwide population-based study using national health insurance database in Korea. PLoS ONE. 2016;11: e0165933. https://doi.org/10.1371/journal.pone.0165933.
6. Jabbour S, Din N, Logeswaran A, Sanchez ST, Ahmad S. Clinical characteristics of patients with chronic Stevens-Johnson syndrome treated at a major tertiary eye hospital within the United Kingdom. Front Med (Lausanne). 2021;8: 644795. https://doi.org/10.3389/fmed.2021.644795.
7. Arantes LB, Reis CS, Novaes AG, Carvalho MR, Göttens L, Novaes M. Stevens-Johnson syndrome and toxic epidermal necrolysis: epidemiological and clinical outcomes analysis in public hospitals. An Bras Dermatol. 2017;92:661–7. https://doi.org/10.1590/abd1806-4841.20176610.
8. Sekula P, Dunant A, Mockehaupt M, Naldi L, Bouwes Bavinck JN, Halevy S, et al. Comprehensive survival analysis of a cohort of patients with Stevens-Johnson syndrome and toxic epidermal necrolysis. J Invest Dermatol. 2013;133:1197–204. https://doi.org/10.1038/jid.2012.510.
9. Park HJ, Kim YJ, Kim DH, Kim J, Park KH, Park JW, et al. HLA allele frequencies in 5802 Koreans: varied allele types associated with SJS/TEN according to culprit drugs. Yonsei Med J. 2016;57:118–26. https://doi.org/10.3349/ymj.2016.57.1.118.
10. Park CS, Kang DY, Kang MG, Kim S, Ye YM, Kim SH, et al. Severe cutaneous adverse reactions to antiepileptic drugs: nationwide registry-based study in Korea. Allergy Asthma Immunol Res. 2019;11:709–22. https://doi.org/10.4168/aair.2019.11.5.709.
11. Neerukonda VK, Stagner AM. Stevens-Johnson syndrome: a review of a vision and life-threatening mucocutaneous disease including histopathology with updates on pathogenesis and genetic risk factors. Seminars Ophthalmol. 2021;36:270–81. https://doi.org/10.1080/08820538.2021.1893764.
12. Ueta M. Results of detailed investigations into Stevens-Johnson syndrome with severe ocular complications. Invest Ophthalmol Vis Sci 2018;59:DE183-DE191. https://doi.org/10.1167/iovs.17-23537.
13. Ma KSK, Chung WH, Hsueh YJ, Chen SY, Tokunaga K, Kinoshita S, et al. Human leucocyte antigen association of patients with Stevens-Johnson syndrome/toxic epidermal necrolysis with severe ocular complications in Han Chinese. Br J Ophthalmol. 2022;106:610–5. https://doi.org/10.1136/bjophthalmol-2020-317105.
14. Mockenhaupt M, Viboud C, Dunant A, Naldi L, Halevy S, Bouwes Bavinck JN, et al. Stevens-Johnson syndrome and toxic epidermal necrolysis: assessment of medication risks with emphasis on recently marketed drugs. The EuroSCAR-study J Invest Dermatol. 2008;128:35–44. https://doi.org/10.1038/sj.jid.5701033.
15. Yang MS, Lee JY, Kim J, Kim GW, Kim BK, Kim JY, et al. Searching for the culprit drugs for Stevens-Johnson syndrome and toxic epidermal necrolysis from a nationwide claim database in Korea. J Allergy Clin Immunol Pract. 2020;8:690-5.e2. https://doi.org/10.1016/j.jaip.2019.09.032.
16. Chatproedprai S, Wutticharoenwong V, Tempark T, Wananukul S. Clinical features and treatment outcomes among children with Stevens-Johnson syndrome and toxic epidermal necrolysis: a 2-year study in a tertiary referral hospital. Dermatol Res Pract. 2018;7(2018): 3061084. https://doi.org/10.1155/2018/3061084.eCollection2018.
17. Iyer G, Srinivasan B, Agarwal S, Kamala Muralidharan S, Arumugam S. Comprehensive approach to ocular consequences of Stevens-Johnson syndrome—the aftermath of a systemic condition. Graefes Arch Clin Exp Ophthalmol. 2014;252:457–67. https://doi.org/10.1007/s00417-014-2568-8.
18. Magina S, Lisboa C, Leal V, Palmares J, Mesquita-Guimaraes J. Dermatological and ophthalmological sequels in toxic epidermal necrolysis. Dermatology. 2003;207:33–6. https://doi.org/10.1159/000070938.
19. Schwartz RA, McDonough PH, Lee BW. Toxic epidermal necrolysis: Part II. Prognosis, sequelae, diagnosis, differential diagnosis, prevention, and treatment. J Am Acad Dermatol 2013;69:187.e1–204. https://doi.org/10.1016/j.jaad.2013.05.002.
20. Morales ME, Purdue GF, Verity SM, Arnoldo BD, Blomquist PH. Ophthalmic manifestations of Stevens-Johnson syndrome and toxic epidermal necrolysis and relation to SCORTEN. Am J Ophthalmol 2010;150:505–10.e.1. https://doi.org/10.1016/j.ajo.2010.04.026.

21. Yip LW, Thong BY, Lim J, Tan AW, Wong HB, Handa S, et al. Ocular manifestations and complications of Stevens-Johnson syndrome and toxic epidermal necrolysis: an Asian series. Allergy. 2007;62:527–31. https://doi.org/10.1111/j.1398-9995.2006.01295.x.
22. Sotozono C, Ueta M, Nakatani E, Kitami A, Watanabe H, Sueki H, et al. Predictive factors associated with acute ocular involvement in Stevens-Johnson syndrome and toxic epidermal necrolysis. Am J Ophthalmol. 2015;160:228-37.e2. https://doi.org/10.1016/j.ajo.2015.05.002.
23. Iyer G, Srinivasan B, Agarwal S. Ocular sequelae of Stevens-Johnson syndrome: a comprehensive approach. Cornea. 2020;39:3–6. https://doi.org/10.1097/ICO.0000000000002532.
24. Panpruk R, Puangsricharern V, Klaewsongkram J, Rerknimitr P, Kittipibul T, Chongpison Y, et al. Clinical parameters and biological markers associated with acute severe ocular complications in Stevens-Johnson syndrome and toxic epidermal necrolysis. Scientific Rep. 2021;11:20275. https://doi.org/10.1038/s41598-021-99370-1.
25. Metcalfe D, Iqbal O, Chodosh J, Bouchard CS, Saeed HN. Acute and chronic management of ocular disease in Stevens-Johnson syndrome/toxic epidermal necrolysis in the USA. Front Med. 2021;8: 662897. https://doi.org/10.3389/fmed.2021.662897.
26. Sotozono C, Ang LPK, Koizumi N, Higashihara H, Ueta M, Inatomi T, et al. New grading system for the evaluation of chronic ocular manifestations in patients with Stevens-Johnson syndrome. Ophthalmology. 2007;114:1294–302. https://doi.org/10.1016/j.ophtha.2006.10.029.
27. Kim DH, Yoon KC, Seo KY, Lee HS, Yoon SC, Sotozono C, et al. The role of systemic immunomodulatory treatment and prognostic factors on chronic ocular complications in Stevens-Johnson syndrome. Ophthalmology. 2015;122:254–64. https://doi.org/10.1016/j.ophtha.2014.08.013.
28. Shanbhag SS, Sangwan VS, Singh A, Donthineni PR, Basu S, Srinivasan B, et al. Clinical aspects of Stevens-Johnson syndrome/toxic epidermal necrolysis with severe ocular complications in India. Front Med. 2021;8: 643955. https://doi.org/10.3389/fmed.2021.643955.
29. Sotozono C, Ueta M, Yokoi N. Severe dry eye with combined mechanisms is involved in the ocular sequelae of SJS/TEN at the chronic stage. Invest Ophthalmol Vis Sci. 2018;59:DES80-DES86. https://doi.org/10.1167/iovs.18-24019.
30. Kodura MA, Prasad D, Upadhyaya S, Jaffet J, Shanbhag SS, Basu S, et. Al. Differential expression of tear film cytokines in Stevens-Johnson syndrome patients and comparative review of literature. Scientific Rep 2021;11:18433. https://doi.org/10.1038/s41598-021-97575-y.
31. Gregory DG. New grading system and treatment guidelines for acute ocular manifestation of Stevens-Johnson syndrome. Ophthalmology. 2016;123:1653–8. https://doi.org/10.1016/j.ophtha.2016.04.041.
32. Thorel D, Ingen-Housz-Oro S, Royer G, Delcampe A, Bellon N, Bodemer C, et al. Management of ocular involvement in the acute phase of Stevens-Johnson syndrome and toxic epidermal necrolysis: french national audit of practices, literature review, and consensus agreement. Orphanet J Rare Dis. 2020;15:259. https://doi.org/10.1186/s13023-020-01538-x.
33. Gueudry J, Roujeau JC, Binaghi M, Soubrane G, Muraine M. Risk factors for the development of ocular complications of Stevens-Johnson syndrome and toxic epidermal necrolysis. Arch Dermatol. 2009;145:157–62. https://doi.org/10.1001/archdermatol.2009.540.
34. Hajj C, Ezzedine K, Thorel D, Delcampe A, Royer G, Hua C, et al. Disabling ocular sequelae of epidermal necrolysis: risk factors during the acute phase and associated sequelae. Br J Dermatol. 2019;181:421–2. https://doi.org/10.1111/bjd.18023.
35. De Rojas MV, Dart JKG, Saw VPJ. The natural history of Stevens-Johnson syndrome: patterns of chronic ocular disease and the role of systemic immunosuppressive therapy. Br J Ophthalmol. 2007;91:1048–53. https://doi.org/10.1136/bjo.2006.109124.
36. Jongkhajornpong P, Lekhanont K, Siriyotha S, Kanokrungsee S, Chuckpaiwong V. Factors contributing to long-term severe visual impairment in Stevens-Johnson syndrome and toxic epidermal necrolysis. J Ophthalmol 2017:2087578. https://doi.org/10.1155/2017/2087578.
37. Basu S, Shanbhag SS, Gokani A, Kedar R, Bahuguna C, Sangwan VS. Chronic ocular sequelae of Stevens-Jonson syndrome in children: long-term impact of appropriate therapy on natural history of disease. Am J Ophthalmol. 2018;189:17–28. https://doi.org/10.1016/j.ajo.2018.01.028.
38. Guegan S, Bastuji-Garin S, Poszepcznska-Guigne E, Roujeau JC, Revuz J. Performance of the SCORTEN during the first 5 days of hospitalization to predict the prognosis of epidermal necrolysis. J Invest Dermatol. 2006;126:272–6. https://doi.org/10.1038/sj.jid.5700068.
39. Chang WC, Abe R, Anderson P, Anderson W, Ardern-Jones MR, Beachkofsky TM, et al. SJS/TEN 2019: from science to translation. J Dermatol Sci 2020;98:2–12. https://doi.org/10.1016/j.jdermsci.2020.02.003.
40. Cheng L. Current pharmacogenetic perspective on Stevens-Johnson syndrome and toxic epidermal necrolysis. Front Pharmacol. 2021;26(12): 588063. https://doi.org/10.3389/fphar.2021.588063.
41. Wang CW, Yang LY, Chen CB, Ho HC, Hung SI, Yang CH, et al. Randomized, controlled trial of TNF-a antagonist in CTL-mediated severe cutaneous adverse reactions. J Clin Invest. 2018;128:985–96. https://doi.org/10.1172/JCI93349.
42. Le HG, Saeed H, Mantagos IS, Mitchell CM, Goverman J, Chodish J. Burn unit care of Stevens-Johnson syndrome/toxic epidermal necrolysis. A survey Burns. 2016;42:830–5. https://doi.org/10.1016/j.burns.2015.12.001.
43. Araki Y, Sotozono C, Inatomi T, Ueta M, Yokoi N, Ueda E, et al. Successful treatment of Stevens-Johnson syndrome with steroid pulse therapy at disease onset. Am J Ophthalmol. 2009;147:1004–11. https://doi.org/10.1016/j.ajo.2008.12.04045.
44. Hirahara K, Kano Y, Sato Y, Horie C, Okazaki A, Ishida T, et al. Methylprednisolone pulse therapy for Stevens-Johnson syndrome/toxic epidermal necrolysis: clinical evaluation and analysis of biomarkers. J Am Acad Dermatol. 2013;69:496–8. https://doi.org/10.1016/j.jaad.2013.04.007.
45. Schneck J, Fagot JP, Sekula P, Sassolas B, Roujeau JC, Mockenhaupt M. Effects of treatments on the mortality of Stevens-Johnson syndrome and toxic epidermal necrolysis: a retrospective study on patients included in the prospective EuroSCAR study. J Am Acad Dermatol. 2008;58:33–40. https://doi.org/10.1016/j.jaad.2007.08.039.
46. Brüggen MC, Le ST, Walsh S, Toussi A, de Prost N, Ranki A, et al. Supportive care in the acute phase of Stevens-Johnson syndrome and toxic epidermal necrolysis: an international, multidisciplinary Delphi-based consensus. Br J Dermatol. 2021;185:616–26. https://doi.org/10.1111/bjd.19893.
47. Torres-Navarro I, Briz-Redon A, Botella-Estrada R. Systemic therapies for Stevens-Johnson syndrome and toxic epidermal necrolysis: a SCORTEN-based systemic review and meta-analysis. J Eur Acad Dermatol Venereol. 2021;35:159–71. https://doi.org/10.1111/jdv.16685.
48. Balkrishnan C, Sharma V, Vyas A. Immunosuppressive therapy in inflammatory ocular surface disease post Stevens-Johnson syndrome. Indian J Ophthalmol. 2011;59:69–70. https://doi.org/10.4103/0301-4738.73701.
49. Chan LS, Soong HK, Foster CS, Hammerberg C. Cooper KD Ocular cicatricial pemphigoid occurring as a sequela of Stevens-Johnson syndrome. JAMA. 1991;266:1543–6.

50. Foster CS, Fong LP, Azar D, Kenyon KR. Episodic conjunctival inflammation after Stevens-Johnson syndrome. Ophthalmology. 1988;95:453–62. https://doi.org/10.1016/s0161-6420(88)33165-951.
51. Kridin K, Brüggen MC, Chua SL, Bygum A, Walsh S, Nägeli MC, et al. Assessment of treatment approaches and outcomes in Stevens-Johnson syndrome and toxic epidermal necrolysis: insights from a pan-European multicenter study. JAMA Dermatol. 2021;157:1182–90. https://doi.org/10.1001/jamadermatol.2021.3154.
52. Valeyrie-Allanore L, Wolkenstein P, Brochard L, Ortonne N, Maitre B, Revuz J, et al. Open trial of ciclosporine treatment for Stevens-Johnson syndrome and toxic epidermal necrolysis. Br J Dermatol. 2010;163:847–53. https://doi.org/10.1111/j.1365-2133.2010.09863.x.
53. Noe MH, Mostaghimi A, Rosenbach M, Shinkai K, Micheletti RG. Selective use of cyclosporine for Stevens-Johnson syndrome/toxic epidermal necrolysis may exclude patients with poor prognostic factors. J Invest Dermatol. 2018;138:2068–72. https://doi.org/10.1016/j.jid.2018.03.1496.
54. Paradisi A, Abeni D, Didona D, Ricci F, Canzona F, Didone B. A new case series on etanercept treatment for toxic epidermal necrolysis. Eur J Dermatol. 2020;30:561–8. https://doi.org/10.1684/ejd.2020.3883.
55. Bachot N, Revuz J, Roujeau JC. Intravenous immunoglobulin treatment for Stevens-Johnson syndrome and toxic epidermal necrolysis: a prospective non comparative study showing no benefit on mortality or progression. Arch Dermatol. 2003;139:33–6. https://doi.org/10.1001/archderm.139.1.33.
56. Trent JT, Kerdel FA. Intravenous immunoglobulin for the treatment of toxic epidermal necrolysis. Arch Dermatol. 2003;139:1081. https://doi.org/10.1001/archderm.139.8.1081-a.
57. Kian W, Zemel M, Elobra F, Sharb AA, Levitas D, Assabag Y, et al. Intravenous immunoglobulin efficacy on pembrolizumab induced severe toxic epidermal necrolysis. Anticancer Drugs. 2022;33:e738–40. https://doi.org/10.1097/CAD.0000000000001162.
58. Kawakita T, Kawashima M, Murat D, Tsobuta K, Shimazaki J. Measurement of fornix depth and area: a novel method of determining the severity of fornix shortening. Eye. 2009;23:1115–9. https://doi.org/10.1038/eye.2008.205.
59. Geerling G, Maclennan S, Hartwig D. Autologous serum eye drops for ocular surface disorders. Br J Ophthalmol. 2004;88:1467–74. https://doi.org/10.1136/bjo.2004.044347.
60. Kohanim S, Palioura S, Saeed HN, Akpek EK, Amescua G, Basu S, et al. Stevens-Johnson syndrome/toxic epidermal necrolysis—a comprehensive review and guide to therapy. I Systemic disease Ocul Surf. 2016;14:2–19. https://doi.org/10.1016/j.jtos.2015.10.002.
61. Kohanim S, Palioura S, Saeed HN, Akpek EK, Amescua G, Basu S, et al. Acute and chronic ophthalmic involvement in Stevens-Johnson syndrome/toxic epidermal necrolysis—a comprehensive review and guide to therapy. II Ophthalmic disease Ocul Surf. 2016;14:168–88. https://doi.org/10.1016/j.tos.2016.02.001.
62. Sharma N, Thenarasun SA, Kaur M, Pushker N, Khanna N, Agarwal T, et al. Adjuvant role of amniotic membrane transplantation in acute ocular Stevens-Johnson syndrome: a randomized control trial. Ophthalmology. 2016;123:484–91. https://doi.org/10.1016/j.ophtha.2015.10.027.
63. Ciralsky JB, Sippel KC. Prompt versus delayed amniotic membrane transplantation in a patient with acute Stevens-Johnson syndrome. Clin Ophthalmol. 2013;7:1031–4. https://doi.org/10.2147/OPTH.S45054. Epub 2013 Max 31.
64. Hsu M, Jayaram A, Verner R, Lin A, Bouchard C. Indications and outcomes of amniotic membrane transplantation in the management of acute Stevens-Johnson syndrome and toxic epidermal necrolysis: a case-control study. Cornea. 2012;31:1394–402. https://doi.org/10.1097/ICO.0b013e31823d02a8.
65. Kim KH, Park SW, Kim MK, Wee WR. Effect of age and early intervention with systemic steroid, intravenous immunoglobulin or amniotic membrane transplantation on the ocular outcomes of patients with Stevens-Johnson syndrome. Korean J Ophthalmol. 2013;27:331–40. https://doi.org/10.3341/kjo.2013.27.5.331.
66. Singh S, Jakati S, Shanbhag SS, Elhusseiny AM, Djalilian AR, Basu S. Lid margin keratinization in Stevens-Johnson syndrome: review of pathophysiology and histopathology. Ocul Surf. 2021;21:299–305. https://doi.org/10.1016/j.jtos.2021.03.011.
67. Yip LW, Thong BY, Tan AW, Khin LW, Chng HH, Heng WJ. High-dose intravenous immunoglobulin in the treatment of toxic epidermal necrolysis: a study of ocular benefits. Eye. 2005;19:846–53. https://doi.org/10.1038/sj.eye.6701653.
68. Kim YJ, Lee HJ, Ryu JS, Kim YH, Jeon S, Oh JY, et al. Prospective clinical trial of corneal reconstruction with biomaterial-free cultured oral mucosal epithelial cell sheets. Cornea. 2018;37:76–83. https://doi.org/10.1097/ICO.00001409.
69. Iyer G, Srinivasan B, Agarwal S, Pillai VS, Ahuja A. Treatment modalities and clinical outcomes in ocular sequelae of Stevens-Johnson syndrome over 25 years—a paradigm shift. Cornea. 2016;35:46–50. https://doi.org/10.1097/ICO.0000000000000680.
70. Kim MK, Lee SM, Lee JL, Chung TY, Kim YH, Wee WR, et al. Long-term outcome in ocular intractable surface disease with Seoul-type keratoprosthesis. Cornea. 2007;26:546–51. https://doi.org/10.1097/ICO.0b013e3180415d35.

Corneal Degenerations

Berthold Seitz and Tim Berger

Abstract

Corneal degenerations are non-hereditary corneal disorders secondary to local or systemic diseases or related to age. They are often associated with chronic light exposure and may occur after inflammation. A late onset with deposition of material, tissue thinning, and vascularization characterizes them. The main age-related forms are bilateral and are represented by arcus lipoides, limbal girdle, Hassall–Henle warts at the peripheral Descemet membrane, and crocodile shagreen. Degenerations with tissue thinning comprise Fuchs–Terrien marginal degeneration, furrow degeneration and corneal dellen. The group characterized by material deposition is composed predominantly by Salzmann nodular degeneration ("Plus disease"), band keratopathy, lipid keratopathy, spheroidal keratopathy and pigment deposition forms. Some of them might induce severe visual impairment while the others are rather innocuous. The correct diagnosis and follow-up are mandatory for the appropriate typically minimal invasive therapy to maintain or restore visual function and prevent corneal pain.

Keywords

Age-related keratopathy · Corneal thinning · Corneal deposits · Corneal nodules · Corneal vascularization · Iron lines

1 Introduction

Degenerations are characterized by a continuing deterioration of a once normal tissue or an organ and frequent loss of functional activity. Degenerations of the cornea are common conditions that, in most cases, have relatively little effect on ocular function and vision. These conditions occur typically with increasing age [1], as a result of past inflammation, and with long-term toxic effects of environmental exposure (e.g. UV light) and in some cases, oxidative stress might be responsible for the onset of degenerative processes [2]. Unlike corneal dystrophies [3], corneal degenerations are not inherited, may be unilateral or bilateral, and often are associated with corneal vascularization. Degenerations tend to involve primarily the peripheral cornea, may overlap the limbus and conjunctiva, but may also concern the (para-)central cornea thus reducing vision at a considerable degree. All attempts to classify corneal degenerations must be arbitrary to some extent.

In this chapter we follow the very reasonable suggestion by Roszkowska and Wylegala who classified corneal degenerations in three groups [4]: **1. Age-related degenerations** (e.g. Arcus lipoides, Vogt white limbal girdle, Crocodile Shagreen, Hassall-Henle warts), **2. Degenerations with tissue thinning** (e.g. Fuchs–Terrien marginal degeneration, Senile corneal furrow degeneration and Dellen), and **3. Degenerations with material or tissue deposits** (e.g. Salzmann nodular degeneration, Pannus corneae, Calcific band keratopathy, Lipid keratopathy, Spheroidal keratopathy, Secondary amyloidosis, Hematocornea and Pigment deposition keratopathies).

B. Seitz (✉) · T. Berger
Department of Ophthalmology, Saarland University Medical Center, Homburg/Saar, Germany
e-mail: berthold.seitz@uks.eu
URL: http://www.augenklinik-saarland.de

B. Seitz et al. (eds.), *Atlas on Cornea*, https://doi.org/10.1007/978-3-031-65422-0_33

Table 1 Degeneration with increasing age—preferably in the periphery of the cornea

Arcus lipoides (= "Arcus senilis" = "Gerontoxon")
Vogt white limbal girdle
Crocodile shagreen degeneration (= Vogt-Mosaik-degeneration)
Hassall-Henle warts

2 Age-Related Degenerations (Table 1)

2.1 Arcus Lipoides (= "Arcus Senilis" = "Gerontoxon")

Arcus lipoides is the most common corneal degeneration. In men, the frequency increases with age and occurs in essentially all men older than 80 years of age. The presentation is delayed by 10 years in women.

Arcus lipoides presents as a gray-to-white, occasionally yellow, band of peripheral corneal opacification. It consists of fine dots, has a clear zone (lucid interval of Vogt) between it and the limbus, and has a diffuse central border with a sharper peripheral border (Figs. 1 and 2). It begins as a gray to yellow arc, first in the inferior cornea, then in the superior cornea. With progressive deposition, the arcs come together and form a complete ring to involve the entire periphery. The depth of deposition begins in the deep stroma and extends into the superficial stroma (Fig. 3). Arcus lipoides is almost always bilateral but can be asymmetric in unilateral carotid vascular disease or chronic ocular hypotony.

Strong evidence exists for an association with increased plasma cholesterol and low-density lipoprotein cholesterol, particularly when it occurs in men younger than 50 years ("**arcus juvenilis**") [5]. Corneal arcus has no visual significance, however arcus juvenilis is associated with a fourfold increased relative risk of mortality from coronary heart disease and cardiovascular disease. Arcus in young patients, therefore, is a useful clinical indication for the need for lipid and cardiovascular evaluation. Young patients who have arcus have an increased risk for type IIa dyslipoproteinemia but a decreased risk for type IV. In older patients, arcus lipoides does not correlate with mortality [6].

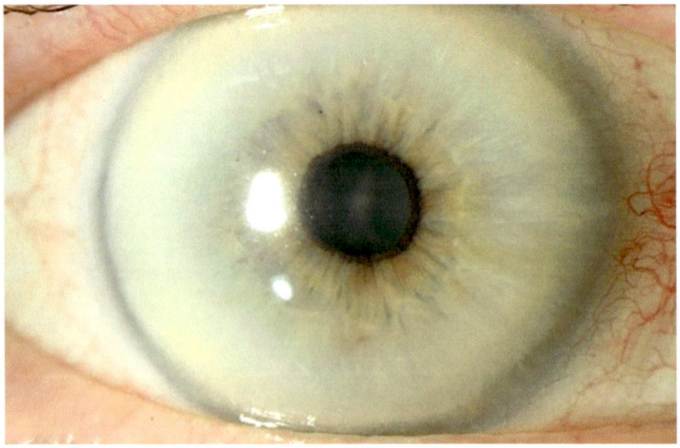

Fig. 1 Arcus lipoides is a corneal degeneration caused by lipid deposits in the peripheral cornea. The slit lamp photograph illustrates an advanced finding in an 80-year-old female patient

2.2 Vogt White Limbal Girdle

Vogt was the first to describe two types of yellowish-white, arc-like opacities in the cornea central to the limbus in the 3 o'clock and 9 o'clock positions (interpalpebral limbus) [7]. The limbal girdle of Vogt is usually more pronounced on the nasal limbus than on the temporal.

Vogt distinguished between two types of limbal girdle, which differ in the presence of a clear interval between the limbus. **Type I** has a lucid interval separating it from the corneal limbus and is more consistent with a mild, early form of calcific band keratopathy. **Type II** lacks a

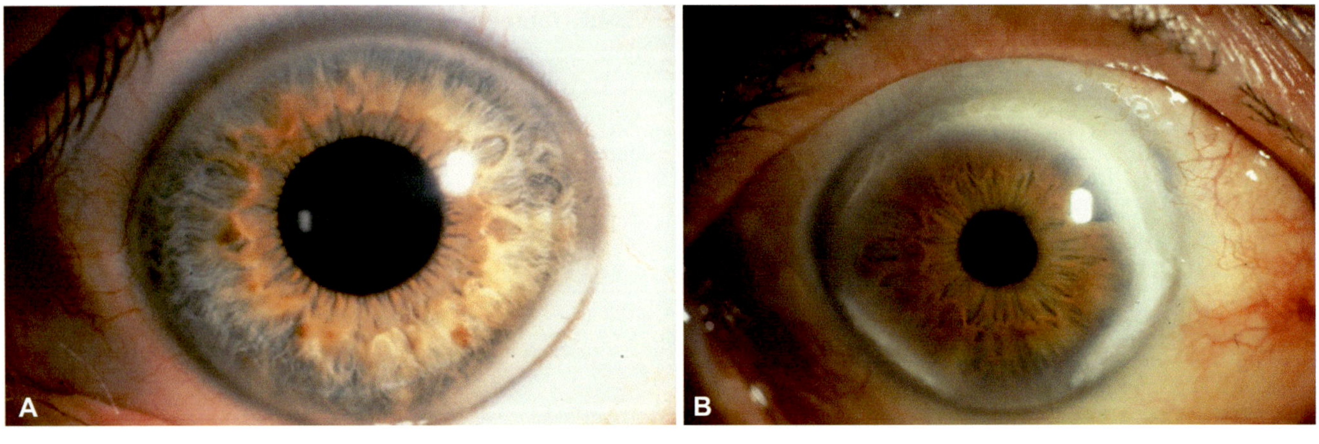

Fig. 2 (**A**) Mild and (**B**) uncomplete forms of arcus lipoides

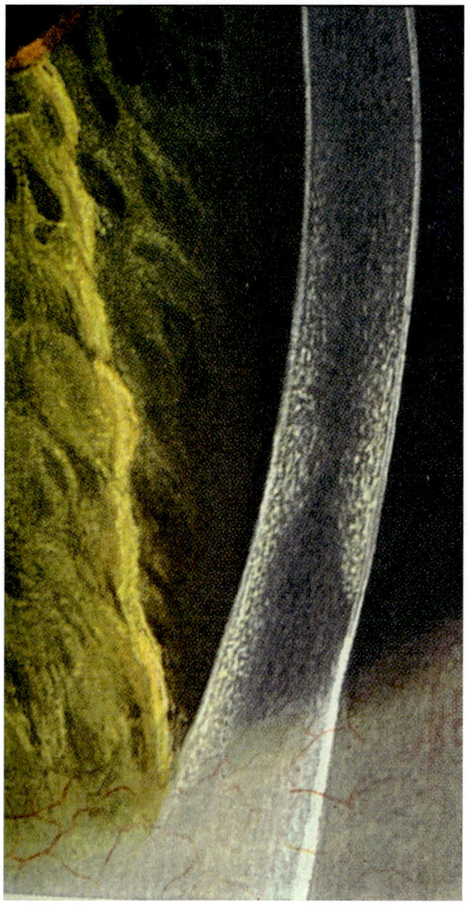

Fig. 3 Arcus lipoides begins in the deep stroma with progression to involve the superficial stroma. Schematic drawing from Vogt's color atlas shows the hourglass appearance

peripheral clear zone and consists of fine, white radial lines, located nasally more often than temporally (Figs. 4, 5, and 6). The prevalence of this fimbriated peripheral corneal opacity increases with age to essentially 100% in those older than 80 years of age [8].

Histologically, Vogt's limbal girdle type II is made up of hyperelastotic and hyaline deposits peripheral to Bowman layer, similar to those seen in a pinguecula and pterygium.

2.3 Crocodile Shagreen

Crocodile Shagreen has been described by Vogt as bilateral polygonal opacities separated by thin clear lines ("crocodile skin"), which are more pronounced in the central cornea (Figs. 7 and 8). However, the peripheral cornea may also be affected. Primarily, the anterior corneal stroma is affected, but in some rare cases the posterior corneal stroma may be involved too. This clinical manifestation appears to be interconnected with the abnormal stromal fiber orientation. By using electron microscopy, the existence of vacuoles could be revealed throughout the corneal stroma, also showing that some of them contained electron dense material [9]. As crocodile shagreen corneal degeneration is quite rare, it may be detected as an incidental finding during a routine slit lamp examination of the eye. Although this degeneration is considered benign, the posterior variation can impair visual acuity in some cases [10].

At this time there is an ongoing discussion whether so-called central cloudy dystrophy of François, which has been classified in category 4 (no clear clinical entity and no genetic proof) by the International Committee on the Classification of Corneal Dystrophies (IC3D) is an entity of its own or it is actually Crocodile Shagreen degeneration [3].

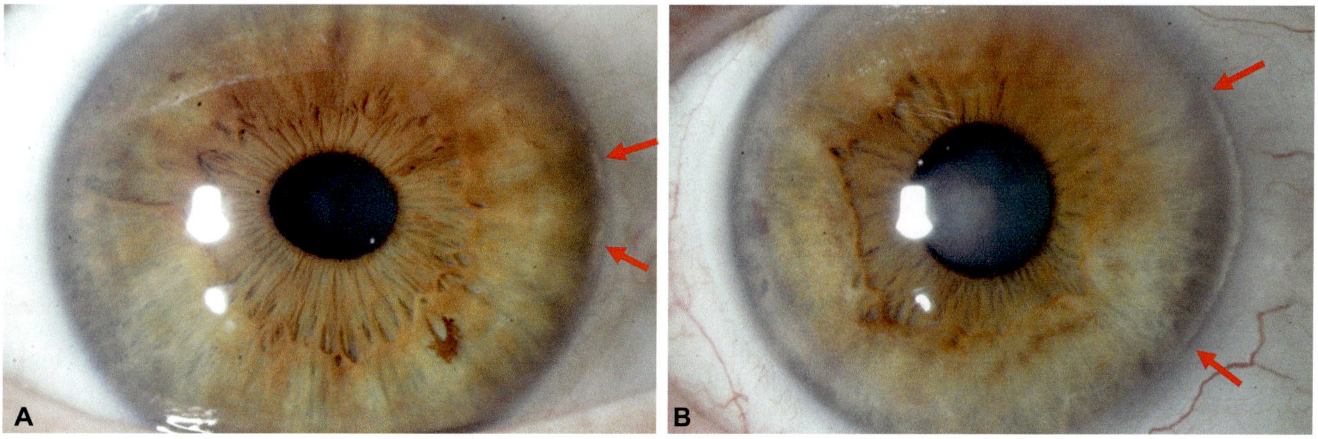

Fig. 4 (**A**, **B**) Vogt white limbal girdle is a symmetrical white band that is parallel to the interpalpebral limbus. It is found more frequently on the nasal limbus than on the temporal limbus, red arrows (**A** right eye, 69-year-old woman, **B** right eye, 74-year-old woman)

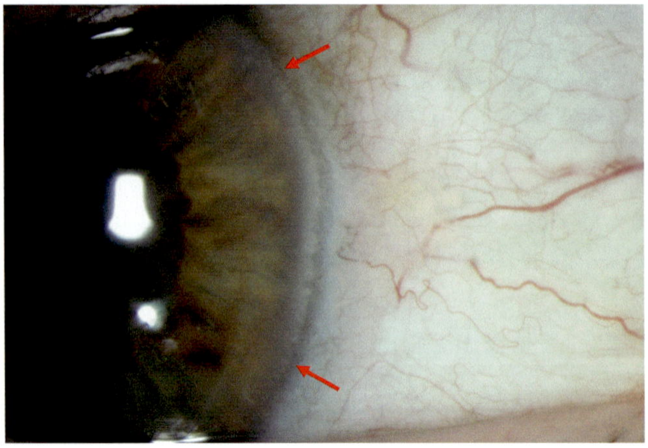

Fig. 5 Vogt white limbal girdle, which is located at the nasal corneal limbus, red arrows (right eye, 70-year-old woman)

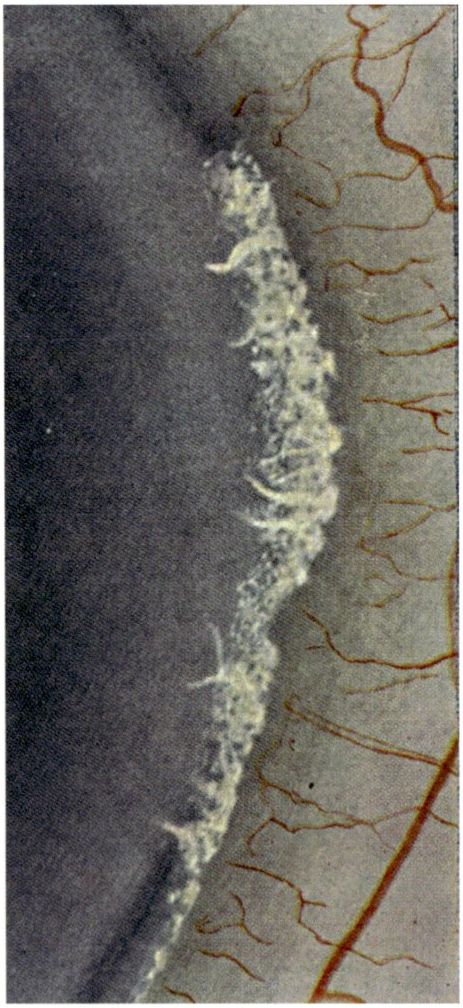

Fig. 6 Vogt white limbal girdle—schematic drawing from Vogt's Color Atlas

2.4 Peripheral Corneal Guttae ("Hassall–Henle Warts/Bodies")

The corneal endothelium undergoes degeneration with age, as manifested by a decreasing endothelial cell density and thickening of the posterior, nonbanded layer of Descemet membrane [11, 12]. The peripheral guttae (excrescences of Descemet membrane) are also known as Hassall–Henle warts or bodies which are composed by the localized deposition of abnormal collagen secerned by the aging endothelial cells. They consist of sporadic hyaline-filled excrescences of Descemet membrane localized generally in the (mid-) periphery of normal adult corneas. This circumstance distinguishes them from Fuchs endothelial dystrophy, which starts in the center and spreads to the periphery, finally causing corneal endothelial decompensation [13]. However, Hassall–Henle warts are histopathologically identical to guttae associated with Fuchs endothelial dystrophy. Due to the limited number and extent of peripheral guttae, the endothelial function and cell density is not compromised.

3 Degenerations with Tissue Thinning (Table 2)

3.1 Fuchs–Terrien Marginal Degeneration

Fuchs and Terrien described this degeneration around 1900 as a non-inflammatory, painless, progressive thinning in the peripheral cornea ("Dystrophia marginalis corneae symmetrica"), but its etiology still remains poorly understood. Fuchs–Terrien marginal degeneration could be observed at any age, but with a prevalence in middle-aged males (fourth decade of life) [14]. The autoimmune mechanism underlying the pathogenesis was hypothesized because of the described association with autoimmune diseases. It occurs mostly bilateral but asymmetric. Usually, the disease begins in the superior area with a local haze (fine punctate opacities) and is separated from the limbus by a clear cornea. Subsequent gradual thinning of the peripheral stroma, typically with an intact epithelial cell layer, is characteristic of this degeneration. After that the degenerative processes spread circumferentially and progressively involve the whole corneal periphery. In the advanced stages, the degeneration becomes circumferential.

The peripheral margin at the thinning has a shallow slope, whereas the central edge is steeper. In the central border of the thinning, progressive neovascularization and lipid deposition (yellow-white zone) may occur (Figs. 9 and 10). Patients are usually asymptomatic but may develop mild irritation. Visual changes might occur because of

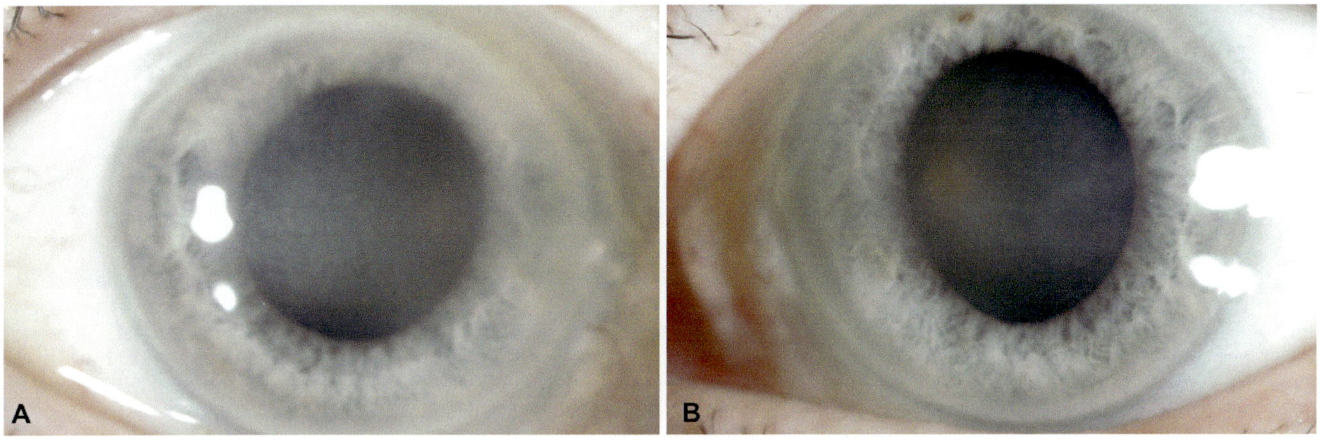

Fig. 7 (**A**, **B**) Crocodile shagreen corneal degeneration in a 75-year-old woman. The degeneration is usually bilateral and is characterized by a corneal opacity with a mosaic-like pattern reminiscent of crocodile skin. Clinically it is indistinguishable from central cloudy dystrophy of François (**A** right eye, **B** left eye)

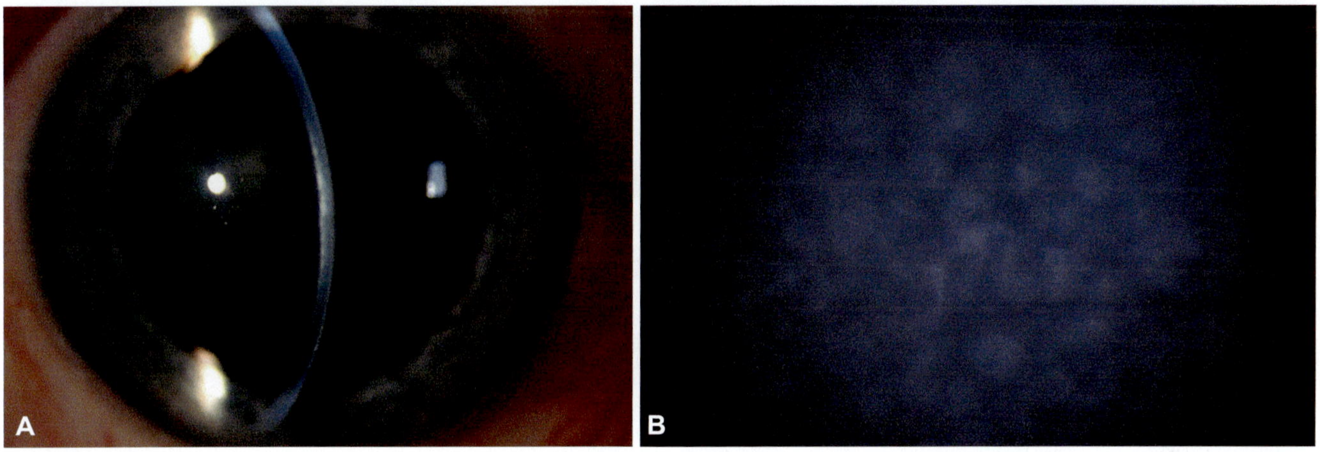

Fig. 8 Crocodile shagreen corneal degeneration in the central posterior cornea. (**A**) Thin slit, (**B**) high magnification

Table 2 Degenerations with tissue thinning—preferably in the periphery of the cornea

Fuchs–Terrien marginal degeneration
Senile corneal furrow degeneration
Dellen

progressive increase in irregular astigmatism (against-the-rule astigmatism or oblique) [14, 15]. A slight inflammation may be present in some rare cases, as noticed by confocal microscopic findings. However, the inflammation can be treated well with topical steroid therapy. According to histopathological studies, an increased lysosomal activity in connection with an absent Bowman layer at the site where thinning occurred, could be shown [15]. For evaluation of peripheral thinning and differential diagnosis with other peripheral corneal diseases, anterior segment optical coherence tomography (AS-OCT) may be helpful. The formation of stromal cavities in the peripheral cornea, probably due to collagen phagocytosis, has been reported in recent AS-OCT findings [16]. In advanced stages of the disease, topographic examination shows irregular astigmatism.

In regards to the differential diagnosis, the peripheral ulcerative keratitis (PUK), Mooren ulcer, pellucid marginal degeneration, and dellen should be taken into consideration. Treatment options include the optical correction of irregular astigmatism and in advanced forms, contact lenses (incl. scleral lenses) are recommended. Corneal perforation is the most feared complication of severe Fuchs–Terrien marginal degeneration and could occur spontaneously or result from any trauma. Therefore, surgical intervention should be considered in cases of extreme thinning [17]. Lamellar ring-shaped or semilunar peripheral corneoscleral grafting can be performed in case of (pre-)perforation (Fig. 11).

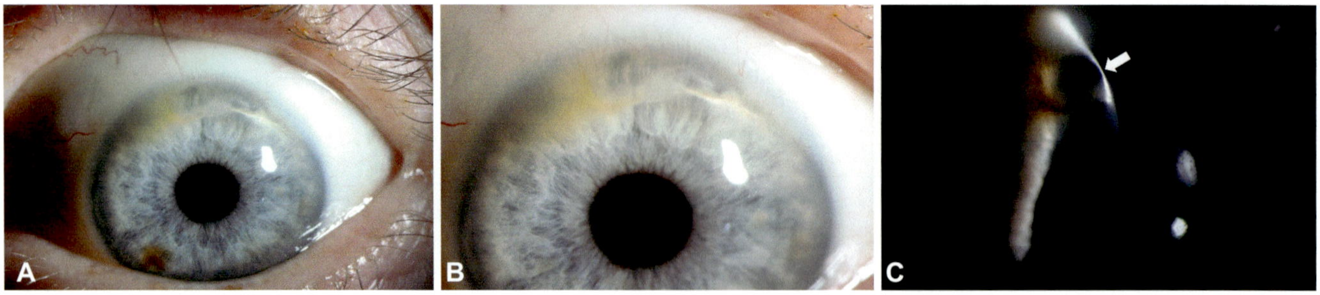

Fig. 9 (**A**–**C**) Fuchs–Terrien marginal degeneration in a 54-year-old man. The mostly bilateral and symmetric degeneration is usually diagnosed in the fourth decade of life. It is characterized by marginal thinning with fine vascularization and a yellow-white area with lipid deposits. It usually begins in the superonasal periphery and can extend in a circular pattern as it progresses. Severe thinning of the corneal stroma (**C** arrow) might occur in advanced stages, carrying the risk of corneal perforation (**A** overview, **B** magnification, **C** thin slit illumination)

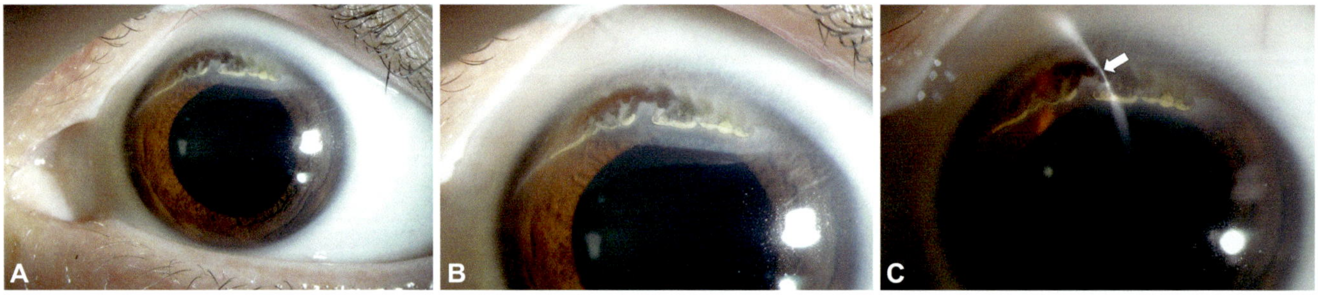

Fig. 10 (**A**–**C**) Fuchs–Terrien marginal degeneration in a 46-year-old woman. Advanced corneal stromal thinning (arrow) is seen in the superior periphery with pronounced lipid deposits (**A** overview, **B** magnification, **C** thin slit illumination)

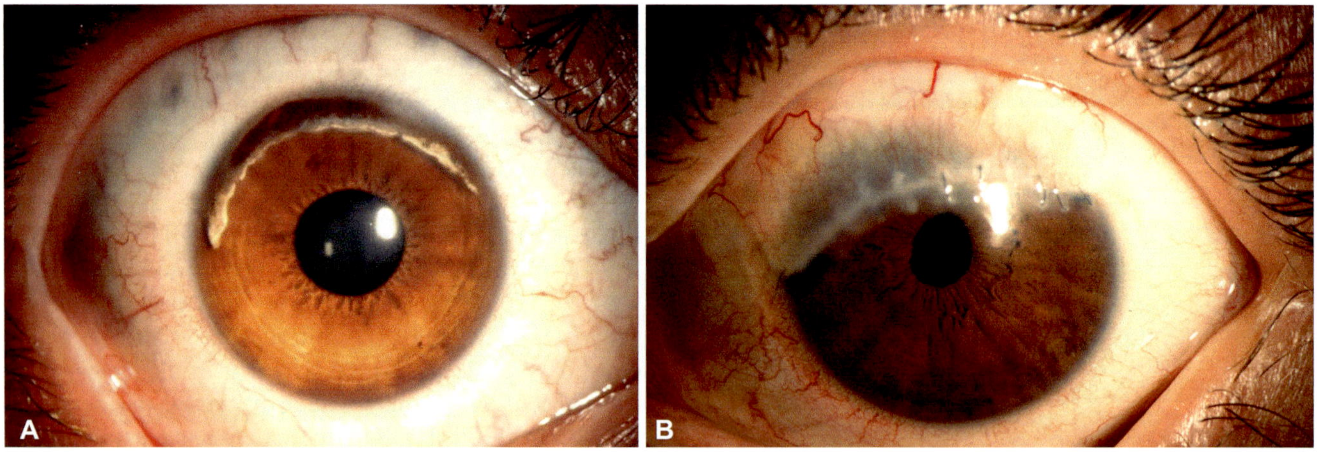

Fig. 11 (**A**) Fuchs–Terrien marginal degeneration, (**B**) 10 months after semilunar penetrating keratoplasty with multiple single sutures—graft is vascularized, the 5 remaining sutures are loose and must be removed immediately

3.2 Senile Corneal Furrow Degeneration

Furrow degeneration is a painless bilateral thinning of peripheral cornea. The thinning is usually shallow. A peripheral corneal furrow can occur between arcus lipoides and the limbus in older adults. Rarely, true thinning with no inflammation, vascularization, or induced corneal astigmatism can occur in this region. Furrow degeneration does not require any therapy, but the location and degree of thinning should be evaluated when considering location for cataract incisions.

3.3 Dellen

Dellen refers to a localized area of corneal thinning in the periphery next to the limbus, usually with an intact epithelial cell layer. When the proper distribution of the tear layer is severely disturbed, it is located near the areas of tissue swelling or inflammation (always adjacent to the elevation). This can often follow some surgical procedures that induce conjunctival chemosis with perilimbal elevation and leads to a localized abnormality of the tear film layer with subsequent localized dehydration and thinning [18–20]. It is frequently associated with pinguecula, pterygia, dermoids, filtering blebs after glaucoma surgery or other elevated bulbar structures. This is a relatively common condition which is reversible. In fact, the appropriate therapy for this disorder is to restore normal tear film spreading and intense lubrication. Moreover, the use of a large-diameter soft contact lens has been proposed as an effective therapeutic solution for the treatment of dellen which occurred after pterygium removal [21].

4 Degenerations with Material or Tissue Deposits (Table 3)

4.1 Salzmann Nodular Degeneration

Salzmann nodular degeneration (SND) is described as a non-inflammatory, slowly progressive disease which is characterized by single or multiple whitish-gray subepithelial corneal nodules. Salzmann described this degeneration in 1925 in association with keratoconjunctivitis. However, over time, several different disorders have been identified that coexist with this disorder. The pathogenesis still remains unknown, but it is thought to be related to ocular surface inflammation or chronic trauma. However, there have been several reports of cases in which the cornea had no previous pathology and the cause of the disease was idiopathic [22].

Table 3 Degeneration with material or tissue deposits—preferably in the midperiphery and the center of the cornea

Salzmann nodular degeneration
Pannus corneae
Calcific band keratopathy
Secondary lipid keratopathy
Spheroidal keratopathy
Secondary amyloidosis
Hematocornea
Silicon oil keratopathy (Fig. 40)
Pigment deposition keratopathies ("Iron lines")

Clinically, the slit lamp examination revealed the typical signs with either single or multiple nodules elevated on the corneal surface and located in the corneal (mid-)periphery but with a normal clear cornea between the nodules which is a characteristic clinical finding (Fig. 12). Routine eye examination in asymptomatic patients may reveal single or few nodules within one or more quadrants in some cases and occasionally the nodules may invade the central zone. With the presence of multiple nodules, a typical circular arrangement occurs and in advanced stages, they may be confluent. Meibomian gland dysfunction and dry eye disease [23], followed by rosacea, phlyctenular keratitis, vernal keratoconjunctivitis, trachoma and interstitial keratitis are ocular surface disorders potentially involved in the pathogenesis of Salzmann degeneration.

Prolonged contact lens wear and preceding corneal surgery, followed by actinic exposure, recurrent erosion and chemical or thermal injury, are the chronic injuries which are most commonly associated with the development of degenerative changes [22, 24, 25].

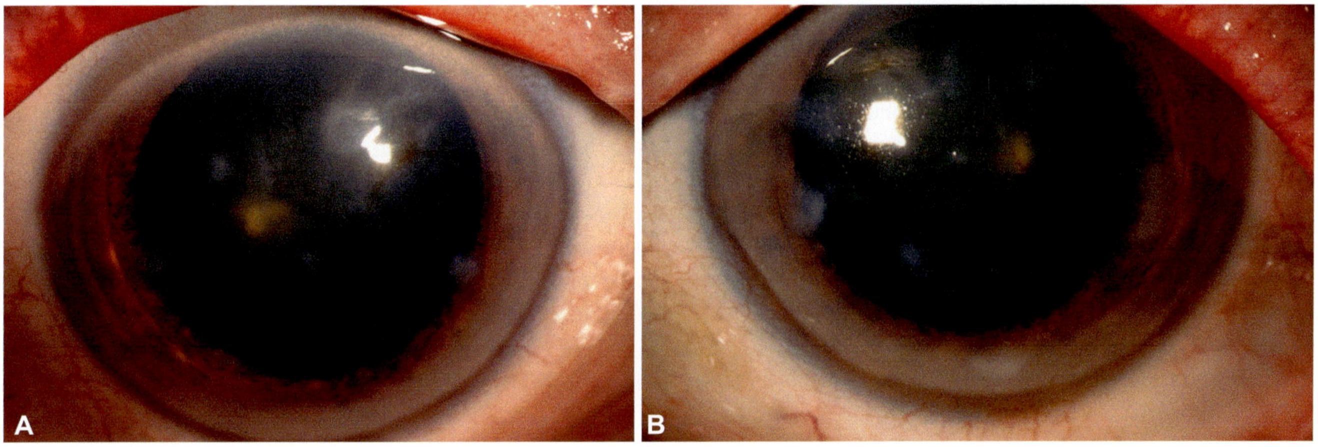

Fig. 12 Multifocal Salzmann nodules with normal clear cornea between the nodules (**A**) right eye, (**B**) left eye

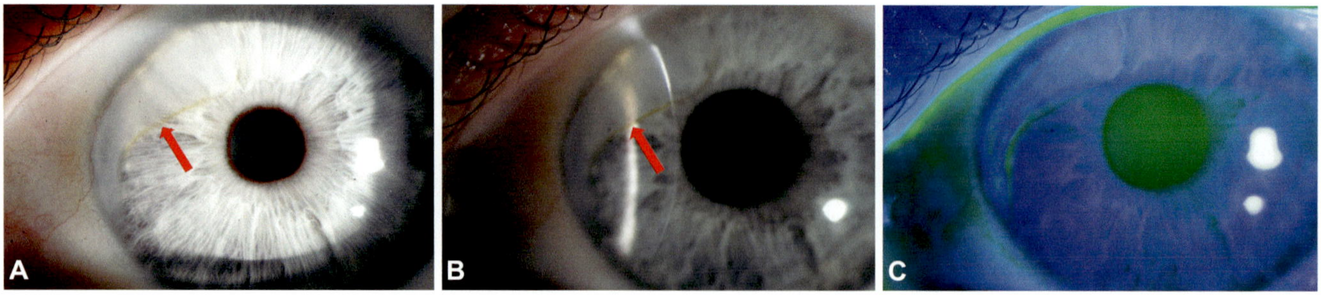

Fig. 13 (**A**–**C**) Salzmann nodular degeneration with adjacent iron line (arrow) in a 31-year-old woman (**A** overview, left eye, **B** magnification). This elevated lesion is causing an asymmetric tear film distribution (**C** fluorescein vital stain)

Therefore, although the etiology remains uncertain, it is hypothesized that SND can be triggered by multiple events that lead to a nonspecific corneal tissue reaction based on individual predisposition. It appears to be more frequent in middle-aged women, and it is bilateral in about 60% of cases. The main symptoms are visual disturbances and photophobia, ocular discomfort, mainly characterized by dryness, and foreign body sensation. In severe forms, characterized by very elevated nodules, painful epithelial lesions can occur. The visual impairment is progressive and is due to secondary induced hyperopia (asymmetric tear film pooling) and astigmatism caused by the elevated nodules (Fig. 13). Severe corneal irregularities in advanced stages generate high irregular astigmatism with severe visual loss. Although the diagnosis of SND is exclusively based on slit-lamp biomicroscopy, several instrumental examinations such as corneal topography, AS-OCT, and confocal microscopy may be useful to provide a better understanding of the corneal alterations and to quantify the amount of visual impairment. AS-OCT may help to differentiate a large vacuolized Salzmann nodule from corneal hydrops [26].

Histopathological studies have revealed that the corneal nodules are located subepithelially but may extend to one-third of the anterior stroma and are formed by a dense connective tissue with hyaline degeneration. The corneal epithelium has an irregular thickness, with extremely increased thinning over the corneal nodules. Bowman layer exhibits disruption, and in the correspondence of the nodules, it is no longer appreciable and frequently replaced by fibrosis [27].

Since 2003 the new term *Peripheral hypertrophic subepithelial corneal degeneration (PHSCD)* has been coined for peripheral corneal nodules as an uncommon, usually bilateral, idiopathic disorder, occurring mostly in white middle-aged women with a distinct phenotype [23, 28–31]. PHSCD can result in progressive flattening of the central corneal topography in the involved meridians (Figs. 14 and 15). This flattening can induce a significant hyperopic and astigmatic shift in refraction. This refractive change can be reversed with superficial keratectomy to remove the degeneration (Fig. 16) [32].

Therapy is related to the symptoms and severity. In early forms, treatment is aimed at reducing the presenting symptoms with conservative therapy concerning eyelid hygiene, lubricants, and anti-inflammatory eyedrops sufficiently to eliminate dry eye symptoms and foreign body sensation. Visual loss is an indication for surgical treatment, which consists of the removal of the nodules and the restoration of corneal surface regularity. In superficial nodules, manual removal with a crescent knife is sufficient and leaves a uniform smooth underlying surface [33]. In the case of deeper ingrowth that involves the anterior stroma, after the nodule's removal, the excimer laser phototherapeutic keratectomy (PTK) is usually performed to smoothen the surface [22, 34–36]. In some cases with deep ingrowth, an anterior lamellar or even penetrating keratoplasty may become necessary. The recurrence of Salzmann nodules after surgical removal can occur with varying prevalence rates (18–21.9%) and periods of time to recurrence (1 month to 6 years) [37, 38]. In recurrent SND, pannectomy and excimer laser PTK is typically augmented by application of Mitomycin-C (0.02%) for 60 to 90 s.

4.2 Pannus Corneae

Fibrous tissue with or without vascularization may be deposited in front of Bowman layer (Table 4) especially in case of long-standing bullous keratopathy due to chronic endothelial decompensation, e.g. in buphthalmos (Fig. 17), after complicated cataract surgery, in Fuchs endothelial corneal dystrophy or PEX keratopathy (Fig. 18).

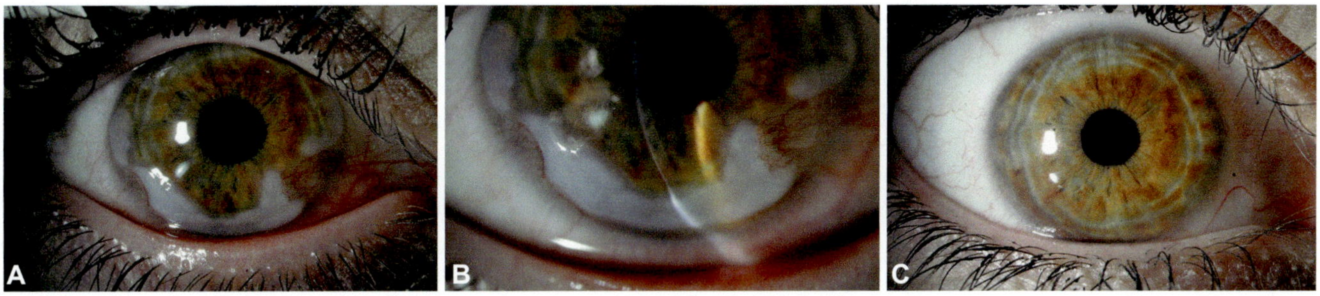

Fig. 14 (**A**, **B**) Peripheral hypertrophic subepithelial corneal degeneration (PHSCD) with a nasal pterygium in a 27-year-old woman. PHSCD is a variant of Salzmann nodular corneal degeneration with identical histopathologic findings (**A** overview, **B** thin slit illumination). (**C**) Corneal findings after pannectomy, pterygium excision and excimer laser-assisted phototherapeutic keratectomy

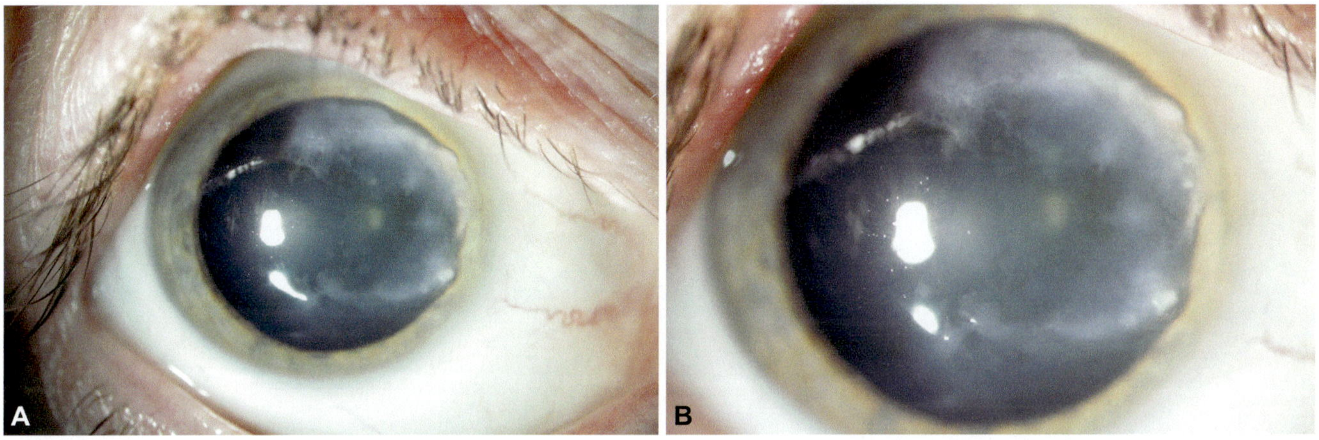

Fig. 15 Peripheral hypertrophic subepithelial corneal degeneration (PHSCD) with atoll-like appearance in a 52-year-old woman (**A** overview right eye, **B** magnification)

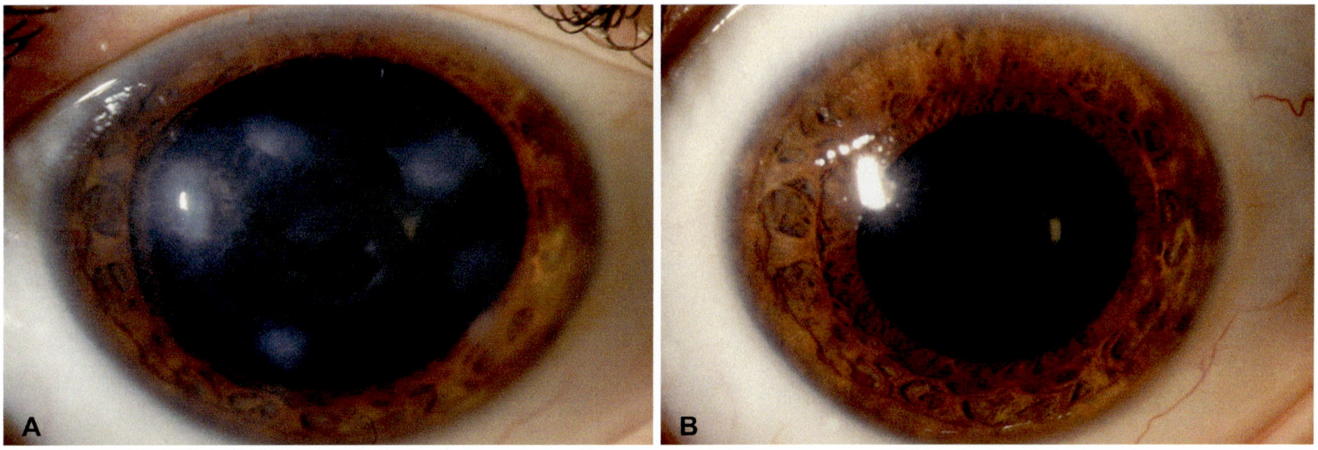

Fig. 16 (**A**) Midperipheral Salzmann nodules inducing asymmetric tear pooling with "optical cornea plana" with high hyperopia and high irregular astigmatism despite normal eye length. (**B**) 6 weeks after Pannus removal and excimer laser PTK (diameter 10 mm, 15 μm tissue removal without masking fluid)

Table 4 Classification of pannus corneae

Degenerative	Non-vascularized
	Vascularized
Inflammatory	Non-vascularized
	Vascularized

4.3 Calcific Band Keratopathy

Calcific band keratopathy is a common corneal degeneration that can occur at any age. It consists of the deposition of calcium salts in the interpalpebral region and typically starts with slight haze at the level of the Bowman layer in proximity to the limbus in the corneal periphery nasally and temporally at the same time. It gradually spreads toward the center and forms a band like whitish-gray plaque [39]. Small, dark, round holes are characteristically seen within the band, which are thought to represent corneal nerves running through Bowman layer. The peripheral edge of the band is separated from the limbus by a clear cornea. Visual acuity decreases as the deposits progress affecting the visual axis (Figs. 19, 20, and 21). It most commonly occurs secondary to chronic corneal diseases, particularly uveitis (Fig. 22), advanced glaucoma, keratitis, or trauma, whereas primary idiopathic forms rarely occur. Band keratopathy can present secondarily with elevated serum calcium or phosphate in systemic diseases, including sarcoidosis, hyperparathyroidism, vitamin D toxicity, metastatic neoplasm to bone, plasmocytoma, M. Waldenström and chronic renal failure with secondary hyperparathyroidism. In children, band keratopathy may be the presenting sign of chronic uveitis as a result of juvenile idiopathic arthritis. Band keratopathy may occur after localized corneal damage from intraocular silicone oil and phosphate forms of corticosteroids or phosphate-containing preservatives in artificial tears [40].

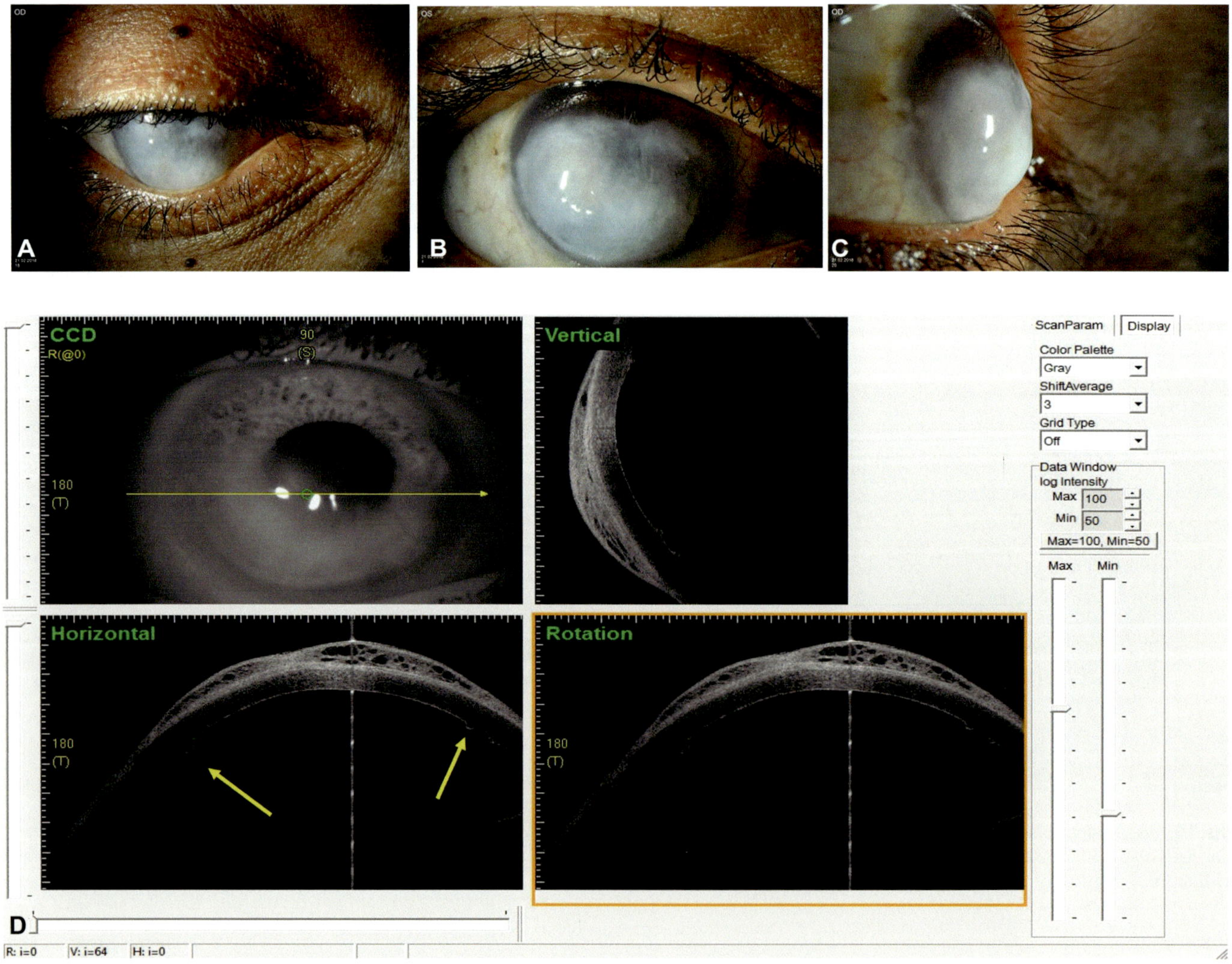

Fig. 17 (**A**–**C**) Prominent degenerative avascular pannus (VA hand motion)—DD: corneal hydrops, (**D**) AS-OCT shows an intact cornea under the vacuolized pannus and retrocorneal prominences indicative for Haab striae in buphthalmos (arrows)

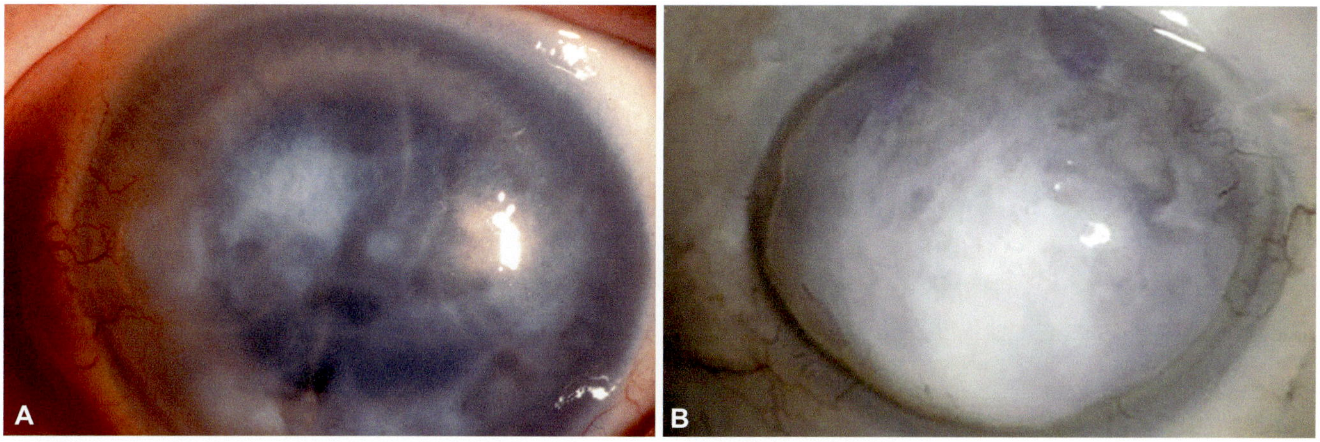

Fig. 18 Pannus degenerativus vasculosus due to long-standing. Fuchs endothelial corneal dystrophy (**A**) and PEX keratopathy (**B**)

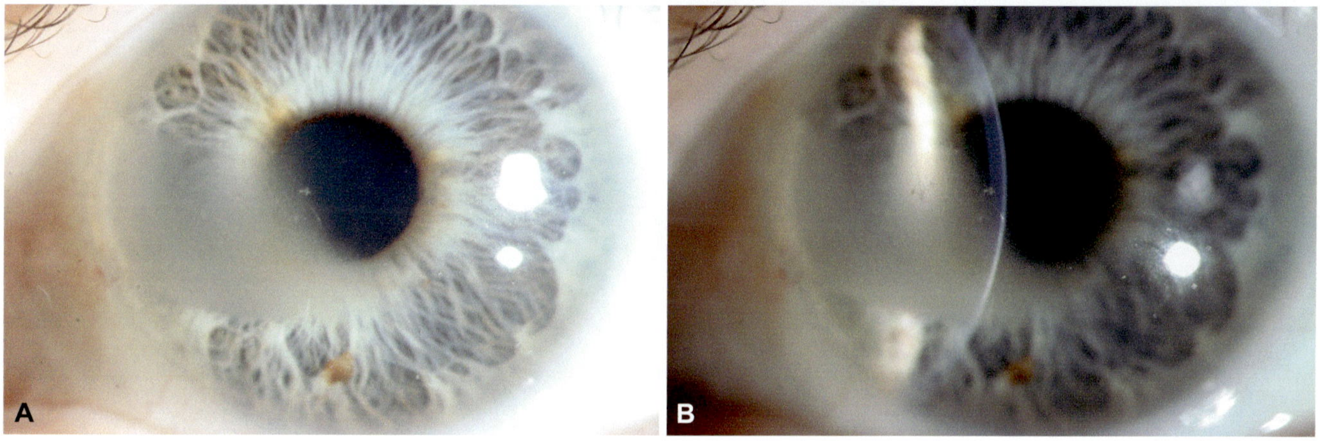

Fig. 19 (**A**, **B**) Subepithelial band keratopathy with involvement of the optical center in a 62-year-old man (**A** left eye overview, **B** thin slit illumination)

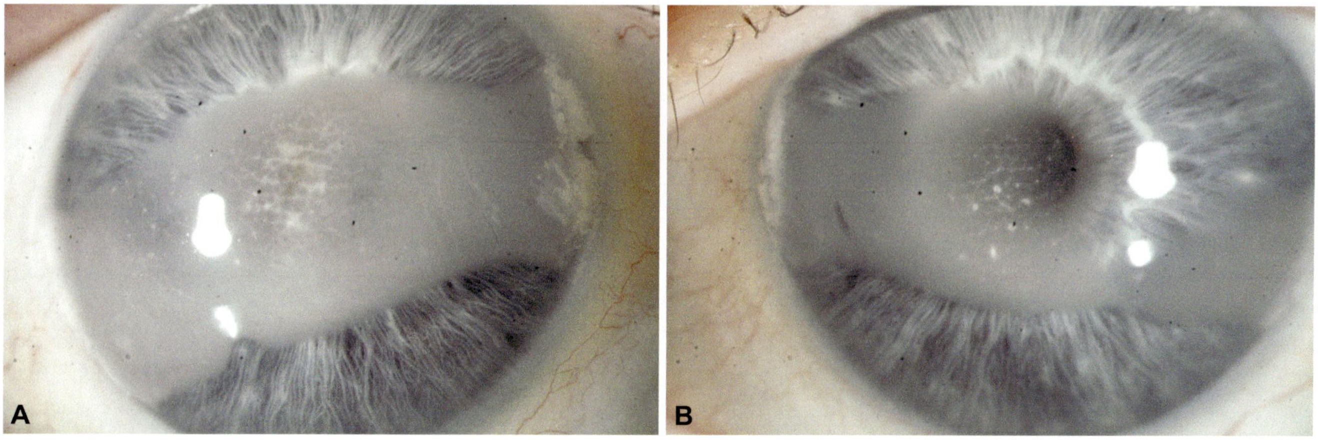

Fig. 20 (**A**, **B**) Severe bilateral band keratopathy with affection of the central cornea in an 83-year-old woman (**A** right eye, **B** left eye)

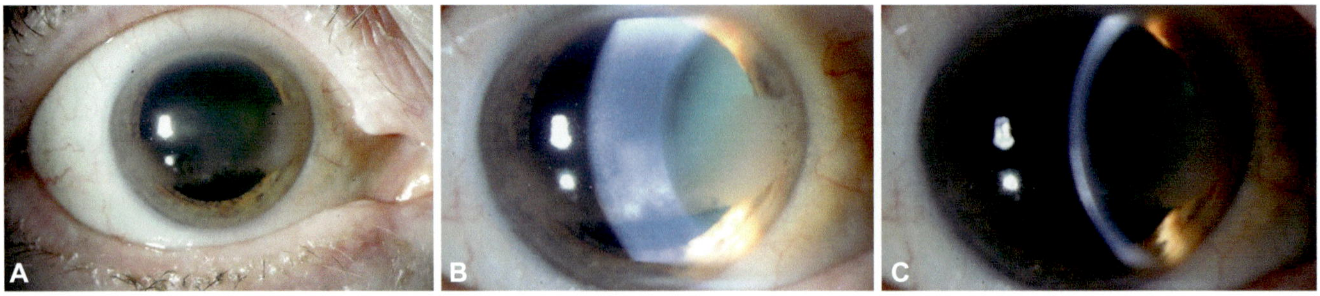

Fig. 21 (**A–C**) Medium severe bilateral band keratopathy with affection of the central cornea in the right eye of a 70-year-old woman with Fuchs endothelial corneal dystrophy (**A** overview, **B** broad beam: the deposits are most pronounced at the nasal limbus, **C** thin slit: very superficial deposition in Bowman layer and anterior stroma)

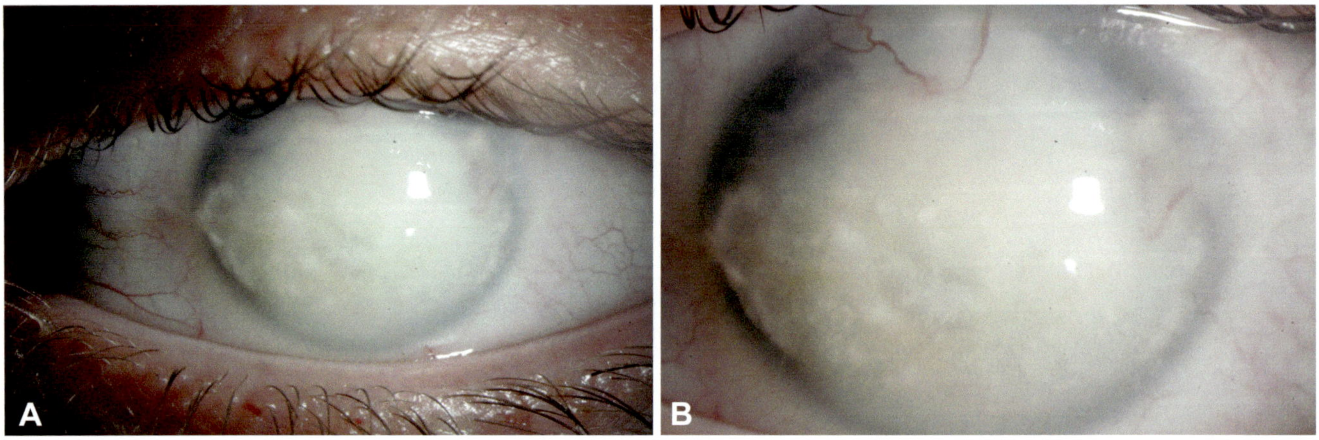

Fig. 22 (**A**, **B**) Severe calcific keratopathy after years of recurrent anterior uveitis in a 25-year-old man (**A** left eye overview, **B** magnification)

Histologically, calcium is deposited as the hydroxyapatite salt in the epithelial basement membrane, basal epithelium, Bowman layer, and anterior stroma. The mechanism of calcium deposition in the cornea is unknown but occurs primarily in the exposed area of the cornea. Deposition of calcium may result from the precipitate tears leave when they evaporate or because the exposed cornea is at a lower pH than other areas. The most severely affected areas are the middle and inferior thirds of the cornea, which are the areas of greatest exposure to the atmosphere.

Patients can have symptoms of pain, foreign body sensation, recurrent corneal erosions, and decreased vision. The rate of development and progression of disease is variable. If band keratopathy causes persistent pain or decreased vision, corneal surgery is indicated. The surgery involves removing the epithelium over the deposits, applying 0.05 mol/L disodium ethylenediaminetetraacetic acid (EDTA) for 10–20 min to chelate the calcium and dissolve it by use of a stylus swab or a brush [41]. Excimer laser phototherapeutic keratektomy PTK also may be used to smoothen the surface after having removed the calcium deposits by EDTA chelating.

Calcareous corneal degeneration differs from band keratopathy in that the calcium deposits extend deeper into the stroma beyond the anterior stroma (Figs. 22 and 23) [42, 43].

4.4 Lipid Keratopathy

Lipid keratopathy may develop spontaneously or as a consequence of a prior ocular injury or inflammation. The primary form has features of a corneal dystrophy, is usually bilateral, and the central lipid, often with cholesterol crystals, may severely decrease vision. It is not associated with vascularization or inflammation.

Secondary lipid keratopathy appears as a white or yellow stromal deposit separated by a narrow, clear zone from corneal stromal neovascularization and may be associated to previous ocular diseases or injury and is much more common. It is usually associated with corneal vascularization (Figs. 24, 25, 26, and 27). The vessels are more permeable and have a lower ability to remove lipids. The most frequent corneal pathologies underlying the secondary lipid

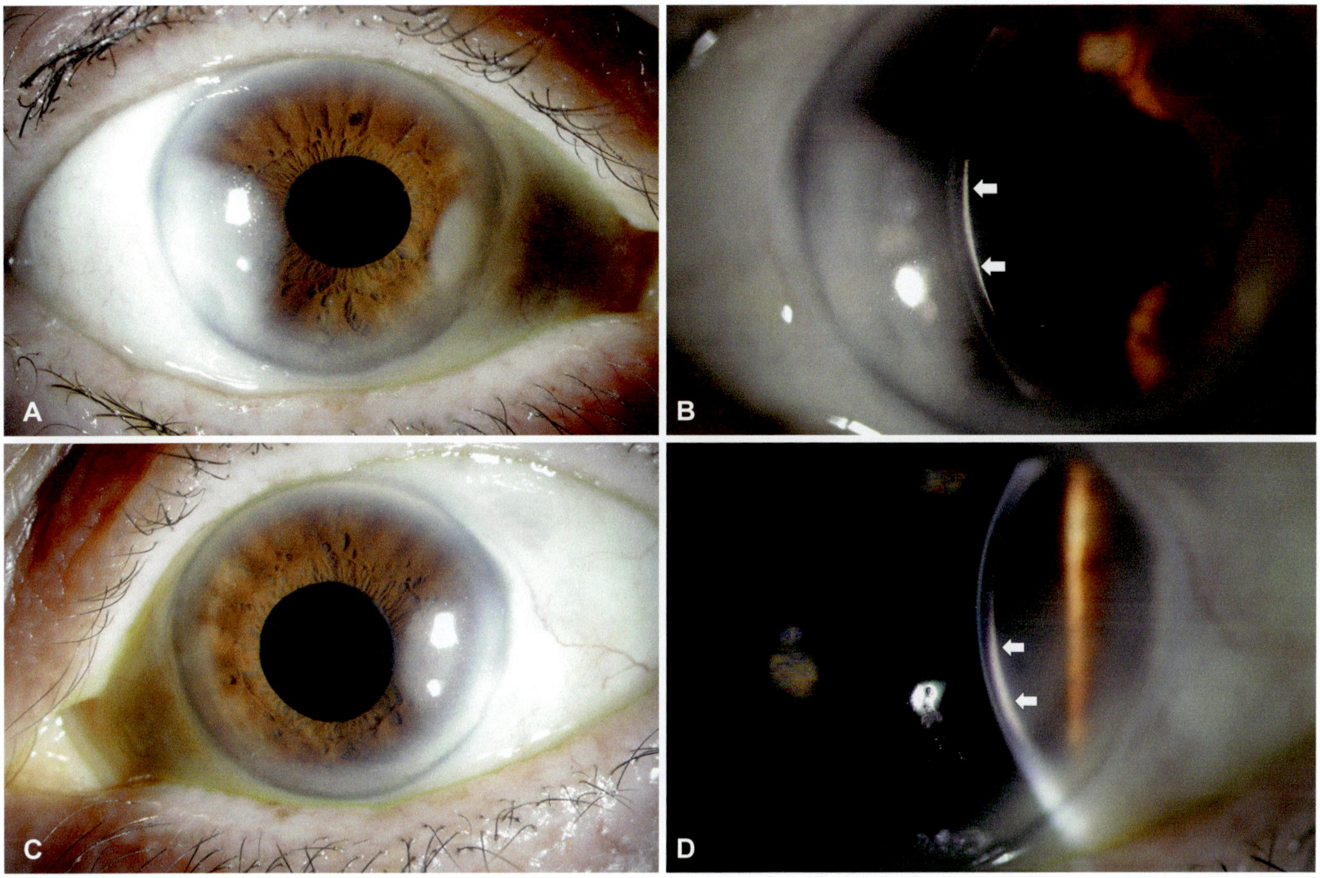

Fig. 23 (**A**, **B**) Calcareous corneal degeneration in an 85-year-old woman. The difference from band keratopathy is that the calcium deposits extend deeper (arrows), beyond the anterior stroma (**A** right eye overview, **B** thin slit illumination, **C** left eye overview, **D** thin slit illumination)

keratopathy are herpetic infections, both simplex and zoster (Fig. 28).

Firstly, treatment should focus on the underlying disease. Subsequently, the abnormal vascularization may be eliminated by means of argon laser photocoagulation or needle point cautery to induce lipid absorption by destroying the feeder vessels. As a final treatment option, corneal transplantation requires a relative quiescence, and the clinical outcome is rather poor due to corneal thinning, hypesthesia, and persistent vascularization [44, 45].

4.5 Spheroidal Degeneration

Spheroidal degeneration is also known as corneal elastosis, Labrador keratopathy, climatic droplet keratopathy, Bietti nodular dystrophy, proteinaceous corneal degeneration, elastotic degeneration, Fisherman keratopathy, and Eskimo corneal degeneration. It was described by Bietti in 1955 and is characterized by oil-like, amber-colored, spheroidal deposits at the limbus and in the peripheral interpalpebral cornea.

It arises typically in outdoor workers, and the main causing factor is ultraviolet exposure. It is more frequent in populations living in zones with high climatic UV light exposure, and the severity is correlated positively with the time of exposure. With time, the corneal opacification increases, and deposits spread toward the center of the cornea. The advanced lesions are associated with localized haze. Sometimes the corneal changes coexist with the same conjunctival deposits. It is twice as prevalent in men as in women. The prevalence varies from 6% in England to greater than 60% in Labrador. It is bilateral and relatively innocuous, although in some cases, visual impairment might occur [46–48].

Histologic examination showed extracellular protein deposits in the anterior corneal stroma with elastotic degeneration. They are formed by UV-degraded protein materials that originated from the plasma through the limbal vessels. Progressively, such deposits slowly replace Bowman layer. In patients with spheroidal degeneration, protection against ultraviolet damage with sunglasses is mandatory. In advanced forms with central involvement, the various grades of visual impairment might occur, requiring appropriate therapeutic

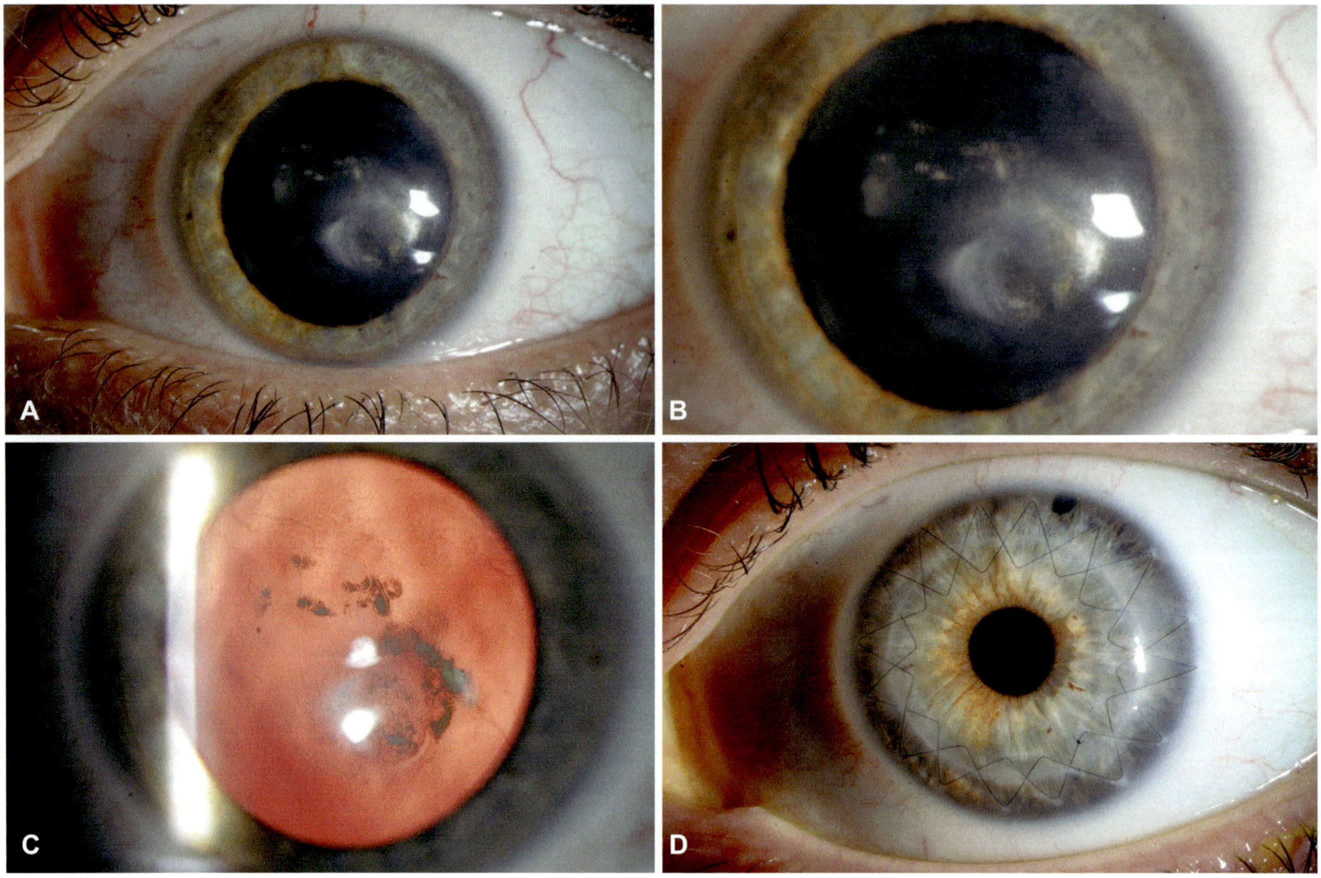

Fig. 24 (**A–C**) Discoid vascularized stromal corneal scar with lipid keratopathy after recurrent herpetic keratitis in a 32-year-old woman (**A** overview, **B** magnification, **C** retroillumination). (**D**) Excimer laser-assisted penetrating keratoplasty was performed for visual rehabilitation

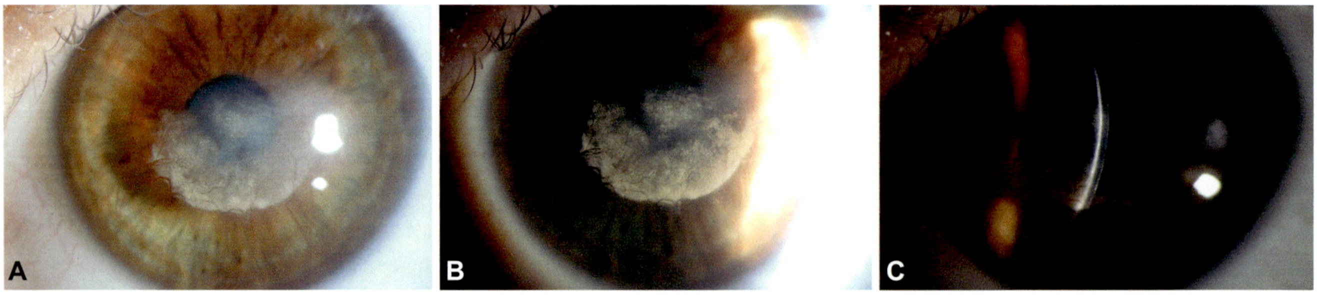

Fig. 25 (**A–C**) Deep stromal vascularized corneal scar of herpetic origin with secondary lipid keratopathy in a 35-year-old-woman (**A** overview, **B** scleral scatter illumination, **C** thin slit illumination)

options such as superficial keratectomy and PTK after which good clinical and visual outcome could be expected.

4.6 Secondary Corneal Amyloidosis (SCA)

Corneal amyloidosis is an infrequent condition that occurs when normally soluble autologous proteins are deposited in tissues as abnormal insoluble fibrils. The amyloid proteins are deposited as insoluble fibrils as a consequence of abnormal protein folding, detected on electron microscopy as non-branching, rigid, and mostly extracellular. Binding of the Congo Red dye in addition to the "apple green" birefringence on polarized light microscopy are diagnostic. Amyloidosis may be classified into two main groups, primary and secondary, each of which is further divided into systemic or localized. Secondary localized corneal amyloidosis is uncommon, and is rarely reported [49]. It has been

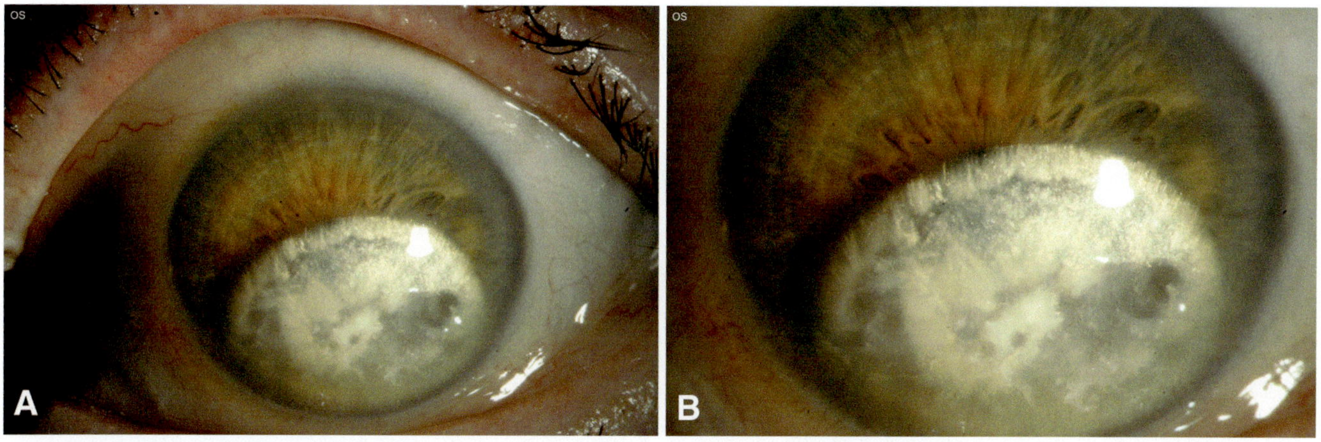

Fig. 26 (**A**, **B**) Severe lipid keratopathy after recurrent herpetic keratitis in the left eye of an 81-year-old woman (**A** overview, **B** magnification)

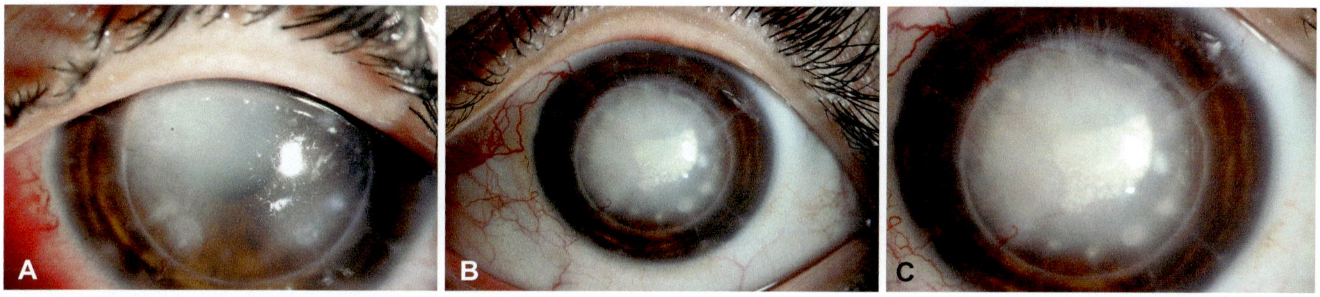

Fig. 27 (**A**–**C**) Severe lipid keratopathy with advanced corneal vascularization in a 21-year-old man after penetrating keratoplasty for keratoconus (**A**). The corneal opacity increased significantly within 6 months (**B**, **C**)

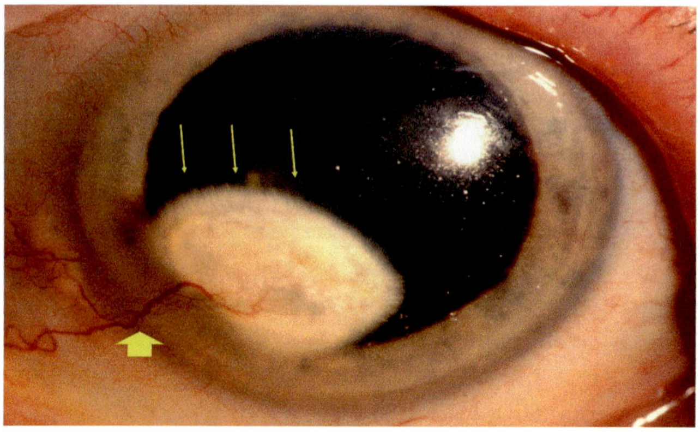

Fig. 28 Midperipheral lipid keratopathy with feeder vessel (yellow bold arrow) after recurrent zoster keratitis in the left eye of a 60-year-old man. Please note the feathery edges towards the clear cornea (arrows)

described in several ocular disorders such as keratectasia [50–53], bullous keratopathy [54], interstitial keratitis [55], eyelid malposition [56], trachoma [57], trauma [49, 58], or inflammatory diseases [59].

Clinically secondary corneal amyloidosis has often a yellowish appearance (Figs. 29 and 30), it may be localized and recur years after surgical removal (Fig. 31).

4.7 Hematocornea (= "Corneal Blood Staining")

Corneal blood staining (CBS) typically occurs after a significant and prolonged hyphema, usually the result of ocular trauma, and especially in cases of chronically elevated intraocular pressure (Figs. 32 and 33). But it may also be the consequence of complicated glaucoma surgery (Fig. 34). The opacification consists of hemosiderin that has become embedded in the corneal stroma. It is initially characterized by small yellow granules within the posterior stroma. A rust-colored opacity of the stroma develops if the hyphema persists. Over time, the blood in the cornea turns yellow and might involve the entire cornea. Predisposing factors that increase the risk of developing CBS include: 1. prolonged duration of hyphema, 2. a large amount of blood

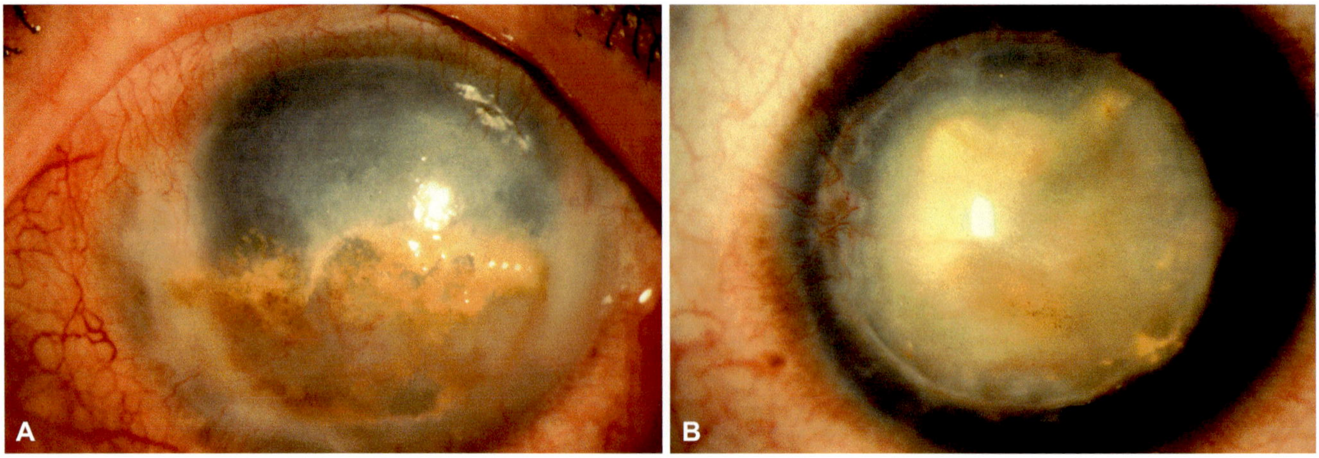

Fig. 29 (**A**) Severe secondary corneal amyloidosis after penetrating injury 20 years ago, (**B**) Severe secondary corneal amyloidosis after penetrating keratoplasty 10 years ago

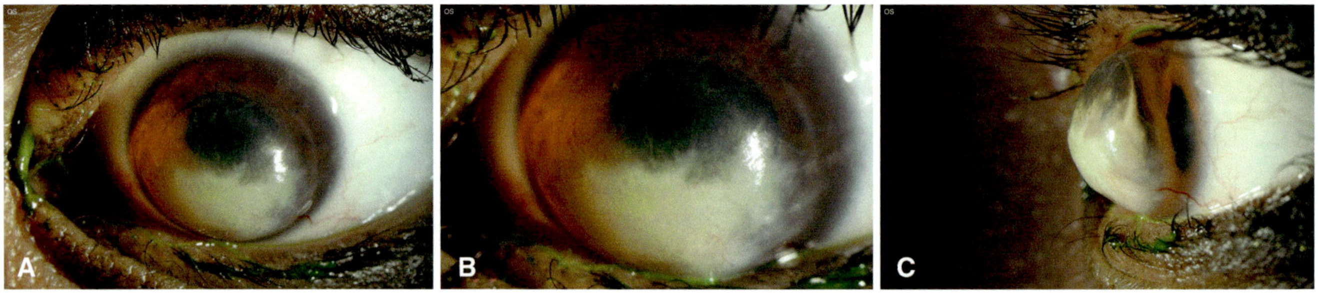

Fig. 30 (**A**, **B**) Secondary corneal amyloidosis in severe graft ectasia after penetrating keratoplasty 16 years ago for keratoconus (**A** overview, **B** magnification), (**C**) Note the side view, which shows pronounced vascularization of the cornea, which could be attributable to the amyloid deposits

in the anterior chamber or total hyphema, 3. dysfunction of corneal endothelium, 4. increased intraocular pressure greater than 25 mm Hg for 6 days, 5. injury to Descemet membrane, 6. Re-bleeding. Continuous overload with hemoglobin leads to necrosis of keratocytes and irreversible corneal blood staining. Prevention is contingent on removal of the hyphema. Clot removal via an anterior chamber wash-out procedure is usually performed before 6 days of raised intraocular pressure (25 mm Hg or greater) and certainly with the first sign of blood staining. It can take months, if not 2–3 years for the cornea to clear, but with patience, it can clear completely. Unfortunately, the periphery clears first followed by the central clearing [60, 61].

4.8 Pigment Deposition Keratopathies ("Iron Lines") [62]

These corneal degenerations consist of deposition of different pigmented substances in corneal layers. Since cornea verticillata may serve as corneal indicator for systemic diseases or systemic medication [63, 64] it will be mentioned in another chapter of this Atlas. The iron deposits are typically present in particular corneal conditions when the regular corneal profile is modified. This can be observed in the cases of pterygium, SND, keratoconus, previous corneal refractive surgery, corneal scars, and filtering blebs [65, 66]. In these conditions, the common finding is related to the high variation of corneal shape, and the deposits are localized typically in the zones where such changes occur. Corneal profile variations generate alteration of the physiological tear film distribution that probably underlies this keratopathy. Histologically, the deposits are formed by intraepithelial hemosiderin in the basal cells.

The most frequent are due to the epithelial iron deposits ("iron lines" according to Naumann). The horizontal running Hudson–Stähli line (Fig. 35) is observed sporadically in normal corneas of middle and older aged individuals, which is found at the junction between the lower and middle third of the cornea, where the eyelids meet when closing. Hudson–Stähli line is typically bilateral and symmetrical. The incidence of the Hudson–Stähli line decreases after the age of 70 for unknown reasons [67].

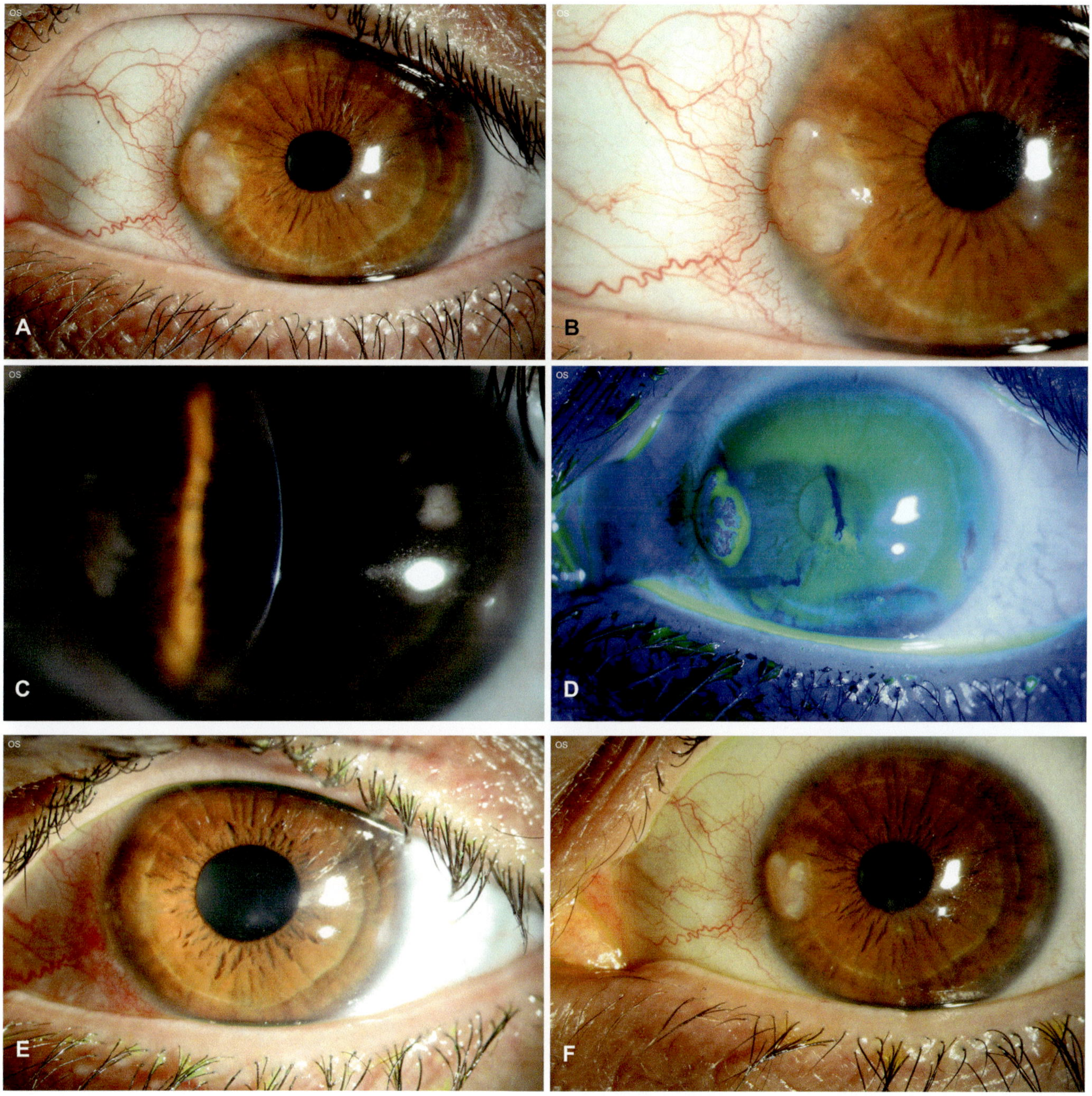

Fig. 31 (**A–D**) Corneal amyloidosis in a 39-year-old man with keratoconus. Note the elevated corneal amyloidosis at the nasal limbus of the left eye. There are also some other small whitish nodules in the cornea (**A** overview, **B** magnification, **C** thin slit illumination, **D** fluorescein vital stain). After surgical removal of the corneal amyloidosis at the nasal limbus (**E**), recurrence of the lesion was observed after 4 years (**F**)

In the advanced forms, the iron deposits separate the advancing head of pterygium (Figs. 36 and 37) or peripheral Salzmann nodule (Fig. 38) exactly where the corneal surface undergoes variations. In this case, the deposits form the so-called Stocker line [68]. In keratoconus or iatrogenic keratectasia after LASIK, circular iron deposits surround the base of the cone where extreme variations of the corneal curvature could be detected (Fig. 39), and they are commonly known as Fleischer ring [69, 70]. Central corneal iron deposits in corneal epithelium are a common side effect of corneal refractive surgery, both incisional and excimer laser. Corneal refractive procedures change corneal curvature by inducing central flattening or steepening [71, 72].

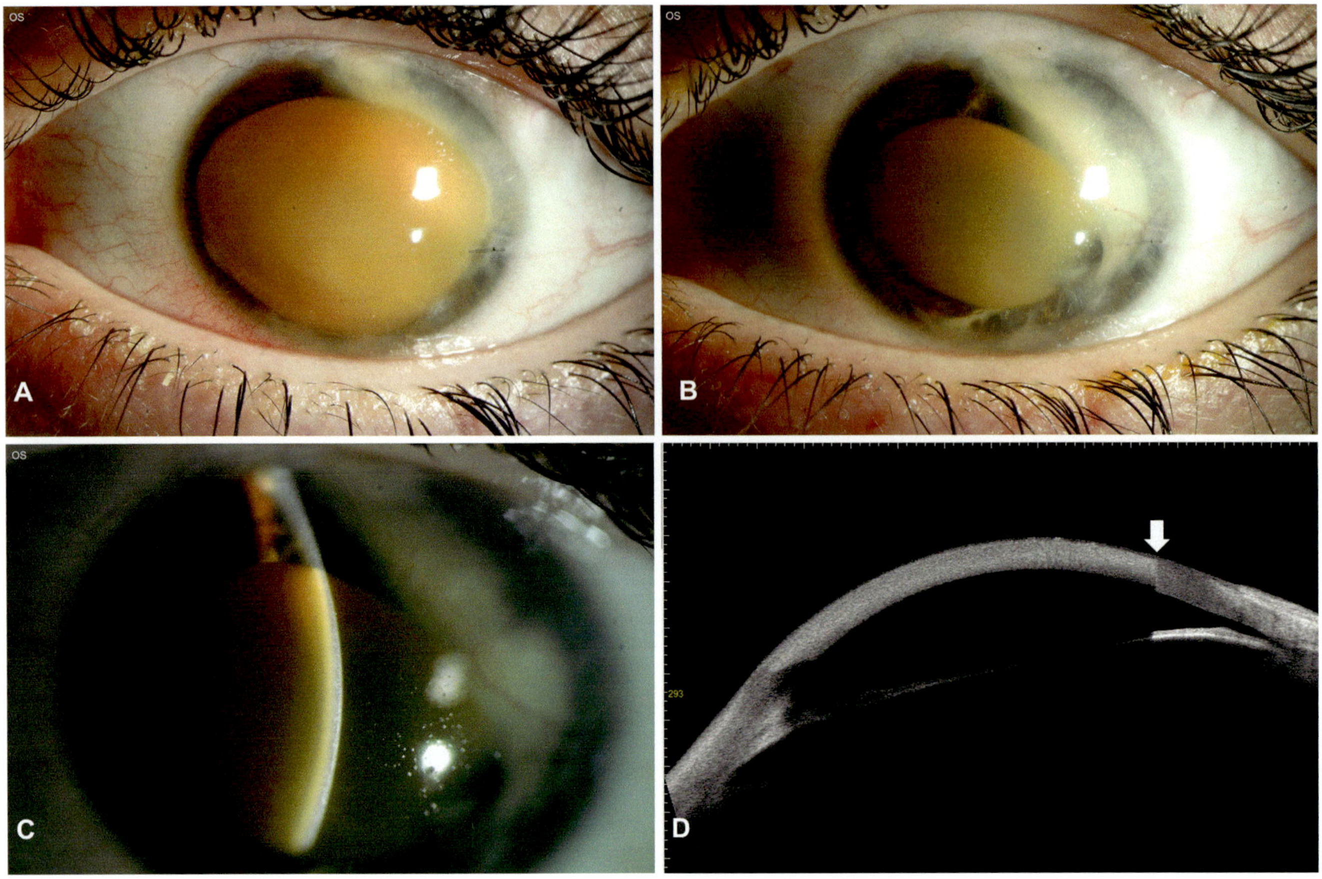

Fig. 32 (**A**) Corneal blood staining after ocular trauma 10 months ago. Generally, the corneal blood staining first resolves in the periphery followed by central clearing, which can take months to years. (**B**–**D**) There is a peripheral clearing of the corneal blood staining within 8 months (**B** overview, **C** thin slit illumination). The anterior segment optical coherence tomography demonstrates a sharp margin of the corneal lesion (**D** arrow)

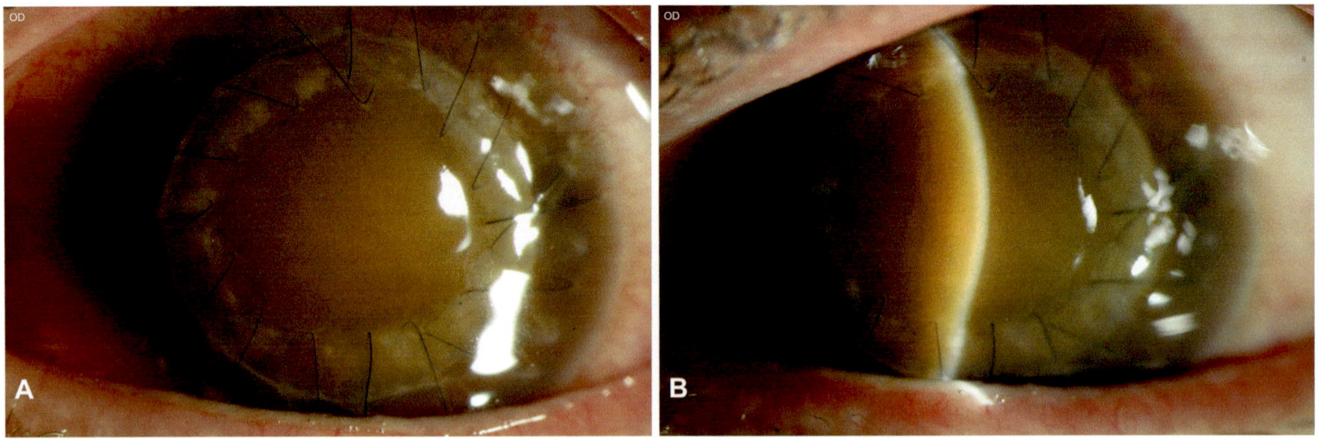

Fig. 33 (**A**, **B**) Corneal blood staining due to ocular trauma in a patient with prior penetrating keratoplasty (**A** overview, **B** thin slit illumination)

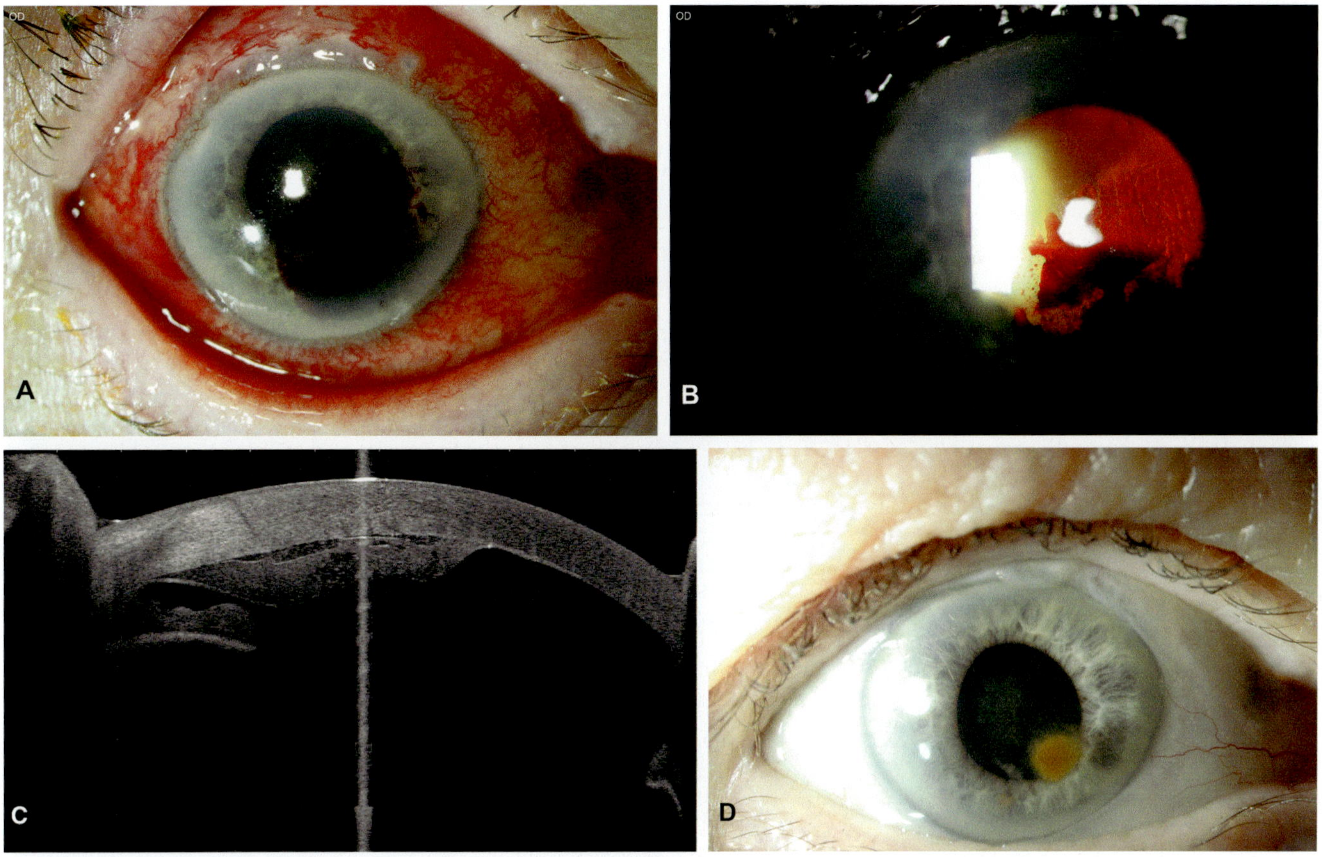

Fig. 34 (**A**–**C**) Injury to Descemet membrane after canaloplasty with blood between posterior stroma and Descemet membrane (**A** overview, **B** retroillumination, (**C**) anterior segment optical coherence tomography). (**D**) After surgical intervention, localized corneal blood staining is seen due to persistent blood residues between the interfaces

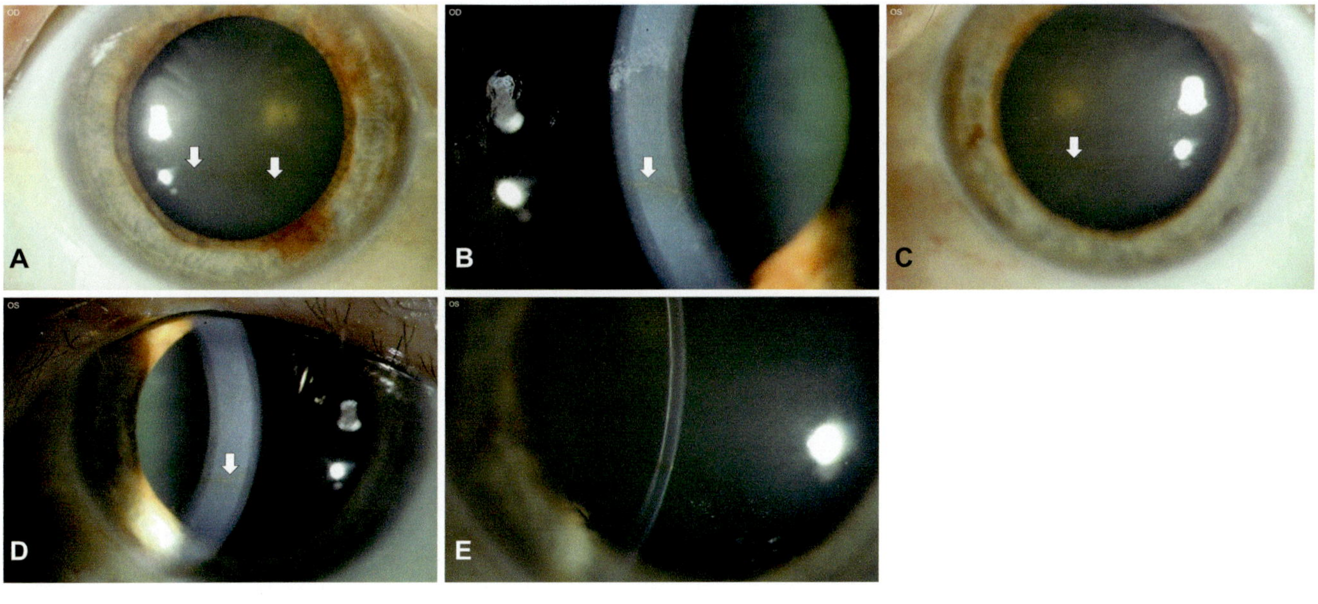

Fig. 35 (**A**–**E**) The horizontal running Hudson–Stähli line (arrows) is located at the juncture of lower and middle thirds of the cornea where the eyelids meet on closure. The Hudson–Stähli lines are typically bilateral and symmetrical (**A**, **B** right eye with overview and broad beam illumination, **C**–**E** left eye with overview, broad beam and thin slit)

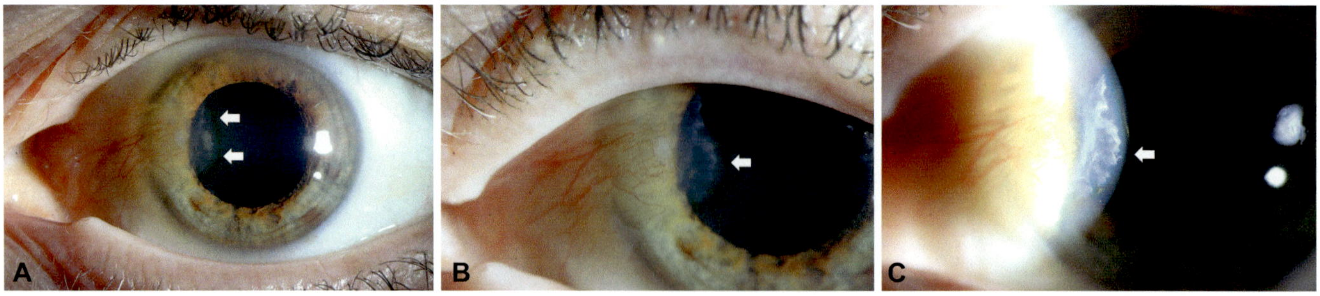

Fig. 36 (**A–C**) Stocker line (arrow) is a brown iron line (hemosiderin deposits) in the cornea at the head of a pterygium. These iron deposits are caused by an irregular tear film distribution (**A** overview, **B** higher magnification, **C** broad slit beam)

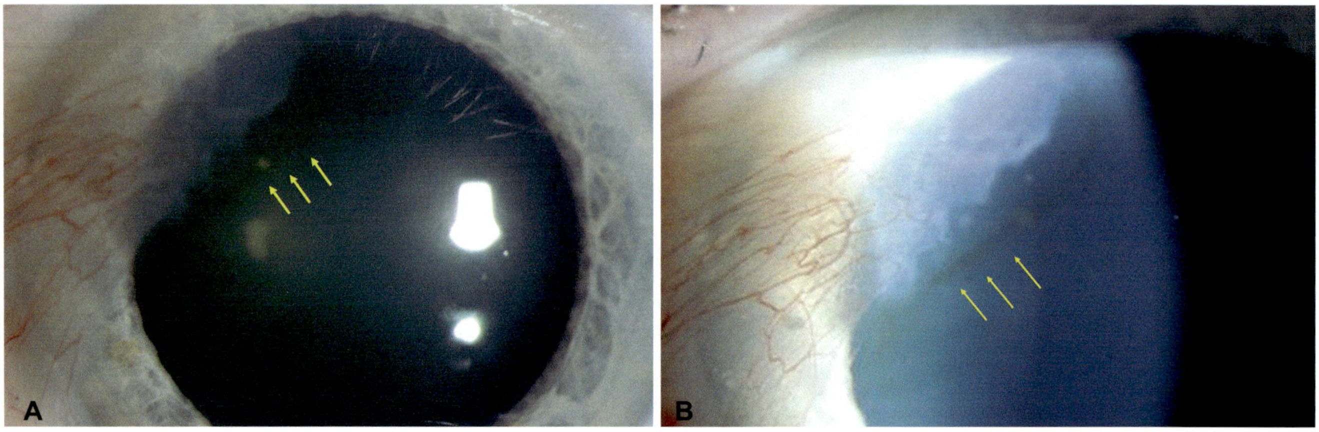

Fig. 37 (**A**, **B**) Stocker line (arrows) at the head of a pterygium (**A** overview, **B** broad slit beam)

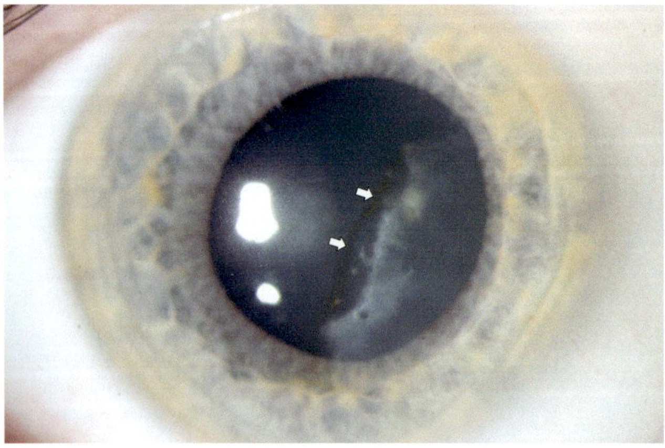

Fig. 38 Salzmann nodular degeneration with an iron line (arrows) caused by irregular tear film distribution

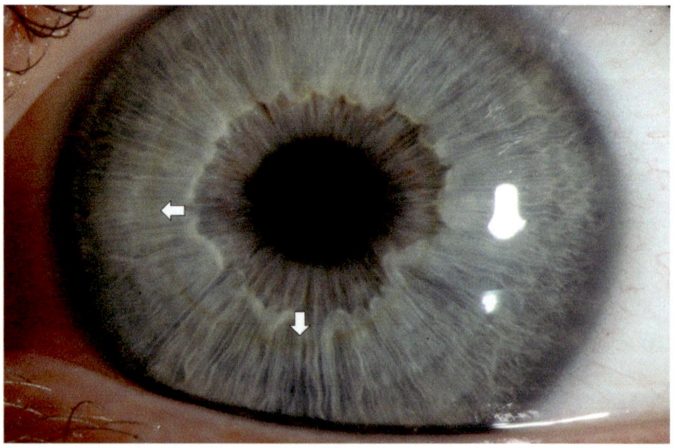

Fig. 39 Brownish Fleischer ring (hemosiderin deposits, arrows) along the base of the cone in a 32-year-old male patient with iatrogenic keratectasia after Laser-in-situ-Keratomileusis (left eye)

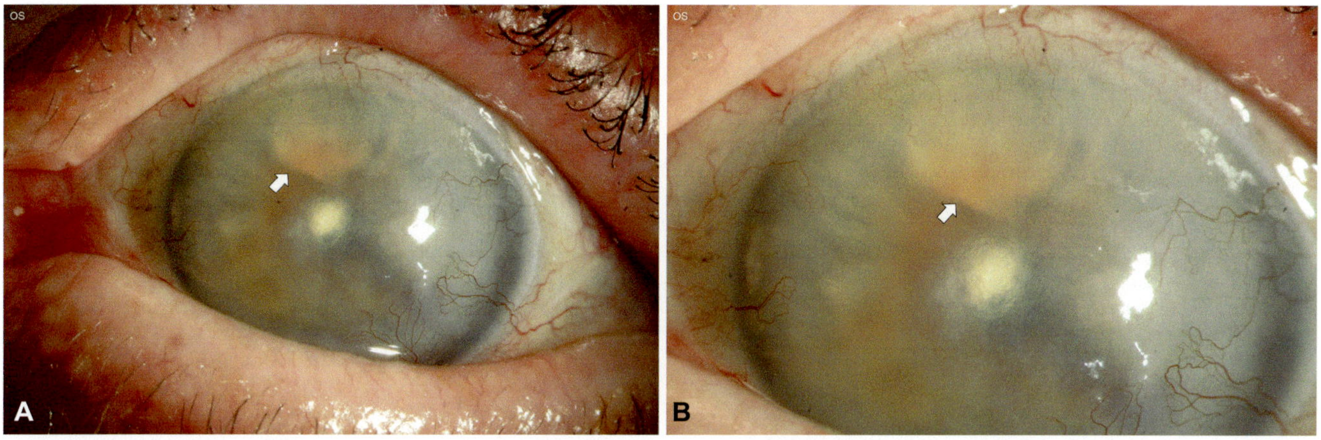

Fig. 40 (**A**, **B**) Silicone oil keratopathy 30 years after vitrectomy with silicone oil tamponade. After incomplete removal of the silicone oil, some of it remained in the anterior chamber, causing endothelial decompensation and progressive vascularization (see Table 3)

5 Conclusion

All attempts to define and classify corneal degenerations must remain artificial and arbitrary to a certain extent. These corneal disorders are not hereditary, have a late onset, may be associated with local or systemic diseases and often arise with aging. In case of local disorders, degenerations occur only in the affected eye, while in case of systemic disorders, the bilateral asymmetric involvement is present. Some forms of degeneration might induce severe visual impairment, and appropriate therapy is necessary to recovery and maintenance of visual acuity. The goal of therapy is to treat the underlying disease first and then treat the corneal changes. Age-related degenerations are bilateral and usually do not affect visual acuity. A correct diagnosis and especially differential diagnosis with respect to corneal dystrophies is mandatory to take the appropriate therapeutic choice thus securing the efficacy of clinical outcomes.

References

1. Kotulak JC, Brungardt T. Age-related changes in the cornea. J Am Optom Assoc. 1980;51(8):761–5.
2. Friedlaender MH, Smolin G. Corneal degenerations. Ann Ophthalmol. 1979;11(10):1485–95.
3. Weiss JS, Rapuano CJ, Seitz B, Busin M, Kivelä TT, Bouheraoua N, Bredrup C, Nischal KK, Chawla H, Borderie V, Kenyon KR, Kim EK, Møller HU, Munier FL, Berger T, Lisch W. IC3D classification of corneal dystrophies—edition 3. Cornea. 2024;43(4):466–527.
4. Roszkowska AM, Wylegala E, et al. Corneal degeneration. In: Babizhayev MA, et al., editors. Studies on the cornea and lens, oxidative stress in applied basic research and clinical practice. New York: Springer Science+Business Media; 2015. p. 23–38.
5. Ang M, Wong W, Park J, Wu R, Lavanya R, Zheng Y, Cajucom-Uy H, Tai ES, Wong TY. Corneal arcus is a sign of cardiovascular disease, even in low-risk persons. Am J Ophthalmol. 2011;152(5):864–71.
6. Chua BE, Mitchell P, Wang JJ, Rochtchina E. Corneal arcus and hyperlipidemia: findings from an older population. Am J Ophthalmol. 2004;137(2):363–5.
7. Vogt A. Textbook and atlas of slit-lamp microscopy of the living eye. (Author's translation). Berlin: Publisher Julius Springer; 1930.
8. Sugar HS, Kobernick S. The white limbus girdle of Vogt. Am J Ophthalmol. 1960;50:101–7.
9. Belliveau MJ, Brownstein S, Agapitos P, Font RL. Ultrastructural features of posterior crocodile shagreen of the cornea. Surv Ophthalmol. 2009;54(5):569–75.
10. Meyer JC, Quantock AJ, Thonar EJ, Kincaid MC, Hageman GS, Assil KK. Characterization of a central corneal cloudiness sharing features of posterior crocodile shagreen and central cloudy dystrophy of François. Cornea. 1996;15(4):347–54.
11. Roszkowska AM, Colosi P, D'Angelo P, Ferreri G. Age-related modifications of the corneal endothelium in adults. Int Ophthalmol. 2004;25(3):163–6.
12. Hillenaar T, van Cleynenbreugel H, Remeijer L. How normal is the transparent cornea? Effects of aging on corneal morphology. Ophthalmology. 2012;119(2):241–8.
13. Bergmanson JP, Sheldon TM, Goosey JD. Fuchs' endothelial dystrophy: a fresh look at an aging disease. Ophthalmic Physiol Opt. 1999;19(3):210–22.
14. Beauchamp GR. Terrien's marginal corneal degeneration. J Pediatr Ophthalmol Strabismus. 1982;19(2):97–9.
15. Pouliquen Y, Dhermy P, Renard G, Goichot-Bonnat L, Foster G, Savoldelli M. Terrien's disease: clinical and ultrastructural studies, five case reports. Eye (Lond). 1989;3:791–802.
16. Hattori T, Kumakura S, Mori H, Goto H. Depiction of cavity formation in Terrien marginal degeneration by anterior segment optical coherence tomography. Cornea. 2013;32(5):615–8.
17. Srinivasan S, Murphy CC, Fisher AC, Freeman LB, Kaye SB. Terrien marginal degeneration presenting with spontaneous corneal perforation. Cornea. 2006;25(8):977–80.
18. Accorinti M, Gilardi M, Giubilei M, De Geronimo D, Iannetti L. Corneal and scleral dellen after an uneventful pterygium surgery and a febrile episode. Case Rep Ophthalmol. 2014;28:111–5.
19. Lin SB, Li ZY, Zhan XK, Cai JH. A case of corneoscleral dellen after medial rectus recession combined with pterygium resection in right eye. Eye Sci. 2012;27(4):198–201.
20. Fenzl CR, Moshirfar M, Gess AJ, Muthappan V, Goldsmith J. Dellen-like keratopathy associated with glaucoma drainage devices. World J Clin Cases. 2014;2(1):1–4.

21. Kymionis GD, Plaka A, Kontadakis GA, Astyrakakis N. Treatment of corneal dellen with a large diameter soft contact lens. Contact Lens Anterior Eye. 2011;34(6):290–2.
22. Das S, Link B, Seitz B. Salzmann's nodular degeneration of the cornea: a review and case series. Cornea. 2005;24:772–7.
23. Riedl JC, Misirkhanova A, Musayeva A, Wasielica-Poslednik J, Pfeiffer N, Gericke A. Risk factors for peripheral hypertrophic subepithelial corneal opacification. Acta Ophthalmol. 2023;101:443–8.
24. Farjo AA, Halperin GI, Syed N, Sutphin JE, Wagoner MD. Salzmann's nodular corneal degeneration clinical characteristics and surgical outcomes. Cornea. 2006;25:11–5.
25. Graue-Hernandez E, Mannis MJ, Eliasieh K, Greasby TA, Beckett LA, Bradley JC, Schwab IR. Salzmann nodular degeneration. Cornea. 2010;29:283–9.
26. Paoletti T, Maamri A, Zemova E, Seitz B. Large Salzmann's nodules or acute keratoconus? Ophthalmologie 2022;119:841–4.
27. Stone DU, Astley RA, Shaker RP, Chodosh J. Histopathology of Salzmann nodular corneal degeneration. Cornea. 2008;27:148–51.
28. Maust HA, Raber IM. Peripheral hypertrophic subepithelial corneal degeneration. Eye Contact Lens. 2003;29:266–9.
29. Jeng BH, Millstein ME. Reduction of hyperopia and astigmatism after superficial keratectomy of peripheral hypertrophic subepithelial corneal degeneration. Eye Contact Lens. 2006;32:153–6.
30. Järventausta PJ, Holopainen JM, Zalentein WN, Paakkanen R, Wennerström A, Seppänen M, Lokki ML, Tervo TMT. Peripheral hypertrophic subepithelial corneal degeneration: characterization, treatment and association with human leucocyte antigen genes. Acta Ophthalmol. 2014;92:71–6.
31. Gore AM, Iovieno A, Connell BJ, Alexander R, Meligonis G, Dart JK. Peripheral hypertrophic subepithelial corneal degeneration: nomenclature, phenotypes, and long-term outcomes. Ophthalmology. 2013;120:892–8.
32. Viestenz A, Bischoff-Jung M, Langenbucher A, Eppig T, Seitz B. Phototherapeutic keratectomy in Salzmann nodular degeneration with "optical cornea plana". Cornea 2016;35:843–6.
33. Roszkowska AM, Colosi P, De Grazia L, Mirabelli E, Romeo G. One year outcome of manual alcohol assisted removal of Salzmann's nodular degeneration. Graefes Arch Clin Exp Ophthalmol. 2009;247:1431–4.
34. Germundsson J, Fagerholm P. Phototherapeutic keratectomy in Salzmann's nodular degeneration. Acta Ophthalmol Scand. 2004;82(2):148–53.
35. Das S, Langenbucher A, Pogorelov P, Link B, Seitz B. Long-term outcome of excimer laser phototherapeutic keratectomy for treatment of Salzmann's nodular degeneration. J Cataract Refract Surg. 2005;31:1386–91.
36. Mahler S, Adams C, Daas L, Langenbucher A, Seitz B. Phototherapeutic keratectomy for Salzmann's nodular degeneration. what effect does the choice of excimer laser have on treatment success? Klin Monbl Augenheilkd 2023;240:1262–8.
37. Severin M, Kirchhof B. Recurrent Salzmann's corneal degeneration. Graefes Arch Clin Exp Ophthalmol. 1990;228:101–4.
38. Yoon KC, Park YG. Recurrent Salzmann's nodular degeneration. Jpn J Ophthalmol. 2003;47:401–4.
39. Jhanji V, Rapuano CJ, Vajpayee RB. Corneal calcific band keratopathy. Curr Opin Ophthalmol. 2011;22(4):283–9.
40. Bernauer W, Thiel MA, Kurrer M, Heiligenhaus A, Rentsch KM, Schmitt A, Heinz C, Yanar A. Corneal calcification following intensified treatment with sodium hyaluronate artificial tears. Br J Ophthalmol. 2006;90:285–8.
41. Najjar DM, Cohen EJ, Rapuano CJ, Laibson PR. EDTA chelation for calcific band keratopathy: Results and long-term follow-up. Am J Ophthalmol. 2004;137:1056–64.
42. Schlötzer-Schrehardt U, Zagórski Z, Holbach LM, Hofmann-Rummelt C, Naumann GOH. Corneal stromal calcification after topical steroid-phosphate therapy. Arch Ophthalmol. 1999;117:1414–8.
43. Messmer EM, Hoops JP, Kampik A. Bilateral recurrent calcareous degeneration of the cornea. Cornea. 2005;24:498–502.
44. Croxatto JO, Dodds CM, Dodds R. Bilateral and massive lipoidal infiltration of the cornea (secondary lipoidal degeneration). Ophthalmology. 1985;92(12):1686–90.
45. Levy J, Benharroch D, Lifshitz T. Bilateral severe progressive idiopathic lipid keratopathy. Int Ophthalmol. 2005;26:181–4.
46. Johnson GJ. Aetiology of spheroidal degeneration of the cornea in Labrador. Br J Ophthalmol. 1981;65(4):270–83.
47. Gray RH, Johnson GJ, Freedman A. Climatic droplet keratopathy. Surv Ophthalmol. 1992;36(4):241–53.
48. Johnson GJ, Overall M. Histology of spheroidal degeneration of the cornea in Labrador. Br J Ophthalmol. 1978;62(1):53–61.
49. Saleh S, Brownstein S, Manusow JS, Jastrzebski A, Lam K, Sassani JW, Mintsioulis G, Gilberg SM. Secondary corneal amyloidosis after perforating corneal trauma: a series of 5 cases and review of the literature. Surv Ophthalmol. 2015;60:590–5.
50. Araki-Sasaki K, Osakabe Y, Fujita K, Miyata K, Hirano K. Collagen fiber changes related to keratoconus with secondary corneal amyloidosis. Int Med Case Rep J. 2018;11:193–9.
51. Stern GA, Knapp A, Hood CI. Corneal amyloidosis associated with keratoconus. Ophthalmology. 1988;95:52–5.
52. Hsu HY, Phillips NJ, Harocopos GJ. Secondary amyloidosis in the hydrops lesion of a patient with pellucid marginal degeneration. Cornea. 2007;26:992–4.
53. Trikha S, Sahu D, Jeffry M, Boase D. Secondary corneal amyloidosis in keratoconus. Cornea. 2011;30:716–7.
54. Suesskind D, Auw-Haedrich C, Schorderet DF, Munier FL, Loeffler KU. Keratoepithelin in secondary corneal amyloidosis. Graefe's Arch Clin Exp Ophthalmol. 2006;244:725–31.
55. Dutt S, Elner VM, Soong HK, Meyer RF, Sugar A. Secondary localized amyloidosis in interstitial keratitis: clinicopathologic findings. Ophthalmology. 1992;99:817–23.
56. Aldave AJ, Principe AH, Lin DY, Yellore VS, Small KW. Lattice dystrophy-like localized amyloidosis of the cornea secondary to trichiasis. Cornea. 2005;24:112–5.
57. Hidayat AA, Risco JM. Amyloidosis of corneal stroma in patients with trachoma: a clinicopathologic study of 62 cases. Ophthalmology. 1989;96:1203–11.
58. Khalifa YM, Bloomer MM, Margolis TP. Secondary localized sectoral keratoconjunctival amyloidosis from ocular trauma. Cornea. 2010;29:1328–9.
59. Tejwani D. Localised corneal amyloidosis associated with herpetic keratitis. Br J Ophthalmol. 2003;87:1049–1049.
60. McDonnell PJ, Green WR, Stevens RE, Bargeron CB, Riquelme JL. Blood staining of the cornea. Ophthalmology. 1985;92:1668–74.
61. Beyer TL, Hirst LW. Corneal blood staining at low pressures. Arch Ophthalmol. 1985;103:654–5.
62. Holbach LM, Hinzpeter EN, Naumann GOH. Kornea und Sklera-B. Degenerationen. In: Naumann GOH, editors. Pathologie des Auges. Berlin Heidelberg: Springer; 1997. p. 521–41
63. Seitz B, Rohrbach JM. The cornea as an indicator of systemic diseases. (Author's translation). In: Pfeiffer N, Cursiefen C, Holz FG, Lagréze WA, editors. Die Augenheilkunde. Springer Reference Medizin. Berlin, Heidelberg: Springer; 2024.
64. Rohrbach JM, Lisch W, Seitz B. The cornea as an indicator for systemic diseases. Ophthalmologe 2018;115:975–86.
65. Rose GE, Lavin MJ. The Hudson-Stahli line. I: An epidemiological study. Eye (Lond). 1987;1:466–70.

66. Rose GE, Lavin MJ. The Hudson-Stahli line. III: Observations on morphology, a critical review of aetiology and a unified theory for the formation of iron lines of the corneal epithelium. Eye (Lond). 1987;1:475–9.
67. Norn M. Hudson-Stahli's iron line in the cornea. Acta Ophthalmol (Copenh). 1990;68:339–40.
68. Hansen A, Norn M. Astigmatism and surface phenomena in pterygium. Acta Ophthalmol (Copenh). 1980;58(2):174–481.
69. Iwamoto T, DeVoe AG. Electron microscopical study of the Fleisher ring. Arch Ophthalmol. 1976;94(9):1579–84.
70. Romero-Jiménez M, Santodomingo-Rubido J, Wolffsohn JS. Keratoconus: a review. Cont Lens Anterior Eye. 2010;33(4):157–66.
71. Seiler T, Holschbach A. Central corneal iron deposit after photorefractive keratectomy. Ger J Ophthalmol. 1993;2:143–5.
72. Yeung L, Chen YF, Lin KK, Huang SC, Hsiao CH. Central corneal iron deposition after myopic laser-assisted in situ keratomileusis. Cornea. 2006;25(3):291–5.

Corneal Trauma

Shady Suffo, Loay Daas, and Berthold Seitz

Abstract

This chapter summarizes the topics of corneal traumas and their treatment with focus on the mechanical corneal injuries. Corneal trauma can be classified into three categories: blunt trauma, partial-thickness laceration and full thickness wound. Depending on the type and the severity of the injury, the treatment of corneal trauma varies from conservative therapy to various types of surgery.

Keywords

Cornea · Injury · Scarring · Corneal suture · Laceration · Perforation

1 Introduction

Corneal injury is very common and was involved in over half of all serious ocular trauma cases in the United States Eye Injury Registry (USEIR) [1]. Chiapella et al. reported in a study that corneal injury accounted for about 10% of all new patient visits to an eye casualty clinic [2].

Scar formation due to a trauma that affects the Bowman layer causes:

- Reduction of the cornea's transparency and the visual acuity
- Photopsia and halos
- Hyperopic astigmatism by altering the cornea's dome shape
- An instable tear film and dry eye by making the normally smooth surface uneven
- A significant and permanent structural weakness [3].

The goal of treating corneal trauma is:

- To reduce the risk of infection
- Achieve rapid wound closure to avoid expulsive bleeding or epithelial invasion
- Restore, as far as possible, the transparency and the shape of the cornea.

2 Blunt Trauma (Contusion)

Direct blunt trauma to the cornea can lead to:

- Focal or diffuse stromal and epithelial edema due to endothelial damage, the so-called corneal endothelial-epithelial-decompensation [4] (Fig. 1A, B). The treatment varies from observation to DMEK [5] or even PKP [6].
- Breaks in Bowman layer/stroma, especially in eyes with previous refractive surgery. In such a case, flap-like wounds require no suture **if not displaced**, just prophylactic antibiotics and mild cycloplegics applied for a few days suffice; **if displaced**; they must be repositioned and sutured. In case of an epithelial ingrowth, the invading epithelium needs to be removed prior to reposition [7, 8] (Fig. 2A–D).

3 Partial-Thickness Laceration

The Seidel test is necessary to rule out a full-thickness wound.

- Non-self-sealing gaped wounds, which are under tension, must be sutured

S. Suffo (✉) · L. Daas · B. Seitz
Department of Ophthalmology, Saarland University Medical Center, Homburg, Germany
e-mail: shady.suffo@uks.eu

B. Seitz et al. (eds.), *Atlas on Cornea*, https://doi.org/10.1007/978-3-031-65422-0_34

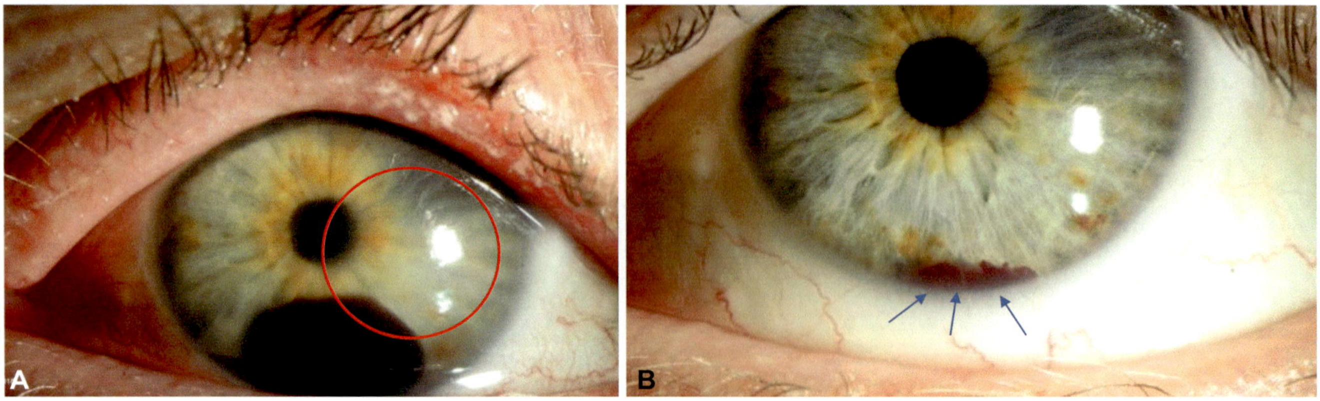

Fig. 1 (**A**) 57-year-old patient with focal corneal edema on the left eye (red circle) and hyphema (partly organised) due to contusion bulbi caused by a soccer ball. (**B**) Spontaneous complete regression of the traumatic corneal edema (Endothelium-epithelium-decompensation) after 5 days. Residual hyphema (arrows) is still present at 6 o'clock

- Small, adapted and clean wounds do not need to be sutured (Fig. 3).

4 Full-Thickness Wound

This type of corneal wound is an emergency case and must be treated as soon as possible to avoid an expulsive choroidal hemorrhage (ECH) [10] and to minimize the risk of endophthalmitis, which increases after 24 h [11].

Like the partial thickness wound, the Seidel test is essential.

- Non-self-sealing wounds should be sutured.
- Self-sealing, clean and not gaped wounds with negative Seidel test do not need to be sutured.

5 How to Suture the Cornea

The most important parameters that must be considered while suturing a corneal wound are the depth and the length of the suture, the distance between the sutures and where to start suturing.

An optimal corneal suture must

- Make the wound watertight
- Minimize postoperative edema
- Minimize scar formation
- Minimize interference with corneal curvature
- Minimize late complications (e.g., anterior synechia formation).

5.1 The Depth of Corneal Sutures

Traditionally, corneal sutures are recommended to be 90% deep: In case of traumatic full-thickness wound, we prefer a full-thickness suture, which effectively blocks the access of the aqueous to the stroma and shortens the time of the cornea clearing, allowing a primary (immediately after wound closure) or secondary early vitreoretinal surgery intervention and minimizes the scar formation (Fig. 4A–D).

5.2 Suture Length

Suture length should be identical on both sides (Fig. 5A, B), unless the wound is oblique [12] (Fig. 6A, B).

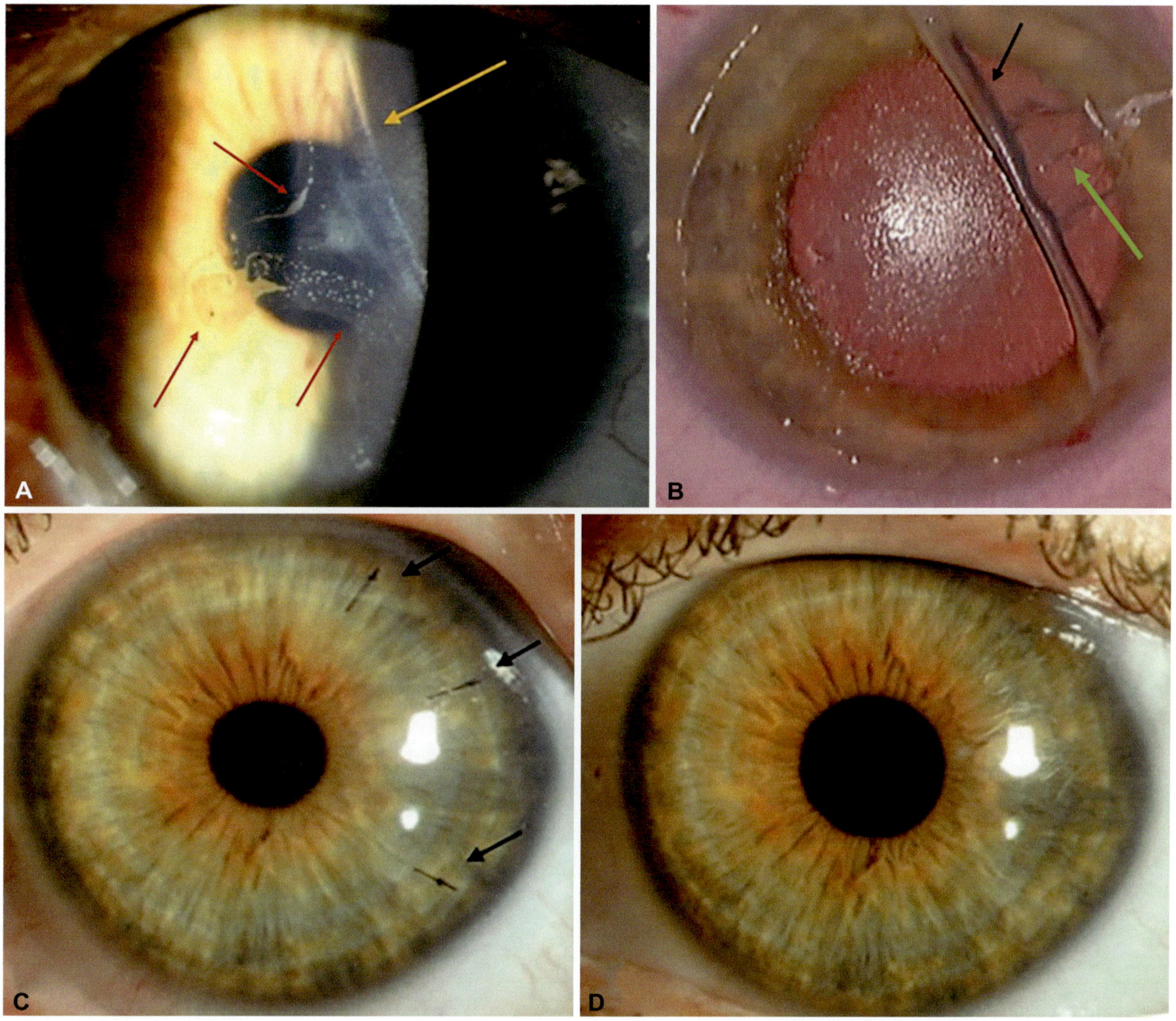

Fig. 2 (**A**) Slit lamp photo shows a dislocated LASIK flap (yellow arrow) with epithelial ingrowth (red arrows) after corneal trauma with a tree branch [9]. (**B**) Intraoperative image while flap elevation (black arrow) and mechanical excision of epithelial cells from the stromal bed (green arrow) and posterior surface of the flap. Through the fundus red reflex the intraoperative mydriasis helps better identifying and removing the epithelial cells. (**C**) At the end, the flap is sutured (black arrows) to avoid a recurrence of epithelial ingrowth. (**D**) Clear cornea with good adapted LASIK-flap after removing the sutures 6 weeks postoperatively

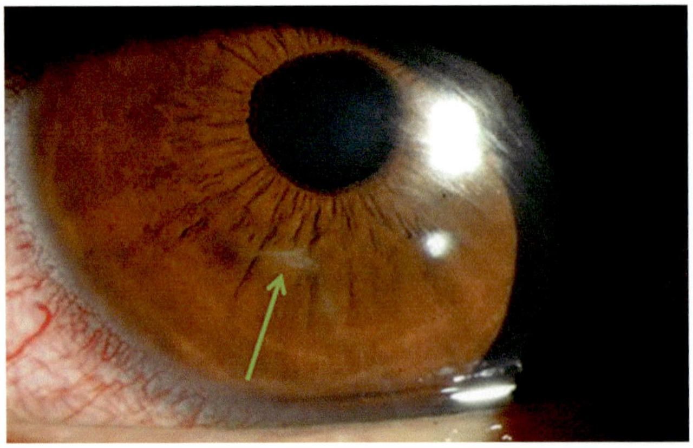

Fig. 3 Small corneal well adapted partial-thickness laceration (green arrow) caused by glass splinter without fistulation. This case requires no surgical intervention

5.3 Order of Sutures Placement

In case of a wound with landmarks such as an angle or limbus involvement, these should be closed first [12] (Fig. 7A, B).

If the wound is long and crosses near to the optical axis, the risk of flattening the corneal dome shape by the scar is high [13]. This effect can be reduced by starting from the two peripheries with long sutures and going progressively shorter as the center is approached [12] (Fig. 8A–C).

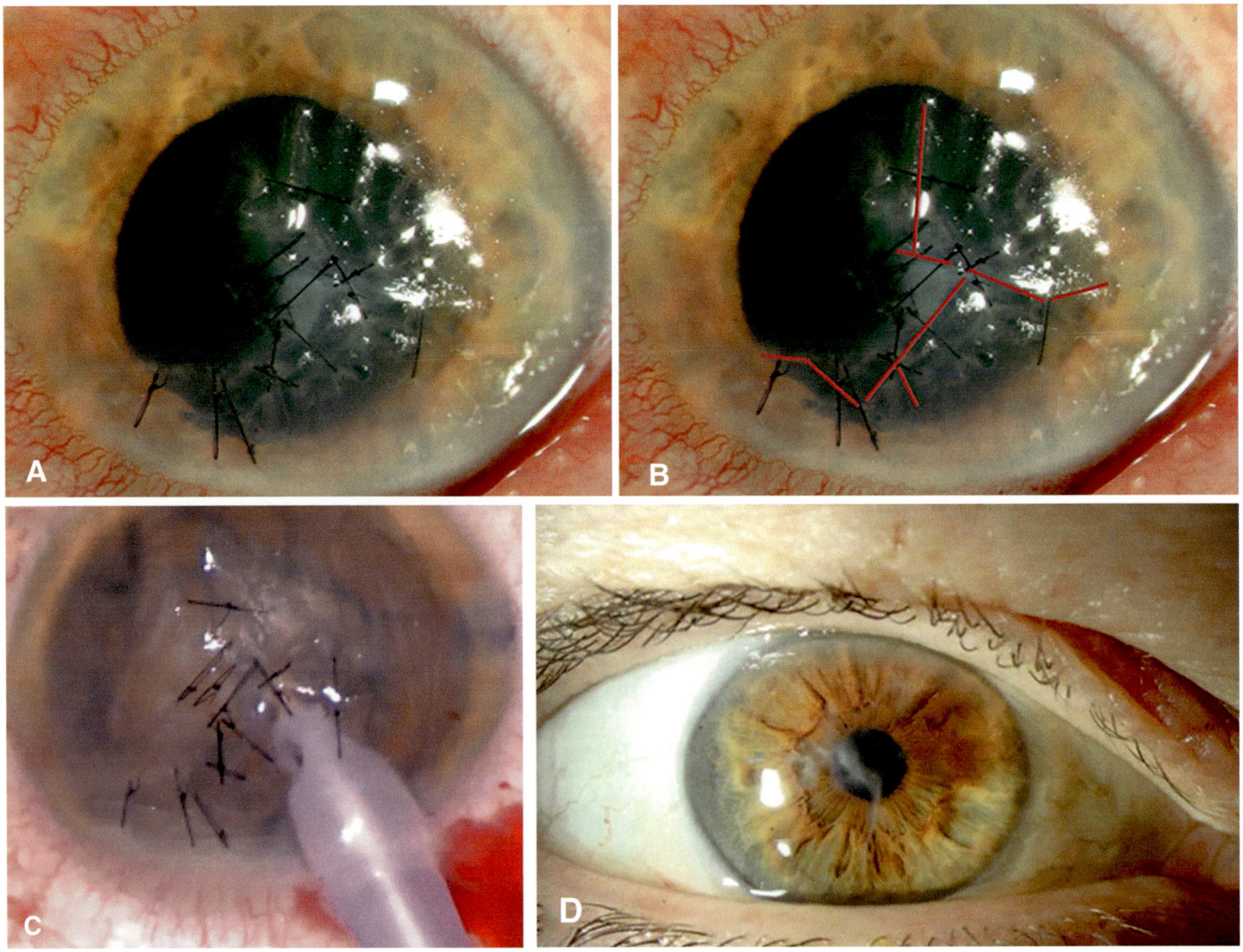

Fig. 4 (**A**) An intraoperative photo after wound closure of a very complicated corneal wound by glass splinters shows a good wound adaptation. (**B**) The red lines show the course of the wound with multiple angles. (**C**) Due to the full thickness sutures, there was a rapid reduction of the edema so that a primary supply of the deeper structures (in this case the traumatic cataract) was possible and (**D**) Finally a minimal scar formation was achieved after 6 months

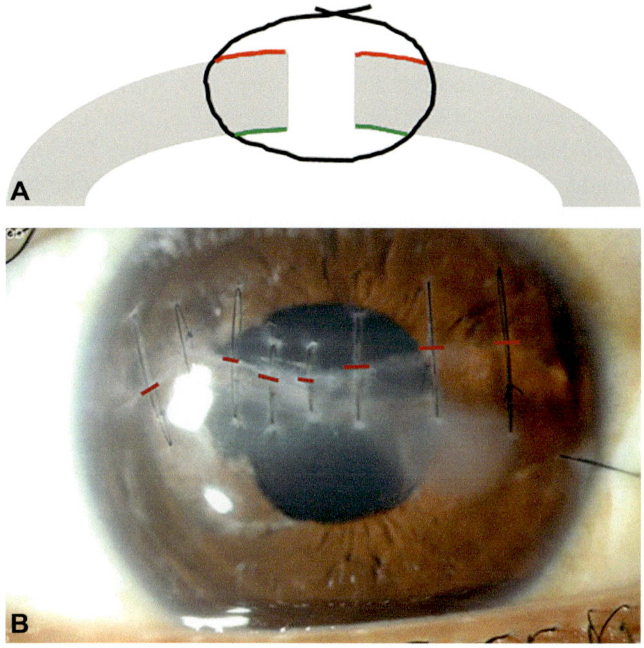

Fig. 5 (**A**) Schematic illustration of a suture readapting a perpendicular corneal wound. If the wound's plane is close to vertical to the surface, the needle's entry and exit points should be at equal distance from the wound on both the epithelial (red lines) and endothelial (green lines) side. (**B**) A perpendicular wound closure achieved with single interrupted sutures. The red dashes demonstrate the epithelial side of the corneal wound. The sutures have a symmetrical length related to the closure line of the corneal wound

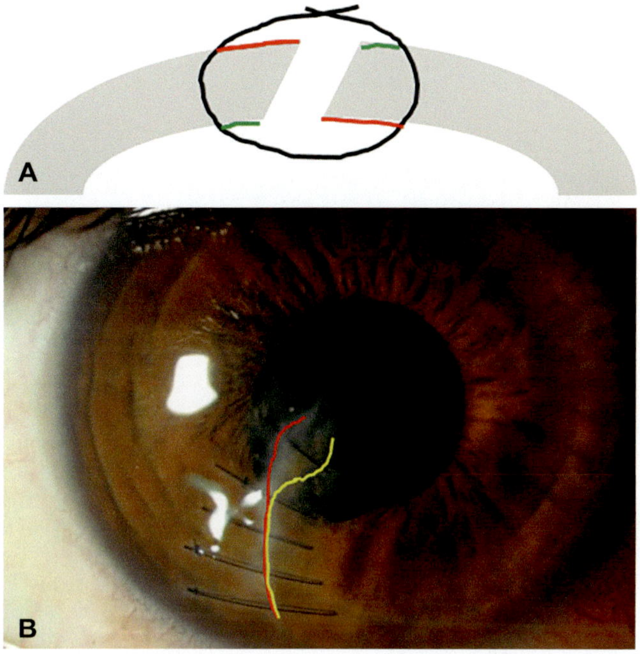

Fig. 6 (**A**) Schematic illustration of a suture for oblique wounds. To create the same compression on either side of an oblique wound, the epithelial length of the suture on one side of the wound must be matched with the endothelial length on the other side (red and green lines). This technique prevents tissue override, which causes a permanent corneal abnormality [12]. (**B**) Corneal wound closure achieved with single interrupted sutures. The wound is oblique in the center and goes in a more perpendicular way to the periphery. The entry and the exit points of the sutures have the same distance to the wound edge in the outer part of the wound but not in the oblique part in the center. The red line demonstrates the epithelial side (entrance) and the yellow line demonstrates the endothelial (penetration) side of the wound. There is no tissue override

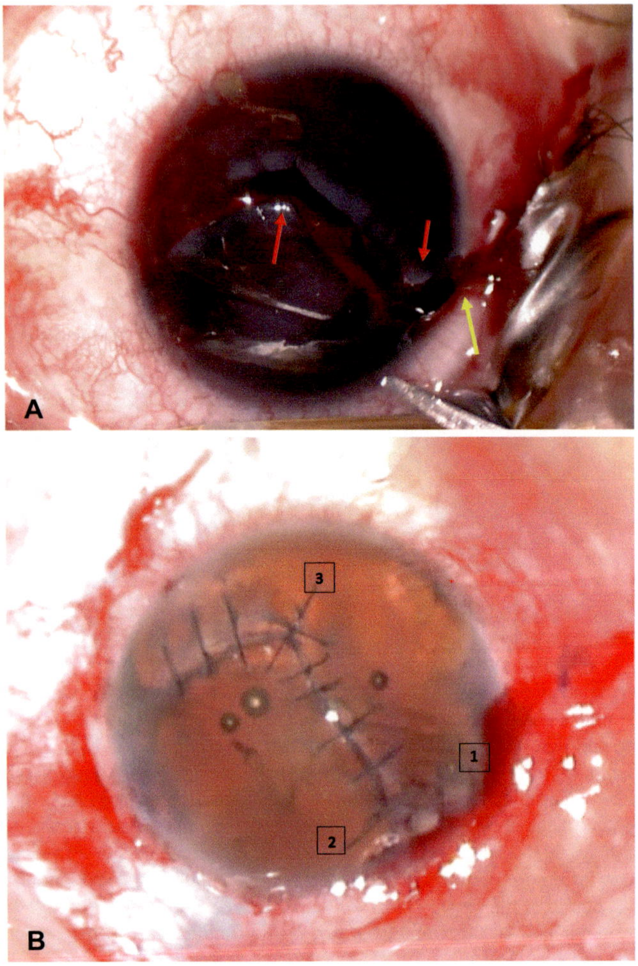

Fig. 7 (**A**) Corneal wound with two angles (red arrows) and limbus involvement (yellow arrow). The limbus must be sutured first, then the two angles. (**B**) The order how the first three sutures are performed. The limbus should be sutured first, then the peripheral angle, followed by the central angle. This intraoperative photo after wound closure shows a good wound adaptation with traumatic aphakia and aniridia. Due to the full thickness bites, there was a rapid reduction of the edema so that a primary supply of the deeper structures was possible

5.4 The Number of the Sutures

To achieve a watertight suture in case of a straight perpendicular wound, the adaptation/compression area of each suture should overlap or at least touch each other. Take into consideration that every suture has an adaptation/compression effect on a part of the wound that equals about half of the suture length itself [12]. We recommend setting every next suture in a distance that equals half of the length of the previous one (Fig. 9).

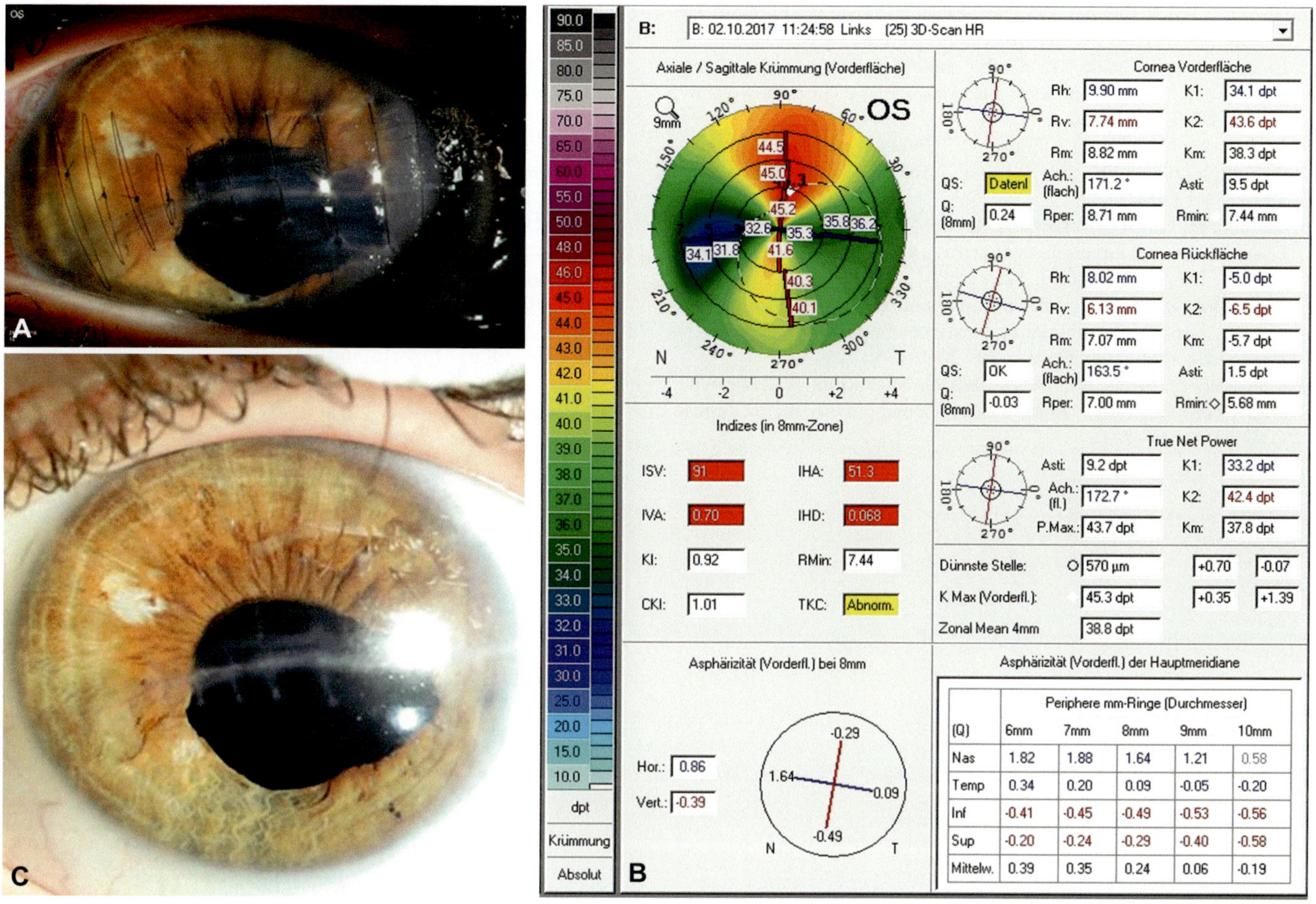

Fig. 8 (**A**) A huge corneal wound from limbus to limbus (without limbal involvement). The wound is adapted with single interrupted sutures that are getting shorter toward the center. (**B**) Postoperative corneal topography of the patient's eye after removing the sutures. In spite of the high astigmatism (9.5 dpt.), it is still regular. (**C**) Postoperative slit lamp photo of the patient's eye after removing the sutures, which shows a minimal scar formation and Dome shape configuration of the cornea

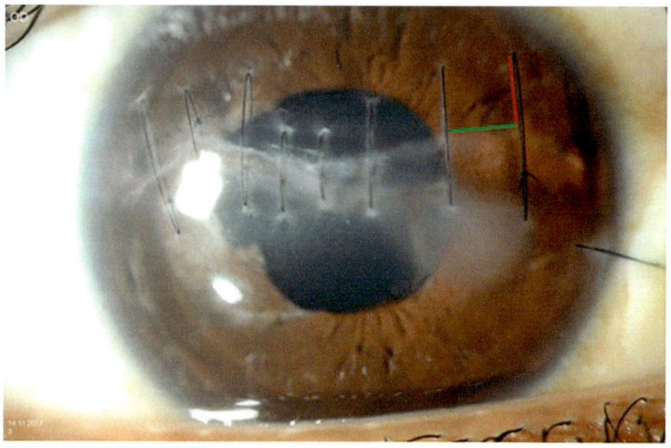

Fig. 9 An irregular corneal wound adapted with single interrupted sutures. The distance between the sutures (green line) is equal to half of the length of the previous one (red line)

6 Conclusion

The cornea is the most commonly injured ocular tissue. Full-thickness wounds must be considered as an emergency case since they represent an increased risk of endophthalmitis and expulsive choroidal hemorrhage. An adequate treatment of the corneal injury is very important to prevent serious visual impairment due to a prominent scar or to delayed vitrectomy because of excessive corneal edema.

References

1. Kuhn F, Mester V, Berta A, et al. Epidemiology of serious ocular trauma. The United States Eye Injury Registry (USEIR) and the Hungarian Eye Injury Registry (HEIR). Ophthalmologe. 1998;95:332–43.

2. Chiapella AP, Rosenthal AR. One year in an eye casualty clinic. Br J Ophthalmol. 1985;69:865–70.
3. Elder, Mark J, Stack RR. Globe rupture following penetrating keratoplasty: how often, why, and what can we do to prevent it? Cornea 2004;23:776–80.
4. Lesher M, Durrie D, Stiles M. Corneal edema, hyphema, and angle recession after air bag inflation. Arch Ophthalmol. 1993;111:1320–2.
5. Melles GR, Ong TS, Ververs B, van der Wees J. Descemet's membrane endothelial keratoplasty (DMEK). Cornea 2006;25:987−90.
6. Seitz B, Daas L, Milioti G, Szentmàry N, Langenbucher A, Suffo S. Excimer laser-assisted penetrating keratoplasty: on 1 July 2019 excimer laser penetrating keratoplasty celebrates its 30th anniversary. Video article. Ophthalmologe. 2019;116:1221–30.
7. Leccisotti A, Fields SV, De Bartolo G, Malandrini A. Traumatic flap complications after femtosecond LASIK. Cornea. 2022;41(5):604–8.
8. Carranza-Casas M, Anaya-Barragán F, Cedillo G, Graue-Hernández EO, Navas A. Management of late traumatic LASIK flap dislocation related to dog scratch 16 years postoperatively. Am J Ophthalmol Case Rep. 2022;25:101–270.
9. Hamon L, Flockerzi E, Ardjomand N, Seitz B, Daas L. A 27-year-old man with "corneal opacity" after branch injury. Ophthalmologe. 2021;118:186–9.
10. Kuhn F, Morris R, Mester V. Choroidal detachment and expulsive choroidal hemorrhage. Ophthalmol Clin N Am. 2001;14:639–50.
11. Barr C. Prognostic factors in corneoscleral lacerations. Arch Ophthalmol. 1983;101:919–24.
12. Kuhn F. Ocular traumatology. Berlin Heidelberg: Springer; 2008.
13. Rowsey J, Hays J. Refractive reconstruction for acute eye injuries. Ophthalmic Surg. 1984;15:569–74.

Chemical Burns

Thomas A. Fuchsluger

Abstract

This chapter provides an in-depth overview into the major aspects of chemical burn management. This comprises common classifications, epidemiology, pathophysiology, diagnosis, examination, therapy on initial contact, rinsing, ectropioning for inspection and cleaning of the fornices and tarsal conjunctiva, drug therapy, surgical treatments, stages of ocular surface recovery after burns and outpatient/inpatient care as well as aftercare.

Keywords

Chemical burns · Dua classification · Reim classification · Alkalis · Acids · Limbal stem cell deficiency · Keratoprostheses

1 Introduction

This chapter on corneal burns will focus on diagnostic evaluation, therapeutic approaches (both conservative and surgical), outpatient treatment and follow-up versus hospital admission and follow-up treatments. These recommendations are consensus and guideline amongst the German Ophthalmological Society (DOG) and the professional Association of German Ophthalmologists (BVA e.V.) [1].

Supplementary Information The online version contains supplementary material available at https://doi.org/10.1007/978-3-031-65422-0_35.

T. A. Fuchsluger (✉)
Department of Ophthalmology, University Medical Center, Rostock, Germany
e-mail: thomas.fuchsluger@med.uni-rostock.de

B. Seitz et al. (eds.), *Atlas on Cornea*, https://doi.org/10.1007/978-3-031-65422-0_35

2 Classifications

Amongst the two most relevant classifications for chemical burns of the cornea and of the ocular surface are the Reim classification (similar to the Roper-Hall classification) [2–6] and the Dua classification [7]. Reim's classification is based on an evaluation of corneal affection and of limbal ischemia (Table 1). Dua's classification is based on an evaluation of limbal impairment (in clock hours) and of percentage of conjunctival affection (Table 2). A randomized control study found superiority of Dua's classification over Roper-Hall's classification with respect to prognosis of severe chemical burns [8]. See Fig. 1 for clinical images of the different grades.

3 Epidemiology

Corneal burns account for 11.5–22.1% of eye injuries [9]. Burns occur most frequently during/as a result of occupational injuries, in domestic environments or as a result of assaults. Alkali-related burns are more frequent than acid-related burns due to the high distribution of alkalis in cleasing supplies and construction materials [10, 11].

4 Pathophysiological Principles

4.1 Alkalis

Alkalis are lipolytic and rapidly penetrate cellular membranes of tissues. They saponify fatty acids of cell membranes and penetrate tissues of lid, conjunctiva, corneal stroma and of limbus and alter these tissues [12].

Table 1 Classification of chemical burns according to Reim

Classification of chemical burns according to Reim				
Initial finding	I	II	III	IV
	Corneal erosion, limbal damage 0, hyperemia	Corneal erosion, limbal damage <1/3, ischemia 1/3, chemosis	Corneal erosion, limbal damage >1/3<1/2, ischemia >1/3<1/2, chemosis	Deep ischemia limbal damage >1/2 dense corneal opacities, conjunctival necrosis, sclera porcelain white, miscolored and atrophic iris, fibrin exsudates
After 1–3 days				
	Regeneration	Recirculation, regeneration	Persisting corneal erosion, pseudopterygium, conjunctivalization, ulceration, neovascularization, scars	Proliferations, conjunctivalization, severe scarring, large ulcerations, tissue melting, cataract, glaucoma

Table 2 Classification of chemical burns according to Dua

Grade	Prognosis	Limbal findings	Conjunctival affection
I	Very good	Zero clock hours limbus damage	0%
II	Good	<3 clock hours limbus damage	<30%
III	Good	3–6 clock hours limbus damage	30–50%
IV	Good to moderate	6–9 clock hours limbus damage	50–75%
V	Moderate to poor	9–12 clock hours limbus damage	75–100%
VI	Very poor	Complete (12 clock hours) limbus damage	Complete (100%)

4.2 Acids

Acids damage tissues through denaturation and by precipitation of proteins. Coagulated proteins serve for the short term as a barrier against further penetration of the acid into the tissue [13]. An exemption is *hydrofluoric acid* as fluoric ions rapidly penetrate the entire thickness of the cornea leading to severe damage of the entire eye [14, 15].

4.3 Mixed Agents

Mixed agents are cleansing products with surface-active substances (tensids) [16].

4.4 Hazard Potential/Prophylaxis

Tissues damaged by chemicals secrete proteolytic enzymes which themselves cause further damage [13, 17, 18]. As virtually all chemical burns occur with concentrated chemicals both protective glasses and decontamination aids are to be held available according to occupational health and safety regulations. Safeguarding equipment protecting against high-pressure leakages have to be placed at the workers' disposal. Scenes of accidents have to be consistently analyzed and protected [13, 17, 18].

Fig. 1 Acute chemical burns with different stages. (**A**, **B**) Acute chemical burn with cement of the right eye of a 38-year-old patient, **grade I** according to Reim. Note conjunctival erosion, conjunctival congestion, and sparing of the limbus and cornea. Examination under blue light after application of fluorescein is essential for good detection of erosions. (**C**, **D**) Acute chemical burn with lime of the left eye of a 41-year-old patient, **grade I** according to Reim. Note corneal erosion and sparing of the limbus. (**E**, **F**) Acute chemical burn with lime cleaner of the right eye of a 39-year-old patient, **grade I** according to Reim. Note corneal erosion, conjunctival congestion and sparing of the limbus. (**G**, **H**) Acute chemical burn with butyl diglycol of the left eye of a 42-year-old patient, **grade II** according to Reim. Note corneal erosion, conjunctival congestion nasally, and limbal involvement (<1/3) ▶

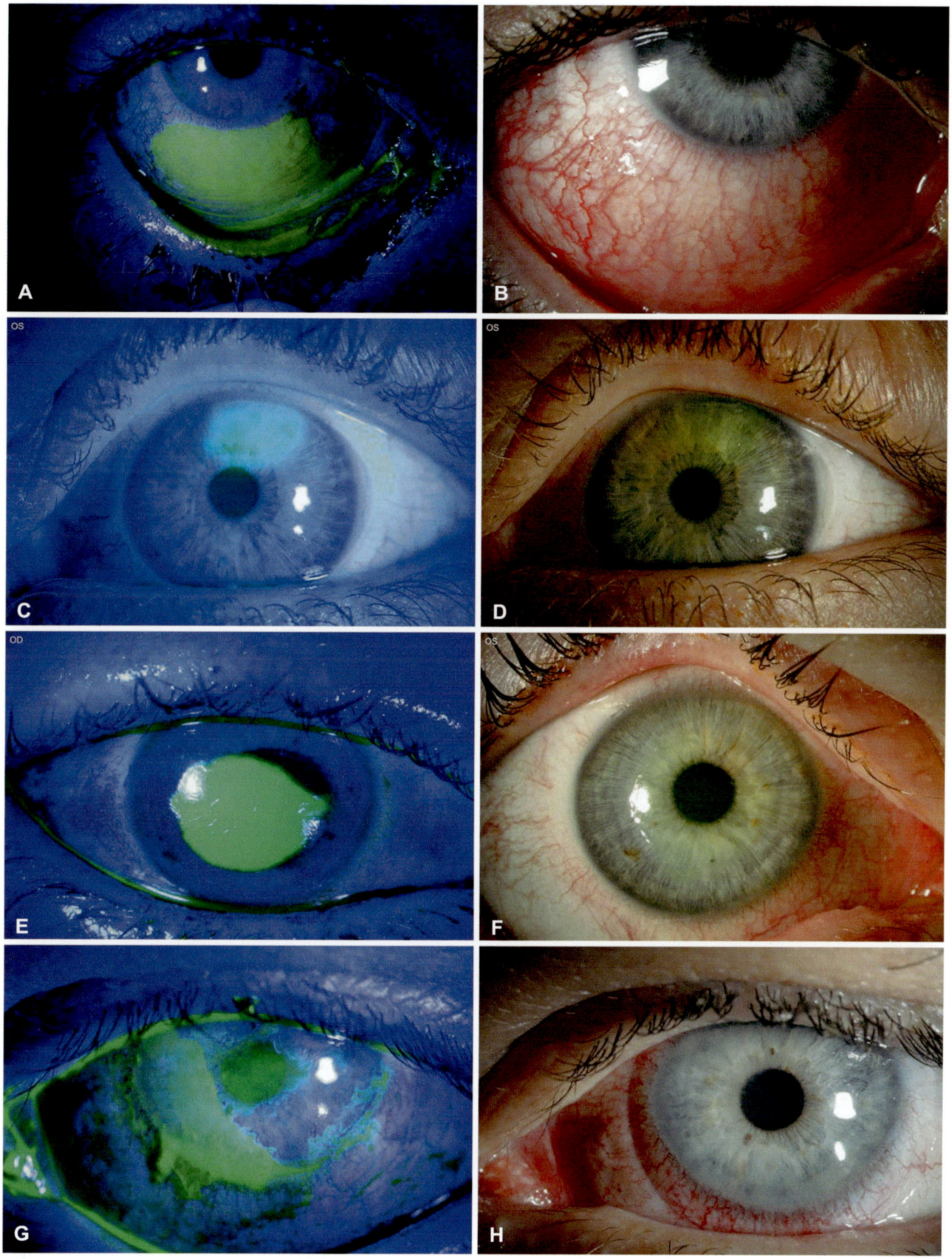
A
B
OS
C
OS
D
OD
E
OS
F
G
H

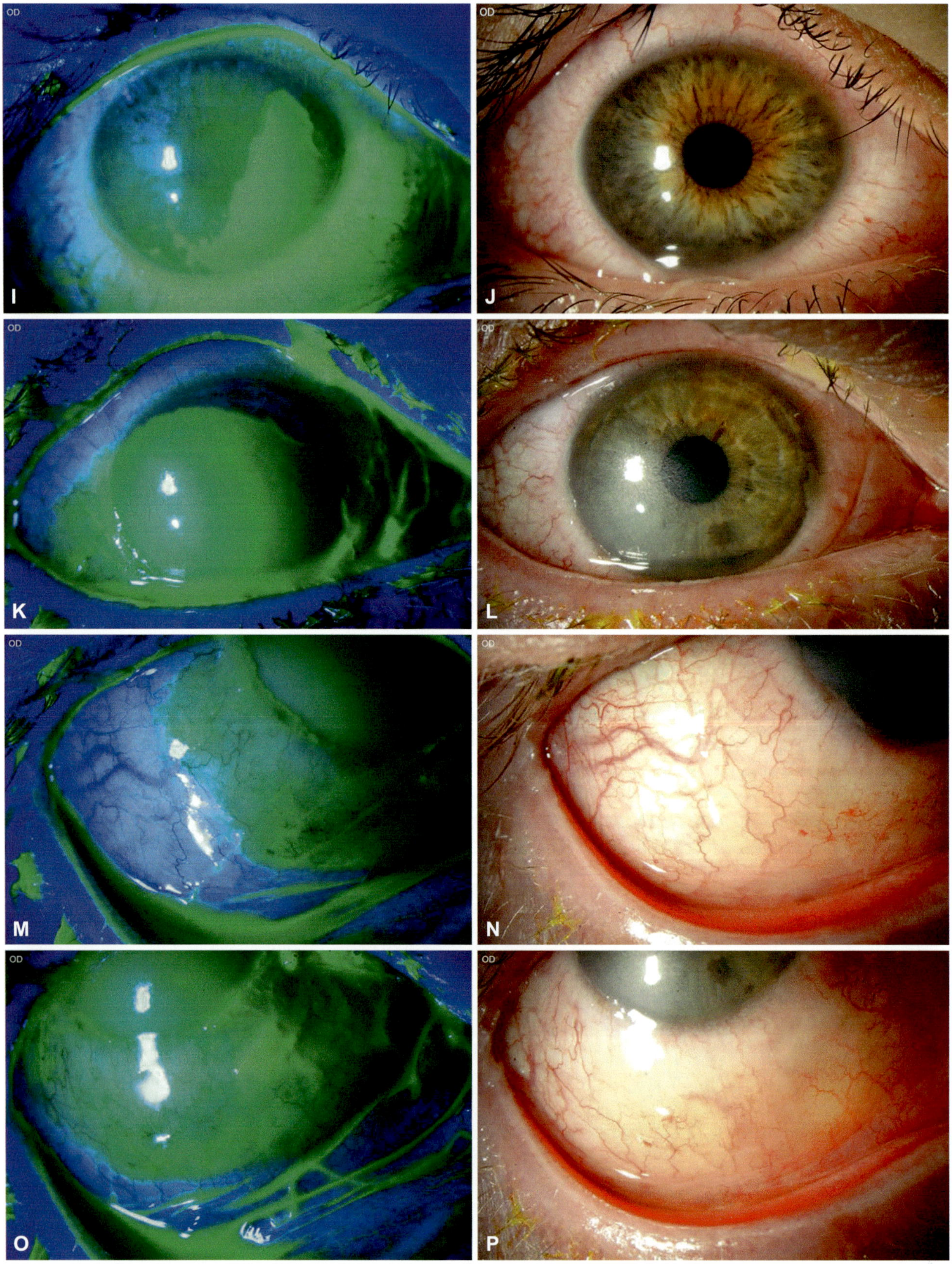

Fig. 1 (**I**, **J**) Acute chemical burn with dishwashing liquid of the right eye of a 27-year-old patient, **grade III** according to Reim. Note corneal erosion, conjunctival erosion, **the absence of** conjunctival congestion in the nasal paralimbal region suggestive of ischemia, and limbal involvement (<1/2 > 1/3). (**K–P**) Acute chemical burn with lime of the right eye of a 62-year-old patient, **grade III** according to Reim. Note corneal erosion, conjunctival erosion, **the absence of** conjunctival congestion in the kaudal nasal and kaudal temporal regions suggestive of ischemia, and limbal involvement (>1/2)

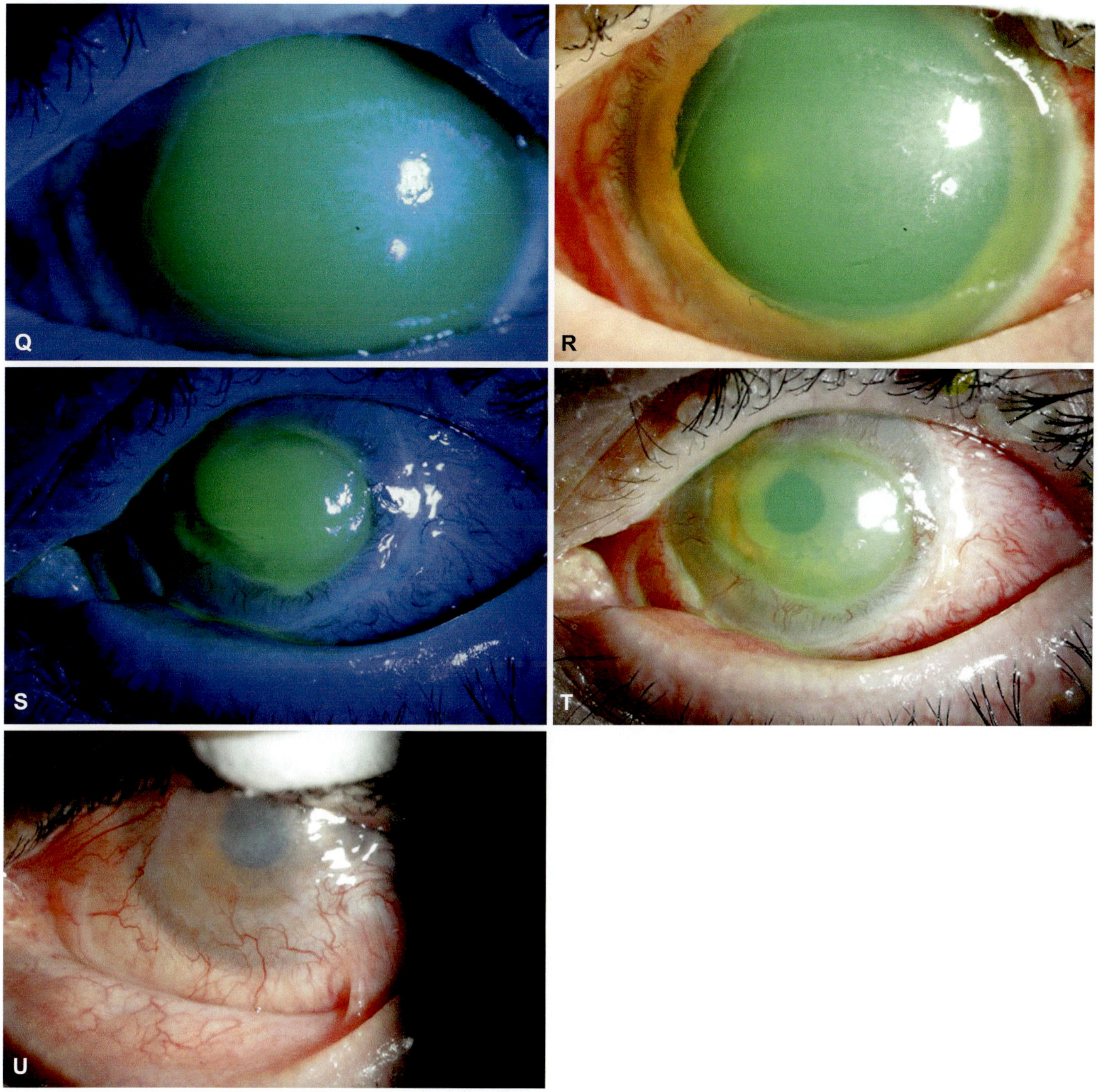

Fig. 1 (**Q**, **R**) A persistent corneal erosion 6 weeks after a chemical burn of the right eye of a 55-year-old patient with cement, **grade IV** according to Reim. (**S**, **T**) The same eye from (**Q**, **R**) 15 weeks after the erosion. Note the development of circular neovascularization in the peripheral region of the cornea and the persistence of erosion. (**U**) The same eye from (**Q**, **R**) 6 months after the erosion. Note the circular vascular pannus, corneal scarring, and development of a symblepharon on the lower lid [Fig. 1 Courtesy of Prof. B. Seitz]

5 Diagnosis

Medical history: Symptoms are unspecific, especially severe ocular burns often show little symptoms and due to severe ischemia little redness [19].

A detailed enquiry of the case history has to include type of chemical (e.g. material safety data sheet), timepoint and location of accident, mechanism of injury (was the chemical under pressure?), eventual flushing and rinsing of the ocular surface (type of washing fluid and duration).

Chemical burn severity depends on five factors:

- contact time of the chemical on the ocular surface
- timepoint of initiation of qualified emergency therapy
- specific toxicity of the chemical (dissociation constant)
- concentration and temperature of the chemical, mechanical pressure of impact
- extension of area in contact with corrosive solution

6 Examination

The initial ophthalmic examination should include:

- Examination of the anterior segments of the eye with a slit lamp including staining with fluorescein: Both the cornea, limbus, palpebral and bulbar conjunctiva including the infoldings should be examined with fluorescein staining using white and cobalt blue light. Inspection should include eyelids and lacrimal puncta. The initial examination should document the extent and depth of the burn (see classification above). In particular, the degree of damage should be documented (with a description of the extent of the damaged marginal loop network), as this is important for therapy and allows statements on the further prognosis [5, 8].
- Visual acuity test if necessary with known correction, if necessary using anesthetic drops.
- Measurement of intraocular pressure in severe burns (even with a corneal epithelial defect, using air or contact tonometry if necessary), as severe burns can lead to intraocular pressure increases in both the acute and chronic stages [20].
- Attempt to evaluate the central fundus of the eye.
- If occlusion of the lacrimal duct is suspected, lacrimal irrigation and intubation of the lacrimal duct if necessary.

During follow-up examinations, the above examinations should be repeated and, if necessary, supplemented depending on the findings and the course of the disease.

7 Immediate Therapeutical Actions on Patient Arrival

When a patient with a chemical burn arrives, the eyes should be **immediately** rinsed and cleansed of any particulate residue. In the case of severe burns, double ectropioning should be performed and the fornices should be inspected, cleaned and rinsed if necessary. The cornea and all burned structures should then be rinsed intensively [19]. In case of burns, do not treat with closed dressing.

8 Rinsing

- The chemical should be flushed out as quickly as possible and, if necessary, removed mechanically, as this is crucial for limiting its exposure time. The goal of irrigation is to remove the agent and restore physiological pH values [19].
- To achieve the highest possible patient comfort and effective performance of the irrigation, topical anesthesia should be administered prior to irrigation. Then, irrigation can also be performed using an eyelid retractor and also using a tube system or an irrigation loop or tray (e.g. Morgan lens) [19].
- In case of very severe pain and for closer inspection and cleaning, para- or retrobulbar anesthesia or short general anesthesia (especially in children) may be considered [19].
- Initial irrigation should be according to the severity of the burn and sufficiently intense, in severe burns until the pH is neutral. This should initially be done with tap water [21].
- Alternatively, rinsing with decontaminating solutions may be used, especially for more severe burns. If neither qualified decontamination solutions nor water are available, rinsing with other liquids, e.g. soft drinks, milk or similar liquids, can also be used for burns [22–24].
- In case of hydrofluoric acid (HF) burns, simultaneous life-threatening skin and inhalation burns should be excluded. Attention should also be paid to possible hazards to the rescuers and, if necessary, measures should be taken for the rescuers' own protection. Eye and skin rinsing should be carried out with the specific hexafluorine solution, or with tap water or calcium gluconate if no special solution is available (however, there is a risk of corneal calcification). Because of the risk of associated systemic hypocalcemia in patients, which is potentially life-threatening, internal medicine co-care and calcium substitution should be provided if necessary [15, 25–27].

Regarding patient comfort, several randomized controlled trials compared the application of different irrigation solutions after chemical burns to the eye. These were small, inadequately powered studies that were evaluated together in two systematic reviews [22, 28]. The authors concluded that immediate rinsing of the eye with tap water was most effective in reducing discomfort. Of the different solutions (NaCl, Ringer's lactactate, NaCl plus bicarbonate, and "Balanced Saline Solution plus (BSS)", none could be classified as clearly superior, with BSS tending to be preferred in a hospital setting. A reduction in the reported complaints was achieved with all rinsing solutions.

9 Ectropioning for Inspection and Cleaning of the Fornices and Tarsal Conjunctiva

In the case of any chemical burn, especially those with solid particles, e.g. with calcareous building materials, the peripheral bulbar conjunctiva, the fornices and the tarsal conjunctiva should be inspected after extensive irrigation, if necessary with the administration of topical local anesthetics, using single or double ectropion. Any foreign bodies present should be removed using cotton swabs, or a field hockey knife if necessary [18] (Video 1).

Please scan to access video content

10 Drug Therapy

The goal of drug therapy is to heal as quickly as possible without or with as little scarring as possible. This includes, among other things, accelerating epithelial closure and collagen synthesis while controlling inflammation [29].

Mild to moderate burns (grades I and II in both classifications) have a good prognosis. Often, drug therapy alone without surgical intervention is sufficient.

For treatment, the following options exist depending on the findings and course, and all eye drops used should preferably be phosphate-free and preservative-free:

- Cortisone-containing eye drops should be used because they reduce an inflammatory response and prevent further corneal tissue loss. Steroids should also be used despite epithelial defects. The dosage of cortisone eye drops should be appropriate to the severity of the burn, initially up to hourly for severe burns (preservative-free eye drops are recommended) [30, 31].
- Topical antibiotic treatment should be applied to an epithelial defect to prevent superinfection [32].
- Wetting eye drops should be used liberally (promoting epithelialization and patient comfort) [32].
- Bandage contact lenses, see DOG-BVA guideline 6a [32].
- Ophthalmic ointments e.g. dexpanthenol can be given to cover the ocular surface with a smoothing ointment film [32].
- Cycloplegics may be used in severe burns to reduce an intraocular irritation and associated pain and to prevent formation of posterior synechiae [33].

The following can be used as further medicinal therapies in case of at least moderate burns

- ascorbic acid (vitamin C) as eye drops and/or tablets [34]
- systemic and/or subconjunctival steroids/NSAIDs [35]
- doxycycline, tetracycline or macrolide antibiotics such as azithromycin orally for corneal burns [32]
- serum eye drops, platelet-rich plasma eye drops, autologous blood therapy to achieve re-epithelialization [36]
- antiglaucomatous therapy for secondary glaucoma (in the acute stage rather systemic therapy)

Ascorbic acid is a cofactor in collagen synthesis and may be decreased as a result of ocular surface burns. Vitamin C can be administered as eye drops (10%, e.g., in hourly doses) or orally (1–2 g, up to 4 times daily in adults). In the rabbit model, severe burns were associated with reduced vitamin C levels in the vitreous. This reduction correlated with corneal stromal ulceration and perforation. Systemic vitamin C administration promoted collagen synthesis and reduced the extent of ulceration [37]. In patients with impaired renal function, care should be taken to adjust vitamin C doses for potential toxicity [38].

Doxycycline or tetracycline or macrolide antibiotics such as azithromycin orally reduce matrix metalloproteinases (MMPs)-initiated degradation processes of collagen type I independently of their antimicrobial properties. Several mechanisms lead to the reduction of MMP-mediated ocular surface inflammation in this regard: restriction of neutrophil collagenase and epithelial gelatinase gene expression, suppression of alpha-1 antitrypsin degradation, and reduction of reactive oxidative substances [39, 40].

11 Surgical Treatments

Surgical treatments may be adjusted depending on the findings and course:

– Debridement of necrotic epithelium, a periotomy/peridectomy may be performed in the first three days after the burn, as necrotic tissue can cause inflammation and prevent re-epithelialization [41].
– Corneoscleral tenonoplasty or sclerocorneal tectal keratoplasty may be performed for severe chemical burn with limbal ischemia [42, 43].
– In rare cases, debridement of necrotic epithelium (periotomy, peridectomy) may be necessary in cases of severe chemosis and ischemia: For this purpose, the chemotic conjunctiva is radially incised under topical anesthesia in the area of the most severe chemosis [44].
– A conformer may be used to prevent symblephara.
– If the chemical burn is at least moderate, a generous amniotic membrane transplantation (AMT) can be performed as a patch, or if necessary as an amnion-encased conformer [45]. This procedure may be repeated.

In the context of severe cauterization, necrosis in the anterior segment of the eye is possible due to the loss of limbal blood supply and, as a result of severe limbal ischemia, the development of a sterile corneal ulcer. After removal of the necrotic tissue, tenonplasty (=relocation of intact conjunctiva and tenon to the limbus) can be performed to restore limbal vascularization and promote re-epithelialization (for medium- and long-term follow-up data, see [42]).

11.1 Amniotic Membrane Transplantation (AMT)

The goal of amniotic membrane transplantation (AMT) is to rapidly restore the conjunctival surface and reduce limbal and stromal inflammation. AMT offers both physical and biological advantages in this regard: Physically, AMT reduces eyelid-related friction on the ocular surface, thereby improving patient sensation. Studies have shown a reduction in pain sensation after AMT in patients with moderate to severe burns [46], as well as a reduction in symblepharon formation. The biological effects of an amniotic membrane include the expression of TGFB1 and epidermal growth factor, both of which are important for wound healing [47–49]. Furthermore, anti-inflammatory properties have been demonstrated [50–52]. In summary, the biological effects of amniotic membrane may reduce inflammatory response, promote epithelial growth, reduce scarring, and reduce neovascularization. A Cochrane Database Review lists a controlled, randomized trial of the use of amniotic membrane in the first seven days after acute burn [9]. Despite of unblinded conditions and unequal baseline parameters in control and treatment groups, patients with moderate burns achieved significantly better visual acuity after AMT than those after sole conservative therapy alone [53–55] (Fig. 2).

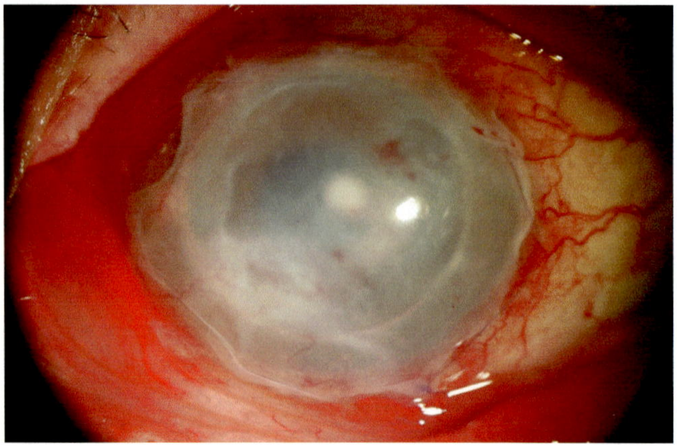

Fig. 2 Amniotic membrane transplantation with continuous 10.0 nylon suture following acute chemical burn after penetrating keratoplasty

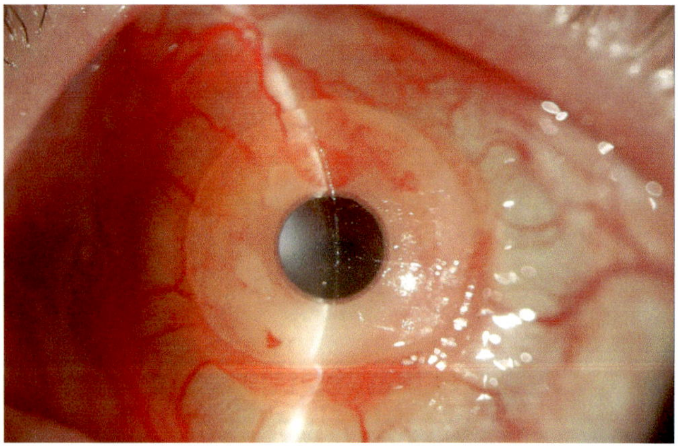

Fig. 3 Boston Type II keratoprosthesis following chemical burn

11.2 Other Microsurgical Options

Limbal stem cell transplantation and/or penetrating keratoplasty (Fig. 2)/keratoprostheses (Fig. 3) may be performed in cases of severe limbal stem cell insufficiency, preferably more than one year after chemical burn at a time when ocular surface inflammation has largely resolved [56, 57].

Limbal ischemia and resulting loss of stem cells capable of epithelial repopulation cause a significant proportion of burn-related injury. Transplantations of limbal stem cells are therefore performed to restore this critical cell population. These stem cells reside in the depth of the limbus, condition epithelial cell proliferation and inhibition of conjunctival overgrowth across the cornea [58]. Limbal

Table 3 .

Stage	Day	Recovery
Initial	0	Clinical findings correspond to the severity of the burn and can be classified according to the extent of limbal damage and corneal and conjunctival involvement
Acute	0–7	Epithelial wound healing begins if sufficient intact limbal stem cells are present. Treatment should aim to promote epithelial growth and suppress the inflammatory response
Early healing stage	7–21	Corneal, conjunctival epithelium and keratocytes proliferate during this phase. Mild burns show complete re-epithelialization while severe burns show persistent epithelial defects. Collagenase activity peaks between days 14 to 21, while collagen synthesis continues. Treatment should maximize collagen synthesis and minimize collagenase activity
Late healing stage	After day 21	In mild burns with intact populations of limbal stem cells, the repair process is complete. In grade II burns with circumscribed stem cell loss, focal conjunctivalization of the cornea may occur. In more severe burns, delayed epithelialization of the cornea occurs. This can lead to either repopulation of the conjunctival epithelium or stromal ulceration and permanent scarring. In severe limbal damage, an eye often cannot be rescued despite optimal therapy management and have to undergo enucleation

autografts can be obtained from the healthy fellow eye provided that only one eye was injured in the burn [59, 60]. Limbal grafts from next of kin were performed in patients with two affected eyes. Postoperatively, the burned eyes showed decreased neovascularization, decreased corneal opacity, and improved epithelialization without the need for systemic immunosuppression [58]. Another option is the use of cadaveric donor eyes. This treatment method requires systemic immunosuppression [57, 61].

12 Stages of Ocular Surface Recovery After Burns

See Table 3 for a summary of ocular surface recovery phases after chemical burns [14, 41].

13 Outpatient/Inpatient Care, Aftercare

- For mild burns, care should be provided on an outpatient basis.
- For moderate burns, the decision whether to treat as an outpatient or an inpatient should be based on the severity of the findings, the required therapy, the patient's ability to implement the required therapy, the pain and the level of subjective suffering.
- In the case of severe burns, inpatient treatment should be considered as first option.
- Ophthalmologic controls should take place in dependence of findings and course for the investigation of possible long-term complications. Long-term complications (trichiasis, entropion etc.) should include glaucoma, dry eye, changes/scarring of the eyelids and ocular surface, scarring of the lacrimal drainage system, and, in the case of esthetically disfiguring findings or severe bilateral visual loss, the psychological consequences for the patient.

13.1 Glaucoma

15–55% of patients with severe ocular surface burns develop glaucoma [20]. The cause is a multifactorial mechanism, which is characterized by contraction of the anterior globe structures after chemical and inflammatory damage, by debris of inflammatory cells in the trabecular meshwork as well as damage to the trabecular meshwork itself [62]. Eyes with higher grade burns (Reim III and IV) show significantly higher intraocular pressure and are more likely to require long-term topical or surgical pressure-lowering therapies than those with grade I–II burns [20]. When prescribing pressure-lowering medications, the goal should be to stabilize intraocular pressure within the normal range.

13.2 Dry Eye

Ocular surface burns can destroy conjunctival goblet cells and in this way lead to reduction or absence of mucus in the tear film. This leads to damaged dispersion of the precorneal tear film. This mucus deficiency results in keratoconjunctivitis sicca (dry eye) [63]. Even in very well-healed ocular surfaces, chronic dryness may be associated with a pronounced disease value due to discomfort, visual impairment, and possible damage to the ocular surface. Here preservative-free lubricants, anti-inflammatory agents and ointments have to be prescribed depending on the severity.

13.3 Damage to the Eyelids or Palpebral Conjunctiva

Direct chemical damage to the conjunctiva may result in scarring, fornix shortening, symblepharon formation, and trichiasis, cicatricial entropion or ectropion. These findings occur week to months after the chemical burn and can be prevented with anti-inflammatory therapies and early amniotic membrane grafts [41, 64, 65].

14 Conclusion

Chemical burns account for 11-22% of all eye injuries. Severity of injury depends on contact time, time point of initiation of qualified emergency therapy ("Rinse immediately!"), specific toxicity as well as concentration and temperature of the chemical and extension of the area in contact with corrosive solution. After cleaning, instant drug therapy includes cortisone-containing eye drops, topical antibiotics, moisturizing eye drops and gels, antiglaucomatous drops, and ascorbic acid topically and orally. Surgical therapy includes early amniotic membrane transplantation after debridement of necrotic tissue or even tenonoplasty. Prognosis reaches from complete resistutio ad integreum to enucleation depending on primary stage and adequacy of treatment.

References

1. AMWF-Register Guideline: 045-018 „Akute Verätzung am Auge", BVA & DOG. https://register.awmf.org/assets/guidelines/045-018l_S1_Akute-Veraetzung-am-Auge_2021-01_1.pdf.
2. Hughes WF Jr. Alkali burns of the eye; review of the literature and summary of present knowledge. Arch Ophthal. 1946;35:423–49. https://doi.org/10.1001/archopht.1946.00890200430010. PMID: 21027052.
3. Roper-Hall MJ. Thermal and chemical burns. Trans Ophthalmol Soc U K. 1962;1965(85):631–53 PMID: 5227208.
4. Reim M. Surgical anatomy, physiology, biochemistry and questions on the inlay technique. Ophthalmologe 1992;89(2):109–18. German. PMID: 1600317.
5. Reim M. Die Brandverletzungen der Augen. In: Bisgwa F, Partecke BD (Hrsg) Verbrennungsmedizin Heute. Hamburg: IN-TRANSFER GmbH; 1999. S 39–46.
6. Reim M, Kuckelkorn R. Verätzungen und Verbrennungen der Augen. Akt Augenheilkd. 1995;20:76–89.
7. Dua HS, King AJ, Joseph A. A new classification of ocular surface burns. Br J Ophthalmol. 2001;85(11):1379–83. https://doi.org/10.1136/bjo.85.11.1379. PMID: 11673310; PMCID: PMC1723789.
8. Gupta N, Kalaivani M, Tandon R. Comparison of prognostic value of Roper Hall and Dua classification systems in acute ocular burns. Br J Ophthalmol. 2011;95(2):194–8. https://doi.org/10.1136/bjo.2009.173724. Epub 2010 Aug 30. PMID: 20805137.
9. Clare G, Suleman H, Bunce C, Dua H. Amniotic membrane transplantation for acute ocular burns. Cochrane Database Syst Rev. 2012 Sep 12;2012(9):CD009379. https://doi.org/10.1002/14651858.CD009379.pub2. Update in: Cochrane Database Syst Rev. 2022 Sep 1;9:CD009379. PMID: 22972141; PMCID: PMC8966384.
10. Haring RS, Sheffield ID, Channa R, Canner JK, Schneider EB. Epidemiologic trends of chemical ocular burns in the United States. JAMA Ophthalmol. 2016;134(10):1119–1124. https://doi.org/10.1001/jamaophthalmol.2016.2645. Erratum in: JAMA Ophthalmol. 2017 Apr 1;135(4):404. PMID: 27490908.
11. Wagoner MD. Chemical injuries of the eye: current concepts in pathophysiology and therapy. Surv Ophthalmol. 1997;41(4):275–313. https://doi.org/10.1016/s0039-6257(96)00007-0. PMID: 9104767.
12. López-García JS, Rivas Jara L, García-Lozano I, Murube J. Histopathologic limbus evolution after alkaline burns. Cornea. 2007;26(9):1043–8. https://doi.org/10.1097/ICO.0b013e31812375fd. PMID: 17893531.
13. Barouch F, Colby KA. Evaluation and initial management of patients with ocular and adnexal trauma. In: Miller JW, Azar DT, Blodi B, editors. Albert and Jakobiec's principles and practice of ophthalmology. 3rd ed. Philadelphia: WB Saunders Elsevier; 2008. p. 5071–92.
14. McCulley JP, Whiting DW, Petitt MG, Lauber SE. Hydrofluoric acid burns of the eye. J Occup Med. 1983;25(6):447–50. https://doi.org/10.1097/00043764-198306000-00008. PMID: 6886845.
15. Spöler F, Frentz M, Först M, Kurz H, Schrage NF. Analysis of hydrofluoric acid penetration and decontamination of the eye by means of time-resolved optical coherence tomography. Burns. 2008;34(4):549–55. https://doi.org/10.1016/j.burns.2007.05.004. Epub 2007 Sep 14. PMID: 17869429.
16. Jähne M. Augenverätzungen durch das Geschirrspülmittel Fit. Dt. Gesundh.-Wesen 29 (1974) 1485–1487. K. Hellmuth unter: https://www.waschbaer.de/magazin/tenside.wirkung-und-umweltaspekte/ (accessed 2023 May 18)
17. Fish R, Davidson RS. Management of ocular thermal and chemical injuries, including amniotic membrane therapy. Curr Opin Ophthalmol. 2010;21(4):317–21. https://doi.org/10.1097/ICU.0b013e32833a8da2. PMID: 20467317.
18. Schrage NF, Struck HG, Gerard M. Recommendations for acute treatment for chemical and thermal burns of eyes and lids. Ophthalmologe. 2011;108(10):916–20. German. https://doi.org/10.1007/s00347-010-2252-2. PMID: 22037724.
19. Sharma N, Kaur M, Agarwal T, Sangwan VS, Vajpayee RB. Treatment of acute ocular chemical burns. Surv Ophthalmol. 2018; 63(2):214–35. https://doi.org/10.1016/j.survophthal.2017.09.005. Epub 2017 Sep 19. PMID: 28935121.
20. Lin MP, Ekşioğlu Ü, Mudumbai RC, Slabaugh MA, Chen PP. Glaucoma in patients with ocular chemical burns. Am J Ophthalmol. 2012;154(3):481–485.e1. https://doi.org/10.1016/j.ajo.2012.03.026. Epub 2012 May 24. PMID: 22633350.
21. Ikeda N, Hayasaka S, Hayasaka Y, Watanabe K. Alkali burns of the eye: effect of immediate copious irrigation with tap water on their severity. Ophthalmologica. 2006;220(4):225–8. https://doi.org/10.1159/000093075. PMID: 16785752.
22. Rihawi S, Frentz M, Schrage NF. Emergency treatment of eye burns: which rinsing solution should we choose? Graefes Arch Clin Exp Ophthalmol. 2006;244(7):845–54. https://doi.org/10.1007/s00417-005-0034-3. Epub 2005 Dec 20. PMID: 16365735.
23. Wiesner N, Dutescu RM, Uthoff D, Kottek A, Reim M, Schrage N. First aid therapy for corrosive chemical eye burns: results of a 30-year longitudinal study with two different decontamination concepts. Graefes Arch Clin Exp Ophthalmol.

2019;257(8):1795–803. https://doi.org/10.1007/s00417-019-04350-x. Epub 2019 May 30. PMID: 31147840.
24. Kompa S, Schareck B, Tympner J, Wüstemeyer H, Schrage NF. Comparison of emergency eye-wash products in burned porcine eyes. Graefes Arch Clin Exp Ophthalmol. 2002;240(4):308–13. https://doi.org/10.1007/s00417-001-0406-2. Epub 2002 Mar 7. PMID: 11981646.
25. Beiran I, Miller B, Bentur Y. The efficacy of calcium gluconate in ocular hydrofluoric acid burns. Hum Exp Toxicol. 1997;16(4):223–8. https://doi.org/10.1177/096032719701600412. PMID: 9154448.
26. Mathieu L, Nehles J, Blomet J, Hall AH. Efficacy of hexafluorine for emergent decontamination of hydrofluoric acid eye and skin splashes. Vet Hum Toxicol. 2001;43(5):263–5 PMID: 11577928.
27. Höjer J, Personne M, Hultén P, Ludwigs U. Topical treatments for hydrofluoric acid burns: a blind controlled experimental study. J Toxicol Clin Toxicol. 2002;40(7):861–6. https://doi.org/10.1081/clt-120016957. PMID: 12507055.
28. Herr RD, White GL Jr, Bernhisel K, Mamalis N, Swanson E. Clinical comparison of ocular irrigation fluids following chemical injury. Am J Emerg Med. 1991;9(3):228–31. https://doi.org/10.1016/0735-6757(91)90082-u. PMID: 1850282.
29. Trief D, Chodosh J, Colby K. Chemical (Alkali and Acid) Injury of the Conjunctiva and Cornea. http://eyewiki.aao.org/Chemical_(Alkali_and_Acid)_Injury_of_the_Conjunctiva_and_Cornea (accessed 2023 May 18).
30. Dohlman CH, Cade F, Pfister R. Chemical burns to the eye: paradigm shifts in treatment. Cornea. 2011;30(6):613–4. https://doi.org/10.1097/ICO.0b013e3182012a4f. PMID: 21242777.
31. Donshik PC, Berman MB, Dohlman CH, Gage J, Rose J. Effect of topical corticosteroids on ulceration in alkali-burned corneas. Arch Ophthalmol. 1978;96(11):2117–20. https://doi.org/10.1001/archopht.1978.03910060497024. PMID: 214063.
32. Pargament JM, Armenia J, Nerad JA. Physical and chemical injuries to eyes and eyelids. Clin Dermatol. 2015;33(2):234–7. https://doi.org/10.1016/j.clindermatol.2014.10.015. Epub 2015 Jan 17. PMID: 25704943.
33. Zoega GM, Kristinsson JK. Chemical injuries of the eye-management of alkali burns. Laeknabladid. 2004;90(6):491–3. Icelandic. PMID: 16819039.
34. Pfister RR, Paterson CA. Ascorbic acid in the treatment of alkali burns of the eye. Ophthalmology. 1980;87(10):1050–7. https://doi.org/10.1016/s0161-6420(80)35126-9. PMID: 7243199.
35. Gross J, Azizkhan RG, Biswas C, Bruns RR, Hsieh DS, Folkman J. Inhibition of tumor growth, vascularization, and collagenolysis in the rabbit cornea by medroxyprogesterone. Proc Natl Acad Sci USA. 1981;78(2):1176–80. https://doi.org/10.1073/pnas.78.2.1176. PMID: 6262756; PMCID: PMC319970.
36. Panda A, Jain M, Vanathi M, Velpandian T, Khokhar S, Dada T. Topical autologous platelet-rich plasma eyedrops for acute corneal chemical injury. Cornea. 2012;31(9):989–93. https://doi.org/10.1097/ICO.0b013e3182114661. PMID: 22759830.
37. Pfister RR, Haddox JL, Yuille-Barr D. The combined effect of citrate/ascorbate treatment in alkali-injured rabbit eyes. Cornea. 1991;10(2):100–4. https://doi.org/10.1097/00003226-199103000-00002. PMID: 2019118.
38. Gabardi S, Munz K, Ulbricht C. A review of dietary supplement-induced renal dysfunction. Clin J Am Soc Nephrol. 2007;2(4):757–65. https://doi.org/10.2215/CJN.00500107. Epub 2007 May 30 PMID: 17699493.
39. Ralph RA. Tetracyclines and the treatment of corneal stromal ulceration: a review. Cornea. 2000;19(3):274–7. https://doi.org/10.1097/00003226-200005000-00003. PMID: 10832682.
40. Smith VA, Cook SD. Doxycycline—a role in ocular surface repair. Br J Ophthalmol. 2004;88(5):619–25. https://doi.org/10.1136/bjo.2003.025551. PMID:15090411; PMCID:PMC1772144.
41. Hemmati H, Colby K. Treating acute chemical injuries of the cornea [Internet]. American Academy of Ophthalmology; 2012. Available: www.aao.org/eyenet/article/treating-acute-chemical-injuries-of-cornea (accessed 2023 May 18).
42. Kuckelkorn R, Kottek A, Schrage N, Redbrake C, Reim M. Long-term results of Tenon-plasty in treatment of severe chemical eye burns. Ophthalmologe. 1995 Aug;92(4):445–51. German. PMID: 7549327.
43. Viestenz A, Seitz B, Struck HG, Viestenz A. Sclerocorneal graft and sequential removal of melted cornea after severe corneal burn with perforation. Clin Anat. 2018;31(1):39–42. https://doi.org/10.1002/ca.22909. Epub 2017 Sep 30. PMID: 28544131.
44. Records RE. Primary care of ocular emergencies. 2. Thermal, chemical, and nontraumatic eye injuries. Postgrad Med. 1979;65(5):157–60, 163. https://doi.org/10.1080/00325481.1979.11715146. PMID: 432147.
45. Eslani M, Baradaran-Rafii A, Cheung AY, Kurji KH, Hasani H, Djalilian AR, Holland EJ. Amniotic membrane transplantation in acute severe ocular chemical injury: a randomized clinical trial. Am J Ophthalmol. 2019;199:209–15. https://doi.org/10.1016/j.ajo.2018.11.001. Epub 2018 Nov 10. PMID: 30419194.
46. Baum J. Thygeson lecture. Amniotic membrane transplantation: why is it effective? Cornea. 2002;21(4):339–41. https://doi.org/10.1097/00003226-200205000-00001. PMID: 11973378.
47. Tseng SC, Di Pascuale MA, Liu DT, Gao YY, Baradaran-Rafii A. Intraoperative mitomycin C and amniotic membrane transplantation for fornix reconstruction in severe cicatricial ocular surface diseases. Ophthalmology. 2005;112(5):896–903. https://doi.org/10.1016/j.ophtha.2004.11.041. PMID: 15878073.
48. Hopkinson A, McIntosh RS, Tighe PJ, James DK, Dua HS. Amniotic membrane for ocular surface reconstruction: donor variations and the effect of handling on TGF-beta content. Invest Ophthalmol Vis Sci. 2006;47(10):4316–22. https://doi.org/10.1167/iovs.05-1415. PMID: 17003421.
49. Gicquel JJ, Dua HS, Brodie A, Mohammed I, Suleman H, Lazutina E, James DK, Hopkinson A. Epidermal growth factor variations in amniotic membrane used for ex vivo tissue constructs. Tissue Eng Part A. 2009;15(8):1919–27. https://doi.org/10.1089/ten.tea.2008.0432. PMID: 19196134.
50. Ueta M, Kweon MN, Sano Y, Sotozono C, Yamada J, Koizumi N, Kiyono H, Kinoshita S. Immunosuppressive properties of human amniotic membrane for mixed lymphocyte reaction. Clin Exp Immunol. 2002;129(3):464–70.https://doi.org/10.1046/j.1365-2249.2002.01945.x. PMID: 12197887; PMCID: PMC1906465.
51. Hao Y, Ma DH, Hwang DG, Kim WS, Zhang F. Identification of antiangiogenic and antiinflammatory proteins in human amniotic membrane. Cornea. 2000;19(3):348–52. https://doi.org/10.1097/00003226-200005000-00018. PMID: 10832697.
52. Li W, He H, Kawakita T, Espana EM, Tseng SC. Amniotic membrane induces apoptosis of interferon-gamma activated macrophages in vitro. Exp Eye Res. 2006;82(2):282–92. https://doi.org/10.1016/j.exer.2005.06.022. Epub 2005 Aug 16. PMID: 16109408; PMCID: PMC3193177.
53. Tandon R, Gupta N, Kalaivani M, Sharma N, Titiyal JS, Vajpayee RB. Amniotic membrane transplantation as an adjunct to medical therapy in acute ocular burns. Br J Ophthalmol. 2011;95(2):199–204. https://doi.org/10.1136/bjo.2009.173716. Epub 2010 Jul 31. PMID: 20675729.
54. Westekemper H, Figueiredo FC, Siah WF, Wagner N, Steuhl KP, Meller D. Clinical outcomes of amniotic membrane transplantation in the management of acute ocular chemical injury. Br J Ophthalmol. 2017;101(2):103–7. https://doi.org/10.1136/bjophthalmol-2015-308037. Epub 2016 May 5. PMID: 27150827.
55. de Farias CC, Allemann N, Gomes JÁ. Randomized trial comparing amniotic membrane transplantation with lamellar corneal graft for the treatment of corneal thinning. Cornea. 2016;35(4):438–44.

https://doi.org/10.1097/ICO.0000000000000754. PMID: 26807898.
56. Samson CM, Nduaguba C, Baltatzis S, Foster CS. Limbal stem cell transplantation in chronic inflammatory eye disease. Ophthalmology. 2002;109(5):862–8. https://doi.org/10.1016/s0161-6420(02)00994-6. PMID: 11986089.
57. Liang L, Sheha H, Tseng SC. Long-term outcomes of keratolimbal allograft for total limbal stem cell deficiency using combined immunosuppressive agents and correction of ocular surface deficits. Arch Ophthalmol. 2009;127(11):1428–34. https://doi.org/10.1001/archophthalmol.2009.263. PMID: 19901207.
58. Huang T, Wang Y, Zhang H, Gao N, Hu A. Limbal allografting from living-related donors to treat partial limbal deficiency secondary to ocular chemical burns. Arch Ophthalmol. 2011;129(10):1267–73. https://doi.org/10.1001/archophthalmol.2011.251. PMID: 21987668.
59. Morgan S, Murray A. Limbal autotransplantation in the acute and chronic phases of severe chemical injuries. Eye (Lond). 1996;10(Pt 3):349–54. https://doi.org/10.1038/eye.1996.72. PMID: 8796161.
60. Barreiro TP, Santos MS, Vieira AC, de Nadai BJ, Hazarbassanov RM, Gomes JÁ. Comparative study of conjunctival limbal transplantation not associated with the use of amniotic membrane transplantation for treatment of total limbal deficiency secondary to chemical injury. Cornea. 2014;33(7):716–20. https://doi.org/10.1097/ICO.0000000000000139. PMID: 24831198.
61. Tsai RJ, Tseng SC. Human allograft limbal transplantation for corneal surface reconstruction. Cornea. 1994;13(5):389–400. https://doi.org/10.1097/00003226-199409000-00003. PMID: 7995060.
62. Paterson CA, Pfister RR. Intraocular pressure changes after alkali burns. Arch Ophthalmol. 1974;91(3):211–8. https://doi.org/10.1001/archopht.1974.03900060219014. PMID: 4814971.
63. Le Q, Chen Y, Wang X, Li Y, Hong J, Xu J. Vision-related quality of life in patients with ocular chemical burns. Invest Ophthalmol Vis Sci. 2011;52(12):8951–6. https://doi.org/10.1167/iovs.11-8355. PMID: 22003122.
64. Kheirkhah A, Ghaffari R, Kaghazkanani R, Hashemi H, Behrouz MJ, Raju VK. A combined approach of amniotic membrane and oral mucosa transplantation for fornix reconstruction in severe symblepharon. Cornea. 2013;32(2):155–60. https://doi.org/10.1097/ICO.0b013e318247983d. PMID: 22735310.
65. Tuft SJ, Shortt AJ. Surgical rehabilitation following severe ocular burns. Eye (Lond). 2009;23(10):1966–71. https://doi.org/10.1038/eye.2008.414. Epub 2009 Jan 23. PMID: 19169226.

Tumours of the Cornea and Conjunctiva

Tim Berger, Ursula Löw, and Berthold Seitz

Abstract

Ocular surface tumours cover a broad spectrum of benign and potentially life-threatening malignant lesions. The cornea is an exceptional tissue in which primary tumours are very unlikely to develop. In most cases, corneal involvement is often secondary to conjunctival neoplasms. This chapter presents the most important tumours with potential corneal involvement, but does not provide a complete summary of all ocular surface tumours.

Keywords

Ocular surface tumours · Corneal tumours · Conjunctival tumours · Solid dermoid

1 Melanocytic Tumours

1.1 Conjunctival Nevus

Conjunctival nevus is the most common benign conjunctival tumour in children and adults and is usually found in the 1st or 2nd decade of life [1, 2].

Nevi are clinically characterized by mixed pigmentation and microcysts. Pigmentation may increase over time, but growth is uncommon. Amelanotic nevi are rare [2]. The predominant location is near the corneal limbus in the interpalpebral area. According to Shields et al. [1] conjunctival nevi typically end abruptly at the corneal limbus and do not involve the corneal epithelium or stroma. Overhang of the cornea by a large conjunctival nevus might occur, but invasion of the cornea is extremely unusual (Fig. 1). Pigmentation of the cornea should therefore primarily indicate a malignant melanocytic lesion. Conjunctival nevi carry a low risk of progression to malignant melanoma (precursor lesion in 7%) [3]. Assessment of vascularization, growth, ulceration, hemorrhage, and change in pigmentation may be helpful. Atypical locations (e.g. palpebral conjunctiva) must also be suspicious for malignant melanoma. Surgical treatment (excisional biopsy) is recommended in cases of unclear dignity [1, 2].

1.2 Primary Acquired Melanosis

Primary acquired melanosis (PAM) typically occurs in middle age and shows a patchy or diffuse pigmented growth pattern with flat appearance and without microcysts [2]. Nonpigmented lesions might also develop. It is important to note that PAM describes a clinical picture and provides no information about the dignity of the lesion. Histopathological examination of these lesions usually demonstrates melanocytes close to the basal cell layers of the conjunctival epithelium and can be divided into PAM with (mild, moderate or severe) and without atypia of the conjunctival epithelium. However, PAM without atypia has a very low risk of developing into a malignant melanoma. Because of the high risk of invasive melanoma, PAM with atypia (precursor lesion in 74%) [3] is also referred to as conjunctival melanocytic intraepithelial neoplasia (C-MIN) with atypia, with the more severe changes being considered melanoma in situ [4]. Corneal involvement usually develops when atypical melanocytes reach the corneal limbus (Fig. 2).

T. Berger (✉) · U. Löw · B. Seitz
Department of Ophthalmology, Saarland University Medical Center, Homburg/Saar, Germany
e-mail: tim.berger@uks.eu

B. Seitz et al. (eds.), *Atlas on Cornea*, https://doi.org/10.1007/978-3-031-65422-0_36

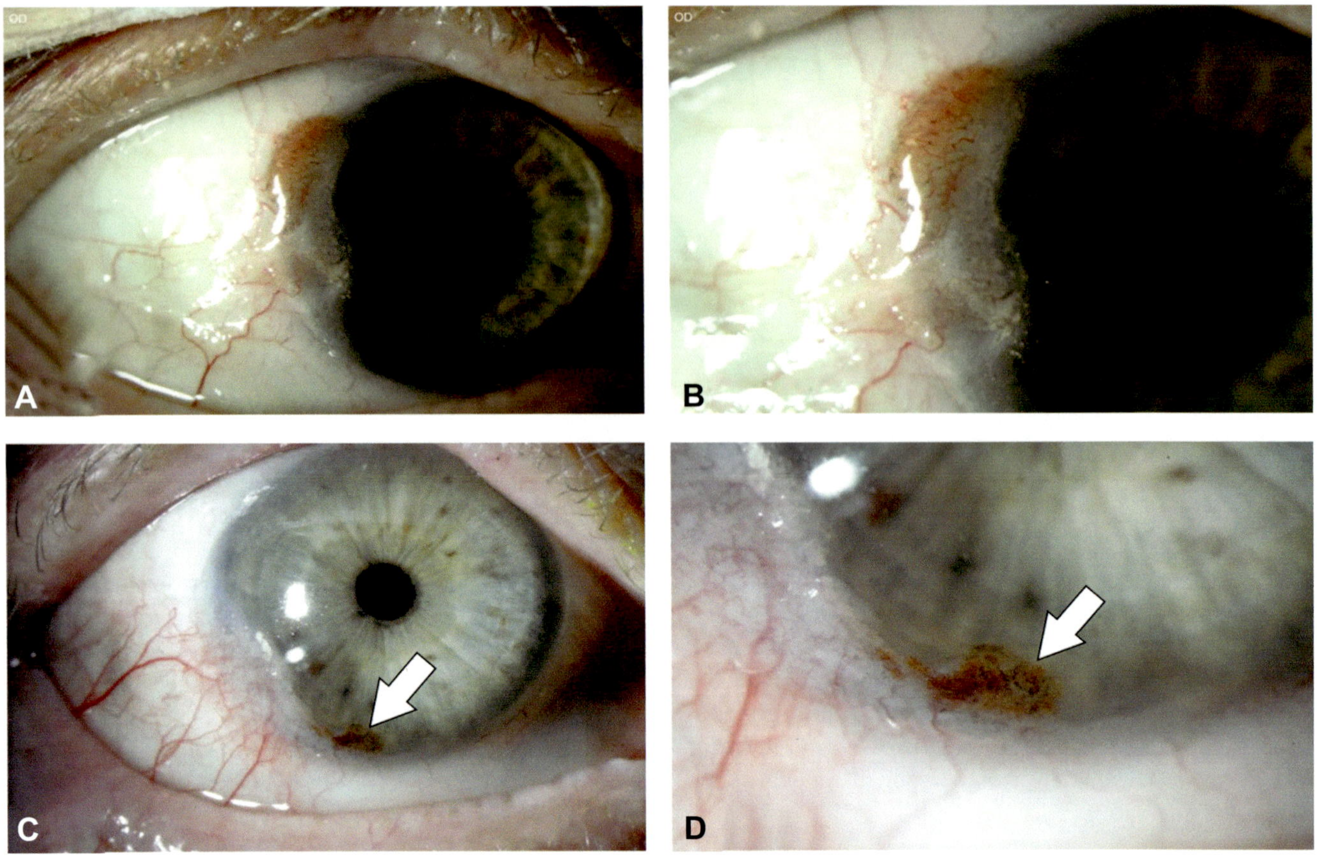

Fig. 1 Compound nevus with corneal involvement and progression to malignant melanoma. (**A**, **B**) Very poorly pigmented compound nevus overlapping the corneal limbus (**A** overview, **B** higher magnification). (**C**, **D**) Recurrence of a pigmented corneal lesion (arrow, histology: malignant melanoma) at seven o'clock with a fibrovascular corneal pannus from seven to nine o'clock six years after excisional biopsy (**C** overview, **D** higher magnification)

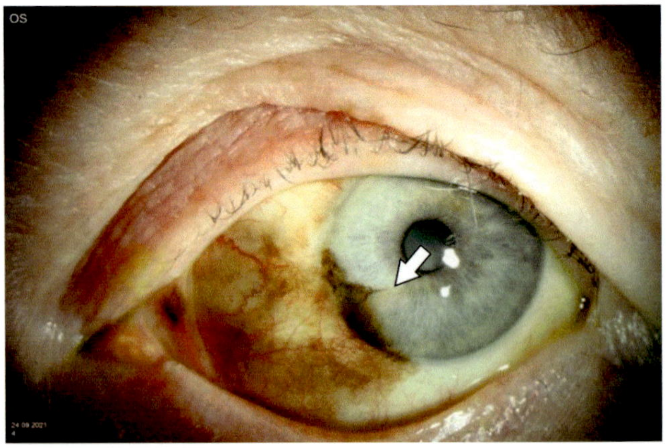

Fig. 2 Primary acquired melanosis of the conjunctiva (histology: melanoma in situ) with secondary involvement of the cornea (arrow)

1.3 Malignant Melanoma of the Conjunctiva

Malignant melanoma of the conjunctiva is a very rare malignancy and occurs mainly in patients over 60 years of age, mostly fair-skinned people. UV radiation seems to be one of the most important risk factors [2, 5, 6].

The clinical presentation is variable and usually appears as an irregularly pigmented, usually prominent, vascularized lesion. Locations range from the corneal limbus, the bulbar conjunctiva, the fornix conjunctiva and the palpebral conjunctiva. The precursor lesion is usually PAM with atypia (in 74%) whereas malignant transformation from conjunctival nevi is observed very rarely in only 7%. De novo development was reported in 19% [3]. Simultaneous inflammatory reaction or increase in thickness of pre-existing lesions such as PAM or conjunctival nevi could be indicative of a malignant transformation [2]. Histopathologically, conjunctival melanoma is characterized by variably pigmented malignant melanocytes. Simultaneous findings such as PAM or a conjunctival nevus might be diagnostically helpful [7]. In rare cases, conjunctival melanoma can spread from the limbal conjunctiva to the cornea (Fig. 3) or the tumour may occasionally predominate on the cornea despite its origin from the conjunctiva (Fig. 4).

In cases of clinical suspicion, treatment of choice is complete excision in no-touch technique as tumour cells are poorly cohesive, posing the risk of intraoperative dissemination (no incisional biopsies!) [8–13]. Simultaneous sclerectomy might be necessary. Intraoperative application of cryocoagulation, topical Mitomycin C (MMC) or alcohol should be considered for the excision margins, especially since the precise extent of the tumor may be difficult to determine. En bloc lamellar keratectomy with excision of the adjacent limbal and conjunctival neoplasm has been advocated in cases of deeper corneal involvement [8, 9]. Large defects of the conjunctiva should be reconstructed, either with autologous conjunctiva of the contralateral eye or amniotic membrane. Since a common cause of tumor recurrence at the limbus is PAM with atypia, the affected cornea is treated with applications of absolute alcohol to the bare Bowman layer (but without disruption!) to devitalize remaining atypical melanocytes [11]. Adjuvant topical chemotherapy, e.g. with MMC (0.02% or 0.04%) or Interferon alpha 2b (IFN-α2b), has been recommended, however the clinical benefit is limited [14–16]. Extensive lesions might require orbital exenteration [7, 11, 17]. Other treatment options include brachytherapy or proton radiotherapy [12].

However, recurrence rate of malignant conjunctival melanoma is quite high with up to 65% at 10 years [18].

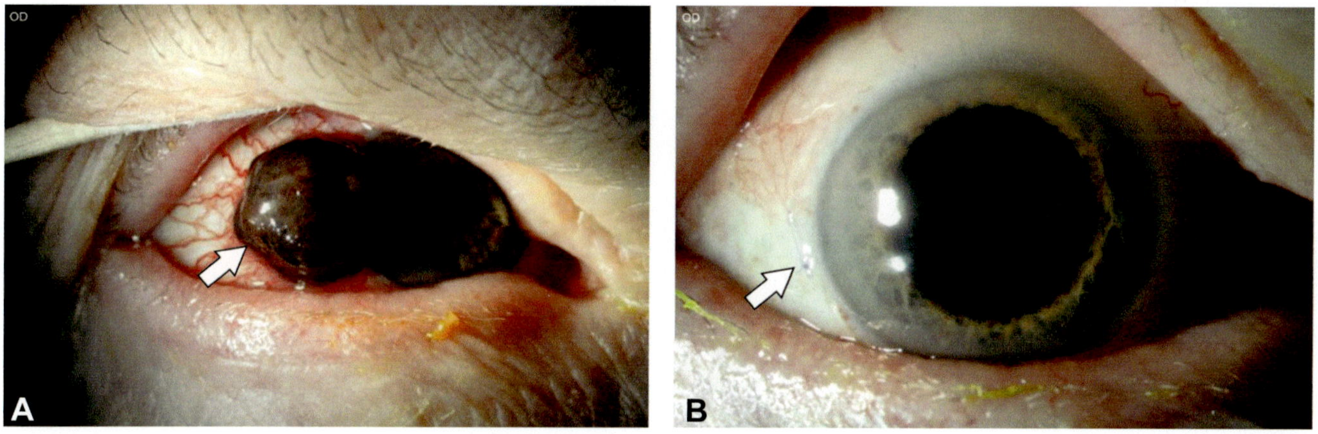

Fig. 3 Prominent malignant melanoma of the conjunctiva. (**A**) Prominent tumour (arrow) with feeder vessels located at the corneal limbus. (**B**) Amniotic membrane (arrow) was used to cover the defect after tumour excision

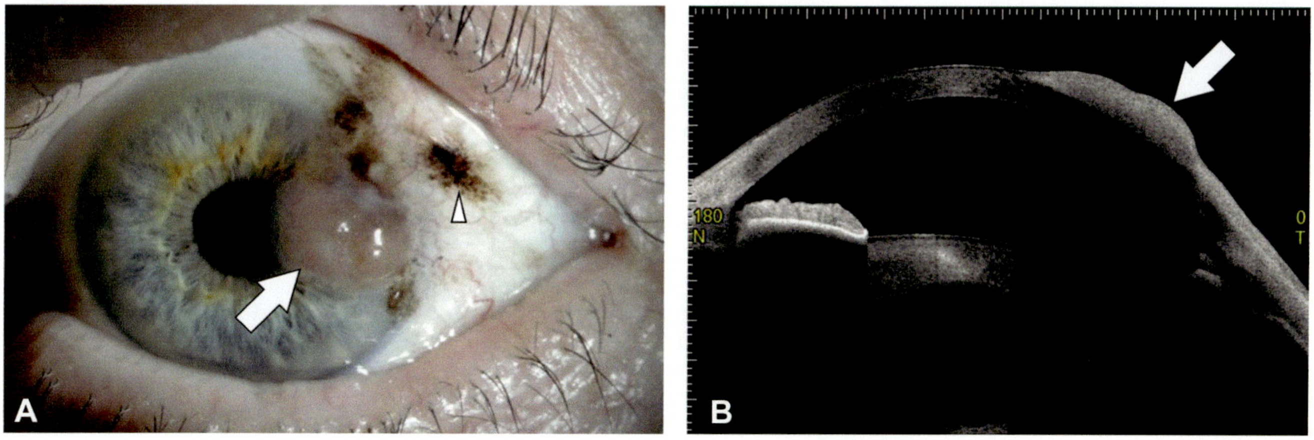

Fig. 4 Malignant melanoma of the conjunctiva with corneal infiltration. (**A**) Poorly pigmented malignant melanoma (arrow) predominant on the cornea, although it originates from the conjunctiva. PAM (arrowhead) is also present, which is presumably the precursor lesion. (**B**) Anterior segment optical coherence tomography demonstrating a large hyperreflective tumour on the cornea (arrow)

Metastasis initially occurs in preauricular and cervical lymph nodes. Haematogenous metastasis develops later, mainly in the lungs, liver, skin and central nervous system, leading to a high mortality of 13% after 10 years [18]. Postoperative staging examinations must be performed at close intervals.

2 Benign Epithelial Tumors

2.1 Conjunctival Papilloma

Conjunctival papilloma is derived from squamous epithelium and has a close association with human papillomavirus (HPV) of the low risk types 6 and 11. It typically occurs in childhood and young adulthood [19].

Clinical suspicion is initially raised by their typical appearance with a flesh-coloured surface and fine vascular channels arranged in a sessile or pedunculated configuration, but the final diagnosis is made by histopathology. Papillomas are localized in the lower fornix (mainly in children) or near the corneal limbus (mainly in adults) and may be solitary or multifocal [20]. Corneal involvement is generally rare in children, but more common in adults (Figs. 5 and 6). Benign conjunctival papillomas may occasionally contain areas of dysplasia (Fig. 7). In severe cases, the cornea may be extensively covered simulating a squamous cell carcinoma. However, the risk of transformation into squamous cell carcinoma is low. Spontaneous regression in children is possible. Therapeutically, surgical excision (no-touch technique to avoid viral spread) may be curative, if necessary combined with cryotherapy (double freeze–thaw). Besides, adjuvant topical treatment with MMC or IFN as well as oral treatment with cimetidine over several weeks is possible [19].

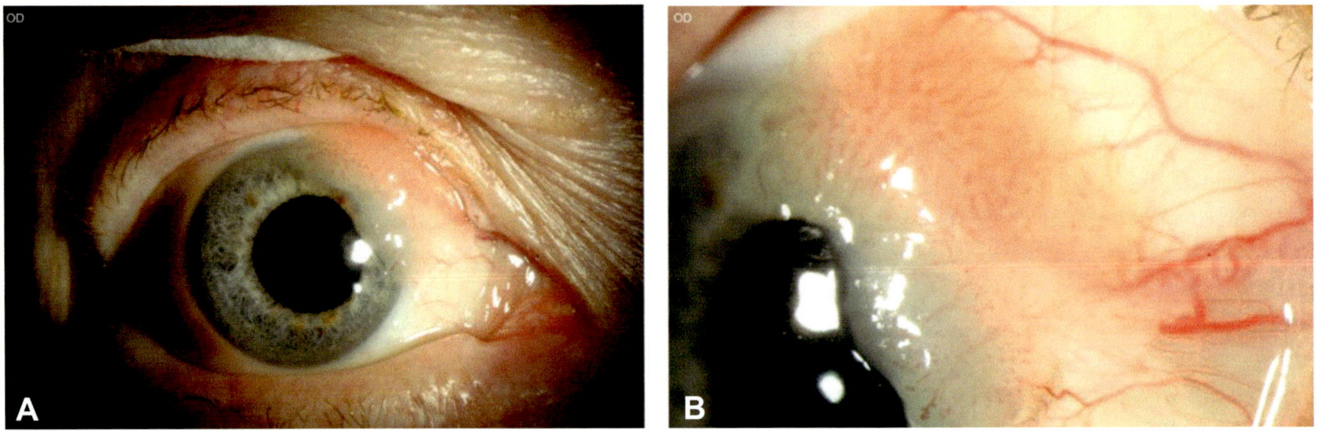

Fig. 5 Conjunctival papilloma extending over the limbus onto the cornea (**A** overview, **B** magnification)

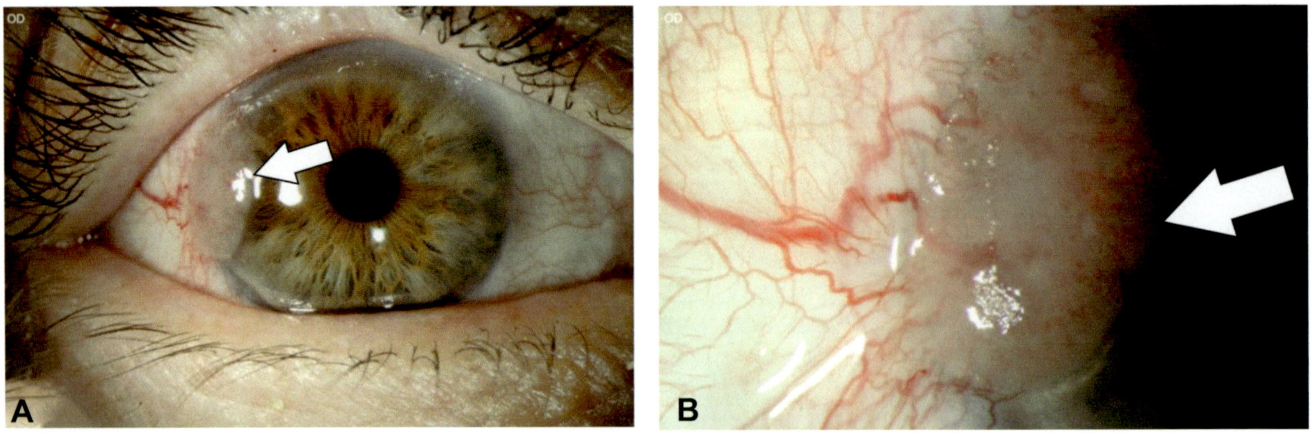

Fig. 6 Conjunctival papilloma with corneal involvement. (**A**, **B**) The vascularized sessile tumour (arrow) partially overlaps the temporal corneal periphery (**A** overview, **B** magnification)

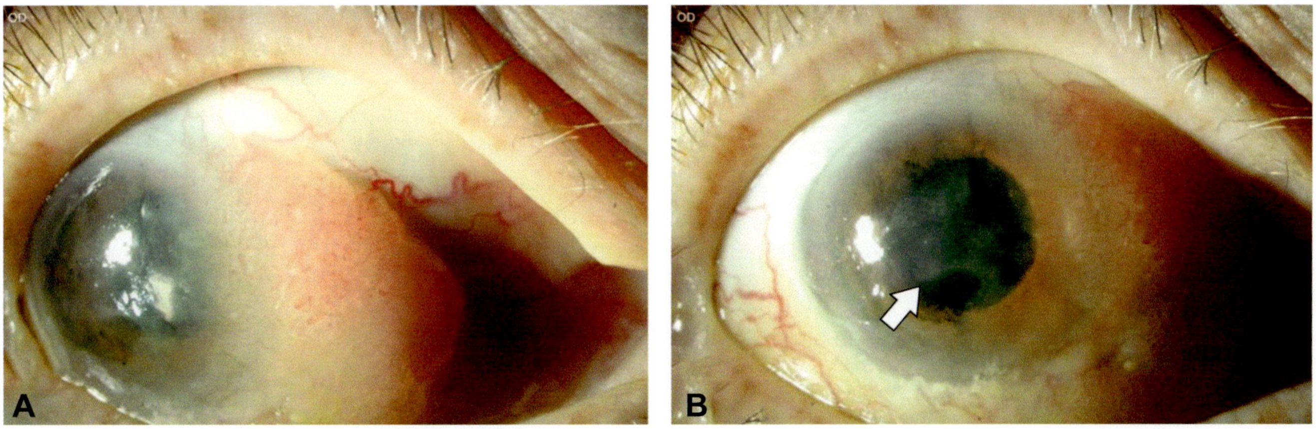

Fig. 7 Sessile conjunctival papilloma (histology: conjunctival papilloma with focal dysplasia) with corneal involvement. (**A**) Prominent tumour with vascular fronds. (**B**) Cornea with greyish epithelial changes (arrow) corresponding to Conjunctival Intraepithelial Neoplasia (CIN)

3 Ocular Surface Squamous Cell Neoplasia

Ocular surface squamous cell neoplasia include the precancerous conjunctival/ corneal epithelial neoplasia (CIN) and squamous cell carcinoma.

3.1 Conjunctival Intraepithelial Neoplasia (CIN)

Carcinomatous intraepithelial neoplasia (CIN) of the conjunctiva and cornea is a circumscribed minimally invasive process limited to the surface epithelium. CIN as well as squamous cell carcinoma predominantly affects mainly older patients over 60 years of age with a predisposition to the male sex. Risk factors for development include UV radiation, HPV infection (high risk types 16 and 18), and abnormal immune status [5].

The clinical presentation is characterized by a fleshy, sessile, and minimally prominent process usually located at the corneal limbus in the interpalpebral area, less common in the area of the fornix or palpebral conjunctiva (Fig. 8) [21]. CIN might present a whitish surface (Fig. 9), that develops as result of secondary hyperkeratosis (Leukoplakia). Tumour margins might be sharp or diffuse. Extensive involvement of the conjunctiva may occasionally occur (Fig. 10).

Low-grade/mild CIN is characterized by atypical proliferation of epithelial cells and partially involves the conjunctival epithelium (1/3 of epithelial thickness), whereas high-grade/severe CIN (Carcinoma in situ, CIS) affects the entire epithelium. However, it must be mentioned that a distinction between mild and severe CIN cannot be made clinically [2].

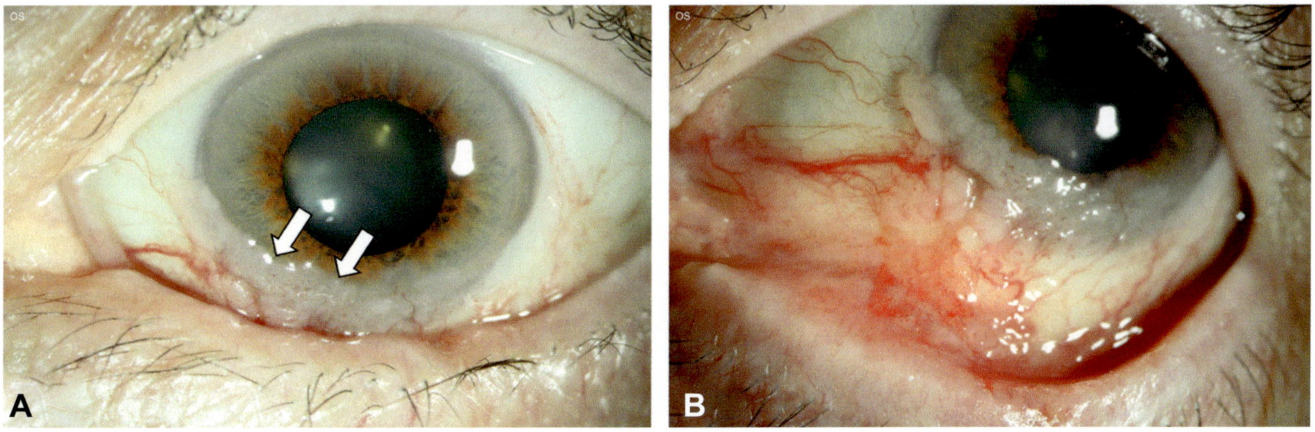

Fig. 8 Carcinoma in situ of the conjunctiva. (**A**, **B**) The tumour extends from the fornix conjunctiva and infiltrates the cornea in the inferior and nasal periphery (arrows) (**A** Overview, **B** Illustration of the lower fornix)

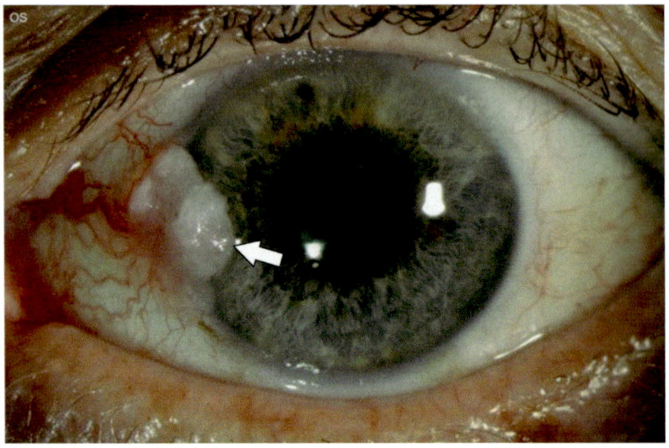

Fig. 9 Carcinoma in situ of the conjunctiva with leukoplakia (whitish appearance) and involvement of the cornea (arrow)

The process can extend to the corneal epithelium where it may appear as a grey superficial opacity of the cornea (Figs. 11 and 12) and is sometimes associated with vascularization, whereas involvement of the basement membrane, Bowman layer and corneal stroma are rare [2].

Even in a relatively unremarkable conjunctiva, suspicious vascularization of the cornea might be indicative of CIN (Fig. 13).

Treatment consists of complete excision, sometimes with combined lamellar sclerokeratectomy followed by cryotherapy if necessary. Other additional treatment options include treatment with topical MMC, 5-Fluorouracil (5-FU) or IFN. There is a high risk of recurrence in cases of incomplete excision [21–24].

3.2 Squamous Cell Carcinoma of the Conjunctiva

Squamous cell carcinoma of the conjunctiva is characterized by involvement of the deeper substantia propria by atypical conjunctival cells. It is mainly located in sun-exposed areas of the bulbar conjunctiva, but might also occur in the palpebral conjunctiva (Fig. 14) [5, 21, 23, 25]. Clinically, squamous cell carcinoma shows a more aggressive course with locally invasive growth, and is typically larger and more prominent than CIN. Histopathologically,

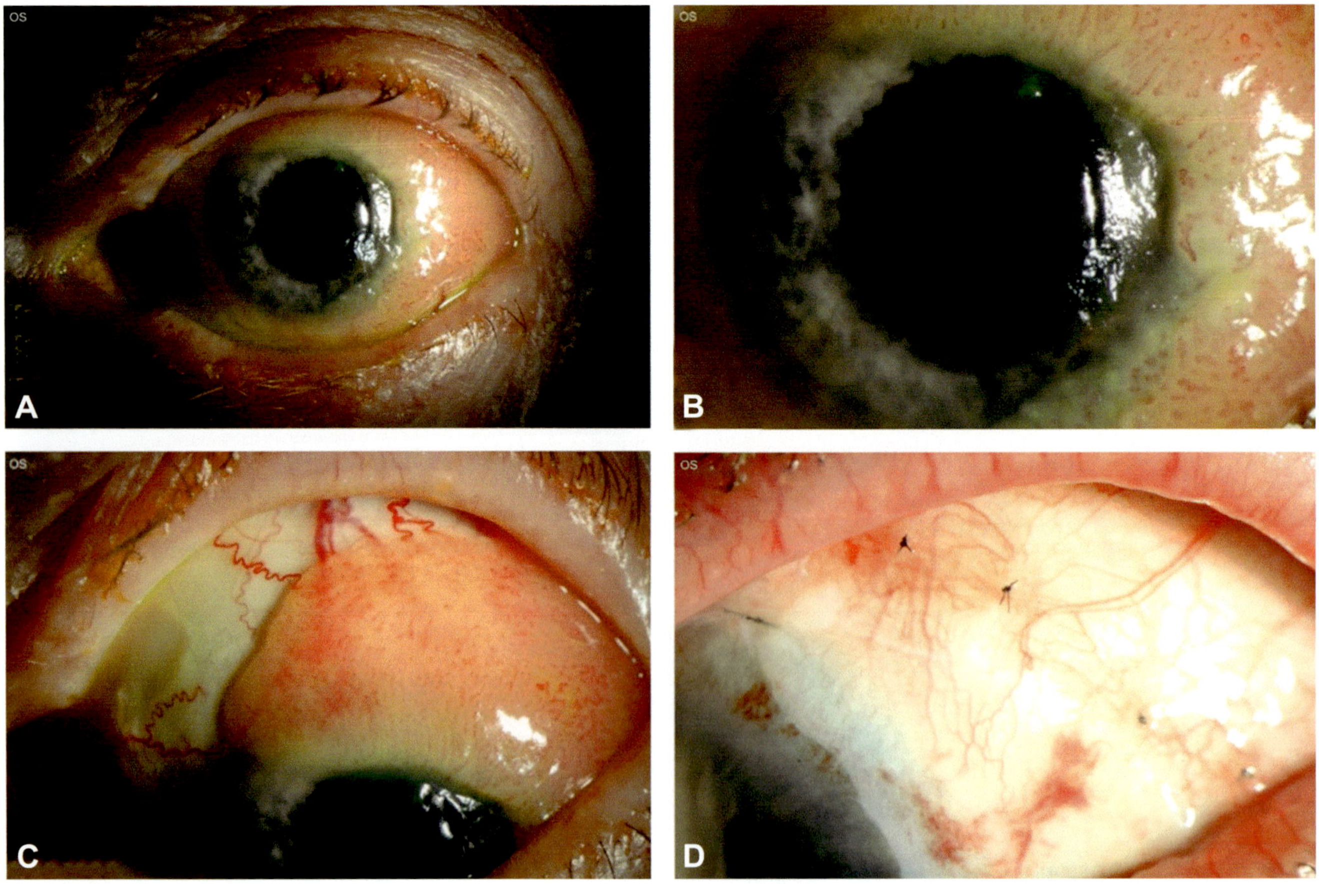

Fig. 10 Sessile papillomatous carcinoma in situ of the conjunctiva. (**A–C**) Severe and extensive conjunctival tumour affecting the cornea (**A** overview, **B**, **C** magnification). (**D**) Early postoperative findings after surgical excision with amniotic membrane transplantation as episcleral graft

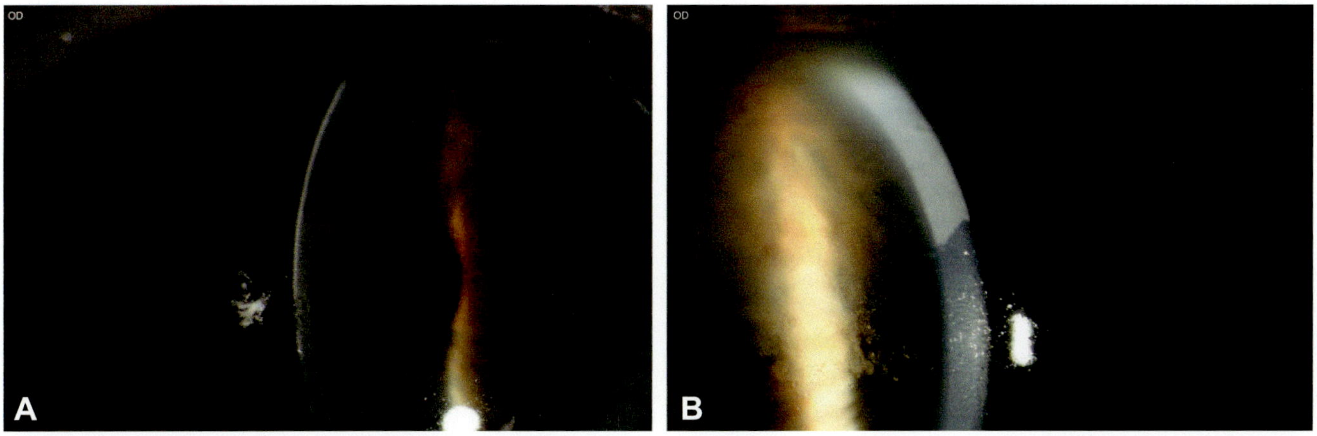

Fig. 11 Corneal intraepithelial neoplasia (CIN). (**A**, **B**) Greyish, slightly prominent opacities (**A**, narrow slit beam) with a distinct demarcation to the healthy epithelium (**B**, moderate slit beam)

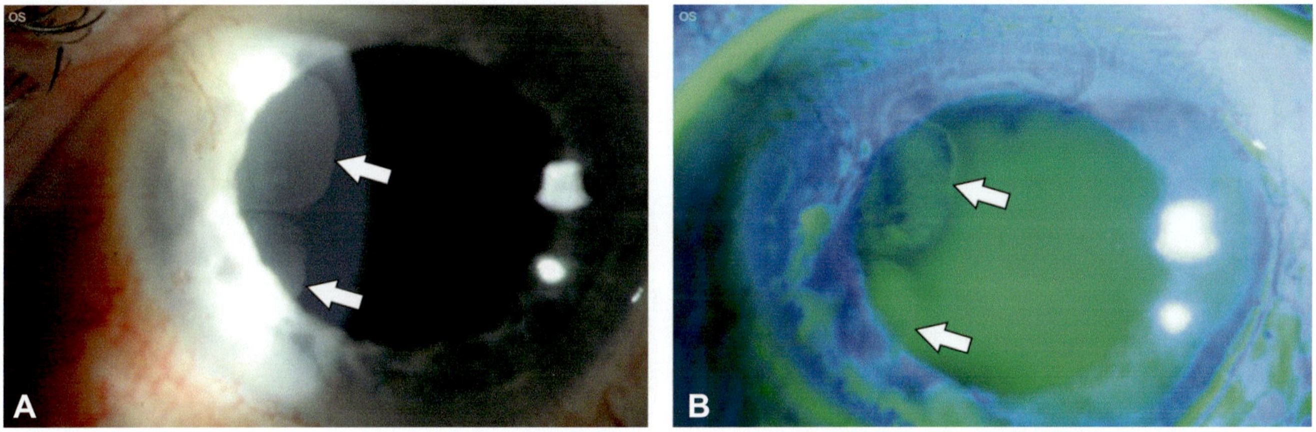

Fig. 12 Corneal intraepithelial neoplasia of the cornea. (**A**, **B**) Well-demarcated superficial opacities (arrows) with vascularization of the cornea (**A**) and asymmetric tear film pooling after application of fluorescein eye drops to demonstrate the tumor margins (**B**)

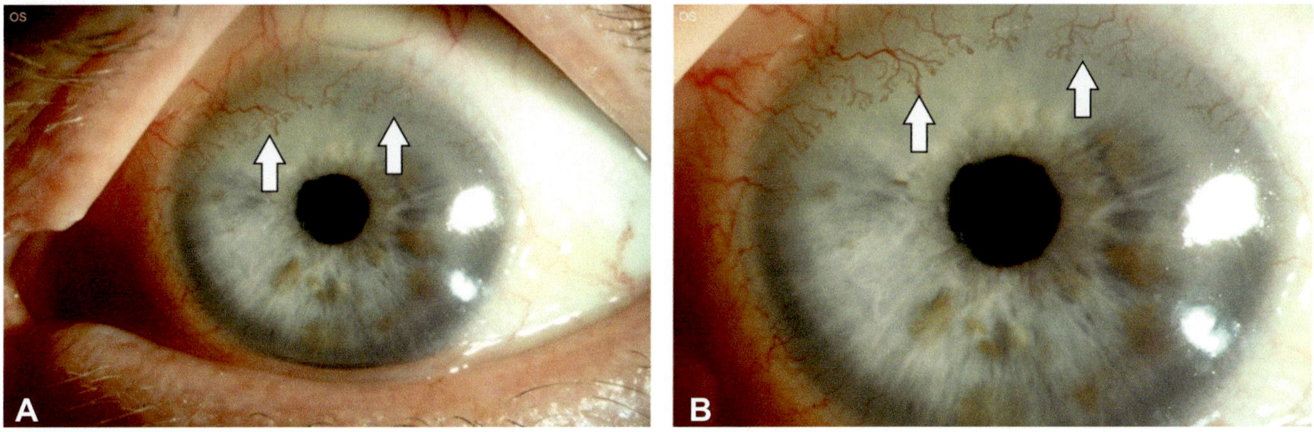

Fig. 13 Carcinoma in situ of the conjunctiva with corneal involvement. (**A**, **B**) Conspicuous corneal vascularisation (arrows) might be indicative of a tumorous lesion (**A** overview, **B** magnification)

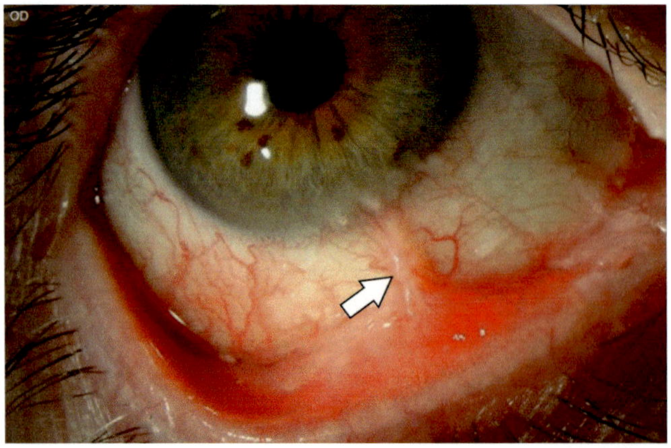

Fig. 14 Conjunctival squamous cell carcinoma with symblepharon extending to the corneal limbus (arrow)

squamous cell carcinoma is a well-differentiated tumour composed of atypical epithelial cells, mitoses and dyskeratosis [2].

The tumour might present with leukoplakia. Severe corneal involvement (Fig. 15) and invasion of the orbit and bulb may occur [26].

Treatment of invasive squamous cell carcinoma includes complete surgical excision (no-touch technique) with safety distance of 4 mm and cryocoagulation of the surrounding conjunctiva and excision margins. In severe cases additional lamellar sclerokeratectomy might be performed. Reconstruction using autologous conjunctiva of the contralateral eye, amniotic membrane or oral mucosa is required for larger tumours [5, 9, 22, 23]. Adjuvant topical treatment with MMC, IFN, or 5-FU has been shown to be useful in terms of recurrence rates. Recurrences usually occur within the first 2 years after excision in up to 56% of cases and depend on the state of the excision margins on histology and the use of adjuvant therapy [23, 24].

Metastasis to the regional lymph nodes (preauricular, submandibular) is possible in 2–3%, whereas risk of hematogenous metastasis is very low [27, 28].

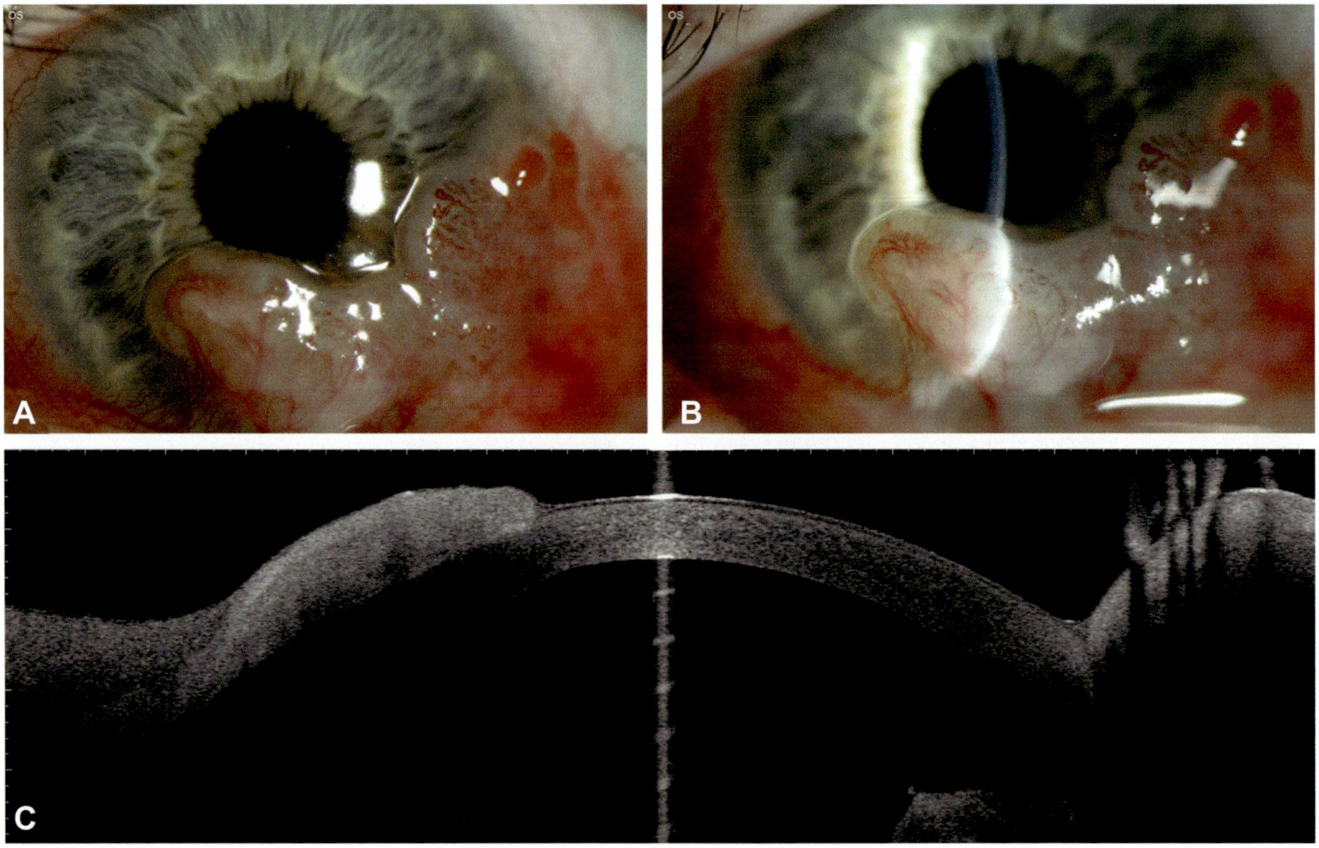

Fig. 15 Conjunctival squamous cell carcinoma with severe infiltration of the cornea. (**A**, **B**) Extensive and prominent tumorous involvement of the cornea. (**A** overview, **B** narrow slit). **C** Anterior segment optical coherence tomography showing a large hyperreflective tumour of the conjunctiva with corneal affection (arrows)

4 Congenital Tumours

4.1 Solid Dermoid of the Limbus and the Cornea

Solid limbal dermoids are the most common congenital tumours of the conjunctiva and belong to choristomas (representing proliferation of cells scattered to an unusual location). A simple choristoma contains one tissue type, whereas complex choristomas contain more than one tissue type such as skin, bone, lacrimal gland, cartilage or other tissues.

Most conjunctival choristomas occur sporadically [2]. Clinically, a solid dermoid is slightly yellowish in appearance (due to lipids) and varies in size (Fig. 16).

Fine hair may be observed on the surface of the dermoid (Fig. 17). Usually, limbal dermoids are located in the temporal inferior quadrant [29].

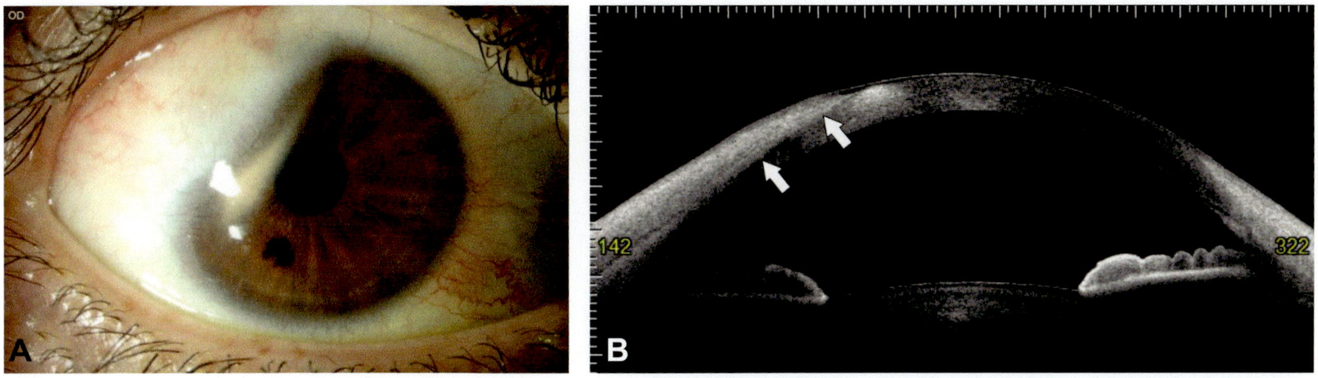

Fig. 16 Flat solid dermoid of the corneal limbus. (**A**) Flat solid limbal dermoid with lipid deposits. (**B**) Anterior segment optical coherence tomography demonstrating a flat limbal dermoid (arrows)

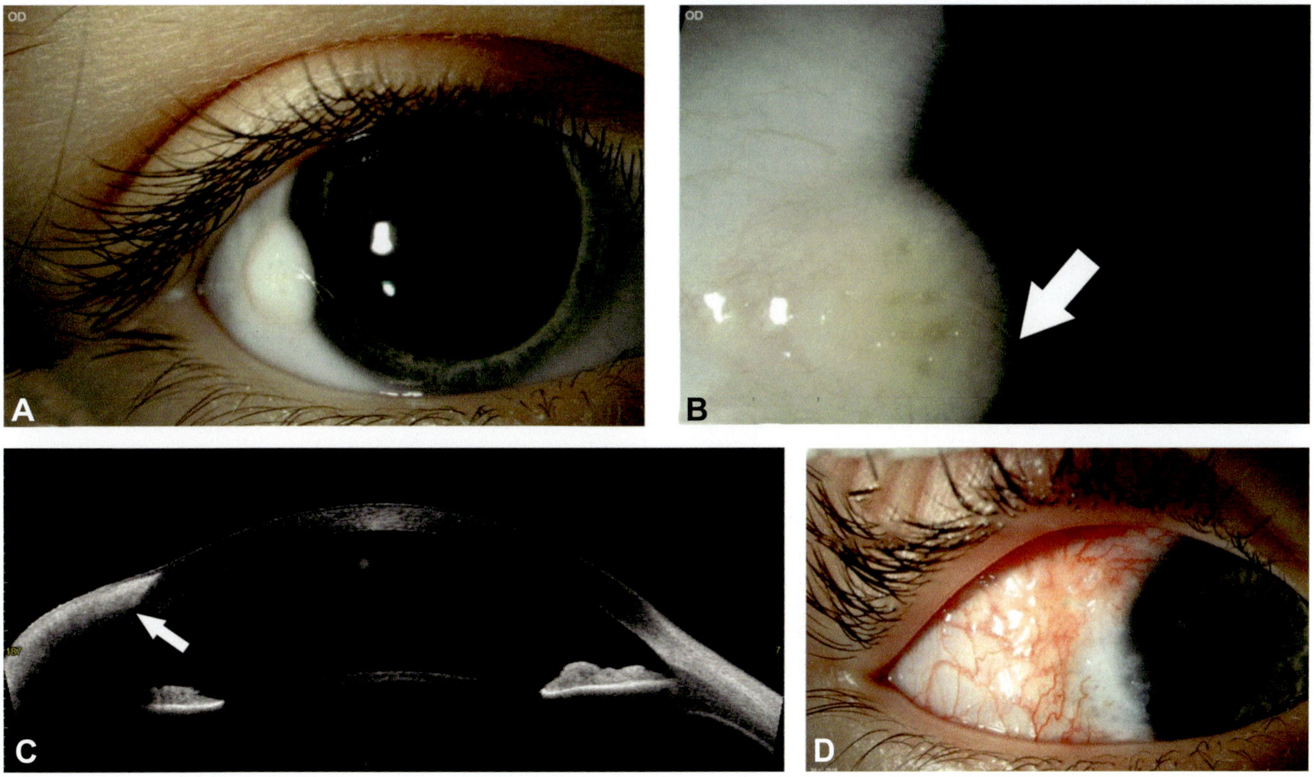

Fig. 17 Solid dermoid of the corneal limbus. (**A**, **B**) A prominent yellowish solid limbal dermoid with hair follicles and fine white hair (**B** arrow) (**A** overview, **B** higher magnification). (**C**) Anterior segment optical coherence tomography for assessing the depth of the tumour (arrow). (**D**) Postoperative findings after lamellar sclerokeratectomy

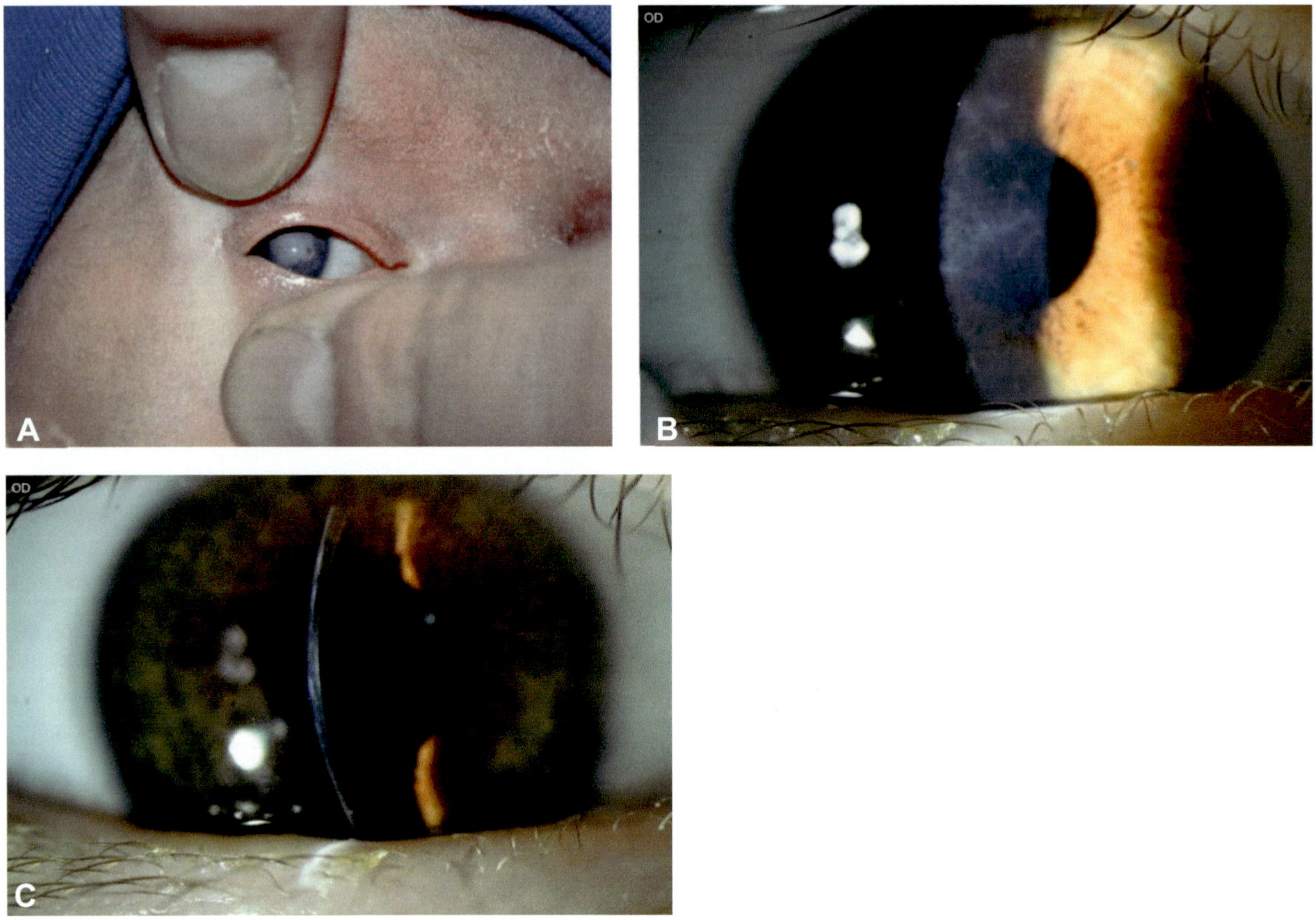

Fig. 18 Dermoid of the central cornea. (**A**) Central dermoid of the cornea in a 3-month-old child. (**B**, **C**) Minor deep stromal corneal scars are present after excision of the central dermoid. At the age of 8 years, the corrected decimal distance visual acuity was 0.5

The method of choice is surgical excision that has the primary goal of avoiding visual loss with amblyopia development in children [30]. Furthermore, large dermoids might induce surface irritation and involve the central cornea (Fig. 18) [29]. Simultaneous amniotic membrane transplantation is possible for large defects.

Recurrence of dermoids are rare (Fig. 19). Severe corneal involvement is a therapeutic challenge and might require lamellar or penetrating keratoplasty [29, 31].

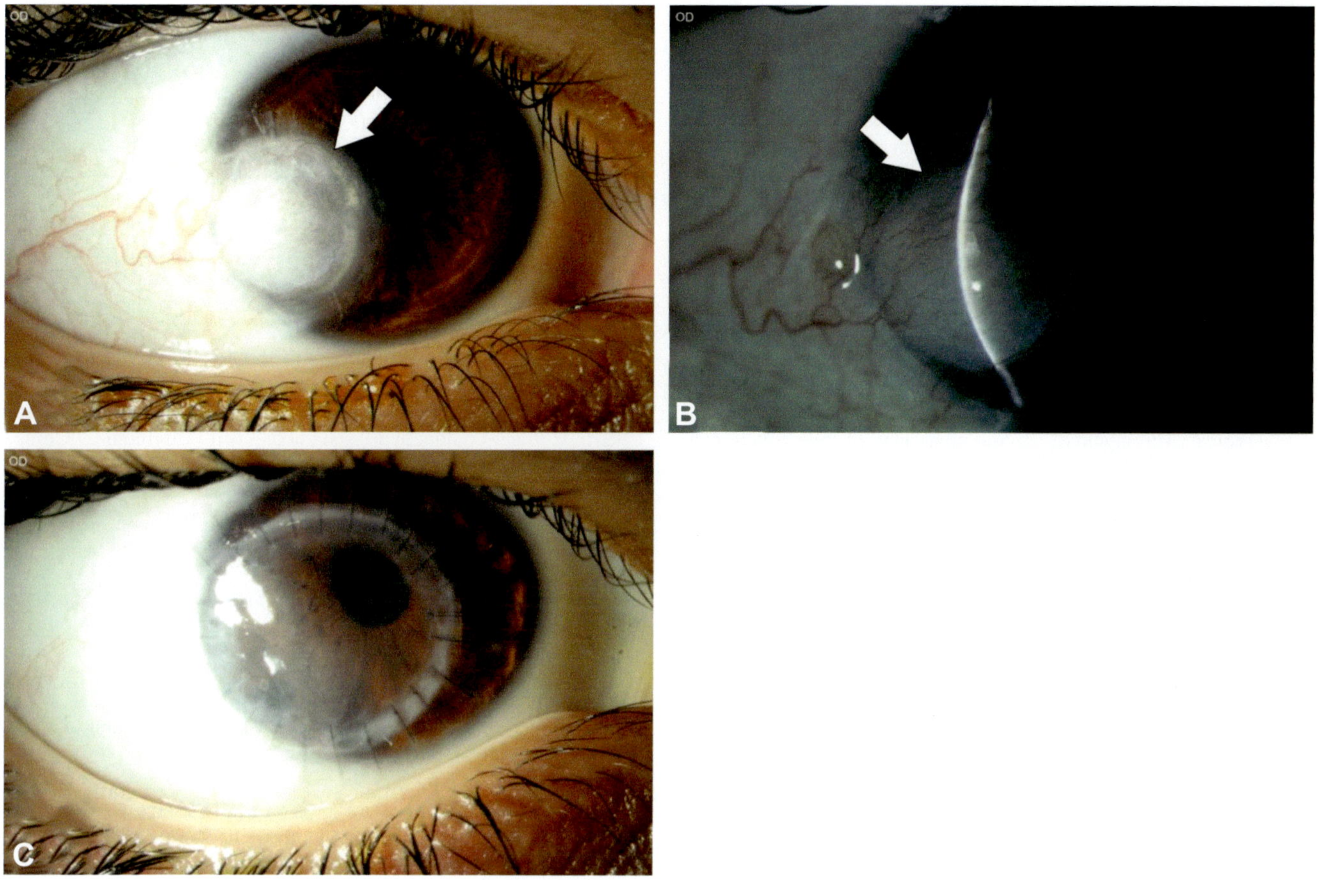

Fig. 19 Recurrent solid dermoid of the corneal limbus. (**A**, **B**) Preoperative findings of a recurrent limbal dermoid after two surgical excisions (**A** overview, **B** narrow slit). (**C**) Decentered penetrating keratoplasty to remove the solid dermoid of the corneal limbus

5 Conclusion

Most "corneal tumors" represent the secondary involvement of the cornea - secondary to conjunctival neoplasms - and should be treated accordingly.

Conflict of Interest The authors have no funding or conflicts of interest to disclose.

References

1. Shields CL. Conjunctival nevi: clinical features and natural course in 410 consecutive patients. Arch Ophthalmol. 2004;122:167–75. https://doi.org/10.1001/archopht.122.2.167.
2. Holbach LM, Pogorelov P, Kruse FE. Differential diagnosis and treatment options for conjunctival tumors. Ophthalmologie. 2007;104:521–39. https://doi.org/10.1007/s00347-007-1551-8.
3. Shields CL, Markowitz JS, Belinsky I, Schwartzstein H, George NS, Lally SE, et al. Conjunctival melanoma: outcomes based on tumor origin in 382 consecutive cases. Ophthalmology. 2011;118:389-395.e2. https://doi.org/10.1016/j.ophtha.2010.06.021.
4. Damato B, Coupland SE. Conjunctival melanoma and melanosis: a reappraisal of terminology, classification and staging. Clin Exp Ophthalmol. 2008;36:786–95. https://doi.org/10.1111/j.1442-9071.2008.01888.x.
5. Auw-Hädrich C, Reinhard T. Conjunctival malignancies. Ophthalmologie. 2019;116:989–1004. https://doi.org/10.1007/s00347-019-00978-6.
6. Hu D-N, Yu G, McCormick SA, Finger PT. Population-based incidence of conjunctival melanoma in various races and ethnic groups and comparison with other melanomas. Am J Ophthalmol. 2008;145:418–23. https://doi.org/10.1016/j.ajo.2007.10.022.
7. Damato B, Coupland SE. Management of conjunctival melanoma. Expert Rev Anticancer Ther. 2009;9:1227–39. https://doi.org/10.1586/era.09.85.
8. Shields JA, Shields CL, De PP. Surgical management of circumscribed conjunctival melanomas. Ophthalmic Plast Reconstr Surg. 1998;14:208–15. https://doi.org/10.1097/00002341-199805000-00012.
9. Shields JA, Shields CL, De Potter P. Surgical management of conjunctival tumors: the 1994 Lynn B. McMahan Lecture. Arch Ophthalmol. 1997;115:808–15. https://doi.org/10.1001/archopht.1997.01100150810025.
10. Wong JR, Nanji AA, Galor A, Karp CL. Management of conjunctival malignant melanoma: a review and update. Expert Rev Ophthalmol. 2014;9:185–204. https://doi.org/10.1586/17469899.2014.921119.

11. Brownstein S. Malignant melanoma of the conjunctiva. Cancer Control. 2004;11:310–6. https://doi.org/10.1177/107327480401100505.
12. Vora GK, Demirci H, Marr B, Mruthyunjaya P. Advances in the management of conjunctival melanoma. Surv Ophthalmol. 2017;62:26–42. https://doi.org/10.1016/j.survophthal.2016.06.001.
13. Shields CL, Chien JL, Surakiatchanukul T, Sioufi K, Lally SE, Shields JA. Conjunctival tumors: review of clinical features, risks, biomarkers, and outcomes—the 2017 J. Donald M. Gass Lecture. Asia-Pacific J Ophthalmol. 2017;6:109–20. https://doi.org/10.22608/APO.201710.
14. Frucht-Pery J, Pe'er J. Use of Mitomycin C in the treatment of conjunctival primary acquired melanosis with Atypia. Arch Ophthalmol. 1996;114:1261–4. https://doi.org/10.1001/archopht.1996.01100140461020.
15. Rodríguez-Ares T, Touriño R, De Rojas V, Becerra E, Capeans C. Topical Mitomycin C in the treatment of pigmented conjunctival lesions. Cornea. 2003;22:114–7. https://doi.org/10.1097/00003226-200303000-00006.
16. Nuessle S, Auw-Haedrich C, Jiang J, Boehringer D, Reinhard T. Real-life data of adjuvant IFN-α2b and MMC in conjunctival melanocytic lesions. Graefe's Arch Clin Exp Ophthalmol. 2022. https://doi.org/10.1007/s00417-022-05832-1.
17. Baum SH, Westekemper H, Bechrakis NE, Mohr C. Conjunctival and uveal melanoma: survival and risk factors following orbital exenteration. Eur J Ophthalmol. 2022;32:612–9. https://doi.org/10.1177/1120672121995131.
18. Shields CL, Shields JA, Gündüz K, Cater J, Mercado GV, Gross N, et al. Conjunctival melanoma: risk factors for recurrence, exenteration, metastasis, and death in 150 consecutive patients. Arch Ophthalmol. 2000;118:1497–507. https://doi.org/10.1001/archopht.118.11.1497.
19. Theotoka D, Morkin MI, Galor A, Karp CL. Update on diagnosis and management of conjunctival papilloma. Eye Vis. 2019;6:18. https://doi.org/10.1186/s40662-019-0142-5.
20. Kaliki S, Arepalli S, Shields CL, Klein K, Sun H, Hysenj E, et al. Conjunctival papilloma: features and outcomes based on age at initial examination. JAMA Ophthalmol. 2013;131:585–93. https://doi.org/10.1001/jamaophthalmol.2013.83.
21. Shields CL, Shields JA. Tumors of the conjunctiva and cornea. Surv Ophthalmol. 2004;49:3–24. https://doi.org/10.1016/j.survophthal.2003.10.008.
22. Basti S, Macsai MS. Ocular surface squamous neoplasia. Cornea. 2003;22:687–704. https://doi.org/10.1097/00003226-200310000-00015.
23. Höllhumer R, Williams S, Michelow P. Ocular surface squamous neoplasia: management and outcomes. Eye. 2021;35:1562–73. https://doi.org/10.1038/s41433-021-01422-3.
24. Seitz B, Fischer M, Holbach L, Naumann G. Differential diagnosis and prognosis of 112 excised epibulbar epithelial tumors. Klin Monbl Augenheilkd. 1995;207:239–46. https://doi.org/10.1055/s-2008-1035375.
25. Westekemper H, Manthey A, Bechrakis N. Diagnosis and therapy of benign and malignant tumors of the conjunctiva. Augenheilkd Up2date 2020;10:223–39. https://doi.org/10.1055/a-1061-9973.
26. Papaioannou IT, Melachrinou MP, Drimtzias EG, Gartaganis SP. Corneal-conjunctival squamous cell carcinoma. Cornea. 2008;27:957–8. https://doi.org/10.1097/ICO.0b013e31816f5ef2.
27. Vempuluru VS, Indusekhar H, Mohamed A, Kaliki S. Metastatic conjunctival squamous cell carcinoma: a study of 5 patients. Int Ophthalmol. 2022;42:3097–108. https://doi.org/10.1007/s10792-022-02309-2.
28. Ramberg I, Heegaard S, Prause JU, Sjö NC, Toft PB. Squamous cell dysplasia and carcinoma of the conjunctiva. A nationwide, retrospective, epidemiological study of Danish patients. Acta Ophthalmol. 2015;93:663–6. https://doi.org/10.1111/aos.12743.
29. Lang SJ, Böhringer D, Reinhard T. Surgical management of corneal limbal dermoids: retrospective study of different techniques and use of Mitomycin C. Eye. 2014;28:857–62. https://doi.org/10.1038/eye.2014.112.
30. Stergiopoulos P, Link B, Naumann GOH, Seitz B. Solid corneal dermoids and subconjunctival lipodermoids: impact of differentiated surgical therapy on the functional long-term outcome. Cornea. 2009;28:644–51. https://doi.org/10.1097/ICO.0b013e3181914305.
31. Lang P, Seitz B, Naumann G. Solid limbal dermoid in an 80-year-old patient. Klin Monbl Augenheilkd. 2004;221:776–80. https://doi.org/10.1055/s-2004-813595.

Recurrent Corneal Erosion Syndrome RCES

Sujata Das

Abstract

Recurrent corneal erosion is characterized by repeated episodes of sudden-onset of pain, watering, foreign-body sensation while waking-up from sleep. This is caused by abnormal epithelial adhesion to the underlying basal lamina. It may be unilateral or bilateral. There may be micro or macro erosions. The diagnosis is made by slit-lamp examination and history. Slit-lamp findings are mild conjunctival congestion with corneal epithelial defect with loose epithelium or focal area of irregular hazy epithelium. It may be associated with trauma, especially nail injury. Other causes include epithelial basement membrane dystrophy, lattice dystrophy, granular dystrophy, and macular dystrophy. Lubricating drops and ointments are helpful in majority cases. In non-responding cases, surgical modalities like phototherapeutic keratectomy, or anterior stromal puncture may be required. Microbial keratitis may occur in occasional cases due to secondary infection.

Keywords

Corneal erosion · Corneal dystrophy · Epithelial basement membrane dystrophy · Trauma · Lubricant · Photo therapeutic keratectomy

S. Das (✉)
Cornea and Anterior Segment Service, L V Prasad Eye Institute, Bhubaneswar, Odisha, India
e-mail: sujatadas@lvpei.org

1 Introduction

Recurrent corneal erosion syndrome (RCES) is a chronic relapsing disease characterized by repeated episodes of sudden onset of pain, redness and watering usually at night or early morning, while waking-up from sleep. This entity has been described more than 100 years ago [1]. Most patients have a history of trauma and/or epithelial basement membrane dystrophy [2–5]. While many respond to conservative management, surgical management is required in non-responsive cases [2–5].

2 Aetiology and Pathogenesis

Many aetiologies have been reported in the literature. Among these, most common are trauma, epithelial basement membrane dystrophy (EBMD) and epithelial recurrent erosion dystrophies (EREDs) [2–8]. Amongst trauma, fingernail injury is the most common injury reported [5, 7]. The other common causes may be due to Reis–Bücklers, lattice, macular, granular dystrophy.

Anomalous structural findings have been described in epithelium, basement membrane and Bowman layer [9]. Abnormality in hemidesmosome formation and function along with focal absence of basement membrane, duplication of basement membrane has been noted [10, 11].

3 Clinical Features and Diagnosis

Patients usually present to the clinic with a history of sudden onset recurrent pain, redness, watering on awakening. This is mostly unilateral and located in the inferior quadrant of the cornea. They may present with irregular loose epithelium with or without epithelial defect (Figs. 1A, B, 2A, 3A, B, 4A–D). In subtle cases, focally aggregated intraepithelial whitish dots were seen during slit-lamp examination.

B. Seitz et al. (eds.), *Atlas on Cornea*, https://doi.org/10.1007/978-3-031-65422-0_37

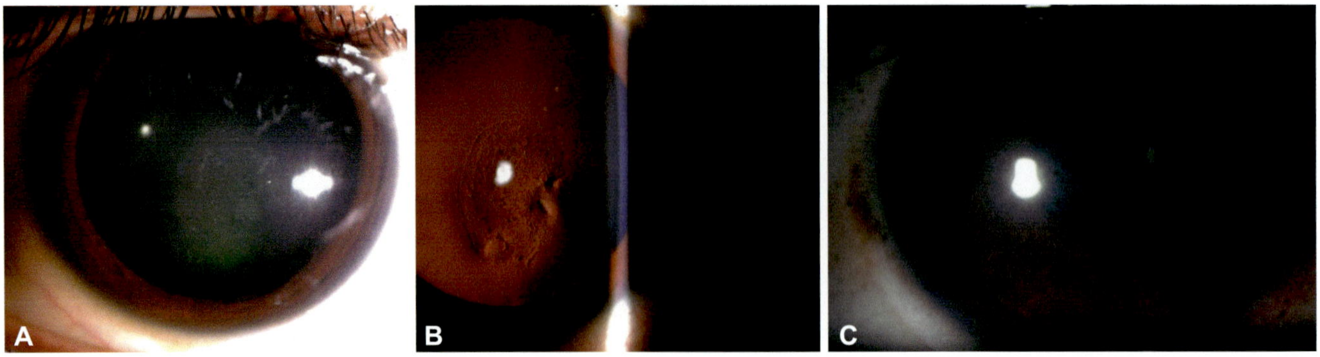

Fig. 1 A 21-year-old male presented with complaints of intermittent foreign body sensation, watering for the last 4–5 months in his right eye. He had a history of trauma with someone's hand 1-year ago. His visual acuity was 20/50 with his glasses. Clinical examination revealed epithelial defect and loose epithelium (**A**, **B**) Epithelium was debrided and bandage contact lens applied. He was reviewed after 3 weeks. His best-corrected visual acuity was 20/20. There was no epithelial defect (**C**)

Detailed slit-lamp examination of the other eye may give clues for diagnosis in cases of EBMD. Broad, angled and retro illumination (Figs. 1B, 4B) (fully-dilated pupil) slit-lamp examination helps in the diagnosis of EBMD and reparative stages of earlier erosion. History and nature of trauma is crucial in diagnosis. The role of confocal microscopy has been described for diagnosis [12].

4 Treatment

Many patients with RCES respond well to lubricating drops, gel and ointment. These need to be used for long term [7]. Bandage contact lens provides symptomatic relief and early healing of epithelial defects (Fig. 1C) [13]. A minimum of six weeks usage has been recommended on the basis of time taken for epithelial remodelling. Matrix metalloproteinase (MMP-**2** and MMP-9) has been upregulated in tears of cases with RCES. Treatment with combination of Doxycycline, inhibitor of MMPs and steroid has been shown to decrease short-term relapses [14]. Autologous serum has been tried as a second line of therapy after failure of conventional treatment [15]. It is effective and safe in reducing the number of recurrences.

Debridement of the loose epithelium fastens early resolution in acute stage. It does not prevent recurrences. Multiple anterior stromal punctures through the abnormal epithelium into anterior stroma using a needle has been used for the treatment of RCES [16]. It induces scar formation between epithelium and stroma. Since deep penetration may induce scarring, it is not used in cases of abnormal epithelium involving the visual axis. To achieve more reproducible results, YAG laser has been used for stromal micropuncture [17]. Phototherapeutic keratectomy (PTK) has been used for recalcitrant cases of RCES [18].

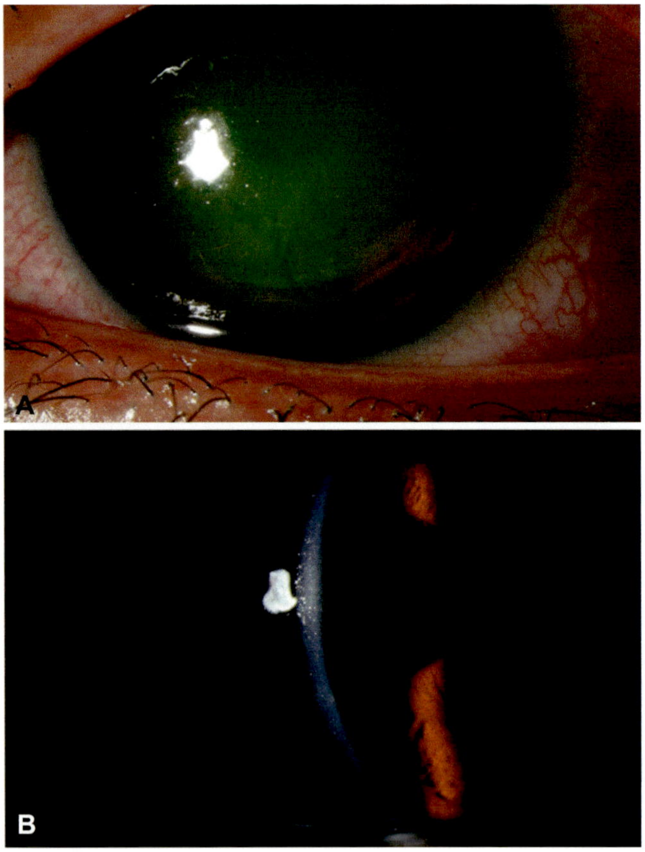

Fig. 2 A 19-year-old boy presented with a history of watering associated with redness and foreign body sensation for 3–4 days. While taking history, the patient revealed that the pain starts in the morning. His visual acuity was 20/30 in the right eye and 20/40 in the left eye. On examination, there was a large corneal epithelial defect with loose epithelium (**A**) Left eye examination revealed epithelial lesions of different shapes (**B**) He was diagnosed to have epithelial basement membrane dystrophy of both eyes and epithelial defect due to recurrent corneal erosion in the left eye. He was prescribed a lubricating drop and ointment. He was lost-to-follow-up

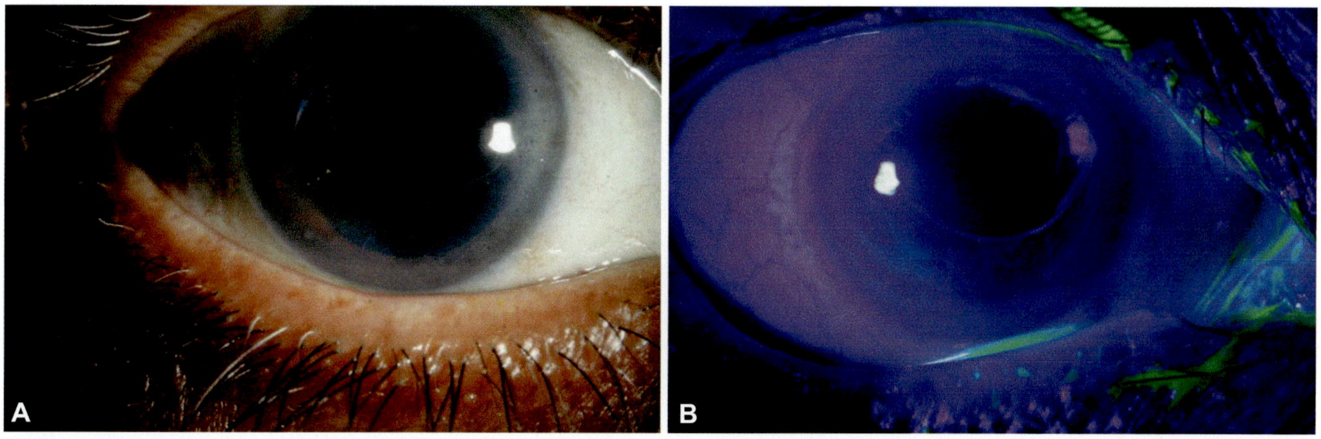

Fig. 3 A 65-year-old female complained of occasional pain and watering in the right eye for 4–5 months. She had undergone cataract surgery in that eye 2 years ago. Her best-corrected visual acuity was 20/20. She had loose epithelium inferiorly from 6 to 8 o'clock (**A**, **B**) On further enquiry, she revealed pain in the right eye while getting-up from bed. She was started lubricating drops and ointment at night

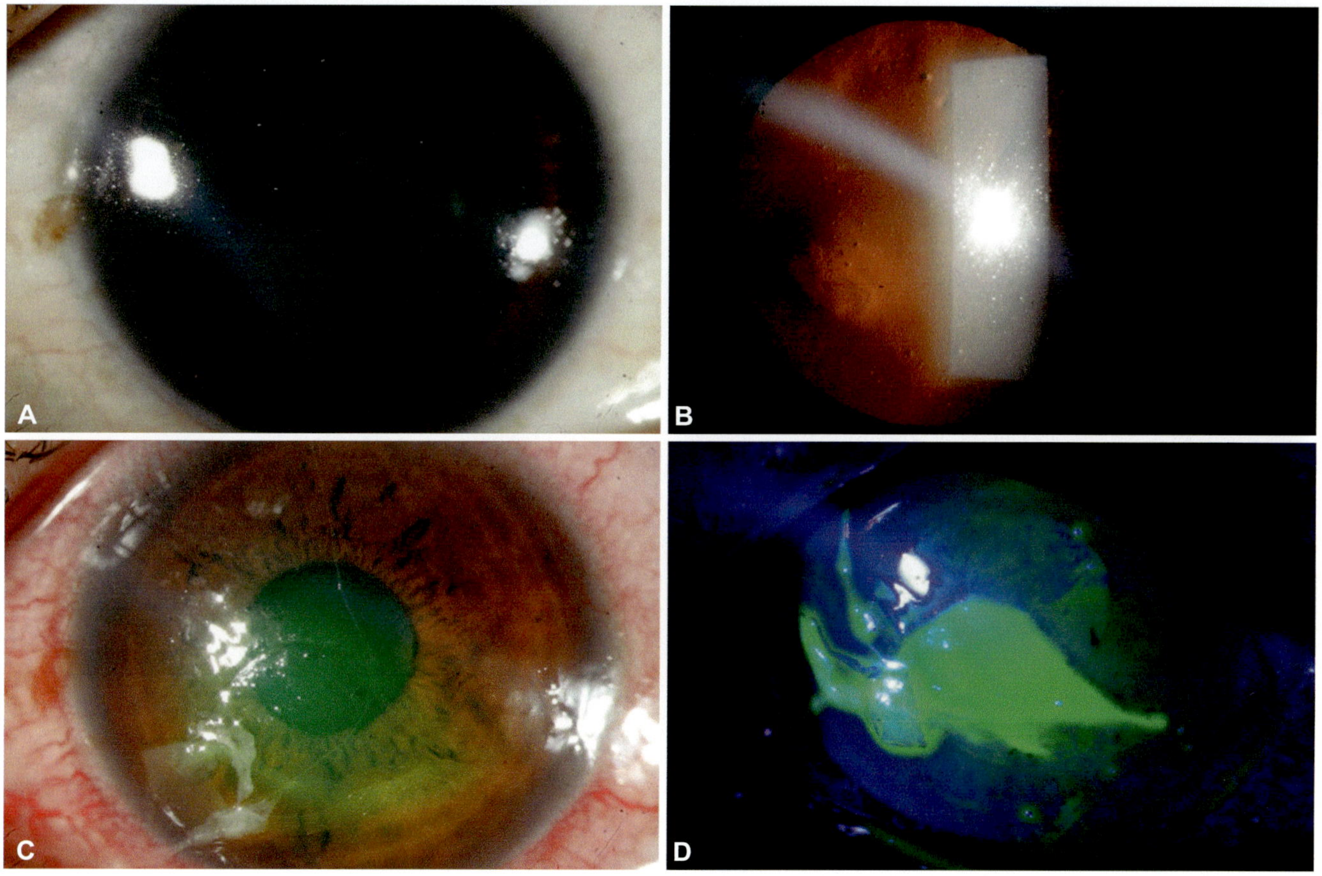

Fig. 4 A 40-year-old male presented with a history of redness and blurring vision of 3 weeks duration following injury with his wife's nail. His best-corrected visual acuity was 20/30. Slit-lamp examination revealed greyish loose epithelium in a localized area without any epithelial defect (**A**, **B**) He was advised lubricating drop in daytime and ointment at night. He presented to the emergency clinic next day with severe pain. There was a large epithelial defect of 6 mm × 4 mm (**C**, **D**) Topical antibiotic drop was added to prior prescription

Success rate is better for recurrent erosion due to trauma than corneal dystrophies. Combined epithelial debridement with diamond burr polishing has a good success rate [19]. Diamond burr polishing prevents recurrence by removing abnormal basement membrane to allow smooth surface for epithelium to grow and by causing fibrosis and scarring. In alcohol delamination method, ethyl alcohol is used to separate the epithelium at the level of the epithelial basement membrane without disrupting Bowman layer and leave a smooth surface for epithelium to reattach [20]. This treatment has shown similar results as PTK.

5 Conclusion

RCES is a relatively common condition. Detailed history and high index of suspicion is required for diagnosis. The treatment is challenging. A rationale stepwise approach helps in management of the condition.

References

1. Hansen E. Om den intermitterende keratitis vesicularis neuralgica af traumatisk opindelse. Hospitalis-Tidende. 1872;51:201–3.
2. Das S, Seitz B. Recurrent corneal erosion syndrome. Surv Ophthalmol. 2008;53(1):3–15.
3. Lin SR, Aldave AJ, Chodosh J. Recurrent corneal erosion syndrome. Br J Ophthalmol. 2019;103(9):1204–8.
4. Ewald M, Hammersmith KM. Review of diagnosis and management of recurrent erosion syndrome. Curr Opin Ophthalmol. 2009;20(4):287–91.
5. Reidy JJ, Paulus MP, Gona S. Recurrent erosions of the cornea: epidemiology and treatment. Cornea. 2000;19(6):767–71.
6. Laibson PR. Recurrent corneal erosions and epithelial basement membrane dystrophy. Eye Contact Lens. 2010;36(5):315–7.
7. Hykin PG, Foss AE, Pavesio C, Dart JK. The natural history and management of recurrent corneal erosion: a prospective randomised trial. Eye (Lond) 1994;8(Pt-1):35–40.
8. Weiss JS, Møller HU, Aldave AJ, Seitz B, Bredrup C, Kivelä T, Munier FL, Rapuano CJ, Nischal KK, Kim EK, Sutphin J, Busin M, Labbé A, Kenyon KR, Kinoshita S, Lisch W. IC3D classification of corneal dystrophies—edition 2. Cornea. 2015;34:117–59.
9. Cogan DG, Donaldson DD, Kuwabara T, Marshall D. Microcystic dystrophy of the corneal epithelium. Trans Am Ophthalmol Soc. 1964;62:213–25.
10. Fogle JA, Kenyon KR, Stark WJ, Green WR. Defective epithelial adhesion in anterior corneal dystrophies. Am J Ophthalmol. 1975;79(6):925–40.
11. Tripathi RC, Bron AJ. Ultrastructural study of non-traumatic recurrent corneal erosion. Br J Ophthalmol. 1972;56(2):73–85.
12. Rosenberg ME, Tervo TM, Petroll WM, Vesaluoma MH. In vivo confocal microscopy of patients with corneal recurrent erosion syndrome or epithelial basement membrane dystrophy. Ophthalmology. 2000;107(3):565–73.
13. Ahad MA, Anandan M, Tah V, Dhingra S, Leyland M. Randomized controlled study of ocular lubrication versus bandage contact lens in the primary treatment of recurrent corneal erosion syndrome. Cornea. 2013;32(10):1311–4.
14. Dursun D, Kim MC, Solomon A, Pflugfelder SC. Treatment of recalcitrant recurrent corneal erosions with inhibitors of matrix metalloproteinase-9, doxycycline and corticosteroids. Am J Ophthalmol. 2001;132(1):8–13.
15. del Castillo JM, de la Casa JM, Sardiña RC, Fernández RM, Feijoo JG, Gómez AC, Rodero MM, Sánchez JG. Treatment of recurrent corneal erosions using autologous serum. Cornea. 2002;21(8):781–3.
16. McLean EN, MacRae SM, Rich LF. Recurrent erosion. Treatment by anterior stromal puncture. Ophthalmology. 1986;93(6):784–8.
17. Geggel HS. Successful treatment of recurrent corneal erosion with Nd:YAG anterior stromal puncture. Am J Ophthalmol. 1990;110(4):404–7.
18. Dedes W, Faes L, Schipper I, Bachmann LM, Thiel MA. Phototherapeutic keratectomy (PTK) for treatment of recurrent corneal erosion: correlation between etiology and prognosis—prospective longitudinal study. Graefes Arch Clin Exp Ophthalmol. 2015;253(10):1745–9.
19. Vo RC, Chen JL, Sanchez PJ, Yu F, Aldave AJ. Long-term outcomes of epithelial debridement and diamond burr polishing for corneal epithelial irregularity and recurrent corneal erosion. Cornea. 2015;34(10):1259–65.
20. Dua HS, Lagnado R, Raj D, Singh R, Mantry S, Gray T, Lowe J. Alcohol delamination of the corneal epithelium: an alternative in the management of recurrent corneal erosions. Ophthalmology. 2006;113(3):404–11.

Corneal Manifestation of Systemic Diseases and Medication

Daniel Kampik and Berthold Seitz

Abstract

Abnormal corneal findings can be indicative of systemic diseases or systemic medications, sometimes making ophthalmologists the first—or even the only—clinicians to detect them. Often asymptomatic, it is important to differentiate between innocuous findings and diseases with lifelong implications for the patient. *Systemic diseases* with corneal involvement are classified into endocrine, metabolic, nutritional, hematologic, dermatologic, skeletal/connective tissue disorders, systemic infectious diseases, and systemic autoimmune/inflammatory diseases. *Systemic medications* with corneal manifestations can be categorized into drug-induced corneal deposits and toxic side effects to the cornea.

Keywords

Cornea · Corneal side effects · Corneal deposits · Systemic diseases · Drug toxicity

1 Introduction

Abnormal corneal findings can be indicative of a systemic disease, sometimes making the ophthalmologist the first person to detect them. Often asymptomatic, it is important to discriminate between innocuous findings and diseases with lifetime impact on the patient. Corneal abnormalities due to systemic medication can be harmless deposits without any consequences or can exert toxic effects on the corneal epithelium requiring dose adjustments.

2 Corneal Manifestations of Systemic Diseases

2.1 Endocrine Disorders

2.1.1 Diabetic Keratopathy (and Neuropathy)

With an estimated global prevalence of 9.3% in 2019, diabetes mellitus is one of the long-term conditions with the highest impact on the well-being of individuals and global health expenditures. Due to an aging population, increased life expectancy of people with diabetes, and lifestyle changes leading to a higher risk of developing diabetes, the number of affected individuals is estimated to increase by 51% by 2045, reaching an estimated 700 million worldwide. While diabetic retinopathy is one of the leading causes of preventable blindness in the adult working population, diabetic changes of the cornea are less severe and therefore often overlooked, despite affecting 47–69% of diabetic patients [1].

Diabetic changes in the ocular surface have been extensively reviewed by Shah et al. [2] and Shih et al. [3]. They include structural changes of epithelium, affecting all diabetes types: poorer epithelial adhesion due to fewer hemidesmosomes, a disruption of the arrangement of anchoring fibrils, and thickening of the epithelial basement membrane. Limbal epithelial stem cells have an altered pattern of putative stem cell marker expression [4]. The stroma features cytoplasmic lipid vacuoles and deposition of amorphous extracellular material. Endothelial cells show increased polymegethism and pleomorphism.

Alterations of the corneal nerves are mostly found in the subbasal nerve plexus. Messmer et al. demonstrated via corneal confocal microscopy that nerve fiber changes correlate with more advanced stages of diabetic retinopathy,

D. Kampik (✉)
Department of Ophthalmology, University Hospital Würzburg, Würzburg, Germany
e-mail: Kampik_D@ukw.de

B. Seitz
Department of Ophthalmology, Saarland University Medical Center, Homburg/Saar, Germany

B. Seitz et al. (eds.), *Atlas on Cornea*, https://doi.org/10.1007/978-3-031-65422-0_38

polyneuropathy, and a history of nephropathy [5]. Changes in confocal microscopy even preceded a decrease in corneal sensation. In diabetic patients, break-up time and tear film secretion are decreased but contain elevated glucose levels.

The combination of structural changes of the epithelium, altered tear film, and loss of corneal neurotrophic function can lead to recurrent corneal epithelial defects with prolonged epithelial healing and eventually to neurotrophic ulcers (Fig. 1). Especially after vitrectomy and other ocular surgery, a compromised epithelium is observed. Initial treatment consists of preservative-free lubricants combined with prophylactic antibiotics. If persistent, autologous serum, insulin eye drops and anti-inflammatory agents as well as bandage contact lenses are indicated. Temporal lid closure by tarsorrhapy or botox injection are additional measures. Amniotic membrane transplantation as patch or graft or a combination of both is sometimes the only effective approach for severe conditions.

2.1.2 Graves' Disease

Graves' disease is an autoimmune disease in which autoantibodies cause hyperstimulation of the thyroid gland (hyperthyroidism) by binding to the thyrotropin receptor. 20–50% of cases are combined with thyroid eye disease (TED) where autoantibodies cause an inflammatory reaction mediated by the activation of orbital fibroblasts in the retrobulbar adipose and connective tissue and/or the extraocular muscles [6, 7]. Antibody-triggered inflammation results in an increase in the volume of the orbital soft tissues, resulting in proptosis, lid retraction, and lid lag on downward gaze, possibly with lagophthalmus, diplopia, and in the worst case, compression of the optic nerve (dysthyroid optic neuropathy, DON). TED can occur simultaneously with Graves' disease but can also start several months earlier or later [8]. In mild cases, TED leads to superficial punctate keratitis due to the enlarged palpebral fissure opening and thus reduced tear break-up time (Fig. 2). Superior limbic keratitis can be caused by mechanical irritation by pressure from the globe against the lids [9]. With a higher degree of protrusion, corneal exposure and surface inflammation, the risk of corneal ulcers increases.

Therapeutic options include intensive surface care (lubrication) with moisture chamber dressing at night, alongside thyrostatic drugs to achieve euthyroid status. Smoking cessation is essential as the number of cigarettes per day is

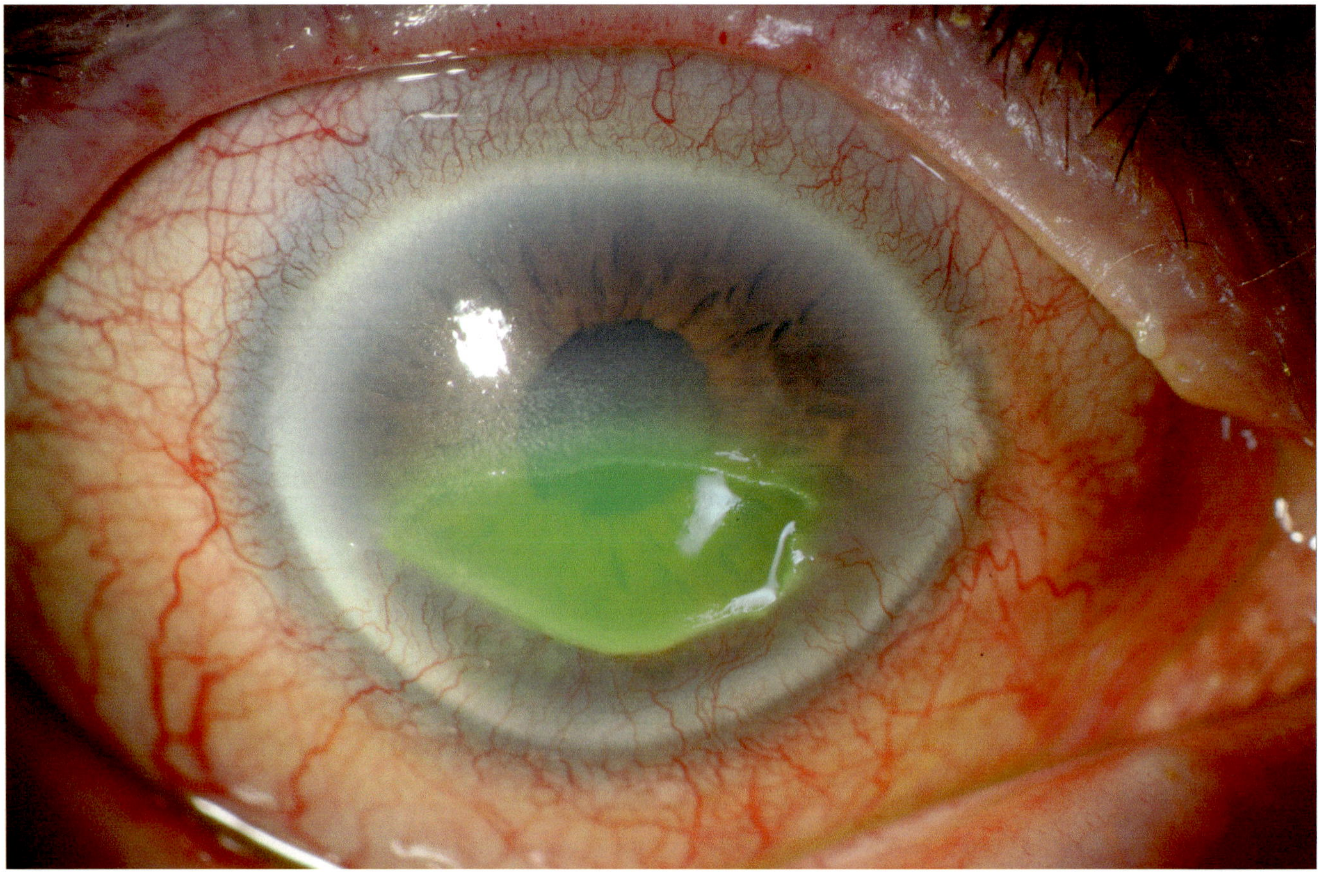

Fig. 1 Neurotrophic keratopathy in a 79-year-old male type II diabetic patient. Note the elevated epithelial borders typical for neurotrophic corneal ulcers, along with superficial neovascularisations

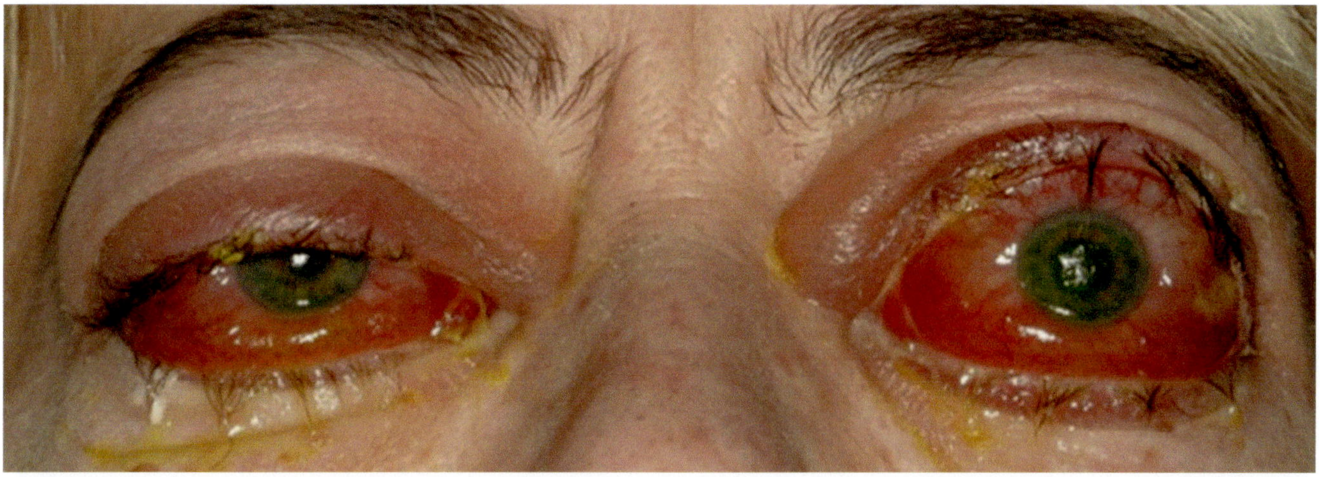

Fig. 2 Proptosis with corneal exposure keratopathy in severe acute thyroid eye disease in a 49-year-old female patient. Orbital decompression of the left eye was planned for the following day

linked to the severity of TED. The intake of selenium is recommended.

For moderate to severe and active TED, high-dose intravenous corticosteroids (intravenous methylprednisolone at cumulative doses of 4.5 g over 3 months) are first-line treatment, in Europe combined with mycophenolate sodium [10].

Second-line therapies include cyclosporine or azathioprine, orbital radiotherapy combined with glucocorticoids, and anti-inflammatory antibodies (teprotumumab—anti-insulin-like growth factor 1 (IGF-1) receptor, rituximab—anti-CD 20, tocilizumab—anti-soluble IL-6 receptor) [11]. Thyroid radiation or surgical thyroidectomy is indicated when euthyroid status is not achieved otherwise. Sight-threatening TED is treated with urgent orbital decompression surgery.

2.1.3 Addison's Disease (Primary Adrenocortical Insufficiency)

Addison's disease is a rare disease characterized by insufficient production of glucocorticoids caused by dysfunction of the adrenal cortex. The production of mineralocorticoids and androgens can also be impaired. The causes can be autoimmune, infectious, neoplastic, or a genetic disorder, but also iatrogenic (pharmacological side effects of prolonged or high-dose corticosteroid therapy). The prevalence of Addison's disease ranges from 100 to 140 per one million.

Cortisol levels are reduced as a result of adrenal hypofunction, leading to increased ACTH production. Typical symptoms include hyperpigmentation of the skin, general weakness and fatigue, weight loss, anorexia, and gastrointestinal complaints. Untreated, it can lead to a life-threatening crisis.

Adrenal hormones can also affect the ocular surface. Cortisol inhibits the release of inflammatory mediators such as cytokines and chemokines [12]. Blepharitis, keratoconjunctivitis, and corneal ulcers can occur [13].

2.1.4 Hyperparathyroidism

Hyperparathyroidism is divided into primary, secondary, and tertiary hyperparathyroidism. In the primary form, the cause of overproduction of parathyroid hormone is in the parathyroid glands themselves, usually as an adenoma (80%) or as primary hyperplasia of the parathyroid glands (about 15%), very rarely due to carcinoma (5%). In the secondary form, a stimulus is present (hypocalcemia), usually triggered by chronic renal failure which results in the increased production of parathyroid hormones. The tertiary form arises from long-standing secondary hyperparathyroidism, and differs from the secondary form by hypercalcemia, due to uncoupling from the intrinsic feedback loop. Hyperparathyroidism may be asymptomatic, but may also manifest with impaired concentration, muscle weakness, generalized pruritus, bone pain, or fractures without adequate trauma [14]. Calcification of soft tissue can occur in a wide variety of body sites, also in the ocular region: uvea, sclera, conjunctiva, and cornea, where it presents as band keratopathy (Fig. 3). The duration of the derailed calcium level seems to play a role: Klaassen-Broekema et al. demonstrated that band keratopathy occurred in 15 of 17 tertiary hyperparathyroidism patients studied over a 6-year observation period [15]. Therapeutic options include vitamin D substitution, calcimimetics, phosphate binders, and in refractory disease, surgical parathyroidectomy [14].

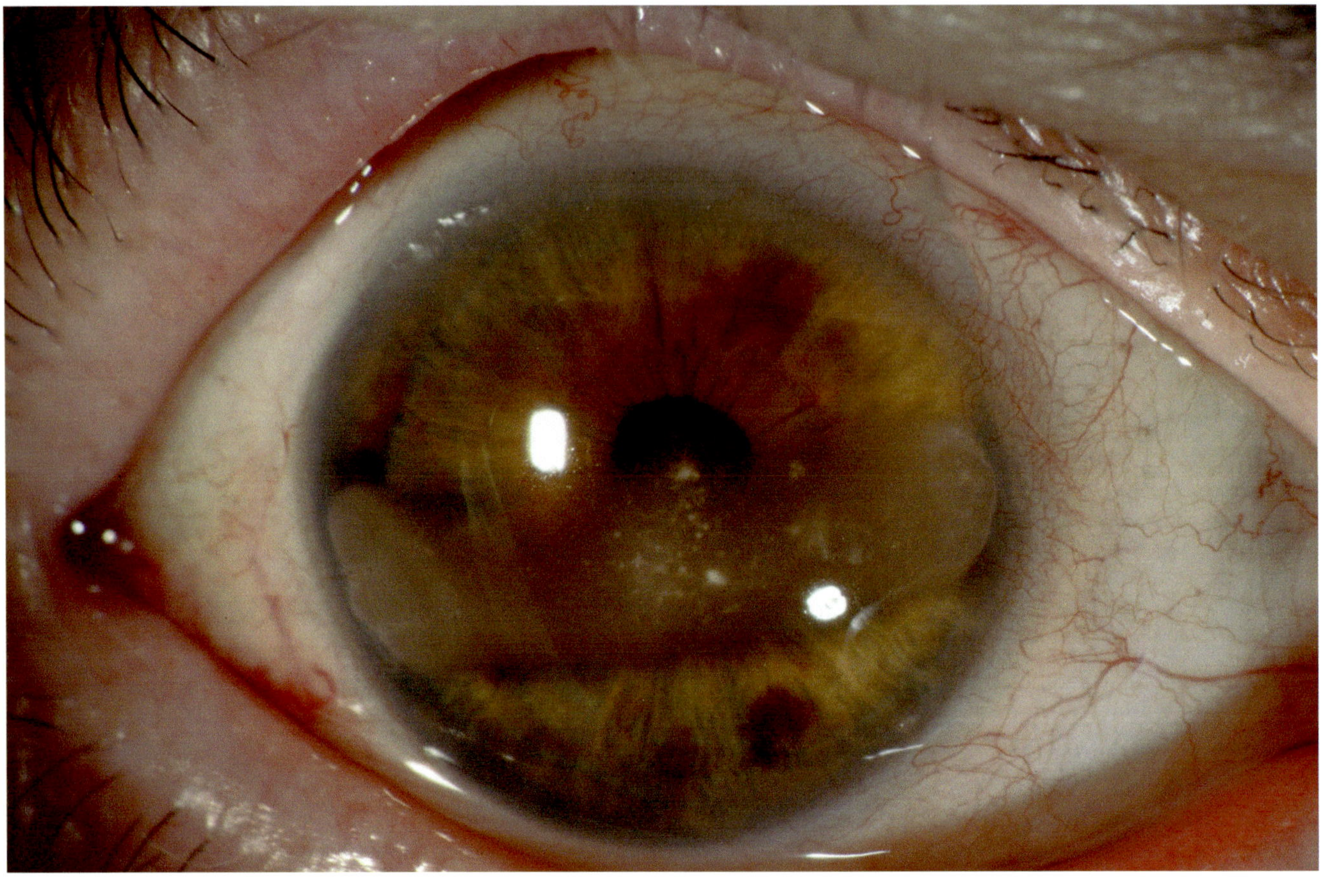

Fig. 3 Band keratopathy can be associated with hypercalcemia due to hyperparathyroidism. Other systemic causes are sarcoidosis, excessive vitamin D uptake, multiple myeloma, and gout

2.2 Metabolic Disorders

2.2.1 Mucopolysaccharidosis

Mucopolysaccharidosis (MPS) is a rare hereditary lysosomal storage disease. A lack or deficiency of lysosomal enzymes causes intra- and extracellular accumulation of glycosaminoglycans (GAG). The disease can be divided into 7 subtypes, all inherited in an autosomal recessive manner, the only exception being type II (Hunter's syndrome), which is inherited in an X-linked manner [16]. Various tissues are affected, including heart valves, arteries, cornea, bones, teeth, liver, cartilage, and the nervous system. The severity of the disease varies depending on its subtype and can lead to death or a very short life expectancy. The disease is associated with a wide variability of symptoms, including neurocognitive dysfunction, respiratory symptoms, middle ear disease and deafness, dental caries, and chronic pain [16–18].

MPS also affects ocular tissues, resulting in glaucoma due to GAG deposition, retinal dysfunction with optic nerve changes, such as disc swelling and optic atrophy, and collagen fibril displacement leading to corneal stromal opacities. The severity of stromal corneal opacities varies between disease types and is associated with varying degrees of visual impairments (Figs. 4 and 5). Current supportive treatment options include bone marrow transplantation and enzyme replacement therapy (ERT) [2, 16, 17, 21]. However, the effect of ERT on the cornea is limited owing to the avascularity of the tissue [22].

2.2.2 Lipidoses (Fabry's Disease, Generalized Gangliosidoses, Multiple Sulfatase Deficiency)

Fabry's disease is an X-linked lysosomal storage disorder. The accumulation of globotriaosylceramide can be caused by more than 965 different mutations that result in reduced or absent α-galactosidase A (GLA) enzyme activity. Even though X-linked, female patients who are heterozygous for GLA mutations can also be affected with variable phenotypes [23].

Accumulation leads to cell, tissue, and organ damage. Patients suffer from progressive renal and cardiovascular dysfunction. Specific systemic complications are

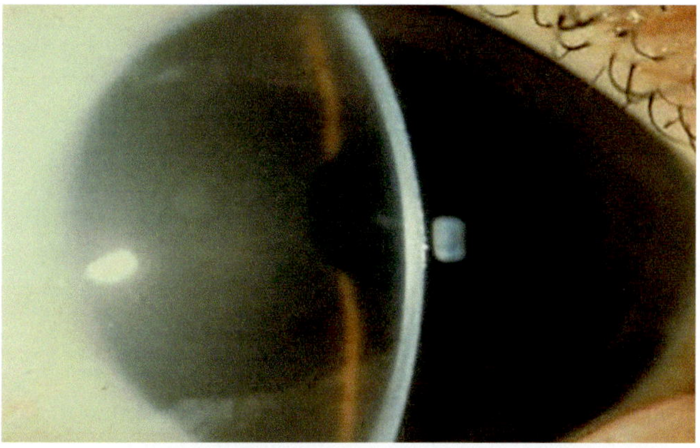

Fig. 4 Mucopolysaccharidosis VI-A (Maroteaux–Lamy syndrome) with diffuse clouding of the corneal stroma (photograph from [19])

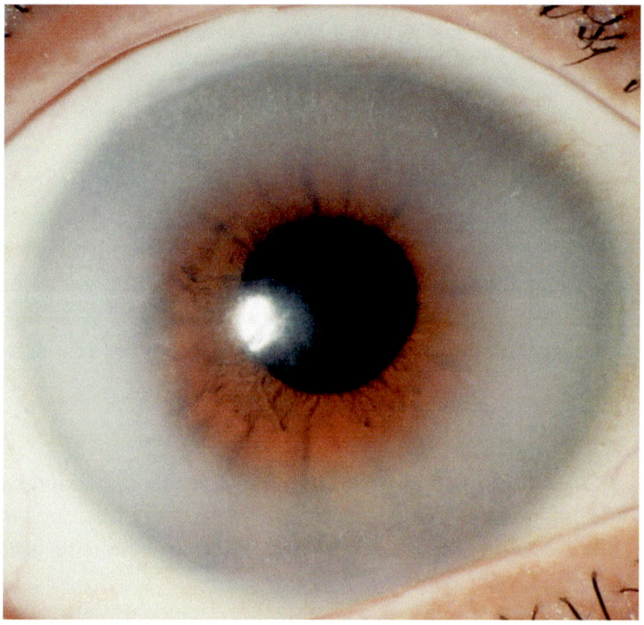

Fig. 5 Mucopolysaccharidosis I-S (Scheie syndrome). Bilateral stromal corneal clouding due to diffuse stromal deposits without a separate lipoid arc (photograph from [20])

angiokeratomas, arrhythmias, and polyneuropathy, including hearing loss, acroparesthesia, and vertigo. Systemic affections, especially ventricular hypertrophy and fibrosis, heart failure, valve disease, angina, and dysrhythmias lead to premature death. Today enzyme replacement therapy is standard of care [23].

There is a substantial delay between symptom onset and diagnosis in male and female patients of about 15 years. Ocular manifestations can be a clue to earlier diagnosis [23, 24]. Previous studies showed an association between ocular findings and more severe disease [25]. The most common ocular sign is cornea verticillata with a prevalence of 42–69% in all age groups (Fig. 6A, B) [25–27]. Other signs are tortuous conjunctival and retinal vessels and posterior spoke-like cataracts [23–25].

2.2.3 Dyslipoproteinemias (Hyper- and Hypolipoproteinemia)

Dyslipoproteinemia does not always cause significant visual impairment in the eye but is important to recognize because it may be associated with an increased risk of other systemic and cardiovascular diseases. A distinction was made between hyperlipoproteinemia and hypolipoproteinemia. Corneal changes occur in both cases.

In hyperlipoproteinemia, the serum levels of lipids and lipoproteins are elevated. This leads to lipid deposition in the limbal cornea and the lid skin. Bilateral corneal arcus and xanthelasmata may develop. Corneal arcus lipoides is usually bilateral [28, 29]. There are five different types of hyperlipoproteinemia [30].

Schnyder's corneal dystrophy (SCD) is also a type of dyslipoproteinemia in which lipids and/or cholesterol are deposited in the cornea [31]. Both corneal arcus and central corneal opacity were observed.

Hypolipoproteinemia is associated with diffuse bilateral corneal opacities. The cause is a deficiency of the enzyme lecithin-cholesterol acyltransferase (LCAT). Hypolipoproteinemia can be divided into three clinical subtypes that manifest in the cornea and are inherited in an autosomal recessive manner: LCAT deficiency, Tangier disease, and fish eye disease [28]. In LCAT deficiency, the corneal findings include a peripheral arcus and nebular opacity in the posterior stroma (Fig. 7) [32]. In fish eye disease, there is a peripherally accentuated dense stromal corneal opacity. In LCAT deficiency and fish eye disease, corneal opacity is usually detected during childhood and adolescence [33]. Tangier disease is characterized by a marked deficiency or absence of HDL. Diffuse dense stromal opacities occur in the cornea, which usually do not affect visual acuity [34].

2.2.4 Wilson's Disease

Wilson's disease (WD) is a hereditary storage disease characterized by a disorder of copper metabolism in the liver. Too little copper is excreted via the bile, so it is deposited in other organs such as the liver or the eye, but also in the brain. WD is inherited in an autosomal recessive manner and often manifests between 5 and 35 years of age with very variable symptoms. Its prevalence is reported to be 1 per 30,000 individuals [35].

Owing to increased copper storage, liver dysfunction up to fulminant liver failure and neuropsychiatric disturbances with movement disorders can occur. In rare cases, the heart and kidneys are affected.

In the cornea, WD manifests with copper deposition in Descemet membrane, resulting in a Kayser–Fleischer ring,

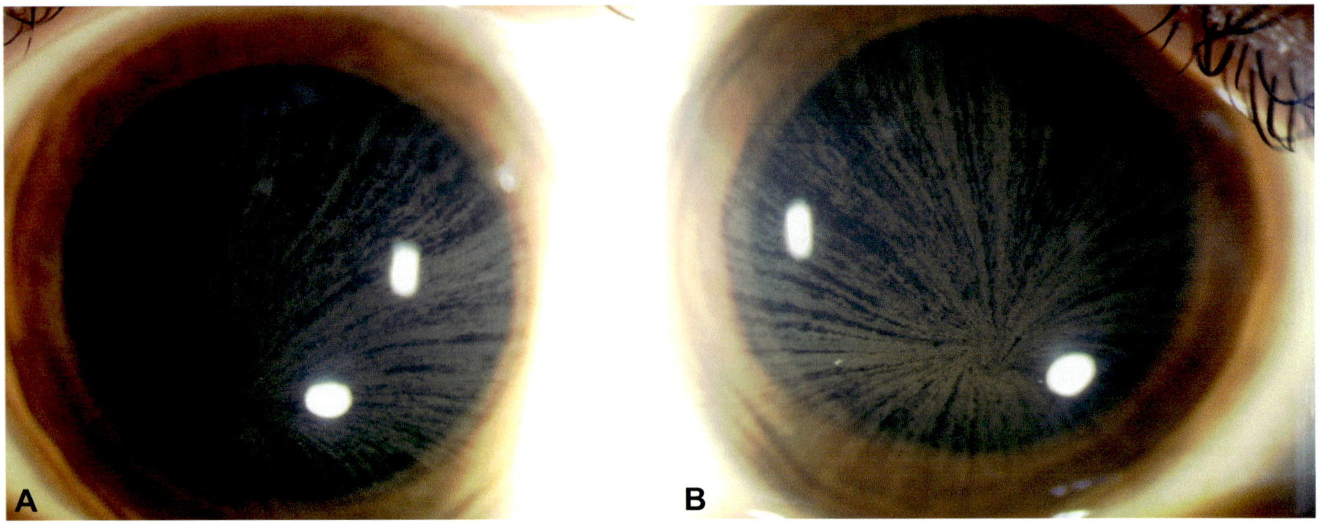

Fig. 6 Cornea verticillata in Fabry's disease. Whorl-like formation of the corneal epithelium in both eyes of this 8-year-old girl led to the diagnosis of Fabry's disease, also in her mother and older brother. DNA sequence analysis of exon 6 of the alpha-galactosidase A gene revealed a causative mutation. (**A**) Left eye (**B**) Right eye

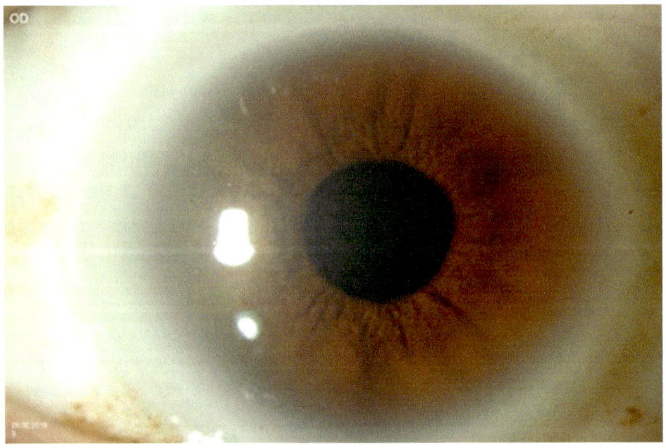

Fig. 7 LCAT deficiency causes a peripheral corneal arcus without clear zone towards the limbus (≠ arcus lipoides) and nebular opacity in the posterior stroma beginning to form during childhood and adolescence

a golden brown to greenish ring in the peripheral cornea (Fig. 8). Copper deposition usually appears in the superior circumference of the cornea, later inferiorly, and in some cases finally forms a ring. Sunflower cataracts may also be present in rare cases [35–38]. Treatment includes a copper-sparing diet and penicillamine to chelate copper from the body.

2.2.5 Amyloidosis

Amyloidosis comprises a group of diseases characterized by abnormal protein folding, leading to the extracellular deposition and accumulation of insoluble fibrils in various tissues. One of the most common systemic forms of amyloidosis is transthyretin amyloidosis (ATTRv), which presents with both systemic and ocular manifestation. Alterations in gelsolin also lead to systemic amyloidosis with ocular manifestations, while alterations in keratoepithelin and lactoferrin

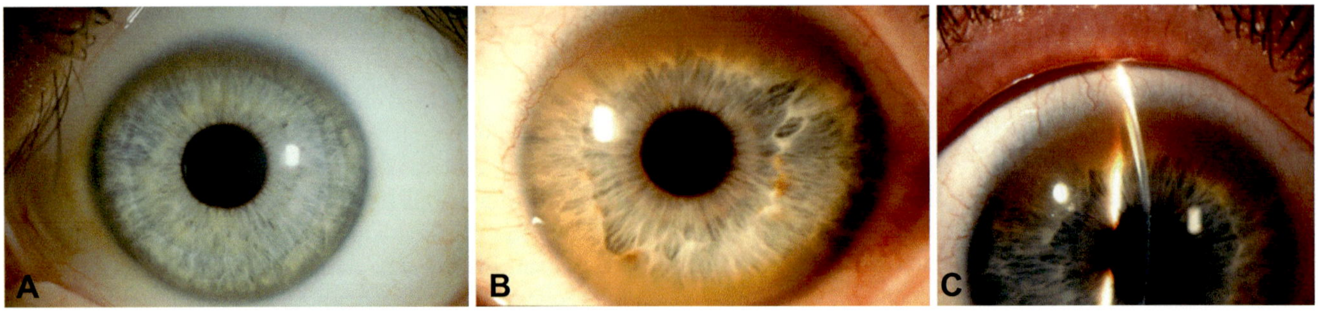

Fig. 8 Kayser–Fleischer peripheral corneal ring in patients with Wilson's disease due to copper deposition in Descemet membrane. (**A**) Early stages often spare the palpebral fissure. (**B**, **C**) Late stage. Slit lamp microscopy reveals the location in Descemet membrane. Treatment with penicillamine can lead to regression

only show isolated ocular manifestations [39]. Diagnosis is made by detecting amyloid deposits in a tissue sample, by in vivo corneal confocal microscopy, or by genetic analysis. Amyloid aggregates can affect all ocular tissues, including the conjunctiva, cornea (Fig. 9), anterior chamber angle, iris, lens capsule, vitreous body, and retina. Clinical signs include corneal or vitreous opacities and, in some cases, open angle glaucoma. In the cornea, reduced density of the nerve plexus can be observed in certain forms of amyloidosis. This can result in neurotrophic keratopathy, dry eye syndrome, and corneal ulcers.

In hereditary gelsolin amyloidosis (AGel), also known as Meretoja syndrome, bilateral lattice corneal dystrophy (originally called lattice corneal "dystrophy" type 2; LCD2) occurs with dry eye syndrome, recurrent erosions, and reduction in visual acuity [31, 40, 41]. Lattice-like corneal opacities are mainly located in the periphery of the middle and anterior corneal stroma (Fig. 10). AGel is inherited in an autosomal dominant manner and associated with the typical triad of slowly progressive ophthalmological, neurological (cranial neuropathy), and dermatological (cutis laxa) manifestations. There is no causal therapy to date [41]. In ATTRv, liver transplantation is often necessary and gene therapies may play an increasingly important role in the future [39].

Amyloidoses associated with disorders of the conformation of lactoferrin (ALac) and keratoepithelin are also associated with various forms of hereditary corneal dystrophy, such as gelatinous drop-like dystrophy [42, 43].

Symptomatic therapy consists of the application of lubricant eye drops and topical cyclosporine in dry eye syndrome. Phototherapeutic keratectomy or even penetrating keratoplasty is indicated in advanced pathologies or perforated corneal ulcer as a secondary complication [2, 39, 41, 44]. Secondary amyloidosis without a hereditary component can occur in the context of chronic inflammatory, degenerative, or neoplastic diseases [39]. In this case, there is no corneal manifestation.

2.2.6 Cystinosis

Crystalline, gold-dust deposition of cystine in the cornea is a feature of cystinosis, an autosomal-recessive lysosomal storage disease [45]. A defect in the CTNS gene leads to cysteine accumulation in various tissues, especially the kidney, and eye, including the conjunctiva, iris, choroid, retinal pigment epithelium, and optic nerve. While

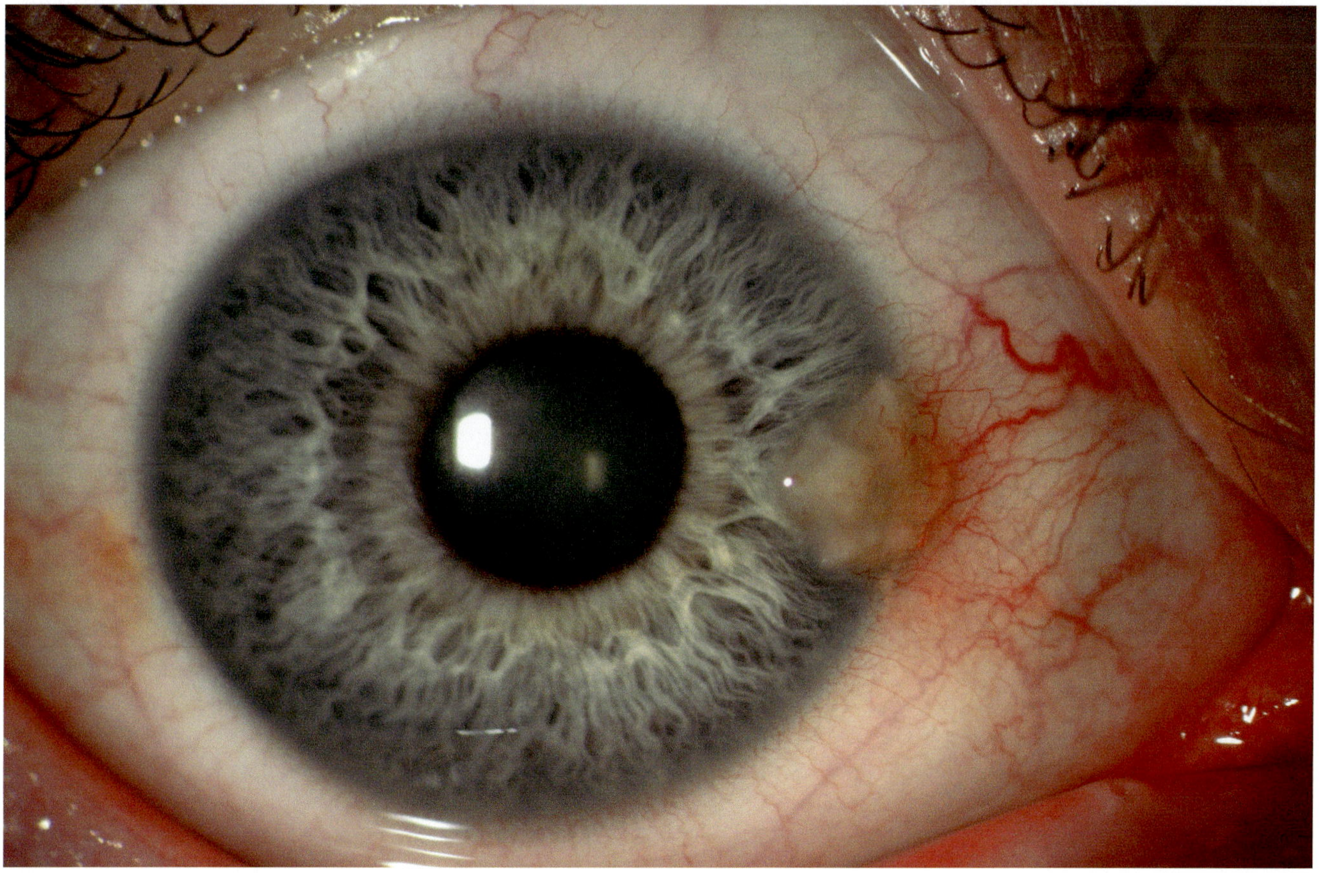

Fig. 9 Secondary amyloidosis at the limbus. Histology (congo red stain) revealed amyloid deposits originating from the conjunctiva and spreading onto the cornea

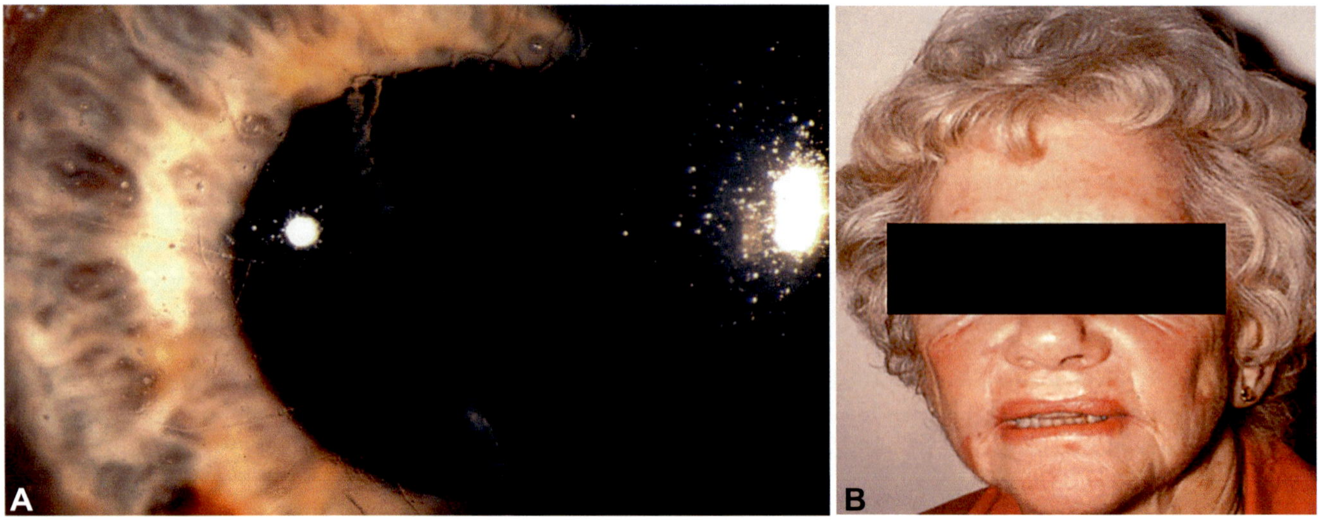

Fig. 10 (**A**) Corneal lattice lines caused by amyloid deposits in the middle and anterior corneal stroma in a patient with hereditary gelsolin amyloidosis (Meretoja syndrome). (**B**) Typical facies is caused by loss of skin elasticity

nephropathic cystinosis has an early onset in newborn or adolescent patients and presents severe manifestations, non-nephropathic cystinosis occurs in adulthood and can even be asymptomatic (Fig. 11).

Initially asymptomatic, corneal deposits can lead to photophobia, blepharospasm, and visual impairment in the first two decades of life. Recurrent erosions, pannus formation, peripheral corneal neovascularization, and limbus stem cell deficiency can follow.

Systemic cysteamine is the standard therapy, alongside cysteamine eye drops, which may dissolve corneal cystine crystals unless a band keratopathy, pannus, or scars have formed. In this case, penetrating corneal transplantation is necessary.

2.3 Nutritional Disorders: Vitamin A Deficiency

Currently, vitamin A deficiency mostly affects people in developing countries and remains a common cause of blindness. Here, it results from the lack of dietary intake of vitamin A. Approximately 140 million children worldwide are still deficient in vitamin A, leading to blindness in about 250,000–500,000 children per year. It is the second most common form of nutritional disorder and the world's leading preventable cause of childhood blindness. In developed countries, vitamin A deficiency is rare and occurs mainly in people with severe malnutrition, gastrointestinal diseases that impair nutrient absorption, or liver diseases.

Vitamin A is essential for the human body and is important for cell differentiation and proliferation. It is an irreplaceable component in the visual circle and gene transcription [44]. Ocular manifestations (xerophthalmia) begin with different stages of night blindness as early symptoms, due to reduced production of the visual pigment rhodopsin. Later stages include conjunctival xerosis, Bitot's spots, corneal xerosis, ulceration, and colliquative necrosis (keratomalacia) (Fig. 12). Retinal dysfunction may also occur [46, 47]. Conjunctival xerosis occurs with the loss of goblet cells, metaplasia in conjunctival epithelial cells, and the formation of a metaplastic, keratinized surface [48]. The conjunctiva appears dry and dull [49]. Bitot's spots are slightly raised whitish foamy lesions that occur mainly on the limbal temporal bulbar conjunctiva, but also on the cornea, resulting from clumps of keratin that develop during conjunctival metaplasia. Bitot's spots contain saprophytic bacteria and can be easily scraped off but form again quickly. Under therapy, they usually disappear within 2 weeks without scarring but can also persist in some cases. They are most common in children with vitamin A deficiencies [46, 50].

The cornea may show superficial punctate keratitis with fluorescein staining in the context of conjunctival goblet cell dysfunction and reduced tear production. This results in the progressive drying of the cornea. In some cases, microcysts are observed in the early stages. In later stages, generalized edema, a dull, dry surface, and usually sharply demarcated corneal ulcers may develop [46, 48–50]. In severe cases, keratomalacia with deep corneal necrosis, which may involve the entire cornea, corneal melting, and

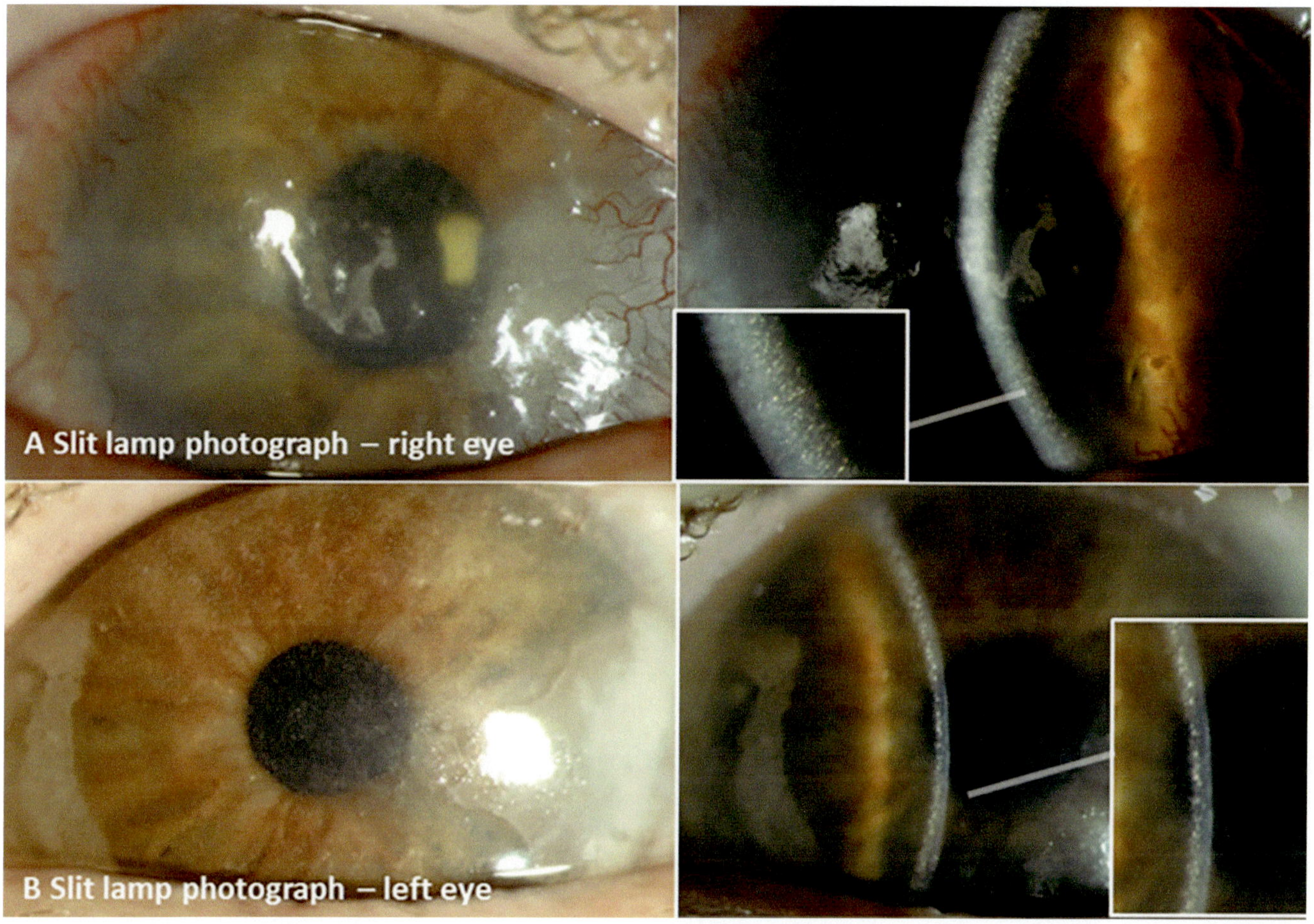

Fig. 11 Corneal findings in a thirty-one-year-old male patient with nephropathic cystinosis. (**A**) Right eye, cystine crystal deposition, central avascular pannus formation, peripheral corneal neovascularization, limbus stem cell deficiency. (**B**) Left eye, cystine crystal deposition, superficial limbal calcifications. Figure from [45]

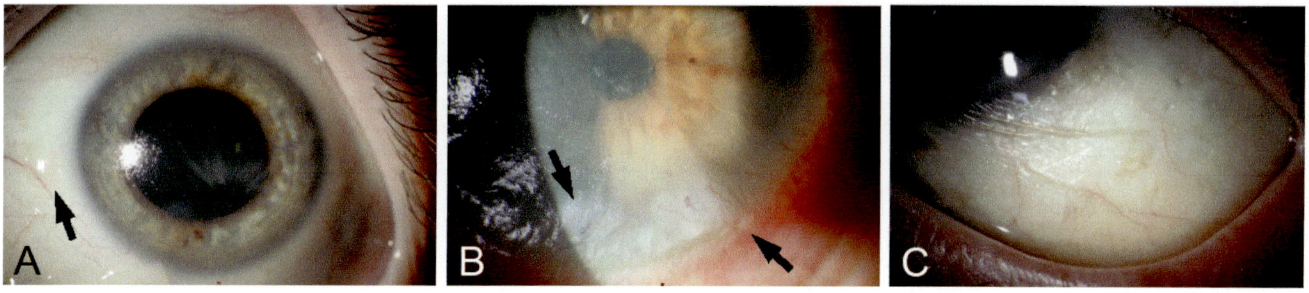

Fig. 12 Corneal stromal opacities in severe vitamin A deficiency due to hepatic dysfunction. (**A**) Bitot's spot forming at the nasal conjunctiva (arrow). (**B**) Limbal infiltrates (arrows). (**C**) The leathery aspect of the conjunctiva is pathognomonic

perforation can occur. Corneal scars, anterior staphylomas, and phthisis bulbi may result.

Xerophthalmia should be treated quickly with vitamin A supplementation. When treated, night blindness resolves within 24–48 h, and corneal xerosis resolves within 2–3 weeks. Late effects such as corneal scars can persist, particularly in the case of corneal ulcers and keratomalacia [46].

2.4 Hematologic Disorders

2.4.1 Graft-Versus-Host Disease

Allogenic hematopoietic stem cell transplantation can provoke an overactive immune reaction of the grafted immune system against host antigens. While this can be a welcome action against remaining leukemia or tumor cells to reduce the risk of relapse (graft-versus-leukemia effect), it can also lead to the destruction of host tissues (graft-versus-host disease, GVHD). Acute GVHD affects the skin, lungs, liver, and the gastrointestinal epithelium. Chronic GVHD, which occurs in over 70% of transplanted patients, can spread to any organ system: musculoskeletal systems, lymphohematopoietic systems, hepatobiliary system, oral mucosa, genitalia, and the eye [51]. Ocular involvement is very common in chronic GVHD (30–85%) and may even be the first sign of GVHD. Dry eye disease is the first and most common manifestation due to infiltration of the lacrimal gland, meibomian glands, and ocular surface by alloreactive T lymphocytes, eliciting a cellular and humoral immune reaction. This can progress to corneal infections and ulcers, corneal and conjunctival fibrosis, corneal neovascularization, neurotrophic keratopathy, and eventually perforation (Fig. 13).

In mild forms, topical steroids, cyclosporine and supportive lubricant therapy for dry eye are effective. Punctal occlusion and bandage contact lenses can help. In moderate to severe forms, systemic immunosuppression with corticosteroids is indicated, but dose and duration must be balanced with the desired effects of a graft-versus-leukemia reaction. Close coordination with the hematologist is essential. Surgical management with amniotic membrane grafting and patching can be necessary in severe cases with ulcers or perforation.

2.4.2 Multiple Myeloma

In multiple myeloma (plasma cell myeloma), abnormal clonal proliferation of plasma cells results in excessive production of immunoglobulins. This can result in hyperviscosity retinopathy, retinal microaneurysms, or retinal detachment. Neoplastic cell masses can infiltrate primarily the bones and skull, but also nearly any other organ.

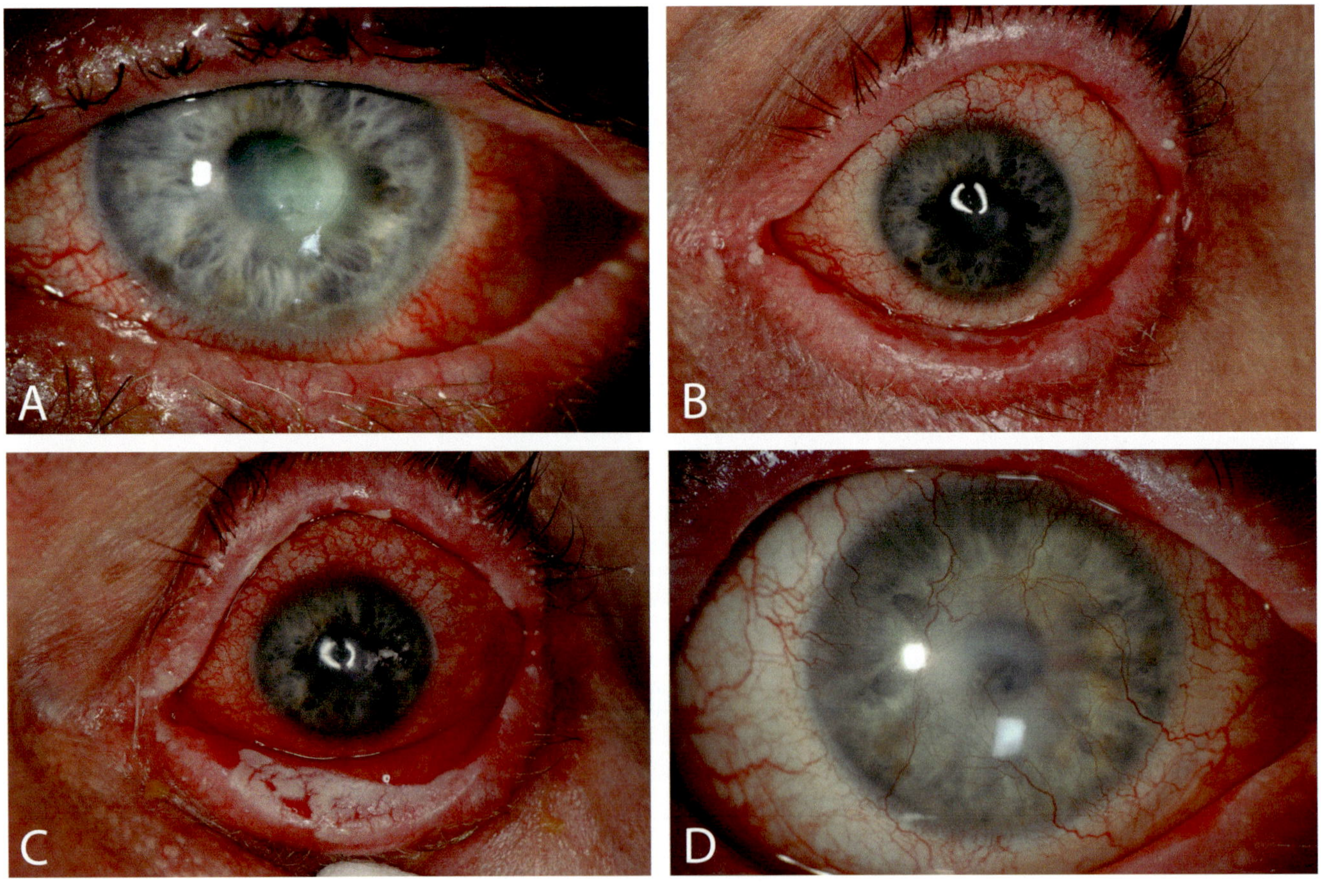

Fig. 13 Ocular graft versus host disease two years after allogeneic stem cell transplantation for chronic lymphocytic leukemia. (**A**) Sterile corneal ulcer, which later perforated, caused by severe tear film insufficiency and meibomian gland disease. (**B**, **C**) Lid margins keratinized over 6 weeks (same eye as (**A**)) despite topical and systemic anti-inflammatory treatment. (**D**) Chronic ocular GvHD shows a vascularized cornea with stromal fibrosis and thinning

Infiltration of the orbit can cause proptosis. In the cornea, subepithelial amorphous crystalline deposits can occur, causing little vision loss but in some cases require corneal transplantation.

2.4.3 MGUS

A precursor of multiple myeloma, monoclonal gammopathy of undetermined significance (MGUS), can lead to paraproteinemic keratopathy where monoclonal protein produced by abnormal plasma cells can deposit in the corneal stroma. The resulting opacities can present in various patterns mimicking corneal stromal dystrophies like Schnyder corneal dystrophy, pre-Descemet, lattice, or granular corneal dystrophy, but also resemble an arcus lipoides or Salzmann nodules (Fig. 14) [52].

2.5 Systemic Infections

2.5.1 Tuberculosis

Tuberculosis is the leading infectious cause of morbidity and mortality worldwide [53]. Systemic infection with *Mycobacterium tuberculosis* affects the lungs in 80% of the patients, while the remaining 20% experience affection of other organs including the eye. Ocular manifestations are most commonly granulomatous uveitis, but also conjunctivitis, scleritis, and episcleritis [53]. In the cornea, infiltrates, ulceration, phlyctenules, and interstitial keratitis can manifest, due to a hypersensitivity against antigens on *Mycobacterium tuberculosis* (Fig. 15) [54].

Treatment includes systemic antibiotic therapy over 6 months and topical steroids.

2.5.2 Lyme Borreliosis

Lyme disease is an infectious illness caused by the spirochete bacterium *Borrelia burgdorferi*. The infection is transmitted to humans through the saliva of ticks. Subsequently, the organisms infiltrate the skin, internal organs, and musculoskeletal system via the lymphatic and hematologic systems. The disease progresses through three stages. The first stage involves localized infection with erythema migrans, the second stage entails disseminated infection with systemic spread to the skin, joints, musculoskeletal system, central nervous system, and other internal

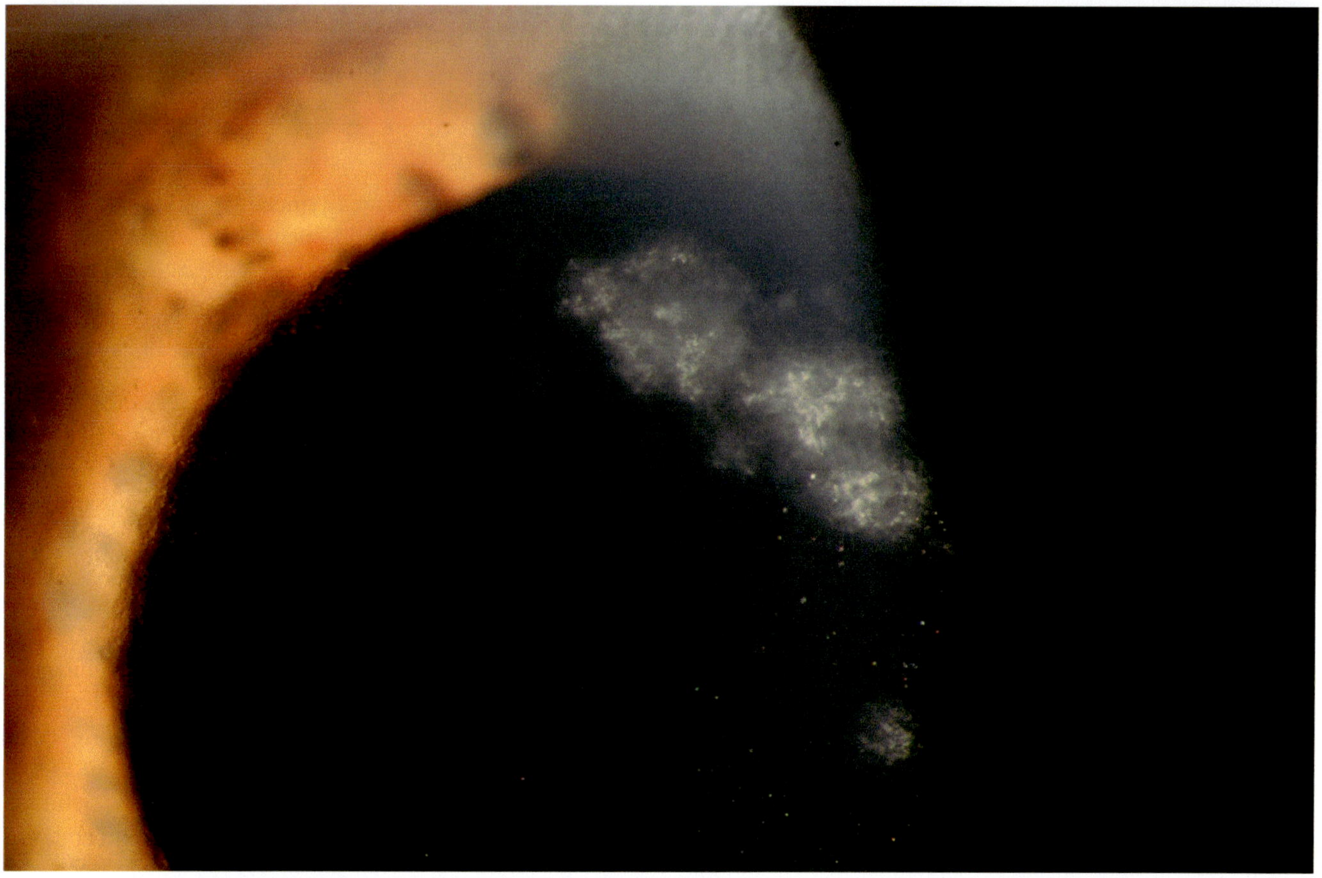

Fig. 14 Superficial crystalline deposits caused by abnormal plasma cells in MGUS (monoclonal gammopathy of undetermined significance), in this case resembling Salzmann nodules

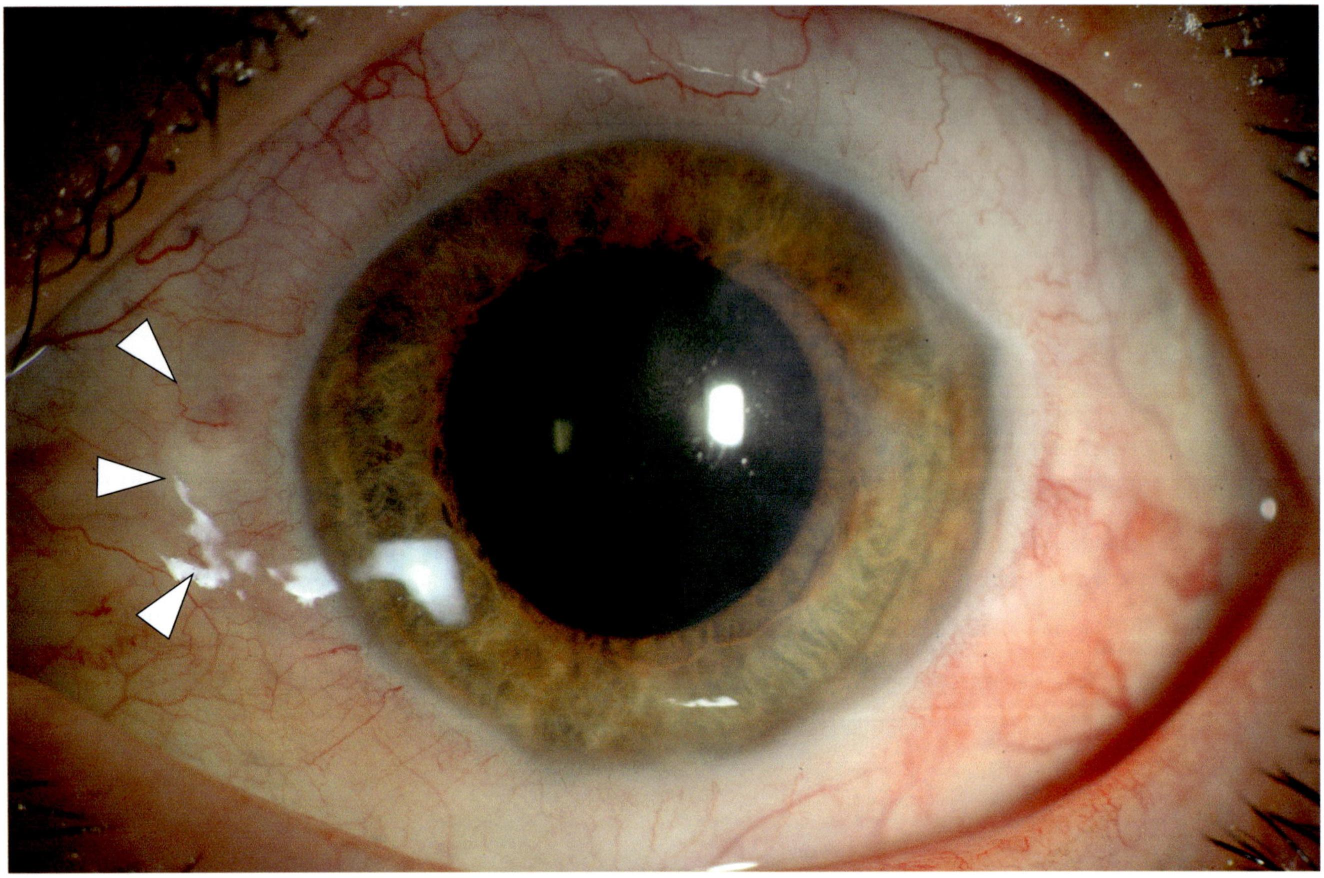

Fig. 15 Gelatinous conjunctival lesions along the limbus (arrowheads) combined with conjunctivitis can be a primary manifestation of tuberculosis even though no other organs are symptomatic

organs including the heart, while the third stage encompasses persistent or progressive infection, often presenting as oligoarthritis of the large joints months after the initial infection [55, 56].

Ocular involvement can occur in all these stages, with ocular manifestations typically observed in the second and third stages, irrespective of whether the site of infection was in direct proximity to the eye [57]. Follicular, unilateral, or bilateral conjunctivitis, interstitial or ulcerative keratitis, scleritis, or episcleritis (very rare), as well as uveitis (most frequently intermediate and pars planitis), may arise (Fig. 16). Retinal involvement with macular edema and vasculitis can also occur. An early form of neuroborreliosis may manifest as double vision, visual impairment, optic nerve neuritis, or cranial nerve palsies (mostly VI or VII) [57–59]. Classic symptoms of ocular manifestations of Lyme disease include photophobia and severe periodic ocular pain [60].

Diagnosis relies on a combination of symptoms and serologic tests, detecting IgM in the early stage or high titers of IgG in later phases. Treatment involves systemic administration of antibiotics typically for 2–4 weeks, such as doxycycline, amoxicillin, penicillin, cefuroxime, ceftriaxone, and azithromycin, along with anti-inflammatory drugs [61].

2.5.3 Syphilis

Syphilis is a sexually transmitted disease caused by the spirochete Treponema pallidum, but also transmission in utero or during delivery is possible. Congenital and less frequent, late acquired syphilis can lead to syphilitic keratitis, a non-ulcerative interstitial keratitis affecting the deeper stroma, often beginning at the superior cornea. Appearance can be variable from one localized infiltrate to multiple nummular infiltrates, attracting corneal superficial and deep neovascularization. New vessels can eventually form a pannus covering the cornea. Descemet folds with stromal edema and microcystic epithelial edema can occur resembling disciform (Herpes simplex) keratitis. Serologic tests are crucial to confirm diagnosis. Treatment with systemic antibiotics (penicillin) is given over three weeks, accompanied by highly dosed topical corticosteroids to reduce inflammation.

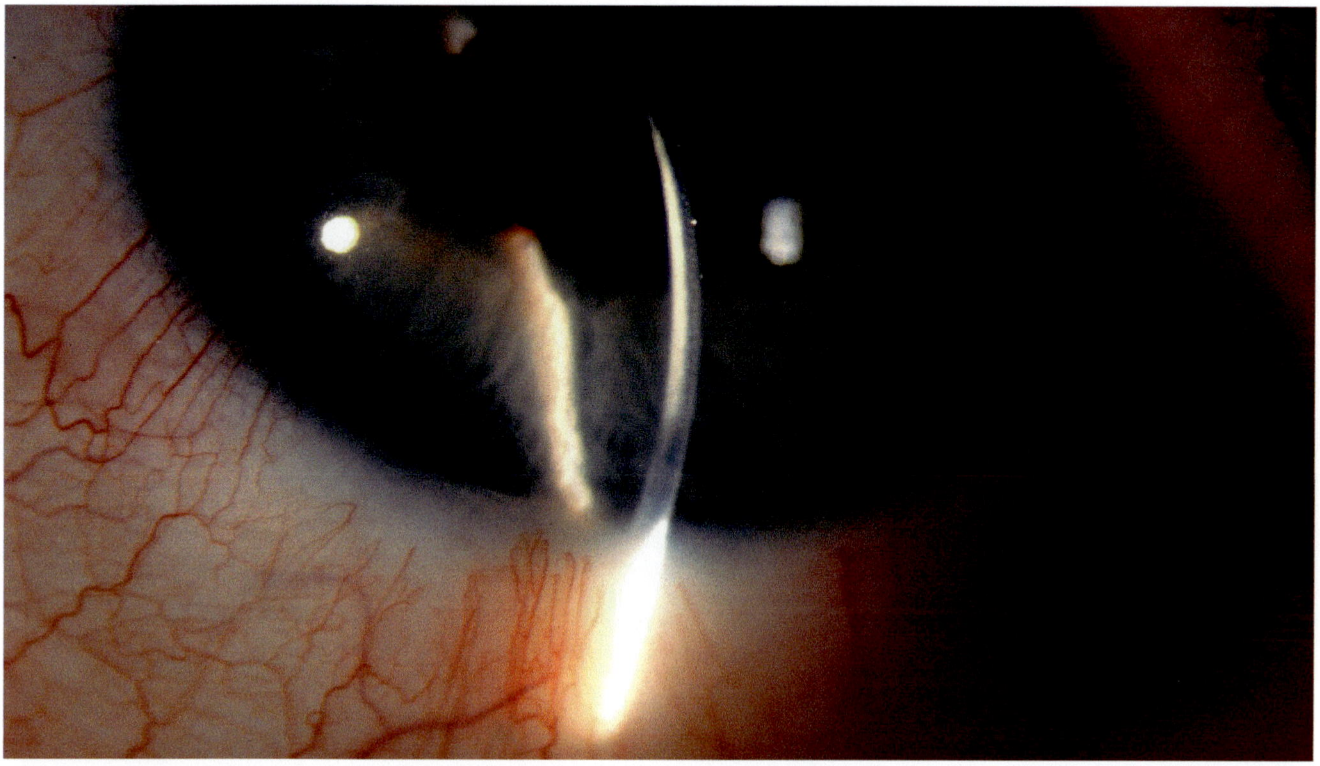

Fig. 16 Focal interstitial keratitis accompanied by follicular conjunctivitis caused by Lyme borreliosis

2.6 Skeletal and Connective Tissue Disorders

2.6.1 Ehlers–Danlos Syndrome

Ehlers–Danlos Syndrome is a rare, genetically variable, heterogeneous group of thirteen connective tissue disorders with multi-organ system involvement [62]. The syndrome is caused by pathogenic variants in many different genes, in particular in various collagen genes, mainly encoding fibrillar collagens, collagen-modifying proteins, or processing enzymes. The main criteria for suspected Ehlers–Danlos syndrome are hyperextensibility of the skin, atrophic scars, and generalized joint hypermobility. Secondary criteria include additional epicanthal folds, generalized joint hypermobility complications, an affected first-degree relative, and mucocutaneous signs such as easy bruising, molluscoid pseudotumors, inguinal, umbilical, and incisional hernia, skin fragility, and soft, doughy skin [63, 64].

Eye involvement varies in the different types. Typical manifestations are eyelid abnormalities like floppy eyelids, infraorbital creases, abnormally slanted palpebral fissures, and ptosis, telecanthus, or hypotelorism. The orbit can show blue sclerae, severe conjunctivochalasis, and xeropthalmia. Patients with craniofacial abnormalities can exhibit double vision, reduced acuity, or stereopsis. In addition, convergence insufficiency is seen [62].

Typically, corneal abnormalities are abnormal corneal thinning and steepness. Myopia, astigmatism, and dry eye disease are common affections [62]. There is an association with brittle cornea syndrome. Due to the abnormal corneal structure, rupture can occur as a result of harmless trauma or spontaneously [65]. Small lens opacities have also been reported in hypermobile Ehlers–Danlos syndrome. In other types, increased lens curvature and lens dislocation are seen [62].

Various but rare vascular complications are known, which can also have significant visual manifestations. In some cases, there is an increased risk of aneurysms. The risk of cervical artery dissection is increased and may lead to ischemia with multiple symptoms such as diplopia, blurred vision, nystagmus, Horner's syndrome, and visual field defects [62, 64].

2.6.2 Marfan Syndrome

Marfan syndrome is an autosomal dominant genetic disorder caused by mutations in the fibrillin-1 gene. Acute aortic dissection is the most common cause of death. There is an increased concentration of TGF-β in the extracellular matrix and degradation of elastin fibers via inflammatory processes. Severe tissue weakness occurs in childhood or adolescence. The aorta, the heart, the eyes, and the skeleton are particularly affected.

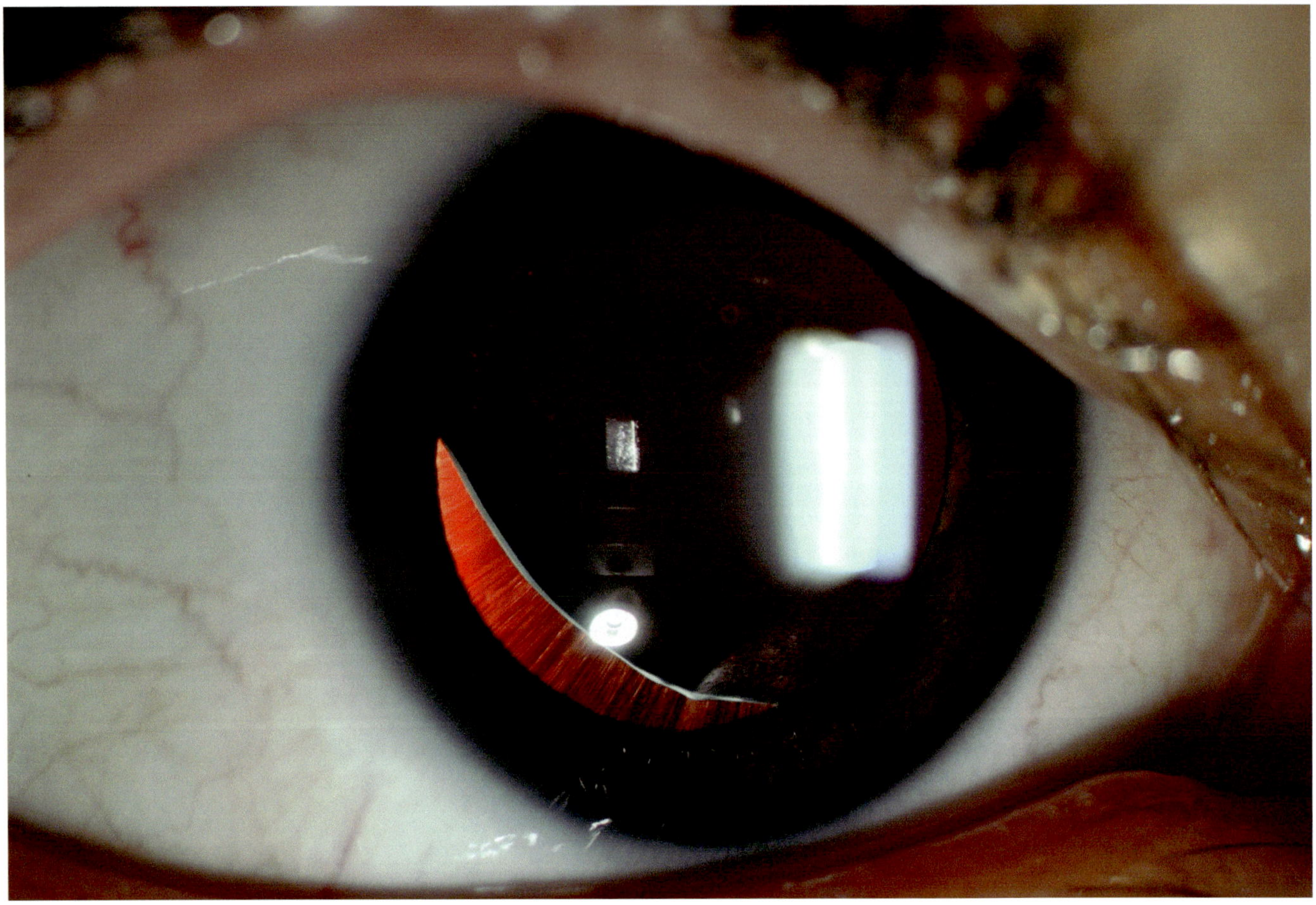

Fig. 17 Ectopia lentis in a patient with Marfan syndrome. The typically flatter corneal curvature and reduced corneal thickness are usually not noticed upon slitlamp examination

Iris transillumination defects, myopia, and ectopia lentis are typical ocular findings in Marfan syndrome (Fig. 17). Megalocornea is also characteristic, but most corneas have normal size with flatter curvature, reduced central corneal thickness, and greater corneal astigmatism. Often, intraocular pressure is measured lower in Marfan syndrome eyes [66].

2.6.3 Goldenhar Syndrome

Goldenhar syndrome or oculo-auriculo-vertebral syndrome is a facio-auriculo-vertebral dysplasia characterized by the triad epibulbar dermoid, accessory auricular appendages, and aural fistula (Fig. 18). Its etiology is not fully understood, but multiple intrauterine risk factors have been identified, such as drugs, maternal diabetes, malnutrition, and smoking.

2.7 Dermatologic Genetic Disorders

2.7.1 Nevoid Basal Cell Carcinoma Syndrome (Gorlin–Goltz Syndrome)

Nevoid basal cell carcinoma syndrome, also called Gorlin–Goltz syndrome, is an autosomal dominant disorder characterized by a predisposition to basal cell carcinomas (BCC), keratocystic odontogenic tumors, and rib abnormalities. BCCs typically present before the age of 30, and commonly affect the lids and periorbital region. Tumors or their scars after surgical removal often damage the cornea and the ocular surface (Fig. 19). In addition to tumors, other skin abnormalities such as milia, epidermoid cysts, chalazia, comedones, and palmar and plantar pits are common [67, 68]. Other neoplasms were described: medulloblastoma, meningioma, ovarian fibroma, ovarian fibrosarcoma,

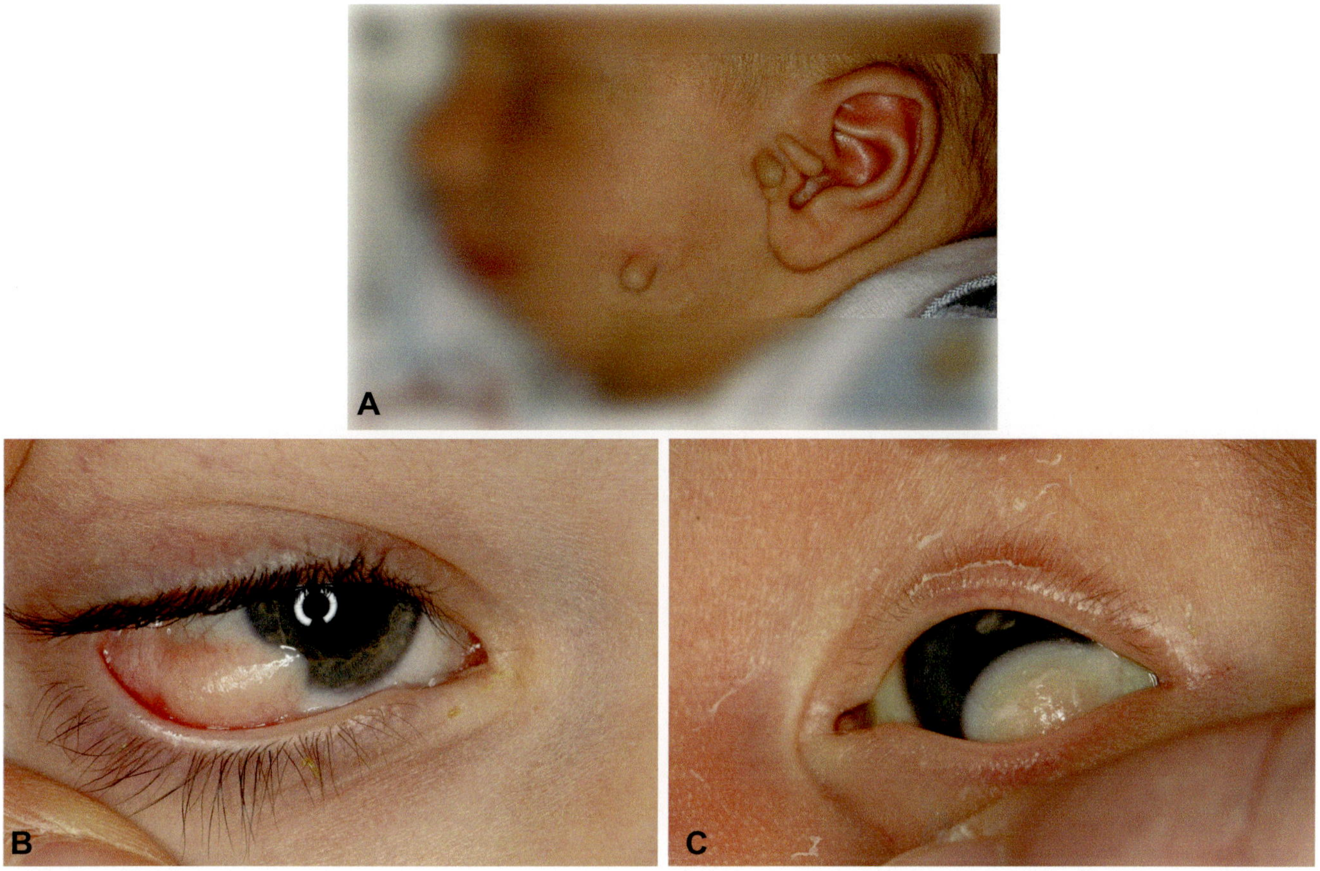

Fig. 18 Goldenhar syndrome in an infant male. (**A**) Typical auricular appendages. (**B**) Right and (**C**) left eye with asymmetric solid limbal dermoid (=choristoma)

fibrosarcoma of the jaws, cardiac fibroma, fetal rhabdomyoma, and lymphatic or chylous cysts of the mesentery. The most frequent mutation is mapped to chromosome 9q22.3 and causes a dysfunction of the hedgehog pathway [69].

First-line treatment is complete surgical excision. Superficial BCC can be addressed by topical therapies (5% imiquimod, 5% fluorouracil), while hedgehog inhibitors like vismodegib or sonidegib are reserved for locally advanced and metastatic BCC [70].

2.7.2 Xeroderma Pigmentosum

Mutations in genes encoding DNA repairing enzymes cause Xeroderma pigmentosum, an autosomal dominant inherited disease characterized by photosensitivity leading to severe burns after minimal sun exposure, and increased incidence of skin malignancies [71]. Early diagnosis of the disease is important to initiate protective measures like avoidance of UV radiation, sun protection with clothes, sunglasses and hats, and application of sunscreen lotions [72]. Strict adherence to these measurements can prevent skin lesions.

Corneal swelling with haze is typical in xeroderma pigmentosum patients, some corneas show vascularisation and scarring. Histologically, all layers of the cornea are affected. Intraepithelial edema, subepithelial bullae, subepithelial fibrosis, and pannus formation can be detected [73]. Partly destruction or complete absence of Bowman layer, but also thickening with fibrosis is possible. Stromal changes include irregular arrangement of collagen lamellae, neovascularisation, and loss of keratocytic nuclei. Descemet membrane was thickened, and endothelial cell density was severely reduced [73].

A compromised endothelial function seems to be a major driver for visual loss, accounting for stromal and epithelial edema, and anterior lamellar keratoplasty is therefore not sufficient for visual rehabilitation.

2.8 Autoimmune/Inflammatory Diseases

2.8.1 Rheumatoid Arthritis

The most common cause of peripheral ulcerative keratitis (PUK) is rheumatoid arthritis (RA), an autoimmune disorder manifesting primarily in the joints, especially of the hands and wrists. Systemic inflammation may affect multiple organs. In the eye, besides corneal ulcers (Fig. 20), keratoconjunctivitis sicca due to lacrimal gland destruction

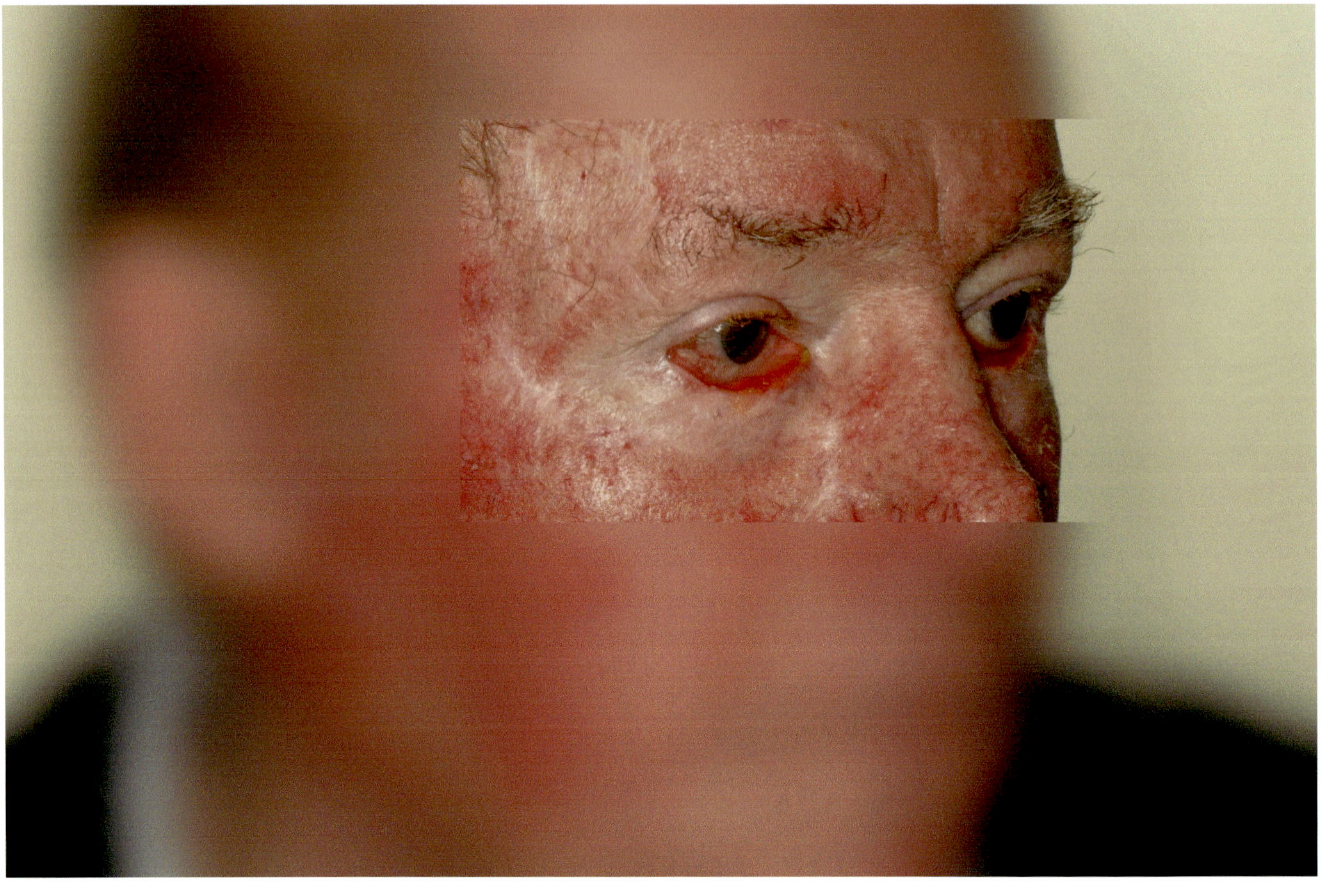

Fig. 19 Multiple basal cell carcinomas and their scars after excision in a 79-year-old patient with Gorlin–Goltz syndrome. Periocular basal cell carcinomas occur in most patients, causing damage to the cornea and ocular surface

(secondary Sjögren's syndrome), uveitis, scleritis, and episcleritis can occur.

Anti-citrullinated protein antibodies (ACPA) and rheumatoid factor are specific markers that help diagnose RA before joint affection is evident. Sufficient systemic treatment is essential for the control of ocular, especially corneal complications. Disease-modifying antirheumatic drugs (DMARDs) like methotrexate, sulfasalazine, hydroxychloroquine, or biologicals against TNF-α or CD20 are the primary treatment. Systemic glucocorticoids can be used to dampen acute flare-up of inflammation especially in vision-threatening complications like PUK. Sufficient and long-term systemic immunosuppression is not only effective in preventing relapses of ocular complications but also lowers mortality [74].

2.8.2 Sjögren's Syndrome

In primary Sjögren's syndrome, lymphocytic cells infiltrate the salivary and lacrimal glands, causing dry mouth and dry eyes. Patients show typical signs and symptoms of keratoconjunctivitis sicca ranging from discomfort to limbal stem cell deficiency, corneal ulcers, and perforation. Up to 5% of patients develop a non-Hodgkin lymphoma of the B-cell series. Serologic markers are antinuclear auto-antibodies anti-Ro/SSA and anti-La/SSB. Secondary Sjögren's syndrome arises in the context of another autoimmune disease, such as systemic lupus erythematodes, rheumatoid arthritis, and progressive systemic sclerosis.

No specific curative therapy is known. Topical tear substitutes, punctal occlusion, and anti-inflammatory eye drops including steroids, cyclosporin, and serum eye drops help alleviate dry eye symptoms and improve quality of life.

2.8.3 Granulomatosis with Polyangiitis

Peripheral ulcerative keratitis (PUK) is the most common corneal manifestation of granulomatosis with polyangiitis (GPA, previously known as Wegener Granulomatosis) [75]. GPA is a rare multi-system autoimmune disorder characterized by a granulomatous necrotizing vasculitis with occlusion of small- and medium-sized vessels. Affected regions besides the orbit are respiratory tract (granuloma formation) and kidneys (glomerulonephritis). PUK in GPA is often accompanied by scleritis and conjunctivitis, but isolated peripheral corneal thinning or keratitis without ulceration

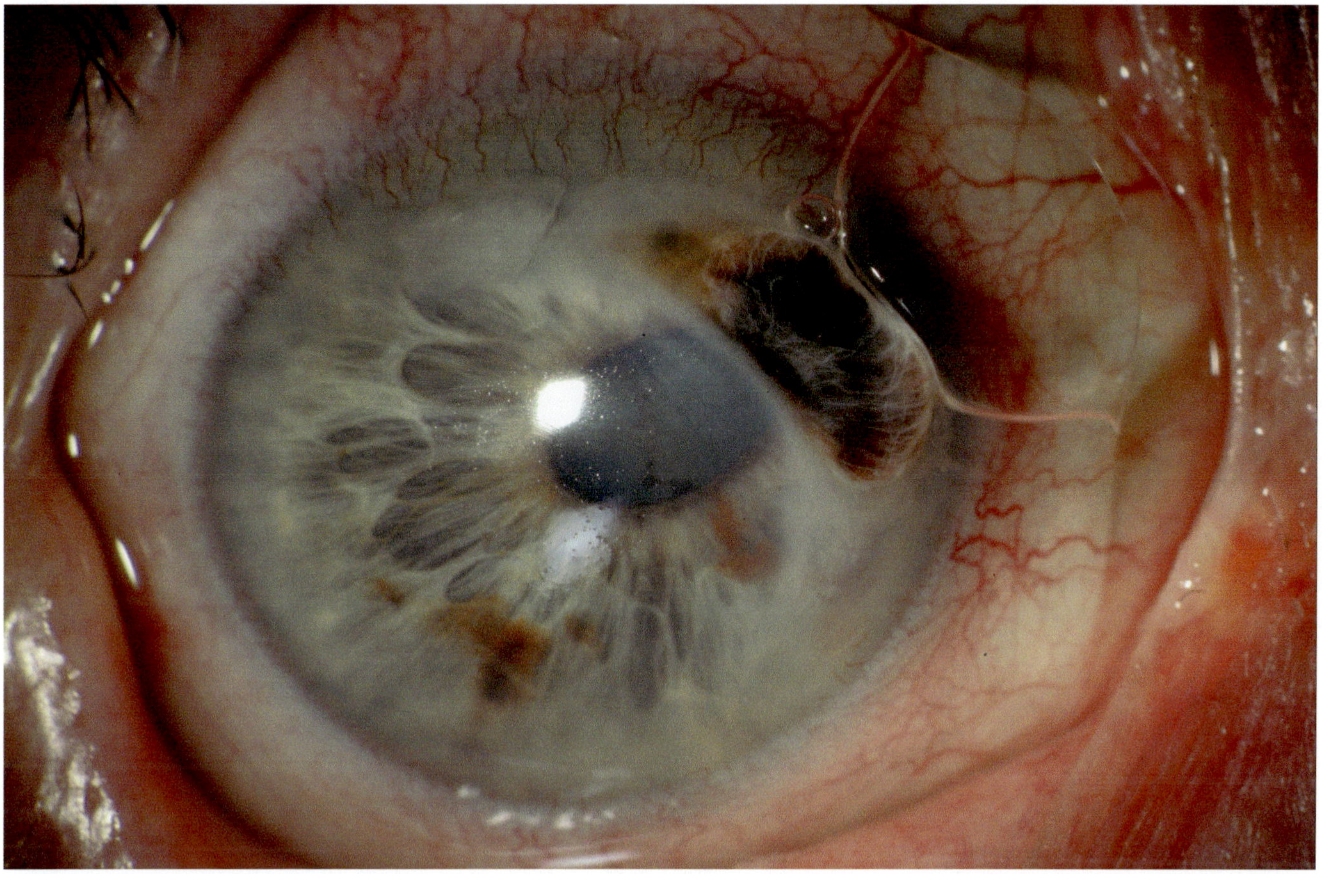

Fig. 20 Perforated peripheral ulcerative keratitis in a 77-year-old female patient with rheumatoid arthritis (temporarily shielded by a bandage contact lens). Note the relatively minor conjunctival injection and absence of intraocular inflammation or hypoyon (air bubbles underneath the contact lens from 2 to 3 o'clock)

can occur (Fig. 21). Uveitis, dacryoadenitis, and vasculitis affecting retinal and optic nerve vessels are isolated or additional manifestations of GPA. Although a systemic disease, unilateral forms are common.

Autoantibodies myeloperoxidase (MPO)-ANCA (or perinuclear (p-)ANCA) and proteinase 3 (PR3)-ANCA (or cytoplasmic (c-)ANCA) are highly specific for GPA, making biopsy of the affected region unnecessary in most cases. The mainstay of therapy is systemic immunosuppression, initially by intravenous corticosteroids. If prolonged therapy is necessary, monoclonal antibodies to CD20 and TNF-alpha are effective. Topical steroids are always added but are by no means sufficient.

2.8.4 Sarcoidosis

Sarcoidosis is a granulomatous inflammatory disease that affects the lungs, skin, and lymph nodes. Uveitis is the most common ocular manifestation (anterior uveitis, followed by intermediate and posterior uveitis) and often the initial clinical manifestation [76]. Affections of the cornea are interstitial keratitis, peripheral ulcerative keratitis, or band keratopathy.

3 Corneal Manifestations of Systemic Medication

3.1 Drug-Induced Corneal deposits

Multiple drugs are known to cause corneal deposits, and affection of all layers of the cornea is possible. Therefore, a complete medical history of drug intake also from the past plays an important role in making the correct diagnosis. Often corneal epithelial keratopathies are related to lysosome dysfunction [77–79].

3.1.1 Epithelial Deposits

The most common presentation of epithelial deposits is verticillate keratopathy seen in the use of amiodarone, aminoquinoline (chloroquine, hydroxychloroquine, amodiaquine), atovaquone, clofazimine, gold, NSAIDs, phenothiazine (chlorpromazine), suramin, tamoxifen and tilorone hydrochloride [77, 79]. Other drugs causing epithelial deposits are Clarithromycin, Vandetanib, Osimertinib, and Cytarabine arabinoside [79].

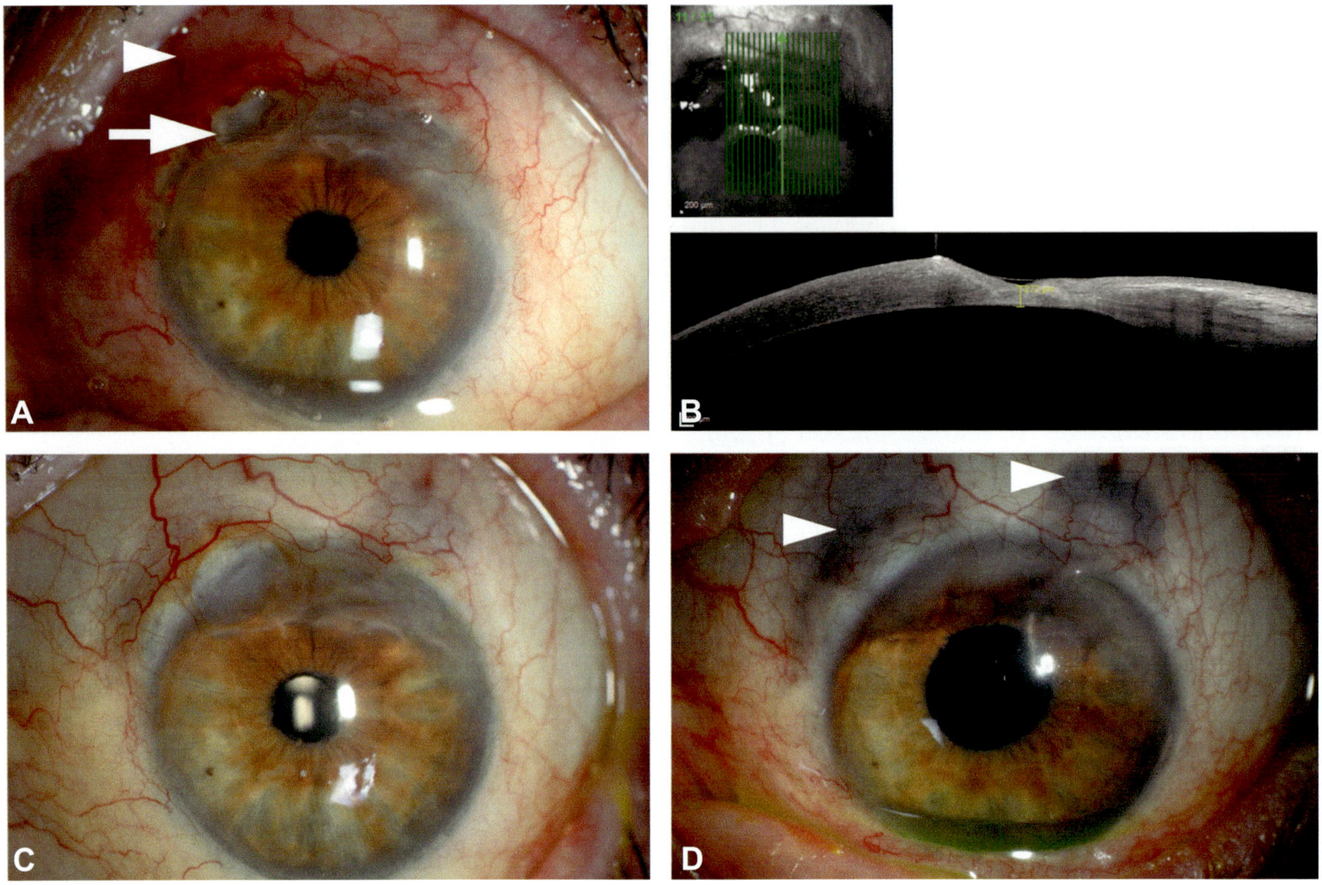

Fig. 21 Peripheral ulcerative keratitis (PUK) in a patient with granulomatosis with polyangiitis (GPA) before (**A**, **B**: Anterior segment OCT) and after initiating systemic immunosuppression (2 months (**C**) and 5 years (**D**) after initiation of therapy). Ulceration with stromal thinning (arrow in **A**) was accompanied by conjunctivitis and scleritis (arrowheads in **A** and **D**)

Amiodarone

Amiodarone is a potassium channel-blocking antiarrhythmic agent developed to treat ventricular fibrillation [79]. Amiodarone is concentrated in tears, and more severe keratopathy has been associated with contact lens wear [77]. It can cause vortex keratopathy, or corneal verticillata, which is a whorl-like opacity in the corneal epithelium (Fig. 22). In slit-lamp examination, this becomes visible in about 98% of patients about 4 weeks after the start of therapy. Lipid deposits within intracytoplasmic inclusions are seen within the cornea under transmission electron microscopy. Keratopathy does not interfere with topography or vision but causes symptoms like eye irritation, halos, and photophobia. Most of these deposits resolve 3–20 months after cessation of the drug [78, 79]. However, amiodarone-associated optic neuropathy, which affects 0.3% of amiodarone patients (mostly males), may be irreversible [80].

Chloroquine

Aminoquinolines are drugs for the treatment of malaria as well as rheumatic diseases. Chloroquine is a drug of this group commonly used. Here, dose-dependent vortex keratopathy, beginning as diffuse punctate deposits, is frequently seen (Fig. 23). Similar to amiodarone, the corneal deposits gradually reverse on cessation of treatment. However, long-term usage can result in irreversible retinopathy by accumulation in the retinal pigment epithelium [78].

Tamoxifen

Tamoxifen is a selective estrogen receptor modulator for the treatment of breast cancer, currently mostly applied as low-dose therapy (10–20 mg/day). Epithelial deposits present as subepithelial white to brown whorl-like deposits,

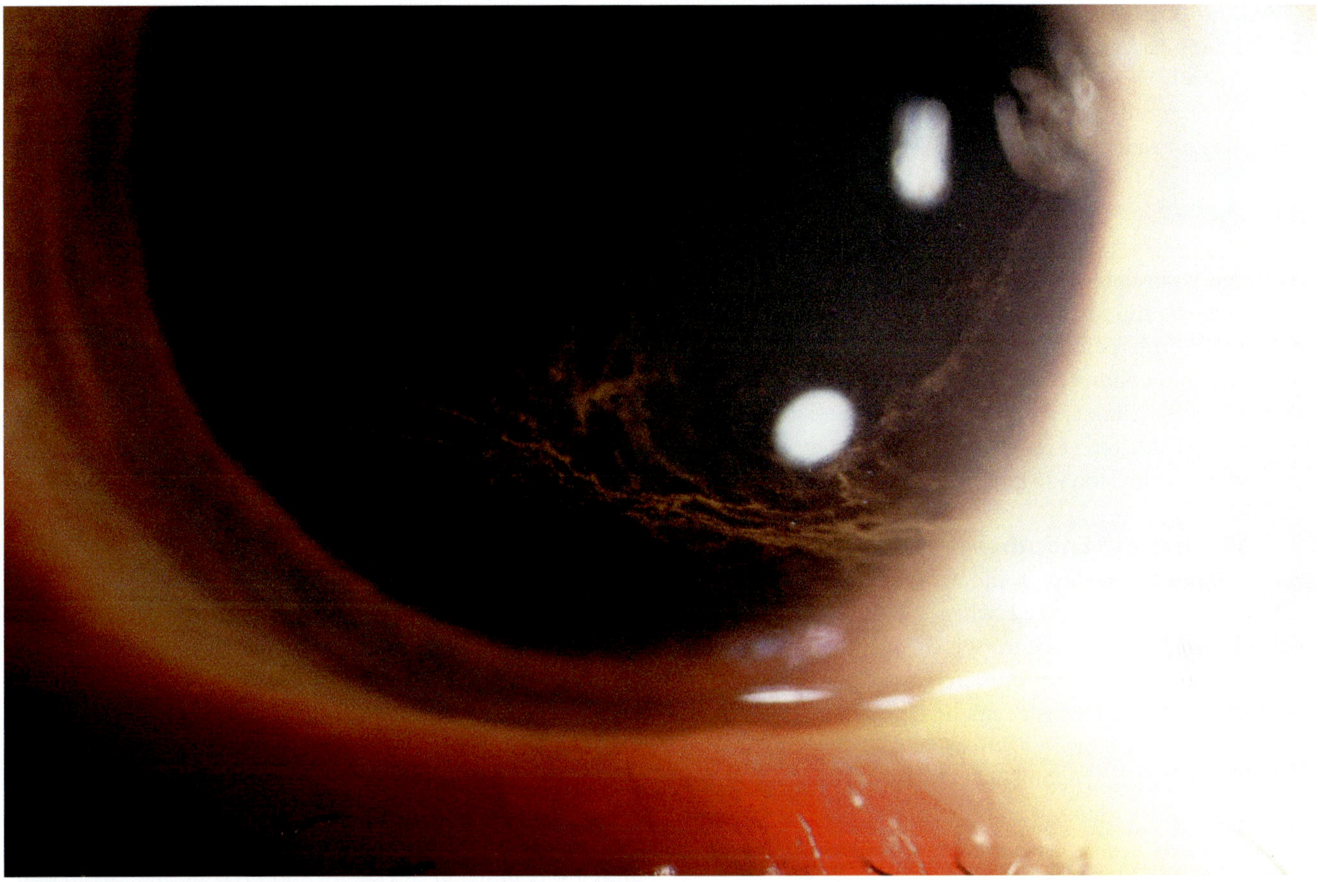

Fig. 22 Early vortex keratopathy, or corneal verticillate, after 5 months of amiodarone treatment, an antiarrhythmic agent. Brown lipid deposits form a whorl-like pattern in the epithelium

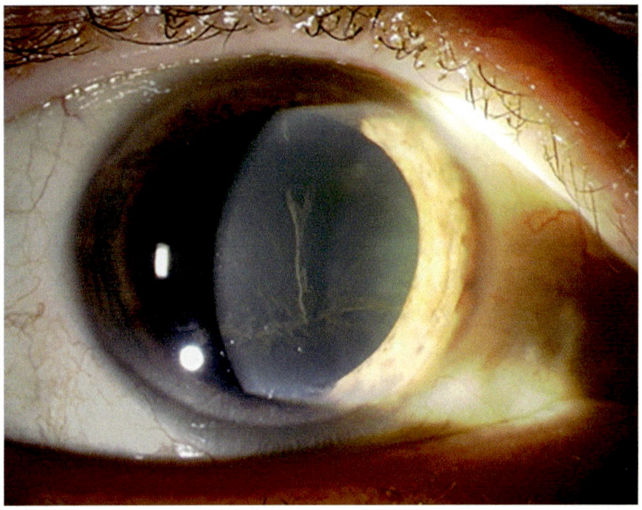

Fig. 23 Chloroquine and other antimalarial agents share a similar appearance of central epithelium deposits forming a vortex keratopathy

subepithelial lines, or streaks in the inferior or central cornea. The findings are often completely regressing after cessation of the drug [77]. It should be noted that while corneal findings do not affect vision, retinal side effects, though rare, can reduce vision and may be irreversible. Crystalline retinopathy features white intraretinal deposits in the paramacular area, macular edema, and punctate retinal pigmentary changes [81]. Optic neuropathy can be associated. When loss of vision is clearly attributable to tamoxifen, the medication should be stopped.

Non-steroidal anti-inflammatory drugs

Non-steroidal anti-inflammatory drugs are drugs used as a standard for pain therapy. Ibuprofen can cause symmetrical epithelial vortex keratopathy. Also with naproxen, a vortex pattern in the superficial cornea is seen, while drug deposits of indomethacin show speckled deposits on the superficial epithelium, Bowman layer, and Descemet membrane.

In addition, retinal toxicities like bull's eye maculopathy, reduced color vision, macular edema, thinning, and retinal pigmentation have been observed. While vortex keratopathy causes no or mildly reduced visual acuity, the deposits of indomethacin can lead to decreased visual acuity [78].

Cytarabine

Cytarabine is an antimetabolite used in acute myeloid leukemia. It shows mild to moderate punctate keratopathy with intraepithelial microcystic opacities, especially in the central cornea, and conjunctival hyperemia [77, 78]. It resolves within 14 days without cessation of the drug. The deposits lead to symptoms like photophobia, foreign body sensation, pain, and blurred vision [78].

3.1.2 Stromal and Endothelial Deposits

Stromal deposits are less common than epithelial deposits. Visual acuity is reduced when the anterior stroma is involved. Stromal deposits are typical for gold salts, indomethacin, clofazimine, isotretinoin, vandetanib, chlorpromazine, and rifabutin. Deposits can be pigmented, crystalline, or refractile [79]. Chlorpromacin as well as rafabutin deposits can also affect the endothelial cell layer [79].

Chlorpromazine

Chlorpromazine is an antipsychotic drug. It can cause dose-related light-induced depositions in the cornea [79]. Corneal deposits normally begin as fine brown, granular opacities in the posterior stroma, Descemet membrane, and endothelium. Only with higher dosages the anterior stroma, subepithelial layer, and epithelium are involved, presenting whorl-like deposits. The changes are reversible in some patients [77, 78].

Rifabutin

Rifabutin is used for the treatment and prophylaxis of *Mycobacterium avium* complex infections, which is especially common in patients with AIDS. The use is associated with bilateral stellate, and refractile endothelial deposits primarily in the periphery but can extend to the central cornea. Another ocular side effect is uveitis with hypopyon. Progression after cessation of the drug is common [77].

3.2 Toxic Effects

3.2.1 Cytostatic Drugs

Ophthalmic complications of chemotherapy are often overlooked and neglected, due to the priority given to other life-threatening effects [82]. However, ocular pain, epiphora, and reduction or even loss of vision can significantly reduce quality of life.

Superficial punctate epitheliopathy is a common side effect of any cytostatic drug, but is especially prevalent in tubulin-binding drugs, i.e., docetaxel and paclitaxel [83, 84]. Damage is caused by the inhibition of DNA synthesis, impeding the constant regeneration of corneal epithelial cells [85]. Symptoms include photophobia, dry eye, foreign body sensation, and reduction of visual acuity. Epiphora might increase the toxicity of drugs secreted into the tear film [86]. Neurotoxic side effects are known for many currently used drugs (platinum-based agents, taxanes, vinca alkaloids, proteasome inhibitors, and thalidomide analogs), increasing dry eye symptoms [87].

Therapy comprises all stages of dry eye therapy as recommended in DEWS II management and Therapy Report [88]. Dose reduction of cytostatic drugs may reduce the severity of corneal side effects. After cessation of therapy, corneal affections usually resolve within two to four weeks.

3.2.2 Antibody–Drug Conjugates

Antibody–drug conjugates (ADCs) are novel cancer therapeutic agents designed to reduce systemic side effects of cytotoxicity by directing the cytotoxin directly to cancerous cells. They are comprised of a monoclonal antibody conjugated with a cytostatic agent by a linker. The ADC's antibody is targeted to specific epitopes on malignant cells. After binding to cancer cells, ADCs are internalized and the linker is degraded by lysosomes, thereby releasing the agent. These are mostly tubulin-inhibiting cytotoxins (maytansinoids, auristatins) or other potent agents that disrupt DNA (calicheamicin, duocarmycin) [84].

Despite high specificity, several ADCs display side effects in non-cancerous tissue including the cornea. The epithelium with its high proliferation rate is prone to damage by the ADC's cytotoxic payload. Unconjugated tubulin-binding drugs (e.g., docetaxel) have been associated with reversible superficial keratopathy (see above). Similar events in ADCs suggest an off-target mechanism, i.e., delivery of unconjugated cytotoxin to the cornea. Especially with ADCs containing monomethyl auristatin F, intraepithelial changes described as "microcyst-like epithelial changes" (MECs) are observed [89]. On slit lamp microscopy, they appear as bilateral microcystic lesions within the corneal epithelium, beginning in the periphery and progressing centripetally, most likely following the migration pattern of maturing cells derived from limbal stem cells (Fig. 24). Intraepithelial cysts are presumed to be apoptotic epithelial cells. While peripherally, MECs can cause a hyperopic shift and irregular astigmatism that can be addressed by rigid gas-permeable contact lenses [90]. When located in the center, vision loss beyond reading vision is possible, accompanied by dry eye symptoms, especially eye

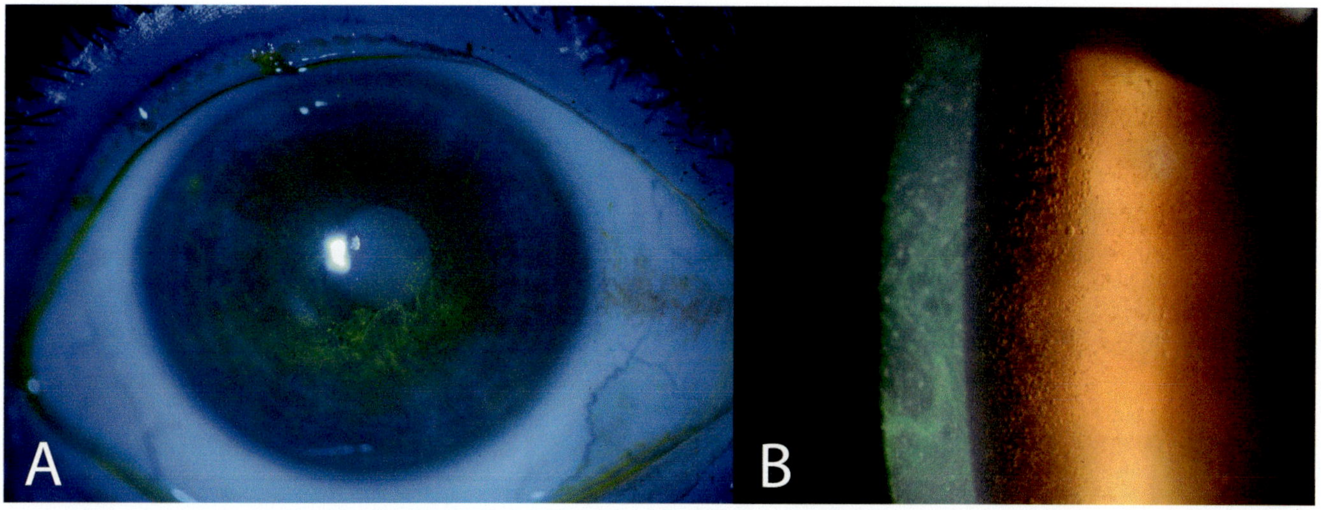

Fig. 24 "Microcyst-like epithelial changes" (MECs) in a patient treated with antibody–drug conjugate belantamab mafadotin for multiple myeloma. The peripheral circular fluorescein staining pattern indicates the affection of peripheral corneal epithelial cells by the cytotoxic payload of the drug, especially transient amplifying cells. Within 2–3 weeks after application of the cytotoxic drug, round vacuoles in the basal epithelial layer become visible, gradually moving toward the center, following the centripetal migration of epithelial cells. Pausing treatment allows recovery by replacement of corneal epithelium

pain, photophobia, and blurred vision. Adverse events are mitigated by dose delay or reduction or, if severe, treatment discontinuation of the ADC. Topical steroids do not affect MECs [89].

Belantamab mafadotin (brand name Blenrep) is an example of an ADC approved for the treatment of relapsed and refractory multiple myeloma. The antibody is directed against the B-cell maturation antigen (BCMA) on myeloma cell surfaces and delivers monomethyl auristatin F as a cytotoxic payload. 72% of patients presented MECs, 29% with a vision loss of more than 3 Snellen lines [89]. Dose modification led to recovery in all cases, but prolonged restoration of vision suggests a slower-than-normal epithelial turnover.

4 Conclusion

The cornea can act as a sentinel, manifesting a diverse array of pathologies in response to systemic diseases and medication. Through diligent clinical observation, ophthalmologists can unravel the interplay between systemic factors and corneal abnormalities, sometimes initiating the diagnosis and therapy of a thus far unknown systemic disease.

References

1. Schultz RO, Van Horn DL, Peters MA, Klewin KM, Schutten WH. Diabetic keratopathy. Trans Am Ophthalmol Soc. 1981;79:180–99.
2. Shah R, Amador C, Tormanen K, Ghiam S, Saghizadeh M, Arumugaswami V, et al. Systemic diseases and the cornea. Exp Eye Res. 2021;204: 108455.
3. Shih KC, Lam KS, Tong L. A systematic review on the impact of diabetes mellitus on the ocular surface. Nutr Diabet. 2017;7(3): e251.
4. Saghizadeh M, Dib CM, Brunken WJ, Ljubimov AV. Normalization of wound healing and stem cell marker patterns in organ-cultured human diabetic corneas by gene therapy of limbal cells. Exp Eye Res. 2014;129:66–73.
5. Messmer EM, Schmid-Tannwald C, Zapp D, Kampik A. In vivo confocal microscopy of corneal small fiber damage in diabetes mellitus. Graefes Arch Clin Exp Ophthalmol. 2010;248(9):1307–12.
6. Chin YH, Ng CH, Lee MH, Koh JWH, Kiew J, Yang SP, et al. Prevalence of thyroid eye disease in Graves' disease: a meta-analysis and systematic review. Clin Endocrinol (Oxf). 2020;93(4):363–74.
7. Wemeau JL, Klein M, Sadoul JL, Briet C, Velayoudom-Cephise FL. Graves' disease: introduction, epidemiology, endogenous and environmental pathogenic factors. Ann Endocrinol (Paris). 2018;79(6):599–607.
8. Marcocci C, Bartalena L, Bogazzi F, Panicucci M, Pinchera A. Studies on the occurrence of ophthalmopathy in Graves' disease. Acta Endocrinol (Copenh). 1989;120(4):473–8.
9. Passons GA, Wood TO. Conjunctival resection for superior limbic keratoconjunctivitis. Ophthalmology. 1984;91(8):966–8.

10. Bartalena L, Kahaly GJ, Baldeschi L, Dayan CM, Eckstein A, Marcocci C, et al. The 2021 European group on Graves' orbitopathy (EUGOGO) clinical practice guidelines for the medical management of Graves' orbitopathy. Eur J Endocrinol. 2021;185(4):G43–67.
11. Antonelli A, Fallahi P, Elia G, Ragusa F, Paparo SR, Ruffilli I, et al. Graves' disease: clinical manifestations, immune pathogenesis (cytokines and chemokines) and therapy. Best Pract Res Clin Endocrinol Metab. 2020;34(1): 101388.
12. Susarla R, Liu L, Walker EA, Bujalska IJ, Alsalem J, Williams GP, et al. Cortisol biosynthesis in the human ocular surface innate immune response. PLoS One. 2014;9(4): e94913.
13. Chopra R, Chander A, Jacob JJ. The eye as a window to rare endocrine disorders. Indian J Endocrinol Metab. 2012;16(3):331–8.
14. van der Plas WY, Noltes ME, van Ginhoven TM, Kruijff S. Secondary and tertiary hyperparathyroidism: a narrative review. Scand J Surg. 2020;109(4):271–8.
15. Klaassen-Broekema N, van Bijsterveld OP. Limbal and corneal calcification in patients with chronic renal failure. Br J Ophthalmol. 1993;77(9):569–71.
16. Nagpal R, Goyal RB, Priyadarshini K, Kashyap S, Sharma M, Sinha R, et al. Mucopolysaccharidosis: a broad review. Indian J Ophthalmol. 2022;70(7):2249–61.
17. Ashworth JL, Biswas S, Wraith E, Lloyd IC. Mucopolysaccharidoses and the eye. Surv Ophthalmol. 2006;51(1):1–17.
18. Stepien KM, Bentley A, Chen C, Dhemech MW, Gee E, Orton P, et al. Non-cardiac manifestations in adult patients with mucopolysaccharidosis. Front Cardiovasc Med. 2022;9: 839391.
19. Naumann GO, Rummelt V. Clearing of the para-transplant host cornea after perforating keratoplasty in Maroteaux-Lamy syndrome (type VI-A mucopolysaccharidosis). Klin Monbl Augenheilkd. 1993;203(5):351–60.
20. Viestenz A, Shin YS, Viestenz A, Naumann GO. Ocular manifestation of mucopolysaccharidosis I-S (Scheie's syndrome). Klin Monbl Augenheilkd. 2002;219(10):745–8.
21. Hampe CS, Yund BD, Orchard PJ, Lund TC, Wesley J, McIvor RS. Differences in MPS I and MPS II disease manifestations. Int J Mol Sci. 2021;22(15).
22. Chen HH, Sawamoto K, Mason RW, Kobayashi H, Yamaguchi S, Suzuki Y, et al. Enzyme replacement therapy for mucopolysaccharidoses; past, present, and future. J Hum Genet. 2019;64(11):1153–71.
23. Beck M, Ramaswami U, Hernberg-Stahl E, Hughes DA, Kampmann C, Mehta AB, et al. Twenty years of the Fabry Outcome Survey (FOS): insights, achievements, and lessons learned from a global patient registry. Orphanet J Rare Dis. 2022;17(1):238.
24. Nilsson M, Kolagari HT, Epstein D, Samolov B, Olsson M, Naess K, et al. Visual outcome, ocular findings, and visual quality of life in patients with Fabry disease. Ophthalmic Genet. 2022:1–9.
25. Kalkum G, Pitz S, Karabul N, Beck M, Pintos-Morell G, Parini R, et al. Paediatric Fabry disease: prognostic significance of ocular changes for disease severity. BMC Ophthalmol. 2016;16(1):202.
26. Pitz S, Kalkum G, Arash L, Karabul N, Sodi A, Larroque S, et al. Ocular signs correlate well with disease severity and genotype in Fabry disease. PLoS One. 2015;10(3): e0120814.
27. van der Tol L, Sminia ML, Hollak CE, Biegstraaten M. Cornea verticillata supports a diagnosis of Fabry disease in non-classical phenotypes: results from the Dutch cohort and a systematic review. Br J Ophthalmol. 2016;100(1):3–8.
28. Barchiesi BJ, Eckel RH, Ellis PP. The cornea and disorders of lipid metabolism. Surv Ophthalmol. 1991; 36(1):1–22.
29. Crispin SM. Lipid deposition at the limbus. Eye (Lond). 1989;3(Pt 2):240–50.
30. Crispin S. Ocular lipid deposition and hyperlipoproteinaemia. Prog Retin Eye Res. 2002;21(2):169–224.
31. Weiss JS, Rapuano CJ, Seitz B, Busin M, Kivelä TT, Bouheraoua N, Bredrup C, Nischal KK, Chawla H, Borderie V, Kenyon KR, Kim EK, Møller HU, Munier FL, Berger T, Lisch W. IC3D Classification of corneal dystrophies—edition 3. Cornea. 2024;43(4):466–527.
32. Viestenz A, Schlötzer-Schrehardt U, Hofmann-Rummelt C, Seitz B, Küchle M. Histopathology of corneal changes in lecithin-cholesterol acyltransferase deficiency. Cornea. 2002;21(8):834–7.
33. Vitali C, Bajaj A, Nguyen C, Schnall J, Chen J, Stylianou K, et al. A systematic review of the natural history and biomarkers of primary lecithin: cholesterol acyltransferase deficiency. J Lipid Res. 2022;63(3): 100169.
34. Burnett JR, Hooper AJ, McCormick SPA, Hegele RA. Tangier disease. In: Adam MP, Everman DB, Mirzaa GM, Pagon RA, Wallace SE, Bean LJH, et al., editors. GeneReviews((R))., Seattle (WA); 1993.
35. Czlonkowska A, Litwin T, Dusek P, Ferenci P, Lutsenko S, Medici V, et al. Wilson disease. Nat Rev Dis Primers. 2018;4(1):21.
36. European Association for Study of L. EASL Clinical Practice Guidelines: Wilson's disease. J Hepatol. 2012;56(3):671–85.
37. Lorincz MT. Neurologic Wilson's disease. Ann N Y Acad Sci. 2010;1184:173–87.
38. Suvarna JC. Kayser-Fleischer ring. J Postgrad Med. 2008;54(3):238–40.
39. Minnella AM, Rissotto R, Antoniazzi E, Di Girolamo M, Luigetti M, Maceroni M, et al. Ocular involvement in hereditary amyloidosis. Genes (Basel). 2021;12(7).
40. Casal I, Monteiro S, Abreu C, Neves M, Oliveira L, Beirao M. Meretoja's syndrome: lattice corneal dystrophy, gelsolin type. Case Rep Med. 2017;2017:2843417.
41. Nikoskinen T, Schmidt EK, Strbian D, Kiuru-Enari S, Atula S. Natural course of Finnish gelsolin amyloidosis. Ann Med. 2015;47(6):506–11.
42. Kawasaki S, Kinoshita S. Clinical and basic aspects of gelatinous drop-like corneal dystrophy. Dev Ophthalmol. 2011;48:97–115.
43. Yuan C, Berscheit HL, Huang AJ. Identification of an amyloidogenic region on keratoepithelin via synthetic peptides. FEBS Lett. 2007;581(2):241–7.
44. Martins AC, Rosa AM, Costa E, Tavares C, Quadrado MJ, Murta JN. Ocular manifestations and therapeutic options in patients with familial amyloid polyneuropathy: a systematic review. Biomed Res Int. 2015;2015: 282405.
45. Flockerzi E, Daas L, Schlötzer-Schrehardt U, Zimpfer A, Bohle R, Seitz B. Ocular changes in nephropathic cystinosis: the course of the gold-dust. Int Ophthalmol. 2019;39(6):1413–8.
46. West KP, Darnton-Hill I. Vitamin A Deficiency. In: Semba RD, Bloem MW, Piot P, editors. Nutrition and health in developing countries. Totowa, NJ: Humana Press; 2008. p. 377–433.
47. WHO. Vitamin A deficiency: WHO; 2009. Available from: https://www.who.int/data/nutrition/nlis/info/vitamin-a-deficiency.
48. Sommer A. Xerophthalmia, keratomalacia and nutritional blindness. Int Ophthalmol. 1990;14(3):195–9.
49. WHO. Xerophthalmia and night blindness for the assessment of clinical vitamin A deficiency in individuals and populations Geneva: World Health Organization; 2014. Available from: http://apps.who.int/iris/bitstream/10665/133705/1/WHO_NMH_NHD_EPG_14.4_eng.pdf?ua=1.
50. Gilbert C. The eye signs of vitamin A deficiency. Commun Eye Health. 2013;26(84):66–7.
51. Soleimani M, Mahdavi Sharif P, Cheraqpour K, Koganti R, Masoumi A, Baharnoori SM, et al. Ocular graft-versus-host disease (oGVHD): from A to Z. Surv Ophthalmol. 2023;68(4):697–712.

52. Lisch W, Saikia P, Pitz S, Pleyer U, Lisch C, Jaeger M, et al. Chameleon-like appearance of immunotactoid keratopathy. Cornea. 2012;31(1):55–8.
53. Shakarchi FI. Ocular tuberculosis: current perspectives. Clin Ophthalmol. 2015;9:2223–7.
54. Arora R, Mehta S, Gupta D, Goyal J. Bilateral disciform keratitis as the presenting feature of extrapulmonary tuberculosis. Br J Ophthalmol. 2010;94(6):809–10.
55. Stanek G, Wormser GP, Gray J, Strle F. Lyme borreliosis. Lancet. 2012;379(9814):461–73.
56. Steere AC, Coburn J, Glickstein L. The emergence of Lyme disease. J Clin Invest. 2004;113(8):1093–101.
57. Mora P, Carta A. Ocular manifestations of Lyme borreliosis in Europe. Int J Med Sci. 2009;6(3):124–5.
58. Huppertz HI, Münchmeier D, Lieb W. Ocular manifestations in children and adolescents with Lyme arthritis. Br J Ophthalmol. 1999;83(10):1149–52.
59. Lindström BE, Skogman BH, Lindström AK, Tallstedt L, Nilsson K. Borrelia ocular infection: a case report and a systematic review of published cases. Ophthalmic Res. 2022;65(2):121–30.
60. Mikkilä HO, Seppälä IJ, Viljanen MK, Peltomaa MP, Karma A. The expanding clinical spectrum of ocular Lyme borreliosis. Ophthalmology. 2000;107(3):581–7.
61. Girschick HJ, Morbach H, Tappe D. Treatment of Lyme borreliosis. Arthritis Res Ther. 2009;11(6):258.
62. Asanad S, Bayomi M, Brown D, Buzzard J, Lai E, Ling C, et al. Ehlers-Danlos syndromes and their manifestations in the visual system. Front Med (Lausanne). 2022;9: 996458.
63. Malfait F, Francomano C, Byers P, Belmont J, Berglund B, Black J, et al. The 2017 international classification of the Ehlers-Danlos syndromes. Am J Med Genet C Semin Med Genet. 2017;175(1):8–26.
64. Ritelli M, Venturini M, Cinquina V, Chiarelli N, Colombi M. Multisystemic manifestations in a cohort of 75 classical Ehlers-Danlos syndrome patients: natural history and nosological perspectives. Orphanet J Rare Dis. 2020;15(1):197.
65. Walkden A, Burkitt-Wright E, Au L. Brittle cornea syndrome: current perspectives. Clin Ophthalmol. 2019;13:1511–6.
66. Salchow DJ, Gehle P. Ocular manifestations of Marfan syndrome in children and adolescents. Eur J Ophthalmol. 2019;29(1):38–43.
67. Gorlin RJ. Nevoid basal-cell carcinoma syndrome. Medicine (Baltimore). 1987;66(2):98–113.
68. Gorlin RJ, Goltz RW. Multiple nevoid basal-cell epithelioma, jaw cysts and bifid rib. A syndrome. New Engl J Med. 1960;262:908–12.
69. Bresler SC, Padwa BL, Granter SR. Nevoid basal cell carcinoma syndrome (gorlin syndrome). Head Neck Pathol. 2016;10(2):119–24.
70. Peris K, Fargnoli MC, Garbe C, Kaufmann R, Bastholt L, Seguin NB, et al. Diagnosis and treatment of basal cell carcinoma: European consensus-based interdisciplinary guidelines. Eur J Cancer. 2019;118:10–34.
71. Leung AK, Barankin B, Lam JM, Leong KF, Hon KL. Xeroderma pigmentosum: an updated review. Drugs Context. 2022;11.
72. Tamura D, DiGiovanna JJ, Khan SG, Kraemer KH. Living with xeroderma pigmentosum: comprehensive photoprotection for highly photosensitive patients. Photodermatol Photoimmunol Photomed. 2014;30(2–3):146–52.
73. Chaurasia S, Mulay K, Ramappa M, Sangwan V, Murthy S, Nair R, et al. Corneal changes in xeroderma pigmentosum: a clinicopathologic report. Am J Ophthalmol. 2014;157(2):495–500 e2.
74. Ogra S, Sims JL, McGhee CNJ, Niederer RL. Ocular complications and mortality in peripheral ulcerative keratitis and necrotising scleritis: the role of systemic immunosuppression. Clin Exp Ophthalmol. 2020;48(4):434–41.
75. Messmer EM, Foster CS. Vasculitic peripheral ulcerative keratitis. Surv Ophthalmol. 1999;43(5):379–96.
76. Heiligenhaus A, Wefelmeyer D, Wefelmeyer E, Rosel M, Schrenk M. The eye as a common site for the early clinical manifestation of sarcoidosis. Ophthalmic Res. 2011;46(1):9–12.
77. Hollander DA, Aldave AJ. Drug-induced corneal complications. Curr Opin Ophthalmol. 2004;15(6):541–8.
78. Raizman MB, Hamrah P, Holland EJ, Kim T, Mah FS, Rapuano CJ, et al. Drug-induced corneal epithelial changes. Surv Ophthalmol. 2017;62(3):286–301.
79. Sahyoun JY, Sabeti S, Robert MC. Drug-induced corneal deposits: an up-to-date review. BMJ Open Ophthalmol. 2022;7(1): e000943.
80. Cheng HC, Yeh HJ, Huang N, Chou YJ, Yen MY, Wang AG. Amiodarone-associated optic neuropathy: a nationwide study. Ophthalmology. 2015;122(12):2553–9.
81. Hager T, Seitz B. Ocular side effects of biological agents in oncology: what should the clinician be aware of? Onco Targets Ther. 2013;7:69–77.
82. Schmid KE, Kornek GV, Scheithauer W, Binder S. Update on ocular complications of systemic cancer chemotherapy. Surv Ophthalmol. 2006;51(1):19–40.
83. Burstein HJ, Manola J, Younger J, Parker LM, Bunnell CA, Scheib R, Matulonis UA, Garber JE, Clarke KD, Shulman LN, Winer EP. Docetaxel administered on a weekly basis for metastatic breast cancer. J Clin Oncol. 2000;18(6):1212–9.
84. Eaton JS, Miller PE, Mannis MJ, Murphy CJ. Ocular adverse events associated with antibody-drug conjugates in human clinical trials. J Ocul Pharmacol Ther. 2015;31(10):589–604.
85. al-Tweigeri T, Nabholtz JM, Mackey JR. Ocular toxicity and cancer chemotherapy. A review. Cancer. 1996;78(7):1359–73.
86. Esmaeli B, Ahmadi MA, Rivera E, Valero V, Hutto T, Jackson DM, et al. Docetaxel secretion in tears: association with lacrimal drainage obstruction. Arch Ophthalmol. 2002;120(9):1180–2.
87. Was H, Borkowska A, Bagues A, Tu L, Liu JYH, Lu Z, et al. Mechanisms of chemotherapy-induced neurotoxicity. Front Pharmacol. 2022;13: 750507.
88. Jones L, Downie LE, Korb D, Benitez-Del-Castillo JM, Dana R, Deng SX, et al. TFOS DEWS II management and therapy report. Ocul Surf. 2017;15(3):575–628.
89. Farooq AV, Degli Esposti S, Popat R, Thulasi P, Lonial S, Nooka AK, et al. Corneal epithelial findings in patients with multiple myeloma treated with antibody-drug conjugate belantamab mafodotin in the pivotal, randomized, DREAMM-2 study. Ophthalmol Ther. 2020;9(4):889–911.
90. Rousseau A, Michot JM, Labetoulle M. Belantamab mafotodin-induced epithelial keratopathy masquerading myopic surgery. Ophthalmology. 2020;127(12):1626.

Immune Reaction After Corneal Transplantation (PKP/DALK/DMEK)

Björn Bachmann

Abstract

Rejection after corneal transplantation is a leading cause of graft failure. The introduction of lamellar transplantation techniques has led to a significant reduction in rejection rates. Epithelial, subepithelial, and stromal rejections are rare immune reactions after penetrating keratoplasty (PKP) or deep anterior lamellar keratoplasty (DALK) and are usually of limited clinical importance. The greater risk for permanent functional graft failure comes from endothelial rejection. Morphologically, they are characterized either by diffusely distributed keratic precipitates on the corneal graft or by a rejection line (Khodadoust line) at the boundary between intact and rejected endothelium. After PKP, rejections with Khodadoust lines often originate from corneal neovascularizations. In contrast to PKP, Khodadoust lines are rare in rejections after Descemet membrane endothelial keratoplasty (DMEK). After reducing the application frequency, prednisolone acetate or dexamethasone eye drops are usually used for 1–2 years for prophylaxis of corneal graft rejection. Overall, there is a very low risk of rejection after DMEK of approximately 2.5% within the first 5 years. Prophylaxis of rejection after DMEK can also be effectively performed with steroids with lower glucocorticoid activity while reducing the risk of intraocular pressure decompensation.

Keywords

Graft rejection · Rejection line · Khodadoust · Steroid · ACAID · High-risk keratoplasty

B. Bachmann (✉)
Department of Ophthalmology, University of Cologne, Cologne, Germany
e-mail: Bjoern.bachmann@uk-koeln.de

1 Introduction

Already before the introduction of corneal endothelial keratoplasty (EK), corneal transplantation was considered the most successful solid organ transplantation. The average survival time after penetrating keratoplasty (PKP) in normal risk recipients is about 15 years whereas corneal endothelial rejection is considered the most common cause of graft failure [1]. After EK, the rejection rate is significantly lower than after PKP.

Khodadoust was a pioneer in identifying the corneal endothelium as an essential structure for rejection after corneal transplantation. He has illustrated the types of immune responses in different animal models by selective transplantation of endothelium and stroma. He was able to identify a rejection line in the corneal endothelium named after him and he also further characterized the much less common corneal stromal and epithelial rejections. In his experiments Khodadoust was also able to demonstrate the local connection of graft rejections with corneal neovascularization which in the meantime has also been demonstrated in many clinical evaluations [2, 3]. Although rejections occur after corneal transplantation, they are rare under normal-risk conditions. The cornea has several strategies, such as avascularity, lack of $MHCII^+$ antigen-presenting cells (APCs) in the center of the cornea, and an immunosuppressive environment which is particularly effective after lamellar corneal transplants [4].

2 Initiation of Allogeneic Immune Responses After Corneal Transplantation

Adaptive cellular T-cell-mediated immune responses are responsible for alloantigen specific rejection after allogeneic corneal transplantation. To initiate such an immune response, which correlates with a type IV hypersensitivity

B. Seitz et al. (eds.), *Atlas on Cornea*, https://doi.org/10.1007/978-3-031-65422-0_39

reaction, the migration of activated antigen loaded APCs from peripheral non-lymphoid tissue to the T-cell zones of the corresponding lymph nodes is required. The migration of resident immunocompetent cells into secondary lymphoid organs is essential for the development of adaptive immune responses [5, 6], and thus represents a crucial step in the context of rejection after allogeneic organ transplantation but also in the defense against infectious pathogens [7, 8]. After allogeneic corneal transplantation, the mechanical stress and the release of endogenous inflammatory mediators lead to a non-specific inflammatory reaction and to the decomposition of the involved tissue and possible pathogenic germs. Mechanical stress, inflammatory mediators, such as TNF-α, and decomposition products of bacteria, such as lipopolysaccharides (LPS), can lead to maturation or activation of resident dendritic cells as some of the main contributors to the process of antigen presentation [9–11]. Activated dendritic cells of non-lymphoid peripheral tissues are the main cellular initiator of T-cell-mediated cellular immune responses. Activation of dendritic cells in peripheral non-lymphoid tissues can be controlled, for example, by the membrane-bound receptors CD14 or Toll-like receptor-4 [12, 13]. Upon activation dendritic cells increase synthesis of the surface molecule MHCII and begin the expression of costimulatory molecules like B7.1 (CD80) and B7.2 (CD86). This constellation of surface antigens is essential for the presentation of antigens to naïve T cells, which in turn initiate the cellular adaptive immune response. The site of antigen presentation essentially occurs in the T-cell rich zones of the draining lymph nodes. Thus, to reach this site, a migration of the formerly sessile, resident dendritic cells into the lymphatic vasculature must occur.

3 Guidance of Activated Antigen Presenting Cells to the Lymph Node

The cornea is physiologically free of blood and lymphatic vessels. Nevertheless, even in non-vascularized low-risk recipient corneas migration of activated dendritic cells into the lymphatic vasculature in the region of the limbus occurs. Sutures after PKP represent a significant risk factor for corneal neovascularization facilitating the migration of activated APCs into the lymphatic vasculature [14].

In vascularized tissues, directional guidance for immunocompetent cells is provided by concentration gradients of chemokines. These small proteins can be secreted into adjacent areas in a tissue- and inflammation-specific manner. The migration towards the lymphatic vasculature is controlled by a concentration gradient of the chemokines CCL-19 and CCL-21. This concentration gradient increases towards the lymphatic vasculature. Activated APCs express the receptor CCR7, which is complementary to CCL-19 and CCL-21 and enables targeted migration along the gradient into the lymphatic vasculature. It was demonstrated that migration of APCs after corneal transplantation in vascularized recipients can be reduced by blocking of CCR7 or the CCR7 ligand CCL21 [15, 16].

The cornea, as an avascular tissue, does not initially reveal any guidance structures that might allow APCs located in the center of the cornea to migrate into the lymphatic vasculature adjacent to the corneal periphery in the region of the limbus. However, $CCR7^{+}$ cells are known to migrate out of the cornea into the cervical lymph nodes after an inflammatory stimulus.

Migration into the lymphatic vasculature describes a pathway also known as the afferent arm of the so-called immune reflex arc [17]. Disruption of the afferent arm of the immune reflex arc results in altered or delayed immune responses, as evidenced by studies in mice with malformation of the lymphatic vasculature [18–20]. It is known that cervical lymph node harvesting significantly prolongs graft survival in mouse models [21, 22]. Furthermore, it has been shown that suppressed lymphangiogenesis after allogeneic corneal transplantation also leads to improved graft survival. Mice with a defect in the gene encoding CCR7, a chemokine receptor that controls the targeted migration of antigen-presenting cells into the lymphatic vasculature [23, 24], exhibit absent or delayed type IV immune responses.

Despite its avascularity and optical clarity, the cornea possesses many potential inflammatory cells. Local immature antigen-presenting cells upon inflammatory stimulation undergo a maturation process with antigen uptake, which enables them to initiate adaptive immune responses by targeted antigen presentation. The central cornea has only immature MHC II negative dendritic cells and macrophages [25]. It is known from studies of other tissues that during such a maturation process, in addition to the upregulation of MHCII, there is also expression of the chemokine receptor CCR7 on the cell membrane outer surface of these cells. This receptor is the only known chemokine receptor that regulates the guidance of immunocompetent cells into the lymphatic system. Even in the physiological state, the number of antigen-presenting cells in the tissues of different organs does not represent a constant quantity, since antigen-presenting cells are subject to a continuous turn over [26, 27]. However, this implies that a controlled, targeted migration must also exist out of the cornea, although the cornea in the physiologically avascular state does not initially reveal any guidance structures. However, it is known that in the inflamed cornea $CD11b^{+}$ and $CD11C^{+}$ antigen presenting cells are present that express CCR7 [28].

4 Immunity and Tolerance

Already hours after transplantation antigen specific dendritic cells arrive in the draining cervical lymph nodes [29]. Allo-antigens in lymph nodes are recognized by host T cells either via the direct pathway, in which intact donor MHC molecules are recognized on donor-derived antigen presenting cells, or via the indirect pathway, in which donor-derived major or minor MHC peptides are recognized on host antigen presenting cells [30, 31]. In prevascularized high-risk recipient corneas, the direct pathway plays a role in allo-antigen recognition by T cells in addition to the indirect pathway [31].

Upon allo-antigen recognition allo-antigen specific $CD4^+$T helper (T_H) and $CD8^+$cytotoxic T cells (CTLs) proliferate and generate graft rejection. The pathway of the rejection is referred to in a simplified description as the immune-reflex arc (Fig. 1), in which the lymphatic vessels represent the afferent arc and the blood vessels represent the efferent arc [17].

CCR7 also mediates the migration of naïve T cells as well as forkhead box P3 $(FOXP3)^+CD4^+CD25^+$ regulatory T (T_{Reg}) cells into the T-cell zone of the lymph nodes. After contact with their target antigen T_{Reg} cells proliferate [32]. Subsets of T_{Reg} cells can either suppress T-cell-mediated inflammation in peripheral tissues (effector-like T_{Reg} cells) or reduce the formation, the number and the differentiation of antigen induced T_H cells as a main contributor to allo-antigen specific immunity [32–34]. The balance between immunity or tolerance depends on the degree of inflammatory response upon antigen stimulation, the pathway by which antigens are processed, and the type and degree of differentiation of cells involved in antigen presentation or recognition [20]. After clonal expansion, allo-antigen-specific Th cells and CTLs use blood vessels for their migration to the graft as the efferent part of the immune reflex arc.

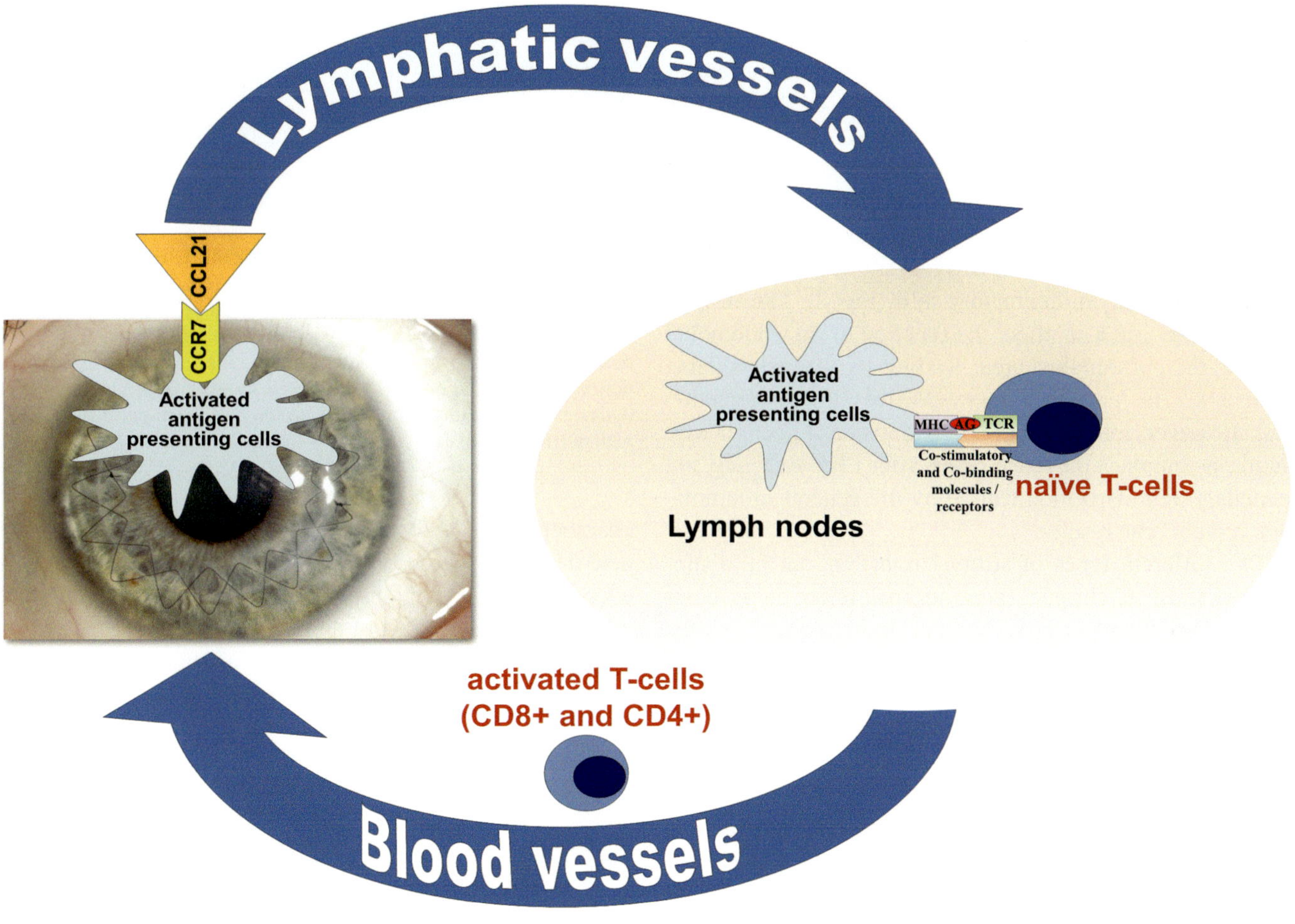

Fig. 1 In this simplified depiction, the immune reflex arc describes the steps leading to corneal graft rejection. After corneal transplantation, activated antigen-presenting cells follow the concentration gradient of the cytokine CCL21 into the lymphatic system (afferent arc) with the corresponding chemokine receptor CCR7 and thus reach the draining lymph nodes. Here, after contact with naïve T cells, proliferation of allo-antigen specific $CD4^+$T helper (TH) and $CD8^+$cytotoxic T cells (CTLs) is induced. These cells then reach the donor cornea via blood vessels (efferent arc) and can thus start the immunological transplant reaction

5 Types of Corneal Graft Rejection

Rejections after corneal transplantation are differentiated according to the tissue involved. The most common rejection with the most clinical significance is endothelial rejection. But there are also rejections of stroma and epithelium of the cornea. The latter is self-limiting and without lasting clinical effects as long as the recipient has his or her own intact limbal epithelial stem cells that allow replacement of the rejected epithelial cells. Since corneal epithelium undergoes a natural turnover, epithelial rejections after standard PKP or DALK are virtually not clinically apparent. However, epithelial rejection remains a serious event after limbal stem cell transplantation. Epithelial rejection after successful limbal stem cell transplantation may be associated with a line of rejection analogous to endothelial rejection, in addition to diffuse opacities and increased corneal neovascularization [35, 36]. The eye is quiet or only slightly inflamed.

Stromal and subepithelial rejections are rare immune reactions occurring after PKP or DALK [37]. The low incidence of such rejections is related to the small number of cells, namely keratocytes, in the grafted stroma; moreover, these donor keratocytes can be replaced by keratocytes from the surrounding recipient cornea. Also type I collagen as an essential component of the corneal stroma does not contribute to allo-antigeneic immune reactions since it is highly conserved even between species. Selective stromal rejection is characterized by a stromal opacification which is caused by inflammatory cells (Fig. 2). The stromal inflammation can also affect the function of the endothelial cells in the surrounding area, leading to stromal oedema without keratic precipitates in selective stromal rejection [38]. However, joint stromal and endothelial rejection with keratic precipitates may also occur after PKP. Scarring and secondary vascularization caused by the general inflammatory stimulus can result.

Two different types of stromal rejection can be distinguished [39]: A chronic focal stromal rejection is characterized by small patchy opacities in or adjacent to the Bowman layer of the graft only. Absence of conjunctival injection may rule out adenoviral infection. A hyperacute stromal rejection occurs suddenly and is characterized by peripheral whitish infiltration involving the entire corneal thickness. An abscess like formation of the infiltration can occur. Typically, there is a simultaneous endothelial rejection.

Endothelial rejection is the principal cause of graft failure after normal-risk PKP and it also occurs at a low rate after normal-risk DMEK [1, 2, 4]. Endothelial rejection can be identified by either diffuse keratic precipitates on the graft or endothelial rejection lines (Khodadoust line) in conjunction with inflammatory cells in the anterior chamber (Fig. 3). At a certain level of inflammation, corneal decompensation occurs, causing either diffuse or focal edema of the cornea. Frequently diffuse precipitates cannot be distinguished from herpes endotheliitis. Since transplanted endothelial cells may also migrate from the graft to the bare stroma or Descemet membrane of the recipient, especially after DMEK, inflammatory precipitates outside the graft also do not always allow a reliable exclusion of rejection.

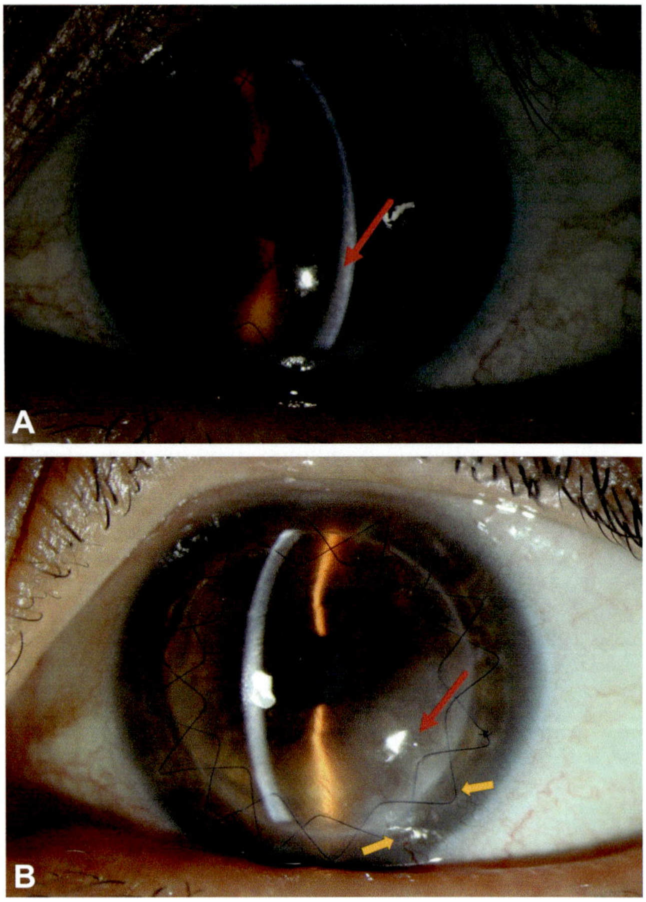

Fig. 2 Stromal rejection after deep anterior lamellar keratoplasty (DALK). There are opacities in the donor stroma (**A**, red arrow) and stromal vascularization in the recipient bed (**B**, yellow arrow) attracted by the sutures and extending into the graft (**B**, red arrow). The opacified area extends to the optically relevant zone. Corneal vascularization would have significantly increased the risk for endothelial graft reaction if penetrating keratoplasty would have been performed in this patient (from [57])

6 Graft Rejection After PKP

The incidence of graft rejection after PKP is reported to be between 17 and 21% reducing the graft survival rate after 10 years from 66 to 40% [1]. Graft rejection accounts for 26% of graft failure after PKP. However, rejection is highly

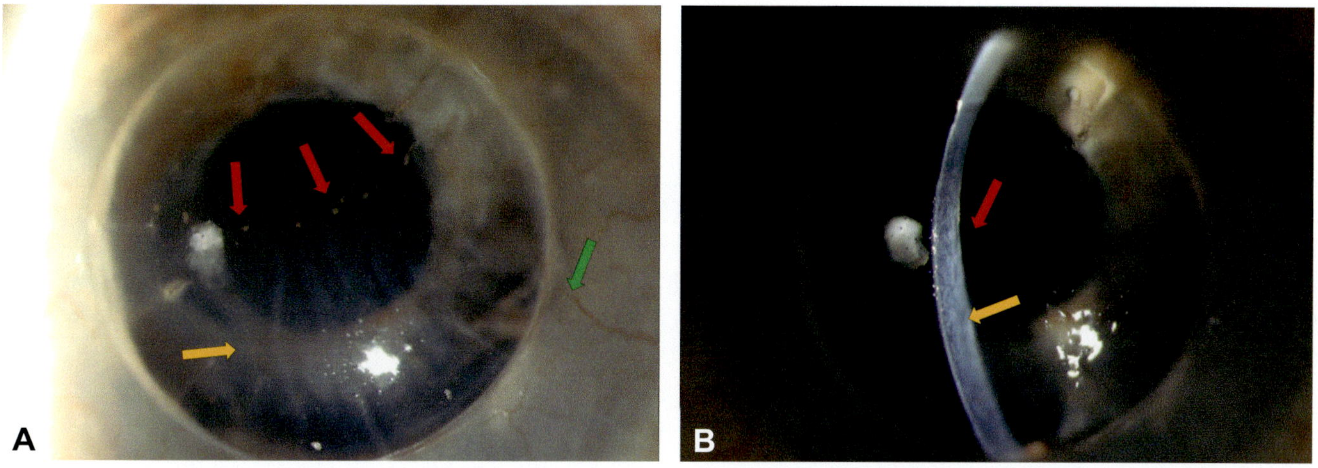

Fig. 3 The corneal graft was placed in a prevascularized recipient bed at high risk for graft rejection. At the time of rejection, clearly visible blood vessels extend to the donor-recipient interface (green arrow in **A**). Typically, the feeding vessels in the adjacent conjunctiva dilate. Endothelial rejection may diffusely affect the entire posterior surface. However, if T lymphocytes are delivered to the graft only via vessels from a specific adjacent area, the rejection crosses the corneal posterior surface coming from that direction. Already rejected endothelial cell areas lead to swelling of the overlying stroma (yellow arrow in **A**, **B**). These areas sometimes look wavy and at their end a rejection line of pigmented immune cells (Khodadoust line; red arrow in **A**, **B**) forms and marks the area where rejection is currently taking place

dependent on the indication, with underlying inflammatory diseases and pediatric transplantation being highly detrimental, as is preexisting vascularization [1, 2]. After first transplantation in keratoconus, in which the cornea is usually free of vessels and in which there is mostly no inflammation of the ocular surface, graft survival is very high at 78% after 10 years, even without systemic immunosuppression [1]. Beyond indication and prevascularization, there are several other risk factors for decreased graft survival, such as donor age, previous cataract surgery, intraocular pressure elevation, but not all are clearly associated with rejection. However, there is an association between graft size in relation to the overall diameter of the recipient cornea as well as to the centration of the graft with the occurrence of rejection after PKP [40]. A relatively large graft and decentration close to the limbus seems to be disadvantageous in terms of rejection (Fig. 4).

7 Graft Rejection After DALK

After DALK, the functional and refractive results are comparable to those after PKP, but not only do significantly more endothelial cells remain but more importantly these

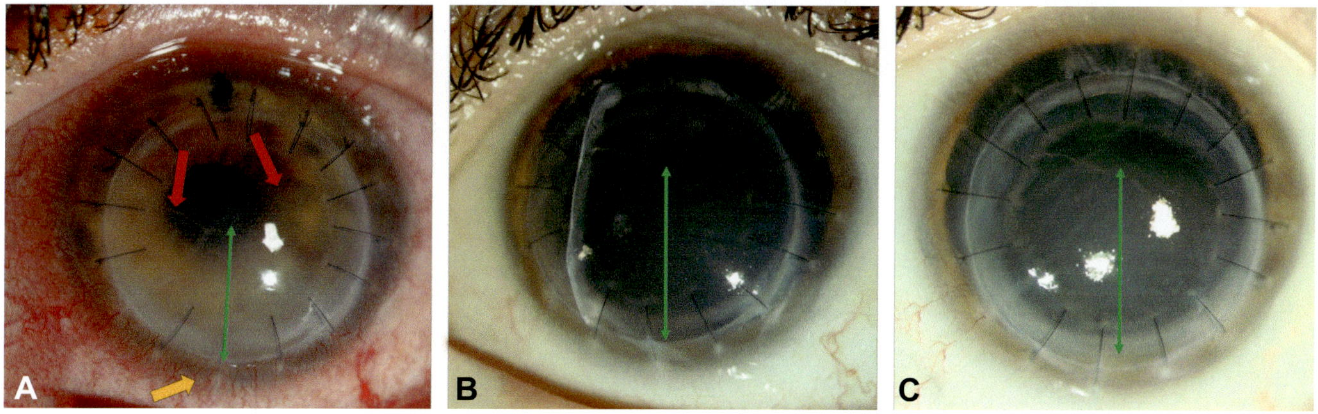

Fig. 4 The graft is decentered downwards and has thus come close to the inferior limbus. From here, blood vessels have grown to the interface (**A**, yellow arrow) causing rejection. The immune reaction has already damaged the endothelial cells of the lower half of the graft (**A**, green arrow). The area with damaged endothelial cells is separated from intact endothelial cells by a rejection line (**A**, red arrows). After immediate initiation of immunosuppressive therapy with corticosteroids, there was a rapid decrease in the local inflammatory response. Still, the affected area of the corneal posterior surface enlarged and the rejection line continued to move further upward (**B**, **C** green arrow) before stabilization could be achieved

are the patient's own endothelial cells [41]. For this reason, only stromal, subepithelial and epithelial rejection can occur [41]. Epithelial rejection is only of clinical significance if transplantation was performed in patients with limbal stem cell insufficiency with attached allogeneic limbus as so-called limbo-DALK [42].

Depending on the DALK indication, stromal rejection occurs in approximately 5.3% of cases and is associated with conjunctival injection, corneal neovascularization, and stromal opacification as well as scarring [37]. Some analysis suggest that stromal graft rejection occurs more frequently after DALK compared to PKP [4]. One possible explanation for this phenomenon is that after PKP, the transplanted endothelial cells induce tolerance through their relationship to the anterior chamber, which is absent after DALK. This mechanism is referred to as Anterior Chamber-Associated Immune Deviation (ACAID) [43]. Many patients with stromal rejection are asymptomatic. There further appears to be a correlation with discontinuation of local steroids and the occurrence of stromal rejection, most of which occur within the first postoperative year [44].

8 Endothelial Rejection After DMEK

Graft rejection has lost its fright since the introduction of DMEK. It barely occurs after DMEK and can only be seen in about 1–2.5% within the first two to five postoperative years [45–47]. In contrast, the rate of graft rejection after DSEK and PKP is 15 fold and 20 fold higher, respectively [48]. The signs for graft rejection are usually weaker than those seen in PKP patients. Many patients just have isolated diffuse keratic precipitates without accompanying corneal edema (Fig. 5). These patients might still have very good vision despite increasing amounts of keratic precipitates over weeks or months and the diagnosis of rejection is frequently made by chance during routine examinations. Commonly the precipitates can be observed on the graft itself but since donor endothelial cells also migrate from the graft onto the neighbouring denuded corneal stroma keratitic precipitates can also be seen outside the graft in the context of DMEK graft rejection [49]. But also corneal edema and the formation of a Khodadoust line can occur in graft rejections after DMEK especially in high-risk situations (Figs. 6 and 7) [50].

9 Prophylaxis and Treatment of Graft Rejections

The mainstay of prophylactic and acute treatment of corneal graft rejections are glucocorticoids. Systemic glucocorticoids are used for short-term immunosuppression, although no advantage over topical steroids has been shown for the course after normal-risk keratoplasty [51]. Often, they can be used to bridge the time until calcineurin inhibitors or mycophenolate mofetil, which can be used for longer-term immunosuppression, take effect. Systemic immunosuppression is generally indicated after high-risk allogeneic corneal transplantation or limbal transplantation to prevent rejection. Systemic immunosuppressants are used immediately after or, when possible, before transplantation. Overlapping systemic immunosuppressive therapy with glucocorticoids should be maintained for several weeks and tapered slowly. Various glucocorticoids have hydrophilic properties, in some rejections, it may be useful

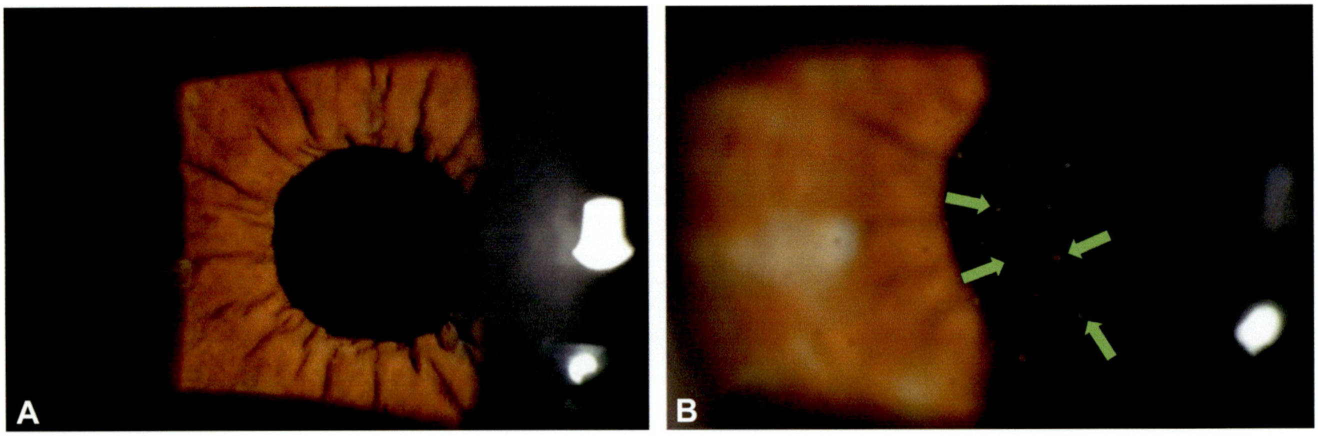

Fig. 5 After Descemet membrane endothelial keratoplasty (DMEK) rejections are generally rare. They occur within the first 5 years in about 2–3% of normal risk patients. Often the rejection is initially very subtle and is then diagnosed by accident during follow-up examinations. Initially, the cornea does not become opacified, and therefore intraocular structures such as the iris are still clearly visible during slit lamp examination (**A**) Only when focusing on the endothelium, diffusely distributed keratic precipitates of different sizes appear (**B**, **green arrows**). A rejection line is rarely found after DMEK. The patient in this example had a visual acuity of 20/20 when rejection was recognized

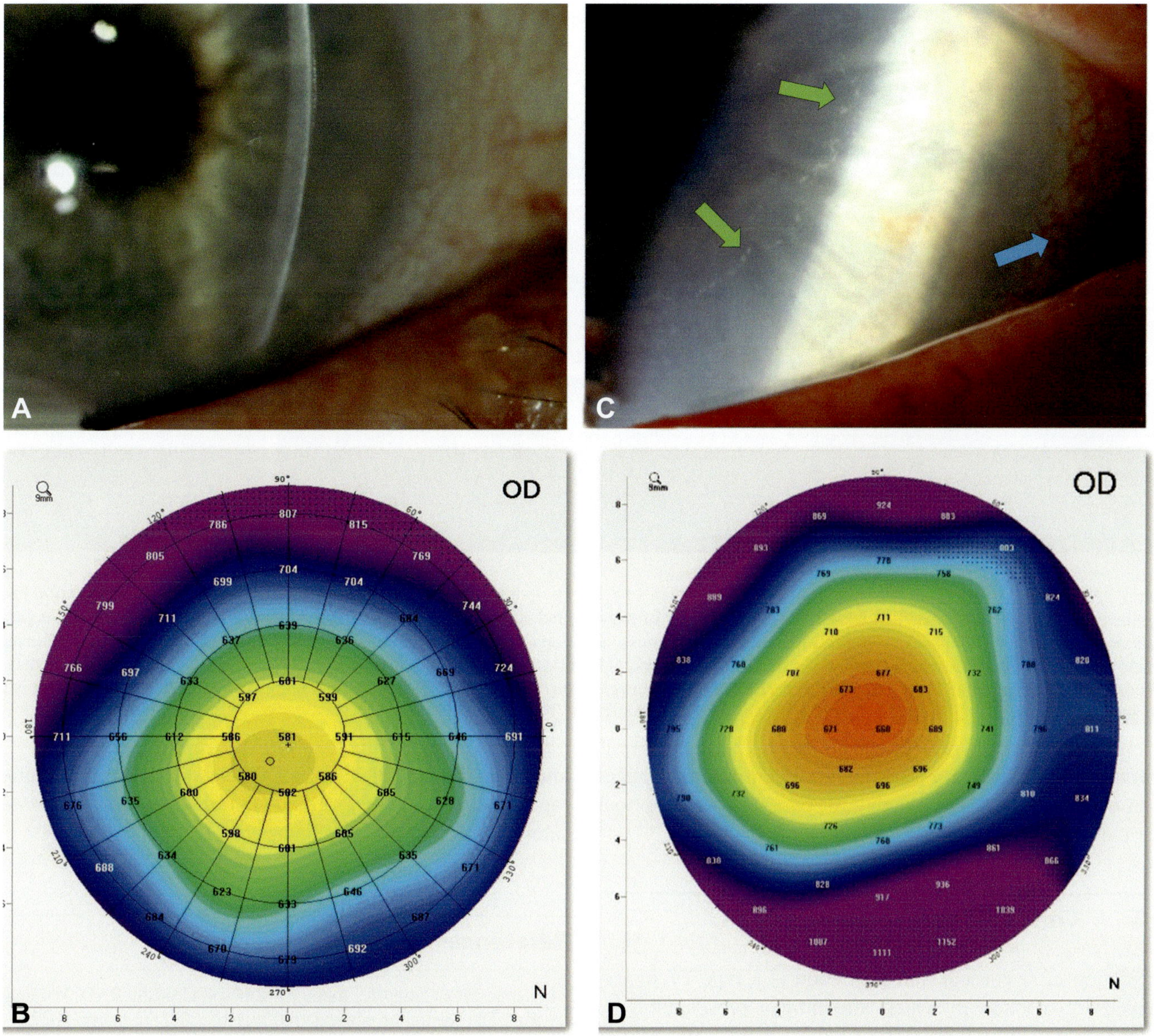

Fig. 6 After successful DMEK with clear cornea and regular corneal thickness (**A**, **B**) a Khodadoust line has developed (**C**, **green arrows**). In the area peripheral to the rejection line, the cornea is thickened (**D**) unlike in early rejections after DMEK without a rejection line, the adjacent conjunctiva is clearly injected (**C**, **blue arrow**)

to bypass the corneal epithelial barrier by peribulbar or intraocular application and create a drug depot. In this way, depending on the choice of preparation, a high, prolonged, and continuous level of action of the glucocorticoid can be maintained.

After keratoplasty, prednisolone acetate eye drops are usually administered, but can be switched to preservative- and phosphate-free dexamethasone eye drops in case of surface defects of the eye. Recommendations for the duration of topical therapy with glucocorticoids differ. Some authors recommend prophylactic treatment at least until 6 months after suture removal, in pseudophakic eyes even longer [52]. It was shown that administration of a single drop prednisolone acetate per day could significantly decrease immune responses when administered for 12 rather than for 6 months after normal-risk PKP [53].

For the prophylaxis of the already very low rejection rate after DMEK, topical application of steroids with lower glucocorticoid activity are effective in preventing graft rejection. In a prospective study loteprednol etabonate had no immunologic disadvantage compared to prednisolone acetate with lower risk of steroid-induced elevation of

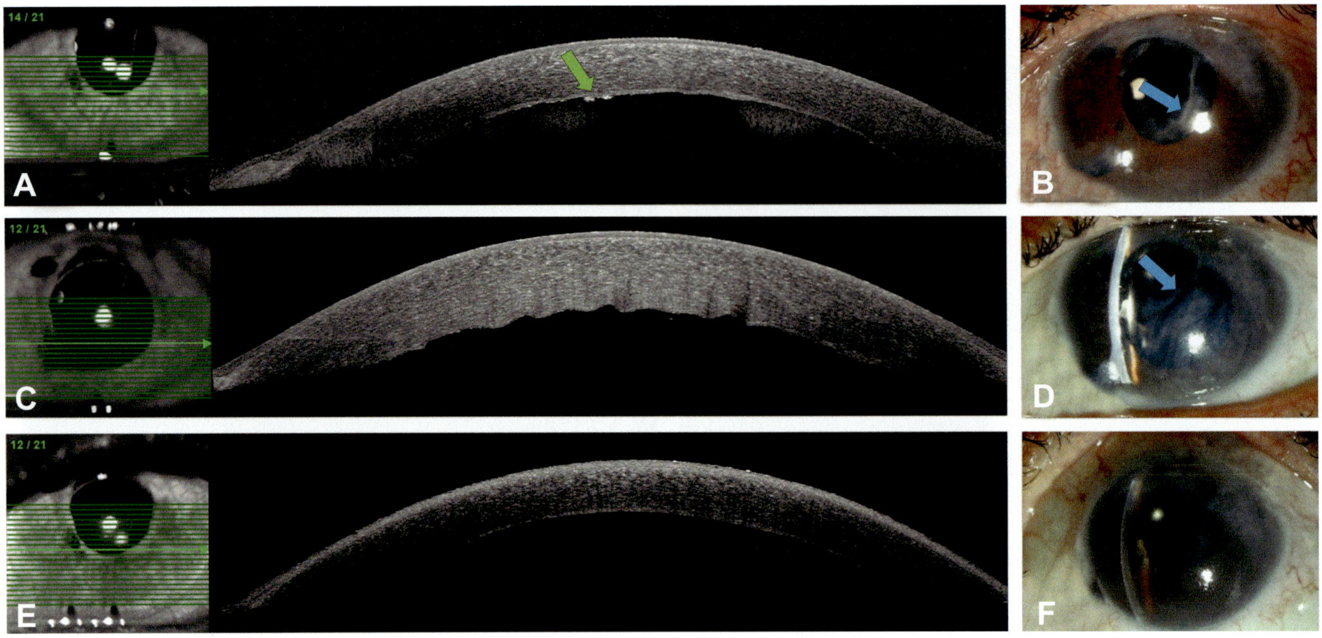

Fig. 7 At the onset of rejection after high-risk DMEK (**A**, **B**) in an eye with multiple previous operations and anterior synechiae, a rejection line is already visible (**B**, blue arrow). However, the cornea is still of regular thickness. Keratic precipitates can also be visualized by optical coherence tomography (OCT; **A**, green arrow). Despite immunosuppressive therapy, the corneal edema increases (**C**) and the rejection line continues to move across the posterior surface of the cornea (**D**, blue arrow). At this stage, inflammation has clearly decreased, as evidenced by a decrease in conjunctival injection and precipitates, which are also no longer seen on OCT sections. With continued immunosuppressive therapy, there is a decrease in corneal edema (**E**) and a disappearance of the Khodadoust line (**F**)

intraocular pressure [54, 55]. However, continuous application of at least one drop per day for two years is important for the prevention of graft rejection [46, 56].

10 Conclusion

Rejection after corneal transplantation is a type IV hypersensitivity reaction in which allo-antigen presentation by either donor antigen-presenting cells (direct pathway) or recipient antigen-presenting cells (indirect pathway) results in the formation of allo-antigen specific $CD4^{+}$T helper (TH) and $CD8^{+}$cytotoxic T cells (CTLs) as the most important promoters of allogeneic cell damage. The immune privilege of the cornea and the anterior chamber as well as the corneal angiogenic privilege contribute to immune ignorance and the development of immune tolerance resulting in a very low rejection rate after low-risk transplantation. In principle, all layers of a corneal graft can be rejected either individually or in combination. Among the different types of alloimmune responses, endothelial rejection has the greatest significance in terms of both numbers and resulting functional impairment. The last two decades have seen an evolution from PKP to lamellar transplantation techniques in which either no donor antigen-presenting cells (DMEK) or no donor endothelial cells (DALK) are transplanted. This, along with a broader and more comprehensive knowledge about rejection prophylaxis after lamellar keratoplasty has led to less frequent rejections and increased safety after corneal transplantation.

References

1. Keane MC, Coffey N, Jones VJ, Lawson C, Mills RAD, Williams KA. The Australian corneal graft registry 2021/22 report. 2022.
2. Bachmann B, Taylor RS, Cursiefen C. Corneal neovascularization as a risk factor for graft failure and rejection after keratoplasty: an evidence-based meta-analysis. Ophthalmology. 2010;117(7):1300-5 e7.
3. Khodadoust AA. Penetrating keratoplasty in the rabbit. Am J Ophthalmol. 1968;66(5):899–905.
4. Hos D, Matthaei M, Bock F, Maruyama K, Notara M, Clahsen T, et al. Immune reactions after modern lamellar (DALK, DSAEK, DMEK) versus conventional penetrating corneal transplantation. Prog Retin Eye Res. 2019;73: 100768.
5. Rennert PD, Hochman PS, Flavell RA, Chaplin DD, Jayaraman S, Browning JL, et al. Essential role of lymph nodes in contact hypersensitivity revealed in lymphotoxin-alpha-deficient mice. J Exp Med. 2001;193(11):1227–38.
6. Lakkis FG, Arakelov A, Konieczny BT, Inoue Y. Immunologic 'ignorance' of vascularized organ transplants in the absence of secondary lymphoid tissue. Nat Med. 2000;6(6):686–8.
7. Kerjaschki D, Regele HM, Moosberger I, Nagy-Bojarski K, Watschinger B, Soleiman A, et al. Lymphatic neoangiogenesis in human kidney transplants is associated with immunologically active lymphocytic infiltrates. J Am Soc Nephrol. 2004;15(3):603–12.

8. Cursiefen C, Cao J, Chen L, Liu Y, Maruyama K, Jackson D, et al. Inhibition of hemangiogenesis and lymphangiogenesis after normal-risk corneal transplantation by neutralizing VEGF promotes graft survival. Invest Ophthalmol Vis Sci. 2004;45(8):2666–73.
9. Roake JA, Rao AS, Morris PJ, Larsen CP, Hankins DF, Austyn JM. Dendritic cell loss from nonlymphoid tissues after systemic administration of lipopolysaccharide, tumor necrosis factor, and interleukin 1. J Exp Med. 1995;181(6):2237–47.
10. Sallusto F, Cella M, Danieli C, Lanzavecchia A. Dendritic cells use macropinocytosis and the mannose receptor to concentrate macromolecules in the major histocompatibility complex class II compartment: downregulation by cytokines and bacterial products. J Exp Med. 1995;182(2):389–400.
11. Gallucci S, Lolkema M, Matzinger P. Natural adjuvants: endogenous activators of dendritic cells. Nat Med. 1999;5(11):1249–55.
12. Cauwels A, Frei K, Sansano S, Fearns C, Ulevitch R, Zimmerli W, et al. The origin and function of soluble CD14 in experimental bacterial meningitis. J Immunol. 1999;162(8):4762–72.
13. Verbon A, Dekkers PE, ten Hove T, Hack CE, Pribble JP, Turner T, et al. IC14, an anti-CD14 antibody, inhibits endotoxin-mediated symptoms and inflammatory responses in humans. J Immunol. 2001;166(5):3599–605.
14. Cursiefen C, Wenkel H, Martus P, Langenbucher A, Nguyen NX, Seitz B, et al. Impact of short-term versus long-term topical steroids on corneal neovascularization after non-high-risk keratoplasty. Graefes Arch Clin Exp Ophthalmol. 2001;239(7):514–21.
15. Jin Y, Shen L, Chong EM, Hamrah P, Zhang Q, Chen L, et al. The chemokine receptor CCR7 mediates corneal antigen-presenting cell trafficking. Mol Vis. 2007;13:626–34.
16. Hos D, Dorrie J, Schaft N, Bock F, Notara M, Kruse FE, et al. Blockade of CCR7 leads to decreased dendritic cell migration to draining lymph nodes and promotes graft survival in low-risk corneal transplantation. Exp Eye Res. 2016;146:1–6.
17. Kaplan HJ, Streilein JW, Stevens TR. Transplantation immunology of the anterior chamber of the eye. II. Immune response to allogeneic cells. J Immunol. 1975;115(3):805–10.
18. Gunn MD, Kyuwa S, Tam C, Kakiuchi T, Matsuzawa A, Williams LT, et al. Mice lacking expression of secondary lymphoid organ chemokine have defects in lymphocyte homing and dendritic cell localization. J Exp Med. 1999;189(3):451–60.
19. Nakano H, Gunn MD. Gene duplications at the chemokine locus on mouse chromosome 4: multiple strain-specific haplotypes and the deletion of secondary lymphoid-organ chemokine and EBI-1 ligand chemokine genes in the plt mutation. J Immunol. 2001;166(1):361–9.
20. Forster R, Schubel A, Breitfeld D, Kremmer E, Renner-Muller I, Wolf E, et al. CCR7 coordinates the primary immune response by establishing functional microenvironments in secondary lymphoid organs. Cell. 1999;99(1):23–33.
21. Yamagami S, Dana MR. The critical role of lymph nodes in corneal alloimmunization and graft rejection. Invest Ophthalmol Vis Sci. 2001;42(6):1293–8.
22. Yamagami S, Dana MR, Tsuru T. Draining lymph nodes play an essential role in alloimmunity generated in response to high-risk corneal transplantation. Cornea. 2002;21(4):405–9.
23. Chan VW, Kothakota S, Rohan MC, Panganiban-Lustan L, Gardner JP, Wachowicz MS, et al. Secondary lymphoid-tissue chemokine (SLC) is chemotactic for mature dendritic cells. Blood. 1999;93(11):3610–6.
24. Dieu MC, Vanbervliet B, Vicari A, Bridon JM, Oldham E, Ait-Yahia S, et al. Selective recruitment of immature and mature dendritic cells by distinct chemokines expressed in different anatomic sites. J Exp Med. 1998;188(2):373–86.
25. Hamrah P, Liu Y, Zhang Q, Dana MR. The corneal stroma is endowed with a significant number of resident dendritic cells. Invest Ophthalmol Vis Sci. 2003;44(2):581–9.
26. Holt PG, Haining S, Nelson DJ, Sedgwick JD. Origin and steady-state turnover of class II MHC-bearing dendritic cells in the epithelium of the conducting airways. J Immunol. 1994;153(1):256–61.
27. Kamath AT, Pooley J, O'Keeffe MA, Vremec D, Zhan Y, Lew AM, et al. The development, maturation, and turnover rate of mouse spleen dendritic cell populations. J Immunol. 2000;165(12):6762–70.
28. Jin Y, Shen L, Chen L, Zhang Q, Dana R. Expression of CCR7 by corneal antigen-presenting cells in inflammation. ARVO. 2005 (Posterpräsentation).
29. Forrester JV, Xu H, Kuffova L, Dick AD, McMenamin PG. Dendritic cell physiology and function in the eye. Immunol Rev. 2010;234(1):282–304.
30. Sano Y, Ksander BR, Streilein JW. Langerhans cells, orthotopic corneal allografts, and direct and indirect pathways of T-cell allorecognition. Invest Ophthalmol Vis Sci. 2000;41(6):1422–31.
31. Huq S, Liu Y, Benichou G, Dana MR. Relevance of the direct pathway of sensitization in corneal transplantation is dictated by the graft bed microenvironment. J Immunol. 2004;173(7):4464–9.
32. Schneider MA, Meingassner JG, Lipp M, Moore HD, Rot A. CCR7 is required for the in vivo function of $CD4^+$ $CD25^+$ regulatory T cells. J Exp Med. 2007;204(4):735–45.
33. Huehn J, Siegmund K, Lehmann JC, Siewert C, Haubold U, Feuerer M, et al. Developmental stage, phenotype, and migration distinguish Naive- and effector/memory-like $CD4^+$ regulatory T cells. J Exp Med. 2004;199(3):303–13.
34. Lee JH, Kang SG, Kim CH. FoxP3+ T cells undergo conventional first switch to lymphoid tissue homing receptors in thymus but accelerated second switch to nonlymphoid tissue homing receptors in secondary lymphoid tissues. J Immunol. 2007;178(1):301–11.
35. Vazirani J, Basu S, Sangwan VS. Allograft rejection after living-related simple limbal epithelial transplantation. Indian J Ophthalmol. 2021;69(2):433–5.
36. Khodadoust AA, Silverstein AM. The survival and rejection of epithelium in experimental corneal transplants. Invest Ophthalmol. 1969;8(2):169–79.
37. Olson EA, Tu EY, Basti S. Stromal rejection following deep anterior lamellar keratoplasty: implications for postoperative care. Cornea. 2012;31(9):969–73.
38. Watson SL, Tuft SJ, Dart JK. Patterns of rejection after deep lamellar keratoplasty. Ophthalmology. 2006;113(4):556–60.
39. Panda A, Vanathi M, Kumar A, Dash Y, Priya S. Corneal graft rejection. Surv Ophthalmol. 2007;52(4):375–96.
40. Tischer N, Zemova E, Maamri A, Pfeiffer M, Reinert U, Sideroudi H, Seitz B. Immune reaction after penetrating keratoplasty depending on graft size and centration. Ophthalmologie. 2023;120(1):36–42.
41. Borderie VM, Sandali O, Bullet J, Gaujoux T, Touzeau O, Laroche L. Long-term results of deep anterior lamellar versus penetrating keratoplasty. Ophthalmology. 2012;119(2):249–55.
42. Schöneberger V, Tahmaz V, Matthaei M, Roters S, Schlereth SL, Schaub F,et al. Allogeneic limbo-deep anterior lamellar keratoplasty (Limbo-DALK)-A novel surgical technique in corneal stromal disease and limbal stem cell deficiency. PLoS One. 2024;19(2):e0298241.
43. Streilein JW, Niederkorn JY. Induction of anterior chamber-associated immune deviation requires an intact, functional spleen. J Exp Med. 1981;153(5):1058–67.
44. Giannaccare G, Weiss JS, Sapigni L, Bovone C, Mattioli L, Campos EC, et al. Immunologic stromal rejection after deep anterior lamellar keratoplasty with grafts of a larger size (9 mm) for various stromal diseases. Cornea. 2018;37(8):967–72.
45. Schrittenlocher S, Schaub F, Hos D, Siebelmann S, Cursiefen C, Bachmann B. Evolution of consecutive Descemet membrane endothelial keratoplasty outcomes throughout a 5-year period performed by two experienced surgeons. Am J Ophthalmol. 2018;190:171–8.

46. Hos D, Tuac O, Schaub F, Stanzel TP, Schrittenlocher S, Hellmich M, et al. Incidence and clinical course of immune reactions after Descemet membrane endothelial keratoplasty: retrospective analysis of 1000 consecutive eyes. Ophthalmology. 2017;124(4):512–8.
47. Schaub F, Bachmann BO, Cursiefen C, Hos D. Midterm follow-up of immune reactions after Descemet membrane endothelial keratoplasty (DMEK). Graefes Arch Clin Exp Ophthalmol. 2019;257(8):1811–2.
48. Anshu A, Price MO, Price FW Jr. Risk of corneal transplant rejection significantly reduced with Descemet's membrane endothelial keratoplasty. Ophthalmology. 2012;119(3):536–40.
49. Hos D, Heindl LM, Bucher F, Cursiefen C. Evidence of donor corneal endothelial cell migration from immune reactions occurring after descemet membrane endothelial keratoplasty. Cornea. 2014;33(4):331–4.
50. Dapena I, Ham L, Netukova M, van der Wees J, Melles GR. Incidence of early allograft rejection after Descemet membrane endothelial keratoplasty. Cornea. 2011;30(12):1341–5.
51. Mayweg S, Reinhard T, Spelsberg H, Reis A, Godehardt E, Sundmacher R. Ranking of systemic steroids after normal-risk keratoplasty. Results of a randomized prospective study. Ophthalmologe. 2005;102(5):497–501.
52. Bachmann BO, Pleyer U, Maier PC, Reinhard T, Seitz B, Cursiefen C. Perioperative/postoperative anti-inflammatory therapy during/after corneal surgery/transplantation. Klin Monbl Augenheilkd. 2019;236(5):653–61.
53. Nguyen NX, Seitz B, Martus P, Langenbucher A, Cursiefen C. Long-term topical steroid treatment improves graft survival following normal-risk penetrating keratoplasty. Am J Ophthalmol. 2007;144(2):318–9.
54. Price MO, Feng MT, Scanameo A, Price FW, Jr. Loteprednol etabonate 0.5% Gel Vs. prednisolone acetate 1% solution after Descemet membrane endothelial keratoplasty: prospective randomized trial. Cornea. 2015;34(8):853–8.
55. Price MO, Price FW, Jr., Kruse FE, Bachmann BO, Tourtas T. Randomized comparison of topical prednisolone acetate 1% versus fluorometholone 0.1% in the first year after Descemet membrane endothelial keratoplasty. Cornea. 2014;33(9):880–6.
56. Price MO, Scanameo A, Feng MT, Price FW Jr. Descemet's membrane endothelial keratoplasty: risk of immunologic rejection episodes after discontinuing topical corticosteroids. Ophthalmology. 2016;123(6):1232–6.
57. Cursiefen C, Siebelmann S, Bachmann B. Complications of deep anterior lamellar keratoplasty. Avoid, recognize and treat. Ophthalmologe. 2015;112(12):961–8.

Neurotrophic Keratopathy: Clinical Picture, Non-surgical and Surgical Treatments

Johannes Menzel-Severing and Gerd Geerling

Abstract

Neurotrophic keratopathy (NK) is a rare corneal condition resulting from impaired corneal sensory innervation. It leads to spontaneous, recurrent epithelial defects that can progress to corneal ulceration and perforation. Causes of NK are manifold. Clinically, NK is divided into three stages. In mild NK, surface irregularities with typical superficial punctate keratitis and decrease or lack of sensitivity in one or more corneal quadrants are seen. Moderate NK is defined by epithelial defects with hypoesthesia or anesthesia of the entire cornea. Severe NK entails additional stromal involvement ("ulcer"), potentially causing corneal perforation. Therapeutically, pre-existing topical therapy should be adjusted to avoid any potential epithelial toxicity. Frequent lubricating eye drops are essential. In case of non-healing or recurrent epithelial defects, a bandage contact lens can provide protection from mechanical abrasion and thereby support resolution of the defect. Recombinant low molecular weight non-peptidic human nerve growth factor (NGF) is another therapeutic option which in clinical trials (Recordati study) has shown to improve epithelial healing in some patients. It however is costly and not readily available in every health system, which is why small molecules that mimic the effect of NGF are being investigated in clinical trials. These conservative options must be weighed individually against surgical measures such as amniotic membrane transplantation or tarsorrhaphy. Keratoplasty is used in patients with severe NK and stromal ulceration. Corneal neurotisation is an invasive, interdisciplinary treatment option that provides a causal treatment for NK and can restore corneal sensitivity.

Keywords

Neurotophic keratopathy · Persistent epithelial defect · Sterile ulceration · Medical treatment · Amniotic membrane transplantation · Keratoplasty · Corneal neurotisation

1 Introduction

Neurotrophic keratopathy is an orphan disease that can cause severe loss of visual acuity and therefore represents a substantial challenge in clinical ophthalmology. The prevalence is estimated at 1–5/10,000 [1]. A plethora of underlying diseases can cause neurotrophic keratopathy (NK) by damaging afferent nerves (Fig. 1) [2]. Etiologies include lesions of the trigeminal nerve (ophthalmic branch) that can be either nuclear lesions (e.g. CNS tumor, ischemia), lesions in the intracranial trajectory (e.g. multiple sclerosis, aneurysm, iatrogenic damage to the trigeminal ganglion, vestibular Schwannoma), lesions in the orbit (e.g. orbital tumors), or lesions in the cornea (e.g. herpes simplex/herpes zoster, refractive surgery, penetrating keratoplasty, contact lens wear) [3]. Diffuse damage of corneal nerves occurs in diabetes mellitus (diabetic polyneuropathy). Systemic or local drugs may also cause corneal hyposensitivity. Hereditary syndromes are rare causes of NK and include Riley–Day syndrome, Möbius syndrome, and Goldenhar syndrome.

NK has a somewhat typical clinical presentation that is relatively independent of the underlying cause (Fig. 2) [4]. The spectrum of neurotrophic corneal damage ranges from superficial punctate keratopathy (mild NK) to the development of a corneal epithelial defect (moderate NK) or

J. Menzel-Severing · G. Geerling (✉)
Department of Ophthalmology, Heinrich Heine University of Düsseldorf, Düsseldorf, Germany
e-mail: Geerling@med.uni-duesseldorf.de

B. Seitz et al. (eds.), *Atlas on Cornea*, https://doi.org/10.1007/978-3-031-65422-0_40

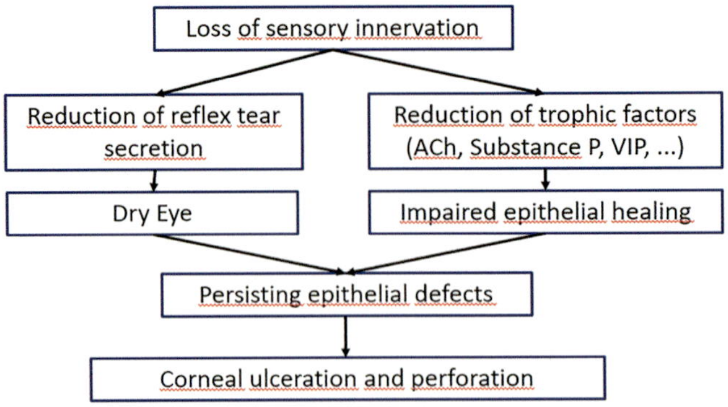

Fig. 1 **Etiology of neurotrophic keratopathy**. Loss of sensory corneal innervation is at the root of neurotrophic keratopathy. It results in reduced aqueous tear secretion and chronic hypo-secretory dry eye. This can cause corneal epithelial defects and/or impair epithelial healing. In addition, epithelial integrity or healing is impaired by the reduction of trophic factors which under physiologic conditions would be provided by sensory corneal nerves. Together, this pathway favours the persistence of epithelial defects, which can progress to corneal ulceration and frank perforation

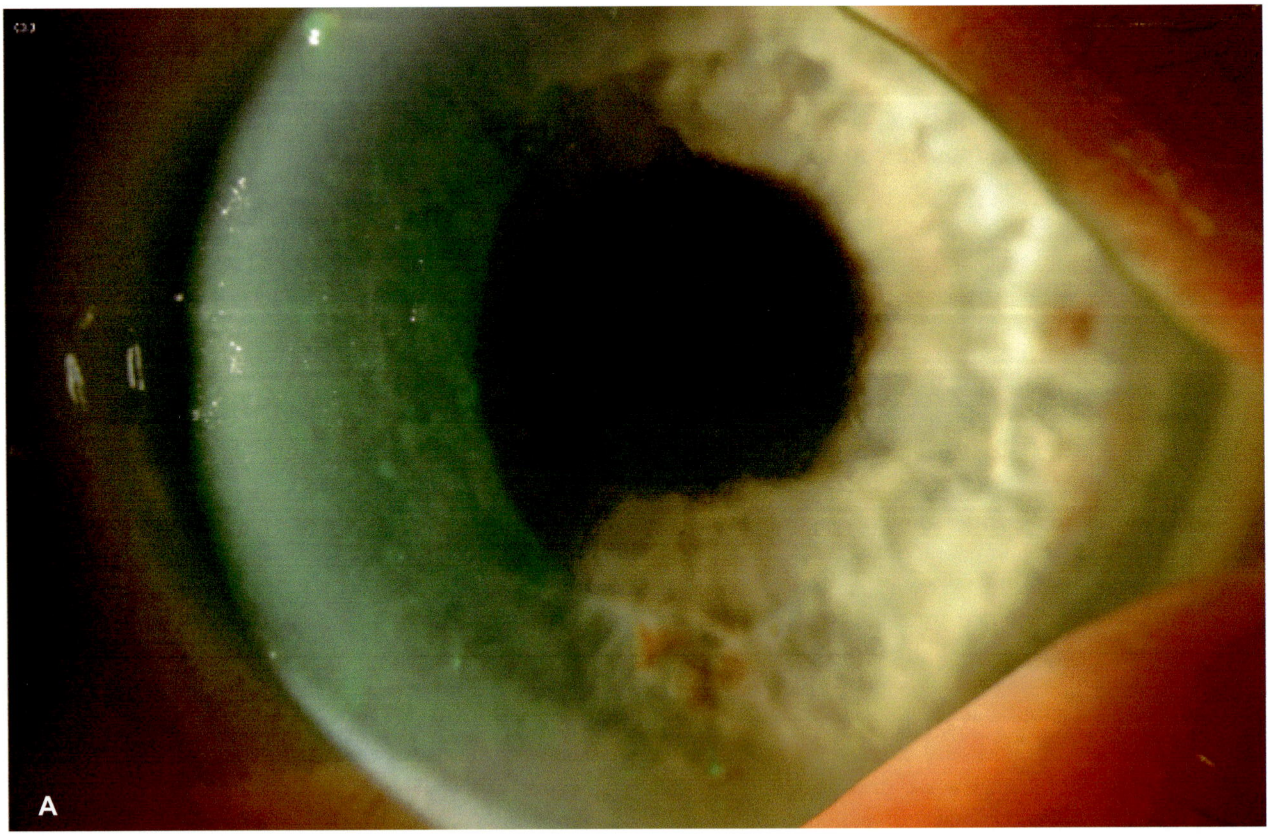

Fig. 2 **Dua classification stage I–III**. Patients with stage I neurotrophic keratopathy feature superficial punctate keratopathy, much like in severe chronic dry eye (**A**) At this stage, the presence of corneal hypoesthesia is crucial in guiding the diagnosis. In stage II, a chronic corneal epithelial defect ensues

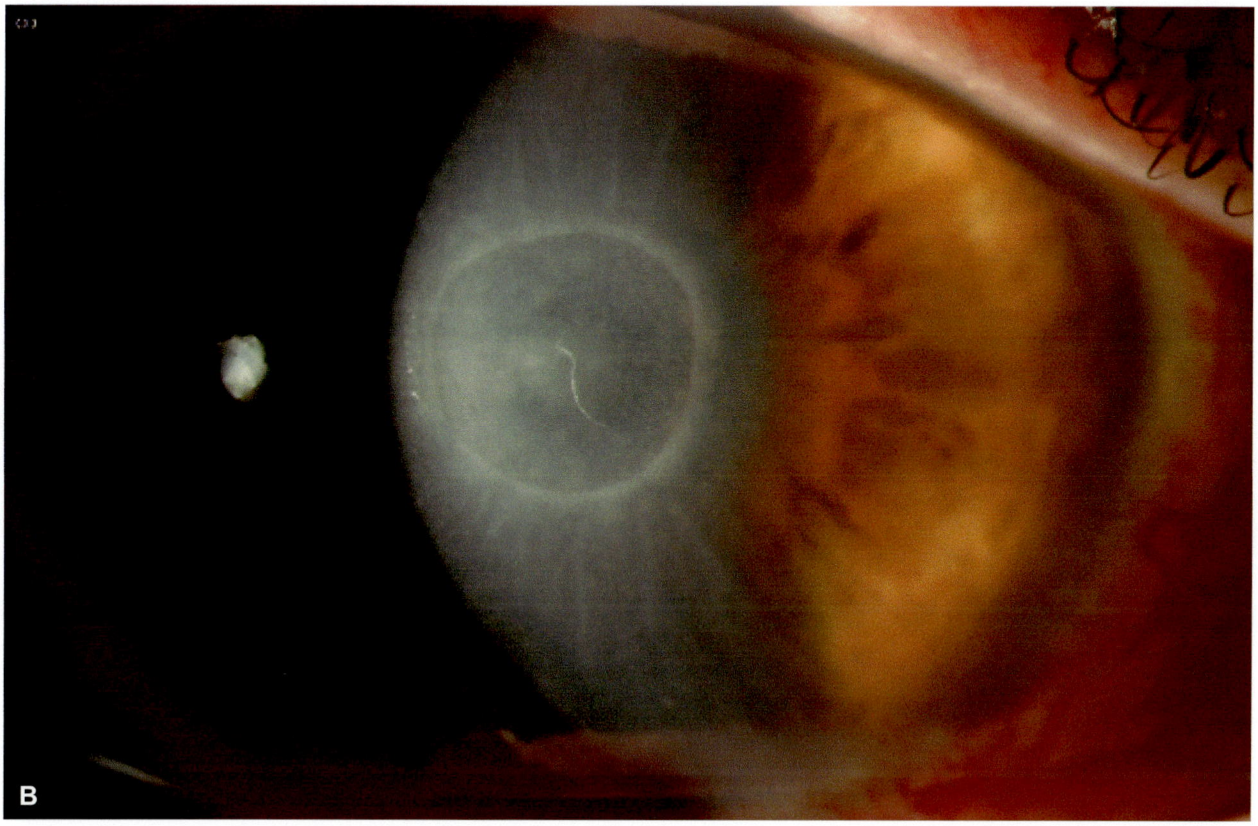

Fig. 2 (**B**) This can often have a rather characteristic appearance with blunt, rolled-up edges and horizontally oriented, oval shape. In contrast, epithelial defects that heal well often show different polygonal shapes. Striate keratopathy/Descemet folds are often present in addition. Inflammatory infiltrates are not a typical feature but may occur, particularly in cases with microbial superinfection. If the epithelial defect persists, lytic enzymes such as matrix metalloproteases contribute to stromal melting, leading to stage III: Corneal stromal ulceration

corneal stromal ulceration (severe NK) with or without perforation (Tables 1 and 2) [3, 5, 6]. In the initial stage, the clinical picture resembles chronic dry eye [7]. Therefore, the diagnosis is often delayed. The presence of surface damage in combination with a reduced corneal sensitivity makes a neurotrophic component of the disease probable (Fig. 3). The progression to more severe corneal epithelial defects is often asymptomatic due to the disturbed pain perception, especially in older patients [8].

Even mild NK should prompt treatment. The therapeutic goal is the preservation or restitution of corneal integrity [9]. In order to attain this goal, timely and stage-appropriate therapy is necessary [10]. As a basic therapy, frequent surface lubrication with preservative-free tear substitutes is required. Any local therapy is—depending on dosage and duration—potentially toxic for the epithelium. All eye drops used by the patient should therefore be preservative-free and phosphate-free, or discontinued

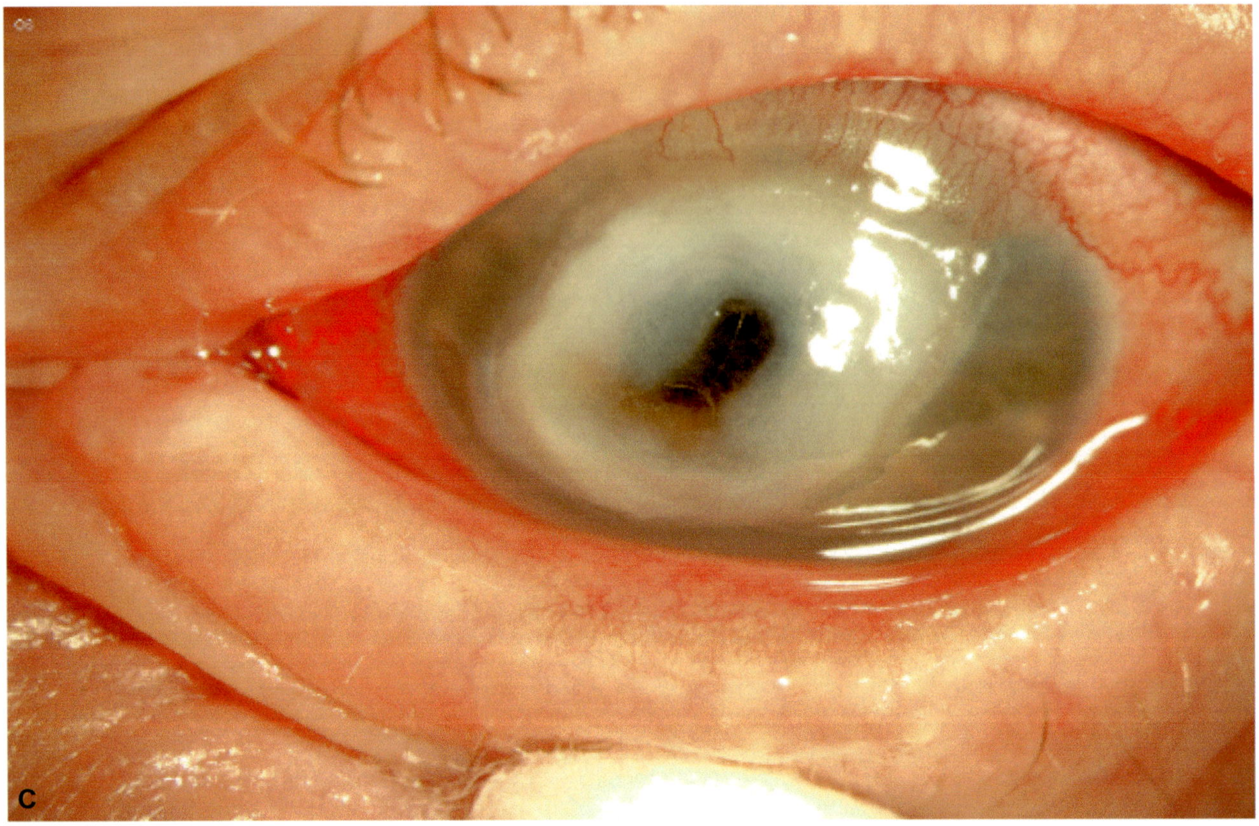

Fig. 2 (**C**) If sufficiently deep, a descemetocele can be seen, as in the eye depicted here. In this situation, corneal perforation may occur spontaneously or following minor trauma

Table 1 Clinical classification of neurotrophic keratopathy according to Mackie [5]

	Neurotrophic keratopathy, clinical stages (Mackie classification)
Stage I	Severe tear film disorder with superficial punctate keratitis, pathologic Schirmer/Jones test
Stage II	Persistent corneal erosions, typically with raised edges, striate keratopathy, stromal edema
Stage III	Corneal ulcer with progressive stromal melting up to perforation

Table 2 Clinical classification of neurotrophic keratopathy according to Dua [3]

	Neurotrophic keratopathy, clinical stages (Dua classification)
Mild	Epithelial irregularity without epithelial defect; tear film instability and symptoms with reduced or absent sensations in one or more quadrants of the cornea
Moderate	Persistent epithelial defect and corneal hypo-aesthesia/anaesthesia
Severe	Stromal involvement from corneal ulcer to perforation, with corneal hypo-aesthesia/anaesthesia

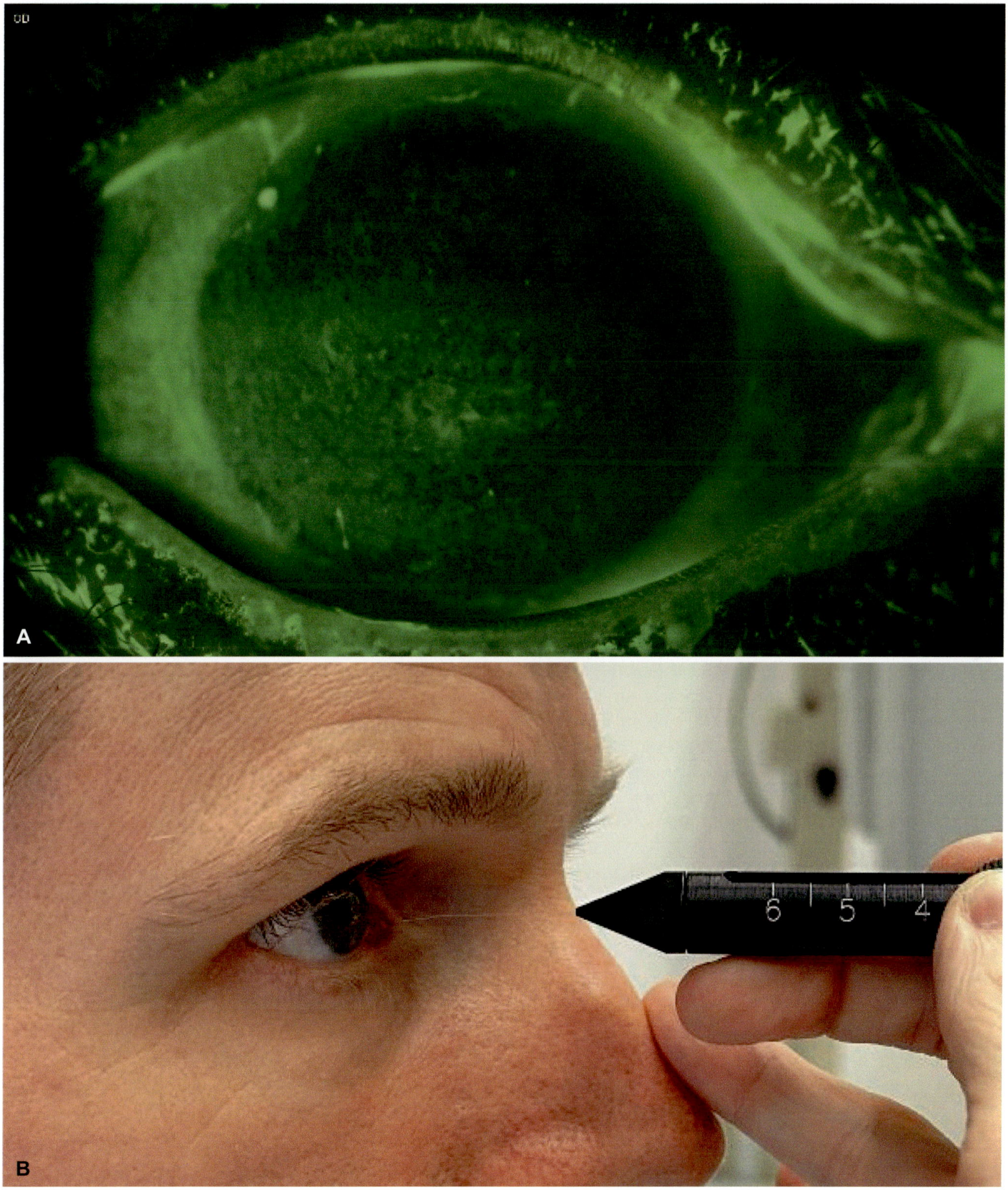

Fig. 3 **Diagnostics**. Fluoresceine staining (**A**) reveals the degree and localization of superficial punctate keratopathy and/or corneal epithelial defects. Corneal sensitivity is tested and quantified using the Cochet-Bonnet Aesthesiometer in all four quadrants of the cornea as well as centrally (**B**) The filament is pulled back in increments of 0.5 cm until the patient reports a sensation

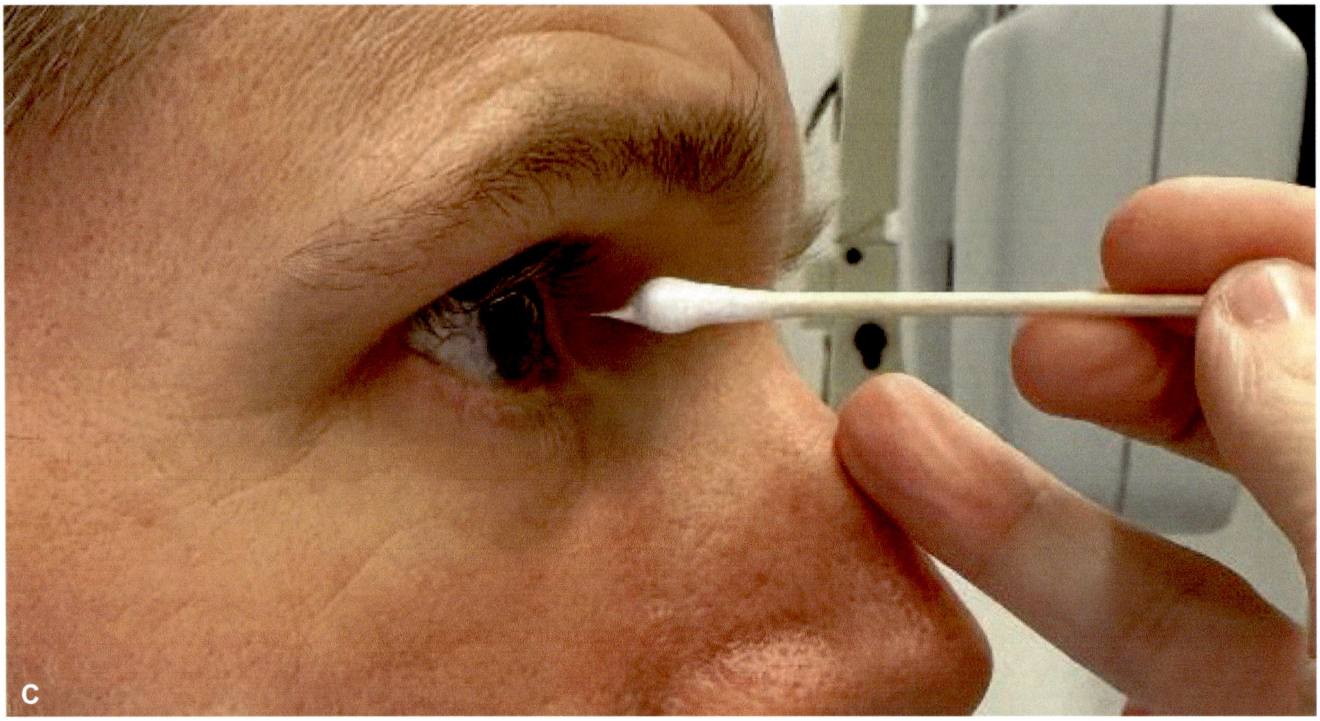

Fig. 3 (**C**) Where this dedicated device is not available, a thin strand from the tip of a clean cotton swab can be used to gain a rough idea of corneal sensitivity

if possible. A therapeutic contact lens, punctal plugs or botulinum toxin ptosis reduce mechanical stress on the corneal epithelium [11] (Fig. 4). Iatrogenic ptosis induced by injection of botulinum toxin in the levator muscle has been advocated, but can lead to a reduction in tear secretion which may be counterproductive. Topical treatment with recombinant human neurotrophic growth factor (NGF) is effective in supporting epithelial healing and may improve corneal sensitivity by increasing sub-basal nerve density, thereby promoting the resolution of persistent epithelial defects in NK, although this remains to be shown in clinical trials [12] (Fig. 5). Small molecules that mimic the effect of NGF are on the horizon as emerging novel therapies for this orphan disease. Eye drops made of autologous serum (AS) are another viable option if available [2]. They can, just like amniotic membrane transplantation (AMT) provide trophic factors, while the latter can simultaneously be used to substitute basement membrane, Bowman layer, and stroma (Fig. 6). Topical application of insulin (25 IU/ml) has also been reported to improve epithelial healing in persisting corneal epithelial defects and may be a good alternative to autologous serum [13]. Tarsorrhaphy can be used alone or in combination with other surgical and non-surgical techniques to reduce corneal exposure in the treatment of non-healing epithelial defects. A conjunctival flap can be

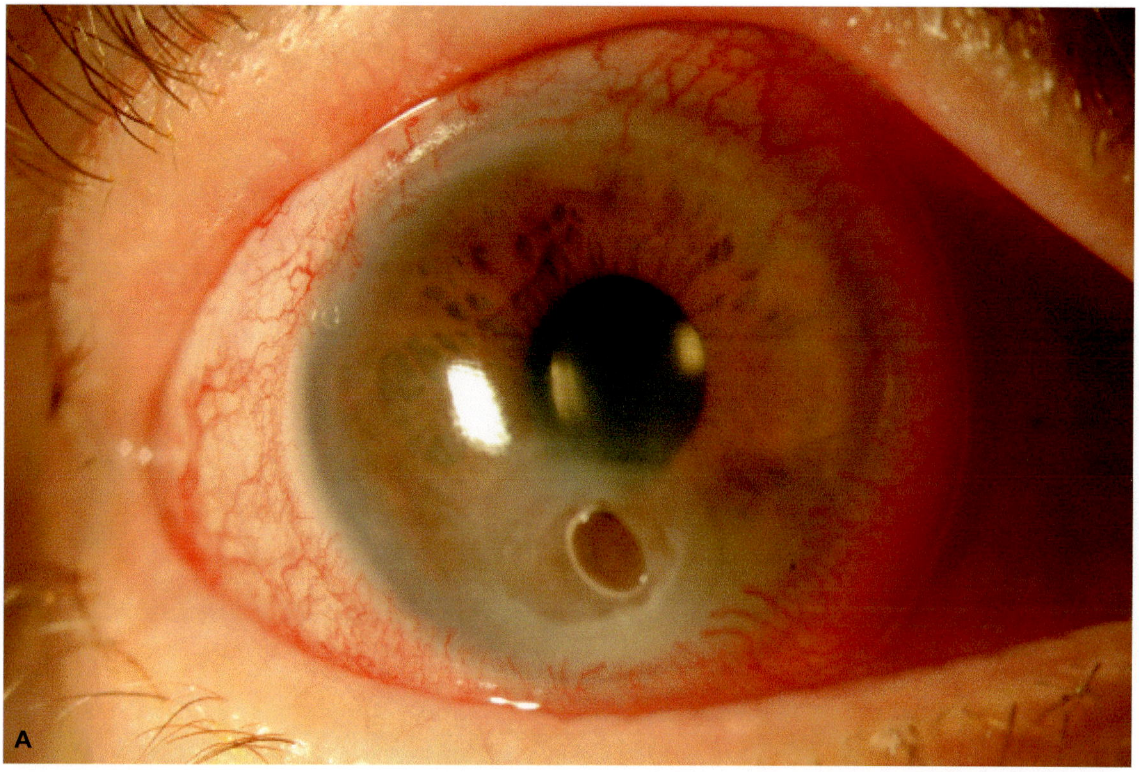

Fig. 4 **Non-surgical techniques**. Bandage contact lenses reduce friction and can be used to improve epithelial healing in corneal epithelial defects (**A**). They should be used in conjunction with frequent application of lubricating eye drops plus unpreserved topical, non-toxic antibiotics without phosphate

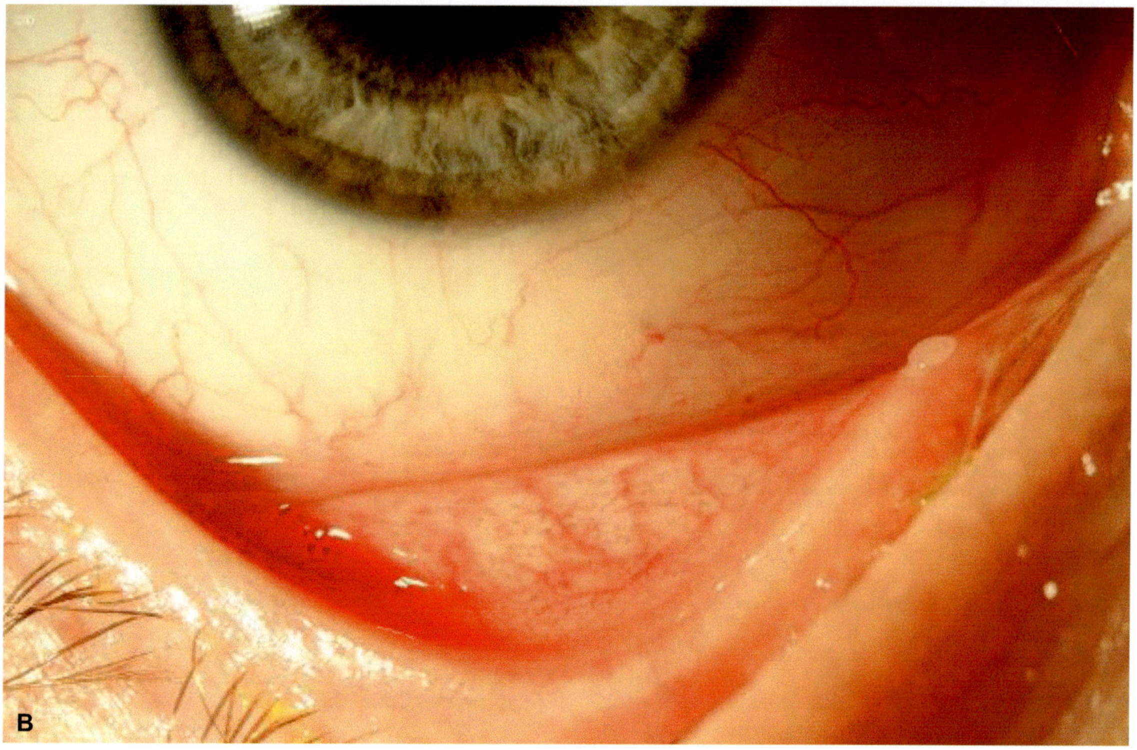

Fig. 4 Punctal occlusion can be achieved by insertion of resorbable punctum plugs, non-resorbable silicone plugs (**B**) or surgically

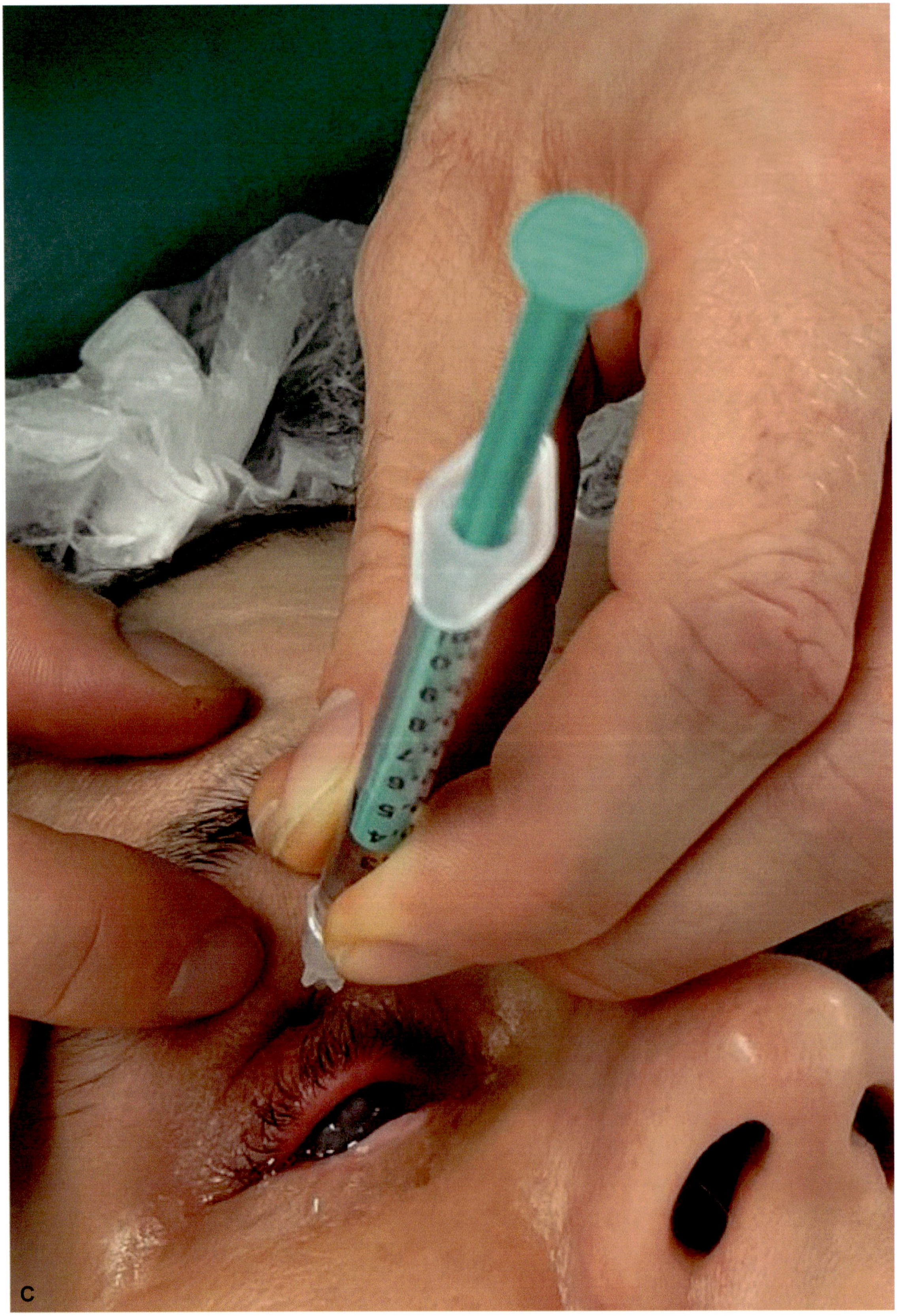

Fig. 4 Botox ptosis (**C**) is a minimally invasive, reversible and effective means of protecting the corneal epithelium from evaporation and frictional forces. However, it may also reduce lacrimal gland secretion. A 27G needle is fully inserted just above the levator muscle and 10 IU of botulinum toxin are injected. The effect may take 48–72 to appear and lasts for about 3 months. Care should be taken to provide sufficient artificial tears to the corneal surface, since tear secretion may be reduced

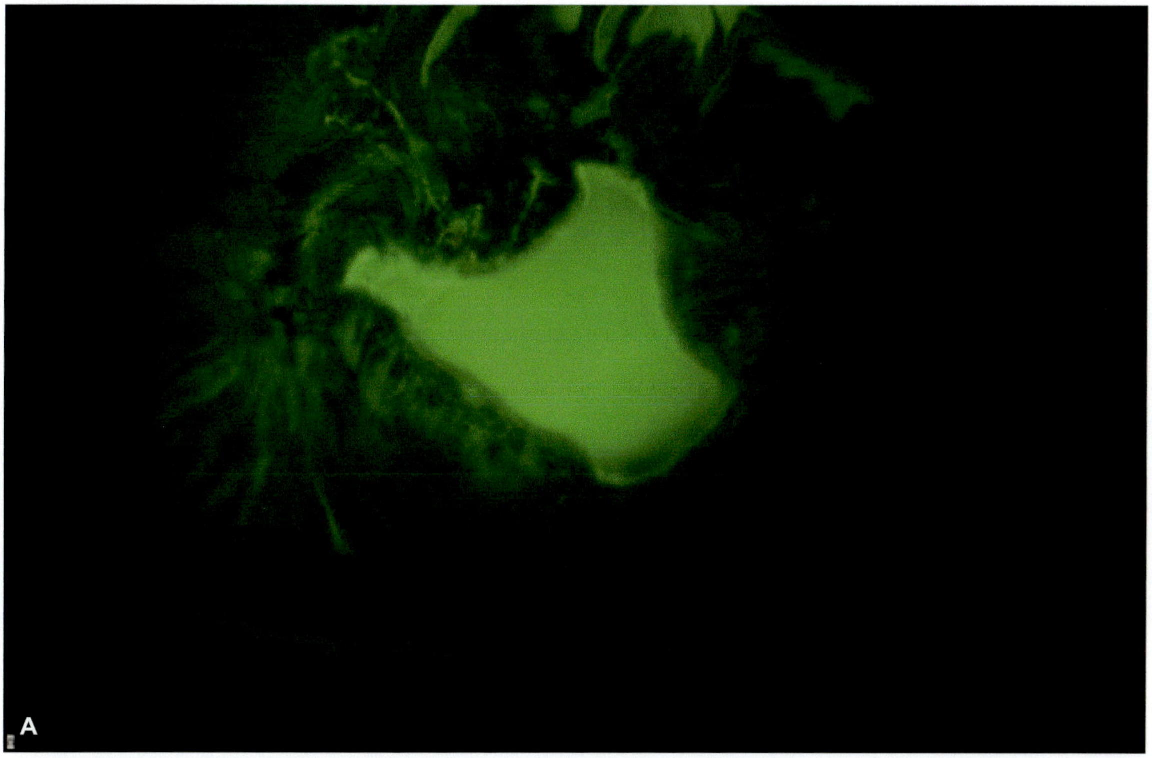

Fig. 5 **Neurotrophic growth factor supplementation**. Neurotrophic growth factor (NGF) features prominently among trophic factors supplied by sensory corneal nerve ends. Its crucial role in supporting corneal epithelial healing is well-established [12]. This has prompted efforts to establish NGF as a therapeutic agent. In clinical trials, about two thirds of patients treated with recombinant human NGF experienced complete epithelial healing within eight weeks. In this patient, a large, non-healing, neurotrophic epithelial defect (**A**; baseline), has become smaller after one week of topical NGF

used to either cover the entire corneal surface in a palliative approach, as conjunctival epithelium provides stable coverage of the corneal defect. Smaller, partial flaps avoid permanent impairment of vision in the affected eye [14] (Fig. 7). Refractory and progressive situations may require tectonic keratoplasty but are frequently complicated by recurrence of disease (Fig. 8). Corneal neurotisation for corneal re-innervation is an advanced, emerging procedure that can be considered if other approaches fail [15] (Fig. 9).

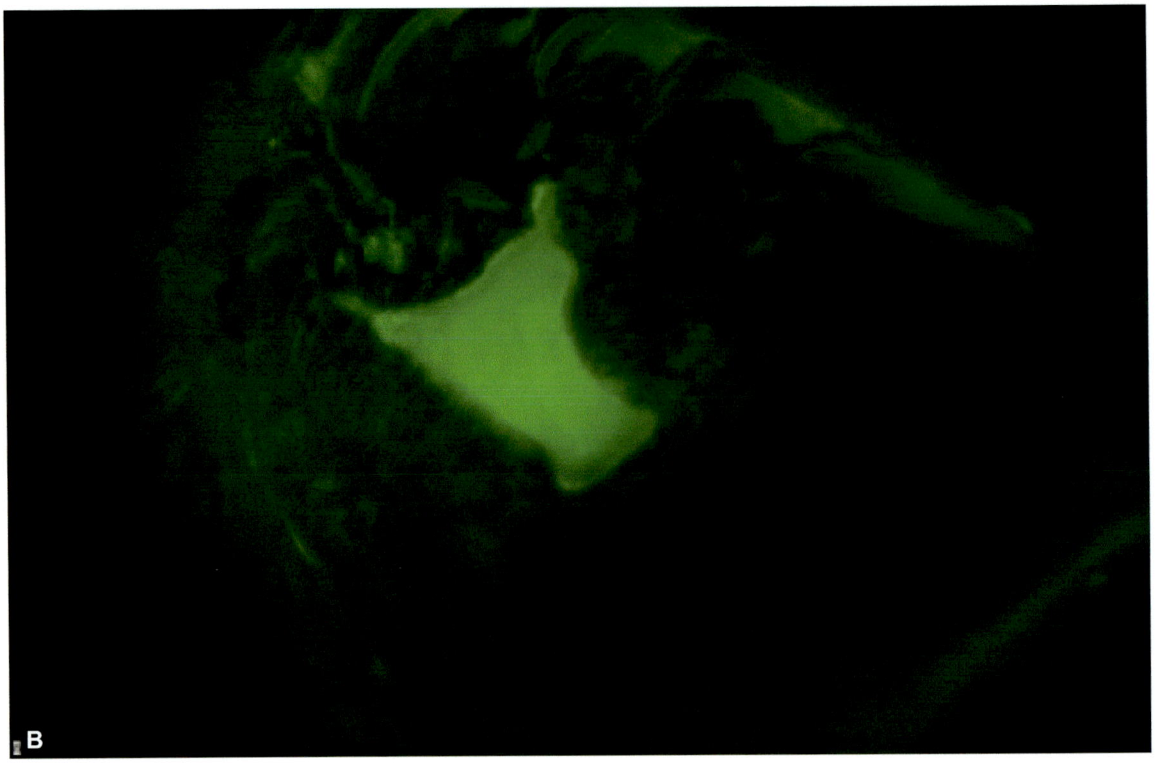

Fig. 5 (**B**) By week eight, complete wound closure is not quite achieved but the overall picture has markedly improved

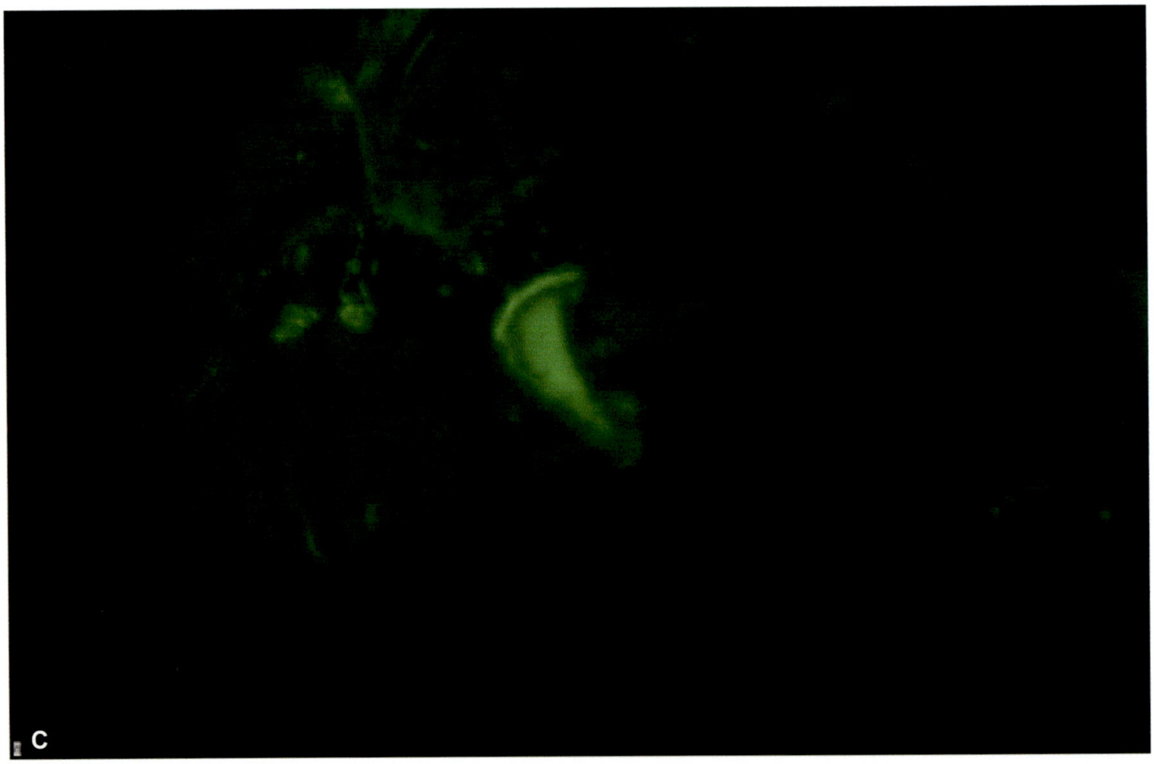

Fig. 5 (**C**) Peptide drugs have the disadvantage of being expensive and not very stable at room temperature. Hence, non-peptidic drugs that bind to neurotrophin receptors and mimic the effects of NGF in corneal epithelial cells are under clinical investigation (e.g. Metalloproteinase-Modulator Thymosin B4 (RGN-259) or polysaccharides that mimic heparan sulfate such as RGTA20)

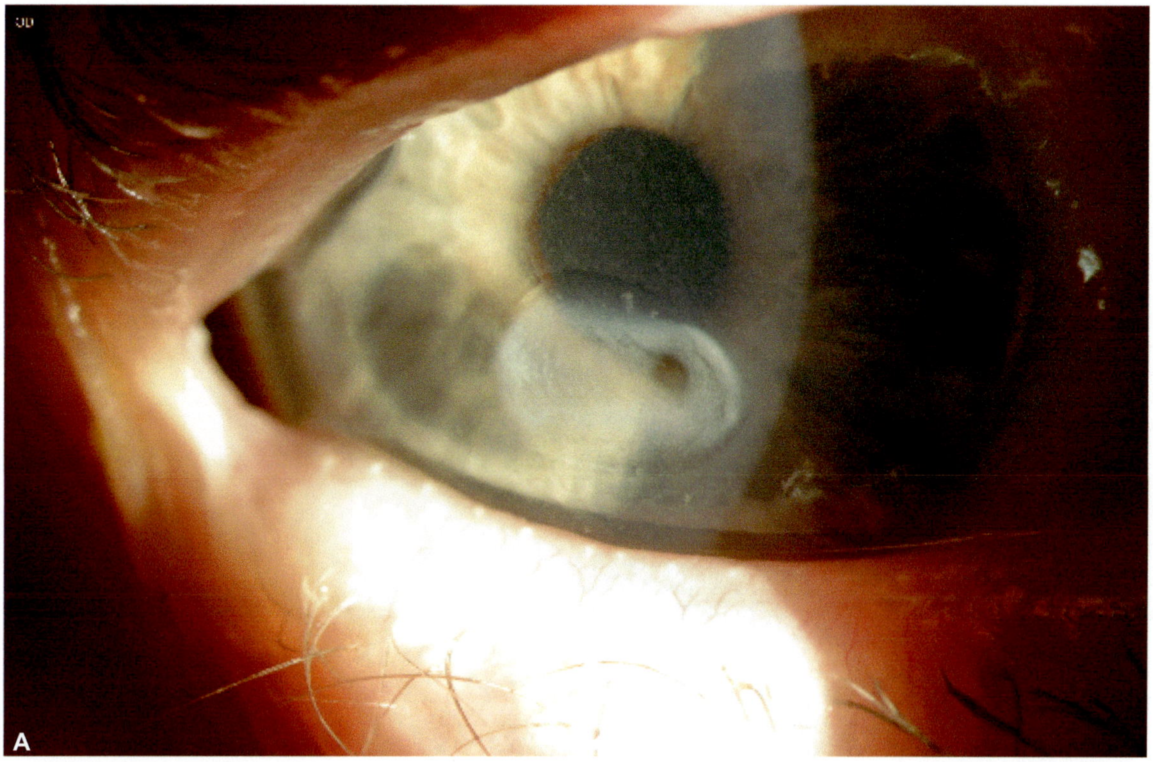

Fig. 6 (**A**) **Amniotic membrane transplantation**. Amniotic membrane can provide structural support for epithelial healing through its basement membrane proteins. In addition, this tissue contributes soluble growth factors with trophic effects on corneal epithelial cells. Here, an amniotic membrane inlay and onlay ("sandwich" [10]) were used in a patient with a deep neurotrophic corneal ulcer and descemetocele

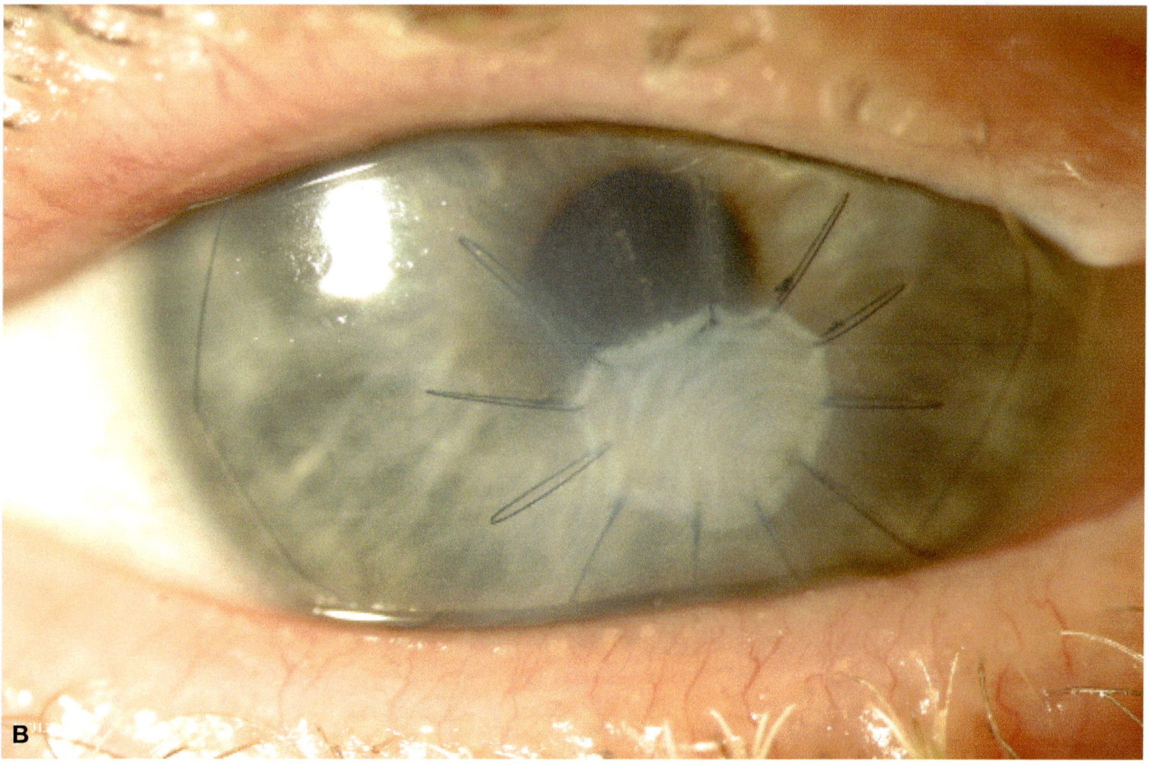

Fig. 6 (**B**) A small graft (that can be multi-layered) is placed within the corneal stromal defect to act as an anchoring support for corneal epithelial cells. A larger graft is placed on top and secured by a circular continuous nylon suture (**B**) It covers the entire cornea, thereby providing mechanical protection against mechanical forces plus growth factors for epithelial healing

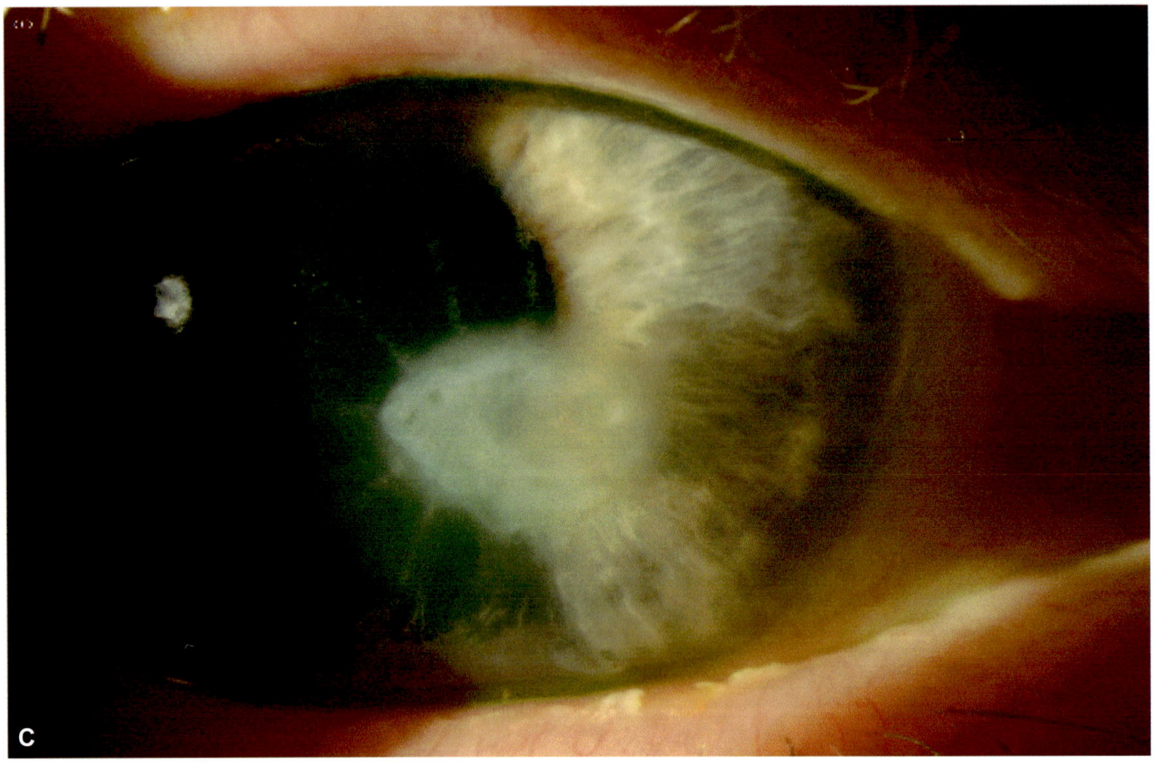

Fig. 6 (**C**) After removal of all sutures and the larger amniotic membrane onlay, the cornea shows a relatively smooth and intact epithelial surface. The smaller amniotic membrane inlay has been incorporated into the corneal stroma and is identified as opaque scar tissue within the area of the previous ulcer [16]

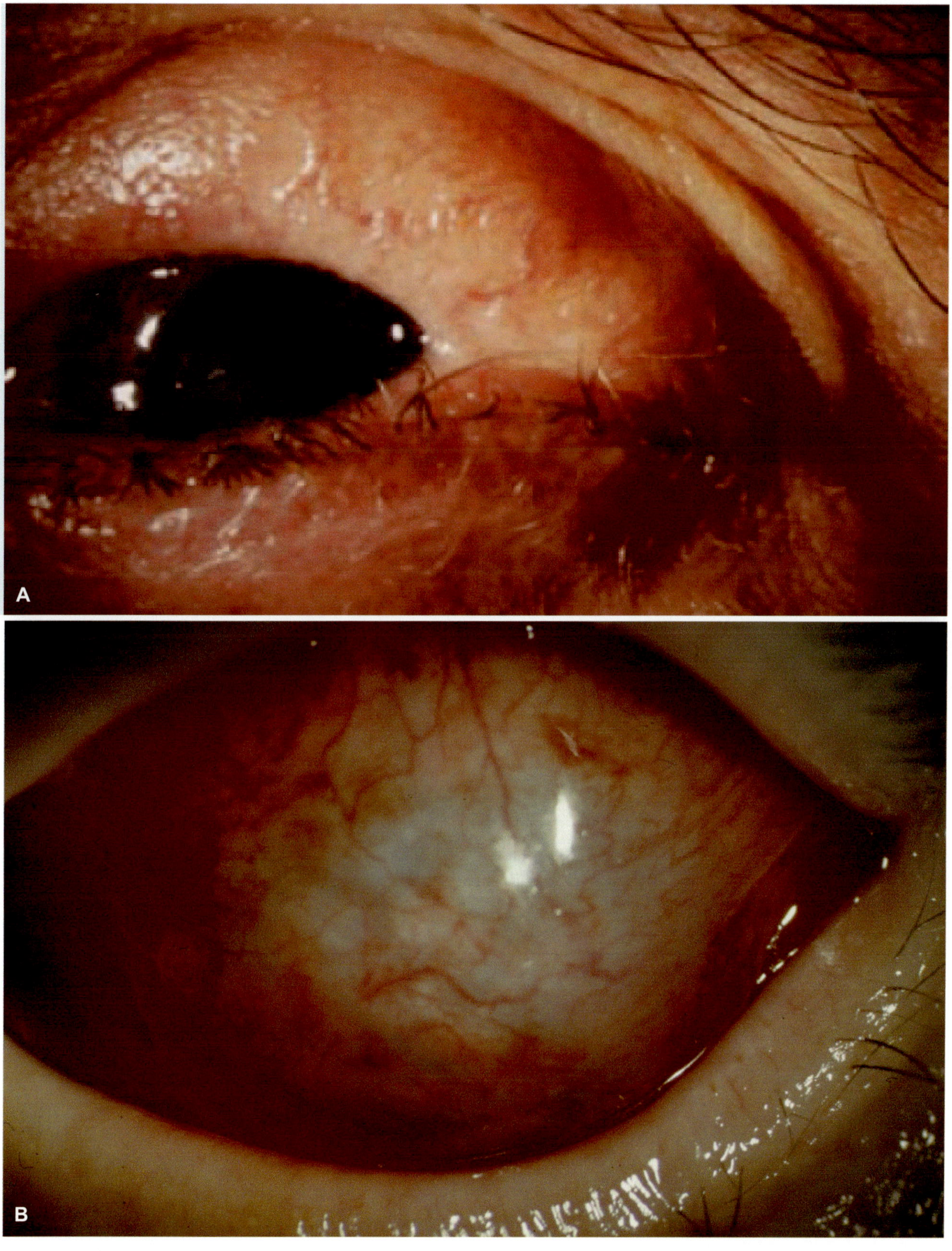

Fig. 7 Tarsorraphy and conjunctival graft. Tarsorrhaphies (**A**) can be classified into permanent or temporary. Despite being a rather simple procedure, tarsorrhaphy (particularly its permanent form) is indicated rarely and only in cases of advanced and refractory neurotrophic keratopathy. An efficacy often is associated with an unacceptable cosmetic result. In situations where recurrent perforations due to most severe uncontrolled NK have reduced visual expectations to zero and treatment goal is to salvage the globe, a bipedicular conjunctival flap according to Gundersen can be used to cover the cornea (**B**)

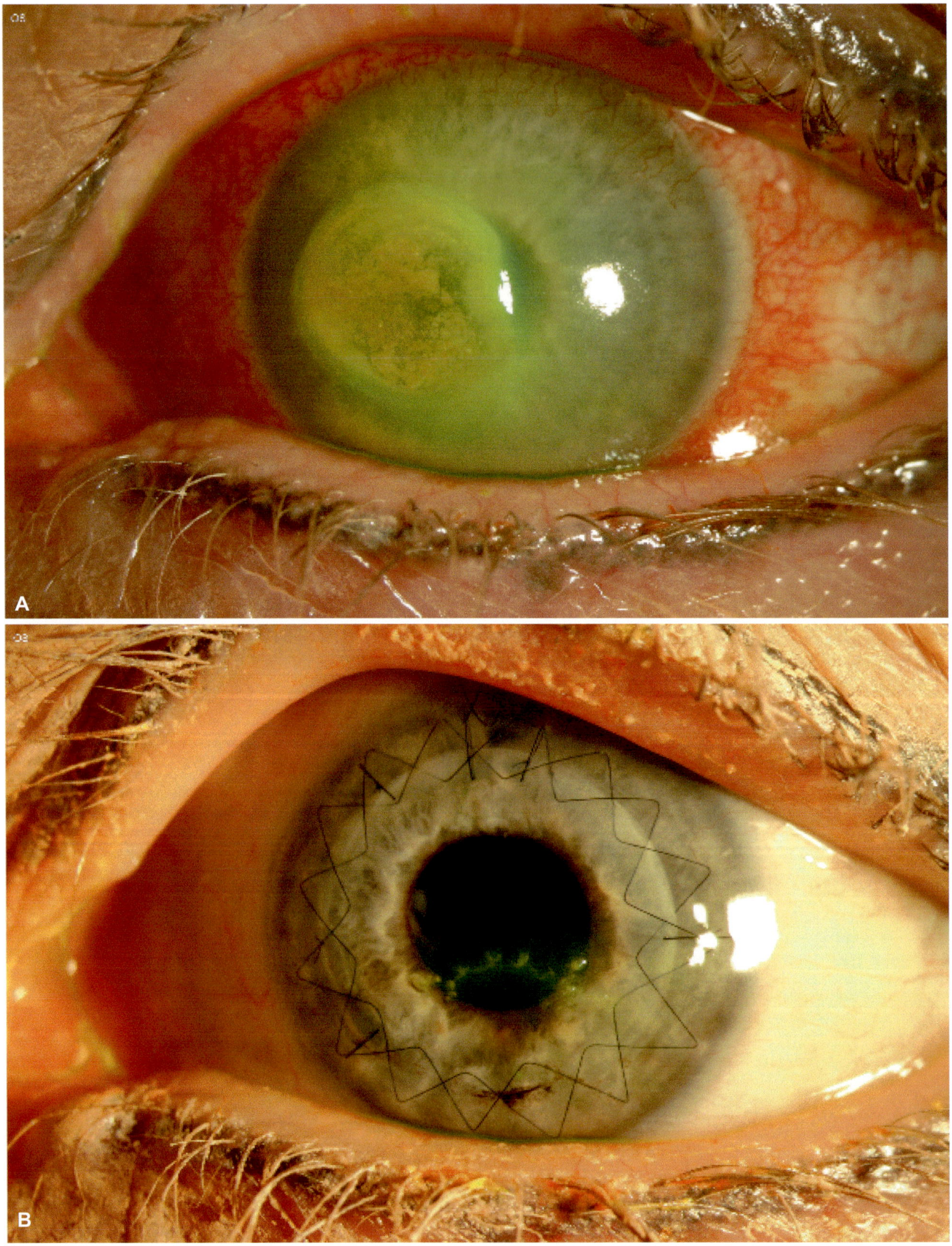

Fig. 8 **Keratoplasty**. In cases of deep and progressive stromal ulceration that threatens the integrity of the globe (**A**), lamellar or penetrating keratoplasty may be required as an urgent procedure. Here, a penetrating graft was sutured in place using a double running suture (**B**). Note the postoperative recurrence of the disease on the surface of the donor cornea (keratoplasty itself is a possible cause of neurotrophic keratopathy, given that all corneal nerves are cut during the procedure). This highlights the need for ongoing attention to the underlying disease (i.e. neurotrophic keratopathy) that persists post-keratoplasty and warrants continuation of intensive therapy

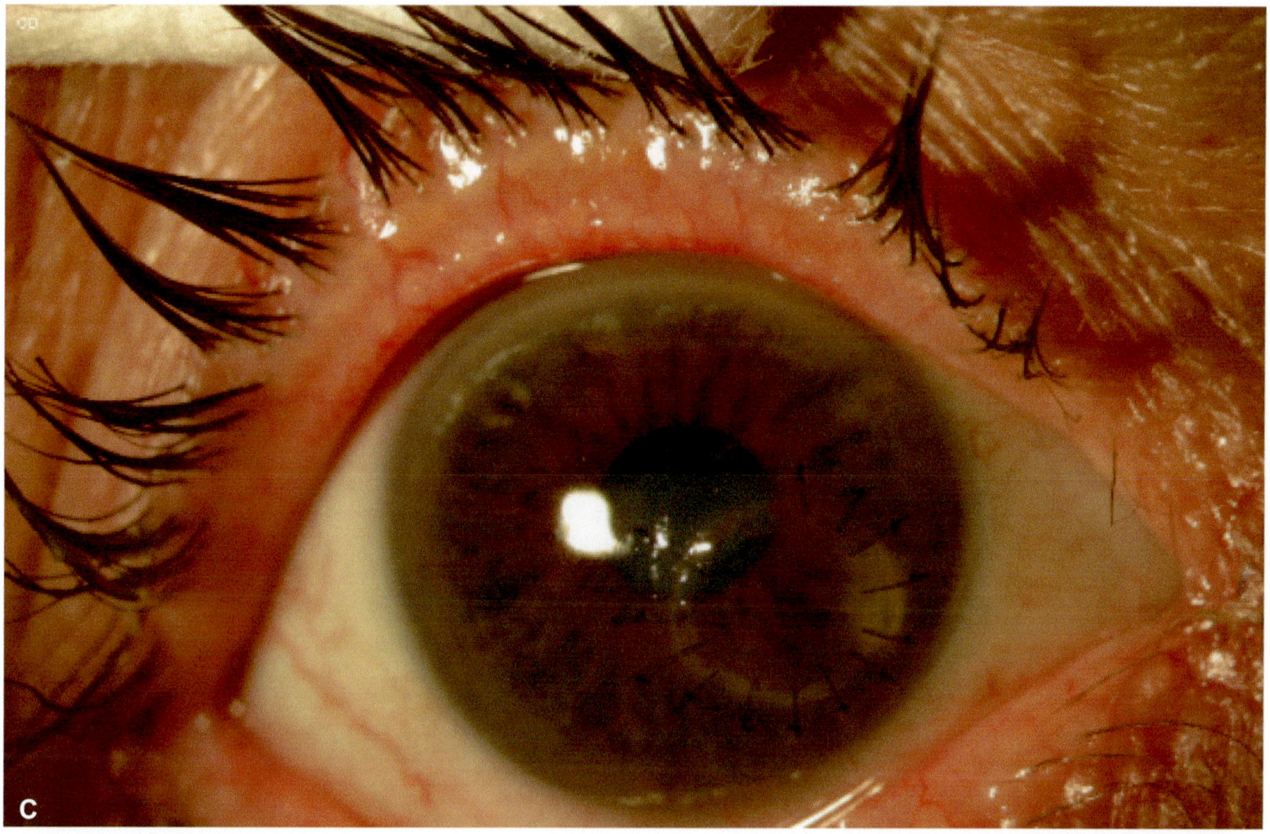

Fig. 8 (**C**) Where corneal defects are small and eccentric, a small-diameter graft ("mini-keratoplasty") may be appropriate as a minimally invasive procedure with a potentially smaller risk of wound-related complications and/or immune reactions

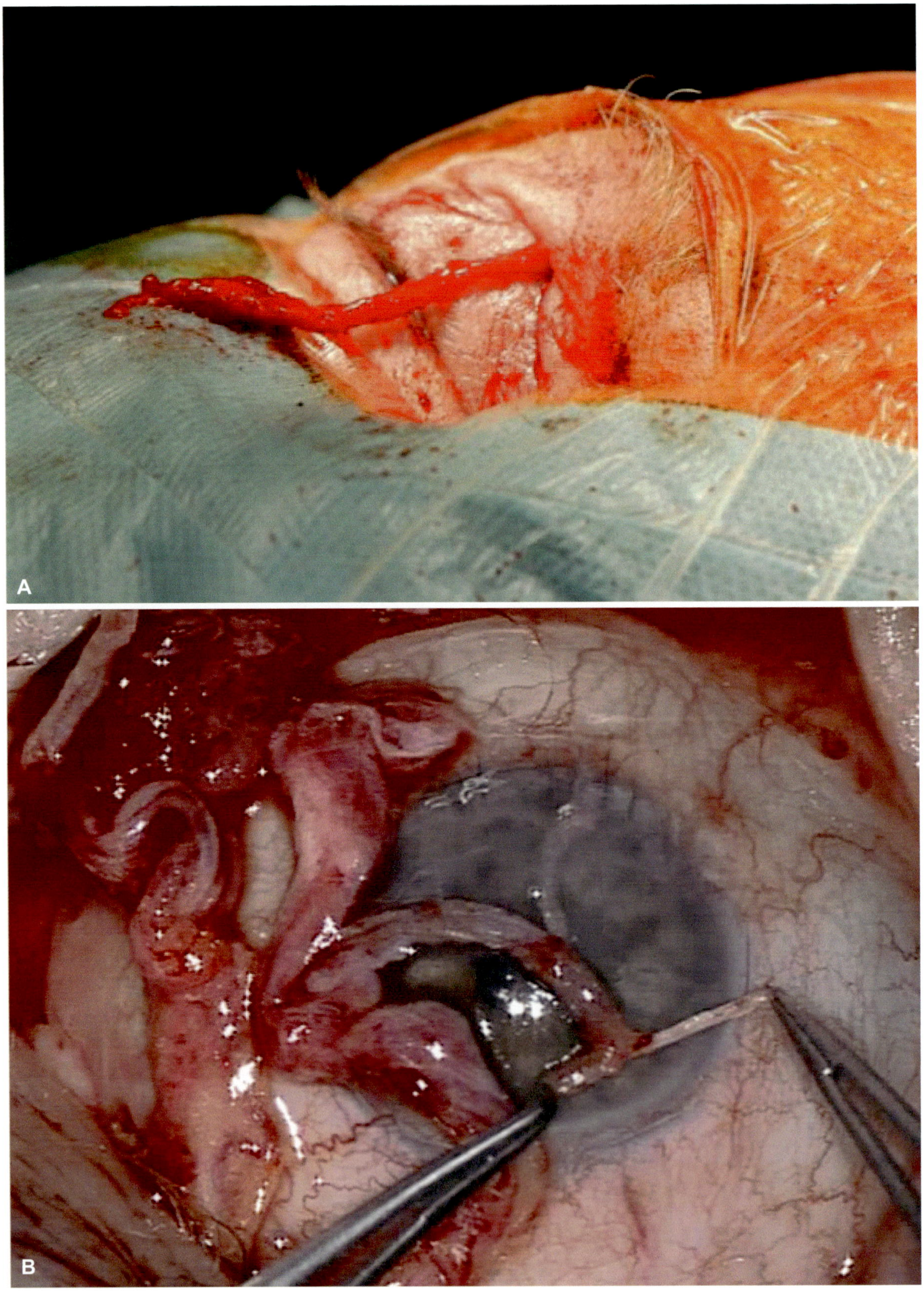

Fig. 9 **Corneal neurotisation**. Corneal neurotisation entails transposition of a sensory nerve to the corneal limbus to re-establish corneal sensitivity and re-introduce trophic support. Here, the supraorbital nerve is passed through a tunnel in the upper lid skin crease between the tarsus and the orbital rim (**A**) Epineurium is removed (**B**) and the different fascicles are placed into perilimbal corneoscleral pockets (**C**; best seen at 4 and 8 o'clock)

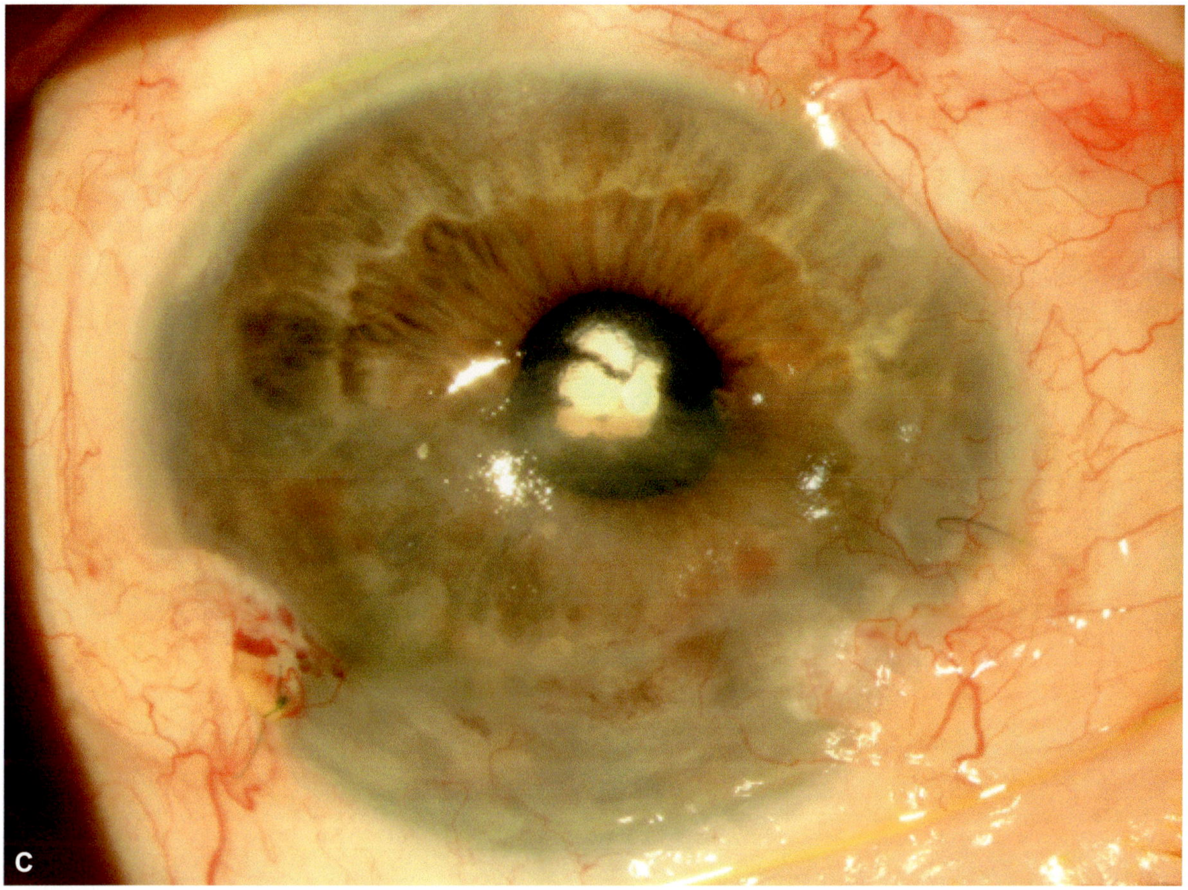

Fig. 9 (**C**) Three months postoperatively, this patient showed an increase in sensitivity centrally as well as in the lower quadrants plus stable corneal epithelium. The patient must be informed that this procedure, performed under general anesthesia, may take several hours and results in at least partial loss of sensation of the forehead, a scar close to the hairline, as well as the possibility of paraesthesias in the surgical area

2 Conclusion

NK is a degenerative corneal disease defined by decreased innervation of the cornea and associated with significant morbidity. Choices of treatment range from ocular lubrication to various pharmaceutical and surgical approaches that may be more or less invasive.

References

1. Roth M, Dierse S, Alder J, et al. Incidence, prevalence, and outcome of moderate to severe neurotrophic keratopathy in a German tertiary referral center from 2013 to 2017. Graefe's Arch Clin Exp Ophthalmol. 2022;260:1961–73. https://doi.org/10.1007/s00417-021-05535-z.
2. NaPier E, Camacho M, McDevitt TF, et al. Neurotrophic keratopathy: current challenges and future prospects. Ann Med. 2022;54:666–73. https://doi.org/10.1080/07853890.2022.2045035.
3. Dua HS, Said DG, Messmer EM, et al. Neurotrophic keratopathy. Prog Retin Eye Res. 2018;66:107–31. https://doi.org/10.1016/j.preteyeres.2018.04.003.
4. Mastropasqua L, Massaro-Giordano G, Nubile M, et al. Understanding the pathogenesis of neurotrophic keratitis: the role of corneal nerves. J Cell Physiol. 2017;232:717–24. https://doi.org/10.1002/jcp.25623.
5. Mackie I. Neuroparalytic keratitis. In: Fraunfelder F, Roy F, Meyer S, editors. Current ocular therapy. Philadelphia: WB Saunders; 1995. p. 452–4.
6. Geerling G, Joussen AM, Daniels JT, et al. Matrix metalloproteinases in sterile corneal melts. Ann N Y Acad Sci. 1999;878:571–4. https://doi.org/10.1111/j.1749-6632.1999.tb07730.x.
7. Jacobi C, Messmer EM. Diagnosis of dry eye disease. Ophthalmologe. 2018;115:433–50. https://doi.org/10.1007/s00347-018-0676-2.
8. Alder J, Mertsch S, Menzel-Severing J, et al. Current and experimental treatment approaches for neurotrophic keratopathy. Ophthalmologe. 2019;116:127–37. https://doi.org/10.1007/s00347-018-0843-5.
9. Seitz B, Grüterich M, Cursiefen C, et al. Conservative and surgical treatment of neurotrophic keratopathy. Ophthalmologe. 2005;102:15–26. https://doi.org/10.1007/s00347-004-1161-7.
10. Seitz B, Resch MD, Schlötzer-Schrehardt U, et al. Histopathology and ultrastructure of human corneas after amniotic membrane transplantation. Arch Ophthalmol (Chicago, Ill 1960) 2006;124:1487–90. https://doi.org/10.1001/archopht.124.10.1487.

11. Merté R-L, Lanzl IM. Botulinum toxin injection for production of ptosis. Ophthalmologe. 2007;104:767–70. https://doi.org/10.1007/s00347-007-1611-0.
12. Mastropasqua L, Lanzini M, Dua HS, et al. In vivo evaluation of corneal nerves and epithelial healing after treatment with recombinant nerve growth factor for neurotrophic keratopathy. Am J Ophthalmol. 2020;217:278–86. https://doi.org/10.1016/j.ajo.2020.04.036.
13. Diaz-Valle D, Burgos-Blasco B, Rego-Lorca D, et al. Comparison of the efficacy of topical insulin with autologous serum eye drops in persistent epithelial defects of the cornea. Acta Ophthalmol. 2022;100:e912–9. https://doi.org/10.1111/aos.14997.
14. Trinh T, Mimouni M, Santaella G, et al. Surgical management of the ocular surface in neurotrophic keratopathy: amniotic membrane, conjunctival grafts, lid surgery, and neurotization. Eye Contact Lens. 2021;47:149–53. https://doi.org/10.1097/ICL.0000000000000753.
15. Lueke JN, Holtmann C, Beseoglu K, et al. Corneal neurotization. Ophthalmologe. 2020;117:248–52. https://doi.org/10.1007/s00347-019-00980-y.
16. Resch MD, Schlötzer-Schrehardt U, Hofmann-Rummelt C, et al. Integration patterns of cryopreserved amniotic membranes into the human cornea. Ophthalmology. 2006;113:1927–35. https://doi.org/10.1016/j.ophtha.2006.03.065.

Therapies

Serum Eye Drops

Hermann Eichler and Heike Lauer

Abstract

Serum eye drops (SED) are a useful adjunctive treatment for patients with severe ocular surface disease, especially those with a compromised tear film [1–3]. Blood serum contains a large number of epitheliotrophic factors that are present in tears [3]. These factors are likely to be responsible for the therapeutic benefits observed with SED therapy [3]. For example, SED should be considered in patients who have refractory or partially responsive acute or chronic severe ocular surface disease [1–4]. Transfusion medicine services in Germany and other European countries have been providing SED since the late 1990s, in UK they are available since 2003 [1–3]. SED are defined as a medicinal product. Therefore, the providing transfusion service needs to apply for an approval at the respective local medical agency. The ophthalmologist is responsible for the indication to perform a SED preparation. The investigation for donor eligibility, the blood donation itself, and the SED preparation and quality control is in the responsibility of the transfusion medicine specialist. To produce SED, the donated blood unit is processed to separate out the serum that than is transferred into sterile dropper bottles and frozen for storage (The innovative and safe process for making autologous serum eye drops. https://www.meise.com/en/products/autologus-serum-eye-drops.html). Frozen SED have a shelf life of several months from the date of donation depending on the label of the providing service.

Keywords

Serum eye drops · Transfusion medicine · Ocular surface disease

1 Step-By-Step Preparation of SED

SED can be produced from either autologous or allogeneic blood donations, delivered either non-diluted or diluted with saline solution. The following step-by-step preparation describes the production of autologous, non-diluted SED (Figs. 1, 2, 3, 4, 5, 6, 7, 8, 9, 10 and 11).

H. Eichler (✉) · H. Lauer
Institute of Clinical Hemostaseology and Transfusion Medicine, Saarland University School of Medicine, Saarland University Medical Center, Homburg, Germany
e-mail: hermann.eichler@uks.eu

B. Seitz et al. (eds.), *Atlas on Cornea*, https://doi.org/10.1007/978-3-031-65422-0_41

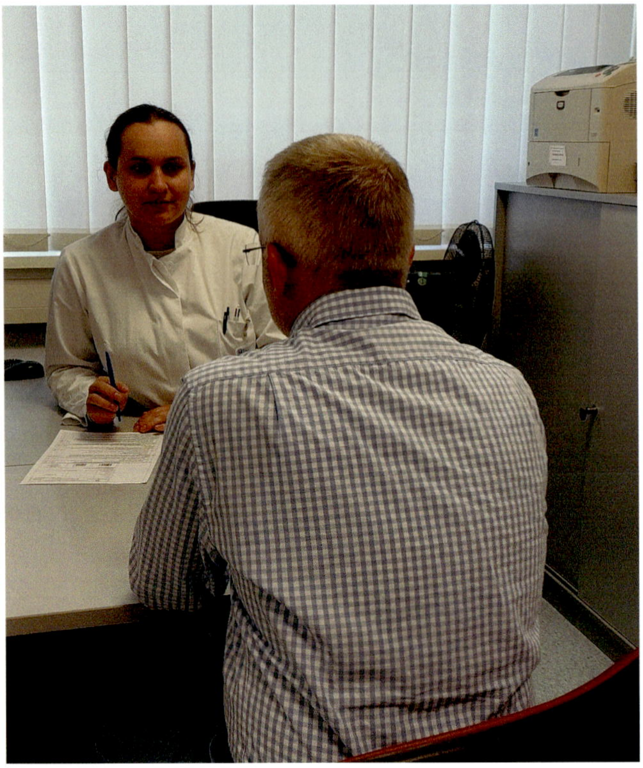

Fig. 1 Patient informed consent and eligibility investigation for blood donation

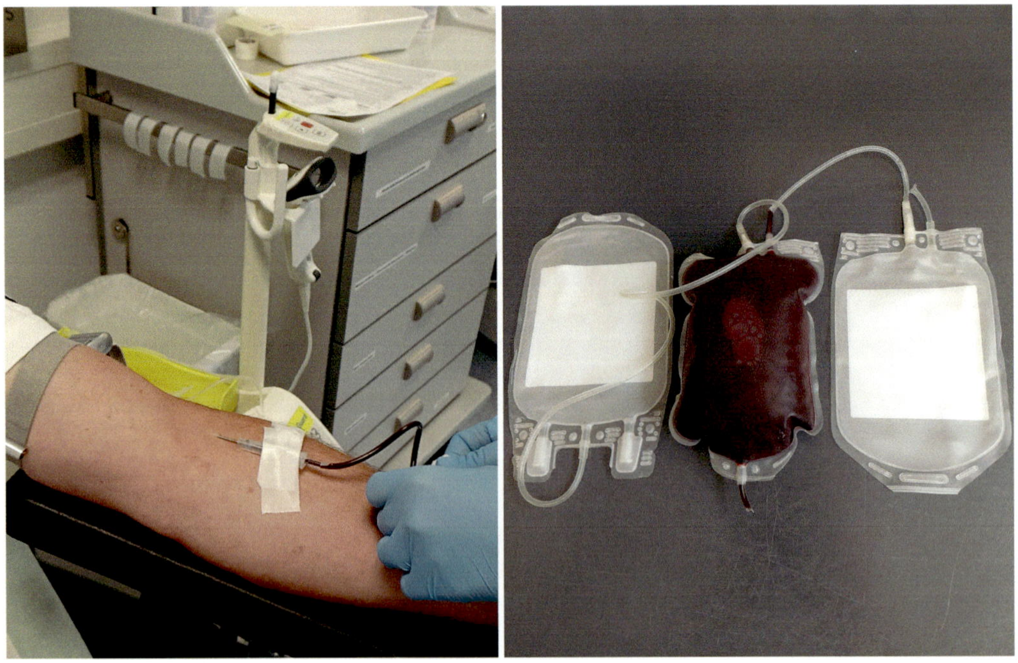

Fig. 2 Venipuncture and donation of 500 ml non-anticoagulated peripheral blood, e.g. by using a special SED blood collection system (4) (triple bags 1 × 500 ml, 2 × 300 ml). Storage of the blood bag system for 2 h at room temperature until complete coagulation

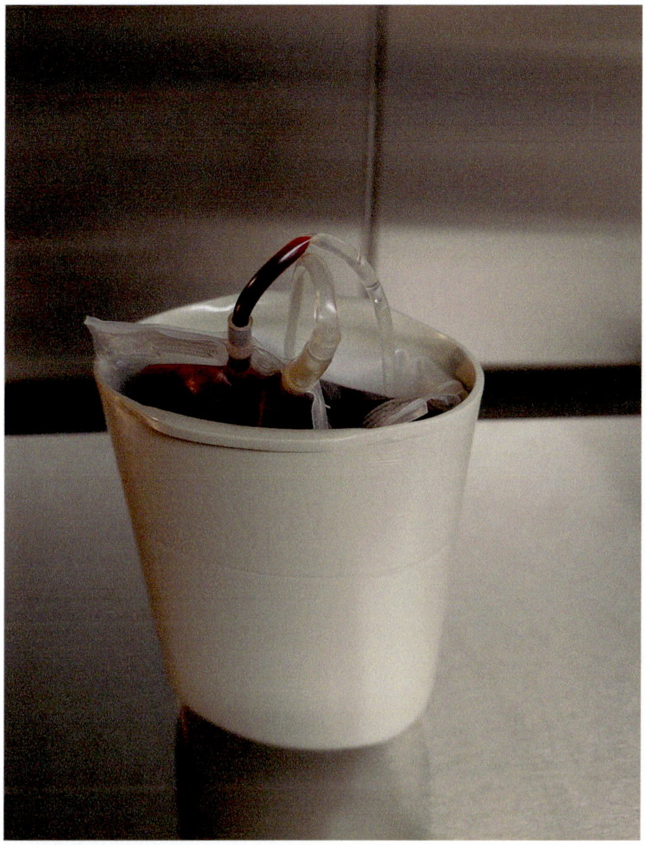

Fig. 3 Overnight storage of the blood bag system at 4 °C for clot retraction in a centrifuge container

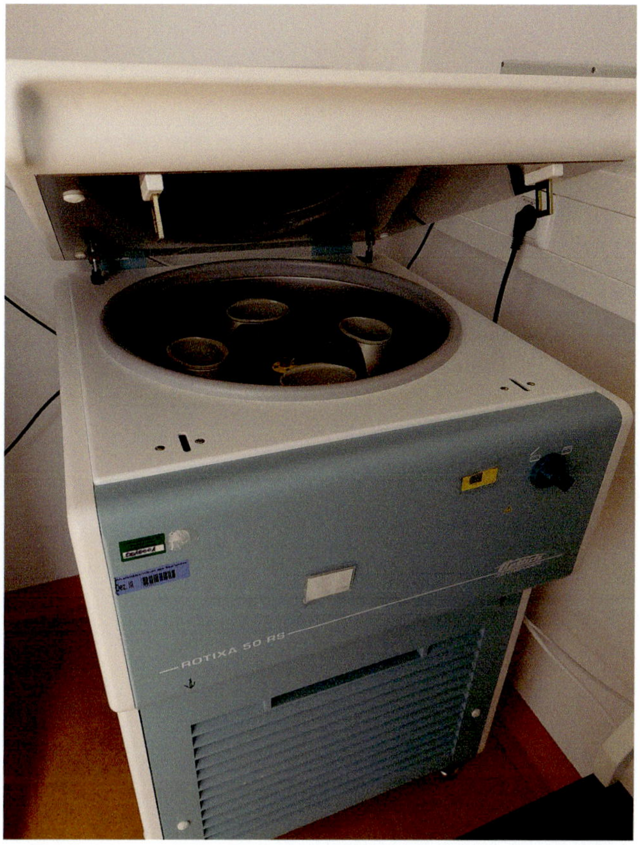

Fig. 4 Centrifugation of the blood bag system at $3,700 \times g$ for 15 min at room temperature

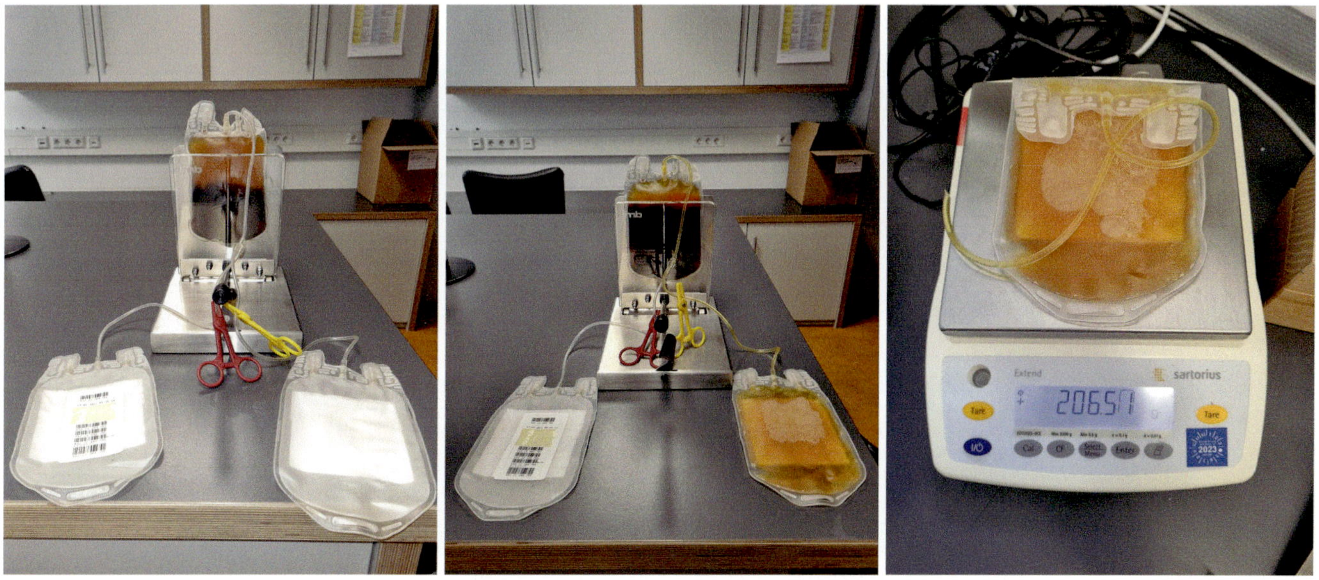

Fig. 5 Transferring the serum into an empty 300 ml bag followed by weighing of the bag

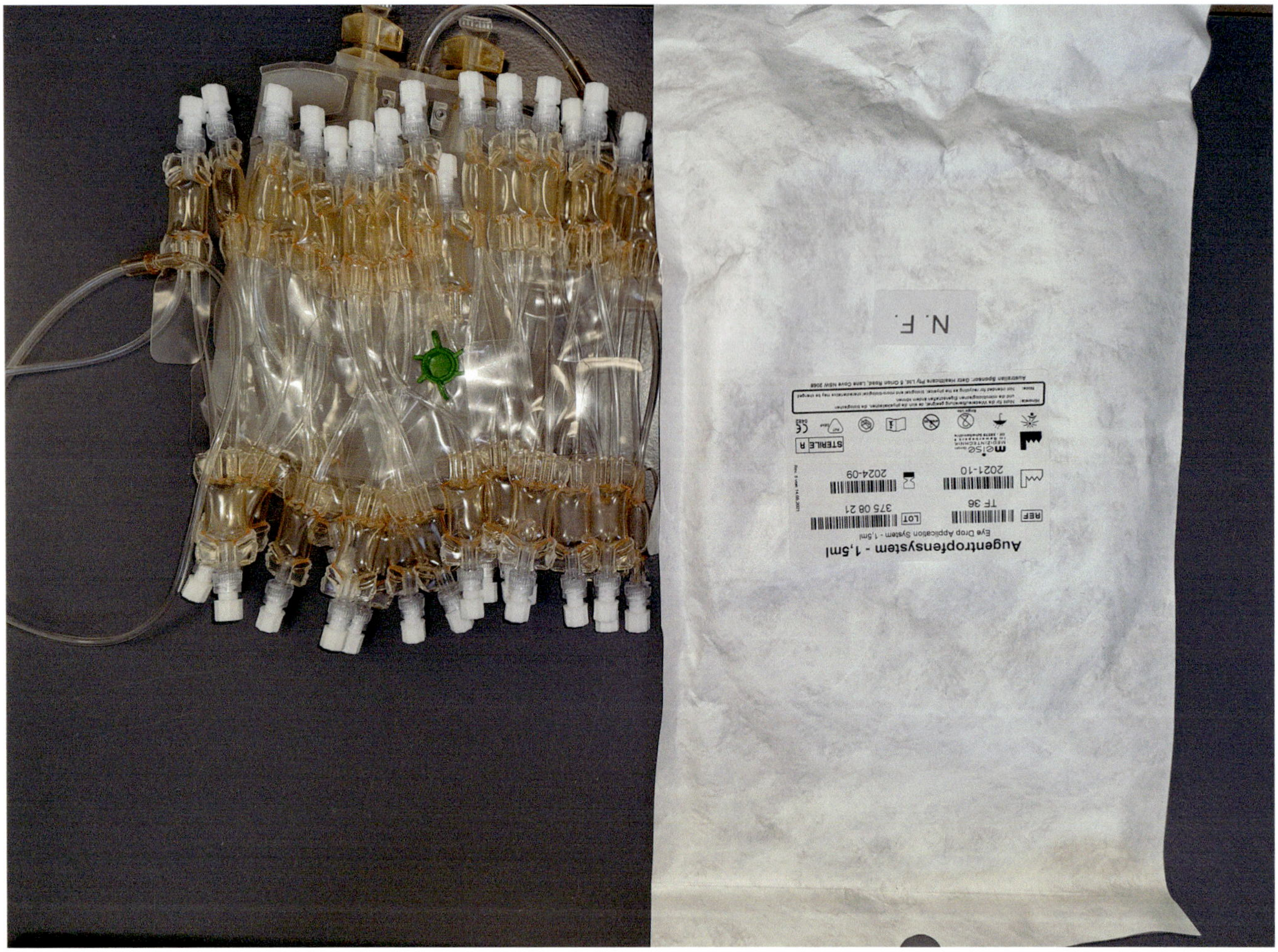

Fig. 6 Use of a special SED system with up to 36 application receptacles (sterile dropper bottles)

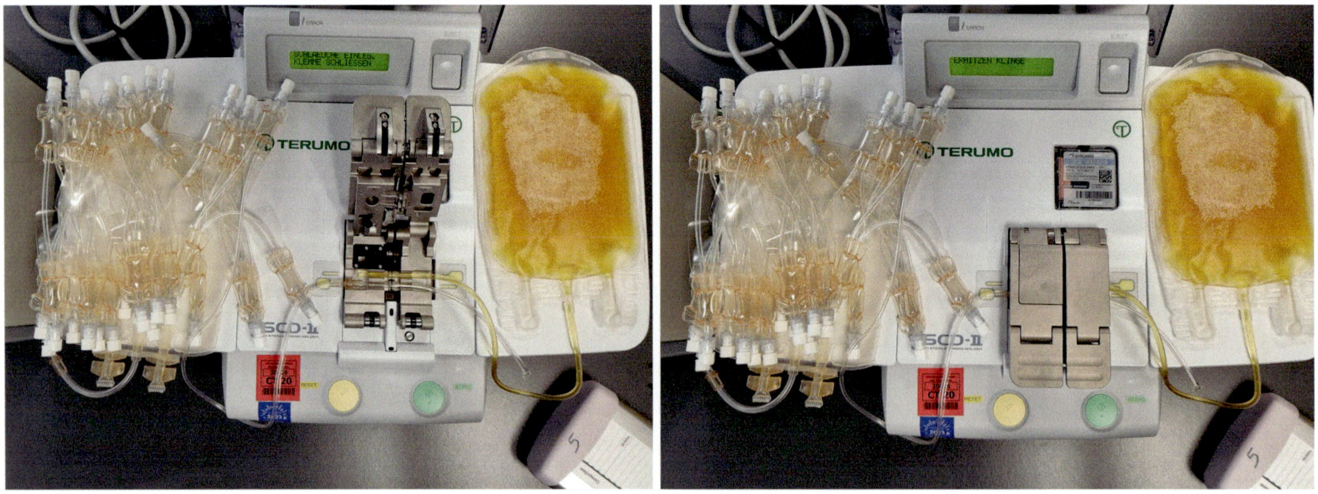

Fig. 7 Use of a sterile-docking device to connect PVC tubings of the serum containing bag and the SED system

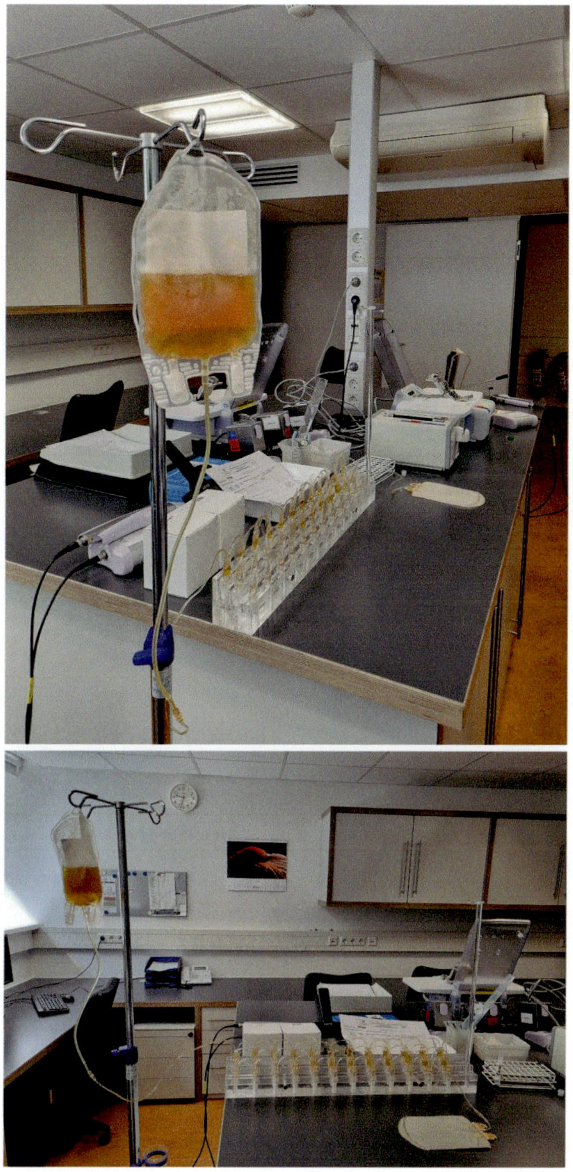

Fig. 8 Transfer of the serum by gravity from the bag into the application dropper bottles. The serum remaining in the transfer bag is used to perform a sterility assay

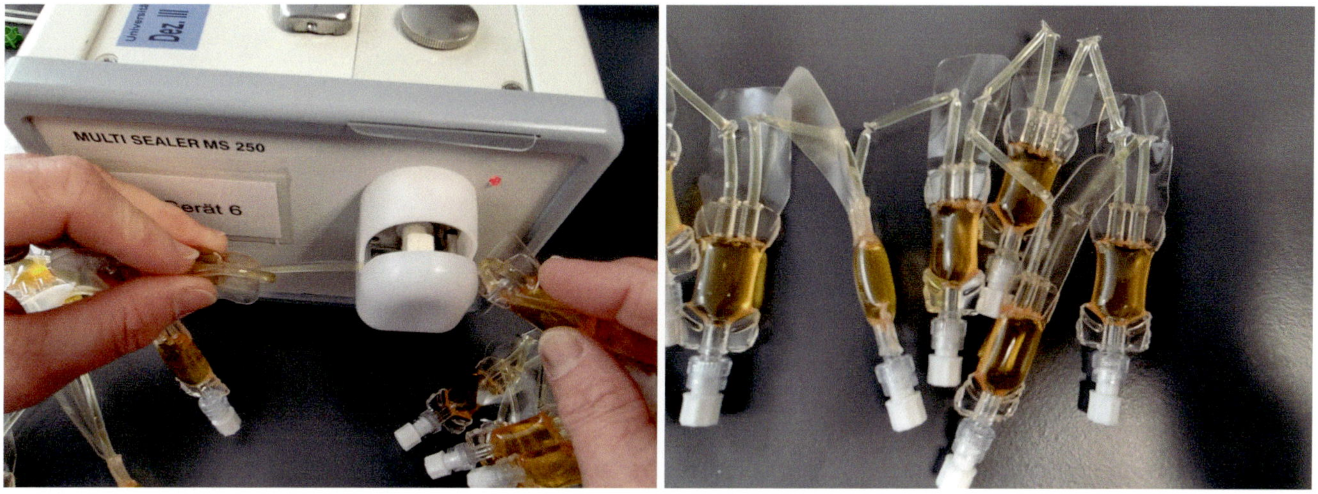

Fig. 9 Sealing the tube line connecting the dropper bottles and separating the dropper bottles from each other

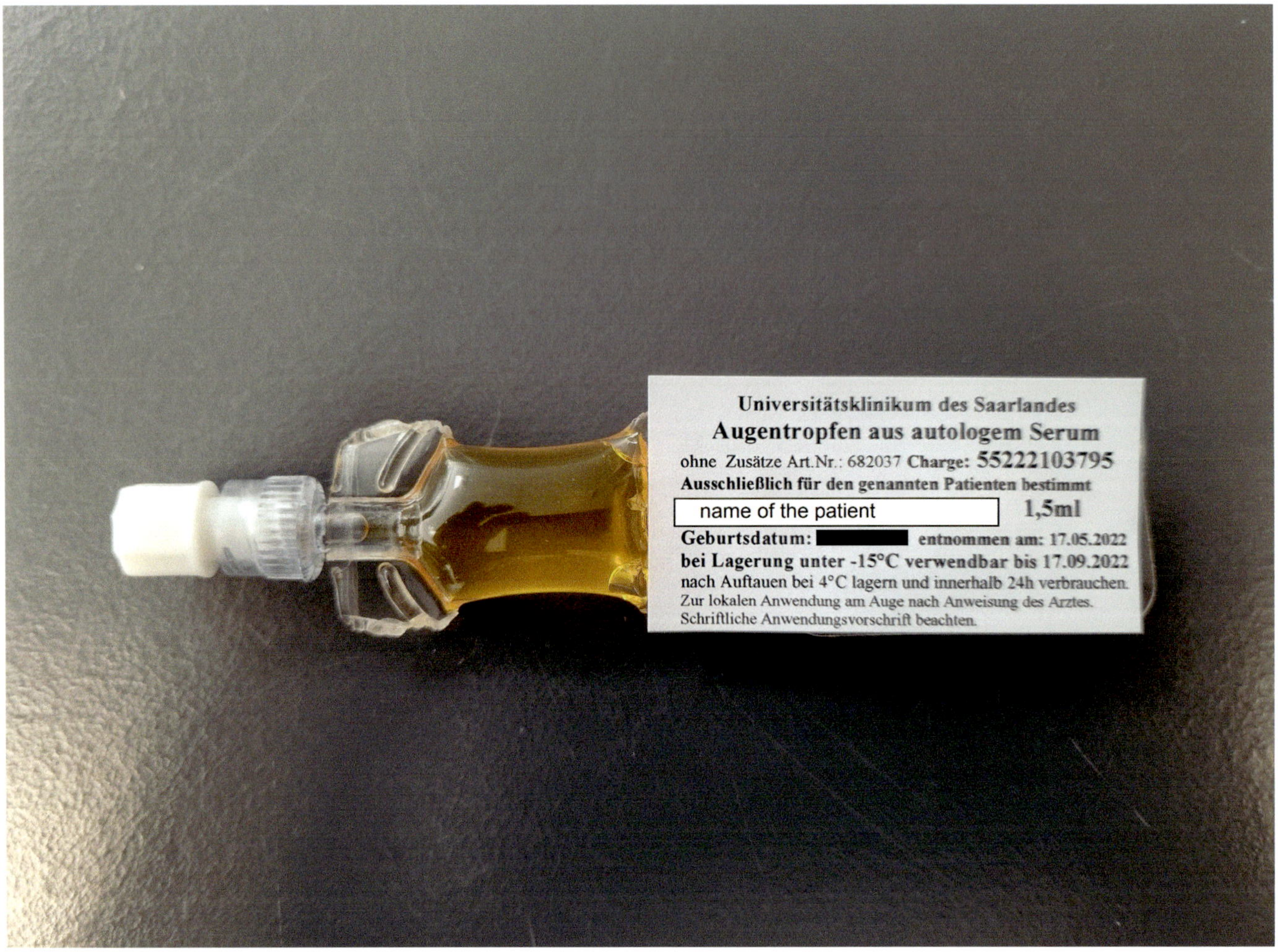

Fig. 10 Labeling of each single dropper bottle

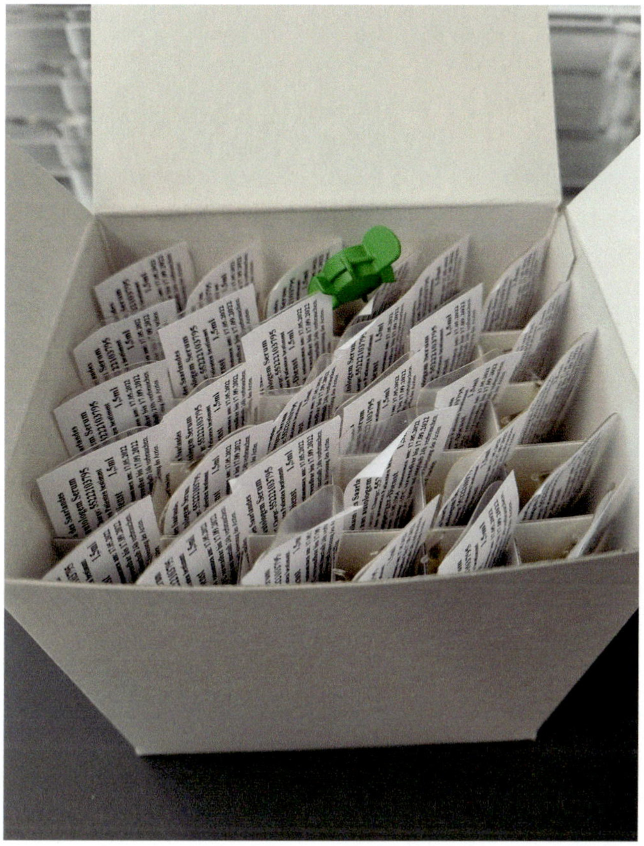

Fig. 11 Packing the labelled dropper bottles into a paper box and placing the box into a freezer at −30 °C for at least 12 h

2 Conclusion

SED are frequently used as a safe, well-tolerated, and effective treatment for ocular surface disease. On the other hand, the quality of evidence for SED treatment published from randomized controlled trials is low, especially for long-term use. Thus, further investigations are needed to assess long-term treatment outcomes.

Funding Financial Support: Nothing to declare.

References

1. Pan Q, Angelina A, Marrone M, Stark WJ, Akpek EK. Autologous serum eye drops for dry eye. Cochrane Database Syst Rev. 2017;2:CD009327.
2. Marks DC, van der Meer PF. On behalf of the biomedical excellence for safer transfusion (BEST) collaborative. Vox Sang. 2017;112:310–7.
3. Rauz S, Koay SY, Foot B, et al. The royal college of ophthalmologists guidelines on serum eye drops for the treatment of severe ocular surface disease: executive summary. Eye. 2018;32:44–8.
4. Weischnur L, Xanthopoulou K, Munteanu C, Leonhard M, Daas L, Seitz B. Autologous serum eye drops for therapy-resistant epithelial defects of the cornea : Impact of underlying disease and simultaneous amniotic transplantation in 990 applications. Ophthalmologie. 2023;120:43–51.
5. The innovative and safe process for making autologous serum eye drops. https://www.meise.com/en/products/autologus-serum-eye-drops.html.

Contact Lenses

Dorothea Kuhn and Ulrike Klühspies

Abstract

Contact lenses play an important role in the therapy of corneal diseases. They can be used as bandage lenses for pain relief and support corneal wound healing. Iris lenses protect the eye from too much glare and enhance the cosmetic situation, especially in an injured eye. Regarding the treatment of keratoconus, contact lenses represent the first step to improve visual acuity. This chapter describes how successful modern contact lens therapy can be and how special contact lens designs are manufactured with the help of different topographic analysis of the cornea. The most common specific contact lenses, used in keratoconus contact lens fitting, are presented. Contact lenses also play a crucial part for visual rehabilitation after keratoplasty. The differing geometries of the cornea after suture removal also require individual solutions. Due to the use of high-oxygen-permeable materials, we have almost unlimited possibilities for fittings with several designs: special rigid keratoconus lenses, individual topographically calculated contact lenses, semi-scleral and scleral contact lenses. The latter enable new possibilities in contact lens fitting after keratoplasty, too. All these types of contact lenses, such as special soft keratoconus contact lenses, hybrid contact lenses and "piggyback" contact lens systems, are shown including fitting examples.

Keywords

Therapeutic contact lens · Bandage lens · Iris lens · Keratoconus · Keratoplasty · Intacs · High-oxygen-permeable material · Rigid gas permeable (RGP) lens · Special rigid gas permeable keratoconus lens · Individual topographic calculated custom-made contact lens · Miniscleral lens · Semi-scleral contact lens · Scleral contact lens · Piggyback contact lens system · Soft gas permeable (GP) keratoconus contact lens · Hybrid contact lens · Visual rehabilitation

Abbreviations

GP Gas permeable
RGP Rigid gas permeable

1 Therapeutic Contact Lenses

Contact lenses have an ambivalent relationship to the cornea:

On the one hand they are used for therapy, but on the other hand they can cause damage to the cornea. Therefore, it is important to always use high-quality materials with the highest possible oxygen permeability, especially when placed on a diseased cornea.

Therapeutic contact lenses include bandage lenses, iris lenses and keratoconus lenses, as well as contact lenses after keratoplasty.

This chapter presents the main lens systems with some interesting cases as examples. The compilation does not claim to be complete but reflects own experiences with the materials we used.

D. Kuhn (✉)
Riedlingen, Germany
e-mail: dr-dorothea-kuhn@t-online.de

U. Klühspies
Department of Ophthalmology, Saarland University Medical Center, Homburg/Saar, Germany

B. Seitz et al. (eds.), *Atlas on Cornea*, https://doi.org/10.1007/978-3-031-65422-0_42

1.1 Bandage Lenses

Highly oxygen permeable, very thin, soft contact lenses made from silicone hydrogel material can accelerate the wound healing of an injured or diseased cornea. These contact lenses act as a bandage under which the epithelial cells can grow and regenerate without disturbance by eye blinking. These contact lenses are subject to an FDA approval process (Figs. 1 and 2).

If there is an underlying epithelial metabolic defect (see Chap. 17 on corneal dystrophies), that causes the production of an inferior basement membrane, optimal adhesion of the epithelium to the Bowman layer is not possible and recurrent erosions occur frequently. In order to prevent recurrences, an extremely high oxygen permeable silicone hydrogel lens can be worn for a maximum of 4 weeks without changing. This option can be continued until the corneal wound has healed smoothly, no recurrence occurs and the lens is tolerated by the cornea. After 4 weeks the dirty lens must be renewed.

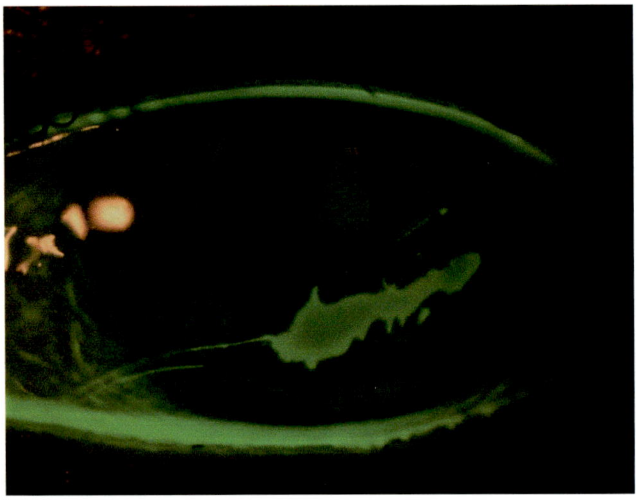

Fig. 1 Therapeutic contact lenses are indicated as bandage lenses in corneal epithelial defects, such as erosio corneae, after abrasion or surgery, burn or cauterization, as well as in special cases such as keratitis bullosa with painful epithelial ruptures or risk of dehydration (keratitis e lagophthalmo, keratitis neuroparalytica, keratitis filiformis) [1]

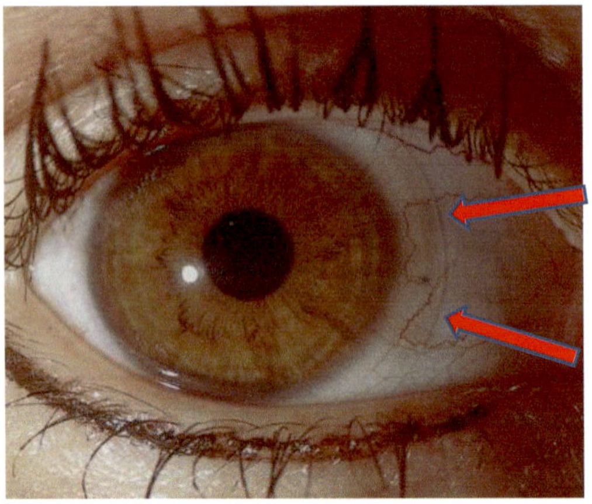

Fig. 2 Therapeutic bandage lenses made from silicone hydrogel. The edge of the lens is marked by the red arrows

1.2 Iris Lenses

Indication: congenital aniridia, acquired iris defects (Fig. 3).

Especially designed iris lenses are used to better tolerate the increased glare caused by aniridia. In cases of a unilateral disease, e.g. after an injury, a rigid gas permeable lens or soft lens is hand-painted according to the template, for example by using a photograph of the healthy eye. The pupil can be placed off-center to improve the cosmetic effect.

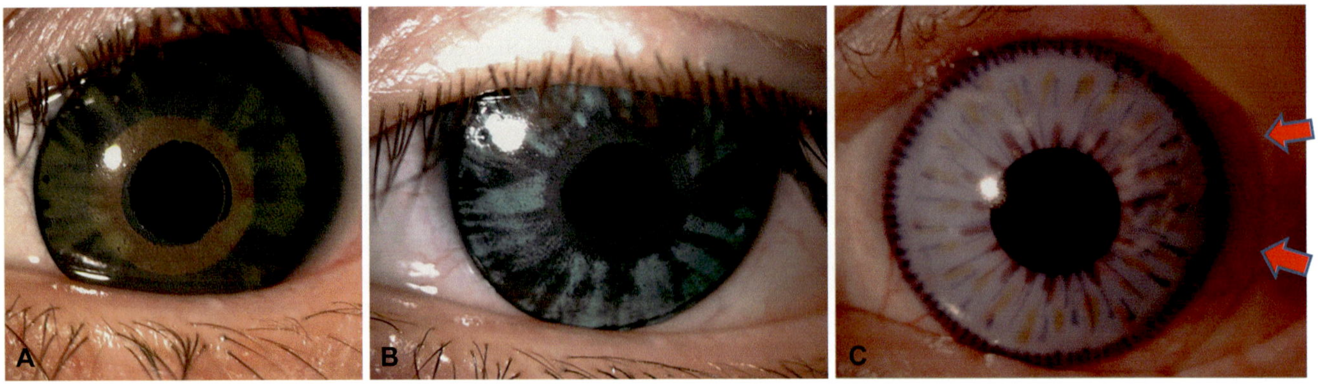

Fig. 3 (**A**) and (**B**) Hand painted rigid iris lenses. (**C**) Hand painted soft iris lens, edge marked by red arrows

2 Keratoconus Lenses

Keratoconus is a crucial indication for contact lenses [2, 3].

Contact lenses usually lead to an improvement in visual acuity, but they cannot prevent the progression of keratoconus. Customization of the lens depends on the stage of the disease, which means that the geometry of the lens becomes more complex with an increasing severity of keratoconus due to the corneal steepening. In order to find the ideal fit, different measuring lenses are often made and worn for trial (Fig. 4).

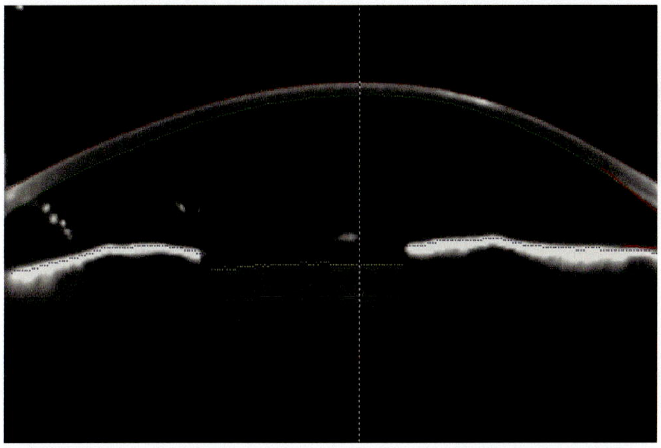

Fig. 4 Corneal scan with the Pentacam: the modern staging of keratoconus refers to the eccentric corneal steepening with corneal thinning and simultaneously more steepening of the posterior corneal surface

2.1 Topographic Diagnosis and Mapping

The parameters of the cornea are measured as a basis for calculating the inner surface of the rigid gas permeable (RGP) contact lens, which is designed on the basis of the topography.

Exemplary for all topography devices on the market, the two most commonly used measurement principles are shown here.

Firstly, there is the placido disc measuring principle using the Oculus Keratograph (Fig. 5).

Advantage: technically simple, inexpensive, good reproducibility for astigmatism and curvature data, possibility of computer-assisted calculation of the first fitting lens.

Disadvantage: only the central corneal surface is measured exactly (the black circle marks the 3 mm zone), no thickness measurement, measurement depends on tear film quality.

The second measuring principle uses the Scheimpflug camera (Fig. 6).

Advantage: Measurement of sagittal and tangential radii of the entire corneal surface, height data of the anterior and posterior corneal surface simultaneously with pachymetry. Important for the fitting are the maximum and minimum radius, the numerical eccentricity and the position of the thinnest part of the cornea. All these parameters can be read directly from the Pentacam image [4] (Figs. 7 and 8).

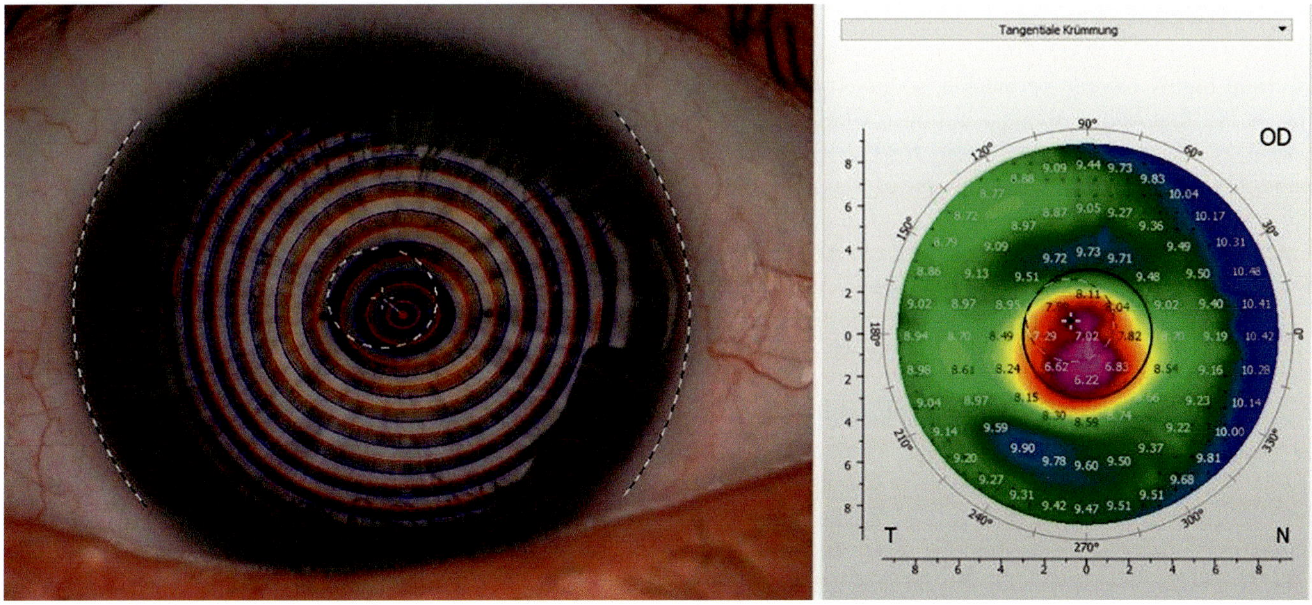

Fig. 5 Keratographic topography

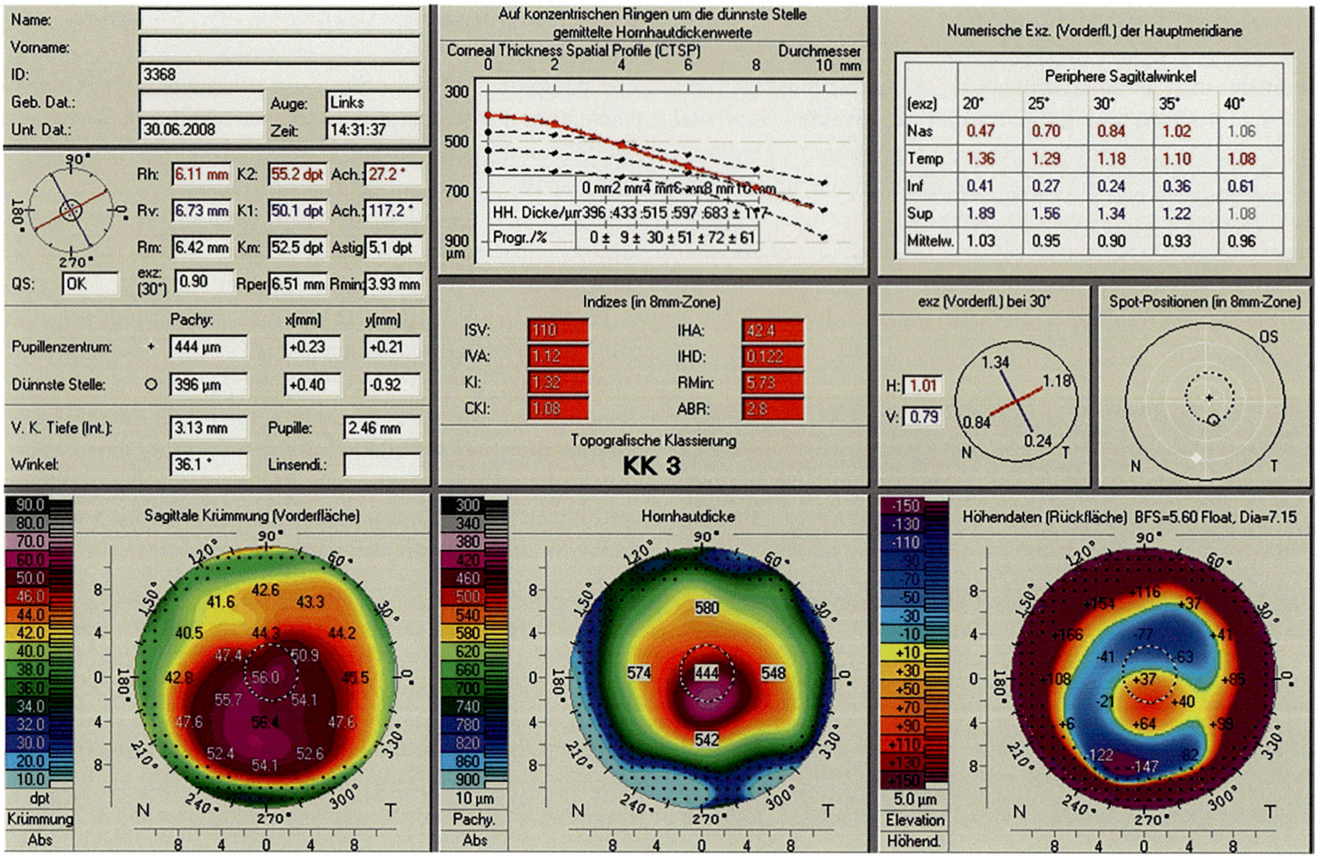

Fig. 6 Pentacam tomography

2.2 Rigid Gas permeable Keratoconus Specialty Lenses

The rigid highly oxygen permeable, so-called RGP contact lens, is the first choice therapy option for keratoconus. In general, contact lenses are not used for therapy in keratoconus, but primarily for rehabilitation of visual acuity [5] (Figs. 9 and 10).

All these lens systems have in common that the center of the lens has a small (= steeper) radius, corresponding to the apex of the cornea, whereas towards the periphery rather larger (= flatter) radii are constructed. The spacing of the flattening curves can also be adjusted according to the topography image. Therefore, the ideal keratoconus lens is always individually manufactured (Figs. 11 and 12).

The fluorescein image shows a central fluorescein lake and a peripheral overlay horizontally. When the fluorescein-stained tear film is exchanged on the apex, the lens can be worn, if it is well tolerated. Ideally, the lens should be irrigated better in the mid-periphery.

Keratokonus Lens Rose K

This lens was developed by Paul Rose, New Zealand. Mr. Rose was able to determine a correlation between the base curve and the size of the inner optic zone during the statistical evaluation of his data: The steeper the base curve, the smaller the optic zone had to be [7] (Figs. 13, 14, 15, 16, 17 and 18).

Regarding keratoconus fitting, no rule can be established. There are cases when a lens with a relatively simple back surface fits well in a difficult cornea and provides good visual acuity. However, in other cases a patient has to try different lens systems in a seemingly "simple" corneal geometry to find the ideal lens [4, 10–13] (Figs. 19, 20, 21 and 22).

In any case, it is important to spare the apex. That means in the apex area, where the cornea is most sensitive, a slight steep fitting or parallel fitting should be aimed for. A highly gas permeable material and an optimal fitting of the lens are crucial for long-term success.

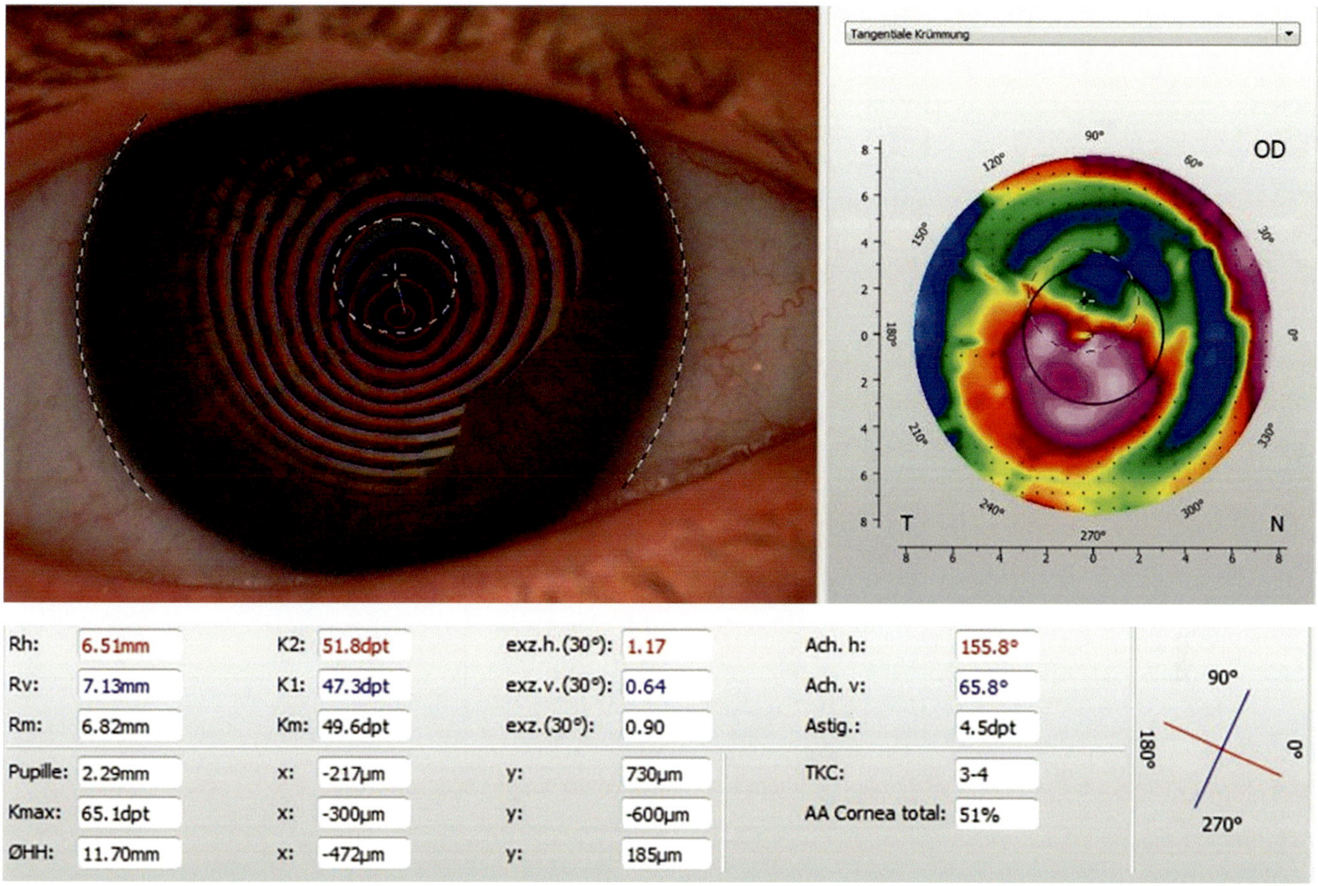

Fig. 7 Location of the main meridians in the central 3 mm area: Rh: horizontal radius of curvature at the center, shown as radius value in mm. K1: horizontal radius of curvature in the center, shown as refractive power in dpt. Kmax: maximum radius of curvature in the center, shown as refractive power in dp. AA: analyzed area: percentage of the effectively measured corneal surface

Since almost any irregularity can be compensated for by rigid contact lenses with modern individual design, amazing visual improvements are often achieved [5].

In addition to the contact lens companies mentioned based on the fitting examples, there are lots of companies which offer the possibility of individual contact lens manufacturing. The most important ones in Germany are Hecht Contactlinsen in Freiburg, MPG + E in Bordesholm, Wöhlk in Kiel, and Jenalens in Jena. In Switzerland, there are Falco in Tägerwilen and the company SwissLens in Prilly, as well as the international company Menicon.

2.3 Soft Keratoconus Lenses

See (Fig. 23).

2.4 Hybrid Lenses

See (Fig. 24).

2.5 Contact Lenses After Intacs

See (Fig. 25).

2.6 Contact Lenses After Crosslinking

During the wound healing phase after epic-off crosslinking, a bandage contact lens can be used until epithelial closure. If the patient has to be able to return to work quickly and wound healing is delayed, there is the possibility of a so-called piggyback system: a highly oxygen permeable

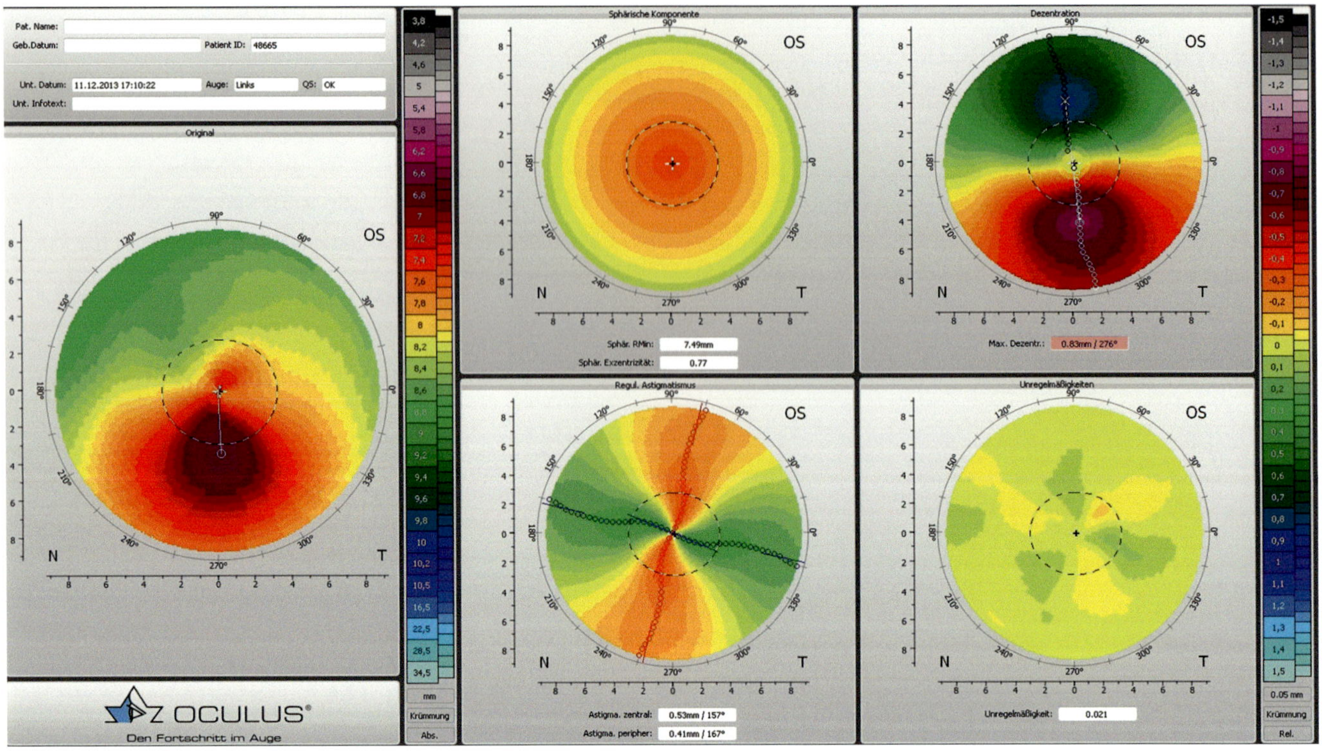

Fig. 8 Pentacam fourier analysis can be used to analyze astigmatism and determine maximum decentration

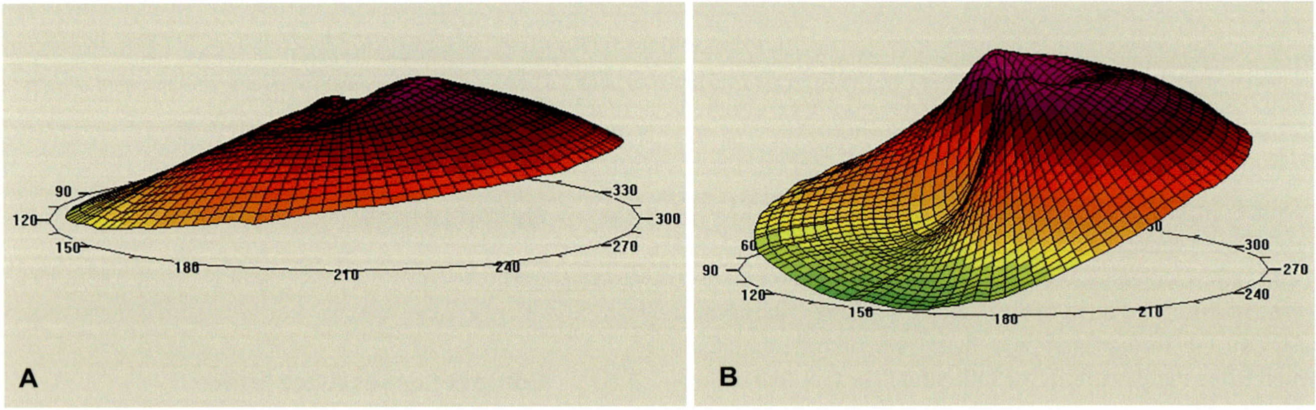

Fig. 9 (**A**) Keratoconus stage 1–2. (**B**) Keratoconus stage 3. (**A**, **B**) Three-dimensional representation of the corneal surface with different degrees of keratoconus. To fit this individual corneal shape, an individual contact lens has to be designed

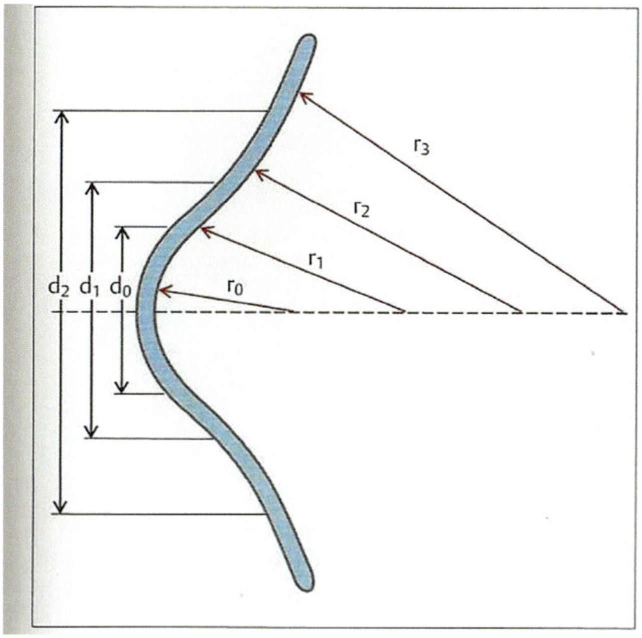

Fig. 10 Contact lens back surface profile for the keratoconus design [6]

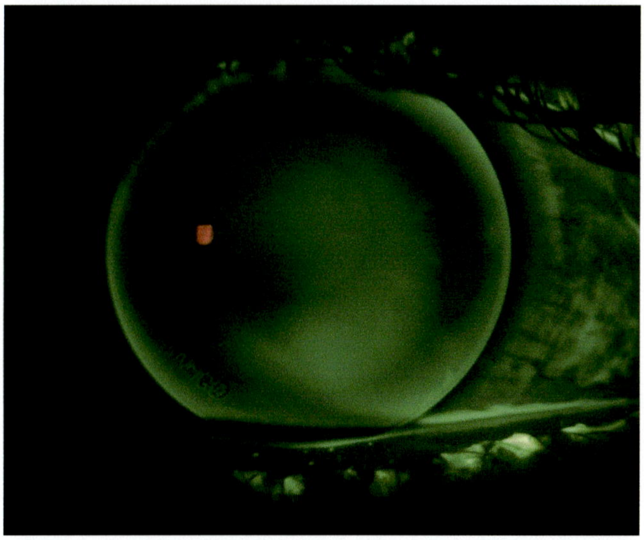

Fig. 11 In keratoconus fitting, special lenses are considered which attempt to map the abnormal irregularly shaped surface of the cornea with the abnormal steepening on the anterior and posterior surfaces. In this case, the aim is to achieve a good centration and pressure distribution in order to protect the sensitive apex. The image shows a special four-curve keratoconus lens "Excellent KK" from the company Appenzeller Kontaktlinsen, Speicher, Switzerland. Staining the tear film with fluorescein has proven useful to check whether the lens is optimally placed. Viewing is then performed with blue light on the slit lamp and with a yellow filter which makes it possible to assess, how well the contact lens glides over the cornea and whether it touches the apex

bandage contact lens on the cornea and on top a rigid gas permeable keratoconus lens, sometimes even the formerly fitted keratoconus lens [16]. The system can be worn at least temporarily and allows early visual rehabilitation [17, 18] (Figs. 26 and 27).

3 Contact Lenses After Keratoplasty

Contact lens fitting can only start a few weeks after complete suture removal [19]. In most cases, significant regular or irregular astigmatism occurs. Difficulties in contact lens fitting are caused by the different curvature of the graft and the host cornea. Sometimes a small diameter contact lens can provide help. But there is also the circumstance that each quadrant behaves differently or that the host cornea is steeper than the graft. In this case, individual solutions are needed, too (Figs. 28, 29, 30, 31, 32 and 33).

In this patient, topography after suture removal showed a keratoconus-like configuration (Fig. 34).

In case the host cornea is steeper than the graft, a special contact lens design is required (Fig. 35).

4 Scleral Lenses

The idea of compensating for corneal irregularities by using a fluid reservoir goes back to Leonardo da Vinci. At the end of the eighteenth century it was taken up again, almost simultaneously, by the French ophthalmologist Eugène Kalt and the German ophthalmologist Adolf Eugen Fick. Since the manufacturing technology at the time was not yet fully developed and the materials were not very permeable to oxygen, problems arose and scleral lenses were forgotten. It is only due to the further development towards extremely oxygen permeable materials that these contact lenses are currently experiencing a renaissance.

The advantages of scleral lenses lie in their size (up to 22 mm) and thus in their contact with the sclera. For the patient this means pain relief and a significant improvement in visual acuity. Due to the large anterior surface of the lens, high irregularities of the cornea can be bridged up to its edge.

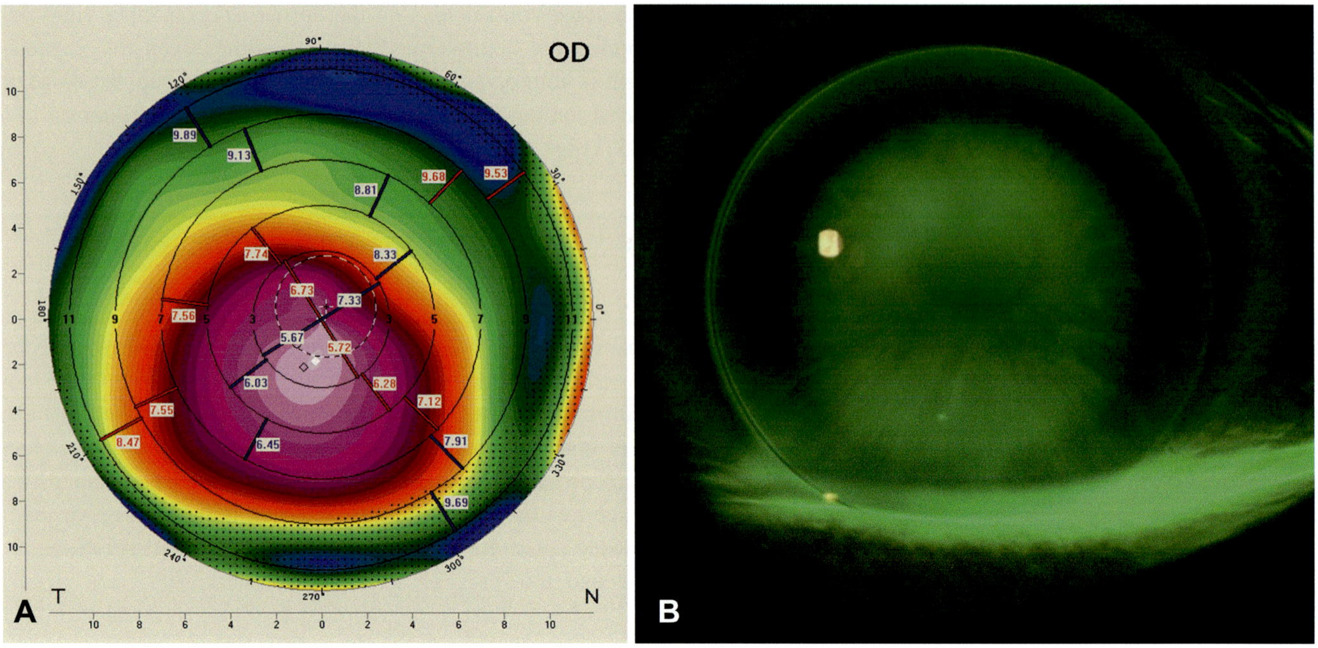

Fig. 12 (**A, B**) High-grade keratoconus with a custom-made keratoconus lens Mk pro from the company Galifa, St. Gallen, Switzerland

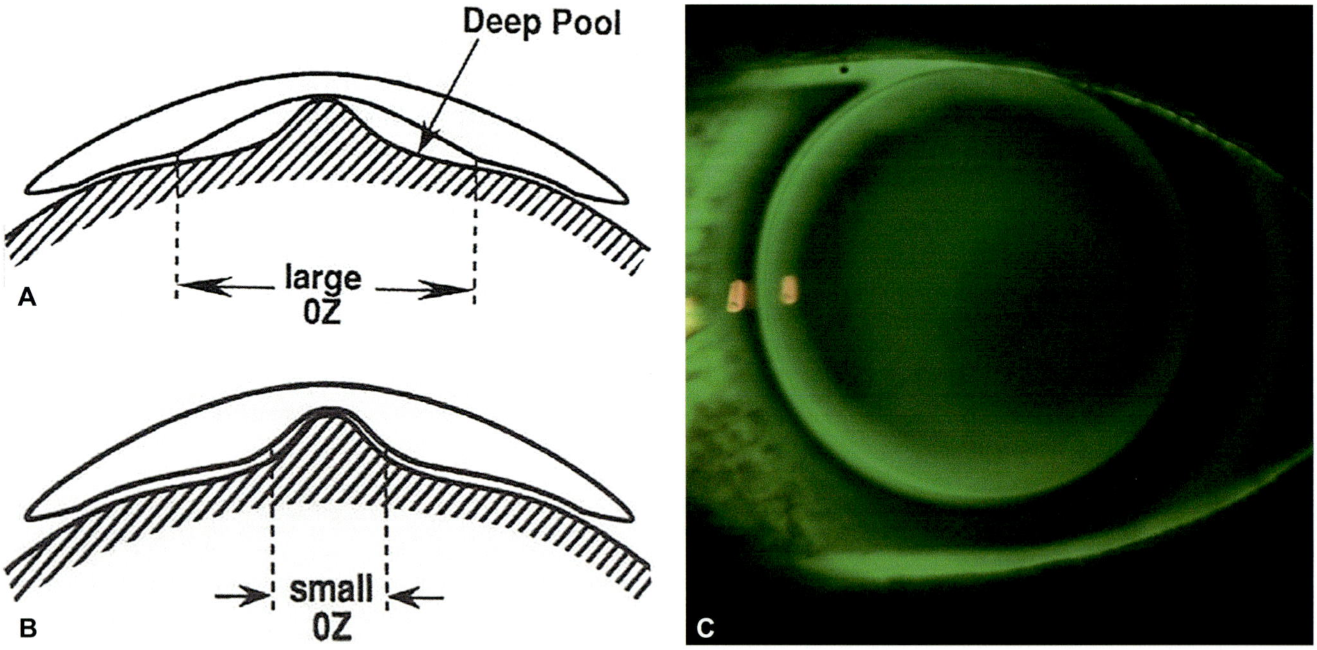

Fig. 13 (**A**) Fitting lenses with a large optic zone results in narrow support zones and deep "pooling" around the apex (accumulation of fluorescein lake, see "Deep Pool" arrow) in advanced keratoconus [8]. (**B**) Reducing the size of the optic zone with the central nipple on the back surface creates a wide peripheral support zone and smoother transitions [8]. (**C**) Shows the fluorescein image of a well-fitted Rose K lens in a patient with stage 2–3 keratoconus. In more advanced stages of keratoconus, the optic zone is sometimes no longer in the center of the pupil as the lens centers on the apex located below the corneal center. This can affect visual acuity and has been considered in the new generation of Rose K2. A very large number of designs can now be manufactured [5, 9]. The Rose K is manufactured by the international company Menicon or by the company Galifa, St. Gallen Switzerland

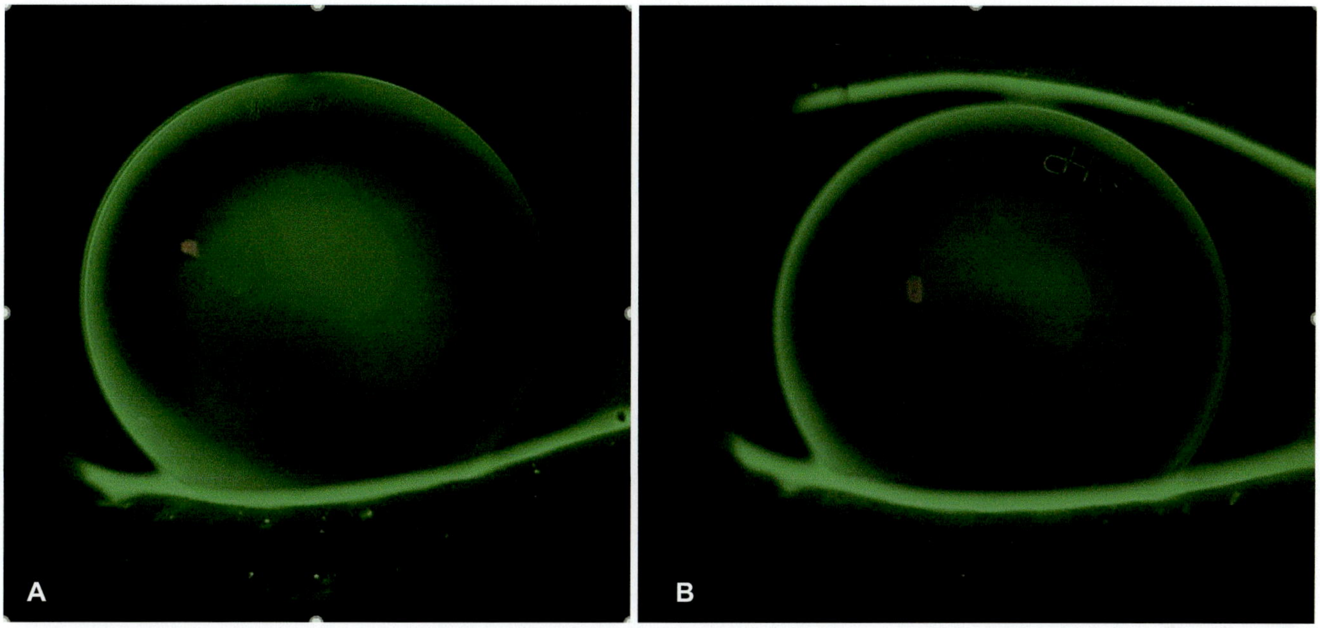

Fig. 14 (**A**) Rose K. (**B**) "Excellent KK". (**A**) Fluorescein image Rose K: central pooling, peripheral light support. (**B**) Fluorescein image "Excellent KK": uniform fluorescein image, therefore uniform support and underwashed with tear film, which is what should be aimed for

The disadvantage is mainly the complex handling. In addition, the tear pool under the lens is not exchanged due to the fixed scleral layer, as it is in the case of the usual dimensionally stable lens systems. Therefore, after a certain time, the fluid under the lens often becomes cloudy. The lens must then be removed and reinserted with fresh fluid. Nevertheless, for many patients the scleral lens brings an enormous improvement to their quality of life, especially in cases of severe keratoconus, irregular astigmatism or after keratoplasty [21–24] (Figs. 36–46).

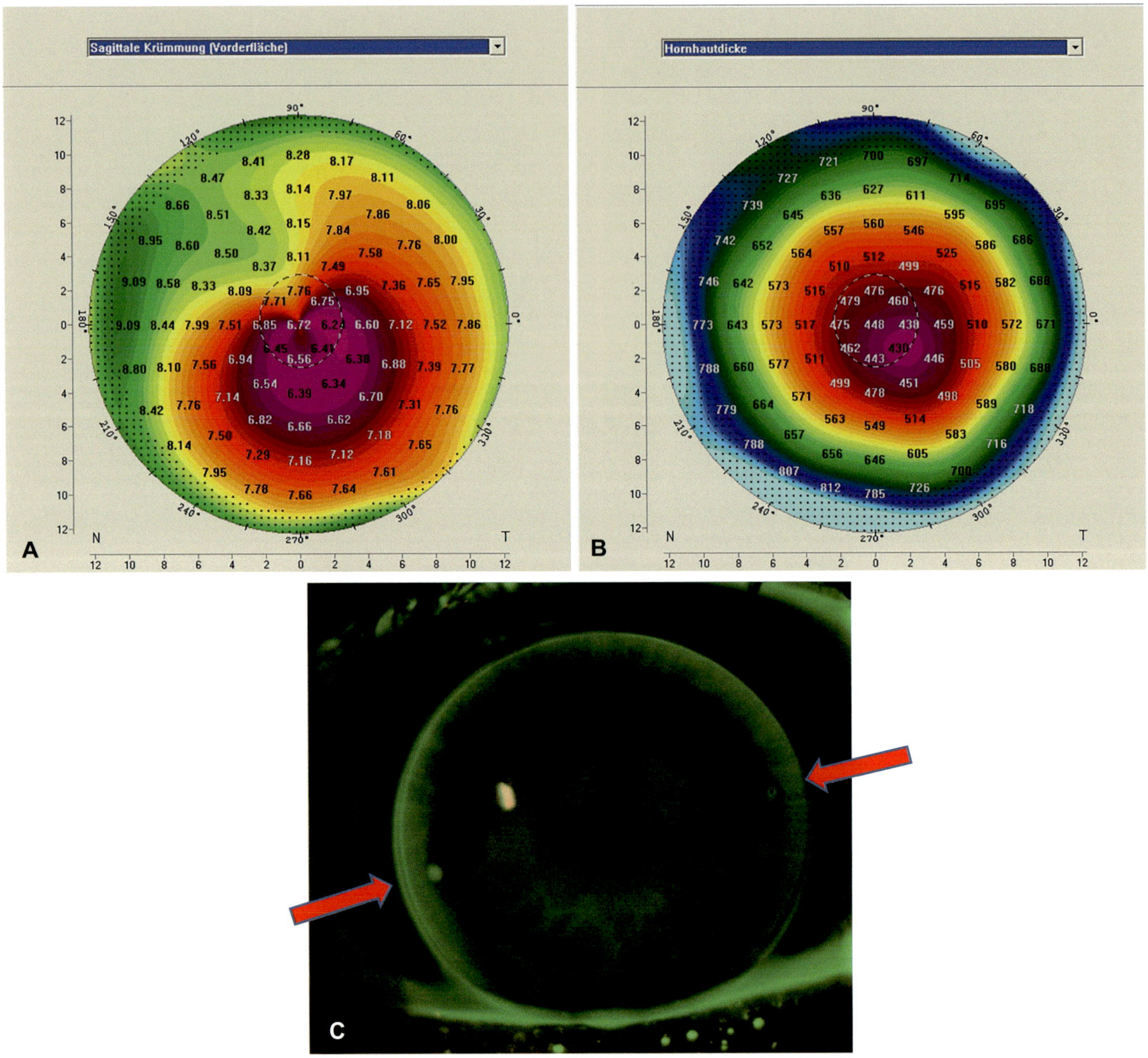

Fig. 15 (**A**) Pentacam tomography. (**B**) Corneal thickness. (**A, B**) In this stage 3 keratoconus the Pentacam analysis shows the topography on the left and the pachymetry on the right. The information helps to recognize, where the apex region is particularly sensitive and the lens must be fitted in a particularly apex-preserving manner. (**C**) In this case, a Rose K with a front prismatic toric design ensured a successful outcome. The arrows mark the axis of the torus. This picture shows how the central nipple on the back surface of the contact lens accommodates the apex, as the fluorescein image shows a uniform undercut

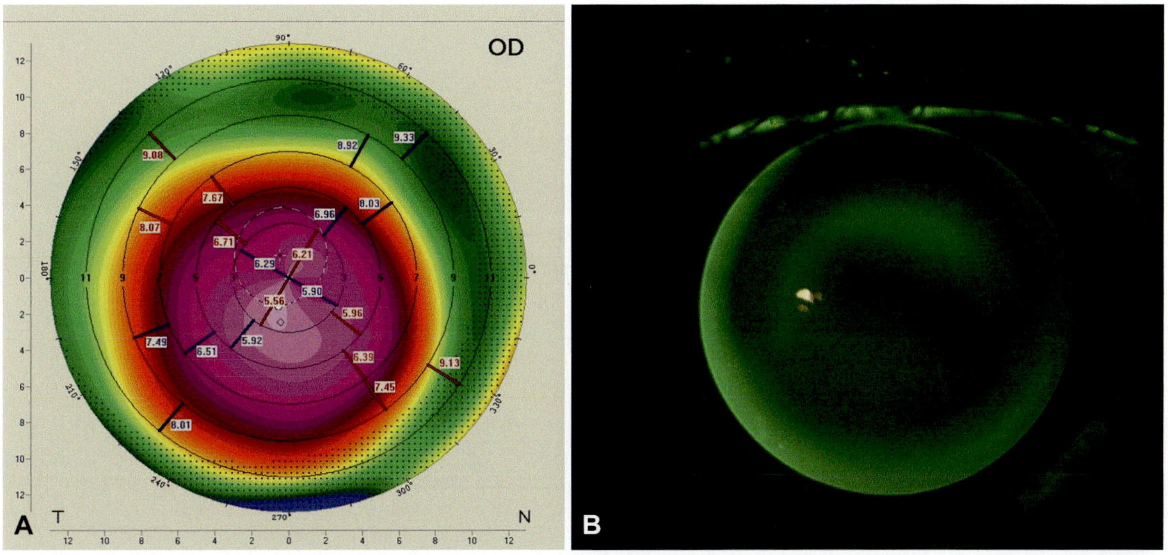

Fig. 16 (**A**, **B**) This large cone could also be fitted well with a Rose K

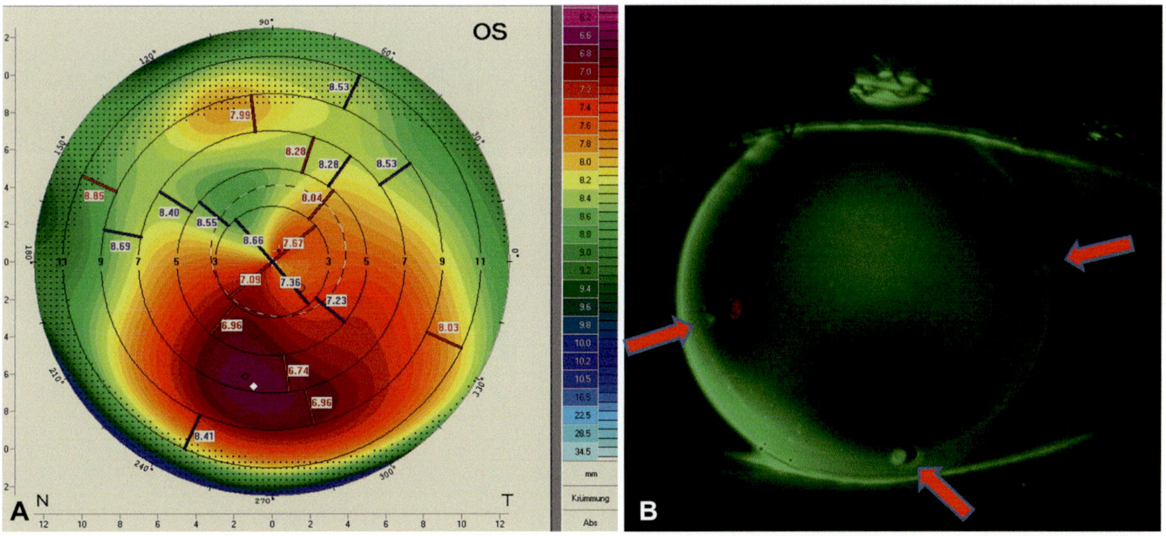

Fig. 17 (**A**) Because of the extreme radial differences in the 4 quadrants of the topography, (**B**) a quadrant-specific lens "Excellent KK" from the company Appenzeller Kontaktlinsen, Speicher, Switzerland, was a successful choice in this case. This lens has different eccentricities, i.e. flattening, in the 4 quadrants. The red arrows indicate the marking points of the quadrants, the 4th point is covered by the upper lid. The cone tip, which is located far below, is irrigated well

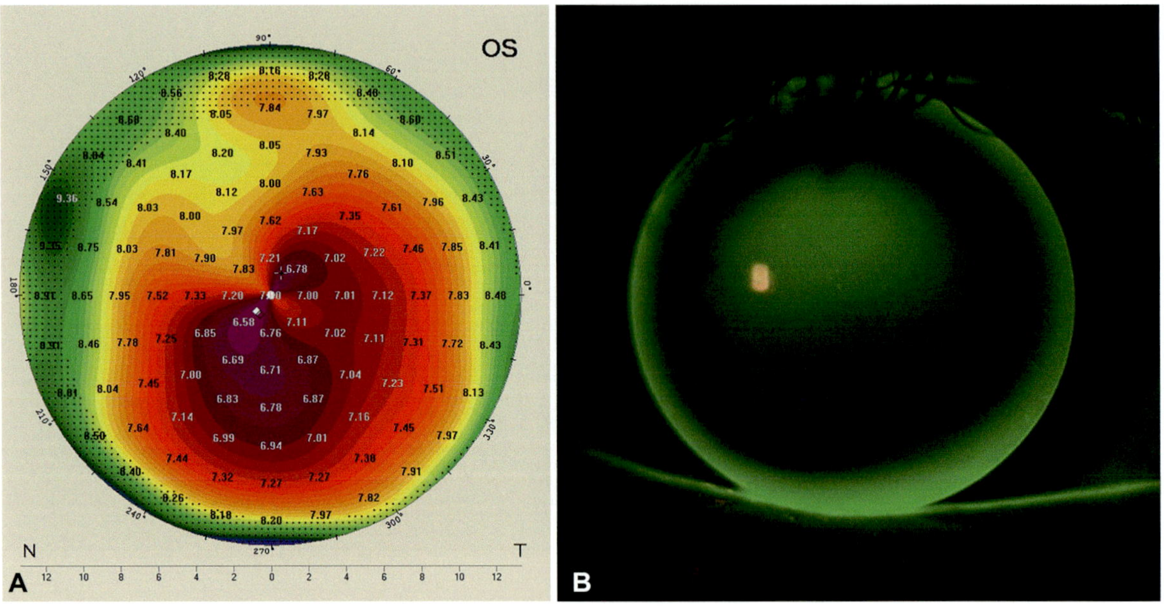

Fig. 18 (**A**) Pentacam tomography and (**B**) corresponding rigid Rose K keratoconus specialty contact lens, fitted with apex touching. Since visual acuity and tolerability were good and there was sufficient exchange of fluorescein-stained tear film in the video, the lens was approved, especially because a quadrant-specific lens did not provide any benefits in this case

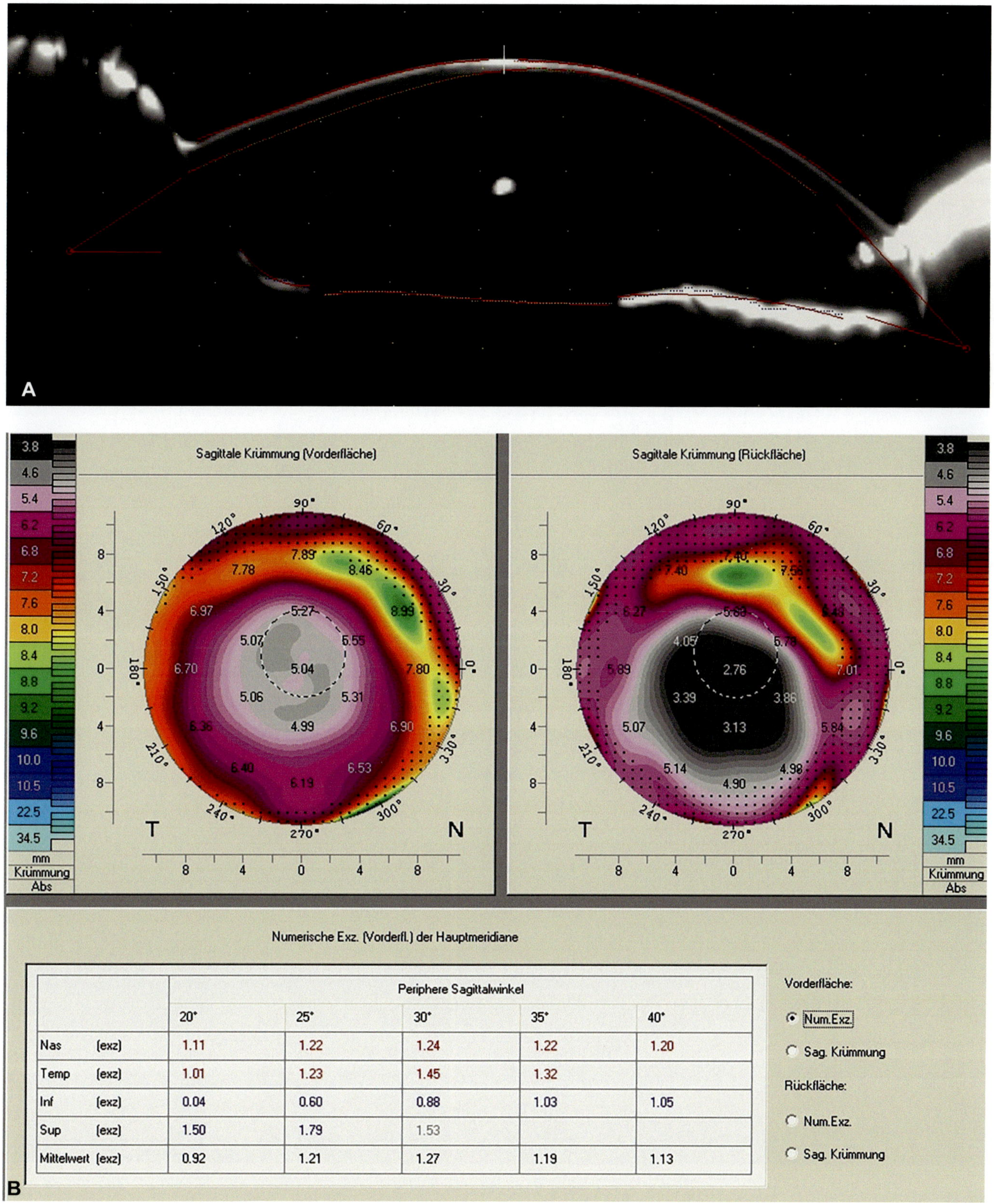

Fig. 19 (**A**) This young patient has keratoconus with an extremely thin cornea in the right eye. In this case, the indication for keratoplasty was given. However, the patient refused surgery and tried contact lens fitting. (**B**) Analysis of the anterior and posterior corneal surface with the Pentacam: extremely steep radii are present on the anterior and posterior surface

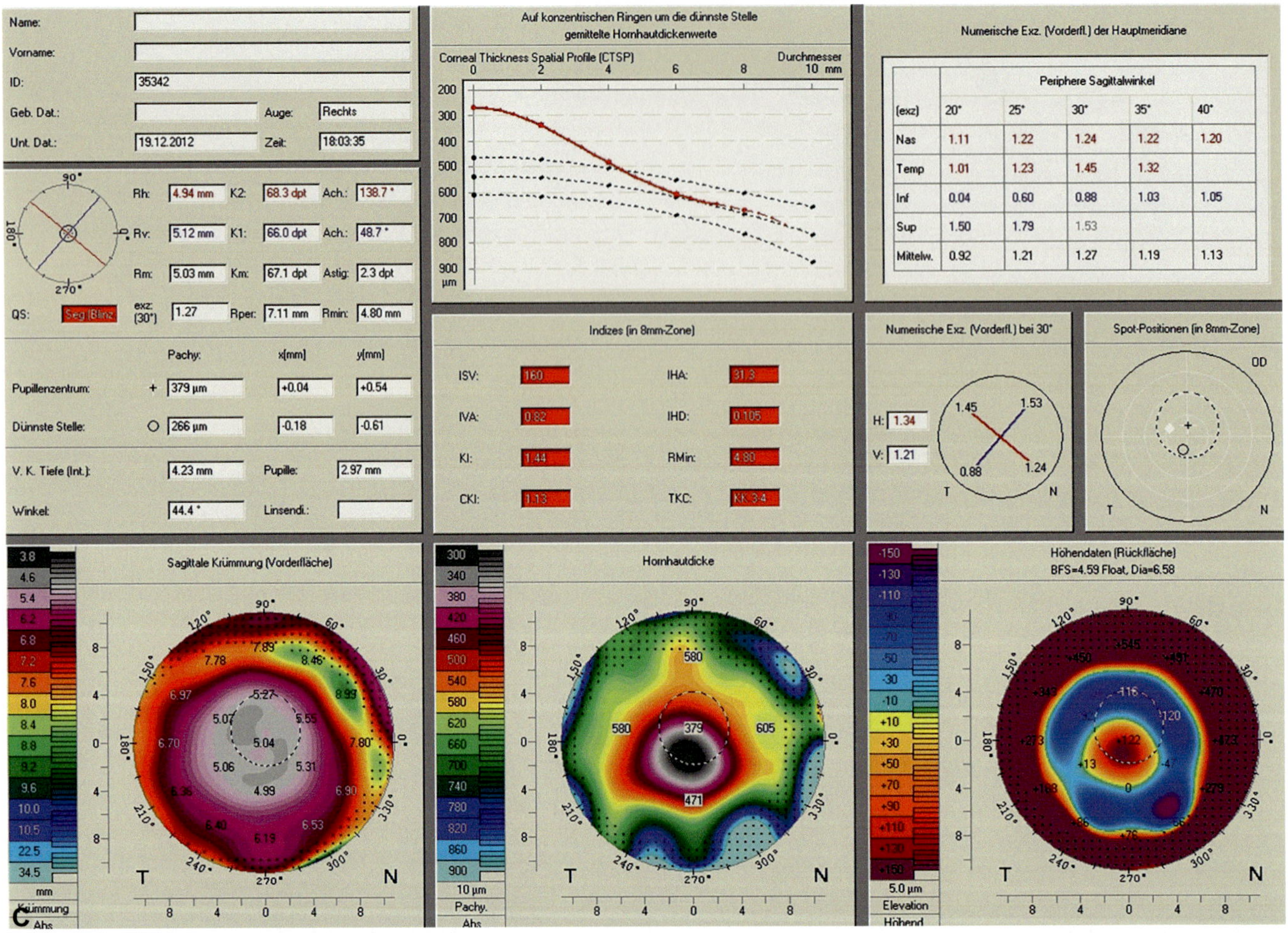

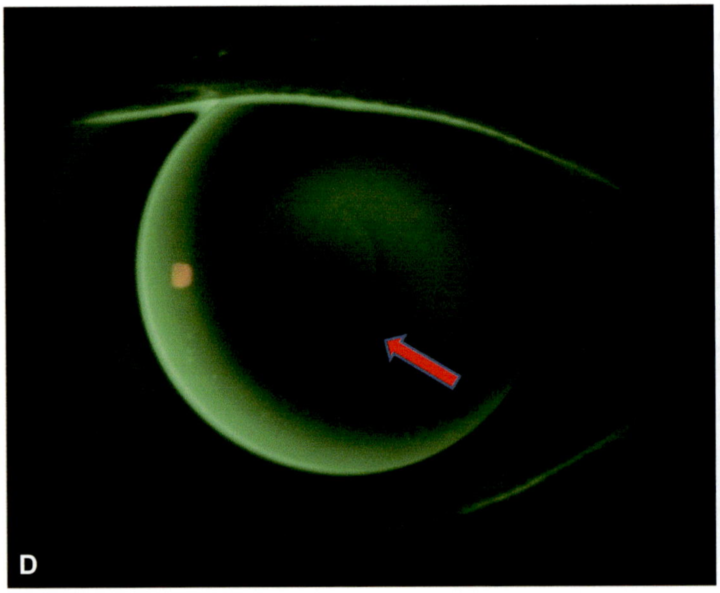

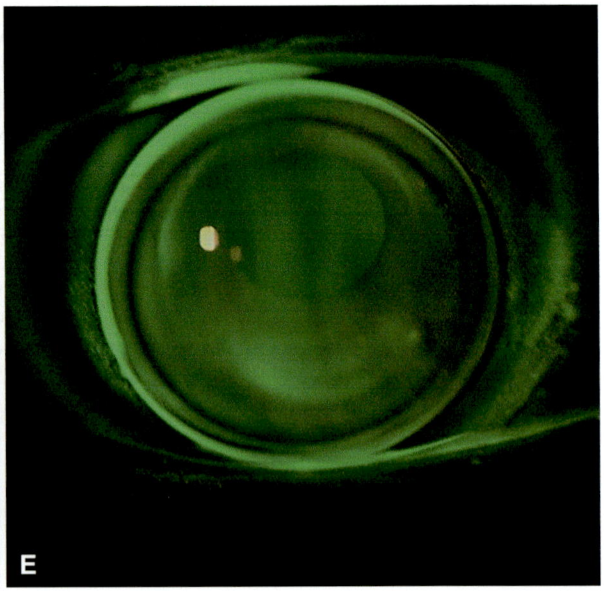

Fig. 19 (**C**) Analysis with the Pentacam: the thinnest point at the lower edge of the apex is 266 µm. These images show an advanced stage of keratoconus. (**D**) First, based on topography calculation, an Excellent KK of the company Appenzeller Kontaktlinsen, Speicher, Switzerland, with a small diameter of 9.1 mm was manufactured. Unfortunately, due to the high eccentricity of the cornea, the lens slipped nasally and rested on the thinnest part of the apex (arrow). (**E**) Therefore, a Rose K was tested as a next step and a better fitting could be achieved, visible in the uniform fluorescein image. Wearing comfort and visual acuity were both good

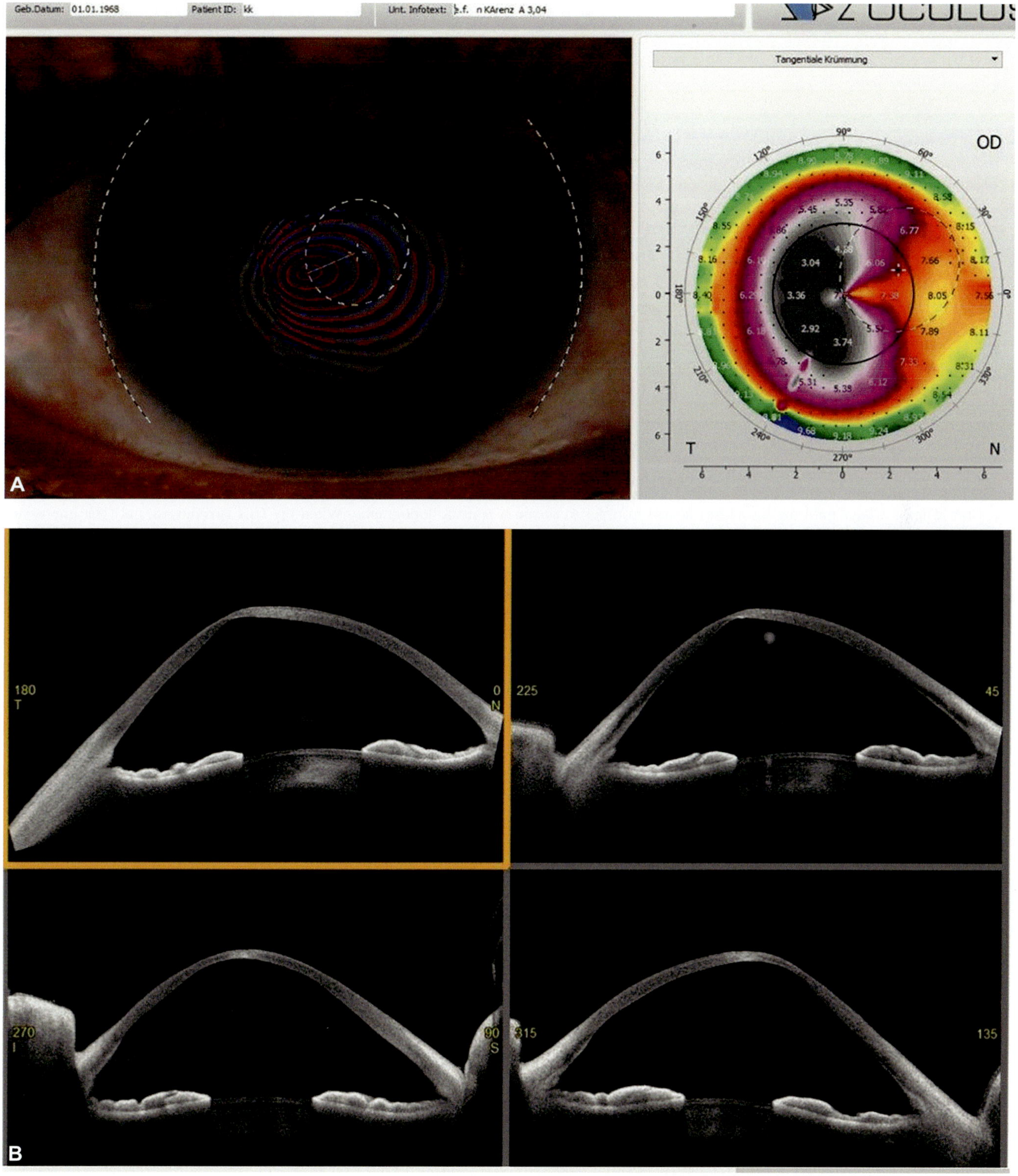

Fig. 20 (**A, B**) Extreme keratoconus (**A**, topography; **B**, anterior segment optical coherence tomography). The patient had worn soft contact lenses for many years without follow-ups. The lenses were the preferred choice due to the lack of a spectacle alternative. Finally, the solution was a penetrating keratoplasty

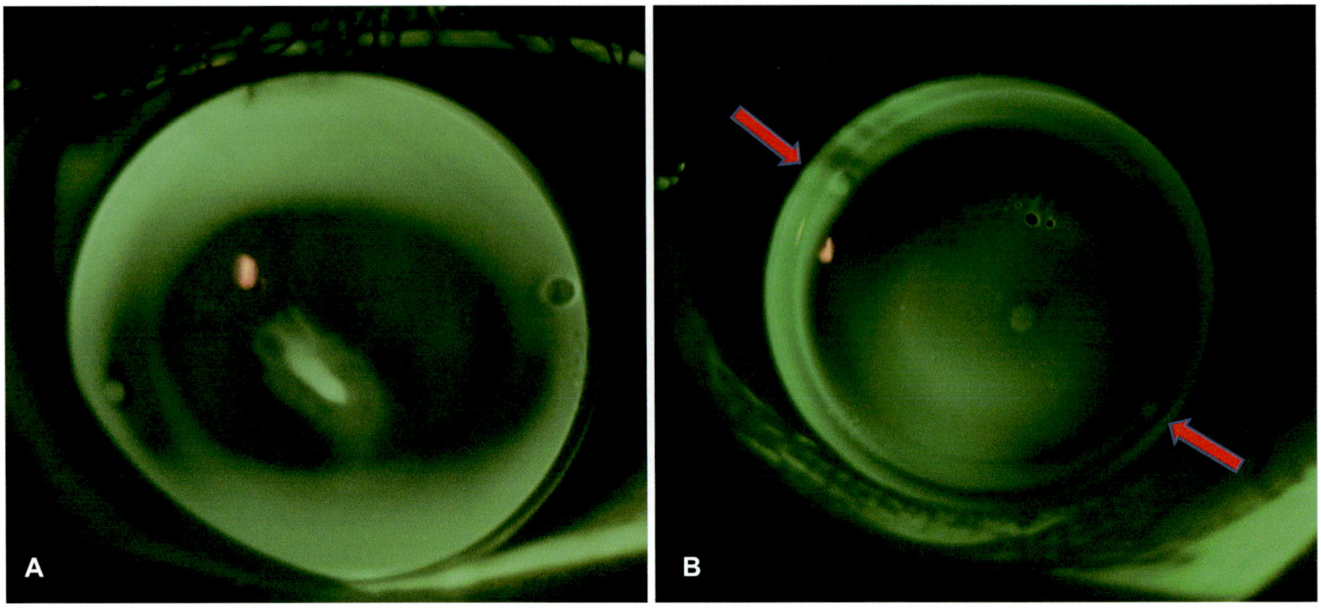

Fig. 21 (**A**) In this case, epithelial defects have occurred at the apex due to the lens being too flat and it is advisable to stop wearing contact lenses for at least 3 days until the lesion has healed in order to obtain a realistic topography. When the lens is removed, only the impression of the lens (warpage) would be obtained and the readjustment would be unsuccessful [14]. (**B**) In this patient, an anterior prismatic custom designed lens, a so-called Mk pro VPT from the company Galifa, St. Gallen, Switzerland, was applied after 3 weeks without contact lens. The red arrows mark the axis points of the torus. The center is intentionally adjusted steeper to preserve the remaining corneal lesion. The fluorescein lake is replaced so that the fitting could be completed and early visual rehabilitation was achieved

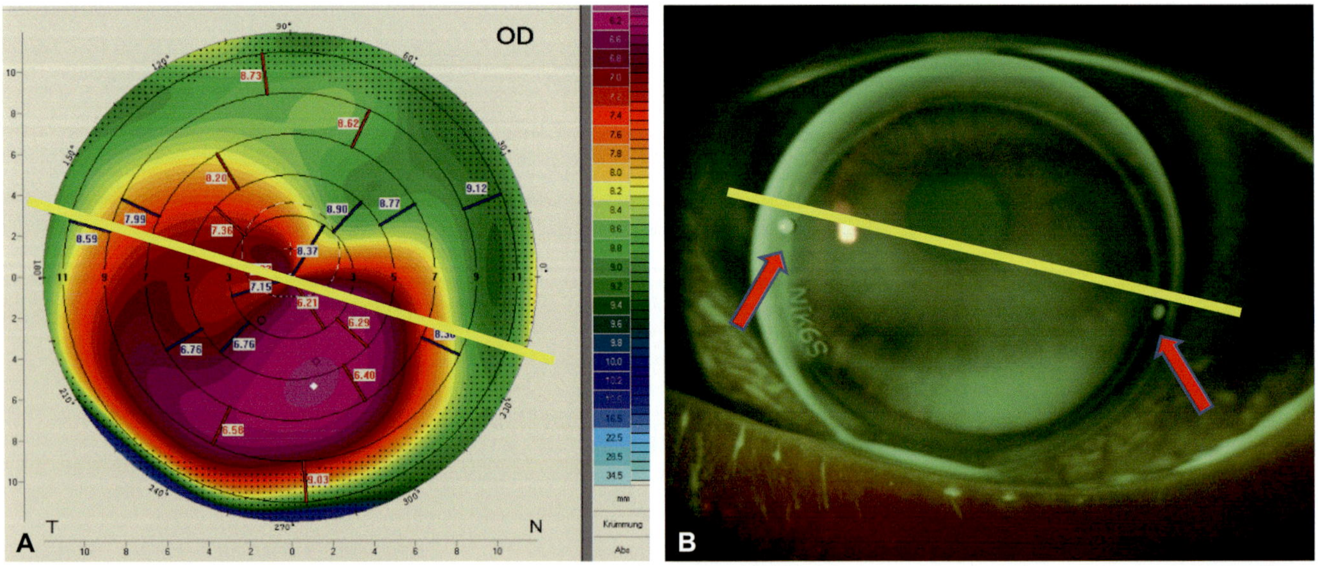

Fig. 22 (**A, B**) In this patient the large cone is located inferiorly and slopes steeply towards the limbus. In such cases, companies offer a special lens shape called asymmetric corneal technology (ACT). Here, the lower lens quadrant is designed steeper to achieve a better fitting. The image on the right shows a fluorescein image of an I-MAP AS VPT from the company Appenzeller Kontaktlinsen, Speicher, Switzerland. The lens was calculated based on topography, hence the name MAP (topographical mapping) and "I" for individual. The axis points of the torus are marked by the arrows and one can see how the lens on the eye corresponds to the axis of the topography (yellow line)

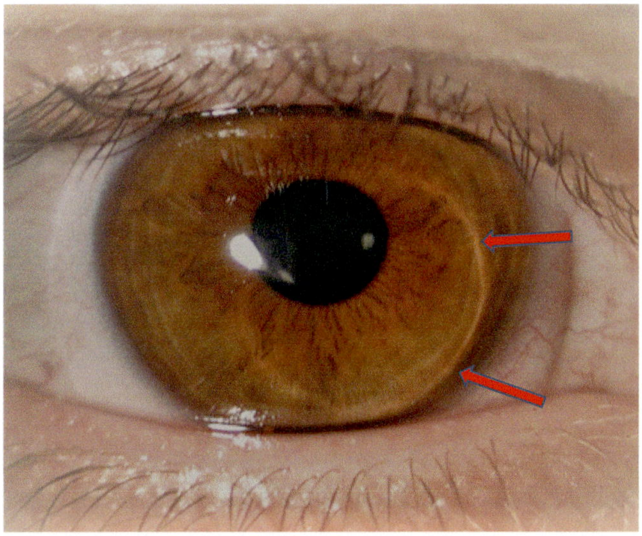

Fig. 23 In case of intolerance of RGP contact lenses, a trial with soft keratoconus lenses, made of highly oxygen permeable silicone hydrogel material, can be a suitable alternative, Visual acuity is usually not as good as with a rigid lens. As the soft lens material must be thicker to bridge the cone, it is prone to debris and corneal vascularization. These contact lenses can be worn for a maximum of ½ year, including check-ups. The red arrows mark the edge of the torus ground into the anterior surface. This image shows a soft keratokonus lens from the company Swisslens, Prilly, Switzerland

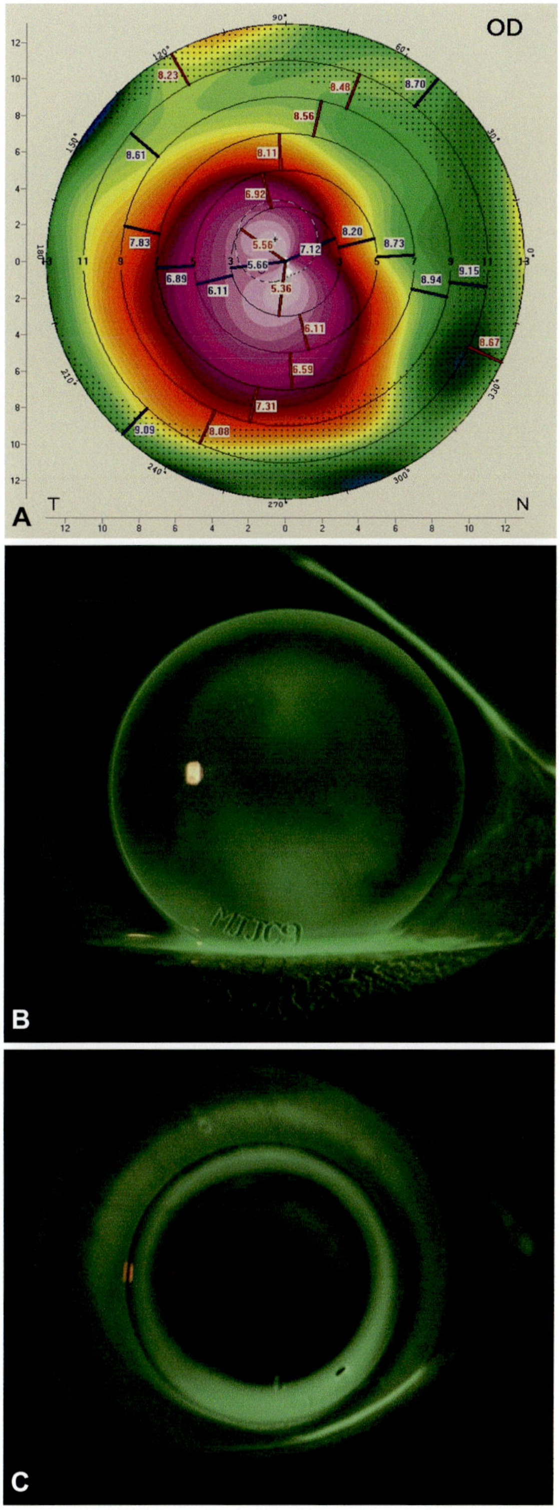

Fig. 24 (**A, B**), This patient's passion is biking. Unfortunately, he often lost his RGP contact lenses while biking although they were well fitted despite the steep cone. (**B**) topography-calculated individual lens I-MAP from the company Appenzeller Kontaktlinsen, Speicher, Switzerland. (**C**) In this case, an experiment with hybrid lenses was carried out and a dimensionally stable lens is centrally fitted onto a soft lens. The Airflex contact lens from the company Swisslens, Prilly, Switzerland (shown here) has the advantage that the fit can be assessed with fluorescein. Because of the high maintenance and the danger of the lens sticking, these lens systems have not been accepted until now, although wearing comfort is very good [13]. A new piggy-back version is under development by the company Hecht Contactlinsen, Freiburg, Germany

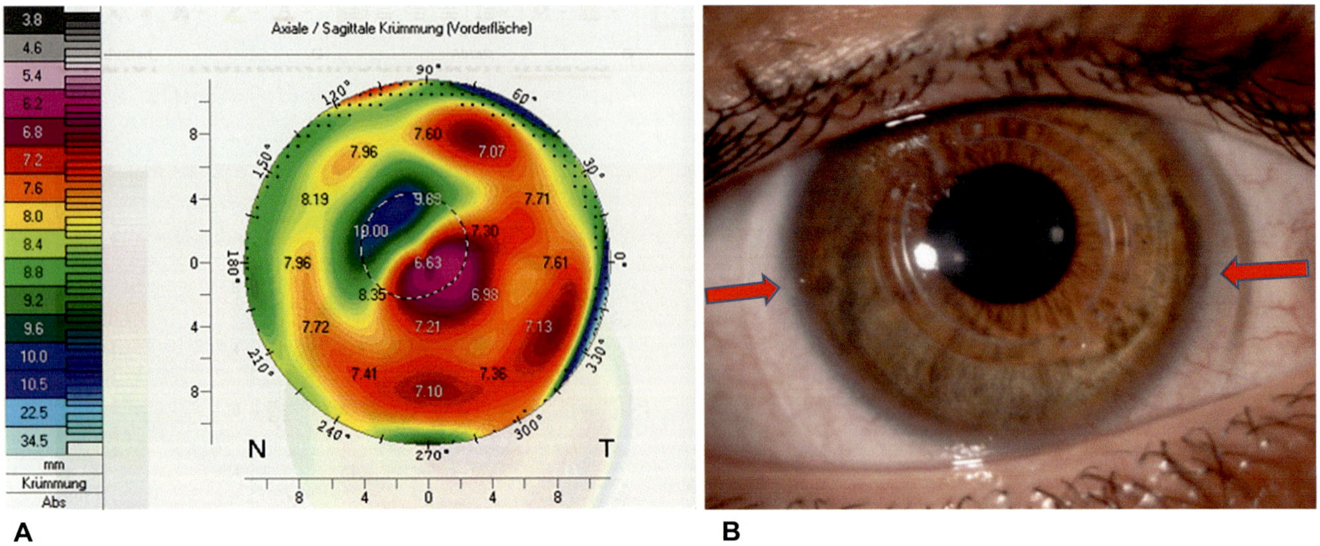

Fig. 25 (**A**) Very high irregularity with Intacs (intracorneal ring segments). A dimensionally rigid lens cannot be constructed with these different radii. An extremely small diameter would be possible, but this would lead to tipping of the lens. For a mini-scleral or scleral lens, the risk was considered too high with the pretreated cornea [15]. (**B**) Since the toric soft contact lens from the company Swisslens, Prilly, Switzerland resulted in a significant improvement in visual acuity, it was dispensed with the indication of a reduction in wearing time (8 h per day). The red arrows indicate the marking points of the toric soft lens

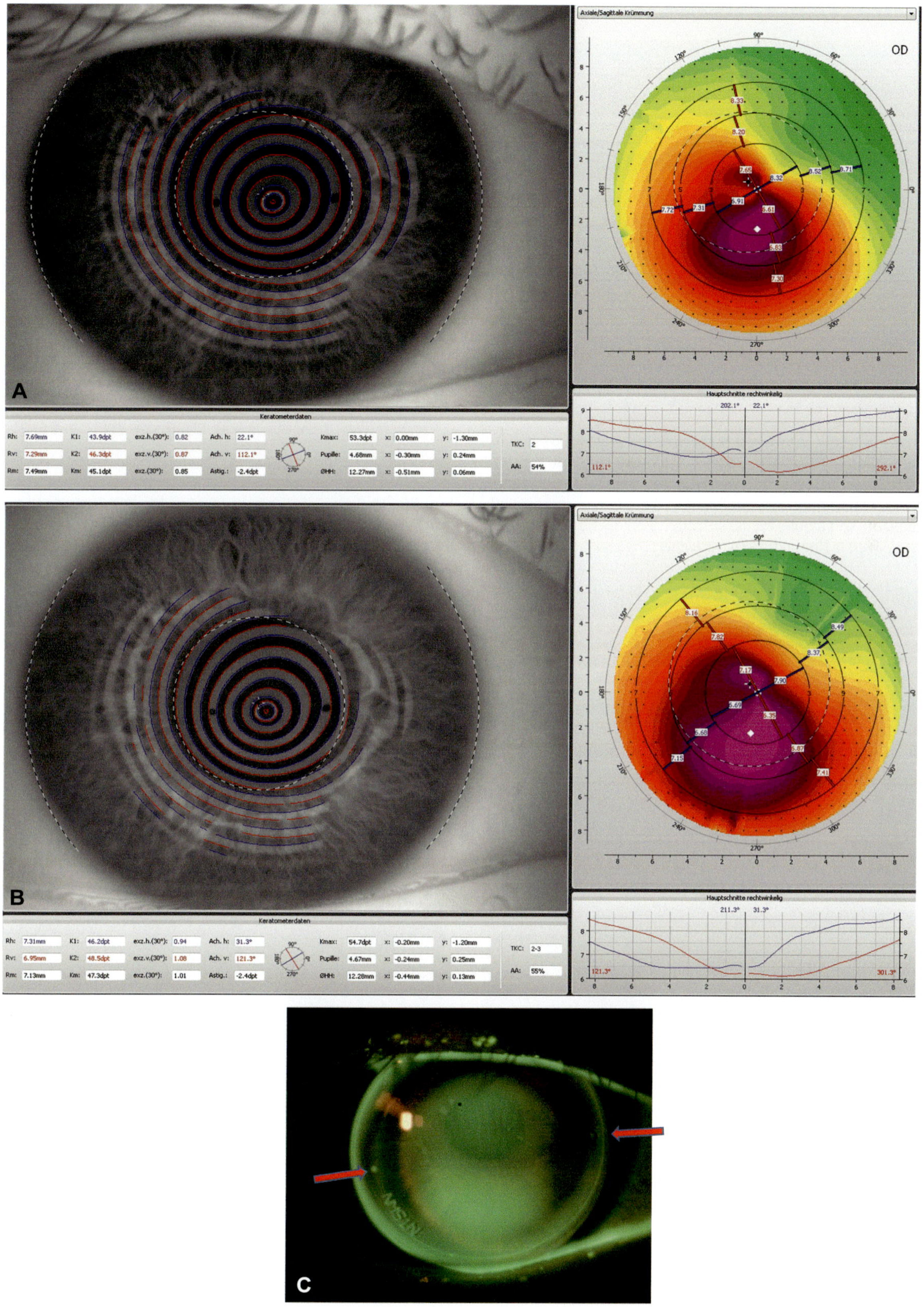

Fig. 26 (**A**) Topography 2010. (**B**) Topography 2011 with a clear progression and the decision for crosslinking. (**C**) After wound healing in the stabilization phase, a slight steep adjustment should be aimed for to preserve the apex. This picture shows a toric Excellent KK from the company Appenzeller Kontaktlinsen, Speicher, Switzerland. The torus is marked by the red arrows

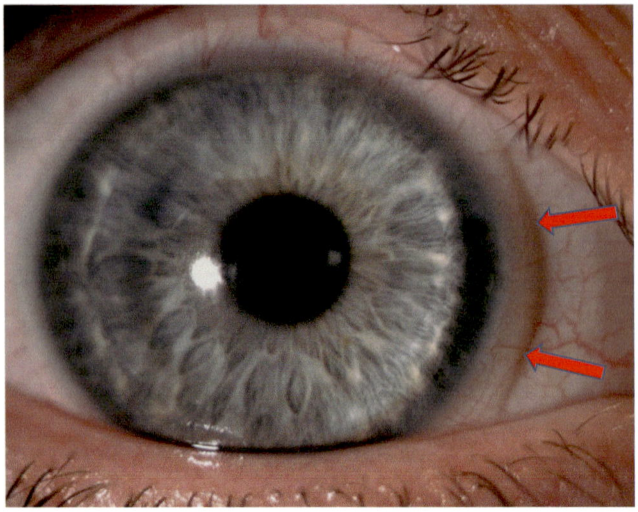

Fig. 27 Trial with soft high-oxygen permeable keratoconus lens for recurrent epithelial defects. The arrows mark the edge of the lens. Attention should be paid to the vessels at the upper limbal margin, as they may be a sign of oxygen deficiency. This image shows a siliconehydrogel soft keratoconus lens, so-called Personelle KK from the company Appenzeller Kontaktlinsen, Speicher, Switzerland

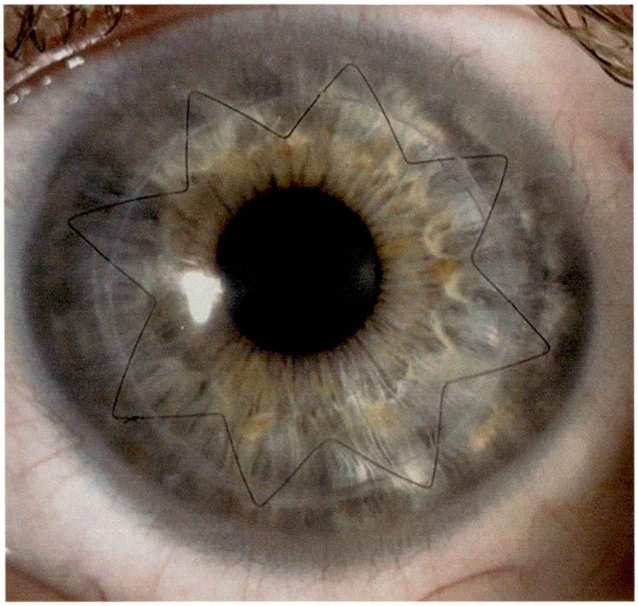

Fig. 28 After corneal transplantation and especially after partial suture removal, there is an urgent desire of the patient to see well again. Contact lens fitting can start at the earliest after the 3rd week in case of sutures in place, when the graft is irritation-free, or after suture removal, when the topography is stable

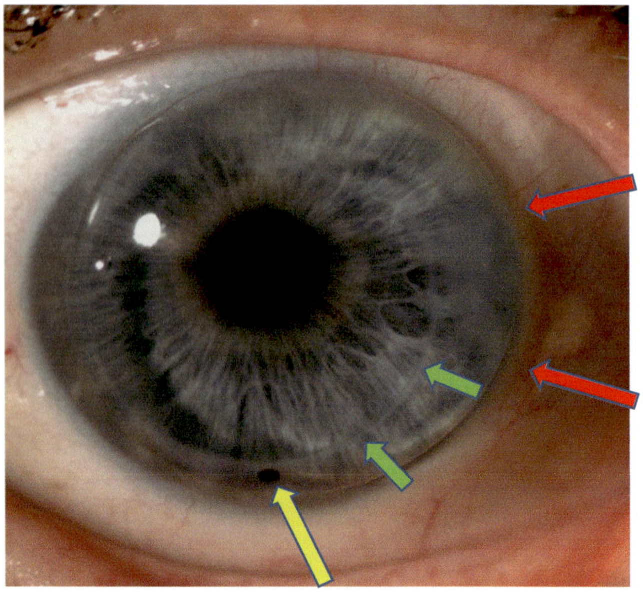

Fig. 29 Problems are usually caused by step formation between the graft and the host cornea. In this image of a right eye the semi limbal lens is nasally decentered (lens edge marked by red arrows) despite the large diameter of 11 mm and prism ballast inferiorly. This has led to recurrent corneal edema between 2 and 4 o'clock due to mechanical irritation. The black dot at the bottom marks the prism ballast and serves as an insertion guide (yellow arrow). The graft margin is visible under the lens (green arrows)

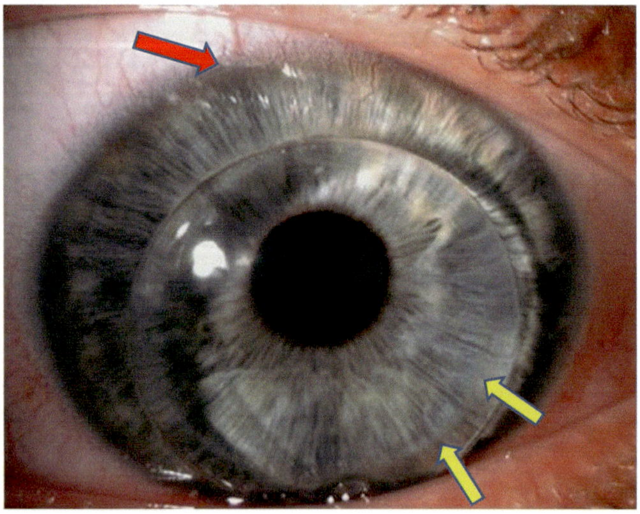

Fig. 30 According to the transplant size, you can choose to fit a small contact lens. An advantage of small lenses is a better oxygen supply of the cornea as it is irrigated with oxygen-rich tear film. A disadvantage may be mechanical irritation due to tipping. In this case, the deep fit rather offers advantages, because the vessels at the upper limbus (red arrow) are spared and a very good visual acuity is still achieved with the large central optic zone of the lens. The yellow arrows mark the graft margin

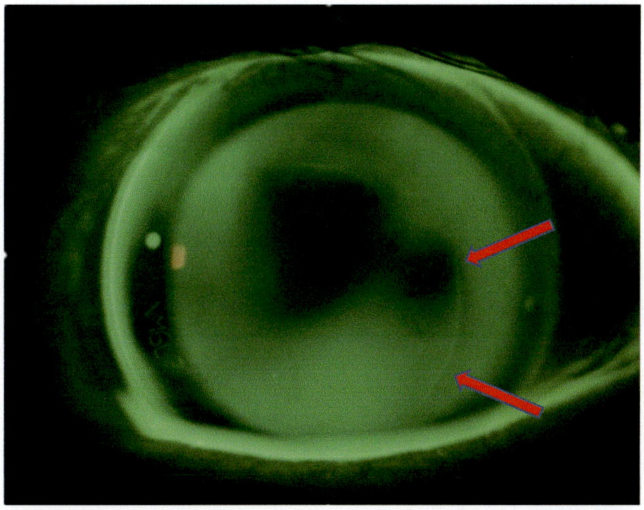

Fig. 31 Another option is to fit a lens with a large diameter, such as a borderline to corneal limbus toric contact lens with a diameter of 11 mm. Due to the advancing mechanization in contact lens manufacturing and material development, increasingly larger diameters are possible. The graft edge is clearly visible in the fluorescein image (red arrows)

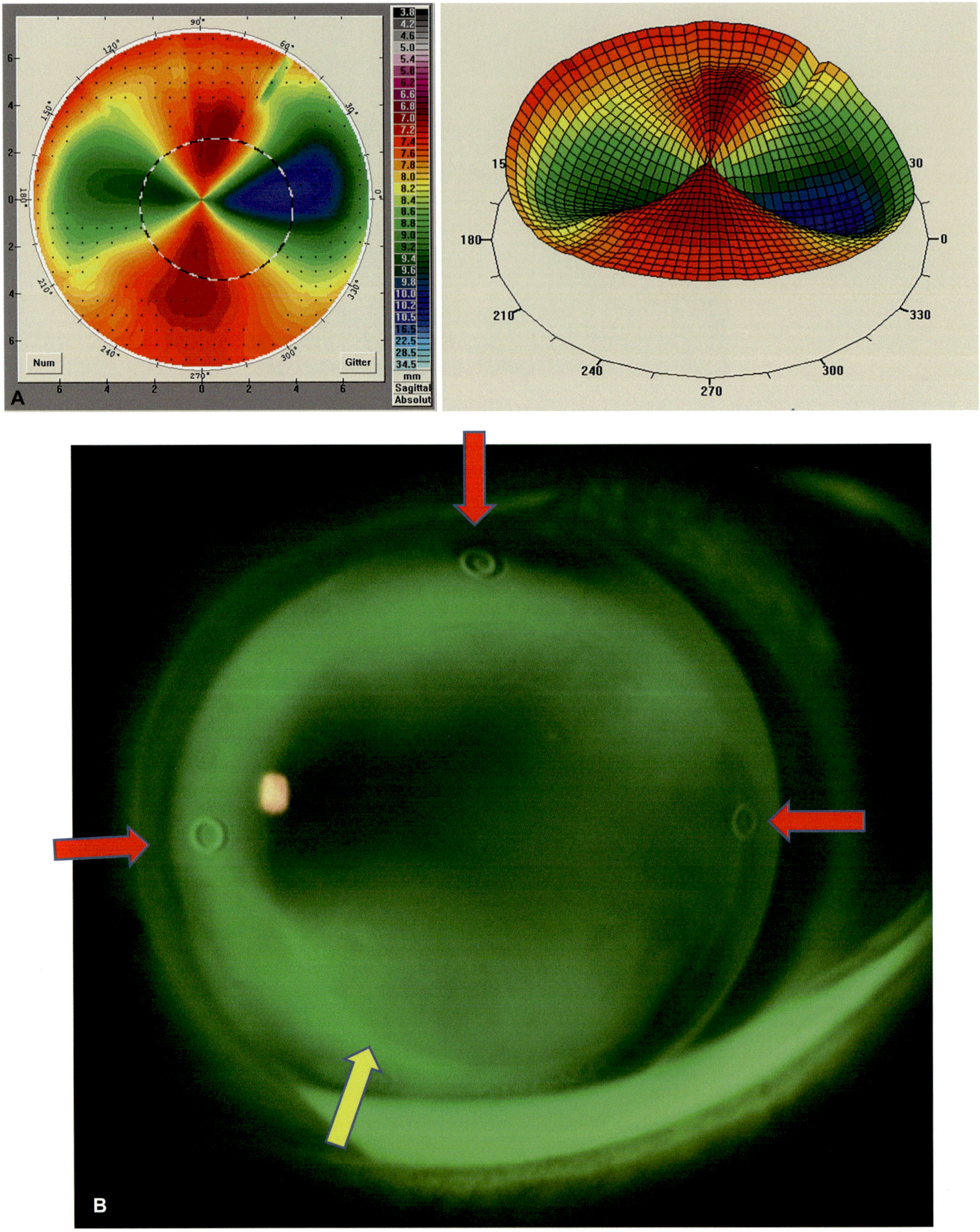

Fig. 32 (**A**) Topography and (**B**) 3-dimensional imaging in a patient after keratoplasty with high irregularity in all 4 quadrants of the cornea. (**C**) The solution is a quadrant-specific contact lens, in this case "Modula Q" (company Galifa, St. Gallen, Switzerland). In all quadrants, marked by 4 dots, (see red arrows, lower dot disappears in the tear pool) a different eccentricity (= flattening) was built in to adapt the contact lens better to the anterior corneal surface. Below the lens, the graft interface is marked by the yellow arrow

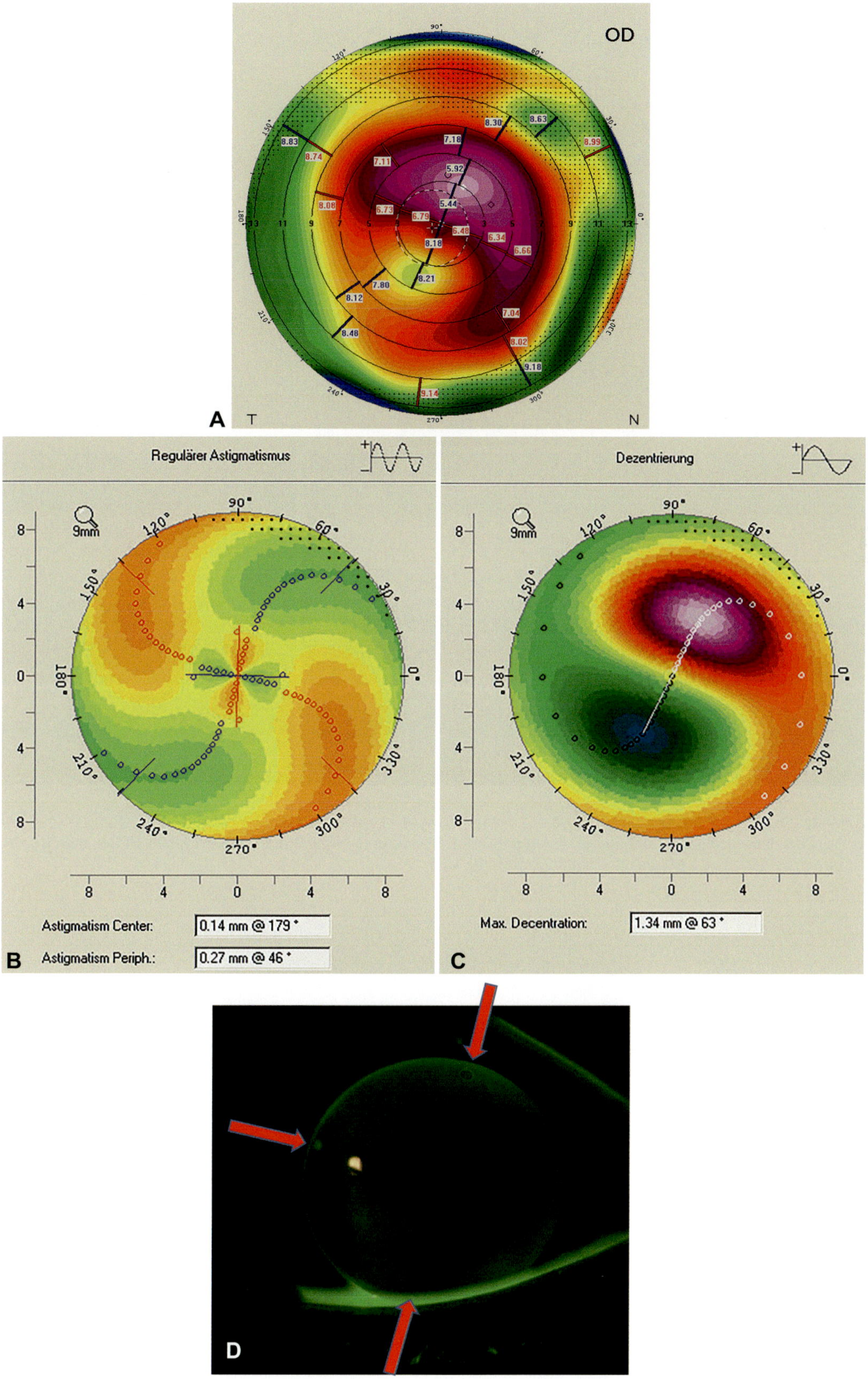

Fig. 33 (**A**) In this patient, the graft also shows high irregularity after keratoplasty. In the Pentacam image, the steeper radii in the graft and the flatter ones of the host cornea (shown in green) are clearly visible. The graft margin is marked by the blue ring. (**B**) The Fourier analysis (left picture) shows a regular astigmatism. (**C**) The analysis of the decentration (right picture) is highly abnormal. Therefore, a special RGP lens was preferred. Alternatively, a scleral lens could be considered. (**D**) The solution was a quadrant-specific custom-made lens Modula Q from the company Galifa, St. Gallen, Switzerland. The red arrows show the marking points of the lens. Below and temporally, the marking points are not visible

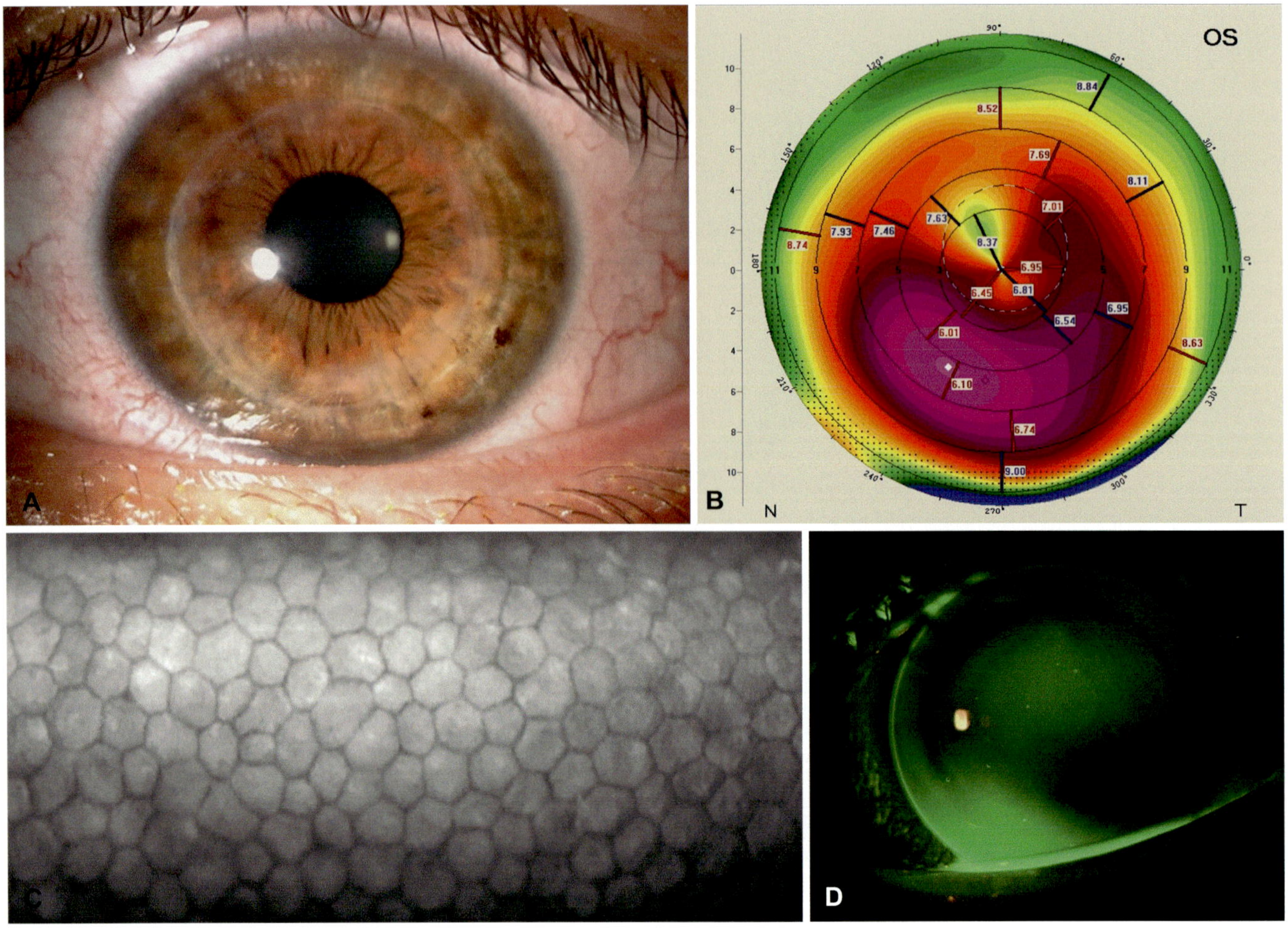

Fig. 34 (**A–C**) Endothelial cell analysis is a must before any contact lens fitting after keratoplasty. If the cell count is below 1000 per mm² [20] and polymegethism is detected, the risk of endothelial decompensation from contact lens fitting increases. (**D**) In this patient, a Rose K2 IC with a diameter of 10.4 mm provided good visual acuity with comfortable wear

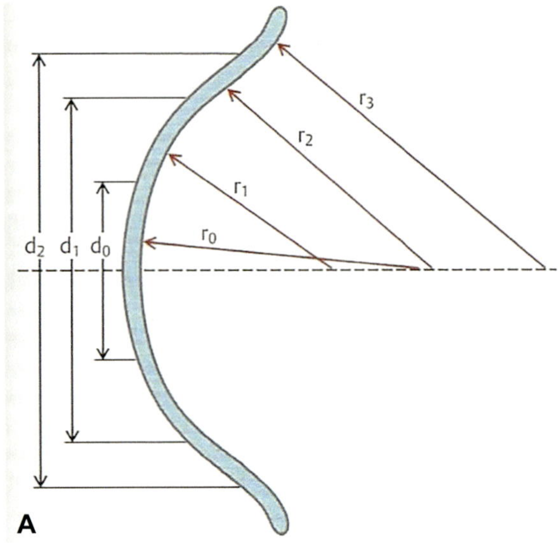

Fig. 35 (**A**) Contact lens back surface for reverse design: peripheral radius r1 is significantly steeper than r0 [6]

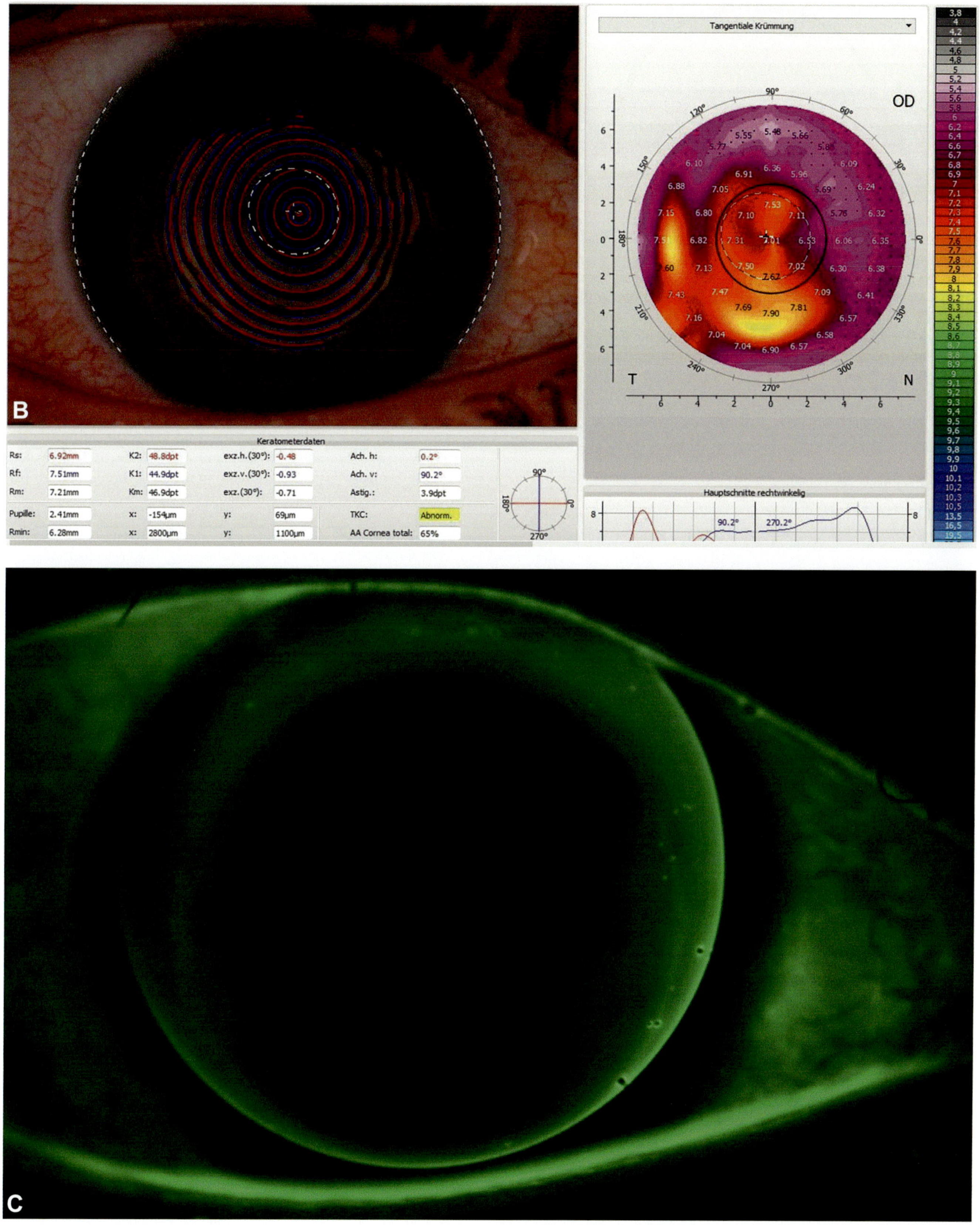

Fig. 35 (**B**) The topography of the right eye of a 41-year-old man who underwent penetrating keratoplasty for keratoconus in 2017 shows the aforementioned situation: the host cornea is steeper than that of the graft. (**C**) In this case, a lens with reverse geometry is a good choice. The fluorescein image shows a KA4 reverse from Hecht Contactlinsen, Freiburg, Germany. The lens moves well, the center is well irrigated with tear film and the slightly protruding edge is not disturbing. The patient achieved a visual acuity of 1.0

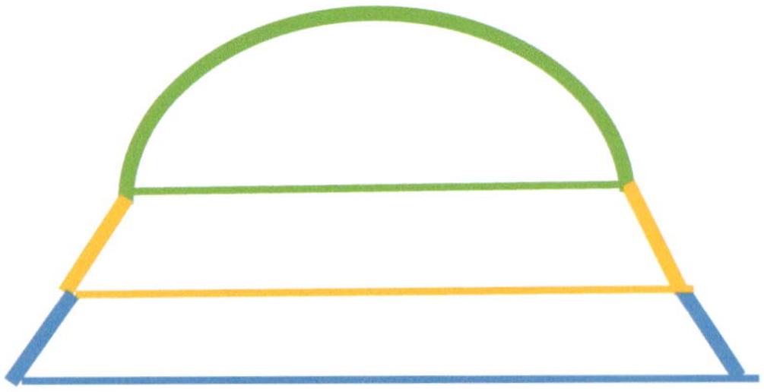

Fig. 36 Schematic of a scleral lens with its 3 zones: central posterior surface zone (green), followed by the limbal zone (yellow) and the scleral zone (blue). The central posterior surface zone is responsible for bridging the cornea, the limbal zone for relieving the peripheral cornea and for bridging the limbus. The scleral zone influences the peripheral support. The diameter depends on the iris diameter and can vary from 14 mm (mini-scleral lens) to 18–22 mm. Scleral lenses can be made toric or quadrant specific according to the amount of irregularity [25]

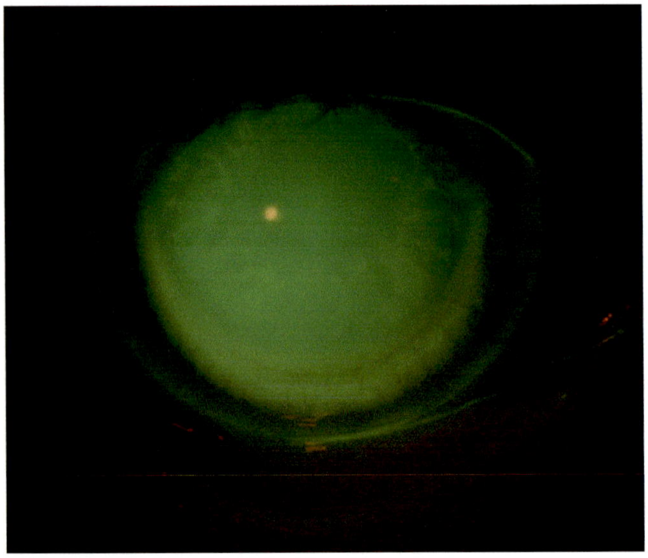

Fig. 37 Scleral lens. In this image, the fluid under the lens is stained with fluorescein. This allows assessment of whether the scleral lens sufficiently bridges the entire cornea (central, peripheral, and limbal) or whether an overlay is seen in certain areas [25]

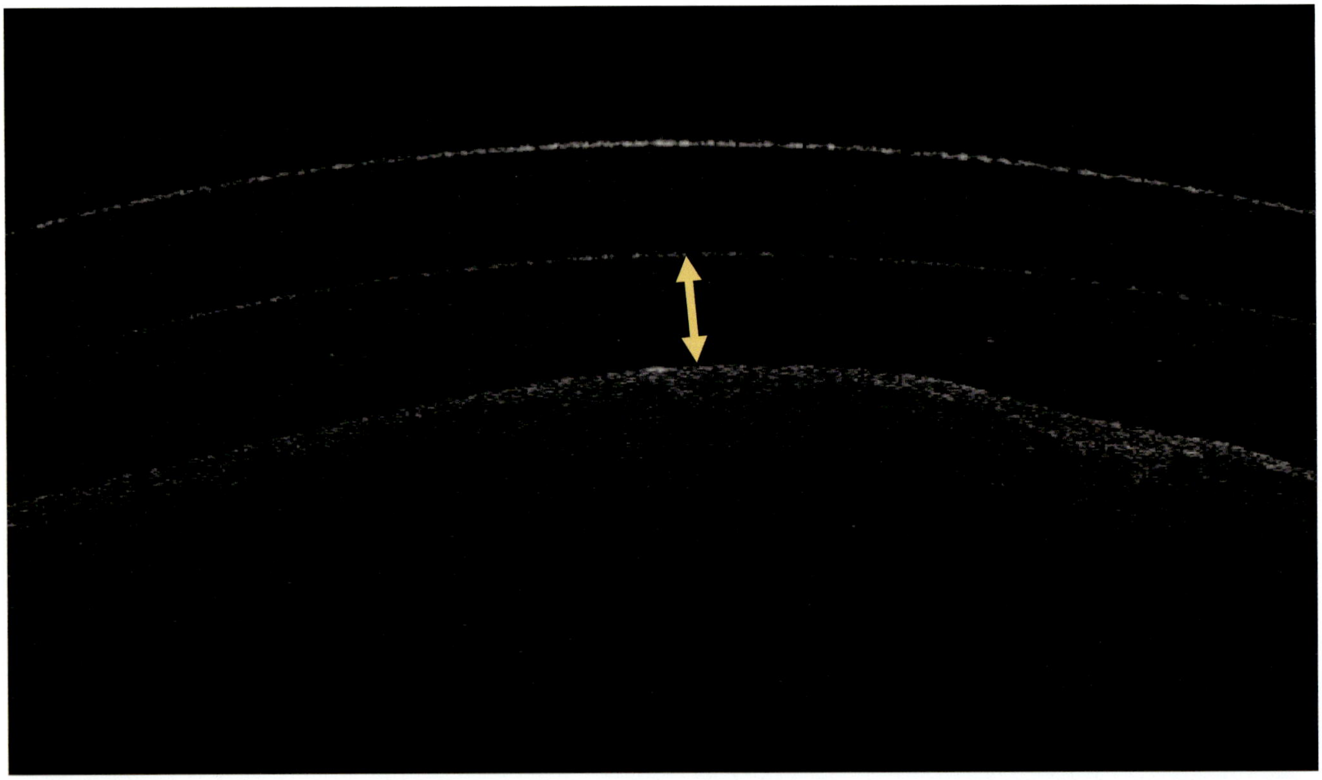

Fig. 38 Anterior segment OCT shows whether there is sufficient fluid (yellow arrow) between the scleral lens (upper two lines) and the cornea below in a pronounced keratoconus. The fluid space should be 350μm on average and is a measure of bridging. It is measured after lens fitting and after 2 h of wear [25]

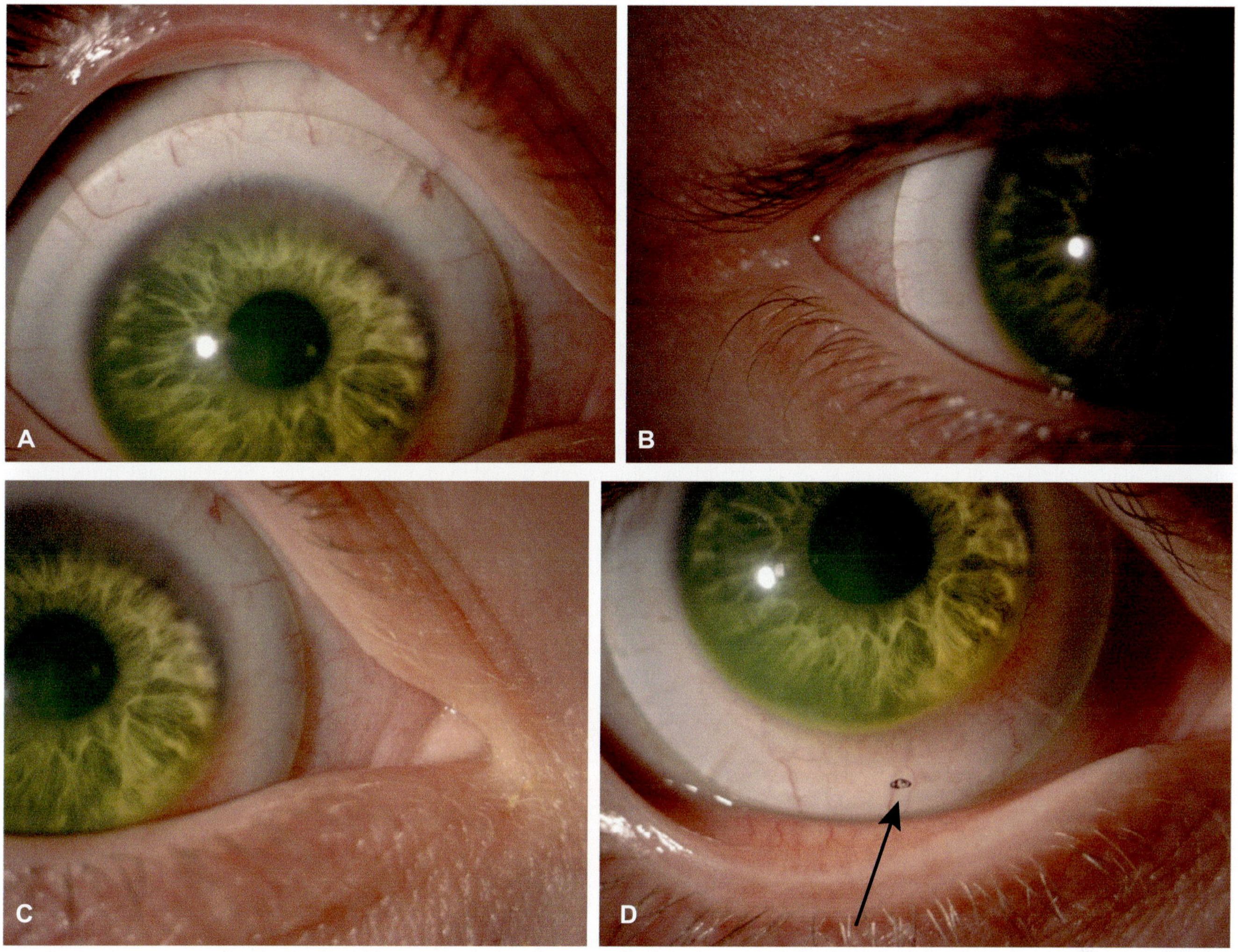

Fig. 39 (**A–C**) In addition to the OCT image, the assessment of the scleral lens fit with the peripheral support in all 4 quadrants is decisive for the quality of the fitting [25]. This is the right eye of a patient with advanced keratoconus, which could not cope with small RGP contact lenses because of the foreign body sensation. An I-Matrix scleral lens from the company Appenzeller Kontaktlinsen, Speicher, Switzerland, was fitted. Particular attention should be paid to the lens overlay and blanching of the scleral vessels. (**D**) The black dot at the lower edge (red arrow) serves as an insertion aid for the anterior prismatic toric I-Matrix lens

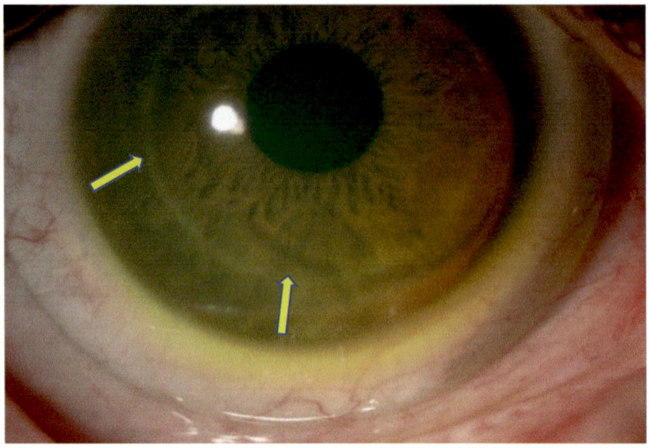

Fig. 40 This image shows a fitting after keratoplasty. Again, it is important to assess the marginal situation: the scleral lens should neither protrude nor lead to compression of the conjunctival vessels (blanching). Fluorescein-stained fluid suggests good bridging, especially in the inferior region. The graft margin is well visible under the lens (yellow arrows)

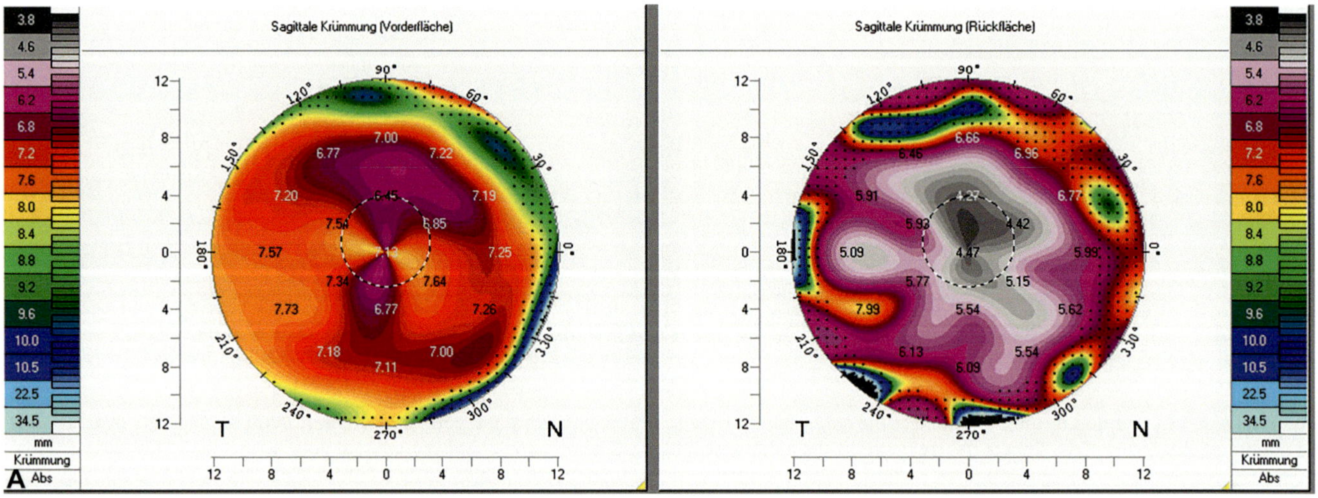

Fig. 41 (**A**) Front and back surface display of the cornea with the Pentacam

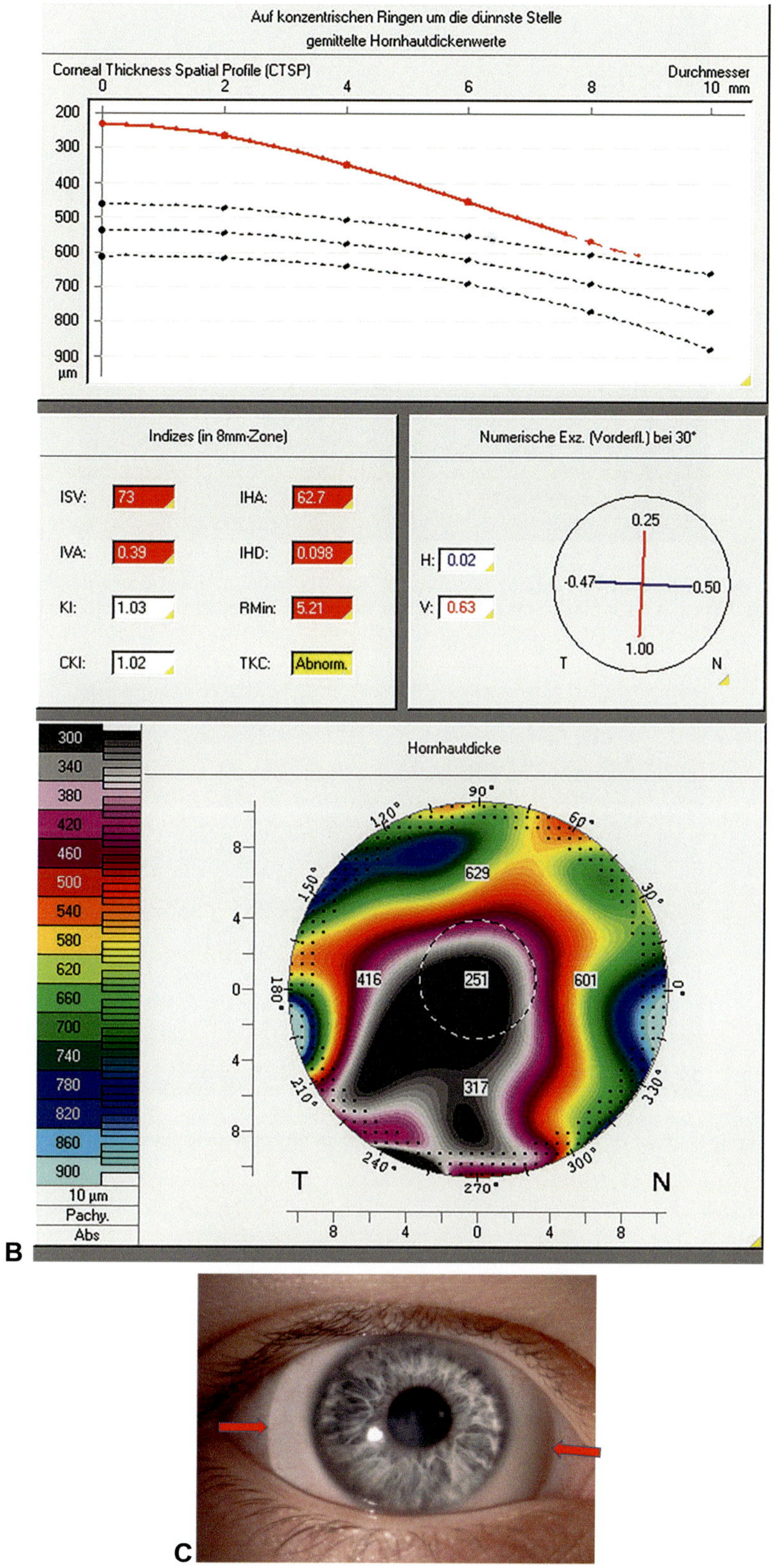

Fig. 41 (**B**) Pentacam Pachymetry. (**A**, **B**) This Pentacam tomography does not look like a typical keratoconus in view of the anterior surface. Only analysis of the posterior surface and pachymetry (Fig. 41B) helped to establish the diagnosis. Since the patient was totally opposed to keratoplasty, an attempt with scleral lenses was made. (**C**) Optimally fitted scleral lens I-Matrix from the company Appenzeller Kontaktlinsen, Speicher, Switzerland, in this patient. The scars are located at the thinnest part of the cornea

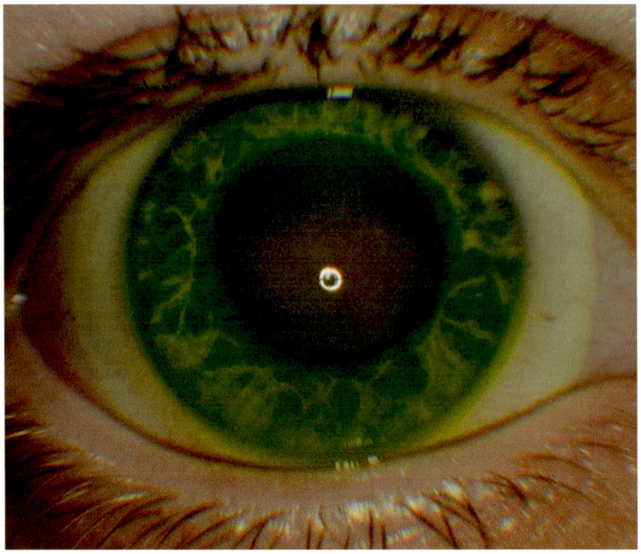

Fig. 42 The fluorescein image shows whether the bridging is sufficient and where the peripheral overlay begins. If the fluorescein overview shows a peripheral overlay on the cornea, it must first be checked whether the overall diameter was selected to match the diameter of the cornea

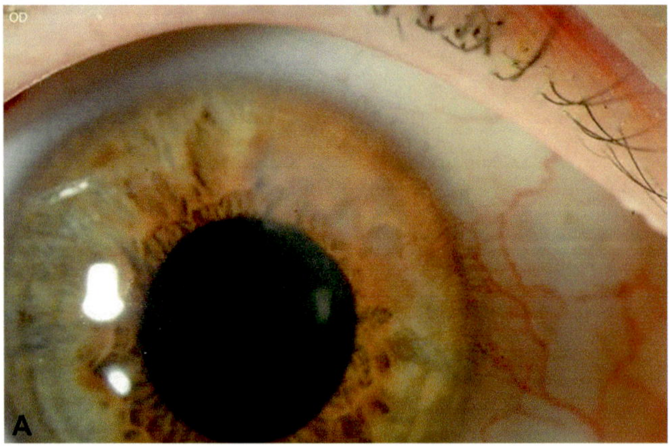

Fig. 43 (**A**) Damage due to wearing because of supposedly RGP contact lens in higher hyperopia without spectacle fitting

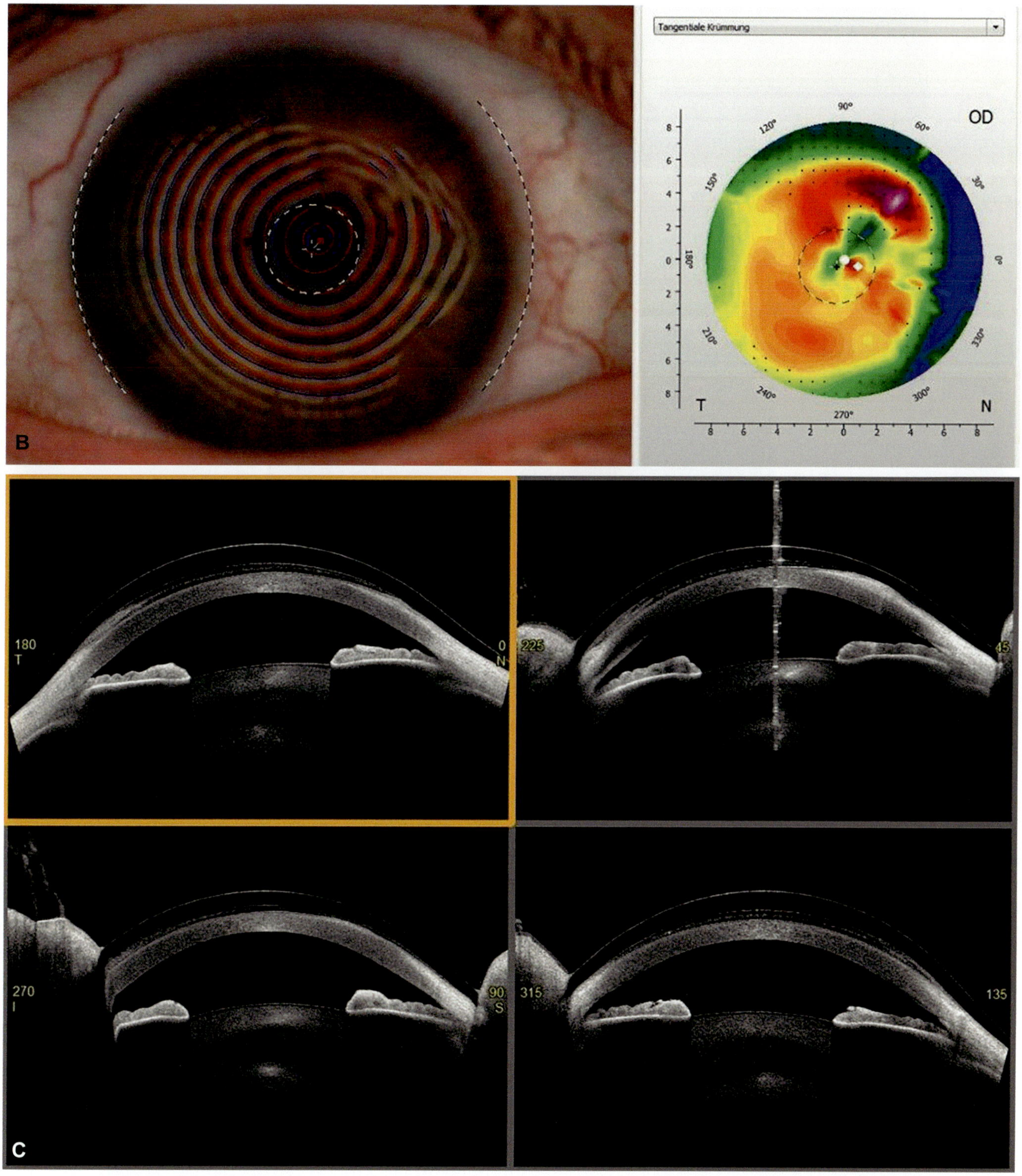

Fig. 43 (**B**) Due to the irregularities, no better visual acuity could be achieved with glasses. (**C**) During fitting small corneal lenses tended to decenter due to the irregularcorneal surface and causing corneal erosions. Subsequently mini-scleral shells (MSK KA4 reverse) from the company Hecht Contactlinsen,Freiburg, Germany, were fitted, which corrected better and were worn with a time limit

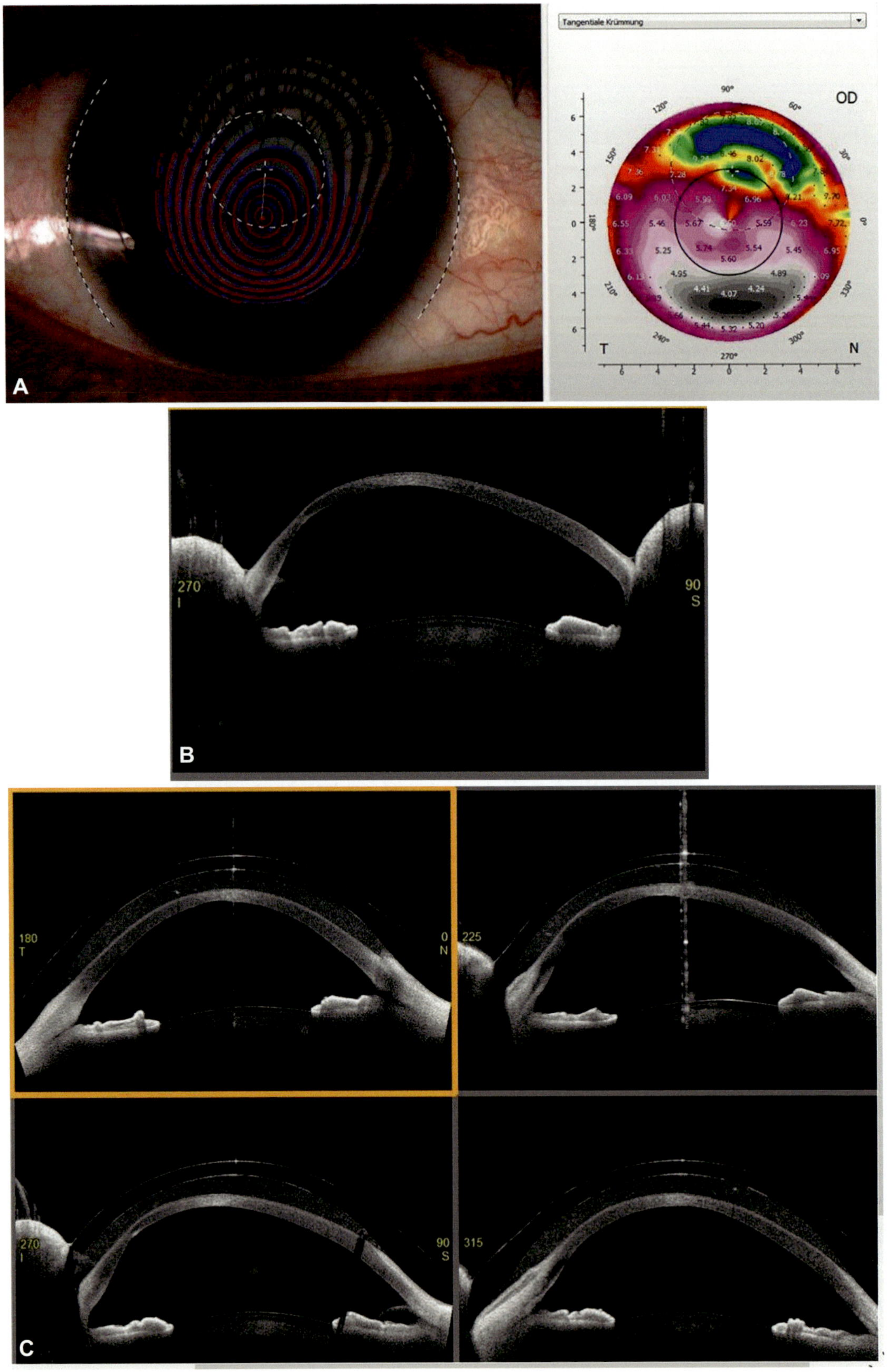

Fig. 44 (**A, B**) Oculus ultimus with severe pellucid marginal degeneration. Visual acuity without glasses was 0.05 difficult to read, there were no glasses available. During the fitting, the corneal lenses decentered too much, so the decision was made to fit scleral lenses. (**C**) In this image, a scleral lens "I-Matrix" from the company Appenzeller Kontaktlinsen was fitted. Anterior segment OCT showed good bridging

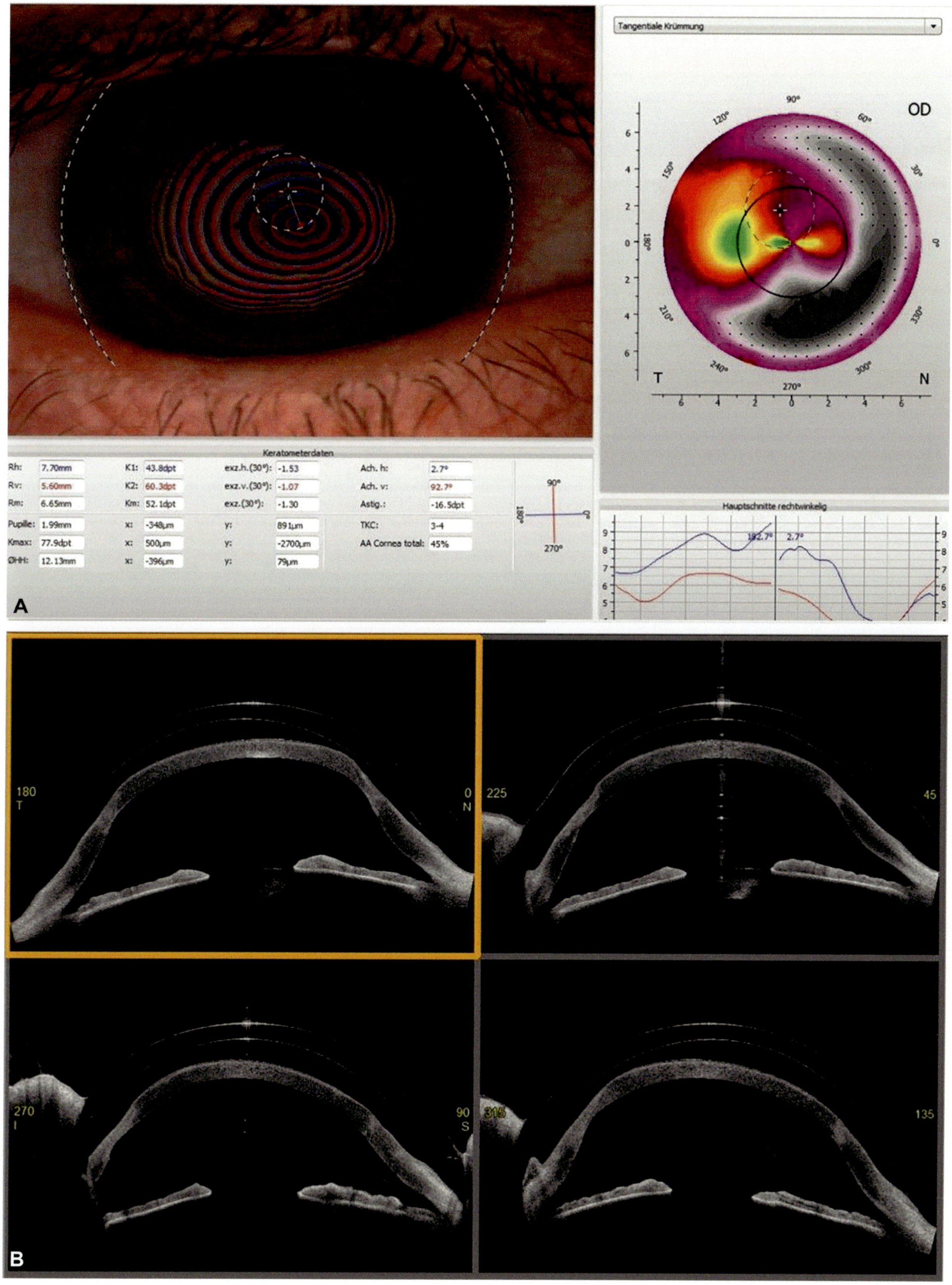

Fig. 45 (**A**) 58-year-old patient post-keratoplasty in 1991. External corneal lenses did not work, the patient refused repeated PKP. (**B**) An I-matrix scleral lens from the company Appenzeller Kontaktlinsen achieved a visual acuity of 0.8, with glasses only 0.4

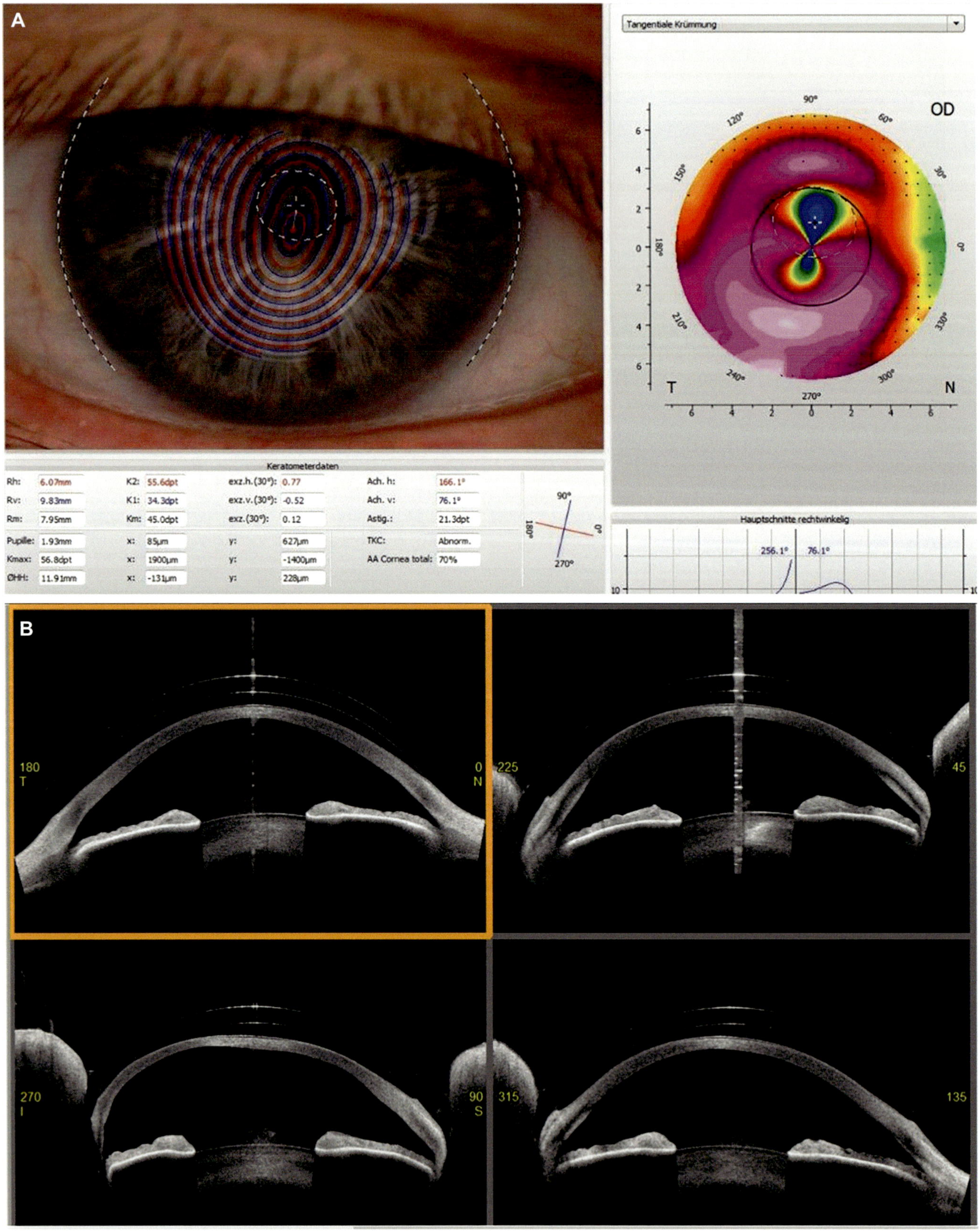

Fig. 46 (**A**) 75-year-old patient with severe pellucid degeneration. The patient presented with an outward-fitted and overaged corneal lens. (**B**) After a new fitting with an I-Matrix scleral lens from the company Appenzeller Kontaktlinsen, the anterior segment OCT showed good bridging

5 Conclusion

As the examples of contact lens fitting show, the rigid highly gas permeable contact lenses give nearly unlimited possibilities. The calculation based on topographic analysis was a decisive step in that direction, just as important as the modern manufacturing technique. Both lead to high individual custom-made contact lenses, almost like an imprint of the cornea, with high wearing comfort and high visual acuity. These are the objectives of lens fitting: best visual acuity and tolerance, together with the best and healthiest care for the cornea. Contact lenses should be used to improve the quality of life for our patients.

Funding The authors assure that the work was created without any financial support or interests and only reflects their own experiences.

References

1. Rashad R, Weed MC, Quinn N, Chen VM. Extended wear bandage contact lenses decrease pain and preserve vision in patients with epidermolysis bullosa: case series and review of literature. Ocul Immunol Inflamm. 2020;28:379–83.
2. Santodomingo-Rubido J, Carracedo G, Suzaki A, Villa-Collar C, Vincent SJ, Wolffsohn JS. Keratoconus: an updated review. Cont Lens Anterior Eye. 2022;45:101559.
3. Seitz B, Daas L, Hamon L, Xanthopoulou K, Goebels S, Spira-Eppig C, Razafimino S, Szentmáry N, Langenbucher A, Flockerzi E. [Stage-appropriate treatment of keratoconus]. Ophthalmologe. 2021; 118:1069–88.
4. Kuhn D. Contact lenses for keratoconus and keratoplasty. Ophthalm. Nachrichten. 2010;6.
5. Klühspies U, Grunder A, Goebels S, Schirra F, Seitz B. Keratoconus lenses: the small correction miracle. Ophthalmologe. 2013;110(830–836):838.
6. Grünauer-Kloevekorn C, Kloevekorn-Fischer U, Kloevekorn-Norgall K, Duncker G. Contact lens fitting: in complicated corneal situations. Stuttgart: Georg Thieme Verlag; 2007. https://doi.org/10.1055/b-002-29642.
7. Ozkurt YB, Sengor T, Kurna S, Evciman T, Acikgoz S, Haboğlu M, Aki S. Rose K contact lens fitting for keratoconus. Int Ophthalmol. 2008;28:395–8.
8. Hoppe O, Kuhn D, Schwarz S. Galifa handbook of contact lens fitting. Köln: Biermann Medizin; 2010.
9. Lim L, Lim EWL. Current perspectives in the management of keratoconus with contact lenses. Eye. 2020;34:2175–96.
10. Downie LE, Lindsay RG. Contact lens management of keratoconus. Clin Exp Optom. 2015;98:299–311.
11. Garcia-Lledo M, Feinbaum C, Alio JL. Contact lens fitting in keratoconus. Compr Ophthalmol Update. 2006;72:47–52.
12. Şengör T, Aydın KS. Update on contact lens treatment of keratoconus. Turk J Ophthalmol. 2020;50:234–44.
13. Zadnik K, Barr JT, Steger-May K, Edrington TB, McMahon TT, Gordon MO. Comparison of flat and steep rigid contact lens fitting methods in keratoconus. Optom Vis Sci. 2005;82:1014–21.
14. McMonnies CW. The biomechanics of keratoconus and rigid contact lenses. Eye Contact Lens. 2005;31:80–92.
15. Moreira LB, Bardal RA, Crisigiovanni LR. Contact lenses fitting after intracorneal ring segments implantation in keratoconus. Arq Bras Oftalmol. 2013;76:215–7.
16. Sengor T, Kurna SA, Aki S, Ozkurt Y. High Dk piggyback contact lens system for contact lens-intolerant keratoconus patients. Clin Ophthalmol. 2011;5:331–5.
17. Isik P, Harbiyeli II, Erdem E, Yagmur M. Improved contact lens fitting after corneal cross-linking in eyes with progressive keratoconus. Cont Lens Anterior Eye. 2022;45:101488.
18. Ozarslan Ozcan D, Ozcan SC. Efficacy of two silicone-hydrogel bandage contact lenses after corneal crosslinking. Clin Exp Optom. 2021;104:505–9.
19. Prazeres S, Malet F, Colin J. Contact lens fitting after keratoplasty for keratoconus. J Fr Ophtalmol. 2008; 31: 849–854.
20. Salmon JF. Kanskis Clinical Ophthalmology:A Systematic Approach. 10th Ed. Urban&Fischer: Elsevier; 2024.
21. Akkaya Turhan S, Özarslan Özcan D, Toker E. Use of a mini-scleral lens in patients with keratoconus. Turk J Ophthalmol. 2020;50:339–42.
22. Baudin F, Chemaly A, Arnould L, Barrénéchea E, Lestable L, Bron AM, Creuzot-Garcher C. Quality-of-life improvement after scleral lens fitting in patients with keratoconus. Eye Contact Lens. 2021;47:520–5.
23. Nguyen MTB, Thakrar V, Chan CC. EyePrintPRO therapeutic scleral contact lens: indications and outcomes. Can J Ophthalmol. 2018;53:66–70.
24. Schornack MM, Patel SV. Scleral lenses in the management of keratoconus. Eye Contact Lens. 2010;36:39–44.
25. Brückner B. Structure and fitting of the i-matrix scleral lens. Contact lenses from Appenzeller Contact lenses. https://www.optikum.at/i-matrix-sklerallinse/. Accessed 3 Sept 2022.

PhotoDynamic Therapy PDT for Keratoconus (CXL) Versus Infectious Keratitis (PACK-CXL)

Kassandra Xanthopoulou, Nóra Szentmáry, Elias Flockerzi, Loay Daas, Tanja Stachon, and Berthold Seitz

Abstract

This chapter presents corneal crosslinking (CXL) and its main features. CXL is based on the principles of photodynamic therapy (PDT) and includes epithelial debridement, the use of a sensibilisator, riboflavin, followed by application of ultraviolet A light (UVA). The induction of formation of cross-links between the collagen fibers of the corneal stroma increases the corneal stiffening and provides corneal stability, thus consisting CXL a basic treatment modality for corneal ectasias. The antimicrobial and cytotoxic properties of riboflavin and UVA have led to the emerging use of CXL in the treatment of further corneal pathologies such as infections, corneal ulcerations and melting. Further investigation in the field of PDT and CXL could show interesting future results in the treatment of infectious keratitis.

1 Introduction: Photodynamic Therapy and Corneal Crosslinking

For the last 20 years, photodynamic therapy (PDT) has been an applied treatment method in different medical disciplines. During PDT, a photosensitizing agent is excited through light of appropriate wavelength leading, either to conversion of the photosensitizer (PS) from its base state (PS^0) to its triplet excited state (^3PS), forming hydrogen peroxide and superoxide radicals, or, to conversion of the oxygen molecule ($^3O_2$) to singlet oxygen ($^1O_2$), which belongs to the reactive oxygen species (ROS) and possesses high biochemical activity. Changing intracellular ROS levels lead to the loss of cell homeostasis, which is followed by a cascade of biological events, impairing cell viability (eucaryotic cells, microorganisms), inducing necrosis or apoptosis of the cells. Thereafter, the amount of ROS is rapidly reduced [1].

Corneal crosslinking (CXL) uses riboflavin (vitamin B2) as photosensitizer, followed by application of ultraviolet A (UVA) light (370 ± 5 nm) irradiation, to induce the formation of cross-links between stromal collagen fibers aiming to increase corneal stiffness [2, 3]. The molecular process includes oxidative pathways and enzymatic glycosylation. The oxidative pathways consist of a type I (non-oxygen mediated oxidative process), resulting from the conversion of a singlet riboflavin molecule into a triplet state after absorving UVA light, and of a type 2 (oxygen mediated) oxidative reaction, including reactive oxygen species, generated through UVA light, which promote the formation of intra- and intermolecular covalent bonds to convert collagen monomers into cross-linked polymers [2, 4].

With increasing resistance of bacteria or fungi against antimicrobial agents it is important to find alternative treatment options in infectious keratitis, such as PDT or Photodynamic Inactivation (PDI) as a potential treatment option.

2 Riboflavin-UVA-CXL in Ectatic Corneal Diseases

CXL was first introduced in 1998 by Spoerl et al. [3] and aims to treat corneal ectasia, thus postponing/preventing the need for (penetrating) keratoplasty. The first treatment of a patient was reported by Wollensak et al. in 2003 [5]. During CXL, corneal epithelium is first removed at the central 7–9 mm zone (epithelium-off, "Epi-off" procedure),

K. Xanthopoulou (✉) · E. Flockerzi · L. Daas · B. Seitz
Ophthalmology Department, Saarland University Medical Center, UKS, Homburg, Saar, Germany
e-mail: kassixanthop@gmail.com

N. Szentmáry · T. Stachon
Dr. Rolf M. Schwiete Center for Limbal Stem Cell and Congenital Aniridia Research Saarland University, Homburg, Saar, Germany
e-mail: nora.szentmary@uks.eu

B. Seitz et al. (eds.), *Atlas on Cornea*, https://doi.org/10.1007/978-3-031-65422-0_43

which is followed by instillation of photosensitizing riboflavin drops for 30 min, then, by irradiation with ultraviolet A light (UVA) of 370 nm wavelength at an irradiance of 3 mW/cm^2 for 30 minutes (min), with a total energy (fluence) of 5.4 J/cm^2. During UVA irradiation, riboflavin instillation continues in 2–5 min intervals [5, 6] (Fig. 1). At the end of the procedure a bandage contact lens is placed upon the cornea and patients will be advised to use antibiotic eye drops 5 times per day as well as lubricants until epithelialization is completed. This is followed by removal of the bandage contact lens and application of tapered topical steroids, with continuation of the lubricants [6]. This protocol was introduced as the standard or ***Dresden protocol*** and until today remains the gold standard CXL method for treating progressive keratoconus, pellucid marginal degeneration and postoperative iatrogenic corneal ectasia [5].

The photoactivated riboflavin causes a stiffening effect on the corneal stroma, increases the corneal resistance to enzymatic degradation and prevents the progression of corneal melting [7, 8]. Based on the Bunsen–Roscoe law of reciprocity, the total energy applied can be maintained by changing the irradiance and the irradiation time, providing shorter protocols in order to reduce patient discomfort, and are known as ***accelerated CXL protocols (ACXL)*** [9] However, exceeding 45 mW/cm^2 irradiance showed no effectiveness in terms of corneal stiffening [10]. The 9 mW/cm^2 irradiance and 10 min protocol is the most comparable with the standard protocol [11, 12] and can provide tomographic stabilization for more than 2 years postoperatively [13, 14].

At the postoperative examination after CXL procedure the demarcation line (Fig. 2) in the posterior part of the corneal stroma is observed and represents the limit between the cross-linked and the non-cross-linked stroma. It can be detected biomicroscopically at the slit-lamp, as well as using anterior segment optical coherence tomography (AS-OCT), as early as 2 weeks after CXL application [15]. By means of in vivo confocal microscopy, a transition area of an edematous zone with low cell density to a deeper zone with less edema and more keratocytes was shown at an approximate depth of 320 μm [16]. The demarcation line ensures that the corneal endothelium remains protected. Its depth within the corneal stroma depends on the concentration of riboflavin and the intensity of UVA light [15, 17]. It remains controversial whether the depth of the demarcation line is analogous to the effectivity of the CXL procedure [18, 19].

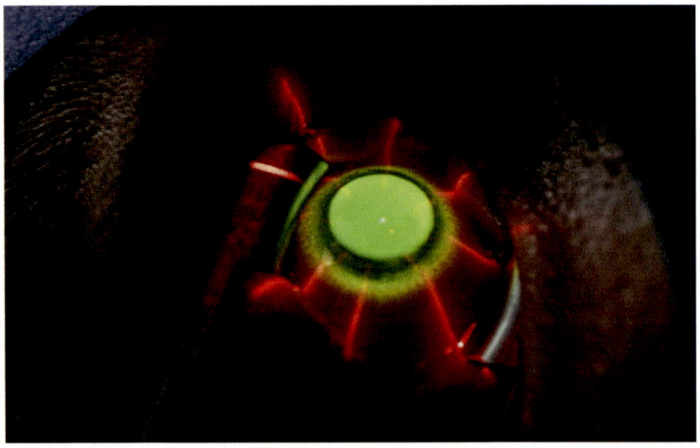

Fig. 1 Crosslinking (CXL) treatment using riboflavin and ultraviolet A (UVA) light in a patient with keratoconus (Image from the Department of Ophthalmology of Saarland University). In this case, an accelerated CXL protocol (10 min, 9 mW/cm^2) was performed

Another interesting feature, observed within the first 6 weeks postoperatively is a "pseudoprogression", which consists of an increase of the tomographic values (anterior keratometry, maximal keratometry), combined with a decrease of the thinnest and apex corneal pachymetry and a deterioration of the visual aquity [13, 14]. This phenomenon is related to the short-term changes of the corneal epithelium, stromal edema and keratocyte apoptosis after CXL and is, though, not representative of the stabilizing long-term effect of the procedure [13, 14, 20].

Concerning the safety of CXL, there is a threshold of 0.35 mW/cm^2 irradiance for endothelial cell damage due to the free radicals [17]. At a corneal thickness of 400 μm, the irradiance level of the endothelium is about 0.18 mW/cm^2 [17]. Therefore, a minimum corneal thickness of 400 μm is recommended in order to avoid damage to the corneal endothelium and further damage of deeper structures such as the lens and retina [21].

In cases of thinner corneas and in order to assure the safety of the procedure and reduce the patient's discomfort and risk of complications, several variants of CXL have been introduced [9]:

- Contact lens-assisted CXL procedure [22], with, however, existence of a barrier to oxygen diffusion into the cornea which might lead to reduced induction of cross-links [23].
- Hypoosmolar riboflavin solution, which results in corneal swelling, thus increasing the corneal thickness and protecting against potential endothelial damage [24].
- "Epithelium-on" ("Epi-on") protocols maintain an intact corneal epithelium to preserve the corneal thickness and protect the endothelium, though with reduced efficacy, compared to Epi-off procedures [25] due to reduced penetration of riboflavin into the cornea.
- Topical chemical enhancers such as tetracain, benzalkonium chloride, ethylenediaminetetraacetic acid and trometanol increase the permeability of tight intraepithelial junctions and promote the penetration of riboflavin through the corneal epithelium [9, 26].
- Iontophoresis CXL induces an electric field to increase diffusion of the negatively charged riboflavin through

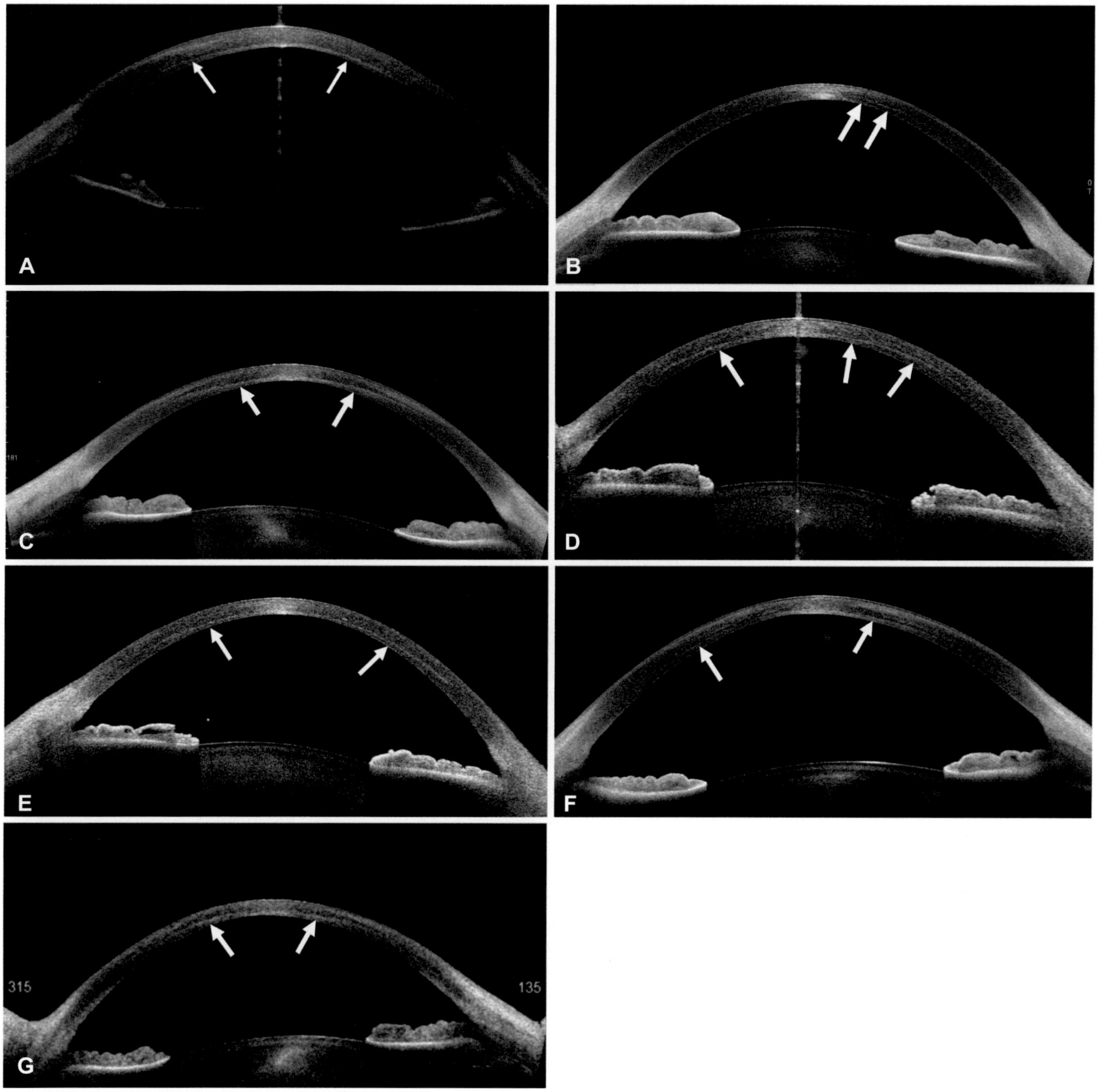

Fig. 2 Demarcation lines (arrows) documented 6 weeks after accelerated corneal crosslinking (10 min, 9 mW/cm^2), with anterior segment optical coherence tomography in cases of progressive keratoconus (Images from the Department of Ophthalmology of Saarland University)

the corneal epithelium into the corneal strom, leads, however, to less reduction of corneal curvature compared to eyes treated with standard CXL [27].

- The "Sub400" CXL protocol presented by Hafezi et al. for thinner corneas (least corneal thickness referred: 214 μm), suggests an adjustment of the UVA light application time and irradiance [28].
- The "M nomogram" introduced by Mazzotta et al. as an adjustment of the UVA power, always maintaining the fluence of 5.4 J/cm^2, with respect to the corneal thickness, after matching the simulated CXL-depth mathematical models with in vivo confocal microscopy and corneal optical coherence tomography [29].

A method of potentially improving the efficacy of CXL, combined with accelerated protocols is the application of pulsed UVA light, thus allowing increased re-diffusion of oxygen between the UVA light pauses, leading to comparable efficacy results and deeper demarcation lines compared to continuous CXL protocols [30, 31]. Furthermore, the use of higher fluence in a shorter time compared to the standard CXL protocol has been proposed in order to achieve a deeper demarcation line [32, 33].

Additionally, several surgical combinations have been presented to achieve better visual outcomes after CXL. The ***Athens protocol*** includes the topographically-guided transepithelial photorefractive keratectomy followed by CXL [34], whereas the ***Cretan protocol*** includes the combination of transepithelial phototherapeutic keratectomy with CXL [35]. The ***enhanced Athens protocol*** proposes a topography-guided transepithelial photorefractive keratectomy with customized CXL to improve the refractive results of the ectatic cornea, with less stromal tissue removal [36]. These methods are questionable.

Nevertheless, CXL also has side effects. It showed a cytotoxic effect on keratocytes from 0.5 mW/cm^2 power density which will be reached at 300 µm corneal depth through illumination with 3 mW/cm^2 [37]. The loss of keratocytes and the myofibroblastic activation in the corneal stroma after CXL may lead to corneal scarring, with a reported incidence of 2.9% [38]. A rate of persisting haze formation of 9% at 1 year follow-up after CXL for keratoconus and a higher haze development rate in eyes with thinner corneas and steeper apex keratometry have been observed [39]. In some cases, it may be permanent [39]. The haze formation can also be attributed to stromal swelling pressure changes, proteoglycan–collagen interactions and glycosaminoglycan hydration [40].

Corneal infections can occur after CXL as a result of corneal debridement and use of bandage contact lenses. Several pathogens have been identified, including Gram-negative organisms (Escherichia coli, Pseudomonas aeruginosa), Gram-positive organisms (Staphylococcus aureus, Streptococcus species), or fungi [9], whereas acanthamoeba keratitis after eye washing under tap water was also observed [40]. Reactivation of herpetic keratitis and newly developed herpes keratitis following CXL have also been reported, thus setting the history of herpes keratitis as a contraindication for CXL [41, 42]. Sterile keratitis [38], epithelial healing problems [9], peripheral corneal ulceration [43] and corneal melting [44] have also been reported.

3 Riboflavin-UVA-CXL in Infectious Keratitis and for Corneal Ulcers

CXL also has further promising applications in other corneal pathologies such as bullous keratopathy [45], corneal ulceration as well as melting (Fig. 3) and infectious keratitis [46–48].

In 1965, the first report that riboflavin could inactivate the ribonucleic acids containing tobacco mosaic virus after exposure to visible or UV light has been published [49]. In 2000, riboflavin has been used to inactivate pathogens

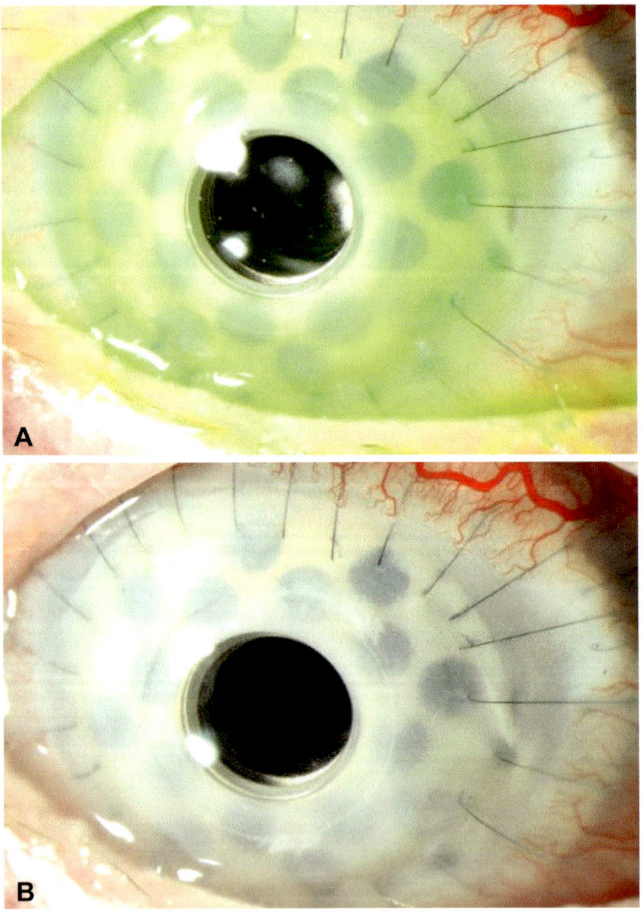

Fig. 3 Persistent extensive corneal erosion and corneal melting of the graft after Boston keratoprothesis implantation following severe Fuchs Stevens Johnson syndrom (due to acetylsalicylic acid use) in a 30-year-old patient (**A**). PACK-CXL (30 min, 3 mW/cm^2) stopped corneal melting and the anterior segment was stable after 3 days ((**B**), images from the Department of Ophthalmology of Saarland University)

in plasma, platelet and red cell products by oxidation, thus causing lesions to chromosomal strands [50] and the successful use of CXL in corneal ulcers of unknown etiology has been first reported [48]. In 2009 CXL has been verified as a potential treatment option for bacterial keratitis [51]. Keratitis caused by Escherichia coli, Pseudomonas aeruginosa, Staphylococcus aureus, Staphylococcus epidermidis, Mikrococcus, Corynebacteria, Propionibacteria or atypical Mycobacteria could be stopped or stabilized by performing CXL [52–54]. In addition, it has been described that corneal infiltates could also be cured using CXL, without the application of topical antibiotics [53, 55].

The use of CXL for treating infectious keratitis was given the term ***photoactivated chromophore for infectious keratitis (PACK-CXL)*** in 2013 [56].

PACK-CXL acts as an inflammatory and antimicrobial agent, causing damage to the DNA/RNA of pathogens, increasing tissue resistance to enzymatic degradation and enhancing the ocular penetration of antifungals [57, 58]. Further mechanisms of CXL treatment for therapy of corneal ulcers include:

- Increase of stromal tensile strength and rigidity of corneal collagen;
- Induction of wound healing by promotion of apoptosis, followed by repopulation;
- Restoration of the normal corneal architecture;
- Reduction susceptibility of the tissue to the pathogen;
- Reformation of the corneal epithelial surface due to the contribution of riboflavin in the development and maintenance of the surface structures of the epithelial cells;
- Chemical alteration of functional groups of nucleic acids in the bacteria, making replication impossible;
- Reduction of the inflammatory reaction as well as of the nociceptive response of corneal nerves that decrease pain [59, 60].

According to several reports, the best visual outcomes were obtained in a case of Moraxella keratitis and Staphylococcus aureus, whereas the worst occured in eyes infected with fungus and especially Mycobacterium, which required corneal transplantation. A faster epithelialization of corneal ulceration was observed in infections with Gram-positive bacteria, followed by Gram-negative bacteria, fungi and acanthamoeba. Corneal melting could be similarly effectively treated: in Gram-negative bacteria, followed by Gram-positive bacteria, acanthamoeba and fungi [59]. It has been described that CXL could not shorten the healing time in cases of infectious keratitis with corneal melting including Staphylococcus and Aspergillus as pathogens among others, could, though, prevent corneal perforation [56].

Additionally, the smaller ulcer size was associated with higher success rates after PACK-CXL in case of bacterial and fungal keratitis, but not in case of acanthamoeba [41]. Treatment of herpes keratitis led to tectonic keratoplasty after corneal melting, thus excluding PACK-CXL as treatment option in viral keratitis [41, 42]. Acanthamoeba keratitis was reported to be efficiently treated with combined PACK-CXL and drug therapy, compared to successful treatment with drug therapy only [41, 61]. However, the treatment of acanthamoeba keratitis still remains a challenge (Figs. 4 and 5).

PACK-CXL can be efficiently used as a standalone procedure in the treatment of superficial keratitis but also as adjuvant therapy in non-resolving cases and can relieve the patients' pain already from the first postoperative day on [62]. A very important exclusion criteria of PACK-CXL is the depth of infiltration, as a depth >250 μm increases the risk of corneal edema due to endothelial damage, thus setting the CXL treatment effectiveness lower, the deeper the infiltration is [59, 63].

Accelerated PACK-CXL (9 mW/cm^2, 10 min) was successfully used in the treatment of infectious keratitis [64], though, caution is advised for shorter treatment protocols given the importance of oxygen levels during the procedure for its efficacy [10].

In case of fungal keratitis, the results remain controversial. PACK-CXL is proposed to be an effective adjuvant therapy combined with antifungal drugs [42, 65]. However, the Cross-Linking-Assisted Infection Reduction (CLAIR) clinical trial showed no additional effect to applied drug therapy in terms of infiltrate or scar size, epithelialization rates or adverse events. The efficacy of different PACK-CXL protocols with 5.4 J/cm^2 fluence was positively discussed as a primary or adjuvant therapy for superficial corneal infections, because approximately half of the energy applied was absorbed in the first 100 μm of the riboflavin-soaked cornea [66]. However, a higher fluence was proposed in cases of fungal keratitis, because of the lack of corneal transparency and involvement of the deeper corneal stroma [66], as well as in case of bacterial keratitis, to increase efficacy [67].

4 Other Photoactivators for PDT

- ***Rose bengal***

An interesting aspect in the treatment of fungal keratitis was the in vitro superiority of rose bengal PDT therapy compared to CXL for the inhibition of fungal isolate growth as well as the in vivo adjuvant application of two sessions PDT with rose bengal in cases of patients with severe

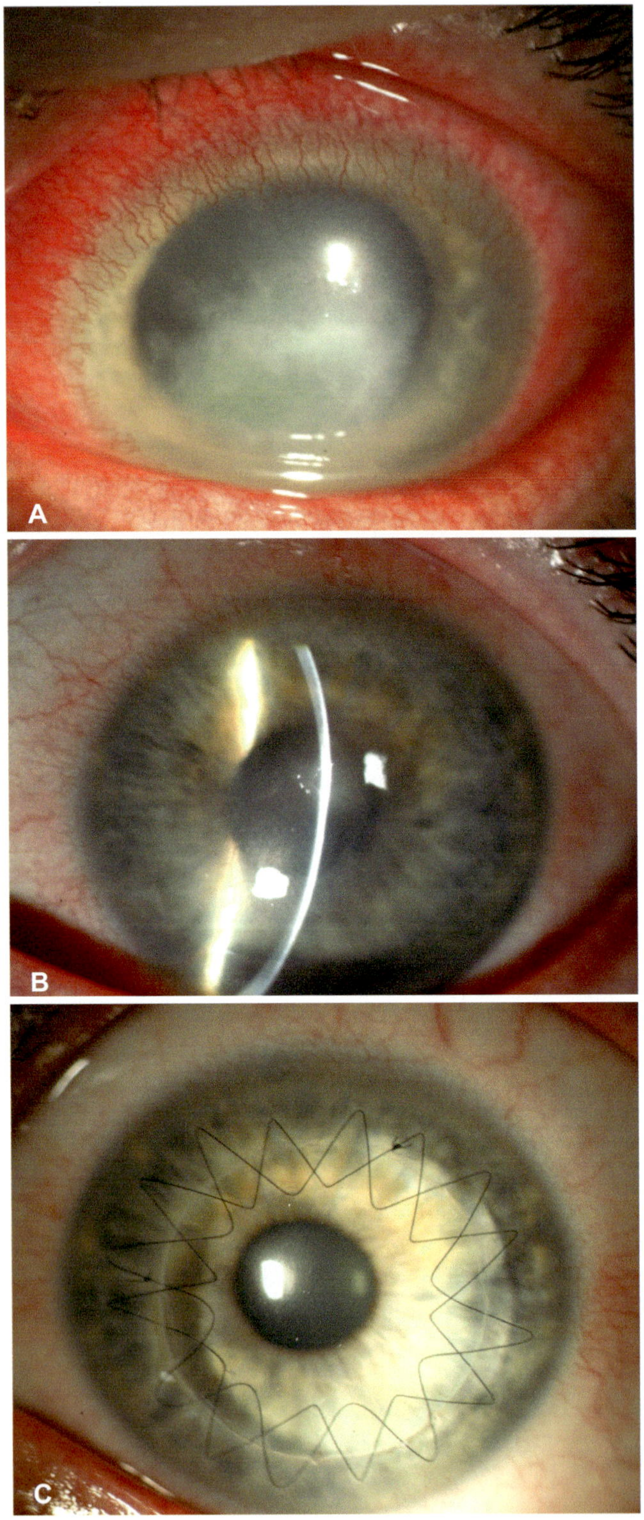

Fig. 4 Acanthamoeba keratitis in a contact lens wearing patient with corneal erosion, ring infiltrate and multifocal stromal infiltrates (**A**). Following 6 months triple-topical therapy, the same eye underwent crosslinking (postoperative image, (**B**)) and 6 months later an optical penetrating excimer laser-assisted keratoplasty was performed with double-running sutures (**C**) (Images from the Department of Ophthalmology of Saarland University)

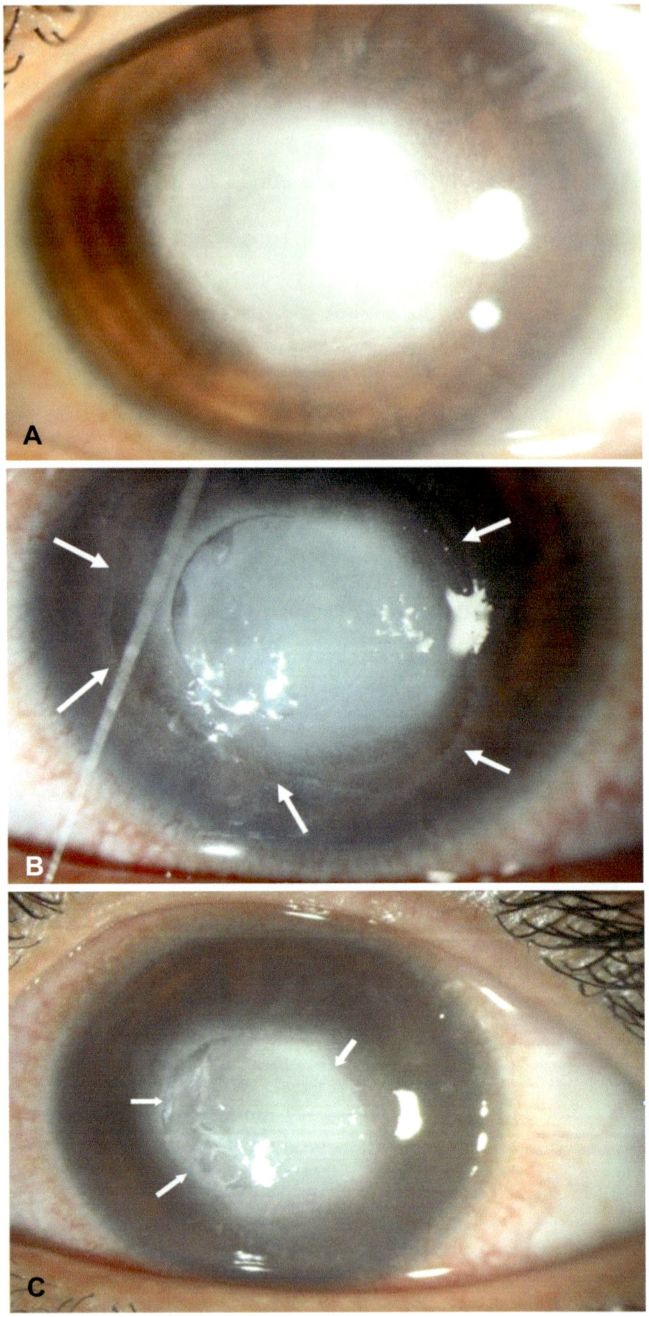

Fig. 5 Acanthamoeba keratitis with corneal ulcer and deep stromal infiltrate 2 days (**A**) before photoactivated chromophore crosslinking for infectious keratitis (PACK-CXL, 30 min, 3 mW/cm^2) and 1 day (**B**) and 7 days (**C**) after PACK-CXL (pre- and postoperatively triple-topical therapy was continued), with signs of infiltrate demarcation and partial epithelialization (arrows, images from Department of Ophthalmology of Saarland University)

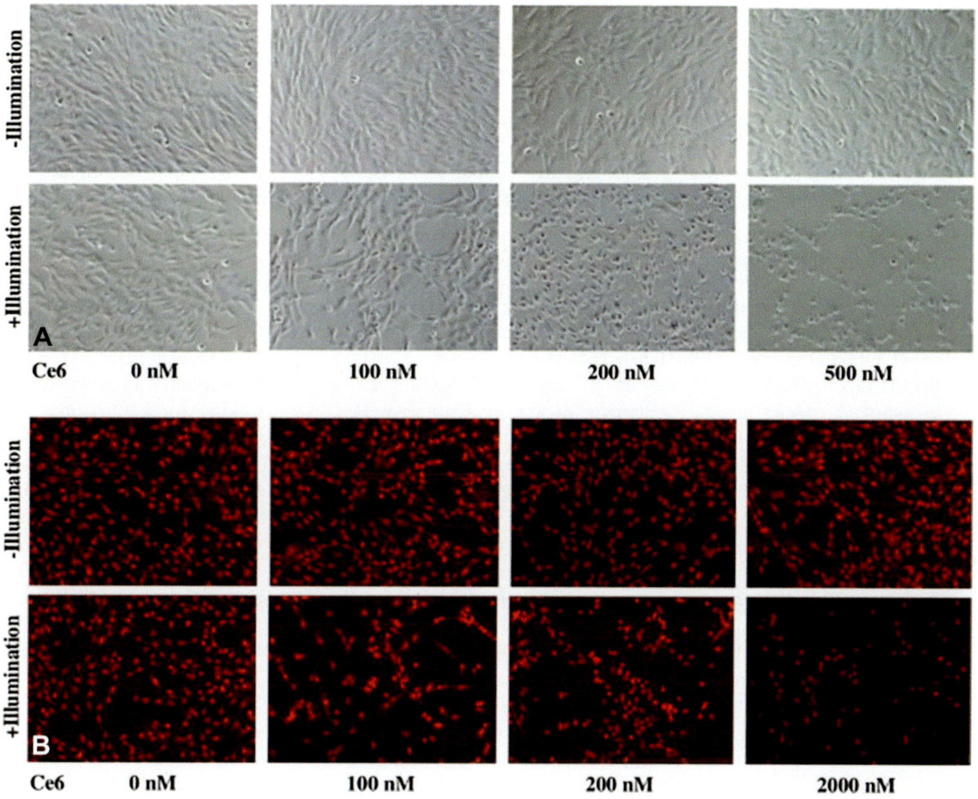

Fig. 6 Inverted phase—contrast photomicrographs and propidum iodide (PI) staining of human keratocytes twenty-four hours after PDI (original magnification 100x). (**A**) Without illumination, the cell morphology remained unchanged with different concentrations of Ce6, while with illumination, cell shrinkage occured, and keratocytes became detached with increasing concentrations of Ce6. (**B**) Twenty four hours after PDI, without illumination, the PI uptake of keratocytes remained unchanged with different concentrations of Ce6, while with illumination, the PI uptake of keratocytes was decreased with increasing concentrations of Ce6 to here. Published data with license from [71]

resistant fusarium keratitis (0.1% rose bengal solution, 30 min, followed by green light radiation, 15 min) [68].

– ***Porphyrin (Chlorin e6)-red light-PDI***

In previous experimental studies we described the effect of the PS Chlorine e6 (Ce6) on human keratocytes and endothelial cells in cell culture, following 13-min 670 nm wavelength illumination. The percentage of apoptotic keratocytes and endothelial cells increased from 250 nM Ce6 concentration and cell viability decreased from 100 nM Ce6 concentration for keratocytes and from 150 nM concentration for endothelial cells [69, 70].

Using 32 μM photosensitizer concentration, 99.99% of *Candida albicans* isolates could be killed, by using >64 μM concentration 99.99% of *Staphylococcus aureus* isolates and with >128 μM concentration 99.99% of *Pseudomonas aeruginosa* isolates could be killed (Fig. 6) [69].

In order to decrease the damage of human cells and to increase the cytotoxicity on microorganisms during PDT, a specific antibody could be used, which binds the PS itself specifically to the microorganisms. This modified PS could damage the microorganisms more effectively and would have a reduced cytotoxicity on eucaryotic cells [72, 73]. This could be one future development.

5 Conclusion

In summary, CXL is effective in stopping progression of keratoconus and iatrogenic corneal ectasia using the Dresden protocol or Accelerated CXL as described above.

With increasing resistance of microorganisms, riboflavin-UVA photodynamic therapy is a potential treatment option for infectious keratitis. PACK-CXL damages microorganisms by inducing free oxygen radicals. Advantages and disavantages of this treatment option are still to be clarified in in vitro and in vivo studies. Until then, PDT remains a potentially adjuvant therapeutic option of treatment for resistant infectious keratitis, with off-label use.

References

1. Fuchs SM, Fluhr JW, Bankova L, Tittelbach J, Hoffmann G, Elsner P. Photodynamic therapy (PDT) and waterfiltered infrared A (wIRA) in patients with recalcitrant common hand and foot warts. Ger Med Sci. 2004;2:Doc08.
2. Gomes JAP, Tan D, Rapuano CJ, Belin MW, Ambrósio R, Guell JL, et al. Global consensus on keratoconus and ectatic diseases. Cornea. 2015;34(4):359–369.
3. Spoerl E, Huhle M, Seiler T. Induction of cross-links in corneal tissue. Exp Eye Res. 1998;66(1):97–103.

4. Raiskup F, Spoerl E. Corneal crosslinking with riboflavin and ultraviolet A. Part II. Clinical indications and results. Ocul Surf. 2013;11(2):93–108.
5. Wollensak G, Spoerl E, Seiler T. Riboflavin/ultraviolet-a–induced collagen crosslinking for the treatment of keratoconus. Am J Ophthalmol. 2003;135(5):620–627.
6. Seitz B, Daas L, Hamon L, Xanthopoulou K, Goebels S, Spira-Eppig C, et al. Stadiengerechte Therapie des Keratokonus. Ophthalmologe. 2021;118(10):1069–1088.
7. Schilde T, Kohlhaas M, Spoerl E, Pillunat LE. Enzymatischer Nachweis der Tiefenabhängigkeit der Vernetzungswirkung von Riboflavin/UVA an der Hornhaut (Enzymatic evidence of the depth dependence of stiffening on riboflavin/UVA treated corneas). Ophthalmologe. 2008;105(2):165–169.
8. Spoerl E, Wollensak G, Seiler T. Increased resistance of crosslinked cornea against enzymatic digestion. Curr Eye Res. 2004;29(1):35–40.
9. Wu D, Lim DKA, Lim BXH, Wong N, Hafezi F, Manotosh R, et al. Corneal cross-linking: the evolution of treatment for corneal diseases. Front Pharmacol. 2021;12: 686630.
10. Wernli J, Schumacher S, Spoerl E, Mrochen M. The efficacy of corneal cross-linking shows a sudden decrease with very high intensity UV light and short treatment time. Invest Ophthalmol Vis Sci. 2013;54(2):1176.
11. Kirgiz A, Eliacik M, Yildirim Y. Different accelerated corneal collagen cross-linking treatment modalities in progressive keratoconus. Eye and Vis. 2019;6(1):16.
12. Shetty R, Pahuja NK, Nuijts RMMA, Ajani A, Jayadev C, Sharma C, et al. Current protocols of corneal collagen cross-linking: visual, refractive, and tomographic outcomes. Am J Ophthalmol. 2015;160(2):243–249.
13. Xanthopoulou K, Milioti G, Daas L, Munteanu C, Seitz B, Flockerzi E. Accelerated corneal crosslinking causes pseudoprogression in keratoconus within the first 6 weeks without affecting posterior corneal curvature. Eur J Ophthalmol. 2022;32(5):2565–2576.
14. Xanthopoulou K, Milioti G, Daas L, Munteanu C, Seitz B, Flockerzi E. Accelerated corneal crosslinking for treatment of keratoconus in children and adolescents under 18 years of age. Klin Monatsbl Augenheilkd. 2023;240(10):1131-1142.
15. Seiler T, Hafezi F. Corneal cross-linking-induced stromal demarcation line. Cornea. 2006;25(9):1057–1059.
16. Mazzotta C, Balestrazzi A, Traversi C, Baiocchi S, Caporossi T, Tommasi C, et al. Treatment of progressive keratoconus by riboflavin-UVA-induced cross-linking of corneal collagen: ultrastructural snalysis by Heidelberg retinal Tomograph II in vivo confocal microscopy in humans. Cornea. 2007;26(4):390–397.
17. Wollensak G, Spörl E, Reber F, Pillunat L, Funk R. Corneal endothelial cytotoxicity of riboflavin/UVA treatment in vitro. Ophthalmic Res. 2003;35(6):324–328.
18. Mazzotta C, Wollensak G, Raiskup F, Pandolfi AM, Spoerl E. The meaning of the demarcation line after riboflavin-UVA corneal collagen crosslinking. Expert Rev Ophthalmol. 2019;14(2):115–131.
19. Spadea L, Tonti E, Vingolo EM. Corneal stromal demarcation line after collagen cross-linking in corneal ectatic diseases: a review of the literature. Clin Ophthalmol. 2016;10:1803–1810.
20. Mazzotta C, Caporossi T, Denaro R, Bovone C, Sparano C, Paradiso A, et al. Morphological and functional correlations in riboflavin UV A corneal collagen cross-linking for keratoconus. Acta Ophthalmol. 2012;90(3):259–265.
21. Spoerl E. Corneal cross-linking and safety issues. Open Ophthalmol J. 2011;5(1):14–6.
22. Jacob S, Kumar DA, Agarwal A, Basu S, Sinha P, Agarwal A. Contact lens-assisted collagen cross-linking (CACXL): a new technique for cross-linking thin corneas. J Refract Surg. 2014;30(6):366–372.
23. Wollensak G, Spörl E, Herbst H. Biomechanical efficacy of contact lens-assisted collagen cross-linking in porcine eyes. Acta Ophthalmol. 2019;97(1):e84–90.
24. Raiskup F, Spoerl E. Corneal cross-linking with hypo-osmolar riboflavin solution in thin keratoconic corneas. Am J Ophthalmol. 2011;152(1):28–32.e1.
25. Li W, Wang B. Efficacy and safety of transepithelial corneal collagen crosslinking surgery versus standard corneal collagen crosslinking surgery for keratoconus: a meta-analysis of randomized controlled trials. BMC Ophthalmol. 2017;17(1):262.
26. Cha SH, Lee JS, Oum BS, Kim CD. Corneal epithelial cellular dysfunction from benzalkonium chloride (BAC) in vitro. Clin Exp Ophthalmol. 2004;32(2):180–184.
27. Wen D, Song B, Li Q, Tu R, Huang Y, Wang Q, et al. Comparison of epithelium-off versus transepithelial corneal collagen crosslinking for keratoconus: a systematic review and meta-analysis. Cornea. 2018;37(8):1018–1024.
28. Hafezi F, Kling S, Gilardoni F, Hafezi N, Hillen M, Abrishamchi R, et al. Individualized corneal cross-linking with riboflavin and UV-A in ultrathin corneas: the Sub400 protocol. Am J Ophthalmol. 2021;224:133–142.
29. Mazzotta C, Romani A, Burroni A. Pachymetry-based accelerated crosslinking: the "M Nomogram" for standardized treatment of all-thickness progressive ectatic corneas. Int J Keratoconus Ectatic Corneal Dis. 2018;7(2):137–144.
30. Dervenis N, Dervenis P, Dragoumis N, Papandroudis A, Zachariadis Z, Balidis M. Accelerated, pulsed collagen cross-linking versus the Dresden protocol in keratoconus: a case series. Med Princ Pract. 2020;29(4):332–337.
31. Mazzotta C, Traversi C, Paradiso AL, Latronico ME, Rechichi M. Pulsed light accelerated crosslinking versus continuous light accelerated crosslinking: one-year results. J Ophthalmol. 2014;2014:1–6.
32. Kanellopoulos J. Long term results of a prospective randomized bilateral eye comparison trial of higher fluence, shorter duration ultraviolet A radiation, and riboflavin collagen cross linking for progressive keratoconus. Clin Ophthalmol. 2012;97–101.
33. Kymionis GD, Tsoulnaras KI, Grentzelos MA, Liakopoulos DA, Tsakalis NG, Blazaki SV, et al. Evaluation of corneal stromal demarcation line depth following standard and a modified-accelerated collagen cross-linking protocol. Am J Ophthalmol. 2014;158(4):671–5.e1.
34. Kymionis GD, Kontadakis GA, Kounis GA, Portaliou DM, Karavitaki AE, Magarakis M et al. Simultaneous topography-Guided PRK followed by corneal collagen cross-linking for keratoconus. J Refract Surg. 2009;25(9):S807-811.
35. Kymionis GD, Grentzelos MA, Karavitaki AE, Kounis GA, Kontadakis GA, Yoo S, et al. Transepithelial phototherapeutic keratectomy using a 213-nm solid-state laser system followed by corneal collagen cross-linking with riboflavin and UVA irradiation. J Ophthalmol. 2010;2010:146543.
36. Kanellopoulos AJ. Management of progressive keratoconus with partial topography-guided PRK combined with refractive, customized CXL-a novel technique: the enhanced Athens protocol. Clin Ophthalmol. 2019;13:581–588.
37. Wollensak G, Spoerl E, Reber F, Seiler T. Keratocyte cytotoxicity of riboflavin/UVA-treatment in vitro. Eye. 2004;18(7):718–722.
38. Koller T, Mrochen M, Seiler T. Complication and failure rates after corneal crosslinking. J Cataract Refract Surg. 2009;35(8):1358–1362.
39. Raiskup F, Hoyer A, Spoerl E. Permanent corneal haze after riboflavin-UVA-induced cross-linking in keratoconus. J Refract Surg. 2009;25(9):S824-828.
40. Dhawan S, Rao K, Natrajan S. Complications of corneal collagen cross-linking. J Ophthalmol. 2011;2011:1–5.

41. Papaioannou L, Miligkos M, Papathanassiou M. Corneal collagen cross-linking for infectious keratitis: a systematic review and meta-analysis. Cornea. 2016;35(1):62–71.
42. Price MO, Tenkman LR, Schrier A, Fairchild KM, Trokel SL, Price FW. Photoactivated riboflavin treatment of infectious keratitis using collagen cross-linking technology. J Refract Surg. 2012;28(10):706–713.
43. Chanbour W, Mokdad I, Mouhajer A, Jarade E. Late-onset sterile peripheral ulcerative keratitis post-corneal collagen crosslinking. Cornea. 2019;38(3):338–343.
44. Labiris G, Kaloghianni E, Koukoula S, Zissimopoulos A, Kozobolis VP. Corneal melting after collagen cross-linking for keratoconus: a case report. J Med Case Rep. 2011;5:152.
45. Ghanem RC, Santhiago MR, Berti TB, Thomaz S, Netto MV. Collagen crosslinking with riboflavin and ultraviolet-A in eyes with pseudophakic bullous keratopathy. J Cataract Refract Surg. 2010;36(2):273–276.
46. Makdoumi K, Bäckman A, Mortensen J, Crafoord S. Evaluation of antibacterial efficacy of photo-activated riboflavin using ultraviolet light (UVA). Graefes Arch Clin Exp Ophthalmol. 2010;248(2):207–212.
47. Martins SAR, Combs JC, Noguera G, Camacho W, Wittmann P, Walther R, et al. Antimicrobial efficacy of riboflavin/UVA combination (365 nm) in vitro for bacterial and fungal isolates: a potential new treatment for infectious keratitis. Invest Ophthalmol Vis Sci. 2008;49(8):3402.
48. Schnitzler E, Spörl E, Seiler T. Bestrahlung der Hornhaut mit UV-Licht und Riboflavingabe als neuer Behandlungsversuch bei einschmelzenden Hornhautprozessen, erste Ergebnisse bei vier Patienten (crosslinking of the corneal collagen by UV-radiation with riboflavin for the mode of treatment melting ulcera of the cornea, first results of four patients). Klin Monatsbl Augenheilkd. 2000;217(3):190–193.
49. Tsugita A, Okada Y, Uehara K. Photosensitized inactivation of ribonucleic acids in the presence of riboflavin. Biochim Biophys Acta.1965;103(2):360–363.
50. Goodrich RP. The use of riboflavin for the inactivation of pathogens in blood products. Vox Sang. 2000;78(Suppl 2):211–215.
51. Ferrari TM, Leozappa M, Lorusso M, Epifani E, Ferrari LM. Escherichia coli keratitis treated with ultraviolet A/riboflavin corneal cross-linking: a case report. Eur J Ophthalmol. 2009;19(2):295–297.
52. Anwar HM, El-Danasoury AM, Hashem AN. Corneal collagen crosslinking in the treatment of infectious keratitis. Clin Ophthalmol. 2011:5:1277-1280.
53. Makdoumi K, Mortensen J, Crafoord S. Infectious keratitis treated with corneal crosslinking. Cornea. 2010;29(12):1353–1358.
54. Makdoumi K, Mortensen J, Sorkhabi O, Malmvall BE, Crafoord S. UVA-riboflavin photochemical therapy of bacterial keratitis: a pilot study. Graefes Arch Clin Exp Ophthalmol. 2012;250(1):95–102.
55. Makdoumi K, Bäckman A, Mortensen J, Magnuson A, Crafoord S. Comparison of UVA-and UVA/riboflavin-induced growth inhibition of Acanthamoeba Castellanii. Graefes Arch Clin Exp Ophthalmol. 2013;251(2):509–514.
56. Said DG, Elalfy MS, Gatzioufas Z, El-Zakzouk ES, Hassan MA, Saif MY, et al. Collagen cross-linking with photoactivated riboflavin (PACK-CXL) for the treatment of advanced Infectious keratitis with corneal melting. Ophthalmol. 2014;121(7):1377–1382.
57. Prajna NV, Radhakrishnan N, Lalitha P, Austin A, Ray KJ, Keenan JD, et al. Cross-Linking-Assisted Infection Reduction: A Randomized Clinical Trial Evaluating the Effect of Adjuvant Cross-Linking on Outcomes in Fungal Keratitis. Ophthalmology. 2020;127(2):159–166.
58. Wei A, Wang K, Wang Y, Gong L, Xu J, Shao T. Evaluation of corneal cross-linking as adjuvant therapy for the management of fungal keratitis. Graefes Arch Clin Exp Ophthalmol. 2019;257(7):1443–1452.
59. Alio JL, Abbouda A, Valle D, del Castillo JM, Fernandez JA. Corneal cross linking and infectious keratitis: a systematic review with a meta-analysis of reported cases. J Ophth Inflamm Infect. 2013;3(1):47.
60. Panda A, Krishna SN, Kumar S. Photo-activated riboflavin therapy of refractory corneal ulcers. Cornea. 2012;31(10):1210–1213.
61. Dart JKG, Saw VPJ, Kilvington S. Acanthamoeba keratitis: diagnosis and treatment update 2009. Am J Ophthalmol. 2009;148(4):487–99.e2.
62. Shetty R, Nagaraja H, Jayadev C, Shivanna Y, Kugar T. Collagen crosslinking in the management of advanced non-resolving microbial keratitis. Br J Ophthalmol. 2014;98(8):1033–1035.
63. Müller L, Thiel M, Kipfer-Kauer A, Kaufmann C. Corneal crosslinking as supplementary treatment option in melting keratitis: a case series. Klin Monatsbl Augenheilkd. 2012;229(04):411–415.
64. Knyazer B, Krakauer Y, Baumfeld Y, Lifshitz T, Kling S, Hafezi F. Accelerated corneal cross-linking with photoactivated chromophore for moderate therapy-resistant infectious keratitis. Cornea. 2018;37(4):528–531.
65. Li M, Yu T, Gao X, Wu XY. Accelerated corneal collagen crosslinking in clinical management of infectious keratitis. J Int Med Res. 2021;48(6):030006052092641.
66. Hafezi F, Munzinger A, Goldblum D, Hillen M, Tandogan T. Repeated high-fluence accelerated slitlamp-based photoactivated chromophore for keratitis corneal cross-linking for treatment-resistant fungal keratitis. Cornea. 2022;41(8):1058–1061.
67. Kling S, Hufschmid FS, Torres-Netto EA, Randleman JB, Willcox M, Zbinden R, et al. High fluence increases the antibacterial efficacy of PACK cross-linking. Cornea. 2020;39(8):1020–1026.
68. Amescua G, Arboleda A, Nikpoor N, Durkee H, Relhan N, Aguilar MC, et al. Rose bengal photodynamic antimicrobial therapy: a novel treatment for resistant fusarium keratitis. Cornea. 2017;36(9):1141–1144.
69. Szentmáry N, Goebels S, Bischoff M, Seitz B. Photodynamic therapy for infectious keratitis. Ophthalmologe. 2012;109(2):165–170.
70. Wang J, Stachon T, Eppig T, Langenbucher A, Seitz B, Szentmáry N. Impact of photodynamic inactivation (PDI) using the photosensitizer chlorin e6 on viability, apoptosis, and proliferation of human corneal endothelial cells. Graefes Arch Clin Exp Ophthalmol. 2013;251(4):1199–1204.
71. Wang J, Stachon T, Eppig T, Langenbucher A, Seitz B, Szentmáry N. Impact of photodynamic inactivation (PDI) using the photosensitizer chlorin e6 on viability, apoptosis and proliferation of human keratocytes in vitro. Graefes Arch Clin Exp Ophthalmol. 2013;251:2725–2731. https://doi.org/1008/s00417-013-2470-9.
72. Demidova TN, Hamblin MR. Photodynamic therapy targeted to pathogens. Int J Immunopathol Pharmacol. 2004;17(3):245–254.
73. Embleton ML, Nair SP, Cookson BD, Wilson M. Antibody-directed photodynamic therapy of methicillin resistant Staphylococcus aureus. Microb Drug Resist. 2004;10(2):92–97.

IntraCorneal Ring Segments ICRS

Loay Daas, Loïc Hamon, Tim Berger, and Berthold Seitz

Abstract

Implantation of intracorneal ring segments (ICRS) is an effective procedure to correct refractive errors of the eye such as myopia and astigmatism. Nowadays, there are several types of ICRS, which differ in thickness, diameter and geometry. This chapter provides an overview of the different types, indications, surgical technique and possible complications of ICRS implantation.

Keywords

Intracorneal ring segment · ICRS · Femtosecond laser tunnel creation · Lamellar channel deposits · In vivo confocal microscopy

1 Types of Intracorneal Ring Segments

Intracorneal ring segments (ICRS) are small, semicircular, biocompatible segments made of polymethyl methacrylate (PMMA) which can be implanted into the cornea, thus altering its geometry for the treatment of a variety of visual disorders, especially corneal ectasia [1, 2] (Fig. 1).

Nowadays, there is a wide range of commercially available ICRS, including Intacs® (SK) (Addition Technology Inc., Des Plaines, IL, USA), Ferrara rings® (AJL Ophthalmic S.A., Minao, Spain), Keraring® (Mediphacos, Belo Horizonte, Brazil) and more recently the asymmetrical rings AJL Pro+(AJL Ophthalmic S.A., Minao, Spain) [3, 4].

ICRS are available in a variety of sizes and shapes to meet the unique needs of the individual patient. Ferrara rings and Keraring present a triangular shape, while Intacs have a hexagonal profile (Fig. 2). The implantation zone (inner diameter from corneal center) is a crucial aspect to consider. For instance, Intacs are typically implanted at 7 mm, while Intacs SK, where the "SK" refers to "Severe Keratoconus", are implanted nearer to the center at 6 mm. This closer proximity to the optical center provides a greater central flattening effect in correcting myopia and astigmatism for individuals with (severe) keratoconus [5–8].

The placement, thickness and geometry of the ICRS are individually adjusted according to the nomograms of the manufacturing companies. These nomograms are based on various parameters such as astigmatism, coma, steep keratometry or preoperative visual acuity. Each ring type refers to its own nomogram [6].

2 Principles of ICRS

ICRS are implanted in the midperipheral corneal stroma outside the central optical zone at a depth of 80%. These implants act as spacers between collagen fibers and induce an arc-shortening effect that flattens the central cornea while preserving its prolate shape. The degree of flattening is directly related to the ICRS thickness and inversely related to the diameter of the implantation site. Consequently, a thicker segment and/or an implantation diameter closer to the optical zone will lead to a greater flattening effect on the cornea [5, 6]. Barraquer et al. proposed an alternative hypothesis ("thickness law") that explains the flattening of the cornea by adding tissue to the corneal periphery, where an equal effect can be achieved as by removing tissue from the central cornea [6].

L. Daas (✉) · L. Hamon · T. Berger · B. Seitz
Department of Ophthalmology, Saarland University Medical Center, Homburg/Saar, Germany
e-mail: loay.daas@uks.eu

B. Seitz et al. (eds.), *Atlas on Cornea*, https://doi.org/10.1007/978-3-031-65422-0_44

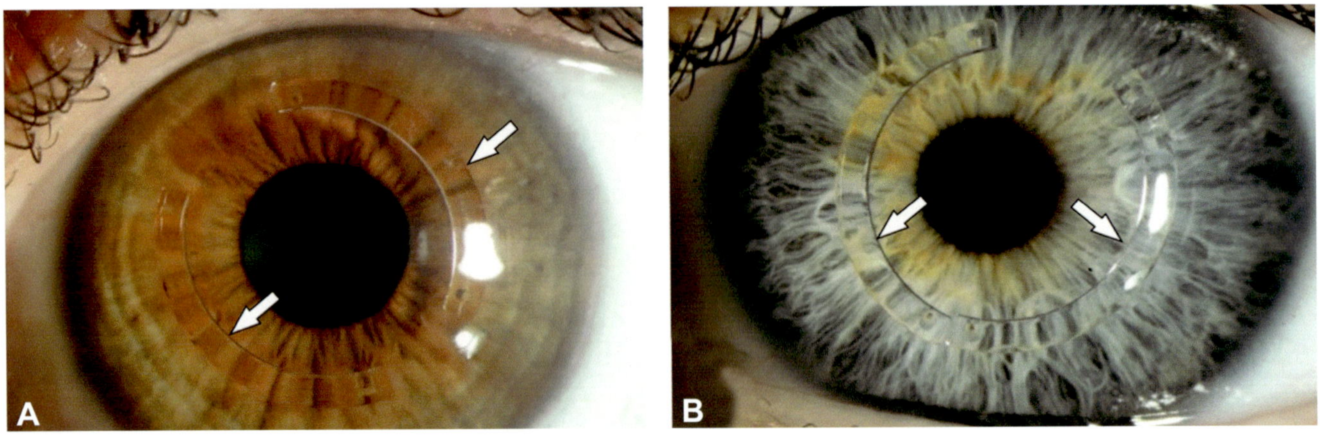

Fig. 1 (**A**, **B**) Normal findings after Intacs SK® implantation (arrows) for keratoconus

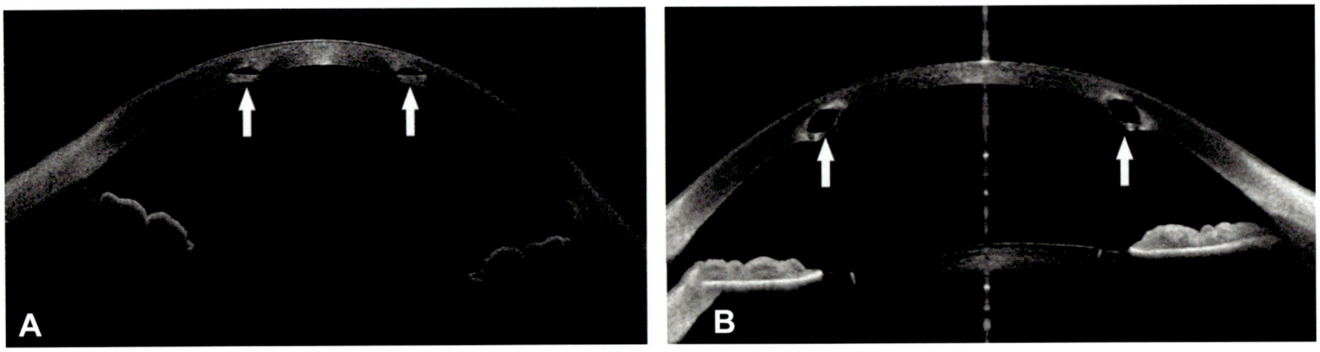

Fig. 2 Illustration of different profiles of intracorneal ring segments (arrows) by anterior segment optical coherence tomography. (**A**) Ferrara rings® with triangular profile. (**B**) Intacs® SK with hexagonal profile

3 Indications and Contraindications

Originally, ICRS were used to correct low myopia (−1.0 to −3.0 dpt) [8]. Nowadays, they are predominantly implanted as treatment for corneal ectatic disorders, such as keratoconus, pellucid marginal degeneration, and post-Laser-in-situ-Keratomileusis (LASIK) keratectasia. Typically, ICRS are indicated for moderate ectatic conditions that are not advanced enough to justify lamellar or penetrating keratoplasty (maximal steep keratometry overall (Kmax) < 62 dpt). Other requirements are contact lens intolerance or poor lens-corrected distance visual acuity. However, ICRS are not a conventional refractive procedure and patients must have realistic expectations, postoperative emmetropia should not be expected [6, 9]. Before implantation, the corneal thickness in the implantation zone (measured by anterior segment optical coherence tomography (AS OCT) should be at least 450 μm [9].

Contraindications include central corneal scarring, advanced keratectasia, corneal hydrops, herpetic keratitis, severe atopic dermatitis and collagen, vascular, and autoimmune diseases [5, 6]. It is important for patients to discuss their medical history and any existing conditions with their local ophthalmologist prior to undergoing intracorneal ring segment implantation. This can help ensure that the procedure is safe and effective for their individual need.

4 Surgery

The ICRS surgical procedure involves implanting ring segments into a corneal channel previously created within the deep corneal stroma either mechanically or with femtosecond laser-assisted techniques, generally under topical anesthesia. The mechanical technique is considered demanding and should only be performed by very skilled microsurgeons. First, marking the pupil or the geometric center of the cornea is necessary for orientation later on. Then a 1.0 mm radial incision is made at a depth of 70–80% with an adjustable diamond knife. At the base of the incision, pocketing dissectors are used to create a small corneal intrastromal pocket on each side. After placing a vacuum-centering guide at the limbus, two semicircular dissectors are used for creating the tunnels under vacuum (clockwise and counterclockwise dissection) followed by insertion of the ring segments into each ostium of the channels [5–8].

In practice, laser-assisted channel creation using the femtosecond laser has become the gold standard, which allows a greater precision and control during the procedure, resulting in improved outcomes and reduced risks for patients. This technique offers wider range of customization, whereby the surgeon is able to tailor the size, shape, and position of the ring segments to meet the individual patient`s needs [5–8]. The femtosecond laser creates a 360° circular channel by using an infrared laser beam at the desired stromal depth (mostly 80%). As with mechanical tunnel creation, the pupil center is marked and the femtosecond laser docking system is adjusted. After the suction ring is placed and centered, the laser creates both the entry incision and the tunnel incision so that the ring segments can be implanted after the system is removed, as with the mechanical method. The femtosecond laser-assisted technique does not only provide a more precise tunnel and keratotomy depth, but also ensures the uniformity of the canal [5–8]. Femtosecond laser assisted tunnel creation also carries a lower risk of postoperative epithelial disorders, stromal edema, and infectious keratitis [10]. The main surgical steps of femtosecond laser-assisted ICRS implantation are shown in Fig. 3.

Postoperatively, a bandage contact lens is placed on the eye for 1 week. Topical steroids (e.g. prednisolone acetate eye drops (ED)) and prophylactic broad-spectrum topical antibiotics (e.g. moxifloxacin ED) are applied alternately, each six times daily for two weeks. After two weeks, antibiotic ED can be discontinued and steroid ED are tapered by one drop weekly. In addition, we recommend the application of preservative-free tear substitute 6 times daily.

5 Complications

While ICRS implantation is generally considered a minimally invasive procedure, there are potential intra- and postoperative complications that can arise.

Although intraoperative complications during ICRS implantation are rare, most of the complications that arise during surgery are associated with the mechanical process of creating the channels [10]. These complications include epithelial defects in the keratotomy area, inadequate

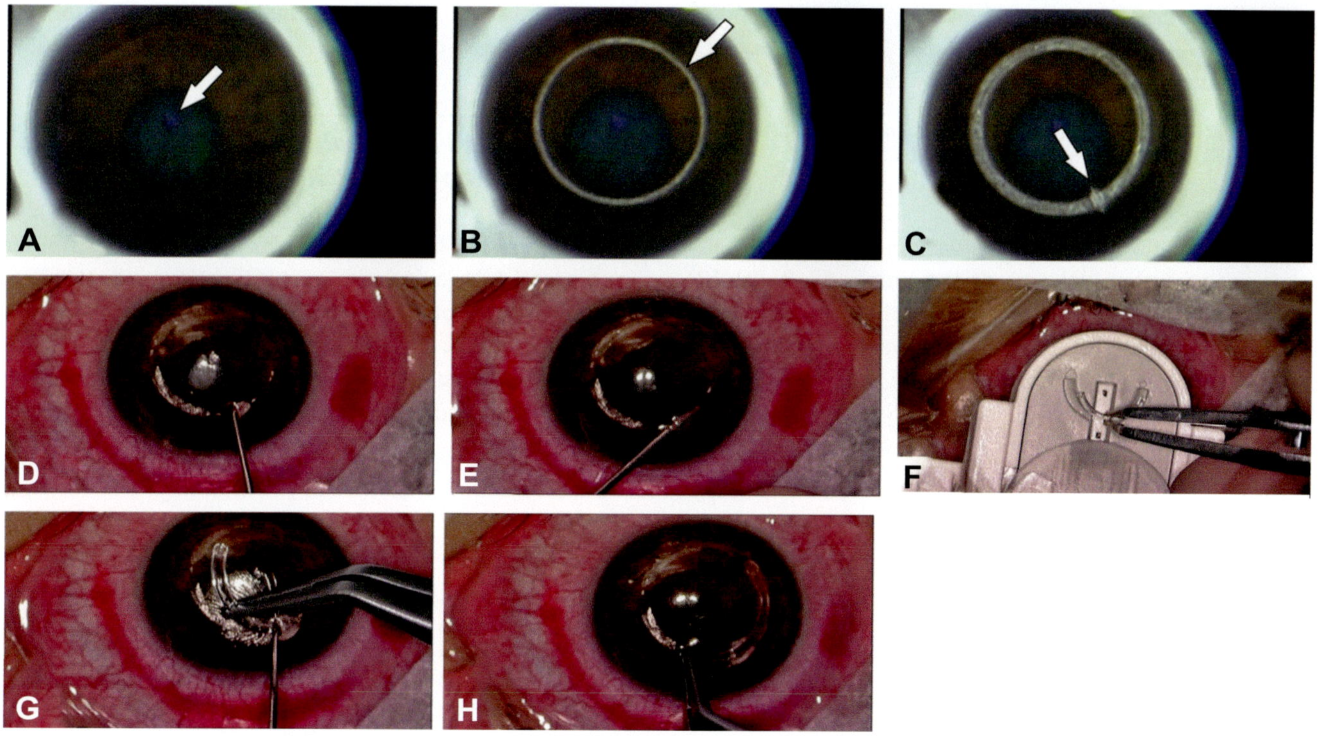

Fig. 3 Surgery steps of femtosecond laser-assisted ICRS implantation. (**A**) A vacuum system is placed on the ocular globe after marking the corneal center (arrow). (**B**) Creating a 360° circular ring (arrow) with the femtosecond laser. (**C**) Small radial incision (arrow) in the implantation site. (**D**) Separation of the upper and lower tunnel planes using a pocketing hook. (**E**) Probing the tunnel. (**F**) Intacs ring segment is removed from the package. (**G**) Insertion of ring segment into the channel ostium. (**H**) Careful pushing of the ring segment forward

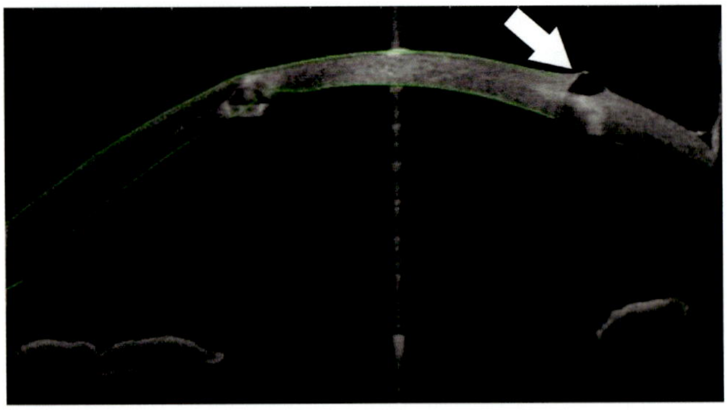

Fig. 4 Anterior segment optical coherence tomography after intracorneal ring segment implantation with mechanical channel creation. One superficial segment shows Bowman layer perforation (arrow)

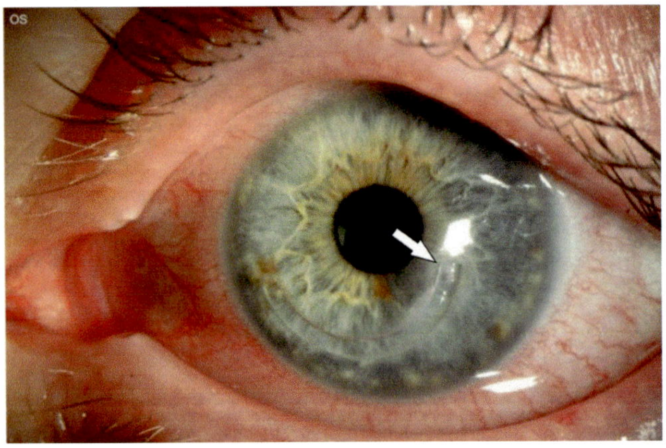

Fig. 5 Intracorneal ring segment with extrusion and infectious keratitis arising from the ostium of the channel (arrow)

channel formation and expansion of incisions towards either the central visual axis or the limbus [5–8, 10–12]. The introduction of the femtosecond laser-assisted technique has led to a reduction in intraoperative complications due to better precision and predictable size and depth of the intrastromal channels [6, 10]. ICRS can also result in complications that are related to the placement of the ring segments such as asymmetrical and/or superficial placement. Superficial channel dissection (Fig. 4) with anterior Bowman layer perforation might occur in cases of insufficient channel depth or uneven placement, resulting in one end of the ring segments lying superficially and the other end lying deep. Anterior chamber perforation during ICRS implantation is a very rare complication [5–8, 10–12].

Potentially severe postoperative complications are infectious keratitis (Fig. 5) and corneal melting that can arise from the superficial placement of rings along the channel [11, 13].

Other postoperative complications include ring segment extrusion (Fig. 6A and B), ring segment migration (Fig. 6C) and breaks of the ring segment (Fig. 6D). Ring segment extrusion is one of the most common causes for explantation and occurs mainly in eyes after mechanical dissection [5, 10]. Corneal neovascularization along the ring segment (Fig. 7A) and epithelial ingrowth (Fig. 7B) at the incision site are also rarely observed [12].

From patient side, nocturnal halos, persistent discomfort, corneal haze with or without focal edema, photophobia, and reduced or fluctuating uncorrected and best corrected visual acuity are occasionally reported [6].

In addition, structural stromal changes such as perisegmental fibrosis (Fig. 8), superficial iron deposits in epithelial cells or lipid lamellar channel deposits (LCD) (Fig. 9) are frequently seen, occurring months to years after the surgery, although these have no clinical relevance [14, 15].

6 Corneal Allogenic Intrastromal Ring Segments (CAIRS)

A new promising approach described by Jacob et al. [16] uses Corneal Allogenic Intrastromal Ring Segments (CAIRS) (Fig. 10) instead of PMMA ICRS. These are formed from human donor corneal tissue and implanted, like PMMA ICRS, into a femtosecond laser created channel. CAIRS allow for a wide range of implantation depths and appear to provide comparable results to PMMA ring segments [17–20].

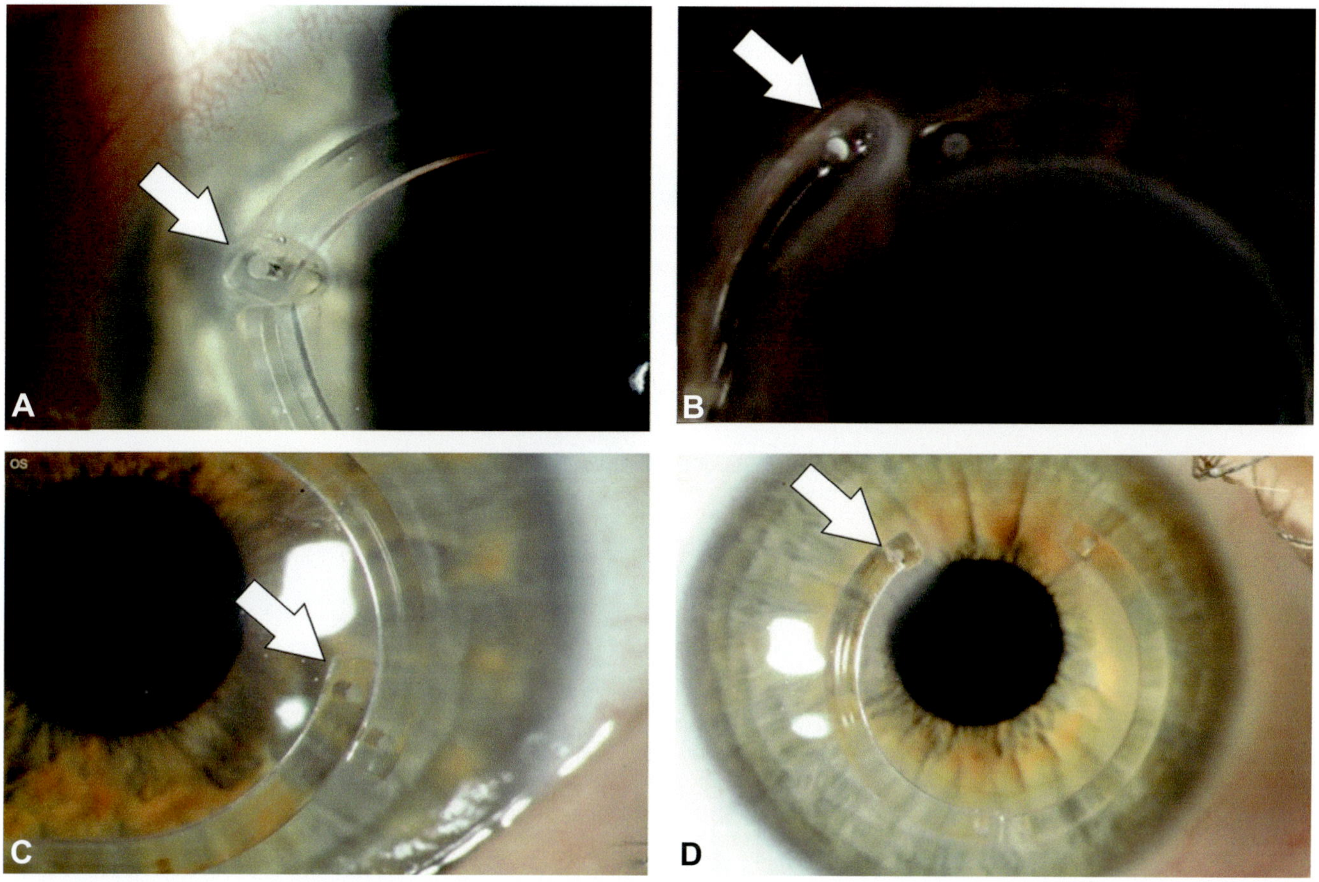

Fig. 6 Several conditions of ICRS displacement. (**A**, **B**) Extrusion of the intracorneal ring segment (arrow). (**C**) Migration (arrow) of the intracorneal ring segment after implantation. (**D**) Break (arrow) of one intracorneal ring segment

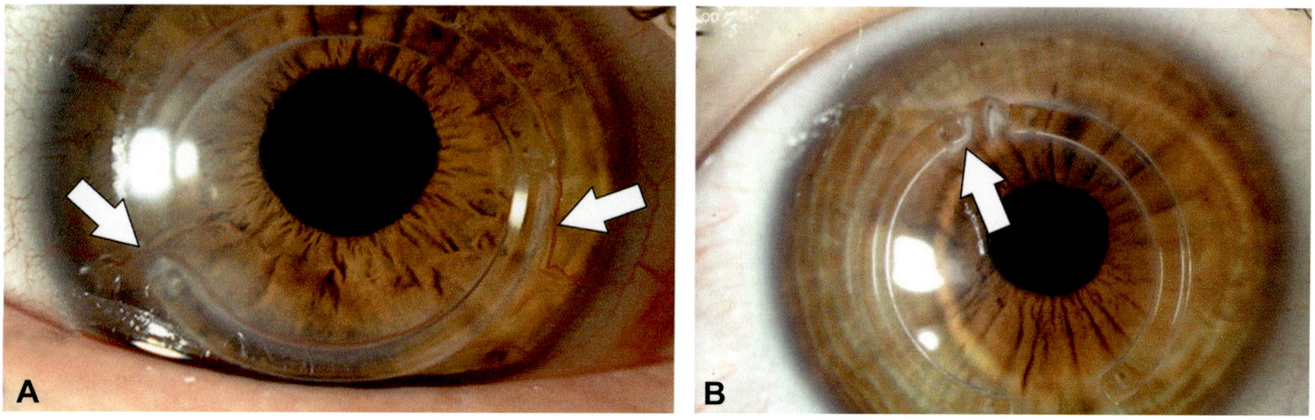

Fig. 7 Complications without displacement of the intracorneal ring segment. (**A**) Vascularization along the intracorneal ring segment (arrows). (**B**) Epithelial ingrowth at the incision site (arrow)

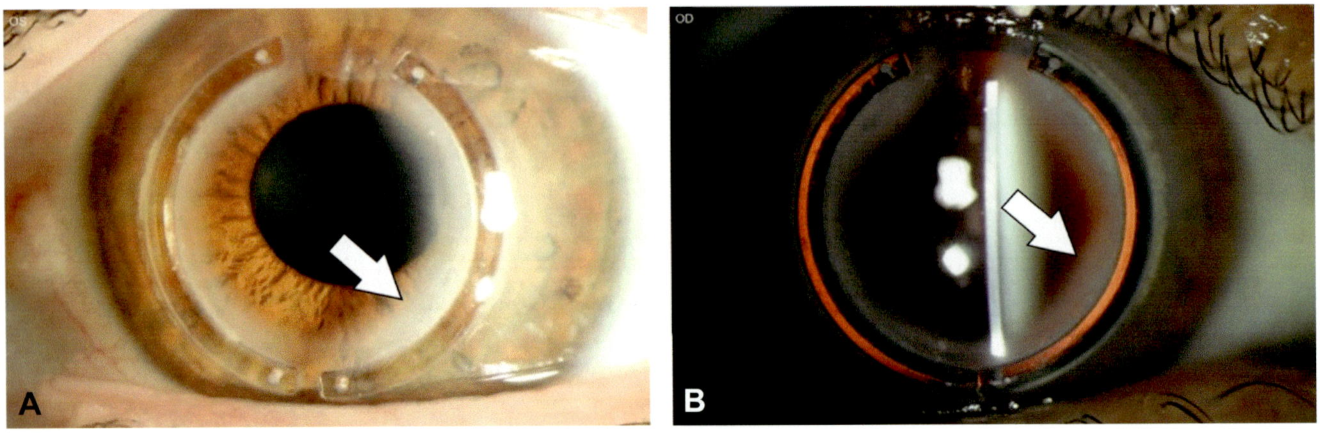

Fig. 8 Perisegmental fibrotic changes (arrow) along the intracorneal ring segments (**A**) Overview. (**B**) Retroillumination

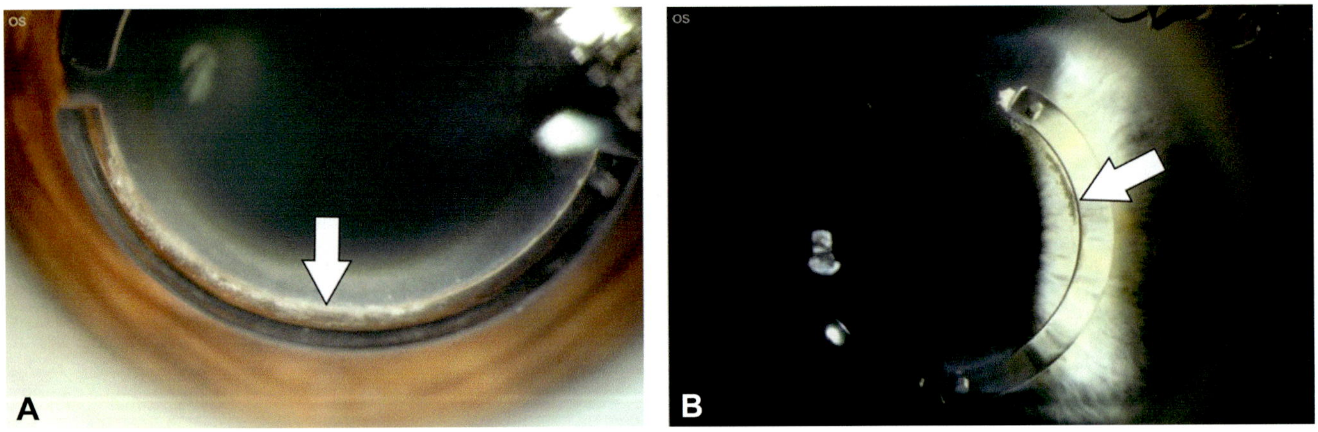

Fig. 9 Lamellar channel deposits and iron line after intracorneal ring segment (ICRS) implantation. (**A**) Lamellar channel deposits are lipid deposits into the small empty channel space between ICRS and stromal tissue (white arrow). It can extend to almost the entire arc length. Iron line is a superficial iron deposit in epithelial cells, inside the ring contour and parallel to the ring (arrow). (**B**) Indirect illumination of the lamellar channel deposits

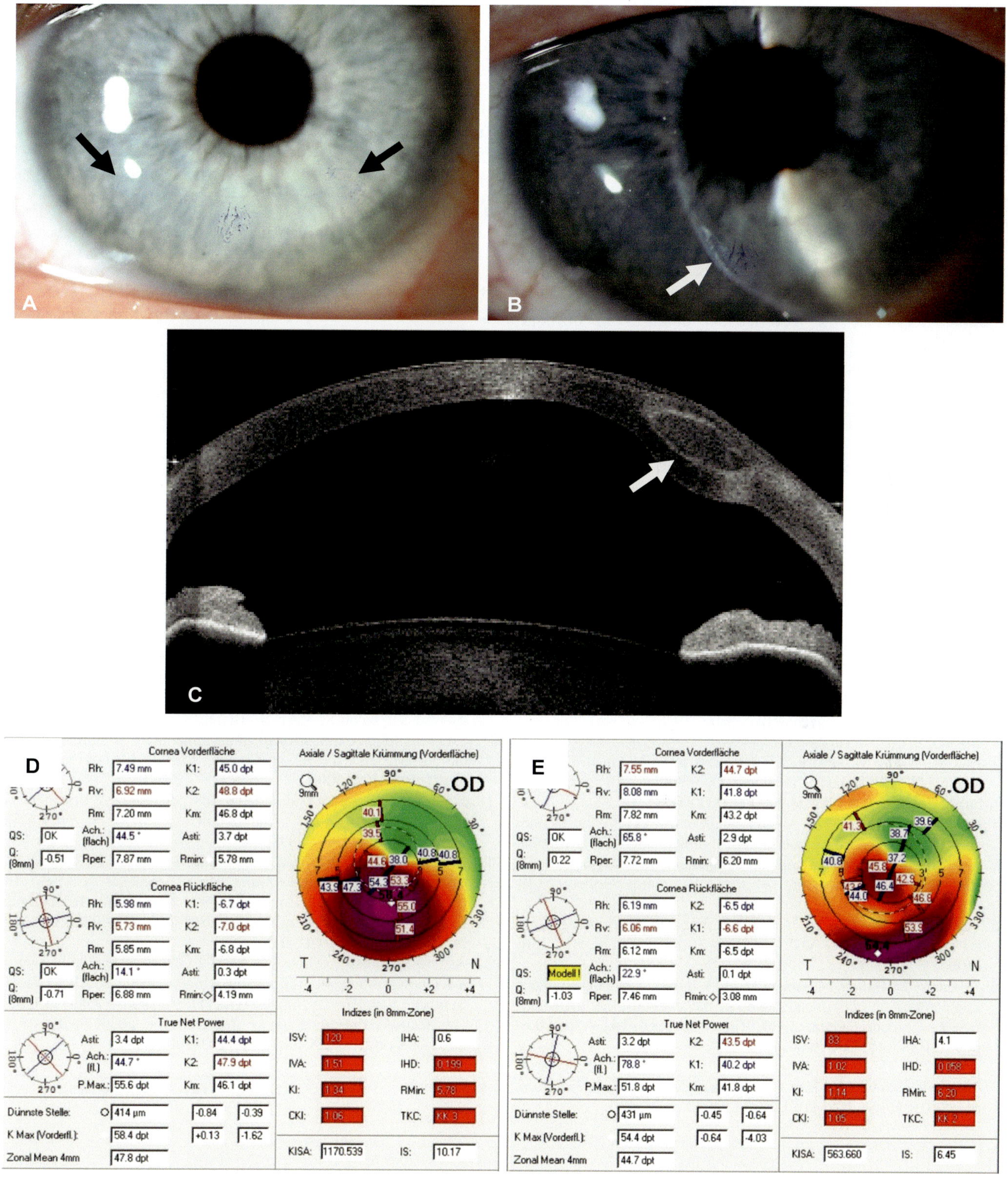

Fig. 10 Corneal allogenic intrastromal ring segments (CAIRS) transplantation in a 43-year-old keratoconus patient. (**A, B**) Slit lamp imaging showing CAIRS in the inferior part of the cornea (white arrows) 3 months after transplantation. (**C**) Anterior segment optical coherence tomography of the same patient after CAIRS transplantation. (**D, E**) Topometric pentacam® display preoperatively (**D**) and 3 months postoperatively (**E**) Note the reduction in K1, K2 and Kmax after the procedure. Preoperatively, the best corrected spectacle visual acuity was 0.4 (-1.0/-5.75/50°), improving to 0.8 (+0.5/-2.50/20°) postoperatively

7 Conclusion

ICRS implantation is a safe and reversible technique that effectively treats ectatic corneas by regularizing the irregular corneal curvature, thus improving visual acuity and quality of life for those mostly young and active patients. ICRS implantation should be considered for patients presenting keratoconus with moderate clinical findings but poor visual acuity or contact lens intolerance.

This procedure offers two key advantages over other treatments. Firstly, it does not require the removal of any corneal tissue, making it less invasive and less risky for patients. Secondly, the geometrical changes in corneal shape induced by the ICRS are reversible: Once ICRS are removed, the cornea will return to its near-original state.

New ICRS profiles such as asymmetric segments could further improve refractive results, especially for patients presenting asymmetrical conus phenotypes.

Funding The authors have no funding or conflicts of interest to disclose.

References

1. El-Husseiny M, Tsintarakis T, Eppig T, et al. Intracorneal ring segments in keratoconus. Ophthalmologe. 2013;110:823–9. https://doi.org/10.1007/s00347-013-2821-2.
2. El-Husseiny M, Daas L, Langenbucher A, et al. Intracorneal ring segments to treat keratectasia-interim results and potential complications. Klin Monbl Augenheilkd. 2016;233:722–6. https://doi.org/10.1055/s-0042-108653.
3. Park SE, Tseng M, Lee JK. Effectiveness of intracorneal ring segments for keratoconus. Curr Opin Ophthalmol. 2019;30:220–8. https://doi.org/10.1097/ICU.0000000000000582.
4. Kammoun H, Piñero DP, Álvarez de Toledo J, et al. Clinical outcomes of femtosecond laser-assisted implantation of asymmetric ICRS in keratoconus with no coincidence of topographic and comatic axes. J Refract Surg. 2021;37:693–9. https://doi.org/10.3928/1081597X-20210712-04.
5. Vega-Estrada A, Alio JL. The use of intracorneal ring segments in keratoconus. Eye Vis. 2016;3:1–7. https://doi.org/10.1186/s40662-016-0040-z.
6. Sakellaris D, Balidis M, Gorou O, et al. Intracorneal ring segment implantation in the management of keratoconus: an evidence-based approach. Ophthalmol Ther. 2019;8:5–14. https://doi.org/10.1007/s40123-019-00211-2.
7. Piñero DP, Alio JL. Intracorneal ring segments in ectatic corneal disease-a review. Clin Exp Ophthalmol. 2010;38:154–67. https://doi.org/10.1111/j.1442-9071.2010.02197.x.
8. Ertan A, Colin J. Intracorneal rings for keratoconus and keratectasia. J Cataract Refract Surg. 2007;33:1303–14. https://doi.org/10.1016/j.jcrs.2007.02.048.
9. Seitz B, Daas L, Hamon L, et al. Stage-appropriate treatment of keratoconus. Ophthalmologe. 2021;118:1069–88. https://doi.org/10.1007/s00347-021-01410-8.
10. Struckmeier AK, Hamon L, Flockerzi E, et al. Femtosecond laser and mechanical dissection for ICRS and MyoRing implantation: a meta-analysis. Cornea. 2022;41:518–37. https://doi.org/10.1097/ICO.0000000000002937.
11. Bautista-Llamas M-J, Sánchez-González MC, López-Izquierdo I, et al. Complications and explantation reasons in intracorneal ring segments (ICRS) implantation: a systematic review. J Refract Surg. 2019;35:740–7. https://doi.org/10.3928/1081597X-20191010-02.
12. Alió JL, Shabayek MH, Artola A. Intracorneal ring segments for keratoconus correction: long-term follow-up. J Cataract Refract Surg. 2006;32:978–85. https://doi.org/10.1016/j.jcrs.2006.02.044.
13. Hofling-Lima AL, Branco BC, Romano AC, et al. Corneal infections after implantation of intracorneal ring segments. Cornea. 2004;23:547–9. https://doi.org/10.1097/01.ico.0000126434.95325.24.
14. Hamon L, Schlötzer-Schrehardt U, Flockerzi FA, et al. Morphological characterization and clinical effects of stromal alterations after intracorneal ring segment implantation in keratoconus. Graefe's Arch Clin Exp Ophthalmol. 2022;260:2299–308. https://doi.org/10.1007/s00417-022-05572-2.
15. Hamon L, Seitz B, Daas L. Intrastromal fibrosis and lipid deposits twenty years after intracorneal ring segments implantation for treatment of mild myopia. J Fr Ophtalmol. 2022;45:147–50. https://doi.org/10.1016/j.jfo.2021.06.018.
16. Jacob S, Patel SR, Agarwal A, et al. Corneal allogenic intrastromal ring segments (CAIRS) combined with corneal cross-linking for keratoconus. JRefract Surg. 2018;34:296–303. https://doi.org/10.3928/1081597X-20180223-01.
17. Awwad ST, Jacob S, Assaf JF, Bteich Y. Extended dehydration of corneal allogenic intrastromal ring segments to facilitate insertion: the corneal jerky technique. Cornea. 2023;42:1461–4. https://doi.org/10.1097/ICO.0000.
18. Jacob S. Custom-shaped CAIRS for personalized treatment of Keratoconus. Indian J Ophthalmol. 2025;73:3-5. https://doi.org/10.4103/IJO.IJO_2589_24.
19. Bteich Y, Assaf JF, Mrad AA, Jacob S, Hafezi F, Awwad ST. Corneal Allogenic Intrastromal Ring Segments (CAIRS) for Corneal Ectasia: A Comprehensive Segmental Tomography Evaluation. J Refract Surg. 2023;39:767-776. https://doi.org/10.3928/1081597X-20231011-01.
20. Asfar KE, Bteich Y, Mrad AA, Assaf JF, Jacob S, Hafezi F, Awwad ST. Corneal Allogenic Intrastromal Ring Segments (CAIRS) Versus Synthetic Segments: A Single Segment Comparative Analysis Using Propensity Score Matching. J Refract Surg. 2024;40:e863-e876. https://doi.org/10.3928/1081597X-20241002-02.

"Muraine Sutures" for Corneal Hydrops

Berthold Seitz, Sonia Razafimino, Fidelis Flockerzi, and Elias Flockerzi

Abstract

Penetrating keratoplasty à chaud is contraindicated in acute keratoconus. In the past the stromal scarring was waited for 3–6 months with the administration of hyperosmolar eye drops. Today, after a prophylactic YAG-iridotomy caudally through the still clear cornea, air is injected into the anterior chamber and multiple deep stromal 10–0 nylon single compression sutures are placed perpendicular to the Descemet tear. Already on the first day postoperatively the cornea is typically much clearer. The histological analysis shows a significantly smaller distance between the ends of the Descemet tear in the range of 100 μm after so-called Muraine sutures compared to more than 1000 μm in the spontaneous course.

Keywords

Corneal hydrops · Corneal edema · Compression sutures · Keratectasia · Acute keratoconus · Air tamponade · Muraine sutures

Supplementary Information The online version contains supplementary material available at https://doi.org/10.1007/978-3-031-65422-0_45.

B. Seitz (✉) · S. Razafimino · E. Flockerzi
Department of Ophthalmology, Saarland University Medical Center, Homburg/Saar, Germany
e-mail: berthold.seitz@uks.eu

F. Flockerzi
Institute for General and Special Pathology, Saarland University Medical Center, Homburg/Saar, Germany

1 Introduction

For more than 16 years, over 3500 patients have been included in our Homburg Keratoconus Center (HKC) [1, 2], some of whom have already returned for 26 follow-up visits (Fig. 1). The stage-appropriate therapy of these patients ranges from contact lenses, crosslinking and intracorneal ring segments to excimer laser-assisted DALK and PKP [3–5].

In corneal ectasias such as keratoconus, keratotorus (= pellucid marginal degeneration PMD) and keratoglobus, a hydrops corneae (so-called "acute keratoconus") can most frequently develop as part of a progression. The result is an immediate and severe reduction in visual acuity (Table 1). The hydrops develops due to a tear in the Descemet membrane resulting in corneal edema with large vacuoles and pseudocysts [6, 7] (Table 2). Very rarely, corneal hydrops can also be the cause of acute secondary graft insufficiency many years after penetrating keratoplasty due to keratoconus [8, 9].

The prevalence of corneal hydrops in keratoconus is 1.6–2.8%. A higher risk is said to exist for keratoconus patients of East Asian origin or with darker skin [11]. Predispositions are considered: Eye rubbing, atopy, allergy, vernal keratoconjunctivitis and trisomy 21. The trigger is often corneal trauma, excessive rubbing with the finger joints or coughing. Posterior curvature changes of the contralateral eye may indicate the incidence of a corneal hydrops [10].

A hydrops corneae is usually self-limiting within 3 to 6 months. Subsequently, a penetrating keratoplasty (PKP) is often necessary due to a scar-related reduction in visual acuity. However, there is also the possibility of an increase in visual acuity due to scar-related flattening and topographical regularization if the scar is located mid-peripherally.

If corneal edema persists, infection, stromal scarring, neovascularization and, in extremely rare cases (e.g. oculodigital phenomenon in Down syndrome) corneal perforation may occur as complications, which is why prompt reduction of the corneal edema is desirable. In particular, severe vascular sprouting with prolonged edema reduces the prognosis of subsequent keratoplasty [12].

B. Seitz et al. (eds.), *Atlas on Cornea*, https://doi.org/10.1007/978-3-031-65422-0_45

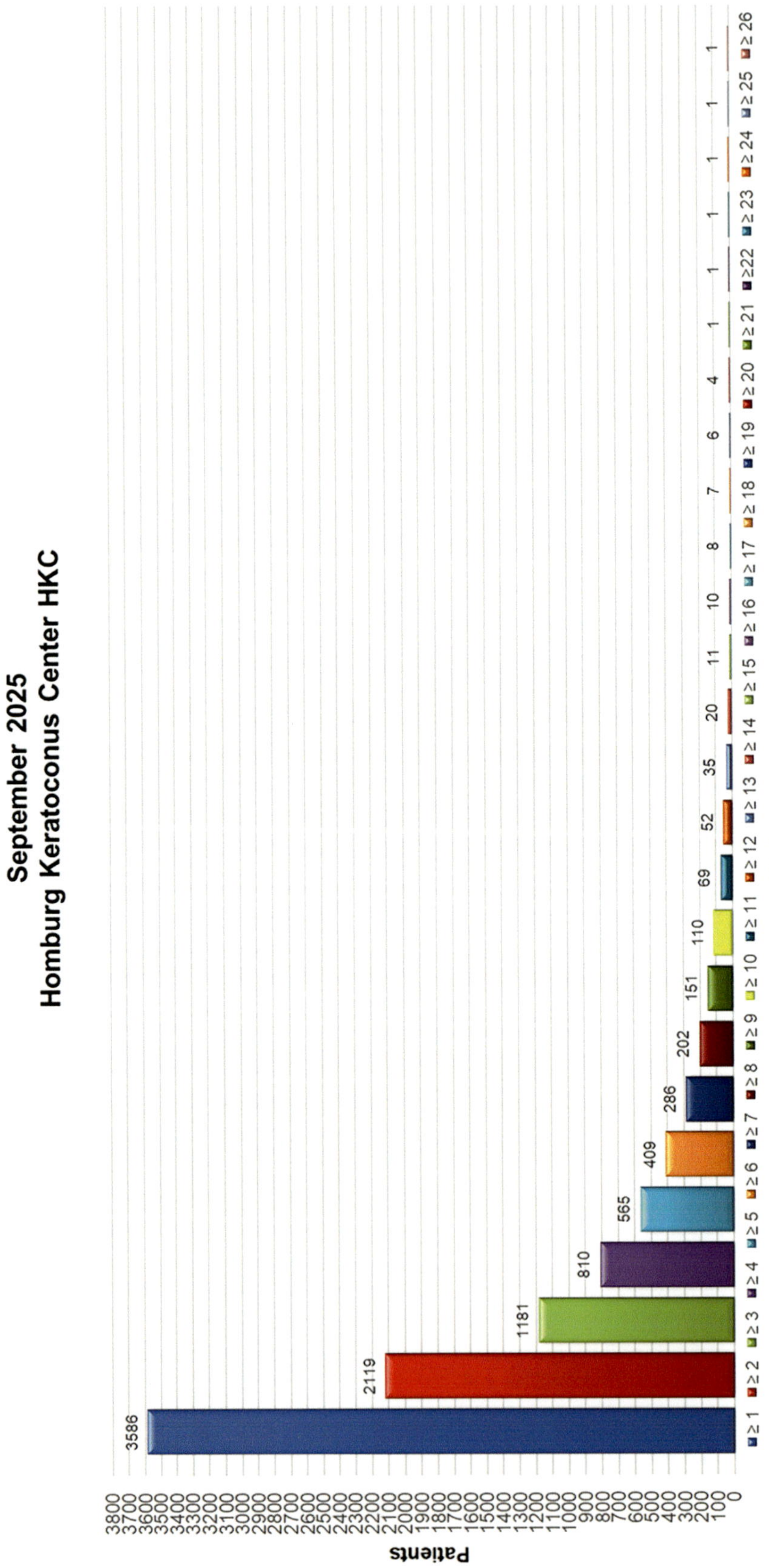

Fig. 1 More than 3500 patients have been included to the Homburg Keratoconus Center *HKC* since 2010 (as of September 2025)

Table 1 Symptoms of corneal hydrops (= „acute keratoconus")

• Almost always unilateral
• Severe, sudden drop in visual acuity
• Photophobia ("fear of light")
• Epiphora („tearing")
• Foreign body sensation
• Pain

Table 2 Findings of corneal hydrops on the slit lamp

• Severe focal stromal edema with vacuoles and pseudocysts
• Focal bullous keratopathy with/without erosio corneae
• Contralateral signs of keratoconus [10]
• No signs of infection (cells in anterior chamber, hypopyon, synechia), DDx: HSV-endotheliitis

2 Therapy

For many decades, the generally accepted "therapy" in Germany was to wait and administer 5% hypertonic NaCl drops, care and, if necessary, pressure reduction (Table 3). Keratoplasty à chaud in the stage of acute keratoconus was and is contraindicated because the risk of suture loosening is very high in the severely edematous corneal tissue. This can result in infiltrates, stromal vascularization, immune reaction and even endophthalmitis [12].

Since January 2017, we have preferred deep stromal predescemetal or penetrating—but never too superficial—compression sutures followed by intracameral air/gas tamponade (so-called "Muraine sutures" [13]). The aim is to readapt the ruptured Descemet edges. The air/gas in the anterior chamber is also intended to prevent the influx of water into the corneal stroma (Table 4).

Table 3 Conservative treatment options for corneal hydrops

• Wait and see
• 5% NaCl eye drops (hyperosmolar)
• Nourishing gel or oitment
• Possible pressure reductions (CAVE: falsely low values with stromal edema!)
• Antibiotic drops in case of epithelial defect
• Steroid eye drops (?)
• Possibly bandage contact lens

3 Surgical Procedure (Video)

Patients are admitted as inpatients and dropped hourly with a hypertonic 5% saline solution to de-swell the corneal edema. If possible, a YAG iridotomy is performed preoperatively in the inferior region of the peripheral iris—ideally at 6 o'clock if the edema allows it—to prevent an air/gas block resulting in an acute increase of the intraocular pressure.

In the operating room, the Descemet tear is visualized under topical or retrobulbar anaesthesia with an air-filled anterior chamber. Multiple (typically 4 to 6) deep stromal, ideally pre-descemetal 10–0 nylon single sutures are placed perpendicular to the Descemet tear. When in doubt, we aim for penetrating sutures—but never stitch too superficial! At the end of the operation, we leave a 90% air/gas filling in the anterior chamber and ask the patients—as with DMEK—to lie on their back for a few days. On the day of surgery, we measure the intraocular pressure every 2 h and, if necessary, release a little air via preexisting paracentesis.

At the follow-up examination 6 weeks postoperatively, a healed, irritation-free cornea with a regular thickness is typically found. At this point, we remove all sutures under topical anesthesia. Any loose corneal sutures are—as always—removed immediately beforehand!

At this point it is decided whether the patient can continue to wear rigid contact lenses (especially in PMD or keratoglobus) or whether we suggest excimer laser-assisted PKP [3, 5]. Due to the Descemet tear, we do not recommend DALK with the exposure of the Descemet membrane, which we consider essential. Femtosecond laser-assisted PKP without liquid interface clearly has worse results than excimer laser PKP, which celebrated its 30th birthday in 2020 [4, 5, 22].

Please scan to access video content

4 Own Clinical Results

Typically, corneal swelling is already significantly reduced on the first postoperative day [20, 21] (Fig. 2)!

Table 4 Surgical treatment options for corneal hydrops

•	Air or gas injection (20% SF_6, 14% C_2F_6, 14% C_3F_8) intracameral (Pneumodescemetopexy) [14–16]
•	Air injection with intrastromal venting incisions [17]
•	Mini-DMEK as Descemet patch [18]
•	Deep compression sutures (predescemetal/full-thickness) + gas/air [13, 19–21]
•	No penetrating keratoplasty in the acute stage!!! [4, 12]

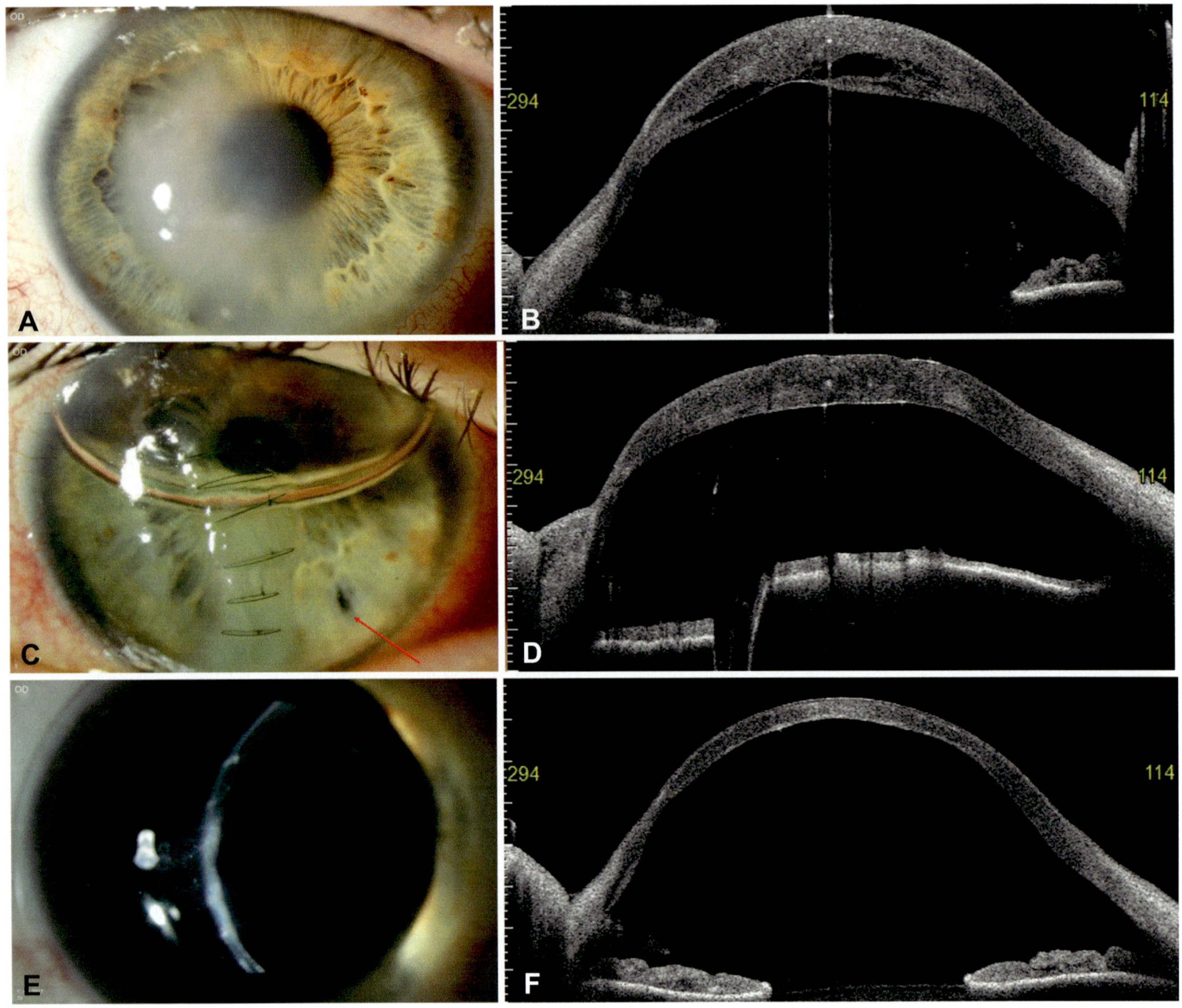

Fig. 2 **Preoperative**: (**A**) A 52-year-old patient presented to our outpatient department for the first time with visual loss in the right eye that had been present for 1 week. Slit lamp microscopy revealed a pronounced corneal edema (hydrops corneae in pellucid marginal degeneration PMD = keratotorus) in the inferior part of the right eye reaching to the center preoperatively. (**B**) The anterior segment OCT (CASIA 2, Tomey Nagoya, Japan) showed a corneal thickness of 1107 μm at the apex. **1st postoperative day**: (**C**) The cornea was already clear on the first postoperative day; YAG iridotomy indicated by red arrow. (**D**) Anterior segment OCT on postoperative day 1: Corneal thickness was reduced to 701 μm and visual acuity was 1/20 reading charts. 20 **weeks postoperatively**: (**E**) The follow-up examination 20 weeks postoperatively showed suture scars and a low corneal thickness of 373 μm. The contact lens visual acuity was stable at 20/50. Upon the patient's request, penetrating excimer laser keratoplasty was not performed. (**F**) Anterior segment OCT 20 weeks postoperatively

We investigated the clinical course in 24 patients who were treated for acute corneal hydrops with a combination of three to six single pre-descemetal sutures (so-called "Muraine sutures") orthogonal to the axis of rupture of the Descemet membrane with simultaneous intracameral air/gas tamponade [20]. Corneal thickness decreased significantly in all our patients quickly (= within a few days!) ($p = 0.001$). The median preoperative corneal pachymetry was 1508 (805–2423) µm and was already significantly reduced to 932 (458–1610) µm on the first postoperative day and to 612 (366–1250) µm 6 weeks after surgery. Visual acuity improved from 1.7 logMAR preoperatively to 0.95 logMAR 6 weeks after surgery. There was no acute increase in intraocular pressure after YAG iridotomy (Figs. 3 and 4).

5 Own Histological Results

All corneal excisions in keratoplasty are examined in our Institute for General and Special Pathology. In case of past acute keratoconus, we endeavor to maintain a histological microtome incision perpendicular to the Descemet rupture during keratoplasty at the scarring site in order to be able to measure the distance between the Descemet edges. The histopathologic processing of our corneal excisions after acute keratoconus with vs. without Muraine sutures showed, for example, a significantly smaller distance of the Descemet margins of 67 µm (Fig. 5) and 147 µm (Fig. 6) after Muraine sutures compared to 1249 µm (Fig. 7) and 1654 µm (Fig. 8) after spontaneous healing.

6 Discussion

Yahia Chérif et al. from Prof. Muraine's working group in Rouen (France) described the intracameral injection of air with pre-descemetal compression sutures perpendicular to the tear. A reduction in corneal edema in acute keratoconus was already seen on the first postoperative day [13]. This work was the reason for integrating this technique of "Muraine sutures" into everyday clinical practice at the Department of Ophthalmology at the Saarland University Medical Center in January 2017.

Rajaraman et al. showed in a retrospective study that an intracameral injection with 0.2 ml perfluoropropane (14% C3F8) combined with compression sutures over the entire corneal thickness led to clearing in 8.8 ± 4.9 days. As a prophylaxis, the patients received acetazolamide 250 mg twice daily for 5 days and had to remain in supine position for 3 days [19].

Miyata et al. performed intracameral injections with 0.1 ml filtered air. 2.4 ± 1.3 injections per eye were performed and patients received acetazolamide 750 mg/d for 3 days as a prophylaxis. This resulted in a persistence of the edema of 20.1 ± 9 days. Without air injection, the time span was 64.7 ± 34.6 days [15].

Panda et al. demonstrated the efficacy of intracameral sulphur hexafluoride (20% SF6) in acute hydrops corneae. The patients received acetazolamide 250 mg 3 times a day and had to maintain supine position. The corneal edema healed within 4 weeks [16].

Basu et al. investigated the results of intracameral perfluoropropane (14% C_3F_8) in the treatment of hydrops corneae. Surgical iridectomies were performed due to postoperative pressure elevations. A supine position had to be maintained for 2 weeks. The time between the start of treatment and completion was 57.2 ± 37.1 days for keratoconus with gas injection and 104 ± 51.4 days for the control group. For keratoglobus and keratotorus, no significant difference to the control group was found [14].

In 2013, Vajpayee et al. performed AS-OCT-guided corneal stab incisions for intrastromal drainage of fluid in combination with intracameral air/gas injection for effective management of five patients with severe acute corneal hydrops [17].

Recently, Bachmann et al. proposed a mini-DMEK as a patch for early sealing of the Descemet defect [18]. However, this technique is likely to be reserved for microsurgical artists, typically with a greatly reduced view into the anterior chamber.

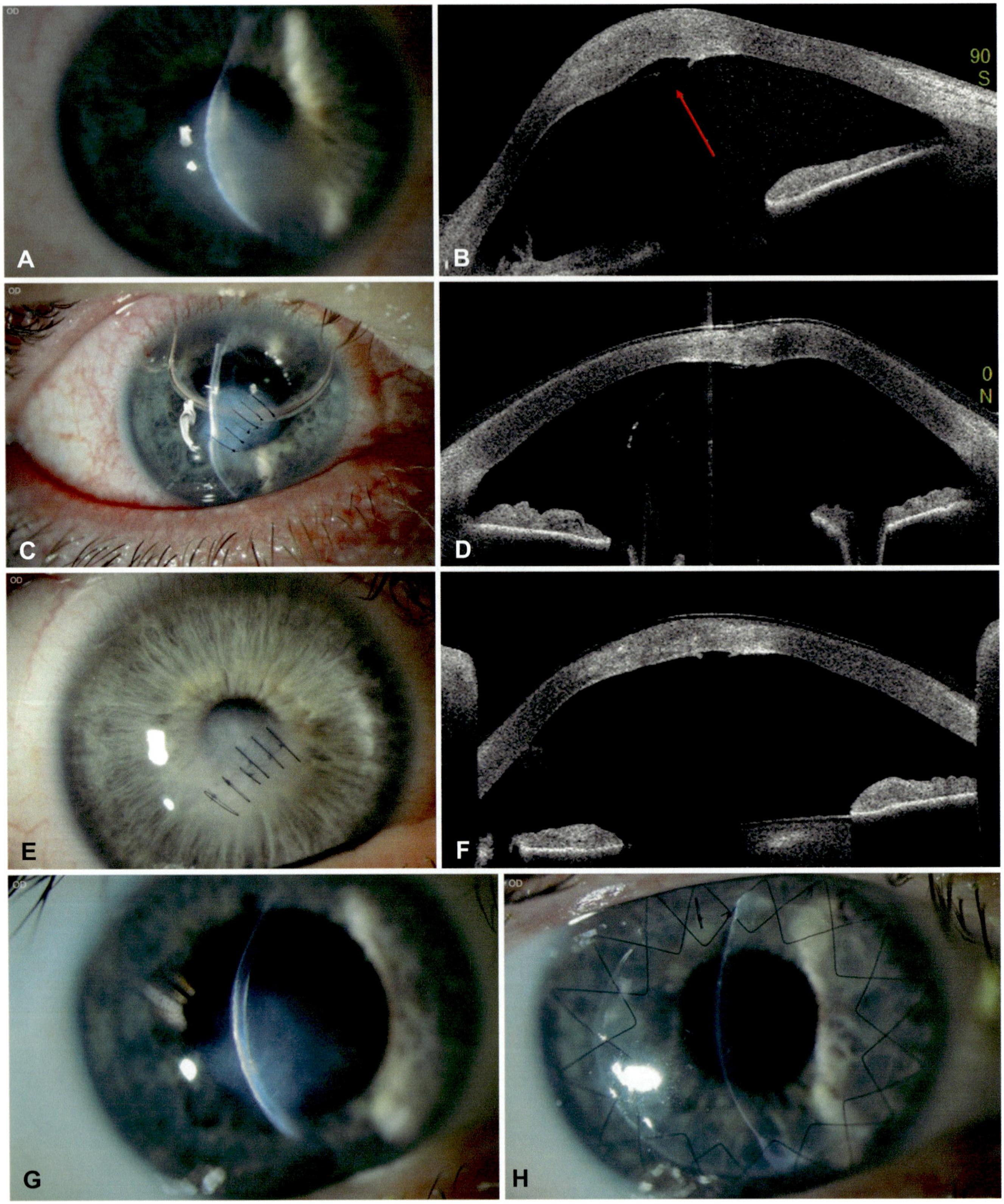

Fig. 3 **Preoperative**: 30-year-old female patient with acute corneal hydrops. (**A**) Clinical picture in the acute stage, (**B**) AS-OCT in the acute stage with Descemet rupture (red arrow), (**C**) On the 1st postoperative day after 6 Muraine sutures perpendicular to the Descemet tear and air in the anterior chamber, the cornea has significantly cleared, (**D**) The AS-OCT showed a clear reduction in corneal swelling on the 1st preoperative day. (**E**) 6 weeks postop before suture removal, (**F**) AS-OCT 6 weeks postop. (**G**) Stable scar 3 months postop before excimer laser PKP. (**F**) 6 weeks after excimer laser PKP (8.0/8.1 mm) with double continuous cross-stitch suture according to Hoffmann

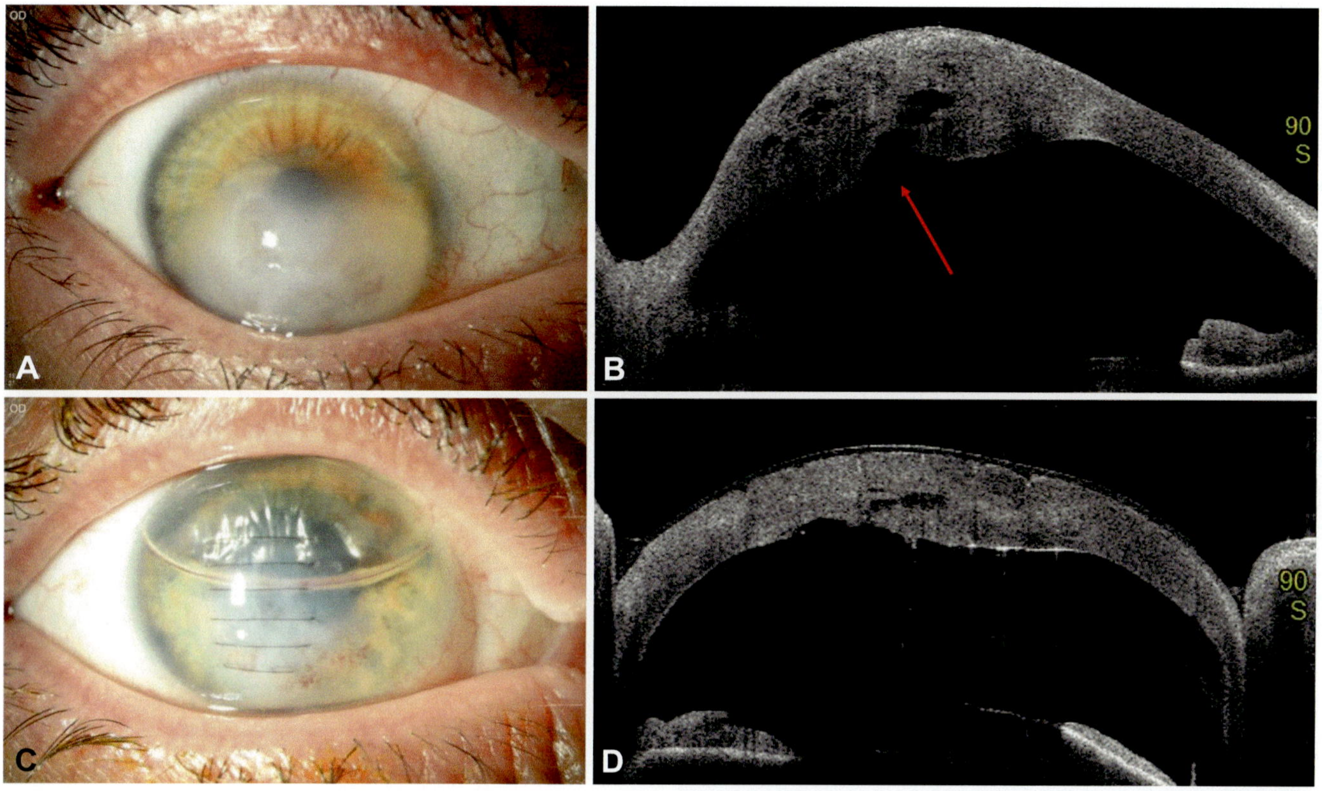

Fig. 4 (**A, B**) 38-year-old patient with excessive acute corneal hydrops. (**A**) Clinical picture in the acute stage, (**B**) AS-OCT in the acute stage with Descemet rupture (red arrow) and dramatic corneal swelling, (**C**) On the 1st postoperative day after 6 Muraine sutures perpendicular to the Descemet tear and air in the anterior chamber, the cornea already partially cleared, (**D**) The AS-OCT showed significant reduction of the corneal swelling on the 1st postoperative day

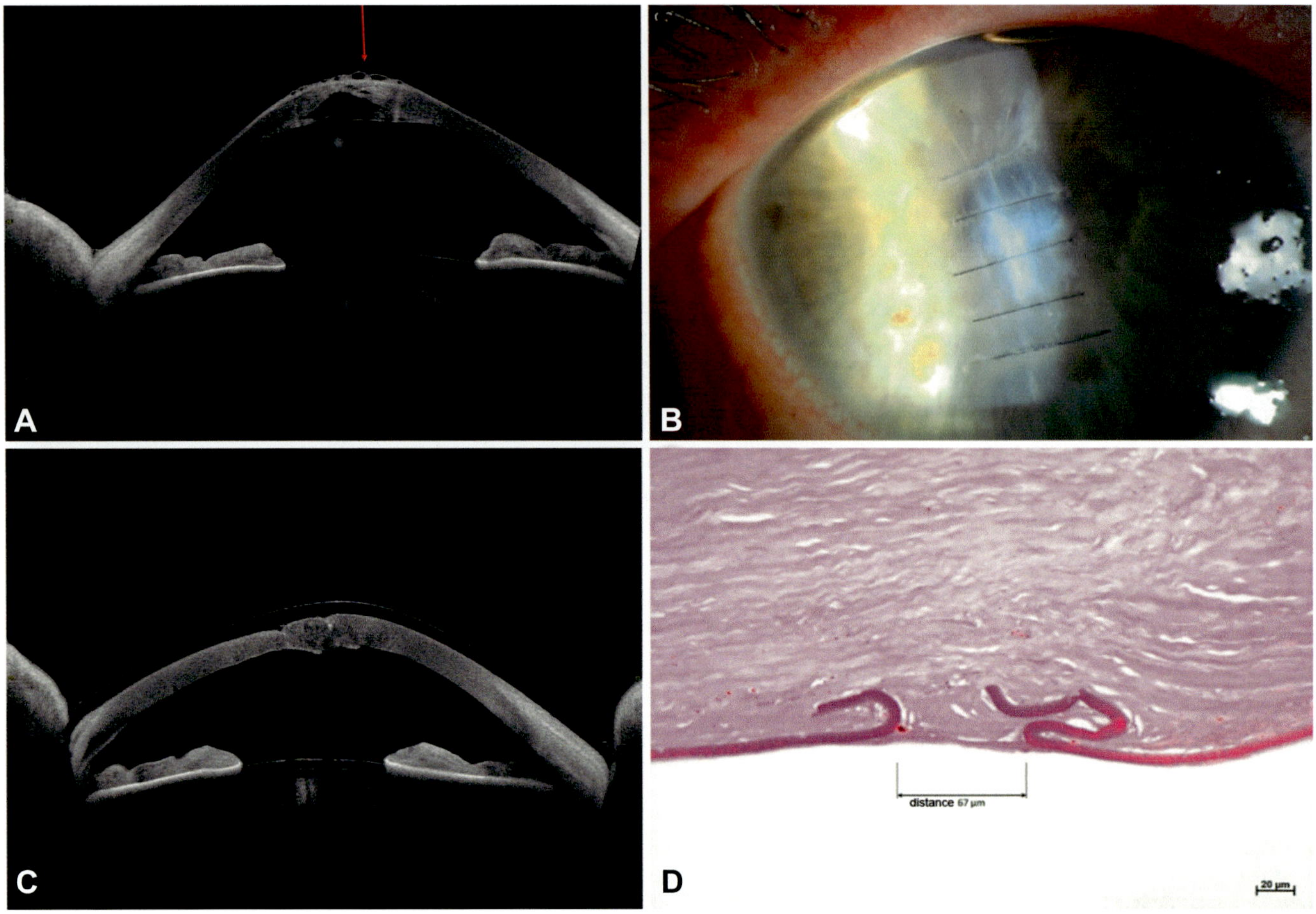

Fig. 5 50-year-old patient with corneal hydrops. (**A**) AS-OCT in the acute stage with bullous keratopathy (red arrow), (**B**) Slit lamp biomicroscopy 3 days after 5 Muraine sutures. (**C**) AS-OCT 3 days after 5 Muraine sutures. (**D**) Histologic image (PAS staining) of a section perpendicular to the Descemet tear after PKP 3 months after corneal hydrops: The distance between the Descemet ends is only 67 µm

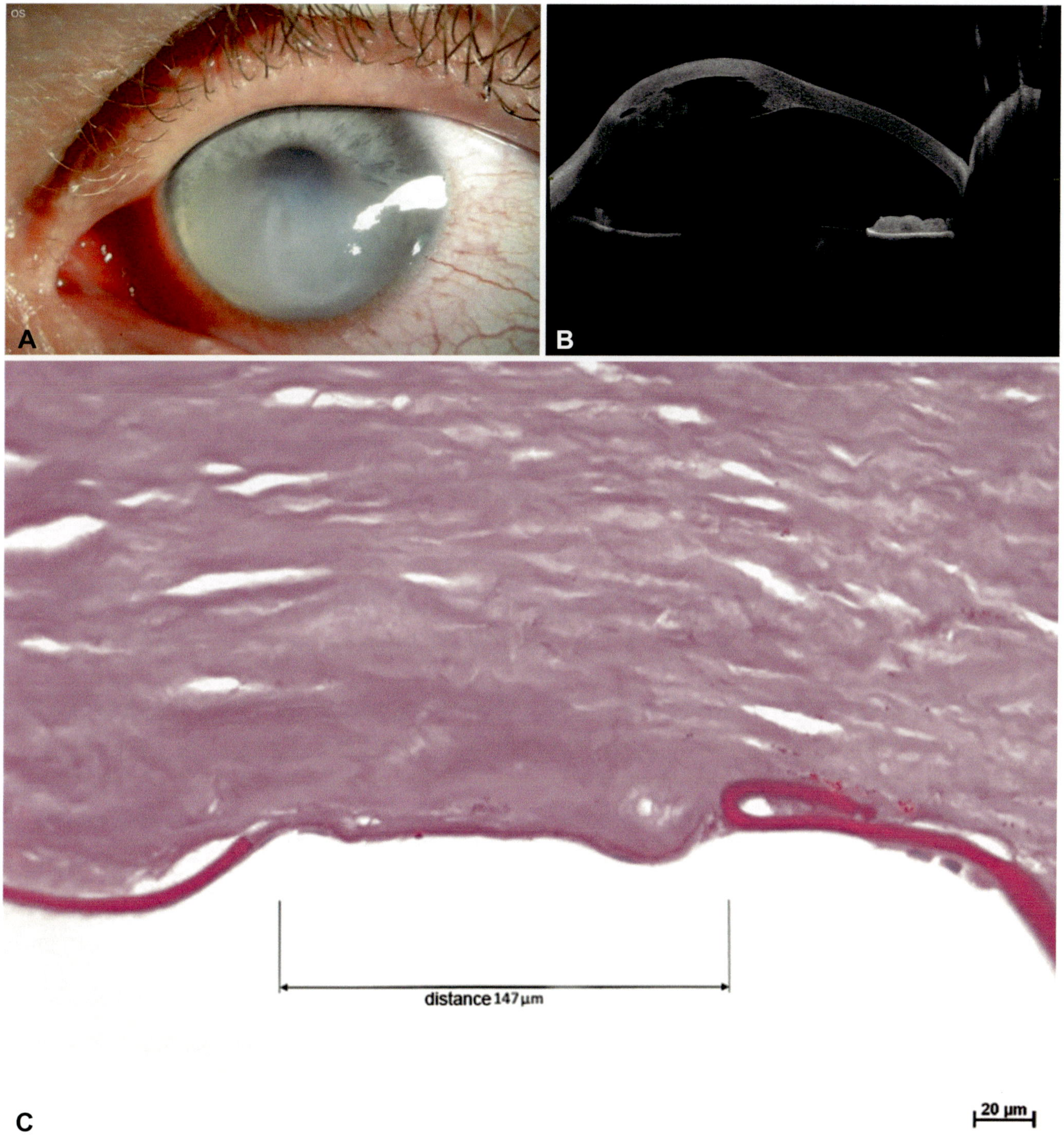

Fig. 6 37-year-old patient with corneal hydrops treated with Muraine sutures. (**A**) Clinical image in the acute stage, (**B**) AS-OCT in the acute stage, (**C**) Histological image (PAS staining) of a section perpendicular to the Descemet tear after PKP 4 months after corneal hydrops: The distance between the Descemet ends is only 147 µm

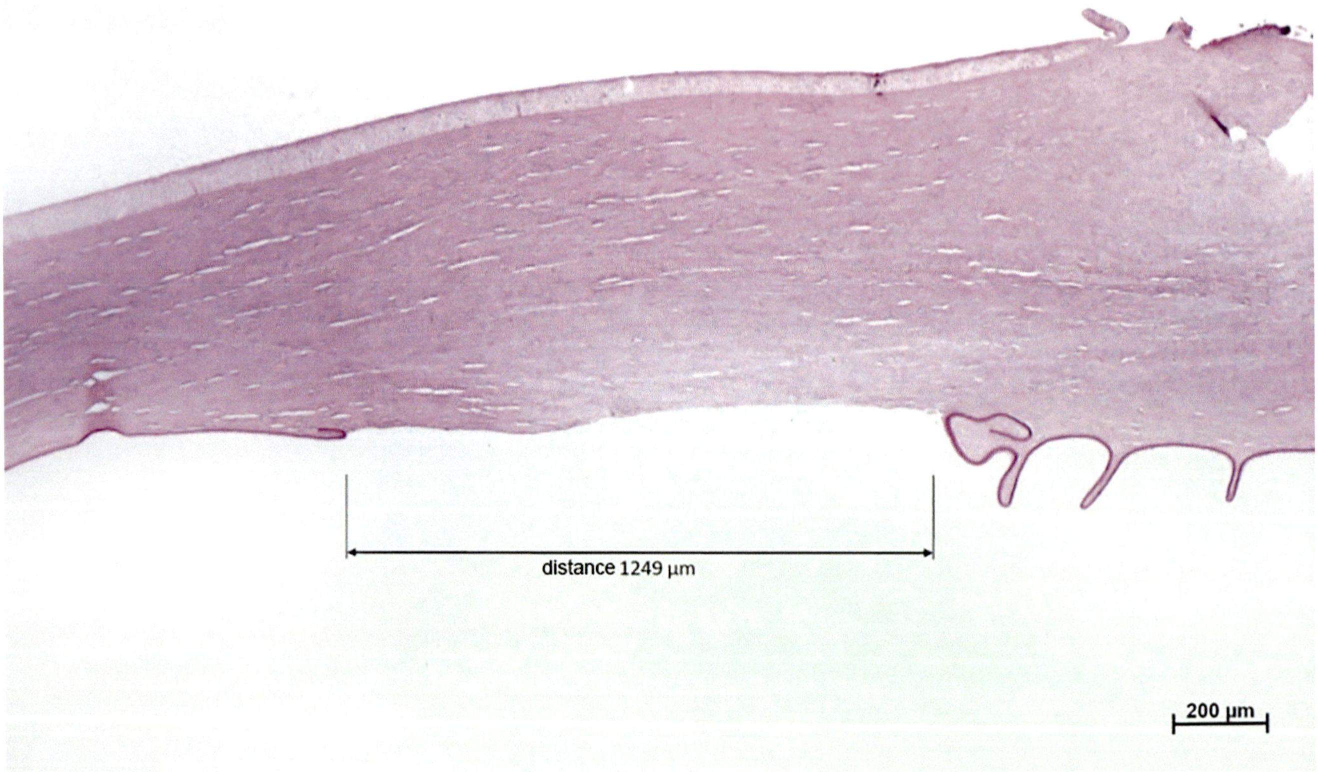

Fig. 7 Histological image (PAS staining) of a section perpendicular to the Descemet tear after PKP due to a corneal scar after spontaneous progression of a corneal hydrops without Muraine sutures: The distance between the Descemet ends is 1249 µm

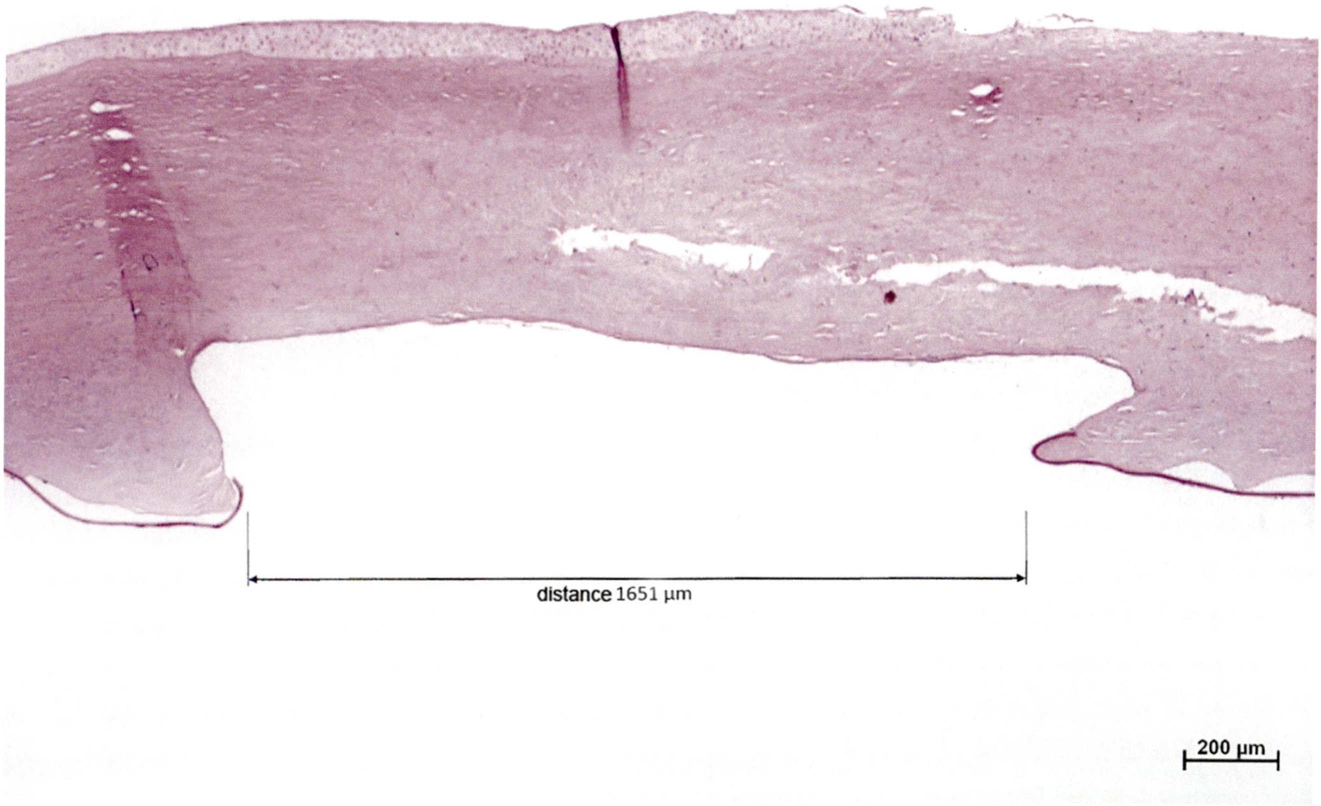

Fig. 8 Histologic image (PAS staining) of a section perpendicular to the Descemet tear after PKP due to a corneal scar after spontaneous progression of a corneal hydrops without Muraine sutures: the distance between the Descemet ends is 1651 µm

7 Conclusion

Our own clinical results show a rapid and significant reduction in corneal thickness and a rapid improvement in visual acuity after deep stromal 10–0 nylon compression sutures and air tamponade. Deep stromal "Muraine sutures" appear to be an effective and safe procedure to promptly reduce corneal swelling in acute corneal hydrops, allowing faster refitting of contact lenses and, if necessary, earlier corneal transplantation [23].

8 Summary for Practical Use

- Acute keratoconus is usually a self-limiting corneal disease, although it is always associated with considerable visual impairment.
- Surgical intervention using very deep 10–0 nylon compression sutures with intracameral air or gas injection leads to a rapid reduction in corneal edema and a faster increase in visual acuity.
- A penetrating keratoplasty can thus either be avoided or, in the case of contact lens intolerance, can be performed more quickly without having to worry about suture loosening as after keratoplasty in the acute stage of hydrops. This is particularly important for young keratoconus patients in terms of professional career and overall life planning.

References

1. Goebels S, Seitz B, Langenbucher A. Diagnostics and stage-oriented therapy of keratoconus: introduction to the Homburg keratoconus center (HKC). Ophthalmologe. 2013;110:808–9.
2. Sideroudi H, Flockerzi E, Daas L, Jullien T, Xanthopoulou K, Hamon L, Seitz B. Baseline characteristics of 1976 patients with ectatic corneal disorders at a single center from 2010 to 2021: a cross-sectional study. Eye Contact Lens. 2023;49:392–8.
3. Alfaro Rangel R, Lepper S, Langenbucher A, Szentmáry N, Seitz B. 8.5/8.6-mm excimer laser assisted penetrating keratoplasties in

a tertiary corneal subspecialty referral center–indications and outcomes in 107 eyes. Cornea. 2020;39:806–11.
4. Seitz B, Szentmáry N, Langenbucher A, Hager T. Viestenz Ar, Janunts E, El-Husseiny M. PKP for keratoconus-from hand/motor trephine to excimer laser and back to femtosecond laser. Klin Monbl Augenheilkd. 2016;233:727–36.
5. Seitz B, Daas L, Milioti G, Szentmáry N, Langenbucher A, Suffo S. Excimer laser-assisted penetrating keratoplasty: on 1 July 2019 excimer laser penetrating keratoplasty celebrates its 30th anniversary. Video article. Ophthalmologe. 2019;116:1221–30.
6. Basu S, Vaddavalli PK, Vemuganti GK, Ali MH, Murthy SI. Anterior segment optical coherence tomography features of acute corneal hydrops. Cornea. 2012;31:479–85.
7. Tuft SJ, Gregory WM, Buckley RJ. Acute corneal hydrops in keratoconus. Ophthalmology. 1994;101:1738–44.
8. Maamri A, Hamon L, Daas L, Seitz B. A 63-year-old male patient with acute visual deterioration after penetrating keratoplasty for keratoconus. Ophthalmologe. 2021;118:728–31.
9. Berger T, Seitz B, Flockerzi E, Suffo S, Flockerzi FA, Berger M, Szentmáry N, Daas L. Surgical management of complicated Descemet's membrane detachment in corneas without prior endothelial keratoplasty. Graefes Arch Clin Exp Ophthalmol. 2024; 262(3):879–89.
10. Bosic V, Mudassar H, Seitz B, Flockerzi E. Is there a predisposition for developing corneal hydrops in keratoconus?-Tomographic and biomechanical analysis of the fellow eyes. Acta Ophthalmol. 2025;103(5):e281–e289.
11. Barsam A, Petrushkin H, Brennan N, Bunce C, Xing W, Foot B, Tuft S. Acute corneal hydrops in keratoconus: a national prospective study of incidence and management. Eye. 2015;29:469–74.
12. Seitz B, El-Husseiny M, Langenbucher A, Szentmáry N. Prophylaxis and management of complications in penetrating keratoplasty. Ophthalmologe. 2013;110:605–13.
13. Yahia Chérif H, Afriat JGM, Delcampe A, Attal P, Gross H, Muraine M. Efficacy and safety of pre-descemet's membrane sutures for management of acute corneal hydrops in keratoconus. Br J Ophthalmol. 2015;99:773–7.
14. Basu S, Vaddavalli PK, Ramappa M, Shah S, Murthy SI, Sangwan VS. Intracameral perfluoropropane gas in the treatment of acute corneal hydrops. Ophthalmol. 2011;118(5):934–9.
15. Miyata K, Tsuji H, Tanabe T, Mimura Y, Amano S, Oshika T. Intracameral air injection for acute hydrops in keratoconus. Am J Ophthalmol. 2002;133:750–2.
16. Panda A, Aggarwal A, Madhavi P, Wagh VB, Dada T, Kumar A, Mohan S. Management of acute corneal hydrops secondary to keratoconus with intracameral injection of sulfur hexafluoride (SF6). Cornea. 2007;26:1067–9.
17. Vajpayee RB, Maharana PK, Kaweri L, Sharma N, Jhanji V. Intrastromal fluid drainage with air tamponade: anterior segment optical coherence tomography guided technique for the management of acute corneal hydrops. Br J Ophthalmol. 2013;97:834–6.
18. Bachmann B, Händel A, Siebelmann S, Matthaei M, Cursiefen C. Mini-Descemet membrane endothelial Keratoplasty for the early treatment of acute corneal hydrops in keratoconus. Cornea. 2019;38:1043–8.
19. Rajaraman R, Singh S, Raghavan A, Karkhansi A. Efficacy and safety of intracameral perfluoropropane (C3F8) tamponade and compression sutures for the management of acute corneal hydrops. Cornea. 2009;28:317–20.
20. Schießl G, Suffo S, Seitz B. Muraine sutures accelerate healing of corneal hydrops in acute keratotorus. Ophthalmologe. 2019;116:665–8.
21. Seitz B, Schießl G, Razafimino S, Flockerzi F, Dahle J, Daas L, Flockerzi E. Muraine sutures for corneal hydrops. Ophthalmo-Chirurgie. 2020;32:267–275.
22. Tóth G, Szentmáry N, Langenbucher A, Akhmedova E, El-Husseiny M, Seitz B. Comparison of excimer laser versus femtosecond laser assisted trephination in penetrating keratoplasty–a retrospective study. Adv Ther. 2019;36:3471–82.
23. Liu Y, Seitz B, Langenbucher A, Nguyen NX, Naumann GOH. Impact of preoperative corneal curvature on the outcome of penetrating keratoplasty in keratoconus. Cornea. 2003;22:409–412.

Amniotic Membrane Transplantation AMT (Patch, Graft, Sandwich)—Techniques and Integration Patterns into the Human Cornea

Miklós D. Resch and Berthold Seitz

Abstract

Amniotic membrane (AM) transplantation (AMT) is a surgically complex technique in ocular surface therapy. The beneficial mechanical and biological qualities of AM provide multiple options for the surgical and pharmacological treatment of corneal and conjunctival diseases. The wide range of indications requires individual surgical plans for the AMT. The AM can serve as a substrate for substituting corneal and conjunctival tissues and can be integrated into the ocular tissues in multiple forms in correlation with the indicating pathology and surgical technique. The various clinical applications for AMT usage in an ophthalmic setting, ranging from commonly used applications to less mainstream approaches can often be identified in postoperative histological examinations (integration patterns).

Keywords

Amniotic membrane · Transplantation · Cornea · Ocular surface · Integration · Conjunctiva

Supplementary Information The online version contains supplementary material available at https://doi.org/10.1007/978-3-031-65422-0_46.

M. D. Resch (✉)
Department of Ophthalmology, Semmelweis University, Budapest, Hungary
e-mail: miklosresch@gmail.com

B. Seitz
Department of Ophthalmology, Saarland University Medical Center, Homburg, Germany

1 Introduction

Human amniotic membrane (AM) was first applied as a substrate in ophthalmology by De Rötth almost a century ago [1]. After a several decade long pause it has become more frequently employed in ocular surface surgery after its use in ophthalmology had been reintroduced in the 1990s by Kim and Tseng [2, 3]. The easy availability and anatomical structure, the better understanding of the multiple benefical properties of AM and the increasing immunological knowledge made it a very improving field of ocular surface disease management even in very challenging cases.

Origin and structure of AM. AM is the innermost, avascular layer of the placenta with an average thickness of 200–500 µm. The AM is of ectodermal origin and consists of epithelium, basement membrane and stroma (Fig. 1). The stroma comprises 98% of the AM and is built of collagenes, elastic fibres and extracellular matrix proteins. The microstructure of AM is highly resembling the cornea and conjunctiva as well. It is elastic like the conjunctiva, but much thinner and not completely transparent in contrast to the cornea due to the irregular organisation of collagen fibres. The AM can be harvested from the placenta during Cesarean section and can be preserved as tissue for transplantation at −80 °C. AM transplantation (AMT) is useful clinically due to its unique structure, biocompatible composition and subsequent biological functions.

Therapeutic mechanisms of AMT. The AM after transplantation can act as a biological contact lens on the ocular surface, it can serve as a barrier and decreases pain by covering the nerve endings of the cornea. Beyond the favourable mechanical properies, the AM has multiple beneficial biological features. The potential role of an AMT in ophthalmology is mainly to support damaged tissue, protect defects from further degeneration or breakdown and to promote wound healing and recellularisation. AM can provide a milieu by several biological properties, including a lack of immunogenicity (reducing the risk of inciting

B. Seitz et al. (eds.), *Atlas on Cornea*, https://doi.org/10.1007/978-3-031-65422-0_46

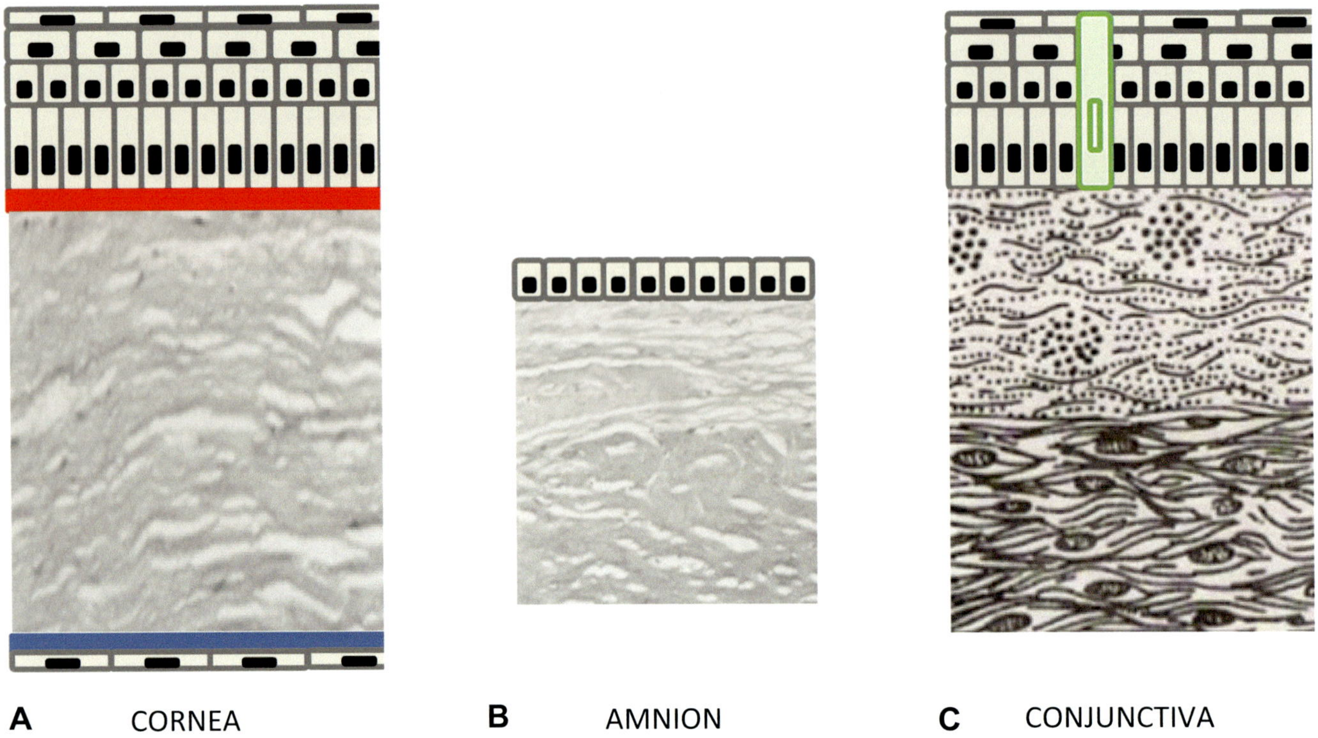

Fig. 1 The schematic structure of the cornea (**A**) AM (**B**) and conjunctiva (**C**) Note the similar structure of the stroma of AM and conjunctiva. The cornea is covered by a multilayered epithelium with basement membrane and Bowman layer (red), AM is covered by a monolayer of cuboid epithelial cells, and in the multliayered conjunctival epithelium, goblet cells are also shown (green). Descemet membrane is blue in the cornea (**A**)

an immune response), preserves and supports stem cells, inhibits neoplastic, inflammatory, angiogenic and fibroblastic cells. Cytokine activities of AM include epidermal growth factor, keratocyte growth factor and neurotrophic substances that support the wound healing. The AM contributes to the regeneration of corneal epithelium, facilitation of migrating epithelial cells and reinforcing basal epithelial cell adhesion to the basement membrane. AM substances also play a role in the promotion of cell differentiation and blockade of apoptosis. AM can control pain, provide anti-microbial benefits and act as a drug reservoir. Several factors are present in AM and in the amniotic fluid including bactricidin, beta-lysin, lysozyme, transferrin, and immunoglobulins [3–5].

2 Indications of AMT

The clinical applications of AMT are covering a wide range of ocular pathologies [6]. The indications can be divided in two groups according to the purpose of the surgery. On one hand, the aim of AMT can be the temporary covering of the ocular surface, on the other hand the the aim of AMT is the permanent integration of AM as new basement membrane into the human cornea. In some cases the combination of the above mentioned two goals are targeted [7].

Temporary cover (patch or onlay). In these cases AM remains on the ocular surface for a few weeks, then absorbs or falls off spontaneously:

- Corneal and conjunctival injuries, e.g. burn or chemical injuries [8, 9]
- Neurotrophic ulcer [10]
- Epithelial defect after keratoplasty [11]
- Band keratopathy [12]
- Excimer laser phototherapeutic keratectomy (PTK), e.g. lattice corneal dystrophy
- Persistent corneal epithelial defects whithout ulceration [13]
- Acute Stevens–Johnson syndrome [14, 15]
- Combination with high risk corneal transplantation [16, 17]
- After antiglaucoma surgery to cover bleb or shunt [18].

Permanent cover, integration (graft or inlay). The AM is integrated into the corneal and conjunctival tissue:

- Tiny perforating or especially not perforating corneal ulcers [19, 20]
- Bacterial keratitis after appropriate antibiotic therapy [20]

- Peripheral ulcerative keratitis [21]
- Symblepharon or fornix reconstruction [22, 23]
- Ocular pemphigoid [24]
- Conjunctival reconstruction after tumor removal [25]
- Corneal or conjunctival scar removal
- Limbal stem cell insufficiency
- Recurrent pterygium [26, 27]
- Conjunctivochalasis
- Strabismus surgery [28].

Multiple layers of AM inlays can be applied for integration according to the lesion size and depth.

The „Sandwich" technique is the combination of patch and graft techniques in case of complex ocular surface lesions with tissue loss and epithelial defect. Indication is getting more and more complex [29].

3 Surgical Techniques

Preparation of AM. AM can be obtained during caesarean section as a part of the placenta after meticulus testing for transmittable infections. Originally AM was used immediately after delivery with the risk of transmitting microbial infections. The current regulations give a detailed description of the preparation and preservation of AM [30]. There are several methods of AM preservation [31]. At some degree, preservation can compromise the integrity of the tissue. The most common technique of preservation is cryopreservation in a storage medium containing cryoprotectants such as glycerol, and freezing to −80 °C [32]. The AM can be preserved via freeze-drying or lyophilisation. Freeze-drying means cooling the AM to −80 °C and then water is removed by sublimation. Lyophilised AM tissue can then be stored at room temperature for long periods, thus facilitating transportation. Cytokines, growth factors and total protein content are affected to some extent by all preservation methods (especially by lyophilisation), but its beneficial qualities are still preserved after cryopreservation [33–36].

Surgical techniques of AMT. Several techniques have been developed due to the flexible options provided by AMT [29]. Traditionally AM pieces are fixed with 10/0 nylon sutures, but fibrin glue or cyanoacrylate glue, or sutureless techniques have been established. In addition, a bandage contact lens fitting can improve AMT survival (Fig. 2).

Patch (onlay) AMT. Used for corneal diseases with non healing epithelial defects with no or only shallow stromal defects. In these cases the AM (ca. 16 mm in diameter) is sutured episclerally covering the whole cornea from limbus to limbus over the peripheral epithelial remnants and the centrally denuded stroma. The current understanding is that the local epithelium

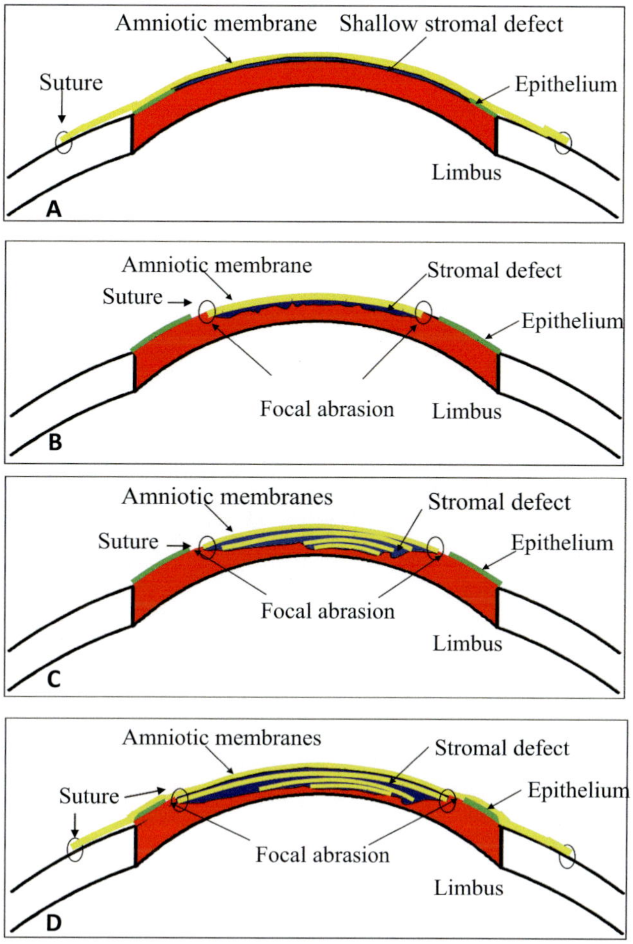

Fig. 2 Schematic drawings of various techniques of AMT. (Adapted from Seitz et al. in Archives 2006) (**A**) Patch = onlay. Used for corneal diseases with non healing epithelial defects with no or only shallow stromal defects. In these cases the AM is sutured episclerally beyond the limbus over the peripheral epithelial remnants and the centrally denuded stroma. The aim is to promote the corneal epithelium to grow under the AM, the epithelial defect is closed and the AM as a natural "contact lens" is dissolving after a few weeks. (**B**) Single layer graft = inlay. Used in case of shallow stromal defects. This graft is fixed in the shallow stromal defect with single interrupted sutures in the periphery of the corneal ulcer. Before transplantation a rim of deepithelialization and/or pannectomy around the stromal defect is prepared to make sure that no epithelium remains under the graft. In this case the corneal epithelium is supposed to grow over the AM, which provides a new basement membrane. (**C**) Multilayer graft = inlay. This technique is applied in case of deep stromal defects. The corneal ulcer is filled up with smaller parts of AM placed on each other layer by layer without sutures before a superficial graft is sutured to the periphery of the ulcer. Accordingly, in these cases the epithelium is supposed to grow over the uppermost layer of this multilayer graft. (**D**) Sandwich = graft(s) + patch. Used in corneal ulcers with unstable epithelium also in the periphery of the cornea, such as in ulcerative bullous keratopathy or in ulcerative herpetic keratouveitis with complete endothelial decompensation or stromal infiltration. A single or multilayer inlay is combined with an onlay as described in 2 (**B**) or (**C**) In these cases the epithelium is supposed not to grow under the patch but grow over the uppermost graft

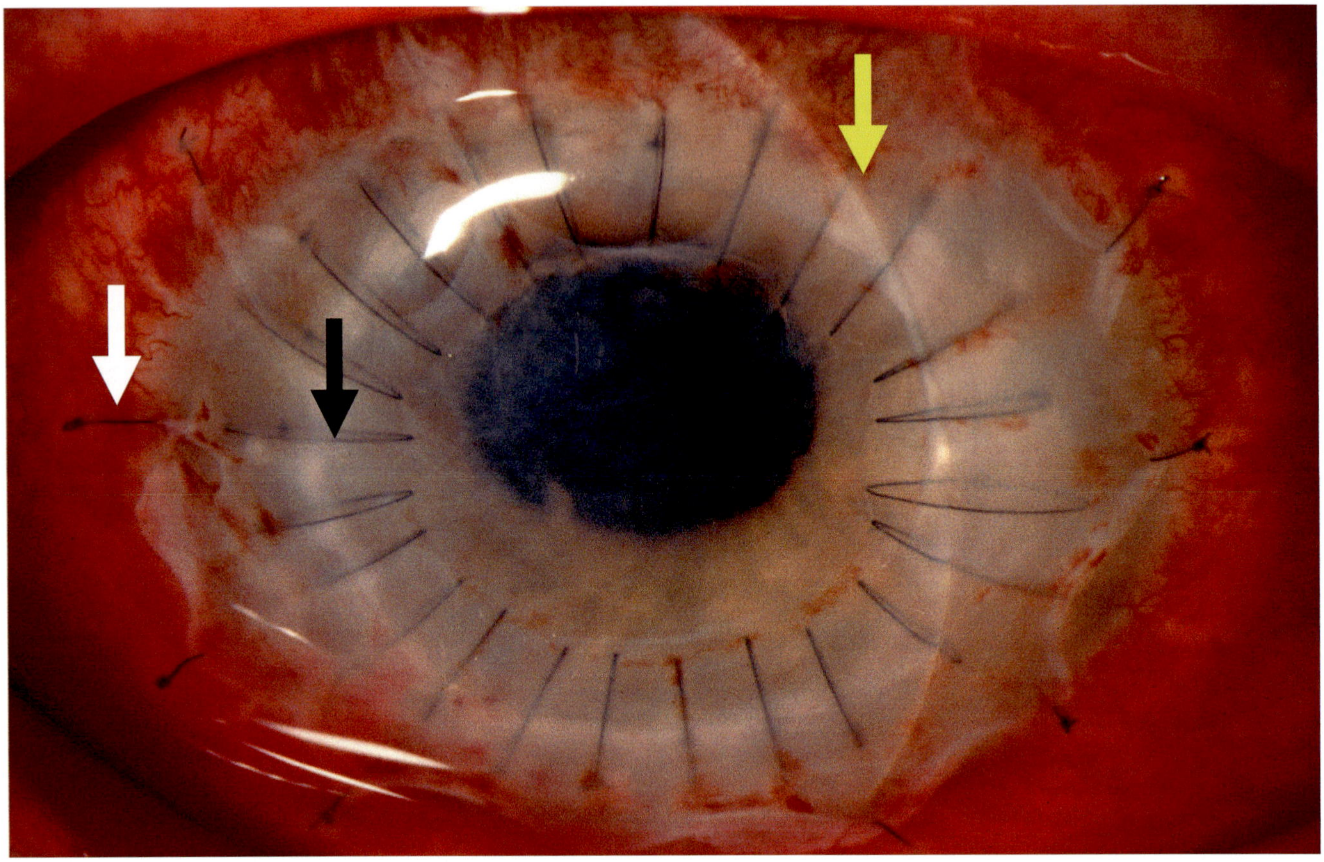

Fig. 3 Postoperative photography after AMT Patch performed simultanously with corneal transplantation. Keratoplasty single sutures (black arrow) for corneal transplant and episcleral single sutures for AM patch (white arrow), yellow arrow points to the edge of the decentered bandage contact lens

should grow under the AM, the epithelial defect is closed and the AM as a natural "contact lens" is dissolving or falling off after a few weeks [37, 38] (Figs. 2A and 3).

Graft (inlay) AMT. Single layer graft = inlay. Used in case of shallow stromal defects. This graft is fixed in the shallow stromal defect with interrupted 10–0 nylon sutures in the periphery of the corneal ulcer. Before transplantation, a rim of deepithelialization and/or pannectomy around the stromal defect is prepared to make sure that no epithelium remains under the graft. In this case the epithelium is supposed to grow over the AM, which provides a new basement membrane [38] (Figs. 2B and 4).

Multilayer graft. Used in case of deep stromal defects. Smaller parts of AM are placed layer by layer into the ground of the ulcer which is filled up without sutures before a superficial graft is sutured to the periphery of the ulcer, again after depithelialization and/or pannectomy of a ring-shaped area around the cornea ulcer. Accordingly, in these cases the epithelium is supposed to grow over the uppermost layer of this multilayer graft, but not between these layers [39] (Figs. 2C and 5).

„Sandwich" technique AMT (combination of inlay and onlay). Sandwich of graft(s) and patch technique is used in corneal ulcers with unstable epithelium also in the periphery of the swollen or inflamed cornea, such as in ulcerative bullous keratopathy or in ulcerative herpetic keratouveitis with complete endothelial decompensation or stromal infiltration. A single or multilayer inlay is combined with an onlay as described in Fig. 2B or C. In these cases the epithelium is supposed to grow under the patch but over the uppermost graft (Figs. 2D and 6).

AMT combined with keratoplasty. Simultaneous AMT and penetrating keratoplasty may improve the prognosis of corneal graft in eyes with risk of epithelial healing problems [17]. The survival of the corneal graft can be improved. Potential advantages of a simultaneous AMT with PKP are epitheliotrophic effects of the AM promoting wound healing and epithelialisation of the graft and therefore allow early topical steroid application. Second, immune modulatory and antifibrotic effects are promoting the healing process. This concept may especially be applied in case of Aniridia-Associated-Keratopathy [40].

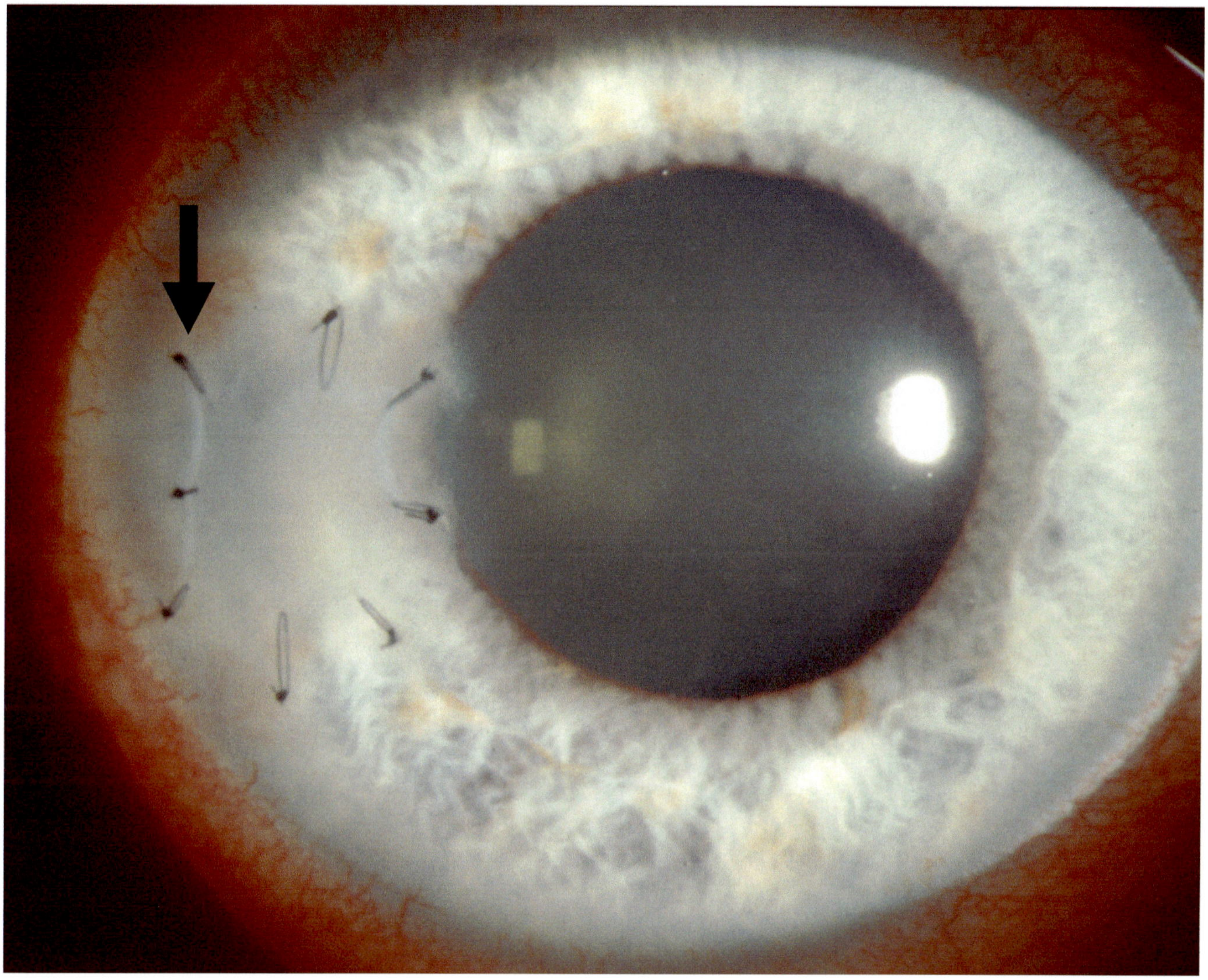

Fig. 4 Postoperative photography after AMT single layer graft. Single corneal sutures (arrow) for AM graft

AMT before keratoplasty. The above mentioned techniques are originally developed to be performed instead of or before keratoplasty. In many cases, AMT can stabilize the corneal structure and prevent perforation. The healed but opaque cornea can be replaced with a corneal graft and visual acuity improvement can be achieved [19].

AMT after keratoplasty. In eyes with ocular surface diseases especially in limbal stem cell deficiency delayed reepithelisation occurs frequently. The slow regrowth of the epithelium leaves an open surface of the graft to be affected by infection and inflammation. The antiinflammatory, antimicrobial and epithelotrophic effects of AMT can increase the survival rate of the transplanted corneas. In addition, it can control the neovascularisation of the cornea by its antiangiogenic effects, and can decrease fibrosis. This can be continued with the application of autologous serum [41].

Conjunctival and fornix reconstruction AMT. In conjunctival fibrotic cases such as after bilateral chemical burns, symblepharon or pemphigoid, there is a lack of transplantable autologous conjunctival tissue, which can be temporarily substituted by AMT (with or without oral mucosa). In these cases, sclera and fornices are covered by single layers of larger AM (Fig. 7). Fibrin glue is very effective in these situations and transpalpebral sutures can ensure the fornix reconstruction. Conjunctival reconstruction after ocular surface tumor resections might require covering the sclera with AM graft tissue that is supposed to be episclerally integrated [22] (Fig. 8).

Bioengineered cell transplantation with AMT. Ultrastructural and immunohistochemical studies showed, that the basement membrane of the AM is very similar to the corneal epithelial basement membrane, which makes it a

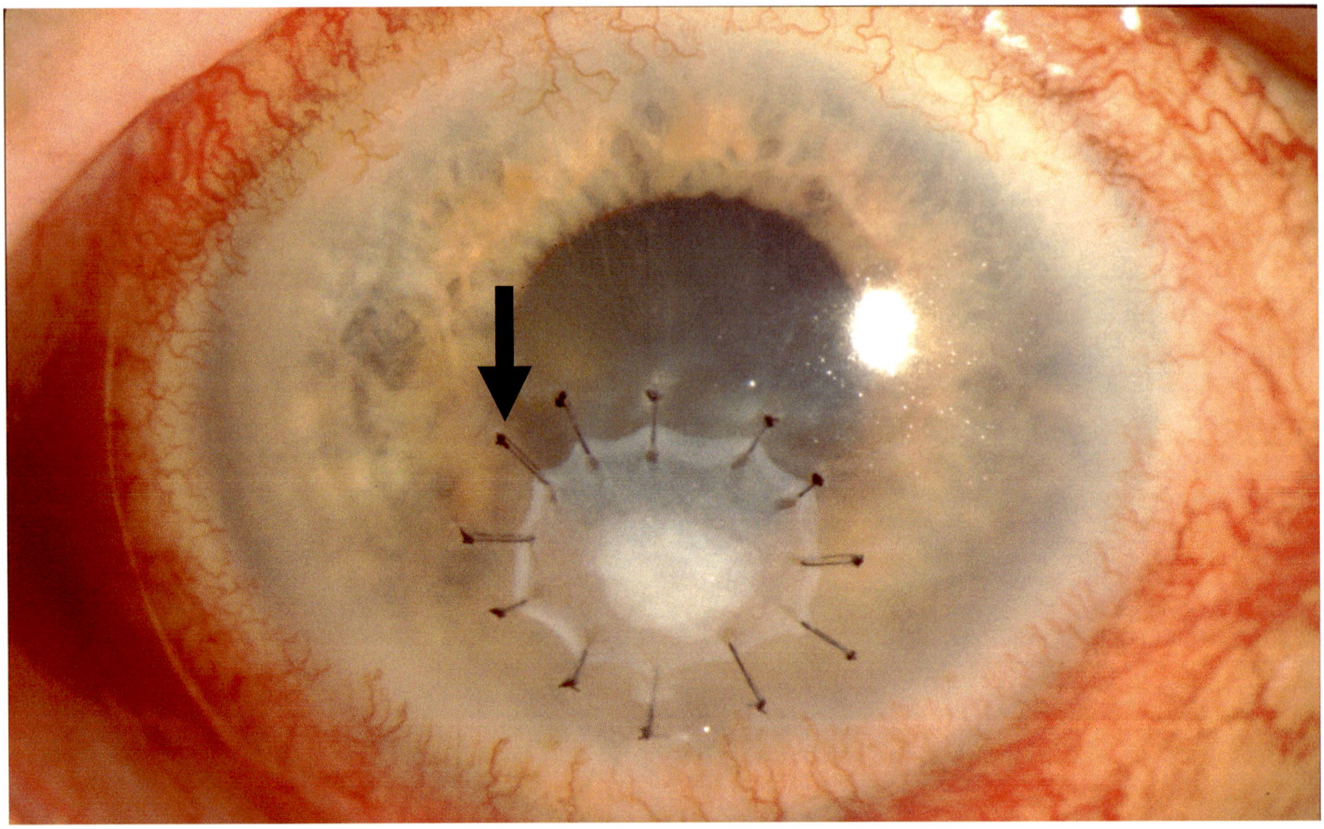

Fig. 5 Postoperative photography after triple layer graft AMT (2-2-4 mm in diameter). Single corneal sutures (arrow) for the uppermost AM graft

good niche to expand the corneal cells on [39]. AMT effectively expands the remaining limbal epithelial stem cells in patients with partial limbal stem cell deficiency. Corneal epithelial cells or limbal stem cells can be cultured on AM ex vivo, AMT is performed after ex vivo stem cell expansion, recovering not only the ocular surface, but the epithelial cell layer [35, 42, 43]. Today simple limbal epithelial transplantation (SLET) is applied for the same purpose [44].

Complications and risks of AMT. Intraoperative risk of corneal penetration has to be handled in situ. Early postoperative complications can occur due to the suture insufficiency, the early absorbance of AM. Potential risks of AMT can be the origin of AM as an allogenic tissue from a single donor, there is always an implicit risk of acquiring infectious diseases through its application. These risks can be minimized in case of adequate donor screening, testing, handling, processing and storage. By keeping the AM pieces in quarantine for 6 months before AMT the risks can be even lowered. The potential risk of prion infection must also be considered. Clinically, the semitransparent AM covering the pathological cornea can hide the fine changes e.g. retrocorneal precipitates or other signs of transplant rejection. Multiple sutures used during AMT can cause infection or neovascularisation, especially after loosening. Intraocular pressure measurement results can be affected by AMT. Late complications of AMT can be fibrosis or neovascularization of the cornea, but usually it is a consequence of the original disease.

Postoperative therapy. Postoperative medication is dependent on the ocular pathology. It is recommended for all patients to receive preservative-free antibiotic eyedrops 5 times a day, artificial tears 10 times a day, and preservative-free cycloplegics twice a day. In addition, all patients with herpetic infection are given topical gancyclovir gel 5 times a day and 5 × 400 mg systemic acyclovir for 4 weeks, and then 2 × 400 mg acyclovir for at least 6 months.

4 Microstructure of the Transplanted AM = "Integration Pattern"

Biomicroscopically, AM remains on the ocular surface for shorter or longer time depending on the surgical technique, pathology, comorbidities and treatment [45, 46]. The patch usually acts like a temporary contact lens and disappears within two weeks. Grafts however can be integrated into the corneal tissue up to several years [47].

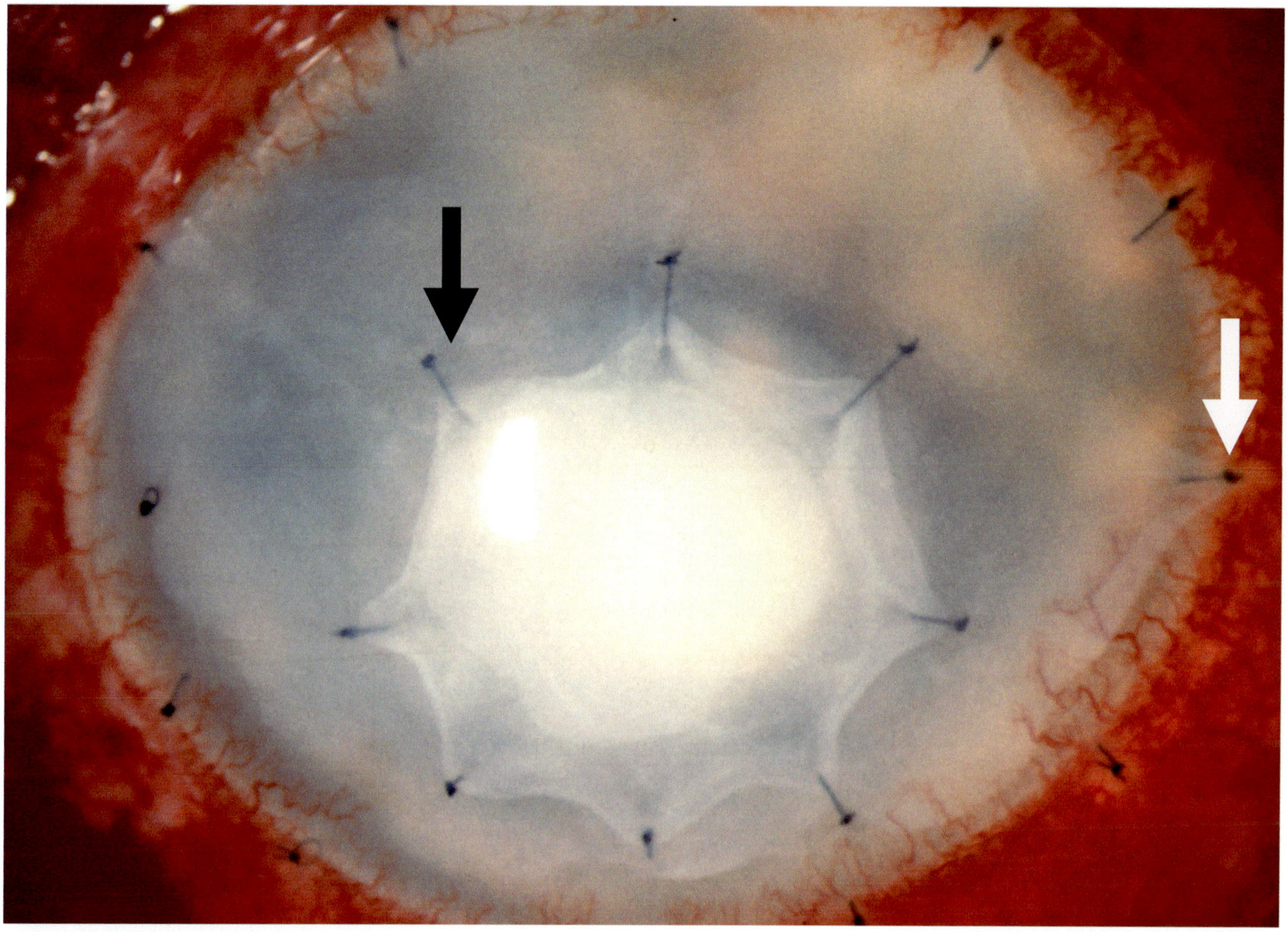

Fig. 6 Postoperative slit-lamp photography after double graft plus patch "Sandwich" technique AMT. Single corneal sutures (black arrow) for the upper AM graft and episcleral single sutures for AM patch (white arrow)

The AM can be integrated into the host corneal tissue after AMT in intraepithelial, subepithelial, or intrastromal patterns, or may remain disintegrated on the corneal surface (Fig. 9). The thicknesses of corneal epithelium and AM are extremely variable [48]. The morphology of the individual pattern seems to depend on the ocular surface disorder, and the AMT technique [29].

Intraepithelial integration of AM. Intraepithelial integration is defined if both the superficial and basal surfaces of the AM are covered by corneal epithelium (Figs. 10 and 11). It is seen if AMT was performed because of persisting epithelial defects or superficial stromal defects. On slit lamp examination intraepithelial remnants of AM are visible. By histology, corneal epithelial cells were found not only on top of the AM, but between AM and Bowman layer or superficial stroma as well. The corneal epithelial cells had strong adhesion structures (hemidesmosomes) to the AM stroma and were connected to each other by desmosomes [49].

Subepithelial integration of the AM. The most common integration pattern is subepithelial integration, defined as corneal epithelium covering only the superficial surface of the AM (Figs. 12 and 13). Subepithelial AM stroma after AMT can usually be visualized by slit lamp. The corneal epithelium becomes hyperplastic at the margin of AM stroma compensating for different thickness, resulting in a regular ocular surface contour. The corneal epithelium is of normal thickness above the AM stroma, but thicker, where no AM is beneath. The AM stroma is residing on the corneal stroma and is overgrown by corneal epithelium. The corneal epithelial cells have usually polymorphous appearance. After multilayered AMT, the integration patterns are of special interest (Figs. 14 and 15). The exact orirgin of the tissue between the AM layers is debated. (Video available as online supplement: QR code).

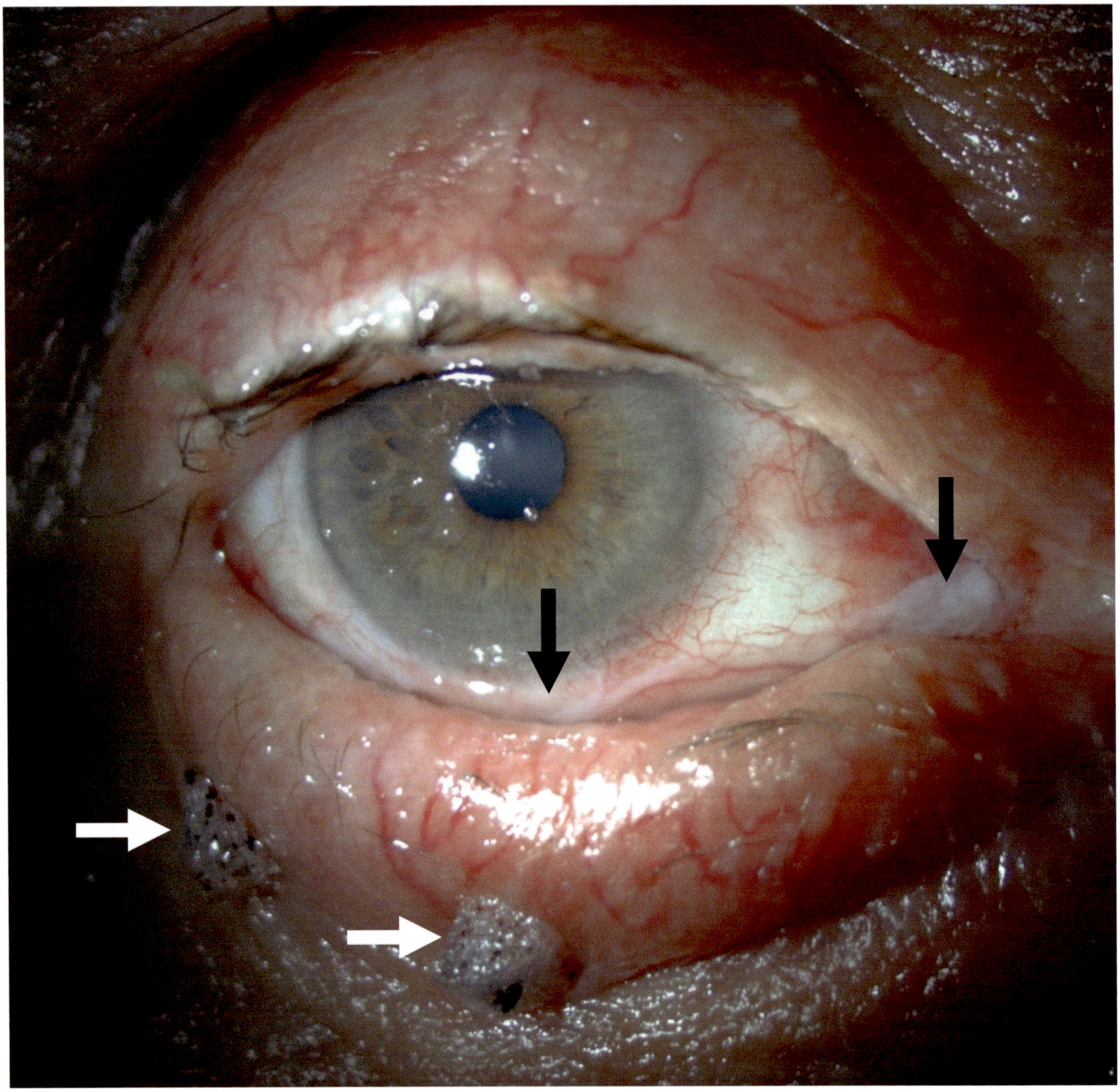

Fig. 7 Postoperative photography after fornix conjunctival reconstruction in a case of complete symblepharon due to ocular pemphigoid. The conjunctival scars are removed, the bulbar and tarsal conjunctiva is substituted with a monolayer of AM (black arrows) fixed with tissue glue and transpalpebral fornix sutures with silicone sponge (white arrows)

Please scan to access video content

Intrastromal integration of the AM. Intrastromal integration is used for cases in which AM stroma was surrounded by corneal stroma, without any contact with the corneal epithelium. This is observed after multilayered (sandwich) AMT, the technique indicated for deep stromal lesions. Biomicroscopic examination revealed that the corneal epithelium was regular and the AM stromal layers were integrated into the corneal stroma. The collagen structure of

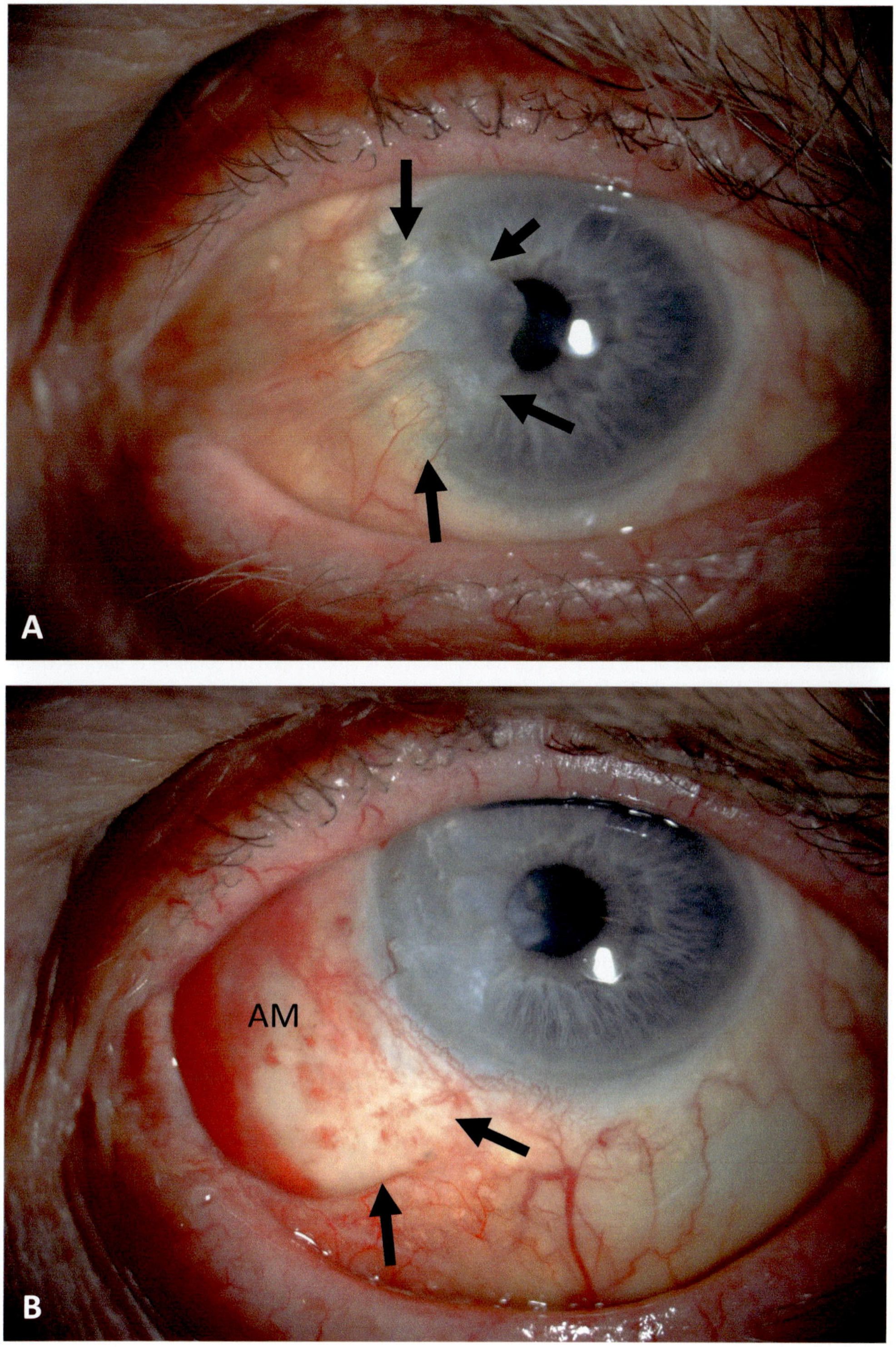

Fig. 8 Conjunctival substitution with AMT in case of conjunctival amyloidosis and pseudopterygium. (**A**) Preoperative image, edge of overgrown conjunctiva is shown with black arows. Note the cream like deposits in the conjunctiva. Autologuous conjunctiva transplantation was not possible, since the conjunctiva was affected by amyloidosis in both eyes. (**B**) Postoperative image at day 3. After removing a significant portion of the conjunctiva, the AM was fixed with tissue glue and is covering the sclera. The edge of the AM is covering the limbus and is secured under the conjunctiva (arrows). Due to the deep stromal involvement, some residual scar tissue has been left in the cornea for 8 to 11 o'clock in the mid periphery

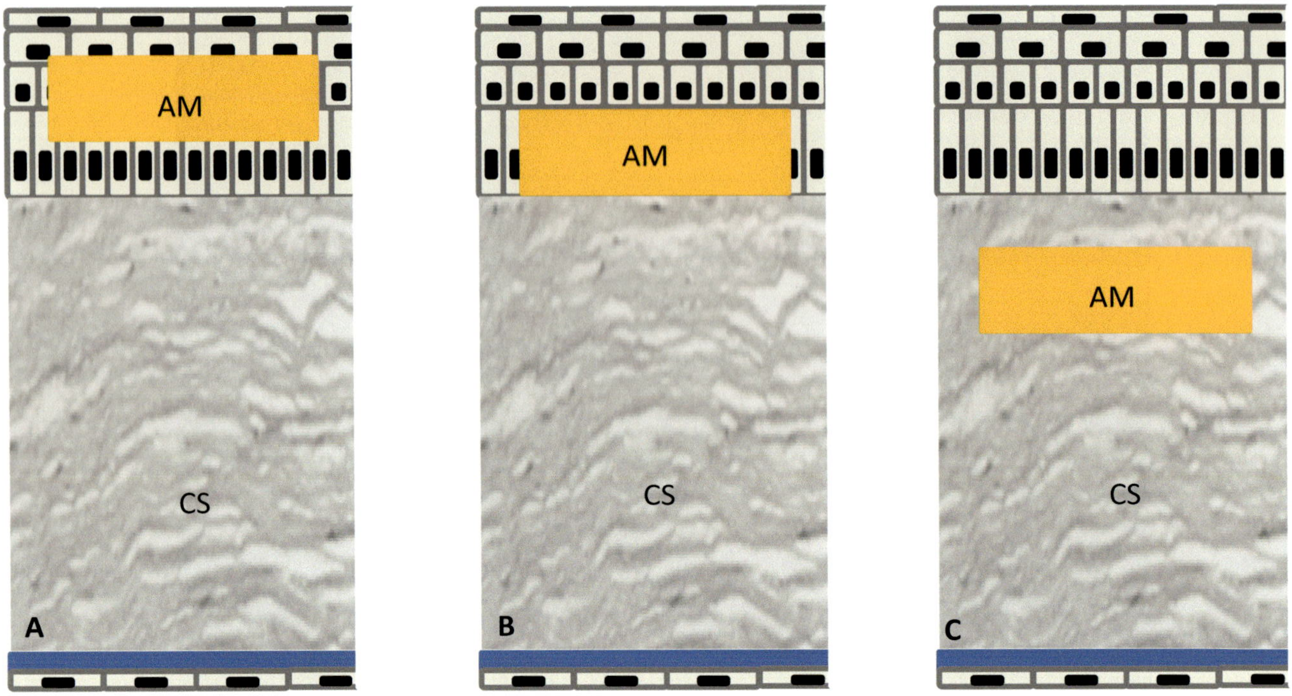

Fig. 9 Schematic drawing of a cross section of the cornea. The Bowman layer is absent, the AM (orange) is integrated into different layers of the cornea: (**A**) Intraepithelial, (**B**) Subepithelial. (**C**) Intrastromal

AM stroma is much less organized compared with the corneal stroma (Figs. 16 and 17). The amniotic stroma is usually acellular and homogeneous compared with the lamellar structure of the corneal stroma with keratocytes in the interlamellar spaces.

The application technique of AMT seems to have a great impact on the morphology of AM integration. The surgical technique is dependent on the type and severity of ocular surface disease. In general, a patch disappears most often during the first one or two weeks after AMT without remnants. Using the sandwich technique the patch is typically lost very early after AMT (similar to a single patch), but all layers of grafts should be integrated into the corneal stroma and remain there for many months or even years [29].

The type of preservation is certainly affecting the structure of AM. Freshly prepared AM (rarely used in ophthalmology) is supposed to have more intact amniotic epithelial cells, than cryopreserved AM, since cryopreservation usually interferes with the survival rate of amniotic epithelial cells. There are commercially available or dried AM on the market, which (in contrast with the cryopreserved) do not contain any viable amniotic epithelial cell or amniotic fibroblast, nor growth factors [35, 49].

5 Pharmacological Impact of AMT

AMT requires complex topical (e.g. antibiotic) treatment during the postoperative period. AMT however interferes with the ocular penetration of topical medications in two ways. On the one hand, the presence of AM limits the penetration of ocular drugs [50], on the other hand it can act as a drug reservoir [51]. Several factors can have impact on transamniotic drug penetration. Corneal thickness in ocular surface disease is rather variable. In case of ulceration, significant thinning of the cornea can be present, whilst significant corneal thickening is usually encountered in ophthalmic inflammatory conditions. On the other hand, excessive presence of fibrotic tissues in cicatricial conditions like ocular pemphigoid or in Stevens–Johnson syndrome may reduce the drug conduit towards deeper ocular tissues [52].

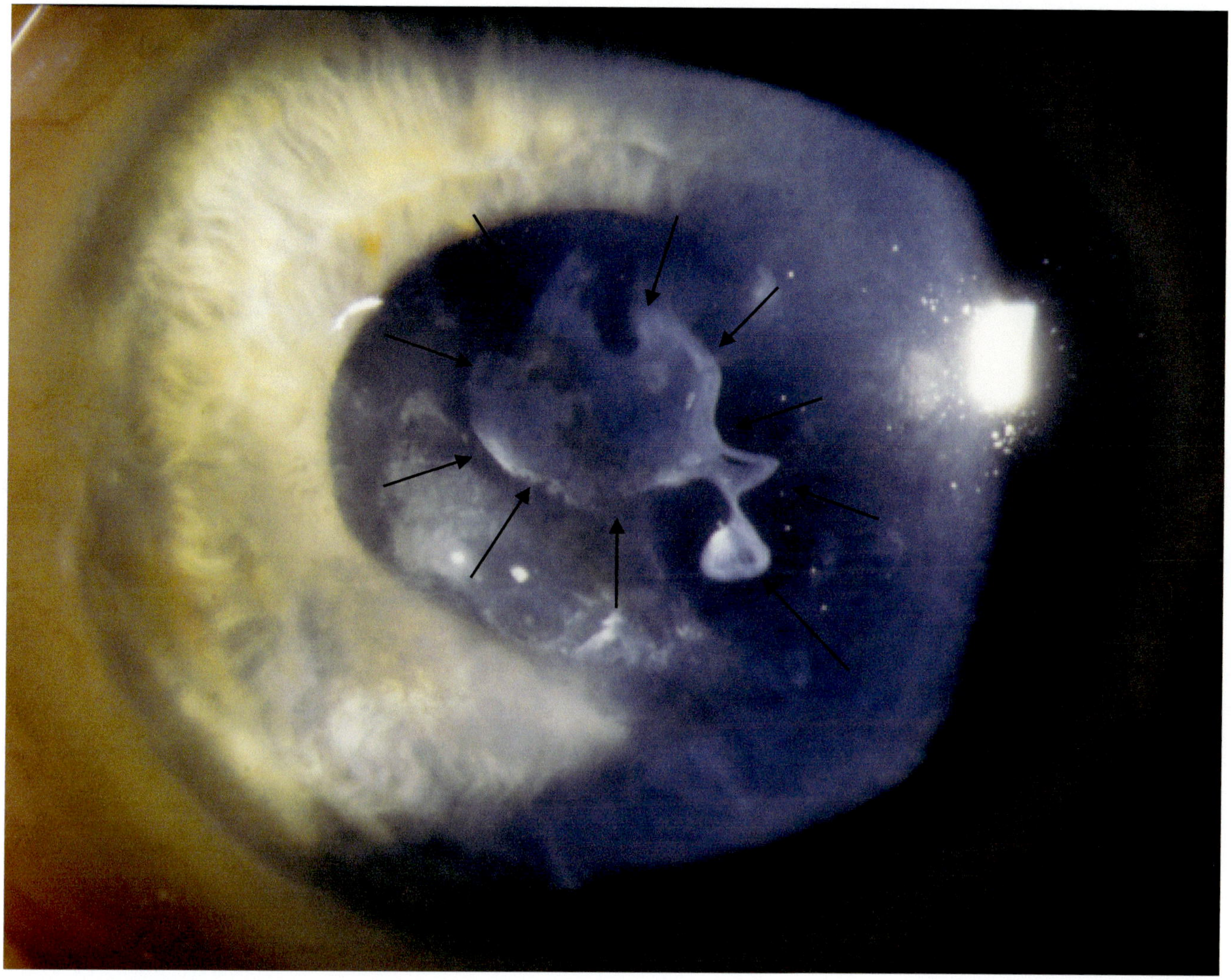

Fig. 10 Intraepithelial AM integration. Biomicroscopic image 12 weeks after transplantation of a single graft AMT. Note that the corneal surface is smooth in the center of the cornea, a whitish thin AM layer is observable within the epithelium (arrows) (Copyright Resch Ophthalmology 2006)

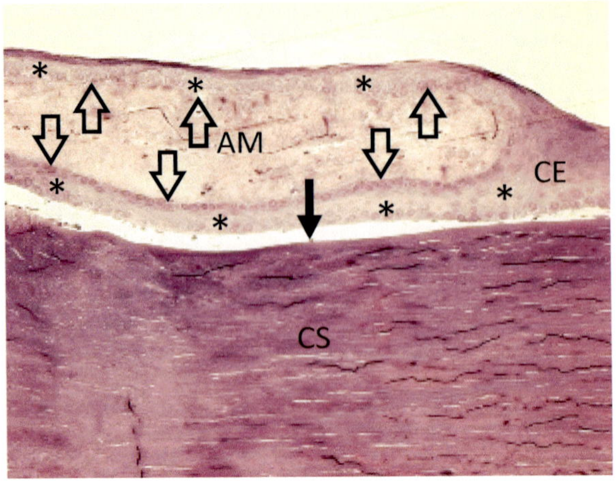

Fig. 11 Intraepithelial integration of AM. Semithin histology (200x). The corneal epithelium (CE) is separated into 2 layers, the AM is covered by corneal epithelium (asterisks) on both sides (arrow heads). The epithelium is artifically detached (arrow) from the anterior corneal stroma (CS)

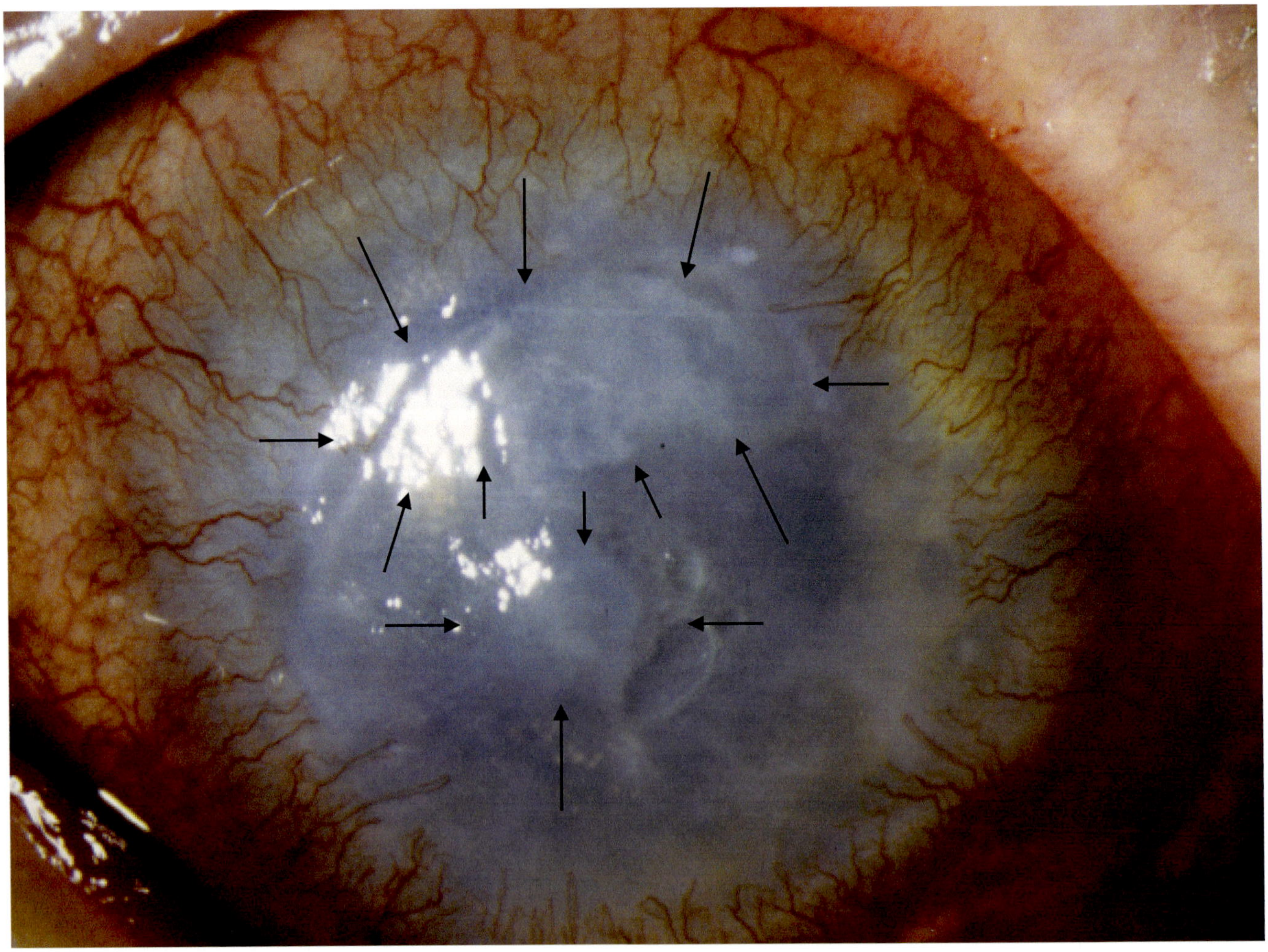

Fig. 12 Subepithelial AM integration. Slit-lamp image 8 weeks after bilocal single layer graft AMT. The opaque cornea is vascularized, the borders of the 2 AM pieces are shown (arrows), the details of AM and corneal stroma cannot be distinguished (Copyright Resch Ophthalmology 2006)

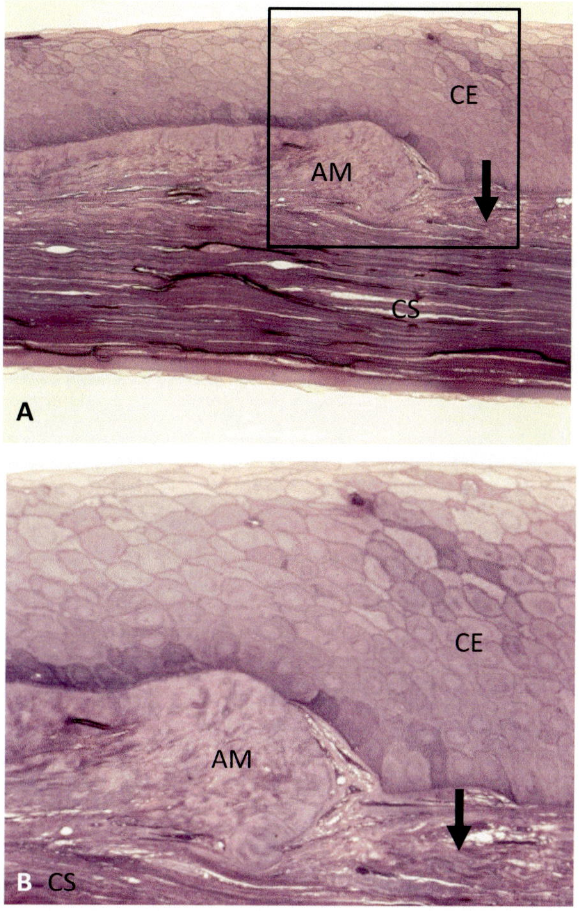

Fig. 13 Subepithelial integration of AM. Light microscopic images of the subepithelial AM stroma 14 weeks after single layer graft AMT. (**A**) (semi thin Sect. 200x) The corneal epithelium (CE) is hyperplastic at the margin of AM stroma, the ocular surface is regular. Number of CE layers is almost normal above AM, but more than 10 layers, where no AM is beneath (arrows). Corneal stroma (CS) is regular. (**B**) larger magnification of the zone shown in black rectangle on image A (400x). The multilayered CE is regular, firmly attached to the almost acellular AM. Area of disorganized, partially absorbed AM is shown with an arrow

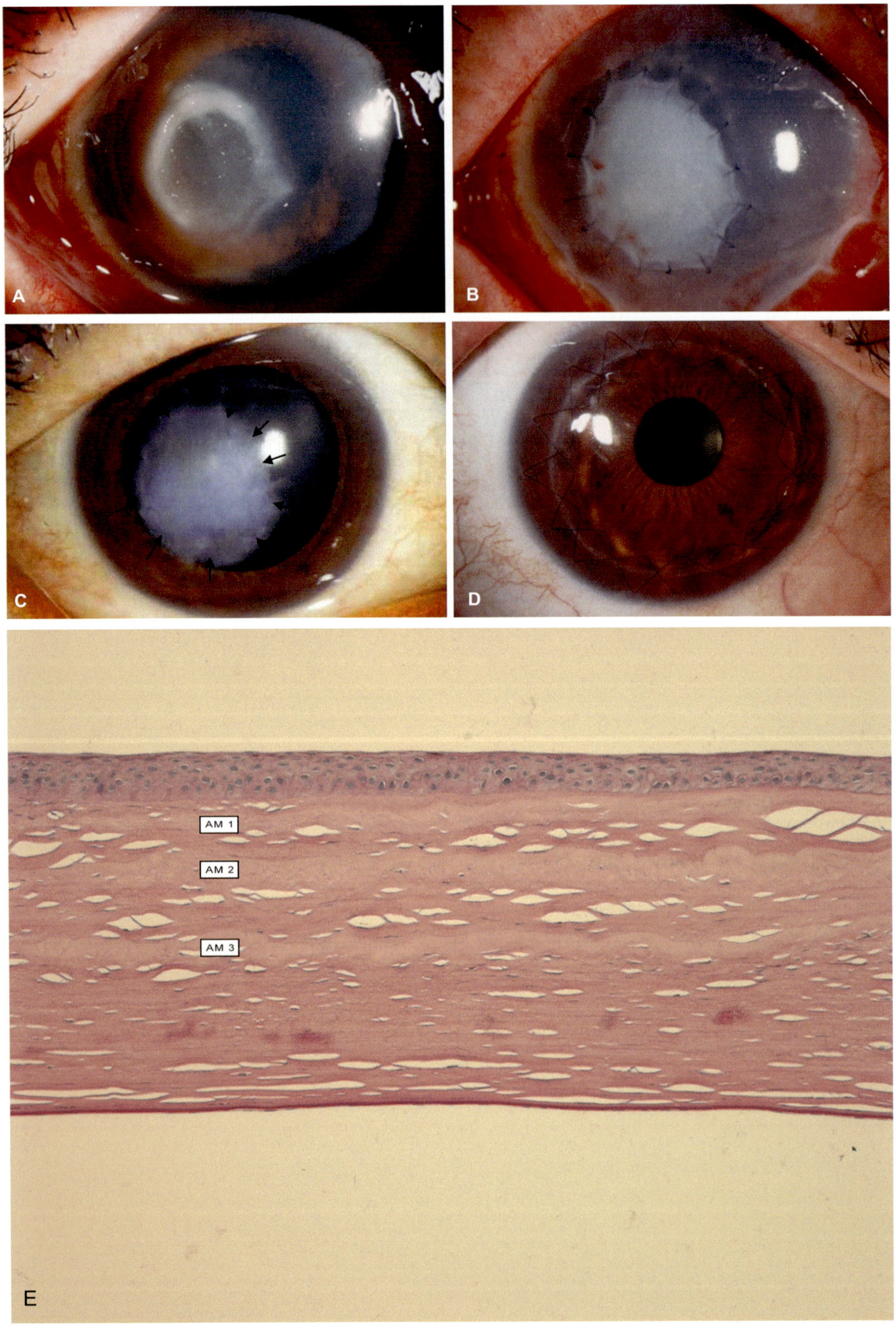

Fig. 14 Corneal transplantation after AMT. (**A**) Pseudomonas aeruginosa ulcer before AMT. (**B**) After triple graft sandwich AMT. (**C**) Subepithelial multilayered integration of AM. (arrows) 18 weeks after AMT. (**D**) After corneal transplantation. (**E**) Stromal integration of three AM graft layers (AM1, AM2, AM3) embedded in collagenous scar tissue

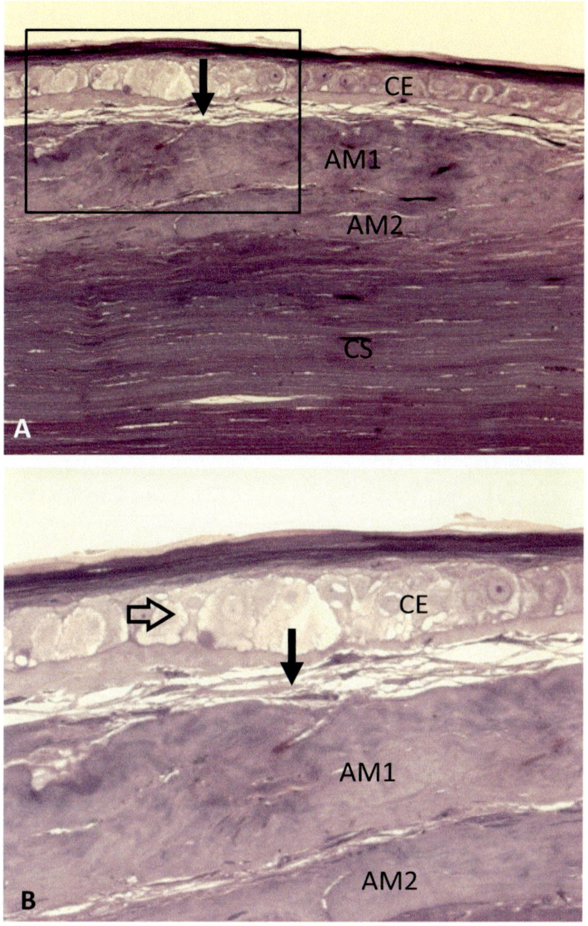

Fig. 15 Subepithelial multilayered integration of AM. Histology of 2 AM layers integrated subepithelially. (**A**) Semi thin 200× section: keratinized corneal surface, only few layers of irregular CE cells with signs of apoptosis. Subepithelially 2 layers of well preserved (AM1 and AM2) are attached to the intact CE. AM1 and 2 contain almost no cells. (**B**) Large magnification of image A (400x) showing the cellular changes with variable CE nuclei (empty arrow)

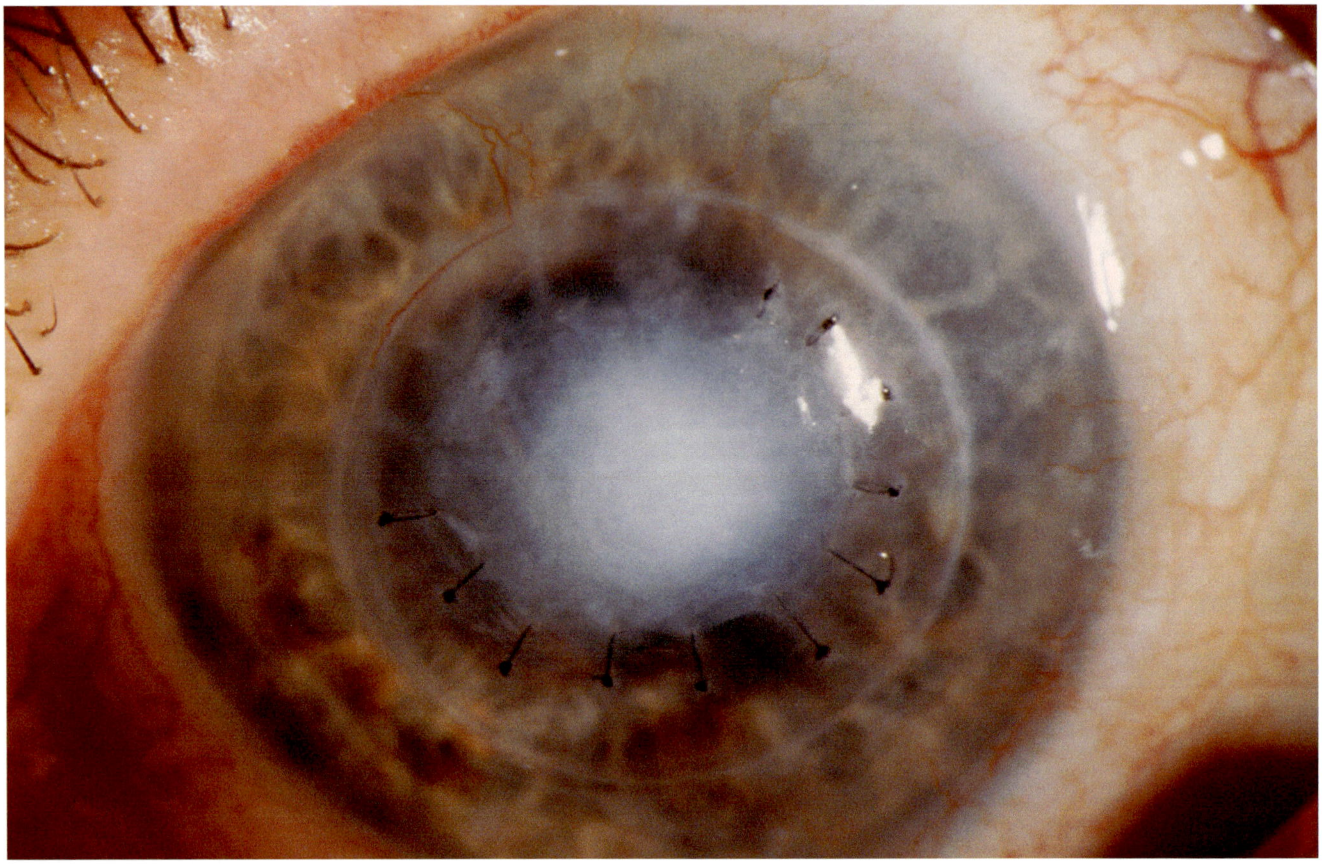

Fig. 16 Biomicroscopic image 6 weeks after five layer graft AMT performed after Descemetocele of previous penetrating keratoplasty. Intrastromal integration was found after repeated corneal transplantation. Some of the corneal sutures were already removed (because of becoming loose)

Fig. 17 Intrastromal integration of mutilayered AM. Histology (PAS stain, 200x) shows the regular epithelial surface, with variable number of epithelial cell (CE) layers, the five layers of intrastromally integrated AM (AM1 to 5) with corneal stromal (CS) tissue among the AM layers. Arrow points to the minimal residual stroma left by the (deep pre-Descemetal) corneal ulcer. Descemet membrane (D) corresponding with the area of the preoperative "desemetocele".

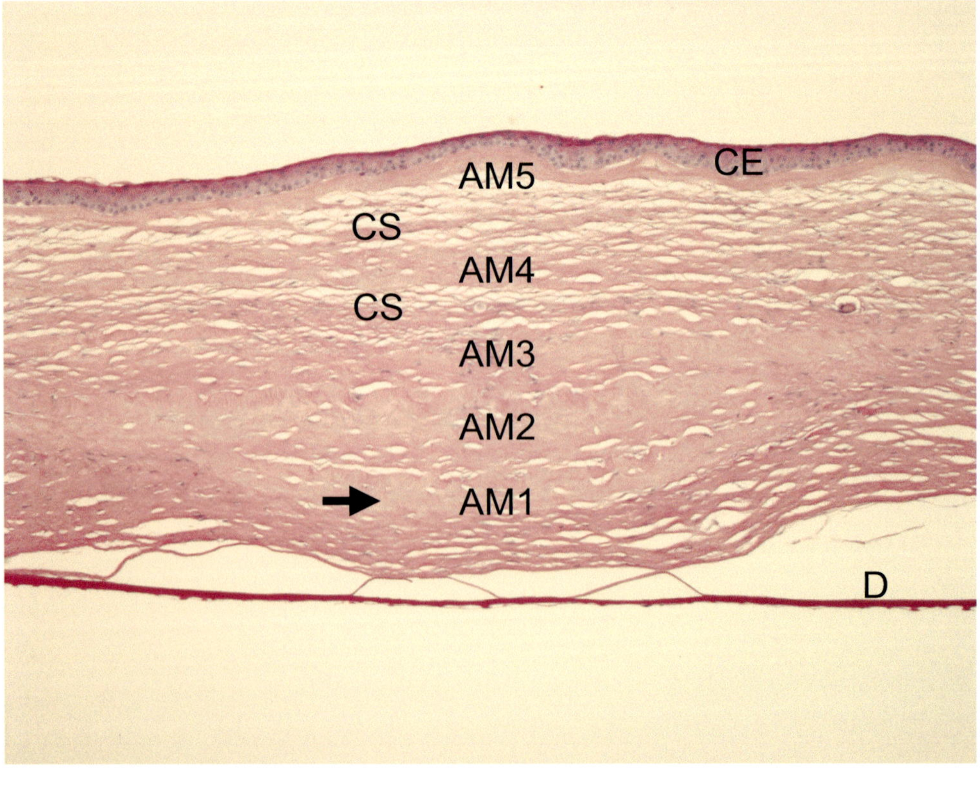

6 Conclusion

The unique anatomical and biological properties of the AM made AMT a multipotent, individualizable surgical alternative and adjuvant therapeutical option in the complex treatment of ocular surface disease. AMT can be performed in several techniques according to the origin, shape, size and depth of the corneal or conjunctival lesion. The increasing information of its mechanisms of action opens up even more future aspects in the management of sight threatening diseases and AMT will certainly remain an essential tool in the armamentarium of ocular surface therapies. AMT is here to stay!

References

1. de Rötth A. Plastic repair of conjunctival defects with fetal membranes. Arch Ophthalmol. 1940;23:522–5.
2. Kim JC, Tseng SC. Transplantation of preserved human amniotic membrane for surface reconstruction in severely damaged rabbit corneas. Cornea. 1995;14:473–84.
3. Tseng SC, Espana EM, Kawakita T, Di Pascuale MA, Li W, He H, Liu TS, Cho TH, Gao YY, Yeh LK, Liu CY. How does amniotic membrane work? Ocul Surf. 2004;2:177–87.
4. Bischoff M, Stachon T, Seitz B, Huber M, Zawada M, Langenbucher A, Szentmáry N. Growth factor and interleukin concentrations in amniotic membrane-conditioned medium. Curr Eye Res. 2017;42:174–80.
5. Stachon T, Bischoff M, Seitz B, Huber M, Zawada M, Langenbucher A, Szentmáry N. Growth factors and interleukins in amniotic membrane tissue homogenate. Klin Monbl Augenheilkd. 2015;232:858–62.
6. Maharajan VS, Shanmuganathan V, Currie A, Hopkinson A, Powell-Richards A, Dua HS. Amniotic membrane transplantation for ocular surface reconstruction: indications and outcomes. Clin Exp Ophthalmol. 2007;35:140–7.
7. Dua HS, Gomes JA, King AJ, Maharajan VS. The amniotic membrane in ophthalmology. Surv Ophthalmol. 2004;49:51–77.
8. Tejwani S, Kolari RS, Sangwan VS, Rao GN. Role of amniotic membrane graft for ocular chemical and thermal injuries. Cornea. 2007;26:21–6.
9. Westekemper H, Figueiredo FC, Siah WF, Wagner N, Steuhl KP, Meller D. Clinical outcomes of amniotic membrane transplantation in the management of acute ocular chemical injury. Br J Ophthalmol. 2017;101:103–7.
10. Khokhar S, Natung T, Sony P, Sharma N, Agarwal N, Vajpayee RB. Amniotic membrane transplantation in refractory neurotrophic corneal ulcers: a randomized, controlled clinical trial. Cornea. 2005;24(6):654–60.
11. Seitz B, Das S, Sauer R, Mena D, Hofmann-Rummelt C. Amniotic membrane transplantation for persistent corneal epithelial defects in eyes after penetrating keratoplasty. Eye (Lond). 2009;23:840–8.
12. Anderson DF, Prabhasawat P, Alfonso E, Tseng SC. Amniotic membrane transplantation after the primary surgical management of band keratopathy. Cornea. 2001;20:354–61.
13. Lee SH, Tseng SC. Amniotic membrane transplantation for persistent epithelial defects with ulceration. Am J Ophthalmol. 1997;123:303–12.
14. Ma KN, Thanos A, Chodosh J, Shah AS, Mantagos IS. A Novel technique for amniotic membrane transplantation in patients with acute Stevens-Johnson syndrome. Ocul Surf. 2016;14:31–6.
15. Singh P, Raj A, Gupta A, Pradhan S, Aftab N, Biswas S. Role of amniotic membrane transplantation in treating acute ocular manifestations in Stevens-Johnson syndrome and its long-term impact. Indian J Ophthalmol. 2022;70:4470–1.
16. Seitz B, Das S, Sauer R, Hofmann-Rummelt C, Beckmann MW, Kruse FE. Simultaneous amniotic membrane patch in high risk keratoplasty. Cornea. 2011;30:269–72.
17. Dietrich T, Sauer R, Hofmann-Rummelt C, Langenbucher A, Seitz B. Simultaneous amniotic membrane transplantation in emergency penetrating keratoplasty: a therapeutic option for severe corneal ulcerations and melting disorders. Br J Ophthalmol. 2011;95:1034–5.
18. Budenz DL, Barton K, Tseng SC. Amniotic membrane transplantation for repair of leaking glaucoma filtering blebs. Am J Ophthalmol. 2000;130:580–8.
19. Hoffmann S, Szentmáry N, Seitz B. Amniotic membrane transplantation for the treatment of infectious ulcerative keratitis before elective penetrating keratoplasty. Cornea. 2013;32:1321–5.
20. Tabatabaei SA, Soleimani M, Behrouz MJ, Torkashvand A, Anvari P, Yaseri M. A randomized clinical trial to evaluate the usefulness of amniotic membrane transplantation in bacterial keratitis healing. Ocul Surf. 2017;15:218–26.
21. Razafimino S, Marjanovic I, Flockerzi E, Seitz B. Conjunctivectomy, multilayer amniotic membrane transplantation and systemic immunosuppression in bilateral peripheral ulcerative keratitis. Ophthalmologe. 2022;119:71–4.
22. Kheirkhah A, Ghaffari R, Kaghazkanani R, Hashemi H, Behrouz MJ, Raju VK. A combined approach of amniotic membrane and oral mucosa transplantation for fornix reconstruction in severe symblepharon. Cornea. 2013;32:155–60.
23. Huchzermeyer C, Gatzioufas Z, Kruse FE, Seitz B. Treatment of severe recurrent symblepharopterygium: combined ipsilateral autologous limbus and homologous amniotic membrane transplantation. Ophthalmologe. 2014;111:839–45.
24. Barabino S, Rolando M, Bentivoglio G, Mingari C, Zanardi S, Bellomo R, Calabria G. Role of amniotic membrane transplantation for conjunctival reconstruction in ocular-cicatricial pemphigoid. Ophthalmology 2003;110:474–80.
25. Agraval U, Rundle P, Rennie IG, Salvi S. Fresh frozen amniotic membrane for conjunctival reconstruction after excision of neoplastic and presumed neoplastic conjunctival lesions. Eye (Lond). 2017;31:884–9.
26. Akbari M, Soltani-Moghadam R, Elmi R, Kazemnejad E. Comparison of free conjunctival autograft versus amniotic membrane transplantation for pterygium surgery. J Curr Ophthalmol. 2017;29:282–6.
27. Taher NO, Alnabihi AN, Hersi RM, Alrajhi RK, Alzahrani RA, Batais WT, Mofti AH, Alghamdi SA. Amniotic membrane transplantation and conjunctival autograft combined with mitomycin C for the management of primary pterygium: a systematic review and meta-analysis. Front Med (Lausanne). 2022;9:981663.
28. Kassem RR, El-Mofty RMA. Amniotic membrane transplantation in strabismus surgery. Curr Eye Res. 2019;44:451–64.
29. Seitz B, Resch MD, Schlötzer-Schrehardt U, Hofmann-Rummelt C, Sauer R, Kruse FE. Histopathology and ultrastructure of human corneas after amniotic membrane transplantation. Arch Ophthalmol. 2006;124:1487–90.
30. Chopra A, Thomas BS. Amniotic membrane: a novel material for regeneration and repair. J Biomim Biomater Tissue Eng. 2013;18:106.
31. Norte-Muñoz M, Botelho MF, Schoeberlein A, Chaves J, Neto Murta J, Ponsaerts P, Agudo-Barriuso M, Costa E. Insights and future directions for the application of perinatal derivatives in eye diseases: a critical review of preclinical and clinical studies. Front Bioeng Biotechnol. 2022;10:969927.
32. Kruse FE, Joussen AM, Rohrschneider K, You L, Sinn B, Baumann J, Völcker HE. Cryopreserved human amniotic membrane for ocular surface reconstruction. Graefe´s Arch Clin Exp Ophthalmol. 2000;238,68–75.

33. Nakamura T, Yoshitani M, Rigby H, et al. Sterilized, freeze-dried amniotic membrane: a useful substrate for ocular surface reconstruction. Invest Ophthalmol Vis Sci. 2004;45:93–9.
34. Jirsova K, Jones GLA. Amniotic membrane in ophthalmology: properties, preparation, storage and indications for grafting. Cell Tissue Bank. 2017;18:193–204.
35. Meller D, Pires R, Tseng S. Ex vivo preservation and expansion of human limbal epithelial stem cells on amniotic membrane cultures. Br J Ophthalmol. 2002;86:463–71.
36. Thomasen H, Pauklin M, Steuhl KP, Meller D. Comparison of cryopreserved and air-dried human amniotic membrane for ophthalmologic applications. Graefes Arch Clin Exp Ophthalmol. 2009;247:1691–700.
37. Letko E, Stechschulte SU, Kenyon KR, et al. Amniotic membrane inlay and overlay grafting for corneal epithelial defects and stromal ulcers. Arch Ophthalmol. 2001;119:659–63.
38. Prabhasawat P, Tesavibul N, Komolsuradej W. Single and multilayer amniotic membrane transplantation for persistent corneal epithelial defect with or without stromal thinning and perforation. Br J Ophthalmol. 2001;85:1455–63.
39. Kruse FE, Rohrschneider K, Völcker HE. Multilayer amniotic membrane transplantation for reconstruction of deep corneal ulcers. Ophthalmology 1999;106:1504–10.
40. Farah CJ, Fries FN, Latta L, Käsmann-Kellner B, Seitz B. An attempt to optimize the outcome of penetrating keratoplasty in congenital aniridia-associated keratopathy (AAK). Int Ophthalmol. 2021;41:4091–8.
41. Weischnur L, Xanthopoulou K, Munteanu C, Leonhard M, Daas L, Seitz B. Autologous serum eye drops for therapy-resistant epithelial defects of the cornea: Impact of underlying disease and simultaneous amniotic transplantation in 990 applications. Ophthalmologie. 2023;120:43–51. German.
42. Grueterich M, Espana EM, Tseng SC. Ex vivo expansion of limbal epithelial stem cells: amniotic membrane serving as a stem cell niche. Surv Ophthalmol. 2003;48:631–46.
43. Shortt AJ, Secker GA, Rajan MS, Meligonis G, Dart JK, Tuft SJ, Daniels JT. Ex vivo expansion and transplantation of limbal epithelial stem cells. Ophthalmol. 2008;115:1989–97.
44. Sangwan VS, Basu S, MacNeil S, Balasubramanian D. Simple limbal epithelial transplantation (SLET): a novel surgical technique for the treatment of unilateral limbal stem cell deficiency. Br J Ophthalmol. 2012;96:931–4.
45. Gris O, Lopez-Navidad A, Caballero F, del Campo Z, Adan A. Amniotic membrane transplantation for ocular surface pathology: long-term results. Transplant Proc. 2003;35:2031–5.
46. Seitz B, Ferreira de Souza R, Hofmann-Rummelt C, et al. Patch, Graft or Sandwich for persistent corneal ulcers–Differentiated technique of amniotic membrane transplantation. Clin Exp Ophthalmol. 2002;30,122.
47. Resch MD, Schlötzer-Schrehardt U, Hofmann-Rummelt C, Sauer R, Kruse FE, Beckmann MW, Seitz B. Integration patterns of cryopreserved amniotic membranes into the human cornea. Ophthalmol. 2006;113:1927–35.
48. Resch MD, Schlötzer-Schrehardt U, Hofmann-Rummelt C, Sauer R, Cursiefen C, Kruse FE, Beckmann MW, Seitz B. Adhesion structures of amniotic membranes integrated into human corneas. Invest Ophthalmol Vis Sci. 2006;47:1853–61.
49. Meller D, Pauklin M, Westekemper H, Steuhl KP. Autologous transplantation of cultivated limbal epithelium. Ophthalmologe. 2010;107:1133–8.
50. Resch MD, Resch BE, Csizmazia E, Imre L, Németh J, Révész P, Csányi E. Permeability of human amniotic membrane to ofloxacin in vitro. Invest Ophthalmol Vis Sci. 2010;51:1024–7.
51. Resch MD, Resch BE, Csizmazia E, Imre L, Németh J, Szabó-Révész P, Csányi E. Drug reservoir function of human amniotic membrane. J Ocul Pharmacol Ther. 2011;27:323–6.
52. Resch MD, Marsovszky L, Csanyi E, Budai-Szűcs M. Nemeth J. Amniotic membrane and the controlled drug release. In: Mamede AC, Botelho MF, editors. Amniotic membrane origin, characterization and medical applications. Springer; 2015. p. 177–192. ISBN 978–94–017–9974–4.

Excimer Laser PhotoTherapeutic Keratectomy PTK—Treatment of Recurrent Erosion Syndrome, Corneal Dystrophies, Degenerations and Scars

Berthold Seitz, Elias Flockerzi, Loïc Hamon, Tim Berger, and Loay Daas

Abstract

In the recent three decades, the treatment of superficial corneal opacities (especially dystrophies, avascular scars, and degenerations) has shifted from corneal transplantation (penetrating keratoplasty PKP) to excimer laser-assisted keratectomy, now commonly referred to as "phototherapeutic keratectomy" (PTK). PTK with the 193-nm excimer laser can lead to significant improvement in vision in these patients, delaying or even completely avoiding primary or repeat keratoplasty. Besides the exact determination of the depth of the deposits at the slit lamp, a preoperative tomographic analysis is advised. In principle, prominent lesions have a good prognosis, while localized lesions (e.g. paracentral foreign body scars) with stromal thinning have a (severely) limited prognosis. In general, PTK should be performed on a "calm eye". Possible interfering problems such as blepharitis and active infections must be brought under control before the procedure. In addition, intraocular inflammation should be controlled. Three basic effects can be targeted with PTK: (1) elimination of corneal opacities (o-PTK), (2) treatment of irregular corneal surface and astigmatism (a-PTK), (3) increase and stabilization of epithelial adherence (e-PTK). These indications may overlap in a number of corneal diseases and apply to varying degrees in a given pathology.

For more than 30 years, PTK has been an indispensable addition to the corneal microsurgical spectrum for selected corneal pathologies also in the future. "*PTK is here to stay!*" A critical patient selection, a detailed preoperative education, a well planned and executed operation ("*PTK is more an art than a science*") and an adequate and consequent follow-up usually help to minimize disappointments and unpleasant postoperative discussions.

Keywords

Phototherapeutic keratectomy · PTK · Recurrent corneal erosion syndrome · Corneal dystrophy · Corneal opacities · Astigmatism · Epithelial adherence

1 Introduction

Excimer laser assisted phototherapeutic keratectomy ("Excimer-PTK") can be used (1) to eliminate superficial corneal **o**pacities (mainly dystrophies, degenerations and scars: o-PTK), (2) to regularize the corneal surface in case of irregular **a**stigmatisms (a-PTK) and (3) to stabilize corneal epithelial adhesion in case of recurrent **e**pithelial defects (e-PTK). In our Department Excimer-PTK is predominantly applied to treat Salzmann nodular degeneration and Epithelial Basement Membrane dystrophy (Fig. 1).

Corneal dystrophies typically lead to a gradual bilateral loss of vision in a primarily "white eye"–but occur in later stages often in association with epithelial defects [1, 2]. Treatment of corneal dystrophies should be stage-specific (Table 1). In recent decades, the treatment of these conditions has shifted from corneal transplantation (penetrating keratoplasty PKP) to excimer laser-assisted keratectomy, now commonly referred to as "phototherapeutic keratectomy" (PTK) [3–5]. PTK with the 193-nm excimer laser can lead to significant improvement in vision in these patients, delaying or even completely avoiding primary or re-keratoplasty.

Supplementary Information The online version contains supplementary material available at https://doi.org/10.1007/978-3-031-65422-0_47.

B. Seitz (✉) · E. Flockerzi · L. Hamon · T. Berger · L. Daas
Department of Ophthalmology, Saarland University Medical Center, Homburg/Saar, Germany
e-mail: berthold.seitz@uks.eu
URL: https://augenklinik-saarland.de/

B. Seitz et al. (eds.), *Atlas on Cornea*, https://doi.org/10.1007/978-3-031-65422-0_47

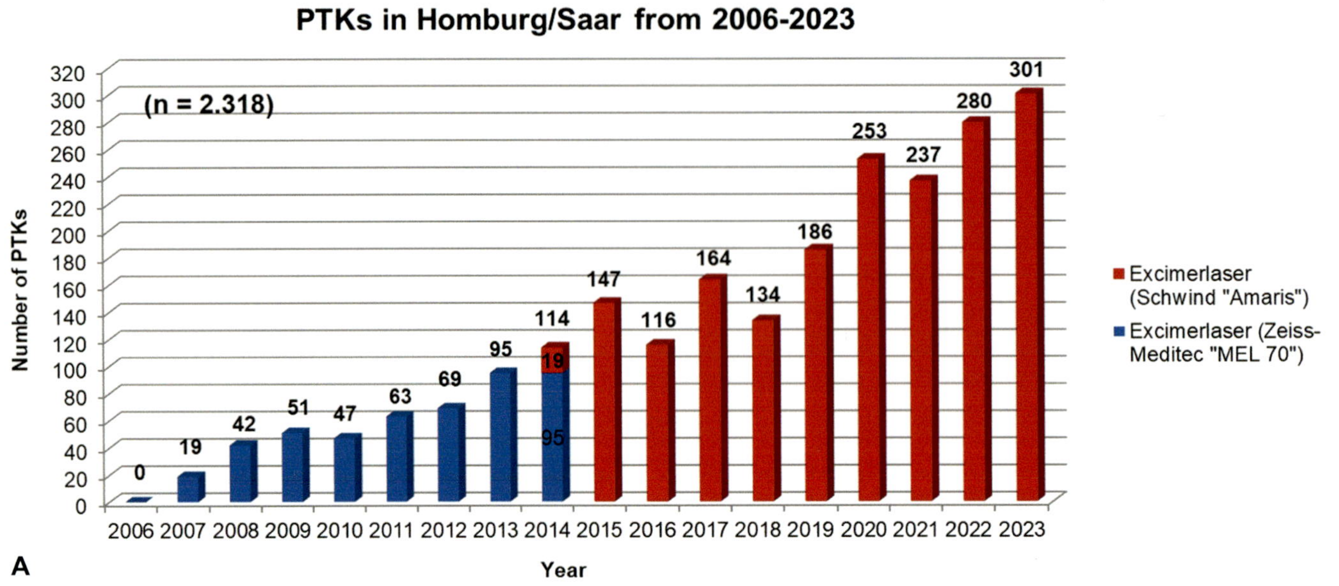

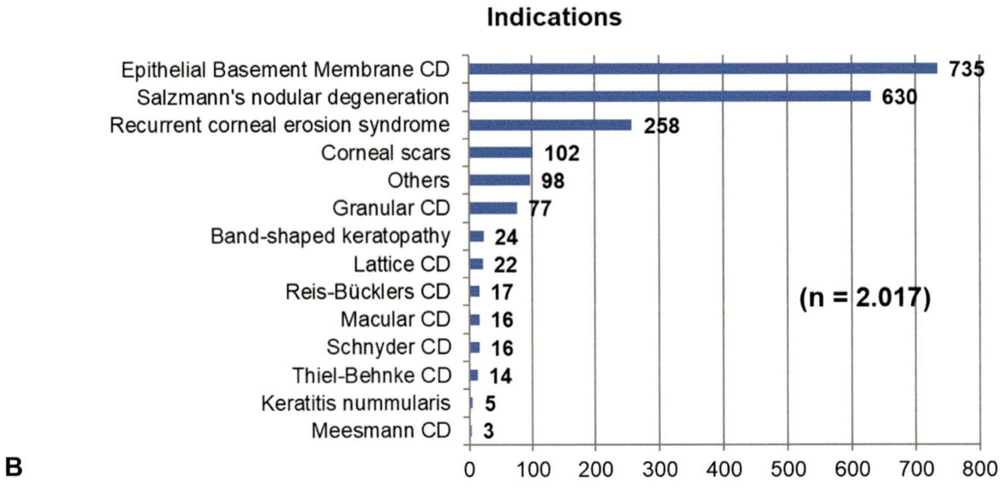

Fig. 1 (**A**) Number of excimer-PTKs per year in the department of ophthalmology at Saarland University medical center in Homburg/Saar, Germany. 2318 PTKs have been performed from 2007 to 2023. (**B**) Salzmann nodular degeneration and epithelial basement membrane dystrophy have been by far the leading indications for excimer-PTK in our department between 2007 and 2022

In predominantly superficial dystrophies of the epithelium, basement membrane and/or Bowman layer (Map-Dot Fingerprint, Meesmann, Lisch, Reis–Bücklers, Thiel–Behnke) recurrent epithelial defects may complicate the clinical picture. If conservative therapy with gels/ointments, application of therapeutic contact lenses and/or conventional corneal abrasion with/without pannectomy are not successful, PTK is nowadays the method of choice (Tables 1 and 2). Besides the exact determination of the depth of the deposits at the slit lamp, a preoperative topographic and—if possible—tomographic analysis is advised. **In principle, prominent lesions have a good prognosis while localized lesions (e.g. paracentral foreign body scars) with stromal thinning have a (severely) limited prognosis** [6]. Paracentral foreign body scars should preferably be treated with oxygen-permeable rigid contact lenses and NOT with Excimer-PTK!

2 Patient Counseling

The efficacy of PTK appears to be dependent on several factors, including (1) the type of corneal disease, (2) the patient's subjective complaints, (3) the preoperative refractive error, (4) the treatment strategy, and (5) the tissue ablation properties of the laser [7, 8]. Specific patient complaints should be given special attention to better determine whether PTK can achieve the desired clinical goals. Of course, the patient should be fully and frankly informed about the different surgical steps and achievable results.

Table 1 Newest classification of corneal dystrophies [31]

Epithelial and Subepithelial Dystrophies
Epithelial basement membrane dystrophy (EBMD)
Epithelial recurrent erosion dystrophies (EREDs)
Meesmann corneal dystrophy (MECD)
Lisch epithelial corneal dystrophy (LECD)

Corneal abrasion

Gelatinous drop-like corneal dystrophy (GDLD) ?

Epithelial-Stromal TGFBI Dystrophies
Reis-Bücklers corneal dystrophy (RBCD)
Thiel-Behnke corneal dystrophy (TBCD)
Granular corneal dystrophy, type 1 (GCD 1)
Granular corneal dystrophy, type 2 (GCD 2)
Lattice corneal dystrophy, type 1 (LCD 1) and variants

Phototherapeutic Keratectomy

Stromal Dystrophies
Schnyder corneal dystrophy (SCD)
Macular corneal dystrophy (MCD) ?
Congenital stromal corneal dystrophy (CSCD)
Fleck corneal dystrophy (FCD)
Posterior amorphous corneal dystrophy (PACD)
Central cloudy dystrophy of Francois (CCDF)
Pre-Descemet corneal dystrophy (PDCD)

Endothelial Dystrophies
Fuchs endothelial corneal dystrophy (FECD)
Posterior polymorphous corneal dystrophy (PPCD)
Congenital hereditary endothelial dystrophy (CHED)
X-linked endothelial corneal dystrophy (XECD)

Table 2 Definition of a corneal dystrophy [2, 32]

• Heredity or familiarity
• Bilateral, generally symmetrical appearance
• Typical morphology and localization in the cornea
• Slow progressive course without signs of vascularization
• Occurence in the 1st or 2nd decade of life
• Intrafamilial consistency of changes and similar course
• No inflammatory cells
• No exogenous causes

A crystal-clear cornea and a visual acuity (VA) of 20/20 is typically <u>not</u> the goal of PTK for superficial corneal dystrophies and scars, but to postpone or even avoid an anterior lamellar ("deep anterior lamellar keratoplasty"–DALK) or PKP. Often, removal of larger central opacities results in significant improvement in visual acuity. Usually, some deposits remain in the mid-stroma without major disadvantages (e.g. in granular and lattice dystrophy) [9]. A dystrophy may recur early after PTK, especially in macular corneal dystrophy [10] and Reis–Bücklers dystrophy [3]. In contrast, recurrence occurs later in Map-Dot Fingerprint dystrophy [11] and granular dystrophy. In case of recurrence, a new PTK can be performed.

Depending on the preoperative refraction, the PTK may lead to an increase in best-corrected visual acuity (BCVA), although uncorrected visual acuity (UDVA) decreases. This may be due to a hyperopic shift after the central PTK. Often, the patient is highly satisfied when the visual acuity increases from 20/100 to 20/30 or even 20/25. <u>In some cases, even a hard/rigid contact lens may be required after PTK to achieve good vision.</u> The patient must be aware of this potential problem in advance and should not be confronted with it for the first time after PTK when a major hyperopic shift has occurred [6].

3 Diagnostic Approaches for Surgical Decision-Making

An appropriate recommendation for the treatment of choice can only be made after an analysis of the horizontal/vertical distribution and pattern of dystrophic or scarring changes. In these cases, indirect illumination and retrograde illumination (with dilated pupils)–always in bilateral comparison–may be required to identify the predominant lesions. In addition to clearly defining patient expectations and reassessing whether they can be met with PTK, the individual corneal pathology itself is most important for surgical decision-making. Contact lens tolerance should be an issue in decision-making prior to surgery. The PTK procedure must always be planned on an individual basis. **Therefore, it is <u>imperative</u> that the microsurgeon HIMSELF/HERSELF takes a close look at the cornea at the slit lamp <u>immediately prior to the procedure,</u> even if he/she would have seen the patient at a previous visit already and has made the indication for surgery**.

To assess vertical extent, it is first necessary to classify the level of the corneal surface at the site of the lesion: (1) **"plus disease"** is defined as an elevated (nodular) lesion compared with the surrounding corneal surface, (2) **"zero disease"** is defined as a lesion within the level of the surrounding corneal surface, and (3) **"minus disease"** is defined as a depressed lesion compared with the surrounding corneal surface. Furthermore, the vertical extent of corneal disease can be divided into (1) anterior to Bowman layer, (2) within Bowman layer, (3) in the anterior and mid-stroma (Table 3).

<u>Scheimpflug analysis</u> (e.g. using Pentacam–OCULUS GmbH, Wetzlar, Germany) provides a thickness profile

Table 3 Classification of corneal opacities [12]

1. Deposition (in front of Bowman layer: „pannus“ with thickening, e.g. Salzmann)
2. Scar (vascularized or non-vascularized—mostly with multi-focal thinning)
3. Infiltrate (mostly fluffy with focal thickening)
4. CEED (corneal endothelial epithelial decompensation) (minor to very severe thickening; with/without bullous keratopathy)
5. Corneal hydrops = acute keratoconus (with extreme thickening)
6. Deposits (often normal thickness) (e.g. dystrophies, e.g. Kayser–Fleischer ring)

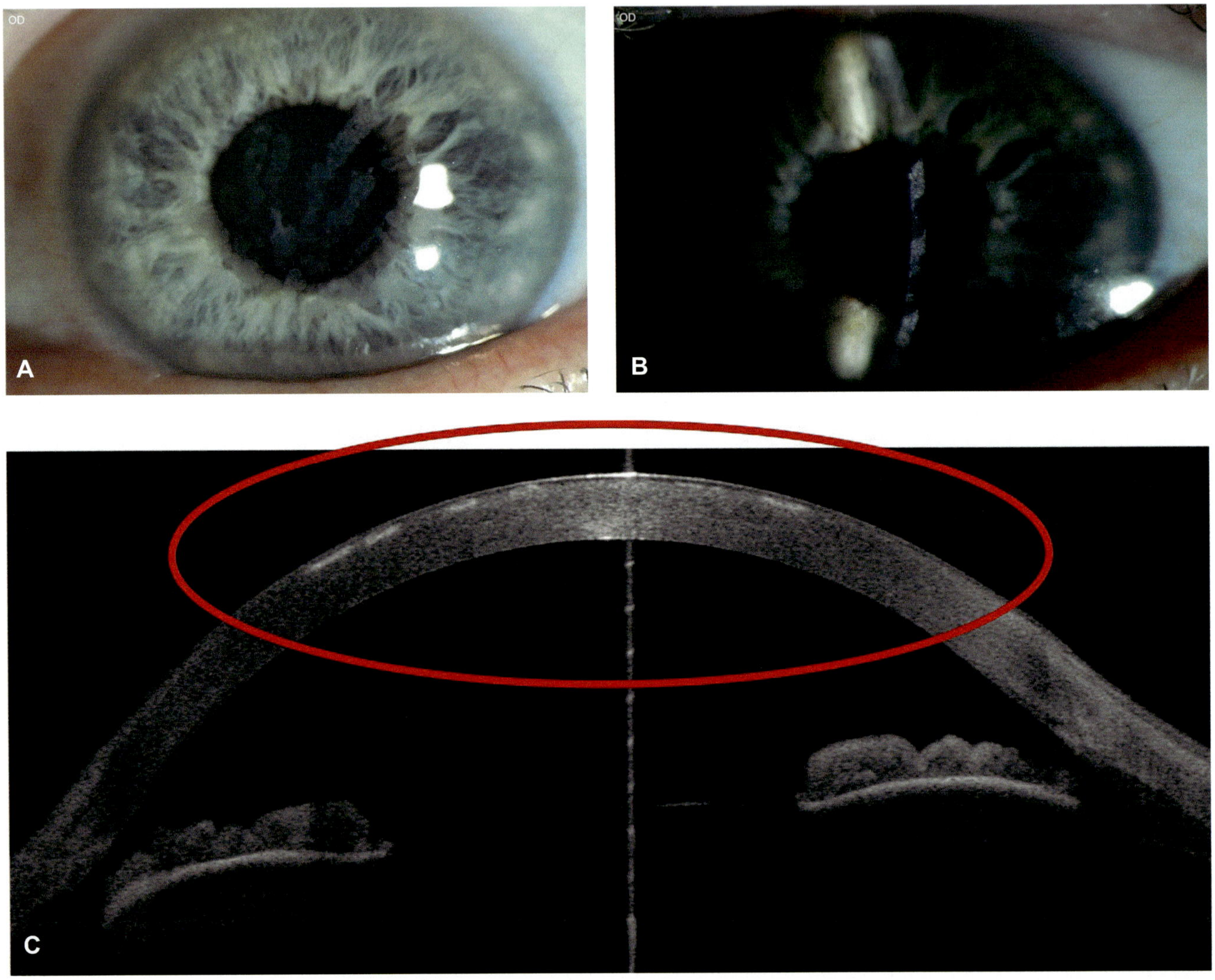

Fig. 2 Granular dystrophy type 2A: (**A**) Overview, (**B**) Slit lamp image. (**C**) AS-OCT shows superficial deposits that are readily accessible to PTK

of the cornea with complete information about the anterior and posterior corneal curvature. To assess the true vertical involvement of the lesion, anterior segment optical coherence tomography (AS-OCT) can be used supportively (Figs. 2, 3, 4, 5 and 6). Nevertheless, high-power slit-lamp examination is still the most important qualitative examination technique for planning the surgical approach [12].

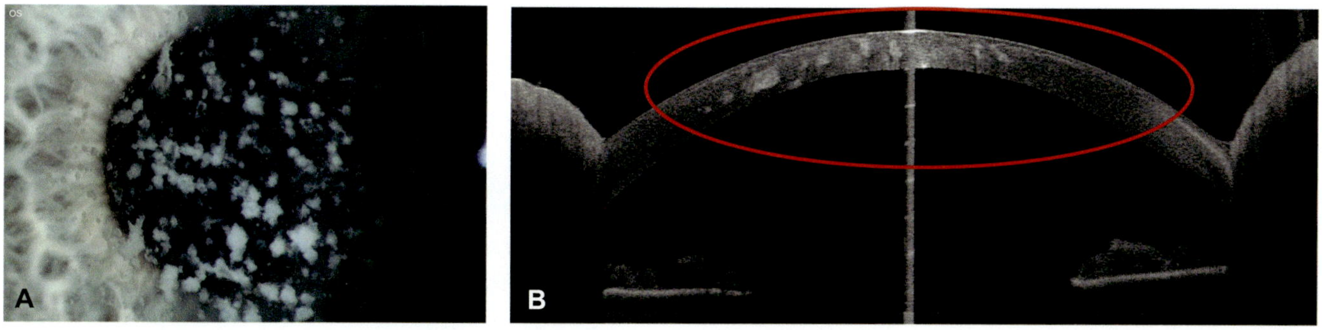

Fig. 3 Granular dystrophy type 1: (**A**) Overview, (**B**) AS-OCT shows mid- and deep stromal deposits, which are not accessible to PTK. In this case, only DALK or PKP is curative

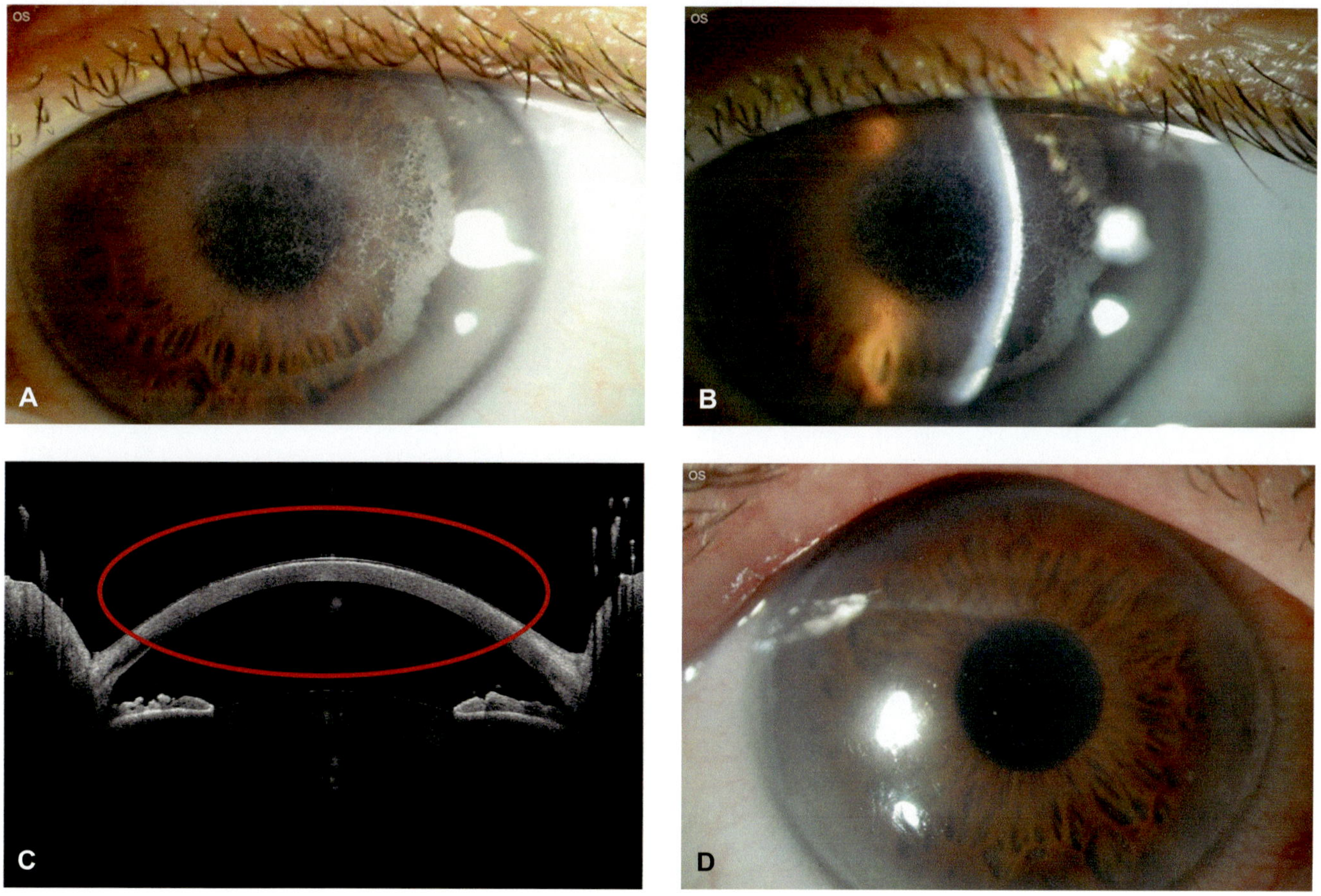

Fig. 4 Schnyder dystrophy: (**A**) Overview, (**B**) Slit lamp image, (**C**) AS-OCT shows superficial deposits that are readily accessible to PTK. (**D**) Clear cornea one day after PTK

4 Strategic Planning and Surgical Techniques

In general, PTK should be performed on a "calm eye". Possible interfering problems such as blepharitis and active infections must be brought under control before the procedure. In addition, intraocular inflammation should be controlled. Three basic effects can be targeted with PTK: (1) elimination of corneal opacities **(o-PTK)**, (2) treatment of irregular corneal surface and astigmatism **(a-PTK)**, (3) increase and stabilization of epithelial adherence **(e-PTK)**. These indications may overlap in a number of corneal diseases and apply to varying degrees in a given pathology (Fig. 7) [4].

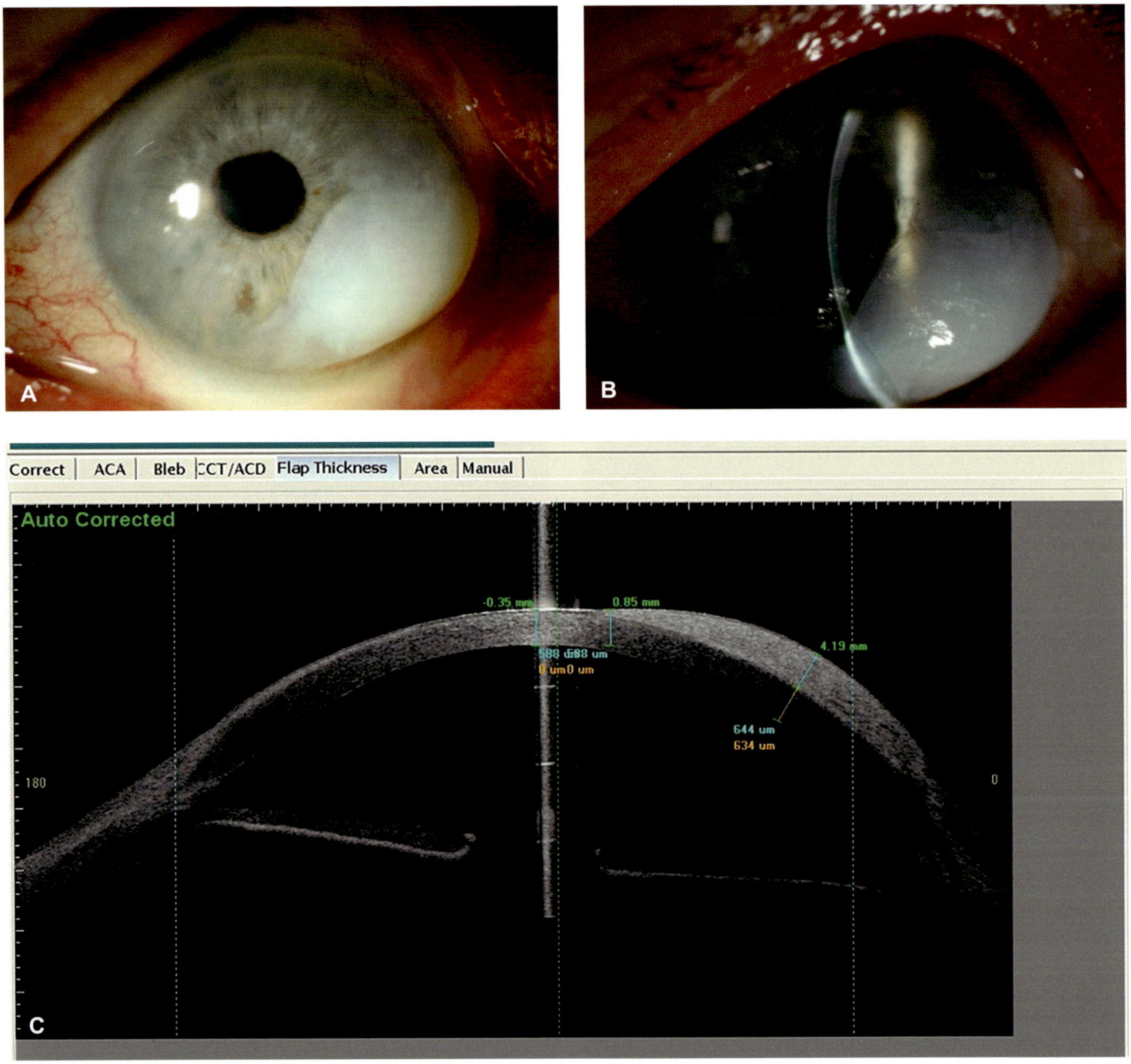

Fig. 5 Large Salzmann nodular degeneration: (**A**) Overview, (**B**) Slit lamp image, (**C**) AS-OCT shows unequivocally that the cornea below the Salzmann nodule is intact and of normal thickness. Thus, a simple pannectomy with simultaneous PTK is possible "without intraoperative worries" [26, 33]

4.1 Removal of Superficial Opacities (o-PTK)

In general, we recommend primarily using the hockey knife to remove as much of the pathological tissue as possible and using the laser to remove as little tissue as possible and especially to smooth the surface (Figs. 8 and 9). This is especially true for all "plus diseases" that are multifocally arranged. A hockey knife is used to identify a splitting zone between abnormal tissue and the Bowman layer or stroma to elevate the tissue edges. For easier visualization and manipulation of the abnormal tissue, the corneal surface is kept dry. Toothed forceps can be used to pull the abnormal material along its natural cleavage surface, while the tip of a dry cellulose sponge can be used as an atraumatic dissection instrument. In cases of severe adhesions, the sharp blade can be used carefully to dislodge adhesions or to remove the remaining abnormal tissue. Care is taken

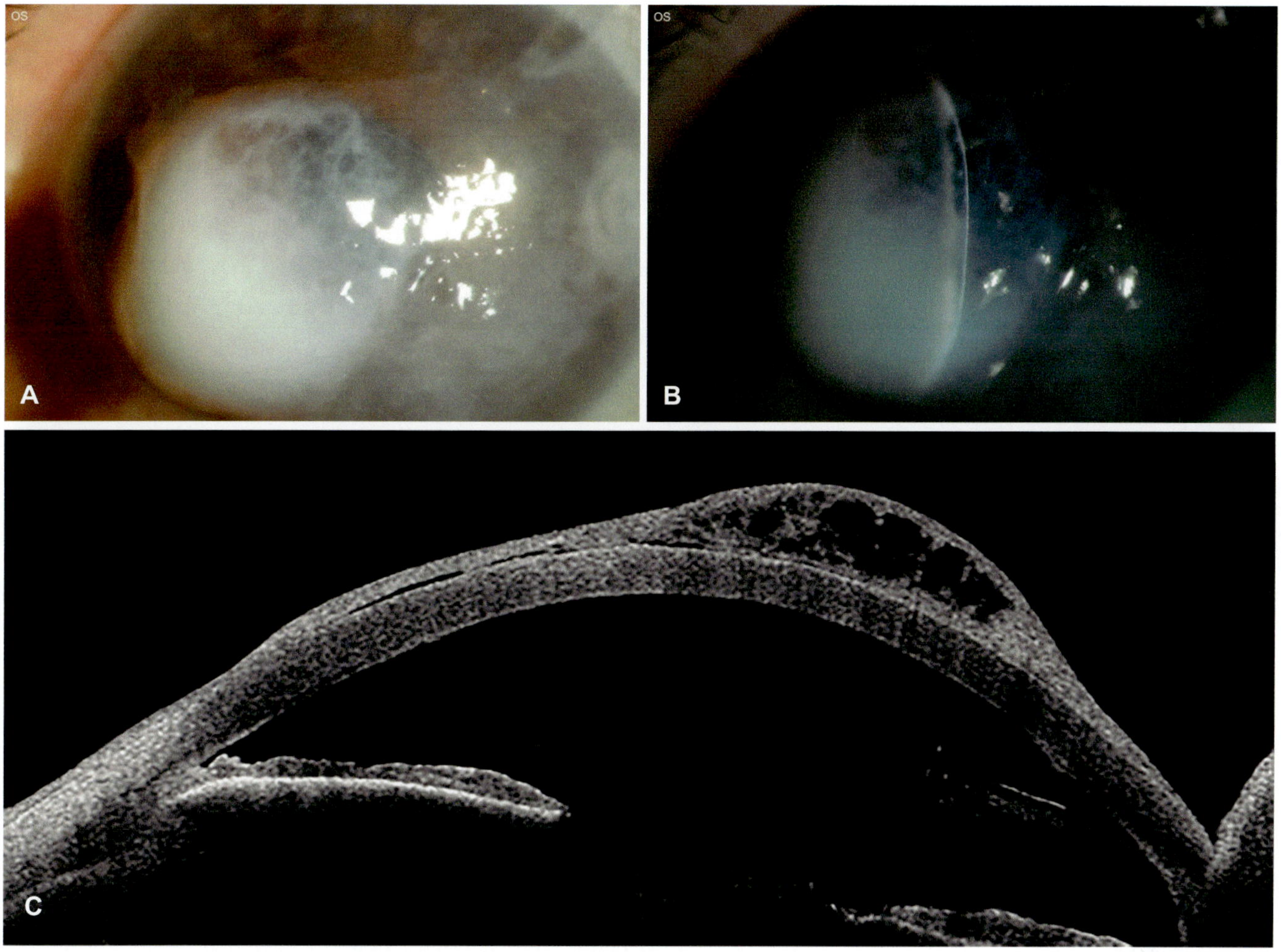

Fig. 6 Giant Salzmann nodular degeneration with cystoid spaces—differential diagnosis "Corneal Hydrops" [34]: (**A**) Overview, (**B**) Slit lamp image, (**C**) AS-OCT shows the pseudocysts confluent spaces within the giant nodule and an intact cornea below the Salzmann nodules

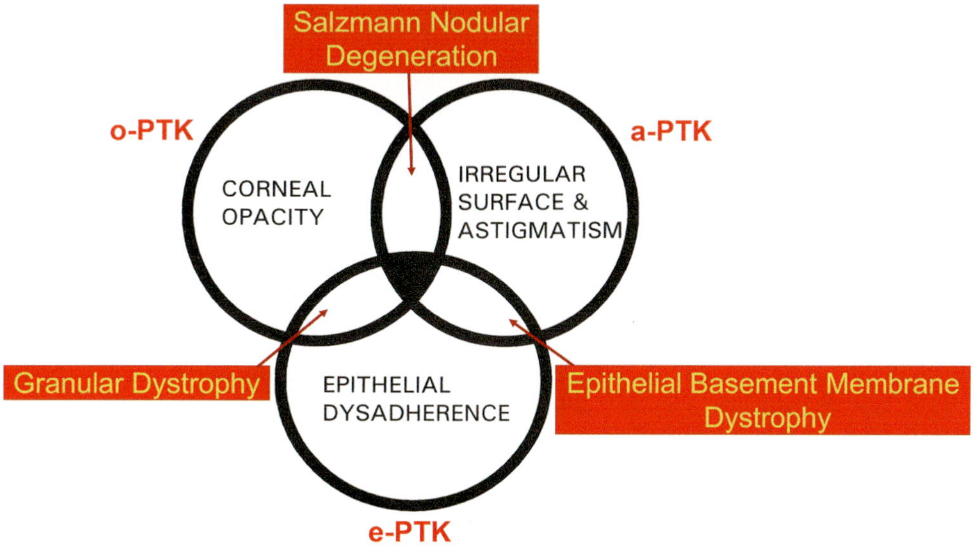

Fig. 7 Indications for phototherapeutic keratectomy (1) corneal opacity (o-PTK), (2) irregular corneal surface and astigmatism (a-PTK), (3) epithelial dysadherence (e-PTK). These indications may overlap in a number of corneal diseases and apply to a specific pathology to varying degrees (modified from Hersh & Wagoner [4])

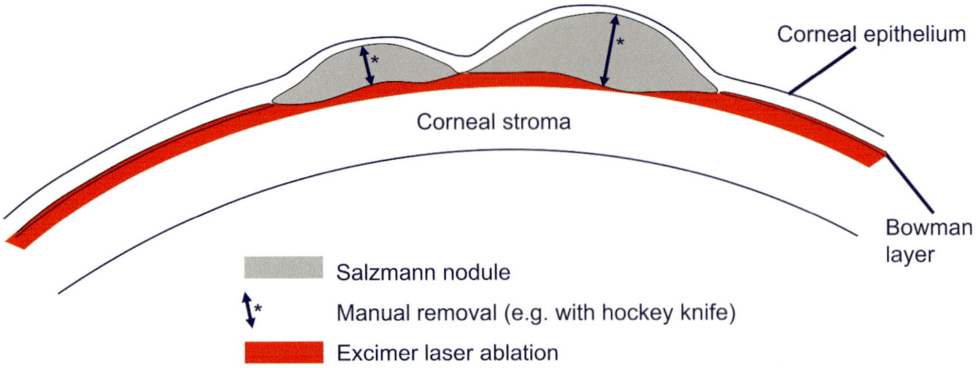

Fig. 8 Technical details in PTK: First, prominent subepithelial tissue is removed manually, preferably with a hockey knife, before excimer laser ablation is performed to remove superficial stromal "opacities" (see Table 3) and especially to smooth the surface (by using masking fluids)

to leave the limbal stem cells intact. Laser ablation is then performed. This technique is referred to as "subepithelial PTK." If the corneal topography is regular–which is very rare–a "transepithelial PTK" may be advisable. In this case, the epithelium masks the irregularities of the superficial stroma, acting as a biological "masking tissue" and contributing to a smoother postoperative stromal surface. However, it is important to be aware of the slight differences in ablation rates in epithelial, stromal, and scar tissue.

4.2 Smoothing of the Surface and Reduction of Irregular Astigmatism (a-PTK)

It is important to note that the excimer laser generally removes an equal amount of tissue over the entire surface it impinges on. Although opacities are removed, surface irregularities remain because the tissue is removed parallel to the surface. Therefore, it is mandatory to use so-called "masking fluids" repeatedly during a session in most PTK procedures. Hyaluronic acid 0.3% (e.g. Vismed®) can be successfully used for this purpose. The viscosity of these fluids is suitable to fill up the "valleys" of an irregular surface and thus "mask" it, while the "peaks" remain exposed to the laser action [13]. Thus, the laser can be used to smoothen the surface while removing scar tissue (Fig. 10). The thickness of the masking fluid layer should be sufficient to smooth the valleys of the corneal surface, but not so thick, that it completely blocks the irradiating laser beam. Usually, two to three rounds with an intended ablation depth of 40 to 50 μm over a suitable masking fluid are sufficient to regularize the corneal stromal surface after extensive mechanical pannus removal [6].

4.3 Improving Epithelial Adhesion (e-PTK)

Recurrent corneal erosions in the context of progressive corneal dystrophies (Fig. 11) or sharp trauma (Fig. 12) should preferably be treated with subepithelial PTK (= treatment of Bowman layer after generous removal of loose and irregular epithelium) [1]. We know from histological and ultrastructural studies that excimer laser ablation leads to a significant proliferation of hemidesmosomes (Fig. 13) and thus improves epithelial adhesion to the underlying stroma [14]. For this reason, dystrophies, such as the Map-Dot Fingerprint variant, which in principle could also be removed only by mechanical abrasion of the cornea, should better be treated with additional excimer laser ablation (e.g. 15 μm) in the sense of PTK in order to smoothen the surface and at the same time stabilize the ocular surface by improving epithelial adhesion. Nowadays stromal puncture using a bended sharp needle should not be performed in the center of the cornea any more (Fig. 14).

4.4 Combination with Mitomycin-C

Combining PTK with a temporary application of 0.02% mitomycin-C (MMC) on a Merocel sponge for 60 to 90 s after laser surgery can prevent scarring and recurrence of certain corneal pathologies, such as granular dystrophy type II and Salzmann degeneration (Fig. 15), especially in the context of congenital aniridia (Fig. 16) [15, 16]. **In PTK on a graft after keratoplasty, MMC application is mandatory to avoid scarring** [17, 18].

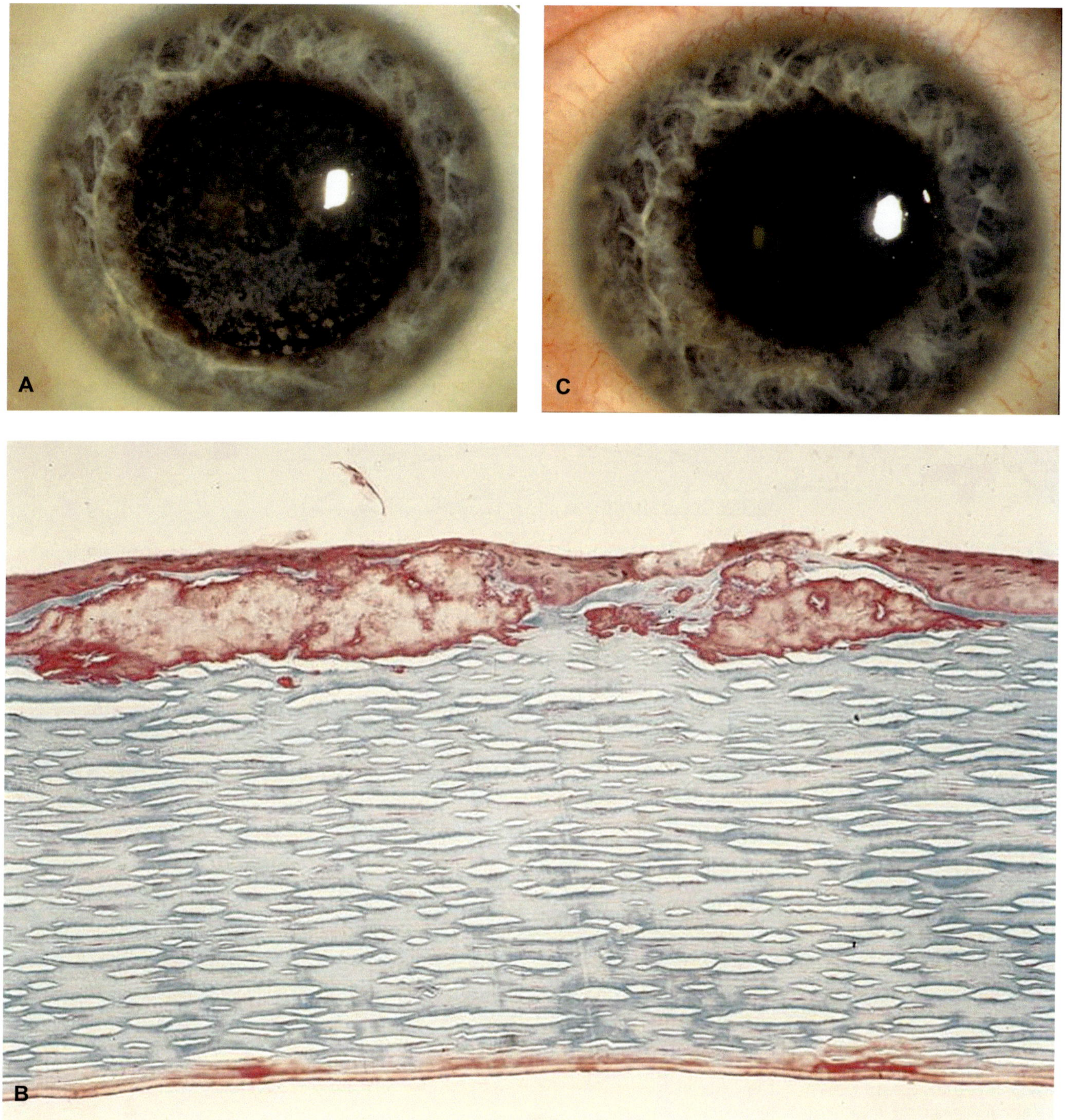

Fig. 9 Granular dystrophy type 1: (**A**) Before PTK, (**B**) Deposits of hyaline in the anterior stroma (other patient), (**C**) Findings after PTK

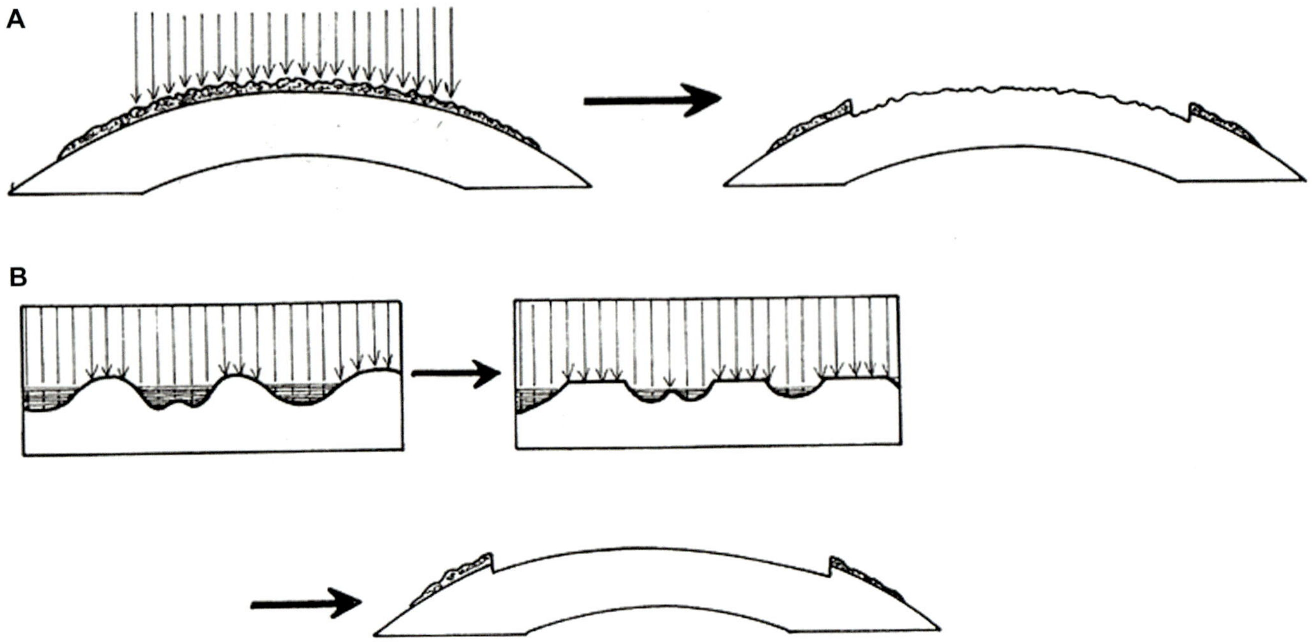

Fig. 10 Application of "masking fluid" to smooth the corneal surface. (**A**) Schematic representation of an irregular corneal surface before/after excimer laser ablation. Note how the irregular corneal surface pattern is preserved even though the superficial scars have been ablated. (**B**) The use of a masking fluid to protect the corneal surface "valleys" by absorbing irradiating laser energy allows the surface to be smoothed as the irregular surface "hills" are removed by photoablation, ideally leaving a smoothed and regularized corneal surface (modified from Hersh & Wagoner [4])

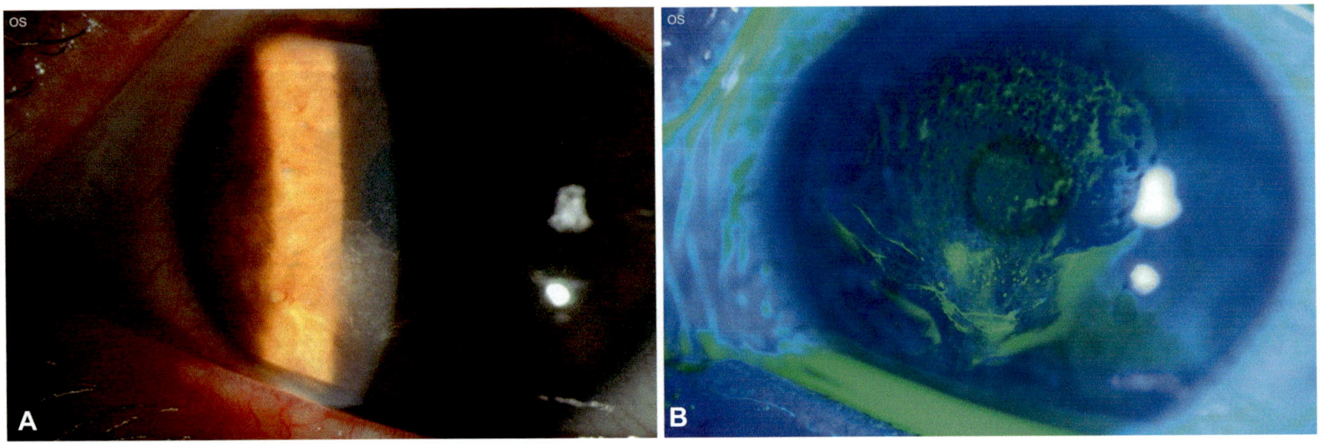

Fig. 11 Recurrent corneal erosions due to epithelial basement membrane dystrophy. (**A**) Slit lamp overview, (**B**) Vital staining with fluorecein and blue light indicates that almost the entire epithelium is loose

4.5 Aftercare

At the end of the operation under topical anesthesia, we rinse with ice-cold Balanced Salt Solution (BSS) and apply a therapeutic contact lens immersed in Diclofenac eye drops (Voltaren ®) for 5 min. Prophylactically, we administer ofloxacin eye drops 5x/d for 1 week as long as the bandage contact lens is worn. After epithelial closure, postoperative local antibiotics are usually no more required. However, lubricants or gels and nonpreserved artificial tears should be used to promote epithelial healing without causing prolonged superficial punctate keratopathy. Usually, topical steroids (e.g. fluorometholone 0.1%) are slowly reduced over several weeks or months. Depending

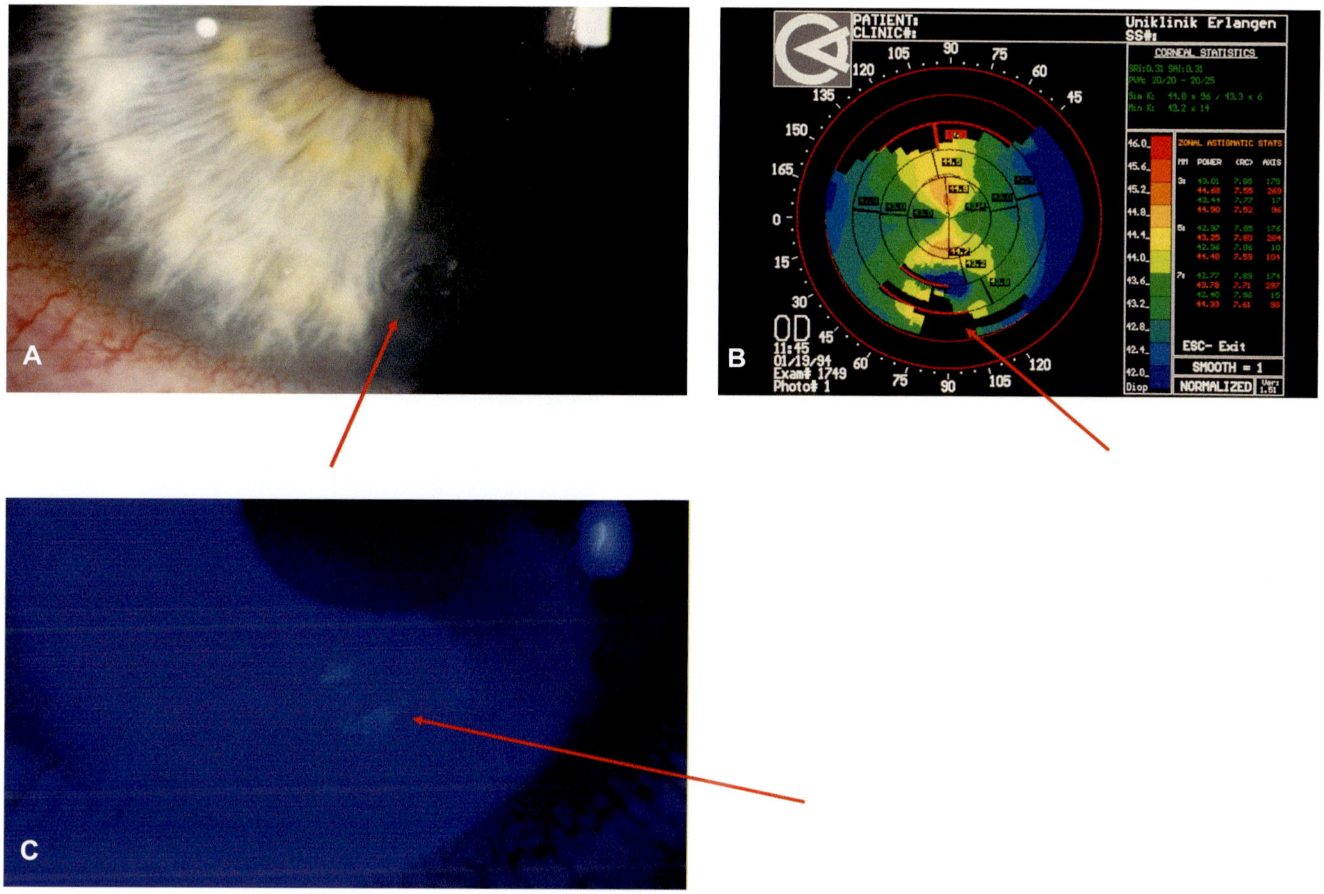

Fig. 12 Recurrent corneal erosions due to sharp trauma (Yucca palm) (**A**) Slit lamp overview (arrow), (**B**) Topography (TMS-5) showing the localized surface disturbance (arrow), (**C**) Vital staining with fluorescein and blue light indicates the localized area of loose epithelium (arrow)

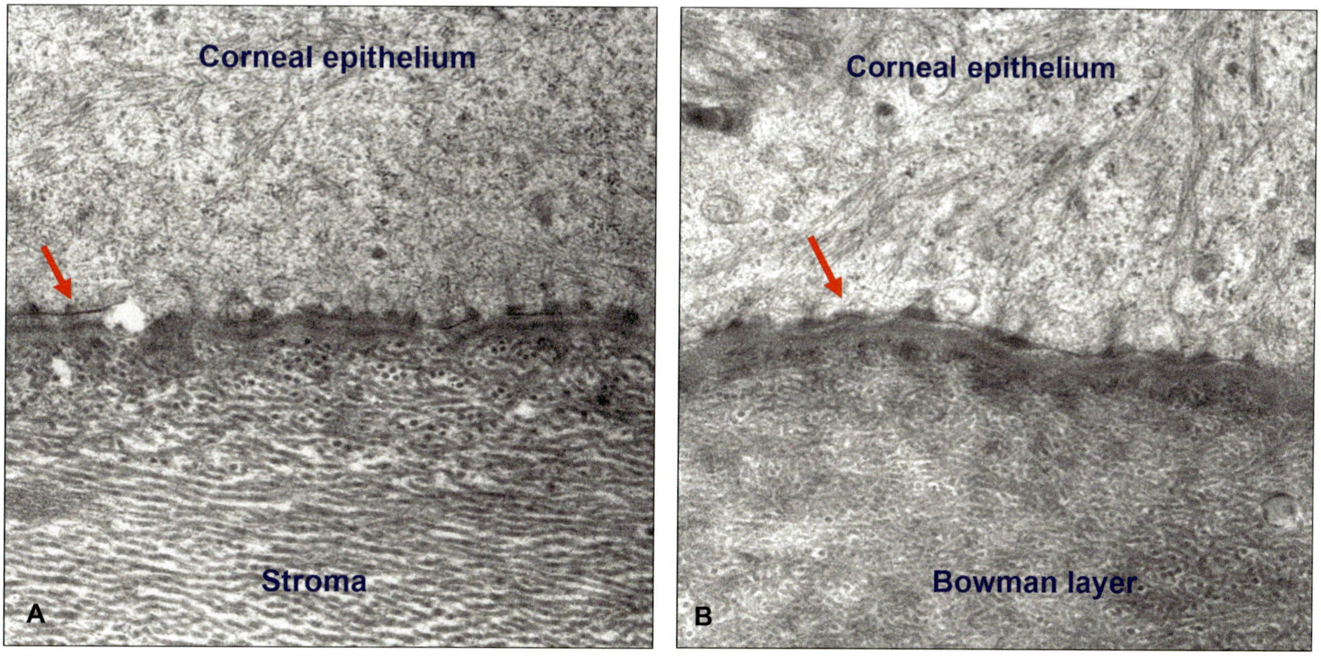

Fig. 13 Augmentation of hemidesmosomes after excimer-PTK in macular corneal dystrophy (transmission electron microscopy). (**A**) After PTK: number of hemidesmosomes 5500 ± 800/mm, (**B**) Without PTK: Number of hemidesmosomes significantly less 3500 ± 900/mm

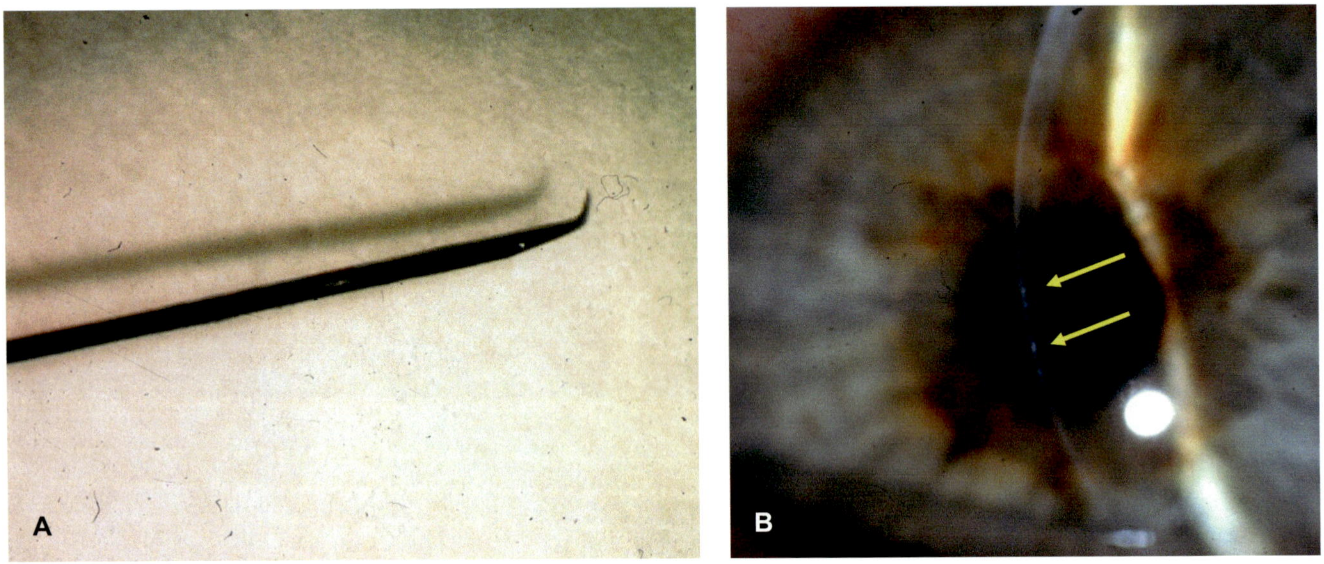

Fig. 14 Central stromal puncture using a bended sharp needle (**A**) will result in central subepithelial scars (arrows) (**B**)

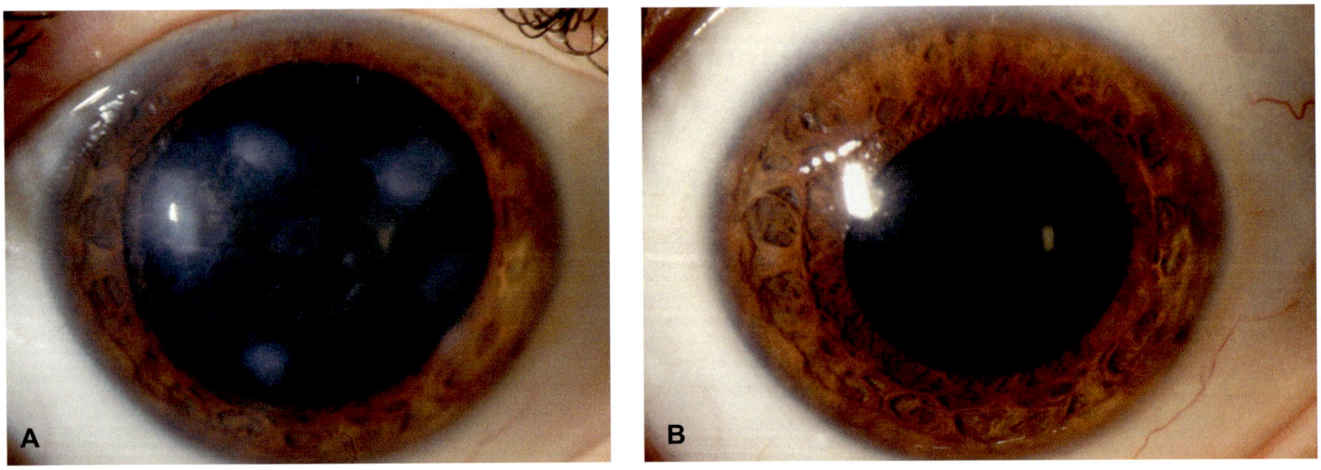

Fig. 15 Asymmetric tear film pooling with "optic cornea plana" due to midperipheral Salzmann nodules [24], (**A**) Visual acuity before PTK (+13.5/−5.0/100°) = 20/100. (**B**) Clear cornea 6 weeks after PTK: uncorrected visual acuity 20/25 to 20/20p

on the depth of ablation, this can be started with an administration 4 × daily and reduced by one drop per day every month.

5 Potential Complications

Eyes with severe ocular surface diseases such as chemical burns, ocular pemphigoid, atopic keratoconjunctivitis, and severe dysfunctional tear syndrome should only undergo PTK with extreme caution, if at all. However, delayed epithelial healing may also occur in eyes with corneal dystrophy only. After Excimer-PTK for lattice corneal dystrophies (Fig. 17) epithelial healing may take significantly longer than with all other diseases (Table 4) [19–21]. This is also true for recurrences of lattice dystrophy on the graft after PKP (Fig. 18) that typically involve only the subepithelial layer of the graft (Fig. 19) [22].

Ablation of the corneal surface results in refractive and topographic changes after PTK. These effects tend to be predictable depending on the type of corneal disease treated and the surgical method used. The expected refractive changes should be considered in surgical decision-making and strategic planning of technical details. Nowadays, with

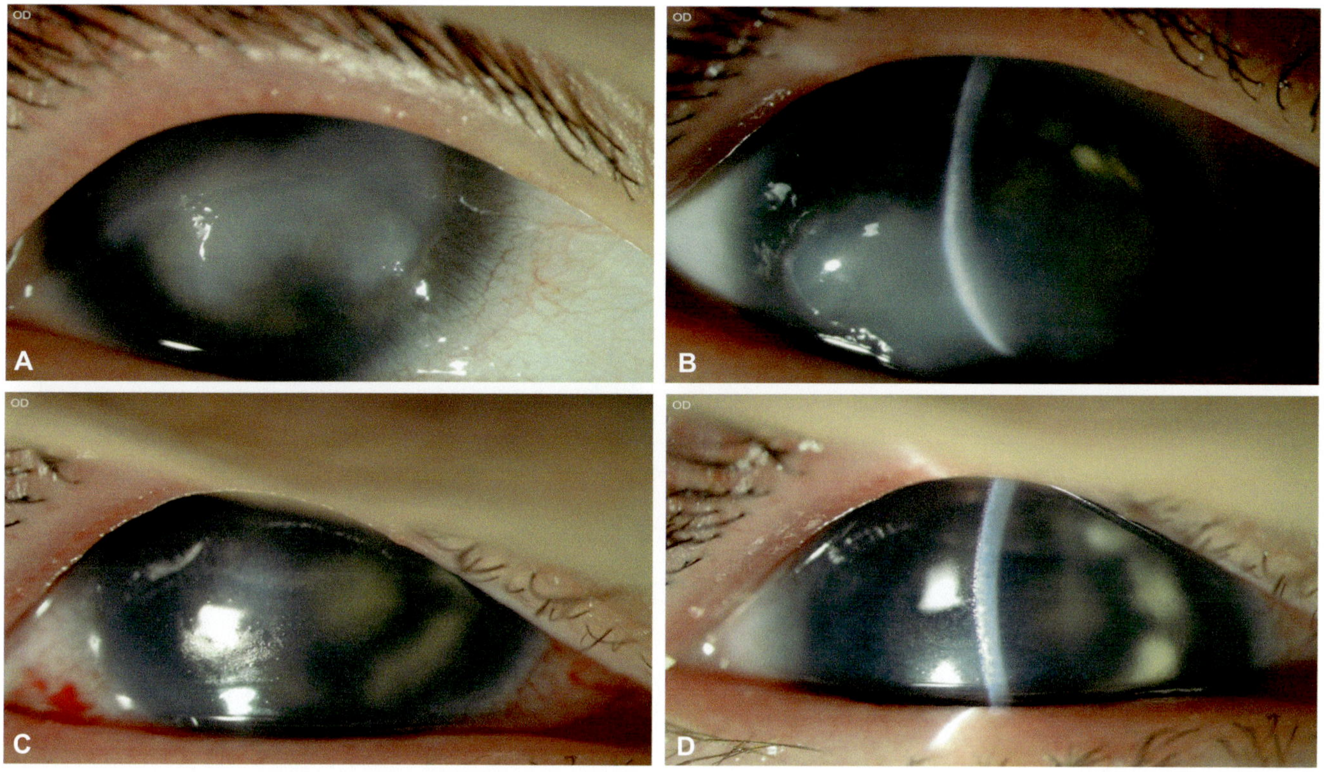

Fig. 16 Large Salzmann nodule in a young patient with aniridia associated keratopathy (AAK). (**A, B**) before Pannectomy and PTK, (**C, D**) after PTK. Note the remaining opacifications of the lens

modern excimer lasers, simultaneous hyperopic/astigmatic or even topography-based refractive ablation can be performed with acceptable results [23].

Clinical practice shows that a so-called "hyperopic shift" is a frequent side effect of PTK procedures (Fig. 20). Typically, on the other hand, a so-called "paradoxical myopia" occurs when (mid-) peripheral pannus is removed with a hockey knife prior to laser treatment (e.g. in Salzmann nodular degeneration) (Fig. 15). Prior to PTK, asymmetric tear film pooling due to midperipheral Salzmann nodules can result in an "optical cornea plana" with high hyperopia and irregular astigmatism [24].

Early after PTK, mild to moderate reticular subepithelial stromal opacification (so-called "haze") is quite common. The intensity seems to depend on the depth of ablation and subsides over the course of a few months. Pre-existing scars are more likely to recur. In these eyes, the use of MMC should be considered [17, 18].

The risk of microbial keratitis due to iatrogenic introduction of an epithelial defect is very low, but is a serious complication that can significantly affect the final visual outcome. After PTK, we routinely administer nonpreserved fluoroquinolone antibiotics because they are much less toxic to the epithelium than aminoglycosides [25].

Immunologic graft rejection after PKP can be induced by any surgical procedure on the eye. PTK may be such a procedure, especially if there is sustained inflammation through a prolonged period of time until epithelial closure. Immunologic graft rejection after PTK may also occur years after PKP. Although it is unclear what triggered the immune reaction (the laser treatment itself, manual epithelial removal, changes in drop application), it is clear that immediate topical and systemic treatment with corticosteroids is essential to prevent or manage this rare complication after PTK. **We also give prophylactic systemic steroids perioperatively for PTK after PK and routinely use**

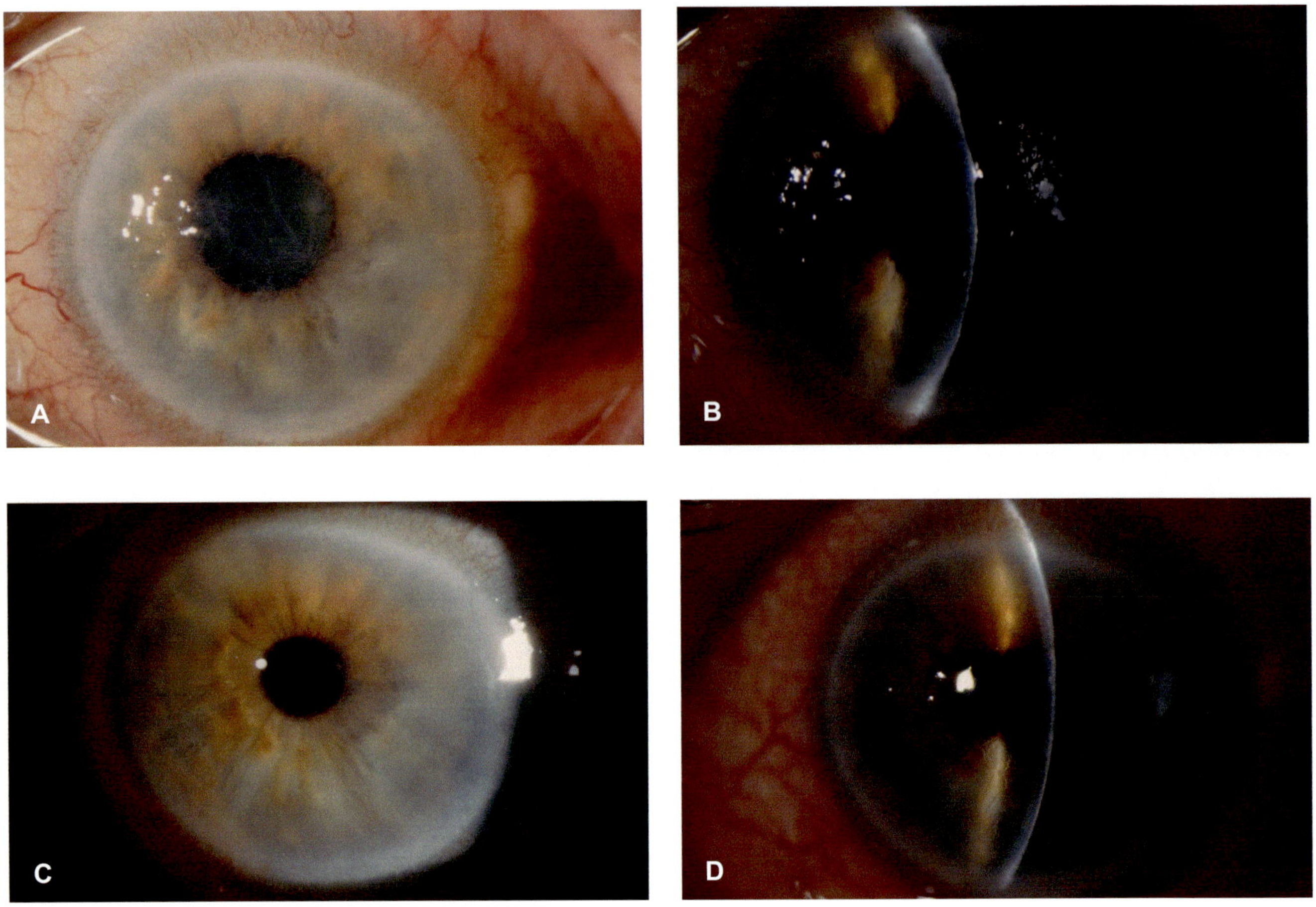

Fig. 17 Lattice corneal dystrophy, (**A, B**) before PTK, (**C, D**) after PTK

Table 4 Mean duration until corneal epithelial closure after excimer-PTK [19]

Lattice dystrophy	(8.6 ± 8.4 days)
EBM dystrophy	(3.0 ± 1.5 days, P=0.009)
Reis–Bücklers dystrophy	(3.7 ± 3.1 days, P=0.03)
Granular dystrophy type 1	(3.1 ± 1.5 days, P=0.001)
Macular dystrophy	(2.7 ± 0.8 days, P=0.01)
Non-herpetic scars	(3.6 ± 2.4 days, P=0.007)
Salzmann degeneration	(3.3 ± 1.3 days, P=0.011)

MMC intraoperatively. If there is a history of herpes, we recommend perioperative prophylaxis with aciclovir orally and ganciclovir gel topically.

Patients with corneal dystrophies undergoing PTK may experience recurrences after the procedure. Conditions such as lattice, granular, and macular corneal dystrophy, epithelial basement membrane dystrophy (Fig. 21) or Salzmann nodular degeneration may recur at varying intervals after PTK [5, 26, 27]. Our clinical impression is that recurrences on the original cornea after PTK behave differently than recurrences of the same dystrophy on the graft after PKP [28]: While granular dystrophy on the PKP/DALK graft recurs quite frequently and rapidly (after a few years), it recurs late after PTK. While macular dystrophy hardly recurs even after three to four decades post-PKP [29, 30], superficial plaque-like opacities recur very quickly (a few years) after PTK in macular dystrophy (Figs. 22 and 23) [10]. In contrast, Map-Dot Fingerprint dystrophy recurs very late (about 10 years) (Fig. 21) [11].

Contraindications against Excimer-PTK include Corneal Intraepithelial Neoplasia (CIN) and systemic collagenosis (Table 5).

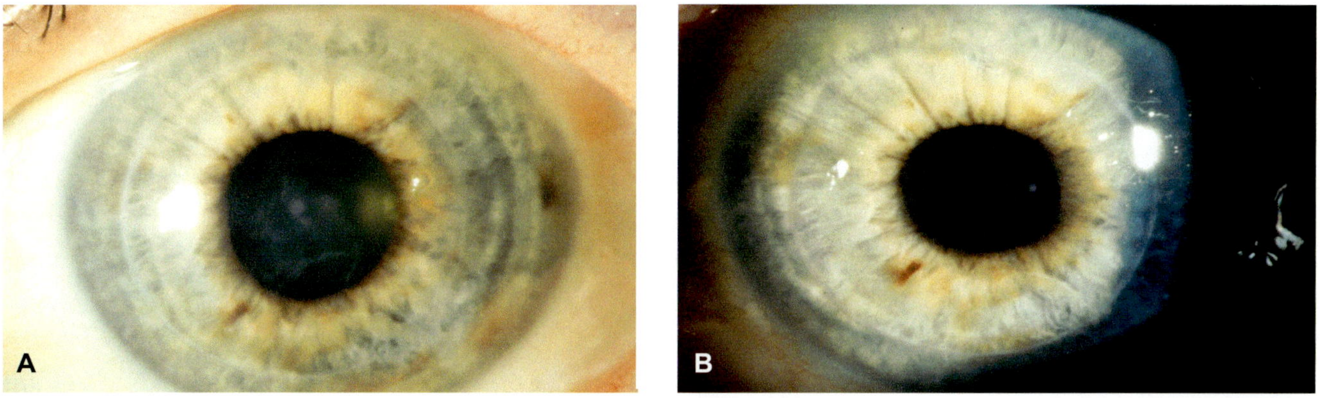

Fig. 18 Recurrence of lattice corneal dystrophy on the graft. (**A**) before PTK, (**B**) after PTK

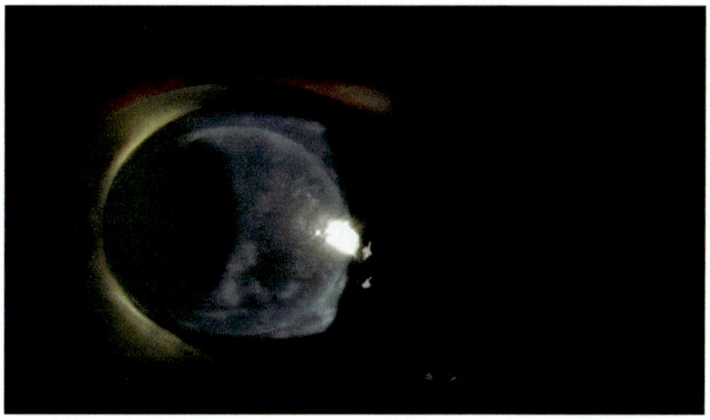

Fig. 19 Recurrence of lattice corneal dystrophy on the graft. The amyloid deposits are found predominantly in the superficial stroma below the epithelium but barely in the stroma [22]

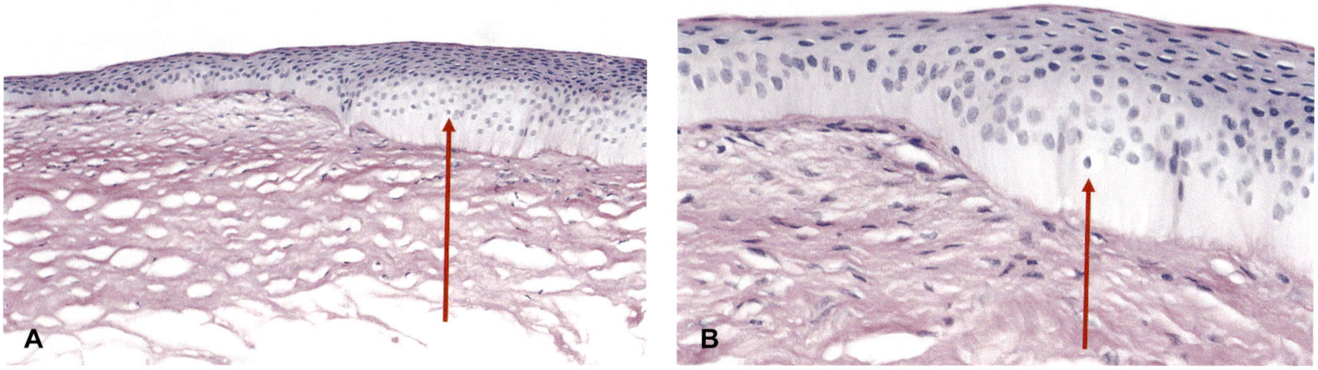

Fig. 20 The so-called "hyperopic shift" is a frequent side effect of PTK procedures. One of the reasons is the hypertrophy and hyperplasia of epithelial cells in the peripheral laser ablation area (arrows)

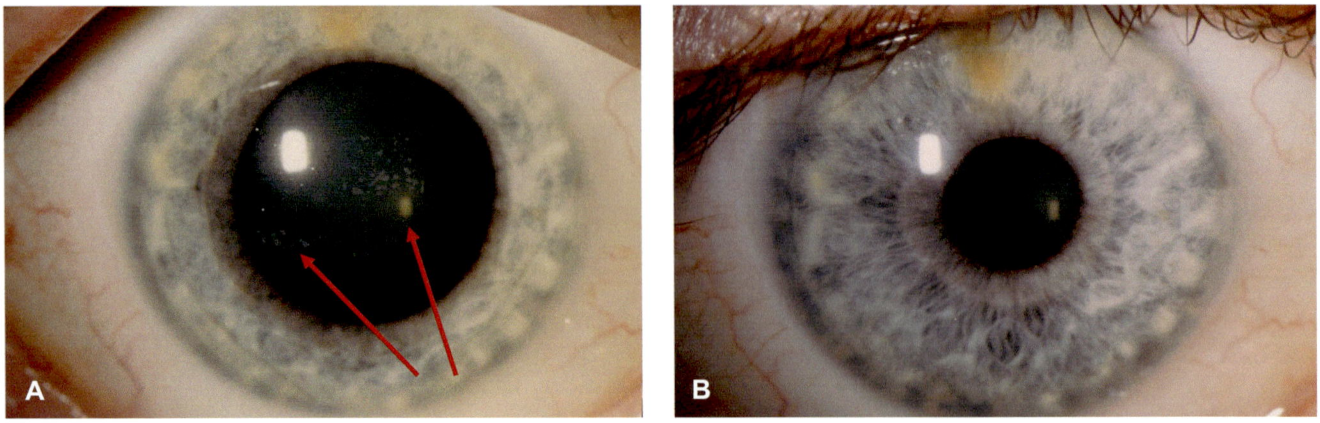

Fig. 21 Epithelial basement membrane dystrophy in a 36-year-old patient. (**A**) before PTK, (**B**) 9 years after PTK without recurrence

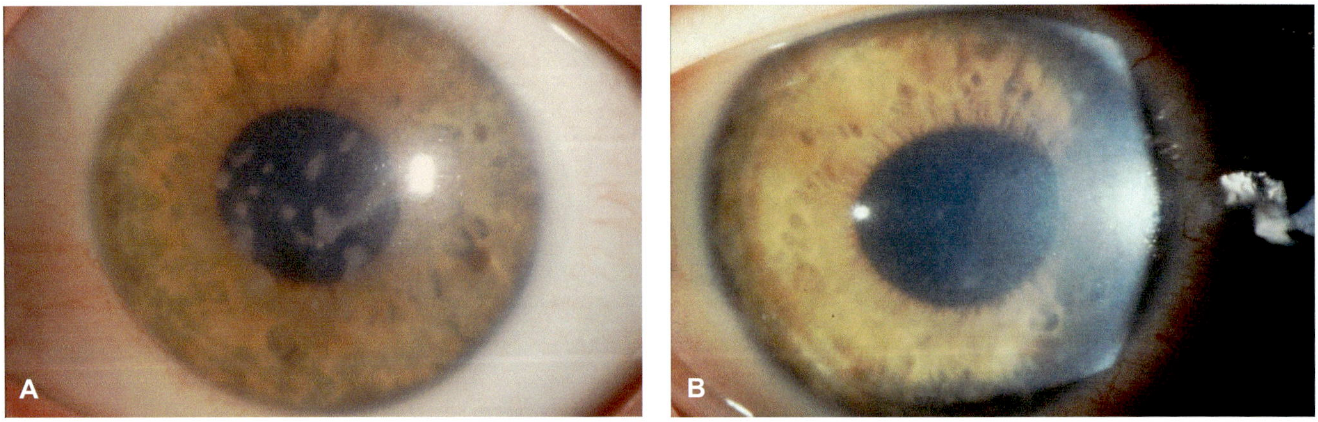

Fig. 22 Macular corneal dystrophy: slit lamp image (**A**) before and (**B**) 6 weeks after PTK (CAVE: Only the superficial plaque-like deposits of acidic mucopolysaccharides can be removed by PTK [10])

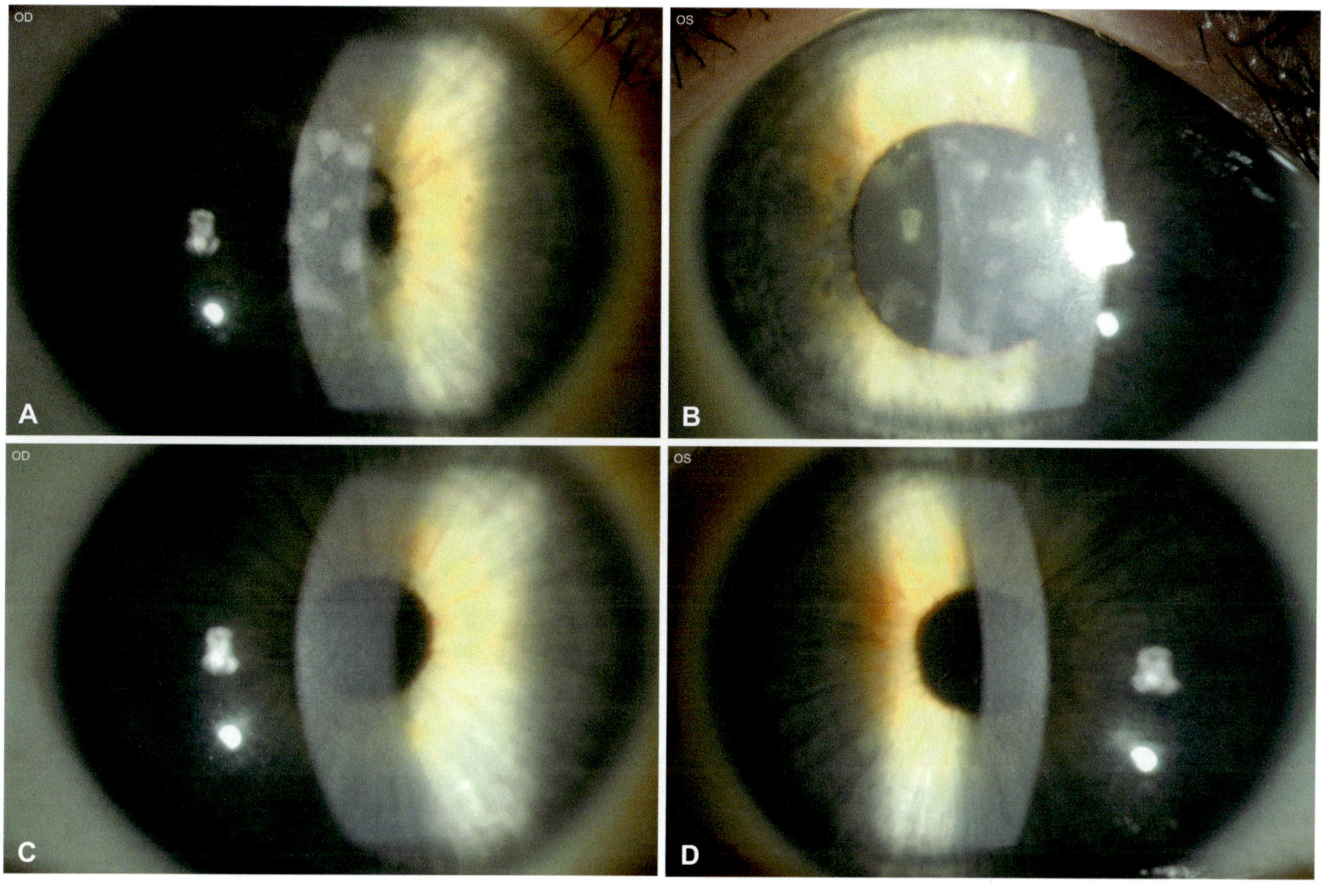

Fig. 23 Macular corneal dystrophy in both eyes of an 18-year-old patient: (**A, B**) slit lamp image before PTK, (**C, D**)slit lamp image 6 weeks after PTK

Table 5 Contraindications for excimer-PTK

→ Vascularized pannus in chronic blepharokeratoconjunktivitis
→ Limbal stem cell deficiency (Fig. 24)
→ Acute infectious ulcer
→ Corneal intraepithelial neoplasia CIN−CAVE: No excimer laser to protect Bowman layer against vertical extension of the tumor !!!!
→ Systemic vasculitis or collagenosis
→ Herpes scars only under acyclovir protection

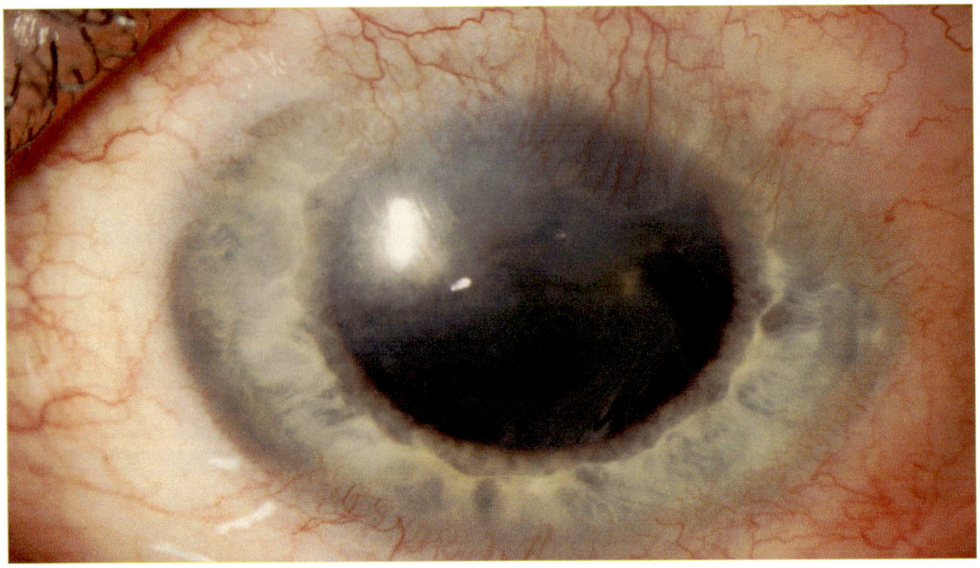

Fig. 24 Vascularized pannus due to limbal stem cell deficiency of unclear origin is a contraindication for excimer-PTK

6 Conclusion

For more than 30 years, PTK has been an indispensable addition to the corneal microsurgical spectrum for selected corneal pathologies also in the future. **"PTK is here to stay!"** A critical patient selection, a detailed preoperative counseling, a well planned and executed operation **("PTK is more an art than a science")** and an adequate and consequent follow-up usually help to minimize disappointments and unpleasant postoperative discussions.

CAVE: „If You Have a Hammer, Everything Looks like a Nail … "

References

1. Seitz B, Langenbucher A, Hafner A, Kus MM, Naumann GO. Phototherapeutic keratectomy for recurrent corneal erosion syndrome (e-PTK). Report on 116 consecutive interventions. Ophthalmologe. 2002;99:703–8.
2. Seitz B, Lisch W, Weiss J. The revised newest IC^{3}D classification of corneal dystrophies. Klin Monbl Augenheilkd. 2015;232:283–94.
3. Fagerholm P. Phototherapeutic keratectomy: 12 years of experience. Acta Ophthalmol Scand. 2003;81:19–32.
4. Hersh PS, Wagoner MD, editors. Excimer laser surgery for corneal disorders. New York: Thieme; 1998.
5. Rapuano CJ. Excimer laser phototherapeutic keratectomy: long-term results and practical considerations. Cornea. 1997;16:151–7.
6. Seitz B, Langenbucher A. Phototherapeutic keratectomy in corneal dystrophies. In: Reinhard T & Larkin F, editors. Essentials in ophthalmology-corneal and external eye disease. Berlin: Springer-Verlag;2007.
7. Adams C, Mahler S, Daas L, Langenbucher A, Seitz B. Phototherapeutic keratectomy for epithelial basement membrane dystrophy: impact of excimer laser systems used on the changes of visual acuity, refraction and astigmatism. Ophthalmologie. 2022; 119:945–51.
8. Mahler S, Adams C, Daas L, Langenbucher A, Seitz B. Phototherapeutic keratectomy for Salzmann's nodular degeneration. What effect does the choice of excimer laser have on treatment success? Klin Monbl Augenheilkd 2023;240:1262–8.
9. Seitz B, Behrens A, Langenbucher A, Fischer M, Naumann GOH. Morphometric analysis of deposits in granular and lattice corneal dystrophy–histopathologic implications for phototherapeutic keratectomy. Cornea. 2004;23:380–5.
10. Hafner A, Langenbucher A, Seitz B. Long-term results of phototherapeutic keratectomy (o-PTK) with 193 nm excimer laser for macular corneal dystrophy. Am J Ophthalmol. 2005;140:392–6.
11. Pogorelov P, Langenbucher A, Kruse FE, Seitz B. Long-term results of phototherapeutic keratectomy for corneal map-dot-fingerprint dystrophy (Cogan-Guerry). Cornea. 2006;25:774–7.
12. Seitz B, Flockerzi E, Daas L. Significance of imaging pathological non-inflammatory findings of the corneal surface for phototherapeutic keratectomy. Z prakt Augenheilkd 2020; 41:125–34.
13. Kornmehl EW, Steinert RF, Puliafito CA. A comparative study of masking fluids for excimer laser phototherapeutic keratectomy. Arch Ophthalmol. 1991;109:860–3.
14. Szentmáry N, Seitz B, Langenbucher A, Schlötzer-Schrehardt U, Hofmann-Rummelt C, Naumann GOH. Histologic and ultrastructural changes in corneas with granular and macular dystrophy after excimer laser phototherapeutic keratectomy. Cornea. 2006;25:257–63.
15. Fries FF, Náray A, Munteanu C, Stachon T, Lagali N, Seitz B, Käsmann-Kellner B, Szentmáry N. A cross-sectional analysis of 556 eyes entering The Homburg Anirida Center. Klin Monbl Augenheilkd. 2024;241:275–282.
16. Seitz B, Käsmann-Kellner B, Viestenz A. Stage-related therapy of congenital aniridia. Ophthalmologe 2014; 111:1164–71.
17. Carones F, Vigo L, Scandola E, Vacchini L. Evaluation of the prophylactic use of mitomycin-C to inhibit haze formation after photorefractive keratectomy. J Cataract Refract Surg. 2002;28:2088–99.
18. Safi T, Seitz B, Flockerzi E, Flockerzi FA, Daas L. Haze after PRK (without use of Mitomycin C) on a pretreated cornea with DALK and LASIK-clinical and histopathological findings. Klin Monbl Augenheilkd. 2023; 240:147–50.
19. Das S, Langenbucher A, Seitz B. Delayed healing of corneal epithelium after phototherapeutic keratectomy for lattice dystrophy. Cornea. 2005D;24:283–7.

20. Förster CG, Langenbucher A, Cursiefen C, Kruse FE, Seitz B. Delayed epithelial healing after keratoplasty for lattice corneal dystrophy. Cornea. 2007;26:1182–3.
21. Resch MD, Schlötzer-Schrehardt U, Hofmann-Rummelt C, Kruse FE, Seitz B. Alterations of epithelial adhesion molecules and beasement membrane components in lattice corneal dystrophy (LCD). Graefes Arch Clin Exp Ophthalmol. 2009;247:1081–8.
22. Lisch W, Seitz B. Lattice corneal dystrophy type 1: an epithelial or stromal entity? Cornea. 2014;33:1109–12.
23. Zhou W, Reinstein DZ, Archer TJ, Nitter T, Feng Y, Mule G, Stojanovic A. The impact of epithelial remodeling on surgical techniques used in topography-guided surface ablation in irregular corneas. J Refract Surg. 2022;38:529–37.
24. Viestenz A, Bischoff-Jung M, Langenbucher A, Eppig T, Seitz B. Phototherapeutic keratectomy in Salzmann's nodular degeneration with "optical cornea plana". Cornea. 2016; 35(6):843–6.
25. Seitz B, Hayashi S, Wee WR, LaBree L, McDonnell PJ. *In vitro* effects of aminoglycosides and fluoroquinolones on keratocytes. Invest Ophthalmol Vis Sci. 1996;37:656–65.
26. Das S, Langenbucher A, Pogorelov P, Link B, Seitz B. Long-term outcome of excimer laser phototherapeutic keratectomy for treatment of Salzmann's nodular degeneration. J Cataract Refract Surg. 2005B;31:1386–91.
27. Das S, Langenbucher A, Seitz B. Excimer laser phototherapeutic keratectomy for granular and lattice corneal dystrophy: a comparative study. J Refract Surg. 2005C;21:727–31.
28. Szentmáry N, Langenbucher A, Hafner A, Seitz B. Impact of phototherapeutic keratectomy on the outcome of subsequent penetrating keratoplasty in patients with stromal corneal dystrophies. Am J Ophthalmol. 2004;137:301–7.
29. Bischoff-Jung M, Flockerzi E, Hasenfus A, Viestenz A, Matoula P, Schlötzer-Schrehardt U, Seitz B. Recurrence of macular corneal dystrophy on the graft 50 years after penetrating keratoplasty. GMS Ophthalmol Cases 2020; 10:Doc34.
30. Küchle M, Cursiefen C, Fischer DC, Schlötzer-Schrehardt U, Naumann GOH. Recurrent macular corneal dystrophy type II 49 years after penetrating keratoplasty. Arch Ophthalmol. 1999;117:528–31.
31. Weiss JS, Rapuano CJ, Seitz B, Busin M, Kivelä TT, Bouheraoua N, Bredrup C, Nischal KK, Chawla H, Borderie V, Kenyon KR, Kim EK, Møller HU, Munier FL, Berger T, Lisch W. IC3D classification of corneal dystrophies-edition 3. Cornea. 2024;43:466–527.
32. Weiss JS, Møller HU, Aldave AJ, Seitz B, Bredrup C, Kivelä T, Munier FL, Rapuano CJ, Nischal KK, Kim EK, Sutphin J, Busin M, Labbé A, Kenyon KR, Kinoshita S, Lisch W. The revised IC3D classification of corneal dystrophies-edition 2. Cornea. 2015;34:117–59.
33. Das S, Link B, Seitz B. Salzmann's nodular degeneration of the cornea: a review and case series. Cornea. 2005A;24:772–7.
34. Paoletti T, Maamri A, Zemova E, Flockerzi F, Seitz B. Large Salzmann's nodules or acute keratoconus? Ophthalmologie. 2022; 119:841–44.

Eye Banking

Loïc Hamon, Adrien Quintin, Tarek Safi, Loay Daas, Isabel Weinstein, and Berthold Seitz

Abstract

In the past, the role of eye banks was limited to collection and preservation of corneal tissues prior to transplantation. In the last decades, continuous improvements of preservation techniques and new approaches of tissue analysis in eye banks extended storage time and provided better tissue quality. Moreover, an increasing number of keratoplasty techniques is challenging eye banks to develop new selection and preparation methods. This chapter gives a comprehensive overview of present and future aspects of eye banking.

Keywords

Eye bank · Cornea · Organ culture · Slit lamp · Endothelial cell count · Donor tomography · Artificial intelligence · Quality management

1 Introduction

Due to the worldwide increasing need for corneal transplantation, eye banks are playing an evermore important role in the collection, cultivation, evaluation and preparation of corneal tissues for corneal surgeons prior to keratoplasty [1].

In this section, we will cover the different roles of modern eye banking.

2 Procurement of Corneal Tissues

In order to minimize the risk of donor-to-host disease transmission, careful donor selection is necessary. Regulatory agencies such as the European Eye Bank Association (EEBA) and the Eye Bank Association of America (EBAA) are continuously working to minimize this risk with well-documented and broadly accepted regulations in the field. A list of contraindications for corneal donation and new testing to exclude potentially transmissible diseases are adapted and updated on a regular basis.

If the donor presents no contraindications for being used as a graft, the eye bank staff can proceed with the collection of the donor corneas [2] using one of the following methods:

Whole globe collection is a simple and quick method of collecting donor tissue. The globe is lifted out of the orbita from the behind with an instrument and the optic nerve and extraocular muscles are cut with scissors, similar to an enucleation procedure. Whole globes need to be prepared at the eye bank prior to surgery. Advantages of this method are the short time of tissue collection and the possibility to prepare scleral tissue, allowing for other surgeries such as sclerocorneoplasty [3] or scleral patches [4].

Corneoscleral explantation (15 mm disc) is a more expensive alternative regarding time and resources. It is performed in the same way as an ophthalmic surgical procedure, in sterile conditions and using surgical equipment (Fig. 1). This method has a much higher acceptance rate

L. Hamon (✉) · A. Quintin · T. Safi · L. Daas · I. Weinstein · B. Seitz
Department of Ophthalmology, Saarland University Medical Center, Homburg, Saar, Germany
e-mail: hamon.loic@outlook.com

L. Hamon · L. Daas · I. Weinstein · B. Seitz
Klaus Faber Center for Corneal Diseases, Including LIONS Eye Bank Saar-Lor-Lux, Saarland University Medical Center, Trier/WestpfalzHomburg, Saar, Germany

L. Hamon
Department of Ophthalmology, Clinique Notre-Dame de Grâce, Charleroi, Belgium

B. Seitz et al. (eds.), *Atlas on Cornea*, https://doi.org/10.1007/978-3-031-65422-0_48

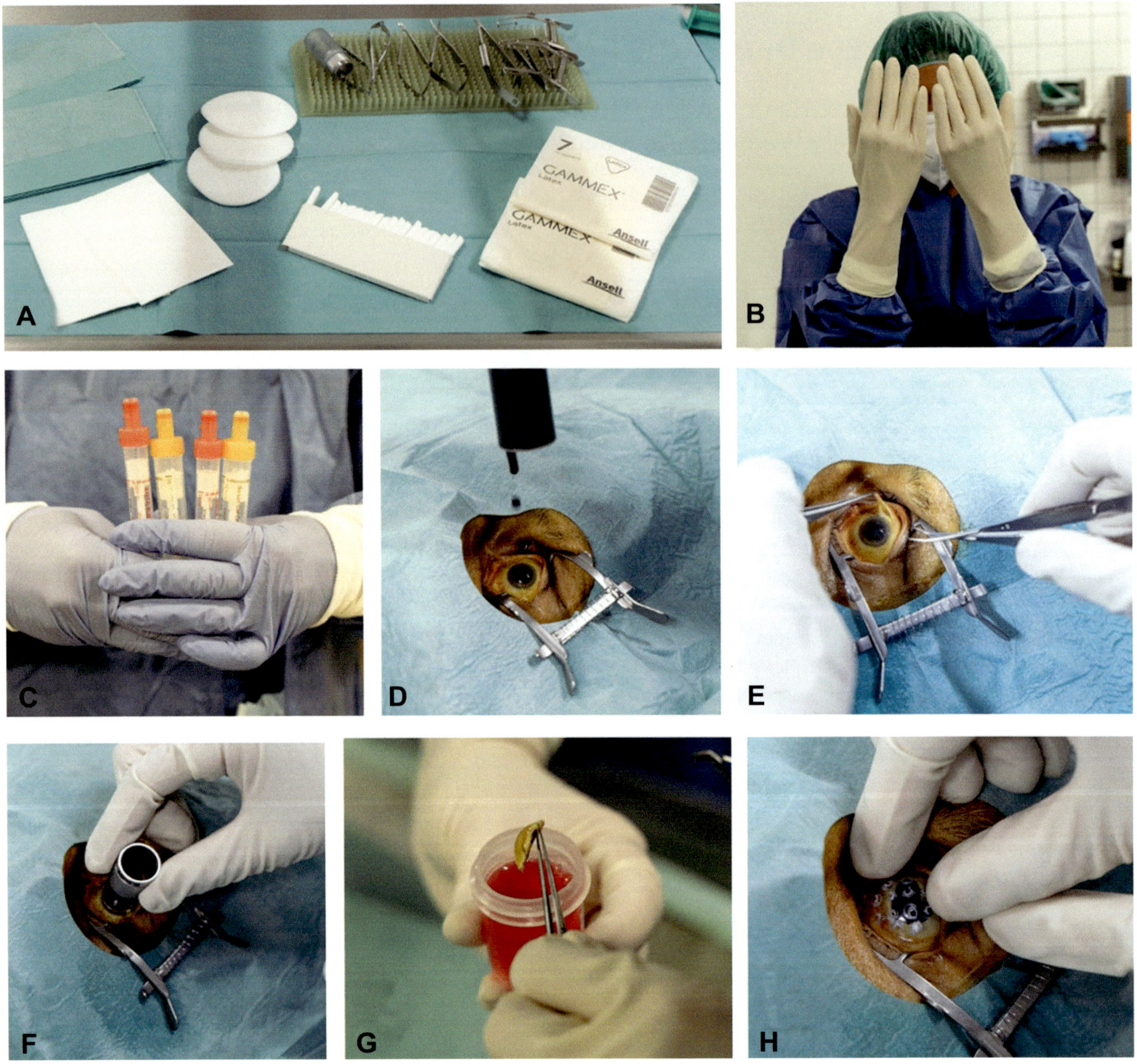

Fig. 1 **Cornea procurement–corneoscleral technique step by step. (A, B)** Material for corneal procurement is prepared sterilely equivalent to an intraocular procedure, and eye bank staff need to wash and sterilize themselves before the procedure. (**C**) If a reserve sample cannot be obtained from the laboratory, blood samples should be taken for donor analysis prior to collection, classically from the subclavian artery. (**D**) Povidone iodine (1.25%) is applied for 5 min before trephination to avoid potential contamination [5]. (**E**) Bulbar conjunctiva is dissected around the limbus before trephination. (**F**) Trephination is performed using a 15 mm diameter round trephine. In order to ensure optimal processing of the graft, trephination should be exact and centered. (**G**) Following trephination, the corneoscleral disc is placed in organ culture medium II (also known as *transport medium*). (**H**) After corneal collection, plastic shells are applied for aesthetic reconstruction and the eyelids are tightly closed and either sutured or glued together. Thus, there is no evidence of the procedure for the relatives

by the donors' relatives as only the corneoscleral disc is explanted [6, 7]. Due to the fact that the corneoscleral disc is also already cut, further manipulation in the eye bank prior to preservation is avoided.

After collection, the whole globes or corneas are taken to the eye bank, where they are preserved, examined and prepared for surgical purposes.

3 Organization and Quality Management System (QMS) in the Eye Bank

An eye bank is bound by the laws, technical norms, guidelines and legislative frameworks of its country which regulate corneal donation, handling, transport and transplantation of donor tissues [1, 8]. The eye bank must be located in a suitable and properly equipped facility. Human tissues should be processed under sterile conditions, ideally with cleanroom concept (Fig. 2). Hereby, tissue quality can constantly be increased and the number of discarded tissues due to contamination concerns can be diminished [9].

A quality management system (QMS) is an essential component of a highly functioning eye bank to ensure a maximum level of quality and safety of human tissues

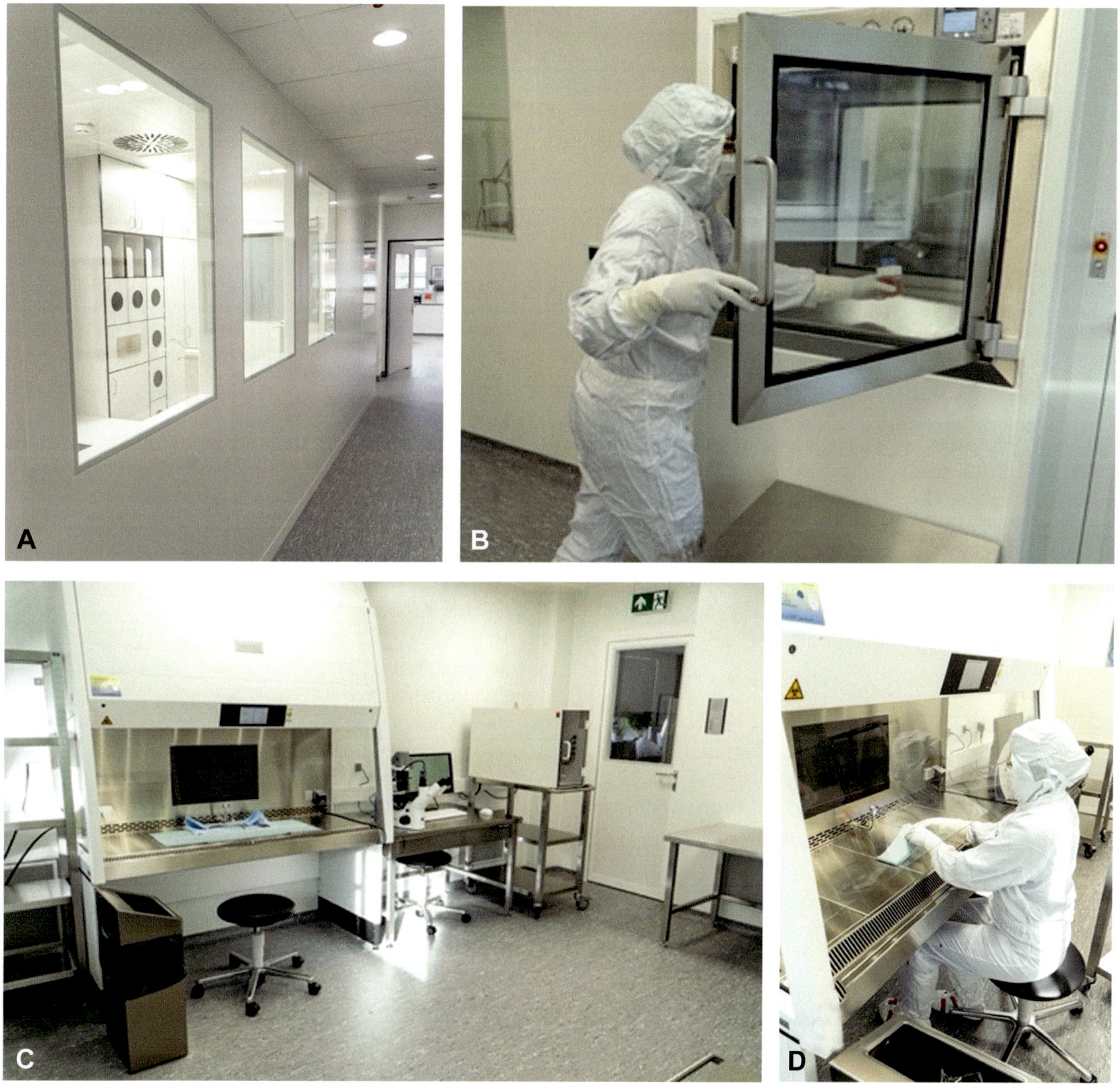

Fig. 2 **Cleanroom in the Klaus Faber Center for Corneal Diseases, incl. LIONS Eye Bank Saar-Lor-Lux, Trier/Westpfalz (Homburg/Saar, Germany).** (**A**) Decontamination area. According to the International Organization for Standardization (ISO) and European Good Manufacturing Practice (EU GMP) guidelines concerning cleanroom standards for manufacturing sterile medical products, eye bank staff dress in several steps through the decontamination area, from room grade E (not controlled and not sterilized) to cleanroom grade B (controlled and sterilized). (**B**) Transfer chambers between the different cleanrooms for corneas and instruments. The chambers are equipped with unilateral flow pressure systems (from the most to the least sterile cleanroom) to ensure the sterility of the areas. (**C**) Laminar flow bench for tissue handling (EU GMP grade A, the cleanest) in cleanroom grade B. (**D**) A staff member sterilely dressed renewing the organ culture medium of organ-cultured corneas under maximum sterile conditions, under laminar flow (EU GMP grade A)

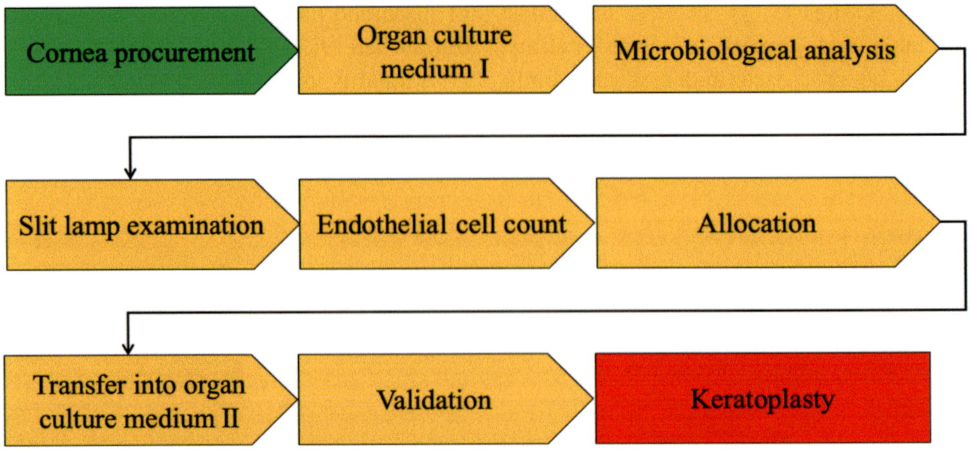

Fig. 3 **Path of a donor cornea** from procurement in the mortuary (*green*) to the operating room (*red*). Between the beginning and the end of its journey, the donor cornea is preserved in the eye bank (*orange*) in isotonic organ culture medium (so-called *medium I* or *preservation medium*), where it undergoes a series of analyses (including microbiological analysis of culture medium, slit lamp examination and endothelial cell count) before being allocated (patient-cornea matching) and approved (= validation) for surgery (mandatory re-verification of all parameters by the physician in charge of the eye bank). Prior to penetrating keratoplasty, donor corneas are transferred into another hypertonic organ culture medium (so-called *medium II* or *transport medium*) in order to deswell to normal corneal thickness. Corneas allocated for Descemet Membrane Endothelial Keratoplasty can remain in *medium I* prior to surgery. Other optional analyses such as a donor tomography can be performed before allocation and included in the validation process if needed

[10]. The International Organization for Standardization (ISO) 9001:2015 standard can be adopted to the entire process in eye banks from donation to transplantation [11] (Fig. 3). Traceability of the donor and the recipient must be ensured and documented throughout the entire process. Internal and external audits need to be held regularly in order to monitor, maintain and improve the quality management system and obtain national and international accreditations.

4 Preservation of Corneal Tissues

Nowadays, corneas are preserved either in hypothermia (especially in North America) or in organ culture (especially in Europe).

Organ culture preservation

Introduced for eye banks by Doughman et al. in the 1970s [12] and then widely popularized in Europe [13], organ culture aims for long-term preservation of the human cornea under simulated physiological conditions. In the eye bank, corneas are suspended in a cell culture container filled with an organ culture medium (modified Minimal Essential Medium—MEM) and supplemented with fetal or newborn calf serum (2–10%), antibiotics and antimycotics (*organ culture medium I*, or so-called *preservation medium*).

After transportation to the eye bank in *organ culture medium II* (so-called *transport medium*), consisting of organ culture medium I supplemented with a macromolecule—mostly dextran T500 4 to 8% [13], donor corneas are transferred under sterile conditions into cell culture containers filled with organ culture medium I and are stored at 30–37 °C for a maximum recommended period of 28 days, with renewal of the culture medium after 7–14 days, depending on the medium composition (Fig. 4).

Medium I being isotonic, the organ-cultured cornea swells to twice its normal thickness during storage [14]. Before penetrating keratoplasty can be performed, the organ cultured cornea has to be re-transferred from *organ culture medium I* into *organ culture medium II* for stromal deswelling. Deswelling time ranges between 1 and 4 days but should be maintained as short as possible to reduce endothelial exposition to dextran, which alters endothelial vitality [15]. The deswelling process being a hyperbolic function, nearly all of deswelling process (at least the clinically relevant portion) is already achieved after only 18 h [16]. This process of deswelling is not required prior to Descemet Membrane Endothelial Keratoplasty (DMEK).

Hypothermic storage

This storage technique at 2–8 °C was developed by McCarey and Kaufman in 1974 [17] and remains by far the most widely used preservation technique for corneoscleral discs in North America [18] (Fig. 5). The original McCarey-Kaufman (M–K) medium consisted of tissue culture medium TC-199, dextran (preventing corneal swelling), bicarbonate and antibiotics (penicillin/streptomycin). In contrary to organ culture, cold storage media usually do not contain antifungal agents. The preservation period

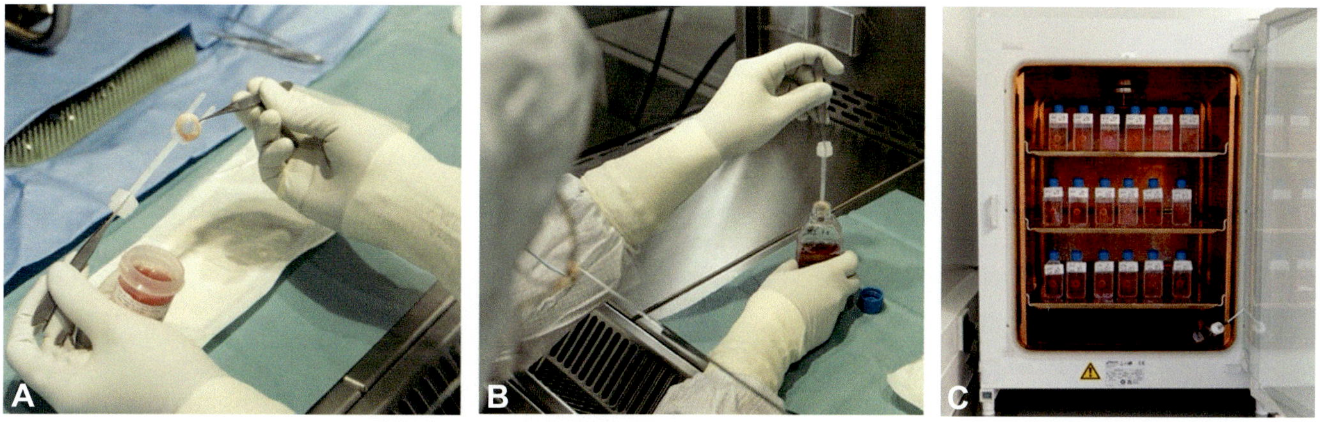

Fig. 4 **Organ-cultured corneas in cell culture flasks**. (**A**, **B**) After procurement, the corneas are transferred from organ culture medium II (*transport medium*-containing dextran) to organ culture medium I (*preservation medium*-without dextran). Corneas are mounted on holders and transferred in sterile conditions under lamina flow. (**C**) Organ-cultured corneas stored in cell culture flasks at +34 °C in an incubator up to 28 days

was formerly very limited. Currently, new culture solutions enable a storage period of 14–16 days [19]. The low temperature drastically reduces the metabolic process of the corneas, thus reducing potential pathogen proliferation, but also interfering with wound healing [20].

5 Tissue Selection and Suitability for Transplantation

Upon arrival at the eye bank, the corneal tissue is assigned an identification code. The tissue is first quarantined and serologic and microbiologic examinations [5] as well as slit-lamp examinations and evaluations of the endothelial cell density (CD) and morphology are performed before the tissue can be declared suitable for transplantation [21].

Before cultured corneas can be transplanted, they have to fulfill certain quality criteria in accordance with current international and/or national standards [1, 8]. These standards vary according to the type and nature of the surgery. Besides necessary examinations, new approaches of tissue analysis have been developed over the last few years, allowing an even better quality of transplanted corneas from modern eye banks [22].

Microbiological testing

In case of organ culture, microbiological testing of the medium sample is performed during the quarantine period at the beginning of the cultivation process [23]. Contaminated tissues are discarded prior to keratoplasty.

In case of hypothermic storage, microbiological testing of samples of the storage solution is generally not performed, as the storage time is too short to receive the results prior to keratoplasty [13]. Moreover, the number of contaminating germs should be low and not grow at this temperature after proper decontamination during retrieval [5] and before storage.

Morphological examination with slit lamp biomicroscopy

Slit-lamp biomicroscopy has been a fundamental method of tissue evaluation and remains the gold standard for determining surgical suitability, allowing an evaluation of all layers of the cornea from both anterior and posterior perspective [24].

The examination is performed through a cell culture container under sterile conditions (Fig. 6). Donor corneas are usually first examined at the beginning of the preservation period to exclude any morphological anomalies and then again at the end of the preservation period for definitive tissue validation and patient's allocation. A cornea with a scar can still be used for posterior lamellar keratoplasty (depending on scar location) or for an emergency tectonic penetrating keratoplasty (so called "keratoplasty à chaud").

Endothelial evaluation and detection of cornea guttata in the eye bank

The evaluation of the endothelial cell layer is of utmost importance to ensure tissue viability and is part of the eye bank evaluation protocol since the early 2000s [8].

Inverted light microscopy is the first-choice technique for organ-cultured corneas (Fig. 7). The endothelial cells are visualized by swelling the intracellular space using a hypotonic solution allowing endothelial layer inspection regardless of the corneal hydration [25]. Application of vital stains, such as trypan blue, may help to discriminate dead or necrotic cells [25].

Specular microscopy can also be used and is the first-choice technique in hypothermic storage. This technique does not require osmotic stimulation of the endothelial

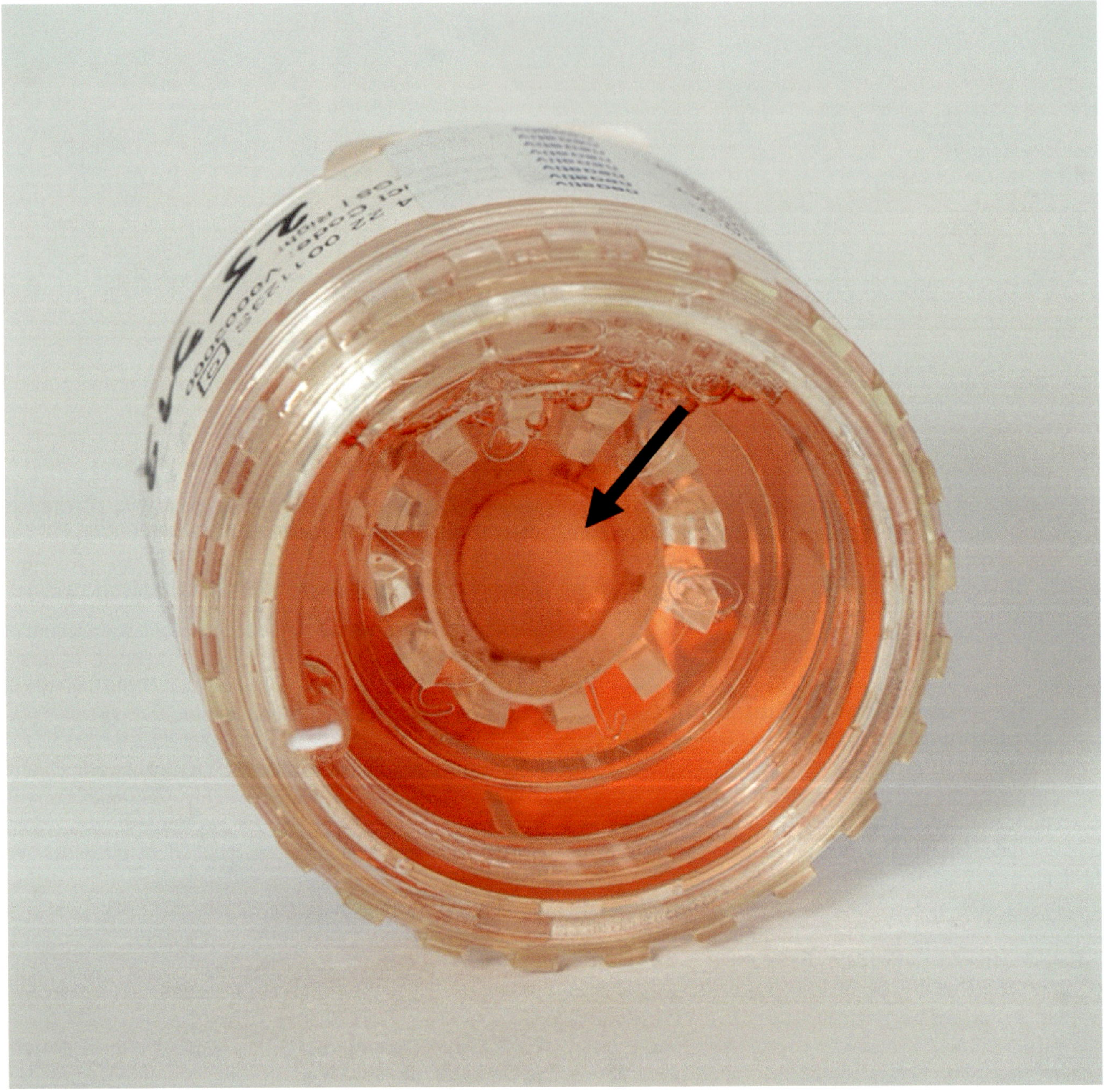

Fig. 5 **Donor cornea prepared for hypothermic storage**. Donor corneoscleral disc (*arrow*) is stored in flat cylindrical containers, allowing morphological inspection with the slit lamp and endothelium inspection by specular microscopy, both under sterile conditions if using special fixation devices [18]

cells, avoiding manipulations and associated endothelial cell loss [26]. However, specular microscopy is usually restricted to the center of the cornea and visualized areas are limited because of a microscope-related fixed magnification.

According to European standards, a minimum endothelial cell density (ECD) of 2000 cells/mm^2 is needed for penetrating or posterior lamellar keratoplasty in order to ensure long term graft survival [8]. A minimum ECD between 1000 and 2000 cells/mm^2 is advised (but not required) for anterior lamellar keratoplasty or tectonic surgery [27]. Corneas with ECD lower than 2000 cells/mm^2, endothelial cell loss of more than 25% during cultivation, cell necrosis, pronounced polymegethism or pleomorphism, pronounced granulation/vacuolization or cornea guttata (CG) have to be discarded for elective penetrating or posterior lamellar surgery [8].

CG detection is neither simple nor standardized using inverted light microscopy as CG is very difficult to detect with

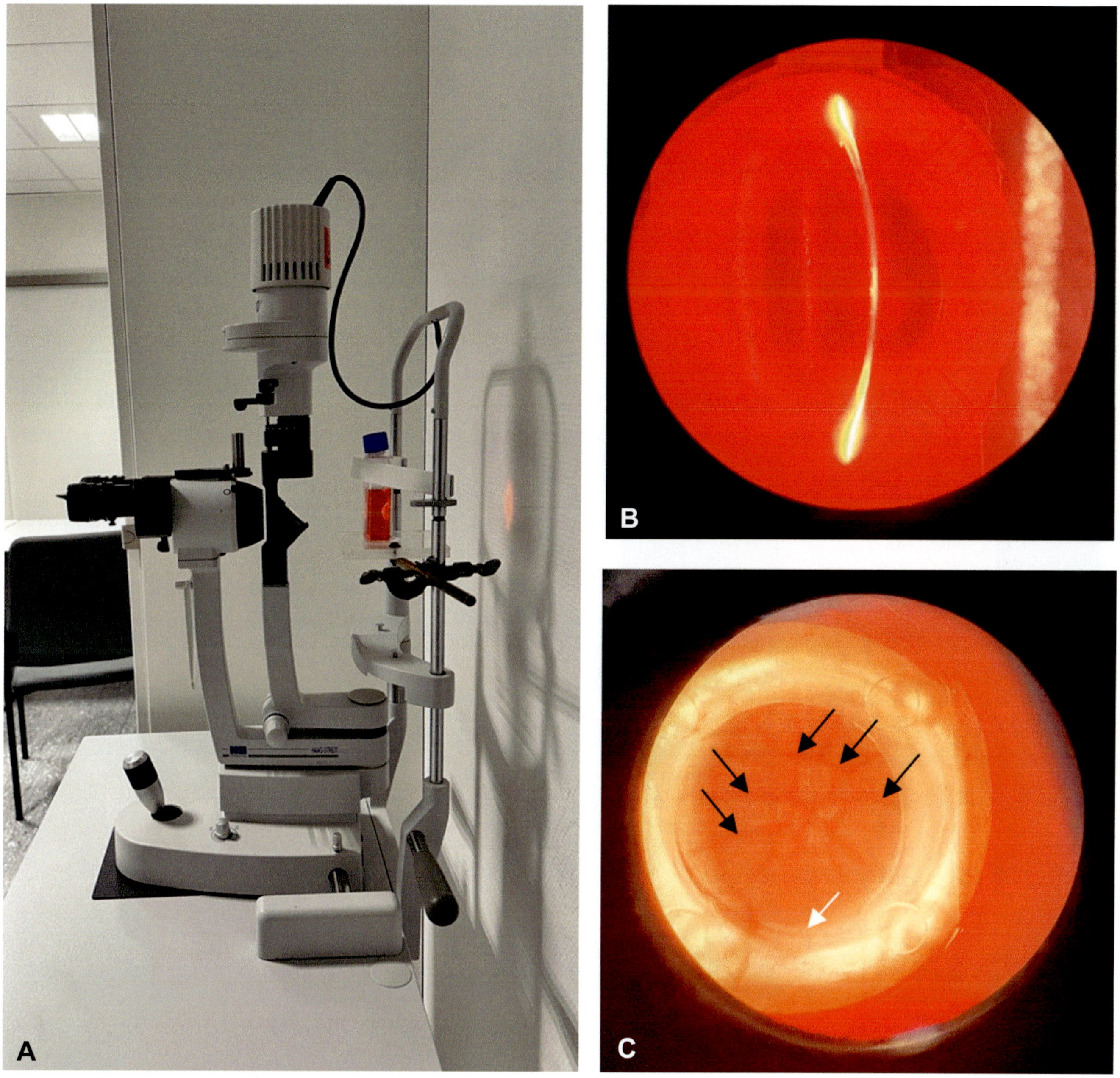

Fig. 6 Slit-lamp examination of a cultured cornea. (**A**) Slit-lamp with support plate for cell culture flask in the eye bank. (**B**) Thin slit lamp photography of cultured cornea in organ culture medium II (containing dextran T500 6%), one day prior to penetrating keratoplasty, presenting no visible defect or scar. (**C**) Overview of cultured cornea in organ culture medium I (without dextran). The cornea is viewed from the back to better evaluate the deep stroma and endothelium and present multiple folds of Descemet membrane (*black arrows*) and an arcus lipoides (*white arow*)

a slit lamp because of corneal swelling and the presence of organ culture medium. Therefore, a relatively high prevalence of CG on transplanted corneas has been reported, with 14.9% and 18.7% after penetrating keratoplasty [28] and DMEK [29], respectively. Safi et al. recently investigated morphological criteria regarding inverted light microscopy that correlated with the presence of CG on transplanted tissues. Those criteria are the presence of less than 50% of the cells in an endothelial picture having a hexagonal or a circular shape, the presence of cell membrane defects and interruptions and the presence of a small thickening of the cell membrane "blebs" [30]. Using these findings, an artificial intelligence-based machine learning algorithm is created to allow automated endothelial cell count (ECC) as well as the detection of abnormalities in specular microscopy images, including areas of necrosis and the presence of CG [31] (Fig. 8).

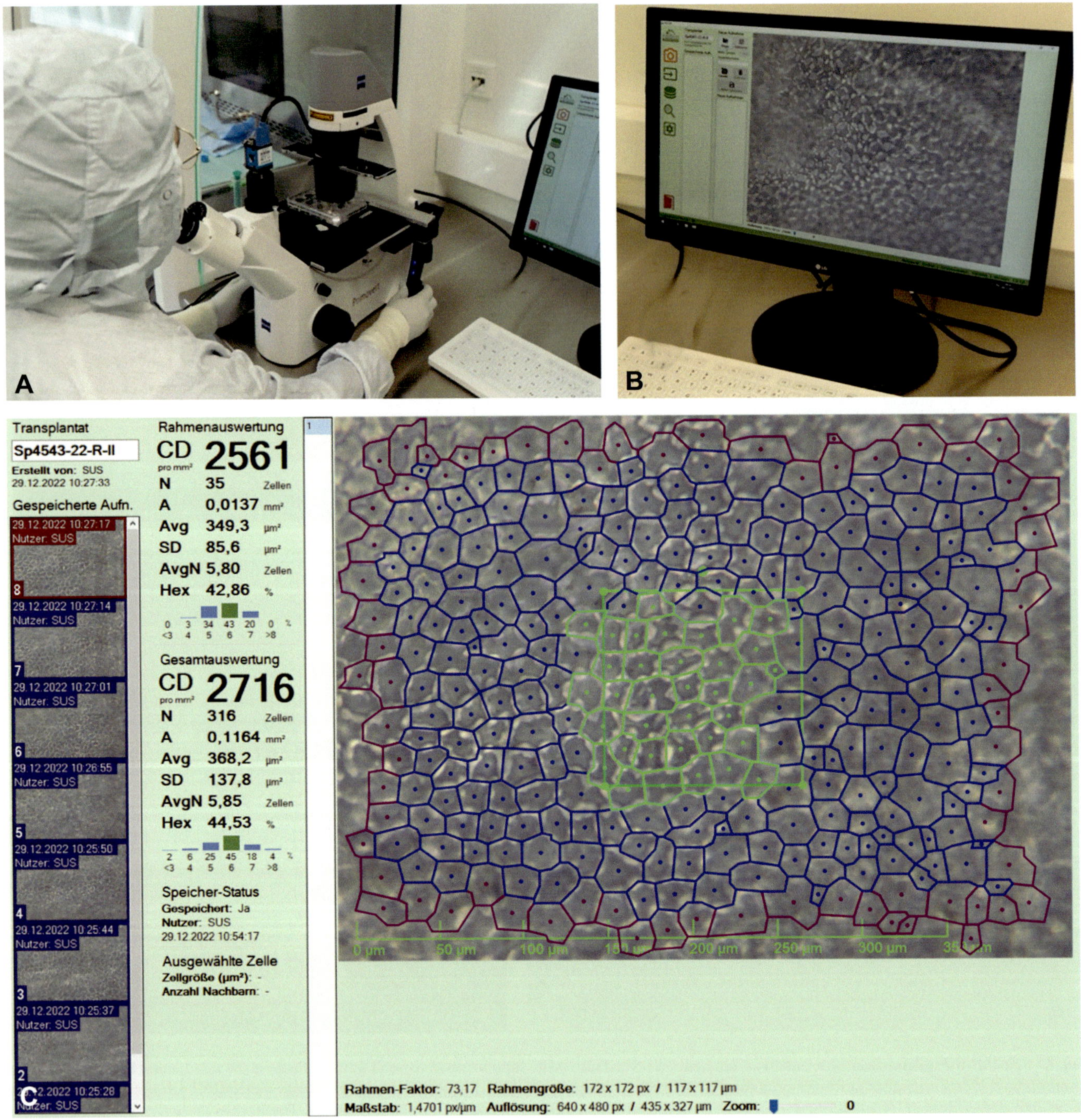

Fig. 7 **Evaluation of corneal endothelium**. The evaluation is performed with an inverted light microscope under sterile conditions in the eye bank. (**A**) A member of the eye bank staff performing endothelial cell count (ECC). (**B**) The examination is displayed on a monitor. The examiner takes a picture of the endothelial cell layer for further analysis. To evaluate donor corneal endothelium, inverted light microscopy should be performed in the center, in the 4 paracentral/midperipheral quadrants and in the periphery of the donor cornea [23]. (**C**) Endothelial cell count using Robin REA XLR (robin GmbH, Haan, Germany). The ECC is performed automatically in the selected area and can be adapted manually by moving or deleting the points in the center of each cell. The cell density (CD) is estimated based on the ECC in the green area. Cells that only partially fit in the area are counted if they cross the lower or left borders of the area and are not counted if they cross the upper or right borders

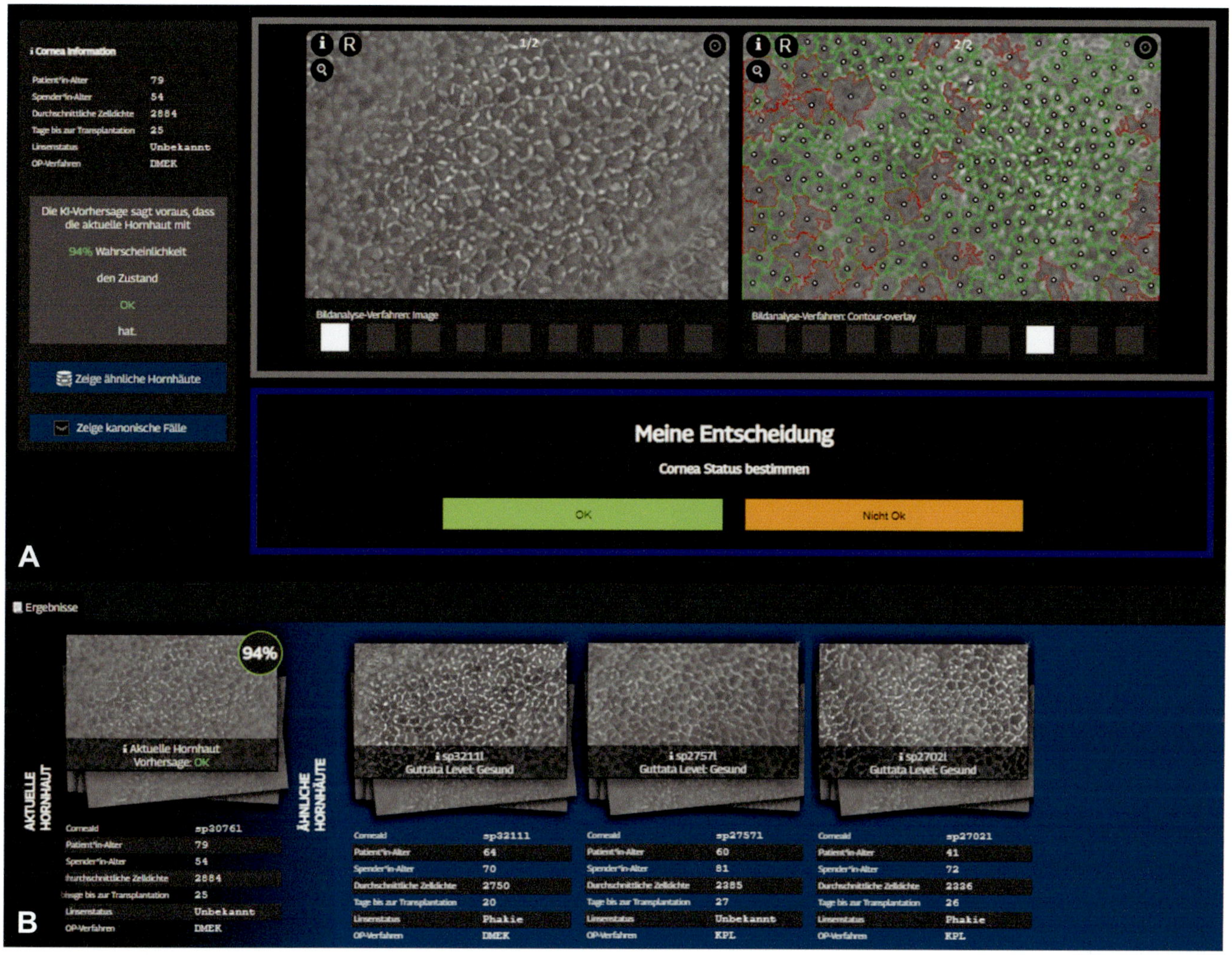

Fig. 8 Artificial intelligence (AI) assisted detection of cornea guttata (CG) in the eye bank. *Kittool* is a decision support tool for the detection of CG integrating 2 components: (**A**) Graphical analytic tools generating several cell representations, such as "honeycomb" representations, for enhanced visualization of endothelial cells. The staff member performing the analysis decides whether the cornea is suitable or not (*blue box*) (**B**) Machine learning classifiers including case-based reasoning (CBR) for AI-based support enable automated CG detection in the eye bank by comparing previous endothelial cell images with known postoperative classification of the graft endothelium after keratoplasty. The CBR model for the detection and classification of CGs in the eye bank is performed using classification of previous endothelial cell images after keratoplasty from the software database [31]

6 Sterile donor tomography

Any corneal microsurgeon performing a high volume of keratoplasties may have inadvertently transplanted a donor corneal tissue with (subclinical) keratoconus or prior keratorefractive surgery, which typically leads to postoperative refractive surprises [32–35]. Given the considerably increased number of keratorefractive procedures performed in the last three decades, eye banks will soon have to more intensively face the problem of identifying donor corneas with abnormal refraction, which cannot always be reliably recognized by slit lamp examination alone [36–38]. One of several methods developed to meet the consequently increasing demand for improved preoperative refractive screening of donor corneal tissues in the eye bank is the sterile donor tomography [39–41].

At our department, 1900 donor corneas have already as of July 2025 been routinely measured preoperatively since 2018, using the swept-source anterior segment optical coherence tomograph (AS-OCT) CASIA 2 (Tomey Corp., Nagoya, Japan) (Fig. 9) [42]. A raster scan is generated from the back surface of the donor cornea, creating a 3D volume data set with a depth resolution of 5.621 μm/voxel in aqueous medium and a lateral resolution of 6 μm/voxel [41]. Thereafter, the measured raw data are loaded into MATLAB (MathWorks Inc., Natick, Massachusetts, USA) and pretreated to remove artifacts due to flask wall and tissue holder, extract background noise, adjust the contrast size, minimize

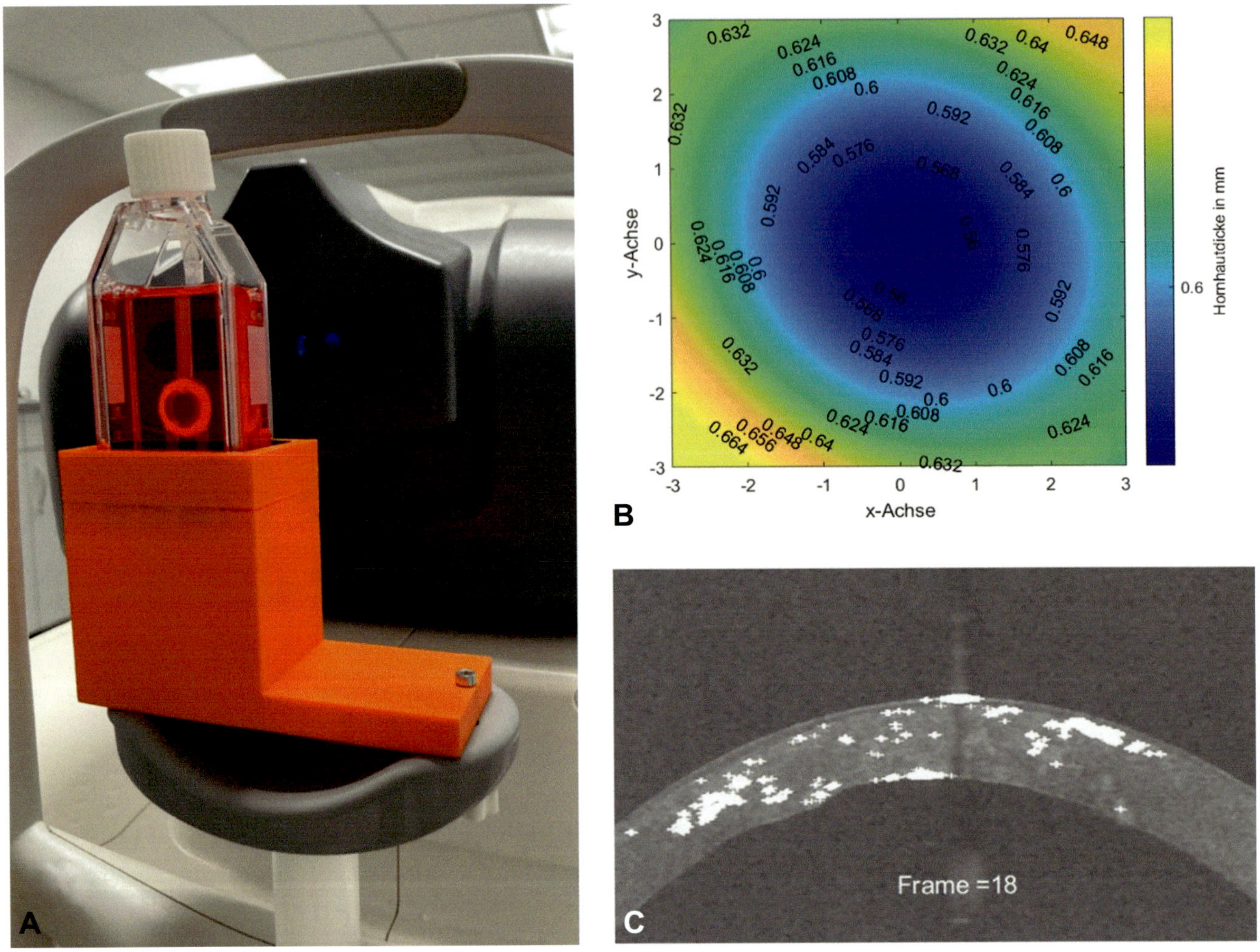

Fig. 9 **Sterile donor tomography in the eye bank**. (**A**) Preoperative measurements of donor corneal tissue are sterilely performed using an anterior segment optical coherence tomography (AS-OCT) through their sealed cell culture flask, mounted on the chin rest of the AS-OCT in a holder previously constructed with a three-dimensional (3D) printer (Ultimaker 2 Go, Ultimaker B.V., Geldermalsen, The Netherlands). (**B**) Self-programmed MATLAB produces a thickness mapping of the donor cornea (thickness displayed in millimetres). Other parameters such as radii of curvature of the anterior and posterior corneal surface are also denoted (not shown). (**C**) Sterile donor tomography of a donor cornea presenting granular corneal dystrophy. The MATLAB software is able to generate images and videos with automated detection of the hyperdensities. Hyalin and amyloid stromal deposits are detected and displayed as white dots

the brightness of the central reflection and identify the edge of the front and back surfaces of the donor cornea [40, 41]. The MATLAB software analyzes corneal thickness as well as anterior and posterior radii of curvature at the steep and flat corneal meridian, from which the refractive power is derived.

In order to allow reliable measurements, sterile donor tomography is ideally performed >12 h after transferring the cornea into *organ culture medium II*, i.e. after more than 12 h of deswelling [16]. To minimize postoperative refractive surprises after keratoplasty, donor corneas with refractive powers that deviate excessively from the mean are relatively contraindicated for penetrating or anterior lamellar keratoplasty. In our department, we have so far set the cut-off at curvature deviations of more than $\bar{x}$ (mean) ± 3 standard deviations (eminence-based) [43] (status January 2023: donor corneas with a total refractive power of < 39.8 D and > 47.7 D). Nevertheless, these donor tissues may still be suited for posterior lamellar keratoplasty, such as DMEK or DSAEK, or for tectonic keratoplasty.

The clinical validity of sterile donor tomography has been investigated by comparing it to keratometry on whole globes in situ of deceased patients before corneal harvesting. The steepest and flattest corneal power as well as the keratometric astigmatism showed to remain unchanged ($p \geq 0.09$) after preserving sclerocorneal discs in *organ culture medium I* (measured using sterile donor tomography) compared to the measurement of the same cornea before explantation using a hand-held refractometer [44]. Other conducted researches have highlighted the repeatability of sterile donor tomography [45].

In the future, sterile donor tomography may permit: (1) harmonization of donor and recipient tomography [41, 46], which could conceivably reduce the residual astigmatism persisting after suture removal for a specific donor-recipient pair; and (2) the improvement of the intraocular lens (IOL) power calculation in a classical triple procedure (keratoplasty + phacoemulsification + IOL implantation) using regression analysis between pre- and postoperative total refractive power of donor corneal tissues [47].

7 Conclusion

To face the increasing demand of corneal tissue and new challenges in terms of tissue selection, the global eye bank activities refocus on large structures with more resources, allowing optimal conditions of preservation as well as a better selection and preparation of tissues. A well-designed quality management system is also essential to ensure the quality and safety of corneal tissue and to face the multiple new challenges of modern eye banking.

In terms of preservation, hypothermic storage, being cheaper but allowing only short-term storage, and organ culture, being more complex and expensive but allowing better control and longer storage, currently remain the two major storage methods in eye banks.

The development of new screening techniques, such as the sterile donor tomography or the AI-based detection of CG, and improvement of existing techniques for tissue preservation, preparation and selection, promises further developments in the field of eye banking in the near future.

References

1. European Eye Bank Association (EEBA). Technical guidelines for ocular tissue (TGOT). EEBA 2020. https://www.eeba.eu/files/pdf/EEBA_Technical_Guidelines_for_Ocular_Tissue_Revision11.pdf. Accessed 6 Nov 2022.
2. Martin C, Tschernig T, Hamon L, Daas L, Seitz B. Corneae from body donors in anatomy department: valuable use for clinical transplantation and experimental research. BMC Ophthalmol. 2020;13(20):284. https://doi.org/10.1186/s12886-020-01546-2.
3. Serfőző A, Suffo S, Viestenz A, Seitz B, Daas L. Central sclerocorneoplasty à chaud in bacterial superinfected mycotic keratitis confirmed by confocal microscopy at the base of recurrent herpetic keratitis. Klin Monbl Augenheilkd. 2022; 239(10):1245–1247. https://doi.org/10.1055/a-1386-5229.
4. Sangwan VS, Jain V, Gupta P. Structural and functional outcome of scleral patch graft. Eye. 2007;21:930–1005. https://doi.org/10.1038/sj.eye.6702344.
5. Li S, Bischoff M, Schirra F, Langenbucher A, Ong M, Halfmann A, Herrmann M, Seitz B. Correlation between microbial growth in conjunctival swabs of corneal donors and contamination of organ culture media. Ophthalmologe. 2014;111:553–9.
6. Lawlor M, Kerridge I, Ankeny R, Dobbins TA, Billson F. Specific unwillingness to donate eyes: the impact of disfigurement, knowledge and procurement on corneal donation. Am J Transplant. 2010;10:657–63. https://doi.org/10.1111/j.1600-6143.2009.02986.x.
7. Wykrota AA, Weinstein I, Hamon L, Daas L, Flockerzi E, Suffo S, Seitz B. Approval rates for corneal donation and the origin of donor tissue for transplantation at a university-based tertiary referral center with corneal subspecialization hosting a LIONS Eye Bank. BMC Ophthalmol. 2022;22:17. https://doi.org/10.1186/s12886-022-02248-7.
8. European Eye Bank Association. Minimum Medical Standards (MMS). EEBA 2020. https://www.eeba.eu/files/pdf/EEBA%20Minimum%20Medical%20Standards%20Revision%205%20Final.pdf. Accessed 06 Nov 2022.
9. Laun D, Suffo S, Kramp K, Bischoff M, Huber M, Langenbucher A, Seitz B. How implementing a quality management system at the LIONS eye bank Saar-Lor-Lux, trier/western palatinate from 2006 to 2016 impacted the rate and reasons for discarding human organ-cultured corneas. Klin Monbl Augenheilkd. 2021;239:717–23. https://doi.org/10.1055/a-1327-3835.
10. Pels E, Rijneveld WJ. Organ culture preservation for corneal tissue. Technical and quality aspects. Dev Ophthalmol. 2009;43:31–46. https://doi.org/10.1159/000223837.
11. Toniolo M, Camposampiero D, Griffoni C, Jones GLA. Quality management in European eye banks. Dev Ophthalmol. 2009;43:70–86. https://doi.org/10.1159/000223840.
12. Doughman DJ, Harris JE, Schmitt MK. Penetrating keratoplasty using 37 C organ cultured cornea. Trans Sect Ophthalmol Am Acad Ophthalmol Otolaryngol. 1976;81:778–93.
13. Pels E, Beele H, Claerhout I. Eye bank issues: II. Preservation techniques: warm versus cold storage. Int Ophthalmol. 2008;28:155–163. https://doi.org/10.1007/s10792-007-9086-1.
14. Müller LJ, Pels E, Vrensen GF. The effects of organ-culture on the density of keratocytes and collagen fibers in human corneas. Cornea. 2001;20:86–95. https://doi.org/10.1097/00003226-200101000-00017.
15. Abdin AD, Daas L, Pattmöller M, Suffo S, Langenbucher A, Seitz B. Negative impact of dextran in organ culture media for pre-stripped tissue preservation on DMEK (descemet membrane endothelial keratoplasty) outcome. Graefes Arch Clin Exp Ophthalmol. 2018;256:213–5. https://doi.org/10.1007/s00417-018-4088-4.
16. Hamon L, Daas L, Mäurer S, Weinstein I, Quintin A, Schulz K, Langenbucher A, Seitz B. Thickness and curvature changes of human corneal grafts in dextran-containing organ culture medium before keratoplasty. Cornea. 2021;40:733–40. https://doi.org/10.1097/ICO.0000000000002543.
17. McCarey BE, Kaufman HE. Improved corneal storage. Invest Ophthalmol. 1974;13:165–73.
18. Moshirfar M, Odayar VS, McCabe SE, Ronquillo YC. Corneal donation: current guidelines and future direction. Clin Ophthalmol. 2021;15:2963–73. https://doi.org/10.2147/OPTH.S284617.
19. Steinemann TL, Kaufmann HE, Lindstrom RL, Beuerman RW, Varnell ED. Intermediate-term storage media (K-Sol, Dexsol, Optisol). In: Brightbill FS, editors. Corneal surgery. St Louis, Mosby Co; 1993. p. 609–13.
20. Armitage WJ. Preservation of human Cornea. Transfus Med Hemother. 2011;38:143–7. https://doi.org/10.1159/000326632.
21. Kramp K, Suffo S, Laun D, Bischoff-Jung M, Huber M, Langenbucher A, Seitz B. Analysis of factors influencing the suitability of donor corneas in the LIONS Cornea bank Saar-Lor-Lux, Trier/Westpfalz from 2006 to 2016. Klin Monbl Augenheilkd. 2020;237:1334–42. https://doi.org/10.1055/a-1141-3703.

22. Batista A, Breunig HG, König A, Schindele A, Hager T, Seitz B, Morgado AM, König K. Assessment of human corneas prior to transplantation using high-resolution two-photon imaging. Invest Ophthalmol Vis Sci. 2018;59:176–84. https://doi.org/10.1167/iovs.17-22002.
23. Thuret G, Carricajo A, Vautrin AC, Raberin H, Acquart S, Garraud O, Gain P, Aubert G. Efficiency of blood culture bottles for the fungal sterility testing of corneal organ culture media. Br J Ophthalmol. 2005;89:586–90. https://doi.org/10.1136/bjo.2004.053439.
24. Clover J. Slit-lamp biomicroscopy. Cornea. 2018;37(Suppl 1):5–6. https://doi.org/10.1097/ICO.0000000000001641.
25. Sperling S. Evaluation of the endothelium of human donor corneas by induced dilation of intracellular spaces and trypan blue. Graefes Arch Clin Exp Ophthalmol. 1986;224:428–34. https://doi.org/10.1007/BF02173358.
26. Schroeter J, Rieck P. Endothelial evaluation in the Cornea bank. In: Bredehorn-Mayr T, Duncker GIW, Armitage WJ, editors. Eye banking. Dev Ophthalmol. Basel, Karger 2009;43:47–62. https://doi.org/10.1159/000223838.
27. Schaub F, Enders P, Adler W, Bachmann BO, Cursiefen C, Heindl LM. Impact of donor graft quality on deep anterior lamellar keratoplasty (DALK). BMC Ophthalmol. 2017;17:204. https://doi.org/10.1186/s12886-017-0600-6.
28. Schönit S, Maamri A, Zemova E, Munteanu C, Safi T, Daas L, Seitz B. Prevalence and Impact of Cornea Guttata in the Graft After Penetrating Keratoplasty in Germany. Cornea. 2022;41:1495-1502.
29. Schmitz LM, Safi T, Munteanu C, Seitz B, Daas L. Prevalence and severity of cornea guttata in the graft following Descemet Membrane Endothelial Keratoplasty (DMEK). Acta Ophthalmol. 2022;100:e1737-e1745.
30. Safi T, Daas L, Kiefer GL, Sharma M, Ndiaye A, Deru M, Alexandersson J, Seitz B. Semi-quantitative criteria in the eye bank that correlate with cornea guttata in donor corneas. Klin Monbl Augenheilkd. 2021;238:680–7. https://doi.org/10.1055/a-1498-1846.
31. Kiefer GL, Safi T, Nadig M, Sharma M, Sakha MM, Ndiaye A, Deru M, Daas L, Schulz K, Schwarz M, Seitz B, Alexandersson J. An AI-based decision support system for quality control applied to the use case donor cornea. In: Degen H, Ntoa S, editors. Artificial intelligence in HCI. HCII 2022. Lecture notes in computer science. Springer, Cham; 2022. p. 257–74. https://doi.org/10.1007/978-3-031-05643-7_17.
32. Fargione RA, Channa P. Cornea donors who have had prior refractive surgery; data from the eye bank association of America. Curr Opin Ophthalmol. 2016;27:323–6. https://doi.org/10.1097/ICU.0000000000000278.
33. Michaeli-Cohen A, Lambert AC, Coloma F, Rootman DS. Two cases of a penetrating keratoplasty with tissue from a donor who had undergone LASIK surgery. Cornea. 2002;21:111–3. https://doi.org/10.1097/00003226-200201000-00023.
34. de Mello Farias RJ, Parolim A, de Sousa LB. Corneal transplant utilizing a corneal graft that had undergone laser surgery-case report. Arq Bras Oftalmol. 2005;68:266–9. https://doi.org/10.1590/s0004-27492005000200022.
35. Mifflin M, Kim M. Penetrating keratoplasty using tissue from a donor with previous LASIK surgery. Cornea 2002;21:537–8; author reply 538–9. https://doi.org/10.1097/00003226-200207000-00024.
36. Kang SJ, Schmack I, Edelhauser HF, Grossniklaus HE. Donor corneas misidentified with prior laser in situ keratomileusis. Cornea. 2010;29:670–3. https://doi.org/10.1097/ICO.0b013e3181c325cc.
37. Mootha VV, Dawson D, Kumar A, Gleiser J, Qualls C, Albert DM. Slitlamp, specular, and light microscopic findings of human donor corneas after laser-assisted in situ keratomileusis. Arch Ophthalmol. 2004;122:686–92. https://doi.org/10.1001/archopht.122.5.686.
38. Vavra DE, Enzenauer RW. Predictive value of slit lamp examinations in screening donor corneas for prior refractive surgery. Arch Ophthalmol 2005;123:707–8; author reply 708–9. https://doi.org/10.1001/archopht.123.5.707-c.
39. Janunts E, Langenbucher A, Seitz B. In vitro corneal tomography of donor cornea using anterior segment OCT. Cornea. 2016;35:647–53. https://doi.org/10.1097/ICO.0000000000000761.
40. Damian A, Seitz B, Langenbucher A, Eppig T. Optical coherence tomography-based topography determination of corneal grafts in eye bank cultivation. J Biomed Opt. 2017;22:16001. https://doi.org/10.1117/1.JBO.22.1.016001.
41. Mäurer S, Asi F, Rawer A, Damian A, Seitz B, Langenbucher A, Eppig T. Concept for 3D measurement of corneal donor tissue using a clinical OCT. Ophthalmologe. 2019;116:640–6. https://doi.org/10.1007/s00347-018-0801-2.
42. Seitz B, Asi F, Mäurer S, Hamon L, Quintin A, Langenbucher A. Anterior segment OCT: application to improve graft selection for corneal transplantation. In: Alió JL, Alió del Barrio JL, editors. Atlas of anterior segment optical coherence tomography. Springer, Cham; 2021. p. 223–36.
43. Quintin A, Hamon L, Mäurer S, Langenbucher A, Seitz B. OCT application for sterile corneal graft screening in the eye bank. Klin Monbl Augenheilkd. 2021;238:688–92. https://doi.org/10.1055/a-1443-5451.
44. Quintin A, Hamon L, Langenbucher A, Seitz B. In situ donor keratometry in deceased patients as a novel screening technique for eye banking. Graefes Arch Clin Exp Ophthalmol 2023. https://doi.org/10.1007/s00417-022-05871-8. [Epub ahead of print].
45. Hamon L, Quintin A, Mäurer S, Weinstein I, Langenbucher A, Seitz B, Daas L. Reliability and efficiency of corneal thickness measurements using sterile donor tomography in the eye bank. Cell Tissue Bank 2021. https://doi.org/10.1007/s10561-021-09980-2. [Online ahead of print].
46. Mäurer S, Seitz B, Langenbucher A. "Harmonization" of donor and recipient tomography in corneal transplantation. Z Med Phys. 2021;31:73–7. https://doi.org/10.1016/j.zemedi.2020.05.006.
47. Quintin A, Hamon L, Mäurer S, Langenbucher A, Seitz B. Comparison of sterile donor tomography in the eye bank and graft tomography after penetrating keratoplasty. Ophthalmologe. 2021;118:1038–44. https://doi.org/10.1007/s00347-020-01256-6.

Corneal Transplantation—Excimer Laser Versus Femtosecond Laser Penetrating Keratoplasty PKP

Berthold Seitz, Elias Flockerzi, Loïc Hamon, Shady Suffo, and Loay Daas

Abstract

This chapter depicts the evolution of laser keratoplasty, which started two decades before the clinical introduction of the femtosecond lasers (FSL) and compares the intraoperative feasibility and postoperative outcome of the excimer and femtosecond laser approaches. Hypothesizing that the properties of the wound bed are of utmost importance for the final optical performance of the graft, Naumann GOH et al. have developed and optimized the technique of non-mechanical corneal trephination using a 193 nm excimer laser along metal masks for penetrating keratoplasty (PKP) since 1986. Starting out with an elliptical trephination the major improvement resulted from the introduction of eight "orientation teeth/notches" at round mask edges minimizing "horizontal torsion". For non-contact donor trephination from the epithelial side, an artificial anterior chamber was used. Prospective clinical studies have shown that the technique of non-contact excimer laser PKP may improve donor and recipient centration, reduce "vertical tilt" and "horizontal torsion" of the graft in the recipient bed, thus resulting in significantly less "all-sutures-out" astigmatism, higher regularity of the topography and better visual acuity. Besides less blood-aqueous barrier breakdown during the early postoperative course after PKP, excimer laser trephination does not induce cataract formation and does not impair the graft endothelium. Likewise, the rate of immunologic graft rejections is not adversely affected by the excimer laser. In addition, trephination of an instable cornea, such as in (pre-) perforated corneal ulcers or after RK or LASIK is facilitated. Clinical results of FSL lamellar or penetrating keratoplasties—requiring variable amounts of applanation thus causing distortion of corneal tissue, especially in keratoconus—are still limited and not yet finally convincing. The evolution of non-mechanical laser keratoplasty started in Erlangen in 1986. Because of undisputed clinical advantages, especially in eyes with keratoconus and instable thin corneas after PKP, noncontact excimer laser trephination with orientation teeth/notches is still favored in Homburg/Saar in daily practice. The FSL-assisted keratoplasty technique has been very exciting but due to major lack of all-suture-out data after introduction of the technique 20 years ago—the superiority of this high price and difficult to maintain option has not been proven, yet! FSL-assisted PKP without liquid interface seems to have major disadvantages in comparison to excimer laser PKP especially in keratoconus.

Keywords

Corneal transplantation · Keratoplasty · Excimer laser · Femtosecond laser · Trephination · Suturing · Astigmatism

1 Introduction

The first successful total penetrating keratoplasty (PKP) was performed by Eduard Zirm on December 9, 1905 in Olmütz, which today is located in the Czech Republic. This means that corneal transplantation is the oldest, most common and most successful transplantation in humans overall [1]. Around 10,000 keratoplasties are performed in Germany per year and around 6000 patients are on a waiting list for corneal transplantation. In the year 2024, 70.6% of all corneal transplants performed in Germany were of the posterior

Supplementary Information The online version contains supplementary material available at https://doi.org/10.1007/978-3-031-65422-0_49.

B. Seitz (✉) · E. Flockerzi · L. Hamon · S. Suffo · L. Daas
Department of Ophthalmology, Saarland University Medical Center UKS, HomburgSaar, Germany
e-mail: berthold.seitz@uks.eu
URL: https://www.augenklinik-saarland.de

B. Seitz et al. (eds.), *Atlas on Cornea*, https://doi.org/10.1007/978-3-031-65422-0_49

lamellar type (98% DMEK), with only 2.4% being anterior lamellar grafts and 27% still being carried out as PKP. This survey is based on the German Keratoplasty Registry, which has been maintained by the Section DOG-Kornea since 2000 [2, 3]. In Homburg/Saar we performed 710 keratoplasties in 2024 (381 PKP, 25 DALK, 304 DMEK) (Fig. 1).

With a better understanding of immunological transplant reactions [4–6] and "secondary glaucomas" after PKP [7]), the demands placed on microsurgeons with regard to corneal transplantation have increased. Today, a crystal-clear cornea after PKP with high and/or irregular astigmatism, especially in combination with high anisometropia, can no longer be considered a successful result in normal-risk keratoplasty. With the increasing experience of the microsurgeon, the *technique of keratoplasty* goes far beyond the replacement of two collagen discs and is crucial for the functional post-operative outcome.

2 Short Overview on Corneal Transplantation [8]

There are a number of indications for which penetrating keratoplasty (PKP) has been and will be the method of choice in the future (Table 1). Besides routine postoperative follow-up the prophylaxis of complications in PKP includes special preoperative and intraoperative aspects to avoid major refractive and/or morphological complications postoperatively (Fig. 2).

Preoperative prophylaxis consists of the therapy of systemic diseases and eyelid abnormalities (Fig. 3), determining individual optimal graft size, avoiding PKP in cases of uncontrolled intraocular pressure, avoiding PKP in cases of acute corneal hydrops (Fig. 4), pretreatment of vascularized cornea, amniotic membrane transplantation before PKP in cases of ulcerative keratitis, quality controlled

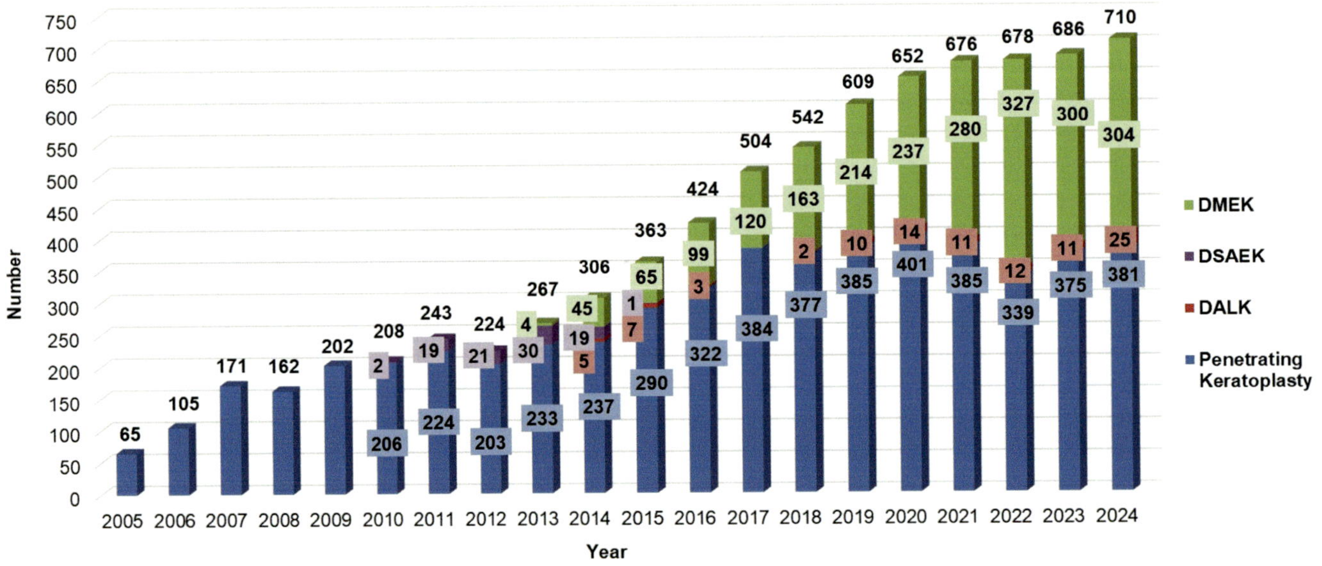

Fig. 1 Keratoplasty is the oldest, the most frequent and most successful human transplannation. Corneal transplantations in Homburg/Saar since 2005—the absolute number has increased more than tenfold from 65 in the year 2005 to 710 in the year 2024

Table 1 Timeless indications for penetrating keratoplasty PKP

• Dystrophies affecting all corneal layers (e.g. macular dystrophy, congenital stromal dystrophy)
• High astigmatism and/or stromal scars after PKP (with/without endothelial decompensation)
• Patients with advanced keratoconus (in any case after acute keratoconus = corneal hydrops with rupture of the Descemet membrane)
• Large (~12 mm) corneoscleroplasty for severe pellucid marginal degeneration or keratoglobus
• Unstable cornea (e.g. after RK, iatrogenic keratectasia after LASIK, Descemetocele, perforated ulcer)
• Aphakia, simultaneous IOL implantation (always with Flieringa ring!)
• Ipsilateral and contralateral autologous keratoplasty (please refer to Autologous Ipsilateral Rotational and Contralateral Keratoplasty)
• Acanthamoeba or fungal keratitis
• Semilunar eccentric corneoscleroplasty
• Block excision with tectonic corneoscleroplasty

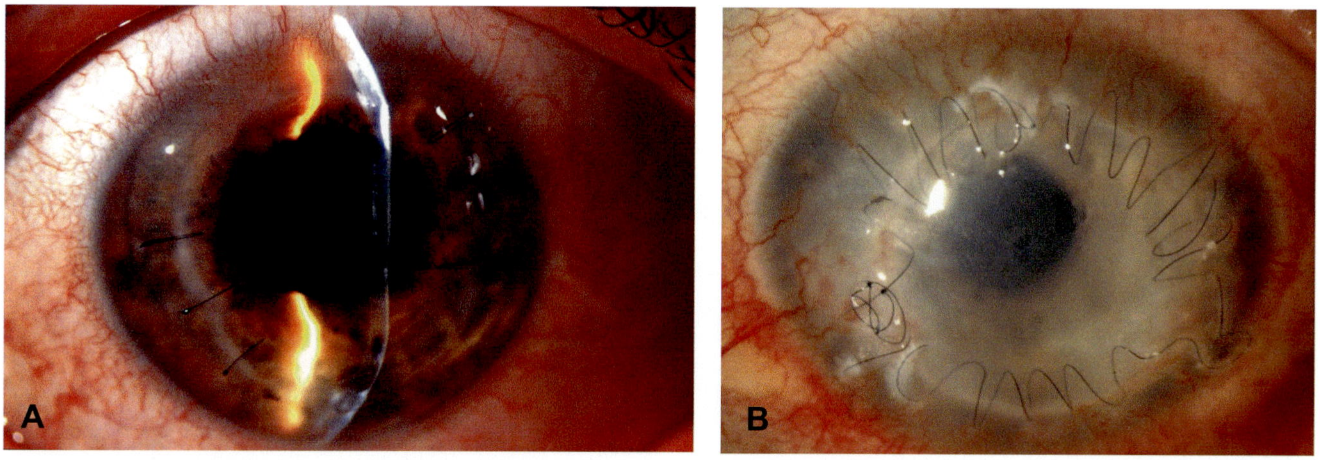

Fig. 2 (**A**) Optical (following wedge resection after Troutman) and (**B**) morphological (decentered graft with loose sutures, infiltrates and acute diffuse endothelial immune reaction) disasters after PKP

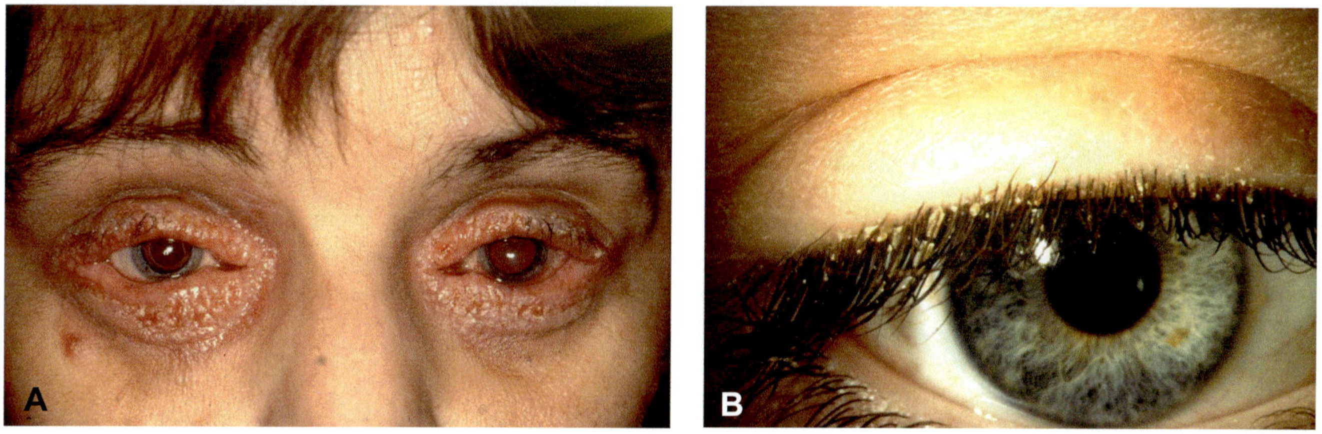

Fig. 3 Severe blepharitis in case of (**A**) neurodermatitis and (**B**) Demodex

organ-cultured transplants [9] including sterile donor tomography (Fig. 5) [10, 11] and avoidance of donor tissue with cornea guttata (Fig. 6) [12–14] as well as preoperative counselling by the surgeon to ensure patient compliance.

Intraoperative prophylaxis consists of controlled arterial hypotension and complete relaxation during general anesthesia, and application of a Flieringa ring in aphakic/vitrectomized eyes (Fig. 7). Ten precautions for intraoperative prophylaxis of astigmatism include:

1. An attempt should be made to determine donor topography for exclusion of previous refractive surgery, keratoconus/high astigmatism, and to allow for "harmonization" of donor and recipient tomography [16].
2. Donor and recipient trephination should be performed from the epithelial side with the same system, which is the prerequisite for congruent cut surfaces and angles in donor and recipient. For this purpose an artificial anterior chamber is used for donor trephination.
3. Horizontal positioning of the head and limbal plane are indispensable for state-of-the-art PKP surgery in order to avoid decentration, vertical tilt, and horizontal torsion (Fig. 8).
4. Orientation structures in donor and host facilitate the correct placement of the first four or eight cardinal sutures to avoid horizontal torsion.
5. A measurable improvement seems to be possible, using the Krumeich guided trephine system (GTS), the second generation Hanna trephine, and the Erlangen/Homburg technique of nonmechanical trephination with the excimer laser.

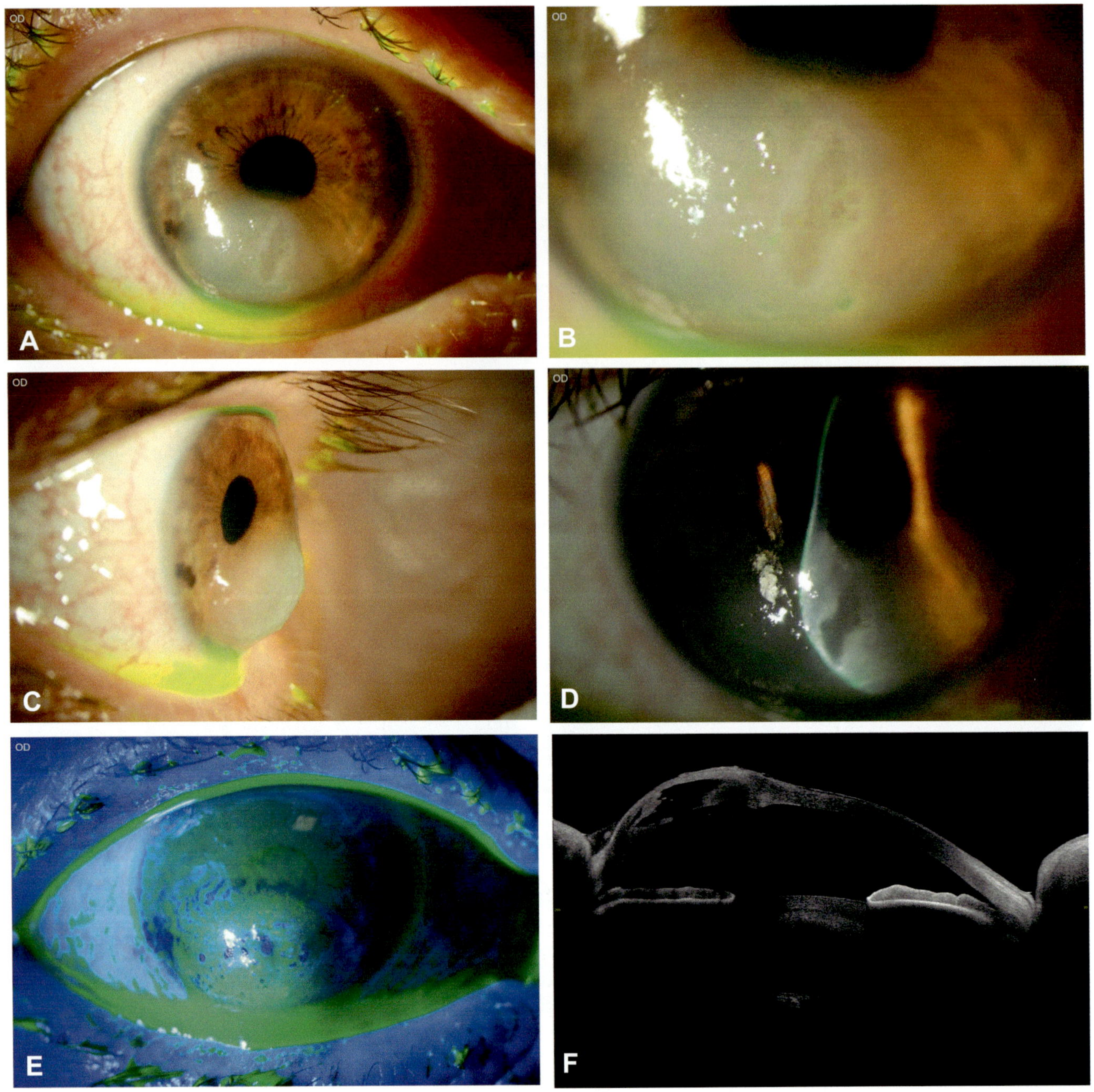

Fig. 4 Corneal hydrops (**A**)/(**B**)/(**C**) Slit lamp overview, (**D**) Slit beam in high magnification, (**E**) Vital staining with fluorescein and blue light: Seidel negative. (**F**) Anterior Segment OCT shows defect in Descemet membrane and confluent stromal vacuols

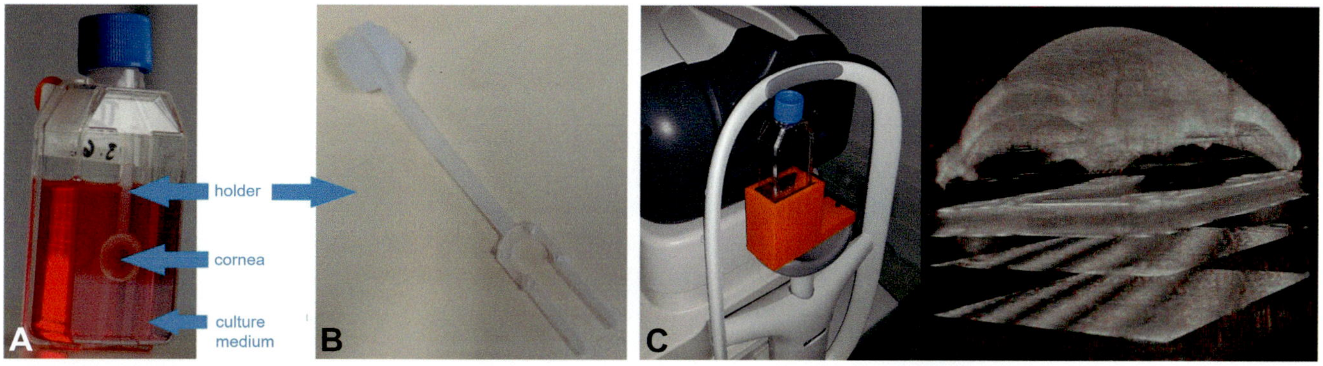

Fig. 5 Sterile Donor Tomography in the eye bank: Donor tissue remains sterile in organ culture flask. Bottle position in front of the OCT device using a chinrest-mounted holder. 3D volume data (anterior/posterior curvature and thickness) of the donor corneoscleral button within a 7.0 mm central zone are grabbed using a raster scan through the posterior surface of the cornea [10, 15]. Curvature/thickness abnormalities (keratoconus, state after PRK/LASIK) are excluded for DALK/PKP but are used for DMEK if the number of endothelial cells is higher than 2200 cells/mm^2

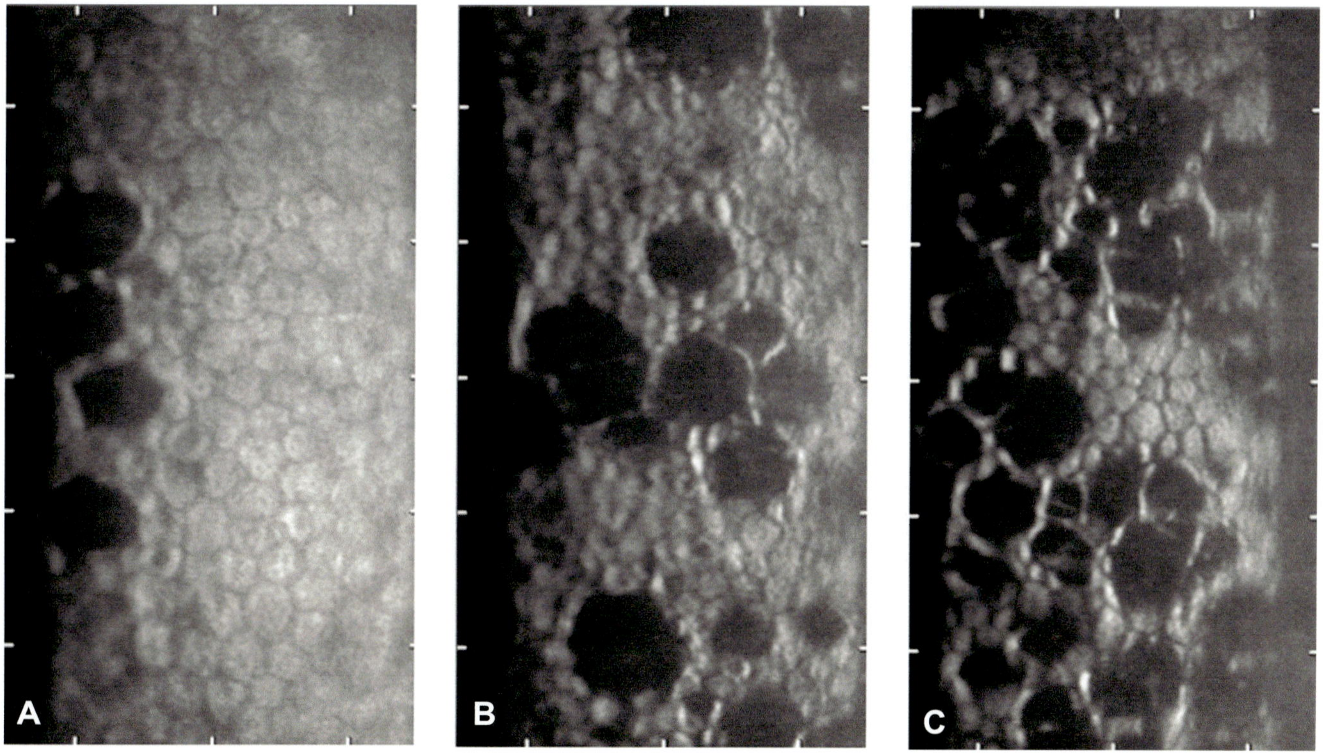

Fig. 6 Mild (**A**), Moderate (**B**) and Severe (**C**) amount of guttae on the graft 6 weeks after PKP. Obviously these guttae have not been detected in the eye bank using inverted specular microscopy

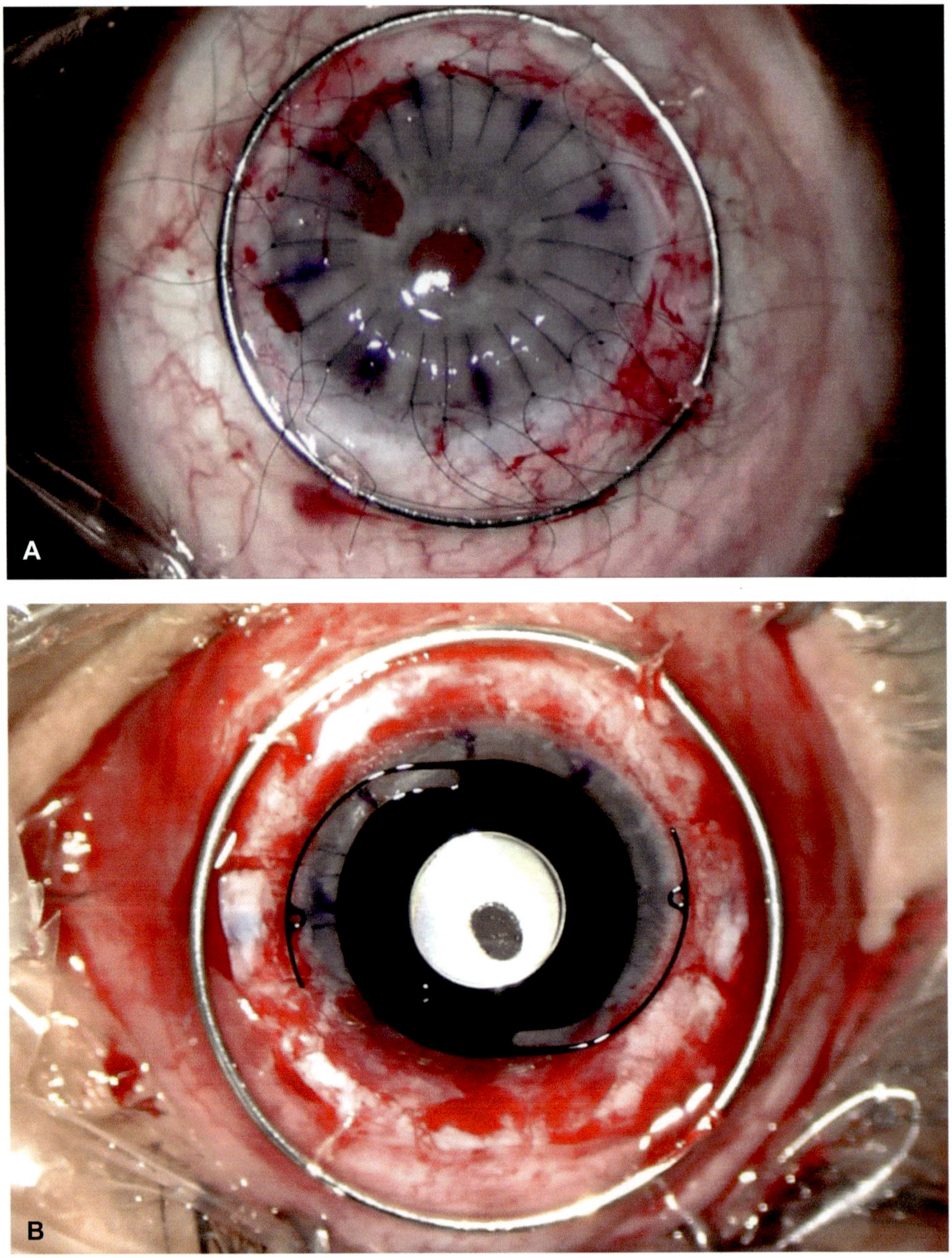

Fig. 7 Flieringa Ring sutured episclerally on an aphakic vitrectomized eye to prevent collapse in the open-eye situation. (**A**) simultaneous retroiridal Verisyse IOL implantation, (**B**) simultaneous sclera-fixated Morcher iris diaphragm lens

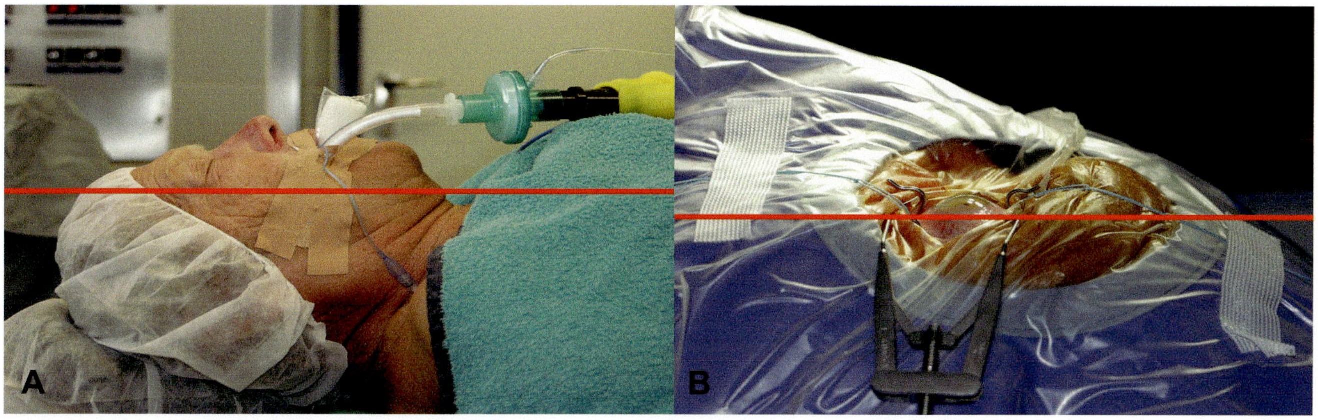

Fig. 8 Horizontal positioning of the (**A**) head and (**B**) limbal plane are indispensable for state-of-the-art PKP surgery in order to avoid decentration, vertical tilt, and horizontal torsion

6. Graft size should be adjusted individually ("as large as possible, as small as necessary").
7. Limbal centration should be preferred over pupil centration (especially in keratoconus).
8. Excessive graft over- or undersize should be avoided to prevent stretching or compression of peripheral donor tissue.
9. As long as Bowman layer is intact, a double running cross-stitch suture (according to Hoffmann) is preferred since it results in higher topographic regularity, earlier visual rehabilitation, and less suture loosening requiring only rarely suture replacement (Fig. 9).
10. Intraoperative keratoscopy should be applied after removal of lid specula and fixation sutures.

Postoperatively, periodical control examinations using fluorescein and blue light are indispensable. All loose sutures have to be removed as early as possible. In cases of herpetic eye disease 2×400 mg of oral acyclovir should be administered for at least 1 year. In cases of therapy-resistant epithelial defects, 100% autologous serum eye drops or amniotic membrane transplantation (patch technique) are valid options. Immune reactions must be diagnosed and treated immediately with high doses of corticosteroids (topically, intracamerally, systemically) [17].

3 Astigmatism and Keratoplasty

3.1 Definition of Astigmatism After Keratoplasty

The cornea provides approximately two thirds of the refractive power of the human eye. Surgical interventions on the cornea can therefore significantly affect the refractive power. Astigmatism after PKP is often irregular, i.e. two or more meridians are separated from one another by an angle, which is not equal to 90°. Two or more steep hemi-meridians are not located opposite one another. The same applies to the flat hemi-meridians. In addition, the refractive power in corresponding hemi-meridians may be different [18]. Especially in the case of irregular astigmatism, patients accept only a smaller subjective cylinder than the objective cylinder measured by keratometry or topography analysis [19]. With high irregular astigmatism, it is only possible to achieve good visual acuity with rigid gas permeable contact lenses as scleral lenses.

In addition to the keratometry, topography analysis is essential today to determine the refractive power distribution over the entire graft. The refractive power and the individual axes of the four hemi-meridians are supplemented by system-specific indices (e.g. SRI "surface regularity index" or SAI "surface asymmetry index" of the TMS topography system) [20].

3.2 Causes of Astigmatism After Keratoplasty

Each individual step, from the selection of the donor, intraoperative trephination and the suture technique to the quality of the post-operative follow-up treatment, can be decisive not only for corneal transparency, but also for the final refractive outcome [21–25].

In addition to tissue-intrinsic factors in the donor and recipient, early astigmatism *with sutures in place* appears to depend strongly on the suture placement technique and the approaches used for intra- and post-operative suture adjustments (the "signature" of the microsurgeon) [26]. After suture removal the corneal curvature normally becomes more regular [19], although the "net astigmatism" can significantly increase [27–29].

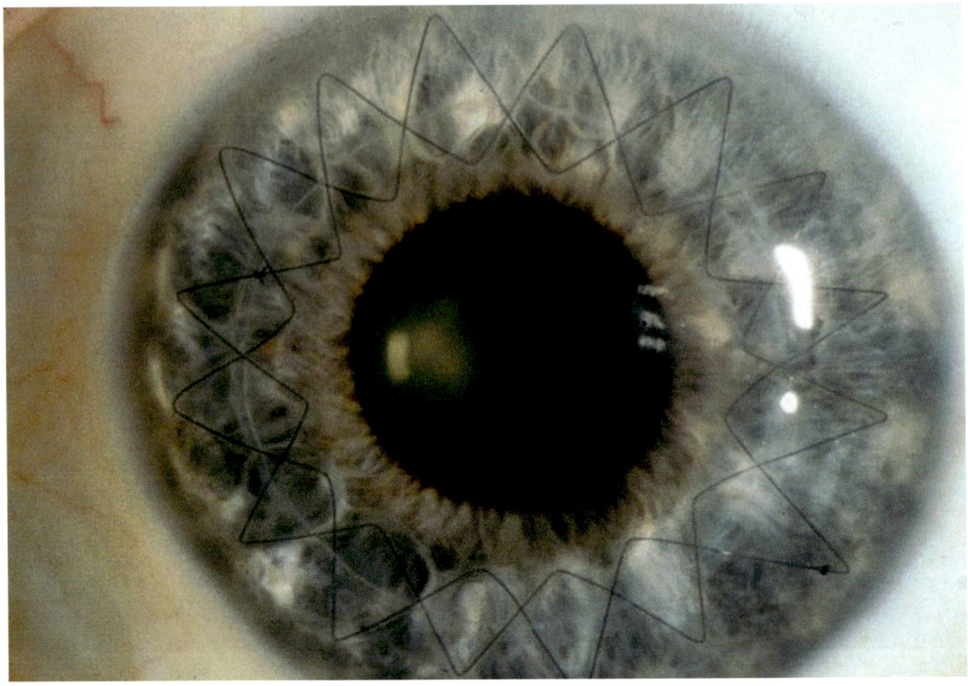

Fig. 9 As long as Bowman layer is intact, a double running cross-stitch suture (according to Hoffmann) is preferred since it results in higher topographic regularity, earlier visual rehabilitation, and less suture loosening requiring only rarely suture replacement

Table 2 Classification of post-PKP Astigmatism

Early postoperatively with sutures in place: • Symmetry of suture positions • Homogeneity of suture tension
Late postoperatively persisting without sutures: • Cut quality • Wound configuration (horizontal/vertical) • Symmetry of graft placement

We have to distinguish between the **early postoperative astigmatism with sutures in place** and the **late persisting astigmatism after suture removal** (Table 2). Concerning the *pathomechanism of the increase in astigmatism* after suture removal, the following suggestions are made:

The low quality of the trephination wound and geometric incongruities (horizontal and vertical) require higher suture tension in order to guarantee a watertight wound closure and pseudo-optimal topography during the early postoperative phase. Asymmetrical regional forces between the donor and recipient can lead to inhomogeneous wound healing processes. The removal of the sutures results in the release of forces due to geometric incongruities and inhomogeneous wound healing. For this reason, horizontal, vertical and topographical discrepancies between the donor and recipient *intra-operatively* appear to be responsible for the increase in astigmatism *after* removal of the sutures. Thus, it is reasonable to conclude that in addition to wound healing, factors associated directly or indirectly with the quality of the wound geometry (quality of the cut, wound configuration (horizontal/vertical), symmetry of the graft fit) have a strong influence on long-term astigmatism *after removal of the sutures* [19, 30–32].

The main intra-operative determinants (Table 3, Fig. 10) for high and/or irregular astigmatism *after suture removal* are [26, 35, 36]:

- decentration (donor and/or recipient trephination)
- "vertical tilt" (incongruent cut angle between donor and recipient)
- "horizontal torsion" (horizontal discrepancy between the donor and recipient form and/or asymmetrical graft fit—"*The second cardinal suture is crucial!*").

4 Trephination Technique

In principle, PKP may be indicated for optical, curative and tectonic reasons. In practice, overlaps between different categories are possible. However, corneal grafts can also be classified according to the type of donor tissue, the vertical/horizontal shape of the graft and the location of the graft within the recipient [22, 26, 37].

Table 3 Intraoperative determinants of high and/or irregular astigmatism after penetrating keratoplasty [35, 36]

"Vertical tilt" due to incongruent wound configuration [26] • Application of different trephines for the donor and recipient • Trephine tilt (i.e. not parallel to the optical axis) • Limbus level not supported horizontally • Slipping of the trephine in the stroma during the incision process • Intraocular pressure too high/too low
"Horizontal torsion" [26] • Asymmetrical placement of the second cardinal suture (Angle unequal 180°) • Incorrect fit of the donor and recipient due to incongruity
Focal overlap or dehiscence of the donor disc in the recipient bed
Excessively over/undersized donor disc
Distortion or compression of the cornea
Trauma to the cornea caused by instruments
Properties of the suture • Suture material • Suture technique (interrupted suture, single running suture, double running suture, combinations) • Length of the stitch • Depth of the stitch • Angle of the stitch to the donor-recipient junction • "Depth disparity" • Tightness of the suture Simultaneous intraocular surgery (e.g. triple procedure, artificial lens replacement, etc.) Flieringa ring and lid speculum Personal experience of the microsurgeon

An "*optimal trephination*" requires:

- full visual control;
- no contact;
- optimal donor and recipient centration;
- identical shape of donor and recipient (typically circular round);
- congruent incision angles;
- 360° symmetrical donor-recipient alignment;
- no completion of the trephination using scissors required;
- no damage to intraocular structures (iris, lens);
- *in the future:* self-sealing donor-recipient apposition ("key-lock principle")

4.1 Donor Trephination

From a 15 mm corneoscleral disc, as provided by the cornea bank, the graft can be produced in two ways:

In the past, it was punched *from the endothelial side* against a firm surface, e.g. paraffin or Teflon block, with the help of special trephines (e.g. "punch trephine"). Particular attention must be paid to ensuring that the excision is performed in a centred position and that the trephine is not tilted, as this would result in an elliptical disc with slanted edges [31]. This risk can be reduced by using "guided donor trephine systems" (e.g. guillotines). In the histological assessment, the cut surfaces without consideration of the cut angles appear to be almost "perfect". However, the deviation in the direction of the cut towards the exterior results in a convergent cut angle due to the smaller diameter on the level of Descemet membrane and a greater diameter on the level of Bowman layer ("undercut", Fig. 11) [25].

Since the introduction of "artificial anterior chambers", microsurgeons have been able to carry out donor trephination *from the epithelial side,* i.e. in the same direction as in the patient. If the pressure in the artificial anterior chamber is kept at its normal level (for example 22 mmHg), the advantages with respect to the congruence of the cutting angles are self-evident.

4.2 Recipient Trephination

In order to increase the overview and reduce Vis à tergo, a Liebermann lid speculum can be used. Almost any viscoelastic agent is suitable for stabilising the anterior chamber during trephination and suture placement.

> A Flieringa ring is not necessary for keratoplasty only or even a triple procedure, however, for aphakic and/or vitrectomized eyes, especially if a secondary sclera-fixated or retroiridal artificial lens implantation is planned.

Investigations by van Rij and Waring have shown that in recipient trephination, the use of all trephine systems results

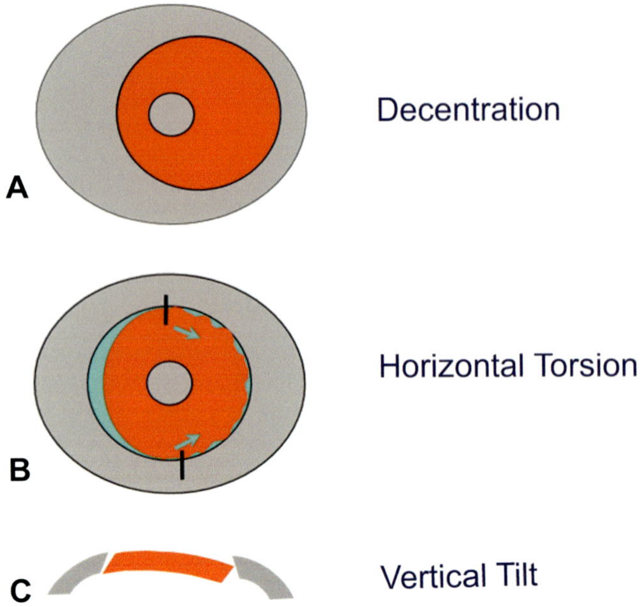

Fig. 10 Main reasons for high astigmatism after keratoplasty. (**A**) Decentring of the donor and/or recipient trephination, (**B**) "horizontal torsion" due to asymmetrical suture placement (**C**) "vertical tilt" due to uneven cutting angle

in openings, which are larger than the nominal trephine size. Furthermore, the diameter at the level of Descemet membrane is greater, resulting in divergent cut angles [25, 38]. This can be explained at least in part by bulging ("ballooning") of the cornea in the trephine opening due to the pressure exerted.

The higher the intraocular pressure, the more divergent angles can be expected in recipient trephination.

This phenomenon of "ballooning" is one of the main disadvantages of the mechanical trephine and can at least partially be prevented by the use of a so-called obturator (exception: keratoconus).

The combination of a donor disc that has been punched from the endothelial side and therefore has convergent cut angles, with a recipient opening with divergent cut angles leads to a triangular-shaped tissue defect at the level of the Descemet membrane. This has to be compensated for intraoperatively by means of increased suture tension, which can result in flattening, vertical tilt and irregular astigmatism (Fig. 12).

4.3 Technical Details of PKP [39]

- *General anaesthesia* has clear safety advantages over local anaesthesia, especially in young keratoconus patients. The arterial blood pressure should be kept as low as possible when the eye is open *("controlled arterial hypotension") and Mivacurium should not be used as a muscle relaxant* [40, 41].
- Typically, the *pupil is constricted with pilocarpine* in order to protect the lens of the phakic eye.

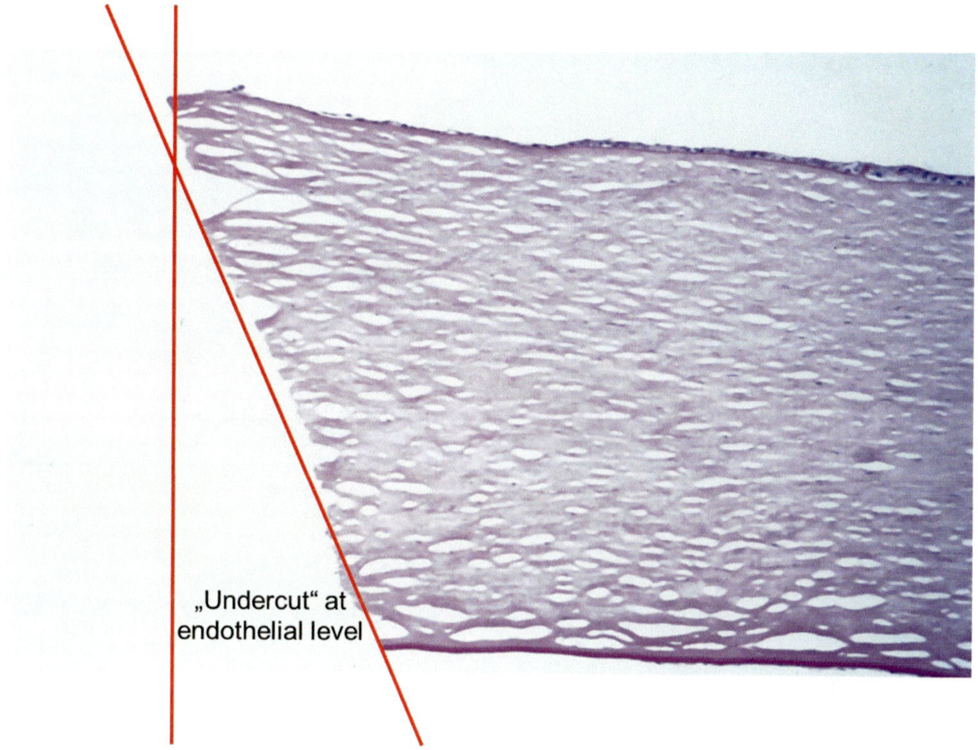

Fig. 11 Donor trephination from the endothelial side: Smooth cutting surface, but "undercut" at the level of the Descemet membrane with convergent incision angle

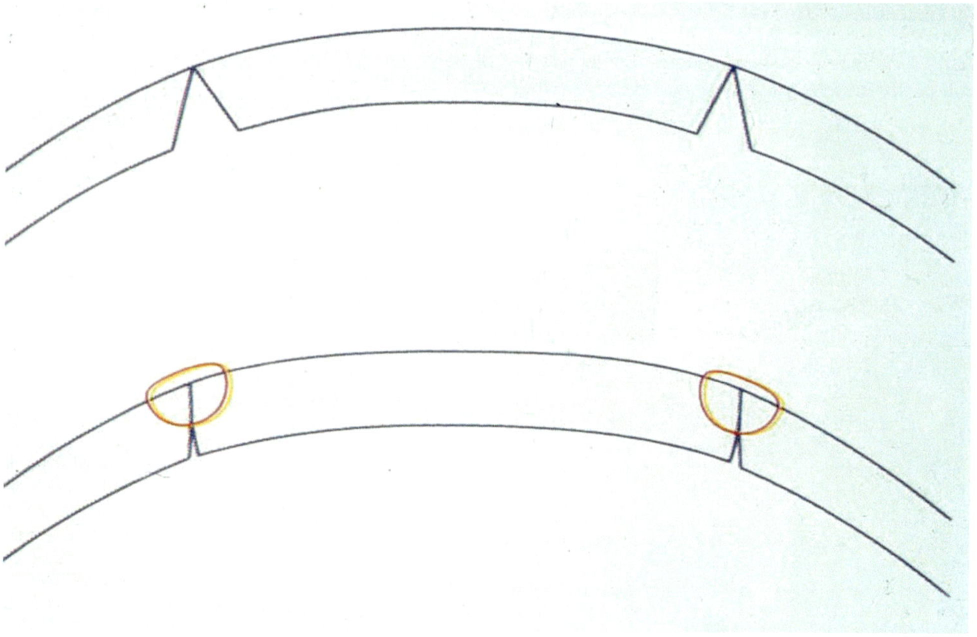

Fig. 12 A triangular defect resulting from divergent incision angles in the patient cornea and convergent incision angles in the donor which is trephined from the endothelial side has to be compensated for by exaggerated suture tension to achieve watertight wound closure. This may result in cornea plana and irregular astigmatism

- Paracentesis at the limbus is recommended before trephination.
- The head and *limbus level* must be *horizontal* during trephination.
- A peripheral iridotomy at 12 o'clock (Fig. 13) prevents pupillary block and therefore an acute glaucoma attack. In case of keratoconus after the administration of atropine, this may appear as a so-called Urrets–Zavalia syndrome with a persistent maximally dilated pupil due to an iris sphincter necrosis (Fig. 14) [42].
- The correct position of the *second cardinal suture* is absolutely crucial for a correct graft alignment.
- *Intra-operative keratoscopy* should be applied *after* removal of the lid speculum and fixation sutures [22, 26, 34, 43].

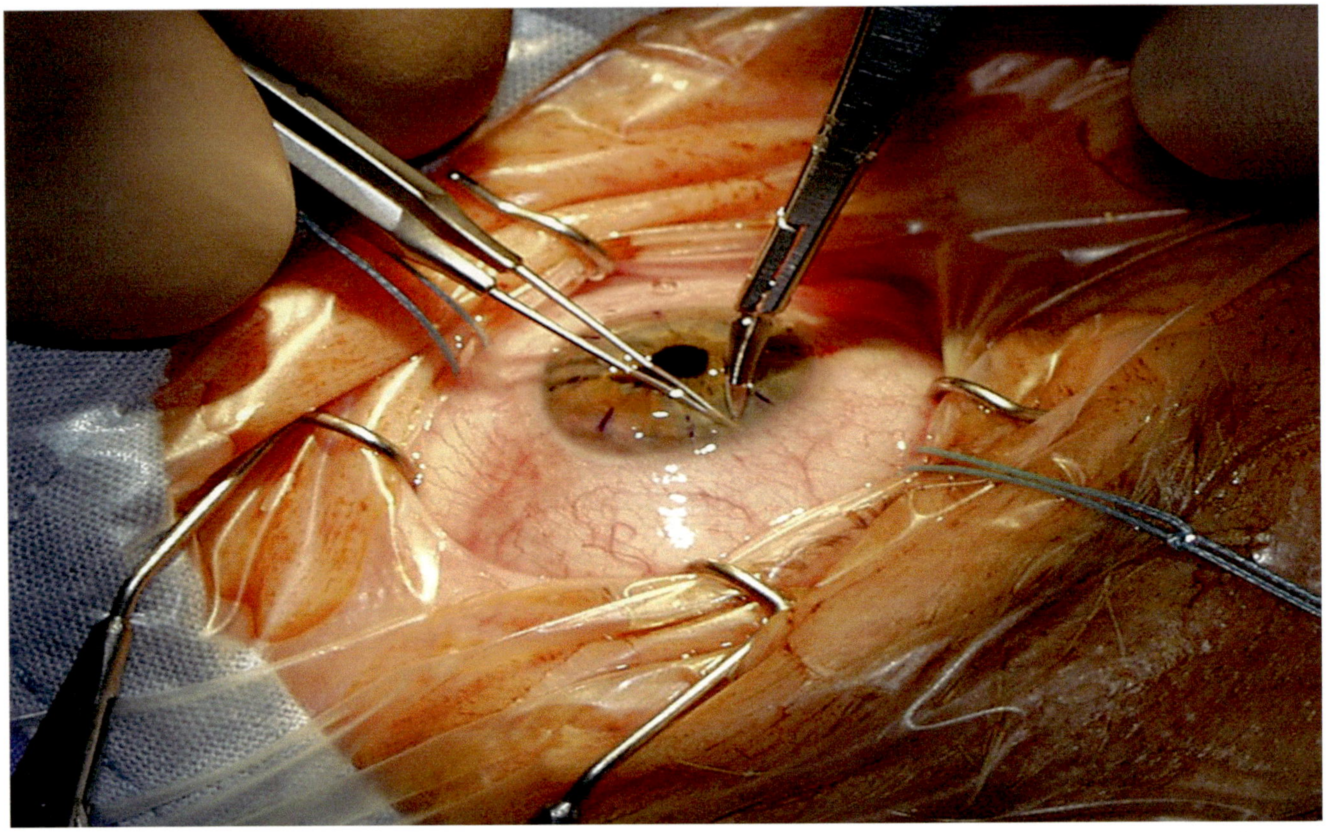

Fig. 13 Manual peripheral iridotomy via open sky at the 12 o'clock position to prevent perioperative pressure rise with iris sphincter necrosis and persistent wide pupil after penetrating keratoplasty

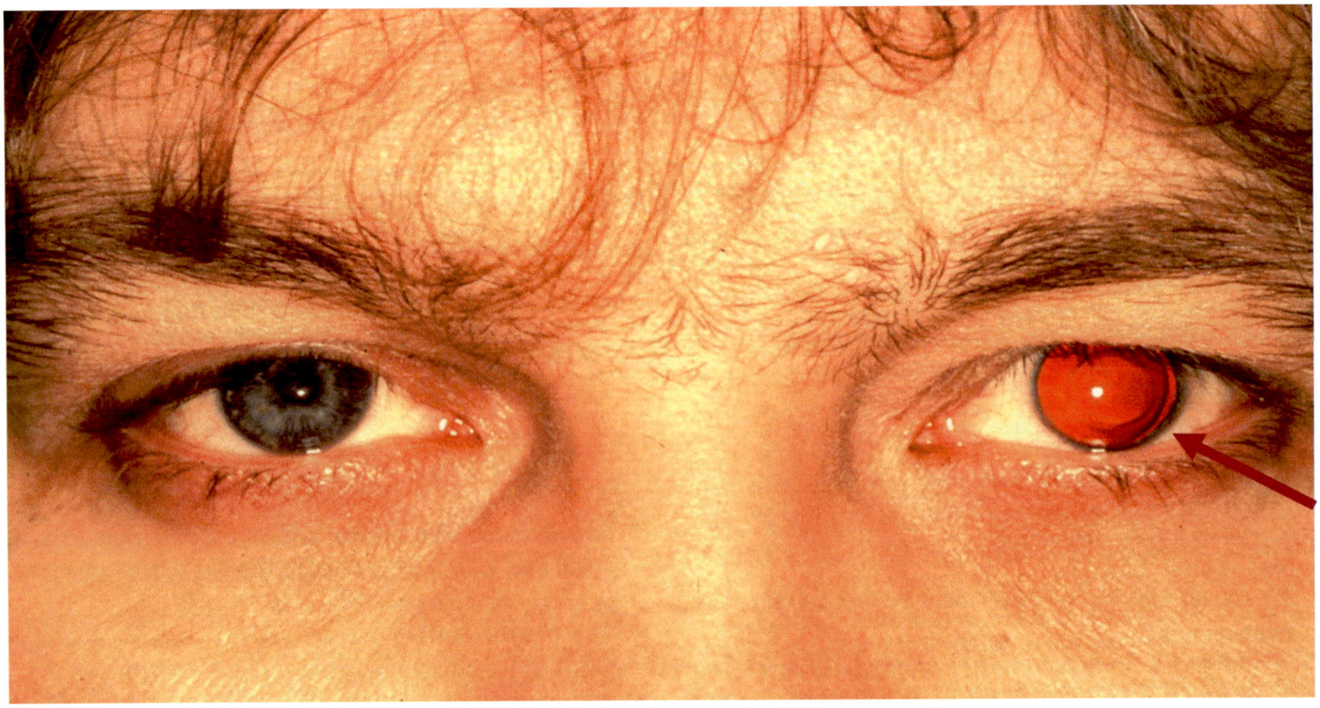

Fig. 14 Wide pupil without light reaction and partial peripheral anterior synechiae after perioperative application of Atropine after penetrating keratoplasty for keratoconus—so-called Urrets–Zavalia syndrome [42]

4.4 Graft Size and Oversize

4.4.1 Graft Size

In a quantitative study, we were able to show that the corneal diameter in keratoconus patients is significantly greater than the diameter in Fuchs patients (mean horizontal diameter of 11.8 mm in keratoconus compared to 11.3 mm in patients with Fuchs dystrophy [44]). In general, larger graft dimensions have a favourable effect on the optical qualities and endothelial cell count, while a low rate of immunological rejection and lower risk of postoperative ocular hypertension is affected by a small graft.

The graft size should be determined on an individual basis: "as large as possible, but as small as necessary".

For many eyes with keratoconus, an 8.0 mm diameter has proven to be a good default for communication with the cornea bank (Arcus lipoides!) [9], while for many eyes with Fuchs dystrophy not suitable for posterior lamellar keratoplasty, a 7.5 mm diameter may be appropriate. Today, diameters from 5.5 to 7.0 mm are only very rarely needed and are usually reserved for small eyes with special immunological implications or à chaud situations.

It has been assumed that a smaller graft is associated with higher astigmatism after keratoplasty. We compared 8.0, 7.5 and 7.0 mm grafts with each other and found the following [19]:

- Smaller grafts are associated with a flatter curvature.
- Smaller grafts are associated with higher topographic irregularity.
- Smaller grafts result in a higher proportion of non-measurable keratometry images.
- Suture removal is associated with a positive tendency towards regularisation of the topography.
- It has not been possible to show a difference with respect to the amount of net astigmatism between smaller and larger grafts, neither for grafts with nor without suture.

We were able to show that the rate of chronic endothelial cell loss after PKP depends on the initial diagnosis [45]. Endothelial migration along a density gradient from the donor to the recipient ring is probably the main reason for this phenomenon in pseudophakic bullous keratopathy. For this reason, eyes with bullous keratopathy are probably better treated with a larger graft, not only in order to improve the optical quality, but also to transplant as many endothelial cells as possible [46]. Nevertheless, the graft size must be determined individually by the microsurgeon for each individual patient before recipient trephination in order to find the best compromise between immunological purposes and optical quality. A slit lamp with a measuring device, such as the Haag-Streit slit lamp, can be helpful. Furthermore, the removal of a vascularised pannus is recommended (in contrast to vascularised stromal corneal scars) before trephination in order to achieve a greater "individually ideal" graft diameter.

In repeat PKP, an attempt should be made to excise the old graft completely and recenter the trephination if the cornea is large enough and a host rim of about 1.5 mm is left [47, 48]. This is of particular importance in eyes with high and/or irregular astigmatism as the reason for repeated grafting (Figs. 15 and 16).

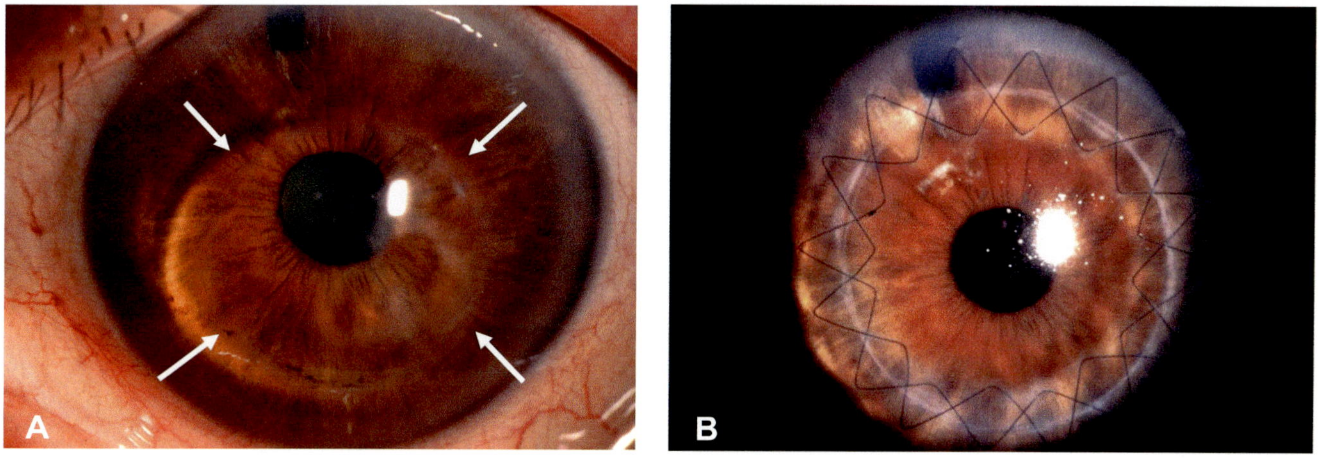

Fig. 15 (**A**) „Repeat keratoconus " after small inferiorely decentered graft (arrows). (**B**) Status after repeat Excimerlaser PKP with optimal centration, optimal graft size (8.5 mm) [49] and optimal suture tension

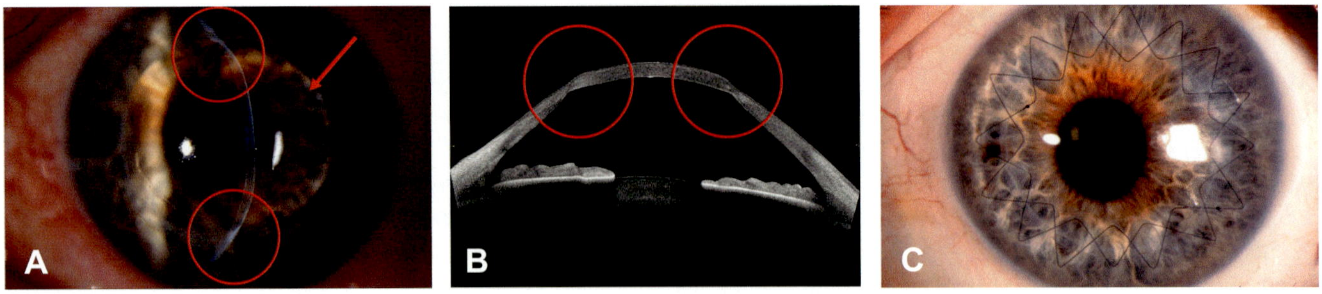

Fig. 16 (**A**) High irregular astigmatism in a small graft with stromal thinning at the graft–host junction (circles) after limbus-parallel keratotomies (arrows). (**B**) Anterior segment OCT shows the "hinge" at the graft–host junction. No indication for DMEK after PKP! (**C**) Status after repeat excimer laser PKP with optimal centration, optimal graft size (8.5 mm) [49] and optimal suture tension

4.4.2 Graft Oversize

In mechanical trephination, the diameter of the recipient bed tends to be larger than the trephine diameter. In contrast, the diameter of the donor disc, which is punched from the endothelial side, tends to be smaller than the trephine diameter, which has a corresponding effect on the spherical equivalent [25, 50]. For this reason, "donor oversizing" of 0.25–0.50 mm is usually carried out in this situation. This is performed on the one hand to prevent the flattening of the graft, and on the other hand to prevent narrowing of the iridocorneal angle where there is a predisposition to secondary glaucoma [29]. In contrast, no oversizing is required with the use of guided trephine systems or laser trephination in which the donor is cut from the epithelial side. In the case of keratoconus, it has been recommended not to carry out donor oversizing (Fig. 17).

Undersizing of the graft for the purpose of simultaneous correction of keratoconus-intrinsic axial myopia will result in irregular astigmatism and is not recommended. The difficulty of achieving a watertight wound closure requires excessive suture tension, with the consequence of irregular astigmatism and a relative cornea plana.

4.5 Pupil or Limbal Centration?

Centration is essential, in terms of both the immunological graft reaction and the astigmatism after keratoplasty [24, 36, 52]. Typically, an attempt is made to reach a compromise between limbus and pupil centration in non-traumatized pupils. However, limbus centration is preferred

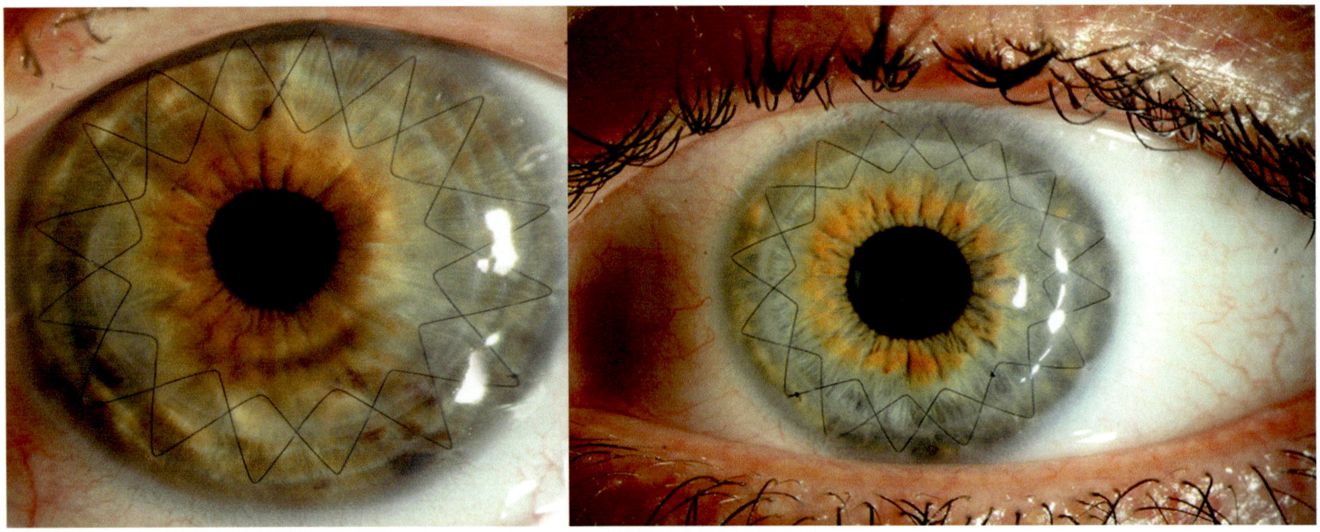

Fig. 17 Excimer laser keratoplasty (8.0/8.1 mm) with typical double-running 10–0 nylon cross-stitch suture, each with 8 stitches (according to Hoffmann [51]) in keratoconus. The donor tissue is trephined from the epithelial side on the corneoscleral button in an artificial anterior chamber—not punched from the endothelial side!

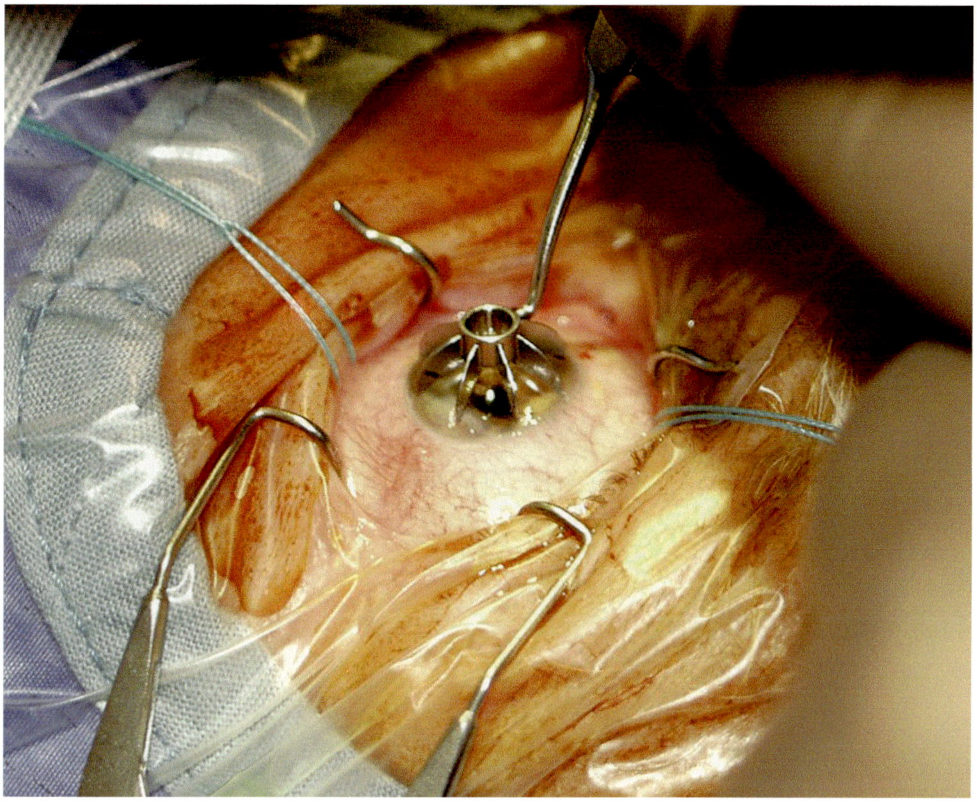

Fig. 18 Radial keratotomy marker with 8 coloured lines for limbal centration on the patient cornea with keratoconus

especially in the case of keratoconus, scars after trauma or irregular astigmatism due to other causes. In such eyes, the centre of the entrance pupil is in fact optically displaced from the position of the actual anatomical pupil [53]. For example, the pupil in the typical keratoconus eye tends to be optically displaced superonasally due to the inferotemporal location of the cone.

We use a radial keratotomy marker with eight lines in order to ensure limbal centration (Fig. 18). Additional central punctate marking can be helpful for certain trephine systems (e.g. Hessburg-Barron trephine, GTS after Krumeich).

4.6 Keratoconus

In keratoconus, a large (typically 8.0 mm or even 8.5 mm) central circular keratoplasty is indicated as soon as rigid oxygen-permeable or scleral contact lenses are no longer tolerated [49]. If nonmechanical excimer laser trephination is used, corneas, which are extremely steep before keratoplasty, do not have worse prognosis than those, which are less deformed [54].

A larger graft diameter in keratoconus contributes towards obtaining a sufficiently thick cornea on the trephination edge, since as a result the cone can usually be completely excised. We advise against centering the trephination at the center of the cone, as this typically necessitates decentering of the trephination with regard to the limbus. This would have unfavourable impacts on the astigmatism [24]. Cauterisation of the cone has been suggested in order to avoid divergent incision angles, but the achieved effect is not reproducible. For this reason, we do not recommend cauterisation of the cone. An obturator should not be used with keratoconus [55] in order not to produce undesirable irregularly elliptical or even pear-shaped host openings (Fig. 19). In this context, "non-contact" excimer laser trephination is preferred over the mechanical method in order to avoid non-circular recipient openings.

In keratoconus, the inhomogeneous corneal thickness typically results in premature perforation at the thinnest point of the cornea, which has to be considered when using conventional trephines in order not to inadvertently traumatize the iris or even the lens.

4.7 Suture Technique

The type of trephination has a major impact on the correct placement of the first four or eight cardinal sutures [23, 34]. The main purposes of these cardinal sutures include:

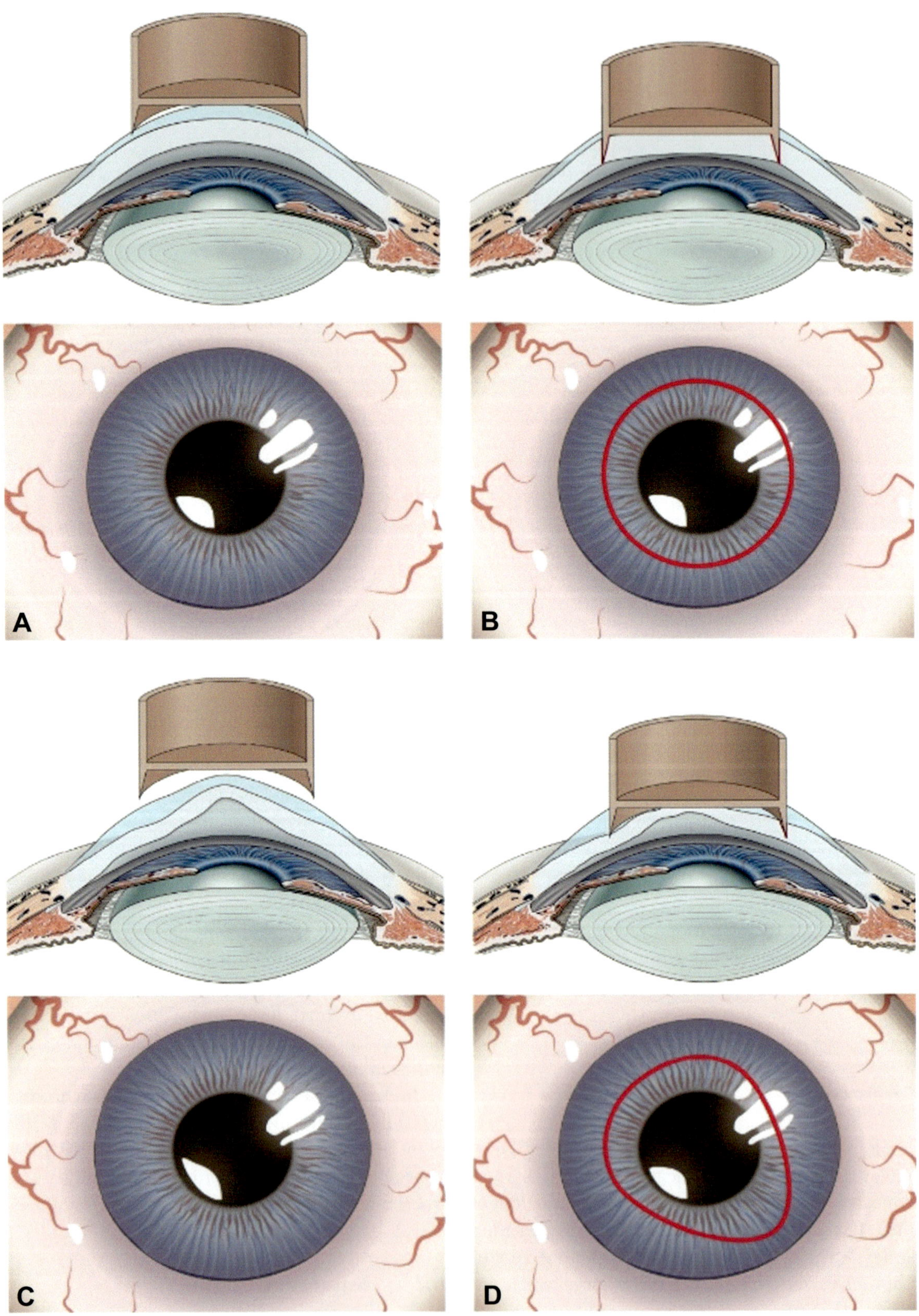

Fig. 19 (**A–D**) In case of keratoconus is has been recommended <u>not</u> to use an obturator in order to avoid elliptical or pear-shaped excision shapes [55]. The same principle of applanation during trephination applies in femtosecond laser application without liquid interface

- The symmetrical horizontal distribution of donor tissue in the recipient bed
- Good adaptation of the donor and recipient wound edge on the level of the Bowman layer
- Stabilization of the anterior chamber to ensure that further suturing is uniform.

> Concerning donor–host alignment, external steps must be avoided, although internal steps sometimes have to be tolerated in the case of very thin recipient corneas (e.g. pellucid marginal degeneration, herpetic scars) or very thick recipient corneas (e.g. longstanding bullous keratopathy).

As far as the correct placement of the second cardinal suture is concerned, unintentional deviations from circular recipient openings can represent a challenge even for the experienced keratoplasty surgeon. After removal of the cardinal sutures, the quality of the trephination and the correct positioning of the graft are the main determinants for a watertight wound closure. The better the trephination, the lower the final suture tension which is necessary to ensure a watertight wound closure after removal of the cardinal sutures. The lower the final suture tension is, the quicker an improvement in visual acuity can be expected. In the case of an intact Bowman layer, a 16-stitch double-running diagonal cross-stitch suture (10–0 nylon) after Hoffmann is typically preferred in Germany [32, 51] (Fig. 20). The faster visual rehabilitation with running sutures—in contrast to multiple interrupted sutures and combined suture techniques—is attributable to the regular topography of the cornea and the avoidance of a relative cornea plana. In addition, with this double running suture the risk of suture loosening is reduced [56].

The new Homburg cross-stitch marker (Fig. 21) ensures the precise localisation of the entry and exit points of the suture [57]. This new instrument allows inexperienced surgeons in particular to feel very confident when performing the running sutures (Video 1). Surgeons with little experience can completely avoid using their still imprecise sense of proportion and significantly shorten the learning curve for this procedure. The use of the Homburg cross-stitch marker for excimer laser PKP in young cornea specialists results in significantly better visual acuity before and after suture removal, significantly lower astigmatism and cylinder value before suture removal, as well as a reduced necessity of early postoperative single interrupted suture addition [58].

Please scan to access video content

> The better the trephination, the more easily a watertight wound closure is achieved.
> If excessive suture tension is required in order to achieve a watertight wound closure, the regularity of the topography and, therefore, the visual acuity after keratoplasty is generally impaired.

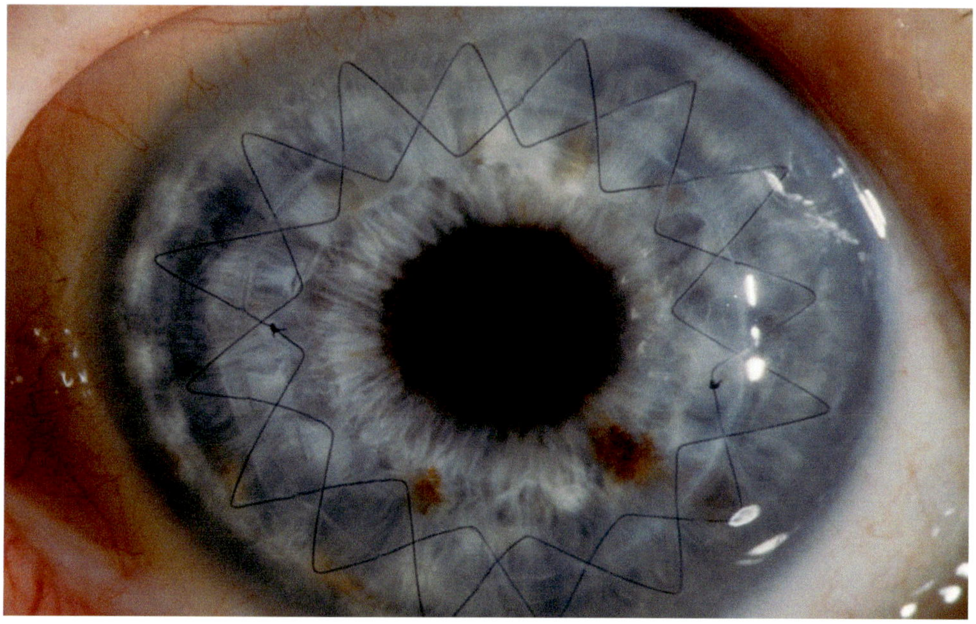

Fig. 20 Excimer laser keratoplasty (8.0/8.1 mm) with typical double-running 10–0 nylon cross-stitch suture, each with 8 stitches (according to Hoffmann [51]) in keratoconus

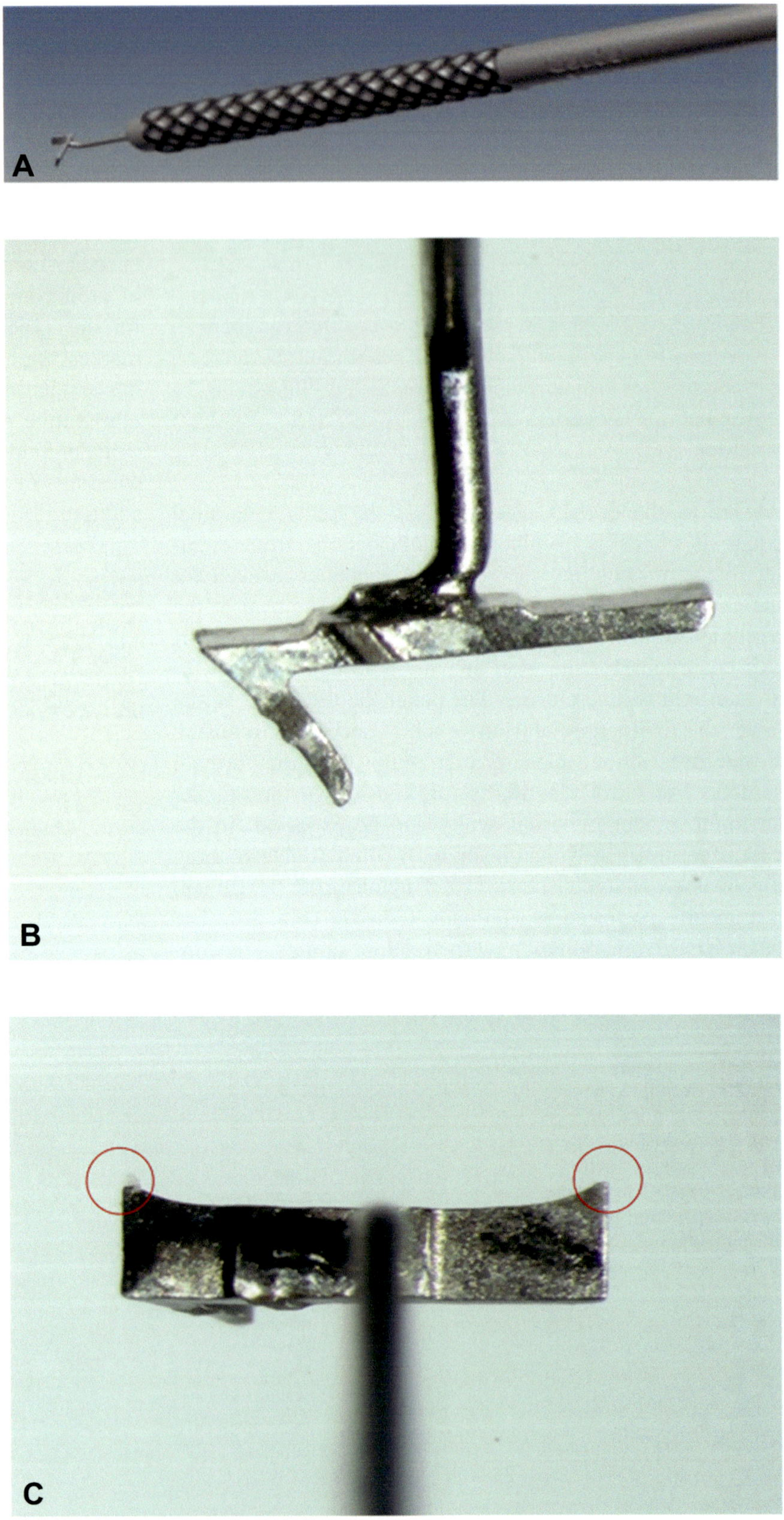

Fig. 21 The new Homburg cross-stitch marker after Suffo (by Geuder) ensures the precise localisation of the entry and exit points of the suture [57]. (**A**) Handle of the marker (**B**) Shape of the Number "7" of the marker, (**C**) Two prominences of the marker which are coloured with blue ink intraoperatively to produce two fine dots, one on the graft and one on the recipient/host cornea

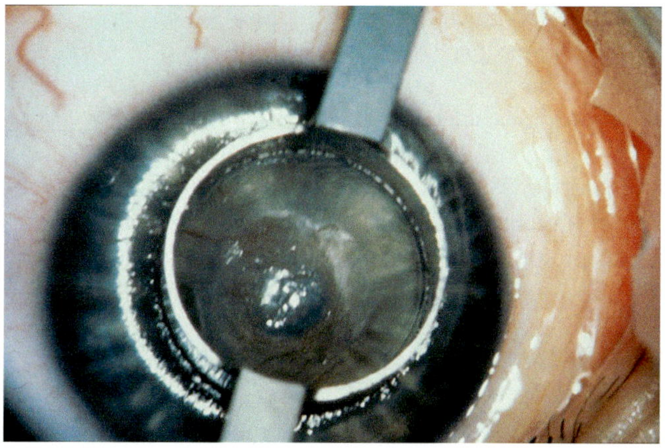

Fig. 22 Conventional mechanical trephination is always associated to some extent with the deformation of corneal tissue, including distortion of the cut edges, and with irregular cutting surfaces as a consequence of the axial and radial forces which are induced by the use of these trephines—"No Incision without Distortion" [26, 34]

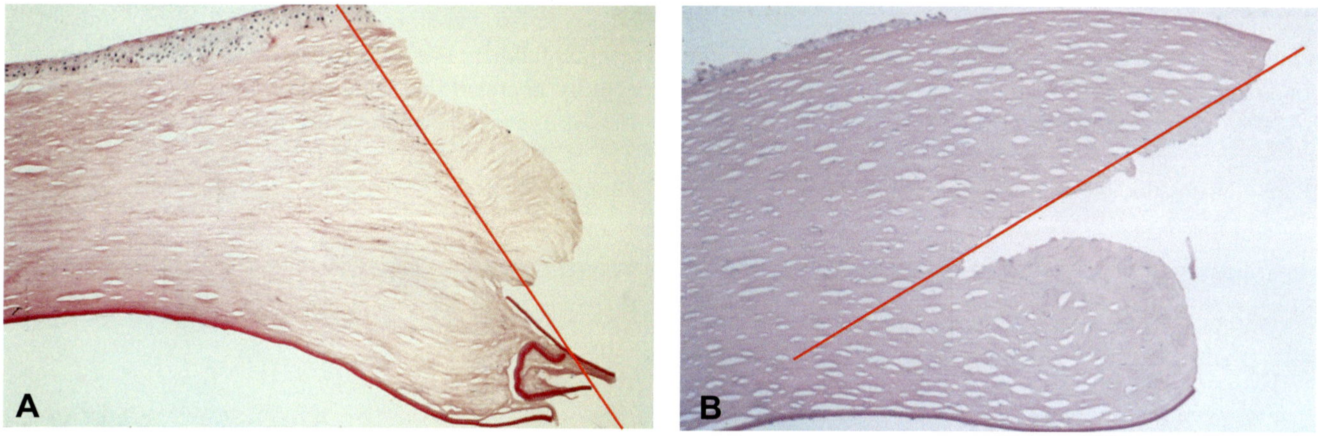

Fig. 23 "Suboptimal" incision edges after mechanical trephination deviate from the perpendicular and are often different in the donor and recipient, (**A**) Divergent recipient trephination in case of repeat PKP—note the remnants of Descemet Membrane from the previous graft, (**B**) "Shark mouth shaped" incomplete recipient trephination with divergent upper part and straight scissors-cut lower part

4.8 Conventional Mechanical Trephines

Unfortunately, conventional mechanical trephination is always associated to some extent with the deformation of corneal tissue (Fig. 22), including distortion of the cut edges, and with irregular cutting surfaces as a consequence of the axial and radial forces which are induced by the use of these trephines [26, 34]. The cut angles deviate from the perpendicular (Fig. 23) and are often different in the donor and recipient, especially when the donor trephination is performed from the endothelial side [23, 29, 31, 50]. The fitting of the donor tissue into an unstable recipient bed is sometimes very difficult to achieve in a perfectly symmetrical manner. After the suturing in of incongruent cut edges and the resulting induction of a vertical tilt [59], the healing of the wound can result in pronounced distortion of the graft topography, especially after suture removal [27, 28, 30]. Moreover, the asymmetrical placement of the cardinal sutures can lead to the uneven distribution of donor tissue in the recipient bed, in particular if the second cardinal suture is not positioned exactly 180° opposite the first stay suture ("horizontal torsion") [26].

If conventional trephines are used, it is recommended that systems should be applied which in the case of donor trephination from the epithelial side provide for the use of an artificial anterior chamber for fixation of the corneoscleral disc. The trephines should always be as sharp as possible in order to keep inappropriate squeezing and shearing forces as small as possible. Disposable items may be advantageous here—also with regard to prion—caused contagious diseases.

4.9 Nonmechanical Excimer Laser Trephination (Video 2)

Please scan to access video content

Following the hypothesis that the characteristics of the wound bed are considerably more important for the astigmatism after suture removal and the optical quality of the graft than various suture techniques or methods of subsequent suture adjustments, the technique of nonmechanical corneal trephination has been developed and optimized in Erlangen since 1986 [60]. Originally, the elliptical shape was proposed on the basis of the idea that an elliptical graft could best be fitted to the natural elliptical human cornea, both from the optical and the immunological perspective [61]. Prof. G.K. Lang published details of the first two patients after elliptical keratoplasty in 1990 [62]. A total of 42 elliptical keratoplasties were performed in humans from 1989 to 1991 [63]. Subsequently, this method was abandoned for optical reasons, because the need for simple interrupted sutures to prevent rotation of the graft in the recipient bed and the need for asymmetric suture tension in these multiple interrupted sutures had ultimately not resulted in improved curvature, neither with nor without sutures [64]. Today, we still use elliptical excimer laser keratoplasty for elliptical ulcers with descemetoceles or penetration for the purposes of keratoplasty à chaud (a typical example of elliptical ulceration would be Acanthamoeba keratitis or pellucid marginal degeneration with eccentric thinning of the cornea at the bottom close to the limbus (Fig. 24) [65].

Since July 01, 1989 more than 6000 eyes have been successfully operated in Erlangen and Homburg/Saar with the MEL70 excimer laser made by Zeiss Meditec and, since 2014, with the AMARIS 1050 RS excimer laser made by Schwind [66, 67].

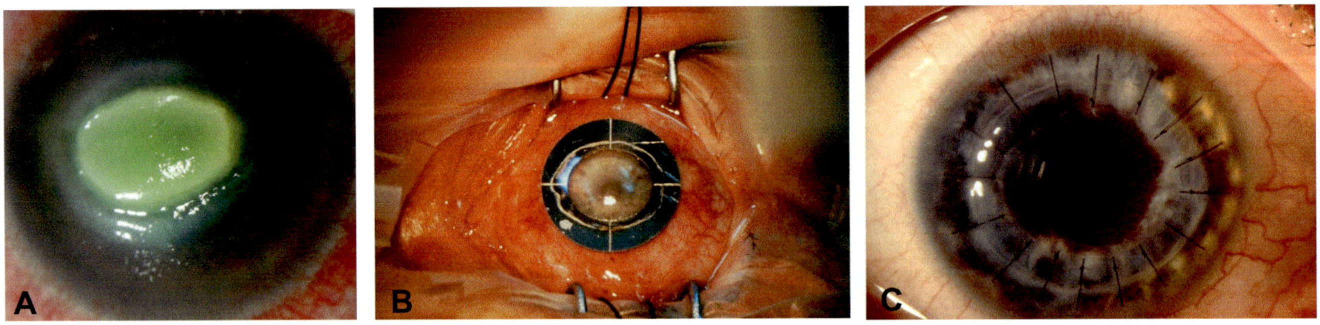

Fig. 24 An elliptical ulceration in Acanthamoeba keratitis may be treated with an elliptical excimer laser keratoplasty with at least 24 single sutures, (**A**) Elliptical ulcer preoperatively, (**B**) Elliptical metal mask directly placed on the patient's cornea, (**C**) Status after PKP with 24 single sutures in place

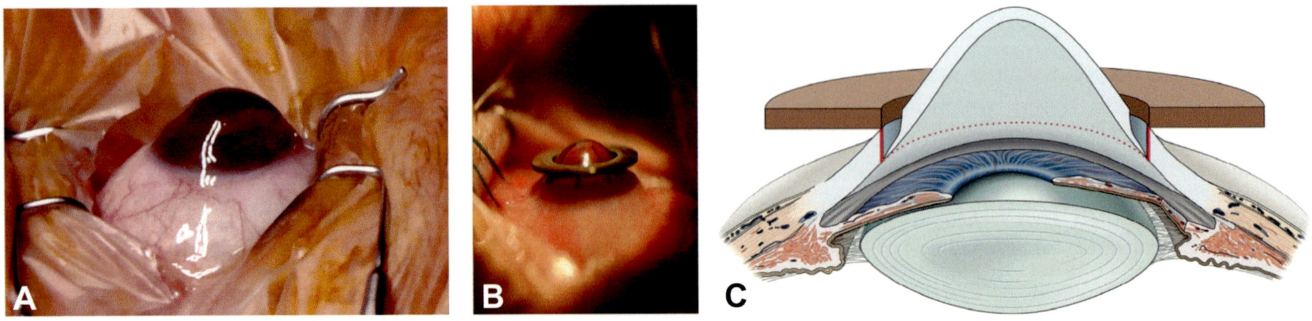

Fig. 25 Severe keratoconus is one of the main indications for excimer laser keratoplasty. (**A**) Very severe keratoconus. (**B**) Metal mask is placed around the cone on the patient's eye without deformation, (**C**) Schematic drawing of excimer laser ablation along the inner edge of the metal recipient mask resulting in a round opening with perpendicular incision angles

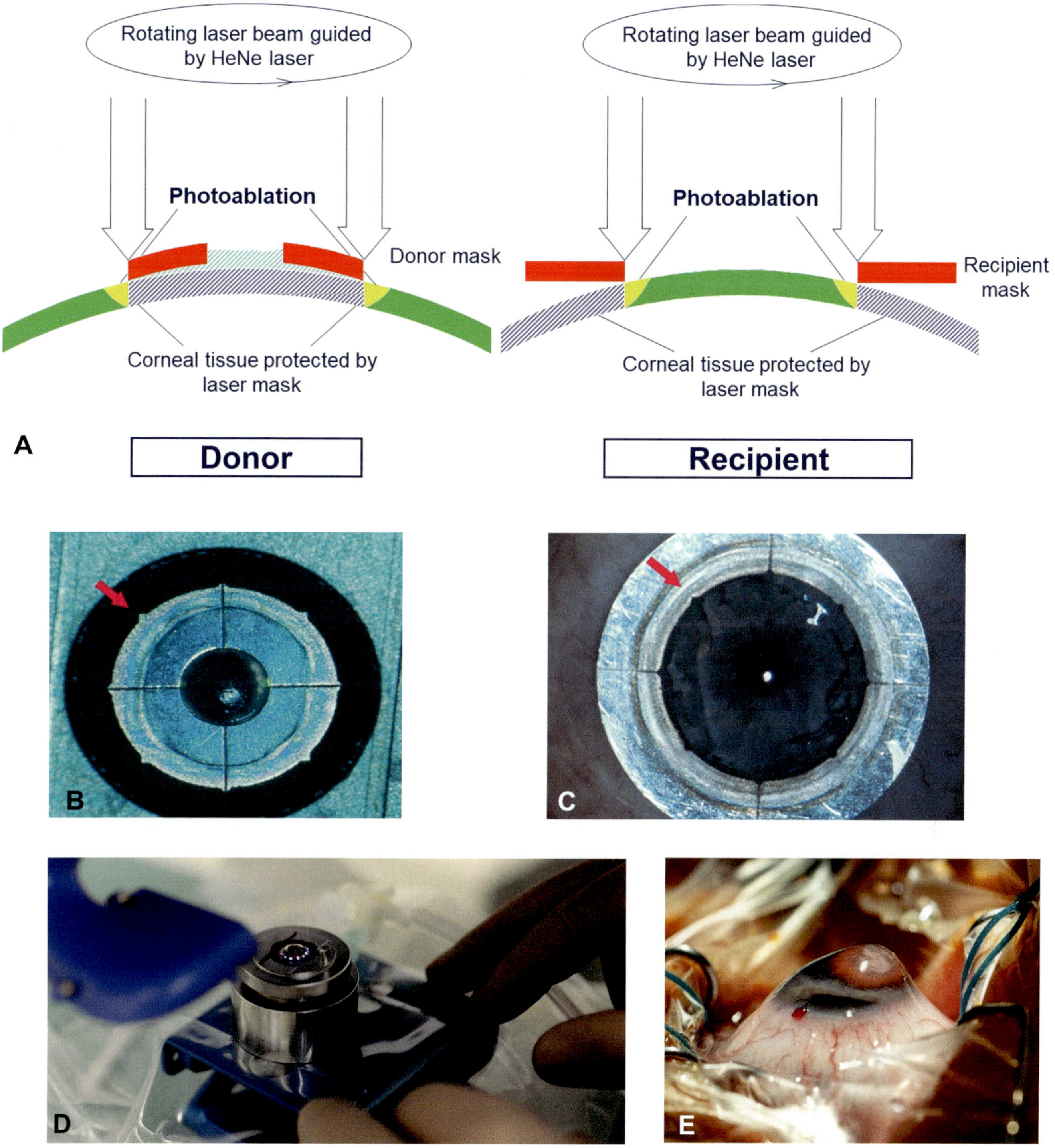

Fig. 26 (**A**) Principle of excimer laser trephination in the donor and recipient (schematic sketch, sagittal view). (**B**) Donor mask (8.1 mm in diameter) with eight "orientation teeth" (red arrow) on the outside lying directly on the corneoscleral disc in the artificial anterior chamber. The laser is guided along the outer edge. (**C**) Recipient mask (8.0 mm in diameter) with eight "orientation notches" (red arrow) on the inside lying directly on the patient's cornea. The laser is guided along the inner edge. (**D**) Pseudo-ring-shaped automated Schwind AMARIS 1050 RS excimer laser ablation profile along the outer edge of a donor mask on a corneoscleral disc in an artificial anterior chamber. (**E**) Side view of a very prominent pellucid marginal degeneration with extreme thinning from 4 to 8 o'clock close to the limbus immediately before trephination

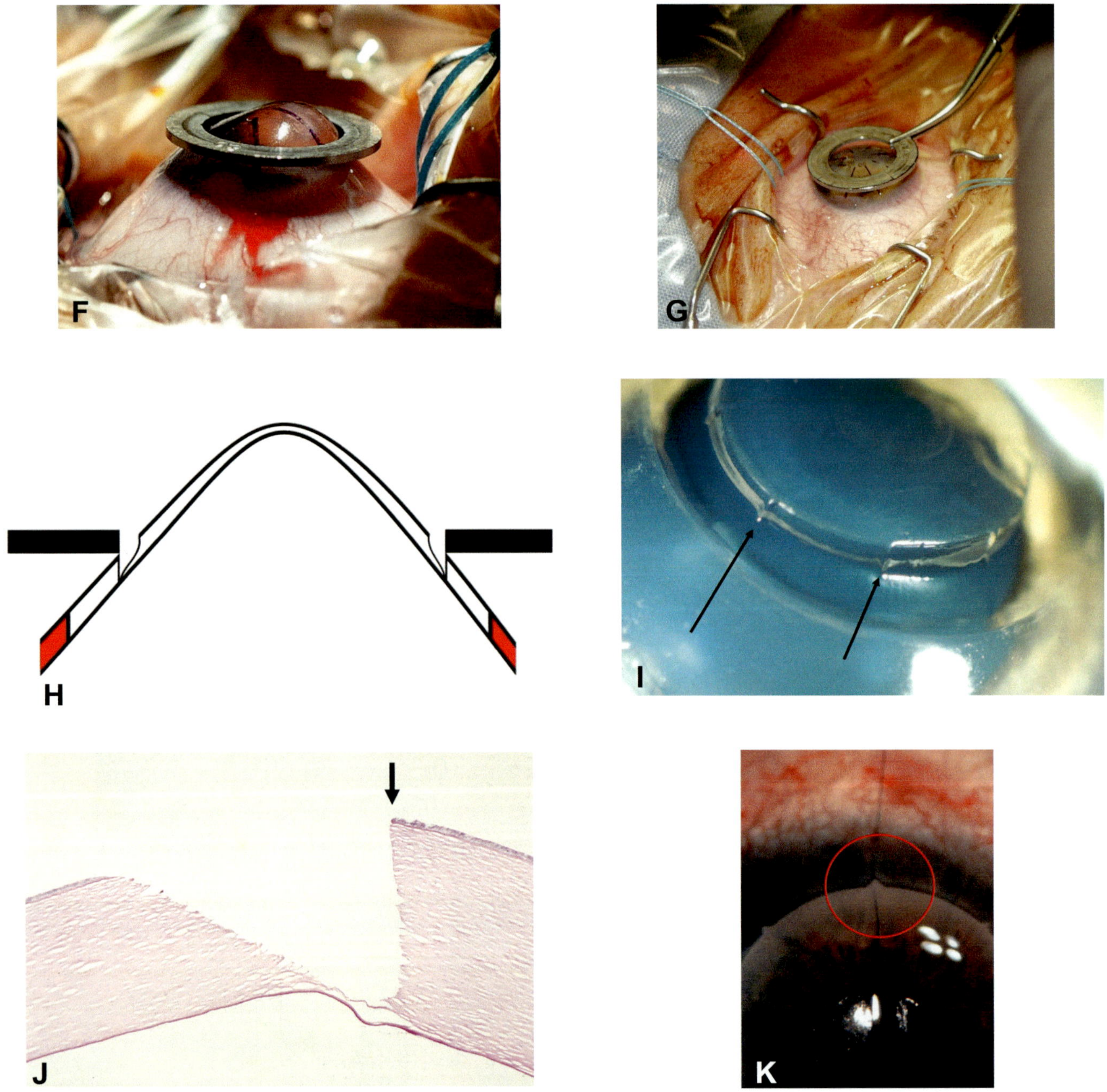

Fig. 26 (**F**) During host trephination with the excimer laser the metal recipient mask (8.5 mm in diameter) is well centered around the protrusion without deformation. The laser is guided along the inner edge of the mask. (**G**) Eight "orientation notches" at the recipient mask are associated with 8 radial keratotomy marks on the patient's cornea. (**H**) Schematic sagittal view of the cone protruding through the central hole of the metal recipient mask allowing a perpendicular round trephination without deformation. (**I**) Donor trephination immediately before penetration with smooth cut edges and orientation teeth *(arrows)*. (**J**) Histology of straight, almost perpendicular incision edges immediately before donor trephination with the excimer laser. (**K**) Exact positioning of the second cardinal suture in penetrating excimer keratoplasty through the use of a small tooth and a corresponding notch to prevent "horizontal torsion" (intra-operatively)

With a share of more than one quarter, keratoconus has always been by far the most common indication for PKP with this "non-contact" excimer laser technique (Fig. 25).

Technique. Before trephination, the limbus is centered along the vertical helium–neon target beam in the donor and patient in order to ensure a reproducible position to the laser beam and therefore symmetric cutting angles in the entire circumference.

Table 4 Advantages of nonmechanical trephination with the 193 nm excimer laser along metal masks with "orientation teeth" [26, 35, 69]

1. No trauma to intraocular tissues
2. Prevention of deformation and compression of the tissue during trephination
3. Reduction of "horizontal torsion" ("orientation teeth")
4. Reduction of "vertical tilt" (almost perfect congruent incision edges)
5. Improvement of recipient and donor centration
6. Possibility of "harmonization" of donor and recipient topography
7. Reduction of anterior chamber inflammation after keratoplasty
8. *Reduction of astigmatism after suture removal*
9. Increase in the regularity of the topography of the cornea
10. *Significantly better spectacle-corrected visual acuity*
11. *Feasibility of trephination of an instable cornea* (e.g. "open eye", descemetocele, status post-radial keratotomy, iatrogenic keratectasia after LASIK)
12. Any shape possible (e.g. elliptical)

For *donor trephination* from the epithelial side, a round open metal mask (diameter 5.6–8.6 mm, central opening 3.0 mm for centering, thickness 0.5 mm, weight 0.2 g, 8 "orientation teeth") is placed on a corneoscleral disc (15 mm) which is fixed in an artificial anterior chamber under microscopic control (Fig. 26 A, B, D, I and J). The pressure within the artificial anterior chamber is adjusted to approximately 22 mmHg using a Maklakoff tonometer.

For *recipient trephination* which is performed clinically with the manually or automated guided laser beam, a corresponding recipient mask is used (diameter 12.9 mm, central opening 5.5 to 8.5 mm, 8 "orientation notches"). Before the start of trephination, centering relative to the limbus is achieved by the association of the eight notches in the mask with the eight linear marks of a blue stained radial keratotomy marker, which has been previously applied under microscopic control (Fig. 26 A, C, E, F, G, and H).

Advantages of nonmechanical trephination. The main advantage of this excimer laser cutting method, which is performed from the epithelial side in donor and recipient, is the avoidance of mechanical distortions during trephination (Table 4). This results in smooth cut edges which are congruent in both the donor and recipient, so that the "vertical tilt" is reduced (Fig. 27) [59]. "Orientation teeth" on the edge of the graft [68] and corresponding notches on the edge of the recipient for undoubted symmetrical positioning of the first eight cardinal sutures reduce the "horizontal torsion" (Fig. 26K). In this way, it is possible to improve the optical quality after transplantation. Furthermore, donor and recipient centration is improved [18, 52]. These beneficial influences on the main intra-operative determinants of astigmatism after keratoplasty (Table 3) result in lower keratometric net astigmatism, higher topographic regularity and improved spectacle-corrected visual acuity after suture removal [32, 35, 69, 70].

In addition to less disruption to the blood-aqueous barrier in the early phase after keratoplasty [71], the laser trephination does not result either in increased cataract formation [72] or higher endothelial cell loss of the graft [46]. In addition, the frequencies of the immunological graft reaction [4] and secondary ocular hypertension were comparable in both techniques [7]. The use of metal masks allows an arbitrary trephination technique [63, 64]. Moreover, the use of the laser allows the trephination of an instable cornea, such as in perforated corneal ulcers (or descemetoceles) or after radial keratotomy or in iatrogenic keratectasia after laser in-situ keratomileusis LASIK [19, 65, 66].

4.10 Practical Considerations for the Microsurgeon

The somewhat longer trephination time (around 90 s with the Schwind laser) is largely compensated for by the practical advantages for the microsurgeon during the subsequent course of the surgery [26, 35, 37, 60, 69]:

- Injury to intraocular structures is impossible with the laser, as tissue ablation ceases as soon as the aqueous humour fills the trephination canal after focal perforation.
- The need to complete the cut using scissors is reduced to a minimum.
- The location of the first eight cardinal sutures is unequivocally specified by the eight "orientation teeth/ notches" (Fig. 26 K).
- Crescent-shaped tissue deficits in the region of the donor-recipient junction (such as in the case of non-circular recipient openings e.g. in keratoconus) are avoided, so that a latent watertight closure is often achieved after just four cardinal sutures.
- During the subsequent suturing procedure, the anterior chamber remains largely stable as a rule.
- The final double-continuous suture only has to be tightened to a very slight extent in order to maintain an anterior-step-free wound adjustment and watertight wound closure—even after the removal of the eight cardinal sutures.
- For this reason, additional interrupted sutures with an unfavourable effect on the graft topography are needed only very rarely at the end of surgery.
- Furthermore, the so-called "barrel-top formation" at the proximal ends of the sutures, which result in a relative

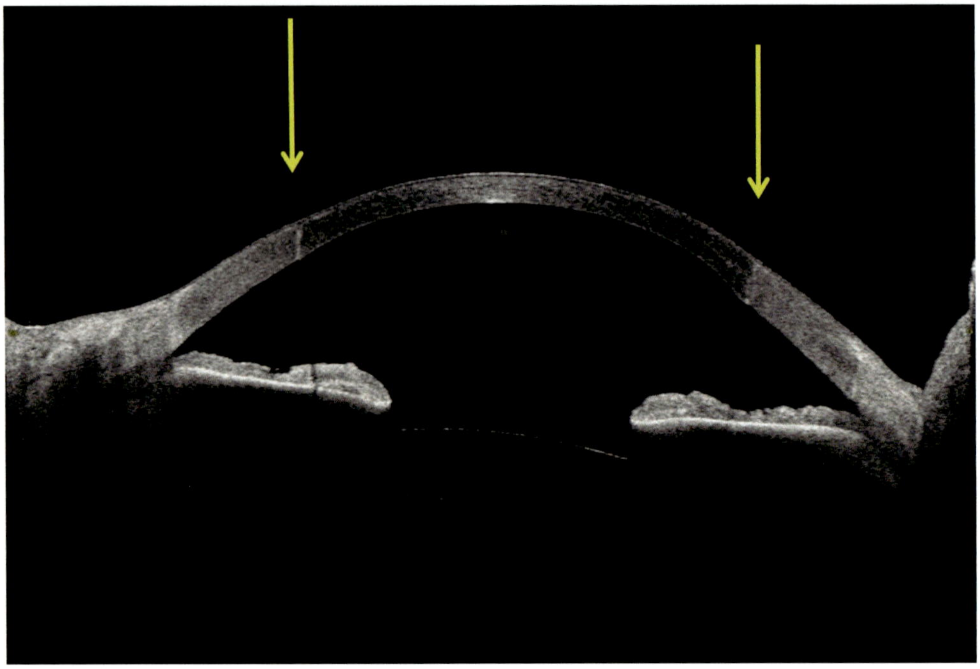

Fig. 27 AS-OCT: tension-free donor–host apposition of perpendicular incisions after excimer laser trephination without step formation/overriding

cornea plana and, therefore, delayed optical rehabilitation, is largely avoided.

- After removal of the eyelid speculum and the fixation sutures, the use of a Placido disc after intra-operative suture adjustment often provides a round projection image.

Nonmechanical trephination using the 193 nm excimer laser along metal masks has significantly improved the results of penetrating keratoplasty after suture removal. The use of the excimer laser also allows controlled trephination of instable corneas, such as in perforated ulcers, iatrogenic keratectasia after LASIK or after radial keratotomies.

4.11 Femtosecondlaser Trephination for PKP

In contrast to the excimer laser, which only allows surface ablation, the *femtosecond laser* (a femtosecond corresponds to 10^{-15} s) enables cutting the cornea within the stroma, so that actual three-dimensional cuts without opening the eye and without thermal damage are possible. With real 3-D incisions, it may be possible to achieve self-sealing wounds. We proposed the "inverse mushroom" (now commonly referred to as the "top hat" configuration) in 2005 in order to achieve a watertight wound closure [73]. FSL-assisted PKP without liquid interface seems to have major disadvantages in comparison to excimer laser PKP, especially in keratoconus (Fig. 28). In a prospective randomized study, we as well as others found that the keratometric astigmatism and incidence of immune

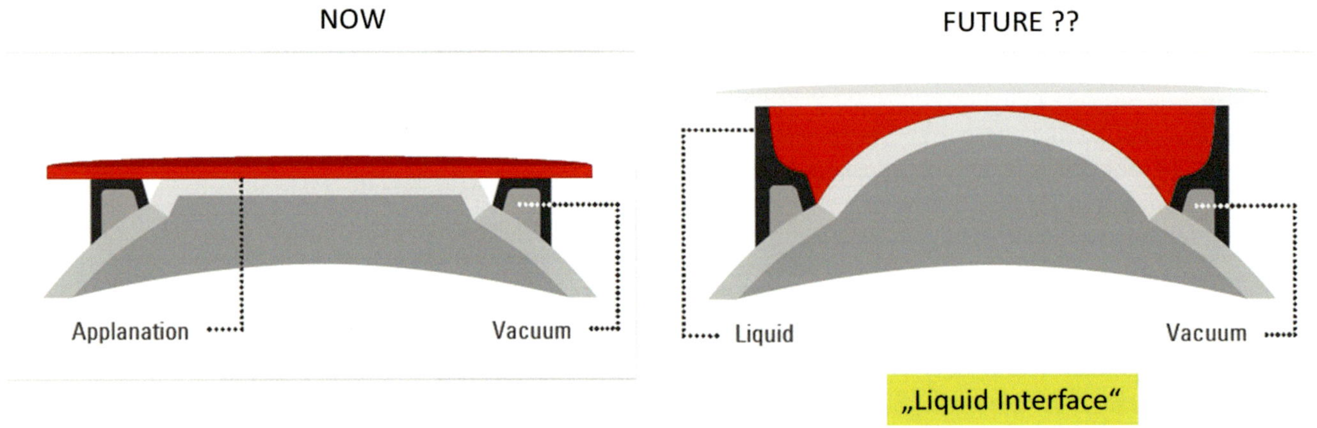

Fig. 28 Conventional FSL trephination with applanation and suction versus application of a so-called "liquid interface" to minimize distortion of the host cornea

reactions after FSL PKP in keratoconus are significantly higher than after excimer laser PKP. After suture removal, mean refractive/topographic (Pentacam and AS-OCT) astigmatism values were significantly lower in the EXCIMER-keratoconus (KC) subgroup (3.0±2.5 D/3.2±2.7 D/3.5±2.9 D) than in the FSL-KC subgroup (7.3±2.8 D/8.1±3.0 D/8.3±3.7 D; $p \leq 0.006$). Mean SRI (Surface Regularity Index) was significantly lower in the EXCIMER-KC subgroup than in the FSL-KC subgroup after suture removal (0.57±0.40 vs. 1.16±0.54; $p = 0.003$) indicating a higher regularity of corneal topography in the EXCIMER-KC subgroup.

The Fundamental Problem of Femtosecond Laser Trephination

Over the last 20 years, femtosecond laser keratoplasty has caused a good deal of excitement. The advantages of femtosecond laser keratoplasty are the arbitrary horizontal and vertical shapes, including the "top hat", "mushroom", "zigzag", "Christmas tree", "octagon", "decagon", "dovetail" [74, 75]. The fundamental problem of every femtosecond laser trephination has been that—even with a curved interface—a certain amount of flattening of the cornea is necessary, which is associated with deformation. Especially in advanced keratoconus, this results in "non-circular" excisions in the patient's cornea and, therefore, "horizontal torsion" as *the* main intra-operative determinant of high/irregular astigmatism after PKP (Fig. 19) [18].

In "regular trephination" during keratoplasty, maximum intraocular pressure values of 135 mmHg are measured with the Intralase, 65 mmHg with the VisuMAX, 205 mmHg with the Femtec and 184 mmHg with the Femto LDV in experimental use [76]. The eight lines which are applied, for example for the Intralase femtosecond laser, in the donor and recipient can sometimes not be brought into alignment intra-operatively in the treatment of keratoconus (Fig. 29).

Some authors claimed that femtosecond laser PKP has advantages in the short-term follow-up concerning refractive cylinder and visual acuity [74, 77–79]. However, there is a large amount of missing data with respect to the potential advantages of femtosecond laser keratoplasty after complete suture removal. Only few groups have published results pertaining to the situation after complete suture removal [80, 81]. After a mean follow-up of 14±5 months, the topographic astigmatism without sutures in the mushroom profile was 6.4±3.0 dpt, and in the top hat profile 5.8±4.6 dpt [80]. The degree of the astigmatism after femtosecond PKP is therefore comparable with that after motor trephination (now withdrawn from the market [35, 69]). Moreover, in the mushroom profile, the rate of the post-operative immune reactions is significantly increased [6].

FSL keratoplasty has been very interesting, but no prospective randomized study had so far been carried out in which both trephination procedures (FSL and excimer laser) for PKP in keratoconus and Fuchs dystrophy have been compared to each other. Such a study has been finished in Homburg/Saar [82]. With FSL-PKP in keratoconus using a double running suture, we found more decentration, more Vis à tergo, and more often the need of single sutures to achieve donor–host apposition without steps and gaps. After suture removal, topographic astigmatism after FSL trephination in keratoconus (8.1±3.0 D) was significantly larger than after excimer laser trephination (3.2±1.7 D). In addition, the surface regularity index (SRI) of the TMS-5 system in keratoconus was significantly unfavorable after FSL trephination (1.2±0.5) than after excimer laser trephination (0.5±0.4). Best spectacle corrected visual acuity after suture removal in keratoconus was 0.8±0.2 after excimer laser and 0.6±0.2 after FSL laser trephination [83]. However, both trephination modalities did not differ concerning endothelial cell count and confocal microscopic features [84, 85]. The advent of the "liquid interface" has opened a favorable new page in the chapter of "Femtosecondlaser trephination for keratoplasty".

Certainly, "manifest cylinder" is not appropriate to compare the outcome of different trephination procedures for PKP [79]. In case of a highly irregular surface, the manifest cylinder will be zero although the benefit for the patient is nil [19]. True benefits of excimer laser versus femtosecond laser trephination for PKP are summarized in Table 5.

On principle, the minimal requirements for comparative studies on various trephination techniques in PKP are:

- visual acuity with spectacle correction (not contact lens visual acuity!) and central refracting power,
- keratometric or topographic astigmatism (not only refractive manifest cylinder!),
- measure of the topographic regularity (e.g. SRI (surface regularity index) or SAI (surface asymmetry index) of the TMS system and ISV (index of surface variance) or IVA (index of vertical asymmetry) of the Pentacam), in each case before and after suture removal.

5 Summary

For penetrating keratoplasty, donor and recipient trephination should be performed with the same system from the epithelial side. The horizontal position of the limbal plane is essential. The graft size should be adapted individually to the cornea size ("as large as possible, as small as necessary") and limbal centration preferred to pupil centration in cases of doubt (especially in keratoconus). Furthermore,

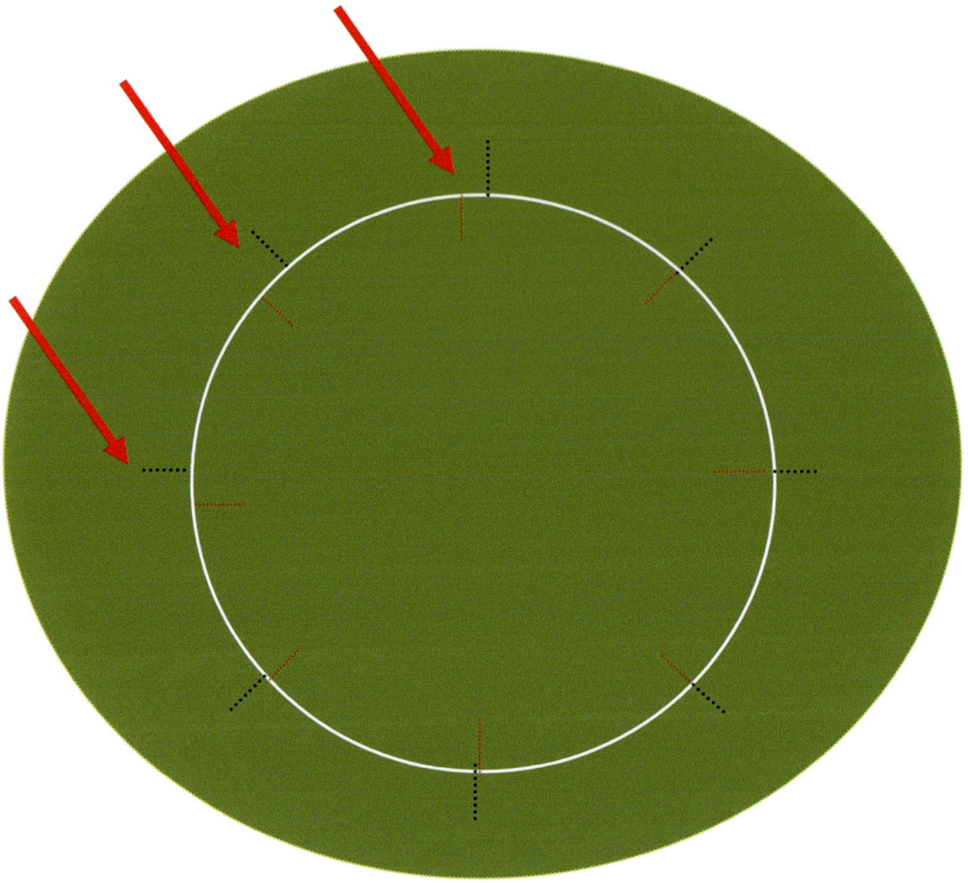

Fig. 29 During femtosecond laser keratoplasty without liquid interface for keratoconus marking lines in donor and host do not match each other due to recipient opening that is not round

excessive graft over- or undersizing should be avoided. At the end of the operation, adjustment of the continuous cross-stitch suture should be carried out using a Placido disk. Nonmechanical excimer laser trephination results in lower astigmatism, higher topographic regularity and better visual acuity (especially in younger patients with keratoconus). In the case of an unstable cornea (e.g. after RK, iatrogenic keratectasia after LASIK, descemetocele, perforated ulcer), trephination by excimer laser application is possible. New "key-lock" variants for the possible self-sealing fit of the donor disc in the recipient bed were looming on the horizon 20 years ago (future "no-stitch keratoplasty") after introduction of femtosecond laser application. However, recent all-suture-out data demonstrate that the potential superiority of this high price and difficult to maintain option cannot be proven! Thus, today the femtosecond laser

Table 5 True Benefits comparing Excimer laser versus Femtosecond laser trephination without liquid interface—Practical Considerations (+++ = very favorable, − − − = very unfavorable)

	Excimer	Femto
"Cumbersome procedure"	+	− −
Centration	+ + +	+
Avoid deformation and compression of tissue during trephination	+ + +	− − −
High IOP during laser action	+ + +	−
Minimizing amount of completion of incision by scissors	(+)	+ +
Location of first 8 cardinal sutures unequivocally given	+ + +	+ +
Stable anterior chamber during suturing	+ +	+ + +
Feasibility of double running suture	+ + +	+ + +
No need for additional single sutures	+ + +	+
Feasibility of trephination with instable cornea	+ + +	− − −
Feasibility of trephination in repeat keratoplasty	+ + +	−
Helpful for DALK	+ +	+ +
Immune reactions	+	− −

application for PKP without liquid interface must be called "**the excitement of yesterday**".

6 Conclusion

Today, the expectations with regard to the results after PKP are limited not only to the achievement of a clear graft. The major criterion that matters to the patient is good visual acuity, preferably without contact lenses, but with a well-tolerated pair of spectacles. For this reason, transplant microsurgeons should not only respect all options for preventing high or irregular astigmatism after keratoplasty. Due to the fact that it is never possible to foresee the refractive outcome in an individual patient after keratoplasty, surgeons should also be familiar with the surgical procedures for correcting refraction errors after PKP (especially in high astigmatism) in order to achieve the best individual result for the patient.

References

1. Zirm E. A successful total keratoplasty. Graefes Arch Clin Exp Ophthalmol. 1906;64:580–93.
2. Flockerzi E, Maier P, Böhringer D, Reinshagen H, Kruse F, Cursiefen C, Reinhard T, Geerling G, Torun N, Seitz B, all German Keratoplasty Registry Contributors. Trends in corneal transplantation from 2001 to 2016 in Germany–A report of the Section DOG-Cornea and its Keratoplasty Registry. Am J Ophthalmol. 2018;188:91–8.
3. Flockerzi E, Turner C, Seitz B, GeKeR Study Group Collaborators: Descemet's Membrane Endothelial Keratoplasty is the predominant keratoplasty procedure in Germany since 2016: A report of the DOG-Section Cornea and its Keratoplasty Registry. Br J Ophthalmol. 2024; 108:646–653.
4. Seitz B, Langenbucher A, Diamantis A, Cursiefen C, Küchle M, Naumann GOH. Immunological graft reactions after penetrating keratoplasty-a prospective randomized trial comparing corneal excimer laser and motor trephination. Klin Monbl Augenheilkd. 2001A;218:710–9.
5. Nguyen NX, Seitz B, Martus P, Langenbucher A, Cursiefen C. Long-term topical steroid treatment improves graft survival following normal-risk penetrating keratoplasty. Am J Ophthalmol. 2007;144:318–9.
6. Szentmáry N, Goebels S, El-Husseiny M, Langenbucher A, Seitz B. Immune reactions following excimer laser and femtosecond laser-assisted penetrating keratoplasty. Klin Monbl Augenheilkd. 2013;230:486–9.
7. Seitz B, Langenbucher A, Nguyen NX, Küchle M, Naumann GOH. Long-term follow-up of intraocular pressure after penetrating keratoplasty for keratoconus and Fuchs' dystrophy: comparison of mechanical and Excimer laser trephination. Cornea. 2002;21:368–73.
8. Seitz B, Szentmáry N, El-Husseiny M, Viestenz A, Langenbucher A, Naumann GOH. The penetrating keratoplasty (PKP)–A century of success. In: Hjortdal J, editor. Corneal transplantation. Springer International Publishing Switzerland; 2016. p. 67–92.
9. Wykrota AA, Weinstein I, Hamon L, Daas L, Flockerzi E, Suffo S, Seitz B. Approval rates for corneal donation and the origin of donor tissue for transplantation at a university based tertiary referral center with corneal subspecialisation hosting a LIONS Eye Bank. BMC Ophthalmol. 2022;22(1): 17.
10. Seitz B, Asi F, Mäurer S, Hamon L, Quintin A, Langenbucher A. Anterior Segment OCT: Application to improve graft selection for corneal transplantation. In: Alío J, Alío del Barrio JL: Atlas of anterior segment optical coherence tomography (Series: Essentials in Ophthalmology), Springer Nature Switzerland AG;2021. p 223–6.
11. Quintin A, Hamon L, Mäurer S, Langenbucher A, Seitz B. Vergleich der sterilen Spendertomographie in der Hornhautbank mit der Tomographie des Transplantates nach perforierender Keratoplastik. Ophthalmologe. 2021;118:1038–44.
12. Safi T, Daas L, Alexandersson J, Ndiaye A, Deru M, Seitz B. Semi-quantitative criteria in the eye bank that correlate with cornea guttata in donor corneas. Klin Monbl Augenheilkd. 2021;238:680–7.
13. Schmitz LM, Safi T, Munteanu C, Seitz B, Daas L. Prevalence and severity of cornea guttata in the graft following Descemet Membrane Endothelial Keratoplasty (DMEK). Acta Ophthalmol. 2022;100:e1737–45.
14. Schönit S, Maamri A, Zemova E, Munteanu C, Safi T, Daas L, Seitz B. Prevalence and impact of corneal guttata in the graft following penetrating keratoplasty. Cornea. 2022;41:1495–502.
15. Mäurer S, Asi F, Rawer A, Damian A, Seitz B, Langenbucher A, Eppig T. Concept for 3D measurement of corneal donor tissue using a clinical OCT. Ophthalmologe. 2019;116(7):640–6.
16. Mäurer S, Seitz B, Langenbucher A. „Harmonization" of donor and recipient tomography in corneal transplantation. Z Med Phys. 2021;31:73–7.
17. Fiorentzis M, Viestenz AR, Viestenz AN, Seitz B. Intracameral dexamethason injection as adjuvant therapy in endothelial immune reaction after penetrating and posterior lamellar keratoplasty: a retrospective clinical observation. Adv Ther. 2017;34:1928–35.
18. Seitz B, Langenbucher A, Naumann GOH. Astigmatismus bei Keratoplastik. In: Seiler T, editor. Refraktive Chirurgie. Stuttgart: Enke-Verlag; 2000. p. 197–252.
19. Seitz B, Langenbucher A, Küchle M, Naumann GOH. Impact of graft diameter on corneal power and the regularity of post-keratoplasty astigmatism before and after suture removal. Ophthalmology. 2003;110:2162–7.
20. Langenbucher A, Seitz B, Kus MM, Vilchis E, Naumann GOH. Regularity of corneal topography after penetrating keratoplasty-comparison between nonmechanical (excimer laser 193 nm) and mechanical trephination. Klin Monbl Augenheilkd. 1996;208:450–8.
21. Hoppenreijs VPT, Van Rij G, Beekhuis WH, Rijneveld WJ, Rinkel-Van DE. Causes of high astigmatism after penetrating keratoplasty. Doc Ophthalmol. 1993;85:21–34.
22. Naumann GOH, Sautter H. Surgical procedures on the cornea. In: Blodi FC, Mackensen G, Neubauer H, editors. Surgical ophthalmology, vol. 1. Berlin, Heidelberg, New York, Tokio, Springer;1991. S. 433–97.
23. Olson RJ. Modulation of postkeratoplasty astigmatism by surgical and suturing techniques. Int Ophthalmol Clinics. 1983;23:137–51.
24. Van Rij G, Cornell FM, Waring GO III, Wilson LA, Beekhuis H. Postoperative astigmatism after central vs eccentric penetrating keratoplasties. Am J Ophthalmol. 1985;99:317–20.
25. Van Rij G, Waring GO III. Configuration of corneal trephine opening using five different trephines in human donor eyes. Arch Ophthalmol. 1988;106:1228–33.
26. Naumann GOH. Part II: Corneal transplantation in anterior segment diseases. The Bowman Lecture (Number 56) 1994. Eye 1995;9:395–421.
27. Filatov V, Alexandrakis G, Talamo JH, Steinert RF. Comparison of suture-in and suture-out postkeratoplasty astigmatism with single running suture or combined running and interrupted sutures. Am J Ophthalmol. 1996;122:696–700.
28. Mader TH, Yuan R, Lynn MJ, Stulting RD, Wilson LA, Waring GO II. Change in keratometric astigmatism after suture removal

more than one year after penetrating keratoplasty. Ophthalmology. 1993;100:119–27.
29. Perl T, Charlton KH, Binder PS. Disparate diameter grafting. Astigmatism, intraocular pressure and visual acuity. Ophthalmology 1981;88:774–80.
30. Cohen KL, Tripoli NK, Pellom AC, Kupper LL, Fryczkowski AW. Effect of tissue fit on corneal shape after transplantation. Invest Ophthalmol Vis Sci. 1984;25:1226–31.
31. Cohen KL, Holman RE, Tripoli NK, Kupper LL. Effect of trephine tilt on corneal button dimensions. Am J Ophthalmol. 1986;101:722–5.
32. Seitz B, Hager T, Langenbucher A, Naumann GOH. Reconsidering sequential double running suture removal after penetrating keratoplasty–a prospective randomized study comparing excimer laser and motor trephination. Cornea. 2018;37:301–6.
33. Seitz B, Langenbucher A, Naumann GOH. The penetrating keratoplasty–A 100-year success story. Ophthalmologe 2005;102:11281139.
34. Seitz B, Langenbucher A, Naumann GOH. Trephination in penetrating keratoplasty. In: Reinhard T, Larkin F, editors. Essentials in ophthalmology-corneal and external eye disease. Berlin: Springer; 2006. p. 123–52.
35. Seitz B, Langenbucher A, Kus MM, Küchle M, Naumann GOH. Nonmechanical corneal trephination with the excimer laser improves outcome after penetrating keratoplasty. Ophthalmology. 1999;106:1156–65.
36. Seitz B, Langenbucher A, Meiller R, Kus MM. Decentration of donor cornea in mechanical and excimer laser trephination for penetrating keratoplasty. Klin Monbl Augenheilkd. 2000;217:144–51.
37. Seitz B, Langenbucher A, Naumann GOH. Perspectives of excimer laser-assisted keratoplasty. Ophthalmologe. 2011;108:817–24.
38. Seitz B, Behrens A, Langenbucher A, Kus MM, Naumann GOH. Experimental 193-nm excimer laser trephination with divergent cut angles in penetrating keratoplasty. Cornea. 1998;17:410–6.
39. Seitz B, El-Husseiny M, Langenbucher A, Szentmáry N. Prophylaxis and management of complications in penetrating keratoplasty. Ophthalmologe. 2013;110:605–13.
40. Fiorentzis M, Morinello E, Viestenz AN, Zuche H, Seitz B, Viestenz AN. Muscle relaxants as risk factor for vis-a-tergo during penetrating keratoplasty: a prospective interventional study. Adv Ther. 2017B;34:2674–9.
41. Morinello E, Wittmann D, Hager T, Seitz B, Volk T, Schneider SO. Anaesthesia influences vis a tergo in corneal transplantations. Anästh Intensivmed. 2018;59:632–9.
42. Urrets-Zavalia A. Fixed dilated pupil, iris atrophy and secondary glaucoma. A distinct clinical entity following penetrating keratoplasty for keratoconus. Am J Ophthalmol. 1963;56:257–65.
43. Belmont SC, Troutman RC, Buzard KA. Control of astigmatism aided by intraoperative keratometry. Cornea. 1993;12:397–400.
44. Seitz B, Langenbucher A, Zagrada D, Budde W, Kus MM. Corneal dimensions in various types of corneal dystrophies and their effect on penetrating keratoplasty. Klin Monbl Augenheilkd. 2000C;217:152–8.
45. Langenbucher A, Seitz B, Nguyen NX, Naumann GOH. Graft endothelial cell loss after nonmechanical penetrating keratoplasty depends on diagnosis: a regression analysis. Graefes Arch Clin Exp Ophthalmol. 2002;240:387–92.
46. Seitz B, Langenbucher A, Nguyen NX, Kus MM, Küchle M, Naumann GOH. Graft endothelium and thickness after penetrating keratoplasty, comparing mechanical and excimer laser trephination-a prospective randomised study. Graefes Arch Clin Exp Ophthalmol. 2001;239:12–7.
47. Graef S, Maier P, Boehringer D, Auw-Haedrich C, Reinhard T. Femtosecond laser-assisted repeat keratoplasty: a case series. Cornea. 2011;30:687–91.
48. Szentmáry N, Seitz B, Langenbucher A, Naumann GOH. Repeat keratoplasty for correction of high or irregular postkeratoplasty astigmatism in clear corneal grafts. Am J Ophthalmol. 2005;139: 826830.
49. Alfaro Rangel R, Szentmáry N, Lepper S, Langenbucher A, Seitz B. 8.5/8.6-mm excimer laser assisted penetrating keratoplasties in a tertiary corneal subspecialty referral center–Indications and outcomes in 107 eyes. Cornea 2020;39:806–11.
50. Javadi MA, Mohammadi MJ, Mirdehghan SA, Sajjadi SH. A comparison between donor-recipient corneal size and its effect on the ultimate refractive error induced in keratoconus. Cornea. 1993;12:401–5.
51. Hoffmann F. Suture technique for perforating keratoplasty. Klin Monbl Augenheilkd 1976;169, 584–90.
52. Langenbucher A, Seitz B, Kus MM, Vilchis E, Naumann GOH. Graft decentration in penetrating keratoplasty-Nonmechanical trephination with the excimer laser (193 nm) versus the motor trephine. Ophthalmic Surg Lasers. 1998A;29:106–13.
53. Langenbucher A, Kus MM, Neumann J, Seitz B. Calculating the localization and dimension of the real pupil in keratoconus with ray tracing of corneal topography data. Klin Monbl Augenheilkd. 1999;215:163–8.
54. Liu Y, Seitz B, Langenbucher A, Nguyen NX, Naumann GOH. Impact of preoperative corneal curvature on the outcome of penetrating keratoplasty in keratoconus. Cornea. 2003;22:409–12.
55. Kaufman HE. Astigmatism after keratoplasty–possible cause and method of prevention. Am J Ophthalmol. 1982;94:556–7.
56. Jonas JB, Budde WM. Loosening of single versus double running sutures in penetrating keratoplasty for keratoconus. Graefes Arch Clin Exp Ophthalmol. 1999;237:522–3.
57. Suffo S, Daas L, Seitz B. The Homburg Cross-Stitch Marker for double-running sutures in penetrating keratoplasty. Klin Monbl Augenheilkd. 2021;238:808–14.
58. Suffo S, El Halabi M, Seitz B, Abdin AD, Munteanu C, Daas L. Penetrating excimer laser keratoplasty with vs without the Homburg Cross-Stitch Marker in inexperienced surgeons. Clin Ophthalmol. 2021;15:4607–14.
59. Langenbucher A, Seitz B, Kus MM, Naumann GOH. Transplant vertical tilt after perforating keratoplasty–comparison between non-mechanical trephination with excimer laser and motor trephination. Klin Monbl Augenheilkd. 1998B;212:129–40.
60. Naumann GOH, Seitz B, Lang GK, Langenbucher A, Kus MM. 193 excimer laser trepanation in perforating keratoplasty. Report of 70 patients. Klin Monbl Augenheilkd. 1993;203:252–61.
61. Lang GK, Schröder E, Koch JW, Yanoff M, Naumann GOH. Excimer laser keratoplasty. Part 2: Elliptical keratoplasty. Ophthalmic Surg. 1989;20:342–46.
62. Lang GK, Naumann GOH, Koch JW. A new elliptical excision for corneal transplantation using an excimer laser. Arch Ophthalmol. 1990;108:914–5.
63. Szentmáry N, Langenbucher A, Kus MM, Naumann GOH, Seitz B. Elliptical nonmechanical corneal trephination: intraoperative complications and long-term outcome of 42 consecutive excimer laser penetrating keratoplasties. Cornea. 2007A;26:414–20.
64. Szentmáry N, Langenbucher A, Kus MM, Naumann GOH, Seitz B. Long-term refractive results of elliptical excimer laser penetrating keratoplasty (EELPK). Curr Eye Res. 2007B;32:953–9.
65. Küchle M, Seitz B, Langenbucher A, Naumann GOH. Nonmechanical excimer laser penetrating keratoplasty for perforated or predescemetal corneal ulcers. Ophthalmology. 1999;106:2203–9.
66. Seitz B, Daas L, Milioti G, Szentmáry N, Langenbucher A, Suffo S. Excimer laser-assisted penetrating keratoplasty: on 1 July 2019 excimer laser penetrating keratoplasty celebrates its 30th anniversary. Video article. Ophthalmologe. 2019;116:1221–30.
67. Pluzsik ML, Seitz B, Flockerzi F, Langenbucher A, Tóth G, Bohle RM, Szentmáry N. Changing trends in penetrating keratoplasty indications in Homburg/Saar between 2011 and

2018–histopathology of 2123 corneal buttons in a single center in Germany. Curr Eye Res. 2020;45:1199–204.
68. Behrens A, Seitz B, Küchle M, Langenbucher A, Kus MM, Rummelt C, Naumann GOH. „Orientation teeth" in nonmechanical laser corneal trephination: 2.94-microm Er:YAG laser vs. 193-nm ArF excimer laser. Br J Ophthalmol. 1999;83:1008–12.
69. Szentmàry N, Langenbucher A, Naumann GOH, Seitz B. Intraindividual variability of penetrating keratoplasty outcome after excimer laser versus motorized corneal trephination. J Refract Surg. 2006;22:804–10.
70. Seitz B, Langenbucher A, Fischer S, Kus MM, Vilchis E, Naumann GOH. The regularity of laser keratectomy depth in nonmechanical trephination for penetrating keratoplasty. Ophthalmic Surg Lasers. 1998;29:33–42.
71. Küchle M, Nguyen NX, Seitz B, Langenbucher A, Naumann GOH. Blood-aqueous barrier after mechanical or nonmechanical excimer laser trephination in penetrating keratoplasty. Am J Ophthalmol. 1998;125:177–81.
72. Behrens A, Seitz B, Langenbucher A, Kus MM, Küchle M, Naumann GOH. Lens opacities after nonmechanical vs. mechanical corneal trephination for penetrating keratoplasty in keratoconus. J Cataract Refract Surg. 2000;26:1605–11.
73. Seitz B, Brünner H, Viestenz A, Hofmann-Rummelt C, Schlötzer-Schrehardt U, Naumann GOH, Langenbucher A. Inverse mushroom-shaped nonmechanical penetrating keratoplasty using a femtosecondlaser. Am J Ophthalmol. 2005;139:941–4.
74. Bahar I, Kaiserman I, Lange AP, Levinger E, Sansanayudh W, Singal N, Slomovic AR, Rootman DS. Femtosecond laser versus manual dissection for top hat penetrating keratoplasty. Br J Ophthalmol. 2009;93:73–8.
75. Gaster RN, Dumitrascu O, Rabinowitz YS. Penetrating keratoplasty using femtosecond laser-enabled keratoplasty with zig-zag incisions versus a mechanical trephine in patients with keratoconus. Br J Ophthalmol. 2012;96:1195–9.
76. Vetter JM, Holzer MP, Teping C, Weingärtner WE, Gericke A, Stoffelns B, Pfeiffer N, Sekundo W. Intraocular pressure during corneal flap preparation: comparison among four femtosecond lasers in porcine eyes. J Refract Surg. 2011;27:427–33.
77. Farid M, Steiner RF, Gaster RN, Chamberlain W, Lin A. Comparison of penetrating keratoplasty performed with the femtosecond laser zig-zag incision versus conventional blade trephination. Ophthalmology. 2009;116:1638–43.
78. Kamiya K, Kobashi H, Shimizu K, Igarashi A. Clinical outcomes of penetrating keratoplasty performed with the VisuMax femtosecond laser system and comparison with conventional penetrating keratoplasty. PLoS ONE. 2014;5(9): e105464.
79. Levinger E, Trivizki O, Levinger S, Kremer I. Outcome of "mushroom" pattern femtosecond laser-assisted keratoplasty versus conventional penetrating keratoplasty in patients with keratoconus. Cornea. 2014;33:481–5.
80. Birnbaum F, Wiggermann A, Maier PC, Böhringer D, Reinhard T. Clinical results of 123 femtosecond laser-assisted keratoplasties. Graefes Arch Clin Exp Ophthalmol. 2013;251:95–103.
81. Chamberlain WD, Rush SW, Mathers WD, Cabezas M, Fraunfelder FW. Comparison of femtosecond laser-assisted keratoplasty versus conventional penetrating keratoplasty. Ophthalmology. 2011;118:486–91.
82. El-Husseiny M, Seitz B, Langenbucher A, Akhmedova E, Szentmáry N, Hager T, Tsintarakis T, Janunts E. Excimer versus femtosecond laser assisted penetrating keratoplasty in keratoconus and Fuchs dystrophy: intraoperative pitfalls. J Ophthalmol. 2015;2015: 645830.
83. Tóth G, Szentmáry N, Langenbucher A, Akhmedova E, El-Husseiny M, Seitz B. Comparison of excimer laser versus femtosecond laser assisted trephination in penetrating keratoplasty. Adv Ther. 2019;36:3471–82.
84. Resch MD, Zemova E, Marsovszky L, Szentmáry N, Bauer F, Daas L, Pattmöller M, El-Husseiny M, Németh J, Nagy ZZ, Seitz B. In vivo confocal microscopic imaging of the cornea after femtosecond and excimer laser assisted penetrating keratoplasty. J Refract Surg. 2015;31:620–6.
85. Tóth G, Butskhrikidze T, Seitz B, Langenbucher A, Hager T, Akhmedova E, El-Husseiny M, Szentmáry N. Endothelial cell density and corneal graft thickness following excimer laser vs. femtosecond laser-assisted penetrating keratoplasty. Graefes Arch Clin Exp Ophthalmol 2019;257:975–81.

Excimer Laser-Assisted Deep Anterior Lamellar Keratoplasty "Excimer-DALK"

Loay Daas, Wissam Aljundi, Shady Suffo, and Berthold Seitz

Abstract

The concept of excimer laser-assisted DALK (Excimer-DALK) has been developed at the Department of Ophthalmology of Saarland University Medical Center and consists of an excimer laser-assisted trephination of 80% of the midperipheral corneal thickness measured with anterior segment optical coherence tomography (AS-OCT).

Keywords

Excimer laser-assisted DALK · Indication · Technique · Naked Descemet

1 Excimer Laser-Assisted Deep Anterior Lamellar Keratoplasty "Excimer-DALK"

In recent years, an increase in lamellar procedures in corneal surgery has been observed, especially in posterior lamellar keratoplasty ("Descemet membrane endothelial keratoplasty" [DMEK]). According to the German Keratoplasty Registry [1], 3.0% of all 9042 corneal transplants in 2020 in Germany were performed as deep anterior lamellar keratoplasty (DALK). This low percentage may be explained by a currently missing standardized surgical technique to perform DALK.

Especially young patients with advanced keratoconus who also suffer from atopic eczema and cannot be treated with a rigid, gas permeable contact lens, riboflavin-ultraviolet-A crosslinking (CXL) or implantation of intracorneal ring segments (ICRS) profit from this method. Prerequisites for performing DALK include an intact corneal endothelium with sufficient endothelial cell density, and an intact Descemet membrane (DALK is not an option after corneal hydrops) [2–4]. DALK is contraindicated in endothelial corneal dystrophies and any form of herpetic keratitis—due to the possible reactivation of herpes in the patient's own endothelium [5].

The concept of excimer laser-assisted DALK (exc-DALK) is developed at the Department of Ophthalmology of Saarland University Medical Center and consists of an excimer laser-assisted trephination of 80% of the midperipheral corneal thickness measured with anterior segment optical coherence tomography (AS-OCT).

All authors certify that they have no affiliation or interest in any organization or entity that has a financial or non-financial interest in the topics or materials covered in this chapter.

No funding or support was received for this contribution.

L. Daas (✉) · W. Aljundi · S. Suffo · B. Seitz
Department of Ophthalmology, Saarland University Medical Center, Homburg, Germany
e-mail: loay.daas@uks.eu

B. Seitz et al. (eds.), *Atlas on Cornea*, https://doi.org/10.1007/978-3-031-65422-0_50

2 Surgical Technique

The steps of a standardized excimer laser-assisted DALK procedure [6] are as follows:

1. *Donor*: In equivalence to excimer laser-assisted penetrating keratoplasty (Excimer PKP): Using excimer laser with mask, a complete trephination of the donor cornea with "orientation teeth" is performed [7].
2. Recipient cornea: An excimer laser trephination of the recipient with congruent "notches" to 80% of midperipheral corneal thickness at the trephination site is performed. The corneal thickness is measured by anterior segment optical coherence tomography (AS-OCT). A successful manual excision of this superficial stromal lamella is followed by intrastromal air injection using a 30-gauge needle according to the "big bubble" technique described by Anwar et al. [8]. After performing the "big bubble", a paracentesis is performed and air is injected into the anterior chamber. The formation of a kidney-shaped intracameral air bubble indicates the successful separation of the deep stromal tissue and Descemet membrane, without perforation. After puncture and deflation of the "big bubble", the intracameral air bubble moves toward the center. If complete exposure of Descemet membrane ("naked Descemet") is successful, the surgical procedure can be continued as DALK. Otherwise, a "conversion" to excimer-PKP with full graft is mandatory.
3. Donor lamella: The donor cornea is fixed without Descemet membrane ("anterior donor lamella") using two continuous sutures according to Hoffmann [9] (Fig. 1).
4. At the end of surgery, an air/gas bubble (approximately 80%) is routinely injected into the anterior chamber to ensure attachment of the patient's own Descemet membrane to the donor lamella. This avoids the development of a so-called "double anterior chamber". To prevent a postoperative rise of intraocular pressure ("air block"), a Nd:YAG laser iridotomy at the 6 o'clock position should be routinely created preoperatively in analogy to the procedure prior to performing DMEK [10, 11].

In a review paper, the American Academy of Ophthalmology (AAO) evaluated DALK to be equivalent to PKP in terms of postoperative visual acuity outcomes [12]. Endothelial cell loss after successful DALK (without intraoperative perforation of the Descemet membrane) (12 months postoperatively: $-12.9\% \pm 17.6\%$) is lower than after PKP ($-27.7\% \pm 11.1\%$) [13]. Endothelial immune reaction of the graft is rarely observed after DALK [14]. Another significant advantage over PKP is that the globe remains intact and is not unroofed as in PKP.

The intraoperative conversion rate to PKP is at least 16.2%. Therefore, a detailed informed consent for both surgeries is absolutely necessary [15]. However, the conversion rate decreases with the expertise of the surgeon.

The excimer laser-assisted technique allows to combine the advantages of DALK (fast visual recovery and less immune reaction) and excimer laser trephination (optimal visual recovery with low postoperative astigmatism) with a low intraoperative perforation rate. Moreover, Excimer-DALK does not result in any disadvantages for the patient in case of conversion to Excimer-PKP.

In our opinion, Excimer-DALK contributes to a certain standardization of deep anterior lamellar keratoplasty.

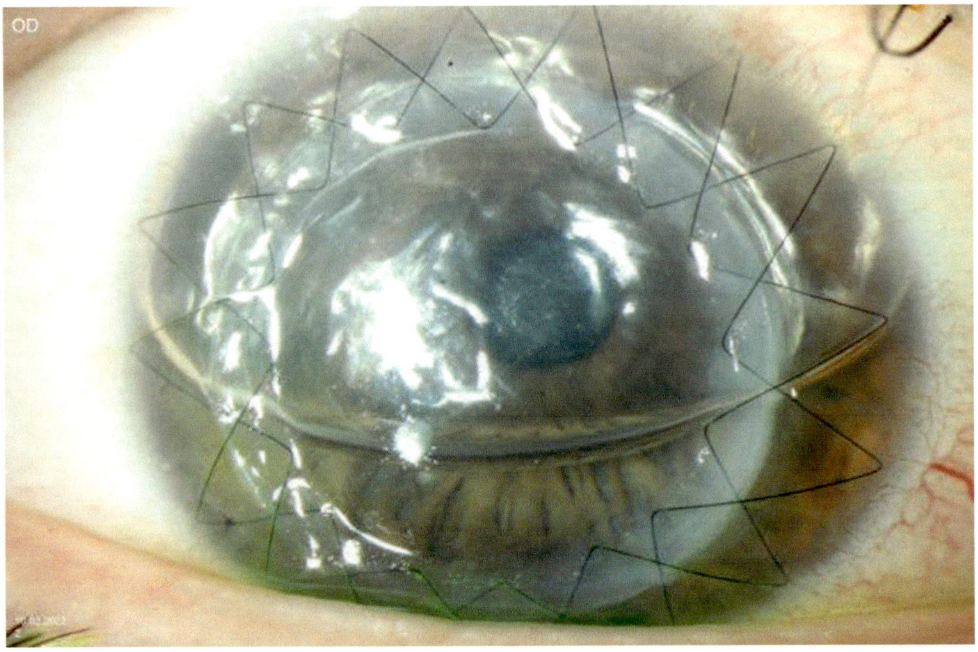

Fig. 1 Slit lamp biomicroscopy photography: 1 day after excimer laser-assisted DALK

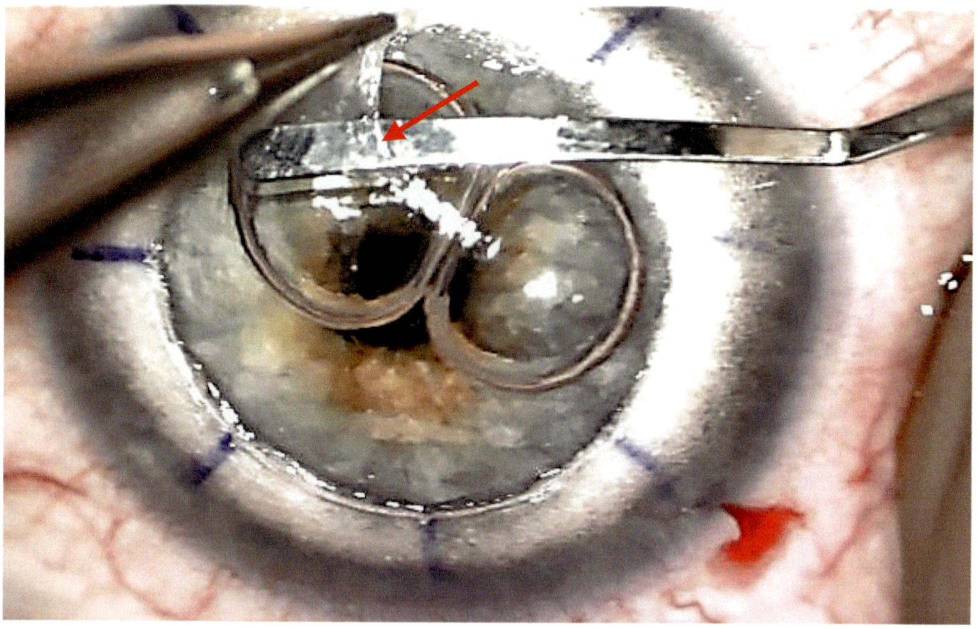

Fig. 2 Intraoperative imaging: complete exposure of Descemet membrane in excimer laser-assisted DALK after successful "big bubble" dissection followed by manual excision of the superficial stromal lamina, but prior to excision of the predescemetal stromal lamina (arrow)

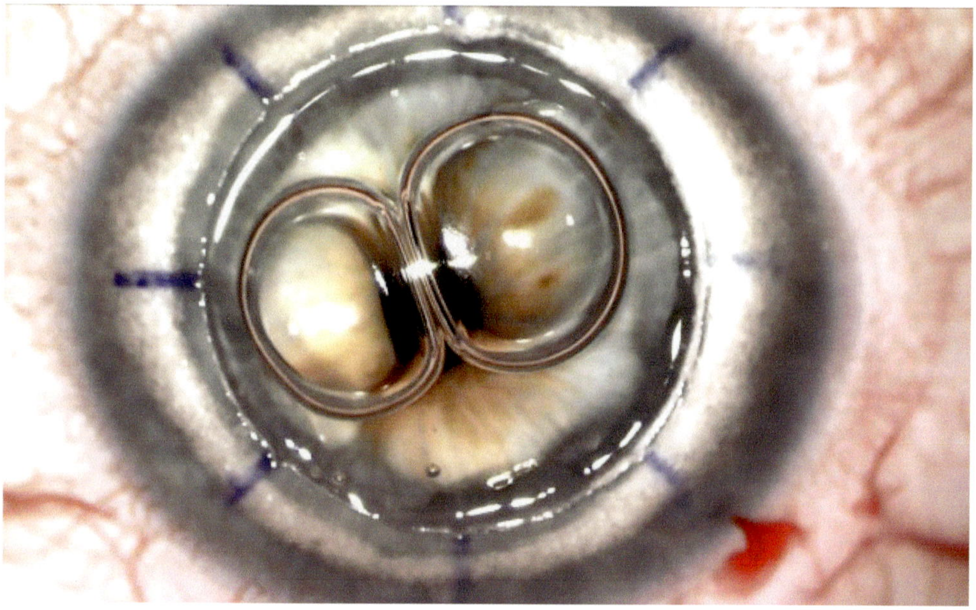

Fig. 3 Intraoperative imaging: complete exposure of Descemet membrane (so-called "naked Descemet") in excimer laser-assisted DALK with successful excision of the predescemetal stromal lamella and crystal clear view into the closed anterior chamber

Furthermore, the "big bubble" represents a safe and more controlled technique to finalize tissue dissection after excision of about 80% of the superficial stromal lamella, especially in absence of an intraoperative AS-OCT. Complete exposure of the Descemet membrane, so-called "naked Descemet" with excision of the predescemetal stromal lamella [16], is an important prognostic factor with regard to postoperative visual acuity outcome (Fig. 2 and 3). If the residual thickness of the recipient bed is less than 80 µm and homogeneous in its thickness, the visual results are shown to be satisfactory. However, postoperative visual acuity development takes longer and may last between 2–5 years according to other studies [17].

3 Conclusion

- The recipient endothelium must be intact for DALK to be an option.
- Contraindications for DALK are acute corneal hydrops, any form of herpetic keratitis or endothelial corneal dystrophy.

- The surgeon should aim for a complete exposure of the Descemet membrane (so-called “naked Descemet”) to achieve best postoperative visual acuity results [18].

References

1. Flockerzi E, Maier P, Böhringer D, Reinshagen H, Kruse F, Cursiefen C, Reinhard T, Geerling G, Torun N, Seitz B. Trends in corneal transplantation from 2001 to 2016 in germany: a report of the DOG-Section cornea and its keratoplasty registry. Am J Ophthalmol. 2018;188:91–8.
2. Seitz B, Cursiefen C, El Husseiny M, Viestenz A, Langenbucher A, Szentmary N. DALK and penetrating laser keratoplasty for advanced keratoconus. Ophthalmologe. 2013;110:839–48.
3. Cursiefen C, Schaub F, Bachmann B. Update: Deep anterior lamellar keratoplasty (DALK) for keratoconus. Ophthalmologe. 2016;113:204–12.
4. Schaub F, Heindl LM, Enders P, Roters S, Bachmann BO, Cursiefen C. Deep anterior lamellar keratoplasty. Experiences and results of the first 100 consecutive DALK from the university eye hospital of cologne. Opthalmology. 2017; 114:1019–26
5. Holbach LM, Asano N, Naumann GO. Infection of the corneal endothelium in herpes simplex keratitis. Am J Ophthalmol. 1998;26:592–4.
6. Daas L, Hamon L, Ardjomand N, Safi T, Seitz B. Excimer laser-assisted DALK: a case report from the Homburg Keratoconus Center (HKC). Ophthalmologe. 2021;118:1245–8.
7. Seitz B, Daas L, Milioti G, Szentmáry N, Langenbucher A, Suffo S. Excimer laser-assisted penetrating keratoplasty: On 1 July 2019 excimer laser penetrating keratoplasty celebrates its 30th anniversary. Ophthalmologe. 2019;116:1221–30.
8. Anwar M, Teichmann KD. Big-bubble technique to bare Descemet’s membrane in anterior lamellar keratoplasty. J Cataract Refract Surg. 2002;28:398–403.
9. Hoffmann F. Suture technique for perforating keratoplasty. Klin Monbl Augenheilkd. 1976; 169:584–90
10. Cursiefen C, Heindl L.M. Perspectives of deep anterior lamellar keratoplasty. Ophthalmologe. 2011; 108:833–9
11. Seitz B, Daas L, Flockerzi E, Suffo S. Descemet membrane endothelial keratoplasty DMEK-Donor and recipient step by step. Ophthalmologe. 2020;117:811–28.
12. Reinhart WJ, Musch DC, Jacobs DS, Lee WB, Kaufman SC, Shtein RM. Deep anterior lamellar keratoplasty as an alternative to penetrating keratoplasty: a report by the American Academy of Ophthalmology. Ophthalmology. 2011;118:209–18.
13. Cheng YYY, Visser N, Schouten JS, Wijdh RJ, Pels E, Cleynenbreugel H, Eggink CA, Zaal MJW, Rijneveld WJ, Nuijts RMMA. Endothelial cell loss and visual outcome of deep anterior lamellar keratoplasty versus penetrating keratoplasty: a randomized multicenter clinical trial. Ophthalmology. 2011;118:302–9.
14. Hos D, Matthaei M, Bock F, Maruyama K, Notara M, Clahsen T, Hou Y, Le VNH, Salabarria AC, Horstmann J, Bachmann BO, Cursiefen C. Immune reactions after modern lamellar (DALK, DSAEK, DMEK) versus conventional penetrating corneal transplantation. Prog Retin Eye Res. 2019;73: 100768.
15. Myerscough J, Friehmann A, Bovone C, Mimouni M, Busin M. Evaluation of the risk factors associated with conversion of intended deep anterior lamellar keratoplasty to penetrating keratoplasty. Br J Ophthalmol. 2020;104:764–7.
16. Dua HS, Faraj LA, Said DG, Gray T, Lowe J. Human corneal anatomy redefined: a novel pre-Descemet’s layer (Dua’s layer). Ophthalmology. 2013;120:1778–85.
17. Sarnicola E, Sarnicola C, Cheung AY, Holland EJ, Sarnicola V. Surgical corneal anatomy in deep anterior lamellar keratoplasty: suggestion of new acronyms. Cornea. 2019;38:515–22.
18. Daas L, Aljundi W, Abdin AD, Munteanu C, Seitz B. Excimer Laser-Assisted Deep Anterior Lamellar Keratoplasty Versus Penetrating Keratoplasty for Patients With Keratoconus: A Retrospective Analysis From the Homburg Keratoconus Center. Cornea. 2025;44:291–299.

Descemet Membrane Endothelial Keratoplasty DMEK

Berthold Seitz, Elias Flockerzi, Shady Suffo, and Loay Daas

Abstract

Descemet membrane endothelial keratoplasty (DMEK) has become the gold standard in Germany for the treatment of corneal endothelial diseases; however, the widespread use of DMEK was initially limited due to problems with donor preparation and the difficulty of correctly and gently unfolding the endothelial Descemet membrane (EDM) in the anterior chamber. This chapter describes the appropriate donor selection followed by the safe donor preparation of the cornea without tearing or even rupturing the EDM, including the indispensable peripheral semicircular orientation marking. Also presented is a step-by-step atraumatic loading of the glass cartridge, the introduction of the EDM roll into the anterior chamber, and its safe step-by-step unfolding based on (1) the sequential use of jets of fluid, (2) repeated tapping on the peripheral/central cornea, (3) controlled flattening of the anterior chamber, (4) use of air bubbles of defined size and finally, the fixation of the EDM in correct orientation to the back of the host cornea with a gas bubble. Since every wrong step with DMEK can have far-reaching consequences for patient and surgeon, this step-by-step pragmatic approach should minimize the incidence of donor tissue damage and failure in patient maneuvers.

Keywords

Posterior lamellar keratoplasty · Donor preparation · Patient maneuvers · Endothelial pathology · Endothelial corneal diseases · DMEK

Supplementary Information The online version contains supplementary material available at https://doi.org/10.1007/978-3-031-65422-0_51.

B. Seitz (✉) · E. Flockerzi · S. Suffo · L. Daas
Department of Ophthalmology, Saarland University Medical Center, Homburg/Saar, Germany
e-mail: berthold.seitz@uks.eu

1 Introduction

After its first description by Gerit Melles from Rotterdam in 2006 [1], DMEK ("Descemet membrane endothelial keratoplasty") has experienced a well-deserved, rapid increase in Germany, particularly in the last 15 years [2–5]. Since the year 2016, DMEK is the predominant keratoplasty procedure in Germany according to a report of the keratoplasty registry of the DOG-section cornea. 99.1% of all posterior lamellar keratoplasties were DMEKs in Germany in 2023 [6]. Overall, Fuchs endothelial dystrophy has become by far the main diagnosis for corneal transplantation in Germany, accounting for around 45% of all keratoplasty cases [7–9].

Although the DMEK method in skilled hands provides morphologic and functional results of unprecedented quality in corneal transplant surgery [10], the widespread use of this minimally invasive method was initially limited due to problems with donor preparation and difficulties with patient maneuvers. Despite the initial descriptions of DMEK pioneers [1, 11–13] suggesting that donor tissue preparation and manipulation in the anterior chamber could be performed routinely, any rupture of the endothelial Descemet membrane (EDM) during attempted preparation results in graft loss with sometimes serious disruption of the organizational procedure. In addition, prolonged and unskillful manipulation of the EDM in the anterior chamber can lead to significant endothelial loss with potential primary or (early) secondary graft failure [14].

The aim of this chapter is to describe DMEK step-by-step from indication and surgical planning to donor preparation, intraoperative manipulation of the graft in the patient and early/late follow-up care [15–17].

B. Seitz et al. (eds.), *Atlas on Cornea*, https://doi.org/10.1007/978-3-031-65422-0_51

2 Indications for DMEK

In principle, indications for posterior lamellar keratoplasty include all diseases of the endothelium with stromal edema, but without permanent stromal scarring (e.g. Fuchs endothelial dystrophy [18], posterior polymorphous dystrophy [19], pseudophakic bullous keratopathy, pseudoexfoliative (PEX) keratopathy, endothelial degeneration of viral etiology [20, 21], endothelial decompensation in Haab's striae in buphthalmus [22] or after forceps delivery (Fig. 1). However, DMEK is also a potential option for the management of secondary graft failure after PKP [23–29] as patients benefit from much faster visual rehabilitation compared to re-PKP and a significantly lower immune response rate. Last but not least, in the hands of particularly experienced DMEK surgeons, "complex diseases" of the anterior segment of the eye can also benefit from DMEK (e.g. after trabeculectomy or pressure-reducing shunt surgery, in ICE [iridocorneoendothelial] syndrome with iris defects, sclera- or iris-fixed intraocular lens [IOL], aphakia and post-pars plana vitrectomy) [30–32].

DMEK is not suitable for pre-descemetal stromal scars (e.g. after interstitial keratitis) (Fig. 2), for long-standing corneal endothelial epithelial decompensation (CEED) with persistent stromal scars (Fig. 3) for a graft after PKP with stromal scars (Fig. 4) and/or high irregular astigmatism with which the patient has never had good vision. In this case, well-centered re-PKP with a larger graft diameter—preferably 8.5/8.6 mm diameter excimer laser-assisted—is still the method of first choice [33, 34].

3 Preparing for Surgery

It is currently unclear how best to preserve endothelial cells during and after EDM graft preparation. There are many factors that have an impact on endothelial survival, such as storage conditions prior to surgery, media used during preparation, as well as the timing of preparation in relation to the time of surgery. In contrast to previous reports [11, 35, 36], we decided partly not to prepare the EDM immediately before surgery, but 1 day prior to surgery, whilst preserving the grafts in an organ culture medium without dextran [37–39]. This way, possible organizational problems in the event of unintentional destruction of the donor tissue can be avoided or solved more easily. Fortunately, our Klaus Faber Center for Corneal Diseases incl. LIONS Cornea Bank Saar-Lor-Lux, Trier/Westpfalz, can always provide us with a replacement cornea promptly in the event of "incidents" in the operating theatre [40].

We ask all patients to have a large peripheral YAG laser iridotomy at the 6 o'clock position (not in the upper quadrant or mid-periphery!) performed in our department or alternatively by an ophthalmologist externally a few weeks before DMEK in order to avoid bleeding or pigment dispersion in the event of an iridotomy on the day before surgery or even during the procedure (Fig. 5). On the evening prior to the operation, we check in retroillumination whether the iridotomy is patent and large enough. If this is not the case, we repeat the YAG iridotomy in pilocarpine miosis. If the peripheral cornea is too cloudy, a kind of "Ando-iridectomy" can be carefully created intraoperatively using the 23 gauge vitrectomy cutter (vitrectome).

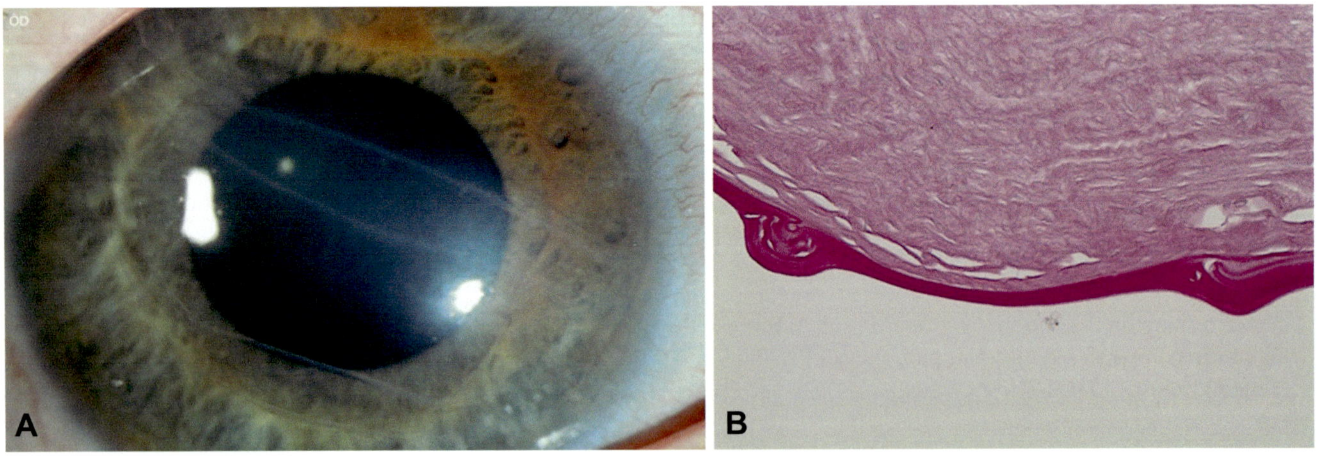

Fig. 1 Endothelial decompensation in case of Descemet striae after forceps delivery ((**A**) Overview, (**B**) Histology PAS staining) is a good indication for DMEK

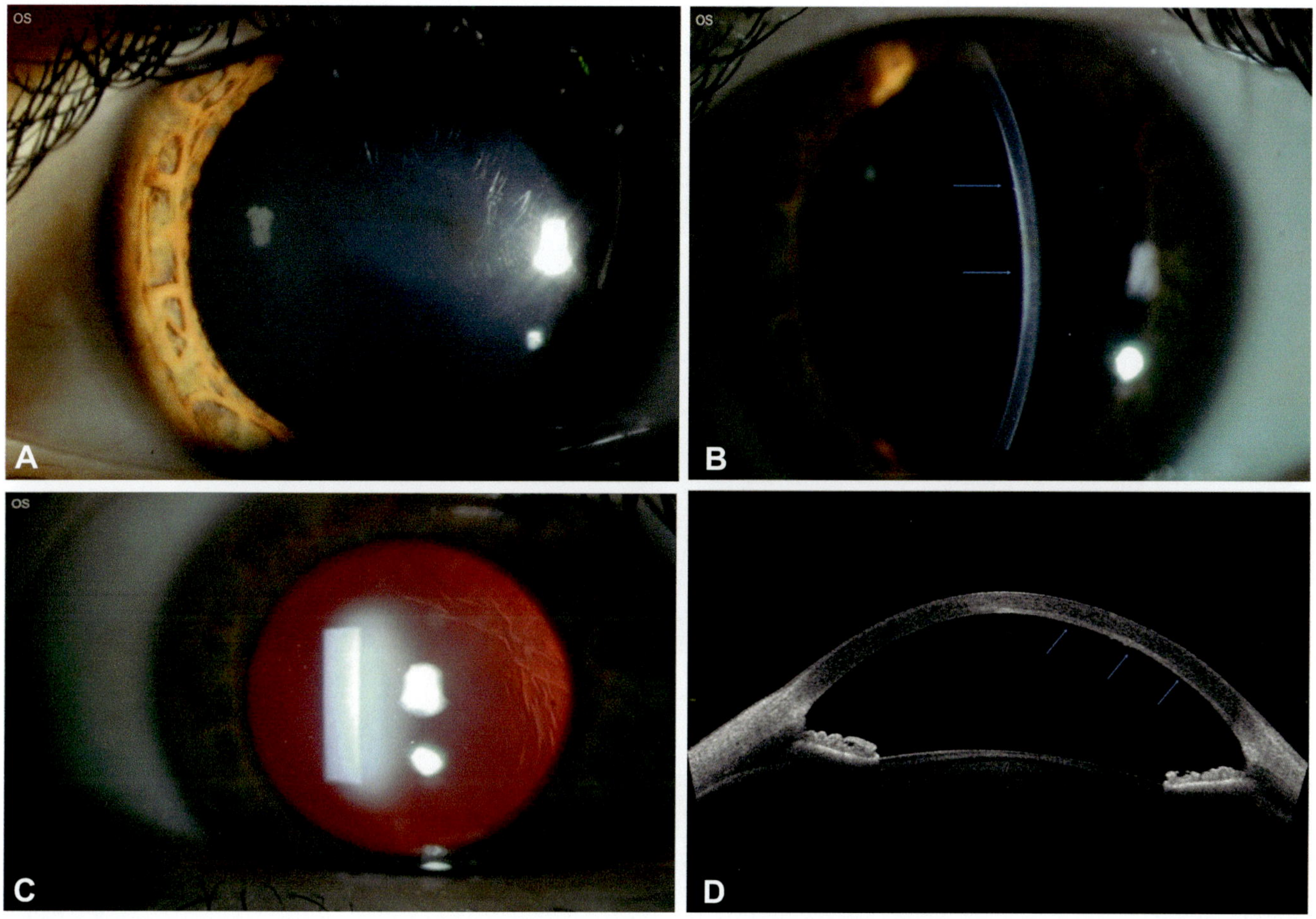

Fig. 2 Predescemetal stromal scars are not an indication for DMEK (**A**) Overview, (**B**) Thin slit, (**C**) Retroillumination. (**D**) AS-OCT: the arrow heads point clearly to the predescemetal stromal scar that cannot be removed by Descemetorhexis during DMEK!

We perform DMEK either sequentially on pseudophakic eyes (first cataract surgery, then DMEK) if cataract is the main clinical picture, or simultaneously with phacoemulsification and posterior chamber lens implantation (so-called "triple DMEK") if corneal edema is the main clinical picture. With triple DMEK, we aim for a refraction of −0.5 to −0.75 dpt in the Haigis formula if we really want to achieve emmetropia. The patient needs to know that this is not "refractive surgery": 40% of patients get a small myopic shift after DMEK and 60% of patients get a hyperopic shift. The refractive change after corneal deswelling varies from −0.5 to+2.0 dpt [41]. We therefore do not recommend the implantation of a multifocal or extended depth of focus IOL in triple DMEK.

To avoid calcification of the central IOL optics, we do not use hydrophilic artificial lenses in triple DMEK [3]. If the lens is clear, DMEK can also be performed in phakic eyes with the aim of preserving accommodation in younger patients [14].

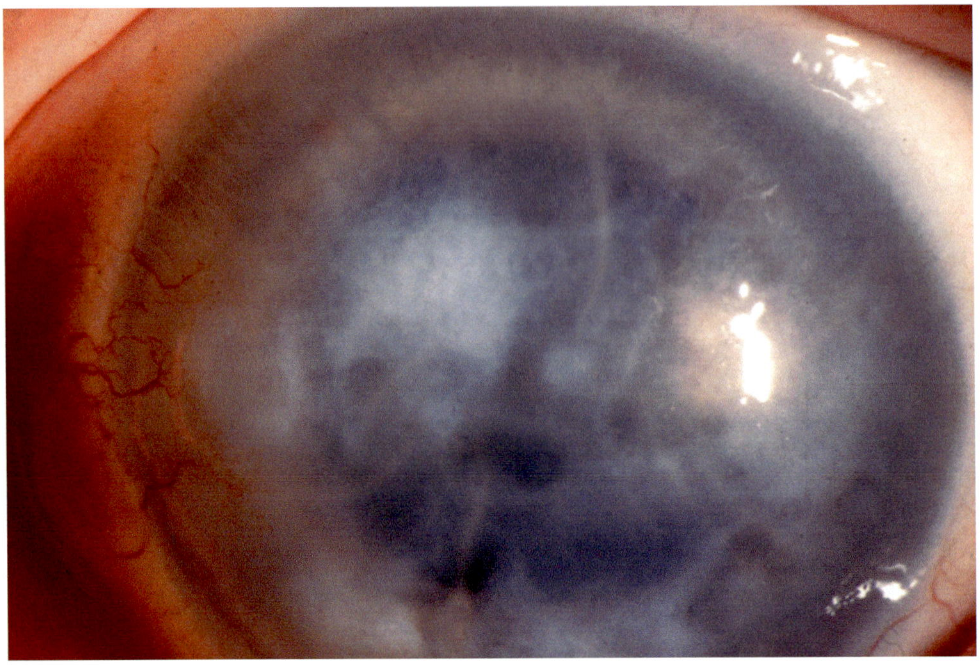

Fig. 3 Long-standing endothelial decompensation with pan-stromal scars is not an indication for DMEK

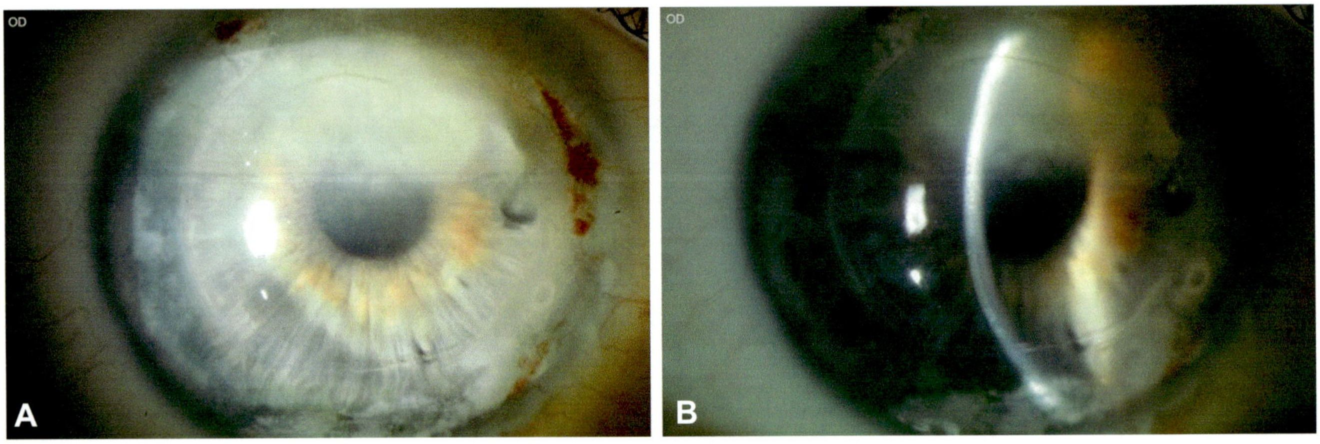

Fig. 4 Endothelial decompensation with stromal scars after PKP are not an indication for DMEK. (**A**) Overview, (**B**) Thin slit

For donor selection, the following details are important for the beginner [42–44]:

- age of the donor > 50 or even 60 years due to easier unfolding in the anterior chamber,
- diabetics should be avoided as donors due to the high risk of rupture during donor preparation [45],
- pseudophakic donors should be prepared by an experienced surgeon due to the increased risk of radial tears in the incision area [46],
- organ culture is to be preferred for EDM preparation.
- Due to the acceptable endothelial cell loss of less than 10% after storage for 1 day [37, 47], we have improved our organization by stress-free graft preparation in the operating room on the day before the planned DMEK and store the so-called "precut tissue" or "prestripped tissue" in organ culture without dextran (medium 1) [39, 48] in a glass vessel until the planned operation on the following day. To allow this sequential procedure the graft size has to be determined in relation to size of the cornea before donor preparation!

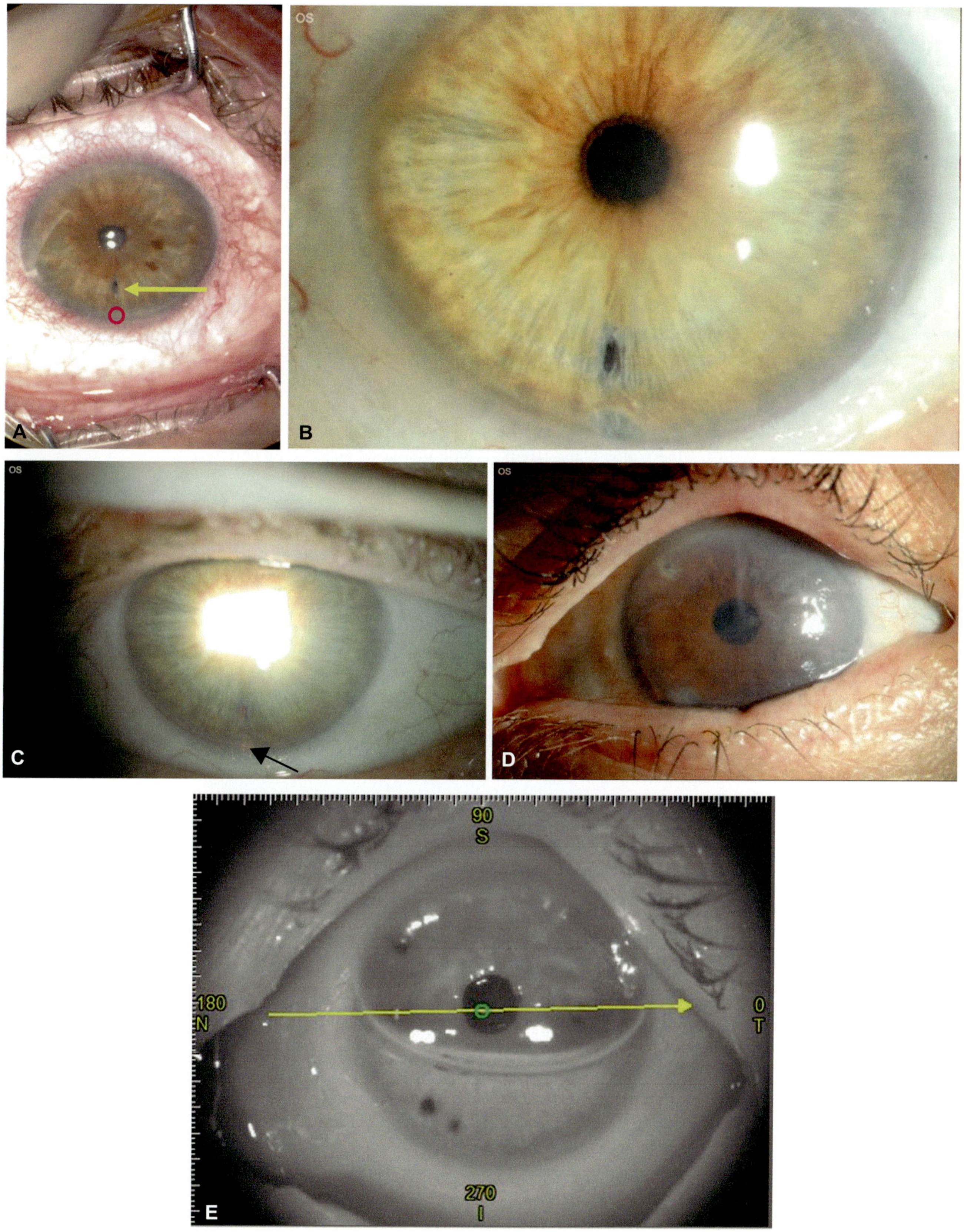

Fig. 5 (**A**) The preoperative YAG laser iridotomy (IT) should preferably be placed peripherally at 6 o'clock (red circle) and not mid-peripherally as shown here (yellow arrow). (**B**) Midperipheral placement of preoperative YAG-IT. (**C**) In retroillumination an open secondary YAG-IT in the periphery at 6 o`clock can be seen (arrow). (**D**) Wrongly placed preoperative YAG-IT at half past seven and 10 o`clock. (**E**). The AS-OCT overview shows another small YAG-IT at 7 o`clock (same patient as in D)

In practice, the pupil for a single DMEK is maximally constricted with Pilocarpine 2%. For triple DMEK, we avoid atropine and adrenaline in the anterior chamber during the cataract procedure so that the pupil can contract as much as possible after implantation of the artificial lens in the capsular bag. If in doubt, we use iris retractors to perform the cataract surgery safely.

4 Donor Preparation Step-By-Step

The surgical nurses prepare a standardized table for the donor preparation (Fig. 6). For stabilization, the 15 mm corneoscleral disc is placed with the epithelium facing downwards on a suction block, which is usually used for trephination of DSAEK tissue (Hanna trephination system; Moria SA, Antony, France) (Fig. 7). After correctly centering (!) the corneoscleral disc, the suction is started using the foot pedal. To improve visibility, Blue Color Caps (BCC, Croma GmbH, Leobendorf, Austria) is used, whereby the coloring takes less than 15 s and may be repeated to clearly mark the edges (Fig. 8). BCC is then replaced by the organ culture medium.

To aid orientation on the surface of the EDM, a very superficial circular marking is typically applied using the 7.5 or 8.0 mm trephine of the Moria DSAEK trephine system (Moria SA, Antony, France), which has the same diameter as the future EDM graft. In buphthalmic eyes or bullous keratopathy with very large corneas, a larger graft diameter may be useful in order to transplant as many endothelial cells as possible.

The marking is applied under haptic control by allowing the trephine to slide down in a controlled manner inside the guide cylinder of the trephine system until it gently touches the surface of the endothelium (Fig. 9). In case of undesired perforation of the DM during this step, the further procedure of donor preparation is more difficult and is associated with increased endothelial cell loss.

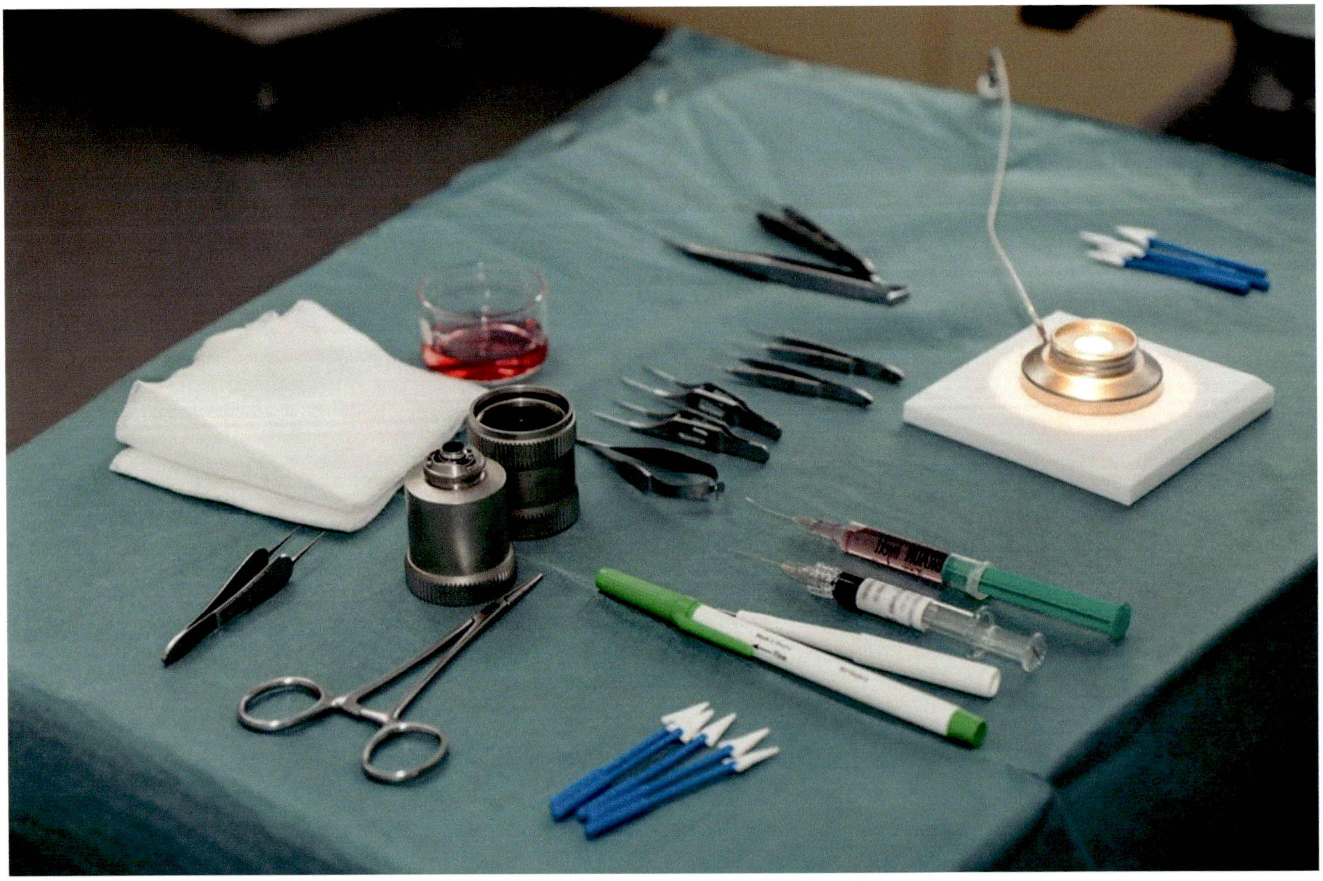

Fig. 6 Operating table with all utensils for donor preparation

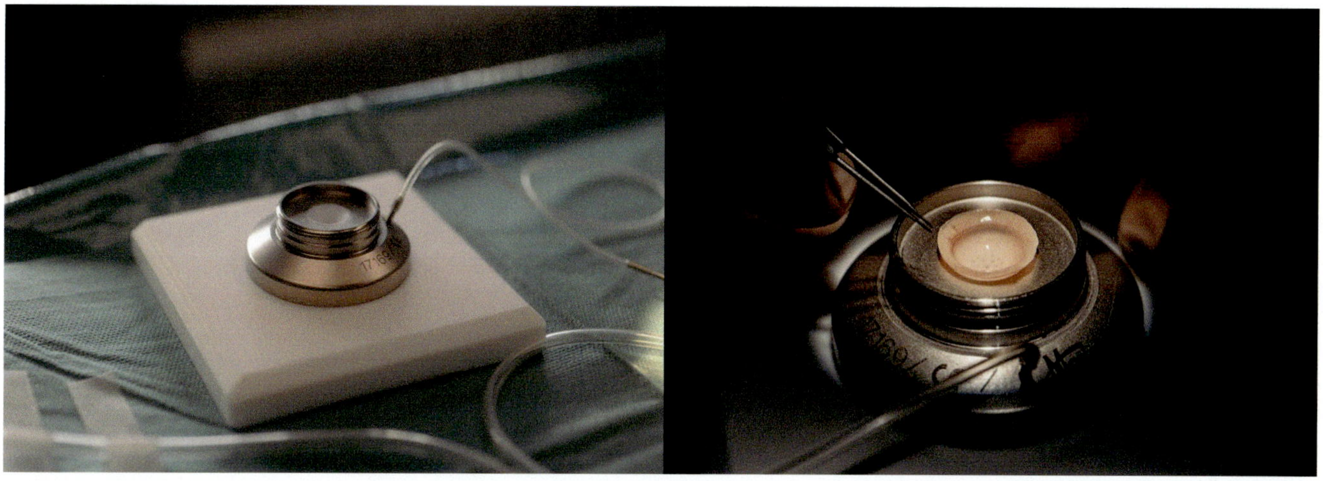

Fig. 7 To prevent displacement during graft preparation, the 15-mm corneoscleral disc is placed with the epithelium facing down on the suction block commonly used for preparation of DSAEK tissue (Hanna trephination system; Moria SA, Antony, France)

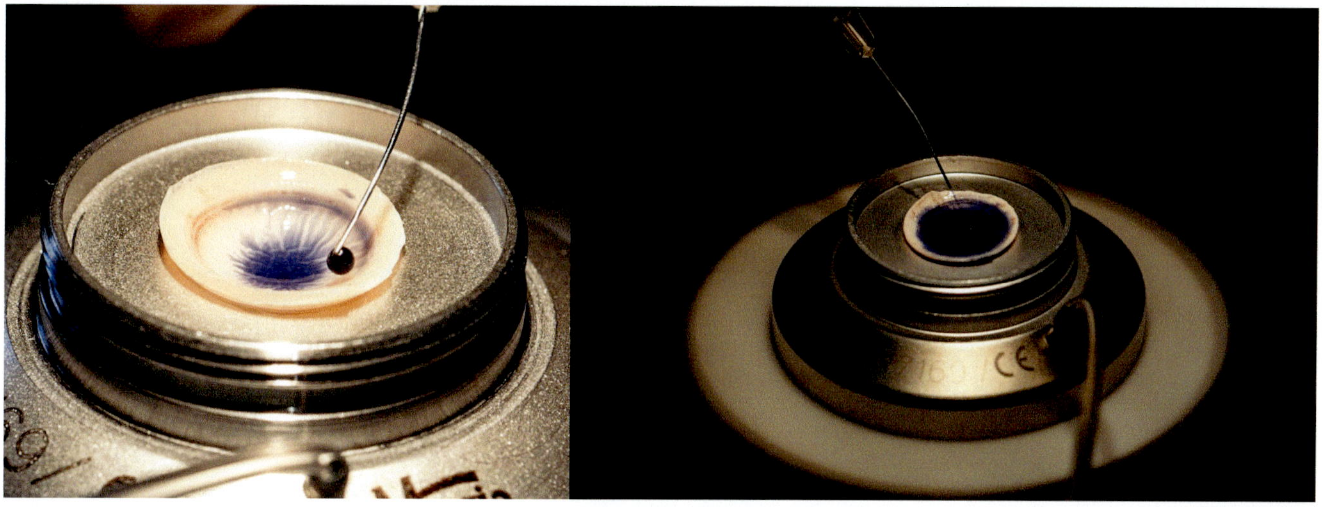

Fig. 8 To improve visualization, Blue Color Caps (BCC, Croma GmbH, Leobendorf, Austria) is dripped into the concave corneoscleral disc, whereby adequate staining takes less than 15 s and may be repeated to clearly mark the edges

The Descemet membrane (DM) adheres firmly to the trabecular meshwork and the peripheral corneal stroma near the limbus. Therefore, at the beginning of the preparation, peripheral lamellar incisions of approx. 1.5 mm in length are made with a razor blade outside the ring-shaped marking in a hexagonal, heptagonal or octagonal manner (Fig. 10). This is necessary to make it easier to grasp the circular edge of the EDM. A right-handed surgeon performs these incisions best in a clockwise direction by turning the suction block to the left. Typically, the DM is not only incised straight with the razor blade, but it also tears in a curved manner (analogous to the capsulorhexis of the lens) (Fig. 11). The incision area is then made more visible by applying BCC Blue Dye again for a few seconds. The DM is grasped radially with very little stretching using tiny, toothless forceps and the peripheral edge of the EDM (preferably starting from the torn edge–not the cut edge!) is lifted in a circular manner analogous to opening an envelope.

Ideally, the edge of the lifted EDM should be about 1 mm outside the round mark to allow manipulation of the edge of the EDM without reducing the number of endothelial cells of the future graft and to be able to react appropriately in case of induced radial tears in the EDM. If small radial tears occur during donor preparation, we grasp one edge of the tear with forceps and complete the radial tear to a semi-circular concave edge (like a capsulorhexis in cataract surgery) and we mark this critical area on the scleral rim with a fine sterile blue pencil.

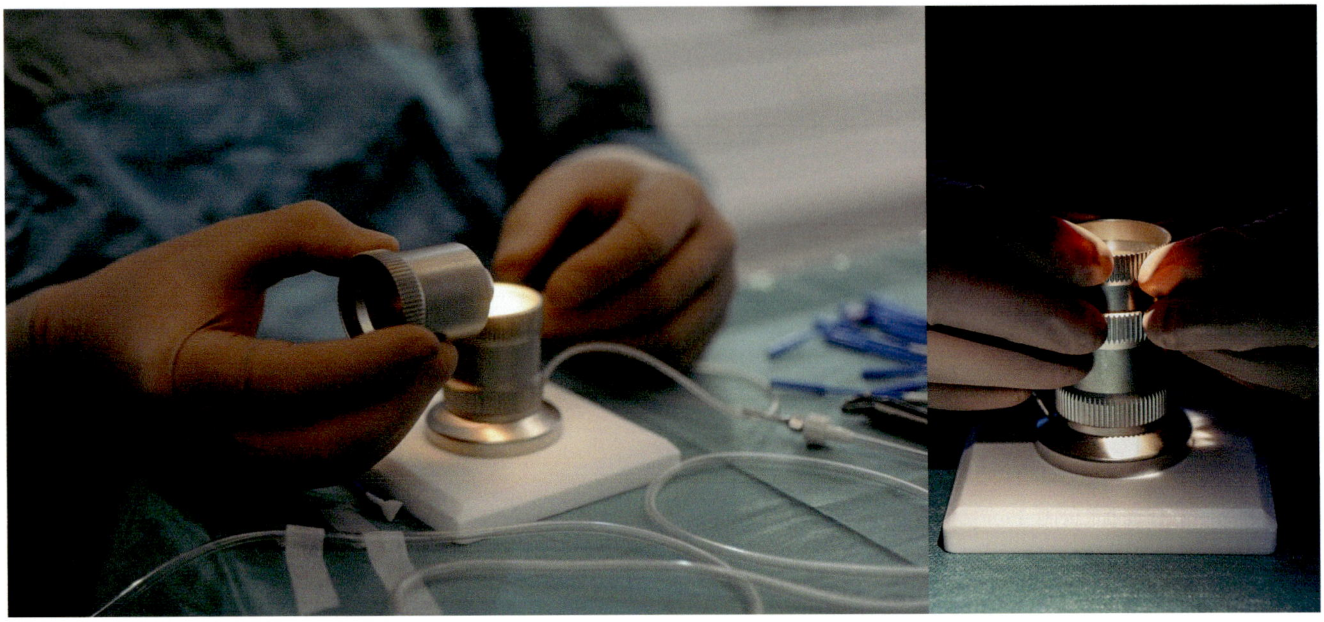

Fig. 9 The marking of the future graft size is made under visual control by carefully sliding the trephine down inside the guiding cylinder of the trephine system until it gently touches the surface of the endothelium. CAVE: Do not perforate!!!

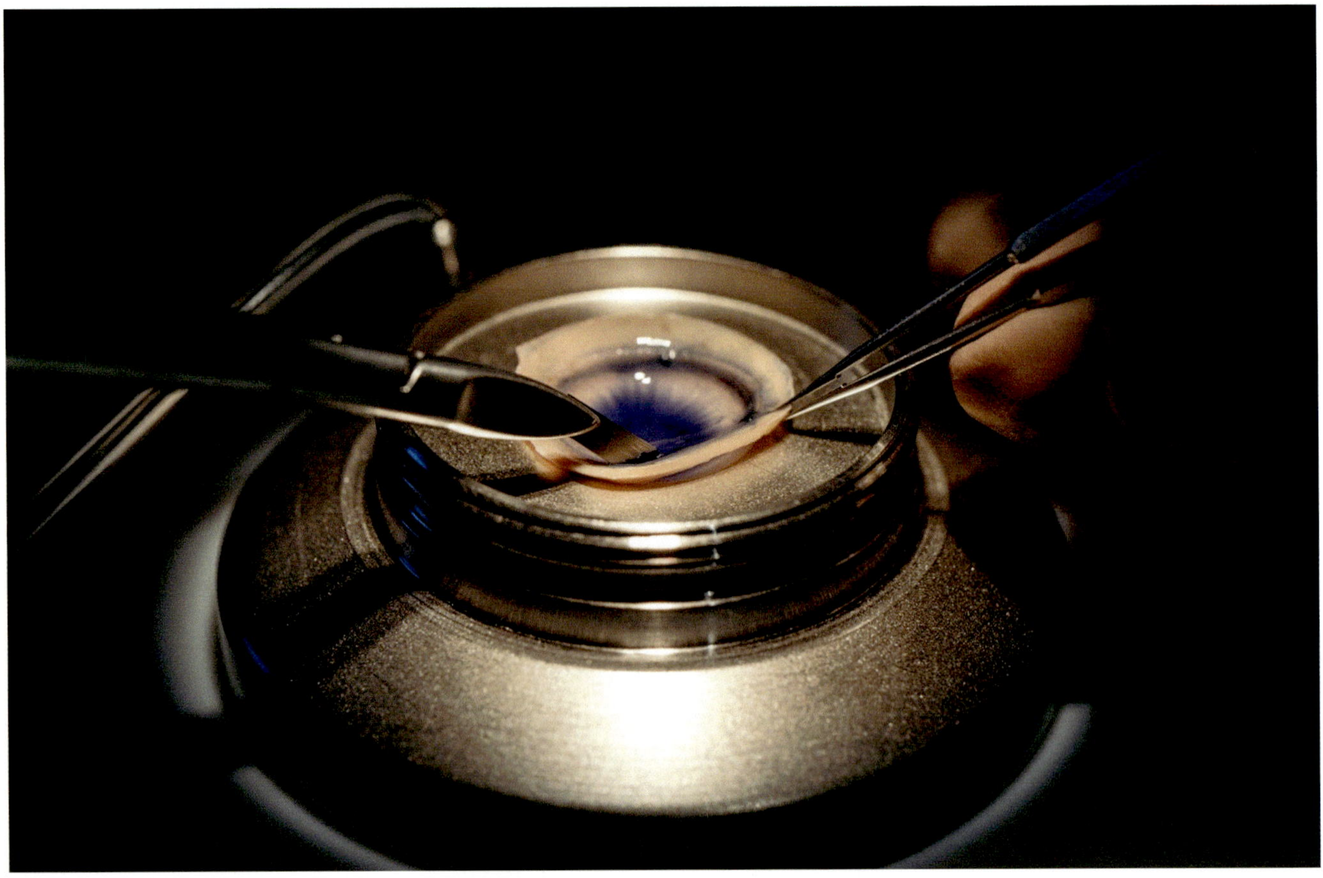

Fig. 10 In order to reach the edge of the EDM, peripheral lamellar incisions of approx. 1.5 mm in length are made outside the mark using a razor blade in a hexagonal, heptagonal or octagonal manner

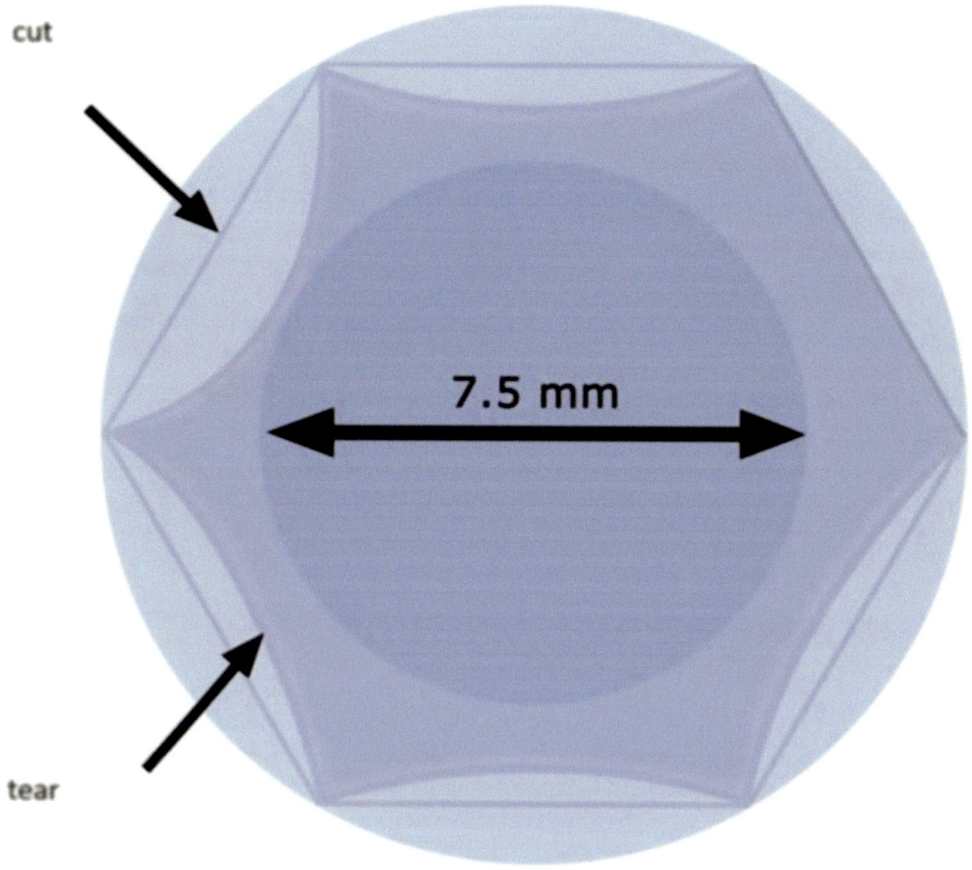

Fig. 11 Schematic: Typically, the DM is not only cut with the razor blade, but it also tears in a curved manner (analogous to the capsulorhexis of the lens). The DM is grasped radially with very little stretching using tiny toothless forceps and the peripheral edge of the DM (preferably the torn area first!) is lifted in a circular fashion, analogous to opening an envelope

After previous phacoemulsification in the donor, the EDM typically tears in the area of the paracentesis and the main incision. In this situation, the process of peripheral EDM elevation must be resumed proximal to the defect, which is often complicated by focal adhesions.

Since the EDM edge outside the round mark is removed anyway, grasping this edge outside the mark with forceps does not lead to endothelial cells loss on the graft, and the EDM can be safely pulled towards the center with one hand. Both lateral edges of the slowly detaching EDM are closely visually monitored in order to immediately stop pulling off if a radial tear becomes visible. Otherwise, the peeling is stopped as planned after just under a third of the entire EDM has been detached. The peripheral EDM is then returned to its original position by grasping the edges to be discarded later. By rotating the suction block about 120°, the EDM can be detached from the stroma in the mid-periphery in the second third. When the EDM is lifted off in the last third, it is important that a small part of the EDM remains attached to the central stroma so that the EDM does not begin to slide uncontrollably. Sometimes the adhesion of the EDM is also so strong in the mid-periphery that only the bimanual technique with 2 forceps prevents recurrent tearing at the focally peripherally grasped areas of the EDM.

After the entire EDM has been unfolded again in the correct anatomical position, the lamellar (!) trephination of the donor cornea is performed with the Moria trephine. The peripheral circular edge of the EDM, which was previously grasped with the forceps, is now discarded. Most importantly, orientation markings are made as described by Bachmann, Cursiefen and Kruse in 2010 [49] to ensure the correct anteroposterior orientation of the EDM during the following surgical steps (Fig. 12A). Using a 1-mm skin trephine, 3 semicircular markings are made on the edge of the EDM so that 2 markings are close to each other and 1 clockwise at a greater distance (Fig. 12B). The formation of radial cracks in the EDM must be avoided.

The suction block is now rotated so that the 3 markings point towards the surgeon. To completely detach the EDM, corneal suture forceps are used to grasp the edge of the EDM opposite the orientation markings. As the majority of the EDM is already detached from the stroma, complete detachment is relatively easy and safe. However, the forceps must again be guided along the concave curvature directly above the endothelium of the corneoscleral disc without touching the endothelium (Fig. 13). After finishing the suction process of the Moria system, the fully detached EDM is transferred into a glass container (12 cm × 1 cm) half-filled with organ culture medium without dextran (Fig. 14).

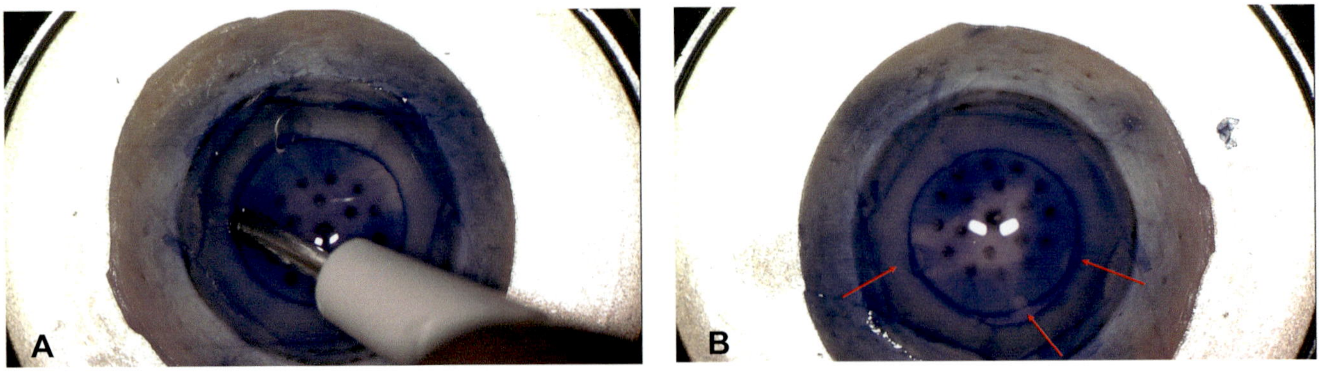

Fig. 12 (**A**) Three semicircular markings (arrows) are made at the edge of the EDM with a 1 mm skin trephine, two close together and one at a greater distance. (**B**) The third mark (thick arrow) on the edge of the EDM is placed clockwise at a greater distance from each other than the first two marks. This ensures the anterior/posterior orientation of the EDM during the subsequent surgical steps, as described by Bachmann et al. in 2010 [49]

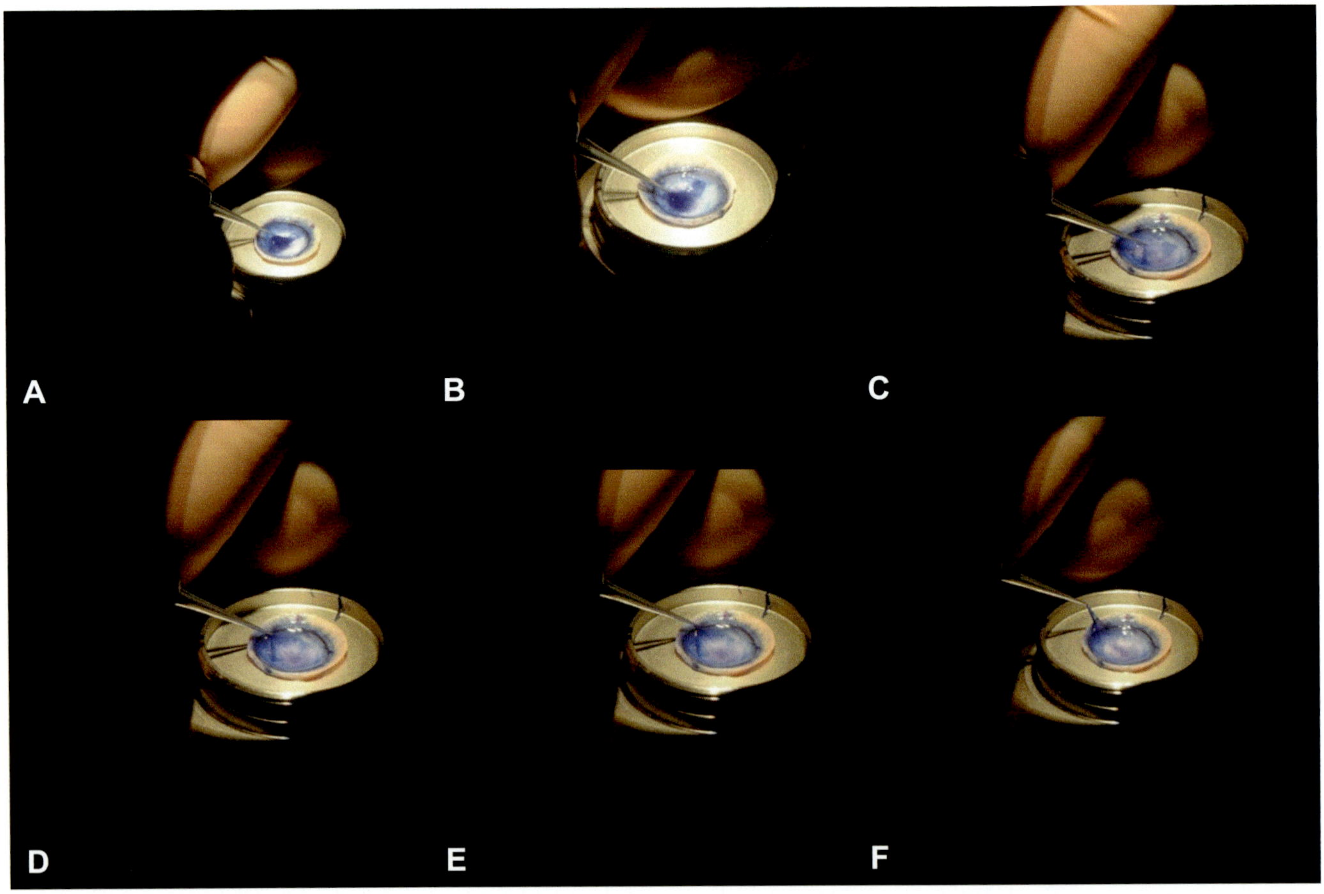

Fig. 13 (**A–F**) To completely detach the EDM, corneal suture forceps are used to grasp the edge of the EDM opposite the orientation markings. The forceps must again be guided along the concave curvature directly above the endothelium of the corneoscleral disc without touching the endothelium

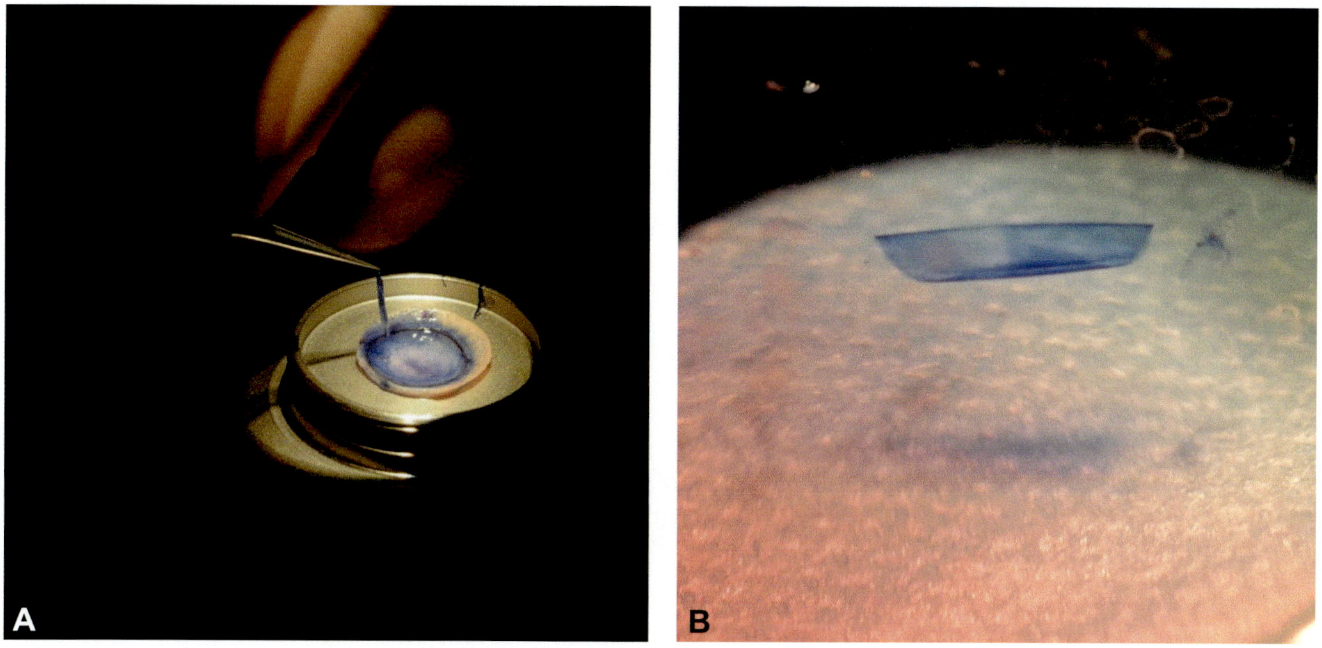

Fig. 14 After finishing the detachment, the rolled EDM is transferred into a glass container (12 cm × 1 cm) half-filled with organ culture medium without dextran using a forceps

For overnight preservation, the EDM is transferred to the original organ culture flask from the eye bank and returned to the corneal incubator.

The safety and speed of preparing the EDM graft is significantly improved through training. This procedure can usually be successfully performed by an experienced DMEK surgeon in 5 to a maximum of 10 min.

5 Recipient and Host Maneuver Step-By-Step

5.1 Recipient Preparation

If the host cornea is very edematous, we drop 5% NaCl (sodium chloride) ½ hourly immediately after the patient gets up and 20% glucose solution intraoperatively. If this does not help sufficiently, we remove the thickened whitish epithelium with a hockey knife, especially if triple DMEK is planned to improve insight into the anterior chamber. The view into the anterior chamber is often much better afterwards and helps to avoid complications. At the end of the operation, these patients receive a therapeutic contact lens with local antibiotic prophylaxis for 2 weeks. First, after drying the corneal surface, an 8.0 mm ring-shaped central marker for a 7.5 mm graft is applied (Fig. 15). After staining the marker, the nurse should dab it on a cloth at least 3 times before touching the cornea so that the ring does not become too wide on the cornea and later impair vision. The donor diameter should always be smaller than the recipient diameter to prevent overlapping of the donor and host DM, as this increases the risk of subsequent graft detachment and thus the need for re-bubbling [3].

A clear corneal phaco incision (width 2.5 mm) (Fig. 16A) and 3 small paracenteses (width 1.8 mm) at a distance of 120° are made at the limbus (Fig. 16B). A relatively short “phaco tunnel” (no longer than 1.5 mm) should ensure that the distance between the inner lip of the tunnel and the contralateral chamber angle provides sufficient space for the centered placement of the graft and that the necessary maneuvers with a cannula through the tunnel are possible. To remove the diseased recipient DM, an anterior chamber maintainer (ACM) is connected to a vitrectomy unit through the paracentesis opposite the tunnel to allow a centered descemetorhexis under air (typically 40 mm Hg pressure) (Fig. 17). This keeps the anterior chamber deep throughout the descemetorhexis. This is very helpful in patients with strong vis-a-tergo (=“positive vitreous pressure”)!

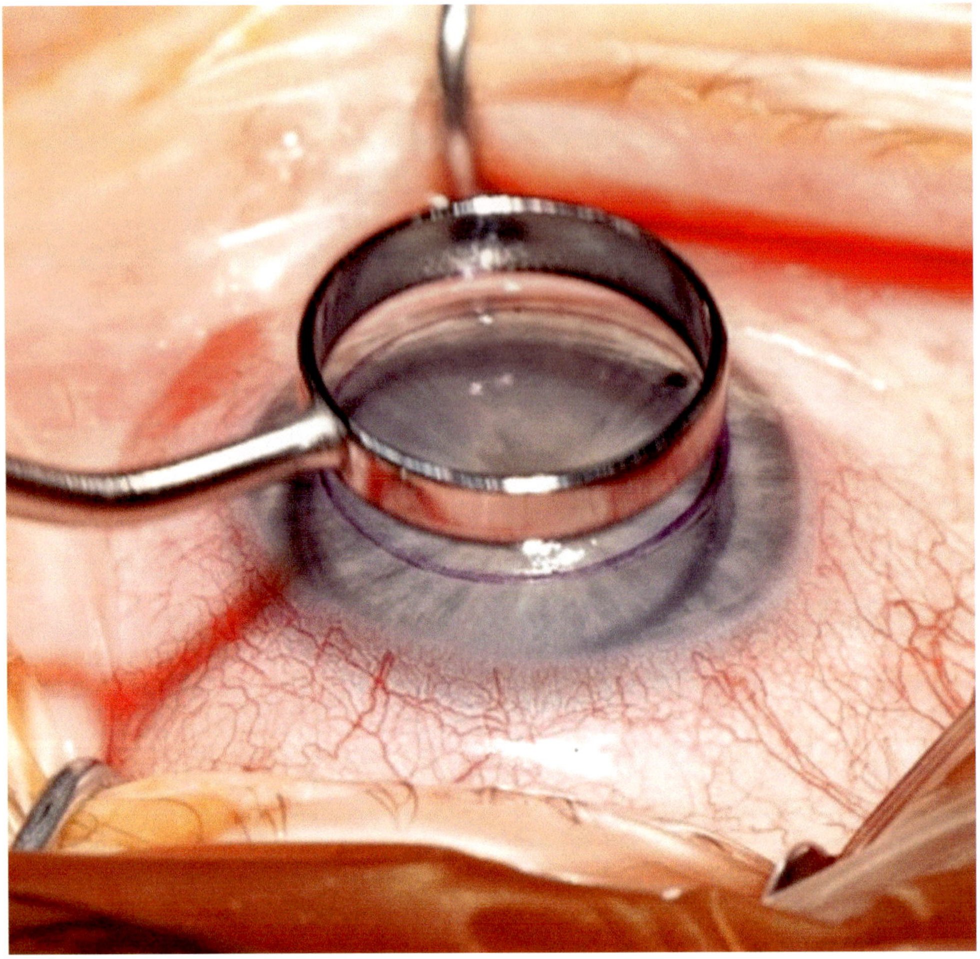

Fig. 15 An 8.0 mm annular marking is applied to the central corneal surface for a 7.5 mm graft to avoid donor–host overlap of DM

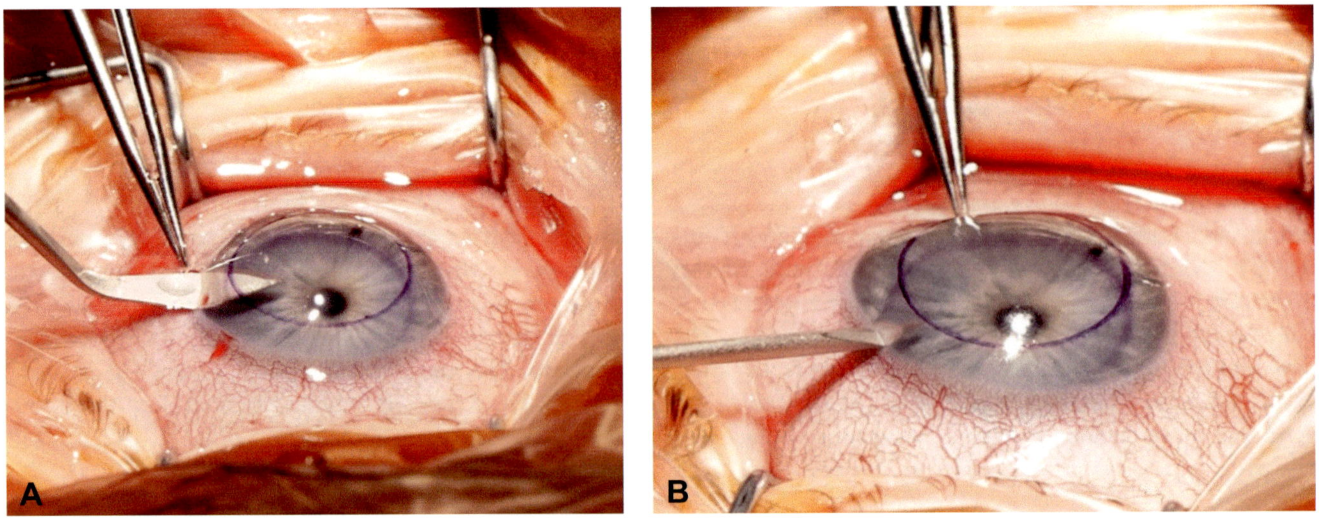

Fig. 16 (**A**) A limbal "phacotunnel" (width 2.5 mm) and (**B**) three small paracenteses (width 1.8 mm) at a distance of 120 degrees from each other are applied to the limbus

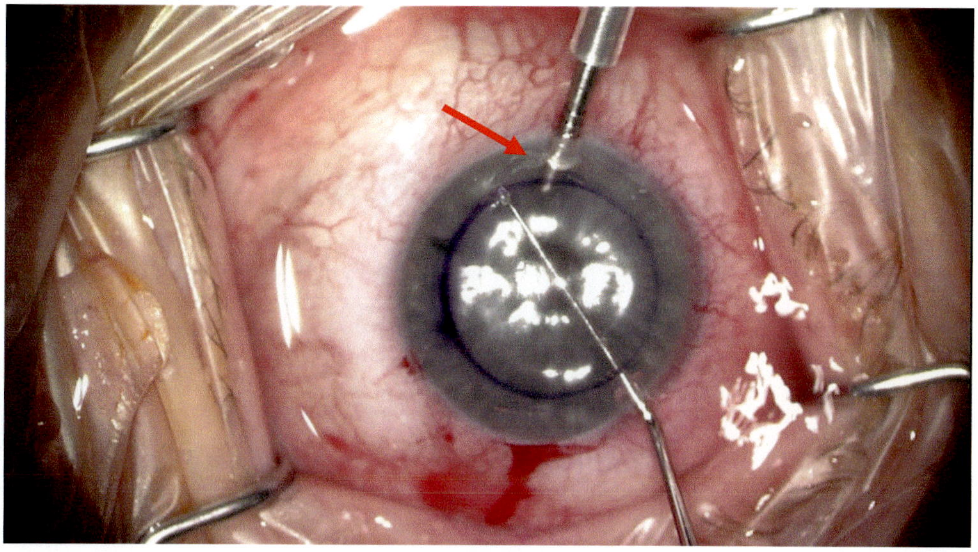

Fig. 17 An "Anterior Chamber Maintainer" ACM (arrow) is placed at the limbus via the nasal paracentesis. This is connected to a vitrectomy unit, which keeps the anterior chamber deep during descemtorhexis with a 40 mmHg air pressure. For the descemetorhexis, an inverted hook (e.g. Price Hook "Reverse Sinskey"; Moria SA) is inserted through a paracentesis opposite the ACM

For the descemetorhexis, an inverted hook (Price Hook "Reverse Sinskey", Moria SA, Antony, France) is inserted through a paracentesis next to the tunnel (Fig. 17). First, a circular incision is made behind the circular mark in the area of the DM. Then the peripheral portion of the EDM is folded over—analogous to the capsulorhexis in cataract surgery—and successively pulled to the opposite edge without causing furrows and defects in the posterior host stroma in the center. The air filling of the anterior chamber—in contrast to water or viscoelastic—best shows the surgeon the areas where remnants of the occasionally lamellar split DM still remain. These can then be completely removed with the wide "scraper" (90° spatula, Moria SA), as used for DSAEK. The paracentesis, which previously contained the ACM, is then securely closed with a 10–0 nylon single suture and the anterior chamber remains filled with air to prevent stromal swelling during preparation of the graft injection cartridge.

The EDM roll, which was prepared the day before or directly prior to the operation, is transferred to a Petri dish (12 cm × 1 cm), half of which is filled with an organ culture medium without dextran. The dark blue dye DORC MEMBRANE BLUE DUAL (DORC, VN Zuidland, Netherlands) is manually injected into the lumen of the roll using a small cannula. The tip of a glass cartridge (disposable DMEK cartridge, Geuder, Heidelberg, G-38635) is connected to a small tube and a 5 ml syringe. It is completely filled with medium and immersed in the medium. Using a spatula, the rolled EDM can be easily maneuvered into the large-lumen posterior opening of the glass cartridge (Fig. 18). To facilitate this procedure, the assisting nurse carefully pulls the plunger of the 5 ml syringe.

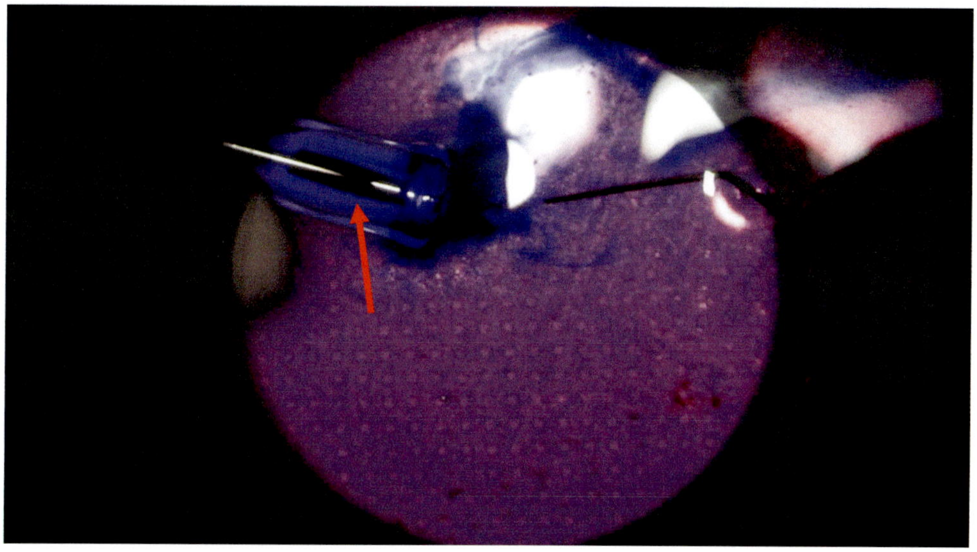

Fig. 18 With the help of a small spatula, the rolled EDM (red arrow) can be easily guided into the large opening of the glass cartridge (Geuder). To facilitate this procedure, the assisting nurse carefully pulls the plunger of the syringe, which is connected to the tip of the cartridge via a small tube

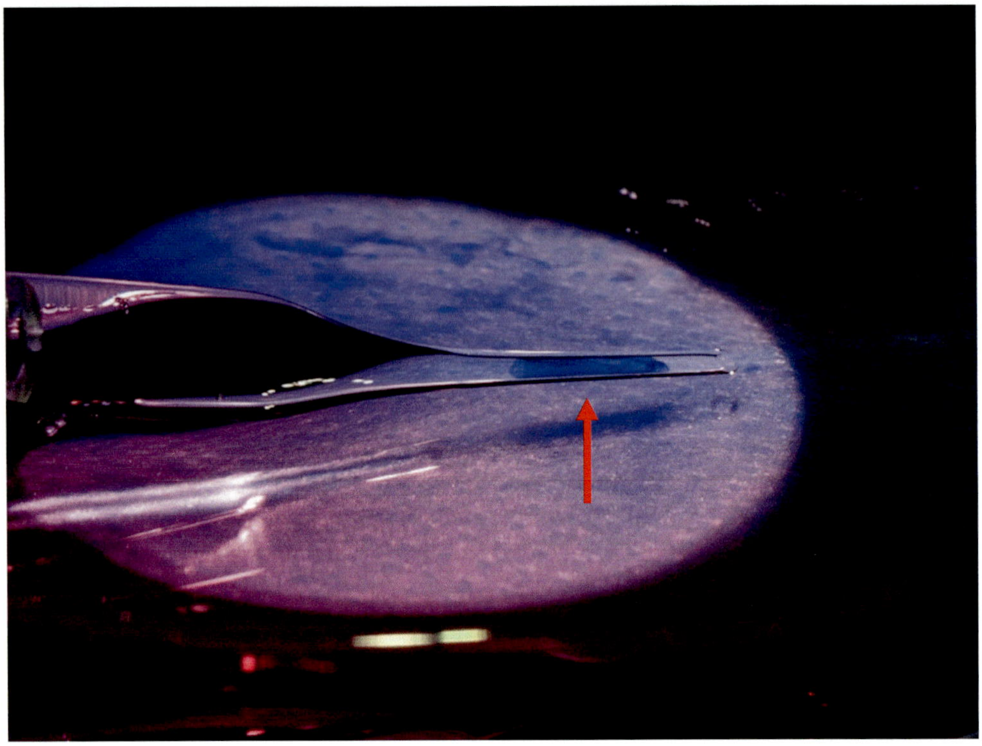

Fig. 19 The EDM roll is advanced to the tip of the glass cartridge (arrow) by carefully turning (not pushing!) the plunger of the 3-ml syringe

Another 3 ml syringe is then screwed into the large opening of the glass cartridge (Luer-Lok tip) and the small tube is removed from the tip of the glass cartridge. The EDM roll is advanced into the tip of the cartridge by carefully turning (not pushing!) the 3 ml plunger (Fig. 19). The dark blue DORC dye is filled into the tip of the glass cartridge via a small, curved cannula until the entire EDM roll is completely covered with the deep blue dye (Fig. 20). Then we wait at least 15 s to be sure that the dye has been well absorbed by the EDM.

5.2 Injection of the Endothelial Descemet Membrane into the Anterior Chamber

To prepare the injection of the EDM roll, the air is completely (!) removed from the anterior chamber and it is completely filled with Balanced Salt Solution (BSS). The tip of the glass cartridge is inserted with the slanted opening facing downwards (!) towards the periphery of the anterior chamber (Fig. 21A) to prevent the graft from disappearing behind the iris—especially in the case of partly dilated pupils in triple DMEK. By pressing the plunger, the EDM roll is injected into the anterior chamber together with the blue liquid—initially without paying attention to the orientation (Fig. 21B). By carefully pressing the inferior lip of the limbal incision with the glass tip, a large amount of the blue dye can be immediately removed from the anterior chamber. The incision is then closed watertight with a 10–0 nylon single suture being sure that the globe has a normal tension during suturing to avoid distortion of the corneal topography and irregular astigmatism (Fig. 22).

5.3 Unfolding and Alignment of the Graft in the Anterior Chamber

Using a Sautter cannula and BSS, the remaining blue dye is now completely flushed out of the anterior chamber. This way, the EDM roll usually tends to open partially so that the surgeon can see the orientation and edges of the graft (Fig. 23A). Observation of the markings on the edge of the

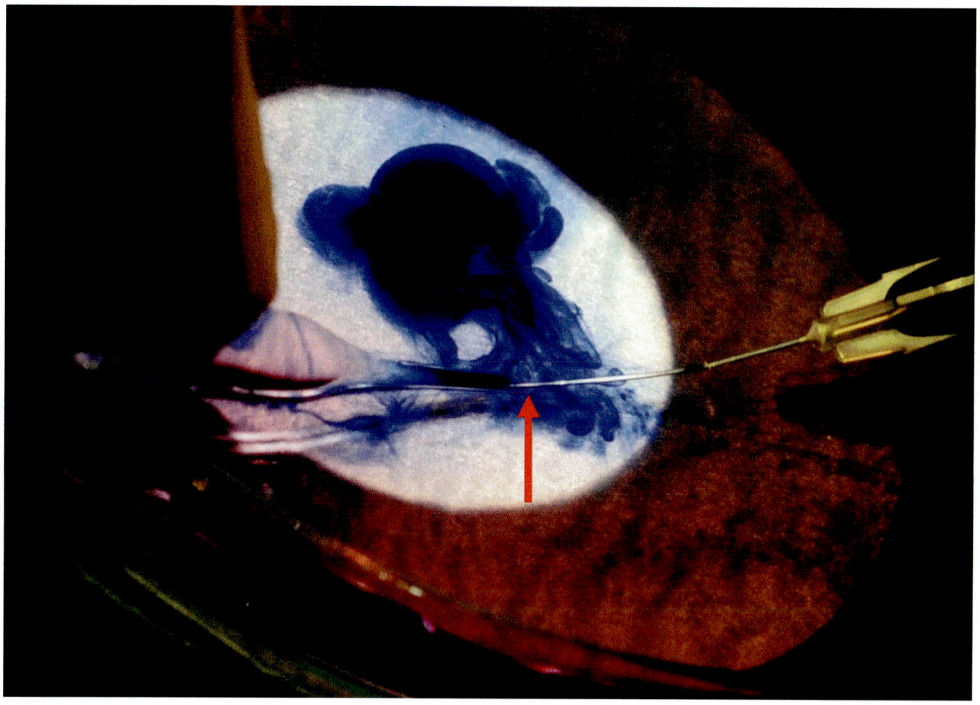

Fig. 20 The dark blue dye DORC MEMBRANEBLUE DUAL (DORC, VN Zuidland, Netherlands) is filled into the tip of the glass cartridge via a small, curved cannula (arrow) until the entire roll is completely covered with the deep blue dye. This step is of utmost clinical importance to ensure that all three markings on the edge of the EDM can be clearly identified later in the anterior chamber

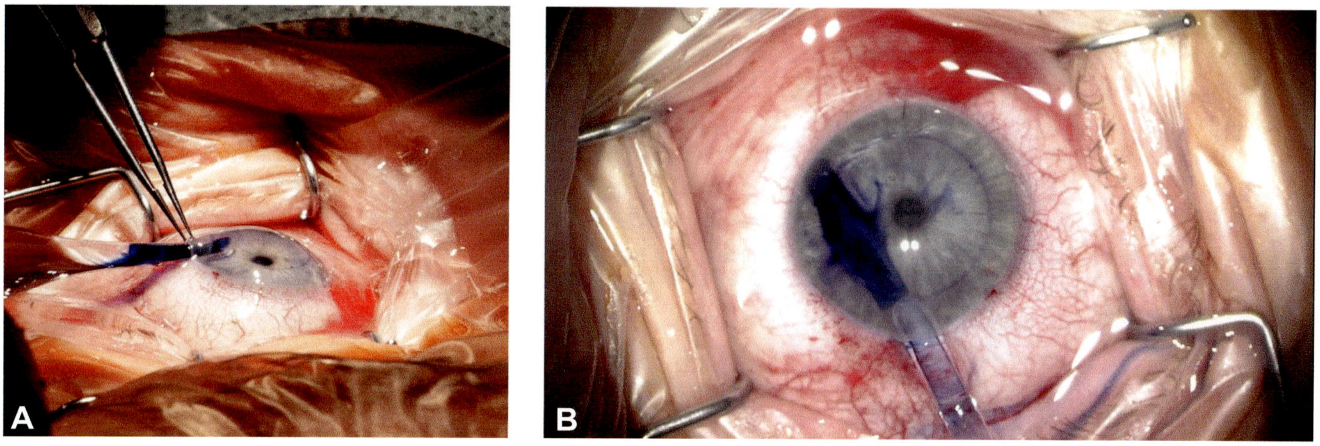

Fig. 21 To prepare the injection of the EDM roll, the air is completely (!) removed and the anterior chamber is filled with BSS. The tip of the glass cartridge is inserted with the slanted opening facing downwards (!) towards the periphery of the anterior chamber ((**A**) sideview) to prevent the graft from disappearing behind the iris. By pressing the plunger, the EDM roll is injected into the anterior chamber together with the blue liquid ((**B**) from above)

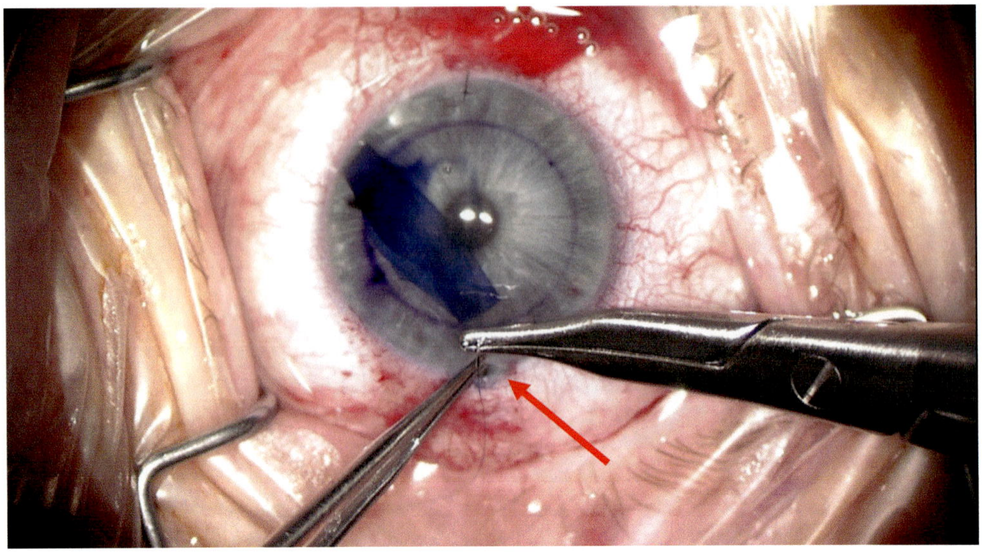

Fig. 22 The „phako incision " is closed watertight with a 10–0 nylon single suture being sure that the globe has a normal tension during suturing to avoid distortion of the corneal topography and irregular astigmatism

EDM in conjunction with observation of the edge of the roll (which curves upwards towards the back of the cornea) makes it in most cases feasible to ensure correct orientation. It is very advantageous if the EDM forms a triangular "Napoleon's hat" at this point. Now, deployment of the graft can be achieved by either tapping the host cornea after repeatedly pressing the bottom of the paracentesis or main incision to flatten the anterior chamber, or by introducing a small air bubble from an insulin syringe, prepared by the nurse, into the inner lumen of the EDM roll (Fig. 23B).

By tapping on the cornea, the air bubble rolling towards the periphery is used to unfold the edges of the EDM one by one. Once unfolded, the edges should be "clamped" in the periphery between the posterior corneal surface and the iris (Fig. 23C). If the EDM cannot be centered indirectly with water bursts, it is sometimes advisable to use a small spatula moving horizontally to center the EDM directly without pressing the graft against the iris. If the anterior chamber is too deep, the membrane can be spread on the surface of the iris by enlarging the air bubble and filling the anterior chamber completely with air, but without too much pressure (Fig. 24). In vitrectomised eyes without vis-a-tergo, unfolding is often only achievable bimanually by consistently holding the anterior chamber flat with the left hand and applying pressure to the central cornea with a 5 mm diameter ring-shaped fine metal instrument (Bores O-Z Marker, Polytech-Domilens, Roßdorf). Careful active aspiration of fluid from the anterior chamber using a Sautter cannula can also help. Alternative techniques and other complex approaches have also been described [30–32, 50].

In any case, the small or larger air bubble must be carefully and completely aspirated using an upward-facing Sautter cannula (lumen of the cannula in the direction of the recipient stroma!). The cornea usually collapses and the EDM remains on the iris—even in young donors, deep anterior chamber or after vitrectomy. The cannula must be removed without affecting the position of the EDM. A cannula connected to a syringe filled with 20% SF6 (sulphur hexafluoride) gas is then inserted under the EDM towards the center of the pupil (Fig. 23D). During this stage, the surgeon's thumb must be away from the plunger to avoid uncontrolled dislocation of the EDM! Due to the controlled gas injection, the EDM usually adheres well to the back of the host cornea like a "jellyfish" (Fig. 23E). Ultimately, the orientation markings ensure correct alignment of the graft and prevent upside-down apposition. After a minute of full gas filling of the anterior chamber a small amount of fluid is administered into the anterior chamber via paracentesis using the Sautter cannula so that the iridotomy is clear at 6 o'clock when looking downwards, allowing a flow of aqueous humor from the production site to the drainage site. We aim for an approximately ½ mm wide circular fluid rim at the limbus, which corresponds to approximately 90% expansive gas filling.

Faux ami: The EDMs of old donors can sometimes be unfolded in the anterior chamber without any problems—but lie "upside down", as the 3 "Bachmann markings" clearly show (Fig. 25).

It is very important to ensure a central position of the EDM in the anterior chamber below the 8.0 mm circular marker before inserting the gas bubble, because the graft—unlike with a DSAEK—often cannot be moved significantly once it is in contact with the host stroma. Sometimes, vigorous tapping with a cross-hook from the limbus to the center in the hemimeridian of the decentration can cause a slight displacement of the EDM. Unfolding typically takes between 2 and a maximum of 10 min after the learning curve has been completed [17].

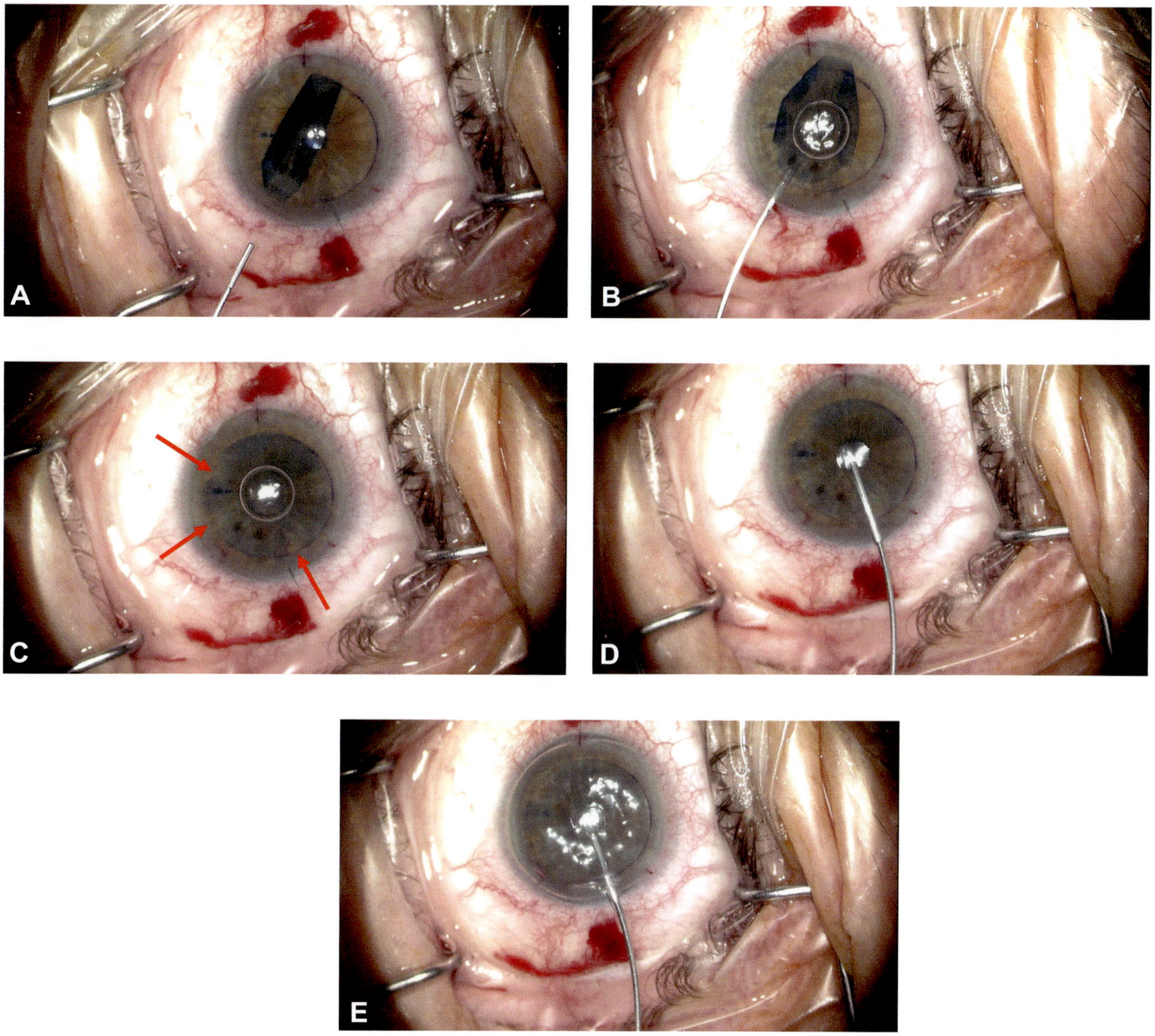

Fig. 23 Unfolding and application of the EDM in the anterior chamber. (**A**) After a few fluid bursts, the EDM points in the right direction. The EDM is locked in this position by applying pressure to the bottom of a paracentesis or the main incision. (**B**) Using an insulin syringe, a small air bubble of defined volume is applied between the EDM and the cornea. Indirectly controlled rolling maneuvers unfold the peripheral edges of the EDM. (**C**) The graft is well centered and in the correct antero-posterior orientation (arrows point to the 3 Bachmann markings) on the iris. (**D**) Once the EDM has unfolded, the cannula connected to a syringe containing 20% SF6 gas must be advanced under the EDM towards the center of the pupil. During this stage, the surgeon's thumb must remain away from the plunger to avoid uncontrolled dislocation of the EDM! (**E**) Due to the controlled gas injection, the EDM usually attaches itself well centered to the back of the host cornea like a "jellyfish"

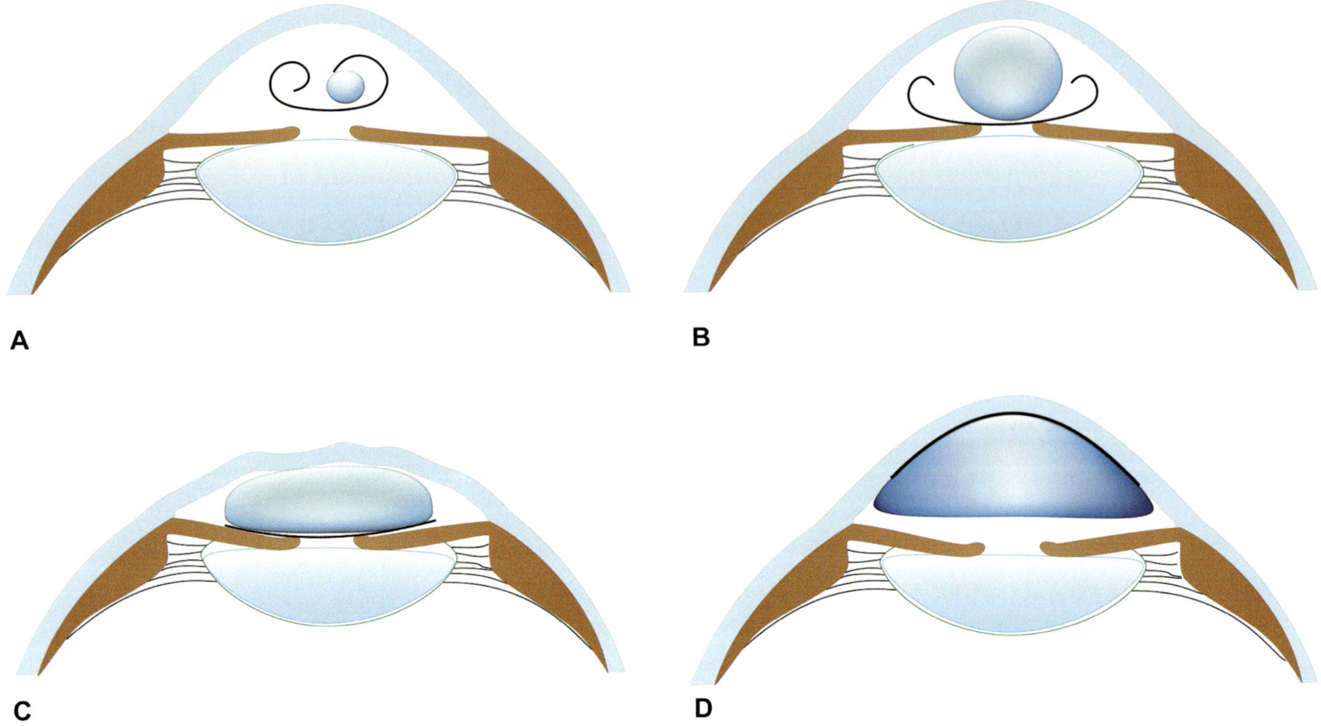

Fig. 24 Suggestion to facilitate unfolding of the graft in vitrectomized eyes. (**A**) To facilitate the unfolding process, a small air bubble is injected into the inner lumen of the rolled endothelial Descemet membrane lamella (EDML). (**B**) The air bubble is enlarged and moved towards the periphery by tapping the cornea to partially unfold the edges of the EDML. (**C**) The anterior chamber is flattened by active aspiration of aqueous humour and BSS by paracentesis, typically collapsing the cornea (complete unfolding of the EDML). (**D**) Removal of the air bubble and injection of 20% sulphur hexafluoride (SF6) under the EDML (final position)

5.4 Perioperative Details

On the day of surgery, we measure the intraocular pressure by applanation every 2 h, for which the patient may stand up, come into the doctor's room and sit down at the slit lamp. If the intraocular pressure rises above 30 mm Hg, some gas can be released by applying mild pressure with the tip of a sterile forceps when the eye is 100% full of gas. If the lower part of the iris is in contact with the posterior surface of the cornea, a new YAG iridotomy (without contact lens) should be performed to widen the apparently too small iris opening. After the operation, the patient is asked to lie on his/her back for two-thirds of the time being awake for 5–7 days or alternately on his/her left and right side and to intermittently stretch the head to allow the gas to press on the inferior part of the graft. Prone position is prohibited for 1 week!

5.5 DMEK After Penetrating Keratoplasty

The classic indication for DMEK after PKP is endothelial graft decompensation with/without bullous keratopathy without stromal scarring [23–29]. This is usually caused by graft fatigue (e.g. in transplanted guttae [51]), endothelial immune reactions and glaucoma drainage implants. Contraindications are stromal scars on the graft (Fig. 4) (also pre-descemetal!) and high and/or irregular

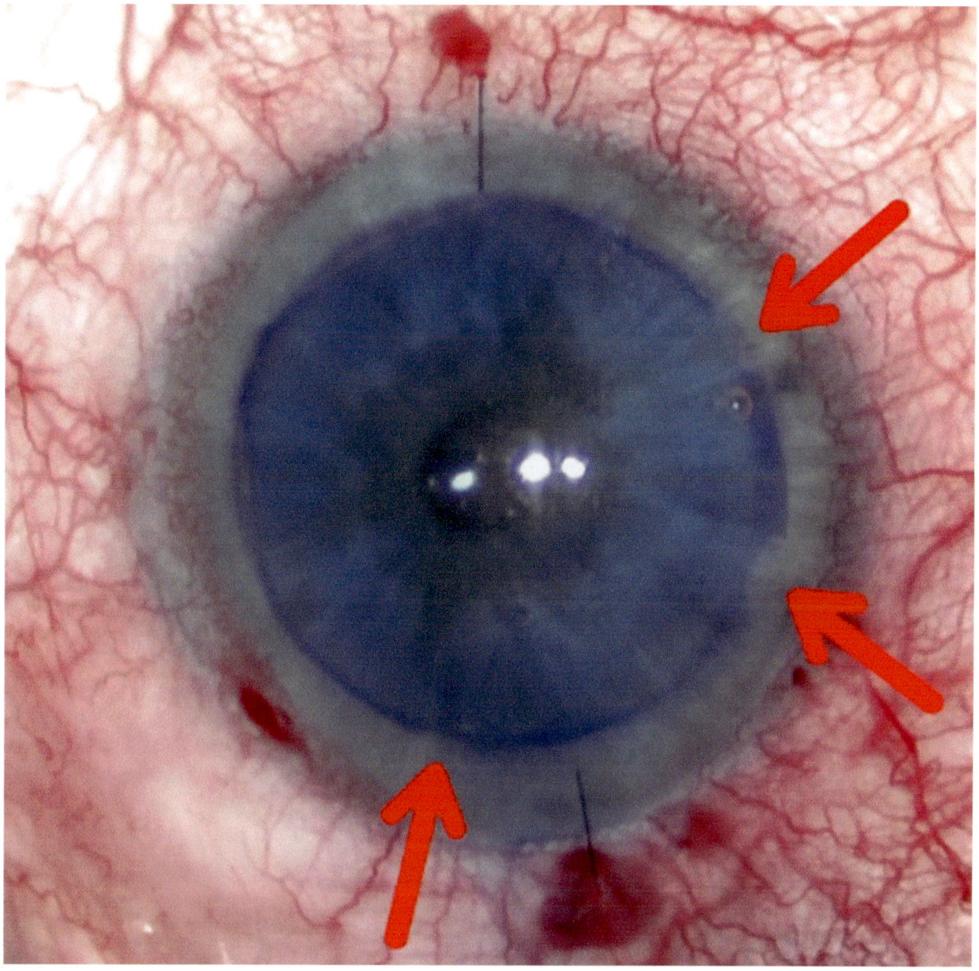

Fig. 25 Faux ami: The EDM of an 85-year-old donor unfolded without any problems in the VK. The 3 Bachmann markings clearly show that the antero-posterior orientation is incorrect and the graft must be rotated upside-down

astigmatism. Re-PKP with a larger (!) graft diameter (preferably as non-contact excimer laser trephination with double continuous cross-stitch suture according to Hoffmann) is the method of choice [28]. Depending on the size of the cornea, the following applies to the size of the new graft: "As large as possible, as small as necessary"-not: "One size fits all". However, in case of incomplete excision of the (e.g. decentered) old graft, a strong increase in astigmatism must be expected after removal of the second suture [34].

Important for the decision DMEK versus Re-PKP is the question to the patient about:

- contact lens tolerance, and
- best visual acuity and subjective satisfaction with the old transplant.

In DMEK, we always remove the Descemet membrane of the PKP graft and use an EDM graft that is 0.5 mm smaller. All patients are informed about the increased likelihood of a delayed re-bubbling, which is often necessary. Anterior segment OCT (optical coherence tomography) is routinely recommended prior to indication in order to search for unfavorable posterior steps at the former graft edges (Fig. 26A–E) (Fig. 27A–G) (Video 1).

Please scan to access video content

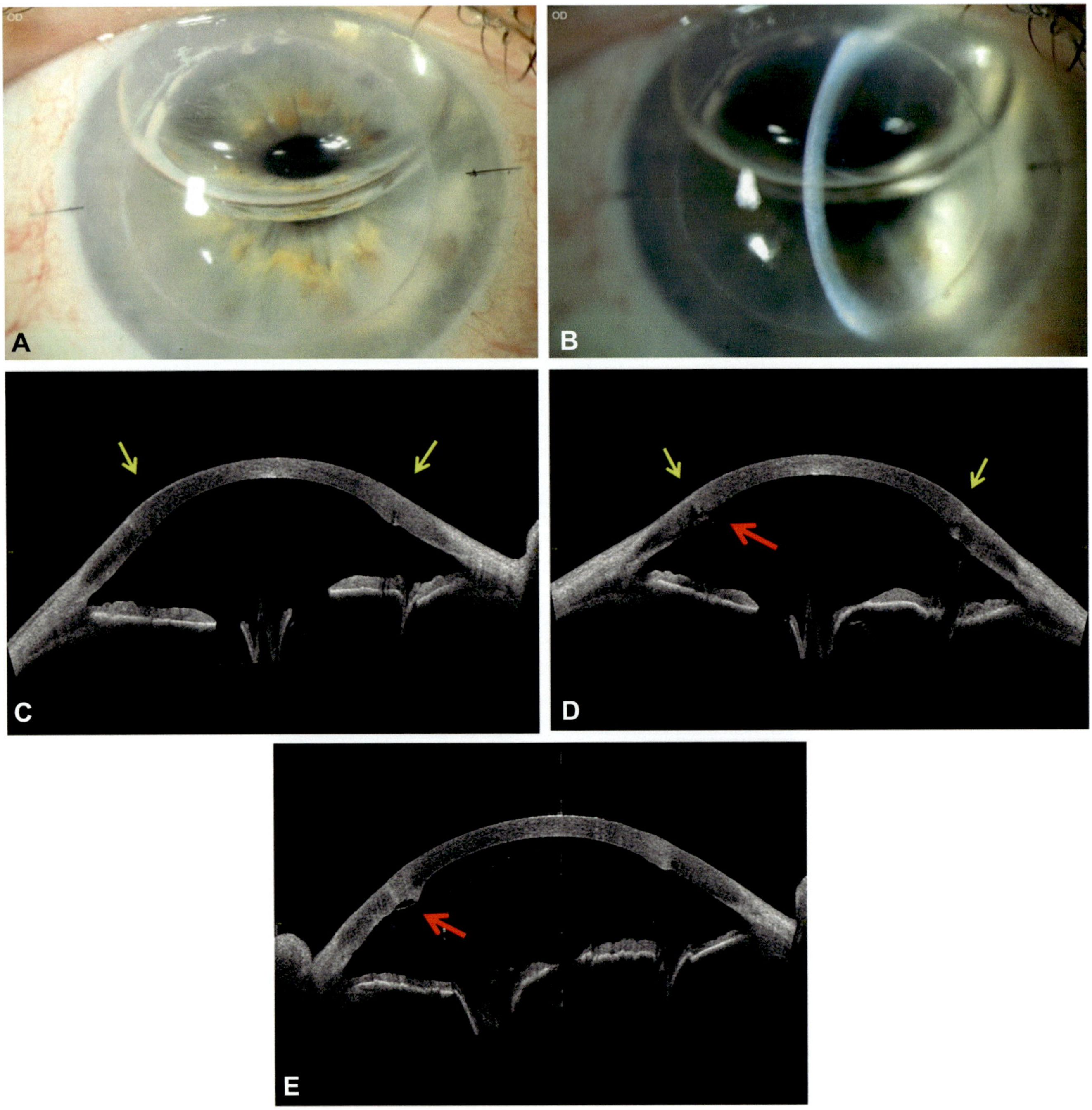

Fig. 26 Slit lamp biomicroscopy ((**A**) overview; (**B**) slit) on day 3 after DMEK (7.5 mm) due to endothelial decompensated excimer laser PKP (8.0/8.1 mm) 11 years previously. The graft is well attached centrally and the 20% SF6 gas bubble fills the anterior chamber to just under 50%. (**C**) Anterior segment OCT (CASIA 2) section from 2 to 8 o'clock: The graft is completely in place, there are no posterior steps in the graft–host interface (yellow arrows). (**D**) Section from 10 to 4 o'clock: partial peripheral graft detachment (red arrow) over a posterior step in the graft–host interface (yellow arrows). Re-bubbling is worth considering here. (**E**) Section from 12 to 6 o'clock: the edge of the EDM nestles around the posterior step. This finding does not require re-bubbling

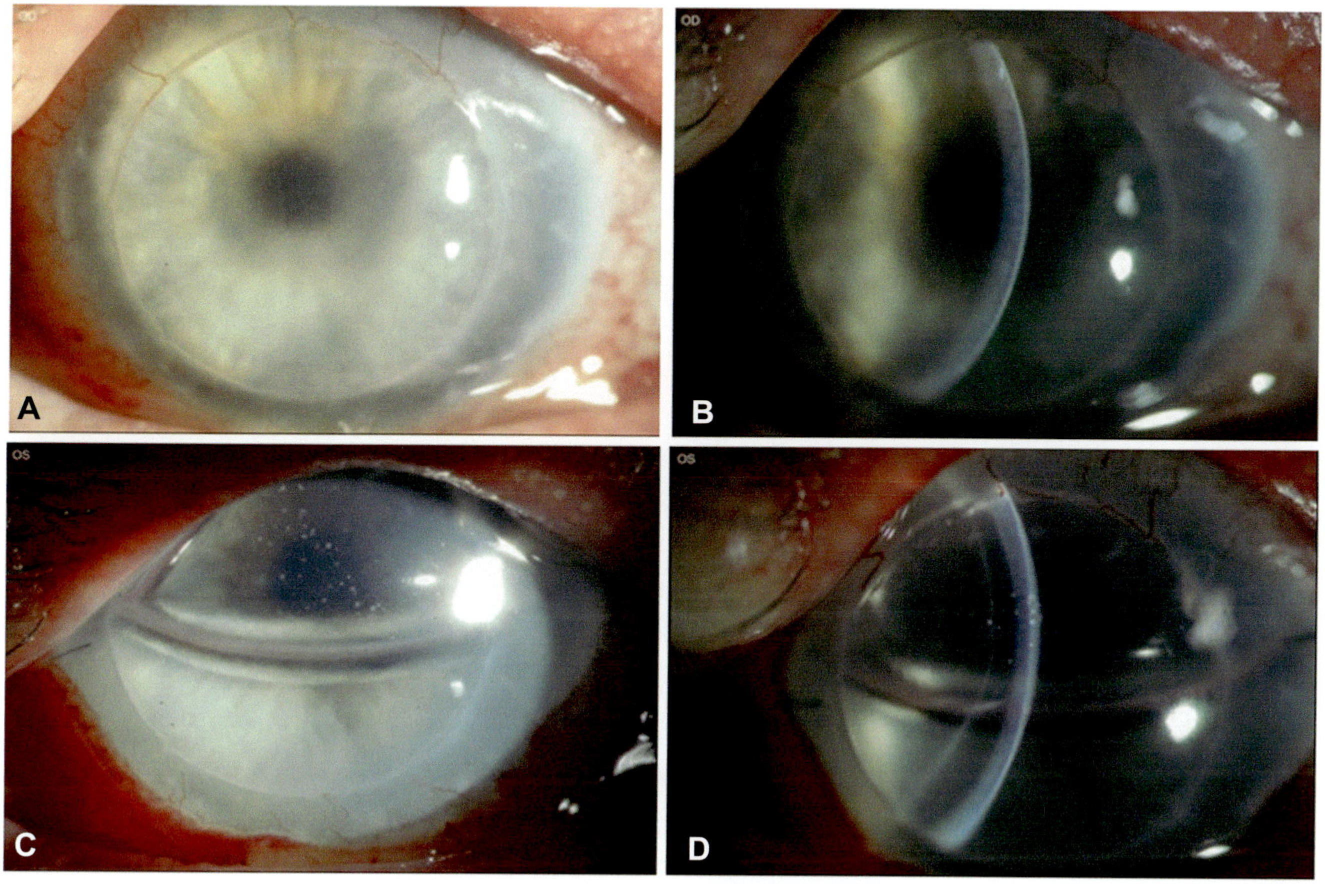

Fig. 27 DMEK 7.5 mm 6 years after failed 8.0 mm penetrating keratoplasty. (**A/B**) Preop overview/thin slit: Visual acuity hand motion, intraocular pressure 14 mmHg, central corneal thickness 1167 μm. (**C/D**) (overview/thin slit) 3 days after DMEK with 20% SF_6 gas bubble still filling half of the anterior chamber, the graft is completely attached

Endothelial cell loss is between 24 and 60% after 1 year [23, 27, 29]. The 4-year survival rate of DMEK versus DSAEK (76% vs. 74%) after a failed PKP was comparable [26]. Previous glaucoma surgery was the only significant risk factor for failure of DMEK after PKP [26].

Quadruple DMEK for endothelial decompensation after implantation of anterior chamber iris claw lens and cataract [52]

Due to a continuous endothelial cell loss, the cornea may decompensate years after implantation of an anterior chamber based iris claw lens. Bullous keratopathy and coexisting cataract can be treated sequentially or—as shown here—with simultaneous release and explantation of the PMMA iris claw lens via "large" incision at 12 o'clock followed by classical Triple-DMEK via small incision from the temporal side (Video 2).

Please scan to access video content

The following known potential postoperative problems with PKP are minimized by the use of DMEK:

- slow and often suboptimal visual recovery,
- high/irregular astigmatism,
- surface problems,
- biomechanical instability,
- endothelial immune reactions,
- suture-associated problems,
- expulsive hemorrhage.

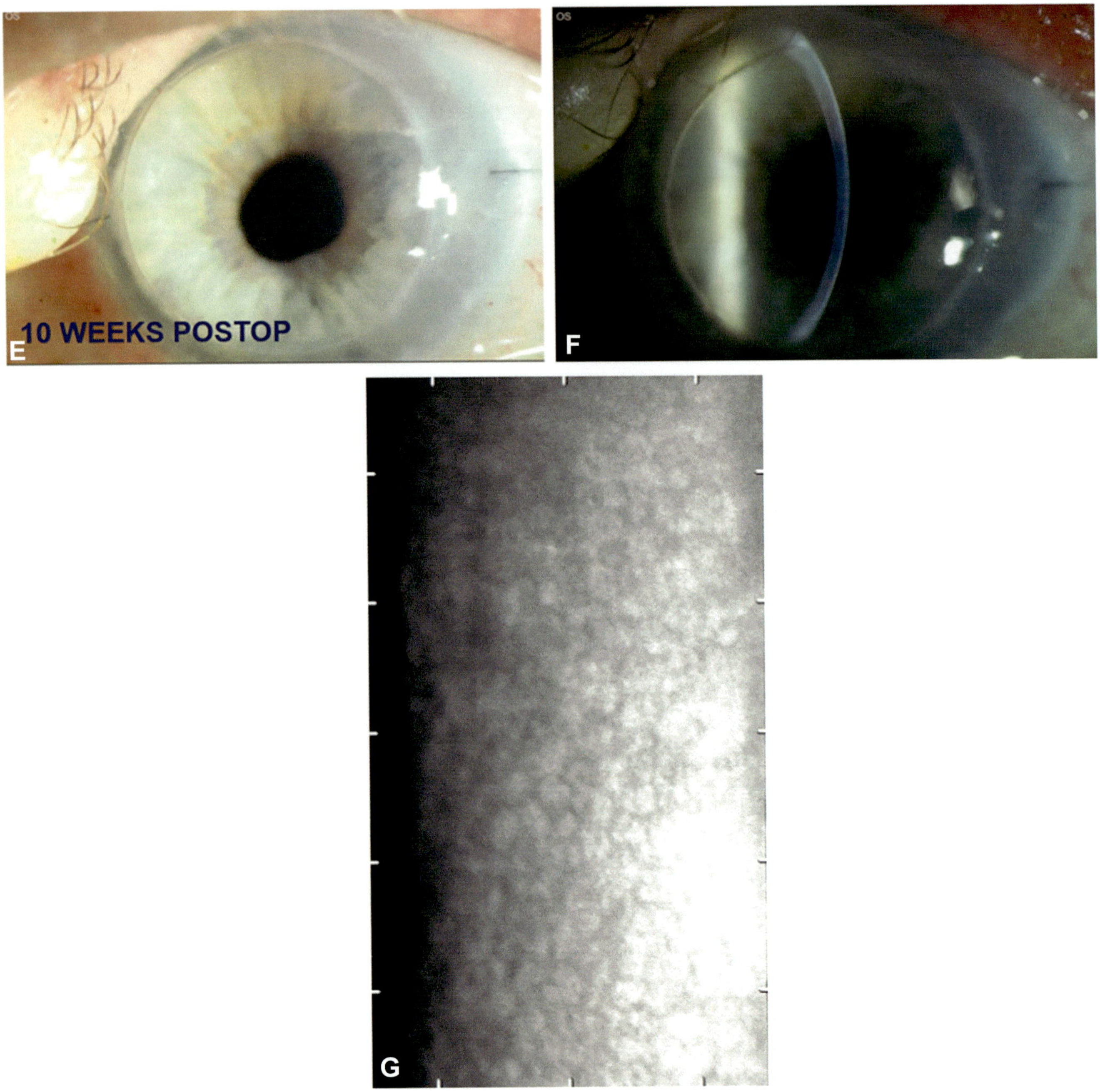

Fig. 27 (**E/F**) (overview/thin slit) 10 weeks postoperatively: visual acuity 20/25, intraocular pressure 9 mmHg, central corneal thickness 581 μm, (**G**) endothelial cell count 1322 cells/mm^2

6 Follow-Up Care

Our current postoperative topical therapy consists of:

- hyperosmolar eye drops 5× for 2 weeks,
- antibiotics 5× for 2 weeks,
- Prednisolone acetate hourly for 1 week to prevent cystoid macular edema [53, 54], then 5 times per day, reduce by 1 drop every 8 weeks—1 drop per day should be continued for at least 2 years [55], in pseudophakic eyes even lifelong if there is no steroid response,
- lubricant as required (typically 5 times a day) due to the accompanying neuroparalytic component after DMEK [3].

To be on the safe side, the patient returns to our department 2 weeks after the operation for a check-up. At this point, we either remove the two single corneoscleral sutures or admit the patient for re-bubbling for 1 night if a (new)

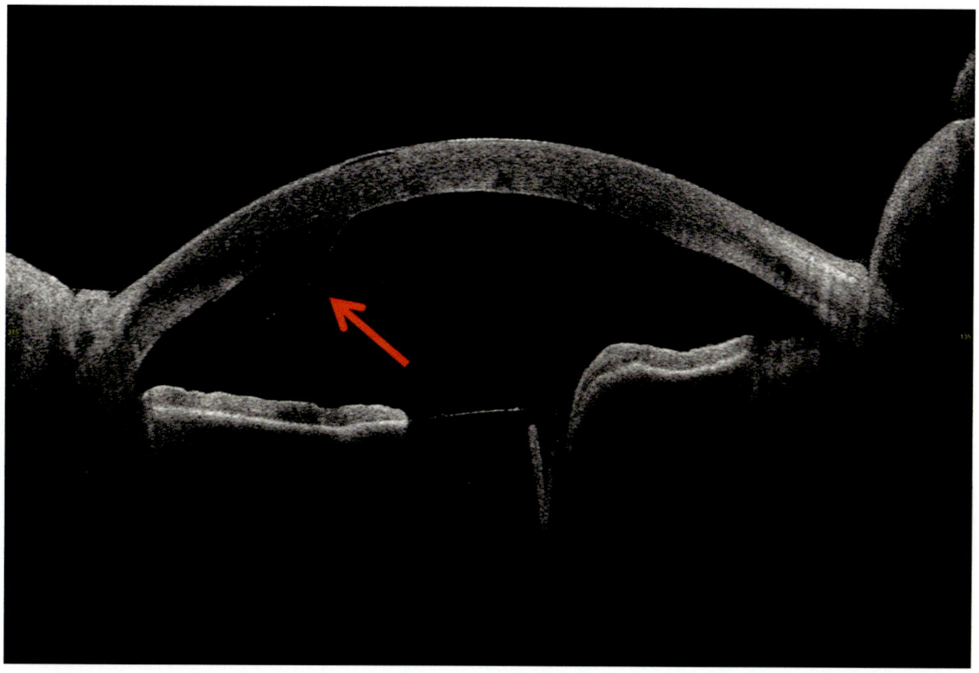

Fig. 28 Anterior segment OCT (CASIA 2): Free peripheral graft detachments (arrow) require re-bubbling because they are often progressive

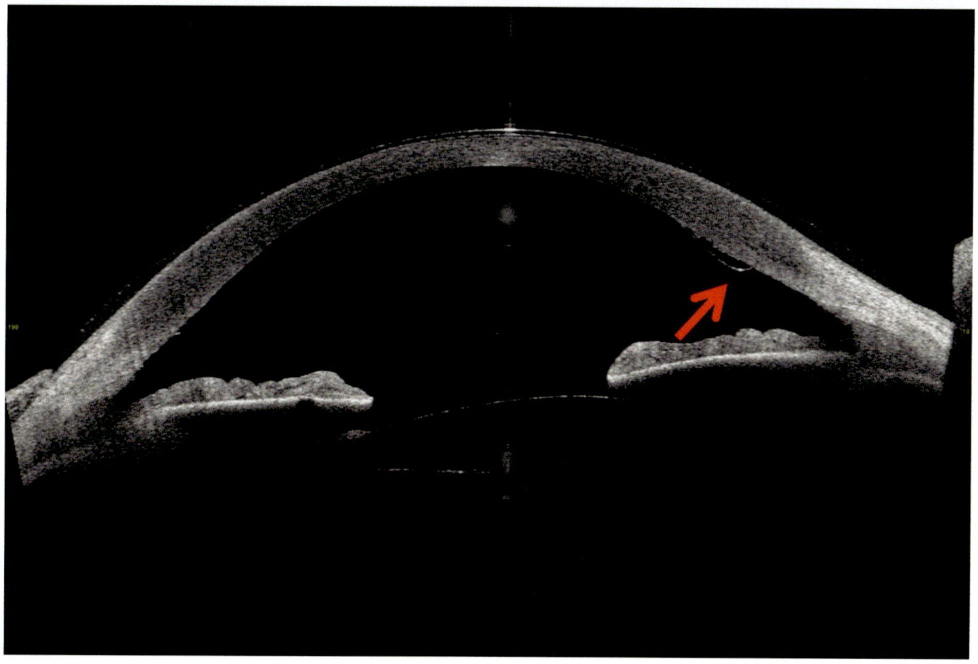

Fig. 29 Anterior segment OCT (CASIA 2): Closed peripheral graft detachments (arrow) do not require re-bubbling because they are often regressive

Table 1 Pre- and postoperative routine corneal diagnostics 2, 6 weeks, 6 months, 1 year, then annually after DMEK

• Best-corrected visual acuity
• Slit lamp biomicroscopy
• Intraocular pressure (IOP)
• Pentacam tomography (curvature/thickness)
• Endothelial cell specular microscopy (number, size, shape of endothelial cells and presence of transplanted guttae [57]
• Anterior segment OCT to assess the peripheral adhesion of the graft over 360°
• Macula OCT to detect cystoid macular edema!

graft dehiscence is present (Fig. 28). Sealed peripheral graft detachments do not require re-bubbling because they are often regressive (Fig. 29) [56].

To reduce the risk of complications, the surgeon should note in the file at the end of DMEK which of the existing paracenteses should be used for de- and re-bubbling. Due to the potential for gas expansion, 90% filling of the anterior chamber with 20% SF6 gas is preferred. It is best to use the pre-existing paracentesis opposite the area of partial EDM detachment for re-bubbling to avoid iatrogenic folding of the graft or enlargement of the descemetolysis. The next outpatient follow-up examinations take place at 2 weeks, 6 weeks, 6 months and 1 year and then annually (Table 1). After 6 to 12 weeks, glasses can already be prescribed—unlike after PKP.

A macular OCT is performed before discharge and during early outpatient follow-up examinations in order to detect cystoid macular edema immediately and treat it if necessary [53, 54].

The rate of immune reactions is realistically between 2 and 3% after 3 years. These are often not noticed by the patients [55, 58]. Therefore, we consistently prescribe 1 drop of prednisolone acetate or dexamethasone phosphate (no fluorometholone, no NSAIDs ["nonsteroidal anti-inflammatory drugs"]) for more than 2 years. In addition to topical and systemic steroids, the intracameral administration of fortecortin has proven effective in the acute stage of graft rejection in our experience [59]. Recurrent graft failures may result from viral endotheliitis which not rarely mask as endothelial immune reaction [21, 60].

The following patient instruction is absolutely necessary on a repetitive basis: If

- visual acuity begins to deteriorate (especially in the morning),
- the patient sees halos around light sources,
- a segmental opacity occurs in the field of vision or
- increased sensitivity to glare,
- the eye is red or painful,

the patient should see an ophthalmologist or come to our department immediately.

7 Conclusion

- Nowadays, DMEK ("Descemet membrane endothelial keratoplasty") is the method of choice in Germany for isolated endothelial defects without stromal scarring.
- The technique described should be easy to understand and simple to repeat, it is reliable and requires as little "individual artwork" as possible.
- In any case, we mark the DMEK donor with 3 asymmetrical semicircles at the edge according to Bachmann, Cursiefen and Kruse in order to be able to determine the graft orientation in the anterior chamber without any doubt.
- To reduce the rate of re-bubbling, we routinely use 20% SF6 (sulphur hexafluoride) gas at the end of the DMEK procedure and then recommend that the patient lies on the back or alternates between lying on either side for several days.
- We recommend DMEK for faster visual recovery in cases of endothelial decompensation of the graft after penetrating keratoplasty (PKP) if there are no stromal scars and the patient was previously satisfied with his graft.

References

1. Melles GR. Descemet membrane endothelial keratoplasty (DMEK). Cornea. 2006;25:987–90.
2. Maier P, Reinhard T, Cursiefen C. Descemet stripping endothelial keratoplasty-rapid recovery of visual acuity. Dtsch Arztebl. 2013;110(21):365–71.
3. Matthaei M, Schrittenlocher S, Hos D, Siebelmann S, Bucher F, Schaub F, Hoerster R, Siggel R, Roters S, Heindl LM, Bachmann B, Cursiefen C. 10 years of Descemet membrane endothelial keratoplasty in Fuchs endothelial corneal dystrophy: What have we learned? Ophthalmologe. 2019; 116:236–42.
4. Flockerzi E, Maier P, Böhringer D, Reinshagen H, Kruse F, Cursiefen C, Reinhard T, Geerling G, Torun N, Seitz B, all German Keratoplasty Registry Contributors. Trends in corneal transplantation from 2001 to 2016 in Germany-a report of the section DOG-Cornea and its keratoplasty registry. Am J Ophthalmol. 2018; 188:91–8.

5. Spaniol K, Hellmich M, Borgardts K, Reinhard T, Joussen A, Bartz-Schmidt KU, Wiedemann P, Seitz B, Schrittenlocher S, Cursiefen C, Bachmann B, Geerling G. DMEK outcome after one year-results of a large multicenter study in Germany. Acta Ophthalmol. 2023;101:e215–25.
6. Flockerzi E, Turner C, Seitz B, GeKeR Study Group Collaborators. Descemet's Membrane Endothelial Keratoplasty is the predominant keratoplasty procedure in Germany since 2016: a report of the DOG-Section Cornea and its Keratoplasty Registry. Br J Ophthalmol. 2024; 108:646–653.
7. Pluzsik ML, Seitz B, Flockerzi FA, Langenbucher A, Tóth G, Bohle RM, Szentmáry N. Changing trends in penetrating keratoplasty indications in Homburg/Saar between 2011 and 2018-histopathology of 2123 corneal buttons. Curr Eye Res. 2020;13:1–6.
8. Seitz B, Lisch W, Weiss J. The revised newest IC^{3}D classification of corneal dystrophies. Klin Monbl Augenheilkd. 2015;232:283–94.
9. Wacker K, Reinhard T, Maier P. Pathogenesis and diagnostic evaluation of Fuchs' endothelial corneal dystrophy. Ophthalmologe. 2019;116:221–7.
10. Anshu A, Price MO, Tan D, Price FW Jr. Endothelial keratoplasty: a revolution in evolution. Surv Ophthalmol. 2012;57:236–52.
11. Kruse FE, Laaser K, Cursiefen C, Heindl LM, Schlötzer-Schrehardt U, Riss S, Bachmann BO. A stepwise approach to donor preparation and insertion increases safety and outcome of DMEK. Cornea. 2011;30:580–7.
12. Price FW Jr, Price MO. Descemet's stripping with endothelial keratoplasty in 200 eyes: early challenges and techniques to enhance donor adherence. J Cataract Refract Surg. 2006;32:411–8.
13. Terry MA, Straiko MD, Veldman PB, Talajic JC, VanZyl C, Sales CS, Mayko ZM. Standardized DMEK technique reducing complications using prestripped tissue, novel glass injector, and sulfurhexafluoride (SF6) gas. Cornea. 2015;34:845–52.
14. Birbal RS, Baydoun L, Ham L, Miron A, van Dijk K, Dapena I, Jager MJ, Böhringer S, Oellerich S, Melles GRJ. Effect of surgical indication and preoperative lens status on Descemet membrane endothelial keratoplasty outcomes. Am J Ophthalmol. 2020;212:79–87.
15. Seitz B, Daas L, Bischoff-Jung M, Szentmáry N, Suffo S, El-Husseiny M, Viestenz A, Milioti G. Anatomy-based DMEK-Wetlab in Homburg/Saar–novel aspects of donor preparation and host maneuvers to teach Descemet membrane endothelial keratoplasty. Clin Anat. 2018;31:16–27.
16. Seitz B, Daas L, Flockerzi E, Suffo S. Descemet membrane endothelial keratoplasty DMEK-Donor and recipient step by step. Ophthalmologe. 2020;117:811–28.
17. Stuhlmacher ES, Suffo S, Munteanu C, Seitz B, Daas L. Assessing the learning curve for DMEK using post-procedural clinical outcomes-Comparison of four different surgeons during two different time periods. J Clin Med. 2023;12(3):811.
18. Seitz B, Hager T. Clinical phenotypes of Fuchs endothelial corneal dystrophy (FECD), disease progression, differential diagnosis, and medical therapy. In: Cursiefen C, Jun A (Hrsg) Current treatment options for Fuchs endothelial dystrophy. Springer International Publishing Switzerland, 2017. S. 25–50.
19. Berger T, Seitz B, Löw U, Flockerzi FA, Schlötzer-Schrehardt, Daas L. Descemet Membrane Endothelial Keratoplasty (DMEK) for severe verrucous posterior polymorphous corneal dystrophy with light and electron microscopic examination. Klin Monbl Augenheilkd. 2024; 241:1081–1090.
20. Asi F, Milioti G, Seitz B. Descemet membrane endothelial keratoplasty for corneal decompensation caused by herpes simplex virus endotheliitis. J Cataract Refract Surg. 2018;44:106–8.
21. Matar C, Seitz B, Daas L. Recurrent DMEK failure. Ophthalmologe. 2021; 118:719–23.
22. Asi F, Daas L, Milioti G, Seitz B. The new-triple Descemet membrane endothelial Keratoplasty (DMEK) as successful surgical option for Haab's striae with corneal decompensation in congenital glaucoma. JCRS Online Case Rep. 2019;7(3):38–41.
23. Alió del Barrio JL, Montesel A, Ho V, Bhogal M. Descemet membrane endothelial keratoplasty under failed penetrating keratoplasty without host descemetorhexis for the management of secondary graft failure. Cornea. 2020; 39:13–7.
24. Ang M, Ho H, Wong C, Htoon HM, Mehta JS, Tan D. Endothelial keratoplasty after failed penetrating keratoplasty: an alternative to repeat penetrating keratoplasty. Am J Ophthalmol. 2014;158:1221–7.
25. Heinzelmann S, Böhringer D, Eberwein P, Lapp T, Reinhard T, Maier P. Descemet membrane endothelial keratoplasty for graft failure following penetrating keratoplasty. Graefes Arch Clin Exp Ophthalmol. 2017;255:979–85.
26. Pasari A, Price MO, Feng MT, Price FW Jr. Descemet membrane endothelial keratoplasty for failed penetrating keratoplasty: visual outcomes and graft survival. Cornea. 2019;38:151–6.
27. Pierné K, Panthier C, Courtin R, Mazharian A, Souedan V, Gatinel D, Saad A. Descemet membrane endothelial keratoplasty after failed penetrating keratoplasty. Cornea. 2019; 38:280–4.
28. Seitz B, Daas L, Wykrota AA, Flockerzi E, Suffo S. Graft failure after PKP and DMEK: What is the best option? Klin Monbl Augenheilkd. 2022;239:775–85.
29. Wykrota A, Hamon L, Daas L, Seitz B. Descemt Membrane Endothelial Keratoplasty DMEK after failed penetrating keratoplasty-case series and review of the literature. BMC Ophthalmol. 2024;24(1):15.
30. Bachmann B, Schrittenlocher S, Matthaei M, Siebelmann S, Cursiefen C. Descemet membrane endothelial keratoplasty in complex eyes. Ophthalmologe. 2019;116:228–35.
31. Weller JM, Tourtas T, Kruse FE. Feasibility and outcome of Descemet membrane endothelial keratoplasty in complex anterior segment and vitreous disease. Cornea. 2015;34:1351–7.
32. Aljundi W, Abdin AD, Suffo S, Seitz B, Daas L. Descemet membrane endothelial keratoplasty (DMEK) in previously vitrectomized eyes: techniques, complications and clinical outcome. Klin Monbl Augenheilkd. 2021;238:1101–7.
33. Alfaro Rangel R, Szentmàry N, Lepper S, Daas L, Langenbucher A, Seitz B. 8.5/8.6-mm excimer laser assisted penetrating keratoplasties in a tertiary corneal subspecialty referral center-indications and outcomes in 107 eyes. Cornea. 2020; 39:806–11.
34. Szentmáry N, Seitz B, Langenbucher A, Naumann GOH. Repeat keratoplasty for correction of high or irregular post keratoplasty astigmatism in clear corneal grafts. Am J Ophthalmol. 2005;139:826–30.
35. Price MO, Giebel AW, Fairchild KM, Price FW Jr. Descemet's membrane endothelial keratoplasty: prospective multicenter study of visual and refractive outcomes and endothelial survival. Ophthalmology. 2009;116:2361–8.
36. Heinzelmann S, Böhringer D, Eberwein P, Reinhard T, Maier P. Graft dislocation and graft failure following Descemet membrane endothelial keratoplasty (DMEK) using precut tissue: a retrospective cohort study. Graefes Arch Clin Exp Ophthalmol. 2017;255:127–33.
37. Safi T, Seitz B, Berg K, Schulz K, Langenbucher A, Daas L. Reproducibility of non-invasive endothelial cell loss assessment on the prestripped DMEK roll after preparation and storage. Am J Ophthalmol. 2021;221:17–26.
38. Berg K, Safi T, Seitz B, Daas L. Non-invasive endothelial cell density measurement of the in toto pre-stripped DMEK roll-Impact of pre- and intraoperative endothelial cell loss on postoperative mid-term clinical outcome. Eye (Lond). 2023;37:2956–62.
39. Abdin A, Daas L, Pattmöller M. Negative impact of dextran in organ culture media for pre-stripped tissue preservation on DMEK

(Descemet membrane endothelial keratoplasty) outcome. Graefes Arch Clin Exp Ophthalmol. 2018; 256:2135–214.
40. Wykrota AA, Weinstein I, Hamon L, Daas L, Flockerzi E, Suffo S, Seitz B. Approval rates for corneal donation and the origin of donor tissue for transplantation at a university based tertiary referral center with corneal subspecialisation hosting a LIONS Eye Bank. BMC Ophthalmol. 2022;22(1):17.
41. Schoenberg ED, Price FW Jr, Miller J, McKee Y, Price MO. Refractive outcomes of Descemet membrane endothelial keratoplasty triple procedures (combined with cataract surgery). J Cataract Refract Surg. 2015;41:1182–9.
42. Heinzelmann S, Hüther S, Böhringer D, Eberwein P, Reinhard T, Maier P. Influence of donor characteristics on Descemet membrane endothelial keratoplasty. Cornea. 2014;33:644–8.
43. Lie JT, Birbal R, Ham L, van der Wees J, Melles GR. Donor tissue preparation for Descemet membrane endothelial keratoplasty. J Cataract Refract Surg. 2008;34:1578–83.
44. Yoeruek E, Hofmann J, Bartz-Schmidt KU. Comparison of swollen and dextran deswollen organ cultured corneas for Descemet membrane dissection preparation: histologic and ultrastructural findings. Invest Ophthalmol Vis Sci. 2013;54:8036–40.
45. Greiner MA, Rixen JJ, Wagoner MD, Schmidt GA, Stoeger CG, Straiko MD, Zimmerman MB, Kitzmann AS, Goins KM. Diabetes mellitus increases risk of unsuccessful graft preparation in Descemet membrane endothelial keratoplasty: a multicenter study. Cornea. 2014;33:1129–33.
46. Trouvain AM, Szurman P, Wahl S, Siegel R, Boden KT, Seitz B, Rickmann A. Impact of previous cataract surgery in corneal donors on the outcome of Descemet Membrane Endothelial Keratoplasty (DMEK). Cornea. 2024; 43:844–852.
47. Bayyoud T, Röck D, Hofmann J, Bartz-Schmidt KU, Yoeruek E. Precut technique for Descemet's membrane endothelial keratoplasty, preparation and storage in organ culture. Klin Monbl Augenheilkd. 2012;229:621–3.
48. Menzel-Severing J, Walter P, Plum WJ, Kruse FE, Salla S. Assessment of corneal endothelium during continued organ culture of pre-stripped human donor tissue for DMEK surgery. Curr Eye Res. 2018;43:1439–44.
49. Bachmann BO, Laaser K, Cursiefen C, Kruse FE. A method to confirm correct orientation of Descemet membrane during Descemet membrane endothelial keratoplasty. Am J Ophthalmol. 2010;149:922–5.
50. Hayashi T, Kobayashi A. Double-bubble technique in Descemet membrane endothelial keratoplasty for vitrectomized eyes: a case series. Cornea. 2018;37:1185–8.
51. Schönit S, Maamri A, Zemova E, Munteanu C, Safi T, Daas L, Seitz B. Prevalence and impact of corneal guttata in the graft following penetrating keratoplasty. Cornea. 2022;41:1495–502.
52. Mergen B, Berger T, Hamon L, Daas L, Seitz B. Anterior chamber intraocular lens removal combined with triple DMEK: Quadruple DMEK for bullous keratopathy. Eur J Ophthalmol. 2024; 34:NP13–NP17.
53. Heinzelmann S, Maier P, Böhringer D, Hüther S, Eberwein P, Reinhard T. Cystoid macular oedema following Descemet membrane endothelial keratoplasty. Br J Ophthalmol. 2015;99:98–102.
54. Hoerster R, Stanzel TP, Bachmann BO, Siebelmann S, Felsch M, Cursiefen C. Intensified topical steroids as prophylaxis for macular edema after posterior lamellar keratoplasty combined with cataract surgery. Am J Ophthalmol. 2016;163:174–9.
55. Hos D, Tuac O, Schaub F, Stanzel TP, Schrittenlocher S, Hellmich M, Bachmann BO, Cursiefen C. Incidence and clinical course of immune reactions after Descemet membrane endothelial keratoplasty: retrospective analysis of 1000 consecutive eyes. Ophthalmology. 2017;124:512–8.
56. Menkene LM, Berger T, Safi T, Hamon L, Munteanu C, Seitz B, Daas L. Analysis of graft detachments and re-bubblings after 450 descemet membrane endothelial keratoplasty procedures. Cornea. 2024; 43:1115–1123.
57. Schmitz LM, Safi T, Munteanu C, Seitz B, Daas L. Prevalence and severity of cornea guttata in the graft following Descemet Membrane Endothelial Keratoplasty (DMEK). Acta Ophthalmol. 2022;100:e1737–45.
58. Anshu A, Price MO, Price FW Jr. Risk of corneal transplant rejection significantly reduced with Descemet's membrane endothelial keratoplasty. Ophthalmology. 2012;119:536–40.
59. Fiorentzis M, Viestenz AR, Viestenz AN, Seitz B. Intracameral dexamethason injection as adjuvant therapy in endothelial immune reaction after penetrating and posterior lamellar keratoplasty: a retrospective clinical observation. Adv Ther. 2017;34:1928–35.
60. Abu Dail Y, Daas L, Flockerzi E, Munteanu C, Smola S, Seitz B. Herpes PCR in aqueous humor samples from patients with and without clinical corneal endothelial graft rejection. J Med Virol. 2024; 96:e29538.

Descemet Stripping Only DSO

Friedrich E. Kruse, Julia M. Weller, Ursula Schlötzer-Schrehardt, and Theofilos Tourtas

Abstract

Descemet Stripping Only (DSO), alternatively termed Descemetorhexis Without Endothelial Keratoplasty (DWEK), is a relatively novel surgical approach for the treatment of Fuchs endothelial corneal dystrophy. The underlying rationale of this procedure is to remove the central area of diseased endothelial cell-Descemet membrane complex to allow the healthier peripheral cells to repopulate the bare corneal stroma, avoiding the need to insert a donor graft. Thus, DSO is currently indicated in patients with early Fuchs dystrophy, central guttae and a healthy endothelial cell reservoir in the periphery. Current evidence suggests that the size of the central descemetorhexis should be limited to 4 mm, allowing central migration of peripheral endothelial cells, resolution of corneal edema and increase in visual acuity in the majority of treated patients. Time to corneal clearance and visual recovery may be accelerated by the use of topical Rho kinase (ROCK) inhibitors as adjunctive treatment after DSO. However, long-term clinical studies have to show whether DSO can provide lasting visual outcomes similar to Descemet Membrane Endothelial Keratoplasty (DMEK), or whether recurrence of guttae and endothelial dysfunction will occur.

Keywords

Descemet Stripping Only · DSO · Descemetorhexis without Endothelial Keratoplasty · DWEK · Descemetorhexis · Fuchs dystrophy · ROCK inhibitor; · Endothelial cell migration

F. E. Kruse (✉) · J. M. Weller · U. Schlötzer-Schrehardt · T. Tourtas
Department of Ophthalmology, Friedrich-Alexander University Erlangen-Nürnberg, Erlangen, Germany
e-mail: friedrich.kruse@uk-erlangen.de

1 The Concept

Ophthalmic surgeons have been performing corneal transplantation for more than a century. Ever since two major problems associated with corneal transplantation have been addressed by numerous researchers in an attempt to improve the outcome of this procedure. One major problem is related to the optical properties which are resulting from the presence of a graft in the donor eye. The second major problem is related to the fact that foreign tissue has to be transferred from a donor to a recipient.

In patients suffering from a pathology which is limited to one of the layers of the cornea the concept of lamellar corneal surgery can be applied. In patients with disorders of the corneal endothelium—namely Fuchs endothelial dystrophy or pseudophakic bullous keratopathy—lamellar surgery has been a game changer regarding the optical properties of the graft: Descemet Stripping Automated Endothelial Keratoplasty (DSAEK) introduced by Gorovoy largely eliminates the problem of postoperative corneal astigmatism [1]. Furthermore, Descemet Membrane Endothelial Keratoplasty (DMEK) as described by Melles even eliminates surgically induced higher order aberrations of the posterior surface of the cornea thus allowing corneal grafts without the induction of refractive errors [2, 3].

Up to now foreign tissue has to be utilized for replacement of the diseased corneal tissue. The risk of immunological graft rejection after DMEK is less frequent than after penetrating corneal surgery or after DSAEK and consequently the use of postoperative steroids can be reduced. However, both immunological problems as well as the possibility of disease transmission by infected corneal grafts, most notably fungal endophthalmitis, persist [4, 5]. Thus, elimination of the need for a transplant would greatly improve the safety of corneal surgery for disorders limited to the corneal endothelium.

The concept of "Descemet Stripping Only (DSO)" relies on the ability of healthy corneal endothelial cells in

B. Seitz et al. (eds.), *Atlas on Cornea*, https://doi.org/10.1007/978-3-031-65422-0_52

the periphery of the cornea of the host to replace diseased cells which are removed from the center during corneal surgery. This concept is based on three findings which reflect a fundamental change in the way corneal specialists understand both Fuchs dystrophy and the biology of the corneal endothelium: First, we have learned that visual impairment in patients with Fuchs dystrophy is due to (confluent) guttae of Descemet membrane prior to the onset of corneal edema [6]. Thus, most patients who seek the help of an ophthalmologist due to problems with glare and contrast sensitivity suffer from cornea guttata rather than from corneal edema. Second, observation at the slit lamp reveals that the process of the formation of guttae (reflected by their number and density) starts in the center of the cornea while Descemet membrane in the periphery remains unremarkable. Thus, a subset of patients with Fuchs dystrophy becomes symptomatic due to central guttae without manifestation of the disease in the periphery. Therefore, for clinical characterization patients with Fuchs dystrophy can be classified in two groups: One in which guttae are evenly distributed over the entire cornea (Fig. 1A) and another (much smaller) group in which the formation of guttae is limited to the central cornea (Fig. 1E). Third, there is increasing evidence that human corneal endothelial cells can migrate on the inner surface of the corneal stroma in the absence of corneal endothelium. Among other findings, the concept of migration of corneal endothelial cells—which is in contrast to the traditional belief of a stationary endothelium—is supported by the surgical concept of using undersized grafts: Melles has proposed to use quarter DMEK tissue for routine surgery and has shown migration of endothelial cells from such grafts onto the denuded corneal surface [7]. Similarly, we have shown by specular microscopy that endothelial cells from the donor repopulate the denuded corneal stroma shortly after DMEK surgery [8].

Taken together, the concept of DSO suggests that patients with central guttae and healthy appearing periphery (Fig. 1E) can be treated by removal of the (central) affected Descemet membrane (Fig. 1F). Following surgery, it is hypothesized that migration of the unaffected healthy cells in the periphery gradually migrate onto the denuded corneal stroma (Fig. 1G) until the space is filled (Fig. 1H) and the integrity of the corneal stroma is restored. In contrast, the majority of the symptomatic patients with Fuchs dystrophy present with confluent guttae extending to the peripheral cornea (Fig. 1A). In these patients the central Descemet membrane is removed (Fig. 1B) followed by placement of a graft of slightly smaller dimensions (Fig. 1C). Shortly after surgery the gap between the graft and the host tissue is filled by migration from the graft (Fig. 1D).

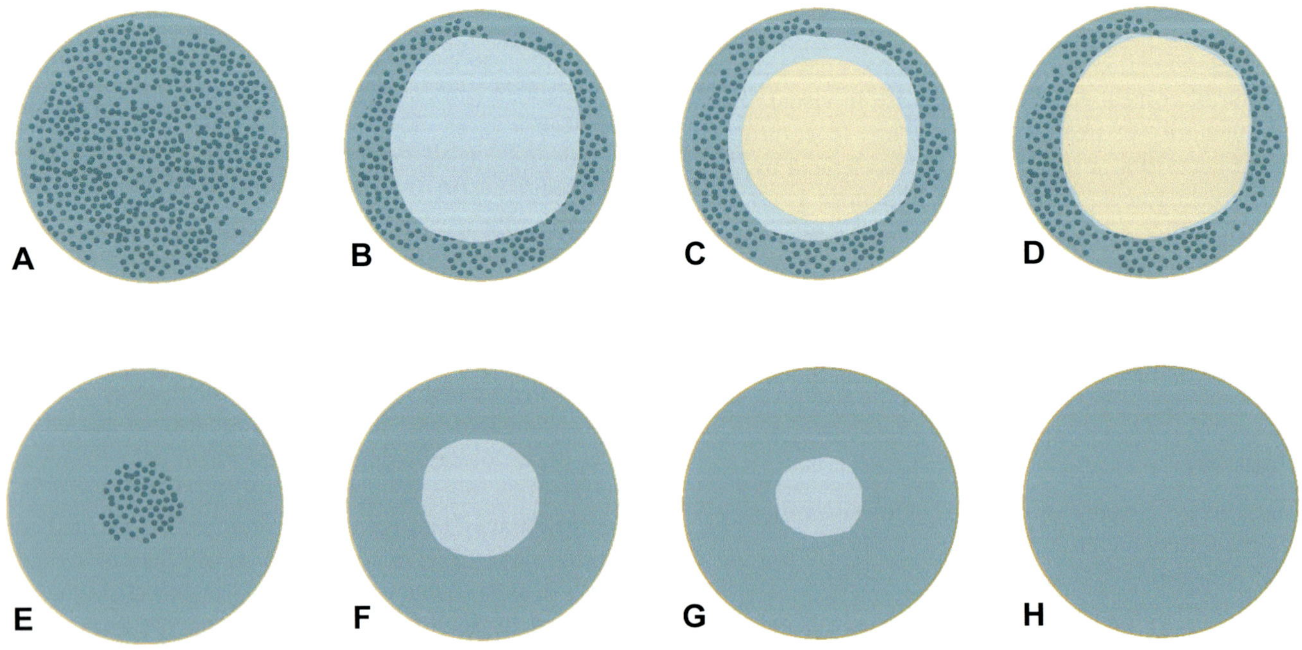

Fig. 1 Schematic diagram illustrating the concept of DSO in two groups of patients with Fuchs dystrophy showing either formation of guttae in the entire corneal endothelium (**A–D**) or limited to the central cornea (**E–H**). In patients with confluent guttae (**A**), the central Descemet membrane (light blue) is removed (**B**), followed by placement of a slightly smaller graft (yellow) (**C**) with its healthy endothelial cells filling the gap between graft and host cornea by migration (**D**). In patients with central guttae (**E**), the central 4 mm of affected Descemet membrane is removed (**F**), followed by migration of healthy endothelial cells from the periphery to the central stroma (**G**) until the space is filled (**H**)

2 Historical Perspective and Nomenclature

Removal of the corneal endothelium was presumably first described in 1953 by Lois Paufique who scraped the posterior surface of 3 patients with advanced Fuchs dystrophy and observed migration upon investigation of corneal buttons following penetrating grafts is these patients [9]. However, this was done in the absence of a clear understanding of the role of the corneal endothelium. Thus, the merit of proposing the concept has to be attributed to Gabriel van Rij who at the occasion of the 2013 EuCornea meeting described a small series of patients in which he had performed Descemet stripping [10]. The use of stripping the central Descemet membrane as a therapeutic measure for Fuchs dystrophy was then simultaneously described by Kathy Colby who used the term "Descemet Stripping Without Endothelial Keratoplasty" and by George Molony who coined the term "Descemetorhexis Without Grafting" [11, 12]. In an effort to standardize nomenclature, Kaufman suggested to use the term "Descemetorhexis Without Endothelial Keratoplasty (DWEK)" [13]. The term "Descemet Stripping Only (DSO)" is currently used by most authors to describe the treatment of patients with Fuchs dystrophy and central guttae by removal of the central Descemet membrane, especially after Kathy Colby in 2022 published an Editorial in the journal Cornea summarizing her experience with DSO [14].

3 Technique

The principle of DSO is simple and solely requires removal of the central Descemet membrane. Based on the biological principle of creating an empty space of corneal stroma devoid of endothelial cells to allow migration of healthy cells onto the stromal surface, removal of the diseased Descemet membrane should be performed as atraumatic as possible. Damage to the corneal stroma inadvertently results in scarring and possible also in delay of migration.

There is only one publication which is exclusively devoted to the technical aspects of DSO describing the "two flap" technique as illustrated in Fig. 2 [15]. Past experience with DSO indicates that the size of removal is important for the outcome of the procedure as illustrated below. Current evidence suggests that the size of the removal should be limited to 4 mm. Therefore, initial step of the surgery is to mark the area of removal. This can be either achieved by use of an ink-marked caliper set at 4 mm or—in our experience more conveniently—by using a 4 mm trephine (Fig. 2B).

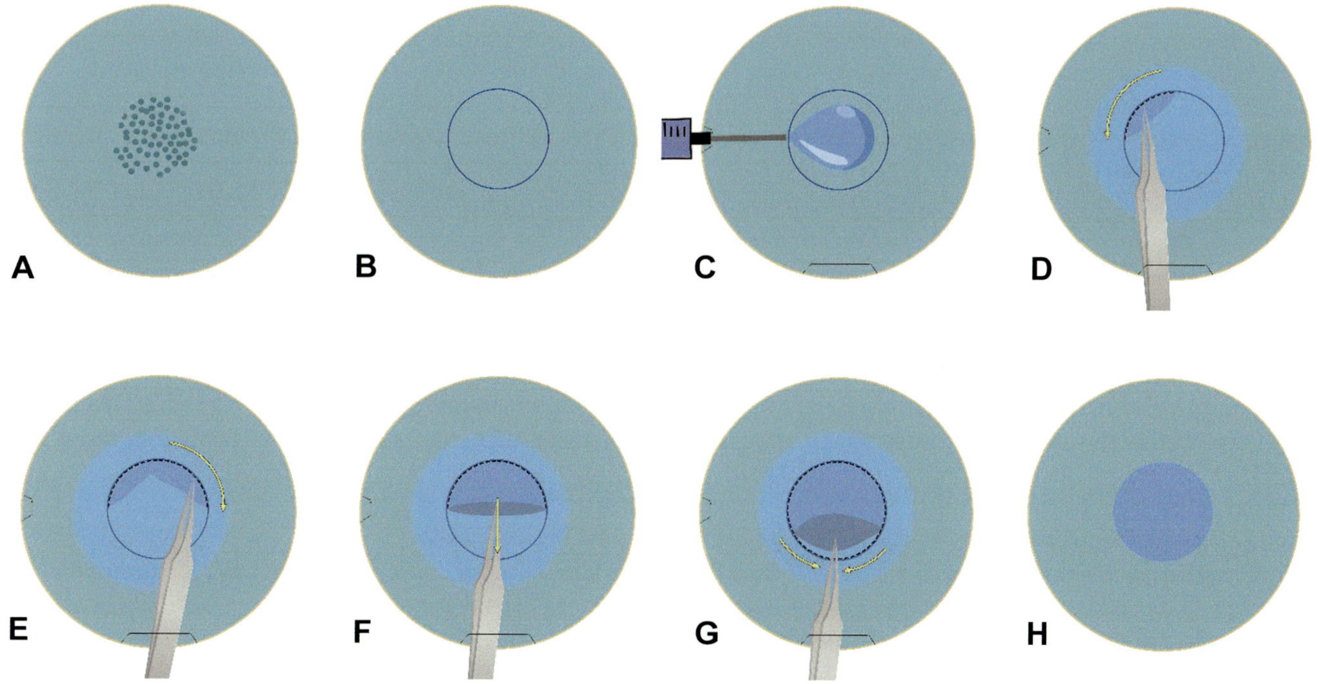

Fig. 2 Schematic diagram illustrating the two-flap technique of DSO according to Cohen et al. (2021). (**A**) Eye with guttae limited to central corneal endothelium. (**B**) Marking of removal area by a 4 mm trephine. (**C**) Creation of a corneal tunnel and injection of cohesive viscoelastic. (**D**) Creation of the first flap using inverted forceps in an anti-clockwise fashion. (**E**) Creation of the second flap in a clockwise fashion. (**F**) Descemet stripping by pulling down from center. (**G**), (**H**) Completion of descemetorhexis by moving in a clock/anti-clockwise fashion

A corneal tunnel is than constructed either in the 12 o'clock position or temporally and a cohesive viscoelastic is injected in the anterior chamber (Fig. 2C). The next step involves creation of a small nick in Descemet membrane to allow is removal. This step seems to be critical and can be performed by either inverted hook or special forceps (Fig. 2C). Such forceps have been described by several surgeons (in alphabetical order: Guell, Govoroy, Hoffnann, Kinoshita, Kobayashi, Pineda, Tan, Villarubia) and manufactured by several specialized companies (e.g. in alphabetical order Corza Medical, U.S.A., Duckworth and Kent, Great Britain; Geuder, Germany; Moria, France; MicroSurgical Technology, U.S.A.). As suggested by Cohen et al. [15] the membrane is than grasped and a flap is created by an anti-clockwise sideward movement over 3 clock hours (Fig. 2D). The membrane is than released and a second flap is created in a clockwise fashion starting from the initial nick and extending also over 3 clock hours (Fig. 2E). The Descemet membrane is then engaged in the center and pulled down (Fig. 2F). Descemetorhexis is finally completed by sideward movements towards the center (Fig. 2G and H).

4 Postoperative Course

Retroillumination is of great help to visualize corneal guttae prior to surgery (Fig. 3A). Following DSO corneal edema usually impairs visualization of the anterior chamber. It can adopt a honeycomb appearance due to the use of an Rho kinase inhibitor in the early postoperative course after DSO (Fig. 3B). After resolution of the corneal edema retroillumination shows a smooth and homogenous appearance of the corneal stroma inside the limitations of the descemetorhexis (Fig. 3C). Specular microscopy allows to monitor ingrowth of healthy endothelial cells onto the denuded corneal stroma (Fig. 3D).

5 Experience

There are several lines of evidence supporting the concept of DSO: First, reports about the removal of the Descemet membrane stem from patients in which the tissue was inadvertently removed during e.g. cataract surgery and resulted in prolonged edema and eventually in healing of the wound [16, 17] (Table 1). Second, the central corneal stroma had been exposed voluntarily or inadvertently after lamellar surgery (mainly DMEK) and healing has been observed by migration originating from the grafted tissue [18–20] (Table 1). Third, initial reports have been published following removal of a relatively large area of Descemet membrane of about 6 mm diameter. Table 2 gives an overview about these reports indicating that removal of a large area of 6 mm was not successful in the majority of patients and resulted due to the failure to repopulate the stroma [21, 22].

Removal of the central 4 mm portion of Descemet membrane results in migration of peripheral endothelial cells to the center and resolution of the corneal edema in the majority of the patients as shown in Table 3. Both the initial reports about 4 mm DSO by Bokar et al. and Moloney et al. described a successful postoperative course [11, 12]. Bokar et al. reported on 13 eyes with Fuchs dystrophy who achieved central endothelial cell counts ranging from 454 to 864 cells/mm^2. Similarly, Moloney et al. reported on 12 patients with a successful course in 9 patients. In a recent meta-analysis Franceshino and coworkers summarized the findings of 11 reports summarizing 127 eyes [24]. They concluded that most patients experienced a significant improvement of visual acuity, endothelial cell count as well as a reduction of corneal thickness. A direct comparison of DMEK with DSO was reported by Huang and coworkers observing 15 patients after DMEK and 12 patients in which the central 4 mm zone was removed by use of an inverse Sinskey hook [25]. Both techniques resulted in a comparable resolution of postoperative corneal edema, increase of visual acuity as well as reduction of corneal pachymetry.

6 Adjunctive Treatment with Rho Kinase Inhibitors

The use of Rho kinase (ROCK) inhibitors as adjunctive treatment after DSO was first described by Moloney and coworkers in 2017 who adopted this idea from the groundbreaking work of Kinoshita and Koizumi in the context of corneal endothelial cell culture [12, 29]. ROCK is a major downstream effector of the small GTPase Rho, which is activated by wounding, growth factors, cytokines and integrin signaling. Upon activation, the two isoforms ROCK-I and ROCK-II phosphorylate various intracellular substrates, such as myosin light chain, and regulate a wide spectrum of fundamental cellular processes, including cell polarity, adhesion, migration, proliferation and survival, mainly via reorganization of the actin cytoskeleton. Previous in vitro and in vivo studies suggested that ROCK inhibitors promote endothelial cell adhesion, proliferation, migration and wound healing [29–31].

Moloney et al. had performed DSO with stripping of the 4 mm central cornea in 12 patients with Fuchs corneal dystrophy and observed delayed clearance in 3 patients [12]. These patients were subsequently treated with topical Ripasudil, a ROCK inhibitor commercially available for the treatment of primary open-angle glaucoma and ocular hypertension, which resulted in resolution of corneal edema and migration of endothelial cells into the center of

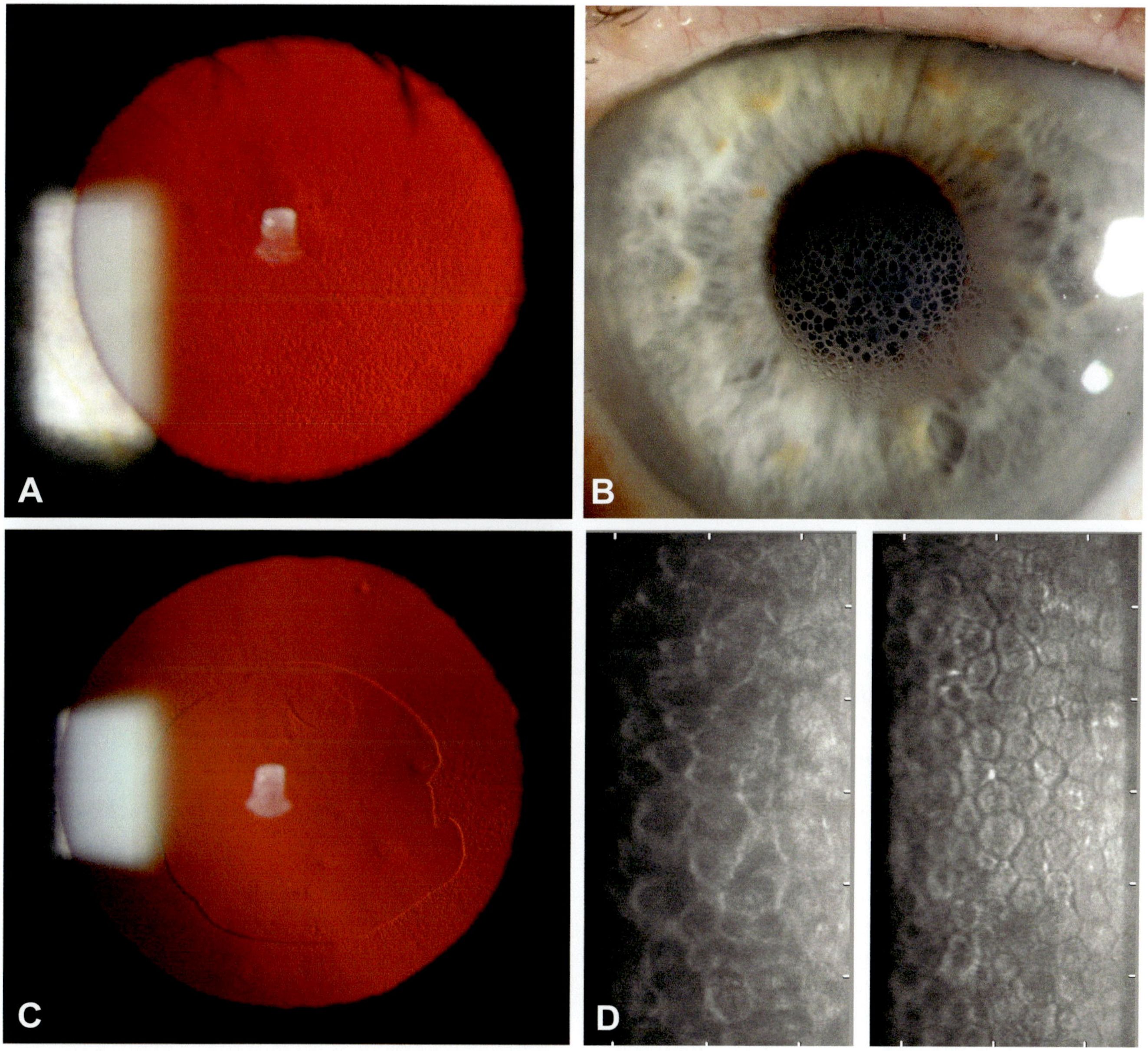

Fig. 3 Clinical outcome of DSO. (**A**) Preoperative retroillumination image of a patient with central guttae. (**B**) Clinical image showing central stromal edema with honeycomb epithelial alterations following ROCK inhibition. (**C**) Postoperative retroillumination image of the same patient with smooth corneal stroma. (**D**) Postoperative specular microscopy images of the central cornea of two patients after DSO

Table 1 Endothelial healing after inadvertent removal of the Descemet membrane in various pathologies prior to the concept of DSO

Reference	Surgical procedure	Success rate	Rescue therapy	Comment
Braunstein et al. [16]	Phaco/IOL (accidentally)	1	–	Visual improvement in the course of 6 months
Pan and Eong [17]	Phaco/IOL (accidentally)	1	–	Visual improvement in the course of 5 months
Balachandran et al. [18]	Graft detachment after DMEK	2/2	–	Endothelial cells on central cornea
Zafirakis et al. [19]	Graft detachment after DSAEK	1/1	–	
Dirisamer et al. [7]	Free floating graft ("DMET")	7/7 (FECD)	–	Not efficient in bullous keratopathy (5 patients)

Table 2 Overview of reports on DSO involving a 6 mm central descemetorhexis

References	Surgical procedure	Success rate	Rescue therapy	Comment
Shah et al. [20]	OD: DSEK graft removed OS: Descemet stripping	1/1	–	
Arbelaez et al. [21]	Descemet stripping	0/3	3/3 (DMEK)	Visual rehabilitation longer than DMEK
Moloney et al. [23]	Descemet stripping 1 × accidentally 1 × scheduled	2/2	–	–
Koenig [22]	6 mm DWEK, 2 patients	0/2	2/2 (DMEK)	ROCK inhibitor recommended

Table 3 Overview of reports on DSO involving a 4 mm central descemetorhexis

Reference	Surgical procedure	Success rate	Rescue therapy	Comment
Borkar et al. [11]	4 mm DWEK, 11 patients	10/13	3/13 (DMEK)	Classification in „Fast responder "/ "Slow responder "
Rao et al. [26]	4 mm DWEK, 3 patients	0/3	3/3 (DMEK)	DMEK for corneal rehabilitation
Moloney et al. [12]	4 mm DWEK, 11 patients	9/12	1: Y-27632 + DMEK 2: Ripasudil for 2 weeks	Topical Ripasudil successful as salvage agent Careful patient selection required
Iovieno et al. [27]	4 mm DWEK, 5 patients	4/5	–	Unpredictable wound healing responses
Davies et al. [28]	4 mm DWEK, 13 patients	14/17	–	Retrospective study; clearance typically after 3 months

the cornea. In addition, the same group reported on 23 eyes in which DSO had been performed together with phacoemulsification [32]. These patients also received topical Ripasudil. 22 out of 23 patients showed clear corneas with a mean time to clear of 4 weeks (between 2 and 8 weeks), but edema was persistent in one eye.

To further substantiate the role of ROCK inhibition after DSO, Macsai et al. performed a monocenter double blind study observing patients after 4 mm stripping [33]. Patients who received Ripasudil showed faster improvement of visual acuity, higher endothelial cell counts in the center as well as less reduction of peripheral endothelial cells as compared to controls. Thus, in the majority of published patients the administration of topical ROCK inhibitors had a beneficial effect on the clinical outcome. However, there are also reports on patients in which ROCK inhibition failed to enhance migration of endothelial cells: while Reinhold and coworkers described prolonged corneal edema with failure to resolve in one patient [34], Arsiwalla and associates reported about mid-term failure after DSO with Ripasudil requiring DMEK as rescue therapy as well [35].

A summary of published data on the effect of ROCK inhibitors on corneal endothelial cells suggests that administration of the drug after DSO (Fig. 4A) enhances migration of presumably healthy endothelial cells from the periphery (Fig. 4B) [31]. In contrast, administration of the drug in eyes in which diseased endothelial cells (and guttae) are still present in the central cornea (Fig. 4C) will not lead to alteration of the diseased tissue (Fig. 4D).

7 Open Questions

DSO is currently in wide spread use especially in the U.S.A. However it remains unclear if DSO (alone or in combination with ROCK inhibition) renders the same results as DMEK which can be considered the gold standard for treatment of endothelial dysfunction. Until the completion of the current ongoing multinational clinical trials, this question remains unanswered. Also despite encouraging mid-term results, the fate of the migrated endothelial cells needs to be determined in long term studies. The recent observation of a recurrence of guttae and endothelial dysfunction after successful DSO [36] feeds the suspicion that presumably healthy cells of patients with Fuchs dystrophy will eventually acquire a pathological phenotype years after translocation from the periphery to the center. We have shown that one of the key elements of Fuchs dystrophy is the production of a false matrix and that this false production can be ameliorated by ROCK inhibition [37, 38]. Thus, prolonged administration of Rho kinase inhibitors might be beneficial to prevent the formation of guttae in the central corneal endothelium following DSO.

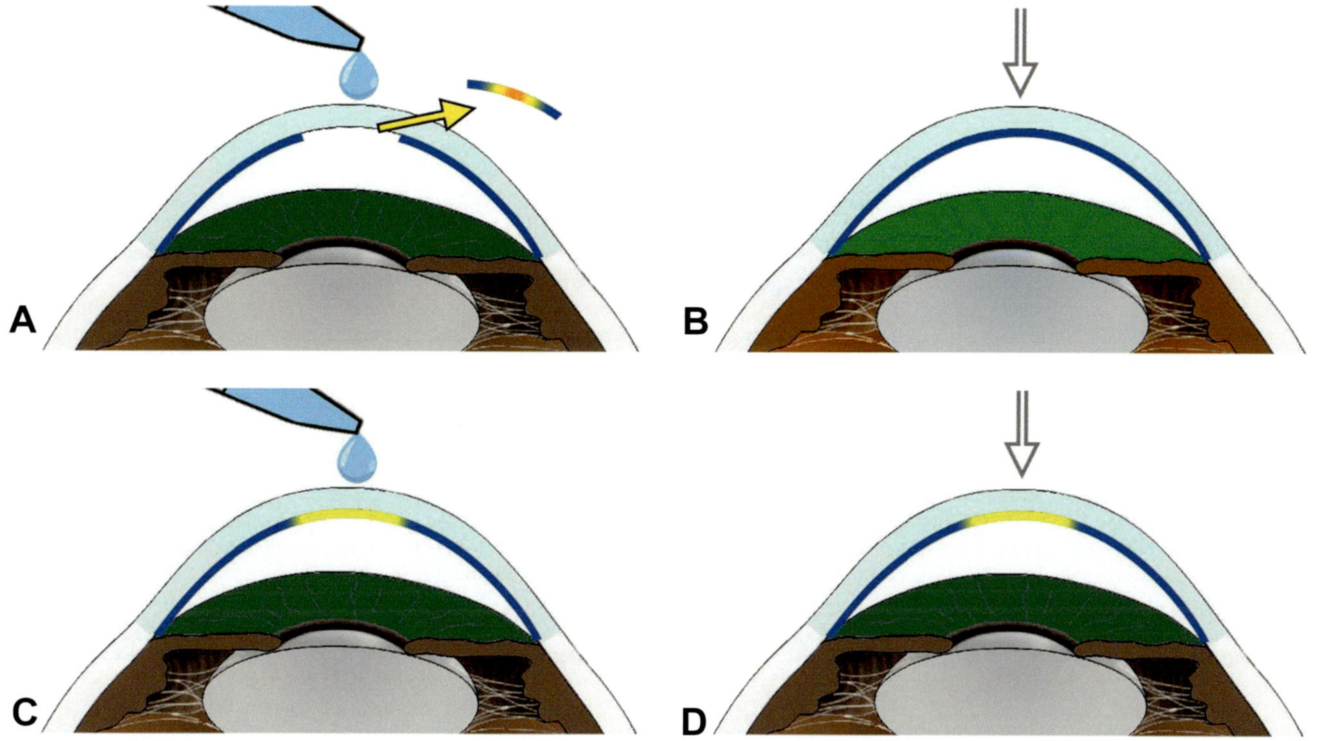

Fig. 4 Schematic diagram illustrating two scenarios of a potential clinical use of ROCK inhibitor eye drops in patients with Fuchs dystrophy. (**A**, **B**) ROCK inhibition post-DSO enhances corneal endothelial wound healing. (**C**, **D**) Without surgical descemetorhexis both guttae as well as pathological endothelial cells persist in the center of the cornea

8 Conclusion

DSO can be used as the initial surgical treatment in the management of patients with early Fuchs dystrophy where peripheral endothelial cell function appears to be preserved. Postoperative topical ROCK inhibitor supplementation will accelerate time to corneal clearance and visual recovery.

References

1. Gorovoy MS. Descemet-stripping automated endothelial keratoplasty. Cornea. 2006;25:886–9.
2. Melles GR, Ong TS, Ververs B, van der Wees J. Descemet membrane endothelial keratoplasty (DMEK). Cornea. 2006;25:987–90.
3. Rudolph M, Laaser K, Bachmann BO, Cursiefen C, Epstein D, Kruse FE. Corneal higher-order aberrations after Descemet's membrane endothelial keratoplasty. Ophthalmology. 2012;119:528–33.
4. Anshu A, Price MO, Price FW. Risk of corneal transplant rejection significantly reduced with Descemet's membrane endothelial keratoplasty. Ophthalmology. 2012;119:536–40.
5. Price MO, Price FW Jr, Kruse FE, Bachmann BO, Tourtas T. Randomized comparison of topical prednisolone acetate 1% versus fluorometholone 0.1% in the first year after descemet membrane endothelial keratoplasty. Cornea. 2014;33:880–6.
6. Watanabe S, Oie Y, Fujimoto H, Soma T, Koh S, Tsujikawa M, Maeda N, Nishida K. Relationship between corneal guttae and quality of vision in patients with mild Fuchs' endothelial corneal dystrophy. Ophthalmology. 2015;122:2103–9.
7. Dirisamer M, Ham L, Dapena I, van Dijk K, Melles GR. Descemet membrane endothelial transfer: "free-floating" donor Descemet implantation as a potential alternative to "keratoplasty". Cornea. 2012;31:194–7.
8. Jacobi C, Zhivov A, Korbmacher J, Falke K, Guthoff R, Schlötzer-Schrehardt U, Cursiefen C, Kruse FE. Evidence of endothelial cell migration after descemet membrane endothelial keratoplasty. Am J Ophthalmol. 2011;152:537–42.
9. Thuret G, Poinard S, Garcin T, Gain P. Who first described descemetorhexis without endothelial keratoplasty (DWEK) for the management of Fuchs' corneal endothelial dystrophy? J Fr Ophtalmol. 2022;45:452–4.
10. Bleyen I, Saelens IE, van Dooren BT, van Rij G. Spontaneous corneal clearing after descemet's stripping. Ophthalmology. 2013;20:215.
11. Borkar DS, Veldman P, Colby KA. Treatment of Fuchs endothelial dystrophy by descemet stripping without endothelial keratoplasty. Cornea. 2016;35:1267–73.
12. Moloney G, Petsoglou C, Ball M, Kerdraon Y, Höllhumer R, Spiteri N, Beheregaray S, Hampson J, D'Souza M, Devasahayam RN. Descemetorhexis without grafting for Fuchs endothelial dystrophy-Supplementation with topical ripasudil. Cornea. 2017;36:642–8.
13. Kaufman AR, Nosé RM, Pineda R 2nd. Descemetorhexis without endothelial keratoplasty (DWEK): proposal for nomenclature standardization. Cornea. 2018;37:e20–1.
14. Colby K. Descemet stripping only for Fuchs endothelial corneal dystrophy: Will it become the gold Standard? Cornea. 2022;41:269–71.

15. Cohen E, Din N, Mimouni M, Trinh T, Gouvea L, AlShaker S, Chan CC, Slomovic AR. The "Two-Flaps" technique for descemet stripping only. Cornea. 2021;40:1211–4.
16. Braunstein RE, Airiani S, Chang MA, Odrich MG. Corneal edema resolution after "descemetorhexis." J Cataract Refract Surg. 2003;29:1436–9.
17. Pan JC, Au Eong KG. Spontaneous resolution of corneal oedema after inadvertent 'descemetorhexis' during cataract surgery. Clin Exp Ophthalmol. 2006;34:896–7.
18. Balachandran C, Ham L, Verschoor CA, Ong TS, van der Wees J, Melles GR. Spontaneous corneal clearance despite graft detachment in descemet membrane endothelial keratoplasty. Am J Ophthalmol. 2009;148:227–34.
19. Zafirakis P, Kymionis GD, Grentzelos MA, Livir-Rallatos G. Corneal graft detachment without corneal edema after descemet stripping automated endothelial keratoplasty. Cornea. 2010;29:456–8.
20. Shah RD, Randleman JB, Grossniklaus HE. Spontaneous corneal clearing after Descemet's stripping without endothelial replacement. Ophthalmology. 2012;119:256–66.
21. Arbelaez JG, Price MO, Price FW. Long-term follow-up and complications of stripping descemet membrane without placement of graft in eyes with Fuchs endothelial dystrophy. Cornea. 2014;33:1295–9.
22. Koenig SB. Planned descemetorhexis without endothelial keratoplasty in eyes with Fuchs corneal endothelial dystrophy. Cornea. 2015;34:1149–51.
23. Moloney G, Chan UT, Hamilton A, Zahidin AM, Grigg JR, Devasahayam RN. Descemetorhexis for Fuchs' dystrophy. Can J Ophthalmol. 2015;50(1):68–72.
24. Franceschino A, Dutheil F, Pereira B, Watson SL, Chiambaretta F, Navel V. Descemetorhexis without endothelial keratoplasty in fuchs endothelial corneal dystrophy: a systematic review and meta-analysis.Cornea. 2022;41:815–25.
25. Huang MJ, Kane S, Dhaliwal DK. Descemetorhexis without endothelial keratoplasty versus DMEK for treatment of Fuchs endothelial corneal dystrophy. Cornea. 2018;37:1479–83.
26. Rao R, Borkar DS, Colby KA, Veldman PB. Descemet membrane endothelial keratoplasty after failed descemet stripping without endothelial keratoplasty. Cornea. 2017;36(7):763–66.
27. Iovieno A, Neri A, Soldani AM, Adani C, Fontana L. Descemetorhexis without graft placement for the treatment of Fuchs endothelial dystrophy: preliminary results and review of the literature. Cornea. 2017;36(6):637–41.
28. Davies E, Jurkunas U, Pineda R 2nd. Predictive factors for corneal clearance after descemetorhexis without endothelial keratoplasty. Cornea 2018;37(2):137–40.
29. Koizumi N, Okumura N, Ueno M, Kinoshita S. New therapeutic modality for corneal endothelial disease using Rho-associated kinase inhibitor eye drops. Cornea. 2014;33(Suppl 11):S25-31.
30. Kinoshita S, Koizumi N, Ueno M, Okumura N, Imai K, Tanaka H, Yamamoto Y, Nakamura T, Inatomi T, Bush J, Toda M, Hagiya M, Yokota I, Teramukai S, Sotozono C, Hamuro J. Injection of cultured cells with a ROCK inhibitor for bullous keratopathy. N Engl J Med. 2018;378:995–1003.
31. Kinoshita S, Colby KA, Kruse FE. A close look at the clinical efficacy of rho-associated protein kinase inhibitor eye drops for Fuchs endothelial corneal dystrophy. Cornea. 2021;40:1225–8.
32. Moloney G, Garcerant Congote D, Hirnschall N, Arsiwalla T, Luiza Mylla Boso A, Toalster N, D'Souza M, Devasahayam RN. Descemet stripping only supplemented with topical ripasudil for Fuchs endothelial dystrophy 12-month outcomes of the sydney eye hospital study. Cornea. 2021;40:320–6.
33. Macsai MS, Shiloach M. Use of topical rho kinase inhibitors in the treatment of Fuchs dystrophy after descemet stripping only. Cornea. 2019;38:529–34.
34. Reinhold A, Eggenschwiler L, Meyer P, Goldblum D. Failed descemet stripping only (DSO) with adjuvant rho-kinase inhibitor therapy in a Fuchs' endothelial dystrophy patient: a case report. Klin Monbl Augenheilkd. 2021;238:376–7.
35. Arsiwalla T, Trinh T, Goolam S, Benito-Pascual B, Devasahayam RN, Moloney G. Medium-term failure of descemet's stripping only and Fuchs' dystrophy with pancorneal guttae. Cornea. 2022;41:1064–7.
36. Kaufman AR, Bal S, Boakye J, Jurkunas UV. Recurrence of guttae and endothelial dysfunction after successful descemet stripping only in Fuchs dystrophy. Cornea. 2023;42:1037–40.
37. Weller JM, Zenkel M, Schlötzer-Schrehardt U, Bachmann BO, Tourtas T, Kruse FE. Extracellular matrix alterations in late-onset Fuchs' corneal dystrophy. Invest Ophthalmol Vis Sci. 2014;55:3700–8.
38. Schlötzer-Schrehardt U, Zenkel M, Strunz M, Gießl A, Schondorf H, da Silva H, Schmidt GA, Greiner MA, Okumura N, Koizumi N, Kinoshita S, Tourtas T, Kruse FE. Potential functional restoration of corneal endothelial cells in Fuchs endothelial corneal dystrophy by ROCK Inhibitor (Ripasudil). Am J Ophthalmol. 2021;224:185–99.

High-Risk Keratoplasty

Claus Cursiefen, Björn Bachmann, Mert Mestanoglu, and Deniz Hos

Abstract

Under uninflamed conditions and in the absence of pathologic corneal blood and lymphatic vessels, corneal transplantation has a "low-risk" of graft rejection. However, grafts that are transplanted into pathologically prevascularized recipients show high rejection rates of more than 50%, hence the term "high-risk keratoplasty" is used in such cases. Conditions that lead to high-risk keratoplasty include infections, trauma, chemical insults, autoimmune conditions, history of inflammation/inflammatory disease, congenital aniridia, ocular surface diseases, prior graft rejection(s) and young recipient age. Here in this chapter, we introduce different examples of high-risk keratoplasty and novel treatment options for (lymph)angioregression to improve graft survival following a high-risk keratoplasty.

Keywords

Chemical injury · Corneal crosslinking · Corneal neovascularization · Fine-needle diathermy · Graft rejection · Graft failure · High-risk keratoplasty · Repeat keratoplasty

C. Cursiefen (✉) · B. Bachmann · M. Mestanoglu · D. Hos
Department of Ophthalmology, University Hospital of Cologne, Cologne, Germany
e-mail: claus.cursiefen@uk-koeln.de

C. Cursiefen · D. Hos
Center for Molecular Medicine Cologne, University of Cologne, Cologne, Germany

1 High-Risk Keratoplasty Conditions

Due to the immune and (lymph)angiogenic privilege of the cornea, corneal transplantations are the most successful solid tissue transplantations in the world. However, if the immune privilege of the cornea is lost due to e.g. severe infection, inflammation, or pathological corneal neovascularization, the success of corneal transplantation decreases significantly. According to the Collaborative Corneal Transplantation Studies (CCTS), high-risk transplantation is defined as (i) a recipient bed with ≥ 2 quadrants of corneal neovascularization and (ii) re-keratoplasty due to graft rejection [1]. In addition, several other conditions are also known to increase the risk of graft rejection. Figures 1, 2, 3, 4, 5, 6, 7, 8 and 9 demonstrate different examples of high-risk corneal transplantation settings with increased risk of graft rejection.

2 Local and Systemic Immunosuppression in High-Risk Eyes

The cornerstone of ocular immunomodulatory treatment in high-risk eyes are corticosteroids [9]. Standard treatment regimen includes both systemic and topical corticosteroid application, usually short-term systemic and long-term topical application. The initial systemic dosage is usually started as 1 mg per kg of body weight, and it is gradually tapered within next weeks, based on individual case management. Topical corticosteroids are used indefinitely after high-risk keratoplasty; however, additional immunosuppressive agents might be required for prevention of graft rejection.

Broad side effect profiles of corticosteroids always require a consideration, especially for long term use. Use of other immunomodulation agents, such as cyclosporine,

B. Seitz et al. (eds.), *Atlas on Cornea*, https://doi.org/10.1007/978-3-031-65422-0_53

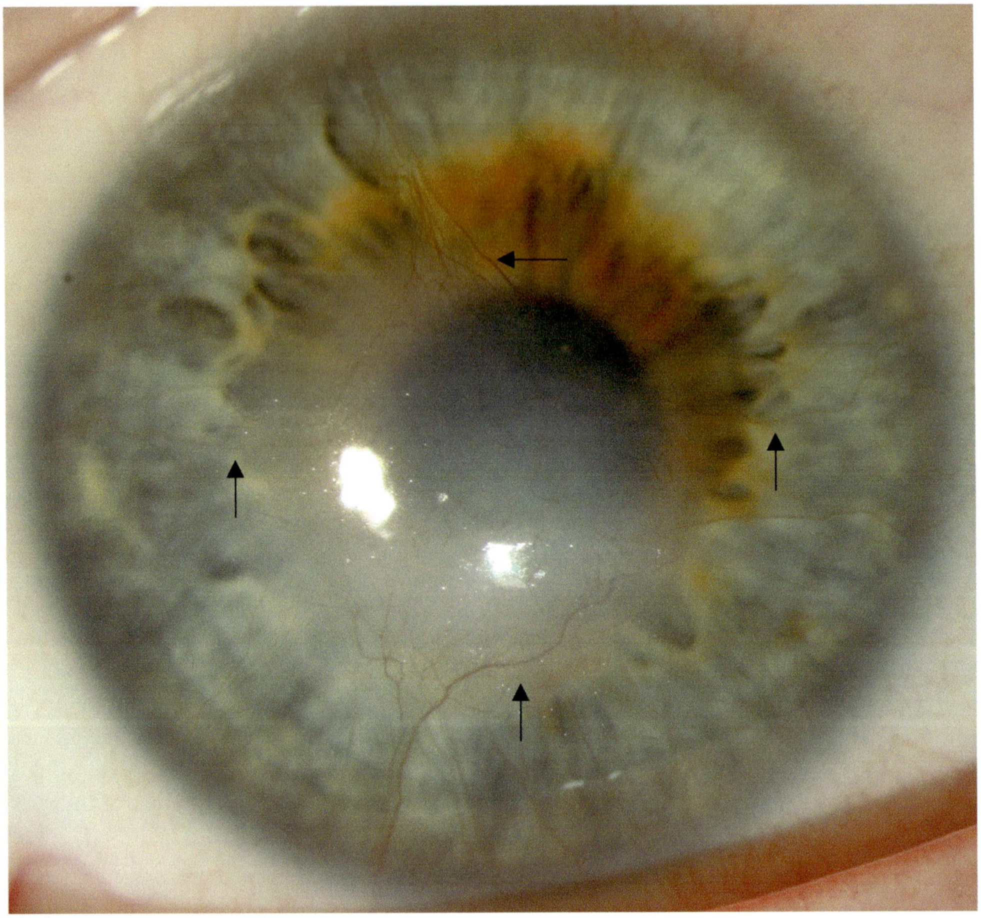

Fig. 1 Cornea of a 28-year-old female patient with corneal neovascularization after contact lens-associated Acanthamoeba keratitis. Blood vessels can be seen in all four corneal quadrants (black arrows). The risk of corneal graft rejection increases with the number of affected corneal quadrants [2]

mycophenolate mofetil and tacrolimus should be considered when corticosteroid use is suspected to cause adverse events, such as delayed wound healing, metabolic syndrome, muscle and skin atrophy, peptic ulcers, osteoporosis and arterial hypertension [10].

Historically cyclosporine and mycophenolate mofetil are the most studied other treatment options in high-risk keratoplasty. A systematic review concluded that 1-year rejection-free graft survival increases after both systemic cyclosporine and mycophenolate mofetil [11], although a retrospective study with 417 patients reported better rejection-free and clear graft survival in mycophenolate mofetil treated patients than cyclosporine treated patients [12]. The side effect profile of mycophenolate mofetil seems also safer in comparison to cyclosporine. Another calcineurin inhibitor, tacrolimus, was also found to be effective in reducing graft rejection and prolonging graft survival in a small cohort that had previous graft failure despite cyclosporine treatment [13]. Nevertheless, it is not yet possible to propose a one-size-fits-all approach for immunosuppression after high-risk keratoplasty with the evidence at hand. The immunosuppressive treatment regimen should be individualized for each case and close follow-up for side effects should be achieved. There is a great need for well-designed clinical trials to optimize immunosuppressive therapy after high-risk keratoplasty.

The effect of human leukocyte antigen (HLA) matching on corneal graft survival is still unclear. A randomized, double-blind, multicenter clinical trial including both normal and high-risk eyes, reported no significant advantage of HLA matching over random graft matching; however, the study was underpowered due to a lower-than-expected event rate [14]. Thus, there is a need for further research to understand in which high-risk conditions HLA-matching might be beneficial. Furthermore, transplantation antigens such as minor histocompatibility antigens e.g., H-Y antigens and ABO group blood matching might play a role in corneal transplantation [1, 15].

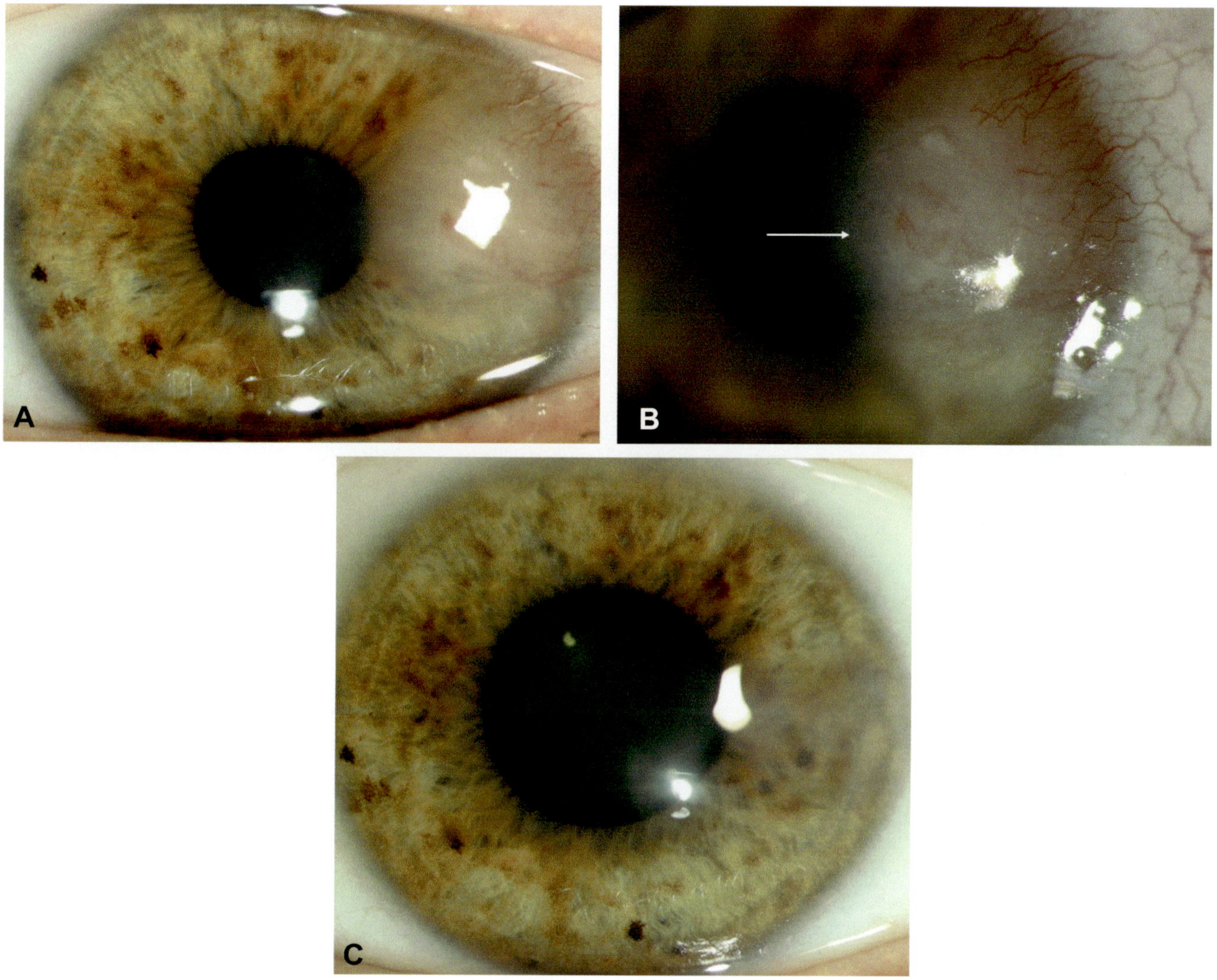

Fig. 2 (**A**) Cornea of a 50-year-old woman with presumed herpetic stromal interstitial keratitis. Herpes simplex virus-1 (HSV-1) is a common cause of corneal neovascularization [3]. As corneal HSV-1 infection can be associated with persistent corneal inflammation, management of corneal neovascularization and any active inflammation/infection should precede keratoplasty. (**B**) same eye in higher magnification. Lipid keratopathy (arrow) is also commonly observed in corneal HSV-1 infection. (**C**) after two rounds of combined fine-needle diathermy and corneal crosslinking including the corneal periphery (together with antiviral and anti-inflammatory therapy), significant vessel regression can be seen. Current visual acuity is 20/20

3 Lymphangioregression Prior to High-Risk Keratoplasty: Options and Techniques

Pathological ingrowth of blood and lymphatic vessels into the cornea leads to faster donor antigen sensitization and increased immune effector cell access to the graft and is an established risk factor for allograft rejection [1, 16, 17]. In fact, lymphatic vessels seem to contribute to mediating immune rejections after corneal transplantation even more than blood vessels [18]. Therefore, the regression of blood and lymphatic vessels within the host cornea prior to transplantation, named "(lymph)angioregressive preconditioning", appears as a potential strategy to improve corneal graft survival in high-risk eyes [19]. In the experimental setting, several approaches such as photodynamic therapy, fine-needle diathermy (FND) and corneal crosslinking were employed to corroborate the feasibility of this novel concept [20, 21]. To translate these findings to the clinic, we conducted a retrospective study with 31 high-risk patients treated with FND combined with subconjunctival bevacizumab for preoperative hem- and lymphangioregression [22]. In this study, eyes treated with FND and bevacizumab prior to high-risk keratoplasty demonstrated short-/

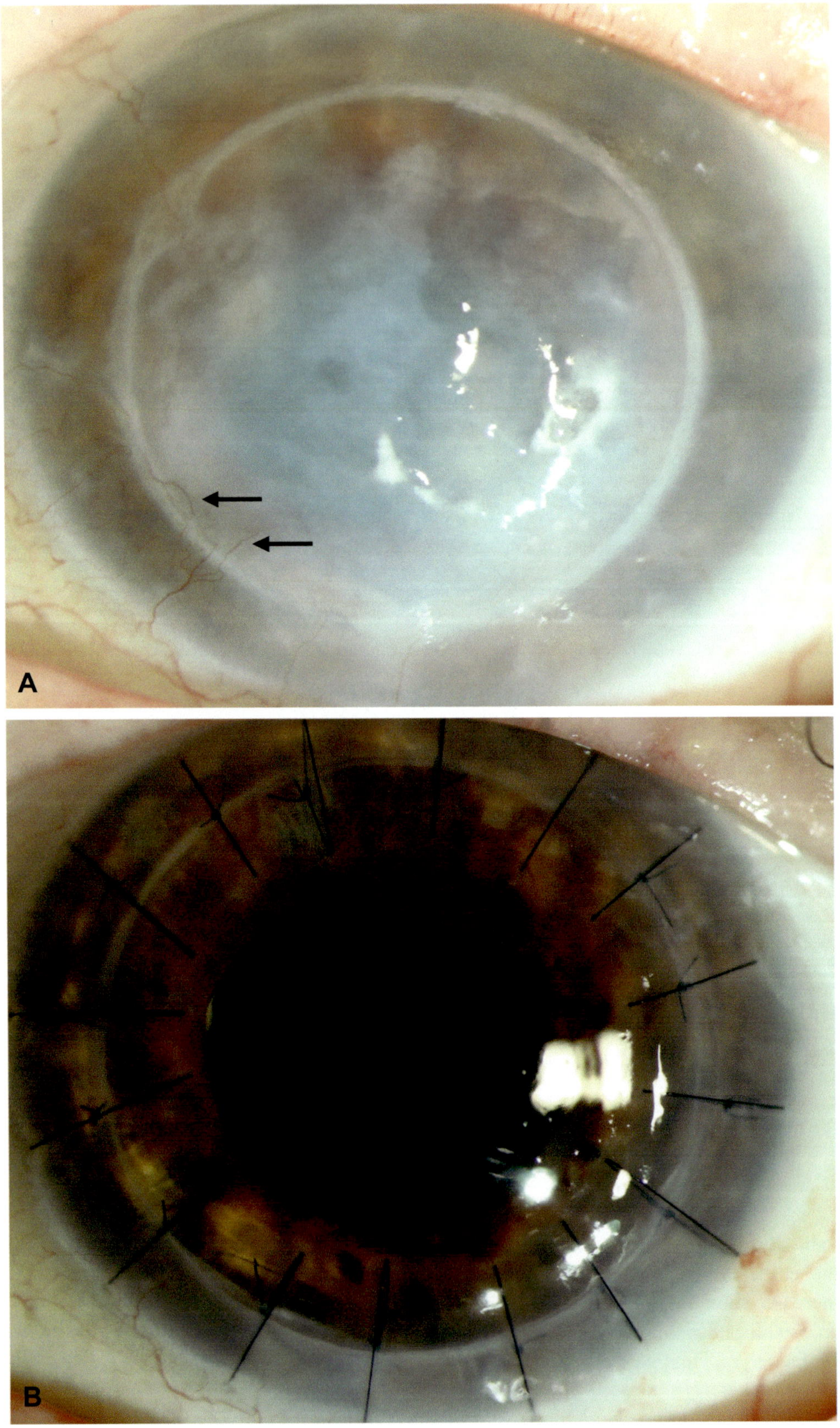

Fig. 3 (**A**) cornea of an 80-year-old male patient with failed prior penetrating keratoplasty. In this case, a corneal graft rejection episode occurred three years post-keratoplasty, followed by corneal ulceration, resulting in graft failure. Diffuse stromal graft scarring and blood vessels invading the graft (arrows) can be seen. Visual acuity of the patient was reduced to hand movements. (**B**) same eye 6 months after repeat penetrating keratoplasty and intravitreal triamcinolone injection, without any signs of graft rejection and the visual acuity of 20/80 despite glaucomatous optic nerve atrophy

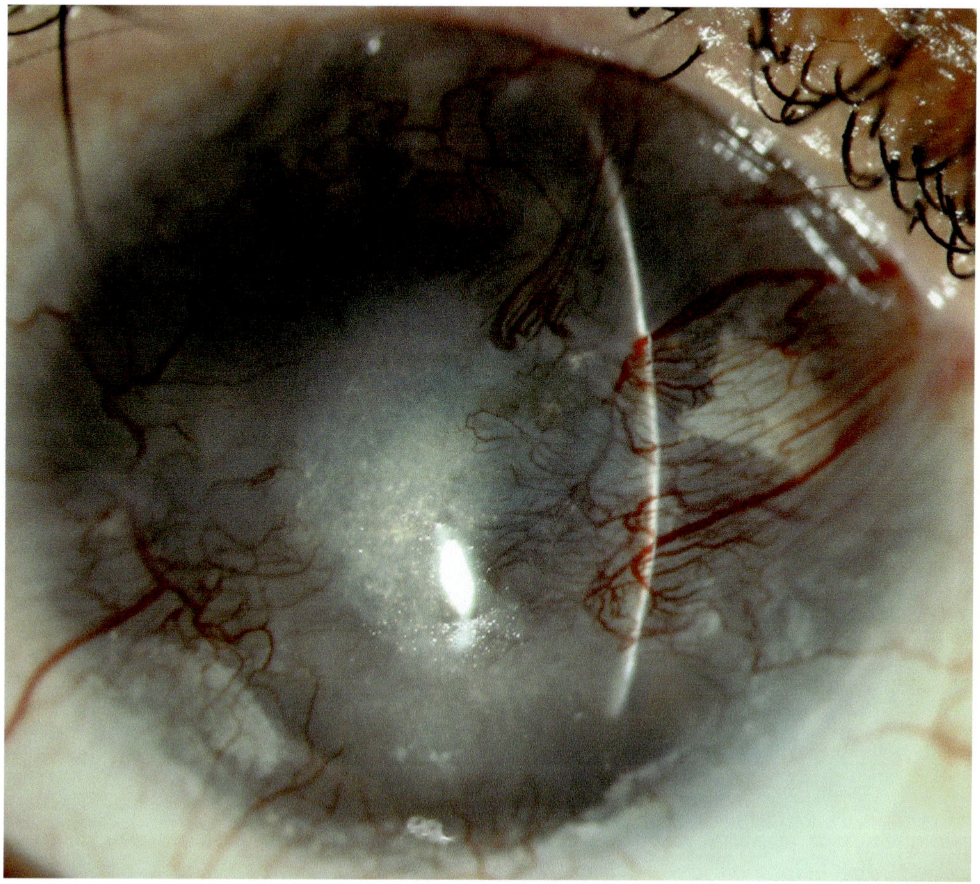

Fig. 4 Right cornea of a 35-year-old patient after severe chemical injury. Chemical injuries with acidic or alkaline compounds can cause severe insults to the ocular surface, initiating (mostly persistent) inflammation [4]. Repeated amniotic membrane transplantations were performed six times due to persisting epithelial defect caused by limbal stem cell deficiency (LSCD) in this patient, followed by fine-needle diathermy of the vessels without long-term success. Almost complete conjunctivalization of the cornea alongside thick tortuous blood vessels can be seen. Symblepharon of the upper lid can be seen at the 3 o'clock position, a sequela of ocular surface inflammation. Corneal transplantation without concomitant treatment of LSCD will not be successful

mid-term rejection rates similar to low-risk eyes (Fig. 10) [22]. However, in a more recent study where we reported the first 3-year follow-up results of this cohort, relatively high immune rejection rates were observed in patients with residual vessels prior to transplantation (46%). In contrast, in eyes with complete vessel regression prior to keratoplasty, rejection-free 3-year graft survival was 75%, implicating that complete vessel regression should be aimed for [23].

Prior experimental studies demonstrated that corneal crosslinking regresses pathological corneal blood and lymphatic vessels and reduces the graft rejection risk after high-risk keratoplasty in mice [20]. More recently, in a small clinical pilot study we demonstrated that (peripheral) corneal crosslinking is a potent method to induce (lymph) angioregression in high-risk eyes with pathological neovascularization (Fig. 11) [24]. A prospective clinical trial to analyze the value of corneal crosslinking in high-risk keratoplasty is currently underway (CrossCornealVision).

An important mediator of (lymph)angiogenesis is VEGF-A [25]. Inhibition of hem- and lymphangiogenesis through VEGF-A modulation improves graft survival after both normal and high-risk setting [25, 26]. Anti-VEGF-A therapy after FND is effective in maintaining hem- and lymphangioregression through prevention of rebound neovascularization induced by FND [27]. A recent multicenter, randomized, prospective clinical trial demonstrated no statistical significance of post-keratoplasty local bevacizumab treatment on overall graft rejection rates after high-risk keratoplasty. However, extended post hoc follow-up analysis at the lead study location showed reduced graft rejection rates in the bevacizumab treated group versus controls [28]. This clinical trial translates the experimental findings on the improvement of graft survival with anti-VEGFs into the clinic and indicates that anti(lymph)angiogenic therapies might be beneficial to achieve improved high-risk graft survival.

Recently we investigated the effect of combined FND and corneal crosslinking on corneal neovascularization

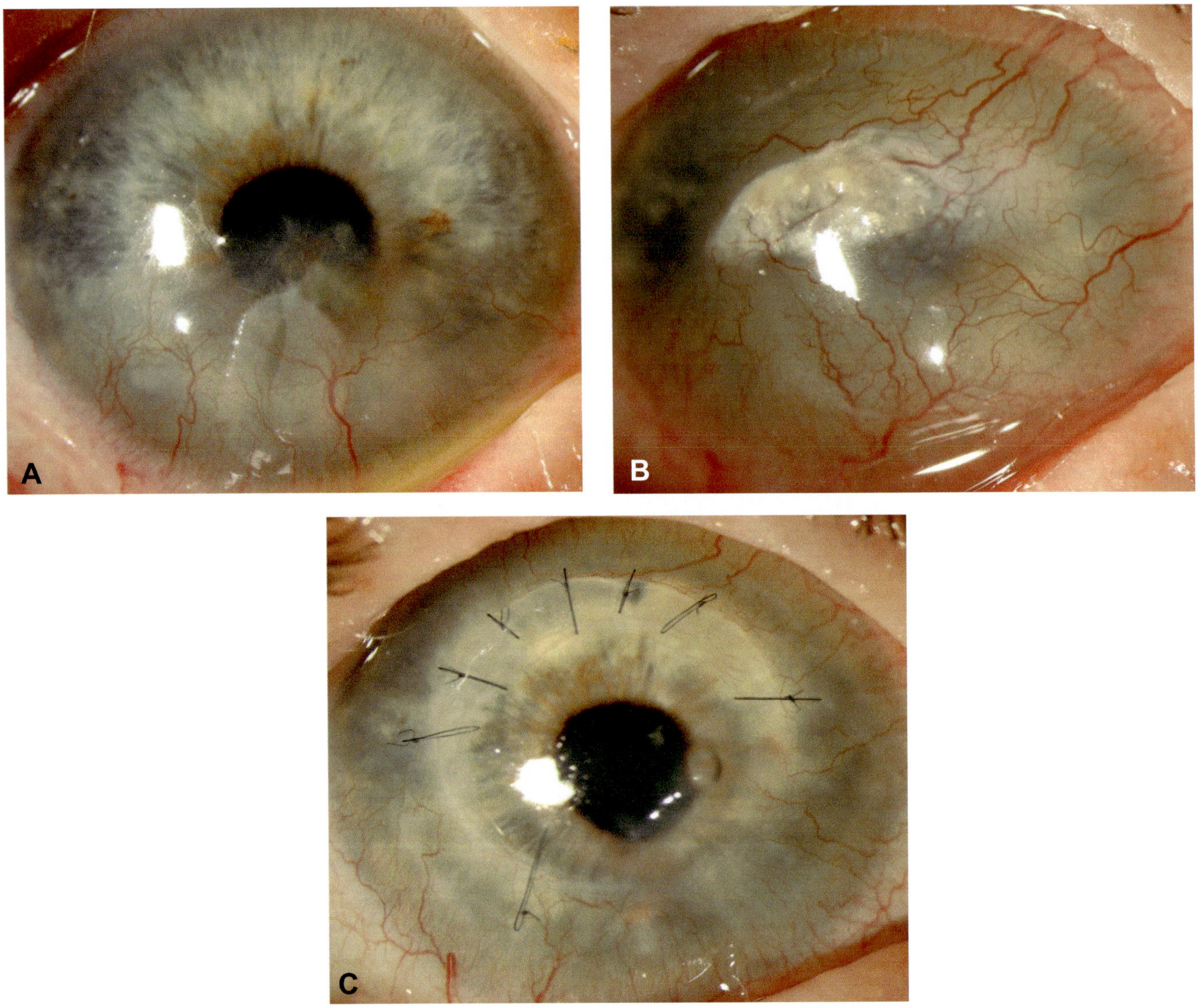

Fig. 5 (**A**) cornea of a 47-year-old patient with limbal stem cell deficiency due to sulfonamide induced toxic epidermal necrolysis (Lyell Syndrome). Here, an imbalance of pro- and antiangiogenic factors leads to conjunctivalization and vascularization of the cornea. (**B**) same eye with disease progression and vascularization including the visual axis with decreased visual acuity to hand movements. Stem cell function still preserved partially from 9 to 11 o'clock, which was relied on for a corneal transplantation. (**C**) penetrating keratoplasty combined with fine-needle diathermy was performed, increasing best-corrected visual acuity to 0.3 4-months after keratoplasty. However, blood vessels are still present, therefore there is a high risk of rejection

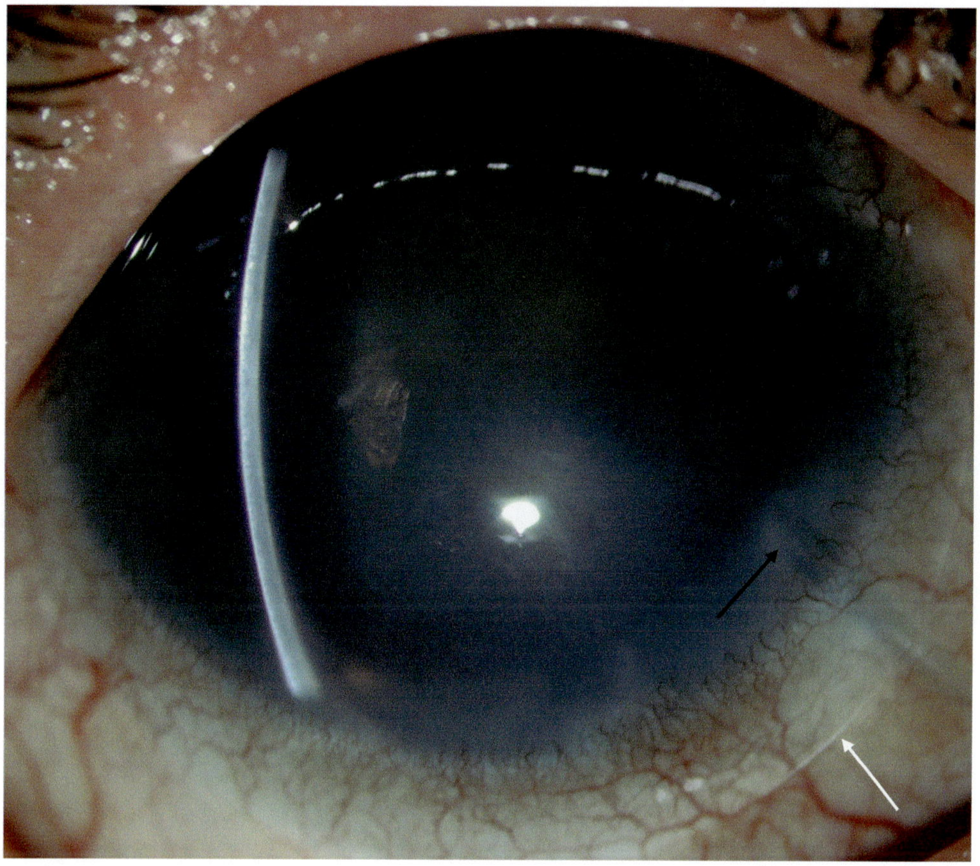

Fig. 6 Right eye of a 38-year-old patient with congenital aniridia and congenital glaucoma after multiple anterior segment surgeries. Congenital aniridia can result in disruption of the limbal stem cell niche (aniridia related keratopathy), leading to loss of corneal immune privilege [5]. Circumferential blood vessel invasion in the peripheral cornea can be seen. Abnormal iridocorneal angle development often leads to glaucoma [6]. In this case, Baerveldt shunt (black arrow) surgery was performed twice, and cyclophotocoagulation three times. Prior anterior segment surgeries are also associated with an increased risk of graft rejection after keratoplasty. Posterior lamellar keratoplasties might therefore offer another treatment option in such complicated cases if stromal scars are not present. This patient underwent Descemet membrane endothelial keratoplasty (DMEK) without any episodes of corneal graft rejection, however, glaucoma-associated endothelial cell failure necessitated two repeat DMEKs during the follow-up. Bandage contact lens is in place (white arrow)

(Figs. 12 and 13), where we aimed to benefit from a synergistic (lymph)angioregressive effect. Early unpublished data from this approach is promising and might pave the way for a novel combination strategy for (lymph)angioregression prior to high-risk keratoplasty.

On a side note, our group previously reported the outcomes of DMEK in vascularized eyes, which would be considered high-risk if penetrating keratoplasty were the treatment of choice [29]. Interestingly, corneal vessel covered areas decreased significantly after DMEK, and rejection rates were relatively low (<5%), indicating that DMEK is a feasible option to treat endothelial dysfunction in vascularized eyes as long as no significant stromal scarring is present (Fig. 14).

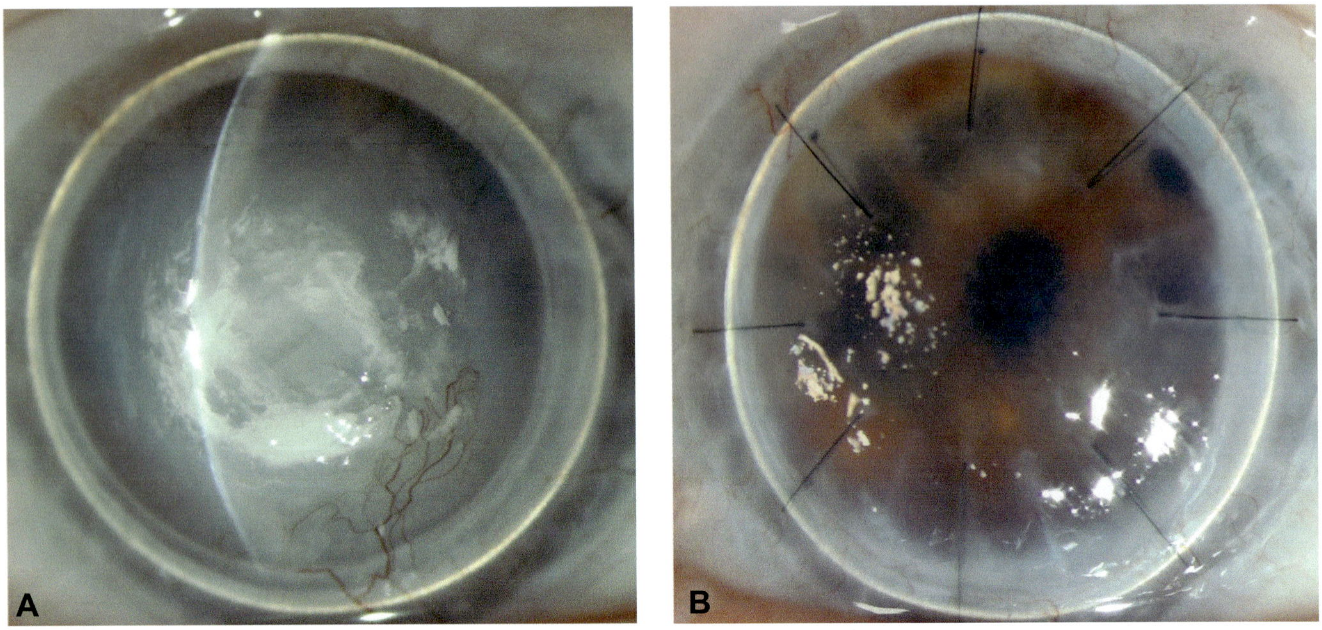

Fig. 7 Repeat keratoplasty in an eye with glaucoma and Krumeich ring. Krumeich ring is a ring-shaped alloy with presumed anti-vascular properties used for corneal surgery. (**A**) Despite Krumeich ring implantation with penetrating keratoplasty, corneal vascularization progressed in this eye with secondary glaucoma due to central retinal artery occlusion. (**B**) same eye 14 months after repeat penetrating keratoplasty, Krumeich ring was left in place to avoid additional stromal trauma. The graft demonstrates secondary failure signs following an immune rejection 4 months after keratoplasty. Previous studies reported no benefit but increased adverse events associated with this ring [7, 8]. Posterior lamellar keratoplasty is planned as DMEK

4 Care After High-Risk Keratoplasty

Postoperative care may considerably influence the outcome of high-risk keratoplasty. With optimal postoperative care, immune reactions can be recognized early, adverse effects can be kept in check and necessary treatment adjustments can be timely implemented.

Patient education for early graft rejection symptoms might allow early diagnosis through emergency visits by patients. More frequently scheduled follow-up visits can be helpful for detecting early inflammation or rejection signs.

The underlying disease causing the high-risk setting, such as herpetic keratitis or atopy, must be adequately controlled. Loosened interrupted sutures might cause local irritation and inflammation and induce vascularization or initiate immune reactions, therefore sutures should be thoroughly evaluated during postoperative visits and all loose sutures would be removed immediately. Another important point is follow-up of the graft vascularization. Allograft rejection risk is increased by postoperative graft vascularization [30]. Retreatment for the regression of the postoperatively developed vessels extending into the graft might prolong graft survival.

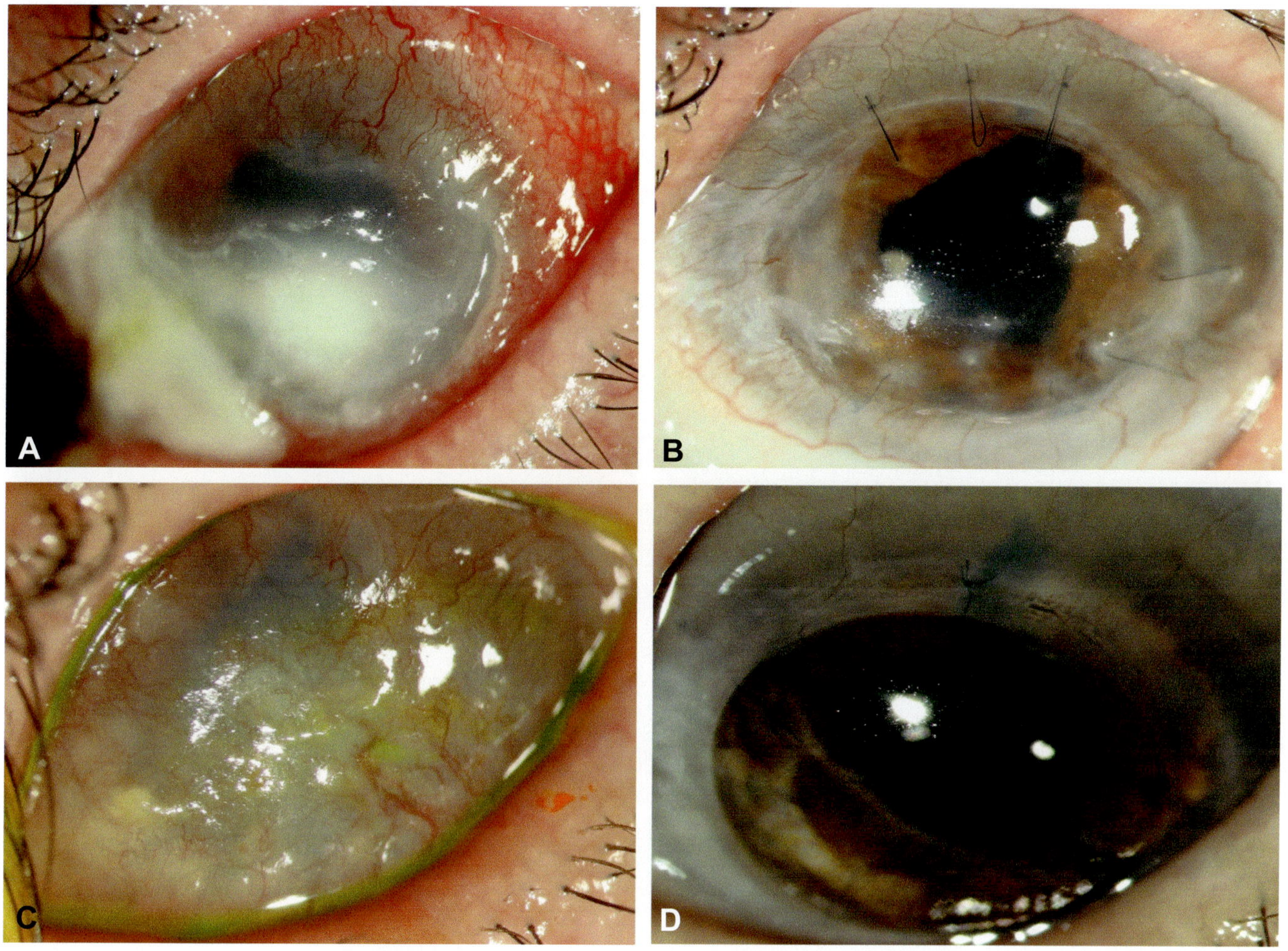

Fig. 8 An example of emergency penetrating keratoplasty (penetrating keratoplasty à chaud = corneal transplantation when the cornea is still inflamed that is mainly performed for preservation of the eye). (**A**) after surgical treatment of granulomatous pansinusitis, this patient developed lagophthalmos, leading to exposure keratopathy progressing further to corneal ulceration, which responded poorly to antibacterial and antifungal therapy. (**B**) Emergency penetrating keratoplasty was performed, followed by orbital reconstruction surgery and canthopexy in separate sessions. (**C**) within one year, the transplanted and rejected graft was highly vascularized, vision decreased to hand movements. (**D**) After one initial round of fine-needle diathermy, HLA-matched repeat keratoplasty in combination with fine-needle diathermy and subconjunctival bevacizumab injection was performed. Best corrected visual acuity (with contact lens) was 20/25 at the last follow-up visit

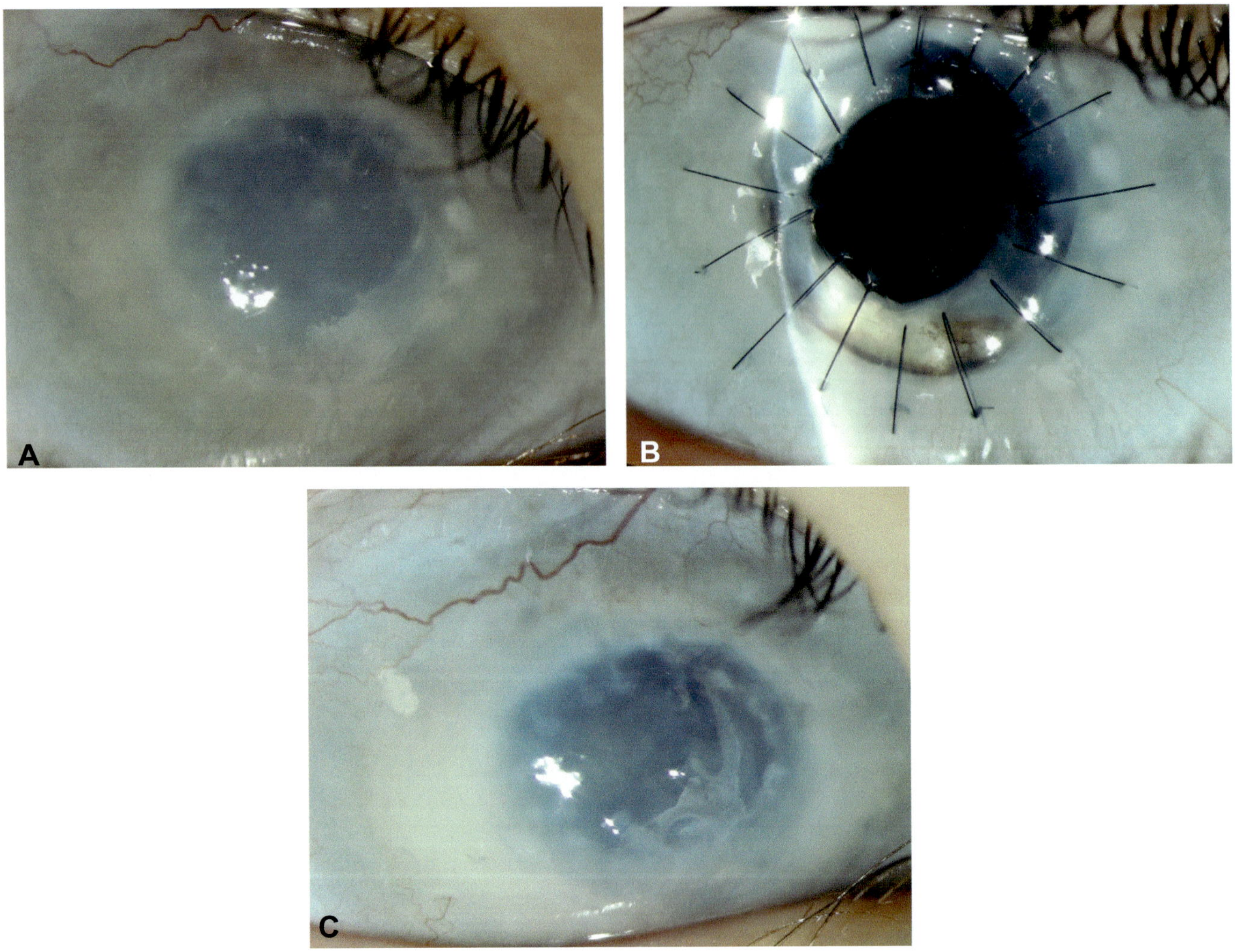

Fig. 9 (**A**) Axenfeld–Rieger syndrome (a group of disorders that mainly affect the development of the anterior segment of the eye), where the transplantation recipient is of young age, which constitutes a risk factor for graft rejection in itself [6]. This child received a penetrating keratoplasty at five years of age. Repeat keratoplasty was performed six months after initial surgery due to immune reaction-related graft failure. (**B**) a third keratoplasty was performed at eight years of age due to graft failure. (**C**) a graft rejection episode occurred one year afterwards, which led to graft failure despite immediate corticosteroid treatment. Current visual acuity is finger counting

5 Tips and Tricks

- Vessel cauterization should precede other interventions when performed in the same session.
- Systemic immunosuppression can be planned, especially in patients with limited visual potential in the other eye.
- Long term topical corticosteroid treatment is crucial in the treatment plan of high-risk eyes.
- Close follow-up of patients with frequent visits is important to intervene when rejection signs, adverse effects or need for retreatment occur.
- DMEK can safely be performed in vascularized edematous corneas (as long as no scars are present centrally), but immune reaction rates are higher than in normal DMEK eyes.

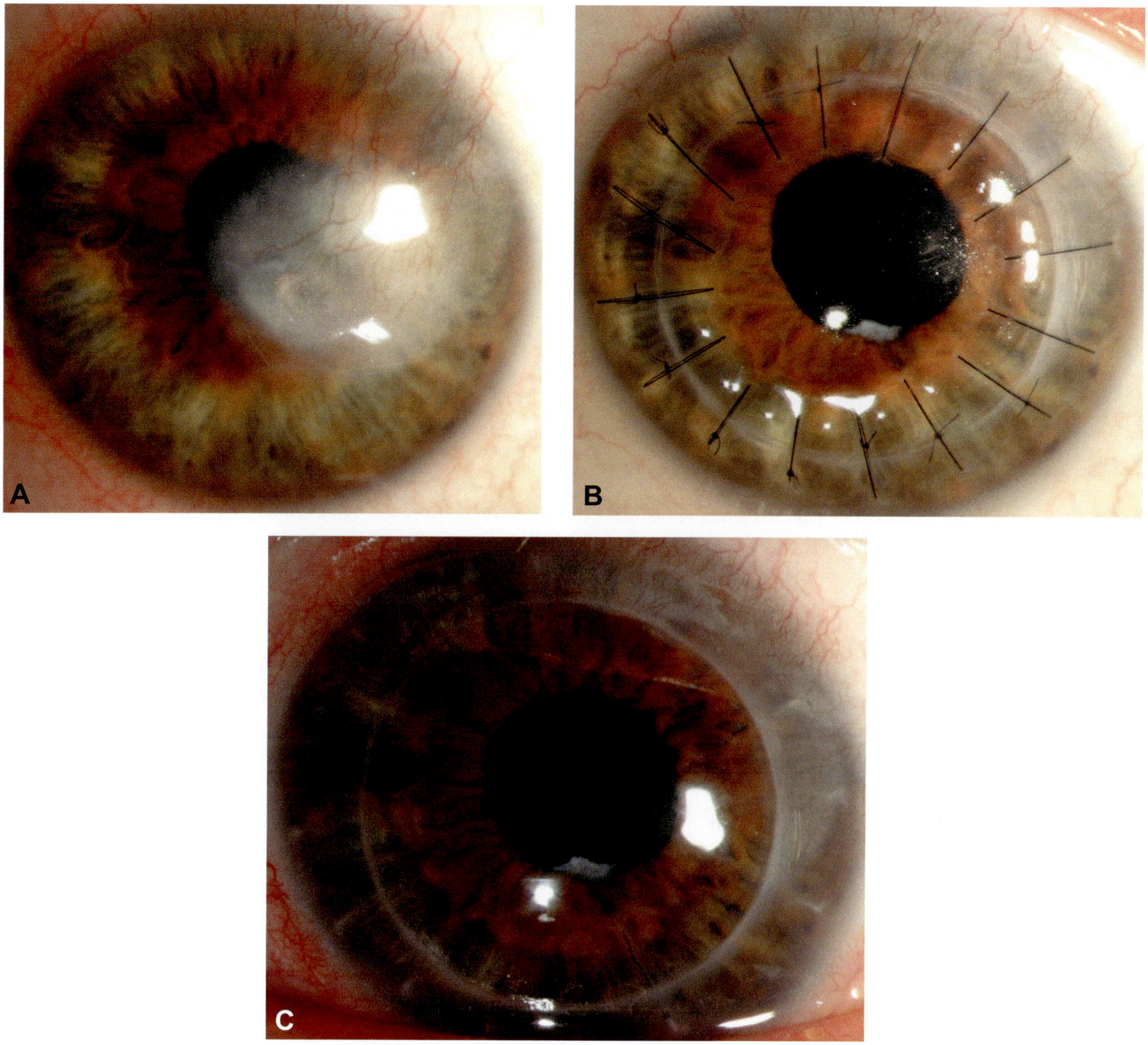

Fig. 10 (**A**) Cornea of a 52-year-old male patient with herpetic keratitis prior to FND and subconjunctival bevacizumab for (lymph)angioregressive preconditioning prior to high-risk keratoplasty. (**B**) 2 months after high-risk keratoplasty with no signs of rejection or revascularization. (**C**) same eye 18 months after keratoplasty

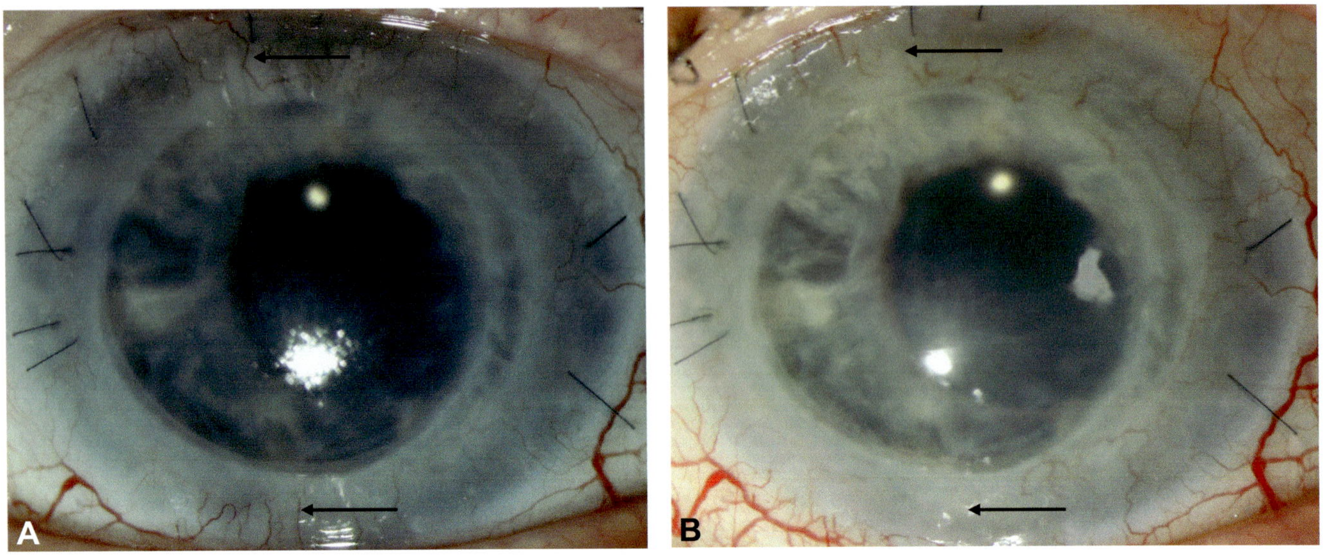

Fig. 11 (**A**) Corneal neovascularization prior to corneal crosslinking for (lymph)angioregression. (**B**) same eye three weeks after treatment. A significant regression of blood vessels can be seen, especially at the 6 and 12 o'clock positions (black arrows)

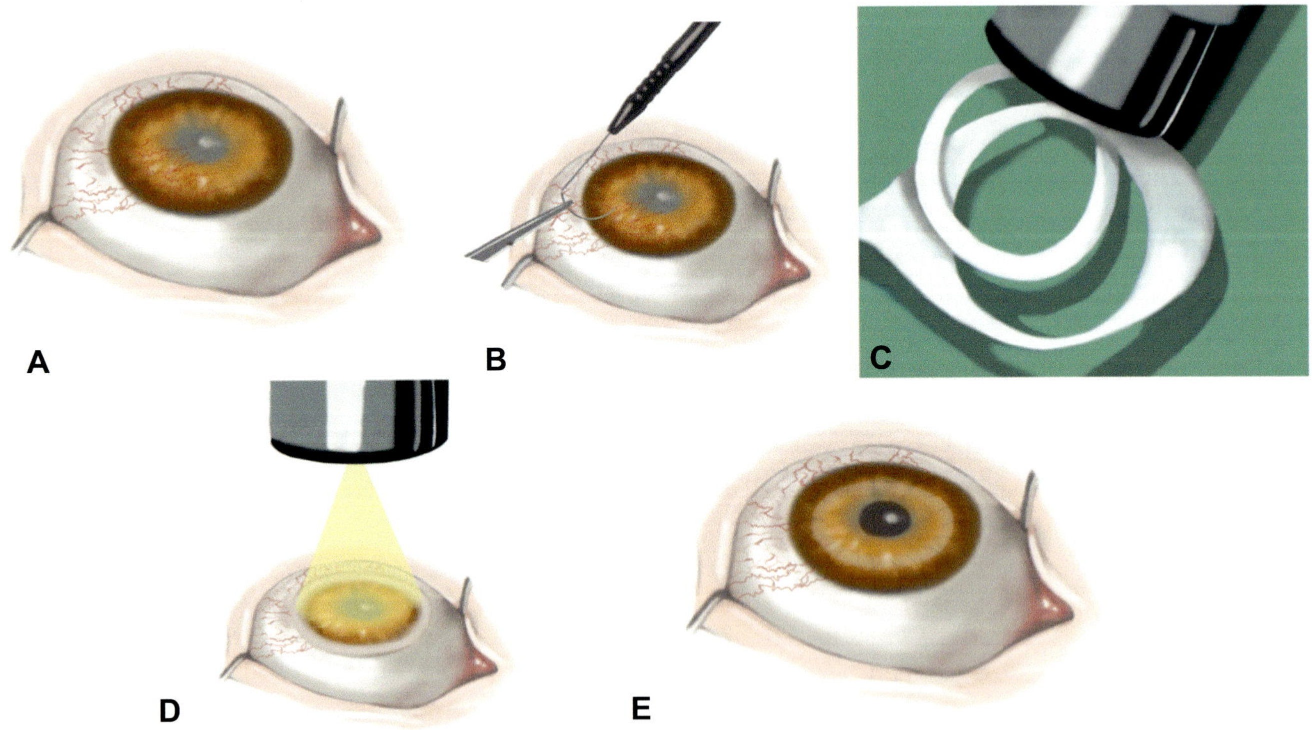

Fig. 12 Schematic description of a novel approach for (lymph)angioregression, namely combined fine-needle diathermy and corneal crosslinking. (**A**) eye with corneal neovascularization. (**B**) application of fine-needle diathermy. (**C**) preparation of a custom-cut limbal protection shield. (**D**) application of peripheral corneal crosslinking. (**E**) keratoplasty as the final procedure

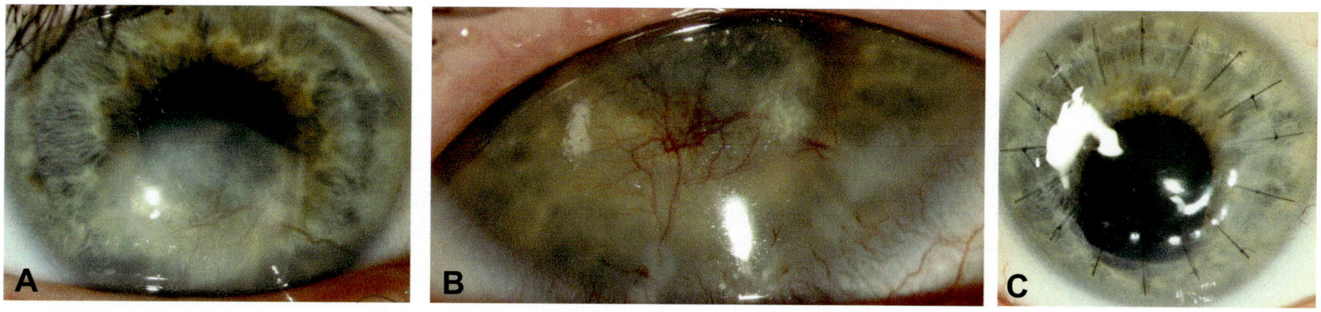

Fig. 13 (**A**) right eye of a 61-year-old male patient that developed a vascularized corneal scar with stromal thinning and lipid keratopathy after blunt eye trauma with a suspicion of herpes infection. Combined FND and CXL with subconjunctival bevacizumab injection was performed for (lymph)angioregression, followed by high-risk keratoplasty. (**B**) 1 day after combined FND and CXL with subconjunctival bevacizumab injection, whitening of the cornea and vessel occlusion due to fine-needle treatment can be observed. (**C**) same eye 12 months after keratoplasty with no apparent revascularization or rejection signs

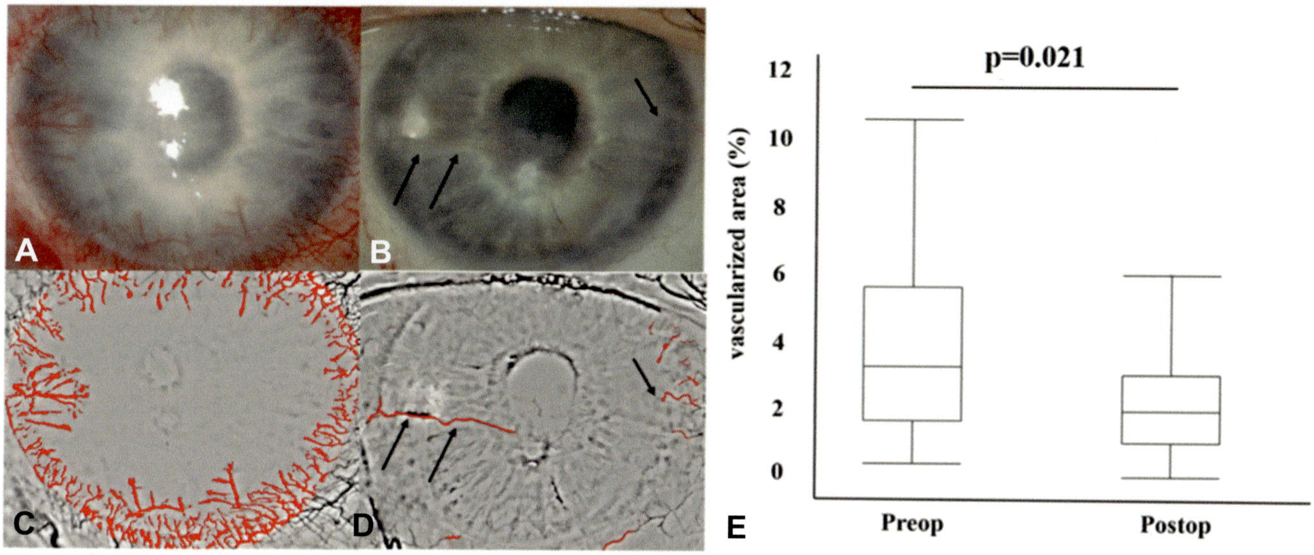

Fig. 14 (**A–E**) High-risk DMEK in vascularized edematous corneas leads to significant regression of corneal vessels [29]

6 Conclusion

Management of high-risk keratoplasty is still an ongoing challenge that requires individualized case-by-case clinical decision-making. Immunosuppressives remain the mainstay of treatment. If there is an underlying disease such as herpetic keratopathy or atopy, it should be kept under control with appropriate treatment. Close monitoring of patients is necessary to optimize postoperative care to reduce possible side effects and detect early rejection reactions. Hem- and lymphangioregressive preconditioning might offer a new solution for longer immune rejection-free graft survival.

Funding German Research Foundation (DFG) FOR2240 "(Lymph)-angiogenesis and Cellular Immunity in Inflammatory Diseases of the Eye" (Cu 47/4-2, Cu 47/6-1, Cu 47/9-1, Cu 47/15-1 to CC, HO 5556/1-2 to DH, www.for2240.de); EU COST BM1302 (CC, DH); CMMC Cologne (CC, DH); EU Horizon 2020 ARREST BLINDNESS (CC); EU COST Aniridia (www.aniridia-net.eu) (CC); BMBF 01KG2127 (DH, CC); Studienstiftung des Deutschen Volkes (MM).

References

1. The collaborative corneal transplantation studies (CCTS). Effectiveness of histocompatibility matching in high-risk corneal transplantation. The Collaborative Corneal Transplantation Studies Research Group. Arch Ophthalmol. 1992;110(10):1392–403.
2. Bachmann B, Taylor RS, Cursiefen C. Corneal neovascularization as a risk factor for graft failure and rejection after keratoplasty: an evidence-based meta-analysis. Ophthalmology. 2010;117(7):1300-5.e7. https://doi.org/10.1016/j.ophtha.2010.01.039.
3. Garcia DD, Shtein RM, Musch DC, et al. Herpes simplex virus keratitis: histopathologic neovascularization and corneal allograft failure. Cornea. 2009;28(9):963–5. https://doi.org/10.1097/ICO.0b013e31819c4e55.
4. Clahsen T, Büttner C, Hatami N, et al. Role of Endogenous Regulators of Hem and Lymphangiogenesis in Corneal Transplantation. J Clin Med. 2020;9(2):479. Published 9 Feb 2020. https://doi.org/10.3390/jcm9020479.
5. Schlötzer-Schrehardt U, Latta L, Gießl A, et al. Dysfunction of the limbal epithelial stem cell niche in aniridia-associated keratopathy. Ocul Surf. 2021;21:160–73. https://doi.org/10.1016/j.jtos.2021.06.002.
6. Ninios K, Jonescu-Cuypers C, Seitz B. Glaukome bei primären Irisveränderungen. Ophthalmologe. 2011;108:585–94. https://doi.org/10.1007/s00347-011-2372-3.
7. Xanthopoulou K, Milioti G, Seitz B. Need for explantation of an intrastromal titan ring after penetrating keratoplasty in two patients. Eur J Ophthalmol. 2022;32(1):35–41. https://doi.org/10.1177/1120672120962031.
8. Birnbaum F, Schwartzkopff J, Böhringer D, Reinhard T. The intrastromal corneal ring in penetrating keratoplasty-long-term results of a prospective randomized study. Cornea. 2011;30(7):780–3. https://doi.org/10.1097/ICO.0b013e318206caa9.
9. Bachmann BO, Pleyer U, Maier PC, et al. Perioperative/Postoperative Anti-Inflammatory Therapy During/After Corneal Surgery/Transplantation. Klin Monbl Augenheilkd. 2019;236(5):653–61. https://doi.org/10.1055/a-0864-4793.
10. Ramamoorthy S, Cidlowski JA. Corticosteroids: mechanisms of action in health and disease. Rheum Dis Clin North Am. 2016;42(1):15–31.
11. Bali S, Filek R, Si F, et al. Systemic immunosuppression in high-risk penetrating keratoplasty: a systematic review. J Clin Med Res. 2016;8(4):269–76. https://doi.org/10.14740/jocmr2326w.
12. Birnbaum F, Böhringer D, Sokolovska Y, et al. Immunosuppression with cyclosporine A and mycophenolate mofetil after penetrating high-risk keratoplasty: a retrospective study. Transplantation. 2005;79(8):964–8.
13. Yamazoe K, Yamazoe K, Yamaguchi T, et al. Efficacy and safety of systemic tacrolimus in high-risk penetrating keratoplasty after graft failure with systemic cyclosporine. Cornea. 2014;33(11):1157–63.
14. Böhringer D, Grotejohann B, Ihorst G, et al. Rejection prophylaxis in corneal transplant: a randomized study of HLA matching (The Fancy Study). Dtsch Arztebl Int. 2018;115(15):259–65.
15. Hopkinson CL, Romano V, Kaye RA, et al. The influence of donor and recipient gender incompatibility on corneal transplant rejection and failure. Am J Transpl. 2017;17(1):210–7. https://doi.org/10.1111/ajt.13926.
16. Hos D, Matthaei M, Bock F, et al. Immune reactions after modern lamellar (DALK, DSAEK, DMEK) versus conventional penetrating corneal transplantation. Prog Retin Eye Res. 2019;73: 100768. https://doi.org/10.1016/j.preteyeres.2019.07.001.
17. Cursiefen C. Immune privilege and angiogenic privilege of the cornea. Chem Immunol Allergy. 2007;92:50–7. https://doi.org/10.1159/000099253.
18. Dietrich T, Bock F, Yuen D, et al. Cutting edge: lymphatic vessels, not blood vessels, primarily mediate immune rejections after transplantation. J Immunol. 2010;184(2):535–9.
19. Hou Y, Bock F, Hos D, et al. Lymphatic trafficking in the eye: modulation of lymphatic trafficking to promote corneal transplant survival. Cells. 2021;10(7):1661. https://doi.org/10.3390/cells10071661.
20. Hou Y, Le VNH, Clahsen T, et al. Photodynamic therapy leads to time-dependent regression of pathologic corneal (Lymph) angiogenesis and promotes high-risk corneal allograft survival. Invest Ophthalmol Vis Sci. 2017;58(13):5862–9. https://doi.org/10.1167/iovs.17-22904.
21. Hou Y, Le VNH, Tóth G, et al. UV light crosslinking regresses mature corneal blood and lymphatic vessels and promotes subsequent high-risk corneal transplant survival. Am J Transpl. 2018;18(12):2873–84. https://doi.org/10.1111/ajt.14874.
22. Hos D, Le VNH, Hellmich M, et al. Risk of corneal graft rejection after high-risk keratoplasty following fine-needle vessel coagulation of corneal neovascularization combined with bevacizumab: a pilot study. Transpl Direct. 2019;5(5): e452.
23. Mestanoglu M, Händel A, Cursiefen C, et al. Three-year follow-up of high-risk keratoplasty following fine-needle diathermy of corneal neovascularization combined with bevacizumab. Graefes Arch Clin Exp Ophthalmol. 2022;260(7):2383–5. https://doi.org/10.1007/s00417-021-05546-w.
24. Schaub F, Hou Y, Zhang W, et al. Corneal crosslinking to regress pathologic corneal neovascularization before high-risk keratoplasty. Cornea. 2021;40(2):147–55.
25. Cursiefen C, Cao J, Chen L, et al. Inhibition of hemangiogenesis and lymphangiogenesis after normal-risk corneal transplantation by neutralizing VEGF promotes graft survival. Invest Ophthalmol Vis Sci. 2004;45(8):2666–73. https://doi.org/10.1167/iovs.03-1380.
26. Bachmann BO, Bock F, Wiegand SJ, et al. Promotion of graft survival by vascular endothelial growth factor a neutralization after high-risk corneal transplantation. Arch Ophthalmol. 2008;126(1):71–7. https://doi.org/10.1001/archopht.126.1.71.
27. Le VNH, Hou Y, Bock F, et al. Supplemental anti VEGF-A-therapy prevents rebound neovascularisation after fine needle diathermy treatment to regress pathological corneal (LYMPH) angiogenesis. Sci Rep. 2020;10(1):3908.
28. Dohlman TH, McSoley M, Amparo F, et al. Bevacizumab in high-risk corneal transplantation: a pilot multicenter prospective randomized control trial. Ophthalmology. 2022;129(8):865–79. https://doi.org/10.1016/j.ophtha.2022.03.024.
29. Hayashi T, Zhang W, Hos D, et al. Descemet membrane endothelial keratoplasty in vascularized eyes: outcome and effect on corneal neovascularization. Cornea. 2021;40(6):685–9. https://doi.org/10.1097/ICO.0000000000002502.
30. Paque J, Poirier RH. Corneal allograft reaction and its relationship to suture site neovascularization. Ophthalmic Surg. 1977;8(4):71–4.

Penetrating Keratoplasty in Children—Special Considerations

Barbara Käsmann-Kellner and Berthold Seitz

Abstract

The younger the children are at the time of corneal transplantation, the worse the survival prognosis of the graft. However amblyopia will become worse while waiting too long. This constellation presents an everlasting dilemma between corneal surgeons and pediatric ophthalmologists. Preoperative considerations are significant in terms of accurate parental education, ensuring adherence to therapy, choosing the appropriate surgical time frame (amblyopia versus graft failure, compliance of the patient). Parental education must include the reduced visual prognosis in young children, exceptions being later acquired corneal pathologies such as inflammatory corneal scars (herpes) and keratoconus. A distinction must be made between morphological care after transplantation and refractive correction as well as amblyopia therapy. The younger the children, the less favourable the prognosis for the transplant and the more often multiple anaesthetic examinations are necessary in order to detect complications such as infiltrates or suture loosening at an early stage. Especially unilateral congenital pathologies often do not lead to a sufficient improvement of amblyopia (refractory amblyopia, poor compliance due to very dominant healthy eye). The prognosis after keratoplasty in childhood is already partly decided by the careful indication (no surgery of a sclerocornea) and the detailed and realistic information of the parents (cooperation with ocular and systemic treatment even if the child has poor compliance, frequent check-ups, reduced chances of amblyopia therapy). The younger the child at the time of transplantation, the more frequent graft failure and the development of complications. Later manifesting diseases in older children (herpetic corneal scars, keratoconus) have a better prognosis.

Keywords

Keratoplasty · Child · Refraction · Amblyopia · Graft failure

1 Background

About 2% of all corneal transplantations are performed in children under 18 years of age (Fig. 1) [1, 2].

The majority of these are children between the ages of 4 and 12 years [3]. Predominantly, these are penetrating keratoplasties. Special problems are the examination conditions before and after surgery, the child's lack of compliance with the administration of therapy, the increased rate of necessary anaesthesia, the increased rate of complications (suture loosening, infiltrates, graft rejection, complications from treatment), and the risk of deprivation amblyopia [1, 4]. These problems are much more common in younger children, which is another reason why the chances of graft survival in young children are much lower than in adults. At the age of 4 years and older, the ability to cooperate is greater and so is the understanding of the children regarding the measures taken. Since the diseases are often bilateral, there is a risk of permanent visual impairment. One must consider pre-, intra- and postoperative requirements. For indications of pediatric keratoplasty and anterior segment surgery in children see Table 1 [1, 2, 5–8] and Figs. 2, 3, 4, 5 and 6.

B. Käsmann-Kellner (✉) · B. Seitz
Department of Ophthalmology, Saarland University Medical Center, Homburg 66424, Germany
e-mail: kaesmann@gmail.com

B. Seitz et al. (eds.), *Atlas on Cornea*, https://doi.org/10.1007/978-3-031-65422-0_54

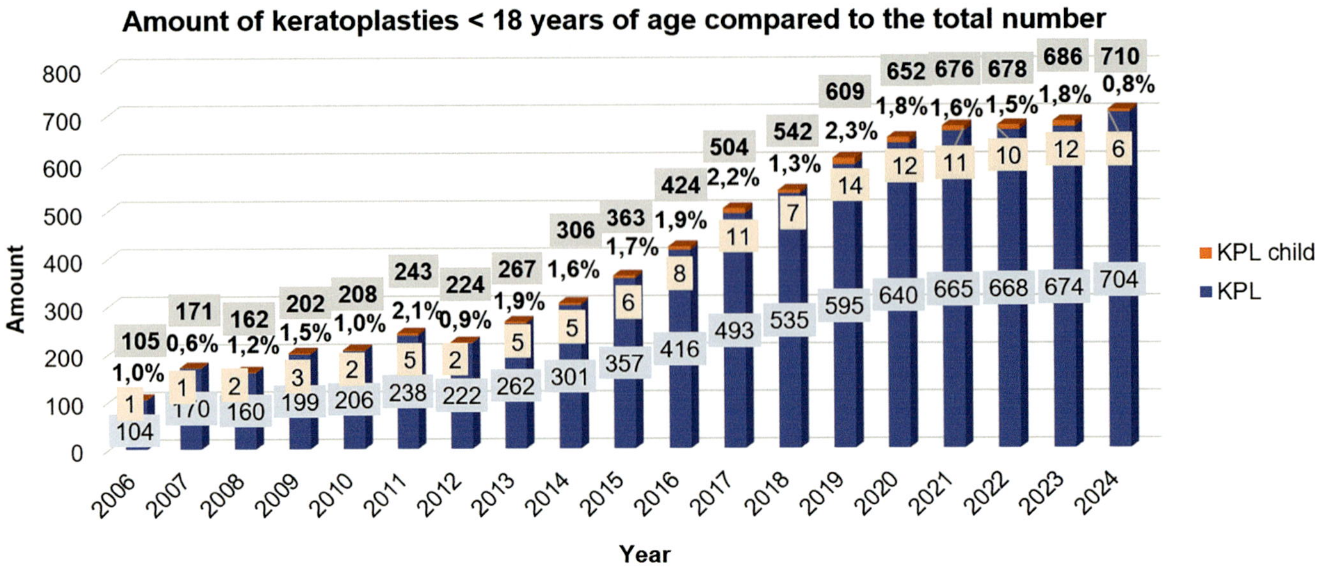

Fig. 1 Number of keratoplasties (KPL) in patients under 18 years and their percentage of all performed keratoplasties, Department of Ophthalmology, Saarland University Medical Center, 2006–2024

2 General Features of the Examination of Children

Table 2 summarizes the essential features in the ophthalmological examination of children. It is evident that the various cooperation-related problems and the limited possibilities of examination with standard ophthalmological diagnostic equipment have a very negative and limiting significance. This is especially the case in conditions after (any) ocular surgery, especially when one depends on an accurate postoperative evaluation [15–22].

3 Considerations Prior to Corneal Surgery Procedures

Careful indication before surgery as well as detailed information for the parents about the complexity of the follow-up are essential to minimize the risk of graft failure and to make the amblyopia therapy as successful as possible. Parents need to know that in the case of congenital findings no normal visual development can be expected even after successful transplantation. The situation is different in the case of acquired (e.g., herpetic scars [9]) or later manifesting (keratoconus [2]) disorders. After completion of the amblyogenic phase, surgery may be delayed in the absence of cooperation to improve the

Table 1 Indications for perforating keratoplasty in children [1–3, 11–14]

Classification	Examples
Congenital	Peters anomaly, stromal corneal dystrophies, buphthalmia, microphthalmia with corneal involvement (sclerocornea), anterior segment dysgenesies, corneal dermoids, CYP1B1 cytopathia, aniridia
Acquired, non-traumatic	–On the basis of a genetic disease: PAX6 associated aniridia associated keratopathy (AAK, 4 grades, Figs. 4 and 5)[a], Keratoconus, Mucopolysaccharidoses –Without genetic basis: Inflammatory (especially herpetic eye disease, Fig. 6, acanthamoeba keratitis, Figs. 16 and 17)
Acquired, traumatic	Perforating or penetrating injuries
Transplant decompensation	Repeat keratoplasties

[a]Limbal stem cell insufficiency in congenital aniridia with consecutive vascularized opacification is not yet fully understood [9, 10]

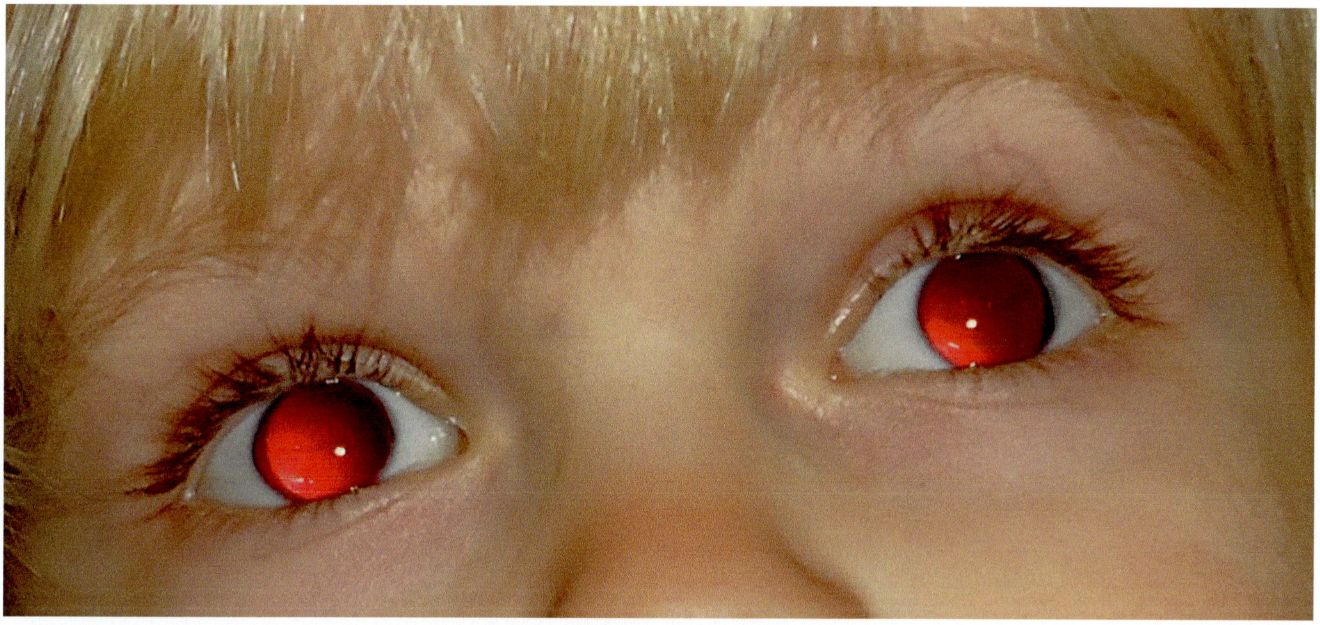

Fig. 2 Boy, 2 years, complete aniridia, divergent squint OS, margin of the lens visible in translucent illumination, no limbal stem cell insufficiency/pannus formation, AAK Grade 0

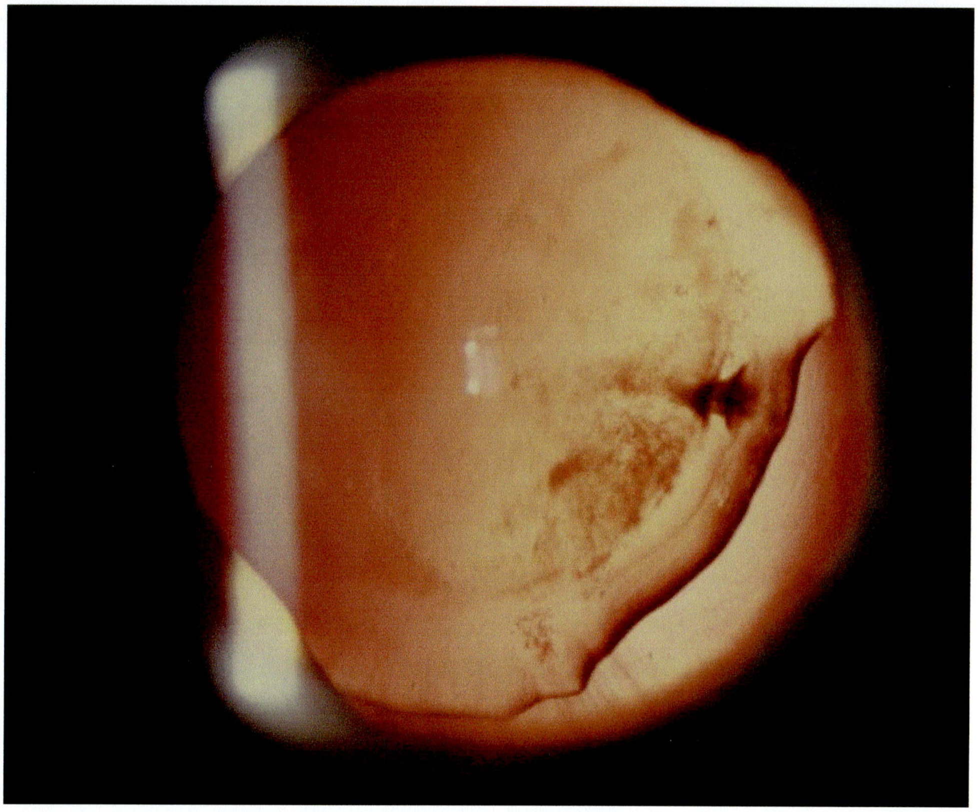

Fig. 3 Girl, 1.5 years, partial coloboma and lens subluxation in congenital aniridia, incipient cortical cataract, visible zonula fibres (5–6 o'clock), indication for lens extraction

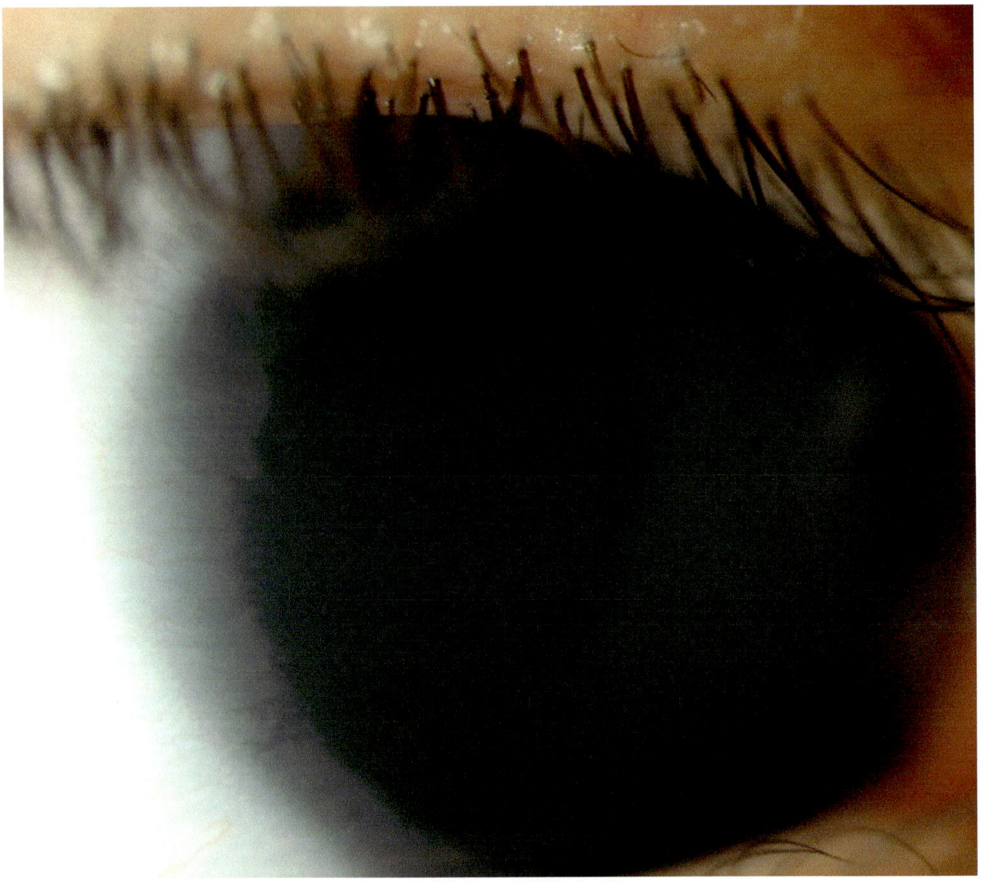

Fig. 4 Boy aged 2 years, congenital aniridia, AAK grade 2, vascularized limbus, progressive growth towards center of cornea

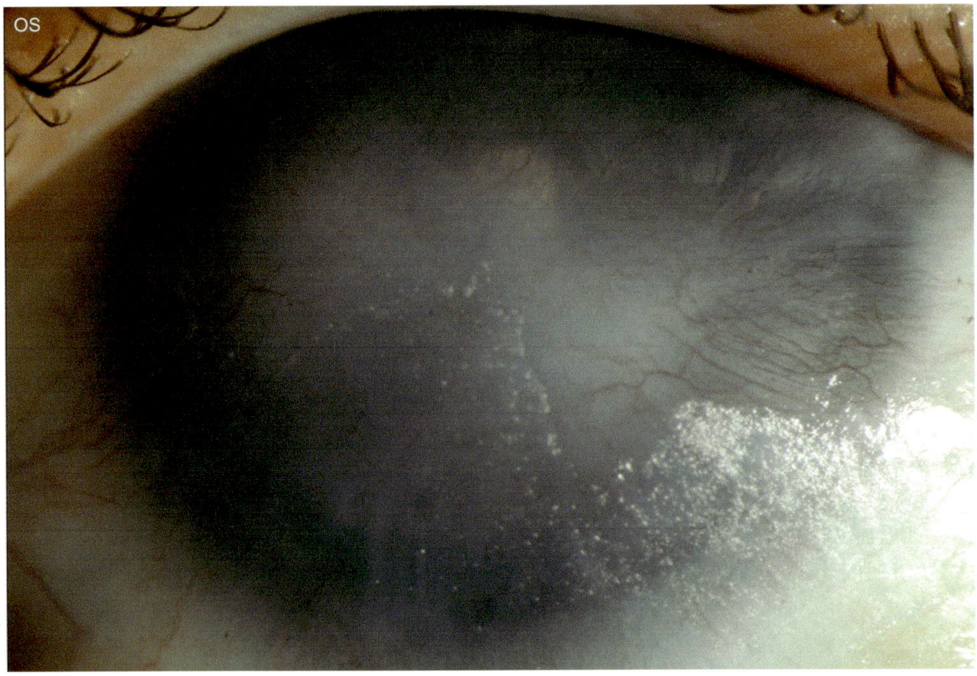

Fig. 5 Girl, aged 11 years, congenital aniridia, AAK grade 4 with opaque corneal center, distinct sicca signs, preoperative documentation

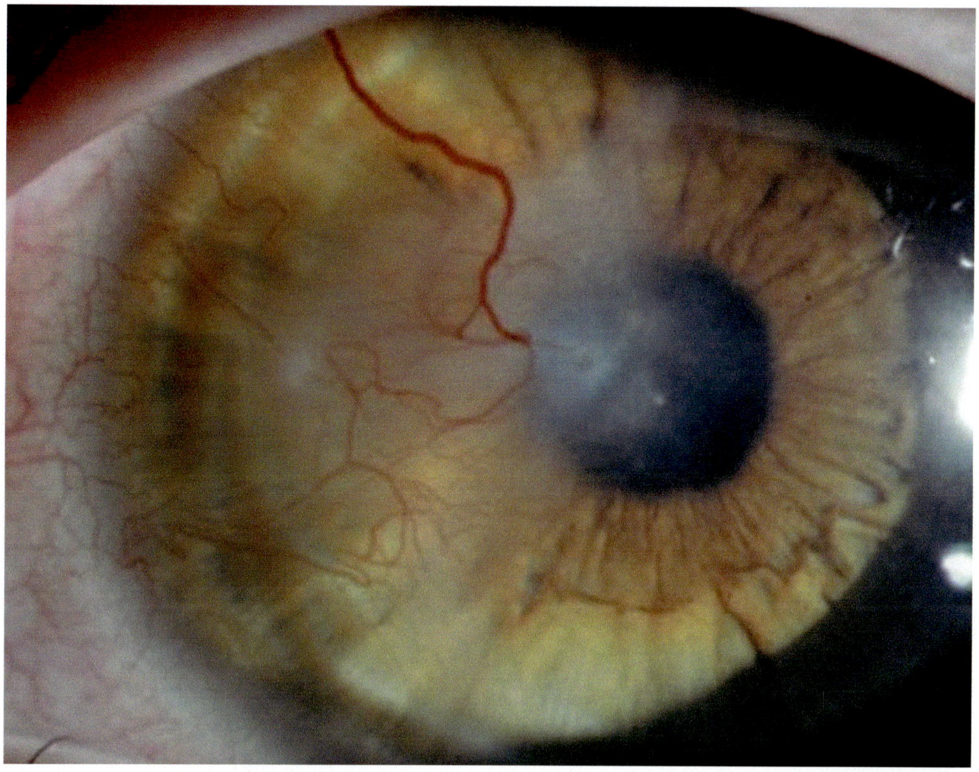

Fig. 6 Boy, 2.5 years, herpetic vascularized corneal scarring with involvement of the centre of the cornea, deep amblyopia, retinoscopy not possible

Table 2 Main features of the examination of children

Area	Special features
Time	–Longer time during examinations –Visual acuity with Preferential Looking, LEA test takes time –Lack of compliance of the child –Longer discussions with parents –More anesthesia examinations needed
Diagnostic tools	–More hand-held devices, but thus also less accurate (hand-held slit lamp) –Retinoscopy essential
Documentation	–Photodocumentation more difficult –Apparative corneal diagnostics not possible/only possible to a limited extent

outlook and not to impair the child too much in its visual, cognitive and motor development.

In younger children, the immune response is more pronounced than in older children. In young children, other surgeries (see Table 3) have also proven successful, such as lamellar keratoplasty, ipsilateral rotational keratoplasty, or even phototherapeutic keratectomy (PTK), which are sparing the endothelium.

The donor should be as young as possible, but at least 4 years old, because transplanting a very young cornea can potentially cause problems for the surgeon and therefore also for the recipient due to the softer tissue (sutures can loosen more easily, inadequate steepening of the graft [2]). For children and adolescents, younger donors should be sought because of their higher endothelial cell numbers, which is important for the survival time of the graft.

Very close collaboration with conservative pediatric ophthalmology both preoperatively and postoperatively is an indispensable requirement for pediatric keratoplasty in the visual plasticity phase to best select occlusion therapy and timing of surgery in the face of amblyopia.

Table 3 Necessary preoperative considerations in KP in congenital corneal opacification [23–27]

Area	Factors	Details
Child	–General health –General development –Often absent compliance with preoperative examinations	–Tolerance to medications and anesthesia examinations –Cooperation during examinations and therapy –Estimation of the severity of postoperative cooperation problems
Parents	–Detailed planning of the surgery –Information about therapy expenses and regular follow-up examinations	–Risk–benefit assessment of the surgery –Ensuring good compliance of the parents
Eyes and visual development	–Collaboration with pediatric ophthalmology essential –Unilateral or bilateral involvement –Time of onset –Visually evoked potentials (VEP) –Intraocular pressure	–Surgery timing, pre- and postoperative care essential –Danger of amblyopia or visual impairment? –Congenital: worse prognosis than acquired corneal opacity –Useful for estimation of potential surgical success –No surgery in case of non-regulated pressure! –If necessary trabeculotomy before corneal surgery
Time of the surgery	–Early OP (<5 years, esp. < 1 year) –Later OP (>5 years)	–Poorer cooperation, poorer transplant survival, strong immunological response, theoretically less amblyopia –Better cooperation, better transplant survival, more pronounced amblyopia
Choice of operation	–Reduction immune response –Reduction endothelial cell loss –Suture technique	–PTK, lamellar keratoplasty, autologous ipsilateral rotational keratoplasty instead of KP –The younger, the more likely single sutures
Choice of graft	–Young donor (but >4 years)	–Endothelial cell count around 3000/mm^2 –No PEX in donor
Immunosuppression	–Interdisciplinary collaboration with pediatric clinic for high-risk KPL (vascularized graft, repeat keratoplasty)	–Clarification of the side effect profile of immunosuppressive drugs –Pediatric control of dosage –Start 3 days before planned surgery

KP: Keratoplasty, OP: Operation, PEX: Pseudoexfoliationssyndrome, PTK: Phototherapeutic Keratektomy, TP: Transplant, VEP: Visually evoked potentials

4 Intraoperative Particularities

The following is a list of the essential pre- and intraoperative requirements [1, 2, 15, 28–33]:

Very experienced corneal surgeon essential, as the following problems can occur [2, 34, 35]

- Pronounced vis à tergo
- Softer tissue
- Iridotomy(ies) to avoid bombata configuration with secondary angle closure glaucoma
- Smaller graft diameters needed
- The younger the child, the more likely to use single sutures
- Suture loosening occurs more often than in older patients
- Lens sparing surgery (lens loss reduces graft survival).

Highly experienced pediatric anesthesiologist [11–15]

- General anesthesia in controlled arterial hypotension with systemic acetazolamide and mannitol as well as adequate muscle relaxation (no mivacurium!)
- Adequate positioning with the upper body elevated by approx. 60°.

5 Care in the Perioperative Phase (0–4 weeks)

In the perioperative period, the focus lies on morphologic controls and controls of the intraocular pressure rather than orthoptic findings and amblyopia [2, 4, 15].

The following complications may arise in the immediate postoperative period:

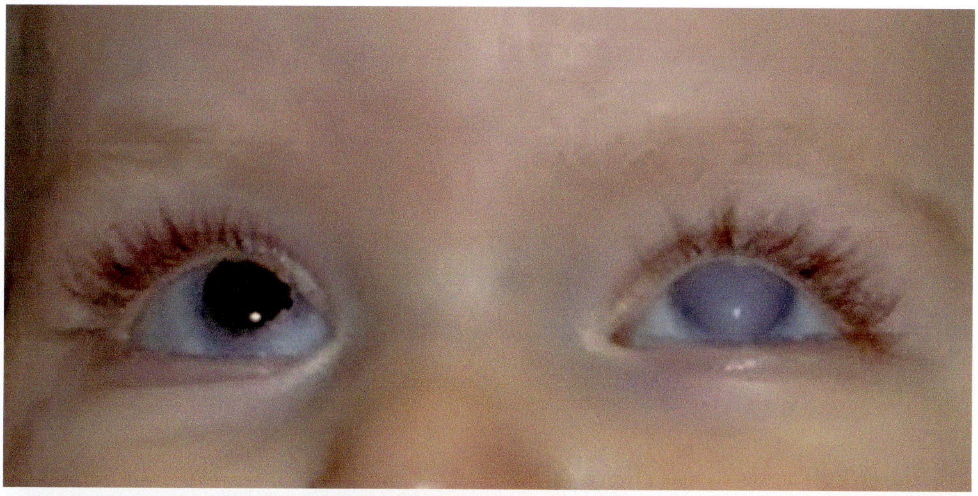

Fig. 7 Girl, 18 months. Aniridia and congenital corneal opacification in CYP1B-related congenital glaucoma. OD penetrating keratoplasty at age 12 months, OS preoperatively. Slit lamp photodocumentation not possible due to lack of cooperation

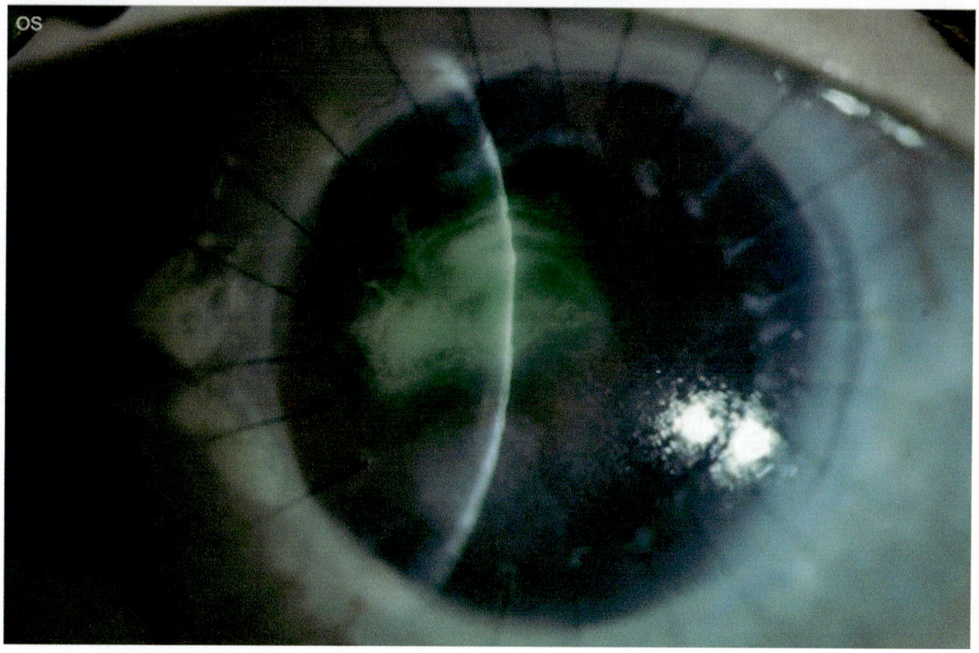

Fig. 8 Boy, aged 10 years: 2nd keratoplasty in buphthalmia. Early postoperative complications: infiltrate formation, endothelial decompensation especially caudally with beginning loss of transparency

(1) Examinations of the child significantly more difficult (Fig. 7—occasionally no slit lamp documentation possible)
   (a) Problematic outpatient´s follow ups
   (b) Anaesthesia examination(s) may be necessary
(2) Local treatment application by parents made more difficult due to lack of compliance by the child
   (a) In addition, parents may refrain from applying the eye drops due to the apprehension of the child
   (b) May jeopardize graft survival
(3) Increase in eye pressure
   (a) Pressure must be regulated because postoperative endothelial decompensation results equally often from pressure decompensation and from immune response [2, 15].
   (b) This is especially relevant in buphthalmia (Fig. 8)
(4) Focal erosions
   (a) Often persistent for a long time
   (b) Risk of development of infiltrates (Fig. 8) and ulcers
(5) Suture loosening and suture infiltrates (Figs. 9 and 10, fibrosis around the single sutures)
   (a) Can lead to neovascularization and stronger endothelial immune response
   (b) More common in congenital than in acquired pathologies
   (c) Examination with fluorescein and blue light obligatory (may also be informative without slit lamp) (Fig. 11, good postoperative findings, intact sutures without vessel formation, Fig. 12 same eye post-suture removal)

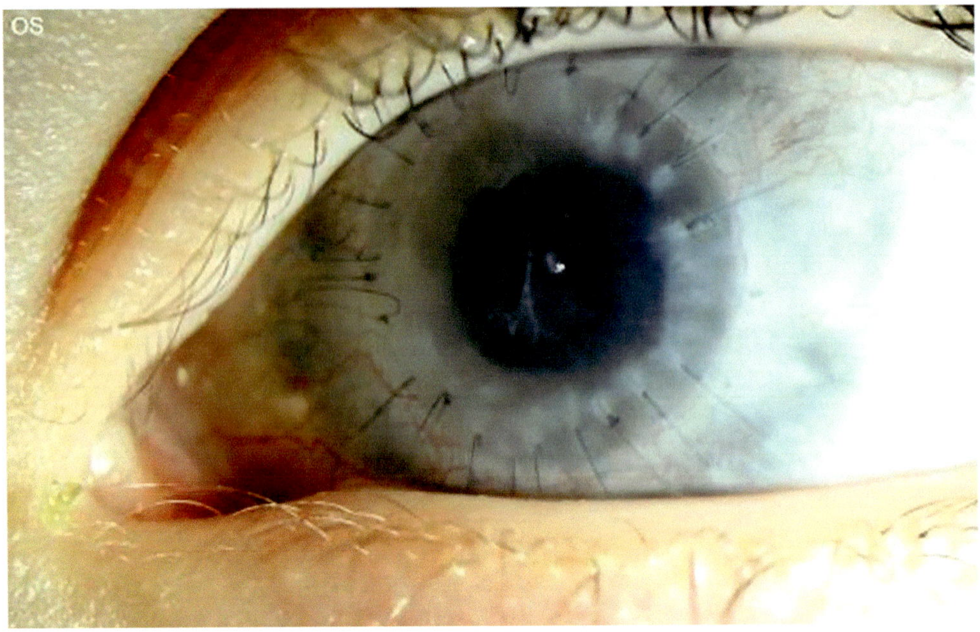

Fig. 9 Boy, 12 months, OS. Aphakia following surgical phakectomy in congenital cataract at age 5 weeks. Aphakia corrected by contact lens. Developed contact lens induced corneal infiltration and ulcus formation plus endophthalmitis. State post pole-to-pole surgery including keratoplasty at age 10 months. Loosening of sutures temporally (already removed) and now nasally. Beginning decompensation of the corneal transplant

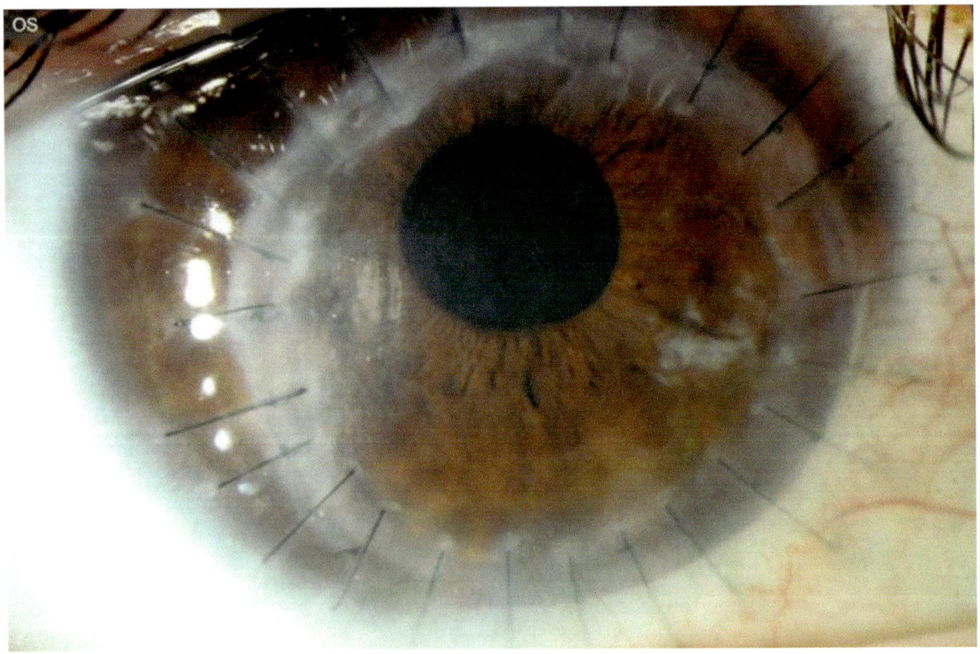

Fig. 10 Girl, aged 4 years, OS. Excentric herpetic ulcer, excentric penetrating keratoplasty 6 months ago. Suture loosening nasally, excision of loose sutures with replacing of sutures, severe corneal fibrosis at the graft–host junction

(6) Warning signs red eye, glare, epiphora, infiltrates ("white spots")
   (a) Inform parents about warning signs and immediate need for re-examination.
   (b) Generously give indication for examination in anesthesia
   (c) Always remove any loose suture/s immediately!!!

Safety glasses should be prescribed at an early stage (even without refraction correction) to get the child used to the wearing of glasses.

6 Refractive, Orthoptic and Morphological Care Postoperatively (From 4th Week Postop)

From the 4th week postoperatively, a first refraction determination by retinoscopy can be performed. Very high and irregular astigmatisms are often found, which complicate the measurement and the refraction correction especially in case of only one-sided findings. Nevertheless, spectacle

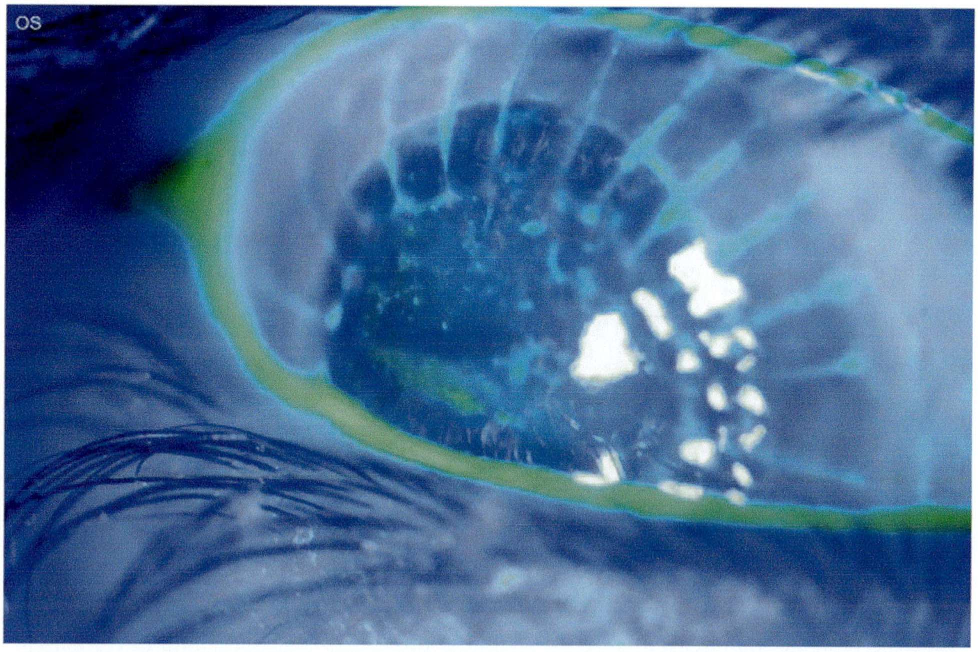

Fig. 11 Girl, aged 2,5 years, OS. Axenfeld–Rieger Syndrome OU with congenital corneal opacification. Fluorescent imaging post-keratoplasty, intact sutures, no infiltrates, superficial keratopathy

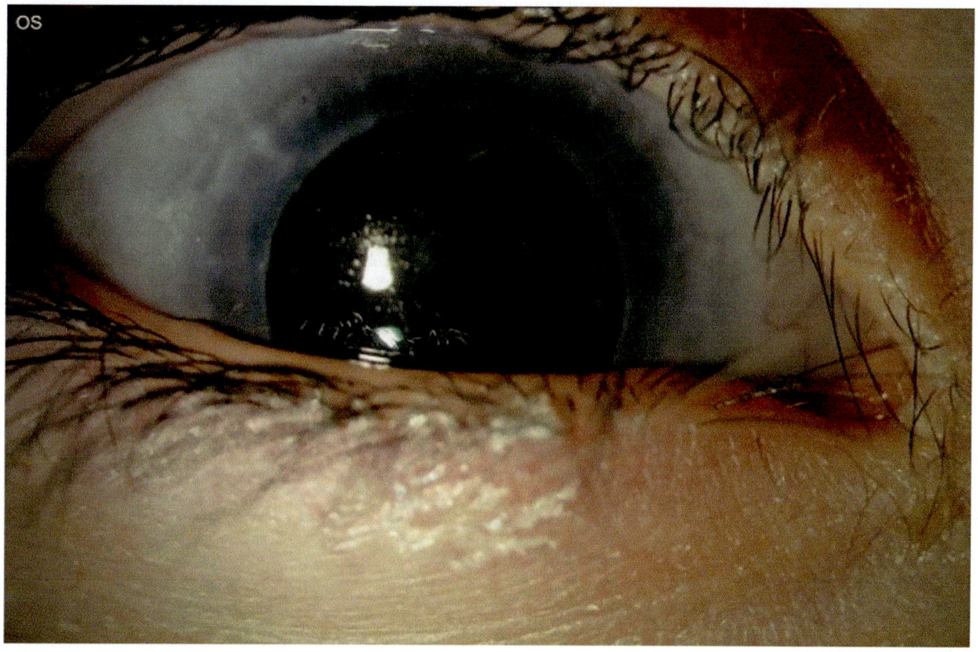

Fig. 12 Same girl as in Fig. 11, now 3 years old, OS. Good findings after suture removal. VA −3.5/−4.0/50 = 0.6 dec

prescription should be done with the implication that the lenses may need to be changed in a few months.

After spectacle prescription also amblyopia therapy should be started (definitely before suture removal!). Especially in unilateral findings longer patching times are necessary in deprivation amblyopia than in simple strabismus amblyopia [15–17]. In the case of bilateral (operated) findings, the adhesive must be applied alternately depending on the visual outcome, if necessary in a different rhythm for each side. Again, careful information of the parents is necessary, because the occlusion therapy after corneal surgery is usually difficult and requires a lot of patience from parents and child.

Even if the main focus is now also on amblyopia therapy, the morphological controls are indispensable and the treating ophthalmologist must be informed exactly about possible complications and their early recognition. The parents need to be informed as well on the necessity of regular eye drops application and about warning signs making an immediate examination essential (more tearing, red conjunctiva, gray-whitish opacity of parts of the cornea (even in very small areas). Parents should as well be trained to palpate the eyes to detect differences between the two eyes or differences to the parental eyes.

After discharge from inpatient treatment, if the healing process is regular, the ophthalmologist should check twice a week for the first 2 weeks, then weekly until the 6th post-operative week. From the 6th postoperative week, the visits to the ophthalmologist can be extended to every 2 weeks up to and including the third postoperative month (with photographic documentation if possible). If the course is regular, from the 4th month controls can take place monthly, from the 6th postoperative month every 2 months until the one-year period after surgery is reached. In the period of short-term controls, orthoptic controls every 2 months are useful. From one year after the operation, 3-monthly morphological controls are necessary, of course with orthoptic control and possible adjustment of the occlusion rhythm. Refraction controls are necessary in the 4th postoperative month as well as after partial removal of the sutures and after complete removal of the sutures (Table 4). At each control, the intraocular pressure should be measured, for example with rebound tonometry, and the cup–disc ratio (CDR) of the optic disc should be documented to detect aniridia-associated or steroid-associated secondary glaucoma at an early stage [36].

A poor postoperative prognosis is seen in vascularized scars, early transplantation and repeat keratoplasties (Fig. 13).

A good prognosis for long-term graft survival is found especially in non-vascularized corneal opacities and surgery after the age of 3 (Figs. 14 and 15).

Occasionally, even highly inflamed corneae such as in Figs. 16 and 17 can yield very good morphological results, although the postoperative astigmatism in single sutures prevents a full cc visual acuity (Fig. 16). This can, however, be better achieved by continuous sutures (Fig. 17).

Parental expectations must be realistically tempered, as both amblyopia and refractive errors can and will affect visual acuity development despite successful surgery [6, 7].

Table 4 Negative and positive prognostic factors for success of childhood corneal transplantation

Prognostic factors	Risk of graft failure
Negative prognostic factors	–Young age (<1 year 50% graft failure) –Congenital pathologies, especially Peters anomaly, sclerocornea –Ocular comorbidities (anterior segment dysgenesis, glaucoma) –Vascularized corneal scars –Additional surgical procedures during keratoplasty (lens, glaucoma) –Poor therapy compliance (medication, occlusion) –Repeat keratoplasties
Positive prognostic factors	–Age over 5 years (visual system more mature, cooperation better) –Acquired pathologies, especially herpetic scars and keratoconus –Suture removal earlier than in adults (from 6 months after keratoplasty) –Absence of vascularization

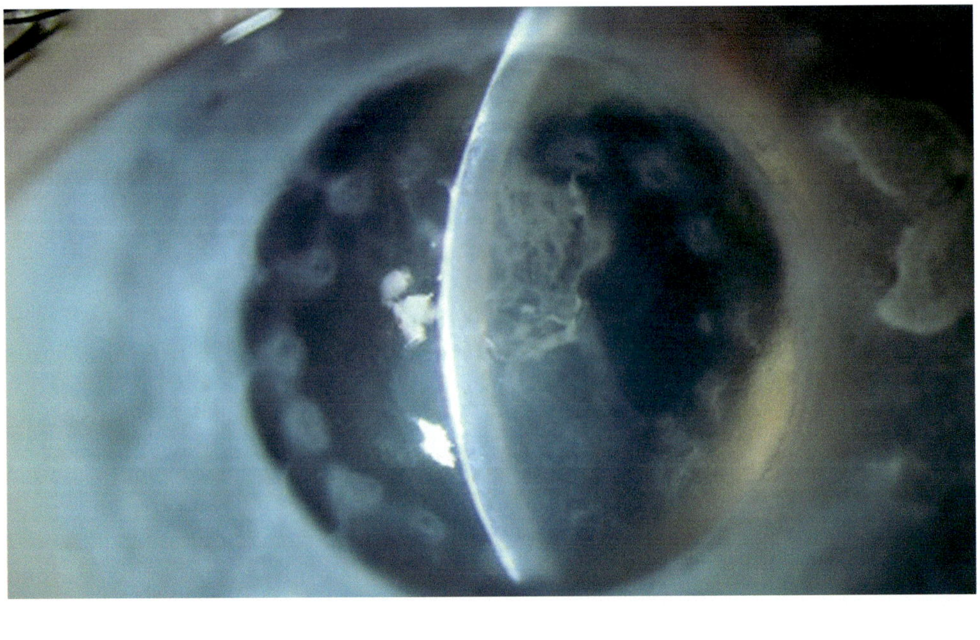

Fig. 13 Boy, 14 years, buphthalmia. Long-term graft failure and calcification in a former re-keratoplasty with HLA-typed donor, 3 years after penetrating keratoplasty

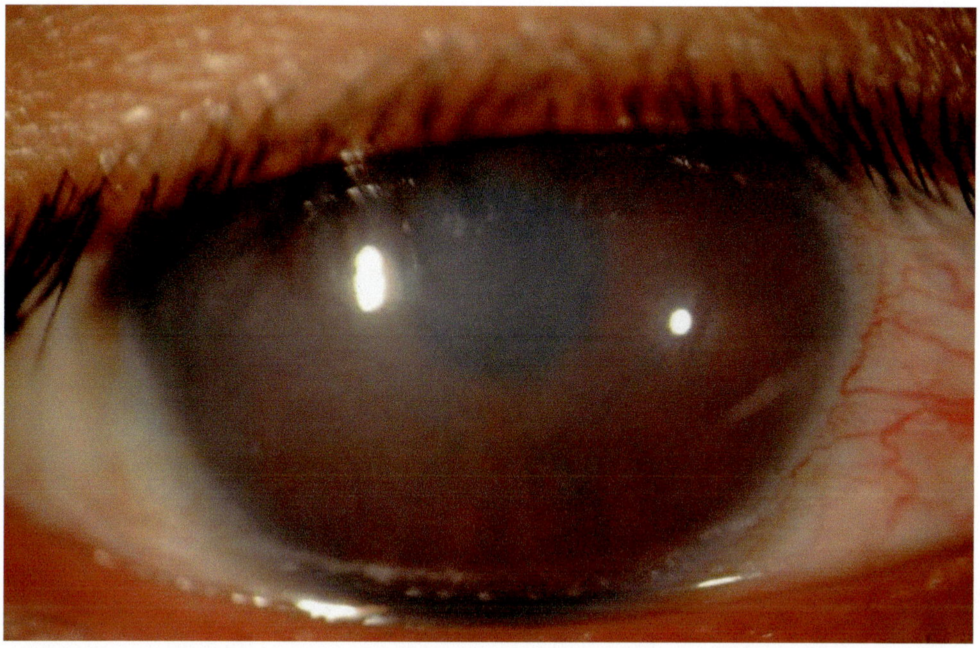

Fig. 14 Boy from Thessaloniki, aged 6 years, non-vascularized corneal opacification in CHSD (congenital hereditary stromal dystrophy), no nystagmus, good prognosis for penetrating keratoplasty

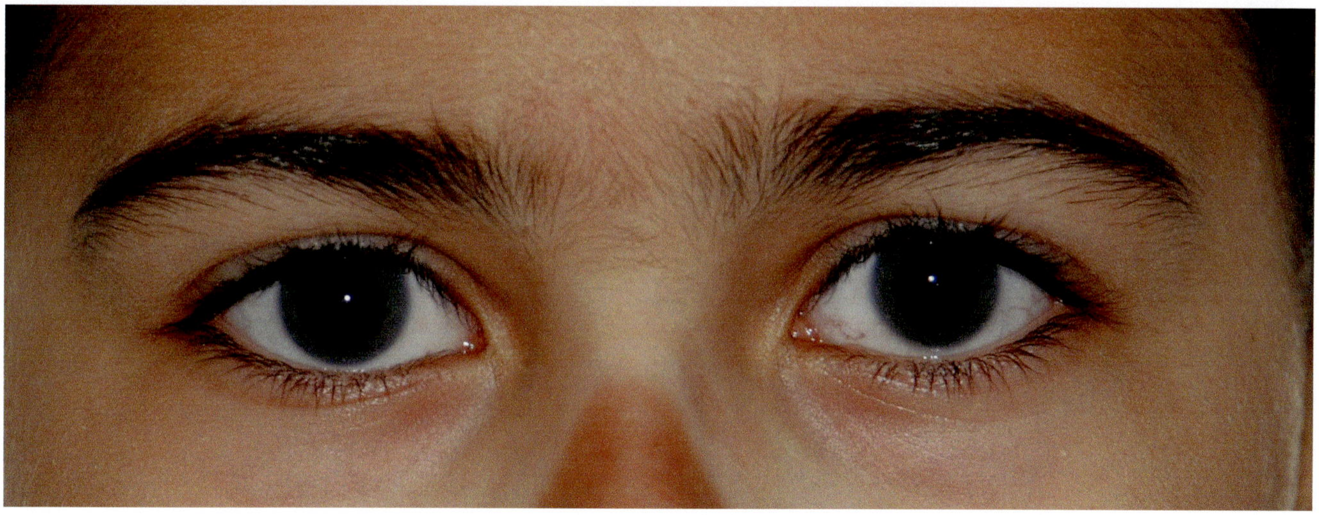

Fig. 15 Same boy as in Fig. 14, CHSD, now 14 years, long term findings following penetrating excimer laser keratoplasty (8.0/8.1) bilaterally, outcome after 8 years and after alternating amblyopia treatment. Visual acuity cc bilaterally 0.7 dec. Image taken with non-mydriatic pupil, the gray peripheral border is the host cornea with congenital hereditary stromal dystrophy

Irregular astigmatism can be better compensated by rigid contact lenses if the child cooperates. Rarely, the question of refractive surgery also may arise.

In addition, the axial length should be measured regularly, because in deprivation amblyopia, myopia is frequently observed, especially in operated children under 2 years of age. Consequences of immunosuppressive and/or anti-glaucomatous therapy can also affect the long-term survival of the graft.

Regarding immunosuppression (e.g. ciclosporin A), regular blood count, kidney and liver value checks in cooperation with the pediatrician for weight-adapted level adjustment are indispensable.

If the children are 3 years old or older, the first magnifying vision aids can be fitted in case of bilateral pathology.

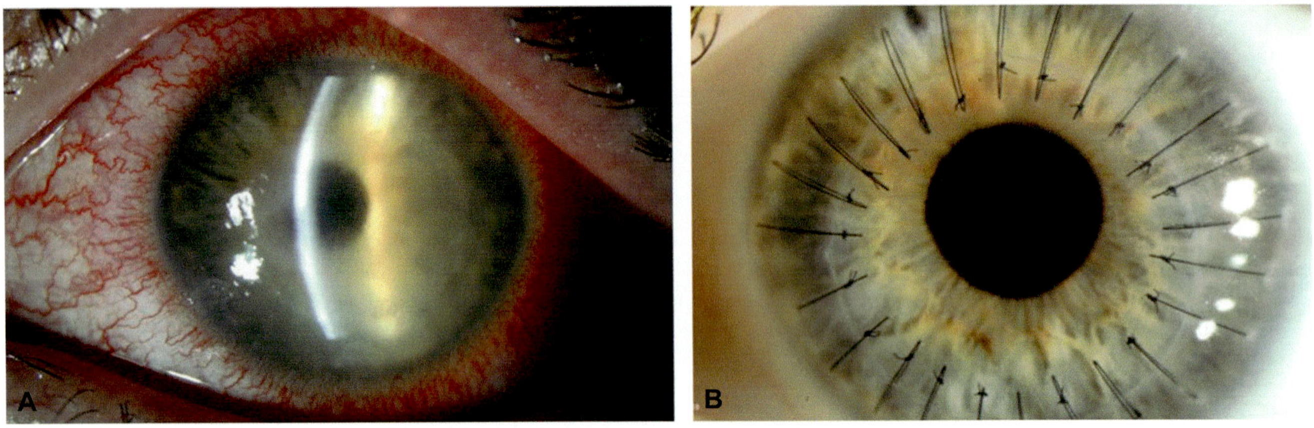

Fig. 16 Girl, 14 years, OU acanthamoeba keratitis, (**A**) OD before penetrating keratoplasty, (**B**) three months following surgery with multiple single interrupted sutures, no inflammation, no vascascularisation. VA OD cc 0.5 dec

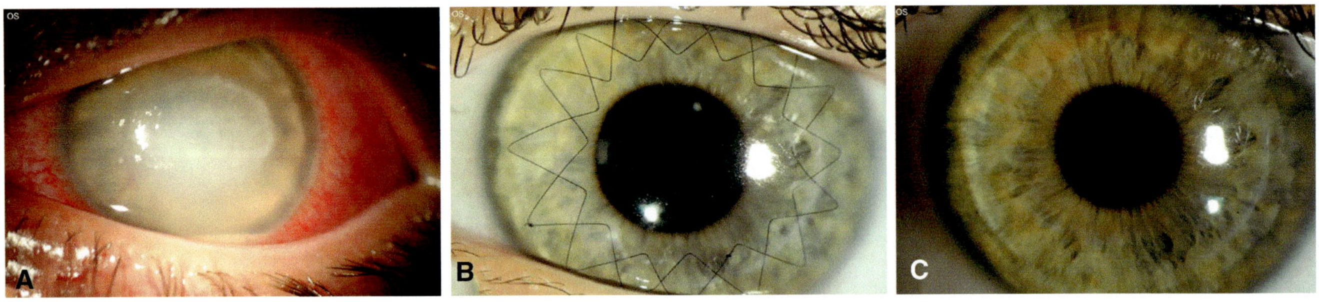

Fig. 17 Boy, presented at age 15 years, OS severe acanthamoeba keratitis after swimming with contact lenses in Southern Californa. First treated conservatively at home town Berlin, transferred to us 6 weeks after the beginning of the infiltration. (**A**) Preoperative finding, hypopyon, severe pain. VA light perception. (**B**) Result 3 months postoperatively, VA 0.3 dec. (**C**) Result 4 years postoperatively, VA with myopic correction 1.0 dec

7 Prognostic Factors and Graft Failure

Prognostic factors determine postoperative morphologic and functional outcome as well as graft survival (Table 4) [7, 17–24].

8 Conclusion

- Corneal surgery in children requires a critical and above all individual indication.
- Already preoperatively, cooperation with the conservative pediatric ophthalmologist is necessary to assess visual development in the phase of visual plasticity as well as to estimate the expected postoperative compliance.
- It should be done as early as necessary (less amblyopia) but as late as possible (better cooperation).
- It is essential to inform the parents comprehensively before surgery regarding realistic expected visual acuity, high effort of follow-up, frequent ophthalmologist visits, possible postoperative complications including the risk of re-transplantation (graft failure, glaucoma), necessary long-term topical therapy and possibly necessary immunosuppression.
- The permanent connection of the child to a good pediatric ophthalmologic-orthoptic section is essential regarding postoperative morphologic controls as well as amblyopia therapy.

Conflicts of Interests B. Käsmann-Kellner and B. Seitz report no conflicts of interest.

References

1. Bachmann B, Avgitidou G, Siebelmann S, Cursiefen C. Pediatric corneal surgery and corneal transplantation. Ophthalmologe. 2015;112(2):110–7.
2. Seitz B, Hager T, Szentmáry N, Langenbucher A, Naumann G. Keratoplasty in children–still a dilemma. Klin Monbl Augenheilkd. 2013;230(6):587–94.

3. Dana MR, Moyes AL, Gomes JA, Rosheim KM, Schaumberg DA, Laibson PR, Holland EJ, Sugar A, Sugar J. The Indications for and Outcome in Pediatric Keratoplasty. Ophthalmology. 1995;102(8):1129–38.
4. Ganekal S, Gangangouda C, Dorairaj S, Jhanji V. Early outcomes of primary pediatric keratoplasty in patients with acquired, atraumatic corneal pathology. J AAPOS. 2011;15(4):353–5.
5. Käsmann-Kellner B, Seitz B. Aniridia syndrome: clinical findings, problematic courses and suggestions for optimization of care ("aniridia guide"). Ophthalmologe. 2014;111(12):1145–56.
6. Käsmann-Kellner B, Moslemani K, Seitz B. Clinical and genetic characteristics of ocular developmental disorders: MAC-spectrum, anterior segment dysgenesis. Klin Monbl Augenheilkd. 2019;236(3):269–85.
7. Nischal KK. A new approach to the classification of neonatal corneal opacities. Curr Opin Ophthalmol. 2012;23(5):344–54.
8. Schlötzer-Schrehardt U, Latta L, Gießl A, Zenkel M, Fries FN, Käsmann-Kellner B, Kruse FE, Seitz B. Dysfunction of the limbal epithelial stem cell niche in aniridia-associated keratopathy. Ocul Surf. 2021;21:160–73.
9. Deng SX, Borderie V, Chan CC, Dana R, Figueiredo FC, Gomes JAP, Pellegrini G, Shimmura S, Kruse FE; and The International Limbal Stem Cell Deficiency Working Group. Global consensus on definition, classification, diagnosis, and staging of limbal stem cell deficiency. Cornea. 2019;38(3):364–75.
10. Deng SX, Kruse F, Gomes JAP, Chan CC, Daya S, Dana R, Figueiredo FC, Kinoshita S, Rama P, Sangwan V, Slomovic AR, Tan D; and the International Limbal Stem Cell Deficiency Working Group. Global consensus on the management of limbal stem cell deficiency. Cornea. 2020;39(10):1291–302.
11. Seitz B, Käsmann-Kellner B, Viestenz A. Stage-related therapy of congenital aniridia. Ophthalmologe. 2014;111(12):1164–71.
12. Gulias-Cañizo R, Gonzalez-Salinas R, Hernandez-Zimbron LF, Hernandez-Quintela E, Sanchez-Huerta V. Indications and outcomes of pediatric keratoplasty in a tertiary eye care center: a retrospective review. Medicine. 2017;96(45): e8587.
13. Karadag R, Rapuano CJ, Hammersmith KM, Nagra PK. Causes of congenital corneal opacities and their management in a tertiary care center. Arq Bras Oftalmol. 2020;83(2):98–102.
14. Nischal KK. Genetics of congenital corneal opacification-impact on diagnosis and treatment. Cornea. 2015;34(Suppl10):p24-34.
15. Lang SJ, Richter C, Richter O, Böhringer D, Geerling G, Reinhard T. Keratoplasty in children and adolescents. Klin Monbl Augenheilkd. 2018;235(3):319–23.
16. Reichl S, Böhringer D, Richter O, Lagrèze W, Reinhard T. Long-term prognosis of Peters anomaly. Ophthalmologe. 2018;115(4):309–13.
17. Lang SJ, Böhringer D, Reinhard T. Keratoplasty in children: indications and results. Ophthalmologe. 2020;117(3):215–7.
18. Lin Q, Li L, Sun Y, Miao S, Li X, Shi W, Pan Z. Penetrating keratoplasty in infants with Peters anomaly: visual and graft outcomes. Cornea. 2021;40(6):720–5.
19. Hoffmann EM, Geerling G. Maximum anterior segment surgery in childhood-folly or feat? Ophthalmologe. 2020;117(3):189.
20. Hager T, Schirra F, Kohnen T, Seitz B, Käsmann-Kellner B. Treatment of cataracts in childhood I: clinical picture und surgical approach. Ophthalmologe. 2012;109(12):1233–45.
21. Hager T, Schirra F, Seitz B, Käsmann-Kellner B. Treatment of pediatric cataracts. Part 2: IOL implantation, postoperative complications, aphakia management and postoperative development. Ophthalmologe. 2013;110(2):179–188; 189–190.
22. Lagrèze WA. Treatment of congenital and early childhood cataract. Ophthalmologe. 2020;117(10):1049–60.
23. Majander A, Kivelä TT, Krootila K. Indications and outcomes of keratoplasties in children during a 40-year period. Acta Ophthalmol. 2016;94(6):618–24.
24. Huang C, O'Hara M, Mannis MJ. Primary pediatric keratoplasty: indications and outcomes. Cornea. 2009;28(9):1003–8.
25. Lowe MT, Keane MC, Coster DJ, Williams KA. The outcome of corneal transplantation in infants, children, and adolescents. Ophthalmology. 2011;118(3):492–7.
26. Serna-Ojeda JC, Loya-Garcia D, Navas A, Lichtinger A, Ramirez-Miranda A, Graue-Hernandez EO. Long-term outcomes of pediatric penetrating keratoplasty for herpes simplex virus keratitis. Am J Ophthalmol. 2017;173:139–44.
27. Toker E, Seitz B, Langenbucher A, Dietrich T, Naumann GOH. Penetrating keratoplasty for endothelial decompensation in eyes with buphthalmos. Cornea. 2003;22(3):198–204.
28. Kim YW, Choi HJ, Kim MK, Wee WR, Yu YS, Oh JY. Clinical outcome of penetrating keratoplasty in patients 5 years or younger: peters anomaly versus sclerocornea. Cornea. 2013;32(11):1432–6.
29. Lin Q, Shi W, Miao S, Zhang Y, Li L, Pan Z. Visual outcomes and prognostic factors of successful penetrating keratoplasty in 0- to 7-Year-old children with congenital corneal opacities. Cornea. 2018;37(10):1237–42.
30. Fiorentzis M, Morinello E, Viestenz A, Zuche H, Seitz B, Viestenz A. Muscle relaxants as a risk factor for vis-à-tergo during penetrating keratoplasty: a prospective interventional study. Adv Ther. 2017;34(12):2674–9.
31. Morinello E, Wittmann D, Seitz B, Hager T, Volk T, Grundmann U, Bomberg H. Anaesthesia during corneal transplantation in children. Acta Anaesth Belg. 2017;234:697–705.
32. Seitz B, El-Husseiny M, Langenbucher A, Szentmáry N. Prophylaxis and management of complications in penetrating keratoplasty. Ophthalmologe. 2013;110(7):605–13.
33. Zuche H, Morinello E, Viestenz A, Fiorentzis MF, Volk T, Seitz B, Viestenz A. The effect of non-depolarising muscle relaxants on ocular pulse amplitude and intraocular pressure. Klin Monbl Augenheilkd. 2015;232(12):1397–401.
34. Farah CJ, Fries FN, Latta L, Käsmann-Kellner B, Seitz B. An attempt to optimize the outcome of penetrating keratoplasty in congenital aniridia-associated keratopathy (AAK). Int Ophthalmol. 2021;41(12):4091–8.
35. Grainger RM, Lauderdale JD, Collins JL, Trout KL, McCullen Krantz S, Wolfe SS Netland PA. Report on the 2021 Aniridia North America symposium on PAX6, aniridia, and beyond. Ocul Surf 2023; 29:423–31.
36. Käsmann-Kellner B, Moslemani K, Seitz B. Optical rehabilitation and pediatric ophthalmological care following keratoplasty for childhood corneal opacities. Ophthalmologe. 2022;119(5):462–70.

Keratoprosthesis

Gerd Geerling and Friedrich Steindor

Abstract

In severe ocular surface disease, where penetrating keratoplasty has a poor prognosis or previous corneal grafts failed, implantation of a keratoprosthesis (KPro) can achieve visual rehabilitation. Prosthetic devices with a biological (Osteo-odonto-keratoprosthesis or Tibia-Keratoprosthesis) and artificial haptic (e.g. Boston KPro type I and II) are available and commonly used. Both approaches show substantial differences in the type of procedure as well as in long-term outcome and complications, such as extrusion, endophthalmitis, glaucoma and retinal detachment. KPros with a biological haptic can be implanted successfully even in severe dry eyes, in which other devices frequently fail.

Keywords

Osteo-odonto-keratoprosthesis · Tibia keratoprosthesis · Boston keratoprosthesis · AlphaCor keratoprosthesis · Corneal blindness

1 Introduction & Indications

Severe ocular surface disorders frequently result from systemic disorders with severe ocular involvement, such as Mucous Membrane Pemphigoid (MMP), Stevens–Johnson Syndrome (SJS), Graft versus Host disease (GvHD) and others. It is often associated with severe ocular dryness, a lack of corneal sensation, complete limbal stem cell insufficiency and intrastromal neovascularization. In these situations, as well as in eyes with failed corneal grafts, penetrating keratoplasty has a very poor prognosis. Many of these conditions affect both eyes and thus leave the patient in a situation of bilateral corneal blindness with little chance for successful visual rehabilitation by means of conventional transplantation surgery. In this situation implantation of a keratoprosthesis (KPro) can be considered [1–4].

A KPro consists of an optic, usually PMMA, as optic pathway and a haptic, to ensure tissue integration or adhesion of the device in the recipient bed. Integration provides a stronger interaction with the recipient tissue and is thus preferred. KPro-Devices are differentiated either according to the haptic material (biological or artificial) or their position in relation to the recipient cornea (epicorneal, intrastromal or transcorneal fixation). Often an oral mucous membrane is used to stabilize the ocular surface over the prosthesis. We here focus predominantly on the currently clinically relevant, i.e. more widely implanted and commercially available types of KPros. These are.

- Transcorneal Boston Keratoprosthesis (Boston KPro, Type 1)
- Epicorneal Osteo-Odonto-Keratoprosthesis (OOKPro)
- Epicorneal Tibia-Keratoprosthesis (TKPro)

Implantation of a KPro with an artificial haptic is usually less invasive, but long-term retention is less favourable compared to KPros with a biological haptic. The latter however involve a more invasive procedure and hence are associated with more substantial changes of anterior segment anatomy. While KPro with a non-biological haptic are complicated by extrusion of the device in association with endophthalmitis, KPros with a biological haptic more often result in retinal detachment. Both types of KPros lead to a high rate of progressive glaucoma. This is—due to the PMMA optic—difficult to monitor, as measurements of

Supplementary Information The online version contains supplementary material available at https://doi.org/10.1007/978-3-031-65422-0_55.

G. Geerling (✉) · F. Steindor
Department of Ophthalmology, University of Düsseldorf, Düsseldorf, Germany
e-mail: geerling@med.uni-duesseldorf.de

B. Seitz et al. (eds.), *Atlas on Cornea*, https://doi.org/10.1007/978-3-031-65422-0_55

IOP using traditional tonometry methods (e.g. Goldmann applanation tonometry) cannot be successfully performed. Therefore, KPros are always considered a last resort and usually limited to patients suffering from bilateral corneal blindness or severe visual impairment (BCVA under 1/20 MV) [1–4] with a very poor prognosis for corneal transplantation.

Indication for KPro Surgery

Before deciding to perform KPro surgery in an eye with corneal blindness, surgeon and patient alike have to understand the potential visual benefit (from best corrected acuity to visual field), the nature of the approach (e.g. staged procedure), potentially severe complications and the required long-term care and follow-up. The patient history, tear quantity and epithelial stability, e.g. judged after vital dye staining decide the choice of implant. Basically, an eye that cannot maintain a stable ocular surface is unsuitable for a Boston KPro and hence requires a device with a biological haptic and replacement of the corneal surface epithelium by an oral mucous membrane graft.

As corneal opacity is always severe, even gross retinal pathology or optic nerve atrophy cannot be ruled out by fundoscopy. Ultrasound B-scan, examination of visually evoked cortical potentials, color vision and entoptic phenomena (e.g. macular chagrin, a phenomenon in which glittering light spots can be seen in the foveal non-vascular area, occuring when a light is rapidly moved over the sclera parallel to the limbus) are used to gain an understanding of the visual prognosis. 23 G vitrectomy with endoscopy assistance allows a direct visualization of retina and optic disc [5] (Fig. 1). It is a minor procedure compared to e.g. OOKPro surgery and thus can help to avoid inappropriate use of resources and patient dissatisfaction [5].

2 Types of KPro

2.1 AlphaCor-KPro

The AlphaCor implant was a device made of a flexible hydrogel material (Poly-HEMA = Poly(2-hydroxyethyl methacrylate)) with 2 distinct parts, a central clear optic and a peripheral opaque circular porous haptic or skirt, intended to facilitate integration into the host cornea. It was available until 2014 as a variant for aphakic and one for phakic eyes [6] and offered the crucial advantages of allowing transprosthetic applanation tonometry. In stage 1 the cornea was deepithelialised, any remaining limbal stem cells removed, a lamellar pocket dissected into the corneal stroma, a posterior central 3 mm keratectomy performed and the AlphaCor KPro inserted in the pocket (Fig. 2A). Finally a thin conjunctival flap was transposed to cover the cornea with vascularised tissue. Three months later (stage 2), when the white skirt was supposedly biointegrated with the host stroma, a central anterior lamellar keratectomy of 3 mm was performed over the optic for visual rehabilitation (Fig. 2B). Longterm problems of the device were extrusion due to poor integration and stromal melt in up to 60% of cases as well as visual loss due to deposition of calcium phosphate on the anterior optic surface in up to 20% of cases [6] (Figs. 2C and 2D). Currently, the prosthesis is no longer available for purchase.

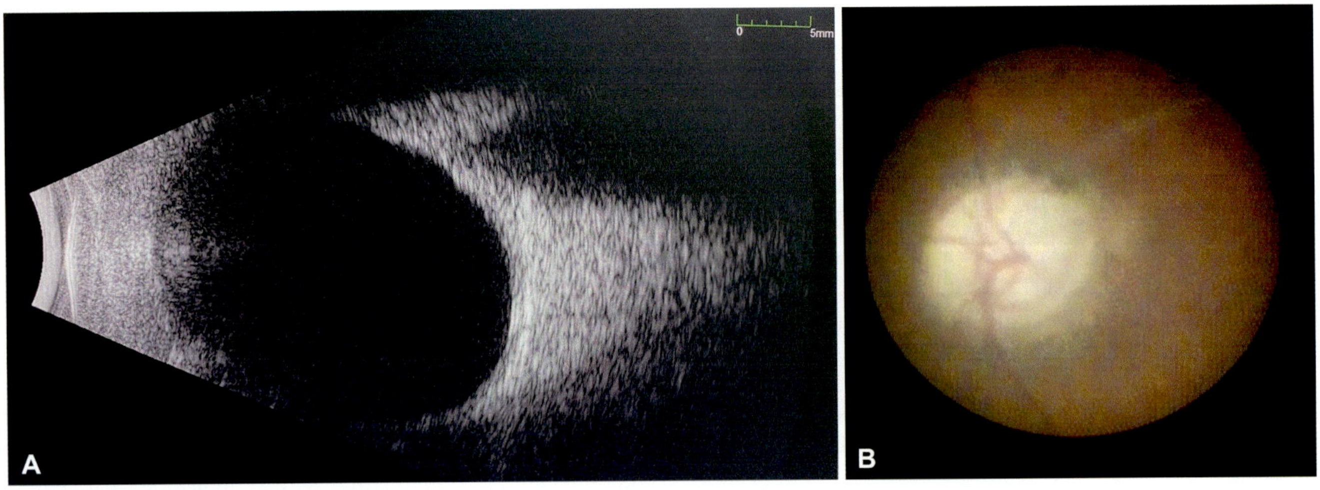

Fig. 1 Left eye of 65-year-old man suffering from limbal stem cell deficiency, corneal opacification and ulceration after severe alkali burn, requesting KPro surgery. Prior to presentation at our clinic, five penetrating keratoplasties including one sclerocorneaplasty and multiple amniotic membrane transplantations had already been performed in each eye. Best corrected visual acuity was light perception in his right and hand movement in his left eye. Ultrasonography (**A**) showed a regular posterior pole. Exploratory pars plana vitrectomy and microendoscopy (**B**) revealed a terminally cupped optic disc and retinal ghost vessel formation of major arterial branches. KPro surgery was therefore declined due to the expected poor outcome

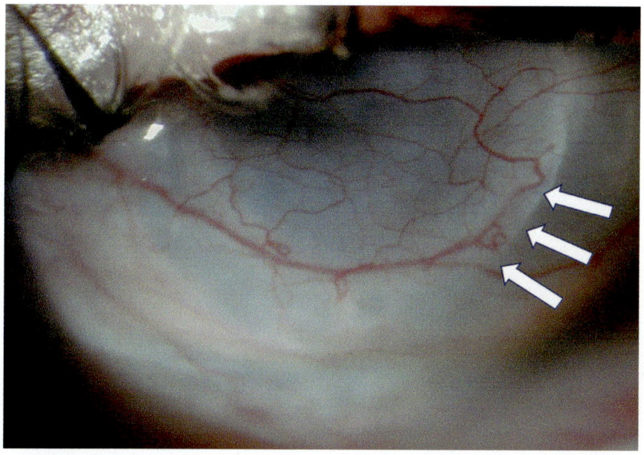

Fig. 2A Left eye of a 55-year-old man following stage 1 Alphacor-KPro surgery. The corneal surface is covered with a conjunctival flap. The intrastromal device can be identified by the white arrows marking the outer border of the skirt

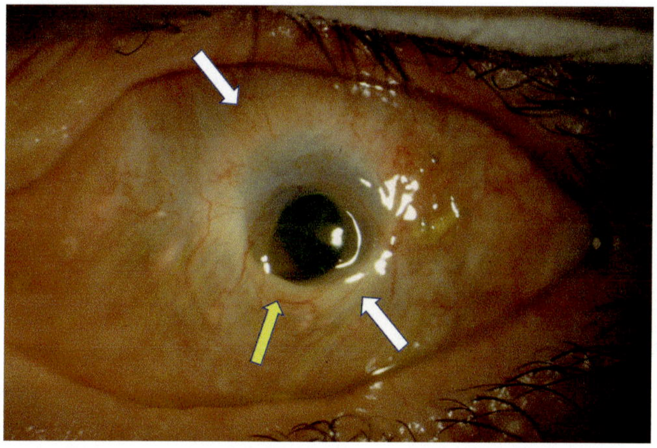

Fig. 2B Same eye 6 weeks after stage 2 Alphacor-KPro surgery. The white arrows mark the skirt. The central optic is exposed after keratectomy. A yellow arrow marks an early anterior stromal melt

2.2 Boston-KPro

The Boston KPro is the currently most commonly used KPro and available in two main variants. Type I is fixed transconjunctivally and available in different powers for pseudophakic and aphakic eyes depending on axial length. It consists of a clear polymethyl methacrylate (PMMA) anterior part and optic, which is inserted into a central trephination in a donor corneal button as carrier. The transcorneal PMMA stem is fixed with a 8.5 mm PMMA or Titanium back plate and a locking ring on the back side of the carrier graft (Figs. 3A and 3B). A smaller size back plate (7.0 mm) is advocated for use in children. The device is commercially available through Massachusetts Eye and Ear Infirmary/Harvard Medical School. Boston-KPro Type I is used in patients with a stable ocular surface. Postoperative routine includes permanent wear of a large therapeutic bandage contact lens and topical vancomycin application as well as 3-monthly conjunctival washes with povidone iodine. For eyes with instable ocular surface epithelium Boston-KPro Type 2 was developed in which the anterior optic stem is elongated and placed through the eyelid [7, 8] (Fig. 3F).

Longterm success has been reported with a visual acuity of more than 0.1 in Snellen decimal in over 90% of cases. The incidence of glaucoma and retroprosthetic membrane are relatively high with 25–60% [12, 13] (Figs. 3B and 3C). Complications include device extrusion, corneal melting in up to 15% (Figs. 3D, 3E and 3F) and relatively often endophthalmitis with up to 15% with a relatively short average follow-up of only 19 months. More than half of the patients require a further surgical procedure in a five year follow-up, e.g. glaucoma surgery in up to 10% (in addition to the already high proportion of more than 50% of patients with preoperative

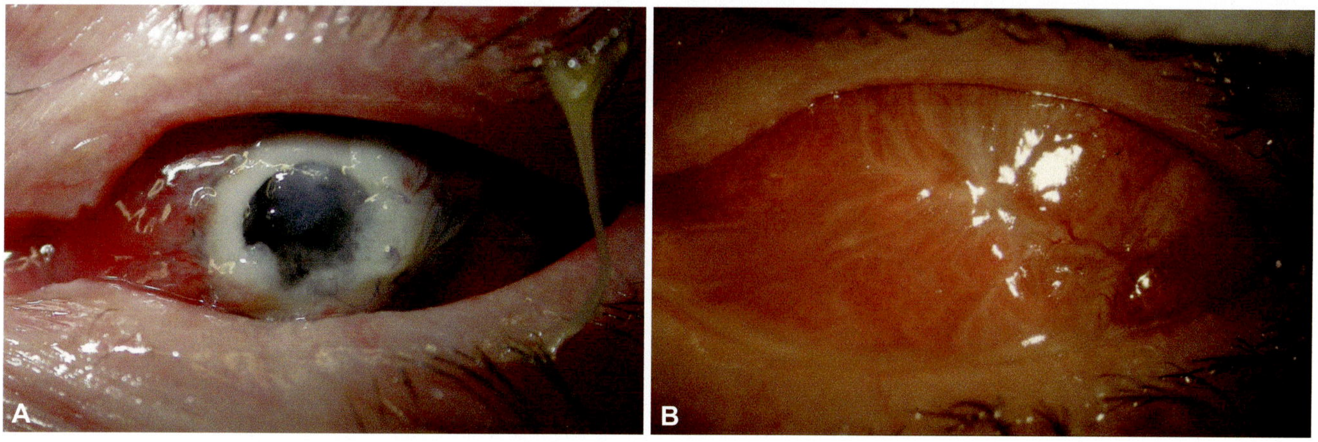

Fig. 2C Six months after implantation severe conjunctival inflammatory and anterior stromal melt are present (**A**) The AlphaCor KPro device was explanted and corneal emergency transplantation and conjunctival flap used to permanently stabilize the eye (**B**) Visual acuity was reduced to light projection

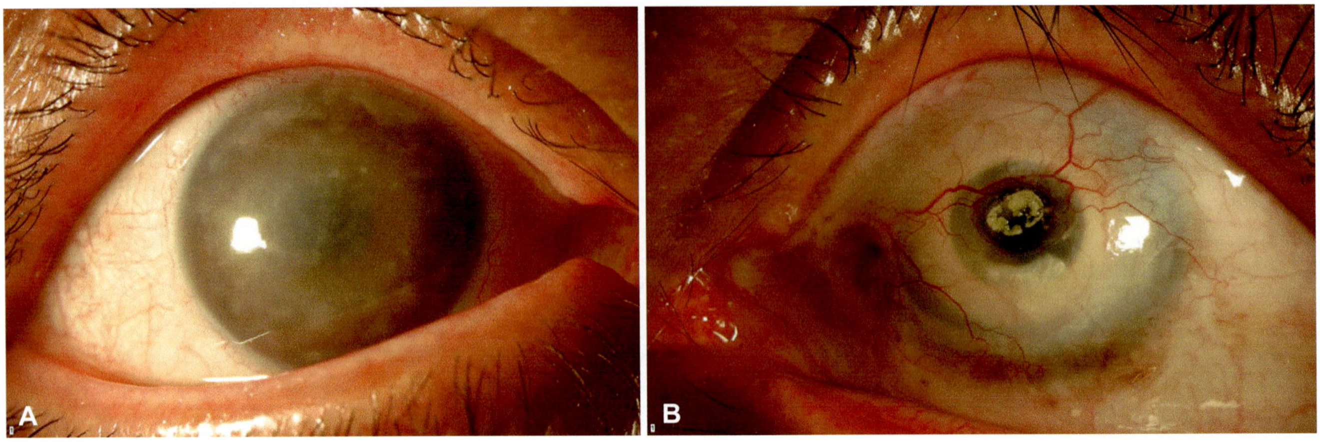

Fig. 2D 42-year-old patient with macular corneal dystrophy. The findings of the right eye are additionally shown (**A**). Left eye of a 42-year-old man more than 5 years after AlphaCor KPro implantation after failed penetrating keratoplasty (a total of four penetrating keratoplasties was performed). The prosthesis is well integrated, but vision—which was initially excellent is reduced to hand movement due to deposits on the optical center (**B**). These are tightly bound to the KPro optic material. The device was exchanged for a Boston Type 1 KPro

or intraoperative glaucoma drainage device, e.g. Ahmed implant) or keratoprosthesis removal and replacement in 10–25% [7–9].

2.3 OOKPro and TKPro

OOKPro was first described in 1963 by Strampelli and subsequently only slightly modified by Falcinelle, Liu and Hille. It is mainly indicated for patients with severe ocular surface diseases, who cannot maintain a stable corneal epithelium, e.g. in Mucous Membrane Pemphigoid with ocular involvement, absolute dry eyes, previous corneal melting or ulceration. The procedure consists of 2–3 stages and alters the natural anatomy irreversibly and most substantially of all KPros, but offers good tissue integration due to a biological haptic, resulting in a better survival rate and lower extrusion rate. First, an autologous healthy canine tooth with a single root and surrounding bone are harvested, usually in collaboration with a maxillofacial surgeon. From this a 4 mm thick osteo-odontal lamina is fashioned and a 3–3.5 mm wide hole is drilled into the dentine to harbour a PMMA optic (OOKPro, Figs. 4A and 4B). When no healthy tooth is available alternatively a 10 mm large disc of cortical and spongiform bone can be harvested from the autologous tibia for the PMMA optic (TKPro, Fig. 4C). The PMMA cylinder is glued into the central hole with bone cement (Palacos®) and placed for 3 months in a suborbicularis oculi pocket, to be covered by fibrous tissues which later serves to fix the device to the recipient bed (Fig. 4B). At the end of stage 1 or in an intermediate stage the corneal and large parts of the conjunctival epithelial surface are removed and replaced by an oral mucous membrane graft (Fig. 4E). In the final stage of the procedure, the device is explanted from its pocket, the mucous membrane mobilised, a central corneal trephination performed, the lens, iris and anterior vitreous removed and the KPro sutured into place. Finally the mucous membrane is perforated, placed over the optic and sutured (Fig. 4F). Additional preoperative assessment includes an X-ray of the tooth and jaw bone or the tibial bone to exclude preoperative donor site pathology [1–5, 10–13]. When available intraoperative cone beam computed tomography can be used intraoperatively before implantation to assess bone integrity (Fig. 4J).

Regarding the long-term outcome, visual acuity of more than 0.2 can be achieved in about two-thirds of the patients and in a smaller proportion of 8–27% even a visual acuity greater than or equal to 0.8 in Snellen decimal can be achieved. The rate of complications especially postoperative glaucoma according to other KPro Types is relatively high with up to 30–50%. Pre- and postoperative glaucoma often requires Ahmed Valve implantation and intraocular pressure measurement is difficult due to solid KPro material [4] (Fig. 4I). (Video of an Ahmed Valve implantation in a patient with OOKPro—see

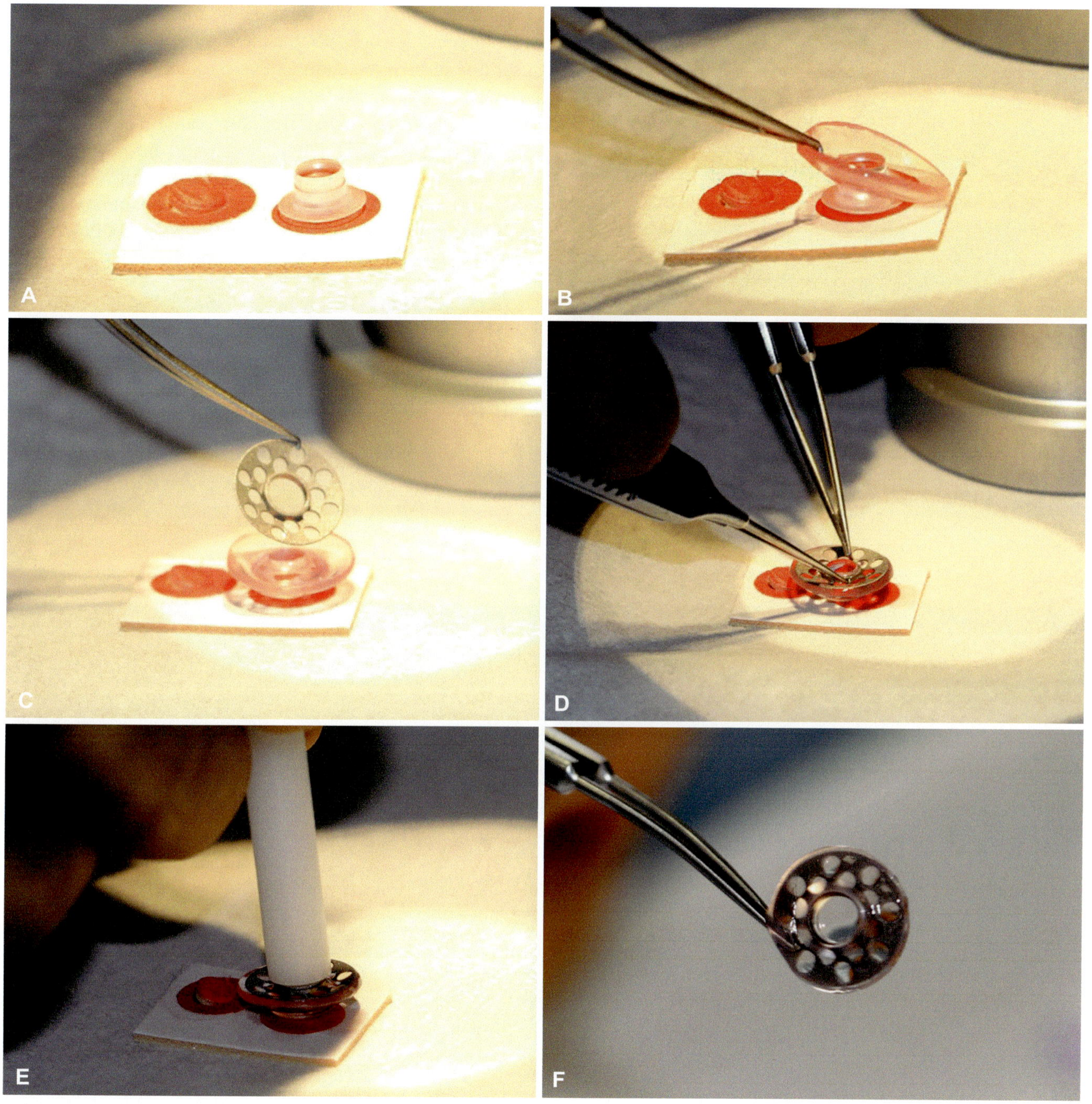

Fig. 3A Assembly of Boston KPro Type I: (**A**) The transparent PMMA cylinder is temporarily placed upside down on a tape. The central optical stem, which will protrude later into the anterior chamber is visible. (**B**) A 7.5–8.0 mm large, corneal full thickness button with a central 3 mm hole is placed on the PMMA stem. (**C**) Next the fenestrated back plate (here titanium) is placed over the PMMA stem and pushed down onto the endothelial side of the corneal donor button. (**D**) A titanium ring is placed posterior to the backplate to the optic. (**E**) A locking ring is pushed down with a plunger until it snaps into place with an audible click, to permanently fix the back plate to the PMMA stem. (**F**) The Boston KPro type I as it is fully mounted onto the corneal full thickness graft, ready to be sutured into an 8.0 mm diameter trephined corneal opening in the recipient.

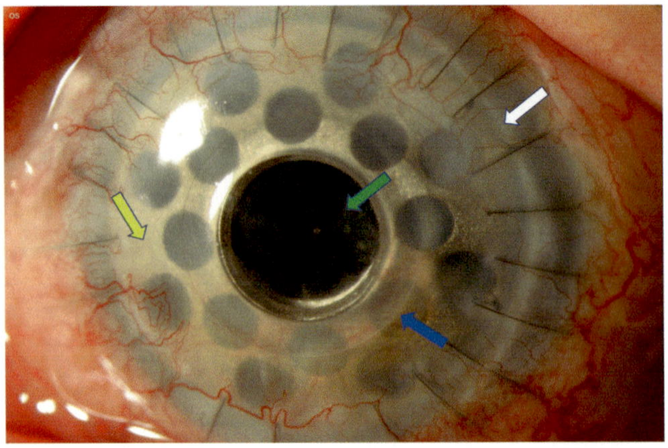

Fig. 3B 18 months after Boston KPro Type I, implanted in exchange for AlphaCor KPro from Fig. 2E. The prosthesis is well centered and integrated, but a retroprosthetic membrane is forming (green arrow). The white arrow marks the interface between host cornea and corneal graft, yellow the fenestrated titanium backplate and blue the edge of the transparent PMMA cylinder

QR Code) In addition retinal detachment, necrosis of the oral mucosa, retroprosthetic membranes, macular edema and bone absorption with extrusion may occur (Fig. 4H). Even KPro explantation may be necessary in up to 12% of cases [4]. Even with a regular course (Fig. 4G), regular thin-slice orbital CT scans should be performed to assess bone absorption (Fig. 4K), which can be treated with oral vitamin D, calcium and bisphosphonates and can ultimately lead to repeated OOKPro or TKPro.

Please scan to access video content

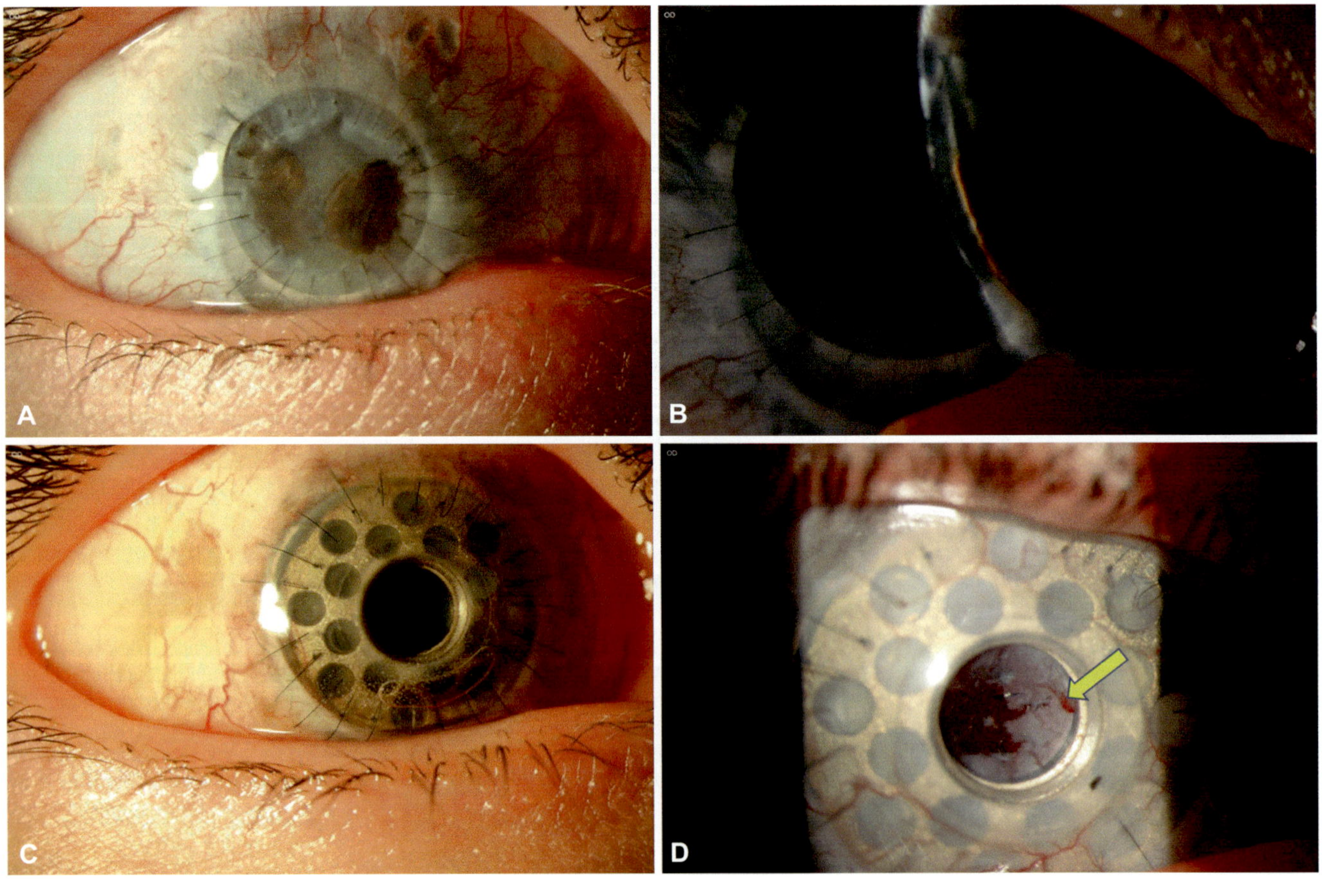

Fig. 3C **Preoperative findings**. 25-year-old female patient with Peters' anomaly and failed repeated penetrating keratoplasty (**A**). The anterior chamber is shallow with broad anterior synechiae (**B**). Four months after Boston KPro Type I the eye is without signs of severe inflammation, but air is accumulating underneath a large contact lens as a sign of tissue retraction (**C**). 29 months after implantation retroprosthetic membrane required YAG-membranotomy. The temporal hemorrhage (yellow arrow) that occurred in the course of laser treatment resolved but visual acuity remained limited to hand movement (**D**)

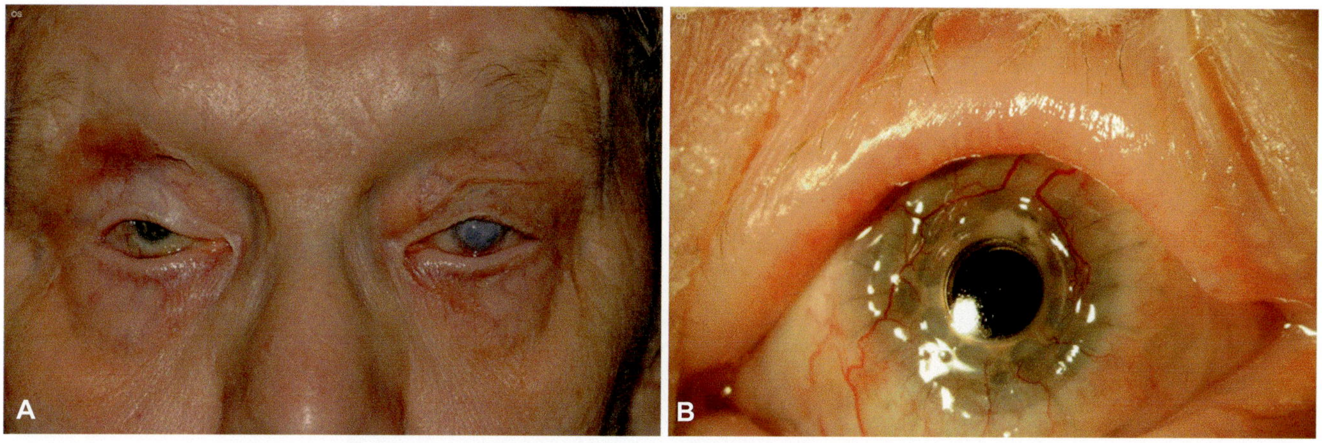

Fig. 3D 88-year-old female patient using a sticky tape to lift her right ptotic eyelid (**A**). 4 years after implantation of a Boston KPro Type I melting of the carrier stroma is seen at 1 o'clock with accumulation of debris or pus underneath the skirt, despite previous treatment with corneal Crosslinking and amniotic membrane transplantation (**B**)

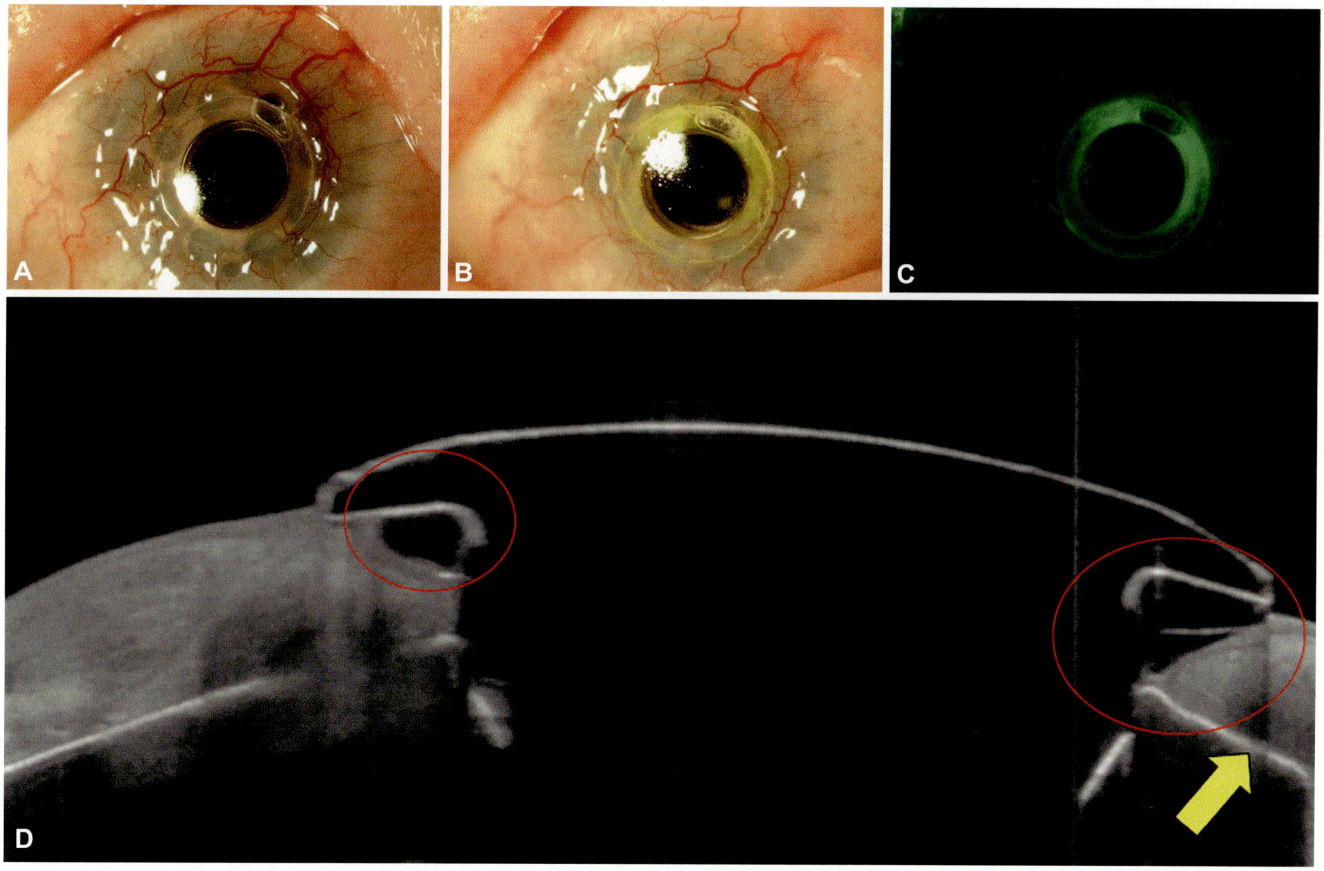

Fig. 3E After removal of the debris (patient from Fig. 3D) air accumulation is seen under the anterior PMMA skirt of the Boston KPro Type I (**A/B**). Circumferential fluoresceine accumulation indicates tissue retraction or melt underneath the skirt (**C**). Subsequently the backplate became exposed and an exchange of the Boston-KPro Type 1 was performed resulting in a best corrected visual acuity of 0.05 in Snellen decimal. The patient was able to cook and lead an independent life—with some support from neighbours—until her death at 88 years of age and 7 years as a KPro patient. Melting can as well be imaged with anterior segment optical coherence tomography which is particularly useful for monitoring of known defects or incipient changes. The red rings mark melting underneath the skirt of the PMMA cylinder (**D**). The yellow arrow marks the dense titanium backplate, which no longer appears to be covered by intact corneal tissue. This patient presented with incipient endophthalmitis and anterior chamber flare (cells 3+). The prosthesis was therefore replaced promptly five and a half years after initial implantation

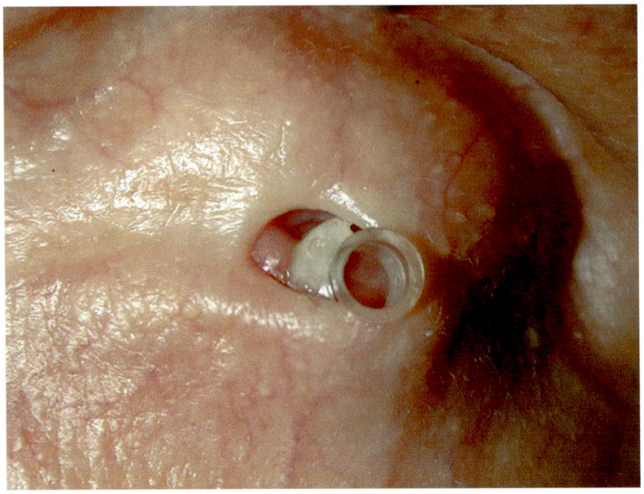

Fig. 3F Left eye with **Boston KPro Type 2** through the lid. The skin has retracted, the carrier cornea has melted away and the eye is phthisical

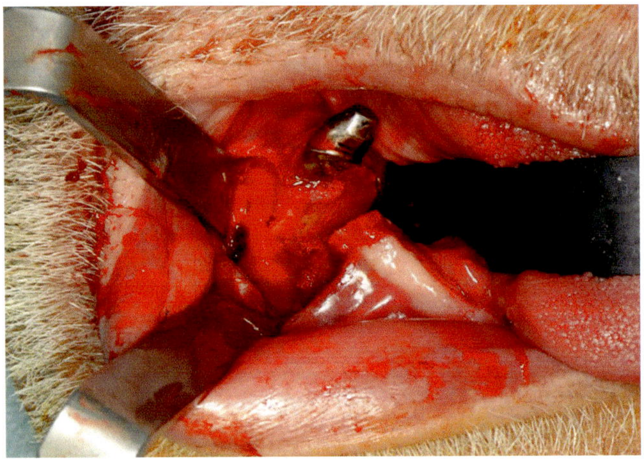

Fig. 4A **Preparation of OOKPro (Stage 1)**. Harvesting of the canine tooth with peridontal mandibular bone**.** The additional bone lamella is important to establish biological integrity, as oral mucosa does not integrate with dentin

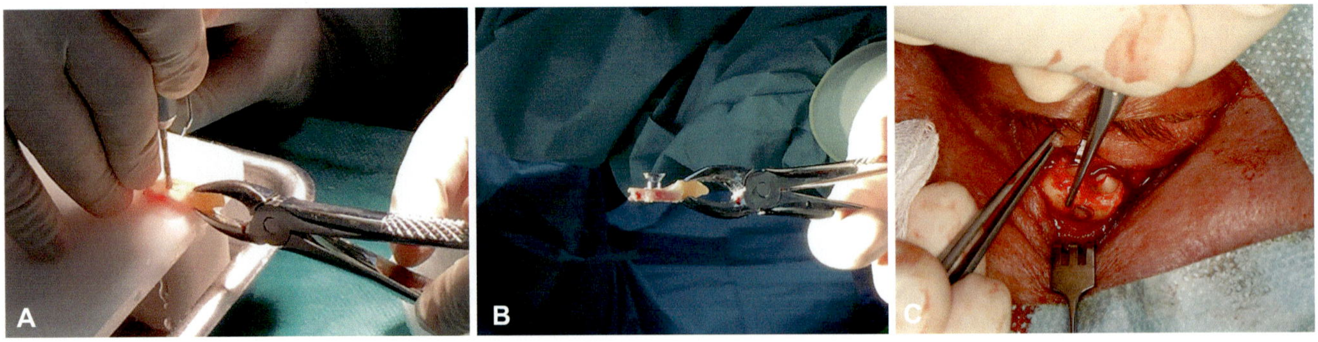

Fig. 4B **(Stage 1): Preparation of OOKPro**. The tooth-bone complex is thinned out, a hole is drilled into the root of the tooth (**A**), the PMMA cylinder with the optical power of cornea and lens is inserted (**B**) and sealed watertight to the osteoodontal lamina with Palacos® glue. After preparation the OOKPro is inserted into a suborbicularis oculi pocket for 3 months to allow formation of a cocoon of fibrous tissue around and firmly attached to the prosthesis (**C**)

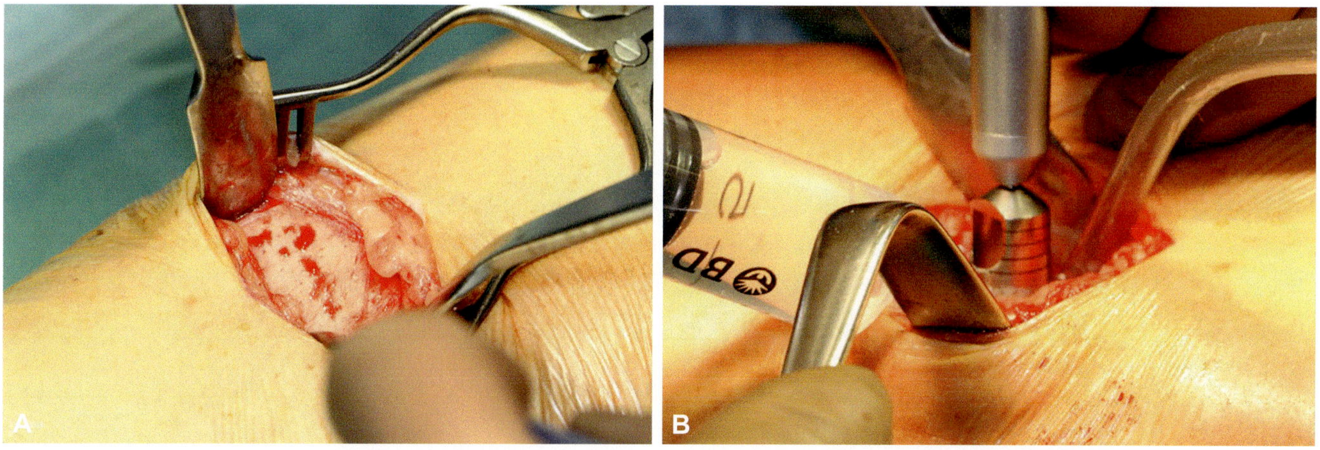

Fig. 4C **Preparation of TKPro (Stage 1)**. Autologous tibial bone is exposed and (**A**) harvested using a motorized trephine (**B**). The periosteum and the wound are closed

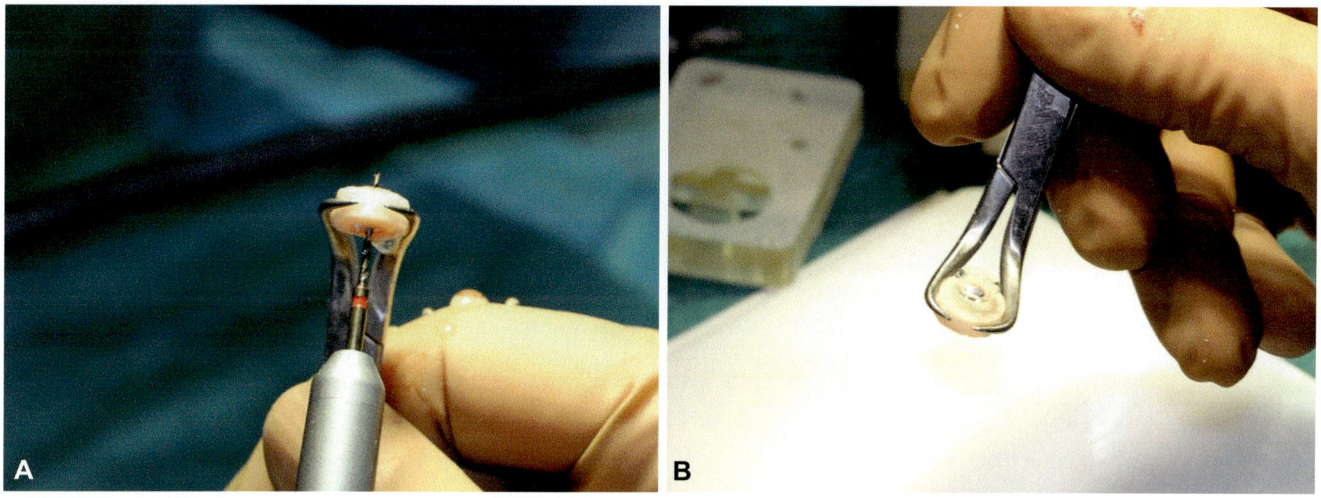

Fig. 4D **Preparation of TKPro (Stage 1)**. The tibial graft (consisting of compact cortical and cancellous bone) is reduced by gentle polishing with a burr to a 4mm thick plate. The cancellous side is facing outwards to allow fibrovascular tissue of the orbicularis to grow in and improve integration into the oral mucosa after implantation. A hole is drilled into the cortico-spongiform tibial graft (**A**) and an identical PMMA cylinder inserted, which is again sealed watertight to the lamina with Palacos® glue (**B**)

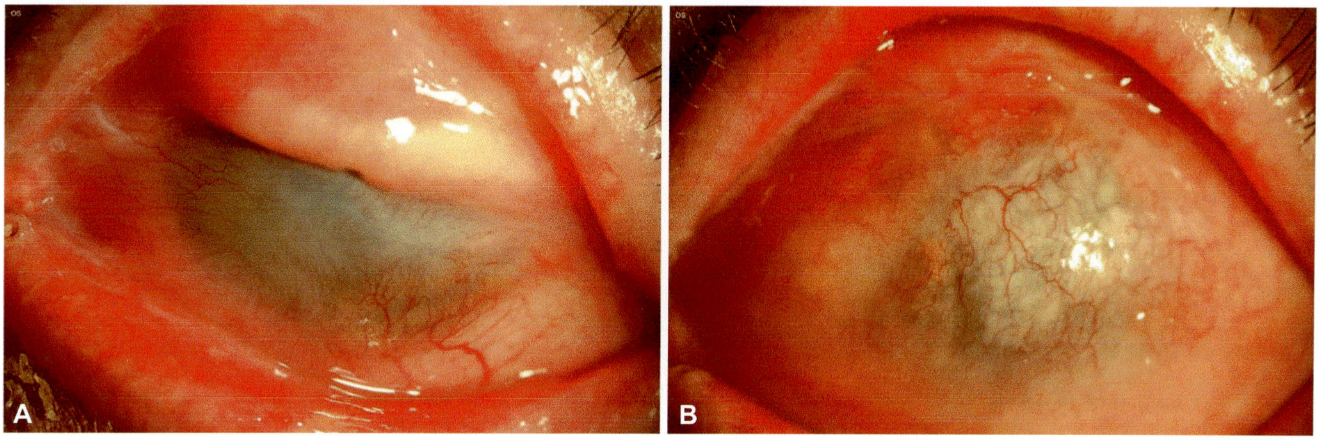

Fig. 4E During or after **preparation the OOKPro** (same eye as Figs. 4A and 4B) ocular epithelial surface including all remaining limbal stem cells itself is replaced by a buccal mucous membrane graft. Left eye of a 61-year-old patient with complete limbal stem cell failure due to severe graft versus host disease. Preoperative visual acuity was 1/20 in the right and hand movement in the left eye (**A**). After a large buccal mucous membrane graft—due to a central thinning of the membrane—cornea and iris are shining through (**B**)

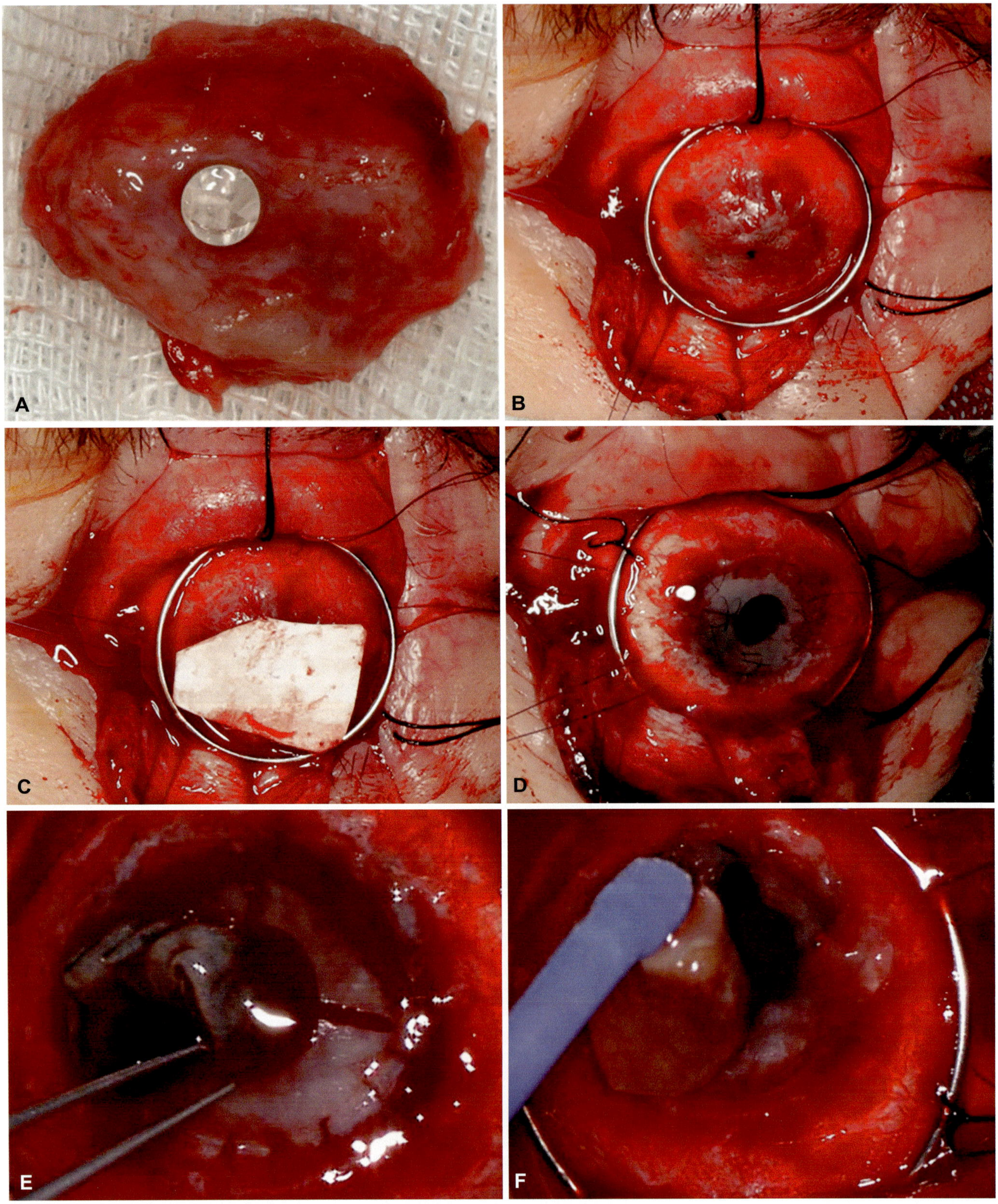

Fig. 4F Implantation of OOKPro (Stage 2). The OOKPro and its cocoon of fibrous tissue are explanted from the submuscular pocket (**A**). The buccal mucosa is incised and reflected (**B**). A sizer—fashioned from surgical paper—in the shape of the OOKpro visualizes its size and reinsures the surgeon, that the prosthesis can be sutured to the sclera within the Flieringa Ring (**C**). The cornea is exposed, an opening 3 or 4 mm is trephined, and radial incisions are made at 3, 6, and 9 o'clock (**D**). Then total iridectomy, lensectomy and anterior vitrectomy are performed (**E–F**) and the OOKPro is implanted

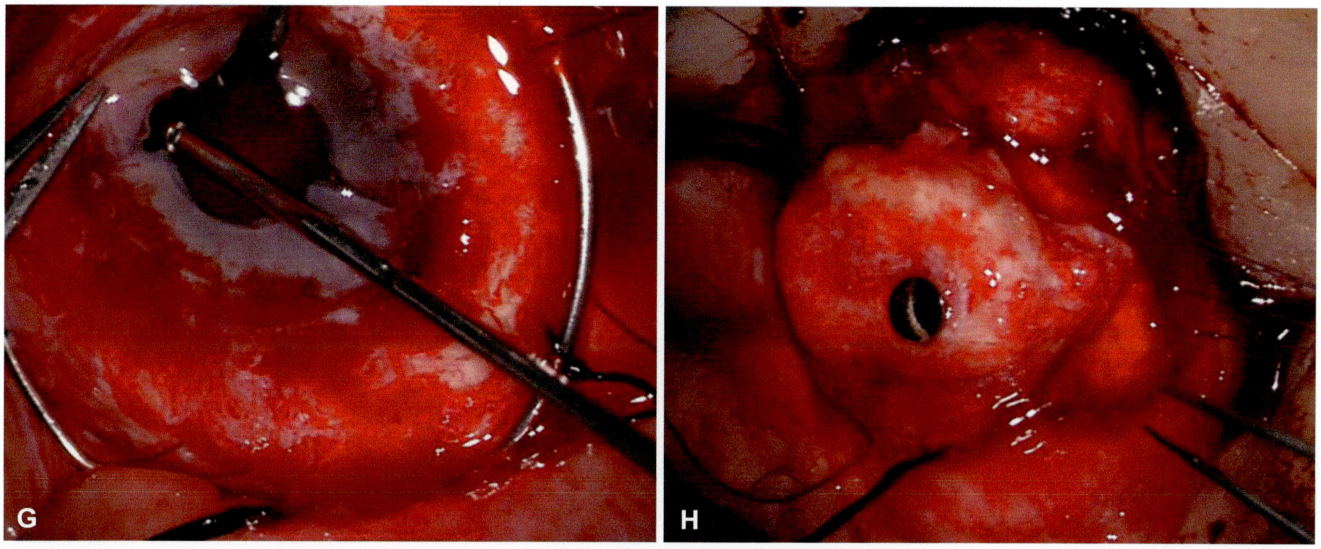

Fig. 4F (**G**) The OOKPro is implanted. (**H**) Finally, the mucosa is sutured back over the OOKpro

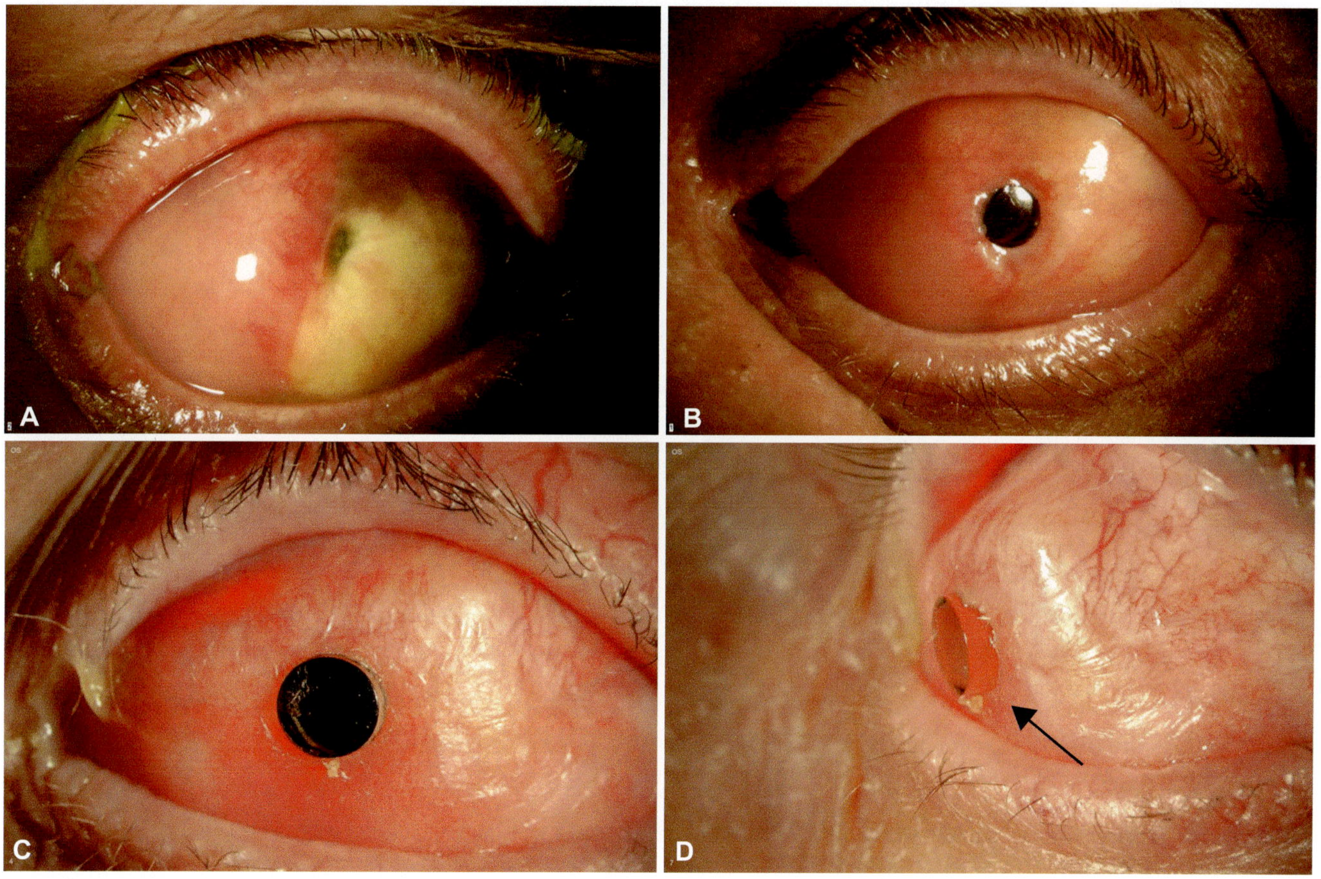

Fig. 4G **Postoperative findings** of the same eye from Fig. 4D. Early after implantation of the OOKPro the mucous membrane shows severe partial ischaemia on the temporal side (**A**). Three months later. The mucous membrane is revascularised and shows good tissue integrity (**B**). 4 years after implantation of the OOKPro the mucous membrane is dry, but firmly attached to the prosthesis (**C**). Visual acuity is 1.0. The optical cylinder is protruding approximately 1 mm in front of the mucous membrane (arrow) (**D**)

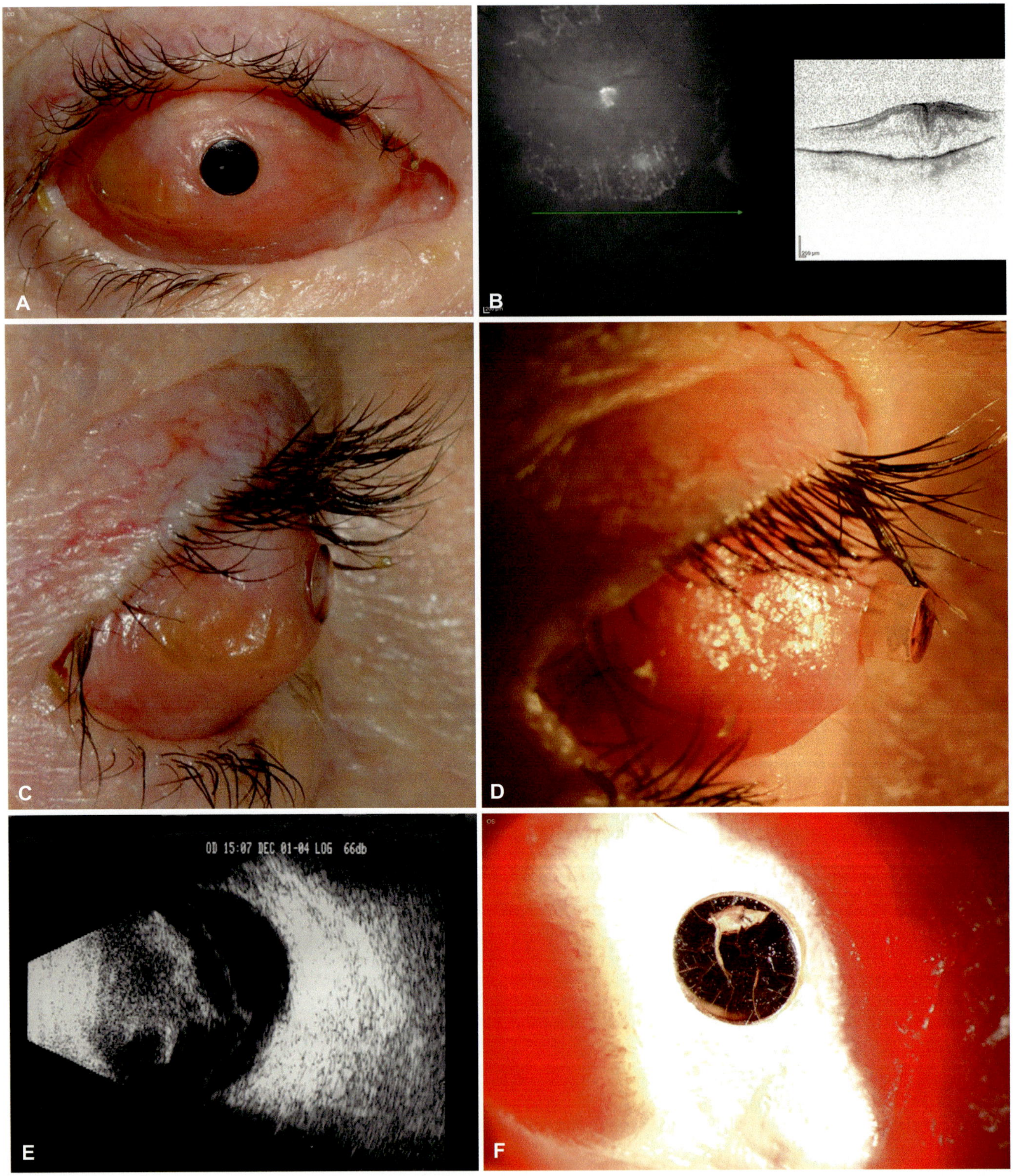

Fig. 4H Complications after KPro with biological haptic. (**A**): Regular postoperative findings in a 59-year-old patient with 12 prior penetrating keratoplasties and secondary glaucoma (CDR 1.0) due to corneal ulceration from rheumatoid arthritis. Three months after TKPro implantation an OCT image shows cystoid macular oedema (**B**), which was successfully treated with oral Acetazolamide. (**C/D**): Side view 3 months after implantation of the same eye. The optical cylinder is hardly extending anterior to the buccal mucous membrane. 45 months later the optical cylinder is protruding approximately 2 mm. CT scans showed signs of bone resorption (Fig. 4K). Visual acuity was stable with 0.2. Annual CT scans are required to monitor bone resorption. (**E/F**): In addition to visual fields, OCT of the optic disc and macula, regular ultrasound examinations are recommended due to an at least 10% risk of retinal detachment (RD), which was detected here two weeks after implantation (**E**). Rhegmatogenous RD can be successfully treated by modern vitrectomy techniques without explantation. Visualisation through the optic of the prosthesis is difficult but sufficient [4]. Scratching or cracking of the optic can occur, as shown here in a patient after a head injury (**F**). Visual acuity is only slightly reduced from 0.4 to 0.3 in Snellen decimal.

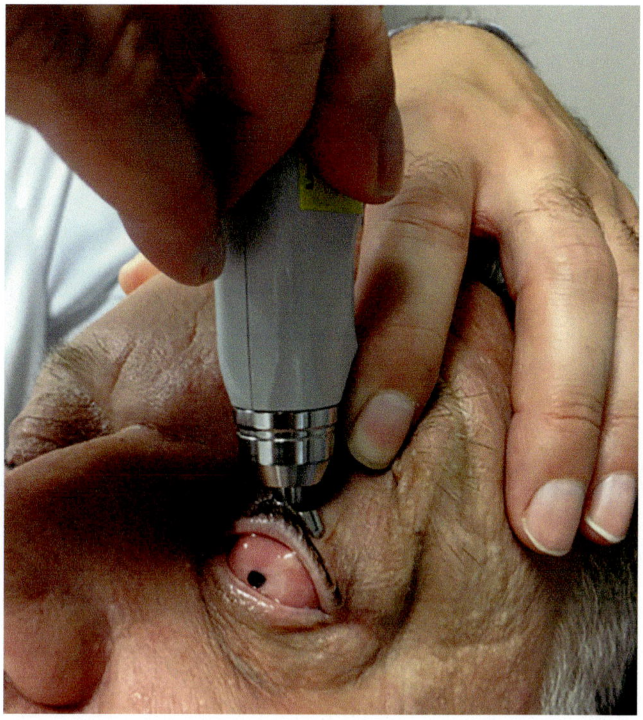

Fig. 41 **Glaucoma monitoring** is of outstanding importance in postoperative follow-up due to the high prevalence of glaucoma in patients before and after keratoprosthesis surgery. In addition to visual field control, OCT of the optic disc and macula, intraocular pressure measurements are difficult due to the solid KPro material. In addition to examiner-dependent and inaccurate manual palpation, transpalpebral impression tonometry (Diaton® (DevelopAll Inc.)) is available. This is performed over the upper eyelid skin, tarsus and sclera with the head tilted backward

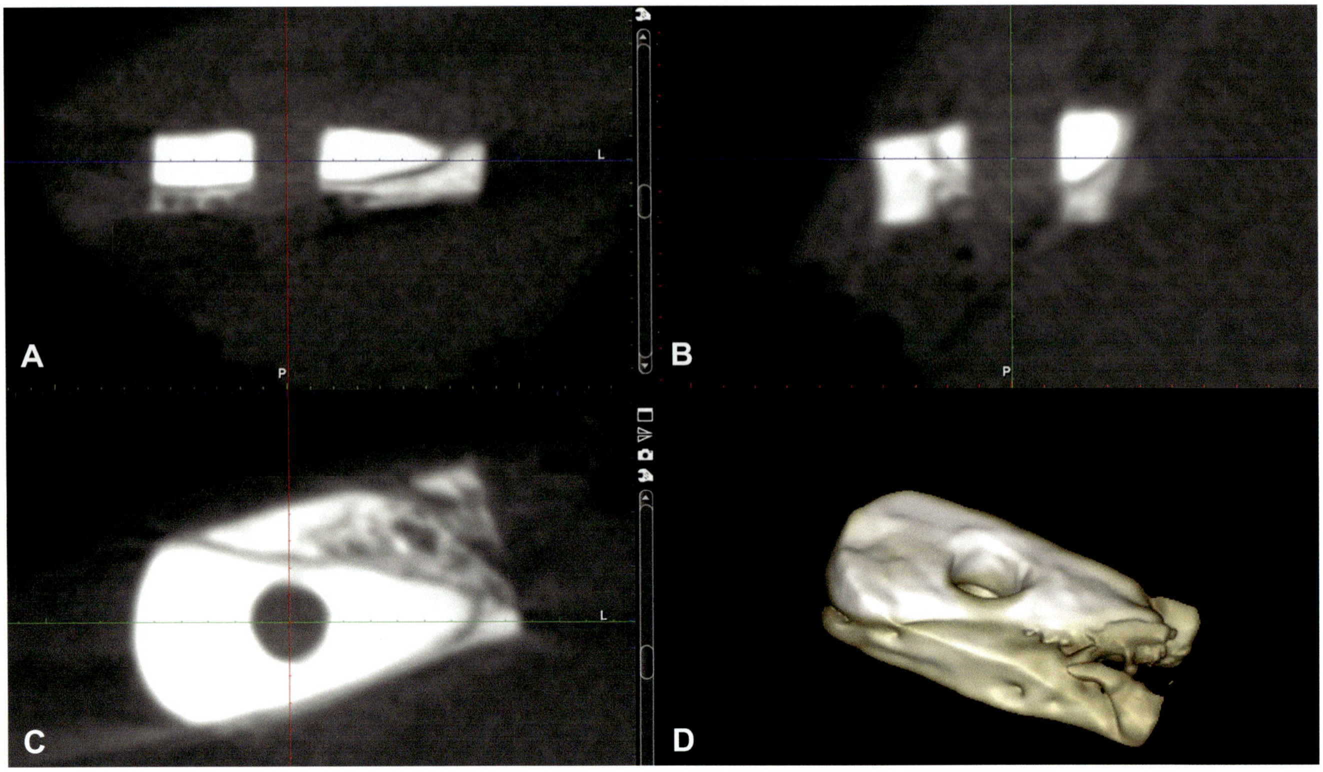

Fig. 4J **Intraoperative Cone beam computed tomography** (a medical imaging technique consisting of X-ray computed tomography which is mainly used in dentistry) can be used to assess the integrity of the OOKPro with its bone intraoperatively and reliably detect possible bone erosions and help the surgeon to decide whether the construct is suitable for implantation. After explantation from the contralateral eyelid, the OOKPro is stored in a sterile container and scanned without risk of contamination. The scan above shows the three-cornered tooth and bone around it. Bone erosion potentially leads to loss of prosthetic integration and risk of endophthalmitis and extrusion. On the top left an axial image of the OOKPro with the upper dense tooth material and the underlying more spongious bone is shown (**A**). Right next to it, the OOKPro is shown in the sagittal plane (**B**). The images below show a coronal image (**C**) as well as a three-dimensional reconstruction (**D**). There, the three-cornered tooth can be differentiated very well from the spongious bone

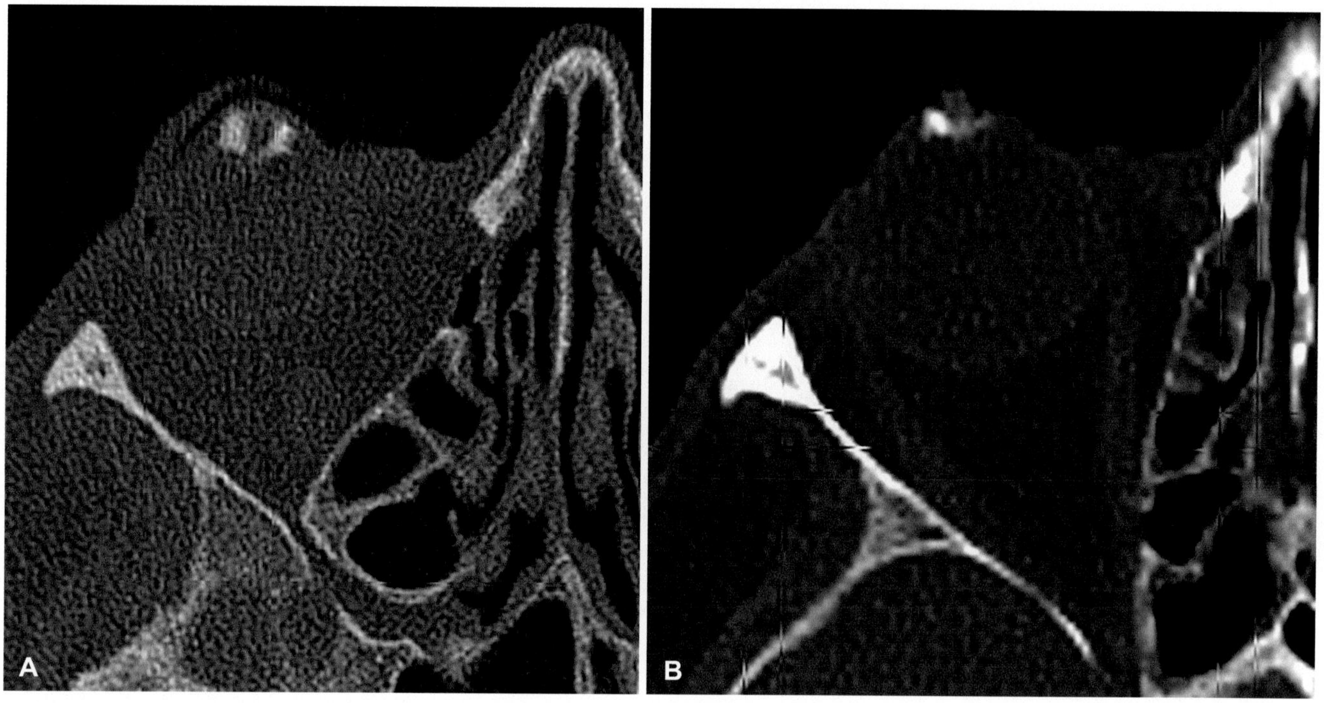

Fig. 4K **Bone resorption** occurs mainly in the longterm after OOKPro or TKPro implantation. Axial CT-slice of the right orbit is shown in A and B (Slice thickness: 3mm, 97mAs, 120 kV), In (**A**) an intact bone mantle around the optic is visible, which in (**B**) has largely resorbed over the course of 4 years after implantation and has led to a progressive protrusion of the optic (shown in Figs. 4D and 4I). Visualization with CT is limited by the resolution of regular CT scanners

3 Conclusion

Keratoprosthesis can be successfully implanted in patients in whom keratoplasty has a very poor prognosis. Prior to surgery, potential visual acuity assessment is vital for appropriate selection of patient and technique. In patients with a stable ocular surface with regular Schirmer's test a Boston KPro type I and in patients with severe dryness a KPro with a biological haptic can achieve excellent long-term visual rehabilititation. As these techniques are performed in low numbers and the eyes carrying such a prosthetic device require permanent screening for postoperative complications, patients should be referred to centers specialised on providing keratoprosthesis services.

References

1. Geerling G, Liu CSC, Dart JKG, et al. Sight and comfort: complex procedures in end-stage Stevens-Johnson syndrome. Eye (Lond). 2003;17:89–91. https://doi.org/10.1038/sj.eye.67002647].
2. Frings A, Schrader S, Hille K, et al. Health-related quality of life after implantation of a keratoprosthesis with biological haptic. Ophthalmologe. 2018;115:34-39.
3. Geerling G, Liu CSC, Collin JRO, et al. Costs and gains of complex procedures to rehabilitate end stage ocular surface disease. Br J Ophthalmol. 2002;86:1220–1. https://doi.org/10.1136/bjo.86.11.1220.
4. Geerling G, Hille K. Keratoprosthesis with Biological Haptic - The Düsseldorf-Offenburg-Experience with Osteo-Odonto- and Tibia-Keratoprosthesis. Klin Monbl Augenheilkd. 2017;234(6):763–769.
5. Korbmacher JP, Borrelli M, Geerling G. Use of Endoscopy in Keratoprostheses with Biological Haptics. Klin Monbl Augenheilkd. 2023; 240(8):1004–1009 https://doi.org/10.1055/a-1807-2197
6. Jirásková N, Rozsival P, Burova M, et al. AlphaCor artificial cornea: clinical outcome. Eye (Lond). 2011;25:1138–46.
7. Greiner MA, Li JY, Mannis MJ. Longer-term vision outcomes and complications with the Boston type 1 keratoprosthesis at the University of California, Davis. Ophthalmology. 2011;118(8):1543–50. https://doi.org/10.1016/j.ophtha.2010.12.032. Epub 2011 Mar 12 PMID: 21397948.
8. Zerbe BL, Belin MW, Ciolino JB; Boston Type 1 Keratoprosthesis Study Group. Results from the multicenter Boston Type 1 Keratoprosthesis Study. Ophthalmology. 2006;113(10):1779.e1–7. https://doi.org/10.1016/j.ophtha.2006.05.015. Epub 2006 Jul 26. PMID: 16872678.
9. Aravena C, Yu F, Aldave AJ. Long-term visual outcomes, complications, and retention of the Boston type I Keratoprosthesis. Cornea. 2018;37(1):3–10. https://doi.org/10.1097/ICO.0000000000001405. PMID: 28990994.
10. Strampelli B. Osteo-odontokeratoprosthesis. Ann Di Ottalmologia E Clin Ocul. 1963;89:1039–44.
11. Falcinelli G, Falsini B, Taloni M, et al. Modified osteo-odonto-keratoprosthesis for treatment of corneal blindness:

long-term anatomical and functional outcomes in 181 cases. Arch Ophthalmol. 2005;123:1319–29. https://doi.org/10.1001/archopht.123.10.1319.
12. Temprano J. Keratoprosthesis with tibial autograft. Refract Corneal Surg. 1993;9:192–3.
13. Hille K, Landau H, Ruprecht KW. Improvement of the osteo-odontokeratoprosthesis according to strampelli: influence of diameter of PMMA cylinder on visual field. Graefes Arch Clin Exp Ophthalmol. 1999;237:308–12. https://doi.org/10.1007/s004170050233.

Pterygium Surgery With/Without Limbus

Philomena A. Wawer Matos Reimer, Johannes J. Wawer Matos, Alexander C. Rokohl, and Ludwig M. Heindl

Abstract

As the cornea, the limbus and the surrounding conjunctiva are equally exposed to the environment and its irritations, especially to ultraviolet light, they are also vulnerable to the development of tissue atypia and dysplasia occasionally transforming into malignant tumors. A very common fibrovascular proliferation of the conjunctiva is the pterygium, which is mostly located in the nasal (more often than in the temporal) interpalpebral zone and is accompanied by irregular astigmatism, visual impairment, dryness and other surface issues. Even if a lot of risk factors for the pterygium are well known, its pathogenesis is still not yet completely understood. Therefore, it remains necessary to improve its understanding to decrease recurrence rate and to optimize its treatment, especially the surgical therapy.

Keywords

Cornea · Corneal limbus · Conjunctiva · Slit-lamp microscopy · Anterior segment OCT of the eye · Ultrasound biomicroscopy

1 Introduction

A pterygium is an abnormal focal fibrovascular proliferation of the conjunctiva, mostly triangularly formed, and extending onto the cornea. It is one of the most common benign tumors of the ocular surface. The term pterygium has its origin in the Ancient Greek word πτέρυξ pteryx (English wing) due to its clinical appearance. Clinical symptoms include foreign body sensations, recurrent conjunctival redness, infections, and visual impairment. Its pathogenesis is consisting of multiple factors and is not conclusively clarified [1–3].

Its prevalence is depending a lot on the observed latitude with a maximum at the so-called "pterygium belt" and consequently varies from 0,3 to 33% [4, 5]. The "pterygium belt" is the region that is localized between approximately 40° north and south of the equator and was described by Cameron in 1965 [5, 6]. It is also common in people with outdoor professions, such as farmers, landscapers, or (professional) surfers ("surfer's eye") [7]. This supports the assumption that the main risk factor is ultraviolet (UV) light. Other risk factors seem to be a genetic predisposition, increasing age, and chronic exposure of the ocular surface to environmental irritations, such as dust or steam.

The UV radiation can not only damage the limbal stem cells directly, but it can activate pro-inflammatory, angiogenetic, and other molecular processes leading to angiogenesis and excessive cell proliferation (Fig. 1) [8, 9]. Predominantly, pterygia appear at the nasal side of the cornea. Underlying mechanisms may be incident UV radiation from the temporal side that is broken by the cornea and then focused on the nasal limbal region (Fig. 2). Furthermore, there may be better protection of the temporal limbal region against the UV radiation from the temporal side by the longer lashes at the temporal edge of the eye on the one hand and the nose on the other hand which stops the nasal incident UV radiation [4, 6].

Histopathologically, a pterygium is marked by a non-keratinizing epithelium. Furthermore, it can be found a loss of goblet cells and/or signs of chronic inflammation like increased angiogenesis and lymphangiogenesis, as well as a compound squamous epithelium in some cases (Fig. 3) [11, 12]. The cap of the pterygium may be firmly attached to the cornea and may sometimes even irrupt the Bowman layer. There is a pathognomonic histopathological sign of

P. A. Wawer Matos Reimer · A. C. Rokohl · L. M. Heindl (✉)
Department of Ophthalmology, University of Cologne
Faculty of Medicine, Cologne, Germany
e-mail: ludwig.heindl@uk-koeln.de

J. J. Wawer Matos
Department of Anesthesiology,
ARCUS Kliniken, Pforzheim, Germany

B. Seitz et al. (eds.), *Atlas on Cornea*, https://doi.org/10.1007/978-3-031-65422-0_56

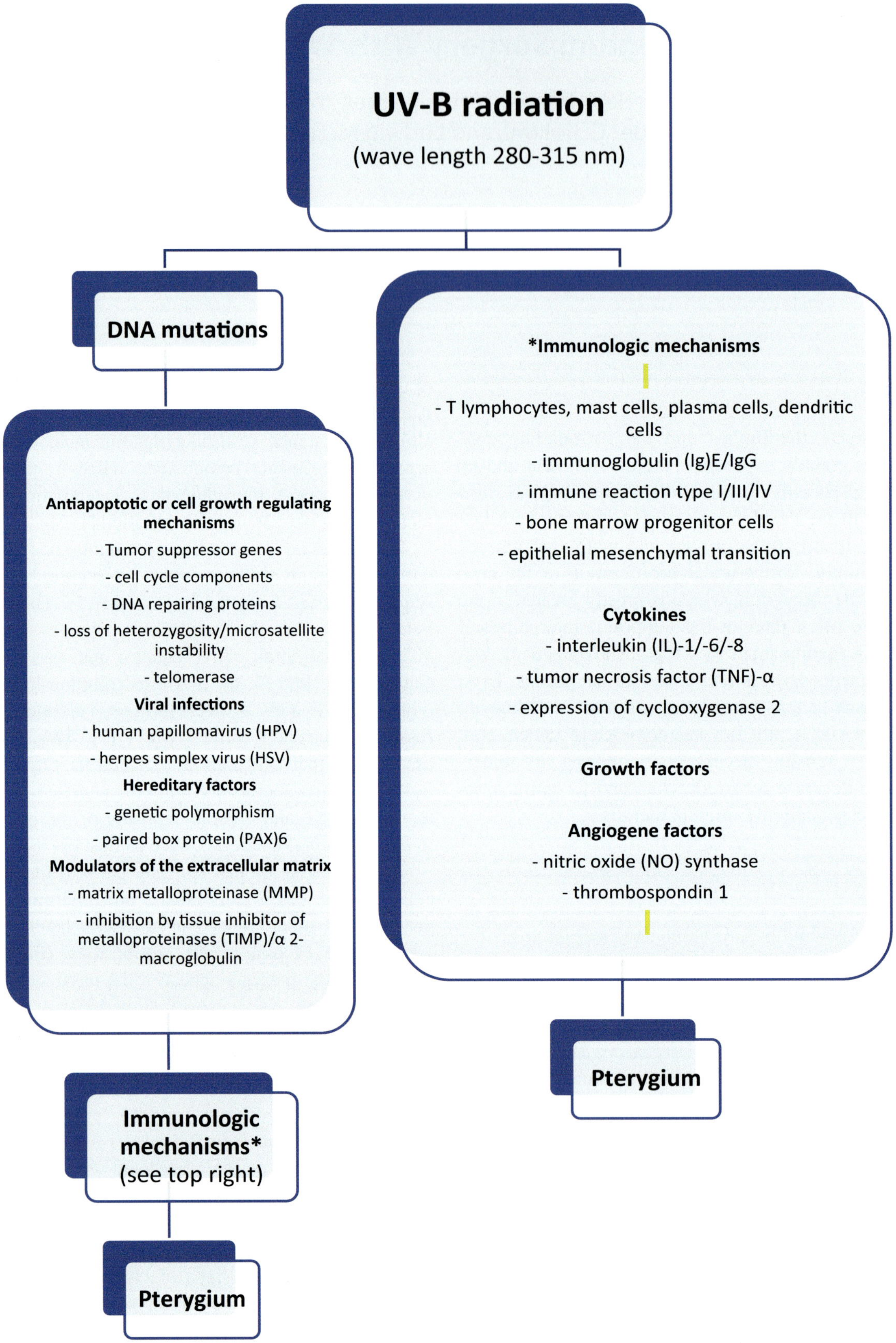

Fig. 1 Pathogenesis concepts of a pterygium's development [8]

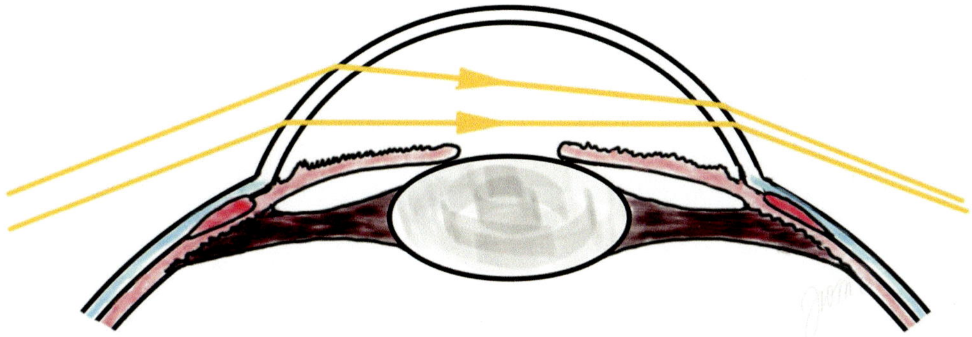

Fig. 2 Theory of pathological UV radiation in pterygium pathogenesis: UV light rays from the temporal side are refracted in the peripheral region of the cornea (left side of the figure) and are then focussed in the nasal limbal region (right side of the figure) where the limbal stem cells are damaged and the incidence of pterygium is increasing at this localization which represents a focal limbal stem cell insufficiency, modified from [10]. © Dr. J. J. Wawer Matos

a pterygium: an elastoid degeneration in the subepithelium which is missing in pseudopterygia [8, 13, 14]. A possible underlying malignancy such as squamous cell carcinoma (SCC) is the reason for the recommended histopathological examination in any case. Studies showed a not inconsiderable rate for undetected SCC is approximately 5% in regions with high UV exposure for example in Australia [1, 15].

2 Diagnostics

A profound slit lamp biomicroscopy is the foundation for all further decisions. Important criteria to assess a pterygium include:

- Localization
- Size
- Vascularization (Fig. 3)
- Dimension and area of corneal involvement
- Presence or absence of Stocker's line

A pterygium is divided into four parts:

- **Cap**: localized at the leading edge, avascular zone, appears like a halo, can merge into Stocker's line which lies towards the cornea (iron which precipitates in the corneal epithelium due to surface irregularity and uneven tear film distribution)
- **Head**: lying peripheral to the cap, vascularized, contains activated fibroblasts, can be firmly attached to the cornea, grows underneath the corneal epithelium onto and later into the Bowman layer
- **Neck**: localized at the level of the limbus corneae
- **Body**: represents the main part and is the interface between the pterygium and the rest of the conjunctiva, loosely overlying [3]

Normally, another clinical criterion is the possibility to underrun and lift the body of the pterygium with a probe [3, 4, 8]. The presence of a Stocker's line (precipitating iron in the tear film) is regularly associated with a lower recurrence rate of a pterygium [3, 8].

There are various classification systems for a pterygium (Table 1).

Furthermore, an eye exam with:

- detailed refraction,
- anterior segment imaging,
  - corneal topography and tomography: astigmatism and extension of the pterygium including e.g. Scheimpflug imaging or anterior segment optical coherence tomography (AS-OCT)
  - ultrasound biomicroscopy (UBM)
- visual acuity testing,
- diplopia testing,
- motility testing
- and evaluation of the lens and the fundus to detect UV-ray-associated involvement is part of a profound screening in diagnosing pterygia [8, 10].

It is important to know that neither the size nor the localization are significant for subjective complaints or visual impairment—even very small pterygia can induce high astigmatism and significant visual impairment [8, 19]. A pterygium can clinically appear in various forms (Figs. 4, 5 and 6).

3 Therapy Concepts

Depending on the clinical examination and the patient's complaints, the decision for a conservative versus an operative approach can be made well-considered.

The conservative concept includes observation and alleviation from symptoms, especially those caused by the

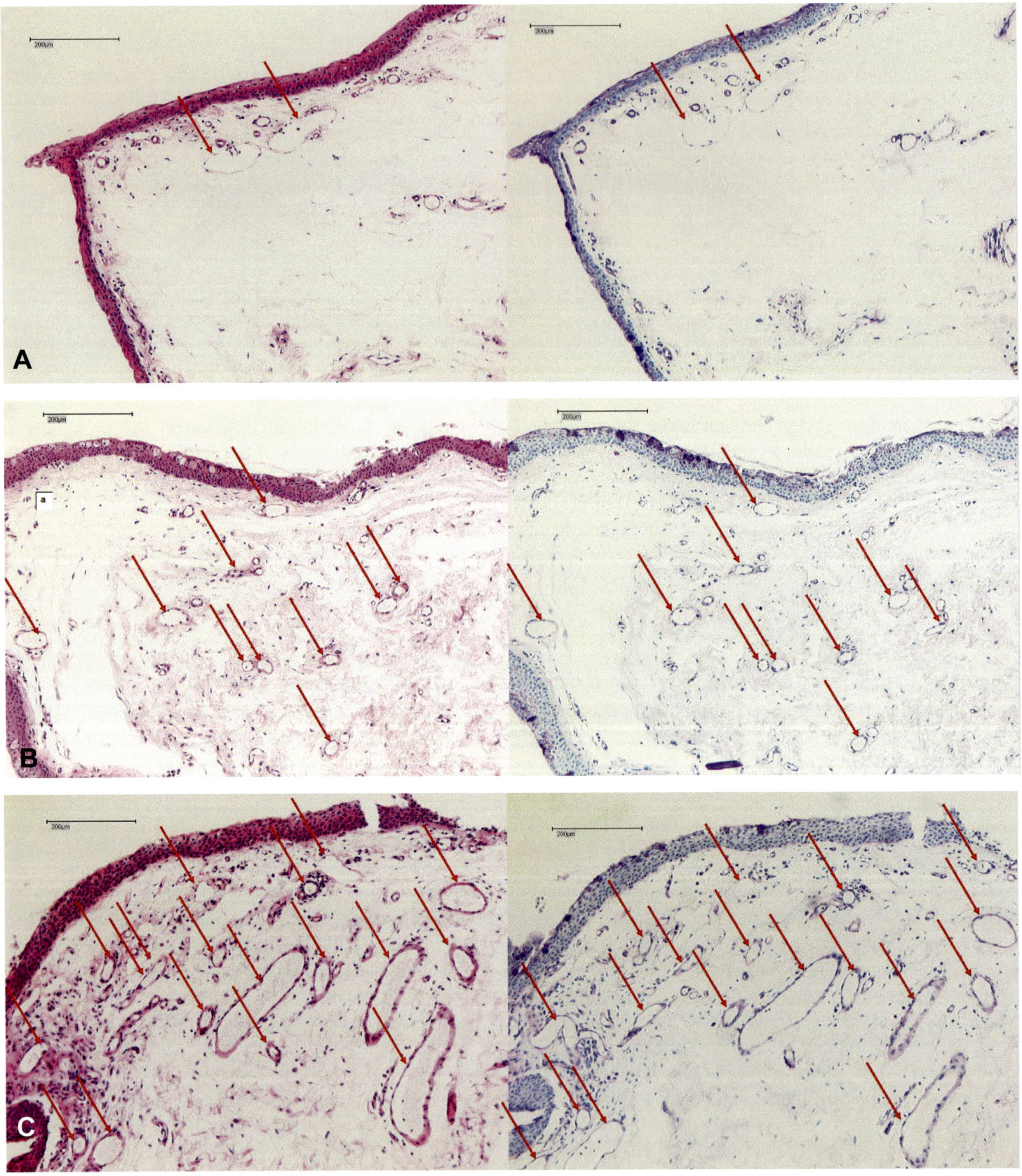

Fig. 3 (**A–C**) Histopathological sections of pterygia shown in H&E (Hematoxylin&Eosin) stain (left, original magnification = 100X) and PAS (Periodic acid-Schiff, original magnification = 100X) stain (right). In literature, it was shown that in clinically severe stadiums of a pterygium (defined by more conjunctival injection, bigger area etc.) there can be found more microvessels (red arrows) [12] © Mrs Martina Becker, histopathological laboratory at University Hospital of Cologne Department of Ophthalmology

Table 1 Classification systems for grading of a pterygium [2, 3, 10, 18]

Grading	Size in millimeters [mm] head-limbus-distance (= height) [2, 3, 16]	Expansion of the pterygium relative to the pupil margin and the optical axis [17]
1	0–2 mm	Maximal expansion of the pterygium is half the distance between limbus and pupil margin (temporal pupil margin in temporal pterygium, nasal pupil margin in nasal pterygium)
2	2–4 mm	The extension of the pterygium is more than half the distance between limbus and pupil margin but does not touch the optical axis
3	>4 mm	The pterygium is growing into the optical axis (reaching the pupillary area in a neutral pupil at medium lighting)

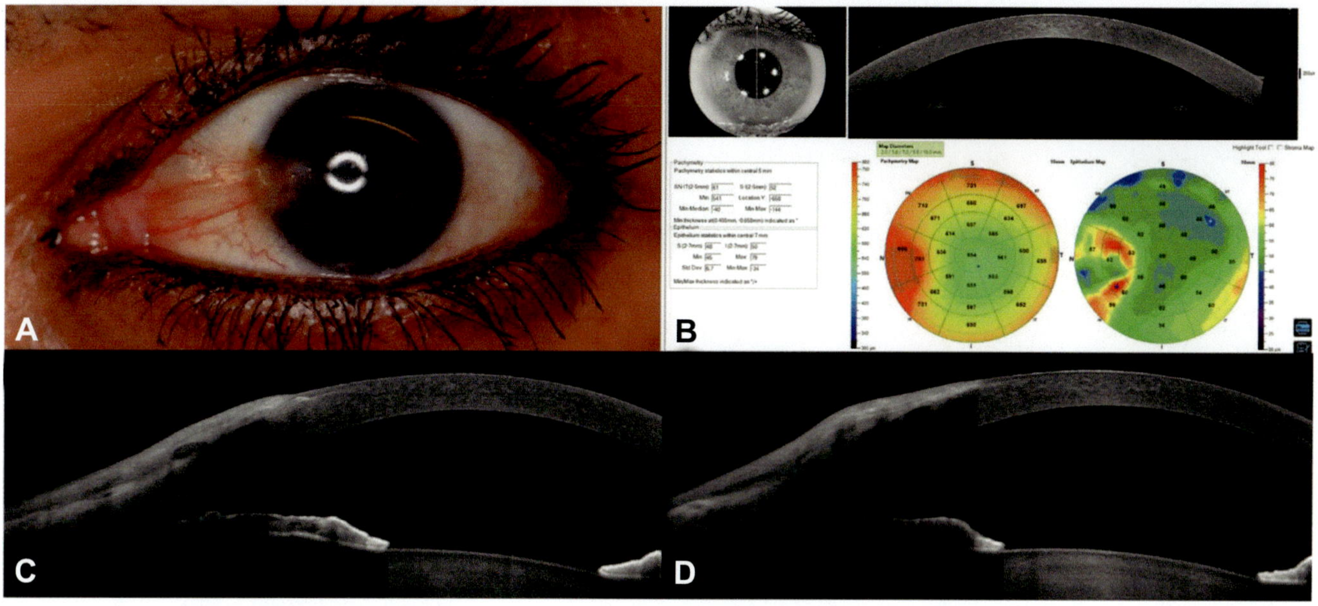

Fig. 4 Pterygium with its typical clinical appearance in a left eye. (**A**) Slit-lamp photo showing the triangularly formed conjunctival mass overgrowing the cornea up to the nasal pupil margin with associated vessel injection inducing redness of the lesion and the surrounding conjunctiva. (**B**) Ultra-high-Speed-Full-Range Spectral Domain OCT imaging with pachymetry (left) and corneal epithelial thickness map (right) showing the distinct induced astigmatism by the pterygium. (**C–D**) Anterior segment-OCT (AS-OCT) images showing the corneal involvement and its clear borders in the depth

disturbed tear film (sicca) with appropriate local therapy. A dermatologic presentation is recommendable as a diagnosed pterygium is a possible indicator of a significantly increased risk for the development of cutaneous malignant melanoma, especially in young patients [20].

A surgical approach is an option if conservative therapy fails and focal exsiccation of the ocular surface is not avoidable, foreign body sensation and other symptoms are not relieved satisfactorily, as well as cosmetic aspects which may bother the patient tremendously because patients also report being socially stigmatized.

If visual impairment, diplopia, and/or pterygium-induced increasing astigmatism are not compensated sufficiently and/or the growth is progressive, an indication for surgery becomes mandatory. To avoid a progression of the growing pterygium into the optical axis which is associated with remaining higher-order aberrations and thus reduced visual acuity after surgery, a causal therapy by surgical excision should not be performed too late [8, 19, 21–23]. In clinical studies it was approved that an increasing head-limbus-distance (= height) of the pterygium has a significant effect on the amount and the irregularity of the pterygium's induced corneal astigmatism before surgery [2]. This might also be a reason for the patients' reduction in visual acuity even if the pterygium does not reach the optical axis yet [2]. If there are associated e.g. eye lid malpositions and/or radiation-induced cataract, it should always be performed a step-by-step surgery "from outside to inside" to get the best results [24].

In general, the surgical pterygium excision can be performed in local anesthesia which provides patients cooperation e.g., eye movement maneuvers. Exceptions that may need general anesthesia are for example reduced patient cooperation, more distinct lesions, and/or previous surgery [21, 25].

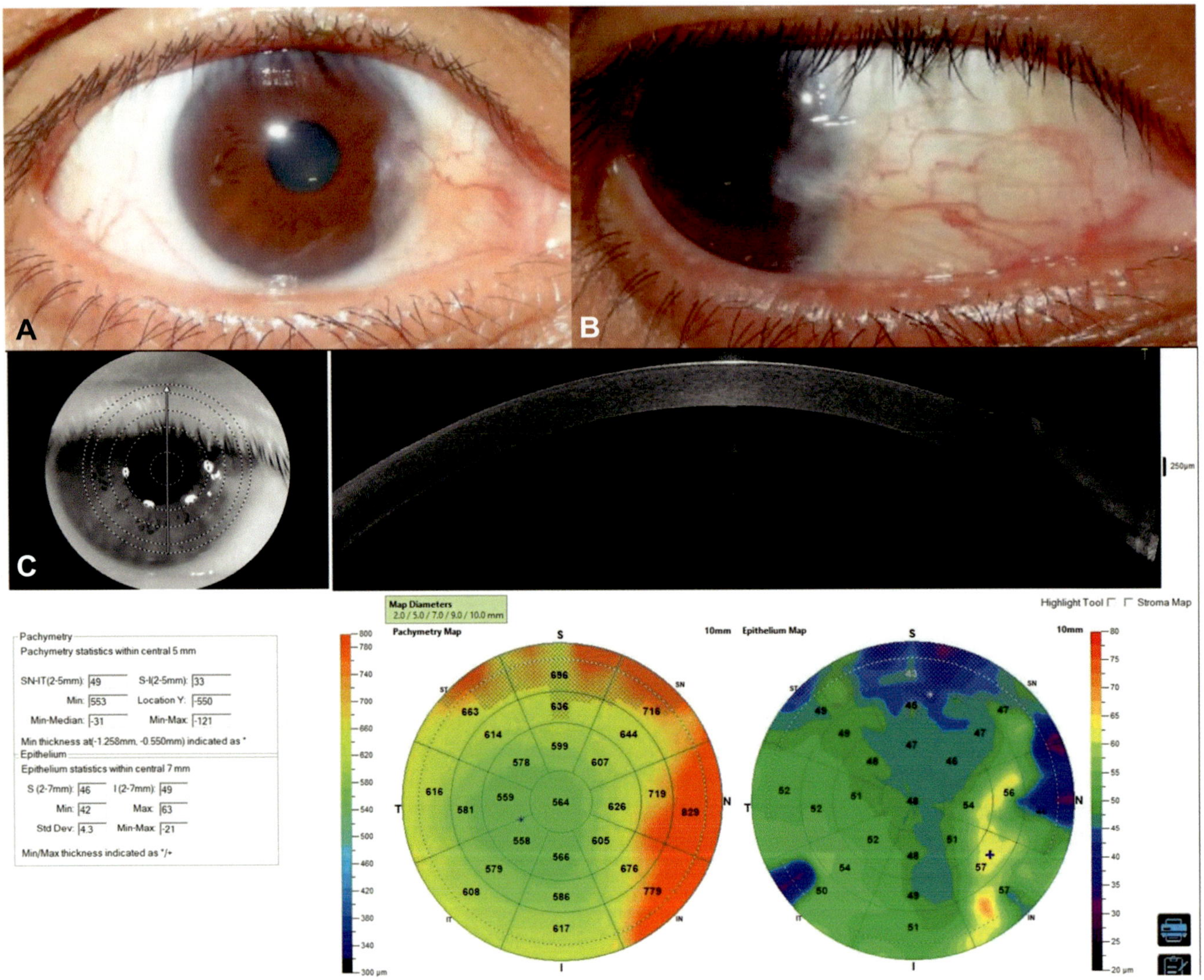

Fig. 5 Pterygium and its clinical appearance in a right eye. (**A, B**) Slit-lamp image presenting a lightly pigmented mass overgrowing the cornea and being accompanied by vessels. (**C**) Ultra-high-Speed-Full-Range Spectral Domain OCT imaging with pachymetry (left) and corneal epithelial thickness map (right) showing the distinct induced astigmatism as a corneal impairment

The current applied surgical techniques include [26]:

- bare sclera technique
- excision with conjunctival suture or glue closure
- excision with adjunctive therapy (antimitotics)
- excision with transplantation/graft techniques
- or combined techniques

4 Bare Sclera Technique

The bare sclera technique was first described by D'Ombrain in 1948 and simply comprises the complete resection of the pterygium with all four parts as well as surrounding conjunctiva and Tenon's capsule leaving an area of bare sclera adjacent to the corneal limbus (Fig. 7) [27, 28]. The tissue loss heals by secondary tissue repair of the cornea and conjunctiva and is filled up with cicatricial tissue. It is not the therapy of choice due to its high recurrence rate lying between 24 and 89% [19, 29]. This led to the development of combined procedures with graft techniques or antimitotics in modern ophthalmic surgery [30, 31].

5 Conjunctival Autograft (CAG)

Instead of dedicating the tissue repair to secondary wound healing, a replacement of the tissue loss after a pterygium excision by a graft of autologous conjunctiva was established. In most cases, conjunctiva of the ipsilateral superior or temporal inferior bulbar conjunctiva without Tenon's capsule can be used easily. The site should

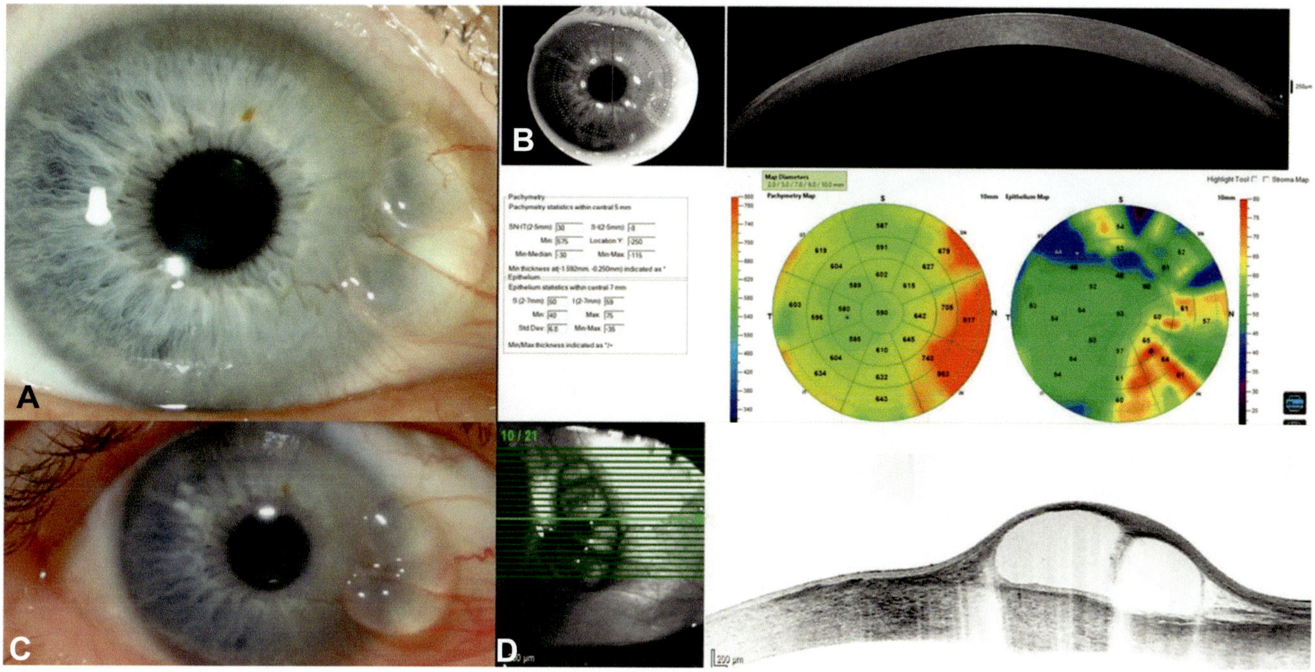

Fig. 6 Cystic Pterygium and its clinical appearance. (**A**) and (**C**) Slit-lamp biomicroscopy showing a pterygium with a huge, chambered cyst and accompanying vessels. (**B**) Ultra-high-Speed-Full-Range Spectral Domain OCT imaging with pachymetry and epithelial thickness illustrates the irregular ocular surface induced by the lesion. (**D**) Anterior Segment OCT images make the huge cyst with its chambers and its clear enclosure to its surrounding tissue visible

be chosen carefully with regard to e.g. glaucoma surgery that might be necessary in the future, for example. If this is not possible, it can be taken from any other quadrant of the same eye or even from the other eye (free graft). The recurrence rate was able to be decreased by the use of an autograft and is about 2.6–39% [32, 33]. There are different ways to attach the autograft (sutures, glue/tissue adhesive, autologous blood), but even though most surgeons agreed to choose this technique as the first-line therapy for primary and recurrent pterygium as well (Figs. 8, 9 and 10) (Table 2).

6 Pterygium-Extended Removal Followed by Extended Conjunctival Transplant (PERFECT) Technique

This type of excision includes a larger excision of the conjunctiva around the pterygium and a larger dissection of the subconjunctival Tenon's capsule from the limbus 10–15 mm peripheral to the limbus and about 2 clock hours below and above the wound margins of the conjunctiva. An appropriate conjunctival graft is excised and placed on the bare sclera. Recurrences are low and occur between 0 to 1.6% but postoperative complications comprise corneal ulcer, strabismus, diplopia, granuloma, or inclusion cysts [38].

7 Conjunctival Limbal Allograft (CLAG)

Using this technique, the pterygium is excised as usual but the conjunctival graft includes a part of the limbus (autologous or allogenic limbal stem cells). Its recurrence rates are low and increase in reappearing pterygia [39–41].

8 Amniotic Membrane Graft (AMG)

Instead of a conjunctival graft, the scleral bed is covered with an amniotic membrane, which is attached with fibrin glue or sutures instead of a conjunctival graft. Pterygium surgery with CAG (Conjunctival AutoGraft) is nevertheless more effective than AMG (Amniotic Membrane Graft) in preventing recurrent pterygia, even in case of recurrence. The recurrence rate in pterygium excision with AMG lies between approximately 6 and 42% [42–45]

9 Adjunctive Agents

The different agents have one thing in common: they inhibit cell proliferation or angiogenesis to reduce pterygium recurrence (Figs. 11 and 12). Most of them are applied intraoperatively to the bare sclera and are well-rinsed after

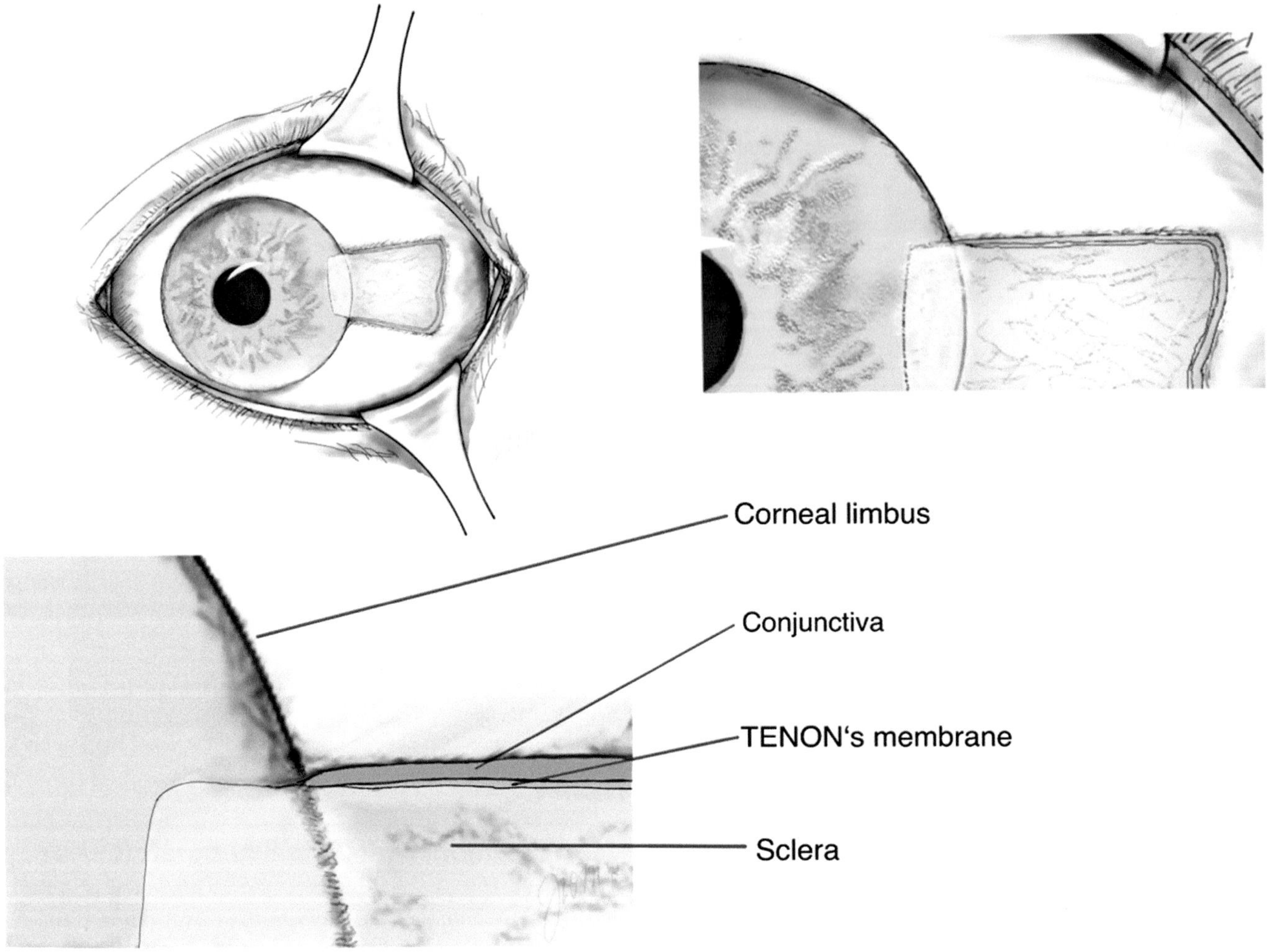

Fig. 7 Last operative step in bare sclera technique in pterygium surgery: after simply excising the lesion, Tenon's edge builds the outer rim, covered by overlapping and less but sufficiently excised surrounding conjunctiva. The Tenon's free zone lies in between them. © Dr. J. J. Wawer Matos

a certain time of exposure. It is also possible to applicate it preoperatively as a subconjunctival application or postoperatively as well injected subconjunctivally or topically in the form of eye drops [46, 47]. They can also be used as adjuvant therapy for dysplastic or malignant differential diagnoses (Table 3).

In general, a postoperative reduction of recurrence can be achieved by a postoperative local anti-inflammatory therapy with corticosteroids and/or ciclosporin A (CsA), as well as intensive therapy with humidifying eye drops for a couple of weeks or months. Steroids need frequent postoperative controls of eye pressure. Systemic therapy with corticosteroids is also recommended in the postoperative period for six days (Table 4). To avoid postoperative pain due to corneal erosion, a contact lens can be used until the corneal epithelium is closed again.

10 Differential Diagnoses of Lesions and Tumors at the Cornea and Limbus

There exist various differential diagnoses to a pterygium, which will be shown in the following [1] (Table 5).

10.1 Limbal Scars and Other Pseudopterygia

The term pseudopterygium includes conjunctival adhesions to the cornea, which are not progressive and are mostly attributed to an injury at the corneal-limbus junction. It is mostly localized in the lower circumference of the eye. In pseudopterygia, it is not possible to lift the body of the fibrovascular mass [51]. In the histopathologic examination of a pseudopterygium, an elastoid degeneration is missing.

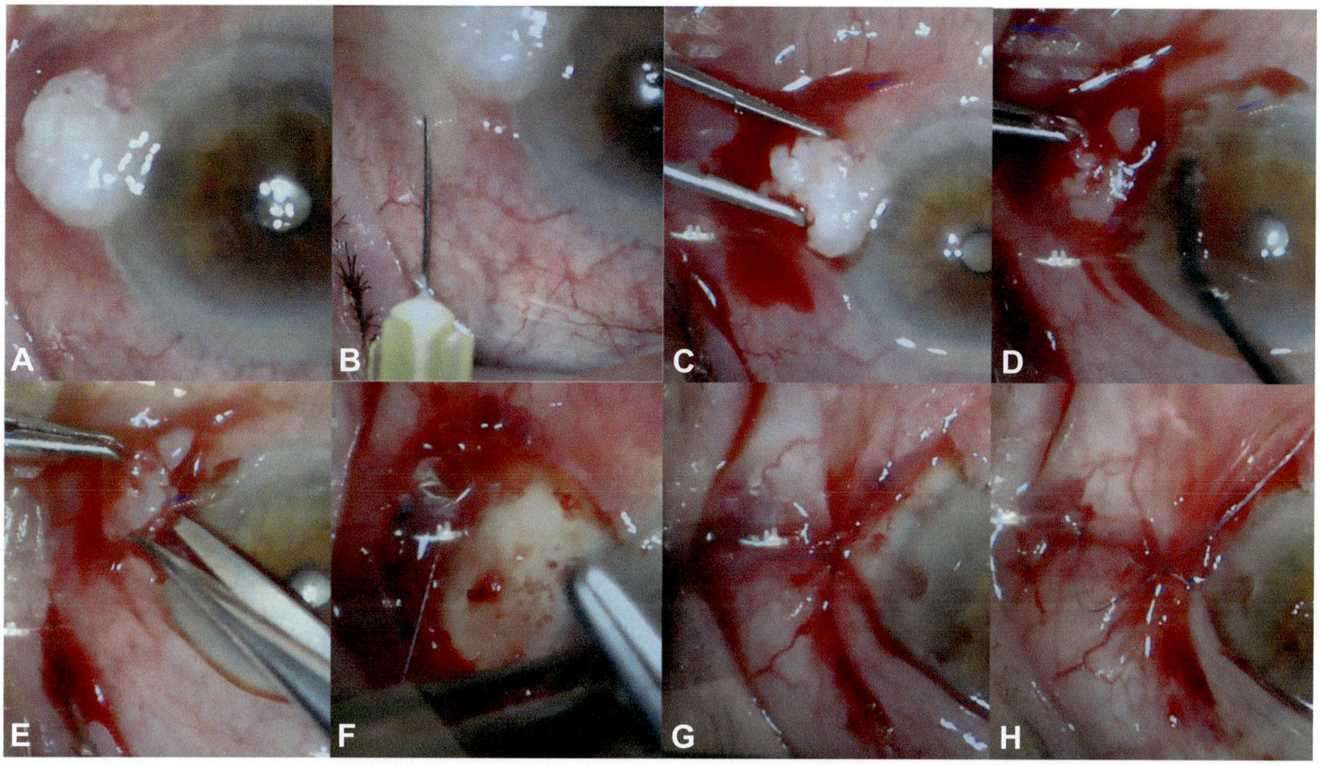

Fig. 8 Pterygium excision with conjunctival graft and suture (**A**) Cystic pterygium under the microscope as initial finding before starting surgery. (**B**) Subconjunctival injection of local anesthesia and vasoconstrictive agent. (**C**) Holding up the pterygium's body. (**D**) Detaching the pterygium from the cornea. (**E**) Excision of the pterygium and surrounding conjunctiva. (**F**) Bare sclera is visible in the excision's area. (**G**) Conjunctival closure with suture. (**H**) Final result after suture

Anamnesis is a key concept that is shown by the presented case: a patient with a huge pseudopterygium in the lower circumference reported trauma with a bow and arrow in his childhood (Fig. 14). Intraoperatively a small perforation lying under the pseudopterygium appeared. Clinically, the so called "(Bowman) *probe test*" can be useful in differentiating a pseudopterygium from a pterygium: it is positive in pseudopterygium if a probe can be passed beneath the lesions' apex [52]. In the following, Table 6 gives an overview how to differentiate between a pseudopterygium and a real pterygium.

10.2 Pinguecula

The term pinguecula is referable to a composition of the Latin word "pinguis" which means "fat" and the word "macula" which means "spot". This is a good description of its clinical appearance: a small, but prominent yellowish conjunctival mass in the nasal and/or temporal edge (Figs. 15, 16, 17, 18, 19 and 20). It should be recommended an examination of the patient's fat metabolism and the exclusion of Gaucher disease [53]. It may disturb the patient due to the irregular surface and consequently inconsistent tear film. A secondary inflammation—so-called pingueculitis—is also possible [54]. This is also the reason why it is considered to be a so-called "pre-pterygium" as well [55]. The histological specimen shows a thickened conjunctival stroma that arises from degenerated collagen fibers [3]. A pingueculitis can be treated with lubricant artificial tears and in acute phases as well with anti-inflammatory agents, e.g., with local steroids and/or CsA which should not be used as a long-term therapy. A pinguecula can also be excised because of cosmetic reasons if the patient insists.

10.3 Solid Limbal and/or Corneal Dermoid

A solid limbal dermoid is a congenital and benign tumor of the ocular surface potentially affecting a patient's visual acuity due to its extension on the cornea but also its corneal infiltration by lipids and consequently arising astigmatism may be induced or the optical axis might be blocked [56]. It is important to check other ophthalmic aberrations e.g. colobomata of the eyelids, anomalies of the lacrimal duct system, or corneal and scleral staphylomata. Furthermore, a pediatric examination due to its association with Goldenhar syndrome is recommended [57]. A limbal dermoid is

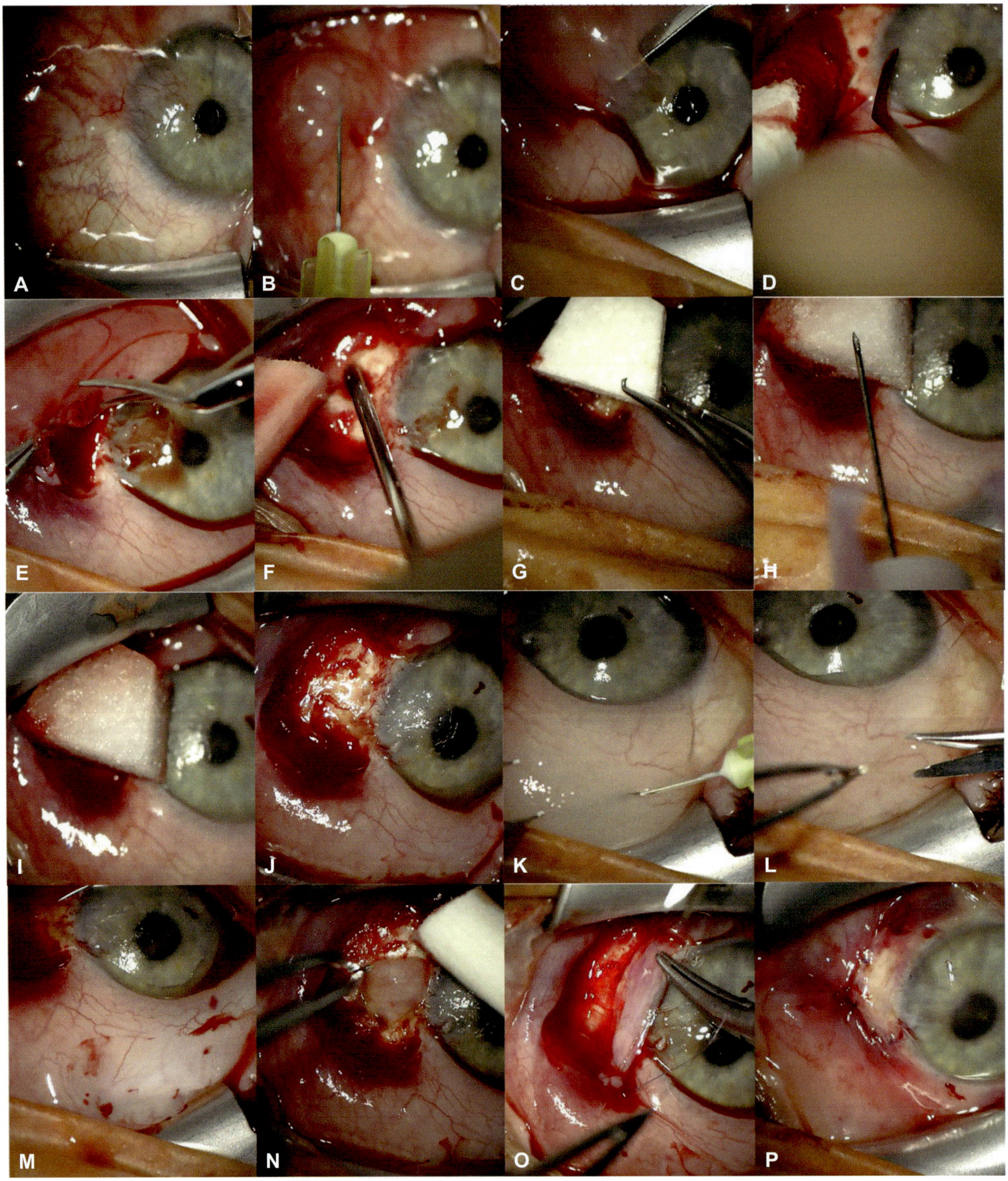

Fig. 9 Pterygium excision with free conjunctival graft, intraoperative mitomycin C (MMC) application and suture (**A**) Intraoperative overview of the pterygium before beginning the surgical excision. (**B**) Subconjunctival application of local anesthesia and vasoconstrictive agent. (**C**) Holding up and detaching the pterygium. (**D**) Peeling off the pterygium of the cornea. (**E**) Excision of the pterygium. (**F**) Cauterization of the bleeding episcleral vessels. (**G**) Positioning of the applicant sponge. (**H**) Soaking the sponge with mitomycin C agent. (**I**) Mitomycin C soaked sponge on the area of the former pterygium. (**J**) Area after (up to) three minutes of application time. (**K**) Subconjunctival application of local anesthesia and vasoconstrictive agent at another quadrant. (**L–M**) Excision of the free conjunctival graft. (**N–O**) Placing the free conjunctival graft into the bare area. (**P**) Final result after suture

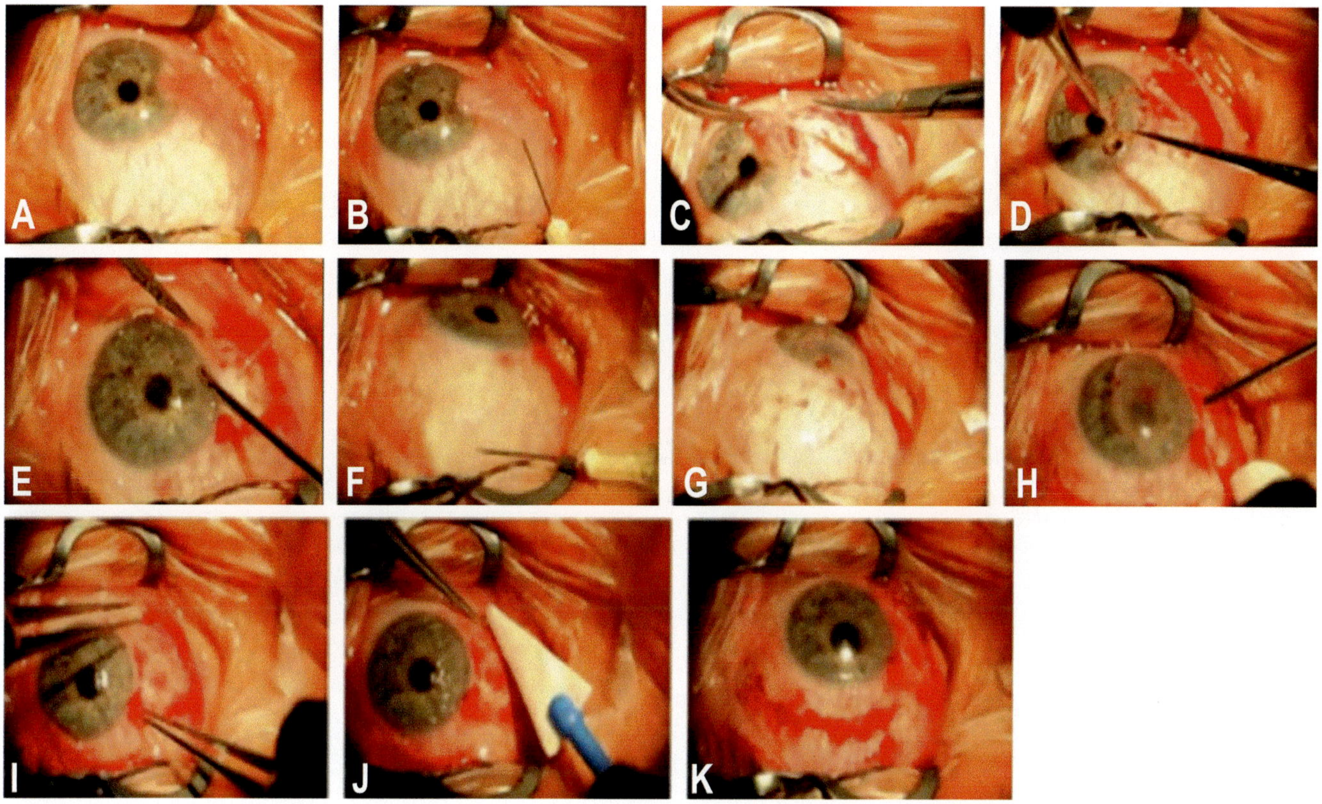

Fig. 10 "Surgical steps of the pterygium resection with conjunctival graft closure and glue adhesion technique (**A**) Finding before section and after local anesthesia with drops respectively Xylocaine Jelly. (**B**) Subconjunctival injection of a mixture of anaesthetic and vasoconstrictor. (**C**) Undermining the pterygium with a scissor, abscising it at the conjunctival end and pulling it towards the cornea. (**D**) Wrenched strongly it can be dissected from the cornea by the use of a hockey knife. (**E**) After an initial equalization with the hockey knife, the resection bed of the cornea is smoothened extra fine with a diamond polisher (not shown) or a diamant-coated hollow needle. To avoid thermic damage this step is realized by continuous irrigation. (**F**) Subconjunctival injection in the upper temporal part of the conjunctiva (meaning between conjunctiva and Tenon's capsule) with anaesthetic/vasoconstrictor mixture. The patient looks nasal-downward. (**G**) A very thin and hole-free conjunctival flap is prepared towards the limbus and turned up onto the cornea. (**H**) The graft is removed approximately 1 mm off the limbus to spare the limbal stem cells and is orientated on the cornea with the epithelial side. The bare scleral resection bed is moistened sparingly with the fibrin glue component. Afterwards, the stromal side of the conjunctival graft is moistened with the thrombin component of the two-component adhesive. (**I**) The graft is turned up rapidly with two tweezers and brought to the final provided position over the resection bed. (**J**) Adaptation by squeezing it with a wedge-formed swab and compressing the edges of the conjunctiva and the graft with a tweezer. (**K**) End of surgery. The graft is well agglutinated. The stromal corneal bed is smooth and rid of pterygium residuals. The point of withdrawal of the graft shows an intact Tenon's capsule", with friendly permission of Prof. Dr. C. Cursiefen [21]

Table 2 Comparison of different adherent techniques [33–37]

Closure technique (Figs. 8–10)	Advantages	Disadvantages	Postoperative complications
Sutures	Low cost, excellent graft stability, easy availability	Prolonged operating time	Patient's discomfort, possible granuloma formation, abscesses, scarring, necrosis, giant papillary conjunctivitis, loosening of the suture
Tissue Adhesive (fibrin sealer protein concentrate and thrombin)	Reduced operating time, reduced postoperative inflammation, estimated less recurrence rate	Higher costs, less availability, Graft displacement/loss, potential risk of blood-born disease transmission, risk of allergic reaction (low)	Graft displacement, graft loss
Autologous blood	Autologous clotting factors (no allergic or immune response)	Prolonged operating time, graft displacement/loss	Graft displacement, graft loss

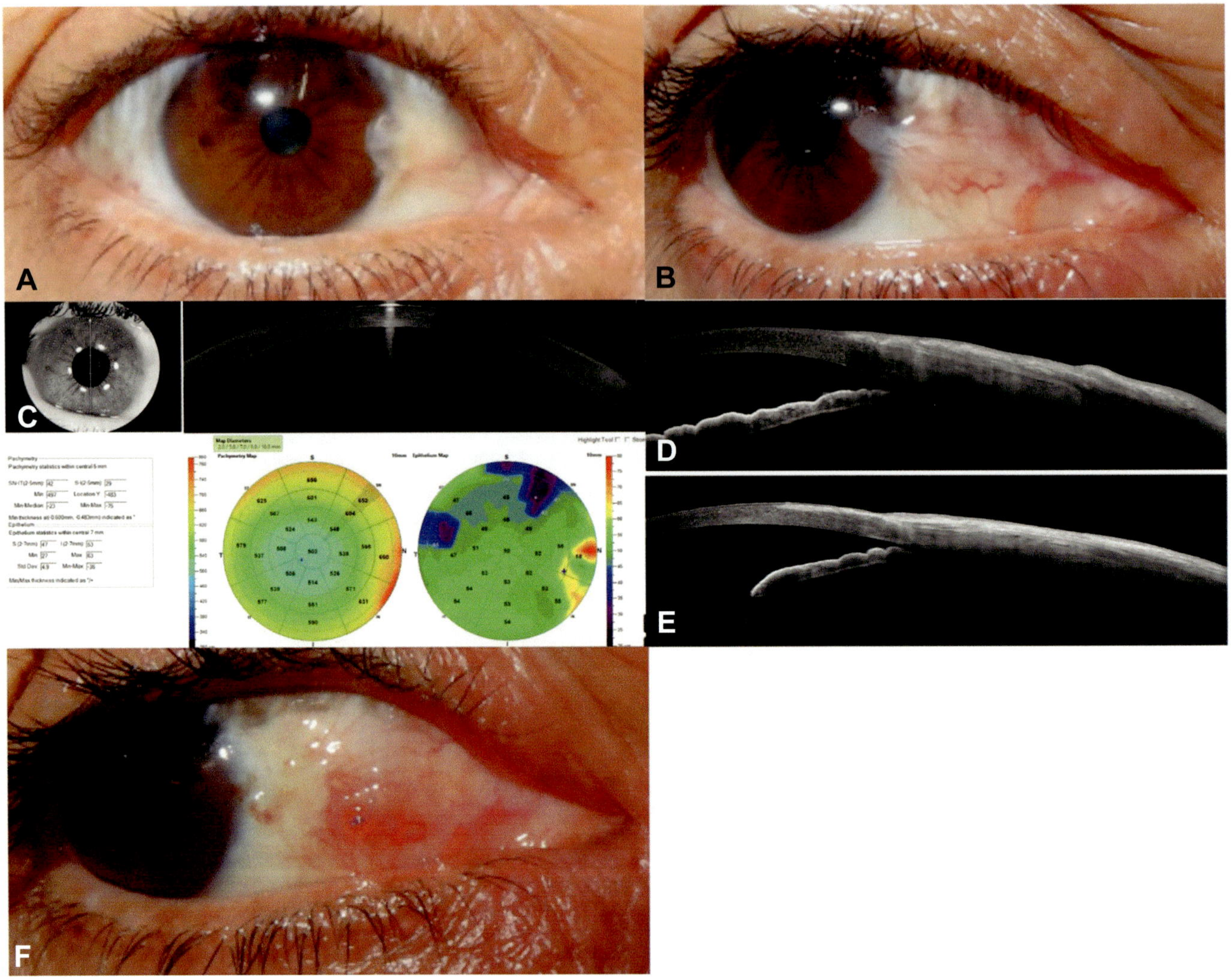

Fig. 11 Pre- and postoperative example of a pterygium excision combined with intraoperative Mitomycin C (MMC) application. (**A, B**) *preoperative* slit-lamp biomicroscopy. (**C**) Ultra-high-Speed-Full-Range Spectral Domain OCT imaging with pachymetry and epithelial thickness showing the induced astigmatism. (**D, E**) *preoperative* AS-OCT images of the pterygium with its irregular surface and its corneal involvement. (**F**) *postoperative* slit-lamp biomicroscopy

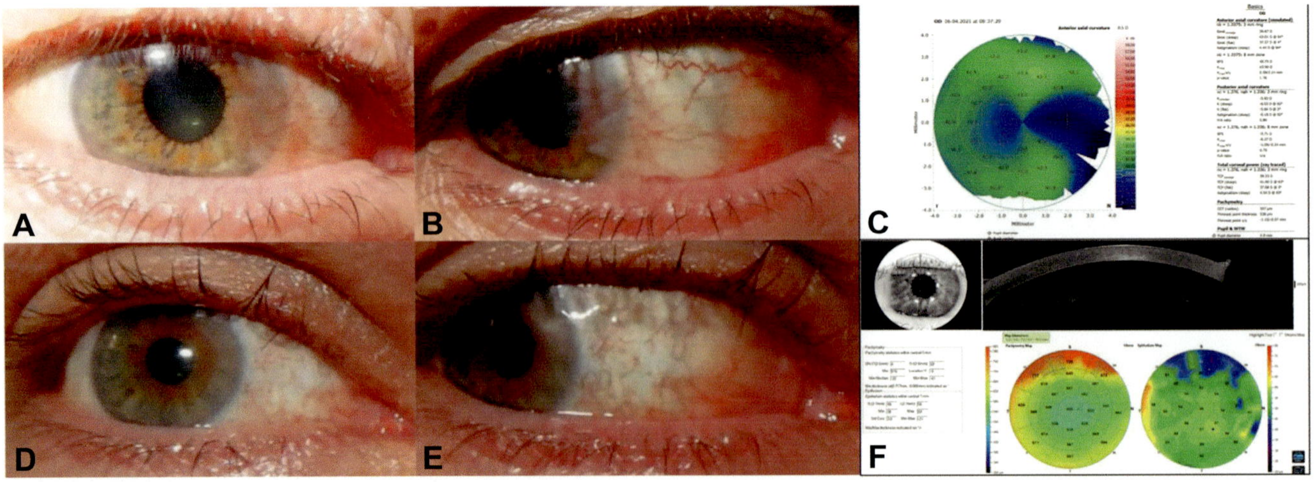

Fig. 12 Pre- and postoperative example of a pterygium excision combined with intraoperative Mitomycin C (MMC) application. (**A–C**) *Preoperative* slit-lamp biomicroscopy and Ultra-high-Speed-Full-Range Spectral Domain OCT imaging with pachymetry and epithelial thickness showing the induced astigmatism at 3–4 o'clock. (**D–F**) Postoperative slit-lamp biomicroscopy and Ultra-high-Speed-Full-Range Spectral Domain imaging with pachymetry and epithelial thickness

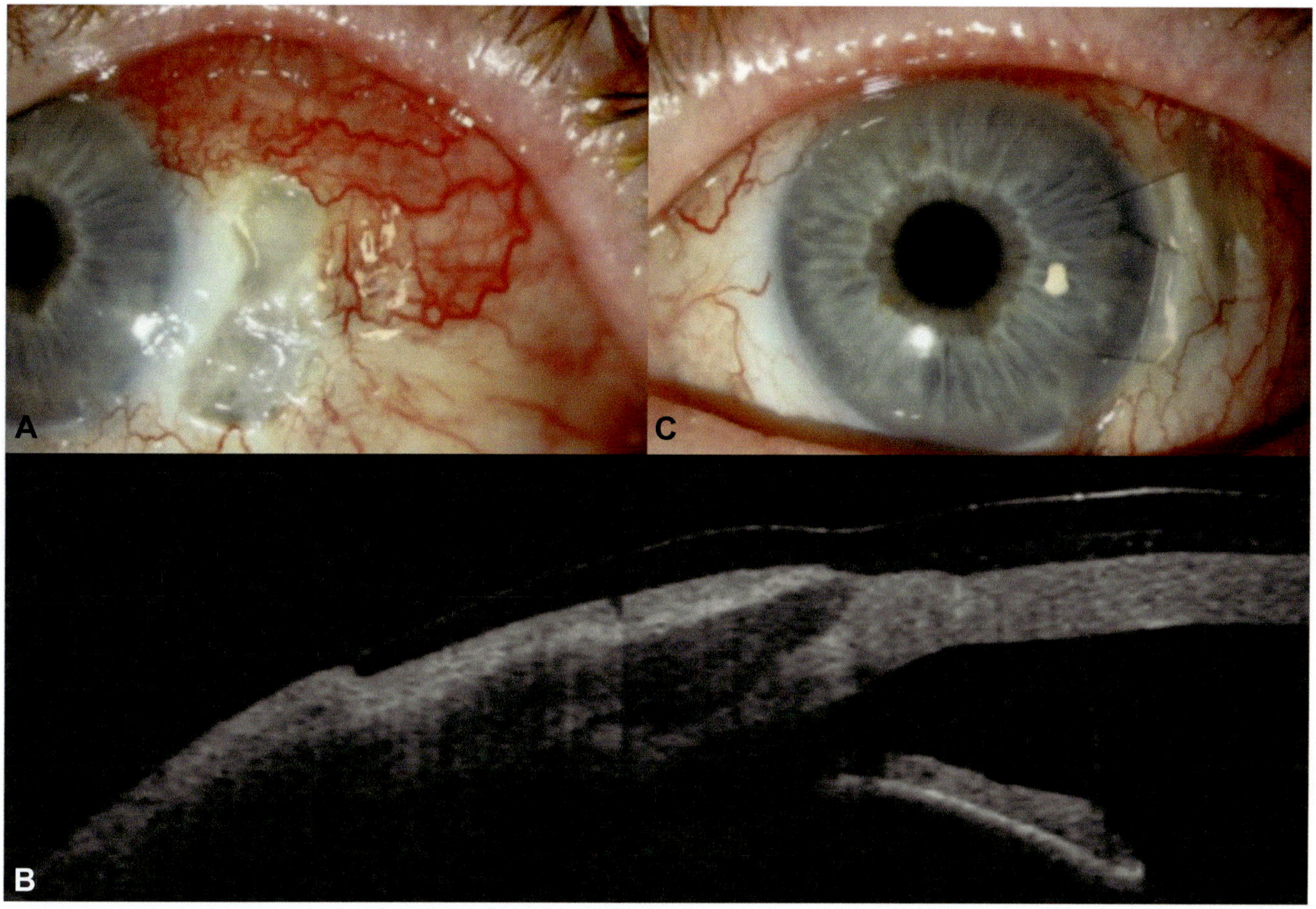

Fig. 13 (**A**) Sclera necrosis after intraoperative application of mitomycin C as part of pterygium excision. (**B**) The anterior-segment OCT shows an early postoperative state with a protecting bandage contact lens and a darker-colored section in the closure defect area in the stroma. (**C**) After a debridement a lamellar corneal graft (residual donor tissue after inhouse graft preparation for Descemet Membrane Endothelial Keratoplasty = DMEK) was put in and covered with conjunctiva. Furthermore, systemic and local immunosuppressive and antibiotic therapy was induced. Modified, with friendly permission from Prof. Dr. Dr. L. M. Heindl [10]

Table 3 Overview of most important and used adjunctive agents [47–50]

Agent	Mechanism	Concentration, application time, and form	Complications
Mitomycin C (MMC)	Antimitotic, anti-proliferative effects on fibroblasts and vascular endothelial cells	0,02–0,04% 3–5 min Subconjunctival or Topical (drops)	Scleral thinning, scleral melts (Fig. 13) to spontaneous globe perforation (postoperative), cataract induction, visual impairment and loss of best visual acuity, iritis
5-Fluorouracil (5-FU)	Antimetabolite, active against fibroblasts (less potent than MMC)	50 mg/ml 3–5 min Subconjunctival or Topical (drops)	Scleral thinning, scleral melts to spontaneous globe perforation (postoperative), cataract induction, visual impairment and loss of best visual acuity, iritis, cosmetic result less satisfactory than MMC with more abnormal conjunctival vasculature
Bevacizumab	Anti-VEGF (endothelial cells)	Subconjunctival or Topical (drops)	Irritation, photophobia, epiphora, redness, discharge, blurred vision, inflammation

Table 4 Possible therapy concept to reduce postoperative inflammation

	Standard therapy after surgical excision of pterygium to reduce postoperative inflammatory reaction
Local therapy	Combined steroid and antibiotic therapy until the epithelium is closed
	After epithelium has healed: – e.g. preservative-free steroids 5 times a day, reducing it every other week, duration depending on the clinical finding (regular measurement of the intraocular pressure is needed) – preservative-free ocular lubricant e.g. at least 5 times a day for 3–6 months
Systemic therapy	Steroids: 150 mg intraoperatively, postoperatively reducing it every second day (100 mg for 2 days, 80 mg for 2 days and 60 mg for 2 days)

Table 5 Overview of the most common differential diagnoses of a pterygium [1, 10]

Pseudopterygium
– Trauma
– Corrosive injury
– Burn
– Fuchs–Terrien marginal degeneration
– (Cicatricial) mucous membrane pemphigoid
– Stevens–Johnson syndrome
Pinguecula
Neoplasia
– Conjunctival intraepithelial neoplasia (CIN)
– Invasive squamous cell carcinoma of the conjunctiva
– Mucoepidermoid carcinoma of the conjunctiva
– Spindle-cell carcinoma of the conjunctiva
Inflammation
– Nodular episcleritis
– Phlyctenular keratoconjunctivitis

clinically characterized by a dome-shaped, misty mass with a keratinized surface and potentially spiked with hair follicles and/or cilia that might also cause irritations (Figs. 21 and 22) [57, 58]. In general, surgical excision is not necessary. If it becomes necessary—due to induced astigmatism, visual impairment, blindness, or patient's insistence (cosmesis)—a resection can be performed in different ways: among others a combined excision with lamellar keratoplasty, resection with conjunctival autografts, resection with penetrating keratoplasty, resection combined with amniotic membrane transplantation or solitary lamellar sclerokeratectomy [56, 58].

10.4 Limbal Squamous Cell Dysplasia and Carcinoma

Squamous neoplasia of the ocular surface comprises a broad range from variable dysplastic lesions to invasive squamous cell carcinoma of the conjunctiva. Squamous cell carcinoma is one of the most common malignant tumors of the ocular surface and can masquerade as a pterygium-like mass. As in pterygia, chronic exposure to UV light is an important risk factor and its prevalence depends as well on the geographic localization reaching from 0,3 to 35 per one million inhabitants. Another important risk factor for the development of squamous cell carcinoma is an infection with the human papillomavirus (HPV) [59, 60]. The variability of the dysplasia can also be seen in its clinical manifestations: vascularized tumors with a gelatinous surface may be white if keratin is on the surface (Figs. 23 and 24). Depending on the extension and the invasion of its surroundings, total excision with adjuvant antimitotic (e.g. Mitomycin C = MMC) treatment is needed (Fig. 25).

10.5 Primary Acquired Melanosis (PAM) of the Limbus and/or the Cornea

Primary acquired melanosis or abbreviated PAM of the cornea is mostly associated with a PAM of the conjunctiva. Whereas melanocytes in the cornea are missing, in the limbus and the conjunctiva melanocytes can appear as local hyperpigmentation and can also extend in/onto the cornea, as well as becoming prominent lesions or accompanied by surrounding inflammation (Fig. 26). The clinical appearance is variable which is different compared to a conjunctival nevus (stationary). Usually, it can be found in people older than 40 years. The histopathological examination often shows its proliferating pigmentation in the corneal epithelium—but it can be found in every cell layer, also in the conjunctiva [3]. It can be surgically removed due to growth or other suspicious changes or the patient's insistence (cosmesis) but in general, it is observed regularly.

10.6 Limbal and/or Corneal Nevi

As nevi can be found highly frequented in the conjunctiva, especially in the limbal region, they are the most common benign tumors of the conjunctiva and can occur congenitally or acquired. They correspond to hamartomas as excessive tissue masses [27]. Mostly, they appear unilaterally. The slit-lamp biomicroscopy reveals a circumscribed variably pigmented, sometimes as well amelanotic, flat to prominent nevus (Fig. 27). Included pseudocysts are possible and pathognomonic for conjunctival nevi compared to PAM/conjunctival melanosis (Fig. 28). Excision can be

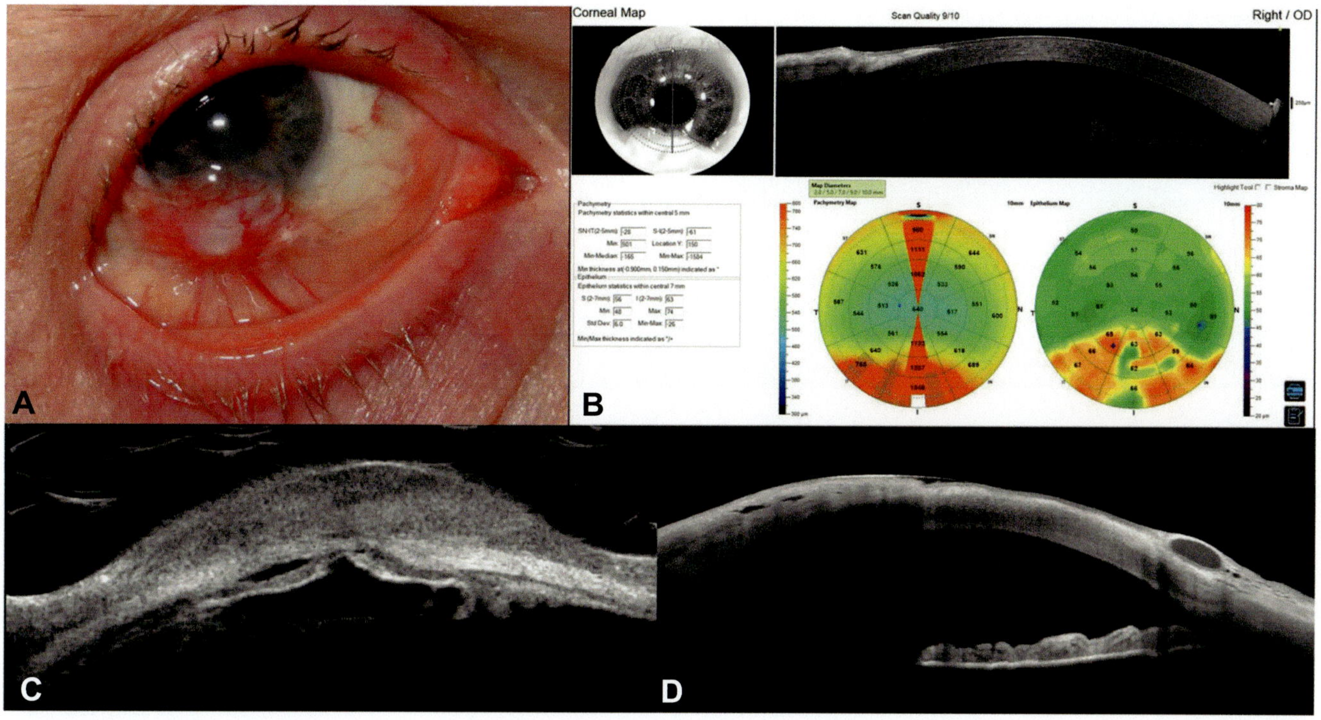

Fig. 14 Pseudopterygium arising after an eye injury in childhood. (**A**) Slit-lamp biomicroscopy. (**B**) Ultra-high-Speed-Full-Range Spectral Domain OCT imaging including pachymetry and epithelial thickness visualizes the pseudopterygium's impact on the irregular ocular surface. (**C**) UBM sonography showing the scar in all layers with an attachment of the iris to the posterior surface of the cornea. (**D**) AS-OCT showing irregular surface and cystoid inclusion

Table 6 Overview of the differences between a pseudopterygium and a pterygium [51]

Title	Pseudopterygium (Fig. 14)	Pterygium
Etiology	Secondary to corneal damage	Degenerative
Location	Anywhere along the 360 degrees	Nasal or temporal limbus
Condition	Stationary	Normally progressive
Form	Anterior portion broad and flat	Head-pointed and well-defined
AS-OCT	Real plane of cleavage	Pseudoline of cleavage
Probe test	Positive	Negative
Histology	Fibrovascular tissue without foci of elastotic degeneration	Elastotic degeneration intermingled with epithelium and stroma

done if there is a visible change, a hint of malignancy, or because of cosmetic reasons. If necessary, a complete or lamellar excision can be done depending on its localization and extension.

10.7 Limbal and/or Corneal Melanoma

Limbal stem cells are capable of regenerating the epithelial layers of the cornea. Approximately 2% of all ocular tumors are conjunctival melanomas, which can grow over the limbal bound onto the cornea, whereas corneal melanomas which appear isolated without any detection of a conjunctival melanoma can be found in 5% of all primary ocular surface melanomas [63].

Melanomas that occur at the limbus—so-called limbal or epibulbar melanomas—are neoplasms that originate from melanocytes at the corneoscleral junction. They must be differentiated from uveal melanomas with an extrascleral extension. There exist various reports about corneal melanomas and multiple theories about their development. In healthy corneal tissue, melanocytes are missing. This fact leads to the current understanding of the pathomechanism which is supposed as a contiguous spreading of melanoma cells from an undetected conjunctival melanoma. It is still discussed in the literature. It is also described as a "corneally displaced conjunctival melanoma" [64]. Furthermore, as well as in other tissues like the skin, melanocytes can change from healthy to atypical to malignant cells. They can arise at the limbus e.g. from corneal primary acquired

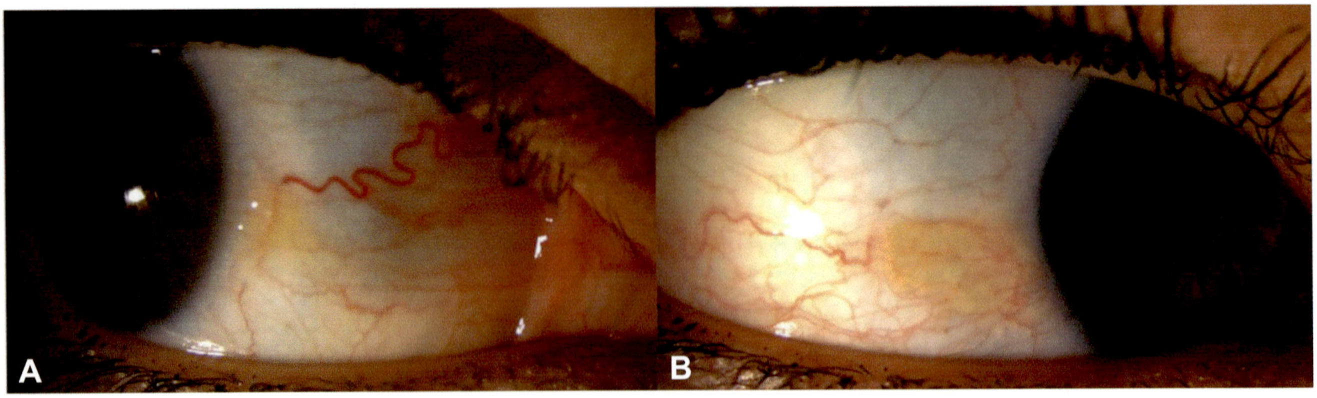

Fig. 15 Typical clinical appearance of pingueculae. (**A, B**) Yellowish lesion at the nasal and temporal limbus of a right eye in slit-lamp photos

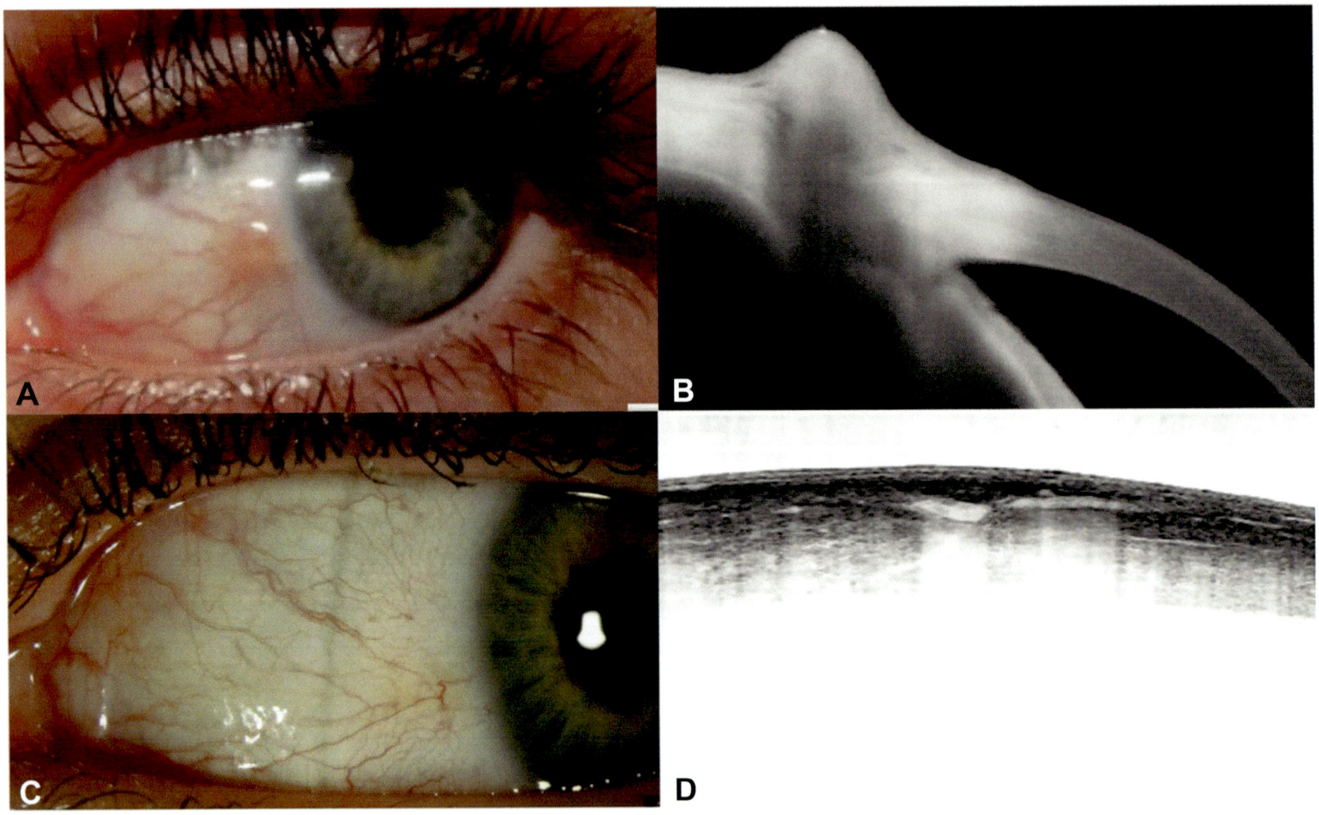

Fig. 16 Pinguecula with pingueculitis in a left eye. (**A**) Slit-lamp biomicroscopy showing the typical yellowish nodule with vessel injection. (**B**) AS-OCT shows the prominent lesion and its boundaries at the limbus. (**C, D**) Slit-lamp biomicroscopy (**C**) and AS-OCT (**D**) showing the healed lesion with flat yellowish alteration after local therapy with anti-inflammatory eye drops for 4 weeks

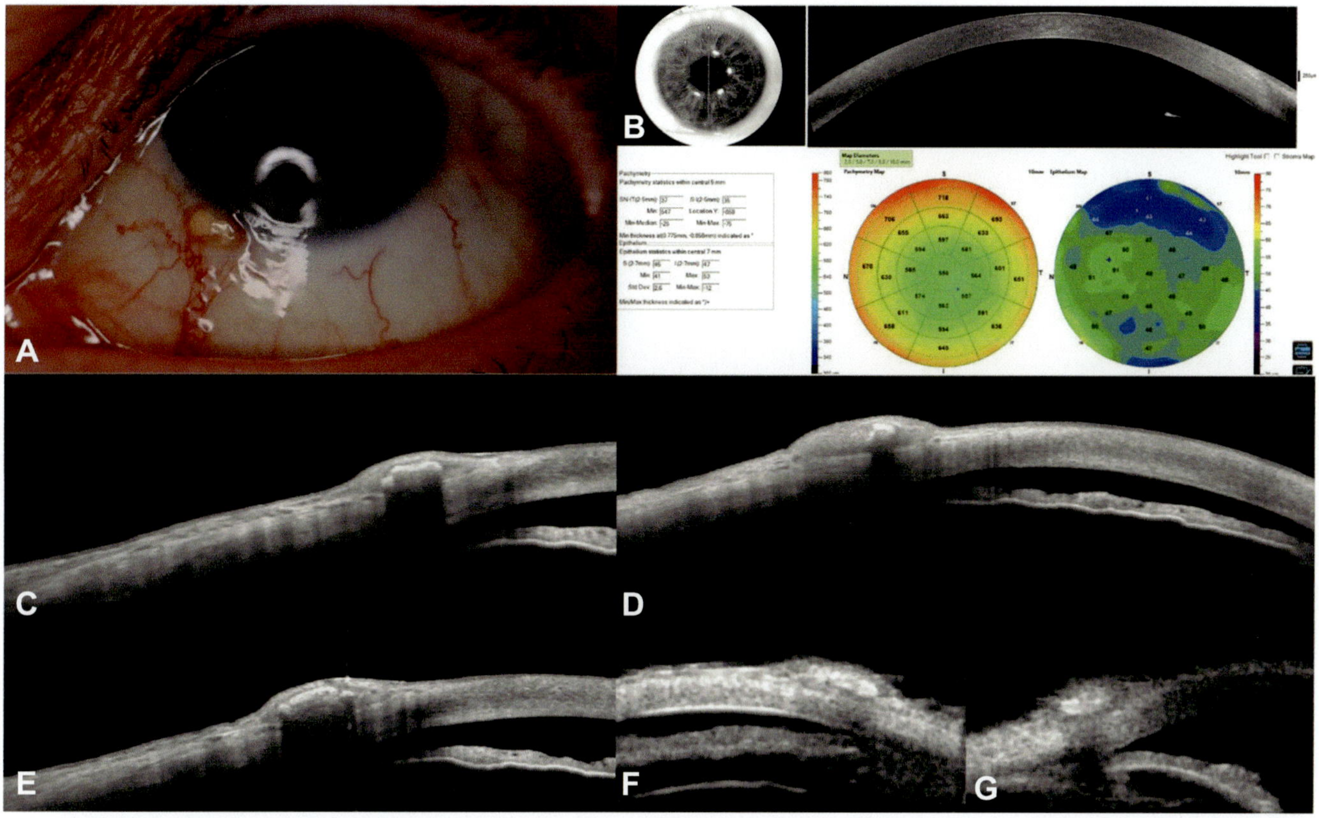

Fig. 17 Pinguecula: Nodular yellowish lesion at 8 o'clock of a left eye. (**A**) Slit-lamp photo. (**B**) Ultra-high-Speed-Full-Range Spectral Domain OCT image with pachymetry and epithelial thickness and absence of induced astigmatism. (**C–E**) AS-OCT images showing a nodular lesion with hyperreflective inclusions and sonic absorption behind it. (**F, G**) UBM showing well-defined, hyperreflective lesion

melanosis (PAM), a nevus, conjunctival dysplasia, or even de novo. It also has been reported, that a limbal stem cell transplantation of a patient with a history of melanoma is not suitable for being a donor for limbal stem cells or sclera [65]. Surgical excision can either be performed by the so-called "no touch" technique with adequate covering e.g. resection combined with a limbectomy and even a lamellar keratoplasty if necessary. Intraoperative cryotherapy is then used as adjuvant therapy (Figs. 29 and 30). A wide or deep extension into the conjunctiva and the orbit can even make an enucleation or exenteration necessary (Fig. 31).

11 Diagnostics

The advantage of corneal and/or conjunctival diseases is, that they are visible. Therefore slit-lamp biomicroscopy is absolutely necessary, especially to outline e.g. the clinical differences and signs of benign vs. malign lesions or the invasion of malignant tumors such as squamous cell carcinoma or melanoma into the cornea which may show a fine gray non-transparency affection of the cornea or tumoral invasion into the anterior chamber [66].

Depending on the lesion, the patient should be asked for any exposure (in private or professionally), any trauma history, tumor history, especially basal cell carcinoma, squamous cell carcinoma, melanoma history, and/or familiar predisposition.

The clinical appearance of neoplasia is variable: the tumor can appear amelanotic, pink, or reddish to melanocytic. Another important sign is the associated angiogenesis not only as a conjunctival injection but also by associated tumor nutrient vessels and especially more prominent feeder vessels as a suggestive sign of malignancy [64]. The local extension can be examined with UBM and anterior segment OCT (AS-OCT).

In general, it should be abstained from taking any biopsy to avoid metastatic spread in the branch canal. If there is a biopsy required, a complete removal in form of total excisional biopsies with epithelectomy is better to be performed [67]. Additional alcoholic debridement and adjuvant cryotherapy are necessary and successful [64]. Regarding the localization, it is difficult to perform an excision with a safety margin. A systemic staging should be performed, as well as periodic examinations and stagings following the guidelines for squamous cell carcinoma and melanoma [68, 69].

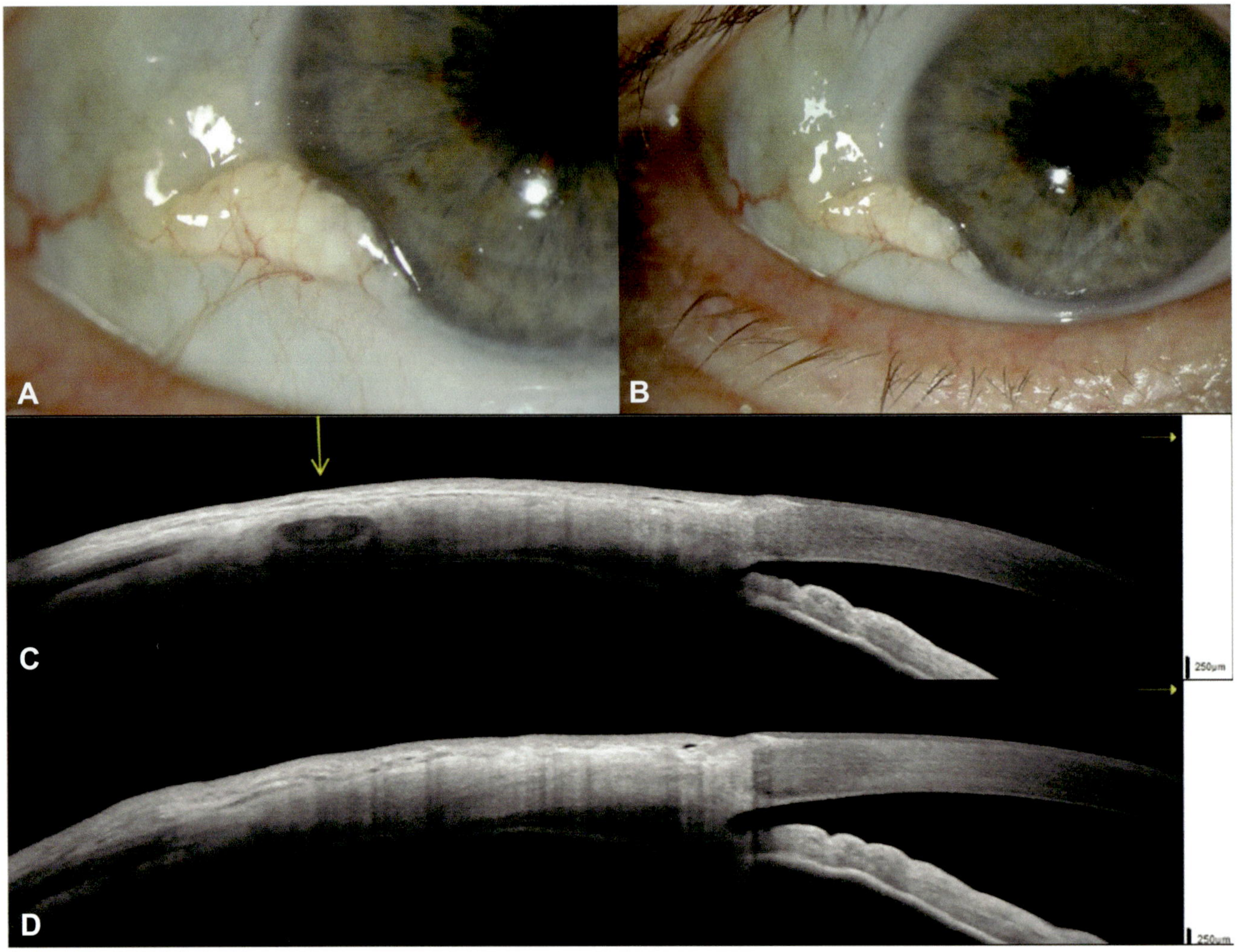

Fig. 18 Serpentiform pinguecula in the right eye at 7–8 o'clock. (**A, B**) Slit-lamp examination presents a white to yellowish prominent, nodular to serpentiform lesion with light nutrient vessels and involvement of the limbus and cornea. (**C, D**) AS-OCT images showing the irregular surface of the lesion with a cystic inclusion

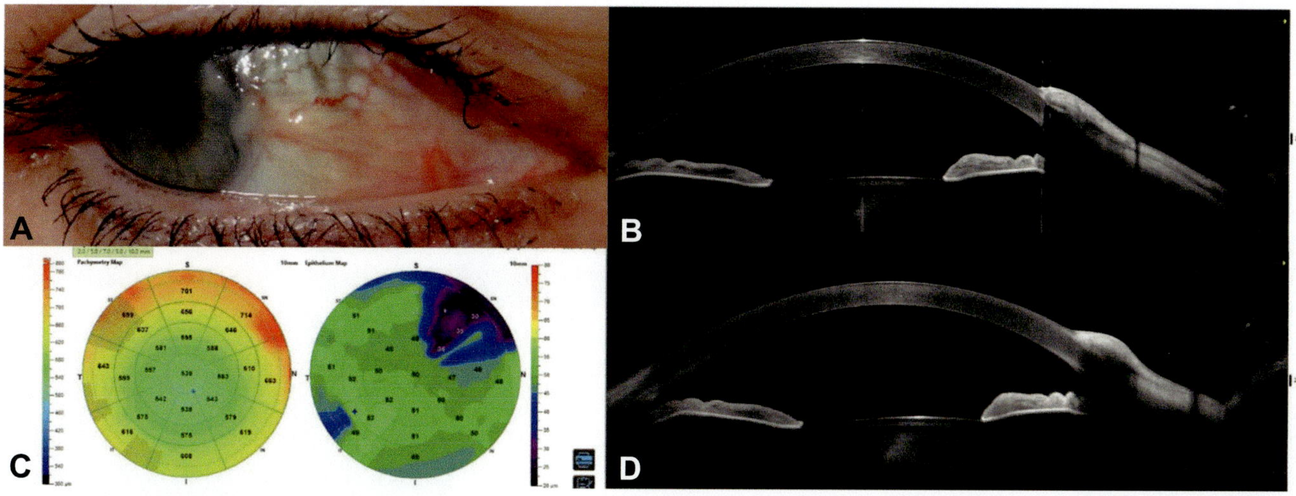

Fig. 19 Combined pinguecula with pterygium shown clinically in (**A**) Slit-lamp biomicroscopy (**B**) and (**D**) AS-OCT with the well-defined lesion at the nasal corneal edge. (**C**) Ultra-high-Speed-Full-Range Spectral Domain OCT imaging showing light changes in pachymetry and epithelial thickness due to the lesion at 2–4 o'clock

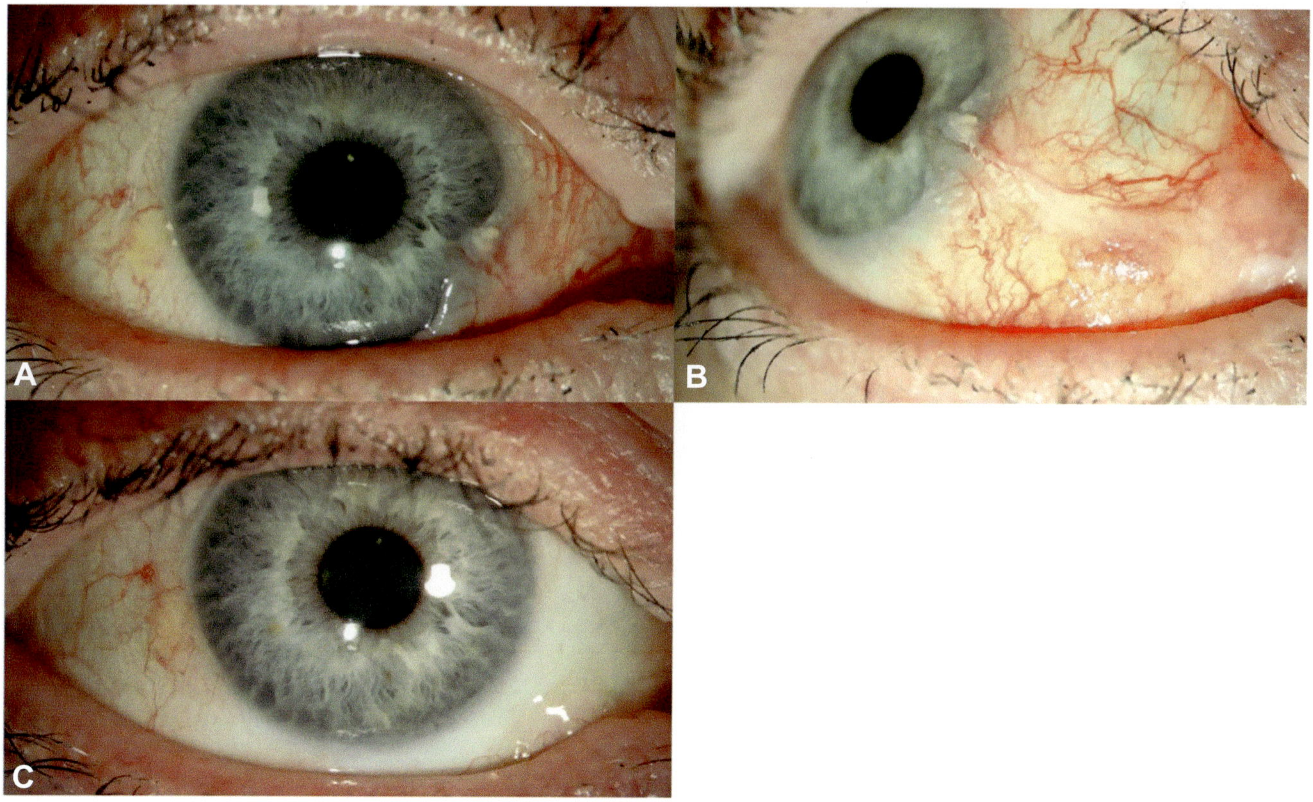

Fig. 20 Temporal and nasal pinguecula with beginning pterygium and corneal involvement nasally. (**A, B**) Preoperative slit-lamp biomicroscopy and (**C**) Four weeks after excisional surgery of the nasal pinguecula with intraoperative application of MMC and conjunctival graft with suture

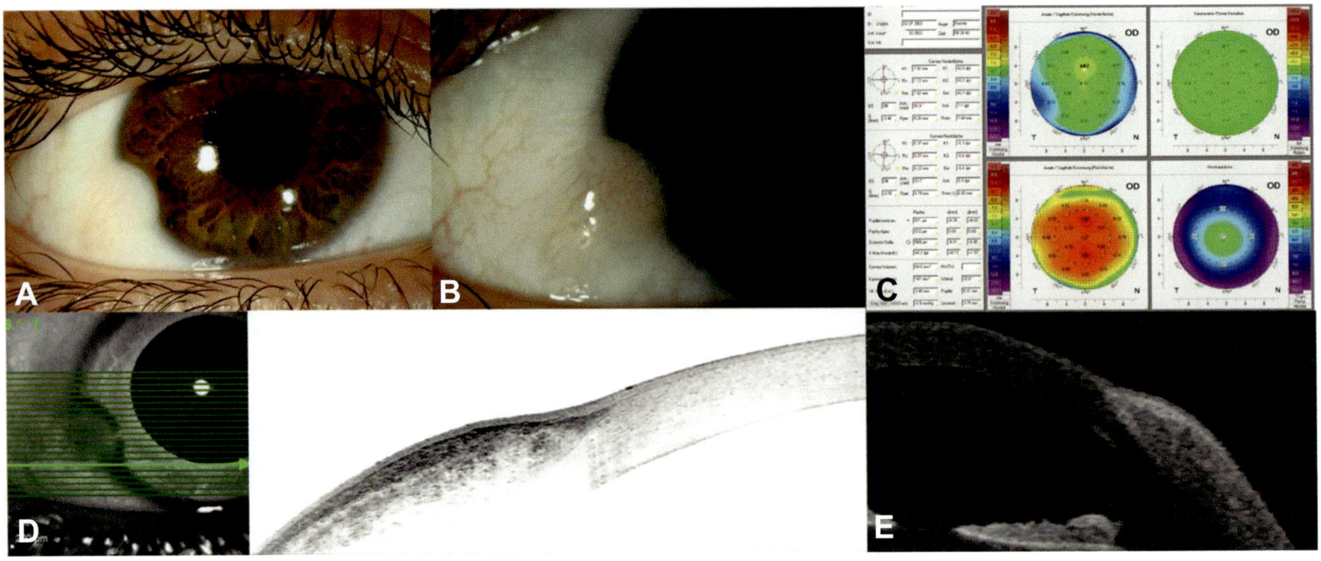

Fig. 21 Limbal dermoid in a right eye at 8 o'clock. (**A, B**) Slit-lamp photography showing a white nodule with light vessels, growing onto the cornea. (**C**) Topography imaging showing corneal part of the dermoid inducing light astigmatism at 8 o'clock. (**D, E**) AS-OCT showing the depth and boundaries of the lesion

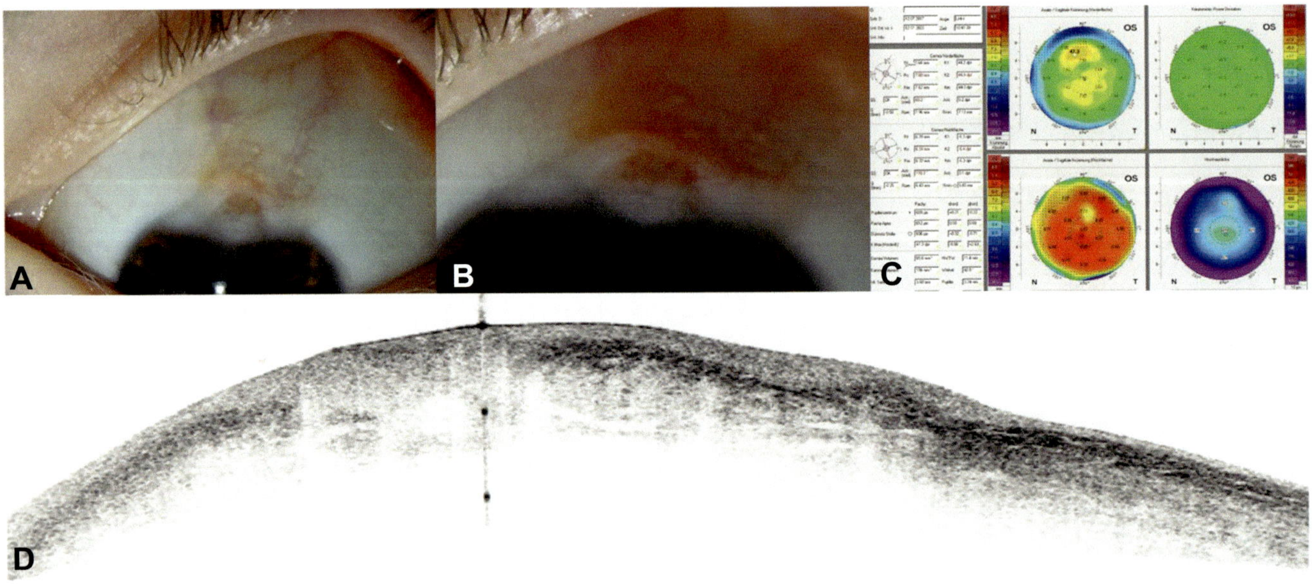

Fig. 22 Limbal dermoid in a left eye at 12 o'clock. (**A, B**) Slit-lamp photography showing a white to pink nodule with light vessels and cysts inside the lesion, growing onto the cornea. (**C**) Topography images showing the corneal part of the dermoid inducing astigmatism at 12 o'clock. (**D**) AS-OCT showing the depth and boundaries of the lesion

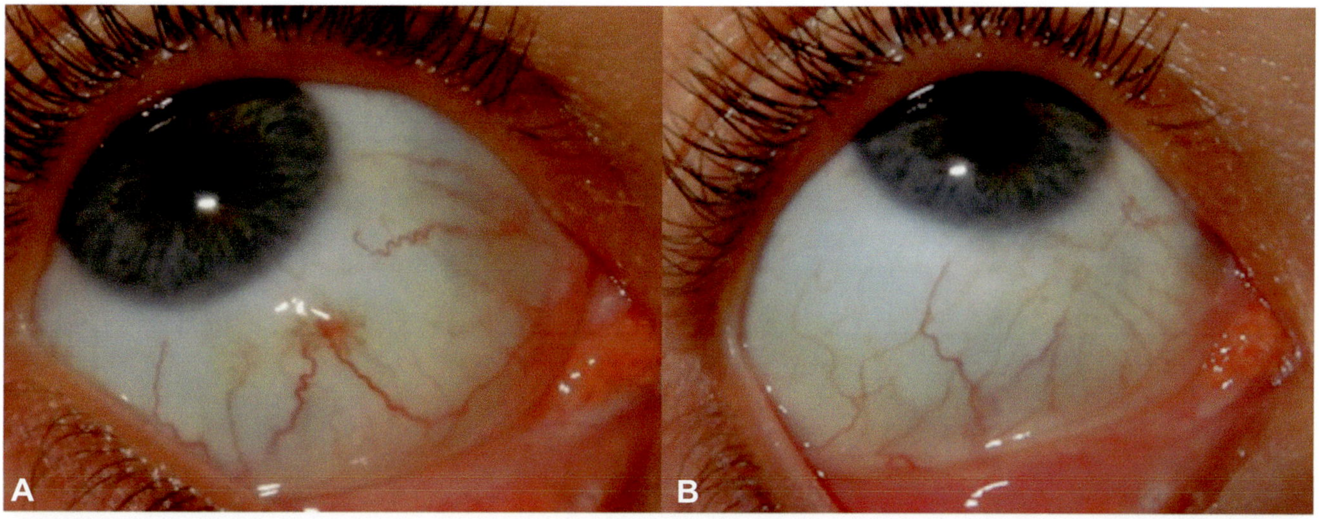

Fig. 23 HPV-associated conjunctival mild dysplasia at the right eye near the limbus. (**A**) Slit-lamp biomicroscopy showing a nodular, yellowish to pink lesion with distinct nutrient vessels and radially ordered small vessel injection in the center of the lesion. (**B**) Slit-lamp biomicroscopy showing the healed lesion eight weeks after excision and one week after two completed cycles of Mitomycin C (MMC) eye drop therapy combined with an intensive ocular lubrication application

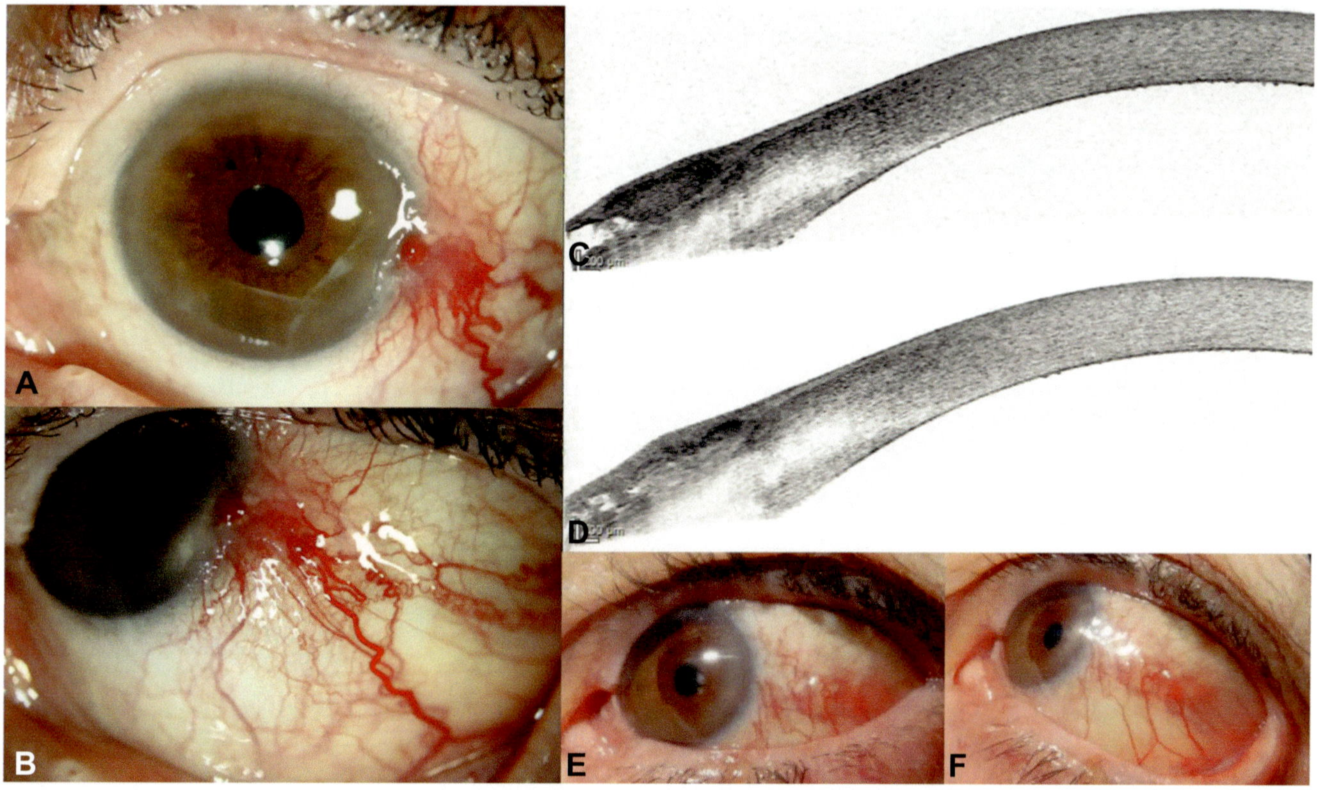

Fig. 24 Squamous cell carcinoma at the left eye's limbus at 3:30 o'clock. (**A, B**) Slit-lamp biomicroscopy showing a reddish prominent nodule with surrounding chemosis and distinct nutrient vessels, as well as one prominent feeder vessel coming from the temporal edge. (**C, D**) AS-OCT. (**E, F**) Slit-lamp biomicroscopy eight weeks after excisional surgery and one week after two completed cycles of Mitomycin C (MMC) eye drop therapy combined with an intensive ocular lubrication application

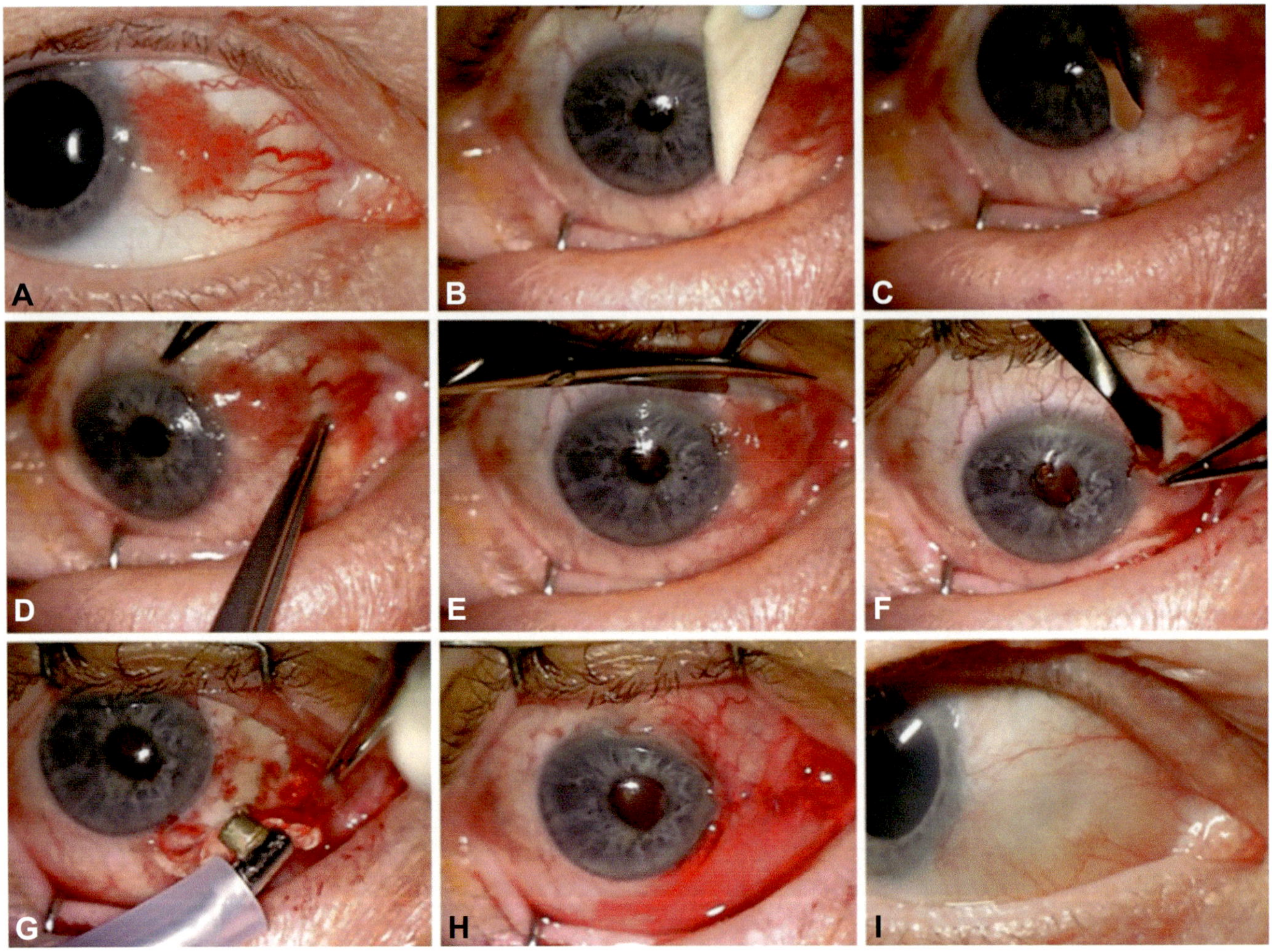

Fig. 25 Surgical excision of a conjunctival squamous cell carcinoma with the "no touch" technique. (**A**) Right eye with a nasal conjunctival squamous cell carcinoma surrounded by prominent feeder vessels. (**B**) Identifying the corneal part of the tumor and drying it using a dry sponge of cellulose. Then absolute alcohol is applicated with a cotton-tipped applicator for 1 min. (**C**) The corneal component of the tumor is removed from the cornea by ablating the epithelium with a #57 Beaver scalpel. The Bowman layer is maintained. (**D**) Identification and cauterization of prominent feeder vessels for minimizing the bleeding. (**E**) Incision of the conjunctiva using a 4-mm-wide surgical margin with blunt-tipped scissors. (**F**) Parallel to the limbus a limbectomy is performed with a sliding movement maintaining a thin scleral base. (**G**) Afterwards, the conjunctiva is lifted and a cryotherapy is performed to the underside of the resected edges. This technique prevents an accidental freezing of the sclera or the ciliary body. (**H**) 7–0 absorbable sutures are used to close the conjunctiva. (**I**) At the six-month follow-up control there is minimal conjunctival scarring without recurrence [61]

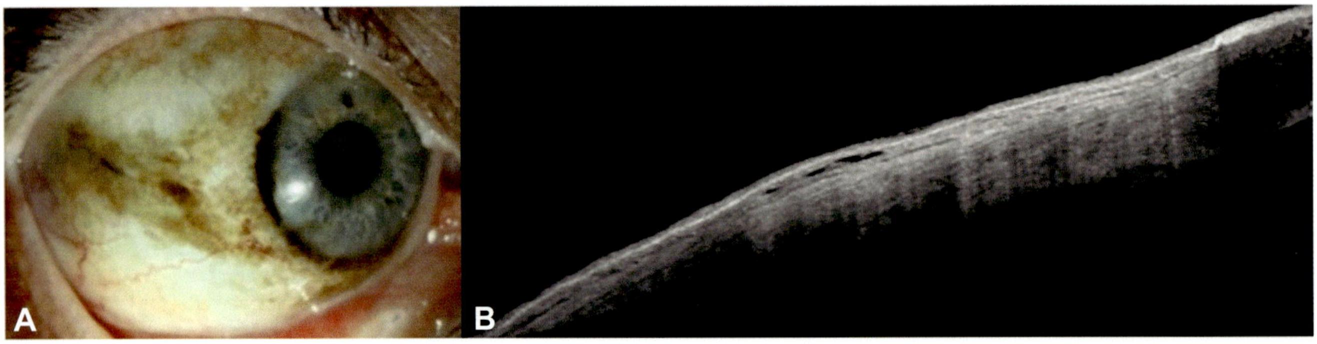

Fig. 26 Unilateral marked findings of an acquired melanosis in a right eye. (**A**) Slit-lamp photography shows a diffuse conjunctival melanosis accumulating in the limbus and corneal periphery mostly from 6–10 o'clock with an additional iris naevus at 12 o'clock. (**B**) AS-OCT image shows hyperreflectivity of the basal epithelial cell layer of the conjunctiva, a small cleavage of the conjunctiva, most likely due to an inflammatory reaction is presented additionally, modified with friendly permission of Prof. Dr. Dr. L. M. Heindl [62]

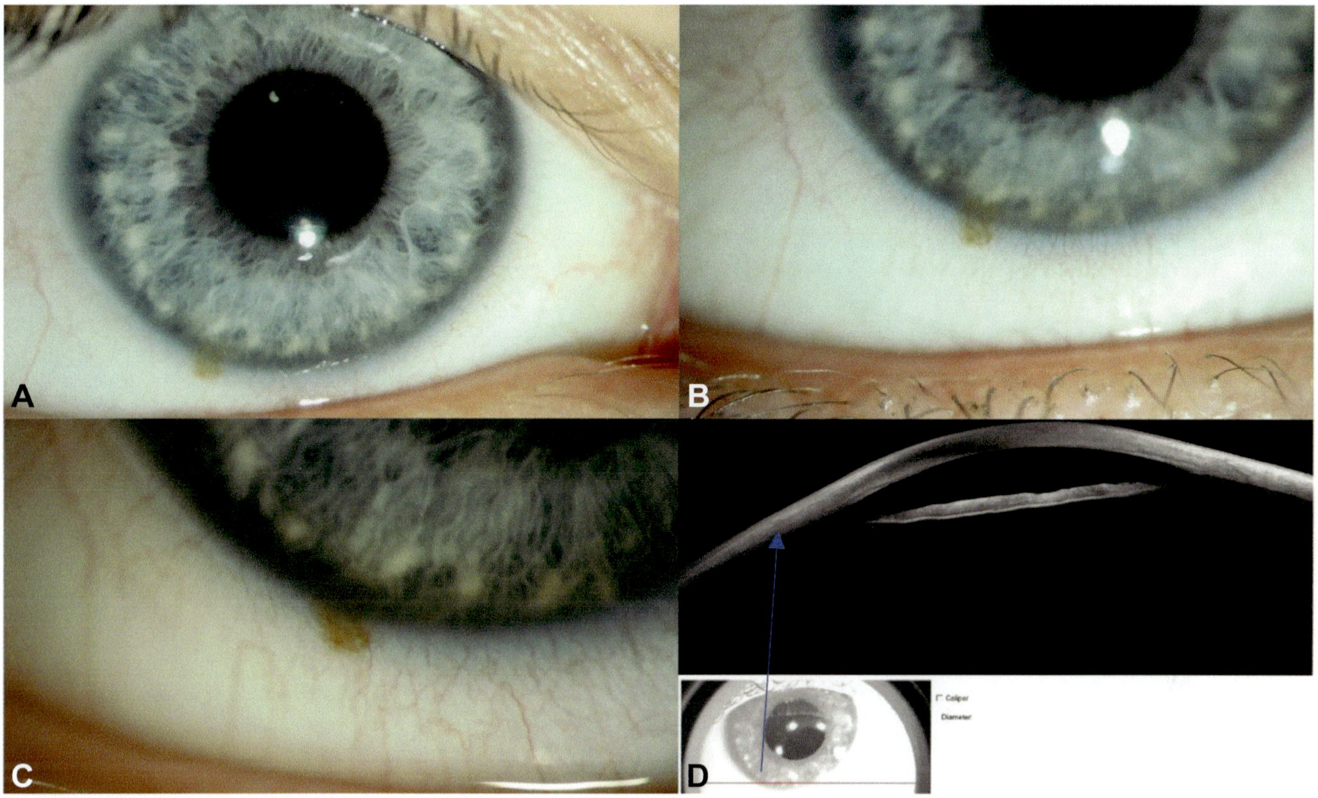

Fig. 27 Small and lightly pigmented nevus in a right eye at the limbus with corneal involvement at 7 o'clock. (**A, B**) Slit-lamp biomicroscopy at the first presentation showing a small nevus with subdued pigmentation and distinct edge sling net. (**C, D**) Slit-lamp photo and AS-OCT at a follow-up examination three years later—still locally limited without infiltration of the surrounding tissue and without significant changes

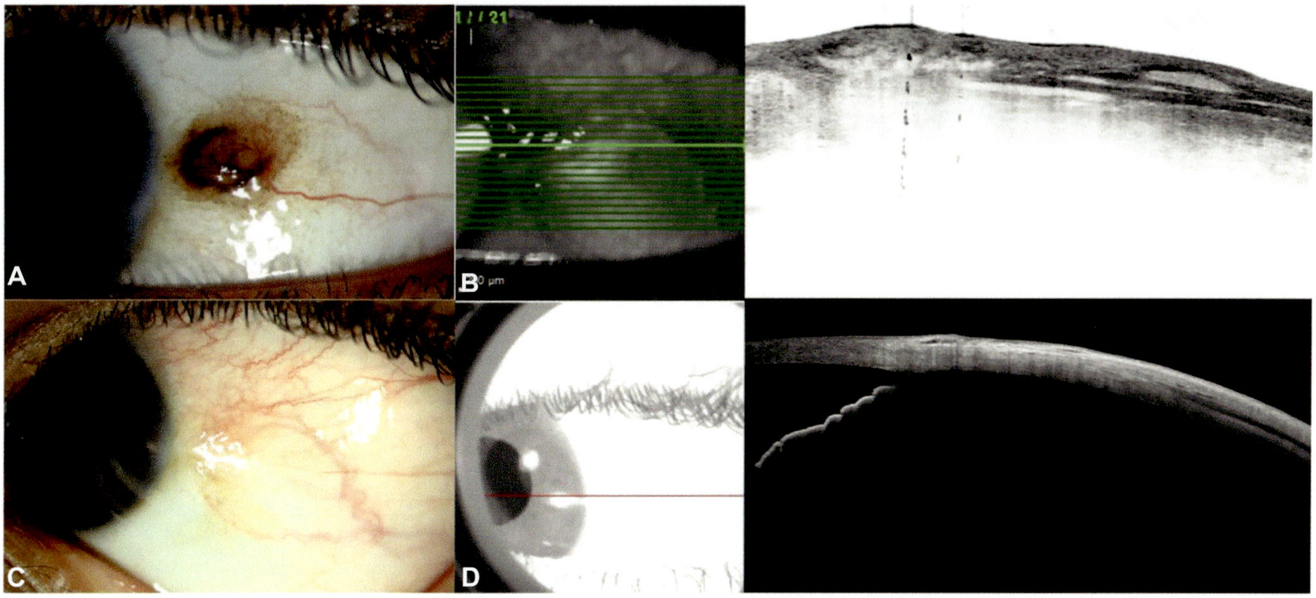

Fig. 28 Prominent nevus at 3 o'clock at the limbus of a left eye. (**A**) Slit-lamp examination shows a round pigmented lesion with a demi-lune higher pigmentation and prominence, a distinct nutrient feeder vessel coming from the temporal edge and cystoid inclusions. (**B**) AS-OCT shows the prominent hyperpigmented lesion with a sonic absorption in the depth and cystoid inclusions as well as associated chemosis. (**C, D**) Postoperative slit-lamp photo and AS-OCT four weeks after surgery with imperceptible residues of the former nevus

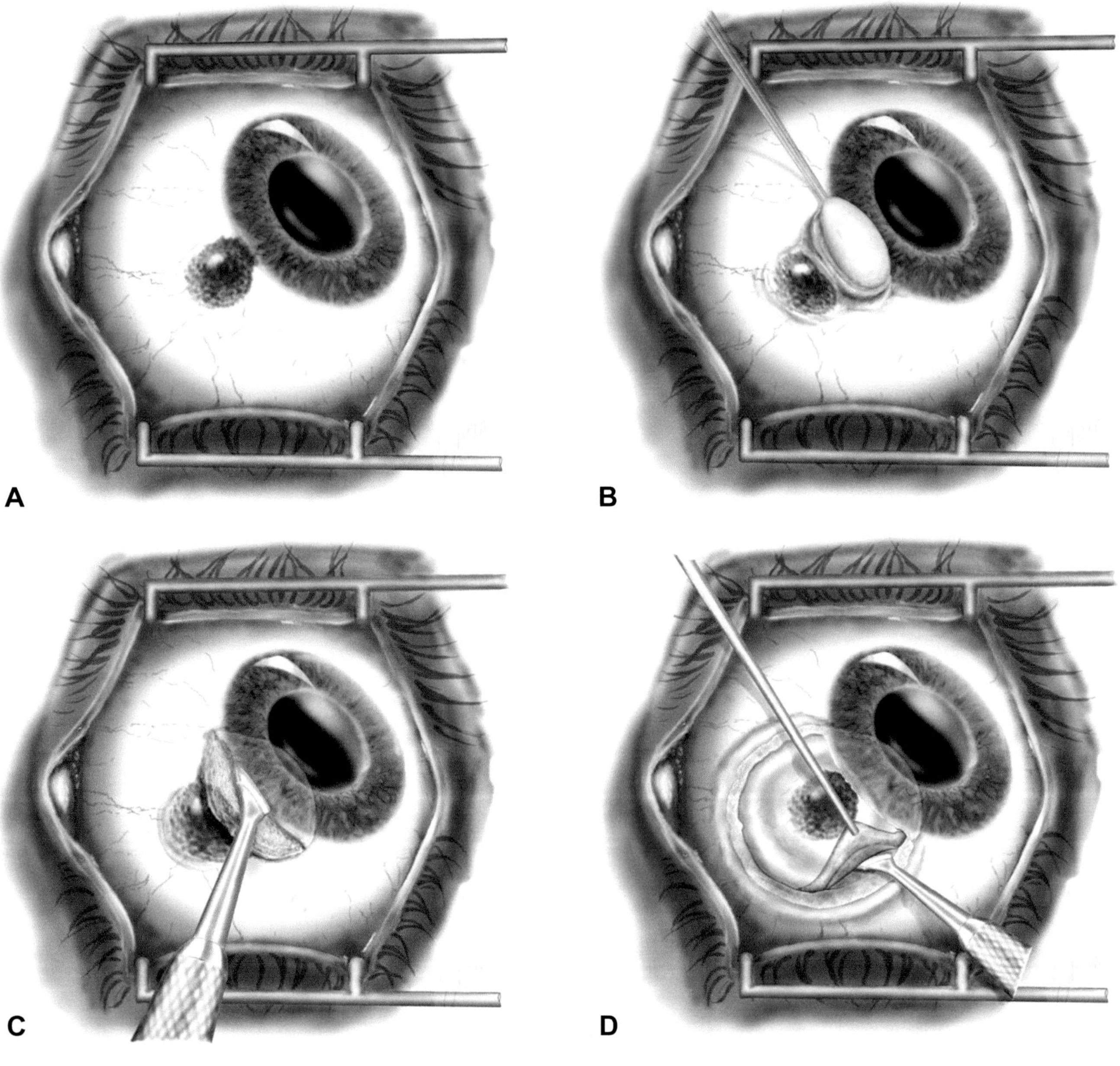

Fig. 29 Surgery with the "no touch" technique of a conjunctival malignancy (e.g. malignant melanoma) with corneal involvement. (**A**) Initial situation in a conjunctival malignancy involving the cornea in a left eye. (**B**) Application of absolute alcohol with a cotton tip applicator to the involved cornea to make the controlled epitheliectomy of the cornea possible. (**C**) Scrolling off the corneal epithelium with a controlled sweeping motion using a beaver blade. (**D**) Approximately 4 mm around the tumor margin the conjunctiva is incised. A thin layer of tumor-free sclera, which lies under the limbal portion of the tumor is excised using a beaver blade © Dr. J. J. Wawer Matos

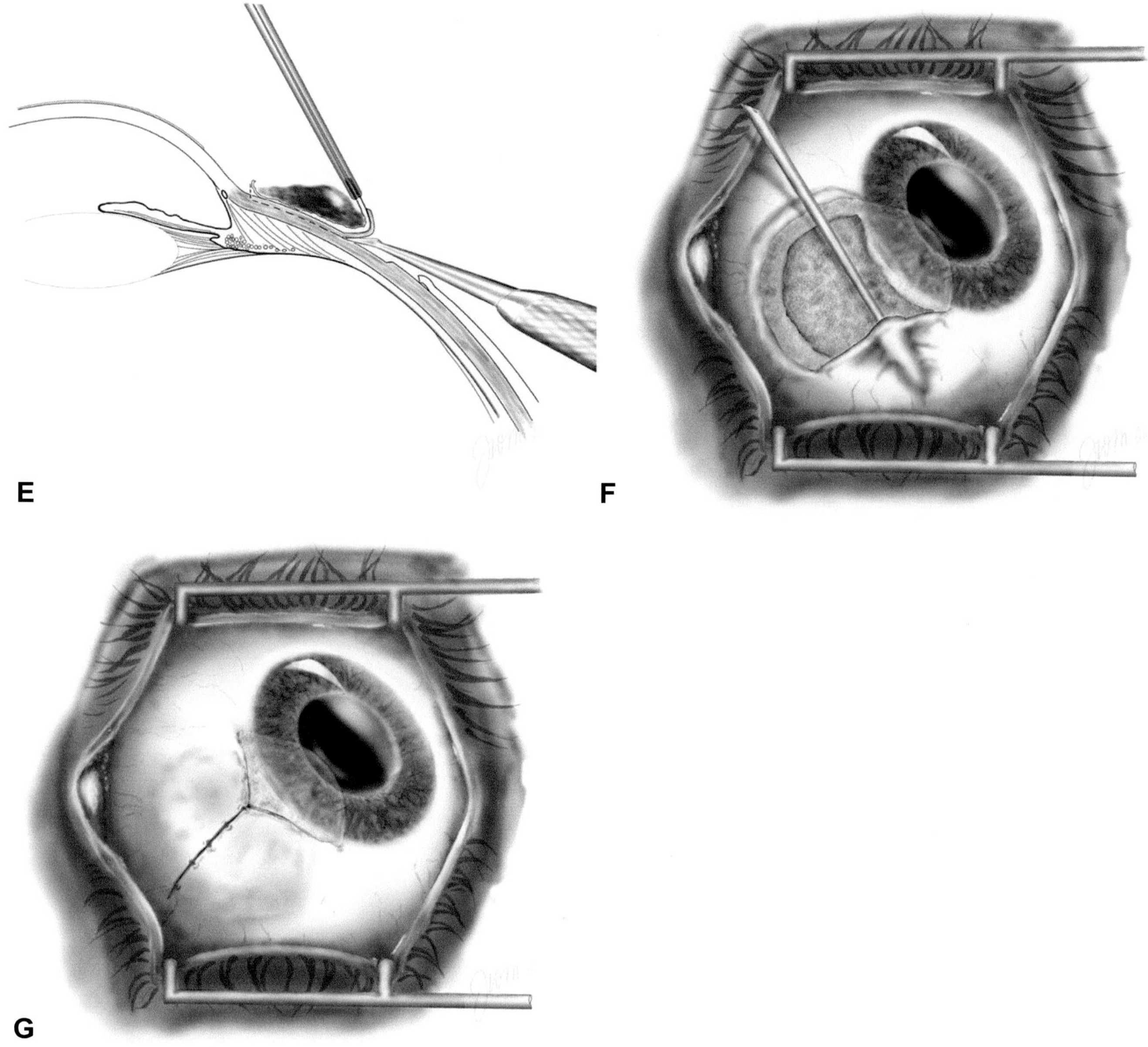

Fig. 29 (**E**) Now the conjunctival malignancy can be removed including the tumor-free margins, the underlying sclera and the limbal corneal epithelium. The excised lesion is fixated on a cardboard and then placed in 10% formalin for histopathological examination. (**F**) Application of cryotherapy to the underside of the conjunctiva, which is surrounding the resection area. (**G**) The conjunctiva is closed with absorbable sutures (e.g. Vicryl 7–0/8–0). Additionally, a soft bondage contact lens can be placed to cover the corneal excision area and reduce pain [66]. © Dr. J. J. Wawer Matos

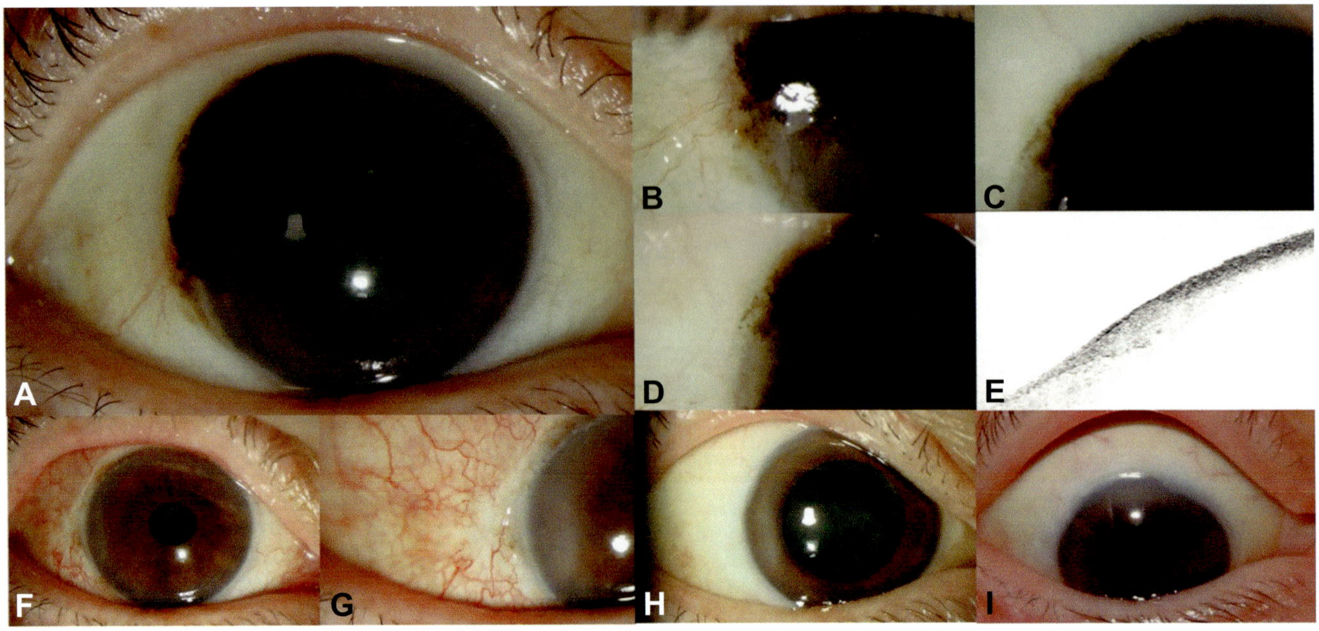

Fig. 30 Conjunctival malignant melanoma with limbal and corneal involvement in a right eye. (**A–D**) Slit-lamp photographs with the highly pigmented lesion growing from the conjunctiva over the limbus onto the cornea with nutrient vessels from the temporal side and opaque to grey corneal halo surrounding the pigmented parts. (**E**) AS-OCT showing the highly pigmented lesion with deep growing through all layers and with sonic absorption behind the lesion. (**F**, **I**) Postoperative slit-lamp photos. (**F**, **G**) Two weeks after excision plus cryotherapy and before starting topical therapy with Mitomycin C (MMC eye drop). (**H**) One week after two completed cycles of MMC therapy and (**I**) six years after surgery and local therapy, no recurrence.

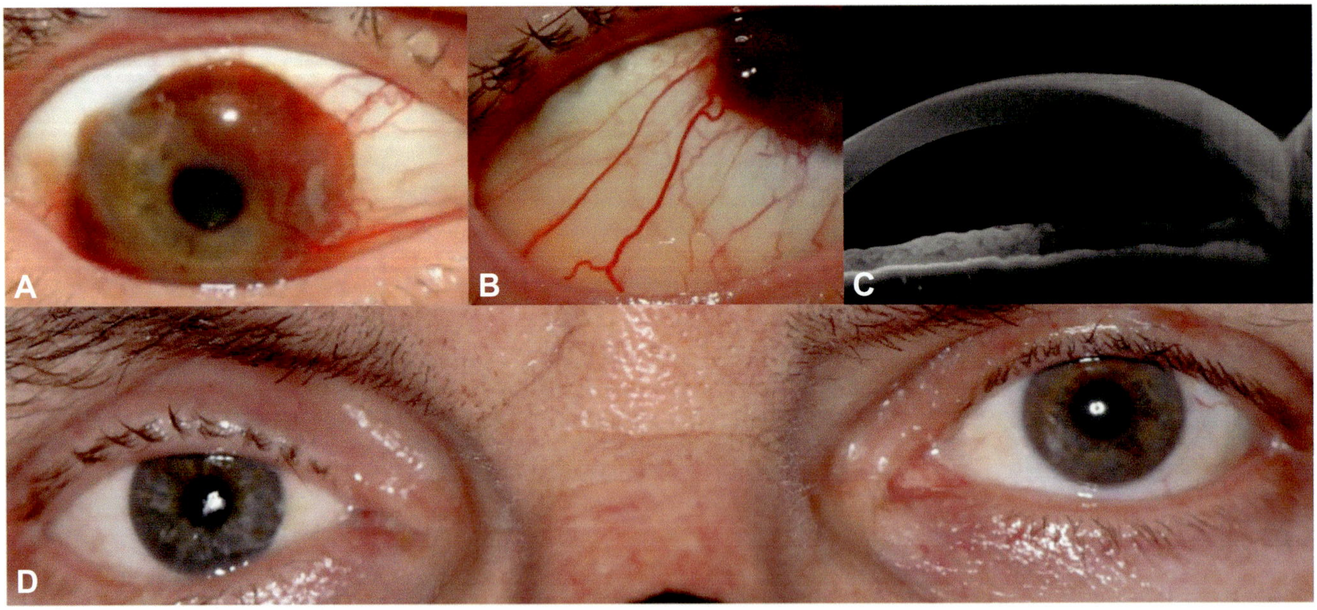

Fig. 31 Conjunctival melanoma arising from PAM, growing over the limbus and onto the cornea in a right eye at first presentation. (**A**, **B**) Slit-lamp photos with the highly pigmented, distinct nutrient vessels/feeder vessels and nodular arising within the lesion, surrounding the tumor there still can be located PAM (e.g. 9 o'clock). (**C**) AS-OCT showing the invasive and highly pigmented lesion with underlying sonic absorption in some parts. (**D**) Postoperative picture after mandatory enucleation due to the tumor's extension and provided with a cryolite glass prosthesis on the right side four weeks after surgery

Table 7 Indications for surgery or topical therapy for tumors at the corneal limbus, cornea, or conjunctiva [61]

Tumor type	Indication for excisional surgery	Indication for other treatments
Pterygium	Failure of local therapy, increasing astigmatism, visual impairment, subjective symptoms, recurrent keratoconjunctivitis, quick and increasing growth	Adjuvant therapy with adjunctive agents to reduce recurrence, but is not mandatory
Pseudopterygium	Astigmatism, visual impairment, subjective symptoms, recurrent keratoconjunctivitis, increasing growth	Watch and wait if there is no ophthalmic impairment
Pinguecula	Therapy-resistant recurrent pingueculitis Cosmetic reasons	Local anti-inflammatory therapy in pingueculitis besides lubricants with e.g. steroids
Limbal dermoid	Increasing astigmatism, visual impairment, subjective symptoms, recurrent keratoconjunctivitis, growth	Watch and wait if there is no ophthalmic impairment
CIN/SCC	Large, but well-circumscribed tumor	Topical chemo- or immunotherapy – Small tumor – Large tumor for chemoreduction or immunoreduction before surgery (neoadjuvant) – Diffuse tumor which is not amenable to get surgery – Positive postoperative margins Plaque radiotherapy – Numerous recurrences – Scleral invasion of the tumor Incisional surgery and possibly necessary enucleation/exenteration – Invasive tumor growth into the orbit
PAM	Lesion's diameter ≥5 mm Documented growth (increasing) thickness Pronounced nodular growth within the lesion (non-/pigmented) Nutrient vessels/prominent feeder vessels to the lesion Involvement of – The cornea – The palpebral conjunctiva Dysplastic nevus syndrome (patient itself or close relatives) Personal history of cutaneous or uveal melanoma	Periodically observation – lesion's diameter <5 mm Lubricants – in associated sicca syndrome
Nevus	Documented growth Atypical localization at – the fornix – the palpebral conjunctiva or – the cornea Atypical age at presentation (≥ middle age) Positive own and/or family history of cutaneous or uveal melanoma Positive own and/or family history of conjunctival melanoma Patient's insistence (cosmesis)	Periodically observation – small and typical nevus
Malignant melanoma	Every case – except absolute medical necessity of enucleation/exenteration	Incisional biopsy/surgery and subsequently possible enucleation/exenteration – deep/large extension, also into the orbit

12 Conclusion

Depending on the anamnesis, the clinical appearance, the extension of the lesion, ancient therapies or operations, the patient's will, and particularly the presumptive diagnosis, every condition requires special treatment. Observation is possible for lesions that do not affect the vision, do not burden the patient, or do not appear malignant. If there is any doubt about benignancy or a suspicious lesion, it is best to be sure about its heritage by excisional biopsy and histopathological examination as a gold standard. Depending on the histopathological result, the use of adjuvant therapy has to be discussed, as well as other diagnostic or therapeutic steps including more extensive surgery e.g. block excision or enucleation. There are different therapeutical and surgical options available and the decision should be taken well-considered, as a shared decision with the patient, and adjusted individually to the patient's situation, clinic/symptoms and medical findings (Table 7).

References

1. Seitz B, Fischer M, Holbach L, Naumann G. Differential diagnosis and prognosis of 112 excised epibulbar epithelial tumors. Klin Monbl Augenheilkd. 1995;207(10):239–46. Verfügbar unter: http://www.thieme-connect.de/DOI/DOI? https://doi.org/10.1055/s-2008-1035375.
2. Seitz B, Gütay A, Küchle M, Kus MM, Langenbucher A. Impact of pterygium size on corneal topography and visual acuity - a prospective clinical cross-sectional study Klin Monbl Augenheilkd. 2001;218(9):609–15. Verfügbar unter: http://www.thieme-connect.de/DOI/DOI? https://doi.org/10.1055/s-2001-17639.
3. Naumann GOH. (Hrsg.). Pathologie des Auges I. 2. Auflage. Berlin, Heidelberg u. a.: Springer-Verlag 1997. S. 443–5.
4. Droutsas K, Sekundo W. Epidemiology of pterygium. a review. Ophthalmologe 2010;107(6):511–2, 514–6.
5. Cameron M. Pterygium throughout the world. Thomas C, Herausgeber. Springfield, Illinois: Thomas; 1965.
6. Coroneo MT. Pterygium as an early indicator of ultraviolet insolation: a hypothesis. Br J Ophthalmol. 1993;77(11):734–9.
7. Chu WK, Choi HL, Bhat AK, Jhanji V. Pterygium: new insights. Eye 2020;34(6):1047–50. Verfügbar unter: https://www.nature.com/articles/s41433-020-0786-3
8. Heindl LM, Cursiefen C. Pterygium. Ophthalmologe 2010;107(6):517–24. Verfügbar unter: http://link.springer.com/, https://doi.org/10.1007/s00347-009-2100-4.
9. Rokohl AC, Heindl LM. Pterygium: new insights into risk factors? Ann Eye Sci. Dezember 2022;7(1):31–31. Verfügbar unter: https://aes.amegroups.com/article/view/6916/html.
10. Rokohl AC, Heindl LM, Cursiefen C. Pterygium: pathogenesis, diagnosis and treatment. Ophthalmologe 2021;118(7):749–63. Verfügbar unter: https://link.springer.com/, https://doi.org/10.1007/s00347-021-01366-9.
11. Notara M, Lentzsch A, Coroneo M, Cursiefen C. The role of limbal epithelial stem cells in regulating corneal (Lymph)angiogenic privilege and the micromilieu of the limbal niche following UV exposure. Stem Cells Int. 2018;2018:8620172.
12. Lin H, Luo L, Ling S, Chen W, Liu Z, Zhong X, u.a. Lymphatic microvessel density as a predictive marker for the recurrence time of pterygium : A three-year follow-up study. Mol Vis. 2013;19(January):166–73.
13. Bradley JC, Yang W, Bradley RH, Reid TW, Schwab IR. The science of pterygia. Br J of Ophthalmol. 2010;94(7):815–20. Verfügbar unter: https://bjo.bmj.com/lookup/doi/, https://doi.org/10.1136/bjo.2008.151852.
14. Chui J, Di GN, Wakefield D, Coroneo MT. The pathogenesis of pterygium: current concepts and their therapeutic implications. Ocul Surf. 2008;6(1):24–43.
15. Hirst LW, Axelsen RA, Schwab I. Pterygium and associated ocular surface squamous neoplasia. Arch Ophthalmol. 2009;127(1):31. Verfügbar unter: http://archopht.jamanetwork.com/article.aspx?, https://doi.org/10.1001/archophthalmol.2008.531.
16. Forbes J, Collin R, Dart J. Split thickness buccal mucous membrane grafts and beta irradiation in the treatment of recurrent pterygium. Br J Ophthalmol. 1998;82(12):1420–3. Verfügbar unter: https://bjo.bmj.com/lookup/doi/, https://doi.org/10.1136/bjo.82.12.1420.
17. Eisenmann K, Zeman F, Helbig H, Gamulescu MA, Barth T. Should mitomycin C be used routinely in pterygium surgery? Ophthalmologe 2020;117(4):367–8. Verfügbar unter: http://link.springer.com/, https://doi.org/10.1007/s00347-019-01009-0.
18. Wolter-Roessler E, Seitz B, Naumann GOH. Pterygoid corneal dystrophy. Klin Monbl Augenheilkd. 2002;219(9):677–81. Verfügbar unter: http://www.thieme-connect.de/DOI/DOI?, https://doi.org/10.1055/s-2002-35166.
19. Hirst LW. The treatment of pterygium. Surv Ophthalmol. 2003;48(2):145–80. Verfügbar unter: https://linkinghub.elsevier.com/retrieve/pii/S0039625702004630.
20. Crewe JM, Threlfall T, Clark A, Sanfilippo PG, Mackey DA. Pterygia are indicators of an increased risk of developing cutaneous melanomas. Br J Ophthalmol. 2018;102(4):496–501. Verfügbar unter: https://bjo.bmj.com/lookup/doi/, https://doi.org/10.1136/bjophthalmol-2017-310686.
21. Sekundo W, Droutsas K, Cursiefen C. Operative techniques for surgical treatment of primary and recurrent pterygia. Ophthalmologe 2010;107(6):525–8. Verfügbar unter: http://link.springer.com/, https://doi.org/10.1007/s00347-009-2099-6.
22. Soriano JM, Janknecht P, Witschel H. Effect of pterygium operation on preoperative astigmatism. Prospective study. Ophthalmologe. 1993;90(6):688–90.
23. Minami K, Tokunaga T, Okamoto K, Miyata K, Oshika T. Influence of pterygium size on corneal higher-order aberration evaluated using anterior-segment optical coherence tomography. BMC Ophthalmol. 2018;18(1):166.
24. Kim SW, Park S, Im CY, Seo KY, Kim EK. Prediction of mean corneal power change after pterygium excision. Cornea. 2014;33(2):148–53.
25. Caccavale A, Romanazzi F, Imparato M, Negri A, Porta A, Ferentini F. Ropivacaine for topical anesthesia in pterygium surgery with fibrin glue for conjunctival autograft. Cornea. 2010;29(4):375–6.
26. Singh G. Pterygium and it's surgery. Smolin and Thoft's The Cornea: Scientific Foundations and Clinical Practice. Philadelphia: Lippincott Williams & Wilkins 2004.
27. Kramer SG, Jaros PA, Deluise VP. Diagnostic and surgical techniques. Surv Ophthalmol. 1988;33(1):41–9.
28. Sheppard J, Mansur A, Comstock T, Hovanesian J. An update on the surgical management of pterygium and the role of loteprednol etabonate ointment. Clin Ophthalmol. 2014;8:1105. Verfügbar unter: http://www.dovepress.com/an-update-on-the-surgical-management-of-pterygium-and-the-role-of-lote-peer-reviewed-article-OPTH.
29. D'Ombrain A. The surgical treatment of pterygium. Br J Ophthalmol. 1948;32(2):65–71.
30. Long T, Li Z. Bare sclera resection followed by mitomycin C and/or autograft limbus conjunctiva in the surgery for pterygium: a Meta-analysis. Int J Ophthalmol. 2015;8(5):1067–73.
31. Aziza Y, Inatomi T, Sotozono C, Kinoshita S. Pterygium excision with modified bare sclera technique combined with mitomycin C. Jpn J Ophthalmol. 2021;65(1):89–96. Verfügbar unter: http://link.springer.com/, https://doi.org/10.1007/s10384-020-00786-5.
32. Prajna NV, Devi L, Seeniraj SK, Keenan JD. Conjunctival autograft versus amniotic membrane transplantation after double pterygium excision: a randomized trial. Cornea. 2016;35(6):823–6.
33. Ratnalingam V, Eu ALK, Ng GL, Taharin R, John E. Fibrin adhesive is better than sutures in pterygium surgery. Cornea. 2010;29(5):485–9.
34. Koranyi G, Seregard S, Kopp ED. Cut and paste: a no suture, small incision approach to pterygium surgery. Br J Ophthalmol. 2004;88(7):911–4.
35. Farid M, Pirnazar JR. Pterygium recurrence after excision with conjunctival autograft: a comparison of fibrin tissue adhesive to absorbable sutures. Cornea. 2009;28(1):43–5.
36. Elwan SAM. Comparison between sutureless and glue free versus sutured limbal conjunctival autograft in primary pterygium surgery. Saudi J Ophthalmol. 2014;28(4):292–8.
37. Xu F, Li M, Yan Y, Lu K, Cui L, Chen Q. A novel technique of sutureless and glueless conjunctival autografting in pterygium surgery by electrocautery pen. Cornea. 2013;32(3):290–5.
38. Hirst LW. Recurrence and complications after 1000 surgeries using pterygium extended removal followed by extended conjunctival transplant. Ophthalmology 2012;119(11):2205–10.

Verfügbar unter: https://linkinghub.elsevier.com/retrieve/pii/S0161642012005520.
39. Ilari L, Daya SM. Long-term outcomes of keratolimbal allograft for the treatment of severe ocular surface disorders. Ophthalmology. 2002;109(7):1278–84.
40. Jap A, Chan C, Lim L, Tan DTH. Conjunctival rotation autograft for pterygium. Ophthalmology. 1999;106(1):67–71.
41. Masters JS, Harris DJJ. Low recurrence rate of pterygium after excision with conjunctival limbal autograft: a retrospective study with long-term follow-up. Cornea. 2015;34(12):1569–72.
42. Jain AK, Bansal R, Sukhija J. Human amniotic membrane transplantation with fibrin glue in management of primary pterygia: a new tuck-in technique. Cornea. 2008;27(1):94–9.
43. Fernandes M, Sangwan VS, Bansal AK, Gangopadhyay N, Sridhar MS, Garg P, u. a. Outcome of pterygium surgery: analysis over 14 years. Eye (Lond) 2005;19(11):1182–90.
44. Tananuvat N, Martin T. The results of amniotic membrane transplantation for primary pterygium compared with conjunctival autograft. Cornea. 2004;23(5):458–63.
45. Clearfield E, Hawkins BS, Kuo IC. Conjunctival autograft versus amniotic membrane transplantation for treatment of pterygium: findings from a Cochrane systematic review. Am J Ophthalmol. 2017;182:8–17.
46. Alsmman AH, Radwan G, Abozaid MA, Mohammed UA, Abd Elhaleim NG. Preoperative subconjunctival combined injection of bevacizumab and mitomycin C before the surgical excision of primary pterygium: clinical and histological results. Clin Ophthalmol. 2017;11:493–501.
47. Kaufman SC, Jacobs DS, Lee WB, Deng SX, Rosenblatt MI, Shtein RM. Options and adjuvants in surgery for pterygium: a report by the American Academy of Ophthalmology. Ophthalmology. 2013;120(1):201–8.
48. Kareem AA, Farhood QK, Alhammami HA. The use of antimetabolites as adjunctive therapy in the surgical treatment of pterygium. Clin Ophthalmol. 2012;6:1849–54.
49. Shenasi A, Mousavi F, Shoa-Ahari S, Rahimi-Ardabili B, Fouladi RF. Subconjunctival bevacizumab immediately after excision of primary pterygium: the first clinical trial. Cornea. 2011;30(11):1219–22.
50. Enkvetchakul O, Thanathanee O, Rangsin R, Lekhanont K, Suwan-Apichon O. A randomized controlled trial of intralesional bevacizumab injection on primary pterygium: preliminary results. Cornea. 2011;30(11):1213–8.
51. Urbinati F, Borroni D, Rodríguez-Calvo-de-Mora M, Sánchez-González JM, García-Lorente M, Zamorano-Martín F, u.a. Pseudopterygium: an algorithm approach based on the current evidence. Diagnostics 2022;12(8):1843. Verfügbar unter: https://www.mdpi.com/2075-4418/12/8/1843.
52. Prabhakar SK. Safety profile and complications of autologous limbal conjunctival transplantation for primary pterygium. Saudi J Ophthalmol. 2014;28(4):262–7. Verfügbar unter: https://www.sciencedirect.com/science/article/pii/S1319453414000356.
53. Eghbali A, Hassan S, Seehra G, FitzGibbon E, Sidransky E. Ophthalmological findings in Gaucher disease. Mol Genet Metab. 2019;127(1):23–7.
54. Song H, Rand GM, Kwon JW. Clinical features of pingueculitis revealed by anterior segment optical coherence tomography findings. Eye Contact Lens Sci Clin Pract. 2019;45(6):394–8. Verfügbar unter: https://journals.lww.com/, https://doi.org/10.1097/ICL.0000000000000574.
55. Rohrbach JM. The pinguecula as a pre-pterygium. Ophthalmologe. 2021;118(11):1161–2. Verfügbar unter: https://link.springer.com/, https://doi.org/10.1007/s00347-021-01500-7.
56. Stergiopoulos P, Link B, Naumann GOH, Seitz B. Solid corneal dermoids and subconjunctival lipodermoids: impact of differentiated surgical therapy on the functional long-term outcome. Cornea 2009;28(6):644–51. Verfügbar unter: https://journals.lww.com/00003226-200907000-00006.
57. Chammout FZ, Souley Y, Ajhoune Y, Reda K, Oubaaz A. Limbal dermoid. J Fr Ophtalmol. 2019;42(2):198–9.
58. Zhong J, Deng Y, Zhang P, Li S, Huang H, Wang B, u.a. New grading system for limbal dermoid: a retrospective analysis of 261 cases over a 10-year period. Cornea 2018;37(1):66–71.
59. Lyall DAM, Srinivasan S, Roberts F. Limbal stem cell failure secondary to advanced conjunctival squamous cell carcinoma: a clinicopathological case report. BMJ Case Rep. 2009;1–7. Verfügbar unter: http://www.ncbi.nlm.nih.gov/pubmed/22121391.
60. Santoni A, Thariat J, Maschi C, Herault J, Baillif S, Lassalle S, u. a. Management of Invasive Squamous Cell Carcinomas of the Conjunctiva. Am J Ophthalmol. 2019;200:1–9. Verfügbar unter: https://linkinghub.elsevier.com/retrieve/pii/S0002939418306718.
61. Rao R, Shields CL. Surgical techniques for conjunctival and corneal tumors. In: Surgical ophthalmic oncology. Cham: Springer International Publishing; 2019. S. 75–83.
62. Rokohl AC, Siebelmann S, Heindl LM. Die optische Kohärenztomografie bei Raumforderungen der Bindehaut und der Augenlider. In: Heindl LM, Siebelmann S, Herausgeber. Optische Kohärenztomographie des vorderen Augenabschnitts. Berlin, Heidelberg: Springer Berlin Heidelberg 2022. S. 43–53. Verfügbar unter: https://link.springer.com/, https://doi.org/10.1007/978-3-662-63273-4_3.
63. Wong JR, Nanji AA, Galor A, Karp CL. Management of conjunctival malignant melanoma: a review and update. Expert Rev Ophthalmol. 2014;9(3):185–204.
64. Yeung A, Uner OE, Wells JR, Grossniklaus HE. Clinical and histopathological features of corneal primary acquired melanosis and melanoma. Ocul Oncol Pathol. 2021;7(2):103–7.
65. Alsara A, Rafi M. Donor-transmitted melanoma after limbal stem cell transplantation. Bd. 7, Avicenna J Med. 2017;75–7.
66. Shields C, Shields J. Tumors of the conjunctiva and cornea. Indian J Ophthalmol. 2019;67(12):1930. Verfügbar unter: https://journals.lww.com/, https://doi.org/10.4103/ijo.IJO_2040_19.
67. Uçakhan-Gündüz Ö, Gündüz K, Karsloğlu MZ, Okçu-Heper A, Kanpolat A. Corneal melanoma: report of three cases. Eye Contact Lens. 2012;38(5):341–4.
68. Leiter U, Heppt MV, Steeb T, Alter M, Amaral T, Bauer A, et al. S3 guideline "actinic keratosis and cutaneous squamous cell carcinoma" - update 2023, part 2: epidemiology and etiology, diagnostics, surgical and systemic treatment of cutaneous squamous cell carcinoma (cSCC), surveillance and prevention]. J Dtsch Dermatol Ges. 2023;21(11):1422–1434.
69. S3 - Leitlinie zur Diagnostik, Therapie und Nachsorge des Melanoms. J Dtsch Dermatol Ges. 2020;18(10).

Surgical Treatment Options of Limbal Stem Cell Deficiency: From Conjunctival Limbal Autografting CLAU to Simple Limbal Epithelial Transplantation SLET

Elias Flockerzi and Berthold Seitz

Abstract

A sufficient limbal stem cell pool is paramount for maintaining a constant renewal of the corneal epithelium. Partial or total limbal stem cell deficiency can be congenital or acquired and leads to overgrowing of the conjunctiva onto the human cornea. Several techniques have been developed in recent years to treat limbal stem cell deficiency and this chapter aims to provide an overview over the existing treatment options.

1 Introduction

The maintenance of an intact epithelium of the human cornea is based upon an intact corneal epithelial stem cell reservoir which has been identified within a protected microenvironment at the limbal Vogt palisades [1]. Congenital or acquired defects affecting this stem cell niche may lead to a limbal stem cell deficiency (LSCD). A total, or 360° circular LSCD has been defined clinically as a combination of (1) the absence of the limbal Vogt palisades, (2) a dull and irregular corneal epithelium, (3) superficial corneal vascularization, (4) persistent defects of the corneal epithelium and (5) conjunctival overgrowth on the corneal surface [2]. The consequence of a complete loss of the corneal-limbal epithelium is the re-epithelialization of the cornea by bulbar conjunctival cells [3]. Histopathologically, impression cytology is the most definitive diagnostic tool to clearly demonstrate and confirm the diagnosis of LSCD by showing conjunctival epithelial and goblet cells invading the corneal surface [4]. A typical example for congenital LCSD is congenital aniridia whereas the most common causes leading to acquired LCSD include alkali burns, autoimmune mucous membrane diseases (e.g. Stevens–Johnson Syndrome), infections (trachoma) or contact lens wear [5]. Different therapeutic approaches have been developed in recent years with the aim to restore the limbal stem cell niche—be it based on autografts from the healthy partner eye or based on allogeneic explants, e.g. from corneal donor buttons.

E. Flockerzi (✉) · B. Seitz
Department of Ophthalmology, Saarland University Medical Center, Homburg, Germany
e-mail: elias.flockerzi@uks.eu

2 Conjunctival Limbal Autografting ("CLAU")

The origins of conjunctival limbal autografting date back to 1977, when Thoft transplanted four conjunctival grafts of 5 mm in diameter from the uninjured eye to the injured partner eye after chemical burn in five cases [6]. The grafts were taken from each of the four quadrants in areas normally covered by the eyelids and anchored at the limbus of the injured partner eye [6]. This technique was later modified by Kenyon and Tseng who aimed for transplanting conjunctiva including limbal epithelium [7]. They proposed sectoral grafts of limbal tissue taken from a healthy partner eye superiorly and inferiorly over about four clock-hours, that extended about 0.5 mm into the clear cornea and about 2mm into the bulbar conjunctiva [7]. After peritomy and pannectomy, the grafts were fixated on the recipient eye and protected by a bandage contact lens or a tarsorrhaphy, which led to epithelial outgrowth resurfacing the entire cornea within seven to 21 days in 21 of 26 cases [7]. The authors also observed a regression of preexisting neovascularization and the arrest of further neovascularization formation and concluded by formulating the universal aim of each corneal limbal stem cell transplantation approach, that should consist of sharing the limbal cell population between the healthy donor and the injured recipient without long-term problems for either [7]. Even though the authors did not describe this, this procedure implies the risk of developing iatrogenic LSCD because of

B. Seitz et al. (eds.), *Atlas on Cornea*, https://doi.org/10.1007/978-3-031-65422-0_57

the comparatively large grafts explanted from the formerly healthy donor eye [8]. However, it has to be distinguished between a purely transplantation of conjunctiva and a transplantation of limbal stem cells using conjunctiva or cornea as a carrier tissue [9]. Modifications of CLAU are the so-called living-related conjunctival limbal allograft (lr-CLAL) that includes harvesting conjunctival grafts carrying limbal stem cells from living-related donors based on the hypothesis that patients with identical or haplo-identical human-leukocyte-antigen matching are less likely to undergo epithelial rejection as opposed to the cadaveric conjunctival limbal allograft (c-CLAL) designating conjunctival grafts carrying limbal stem cells obtained from corneal donors [9, 10]. The aim of all these procedures was to minimize the graft size and thus the damage to the healthy partner eye ("as small as possible, but as large as necessary"). One CLAU study reported the successful reconstruction in total LSCD by using only one 60° (two clock-hours) conjunctival limbal graft together with two amniotic membranes: one as a permanent graft underneath and one as a temporary patch covering it [11].

3 Cultivated Limbal Epithelial Transplantation ("CLET")

The principle of Cultivated Limbal Epithelial Transplantation (CLET), as first published by Pellegrini et al. in 1997, has been based on an even smaller tissue sample taken from the healthy partner eye: Less than one clock-hour of donor limbus was excised (1 mm^2), cultivated, prepared as grafts containing 2×10^6 cells each 16 to 19 days after biopsy, mounted on a petrolatum gauze or the inner side of a soft contact lens and placed upon the recipient eye after peritomy and pannectomy [3]. The recipient eye was patched for three days and the contact lens was removed two weeks later [3]. This procedure enabled minimizing the risk of iatrogenic injury to the healthy eye by harvesting a smaller amount of tissue and became the first stem cell-based therapy to receive approval for application throughout the European Union under the trade name "Holoclar®" [5] (Figs. 1, 2, 3 and 4). A meta-analysis reported a successful re-epithelialization in 72% (n = 720) of cases and improved visual acuity in 63% (n = 539) of cases after the application of standard CLET technique

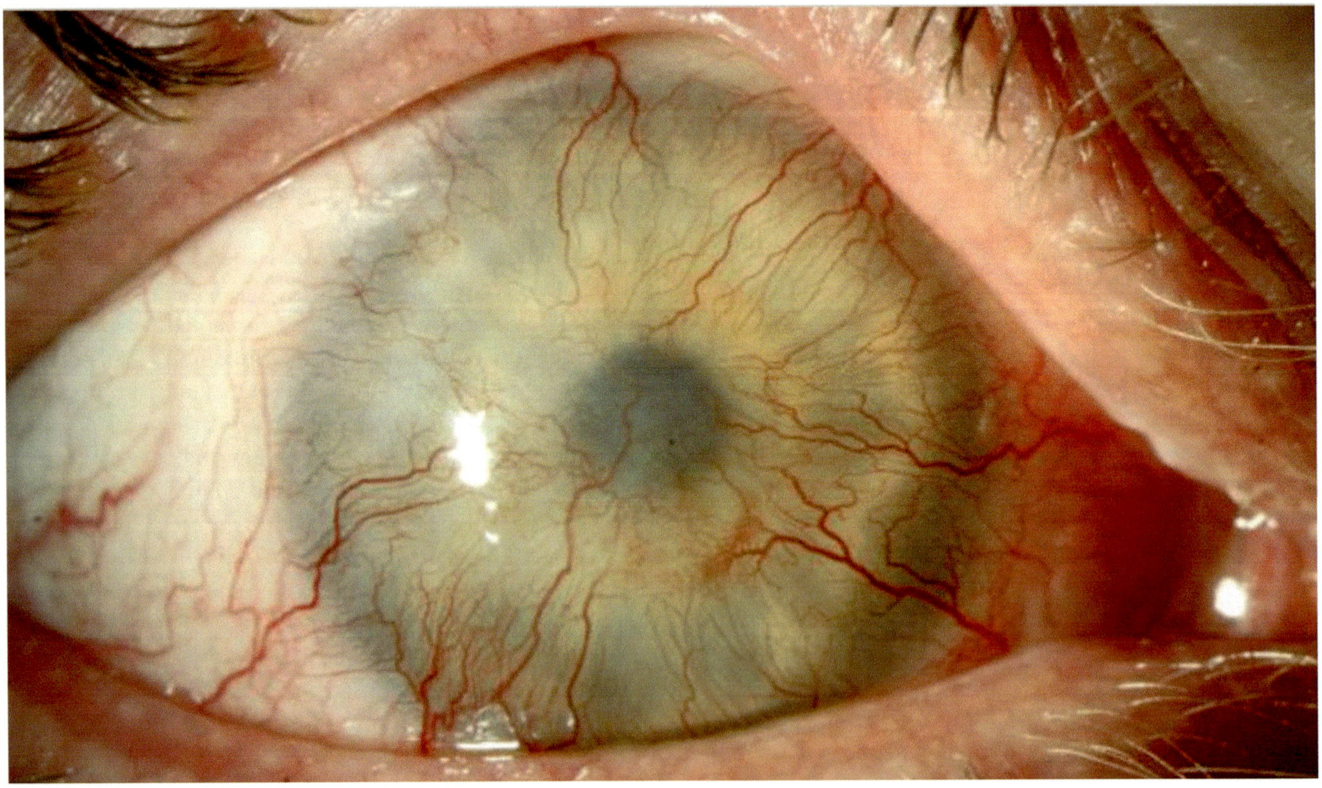

Fig. 1 Right eye of a 52-year-old male phakic patient after alkali burn seven years before

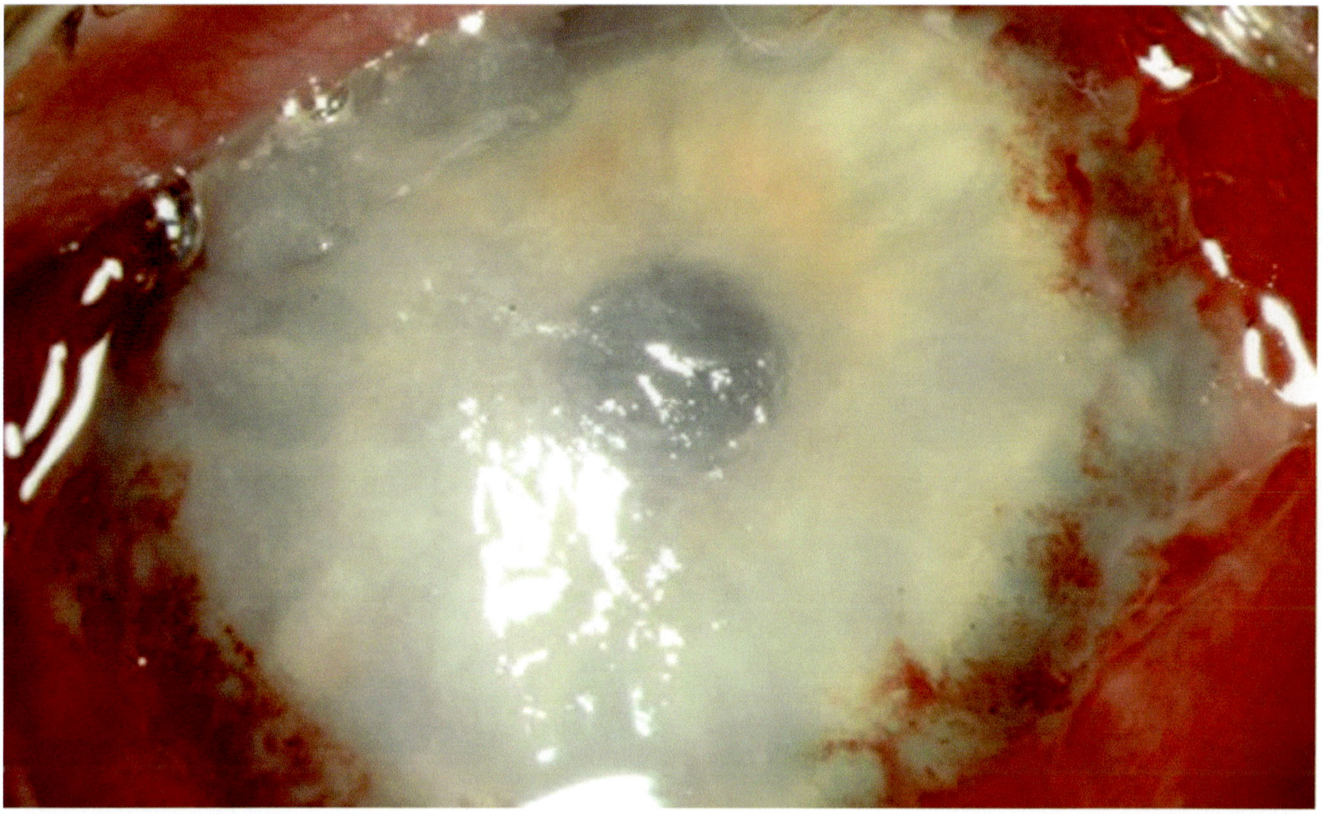

Fig. 2 Same eye one week after peritomy, pannectomy and Holoclar® implantation

[12]. However, the need for ex vivo expansion of stem cells in CLET was at the same time a limitation putting the procedure out of reach of most cornea-blind individuals living in the developing world [1] and making it accessible to only a few centers around the world [13].

4 Simple Limbal Epithelial Transplantation ("SLET")

This obstacle was overcome by the introduction of an equally minimally invasive approach by Sangwan in 2012, which has been called Simple Limbal Epithelial Transplantation ("SLET") [2]. SLET has been proposed as treatment option mainly for unilateral ocular burns (Fig. 5) and—with restrictions—for ocular surface squamous neoplasia or recurrent pterygia and the health of the donor limbus has been reported to be the main factor determining the outcome after undergoing SLET [8]. Anterior segment optical coherence tomography may be helpful to estimate in which depth a clear corneal stroma can be found (Fig. 6). The initial describers marked a 2×2 mm area on the superior limbus, opened the conjunctiva and conducted a shallow dissection towards and 1 mm into the clear cornea [2] (Figs. 7, 8, 9 and 10). After peritomy and pannectomy (Figs. 11, 12 and 13), possibly in multiple layers (Figs. 14, 15 and 16), an amniotic membrane graft was placed upon the recipient (Figs. 17 and 18) and secured with fibrin glue [2]. The donor tissue was thereafter cut into eight to ten small pieces that were arranged in a circular pattern around the center of the cornea, fixed also with fibrin glue (Figs. 19, 20, 21 and 22) and covered by a bandage contact lens [2]. It has been reported that the superior limbus should be preferred as explantation site because there is a larger number of Vogt palisades in this region [8]. Contraindications for SLET include (1) dry ocular surface (Schirmer II < 10 mm or visible keratinization), (2) an eye without visual potential, (3) a disorganized anterior segment (leukoma, symblephara, staphyloma anterius), (4) uncorrected adnexal pathologies (lagophthalmos, entropion, ectropion) [8] or (5) bilateral autoimmune mucous membrane diseases like Stevens–Johnson syndrome or ocular pemphigoid [5]. Whereas Sangwan et al. reported a confluent and stratified corneal epithelial layer by six weeks and an incorporation of the stromal element of the graft within the underlying cornea by six months [2], other studies reported that the epithelialization after SLET started from the limbal transplants over the amniotic membrane on the second postoperative day and completed over the whole cornea within two weeks [5, 14]. The success of SLET is defined as

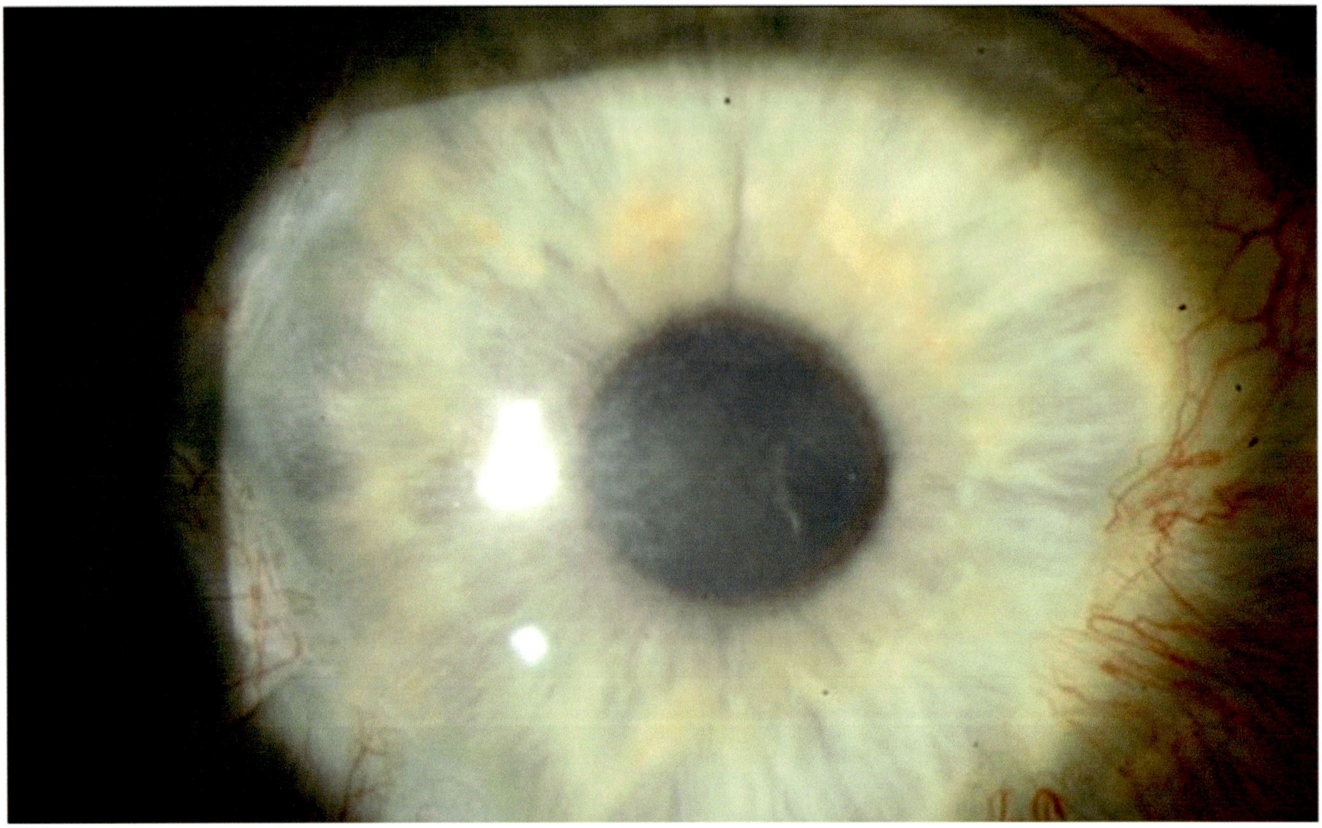

Fig. 3 Same eye six months after peritomy, pannectomy and Holoclar® implantation

complete epithelial healing and decrease of neovascularization. One recent multicenter study reported a success rate of 83% in 68 eyes of 68 patients after a median follow-up of 12 months [15]. Four major SLET reports [1, 13, 15, 16] described the results of 253 cases of unilateral LSCD that underwent SLET and found a treatment success in 78% (197/253) after a mean follow-up of 1.5 years. SLET has also been reported to have a much better success rate than CLET in children (71% versus 37%) [1]. Most failures have been reported to occur within the first six months [2, 8] and the main predictor for failure were the presence of preoperative symblephara and the combination of SLET and penetrating keratoplasty [1, 8, 16].

SLET has also been described as a salvage therapy option after failed CLET and subsequently achieved similar results as in eyes not pretreated with CLET [16]. In recent years, allogeneic SLET grafts have also been used for the treatment of patients with bilateral LSCD. One first study harvested limbal tissue from corneal donor buttons, cut it into small pieces and fixed it with fibrin glue onto an amniotic membrane that was fixed as a graft on the recipient's eye [17]. This was performed in 18 eyes of 17 patients out of which ten patients were children: It took a mean of 22.5 days until epithelialization and none of the eyes developed signs of allorejection, although systemic immunosuppression was deliberately avoided [17]. Chimerism analysis proved that both donor and recipient cells were responsible for epithelialization and the authors concluded that any form of epithelial cover to the cornea would be preferable to no cover at all [17] because, obviously, even allogeneic explants have an anti-inflammatory effect on the ocular surface [5].

One further comparative study investigated living-related SLET (n = 16 eyes of 16 patients) versus cadaveric allogeneic SLET (n = 14 eyes of 13 patients) and one year later, there was a significant improvement in both groups considering corneal conjunctivalization, vascularization and opacification [8]. In view of the five-year survival analysis, there was a slight advantage of living-related (90 ± 4%) over cadaveric allogeneic SLET (82 ± 7%). Besides topical steroids that should be continued once or twice without tapering off, all the patients received systemic pulse intravenous immunosuppression starting with 500 mg intravenous methylprednisolone on the day of surgery, after one week,

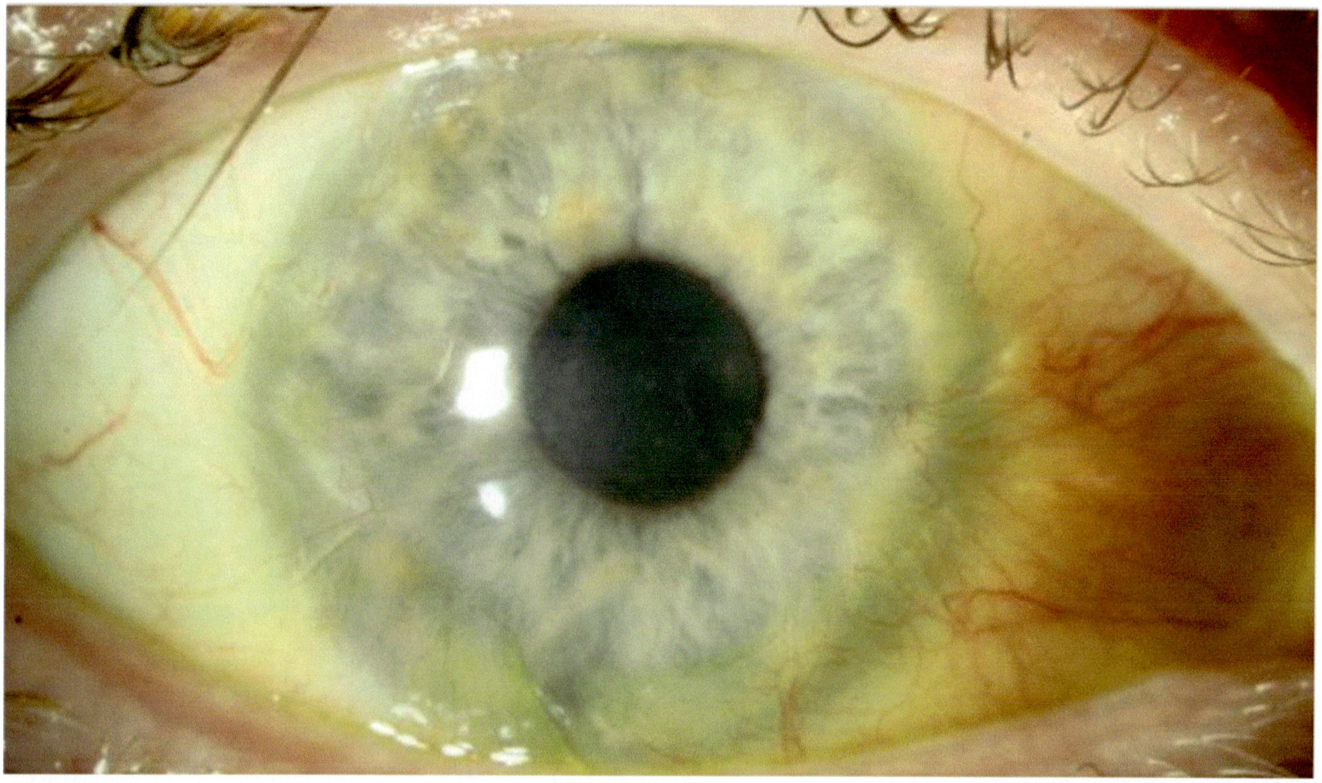

Fig. 4 Same eye one year after peritomy, pannectomy and Holoclar® implantation. Best spectacle-corrected distance visual acuity increased from 20/400 preoperatively to 20/40 one year later. Topical therapy consists of topical Dexamethasone and Cyclosporine 0.1% eyedrops once daily and lubrication

than every six weeks for the first six months, every two months from month seven to 12, every three months from month 13 to 24 and every six months from month 24 on [8].

One recent study used mycophenolate mofetil as systemic immunosuppression (1-2 g/d) and compared the results of seven allogeneic SLET procedures with seven allogeneic SLET and simultaneous penetrating keratoplasty procedures [18]. Ten of 14 eyes showed a completely healed epithelium after 12 months and the authors concluded that neither the age of the corneal donor, the death-to-harvest time nor the time of culture of the corneal donor button had a major impact on the epithelialization of the corneal surface [18].

All the studies mentioned above have in common the use of fibrin glue and amniotic membranes as grafts that carry the precious limbal stem cell grafts. On the one hand, in vitro studies revealed that fibrin glue inhibits cell migration, which might prevent the ingrowth of conjunctival tissue in the early postoperative SLET period and facilitate the expansion of epithelial cells from the limbal stem cell explants [5]. On the other, the amniotic membrane provides a thick basement membrane and an avascular stroma [4] containing anti-inflammatory cytokines, growth factors and thus plays a major role in controlling inflammation in the early postoperative SLET period [5]. Not least in view of the positive effects of amniotic membranes on corneal wound healing, the authors recommend—deliberately deviating from the original publication—an additional layer of amniotic membrane after fibrin glue fixation of the limbal stem cell grafts onto the amniotic membrane graft, that covers both the amniotic and the limbal stem cell grafts as a protective patch for four to six weeks (Figs. 23, 24 and 25). A temporary lateral tarsorrhaphy can be made to protect the surface of the eye and to ensure sufficient eyelid closure (Fig. 26). Simple limbal epithelial transplantation can achieve promising results with epithelialized corneas and a good recovery of visual acuity (Figs. 27 and 28). It has been recommended to wait at least two months after SLET before performing penetrating keratoplasty [13], if necessary.

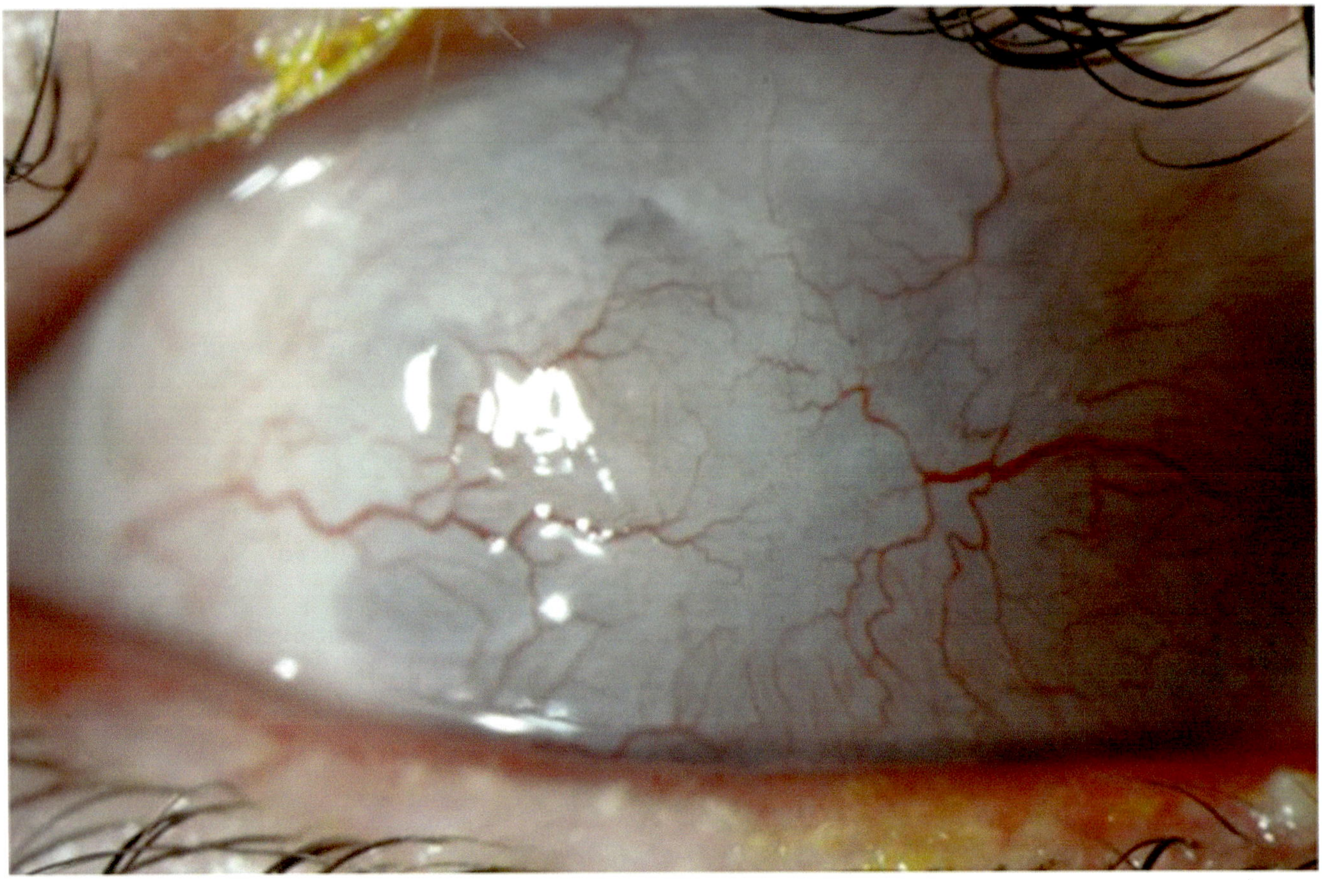

Fig. 5 Right eye of a 12-year-old male phakic patient one year after firework-associated burn

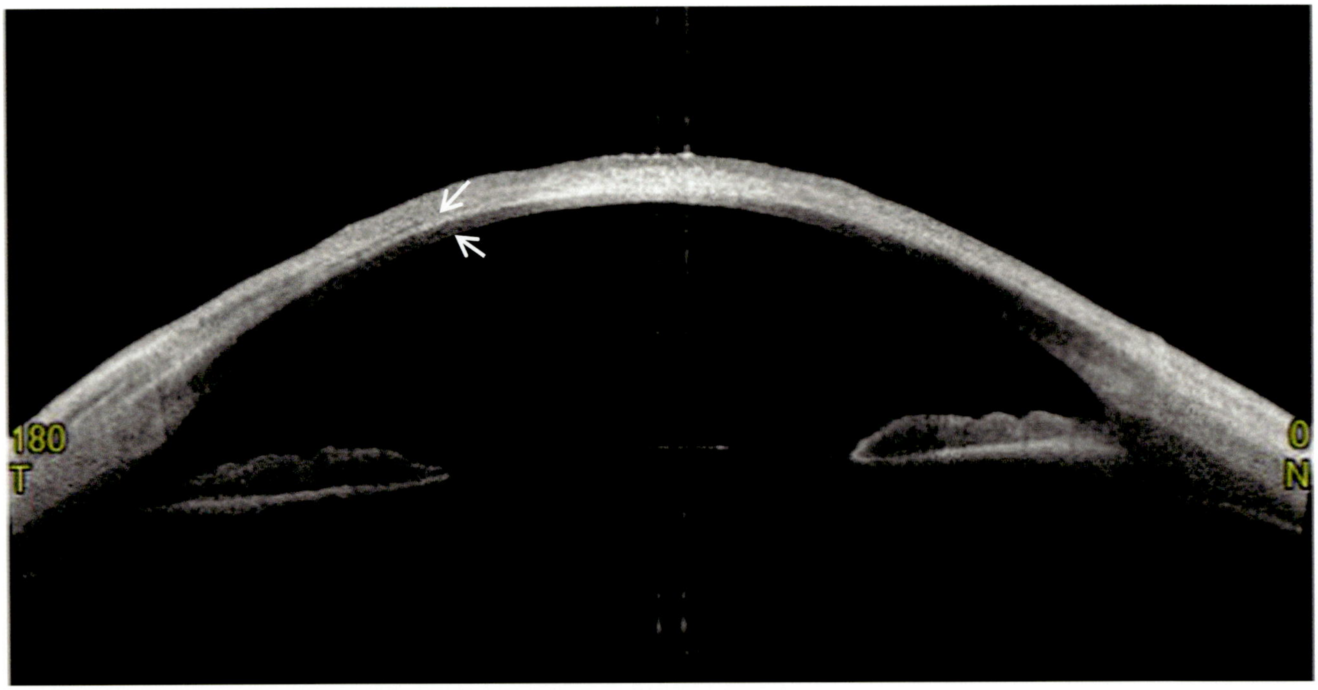

Fig. 6 Anterior segment optical coherence tomography of the same eye showing deep stromal scarring with a very thin remaining clear stroma (arrows)

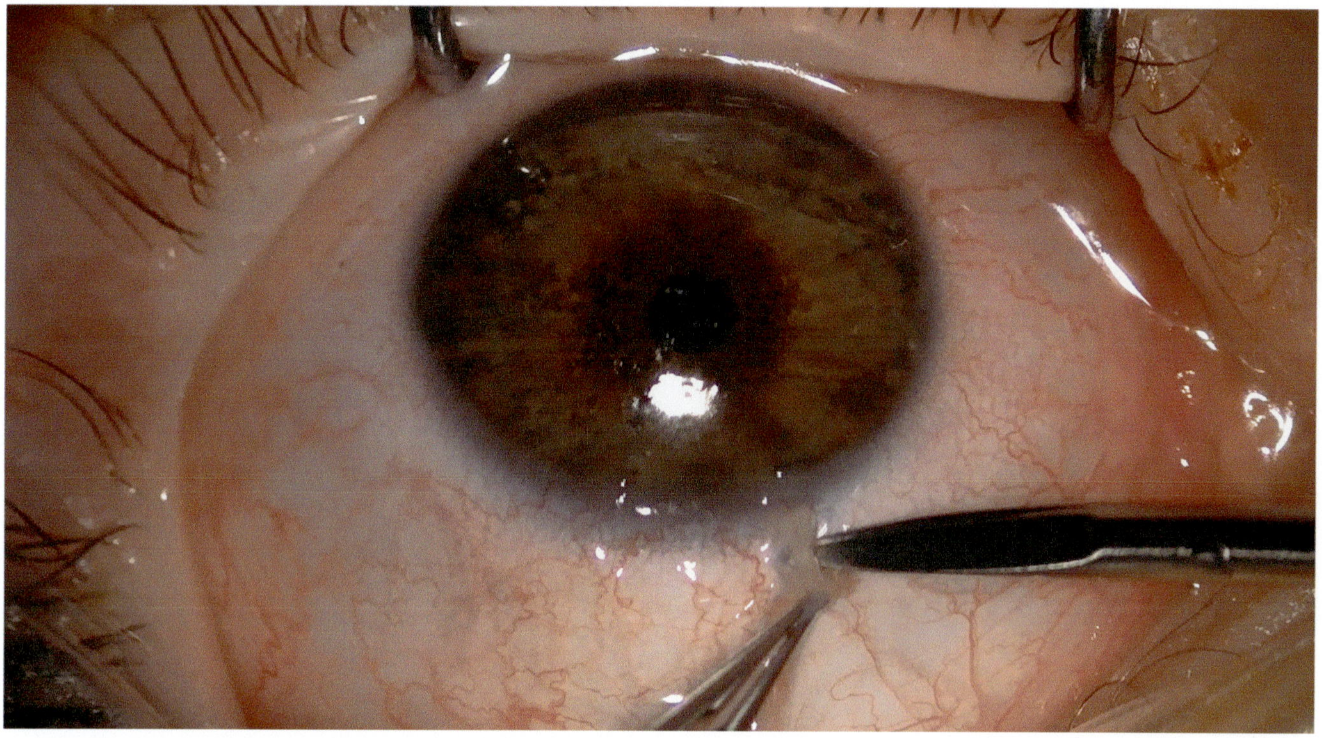

Fig. 7 Simple Limbal Epithelial Transplantation SLET intraoperatively: Step 1: Limbal graft preparation in the healthy partner eye. Opening of the conjunctiva

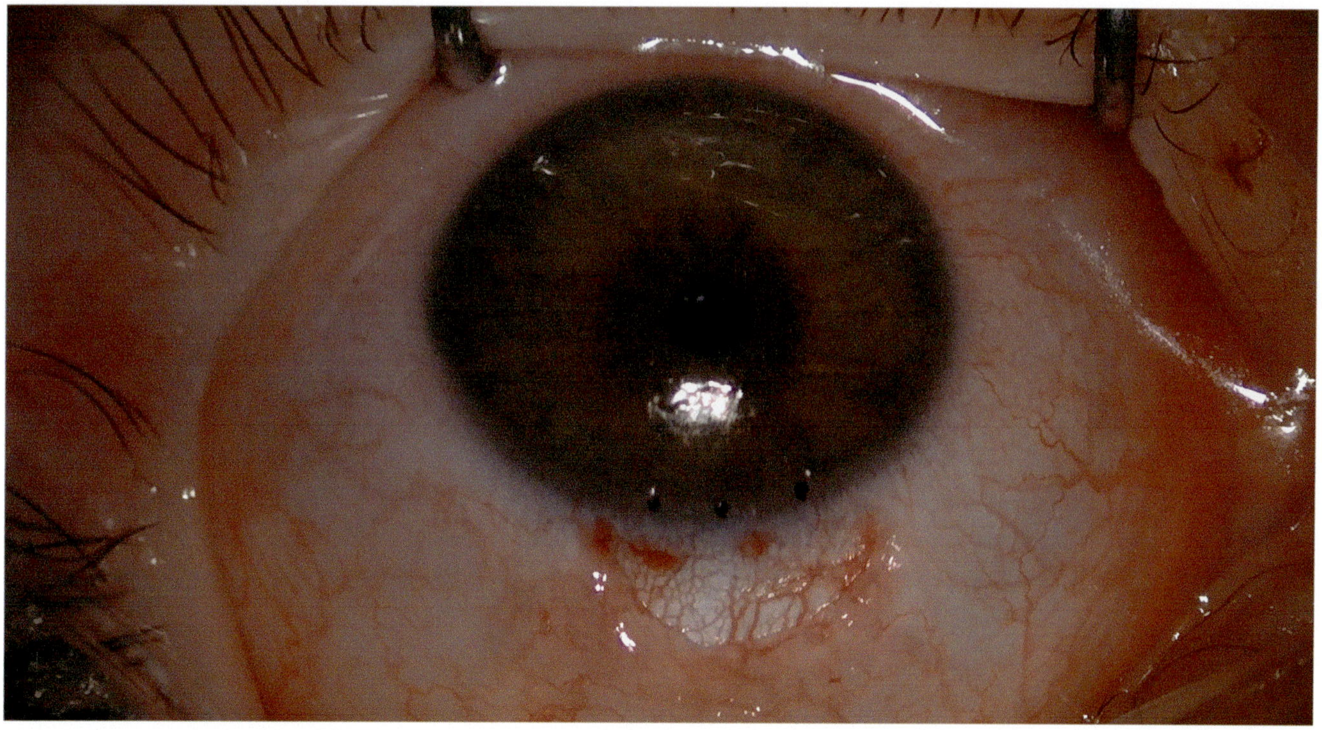

Fig. 8 Simple Limbal Epithelial Transplantation SLET intraoperatively: Step 1: Limbal graft preparation in the healthy partner eye. Marking of the superior limbus explantation area

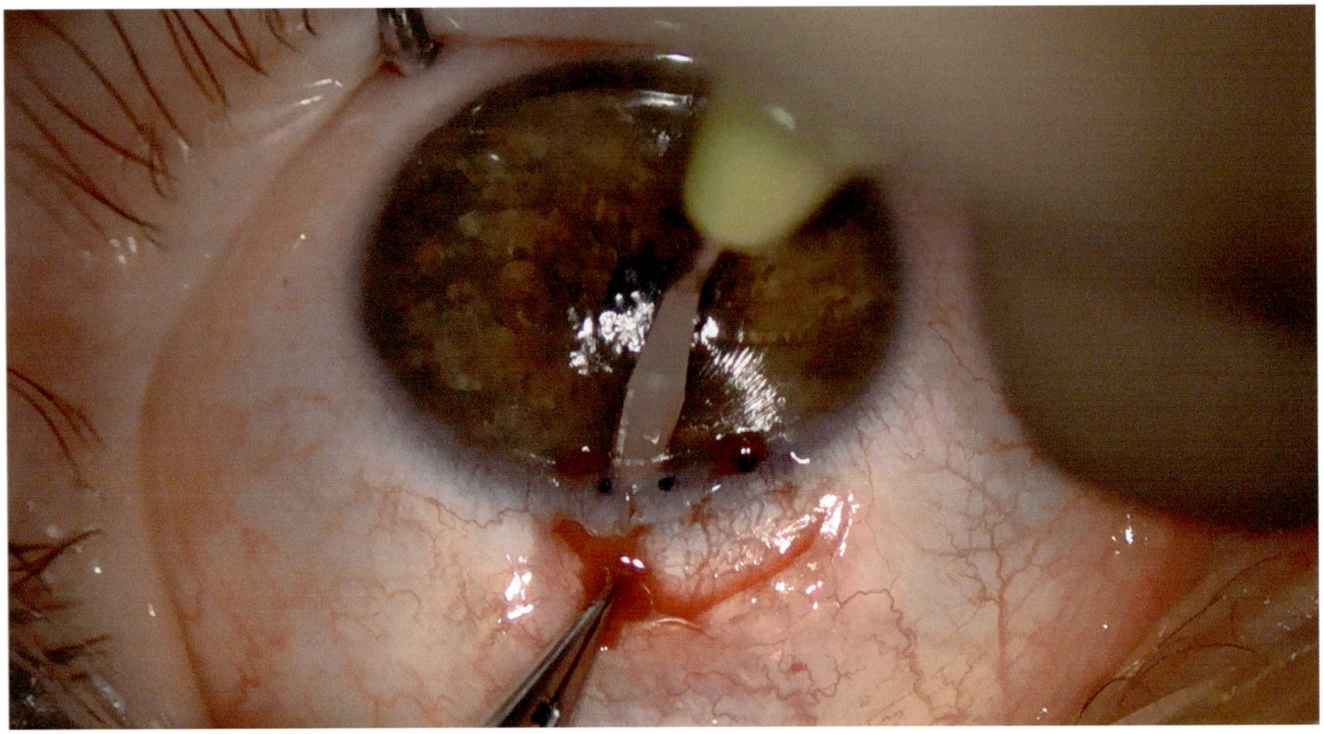

Fig. 9 Simple Limbal Epithelial Transplantation SLET intraoperatively: Step 1: Limbal graft preparation in the healthy partner eye. Lamellar dissection of the limbal autograft

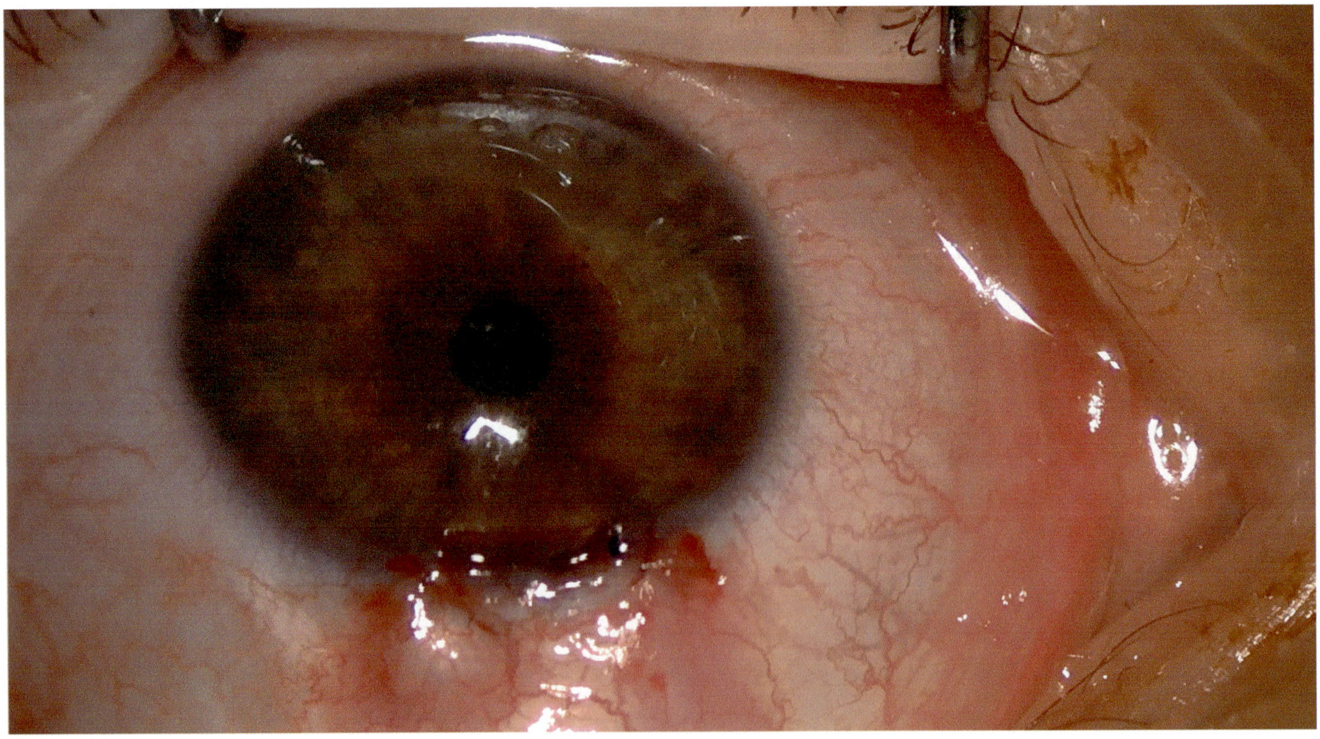

Fig. 10 Simple Limbal Epithelial Transplantation SLET intraoperatively: Step 1: Limbal graft preparation in the healthy partner eye. Re-adapted conjunctiva after limbal autograft explantation

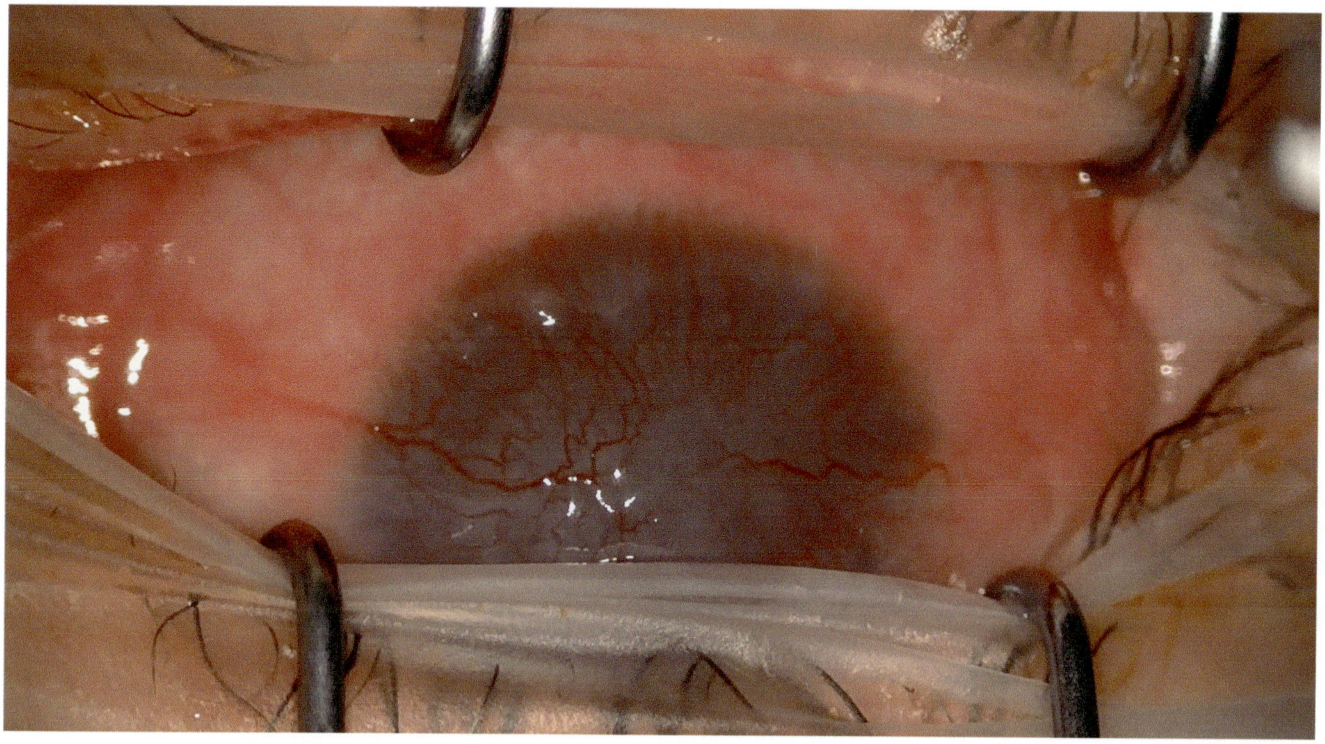

Fig. 11 Simple Limbal Epithelial Transplantation SLET intraoperatively: Step 2: Preparation of the recipient eye. The eyelid speculum cannot be opened completely because of symblephara, which is a negative prognostic factor

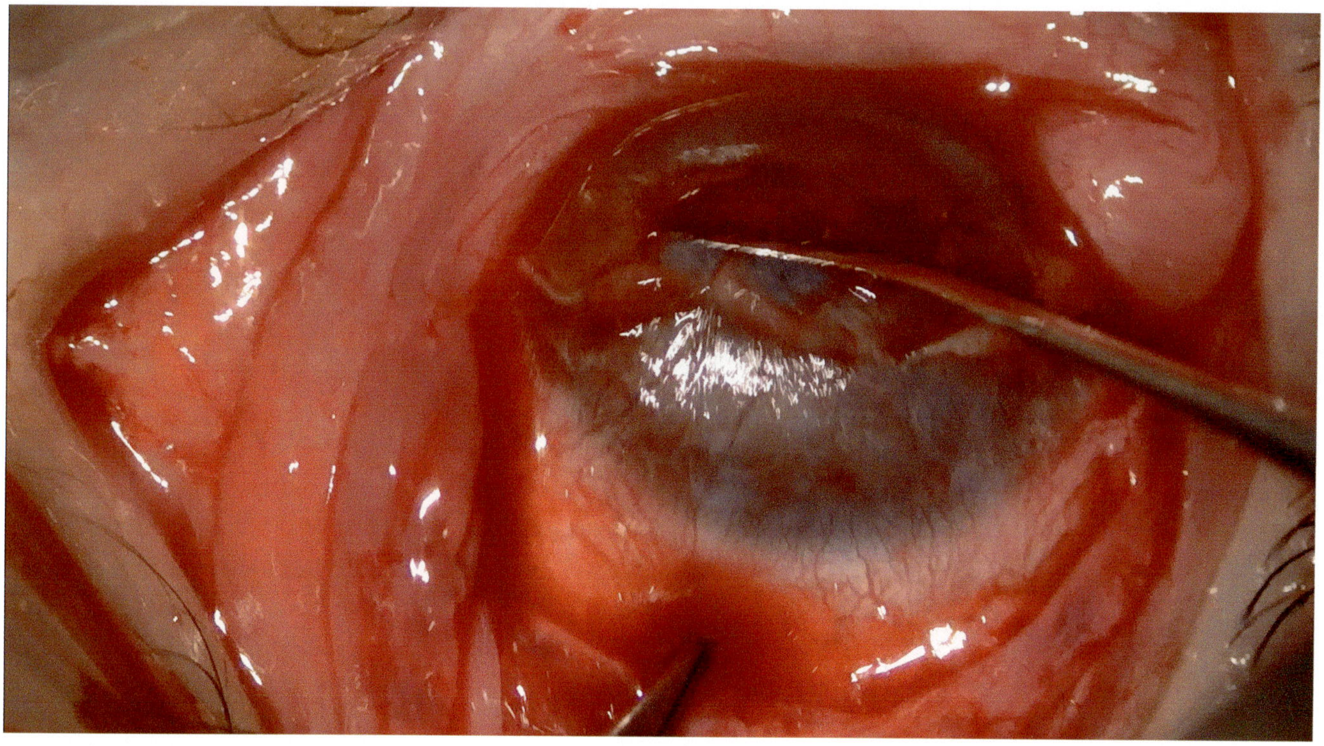

Fig. 12 Simple Limbal Epithelial Transplantation SLET intraoperatively: Step 2: Peritomy and pannectomy

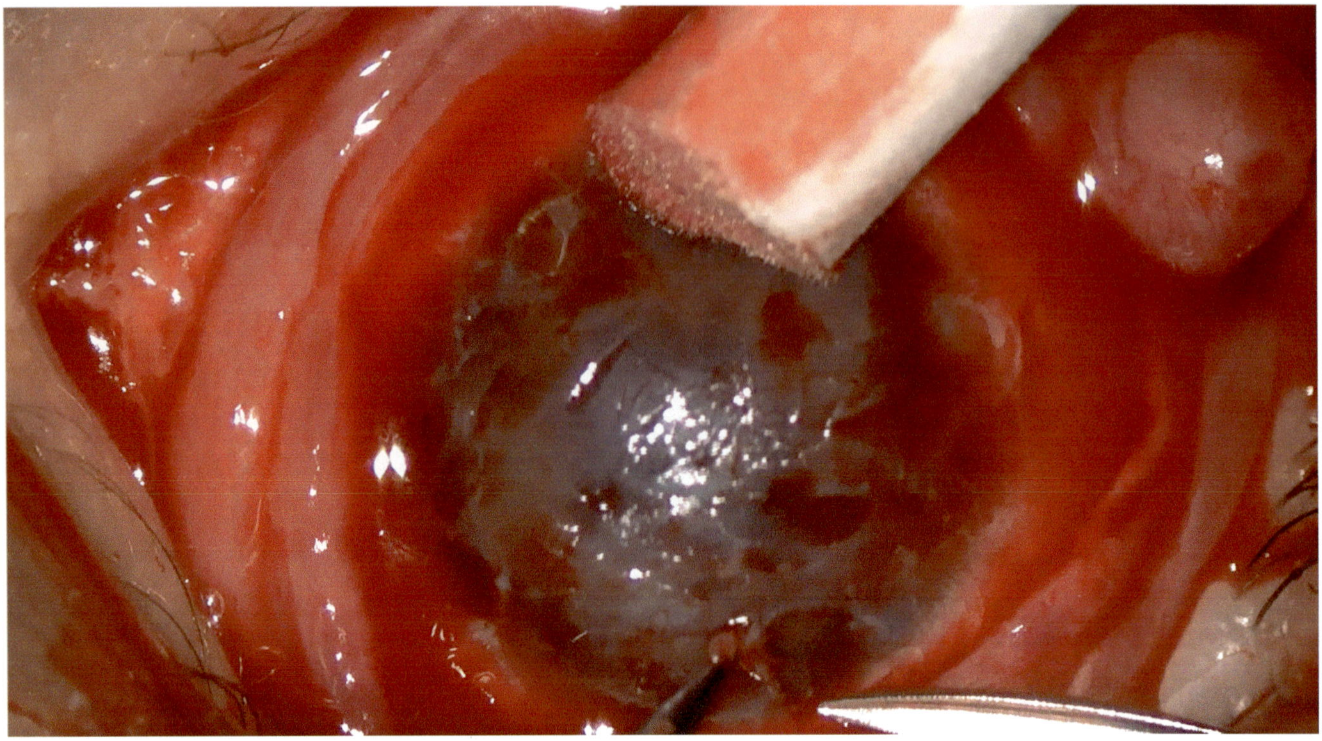

Fig. 13 Simple Limbal Epithelial Transplantation SLET intraoperatively: Step 3: Preparation until a clear cornea becomes visible

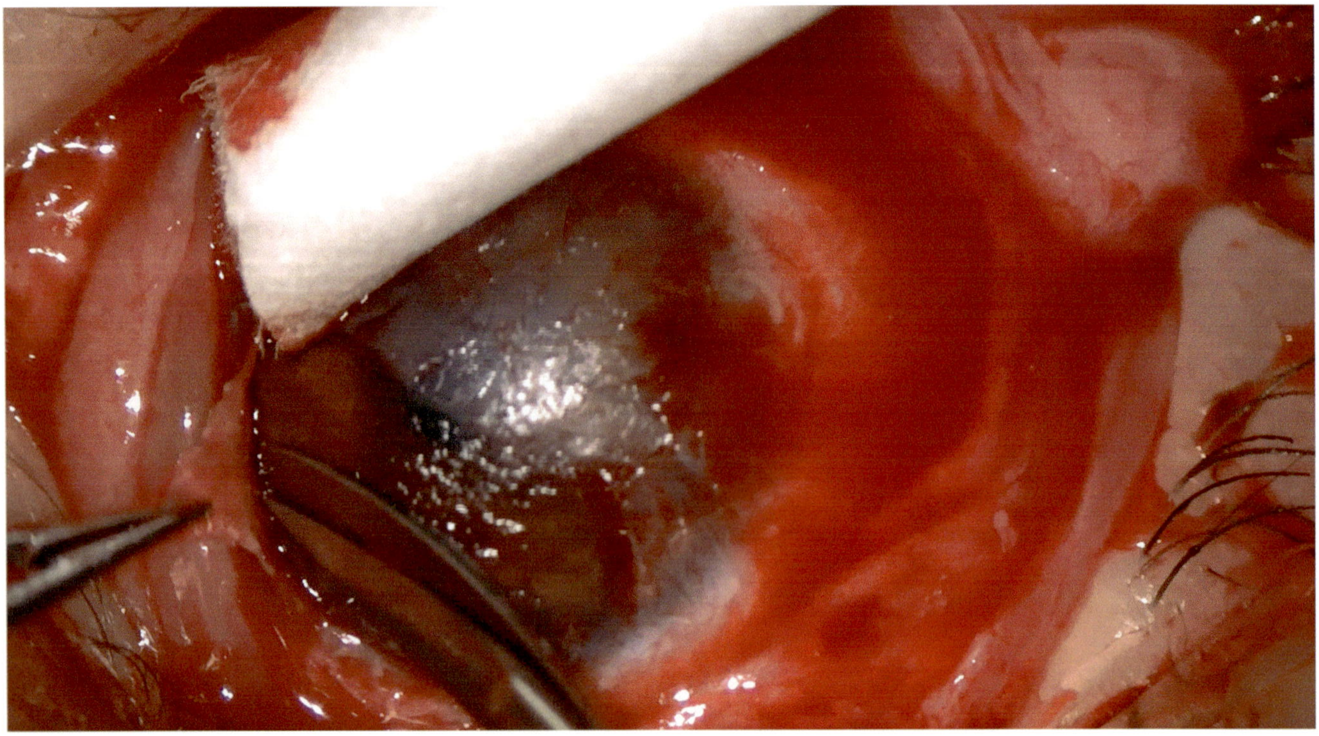

Fig. 14 Simple Limbal Epithelial Transplantation SLET intraoperatively: Step 3: Deeper lamellar preparation until a clear cornea becomes visible

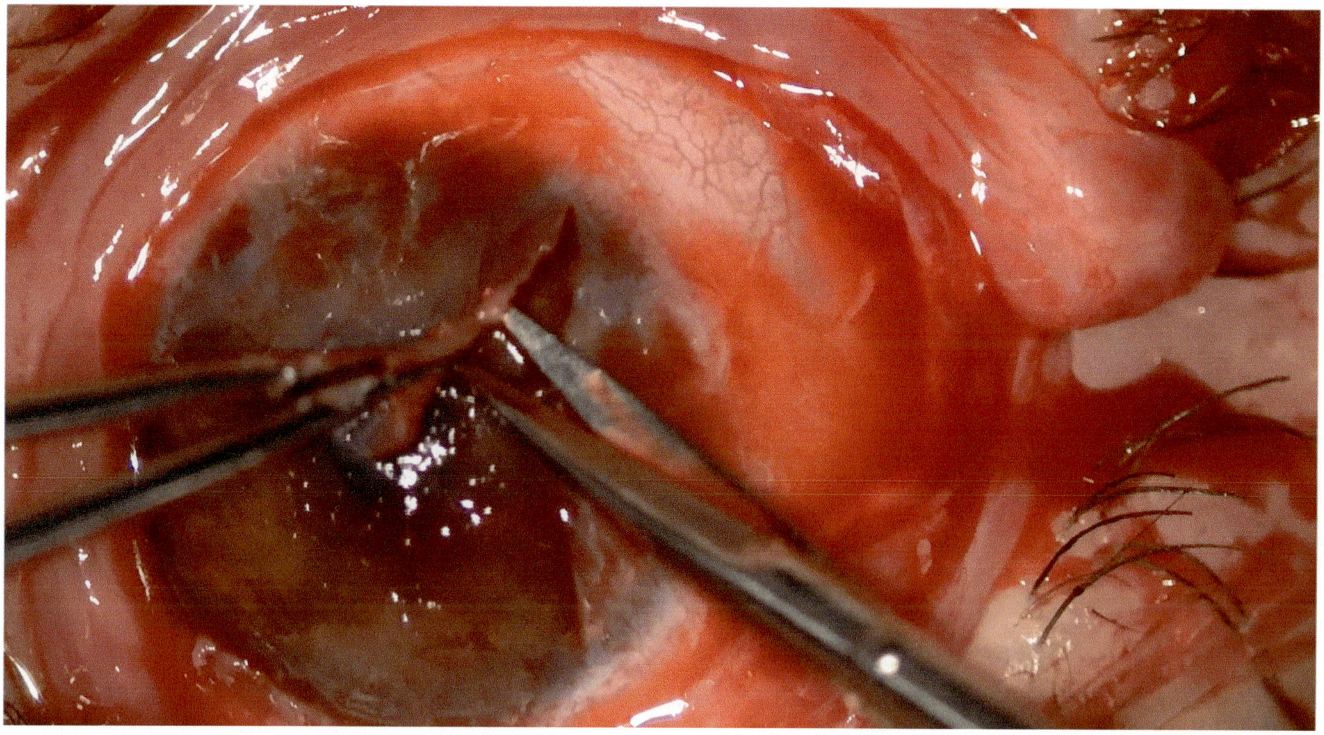

Fig. 15 Simple Limbal Epithelial Transplantation SLET intraoperatively: Step 3: Further lamellar preparation

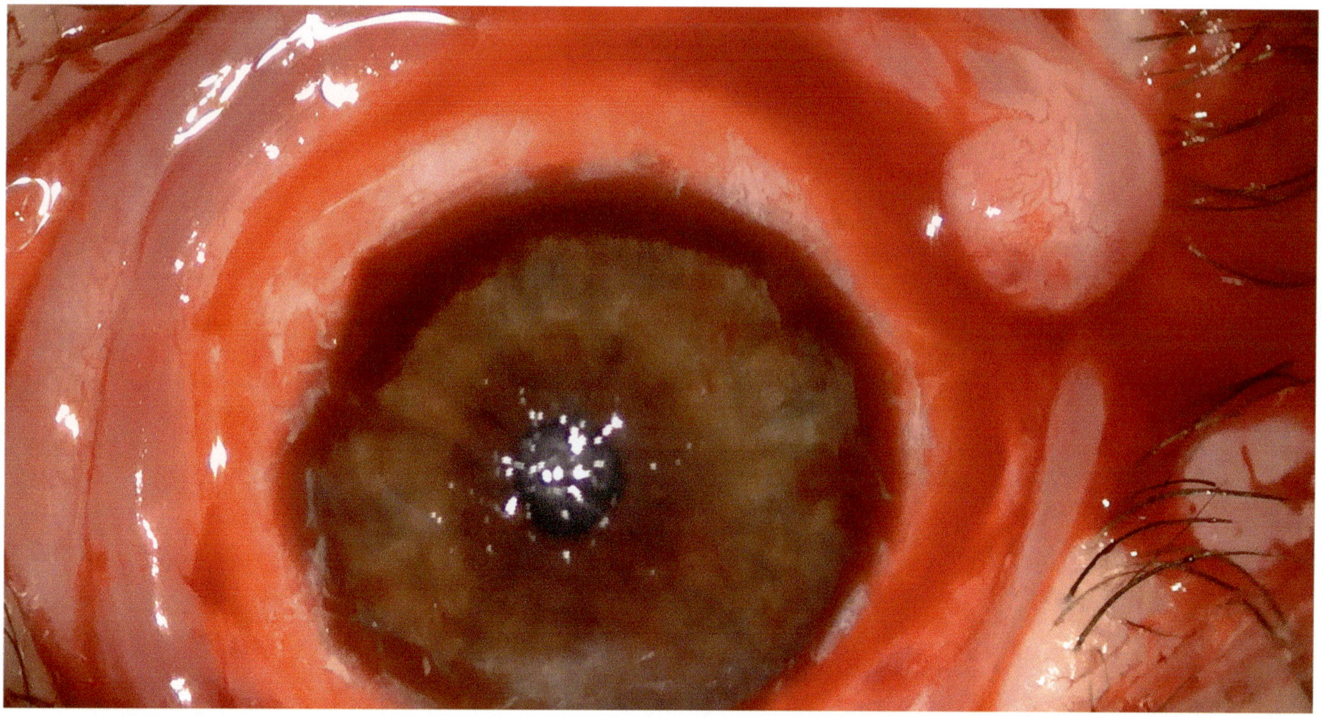

Fig. 16 Simple Limbal Epithelial Transplantation SLET intraoperatively: Step 3: Clear cornea after finishing deep lamellar preparation

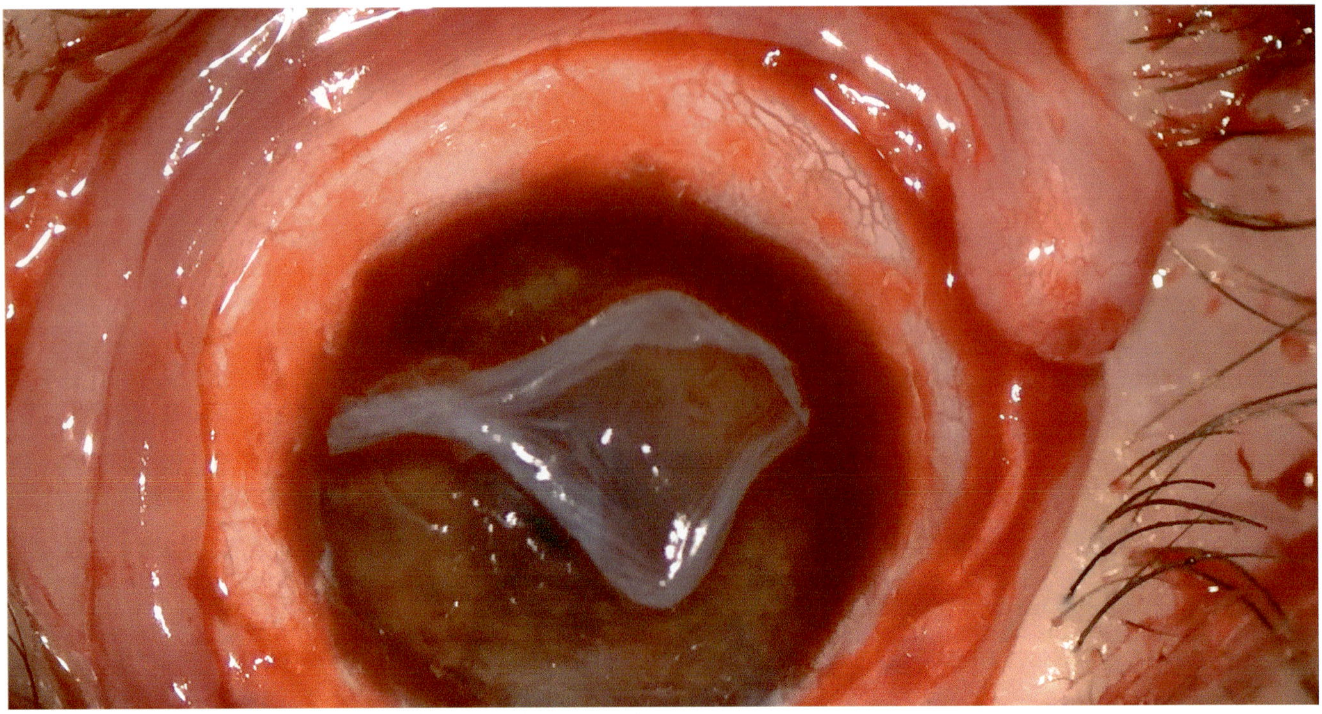

Fig. 17 Simple Limbal Epithelial Transplantation SLET intraoperatively: Step 4: Amniotic membrane transplantation as graft

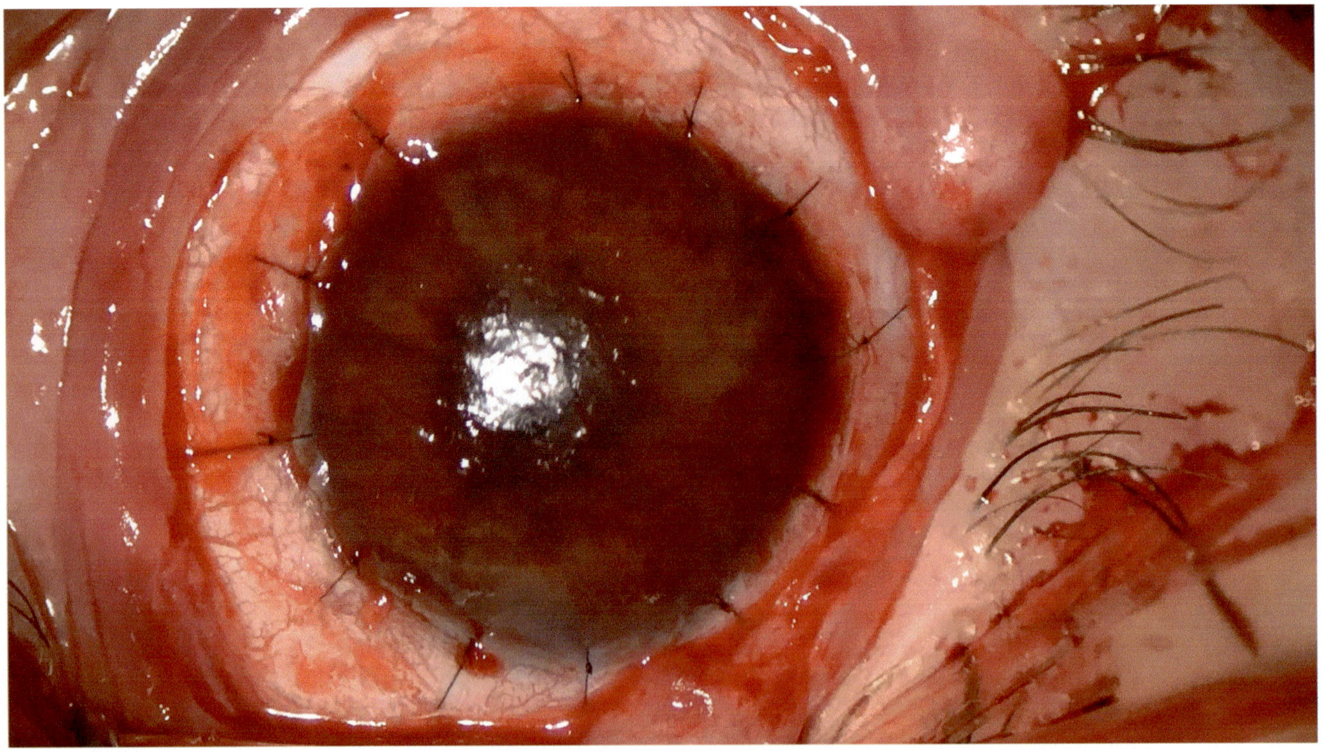

Fig. 18 Simple Limbal Epithelial Transplantation SLET intraoperatively: Step 4: Amniotic membrane transplantation as graft–episcleral suturing

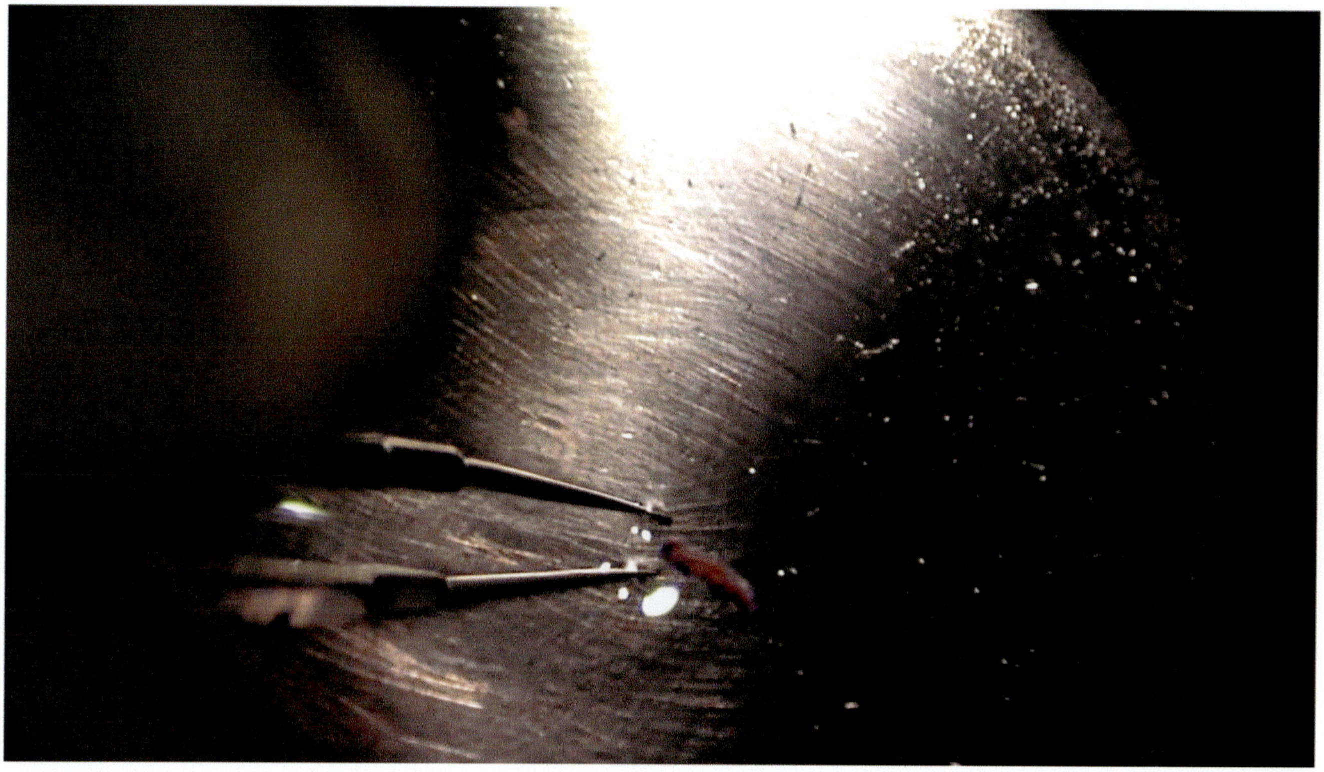

Fig. 19 Simple Limbal Epithelial Transplantation SLET intraoperatively: Step 5: Graft preparation (stored in buffered saline solution)

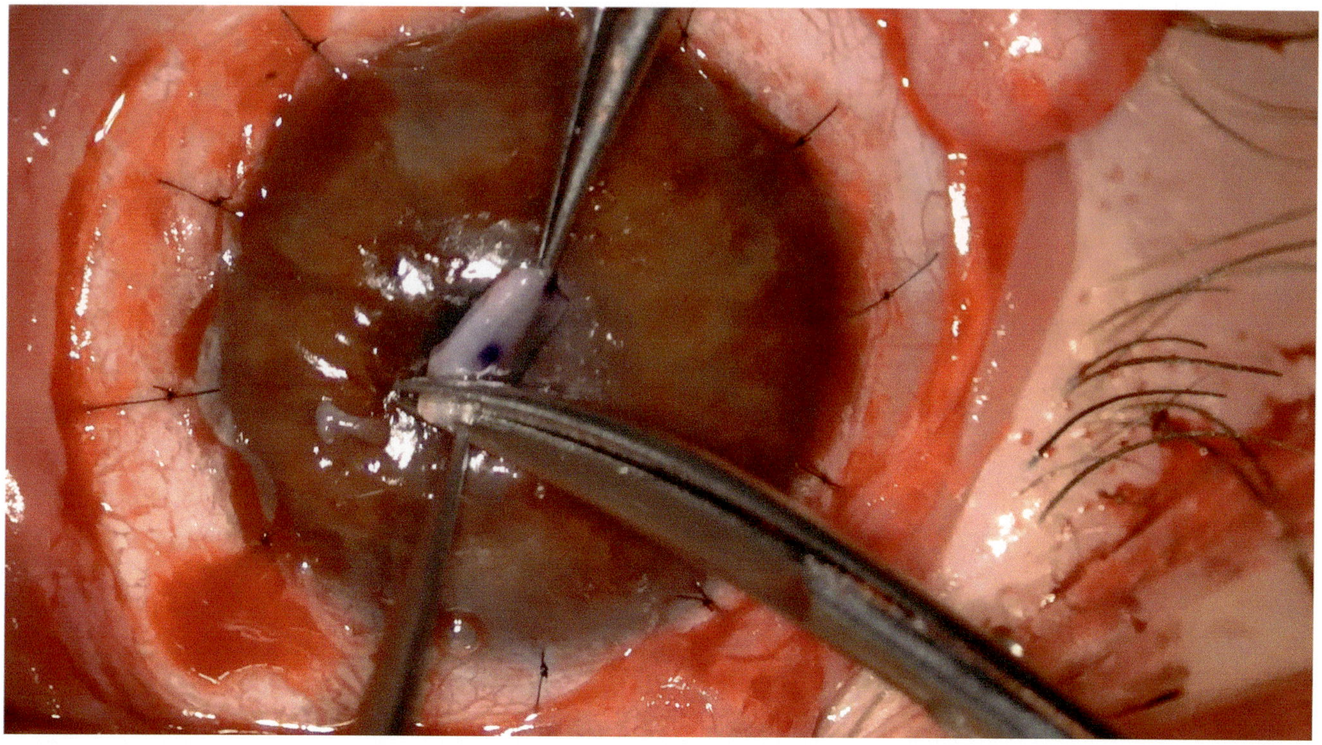

Fig. 20 Simple Limbal Epithelial Transplantation SLET intraoperatively: Step 5: Graft cut into small pieces onto the amniotic membrane covering the recipient cornea

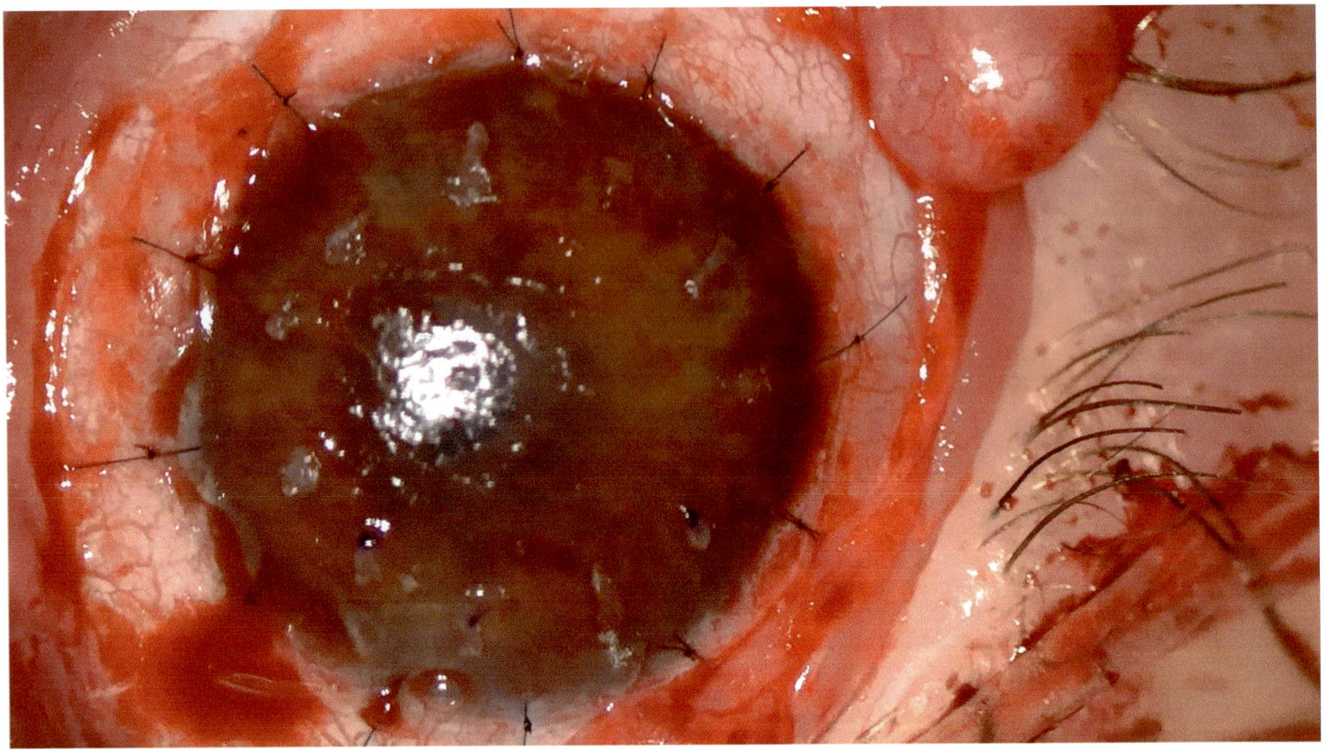

Fig. 21 Simple Limbal Epithelial Transplantation SLET intraoperatively: Step 5: Limbal stem cell grafts aligned in a circular pattern onto the amniotic membrane graft covering the recipient cornea

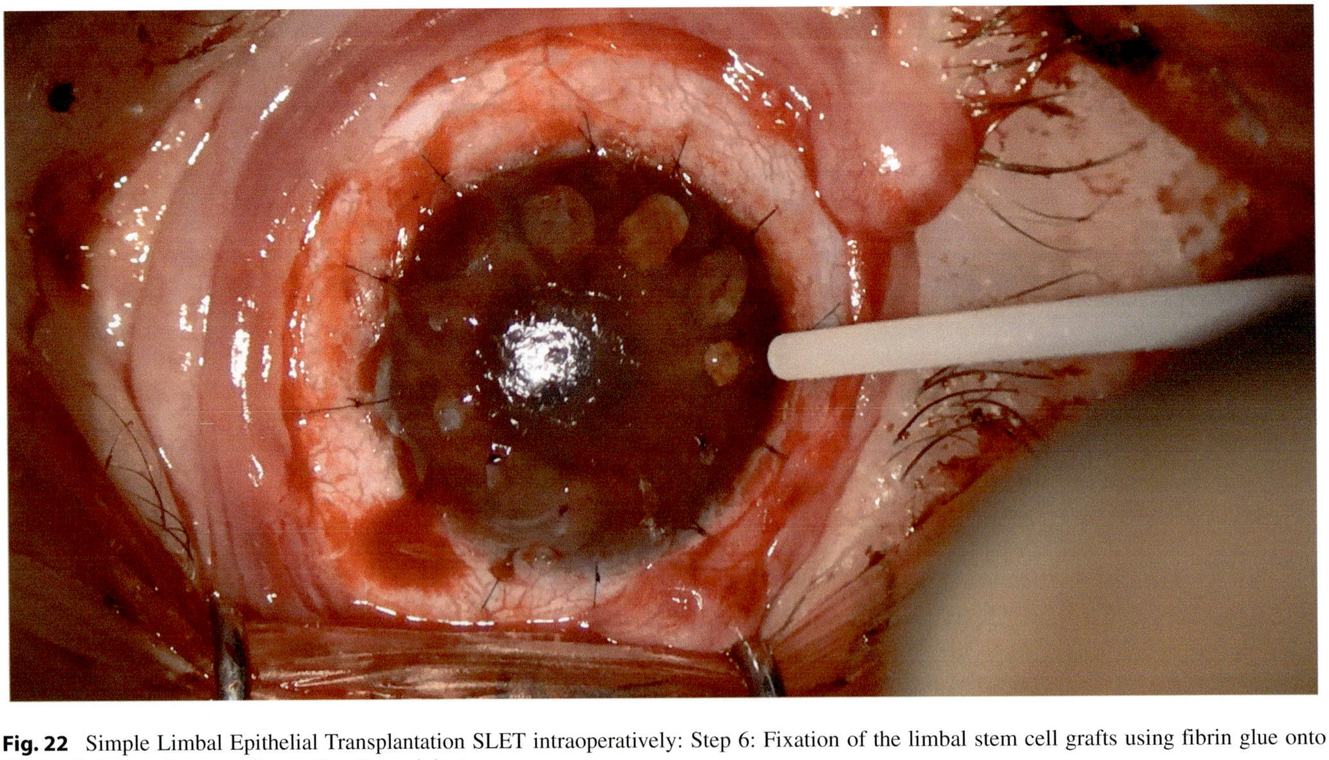

Fig. 22 Simple Limbal Epithelial Transplantation SLET intraoperatively: Step 6: Fixation of the limbal stem cell grafts using fibrin glue onto the amniotic membrane graft covering the recipient cornea

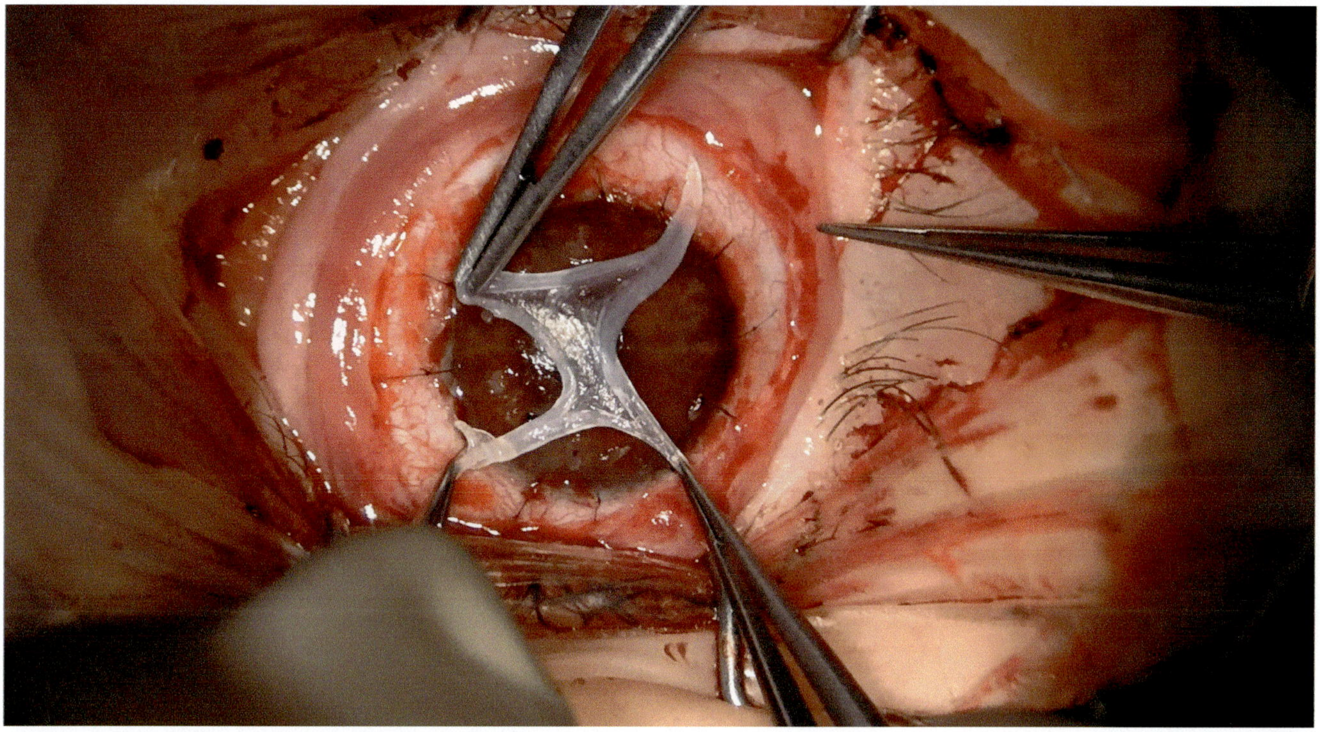

Fig. 23 Simple Limbal Epithelial Transplantation SLET intraoperatively: Step 7: Covering the fixated limbal stem cell grafts with another amniotic membrane patch

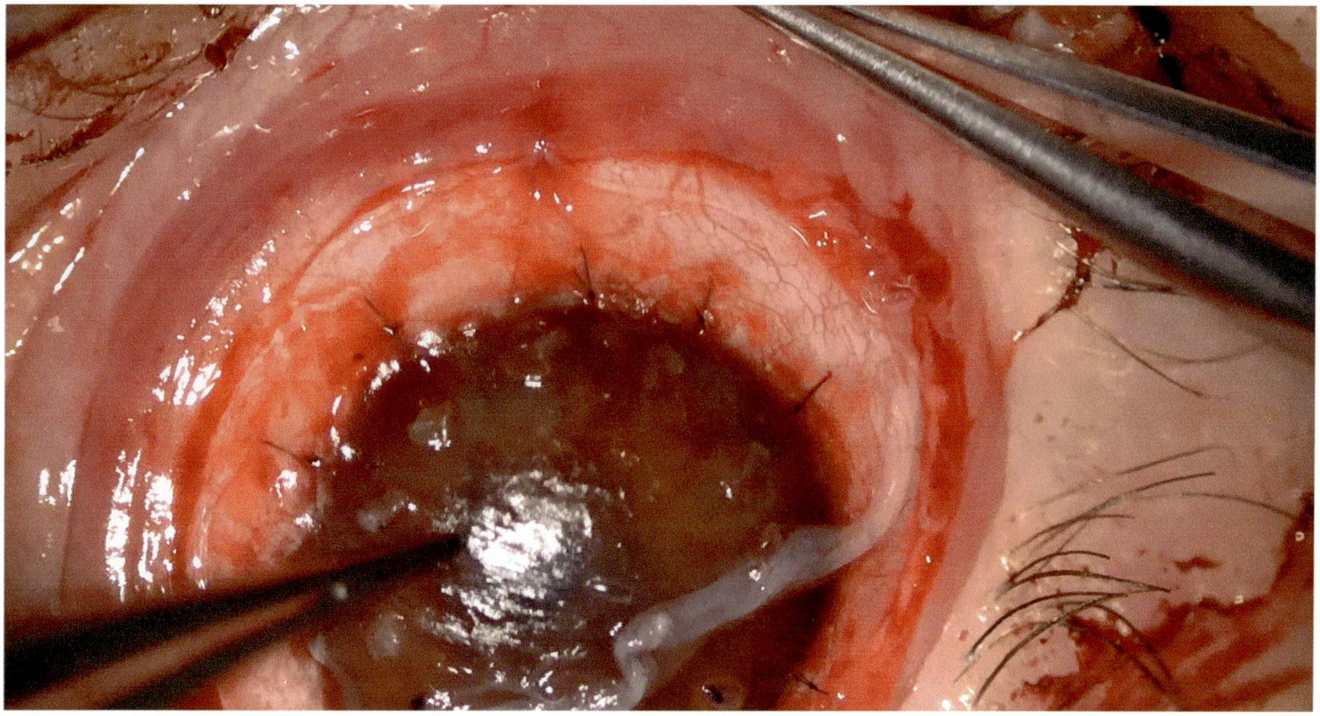

Fig. 24 Simple Limbal Epithelial Transplantation SLET intraoperatively: Step 7: Fixation of the protecting amniotic membrane patch by end-to-end anastomosis with the conjunctiva

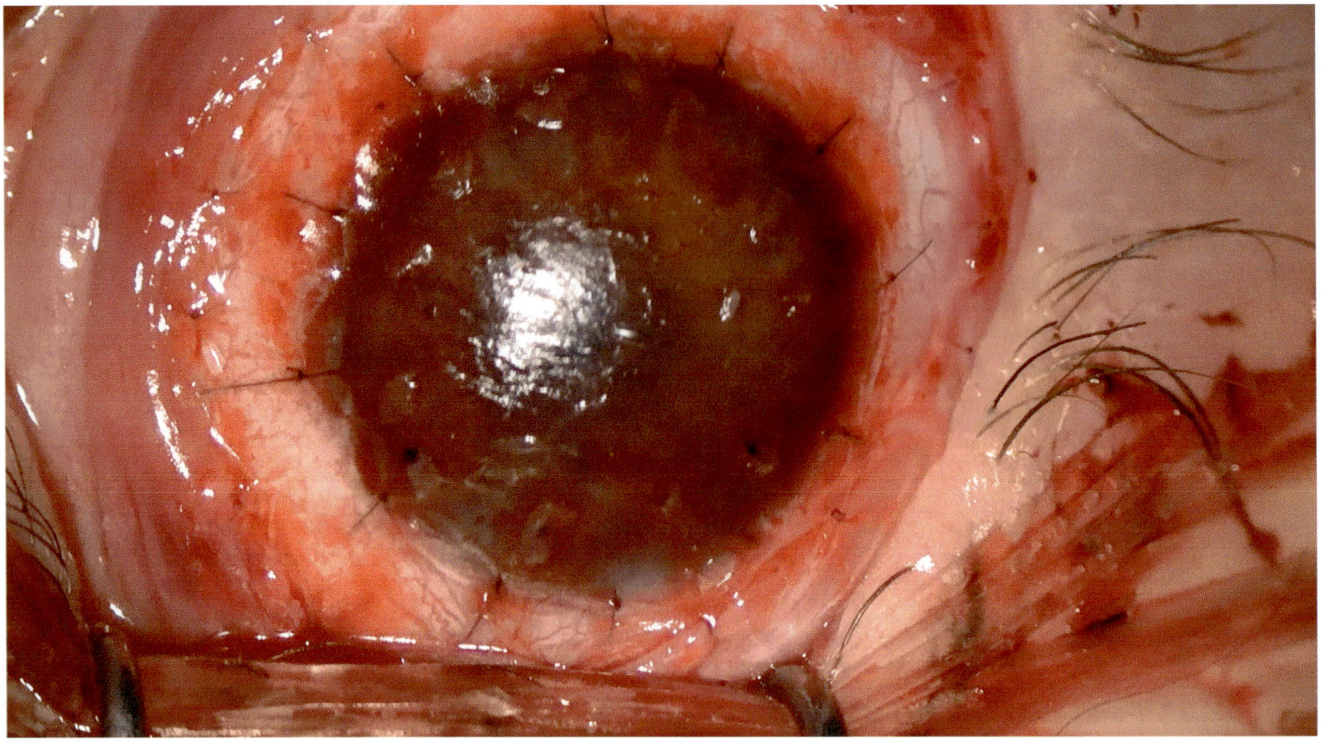

Fig. 25 Simple Limbal Epithelial Transplantation SLET intraoperatively: Step 7: Amniotic membrane patch circularly attached

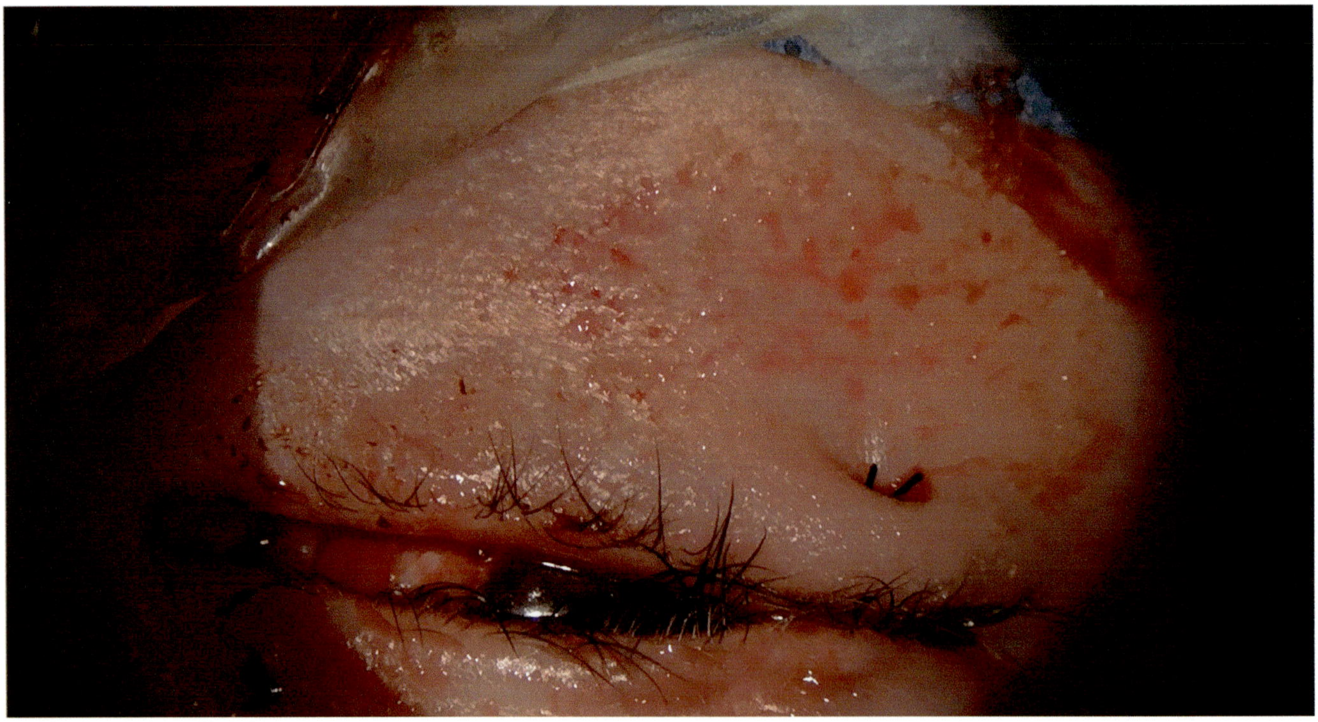

Fig. 26 Simple Limbal Epithelial Transplantation SLET intraoperatively: Step 8: Temporary lateral tarsorrhaphy using silk 7–0 suture after inserting a bandage contact lens

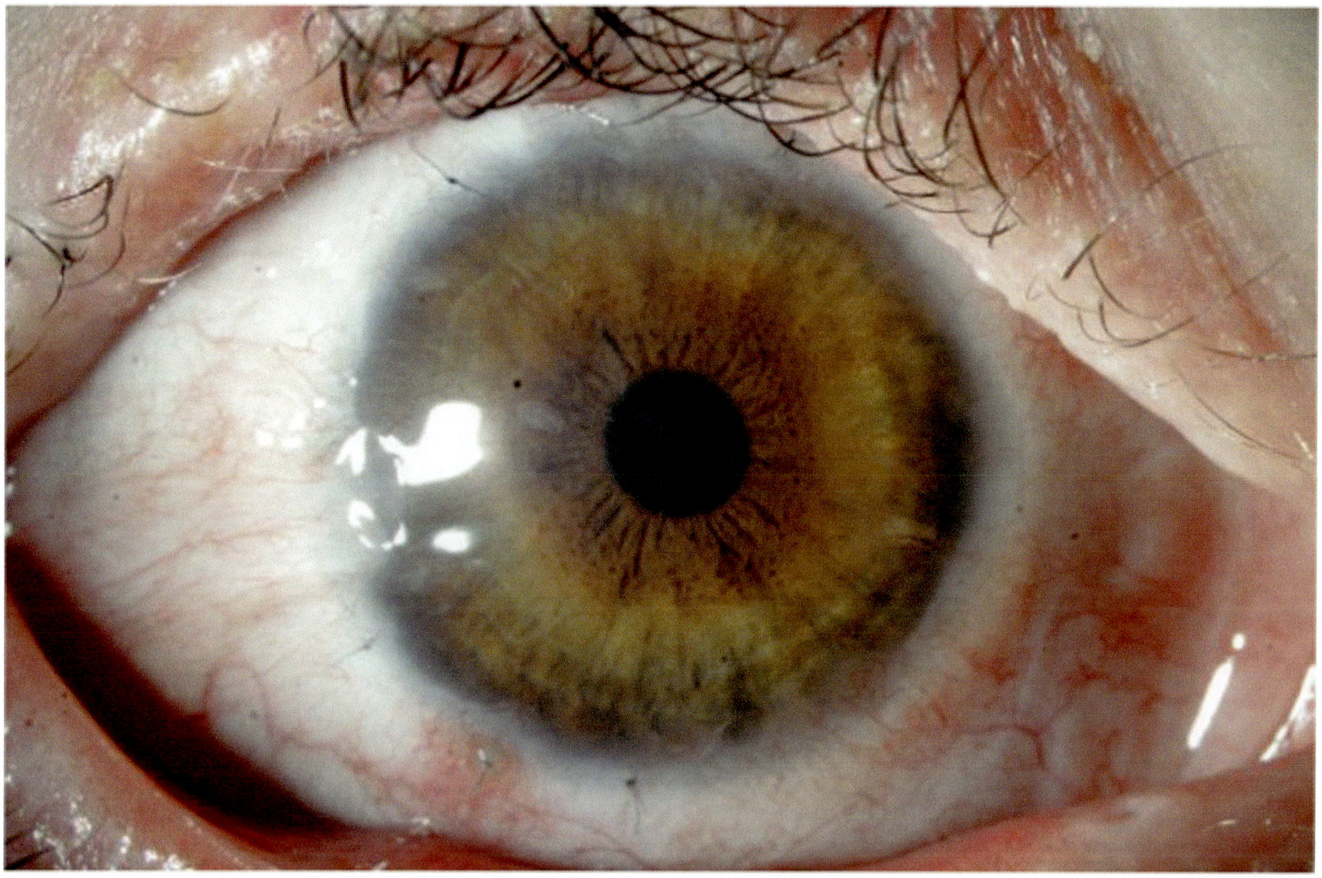

Fig. 27 Simple Limbal Epithelial transplantation SLET postoperatively: Findings six months after surgery. Epithelial closure, uncorrected visual acuity: 20/50 (0.4)

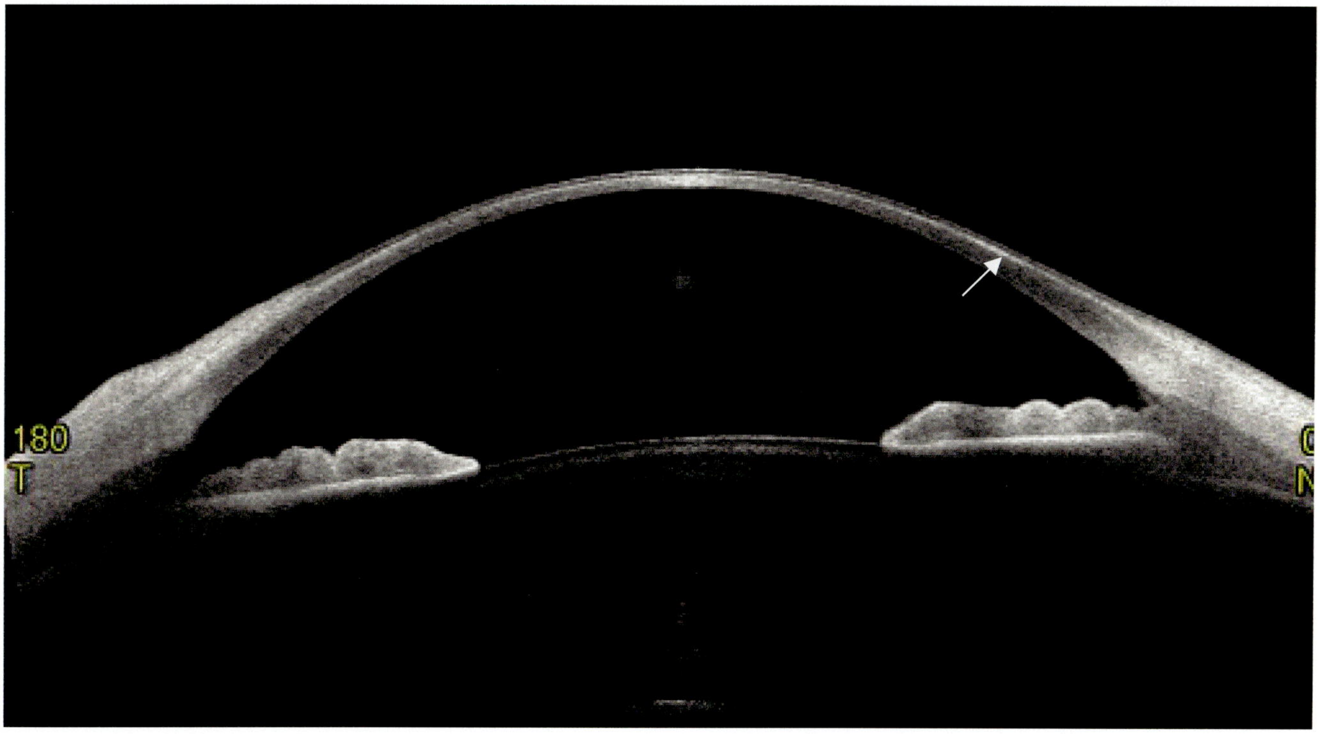

Fig. 28 Anterior segment optical coherence tomography six months after SLET. Thinnest corneal thickness at 182 µm, integrated amniotic membrane graft (arrow)

5 Conclusion

Limbal stem cell deficiency is characterized by invading conjunctival epithelial and goblet cells on the corneal surface. The most common cause leading to acquired LSCD is alkali burn. Therapeutic options have evolved in recent years from purely conjunctival grafting towards ex vivo expansion of limbal epithelial stem cells. A less expensive option is the direct transplantation of limbal epithelial stem cells from the healthy fellow eye to the affected eye, which can be achieved in one surgical session and is often performed in preparation for a later scheduled penetrating keratoplasty. However, care should be taken to allow at least a two-months interval [13] to allow migration of the limbal stem cells on the corneal surface and thus avoid a complete excision during the penetrating keratoplasty.

References

1. Basu S, Sureka SP, Shanbhag SS, et al. Simple limbal epithelial transplantation: long-term clinical outcomes in 125 cases of unilateral chronic ocular surface burns. Ophthalmology. 2016;123(5):1000–10.
2. Sangwan VS, Basu S, MacNeil S, et al. Simple limbal epithelial transplantation (SLET): a novel surgical technique for the treatment of unilateral limbal stem cell deficiency. Br J Ophthalmol. 2012;96(7):931–4.
3. Pellegrini G, Traverso CE, Franzi AT, et al. Long-term restoration of damaged corneal surfaces with autologous cultivated corneal epithelium. Lancet. 1997;349:990–3.
4. Espana EM, Di Pascuale M, Grueterich M, et al. Keratolimbal allograft in corneal reconstruction. Eye (Lond). 2004;18(4):406–17.
5. Jackson CJ, Myklebust Ernø IT, Ringstad H, et al. Simple limbal epithelial transplantation: current status and future perspectives. Stem Cell Translat Med. 2020;9(3):316–27.
6. Thoft RA. Conjunctival transplantation. Arch Ophthalmol. 1977;95(8):1425–7.
7. Kenyon KR, Tseng SCG. Limbal autograft transplantation for ocular surface disorders. Ophthalmology. 1989;96(5):709–23.
8. Shanbhag S, Patel C, Goyal R, et al. Simple limbal epithelial transplantation (SLET): review of indications, surgical technique, mechanism, outcomes, limitations, and impact. Indian J Ophthalmol. 2019;67(8):1265.
9. Holland EJ, Schwartz GS. The evolution of epithelial transplantation for severe ocular surface disease and a proposed classification system. Cornea. 1996;15(6):549–56.
10. Tan DTH, Ficker LA, Buckley RJ. Limbal transplantation. Ophthalmology. 1996;103(1):29–36.
11. Kheirkhah A, Raju VK, Tseng SCG. Minimal conjunctival limbal autograft for total limbal stem cell deficiency. Cornea. 2008;27(6):730–3.
12. Holland EJ. Management of limbal stem cell deficiency: a historical perspective, past, present, and future. Cornea. 2015;34(10):9–15.
13. Gupta N, Joshi J, Farooqui J, et al. Results of simple limbal epithelial transplantation in unilateral ocular surface burn. Indian J Ophthalmol. 2018;66(1):45–52.
14. Mittal V, Jain R, Mittal R. Ocular surface epithelialization pattern after simple limbal epithelial transplantation: an in vivo observational study. Cornea. 2015;34(10):1227–32.
15. Vazirani J, Ali MH, Sharma N, et al. Autologous simple limbal epithelial transplantation for unilateral limbal stem cell deficiency: multicentre results. Br J Ophthalmol. 2016;100(10):1416–20.
16. Basu S, Mohan S, Bhalekar S, et al. Simple limbal epithelial transplantation (SLET) in failed cultivated limbal epithelial transplantation (CLET) for unilateral chronic ocular burns. Br J Ophthalmol. 2018;102(12):1640–5.
17. Iyer G, Srinivasan B, Agarwal S, et al. Outcome of allo simple limbal epithelial transplantation (alloSLET) in the early stage of ocular chemical injury. Br J Ophthalmol. 2017;101(6):828–33.
18. Riedl JC, Musayeva A, Wasielica-Poslednik J, et al. Allogenic simple limbal epithelial transplantation (alloSLET) from cadaveric donor eyes in patients with persistent corneal epithelial defects. Br J Ophthalmol. 2021;105(2):180–5.

Autologous Ipsilateral Rotational and Contralateral Keratoplasty

Adrien Quintin and Berthold Seitz

Abstract

Corneal opacities can cause severe and permanent impairment of the visual acuity if centrally located. Homologous penetrating keratoplasty (HPK) is usually the standard therapeutic option to treat patients with such clinical conditions. However, autologous penetrating keratoplasty (APK) can sometimes be a more suitable alternative depending on the clinical presentation, the patient's compliance and even the infrastructural and geographical situation, without risk of immunological graft rejection. This chapter summarizes the topic of autologous penetrating keratoplasty (APK), and reports surgical techniques, indications and (dis)advantages of two subtypes of APK: ipsilateral rotational and contralateral APK. In ipsilateral rotational APK, an eccentric trephination is performed, whereby a central corneal opacity lies at the edge of the excision margin. The corneal button is then rotated, bringing the scar toward the limbus and the clear cornea towards the visual axis. A contralateral APK could be performed in a more particular clinical presentation with a central corneal opacity in a functionally better eye with good visual prognosis, and a clear cornea in the nearly blind fellow eye with poor or no visual prognosis. During this procedure, the clear cornea from the (nearly) blind eye with a non-corneal pathology is transplanted into the potentially better-seeing eye with the corneal pathology. As part of this procedure, a HPK must first be performed in the (nearly) blind donor eye. The option of an autologous penetrating keratoplasty (APK) should always be considered in particular clinical situations before corneal microsurgeons move on directly towards homologous keratoplasty (HPK).

Keywords

Contralateral autologous keratoplasty · Ipsilateral rotational autologous keratoplasty · Penetrating corneal transplantation · Central corneal scar

1 Background

Full-thickness corneal opacities such as scars after bacterial or herpetic inflammation or due to perforating lesions can cause severe and permanent impairment of the visual acuity if they are centrally located. Homologous penetrating keratoplasty (HPK), first successfully performed by Eduard Zirm in 1905 [1], is usually the standard therapeutic option to treat patients with such clinical conditions. However, autologous penetrating keratoplasty (APK) can sometimes be a more suitable alternative depending on the clinical presentation, the patient-dependent features (age, compliance, etc.), and even the infrastructural and geographical situation. According to the literature, APK represents 1% among all corneal transplantations [2].

A major risk factor that jeopardizes the transparency of the corneal graft is an immune reaction. The incidence of this risk increases with larger diameter grafts [3], with highly vascularised recipient corneas, and after multiple graft rejections. Indeed, when the cornea is highly vascularised, or has been rejected previously, it breaks down its initial "immunological privilege", which is normally responsible for the remarkable success of HLA-incompatible corneal transplantation [4]. Immunologically "high-risk" corneas are defined as those in which a graft has been previously rejected ≥ 2 times and/or those with

A. Quintin (✉) · B. Seitz
Department of Ophthalmology, Saarland University Medical Centre, Homburg, Germany
e-mail: Adrien.Quintin@outlook.com

B. Seitz et al. (eds.), *Atlas on Cornea*, https://doi.org/10.1007/978-3-031-65422-0_58

two or more quadrants of vascularisation. It has indeed been demonstrated previously that the frequency of rejection increases with both the number of vascularised quadrants and the total number of blood vessels crossing the recipient/donor interface [5]. Early detection of these immune reactions requires regular follow-ups. If these regular and necessary follow-up examinations cannot be easily performed because of the patient's age (e.g. young children and infants), low patient compliance or a geographically low density of ophthalmologists, conventional HPK may not be recommended [6].

For these reasons, the options of tissue (and especially HLA) typing, as well as autologous penetrating keratoplasty in special clinical circumstances, should always be considered first for "high-risk" corneas before corneal microsurgeons move on straight towards HLA-incompatible HPK. The variants of APK are described and elaborated in the current chapter.

Due to the autologous origin of the corneal graft, there is no threat of an immunological reaction in autologous penetrating keratoplasty. Despite this advantage, the operation does not prevent the risk of graft failure. The only factor that endangers the transparency of the graft is the loss of corneal endothelial cells due to the initial corneal trauma and the operation itself, also impacted by the patient's age. Bertelmann et al. reported a lower endothelial cell loss in autografts (15%) compared to allografts (40%) 1 year postoperatively [7], which might be attributed to a reduced migration of endothelial cells from the graft to the host in APK [8]. Since this possible postoperative endothelial decompensation cannot be avoided by regular clinical examinations, patients typically do not require as many postoperative follow-up examinations after APK compared to HPK [6].

The healing of the trephination wound is faster after autologous keratoplasty as topical steroids need to be administered less frequently, which means that complications associated with long-term steroid use, such as cataract formation and increased intraocular pressure, are less frequent.

However, the risk of postoperative fistulation is higher with APK, as there is no positive difference between the trephination opening and the autograft, as compared to HPK where the diameter of the graft is usually oversized by 0.1 to 0.3 mm [9]. However, similar to the Krumreich guided trephine system, the same diameter of opening and autograft can be achieved by "donor" trephination from the epithelial side under physiological intraocular pressure [10].

Unfortunately, an additional weakness of this surgical procedure is the impossible use of non-mechanical corneal trephination with the excimer laser because of the loss of tissue intrinsic to the action of the laser along the corneal tissue-protecting mask [11, 12]. Indeed, in APK, the donor trephination is at the same time a recipient trephination, making the cutting edges between graft and recipient incongruent to each other if an excimer laser is used. Indeed, the use of the excimer laser and metal masks lead to a perpendicular incision under the mask's edge but to a parabolic slope on the opposite unprotected side. In comparison to excimer laser trephination, mechanical trephination is however associated with a poorer refractive outcome, in particular with a higher postoperative keratometric astigmatism, a less regular topography and a lower visual acuity after suture removal [12, 13]. Femtosecond laser trephination could also be applied, as it does not induce tissue loss. However, femtosecond laser trephination is associated with a mandatory flattening of the cornea. This in turn may contribute to a non-circular excision, and hence to horizontal torsion, the major intraoperative determinant of high/irregular astigmatism [14, 15]. Nevertheless, a liquid interface could be applied to reduce corneal applanation today.

Two variants of autologous penetrating keratoplasty (APK) exist:

→ Ipsilateral rotational APK
→ Contralateral APK

These variants are described in detail below:

2 Ipsilateral Rotational Autologous Penetrating Keratoplasty

In ipsilateral rotational autologous penetrating keratoplasty (APK), an eccentric trephination is performed, with a central corneal opacity situated at the edge of the excision margin. The corneal button is then rotated, bringing the scar toward the limbus and clear cornea towards the visual axis (Figs. 1 and 2). Due to the autologous origin of the corneal graft, there is no threat of an immunological reaction. Kraupa first reported this method in 1914 [16].

For a more beneficial visual result, the corneal opacity should, if possible, be rotated under the upper eyelid to minimise postoperative glare [11].

Jonas et al. [11] presented the following formula to determine the size of the trephine, as a function of the individual size of the cornea and the distance "*e*" from the margin of the opacity to the center of the cornea:

$$Diameter_{trephine} = \frac{3}{4} Diameter_{cornea} - \frac{e}{2}$$

In such cases, preoperative photographs of the cornea are useful and recommended. On the one hand, this equation optimises the postoperative distance between the centre of the cornea and the rotated opacity. However, it also optimises the distance between the centre of the cornea and

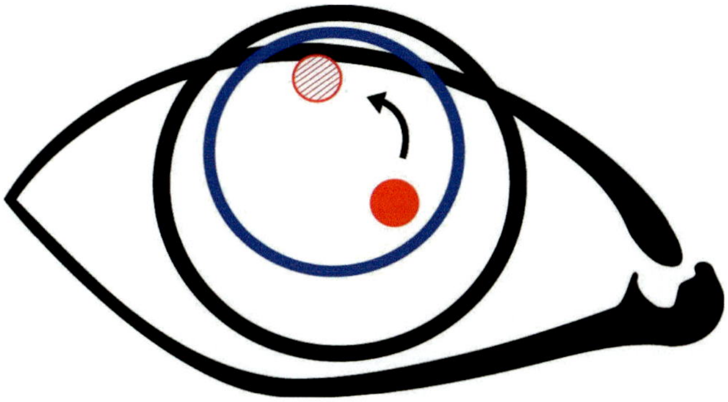

Fig. 1 Ipsilateral rotational autologous penetrating keratoplasty (schematic). First, an eccentric trephination is performed, with the keratoplasty central corneal opacity (*red, full*) situated at the edge of the excision margin (*blue*). Secondly, the corneal button is rotated (*arrow*), bringing clear cornea towards the visual axis, and the scar (*red, diagonal pattern*) in the direction of the limbus. If possible, the corneal opacity should be rotated under the upper lid in order to reduce postoperative glare and achieve a more favourable visual result

the excision edge. These two factors are critical for achieving the largest clear optical zone possible after rotation. To ensure a lower postoperative keratometric astigmatism and better postoperative visual acuity, the opacity should preoperatively not extend by more than 20% of the corneal diameter beyond the centre of the cornea, providing a postoperative clear optical zone of at least 30% of the corneal diameter [11].

Clinically, it must be taken into consideration that involvement of the limbus causes stress on the angle structures with a higher risk of developing secondary glaucoma [17] and increases the likelihood of corneal vascularisation. In addition, sutures near the limbus have a tendency to loosen and induce corneal epithelial defects or infectious keratitis if left undetected. For this reason, interrupted 10–0 nylon sutures should usually be used [17]. However, interrupted sutures are associated with a lower topographic regularity and a later visual rehabilitation in comparison to the double cross-stitch suture according to Hoffmann [18, 19].

Ipsilateral rotational APK is especially beneficial for patients at high risk of immunological reactions, as well as those who are difficult to control, treat, and/or comply with topical medication (e.g. paediatric patients). In fact, ipsilateral rotational APK should be considered in all patients with a central non-progressive corneal opacity, in whom the risk of graft failure can be considerably reduced due to the lack of immunological reactions, provided that the patient is willing to accept the inconvenience of a relatively lower postoperative visual acuity, typically requiring contact lens fitting, in exchange for this benefit [20].

Ipsilateral rotational APK indeed results in lower postoperative visual acuity compared to HPK due to higher and more irregular postoperative refractive and keratometric astigmatism. This is attributed to the eccentric trephination with proximity of one edge to the visual axis, and to the rotation of the autograft, taking the disparity of the paracentral and peripheral corneal thickness as well as the

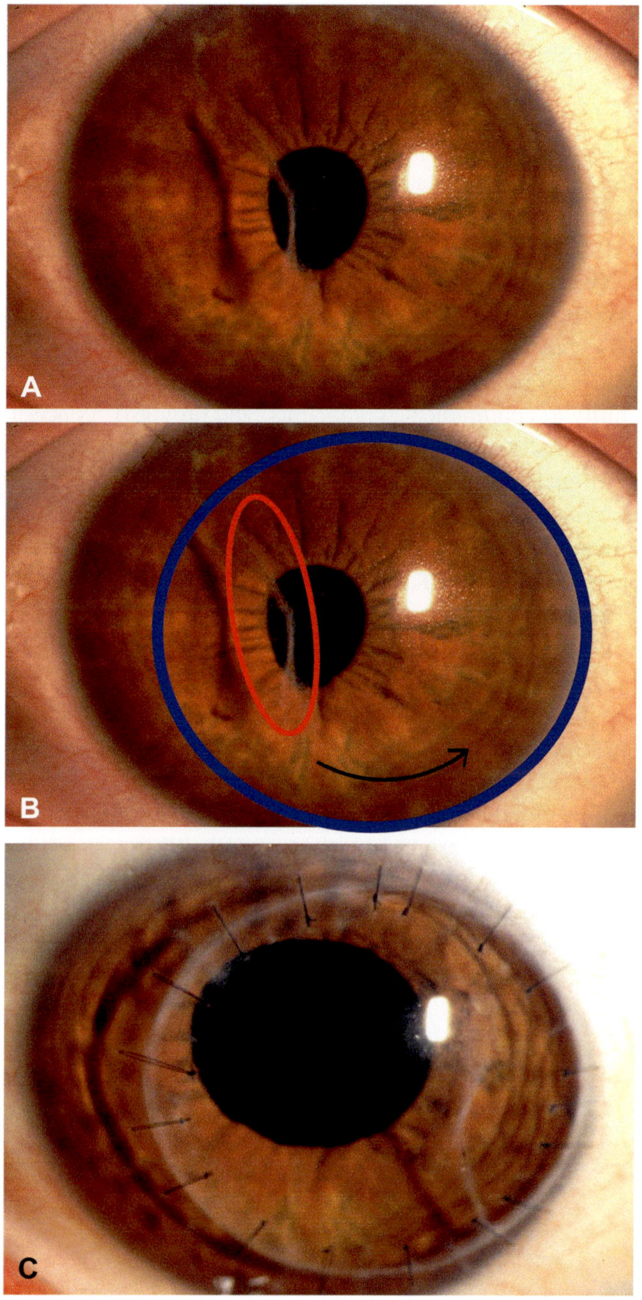

Fig. 2 Ipsilateral rotational autologous penetrating keratoplasty. (**A**) Clinical presentation of an eye with a (para)central stromal corneal scar. (**B**) Schematic representation of the planned ipsilateral rotational autologous penetrating keratoplasty, with the (para)central corneal opacity (*red*) situated at the edge of the eccentric trephination margin (*blue*). The corneal button is then to be rotated (*arrow*). (**C**) Postoperative clinical presentation, with clear cornea at the visual axis and with the stromal corneal scar being located in the mid-periphery

different central, paracentral and peripheral corneal topography (respectively spherical, ellipsoidal and parabolic) into account [6]. The latter is also the underlying cause of the often reported contact lens intolerance.

The eccentric trephination with one edge close to the limbus also enhances the risk of anterior synechiae, which has been found to increase the overall risk of graft failure [21].

Notwithstanding the restricted visual potential, ipsilateral rotational APK is still indicated for young infants and toddlers with central corneal opacities. In these young patients, the risk of immune reactions is high and patient cooperation (ability to communicate complaints) and prognosis concerning clear allograft survival is poorer the earlier the surgery is performed [22]. On the other hand, keratoplasty should be performed quickly to reduce the risk of amblyopia ("as early as necessary, but as late as possible") [22]. Indeed, with ipsilateral rotational APK, a prompt (because no donor material is required) and long lasting (because of the expected clear survival of the autograft without risk of immune reactions) therapy against amblyopia can be accomplished. This precise therapeutic outcome after APK may outweigh the limited functional outcomes after HPK in young children who are difficult to treat and in whom the allograft is likely to become cloudy within a short time, despite the limited visual outcomes of ipsilateral rotational APK [9].

3 Contralateral Autologous Penetrating Keratoplasty

In more particular clinical presentations with a central corneal opacity in a functionally better (best) eye with good visual prognosis ("oculus unicus functionalis "), a contralateral APK could be a potential surgical alternative. During this procedure, a clear cornea from a (nearly) blind eye affected by a non-corneal pathology—such as amblyopia or retinal disease—is transplanted into the potentially better-seeing eye affected by a corneal pathology.

As part of a contralateral APK, an HPK has to be performed first in the (almost) blind donor eye in order to obtain the autologous clear graft, which is temporarily preserved on a viscoelastic bed or alternatively in an eye bank preservation medium in a sterile environment until the HPK is completed. After watertight closure of the partner eye with HPK, the APK is completed (Fig. 3).

Because of the double conducted keratoplasty, many benefits of ipsilateral rotational APK no longer apply to contralateral APK. Indeed, contralateral APK still requires donor material and still necessitates regular follow-up examinations.

This is however not the case for a specific subtype of contralateral APK, in which both corneas (from the right and left eye) are autologously switched (to the left and right eye, respectively) (Fig. 4). In theory, this contralateral bilateral APK can only be performed when the eye affected by the non-corneal pathology has no remaining visual acuity (nulla lux) and no visual prognosis. In practice, this method is rarely used because of the obligatory prolonged intraoperative open-sky situation in one eye.

In a second specific subtype of contralateral APK, as an alternative to bilateral contralateral APK, the contralateral blind eye is enucleated, after which its cornea is used for autologous penetrating keratoplasty on the fellow eye affected by a corneal pathology, with better visual potential [23] (Fig. 5).

Postoperative astigmatism and visual acuity after contralateral APK are, due to the central position of the corneal graft, comparable to that achieved after HPK and better than after ipsilateral rotational APK.

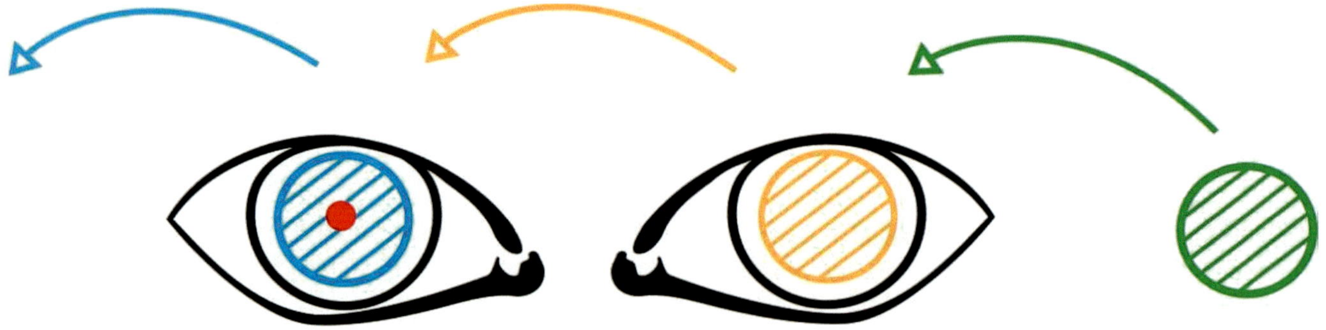

Fig. 3 Contralateral autologous penetrating keratoplasty (APK). First, homologous penetrating keratoplasty (HPK) (*green*) is first conducted in the nearly blind donor eye affected by a non-corneal pathology. The removed clear cornea (*orange*) is temporarily preserved as an autologous graft in a sterile environment. In a second step, the autograft (*orange*) is then transplanted into the potentially better-seeing eye affected by a corneal pathology (*blue*, *opacity red*). The excised corneal tissue is transferred for histological evaluation (*blue arrow*)

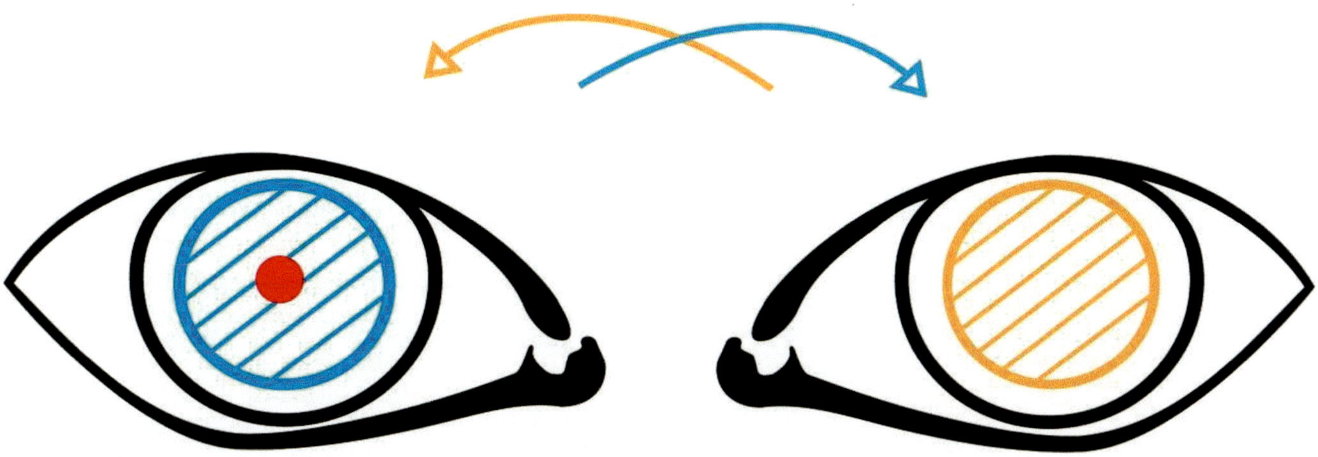

Fig. 4 Bilateral contralateral autologous penetrating keratoplasty (APK). Both the opacified (*red*) cornea (*blue*) of the potentially better-seeing eye and the clear cornea (*orange*) of the blind eye are autologously exchanged. This technique unfortunately involves an obligatory prolonged open-sky situation in one (the blind) eye

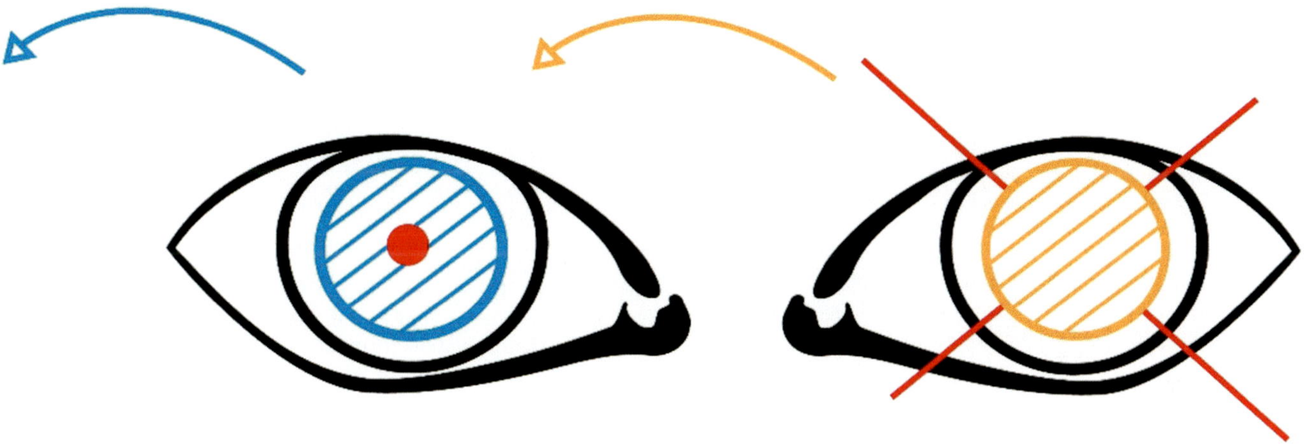

Fig. 5 Contralateral autologous penetrating keratoplasty (APK) after enucleation of the autologous donor eye. A blind eye (with no visual prognosis) with non-corneal pathology is enucleated (*red cross*), after which its clear cornea (*orange*) is employed for autologous penetrating keratoplasty on the fellow eye affected by a corneal pathology (*blue*, *opacity red*), with better visual potential. The excised corneal tissue is transferred for histological evaluation (*blue arrow*)

4 Conclusion

In light of the aforementioned higher keratometric astigmatism and lower postoperative visual acuity that typically requires contact lens fitting, *ipsilateral rotational APK* should be reserved for patients with an increased risk of immunological reactions and poor controllability, treatability and/or compliance with topical medications (e.g. paediatric patients). Furthermore, it can be a preferred option in unconventional clinical situations with either shortage of donor material or without the possibility of regular postoperative follow-ups, e.g. in developing countries with scarceness of ophthalmologists [20].

Compared with the larger number of ipsilateral rotational APK conducted, the discussed contralateral variant constitutes a rather uncommon alternative due to the unusual initial clinical presentation required for surgical indication. Nevertheless, *contralateral APK* should be the preferred operation in these particular unconventional clinical situations for patients with (1) corneal opacity in the potentially better seeing eye and (2) a clear cornea in the fellow eye with poor or no visual acuity and prognosis, especially in patients with a greater risk of graft rejection, i.e. for "high-risk" corneas ($\geq$ 2 times previously grafted and/or corneas with $\geq$ 2 quadrants of vascularisation), given the otherwise high failure rate after conventional HPK [20].

The option of an ipsilateral rotational and contralateral autologous keratoplasty should always be considered in particular clinical situations before corneal microsurgeons move on to homologous keratoplasty straight away [20].

References

1. Zirm E. A successful total keratoplasty. Graefes Arch Clin Exp Ophthalmol. 1906;64:580–93.
2. Akhmedova E, Goebels S, Löw U, Bauer F, Szentmáry N, Seitz B. Autologous contralateral keratoplasty in a patient with disciform herpetic corneal scar and contralateral macular toxoplasmotic scar. Klin Monbl Augenheilkd. 2015;232(6):785–7. https://doi.org/10.1055/s-0034-1396177.
3. Seitz B, Langenbucher A, Küchle M, Naumann GOH. Impact of graft diameter on corneal power and the regularity of post-keratoplasty astigmatism before and after suture removal. Ophthalmology. 2003;110(11):2162–7. https://doi.org/10.1016/S0161-6420(03)00659-6.
4. Hill JC. High risk corneal grafting. Br J Ophthalmol. 2002;86(9):945. https://doi.org/10.1136/bjo.86.9.945.
5. Khodadoust AA. The allograft rejection reaction: the leading cause of late graft failure of clinical corneal grafts. In: Porter R, Knight J, editors. Corneal graft failure. Amsterdam: Elsevier; 1973. p. 151–64.
6. Jonas JB, Rank RM, Budde WM. Autologous ipsilateral rotating penetrating keratoplasty. Am J Ophthalmol. 2001;131(4):427–30. https://doi.org/10.1016/s0002-9394(00)00857-6.
7. Bertelmann E, Hartmann C, Scherer M, Rieck P. Outcome of rotational keratoplasty: comparison of endothelial cell loss in autografts vs allografts. Arch Ophthalmol. 2004;122:1437–40. https://doi.org/10.1001/archopht.122.10.1437.
8. Reinhard T, Böhringer D, Hüschen D, Sundmacher R. Chronic endothelial cell loss of the graft after penetrating keratoplasty: influence of endothelial cell migration from graft to host. Klin Monbl Augenheilkd. 2002;219(6):410–6. https://doi.org/10.1055/s-2002-32876.
9. Birnbaum F, Reinhard T, Ulbricht T, Hausser J, Sundmacher R. Functional results after autologous rotational keratoplasty. A retrospective study. Ophthalmologe. 2004;101(1):54–8. https://doi.org/10.1007/s00347-003-0876-1.
10. Belmont SC, Zimm JL, Storch RL, Draga A, Troutman RC. Astigmatism after penetrating keratoplasty using the Krumeich guided trephine system. Refract Corneal Surg. 1993;9(4):250–4.
11. Jonas JB, Panda-Jonas S. Calculation of size and location of autologous ipsilateral rotating keratoplasty. Graefes Arch Clin Exp Ophthalmol. 1994;232:538–44. https://doi.org/10.1007/BF00181997.
12. Seitz B, Langenbucher A, Kus MM, Küchle M, Naumann GOH. Nonmechanical corneal trephination with the excimer laser improves outcome after penetrating keratoplasty. Ophthalmology. 1999;106(6):1156–65. https://doi.org/10.1016/S0161-6420(99)90265-8.
13. Szentmáry N, Langenbucher A, Naumann GOH, Seitz B. Intra-individual variability of penetrating keratoplasty outcome after excimer laser versus motorized corneal trephination. J Refract Surg. 2006;22(8):804–10.
14. Seitz B, Langenbucher A, Naumann GOH. Astigmatism in keratoplasty. In: Seiler T, editor. Refraktive Chirurgie. Enke: Stuttgart; 2000. p. 197–252.
15. Tóth G, Szentmáry N, Langenbucher A, Akhmedova E, El-Husseiny M, Seitz B. Comparison of excimer laser versus femtosecond laser assisted trephination in penetrating keratoplasty: a retrospective study. Adv Ther. 2019;36(12):3471–82. https://doi.org/10.1007/s12325-019-01120-3.
16. Kraupa E. Transposition durch Lappendrehung, eine neue Methode der Keratoplastik. Zentralbl Ges Ophthalmol. 1914;1:132–3.
17. Panda A, Sudan R, Nainiwal S. Autologous ipsilateral rotating penetrating keratoplasty. Am J Ophthalmol. 2002;133(4):590; author reply 590–1. https://doi.org/10.1016/s0002-9394(01)01413-1.
18. Seitz B, Langenbucher A, Naumann GOH. The penetrating keratoplasty. A 100-year success story. Ophthalmologe. 2005;102(12):1128–6, 1138–9. https://doi.org/10.1007/s00347-005-1291-6.
19. Seitz B, Szentmáry N, El-Husseiny M, Viestenz A, Langenbucher A, Naumann GOH. The penetrating keratoplasty (PKP): a century of success. In: Hjortdal J, editor. Corneal Transplantation. Cham, Switzerland: Springer; 2016. p. 69–92.
20. Quintin A, Serfözö A, Daas L, Suffo S, Seitz B. Autologous contralateral and ipsilateral rotational penetrating keratoplasty—a case series and mini-review. Klin Monbl Augenheilkd 2025;242(1):52–61.
21. Martinez JD, Galor A, Perez VL, Karp CL, Yoo SH, Alfonso EC. Endothelial graft failure after contralateral autologous corneal transplantation. Cornea. 2013;32(6):745–50. https://doi.org/10.1097/ICO.0b013e31826dff17.
22. Seitz B, Hager T, Szentmáry N, Langenbucher A, Naumann GOH. Keratoplasty in children–still a dilemma. Klin Monbl Augenheilkd. 2013;230(6):587–94. https://doi.org/10.1055/s-0032-1328653.
23. Onishchenko AL, Kolbasko AV, Tatarnikova GN, Mamontova ÉG. Urgent therapeutic penetrating autokeratoplasty for a purulent corneal ulcer in the only functional eye. Vestn Oftalmol. 2014;130(4):68–70.

EDTA Chelating for Corneal Calcific Band Keratopathy and Calcareous Corneal Degeneration

Elias Flockerzi, Loay Daas, and Berthold Seitz

Abstract

This chapter summarizes the topic of corneal calcifications and their treatment. Corneal calcifications occur mainly after chronic intraocular inflammation. They can be located superficially in the sense of a corneal calcific band keratopathy. The standard treatment consists of the abrasion of the epithelium and a combination of Ethylene-Diamine-Tetraacetic Acid (EDTA) chelation and mechanical debridement. Phototherapeutic keratectomy can be added to further smoothen the corneal surface. Pancorneal calcifications are rare, but have been described in the context of the so-called calcareous corneal degeneration, which requires penetrating keratoplasty for complete removal and visual rehabilitation.

Keywords

Corneal calcific band keratopathy · Calcification · EDTA · Calcareous corneal degeneration

1 Introduction

Ethylene-Diamine-Tetraacetic Acid (EDTA) was first discovered and synthesized by the Austrian chemist Ferdinand Münz in 1935 as a substitute for citric acid to reduce Germany's dependency on the import of foreign chemicals [1]. In 1952, the chemist and ophthalmologist Morton W. Grant from Massachusetts reported "a clinically useful method for dissolving calcific corneal opacities by means of a solution of the neutral sodium salt of ethylenediaminetetraacetic acid" [2]. Since that time, EDTA chelation has become the standard treatment of corneal calcifications. When considering corneal calcifications, there exist two entities that have to be differentiated: (1) corneal calcific band keratopathy (BK) and (2) calcareous corneal degeneration (CCD).

2 Corneal Calcific Band Keratopathy (BK)

Corneal calcific BK was first described by Dixon in 1848 [3] and remains an issue until nowadays in daily ophthalmologic practice. It designates (sub-)epithelial calcium deposits within the human cornea, that descend to the Bowman layer and the superficial corneal stroma [3, 4]. Although a few rare cases of inherited forms have been described [5, 6], most cases have been reported following chronic ocular inflammation or systemic hypercalcemia [3]. Corneal calcific BK has also been characterized as the end product of a large number of inflammatory and degenerative processes within the cornea or even the whole eye [4]. The mechanism of developing BK has been investigated in different studies including animal models. An experimental rabbit model published in 1969 reported that a combination of inducing uveitis by injecting ovalbumin into the vitreous and vitamin D intoxication resulted in BK [7]. Surgical closure of the rabbits' eyelids, however, prevented the formation of BK [7]. Up to nowadays, the mechanism of BK formation has been hypothesized to consist of multiple minor milieu changes including (1) an increased water evaporation from the surface of the eye and (2) a loss of carbon dioxide (CO_2) resulting in (3) a secondary hyperosmolarity, (4) an increasing pH value and (5) increasing levels of calcium and phosphate concentration in the interpalpebral area of the cornea [3, 4, 7]. It has also been reported in line with these hypotheses, that BK develops

E. Flockerzi (✉) · L. Daas · B. Seitz
Department of Ophthalmology, Saarland University Medical Center, Homburg, Germany
e-mail: elias.flockerzi@uks.eu

B. Seitz et al. (eds.), *Atlas on Cornea*, https://doi.org/10.1007/978-3-031-65422-0_59

more frequently in dry eye patients [3, 8]. In addition, damage to the corneal endothelium seems also to play a role in the development of BK: Another rabbit model showed that BK developed after damaging the corneal endothelium with potassium permanganate [9].

Corneal calcific BK typically develops in a centripetal manner extending from the periphery of the interpalpebral part of the cornea towards the corneal center (Fig. 1).

A remaining clear zone between the limbus and the calcifications might be attributable to the limbal vascularization that is assumed to clear higher calcium concentrations [4] (Fig. 2).

Diseases associated with BK include ocular diseases on the one hand, but also systemic diseases associated with a disturbance of the calcium-phosphate balance on the other. Ocular diseases associated with BK include recurrent corneal ulcers (Fig. 3A), chemical burns, uveitis and phthisis bulbi (Fig. 3B) [3].

In addition to the documented association with chronic ocular inflammation, there exist also series of case reports that suggest a connection with substances applied onto or introduced into the eye. First, BK development has been reported to be a possible adverse effect of topical steroid-phosphate or phosphate buffered hyaluronate preparations applied in form of eyedrops [10–12]. Second, another rabbit model reported that nine of 19 eyes developed BK after injection of chondroitin sulfate-sodium hyaluronate (Viscoat®, Alcon Deutschland GmbH, Freiburg, Germany) in the anterior chamber [13] and third, BK has been attributed to silicone oil instilled into the eye after retinal detachment, touching the endothelium, thus reducing fluid flow across the cornea and therefore inducing pH changes [14].

If BK already manifests itself in childhood, juvenile rheumatoid arthritis (Morbus Still) is likely to be the cause [4]. It is also associated with rheumatoid arthritis in adults, sarcoidosis and diseases that go along with hypercalcemia as primary hyperparathyroidism, nephrocalcinosis or vitamin D intoxication [4]. Therefore, serum calcium or phosphate levels should be determined in unclear cases or in cases of frequent recurrences [15]. An adjustment of serum levels by medication or diet, however, does not lead to the regression of corneal deposits [3]. One study reported that the most commonly identified underlying diagnosis of developing BK in 24 of 89 cases was long-term topical glaucoma therapy [16]. Another study investigated the underlying causes of BK in 286 eyes of 230 patients and concluded that the most common causes were chronic corneal edema (n = 80), idiopathic BK (n = 74), phthisis bulbi (n = 47), herpes simplex or herpes zoster (n = 26), chronic uveitis (n = 19), trauma (n = 11), end stage renal disease (ESRD, n = 9), chronic corneal ulcers (n = 6) and chemical burn (n = 6) [15].

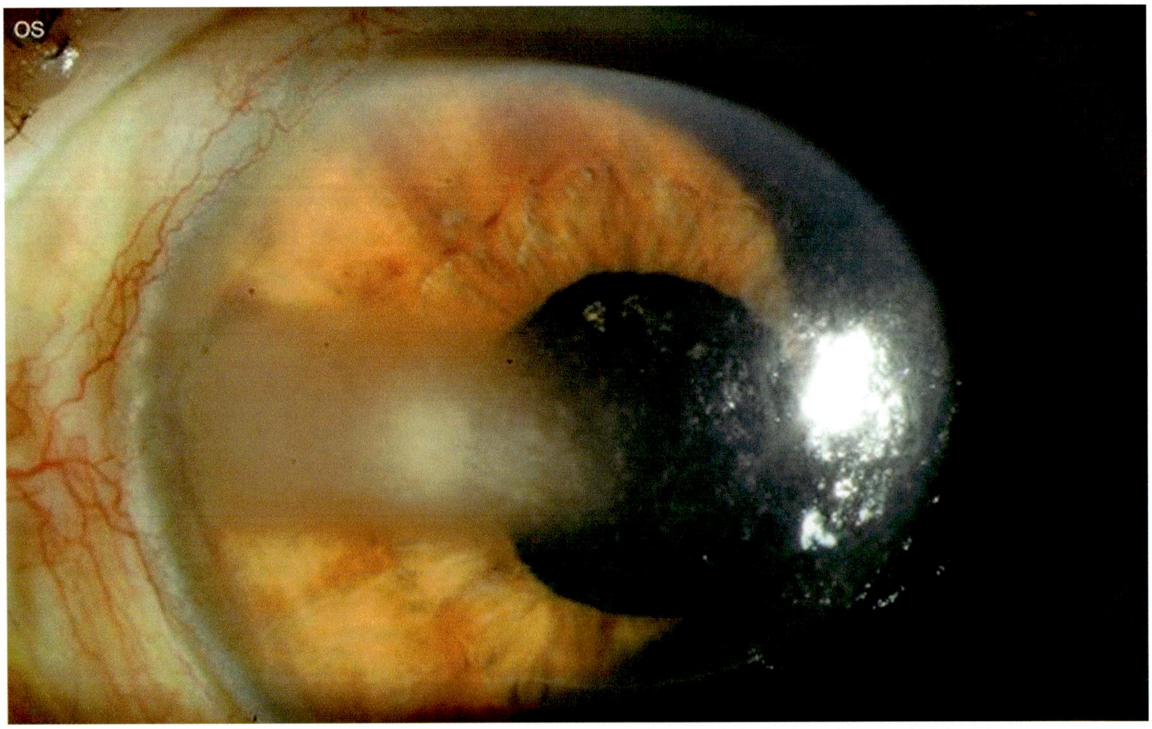

Fig. 1 Corneal calcific band keratopathy developing in a centripetal manner from the periphery of the interpalpebral part of the cornea towards its center. Right eye of an 84-year-old female pseudophakic patient with proliferative diabetic retinopathy

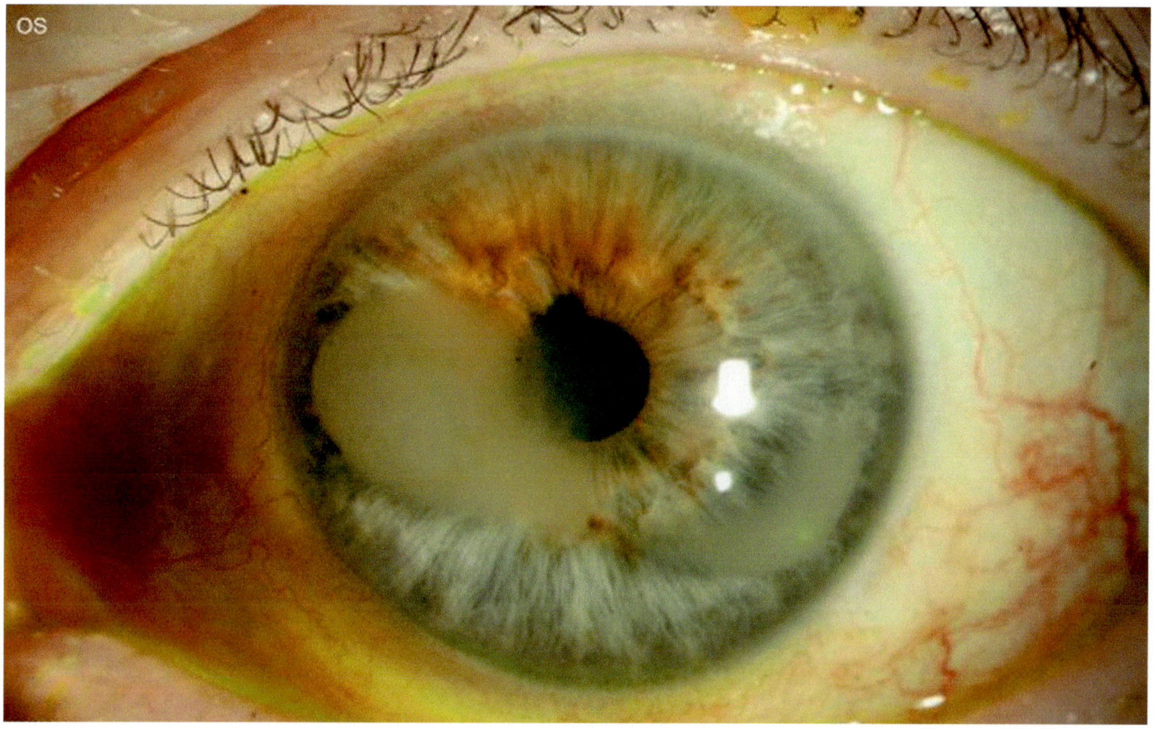

Fig. 2 Remaining clear zone between the limbus and the calcifications and centripetal development in corneal calcific band keratopathy. Left eye of a 78-year-old male phakic patient with non-proliferative diabetic retinopathy

Because renal diseases are closely linked to disturbances of the electrolyte balance and often go along with elevated serum phosphate levels, ESRD patients have been reported to be 11.56 times more likely to develop BK than others [17].

The main indications for surgical treatment of BK are visual impairment and mechanical irritation with foreign body sensation because of recurrent corneal erosions (Fig. 4A) and erupting calcification fragments (Fig. 4B).

Surgical options include (1) mechanical debridement after superficial keratectomy, (2) mechanical debridement after superficial keratectomy in combination with EDTA chelation, (3) EDTA chelation after superficial keratectomy in combination with phototherapeutic keratectomy or amniotic membrane transplantation [3] and (4) EDTA chelation after lifting an epithelial flap using 19% ethanol solution as used in laser-assisted subepithelial keratectomy (LASEK) in refractive surgery [18]. We recommend the abrasion of the epithelium and a combination of EDTA chelation and mechanical debridement using a forceps or surgical blade, which is the standard therapy in our ophthalmologic department with an estimated duration of surgery of 10 to 15 minutes. This is slightly shorter compared to a mean surgery duration of 20 min reported in literature and a range from 10 to 45 minutes [16]. After topical anaesthesia, a lid speculum is inserted and the corneal epithelium is removed using a Hockey knife. Then, EDTA is applied on the cornea using surgical sponges soaked in EDTA. Postoperative treatment includes a bandage contact lens for one to two weeks, topical unpreserved antibiotics and artificial tears without phosphate buffers (Fig. 5A, B).

It has also been suggested to perform the treatment via phototherapeutic keratectomy. Smooth BK has been reported to be treated with phototherapeutic keratectomy without abrasion of the epithelium whilst phototherapeutic keratectomy was preceded by mechanical removal of calcified plaques in rough BK [19]. However, the authors plead for dividing the surgical treatment of corneal calcific BK into different steps by using the different and most appropriate tools in each step: Thus, the calcifications are first exposed by superficial keratectomy, then removed with EDTA and finally—if necessary—the cornea is smoothened by phototherapeutic keratectomy. When performing phototherapeutic keratectomy, it has to be kept in mind that it may go along with a hyperopic shift and that it did not show superiority over other treatment options in terms of preventing BK recurrence [3]. Data on recurrence rates vary, which is also attributable to the inconsistent definition of recurrence, which sometimes designates a BK stage that requires a new treatment. From this point of

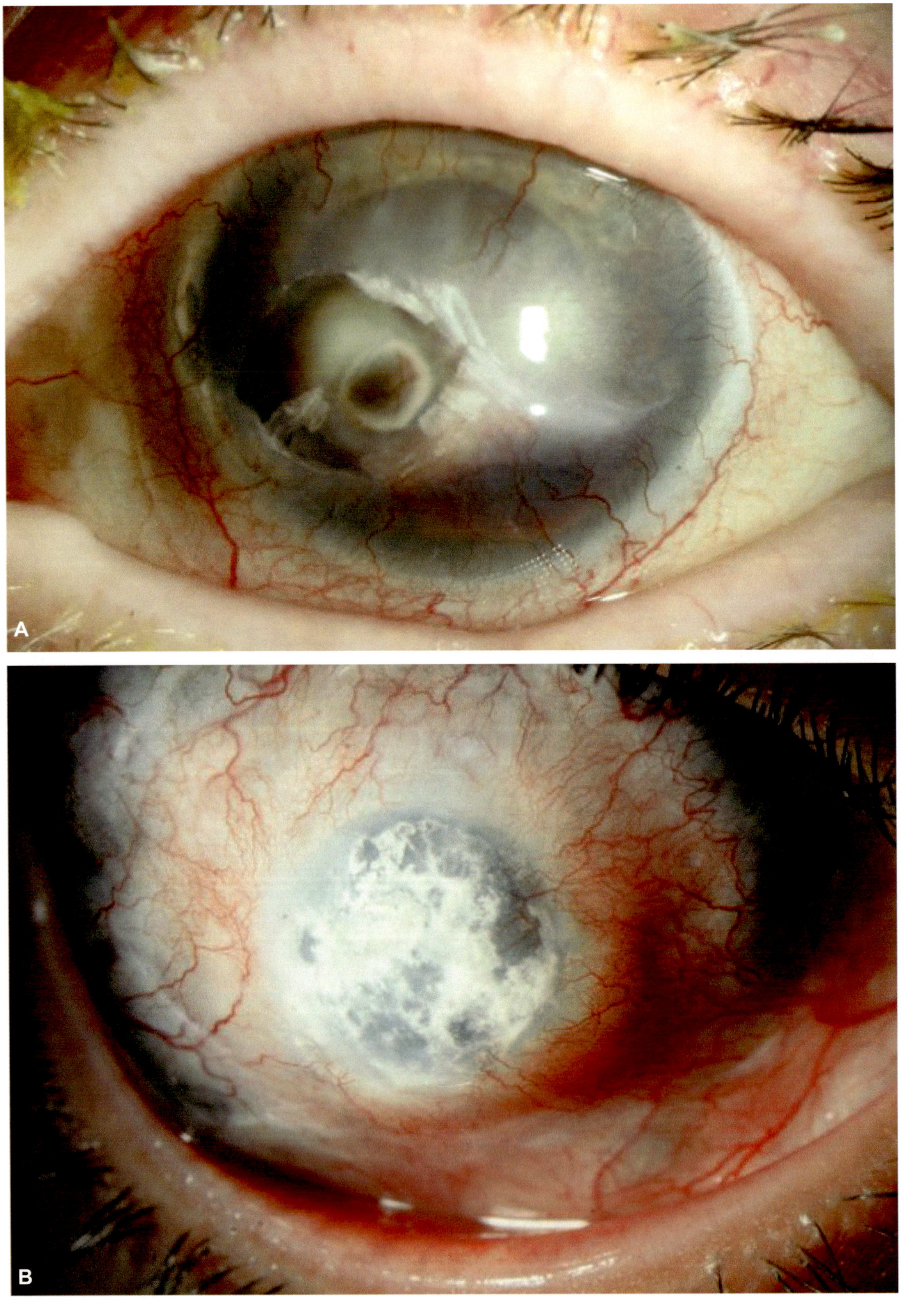

Fig. 3 Ocular diseases associated with corneal calcific band keratopathy include recurrent corneal ulcers (**A**) and phthisis bulbi (still large bulbus in this case because of former buphthalmos, (**B**). (**A**) left eye of a 93-year-old female phakic patient with primary open angle glaucoma and perforated herpetic ulcer under bandage contact lens after recurrent herpetic keratitis. (**B**) right eye of a 24-year-old male aphakic patient after repeated penetrating keratoplasties and vitrectomies because of initially penetrating ocular trauma

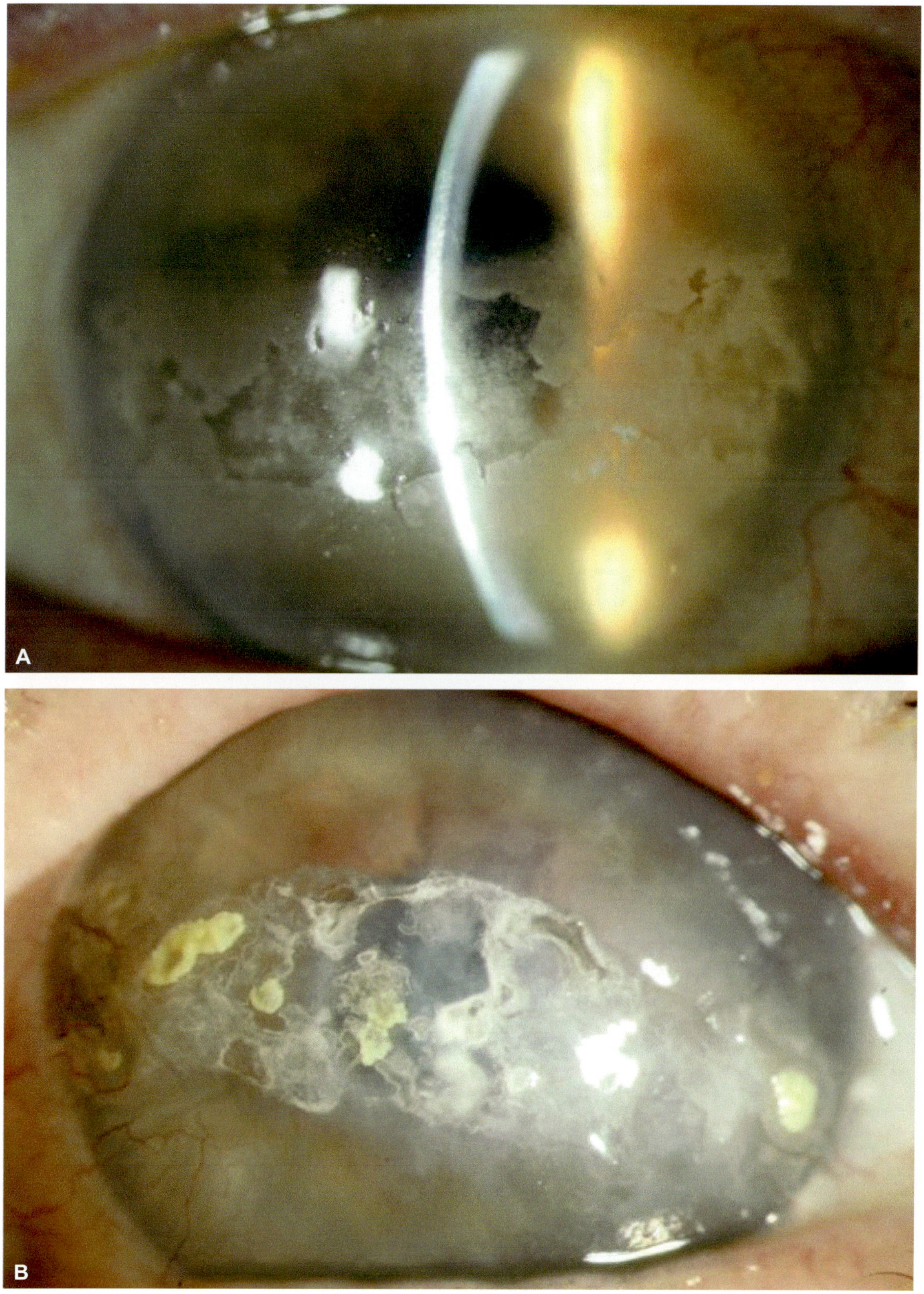

Fig. 4 Main indications for surgical treatment are visual impairment and mechanical irritation from recurrent erosions (**A**) or erupting calcification fragments (**B**). (**A**) right eye of a 72-year-old female pseudophakic patient with proliferative diabetic retinopathy, Fuchs endothelial corneal dystrophy and primary open angle glaucoma. (**B**) left eye of an 88-year-old female pseudophakic patient with Fuchs endothelial corneal dystrophy, Retinitis pigmentosa and secondary open angle glaucoma because of pseudoexfoliation syndrome

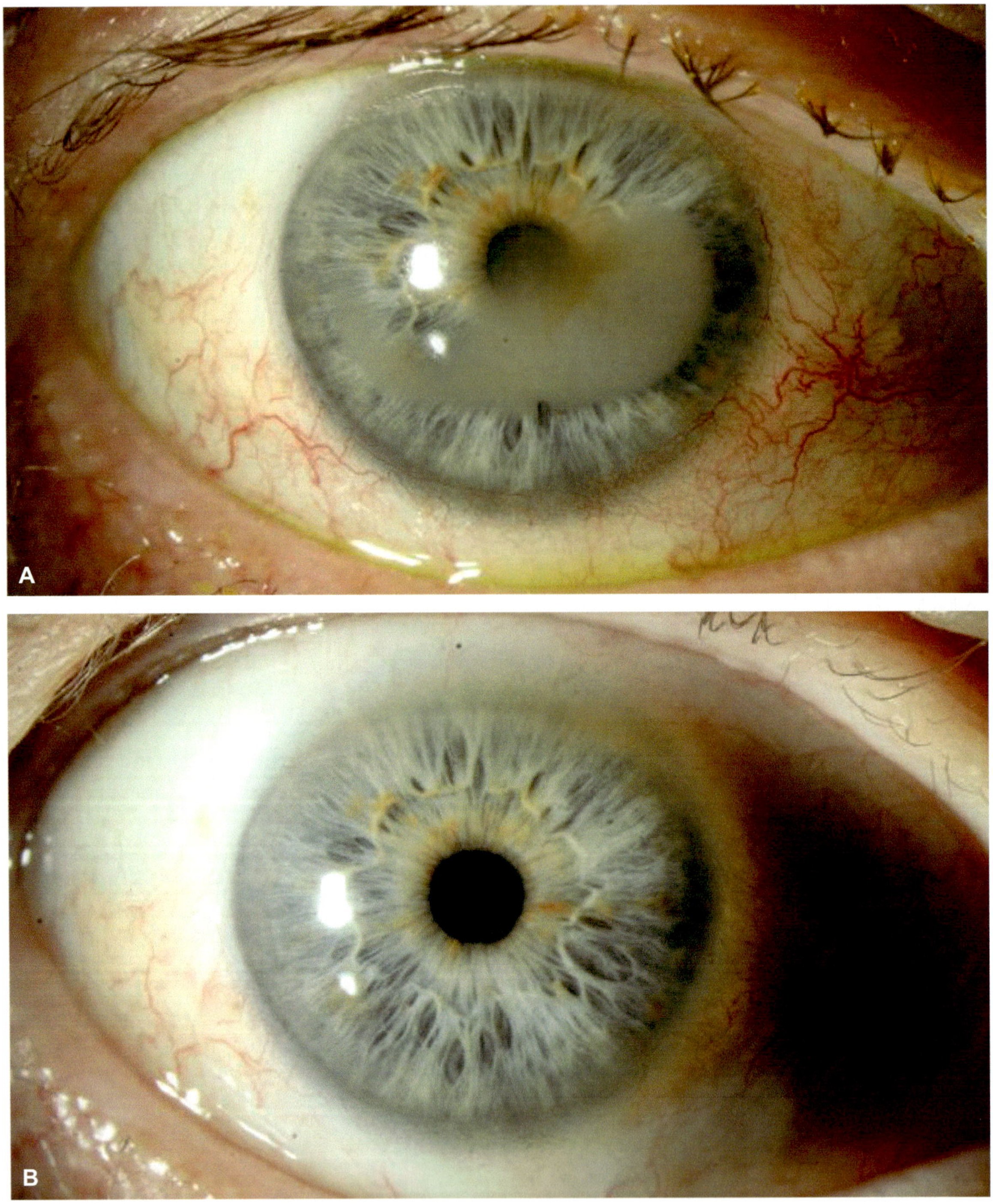

Fig. 5 (**A**) Calcific corneal band keratopathy in a right eye of a 77-year-old male phakic patient without ocular diseases. (**B**) clear cornea six months after epithelial abrasion and EDTA-chelation

view, recurrence rates range from 4.5% [16] to 17.8% [3]. However, there is consent that the highest recurrence rate occurs in eyes that are filled with silicone oil permanently [3]. The simultaneous amniotic membrane transplantation as patch may be useful in cases of delayed epithelial healing such as limbal stem cell deficiency after chemical burns (Fig. 6A, B, C).

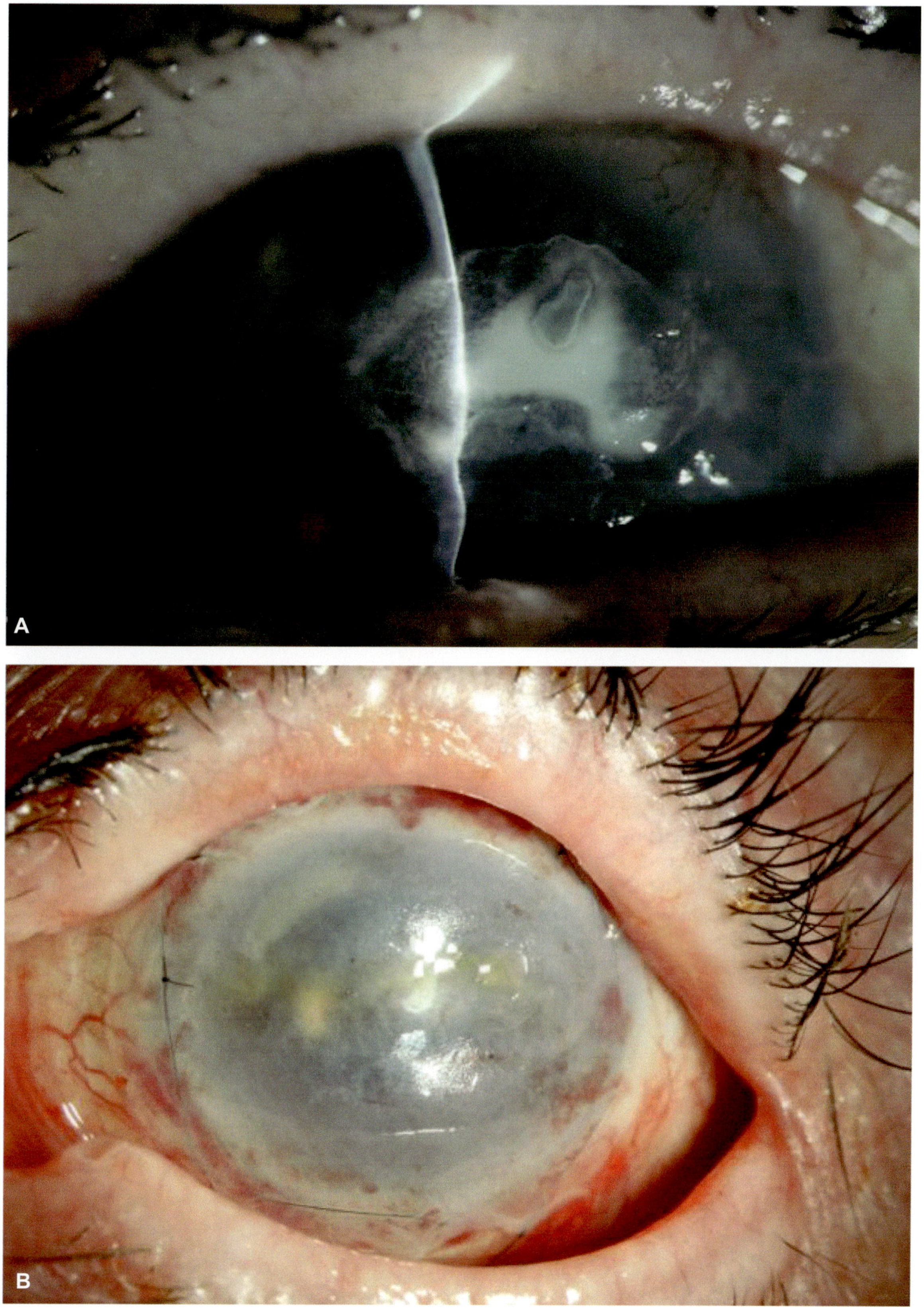

Fig. 6 (**A**) corneal calcific band keratopathy in the left eye of an 84-year-old female pseudophakic patient with primary open angle glaucoma and dry age-related macular degeneration. (**B**) first day after surgery including (1) superficial keratectomy, (2) EDTA-chelation, (3) mechanical debridement using forceps and surgical blades, (4) phototherapeutic keratectomy (20 μm without and 30 μm with masking fluid over 10 mm in diameter), (5) amniotic membrane transplantation as patch (15 mm in diameter, fixed with 10–0 nylon suture) and (6) bandage contact lens (**C**)

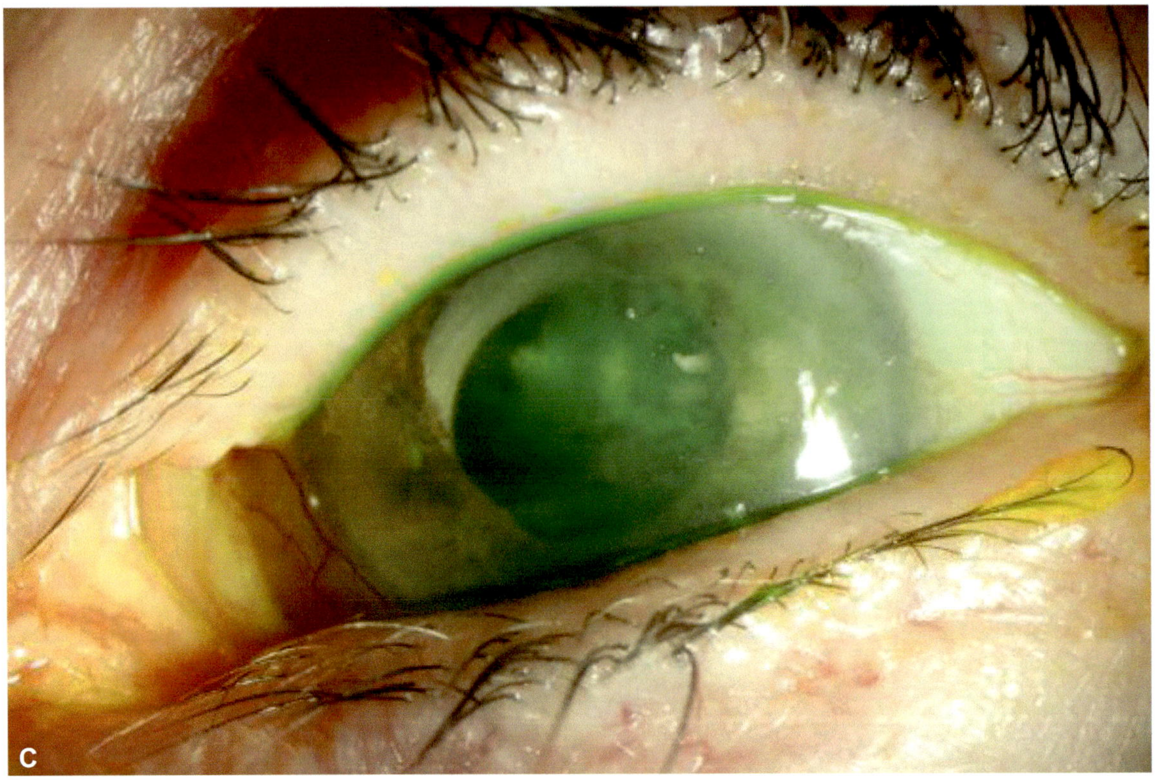

Fig. 6 (**C**) postoperative finding after complete epithelialization

3 Calcareous Corneal Degeneration (CCD)

Calcareous corneal degeneration (CCD) represents another entity that has to be differentiated from BK. It is characterized by the affection of deeper layers of the cornea and also intraocular bone formation [4]. The calcifications extend throughout the whole corneal stroma down to the Descemet membrane resulting in a pancorneal extracellular calcium deposition [8] requiring penetrating keratoplasty for complete removal [20]. Reports of bilateral cases exist and it has been associated with persistent epithelial defects, severe keratoconjunctivitis sicca, chronic keratoconjunctivitis [21], alkali burns (Fig. 7), necrotizing intraocular tumors, in a post-traumatic sequela and in patients with severe acquired immunodeficiency syndrome [8]. Nevertheless, CCD and BK may coexist, which implicates that they both have a common underlying pathogenic mechanism [22] that may be summarized as follows: Mild and chronic corneal injury may lead to BK whereas severe and multifactorial corneal injuries may lead to a pancorneal full-thickness calcium deposition [22].

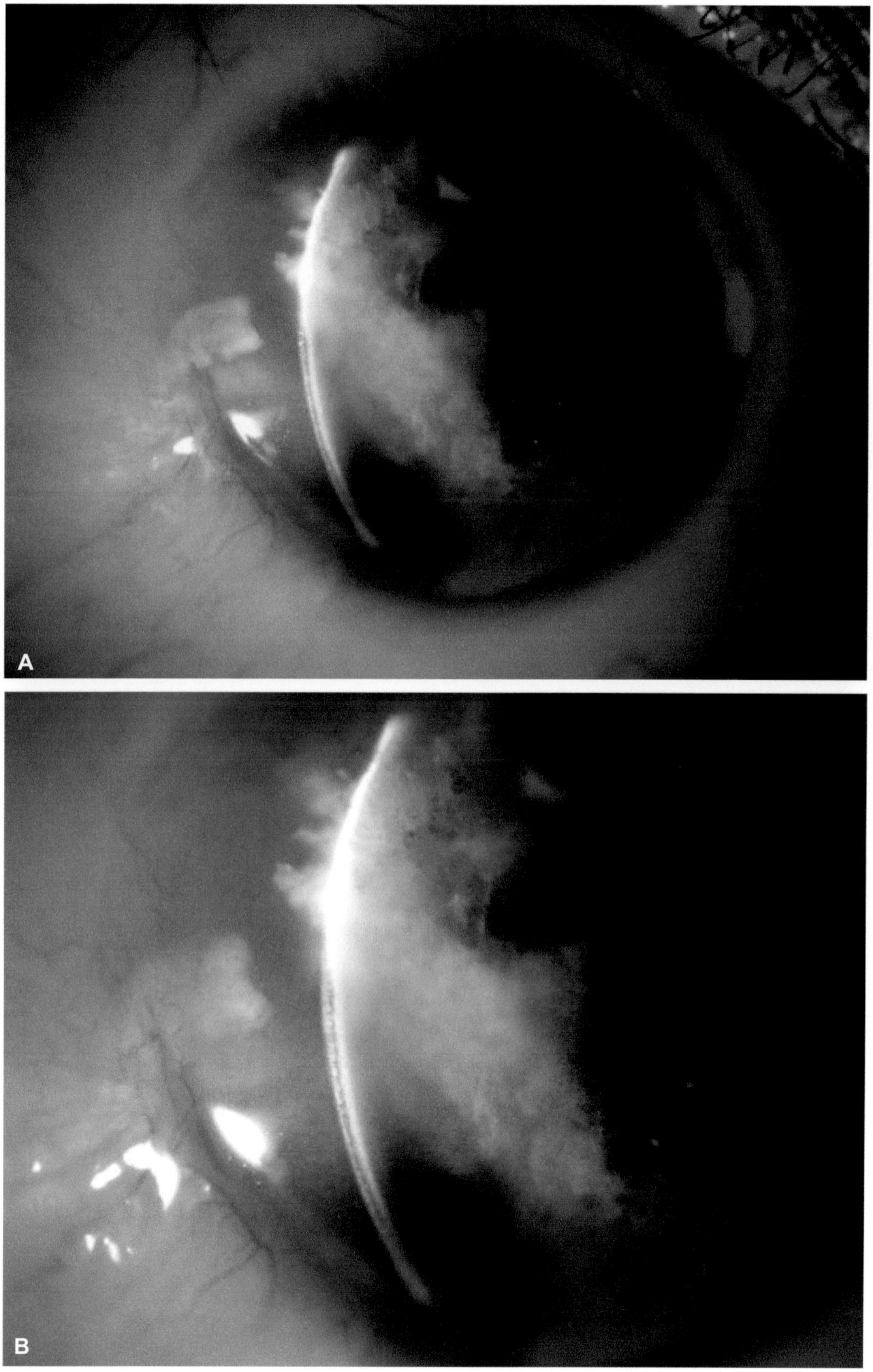

Fig. 7 Calcareous corneal degeneration in the right eye of a 41-year-old male phakic patient 13 years after alkali burn. (**A**) slit lamp photograph showing superficial calcifications in the upper part and clear epithelium and anterior stroma with deep stromal calcification layer in the lower part. (**B**), magnification of (A).

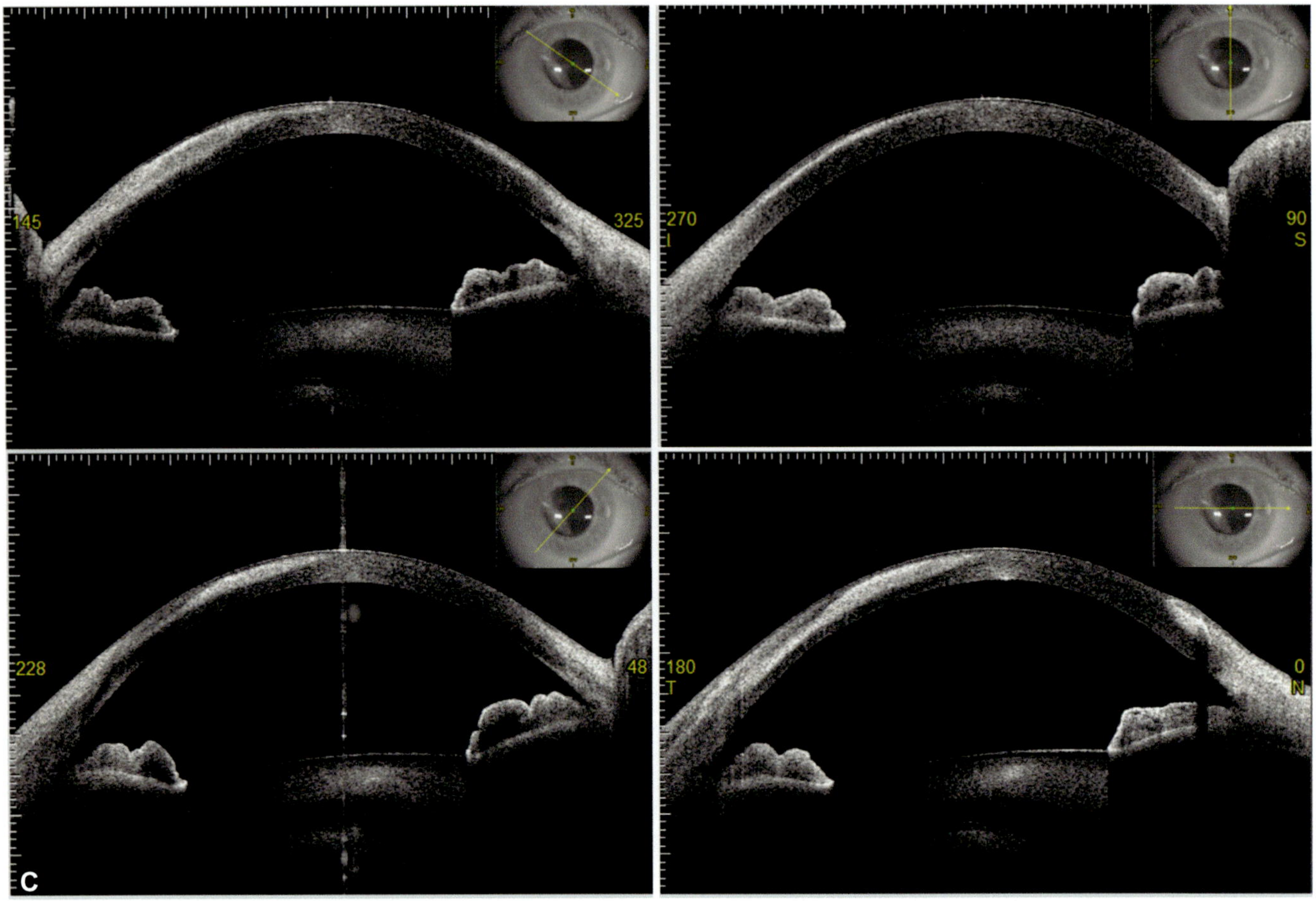

Fig. 7 (**C**) anterior segment optical coherence tomography (Casia 2®, Tomey, Nagoya, Japan) showing a subepithelial and intrastromal calcification layer

4 Conclusion

The differential diagnosis of corneal calcifications includes corneal calcific band keratopathy and calcareous corneal degeneration. Corneal calcific band keratopathy is by far the more common entity. It is located superficially, easily amenable to treatment with epithelial abrasion and EDTA-chelation but sometimes tends to recur. Calcareous corneal degeneration is much rarer, must also be considered in the differential diagnosis of deep stromal deposits and requires corneal transplantation for complete removal.

References

1. Paolieri M. Ferdinand Münz: EDTA and 40 years of inventions. Bull Hist Chem. 2017;42(2):133–40.
2. Grant WM. New treatment for calcific corneal opacities. AMA Arch Ophthalmol. 1952;48(6):681–5.
3. Jhanji V, Rapuano CJ, Vajpayee RB. Corneal calcific band keratopathy. Curr Opin Ophthalmol. 2011;22(4):283–9.
4. O'Connor GR. Calcific band keratopathy. Trans Am Ophthalmol Soc. 1972;70:58–81.
5. Taylor PJ, Coates T, Newhouse ML. Episkopi blindness: Hereditary blindness in a Greek cypriot family. Br J Ophthalmol. 1959;43(6):340–4.
6. Alexandridis A, Stefani F. Treatment of band keratopathy. Klin Monbl Augenheilkd. 1980;176(6):968–71.
7. Doughman DJ, Olson GA, Nolan S, et al. Experimental band keratopathy. Arch Ophthalmol. 1969;81(2):264–71.
8. Messmer EM, Hoops JP, Kampik A. Bilateral Recurrent Calcareous Degeneration of the Cornea. Cornea. 2005;24(4):498–502.
9. Obenberger J, Babický A. Experimental Corneal Calcification in animals. Ophthalmic Res. 1970;1:187–92. https://doi.org/10.1159/000264516.
10. Taravella MJ. Calcific band keratopathy associated with the use of topical steroid-phosphate preparations. Arch Ophthalmol. 1994;112(5):608–13.
11. Bernauer W, Thiel MA, Kurrer M, et al. Corneal calcification following intensified treatment with sodium hyaluronate artificial tears. Br J Ophthalmol. 2006;90(3):285–288.
12. Bernauer W, Thiel M, Rentsch K. Phosphate concentrations in Antiglaucoma medication. Klin Monbl Augenheilkd. 2007;224(4):249–51.
13. Nevyas AS, Raber IM, Eagle RC, et al. Acute band keratopathy following Intracameral Viscoat. Arch Ophthalmol. 1987;105(7):958–64.
14. Bennett SR. Band keratopathy from emulsified Silicone Oil. Arch Ophthalmol. 1990;108(10):1387.

15. Najjar DM, Cohen EJ, Rapuano CJ, et al. EDTA chelation for calcific band keratopathy: results and long-term follow-up. Am J Ophthalmol. 2004;137(6):1056–64.
16. Al-Hity A, Ramaesh K, Lockington D. EDTA chelation for symptomatic band keratopathy: results and recurrence. Eye (Lond). 2018;32(1):26–31.
17. Weng S-F, Jan R-L, Chang C, et al. Risk of band keratopathy in patients with End-Stage Renal Disease. Sci Rep. 2016;6:28675.
18. De Ortueta D, Schreyger F, Baatz H. Band Keratopathy: A Modified Treatment. Eur J Ophthalmol. 2006;16:618–20.
19. O'Brart DP, Gartry DS, Lohmann CP, et al. Treatment of band keratopathy by excimer laser phototherapeutic keratectomy: surgical techniques and long term follow up. Br J Ophthalmol. 1993;77(11):702–8.
20. Bordin G, Dornelles F, Martins J, et al. Primary calcareous degeneration of the cornea. Indian J Ophthalmol. 2017;65(10):1027–30.
21. Corneal S-S, Therapy S-P. Arch Ophthalmol. 1999;117(10):1414–8.
22. Lavid FJ, Herreras JM, Calonge M, et al. Calcareous corneal degeneration: report of two cases. Cornea. 1995;14(1):97–102.

Suture-Related Complications After Keratoplasty

Loay Daas, Yaser Abu Dail, and Berthold Seitz

Abstract

This chapter provides an overview on suture-related complications after keratoplasty. The correct choice of suture technique in keratoplasty plays an important role in the postoperative visual outcome and graft survival. Keratoplasty can be plagued with several suture-related complications, including suture loosening and breakage, as well as suture-related infection, neovascularization and melting.

Keywords

Suture removal · Suture rupture · Suture-related complications · Corneal infiltrates · Corneal neovascularizaion · Corneal melting

1 Introduction

Corneal transplantation was first introduced by Eduard Zirm 1906 and is the most widespread and successful human transplantation [1]. Recent developments in microsurgery and the accumulated expertise of microsurgeons have transformed penetrating keratoplasty (PKP) from a simple exchange of two corneas into an optical procedure aimed at achieving good postoperative visual acuity and reducing complications. A major factor influencing the postoperative outcome is the correct choice and execution of the suturing technique, including time and modality of the suture removal [2].

L. Daas (✉) · Y. Abu Dail · B. Seitz
Department of Ophthalmology, Saarland University Medical Center, Homburg, Germany
e-mail: loay.daas@uks.eu

2 Choice of Suture Technique

PKP is dominantly performed using one of three suture techniques: the double running continuous suturing (DCS) according to Hoffmann [3], the single interrupted suturing (SIS) using multiple sutures and simple continuous suture (SCS) [4, 5].

If the Bowman layer is intact, DCS is recommended as it results in higher topographic regularity and faster visual rehabilitation compared to SIS, as well as a reduced rate of suture loosening [6–9] (Fig. 1). All knots should be buried in the stroma to avoid mechanical irritation and the eventual development of neovascularization and infiltration, potentially resulting in endophthalmitis.

In all conditions where the Bowman layer is disrupted, or in cases where there is a risk of melting (infectious and autoimmune corneal diseases), the use of SIS (typically at least 24 in number) is preferred to minimize the need for replacing the sutures after surgery if some of them become loose (Fig. 2). In these cases, all knots are ideally buried in the donor`s tissue right below the Bowman layer.

DCS offers the visual advantages of SCS with additional safety against graft dehiscence [10], which is why it is our method of choice whenever applicable.

3 Suture Removal

We recommend removing the first of the two running sutures or the first half of the interrupted sutures after 12 months. The second running suture or the second half of the single interrupted sutures are routinely removed after 18 months (Fig. 3). When removing the suture, the knot must be pulled out **without passing through the interface**.

Topical antibiotics and steroids are routinely used in all major keratoplasty centers after suture removal. However, the dose and duration may vary [11]. We recommend using

B. Seitz et al. (eds.), *Atlas on Cornea*, https://doi.org/10.1007/978-3-031-65422-0_60

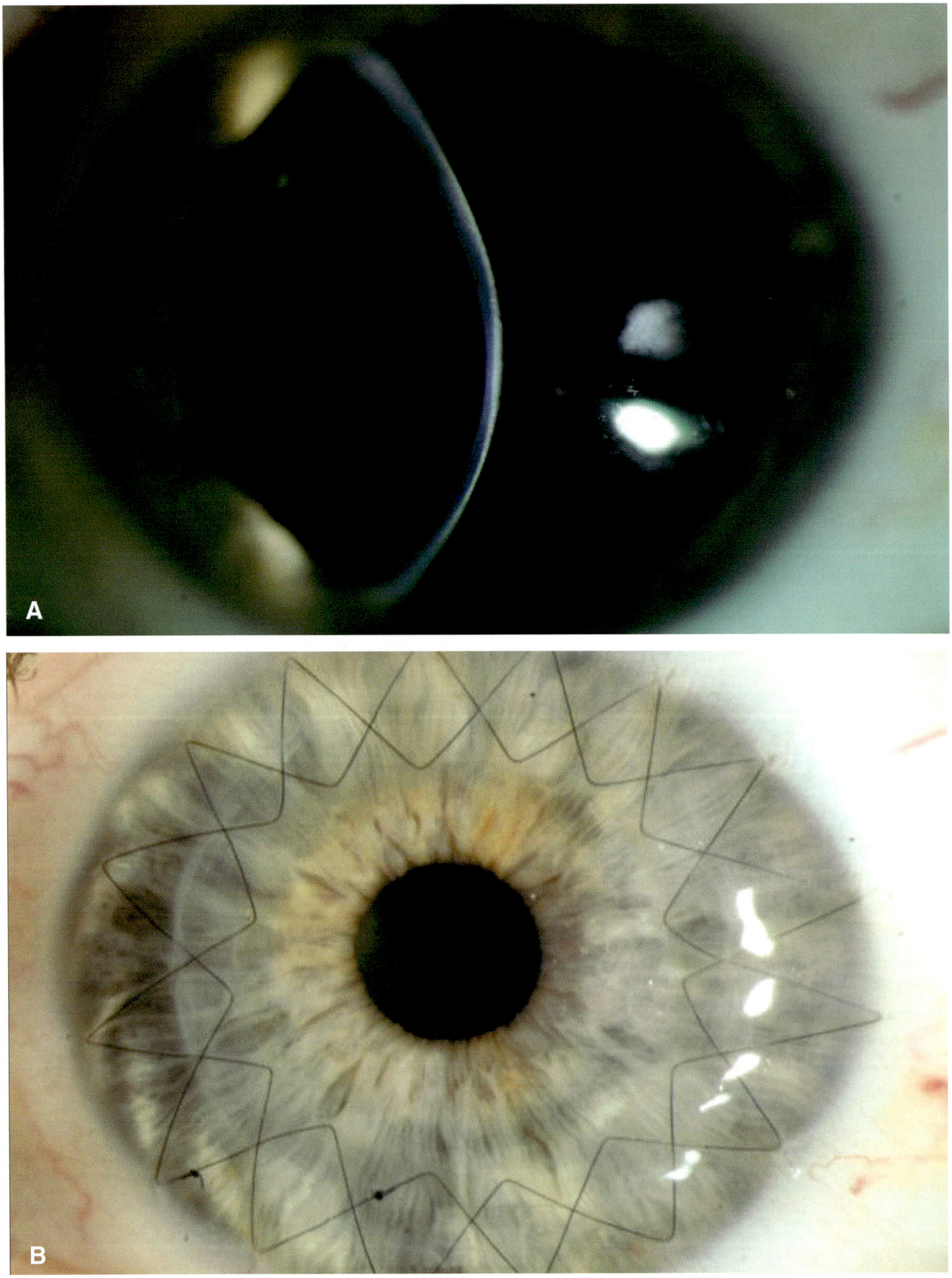

Fig. 1 (**A**) The left eye of a 54-year-old keratoconus patient with central scarring of the cornea. (**B**) Same eye after an excimer laser penetrating keratoplasty with double running sutures

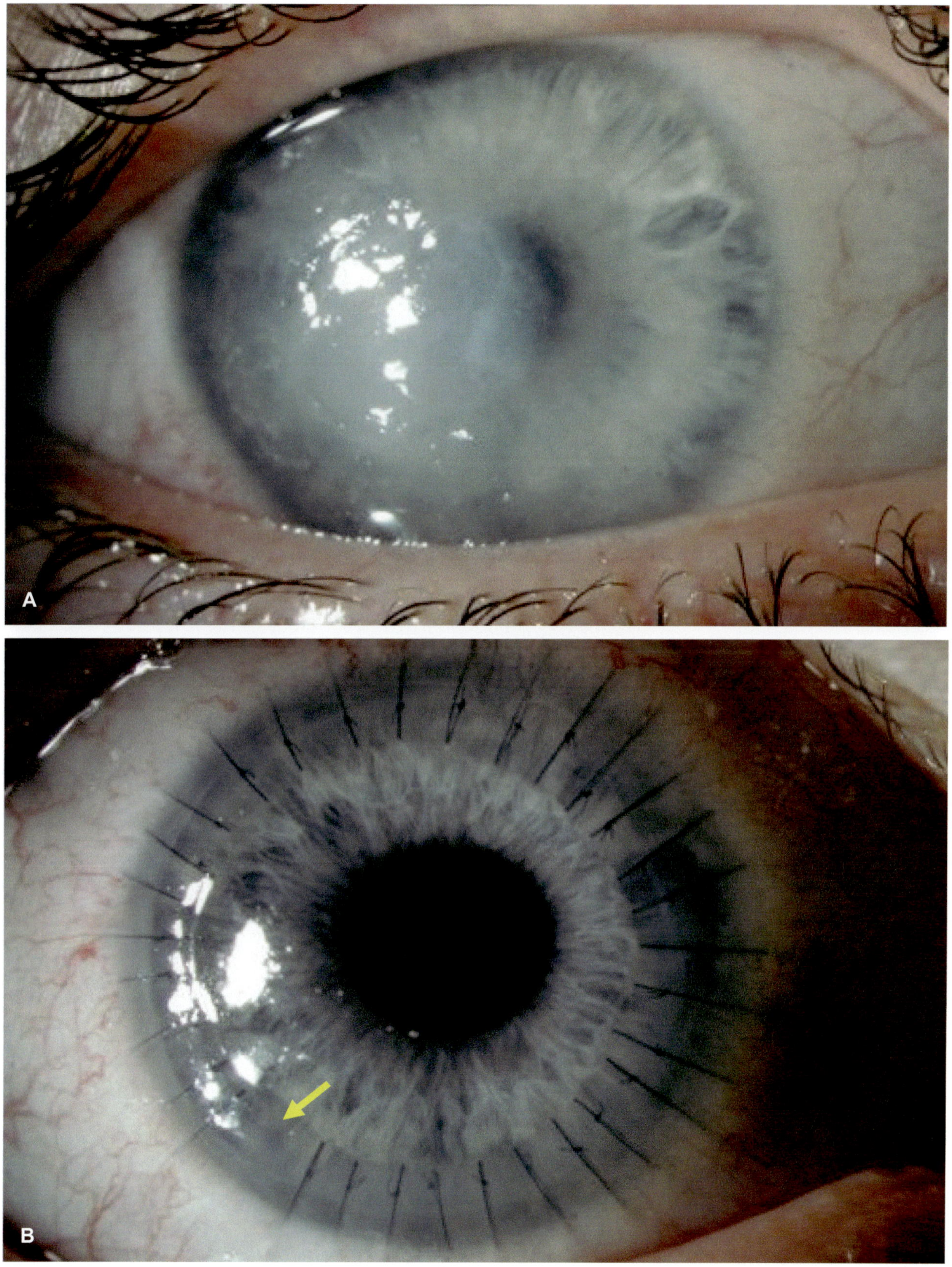

Fig. 2 (**A**) A 28-year-old patient with contact lens-associated acanthamoeba and mycotic keratitis in the right eye. (**B**) Same eye 4 weeks after a penetrating keratoplasty. The graft was fixed with single interrupted sutures because of the higher risk of postoperative corneal infiltration and neovascularization. One loose suture was removed at 7 o'clock postoperatively without the need for replacement (arrow)

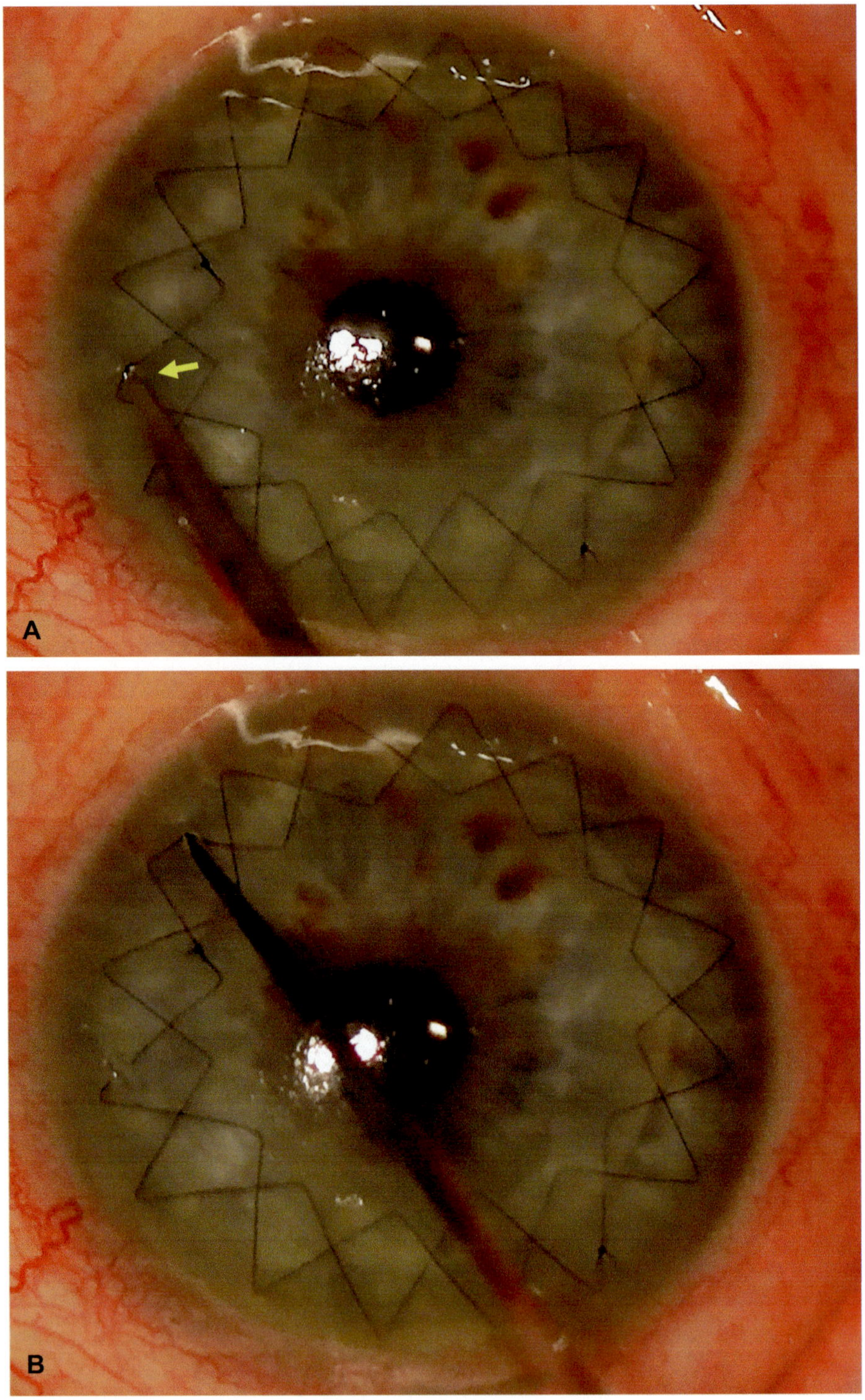

Fig. 3 (A, B) First, the superficial part of the suture on both sides of the knot is cut with the sharp side of a Graefe knife distal to the knot so that the suture end is long enough for later extraction

Fig. 3 (C, D) Then, using the blunt side of the knife, the suture is gently pulled out at the superficial site adjacent to the previous cut site. (**C**) The superficial part of the thread should then be cut and pulled in an alternating fashion (**D**)

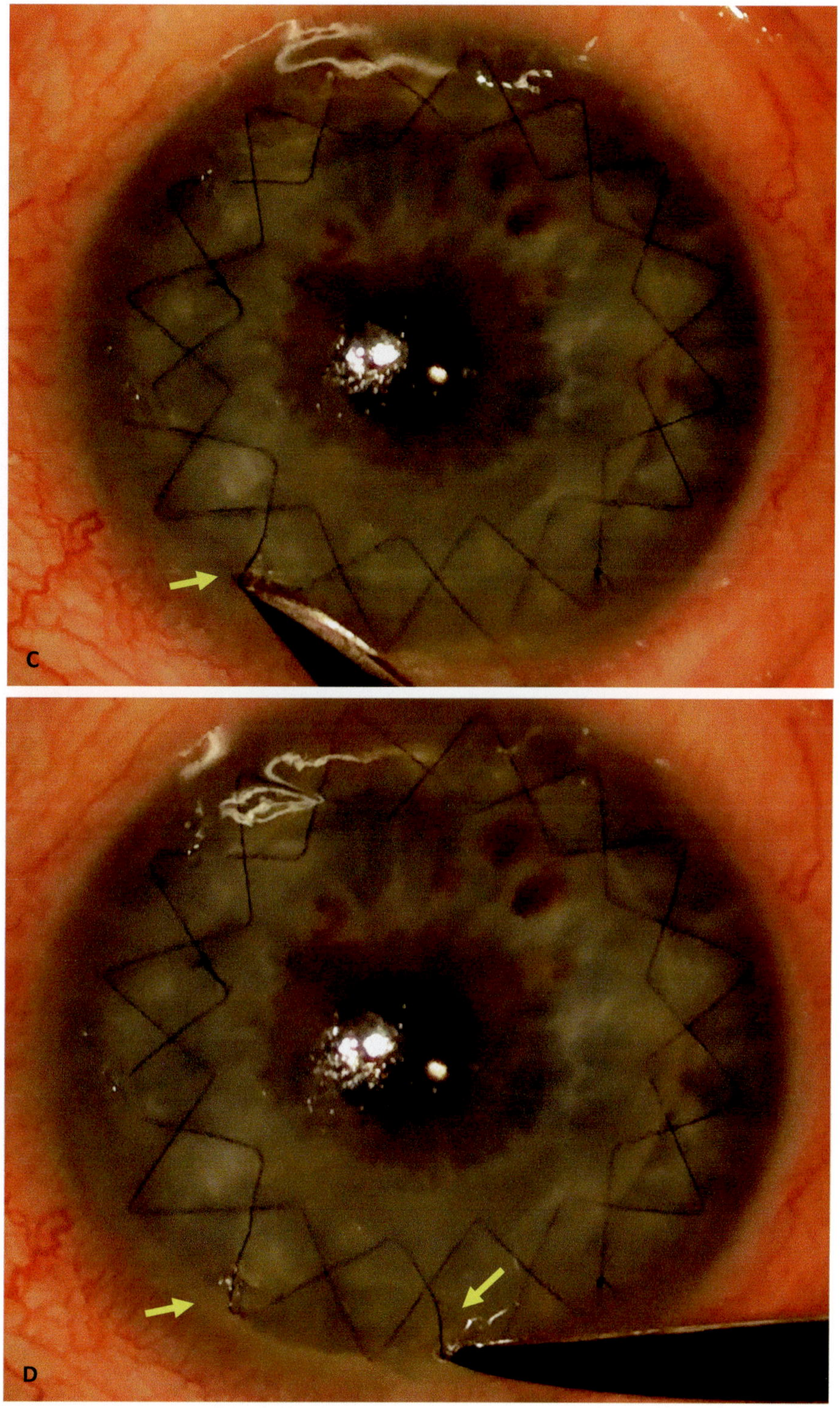

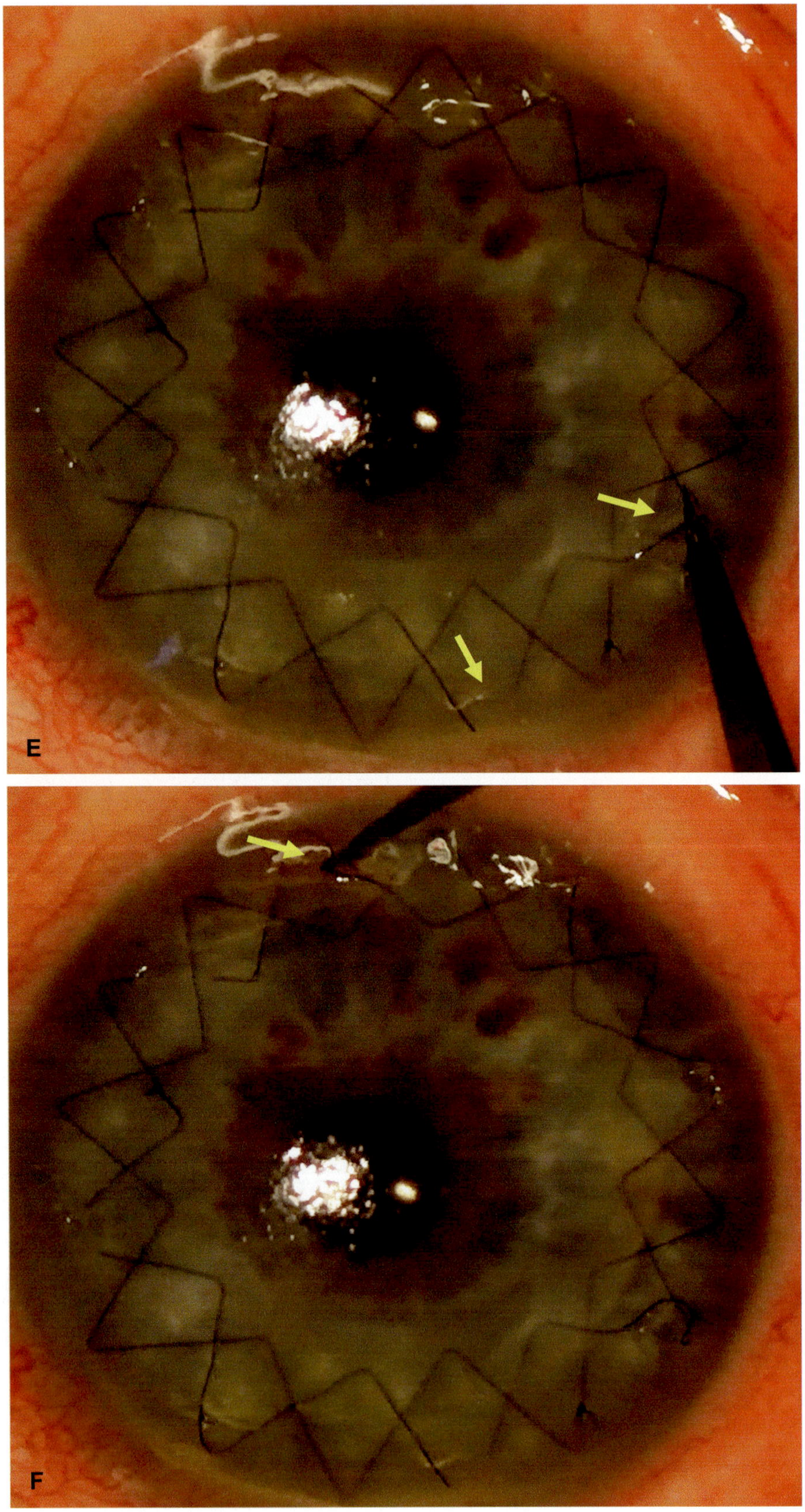

Fig. 3 (E, F) The superficial part of the thread should then be cut and pulled in an alternating fashion

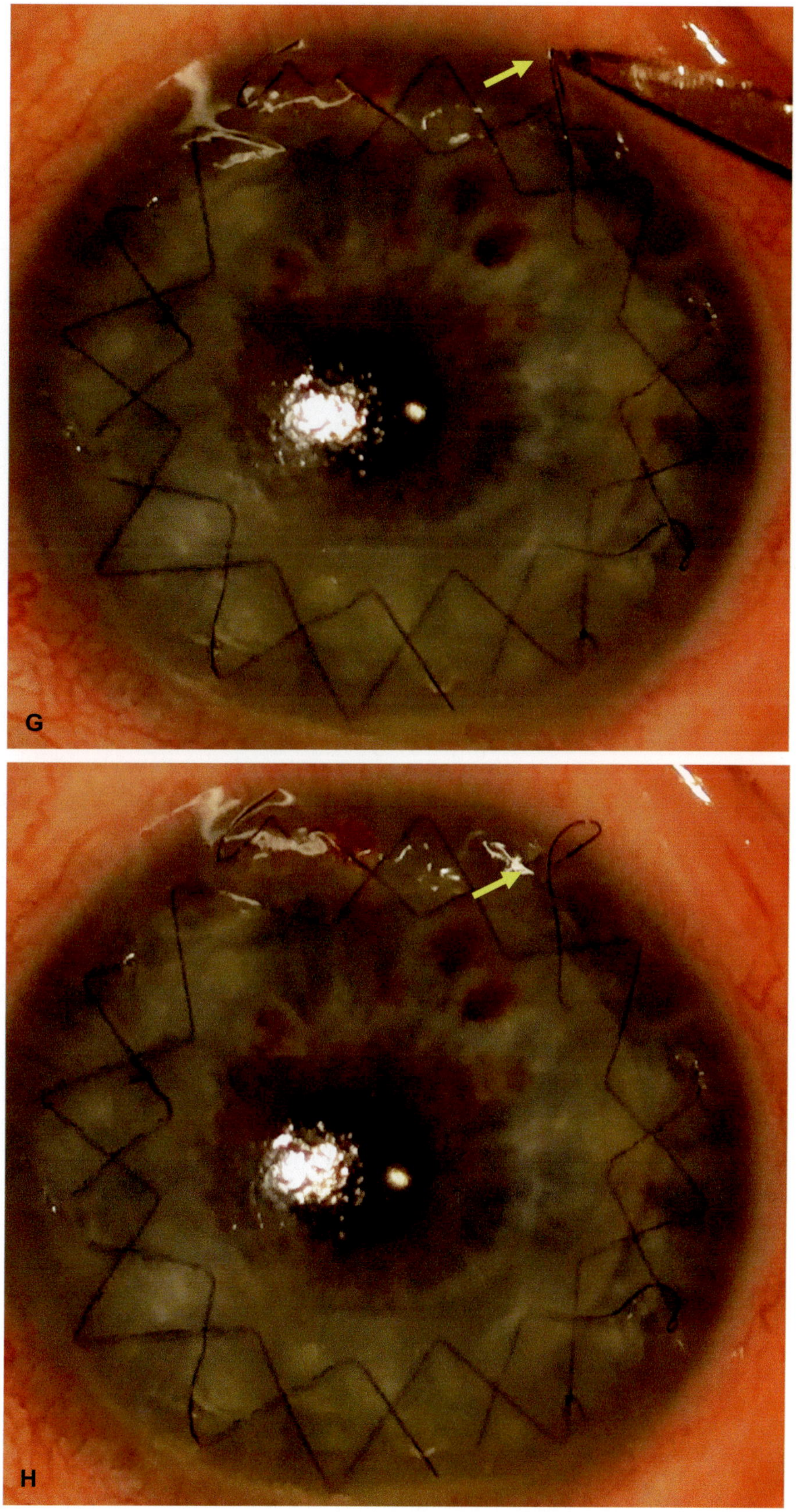

Fig. 3 (G, H) The superficial part of the thread should then be cut and pulled in an alternating fashion

Fig. 3 (I, J) Subsequently, the thread pieces should be carefully removed with a forceps by finally pulling out the partially extracted parts

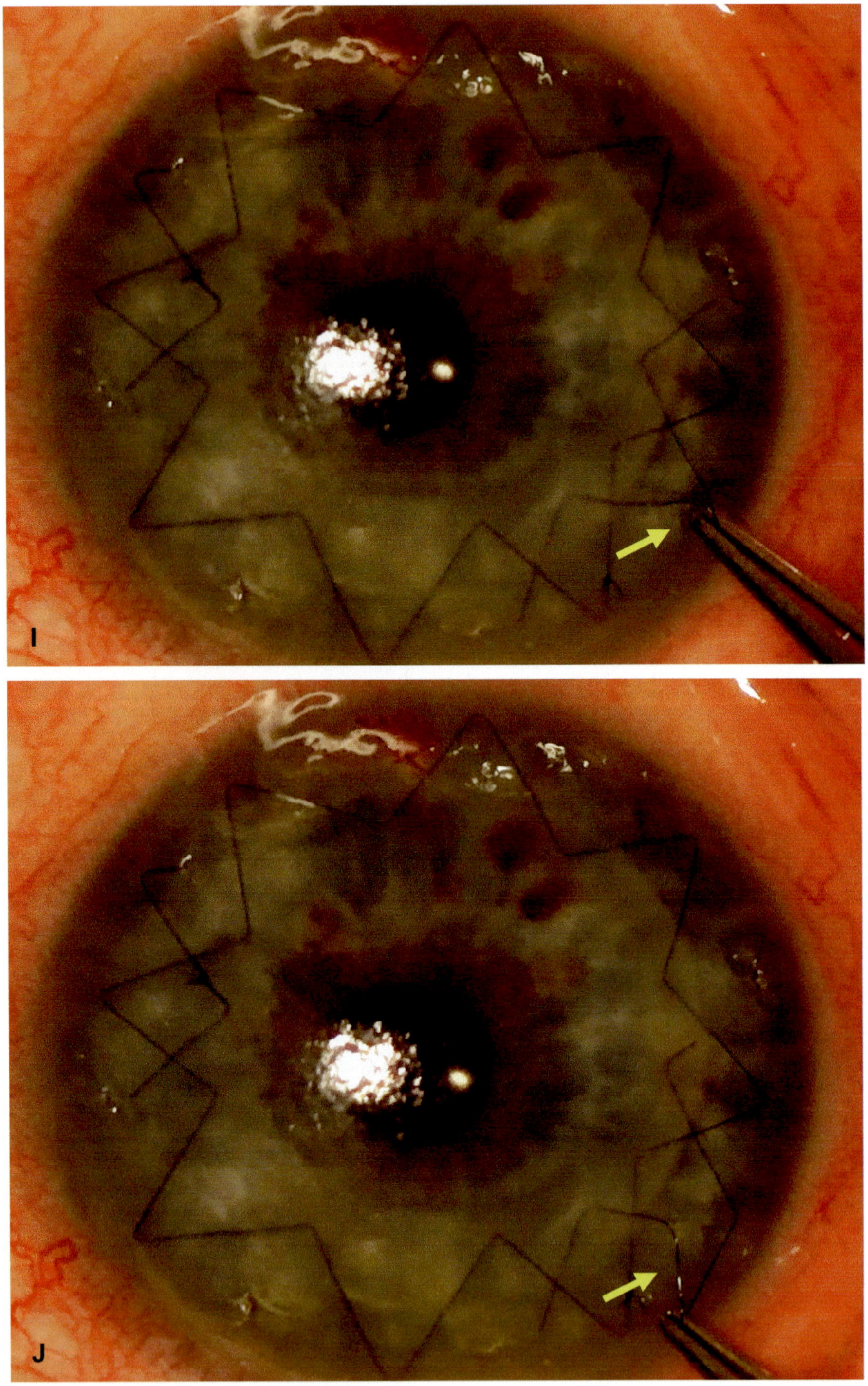

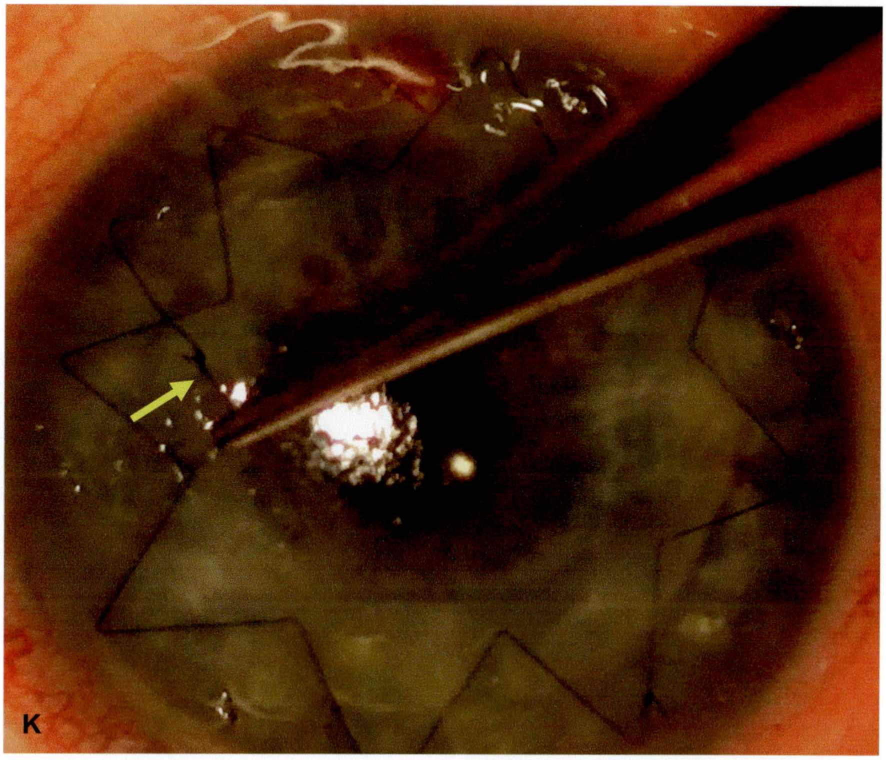

Fig. 3 (K) At last, the knot should be pulled out primarily without passing through the interface

ofloxacin eye drops 5 × daily for 1 week and prednisolone acetate eye drops 5 × daily for 1 week and tapering them off over 5 weeks. Systemic steroids should also be considered in cases with a high risk of graft rejection.

4 Suture-Related Complications After Keratoplasty

Several suture-related complications can occur postoperatively. Their timely recognition and treatment are of great importance for the survival of the graft and even the preservation of the eye [10, 12, 13]. We recommend regular postoperative examination by slit lamp microscopy in combination with the use of fluorescein-natrium and blue light, as these improve the visibility of erosions and mucus accumulation along the loose suture (Fig. 4). The most common postoperative complications associated with sutures are listed below:

- Therefore, **they should be removed immediately**, along with prophylactic topical therapy with antibiotics for one week. Risk factors for postoperative suture loosening are: disruption of Bowman layer, keratoplasty in children (26–34%)[14], stromal vascularization, underlying rheumatoid disease, and a single continuous suture [10].
- **Suture-related corneal infections** (Fig. 5): Suture-related infectious keratitis can have serious consequences such as graft failure, endophthalmitis and even loss of the eye [10, 12, 13, 15]. Therefore, its timely detection and treatment is crucial. Loose sutures, contact lens wear and broken sutures are risk factors for infectious keratitis [10]. The clinical manifestations vary depending on the organism and the stage of the infection [12, 13, 16]. Empirical therapy with broad-spectrum antibiotics as well as antifungals and/or therapy against acanthamoeba should be given immediately, depending on the clinical symptoms and history, until the results of the culture are available.

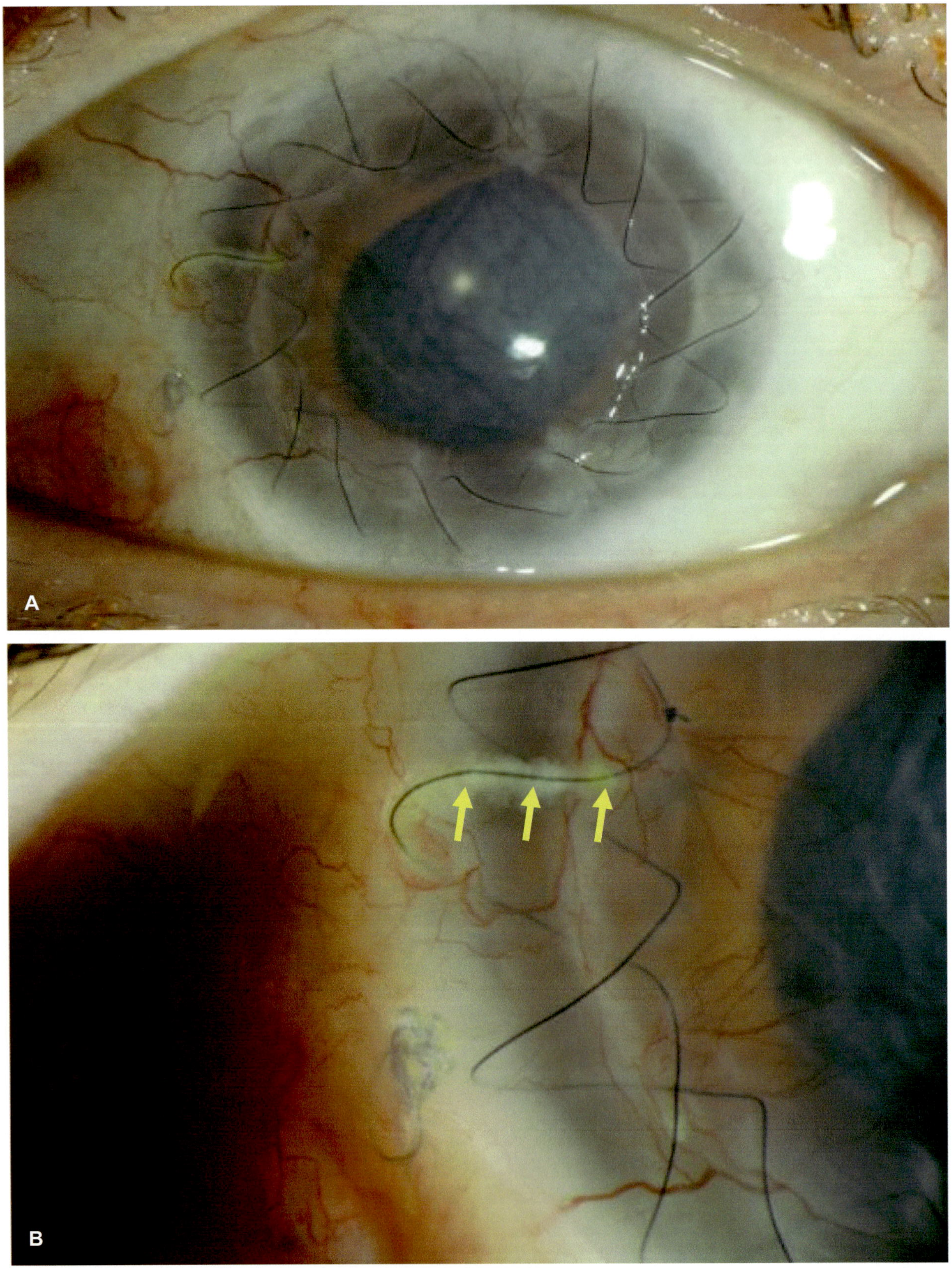

Fig. 4 (**A**) Suture loosening of double continuous sutures in a 66-year-old patient after silicone oil-associated keratopathy. (**B**) The same eye with magnification after staining with fluoresceine. The loose suture shows a yellow color and mucus accumulation along it. Note the positive staining under blue light

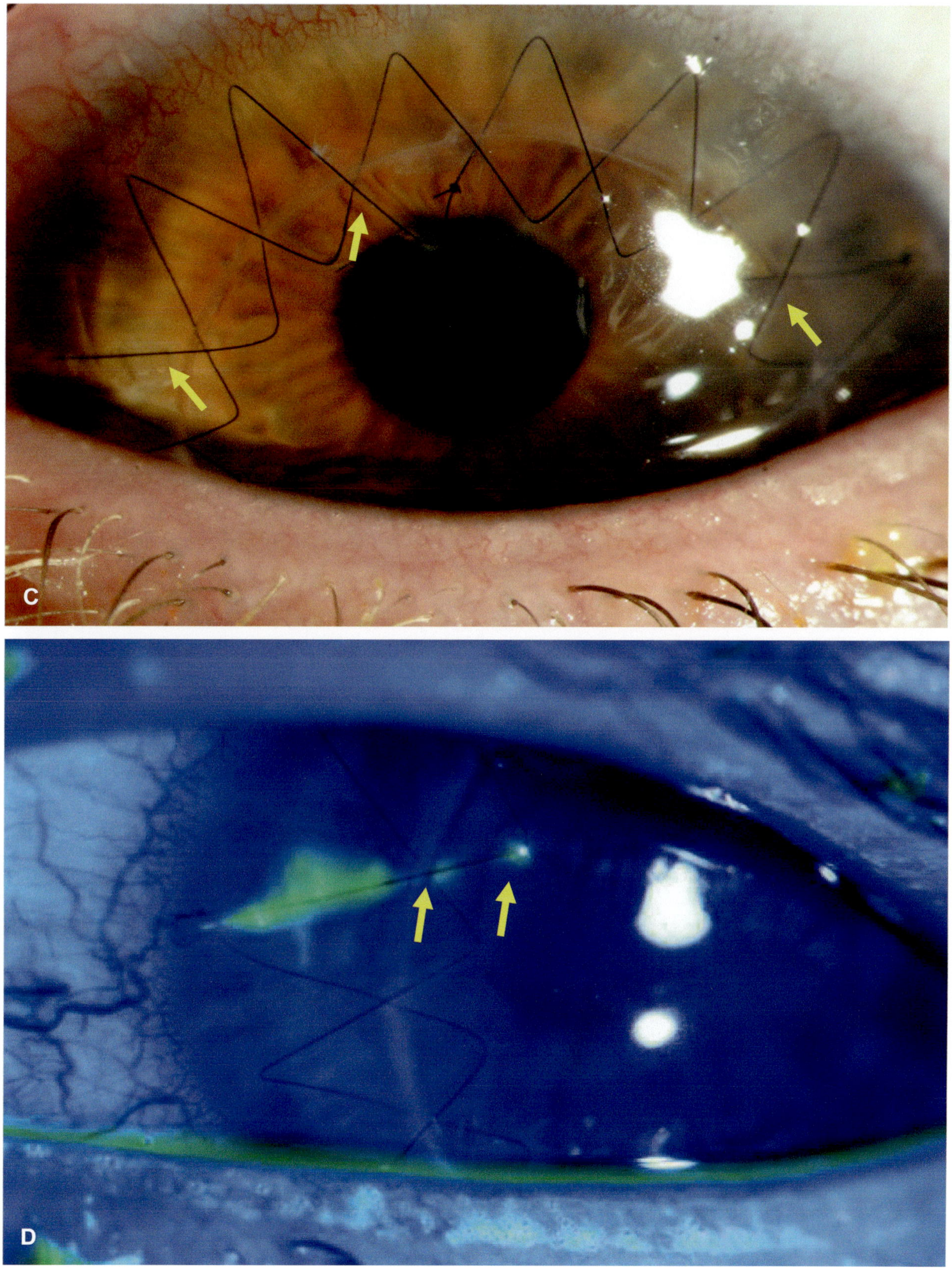

Fig. 4 (**C, D**) An apparently intact suture under normal light. Staining with fluoresceine and examination under blue light reveals the loose suture

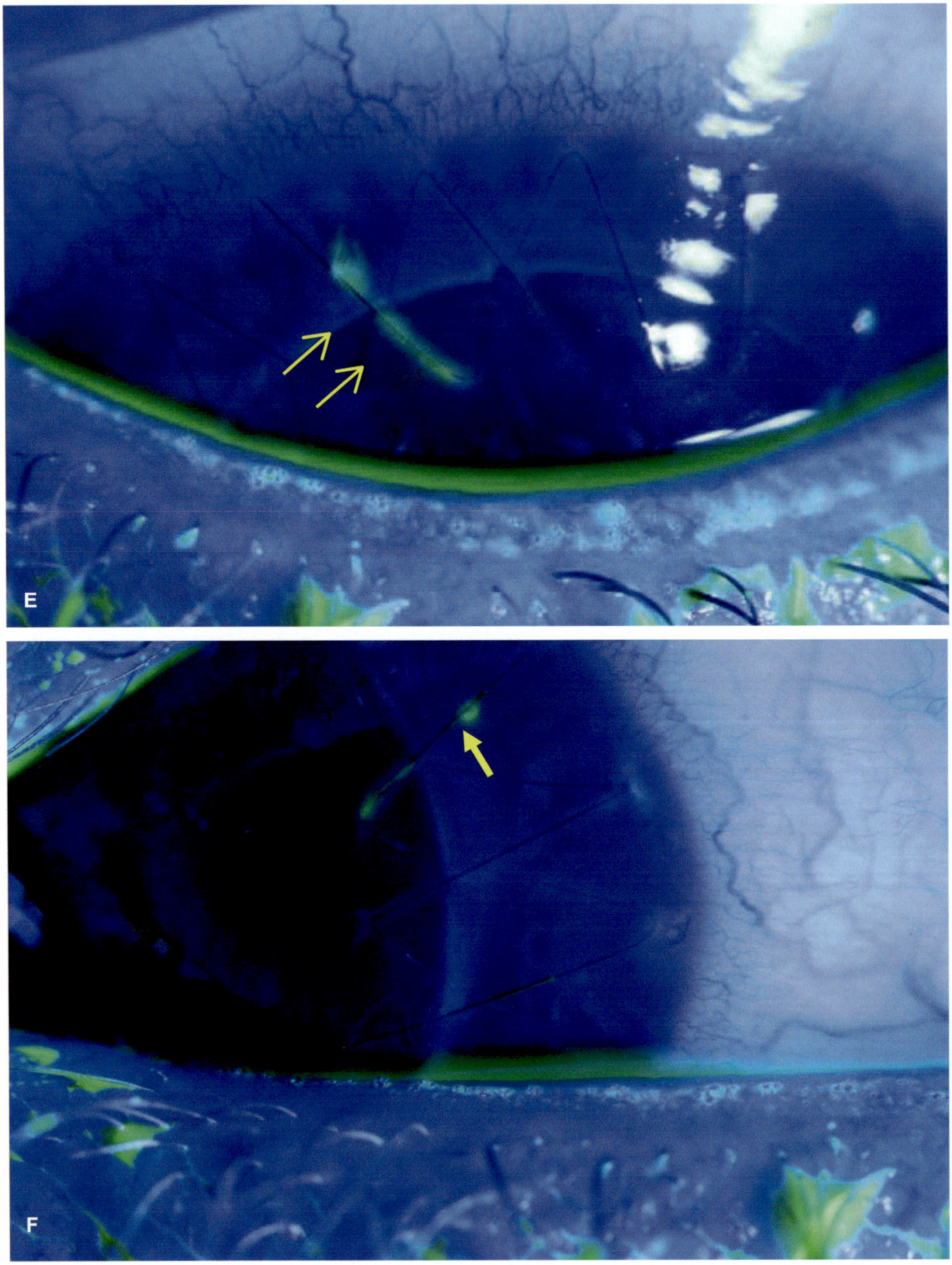

Fig. 4 (**E**, **F**) An apparently intact suture under normal light. Staining with fluoresceine and examination under blue light reveals the loose suture

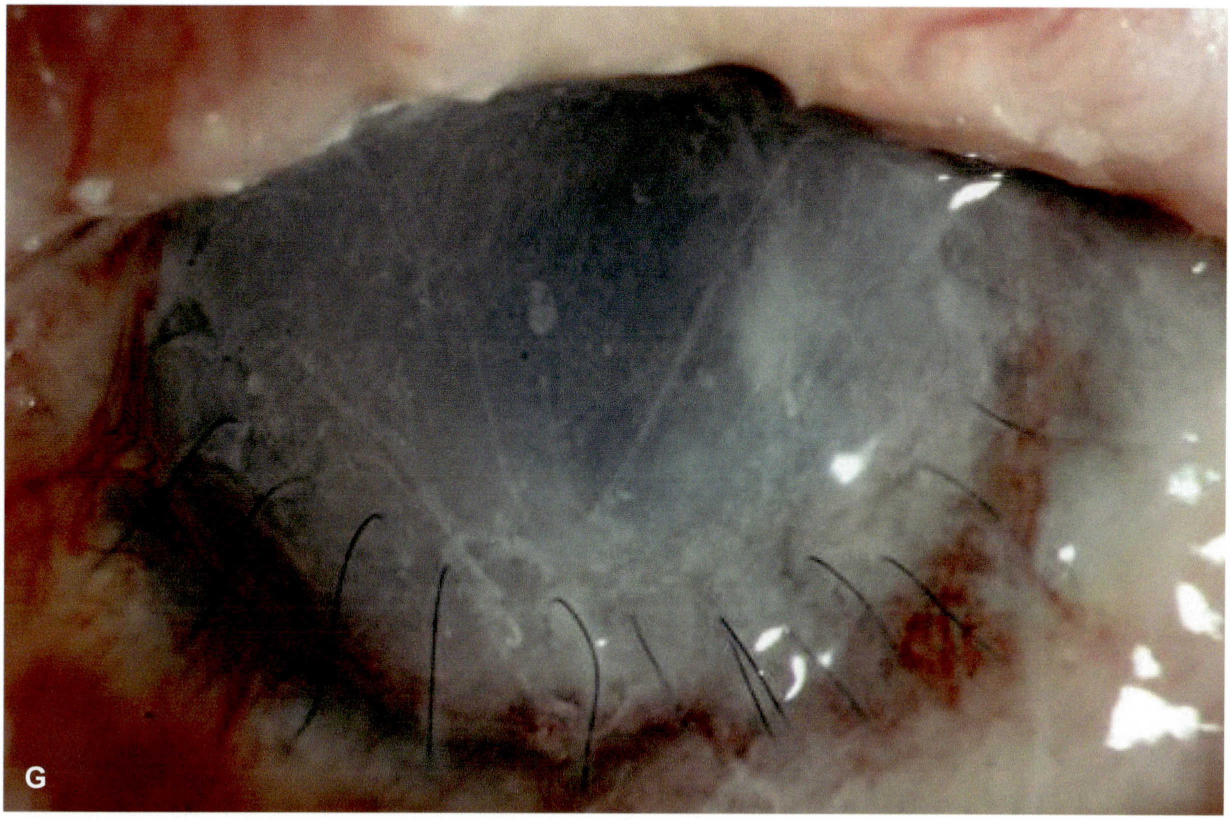

Fig. 4 (**G**) Multiple loose sutures in a patient with rheumatoid arthritis after amniotic membrane transplantation as patch

- **Subepithelial immune infiltrates** (Fig. 5F): These are sterile, small, and well demarcated corneal micro-abscesses along the suture. Immune infiltrates often occur early postoperatively, probably in response to suture material and contaminants such as talc from surgical gloves and appear typically in the highly vascularized host cornea [2] and respond well to high-dose topical steroid therapy.
- **Corneal melting in the entrance area of the suture** (Fig. 6): Systemic rheumatic diseases are an important risk factor for postoperative corneal melting [17]. Immediate suture removal and intensive therapy with topical and systemic steroids as well as close observation are indicated. In addition, systemic assessment and therapy are essential to rule out and control autoimmune diseases [17]. Typically, in such cases, keratoplasty should only be performed if sufficient systemic immunosuppressive therapy is administered.
- **Development of neovascularization along the suture** (Fig. 7): Neovascularization is associated with higher risk of graft rejection. Therefore, early removal of the suture is to be considered in case of vessel growth along the suture. **Certainly, a loose suture has to be removed immediately.** Additionally, the dose of typical steroids should be increased. Topical VEGF-antagonists are of minor help.

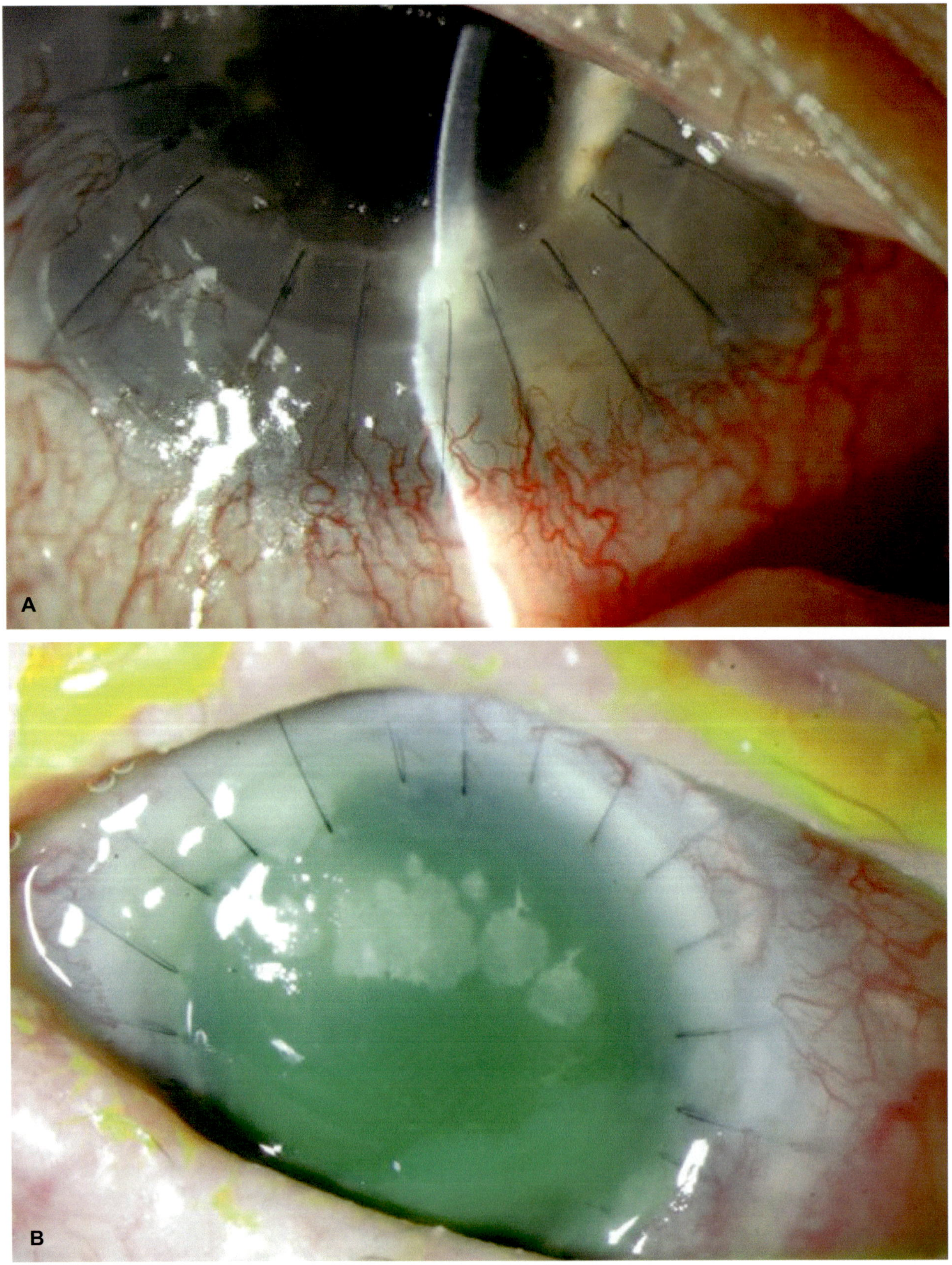

Fig. 5 (**A**) Corneal infiltrate at the entrance area of the suture on the graft. (**B**) Crystalline keratopathy with corneal infiltrate in the suture area

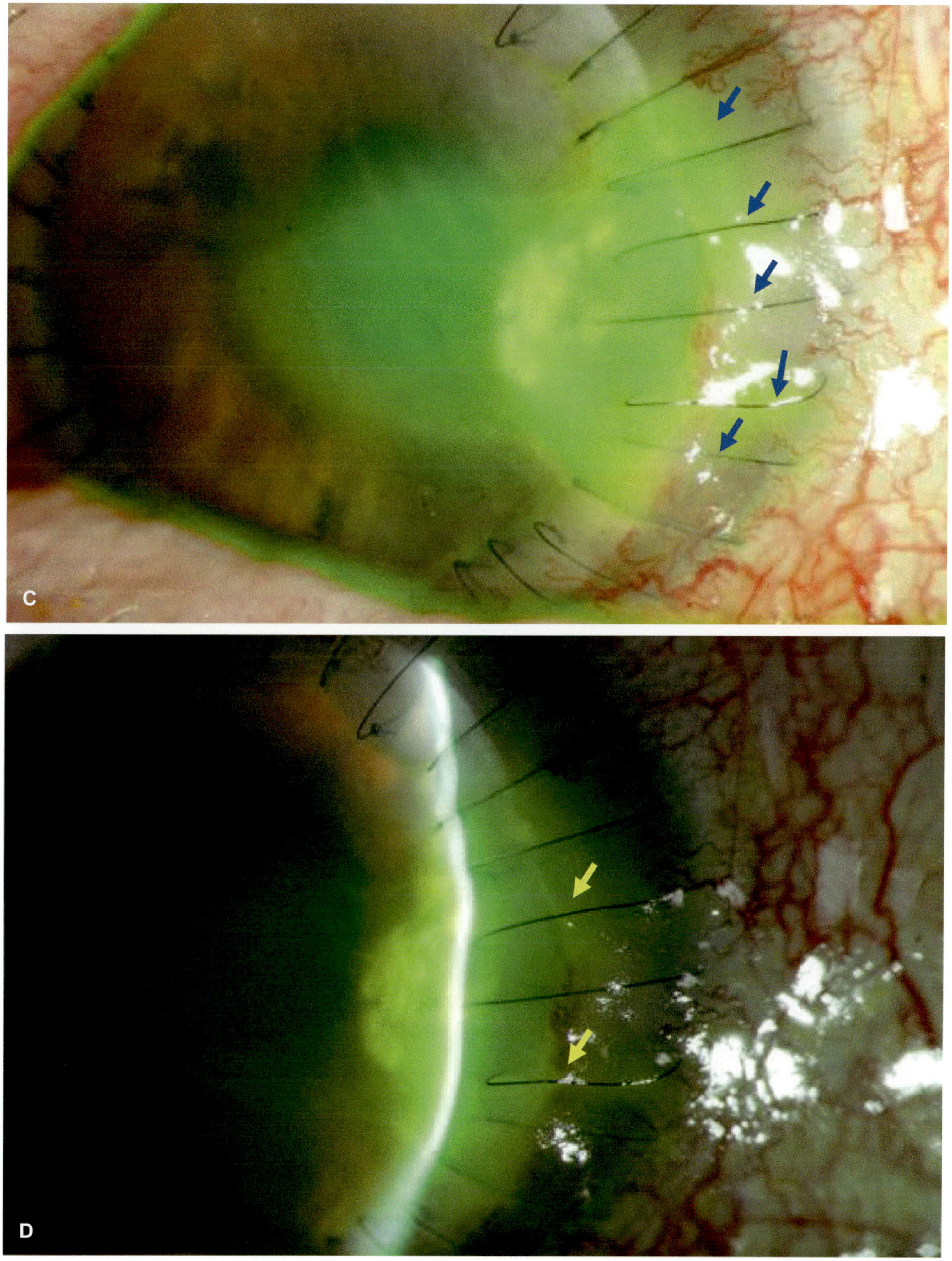

Fig. 5 (**C**, **D**, **E**) Beginning abscess formation in the sutures area with loose sutures

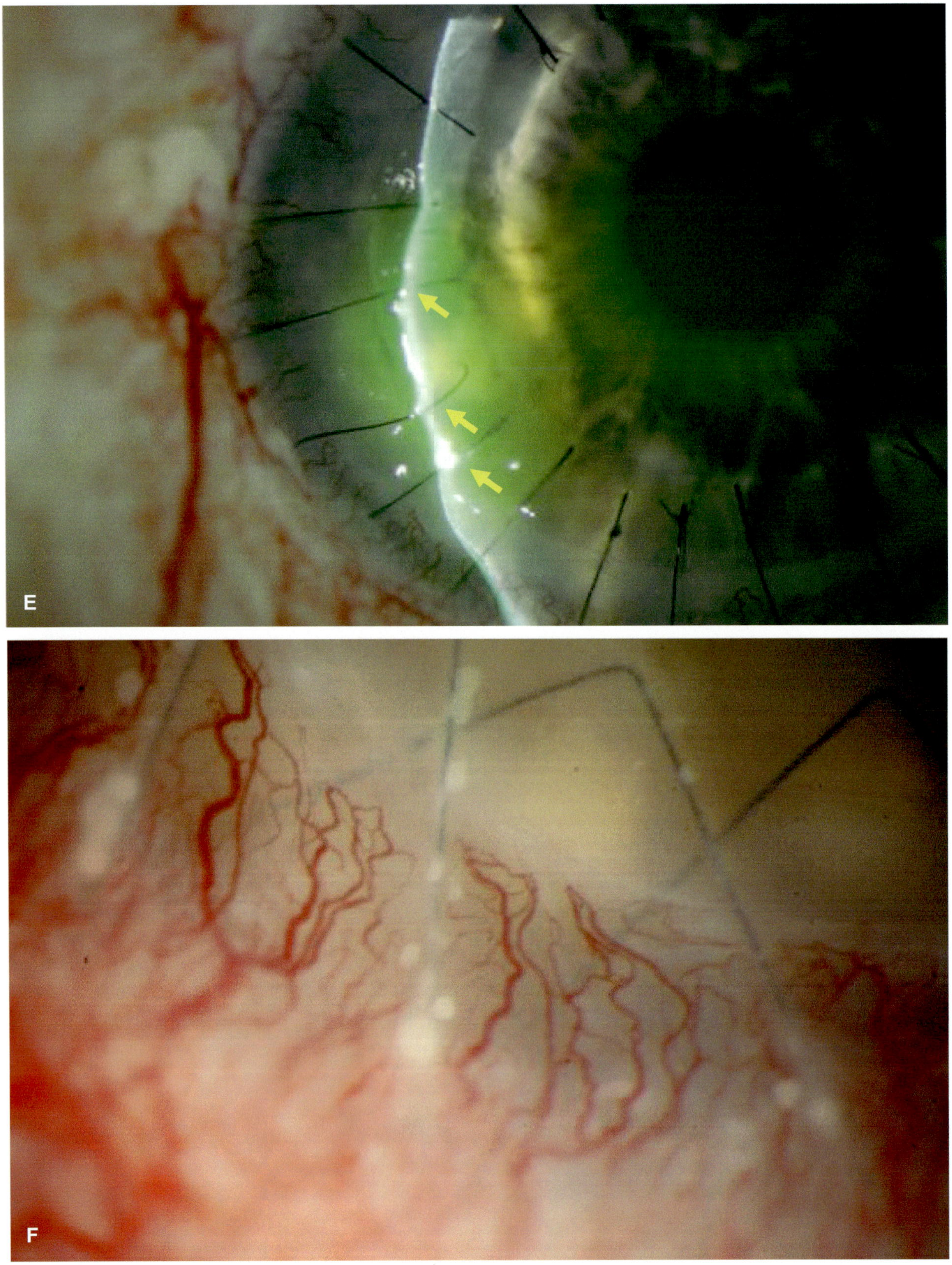

Fig. 5 (**F**) Multiple sterile corneal infiltrates after penetrating keratoplasty (typically in the highly vascularized host cornea without or with too little use of topical steroids

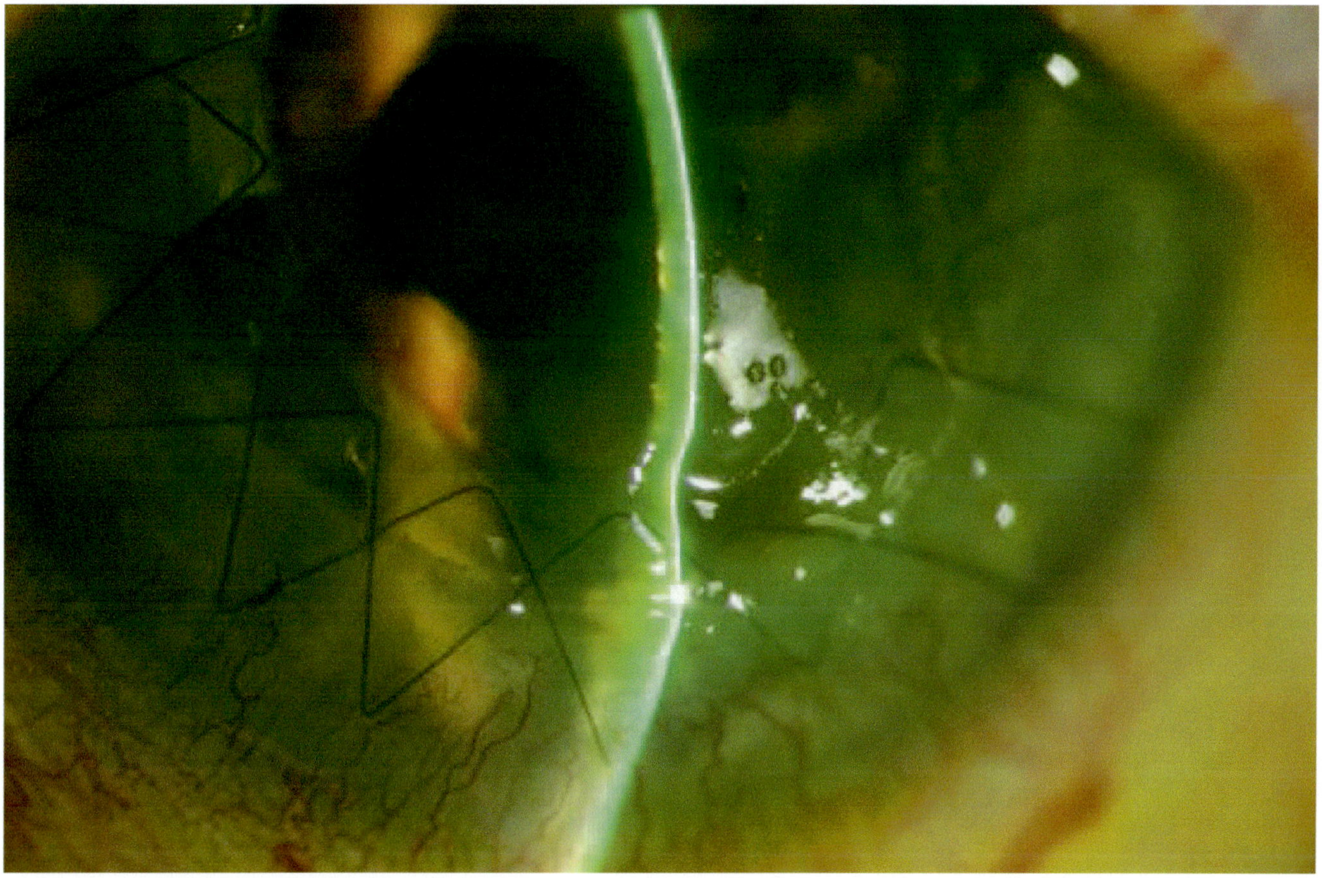

Fig. 6 Corneal melting in the entrance area of a continuous suture

- **Suture rupture** (Fig. 8): Like loose sutures, ruptured sutures also have to be removed immediately to avoid infectious keratitis.
- **Dehiscence and step formation during or after suture removal** (Fig. 9): Although premature suture removal may be associated with graft dehiscence due to incomplete wound healing, dehiscence remains a risk at all points after keratoplasty [10]. Other predisposing factors for dehiscence and step formation include trauma, and bullous keratopathy. Here, the first suture should never be removed before one year has passed. Additionally, the suture knot should—whenever possible—not be passed through the interface, as this would create unnecessary strain on the freshly healed wound [10].

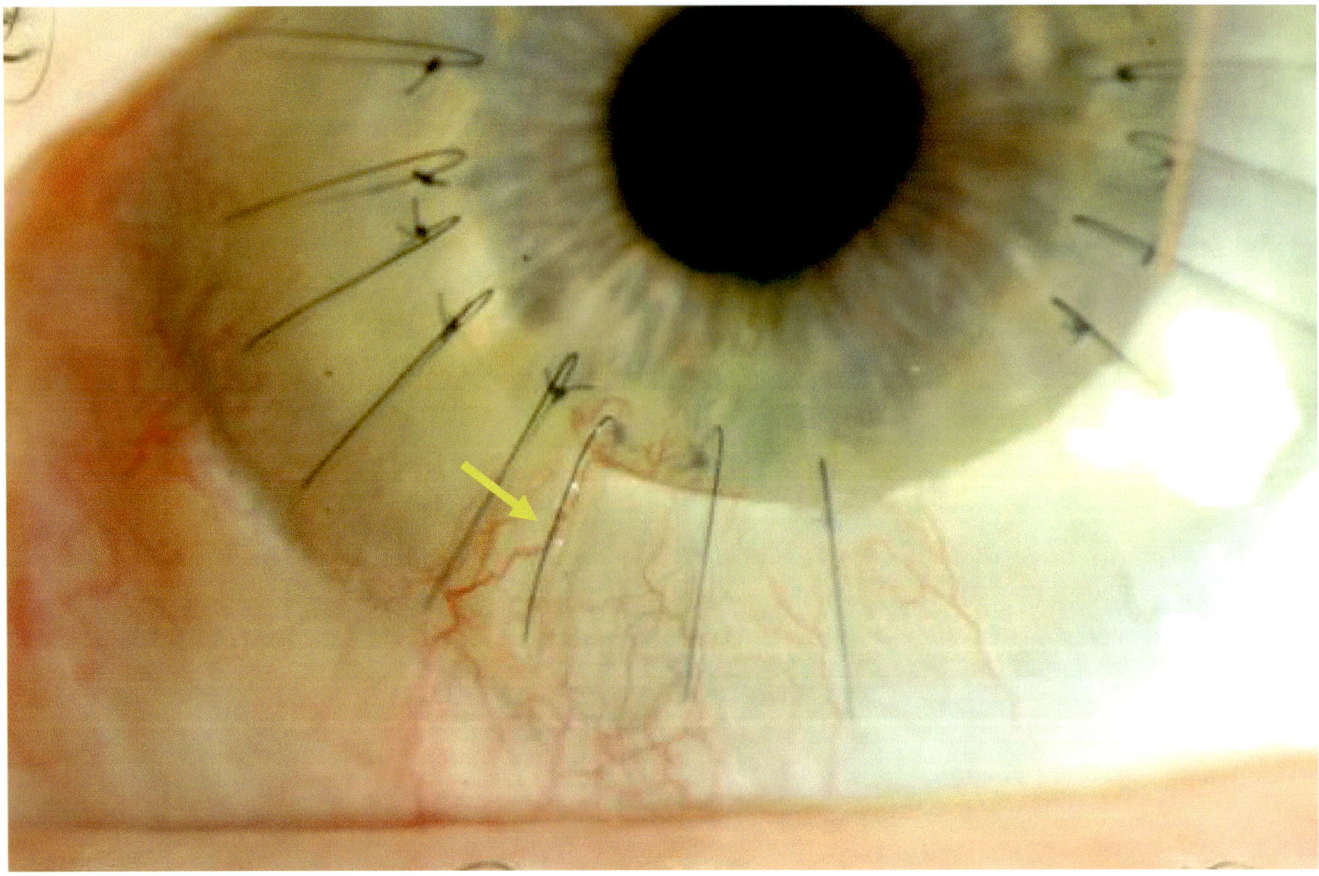

Fig. 7 New vessel growth along an interrupted loose suture

- **High and/or irregular astigmatism after suture removal**: Removal of the sutures releases the forces created by geometric non-uniformity and inhomogeneous wound healing, which could lead to increased regular and irregular astigmatism after suture removal [18]. Therefore, to reduce astigmatic increase as well as the required suture tension for wound closure and to achieve better visual acuity with sutures in place and after suture removal, a trephination method should be used in PKP, which allows tension-free symmetrical fitting of a perfectly circular donor disc into a circular recipient bed with matching, unproblematic watertight incision margins. For more than 30 years, optimal trephination is most likely to be achieved by non-contact excimer laser-assisted trephination [2, 19–25]. Excimer laser-assisted trephination avoids mechanical deformation during trephination and results in smooth incision edges in both the donor and recipient cornea, thereby reducing "vertical tilt". Additionally, the "teeth" in the donor and the corresponding notches in the recipient can guide the accurate positioning of the first eight cardinal sutures and avoid intraoperative "horizontal torsion", thus improving optical quality after PKP [26–28]. The suture technique also

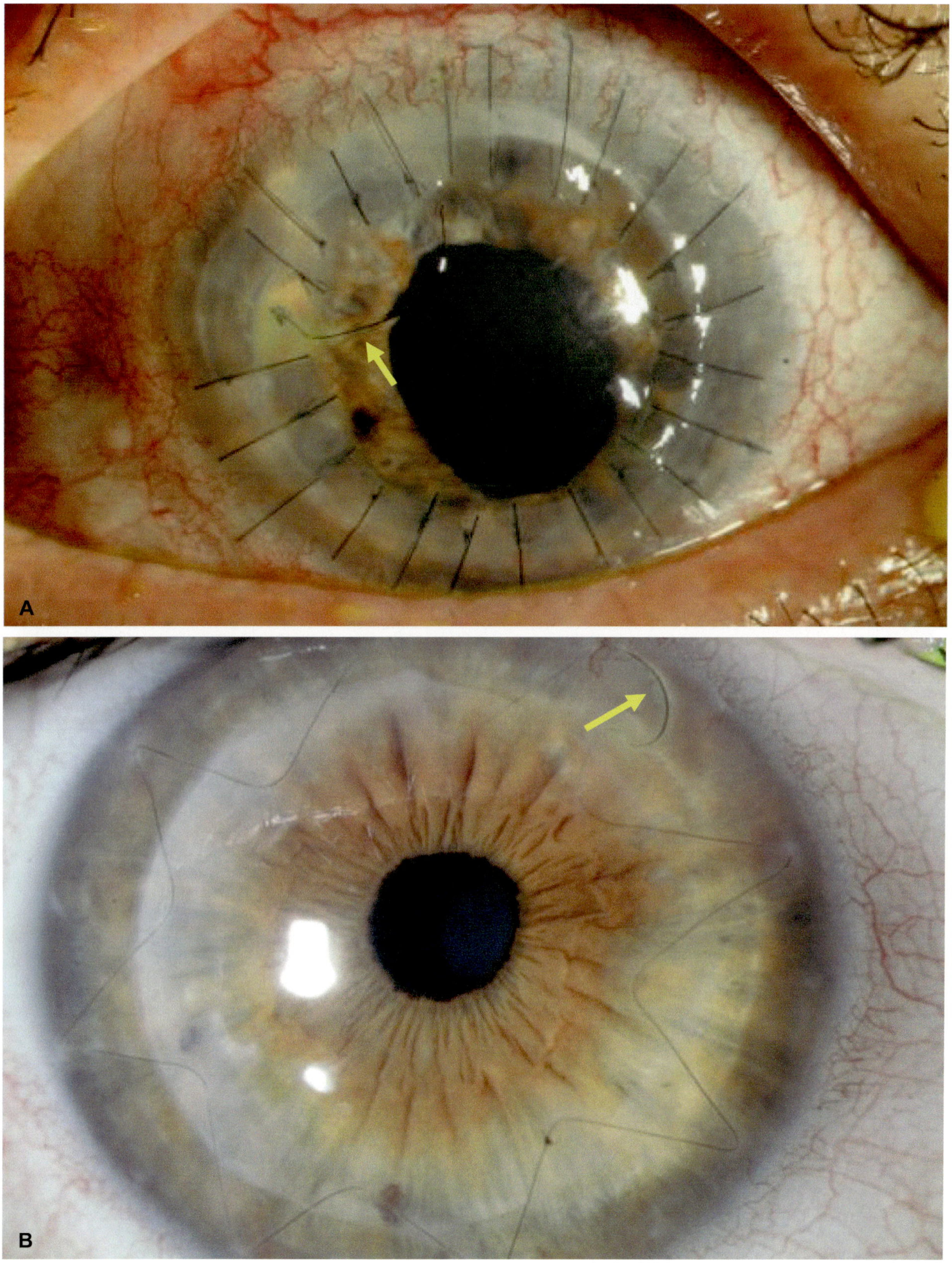

Fig. 8 (**A**) A ruptured, interrupted suture. (**B**) A ruptured, continuous suture with positive staining with fluoresceine and blue light (see Fig. 8C). All these sutures have to be removed immediately upon detection

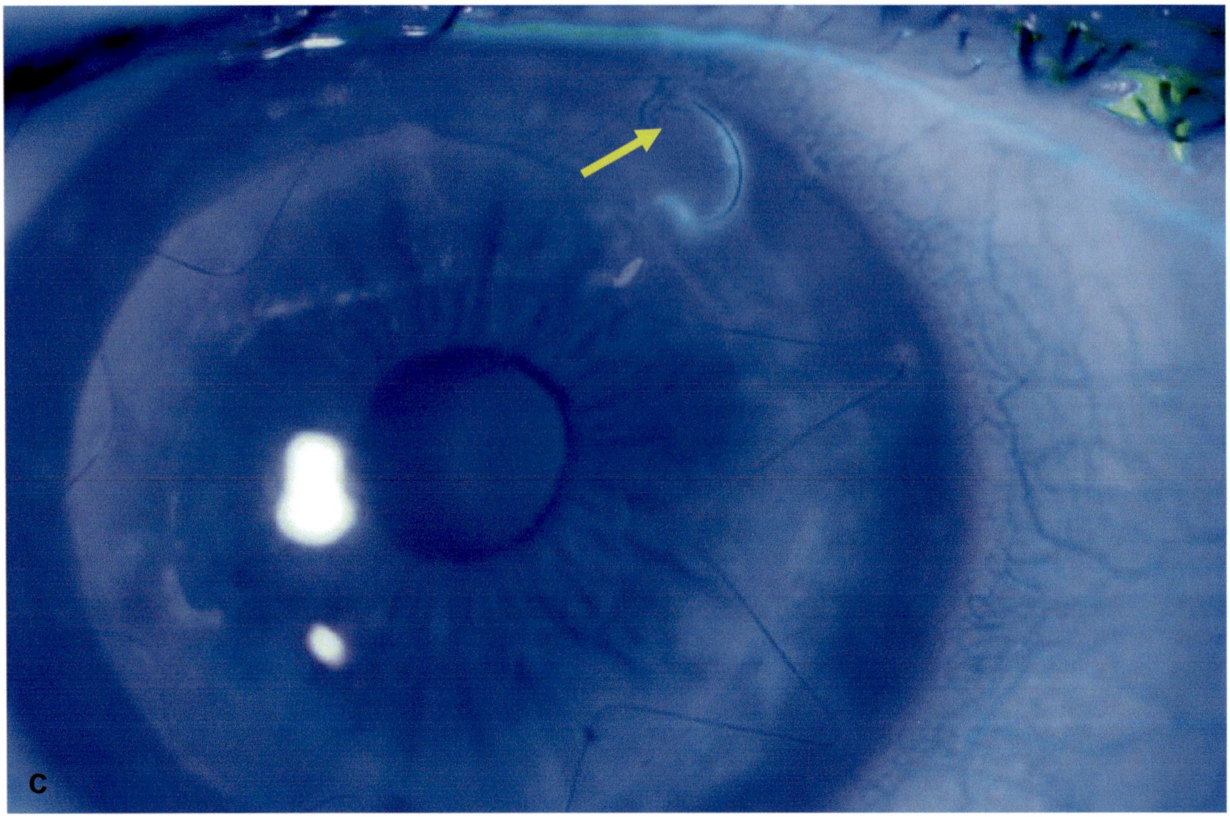

Fig. 8 (**C**) A ruptured, continuous suture with positive staining with fluoresceine and blue light

significantly influences postoperative astigmatism. Most studies show lower topographic astigmatism when using DCS compared to SIS [8, 29]. High regular astigmatism can be treated with various refractive procedures, including limbal parallel keratotomy and toric intraocular lenses in the bag or add-on. Irregular astigmatism requires the use of rigid contact lenses. In case of contact lens intolerance or persistent reduced visual acuity, a repeat keratoplasty with larger diameter should be considered [30].

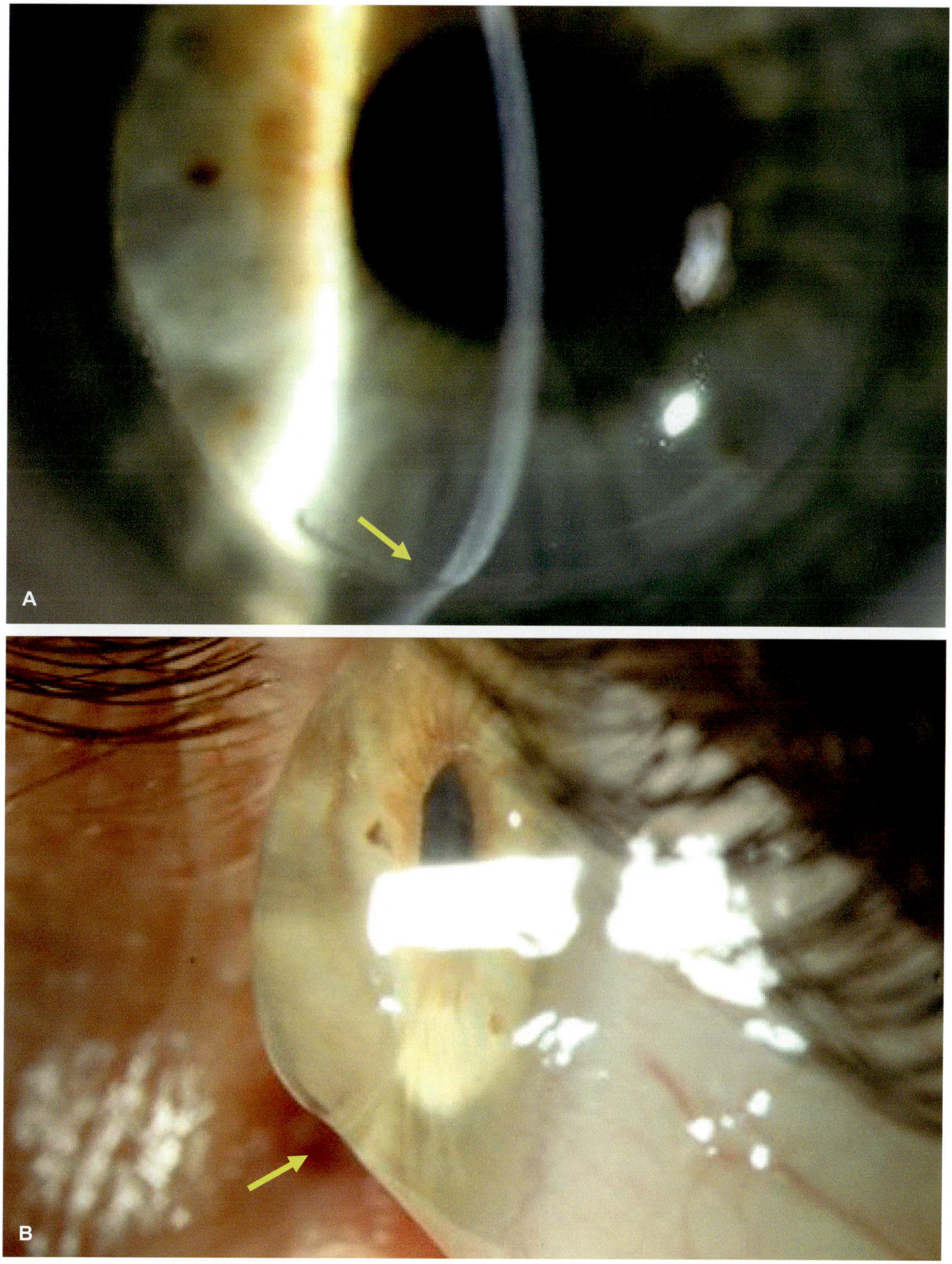

Fig. 9 (**A**–**C**) Chronic step formation at 6 o'clock in a 59-year-old keratoconus patient after penetrating keratoplasty. (**C**) Anterior segment OCT (AS-OCT) shows the finely healed positive step

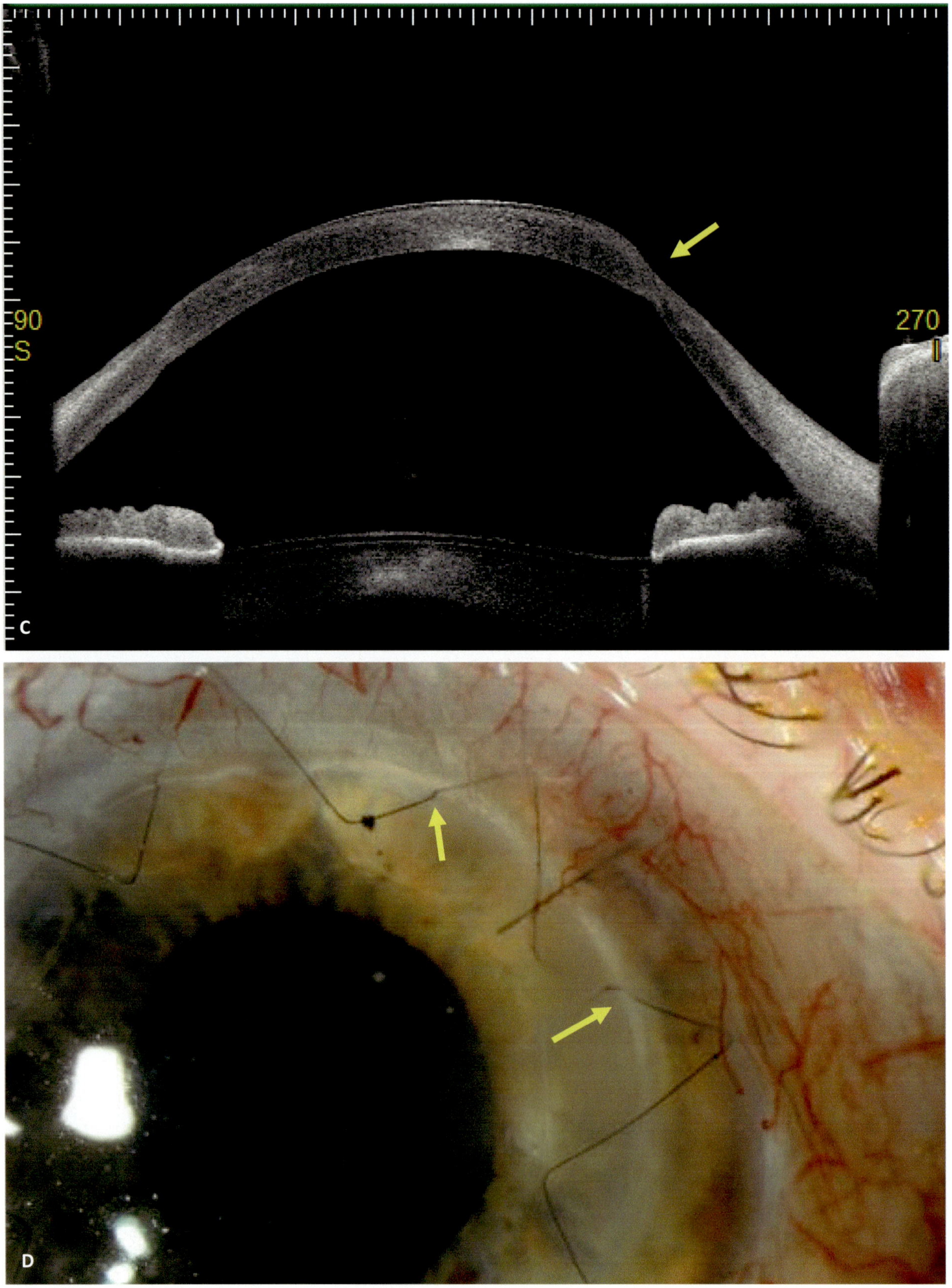

Fig. 9 (**D**, **E**) Step formation in a 79-year-old patient with bullous keratopathy after removing the first continuous suture, notice the slightly bent suture in the interface in (**D**) and the prominent acute "plus step" formation in (**E**) (arrows)

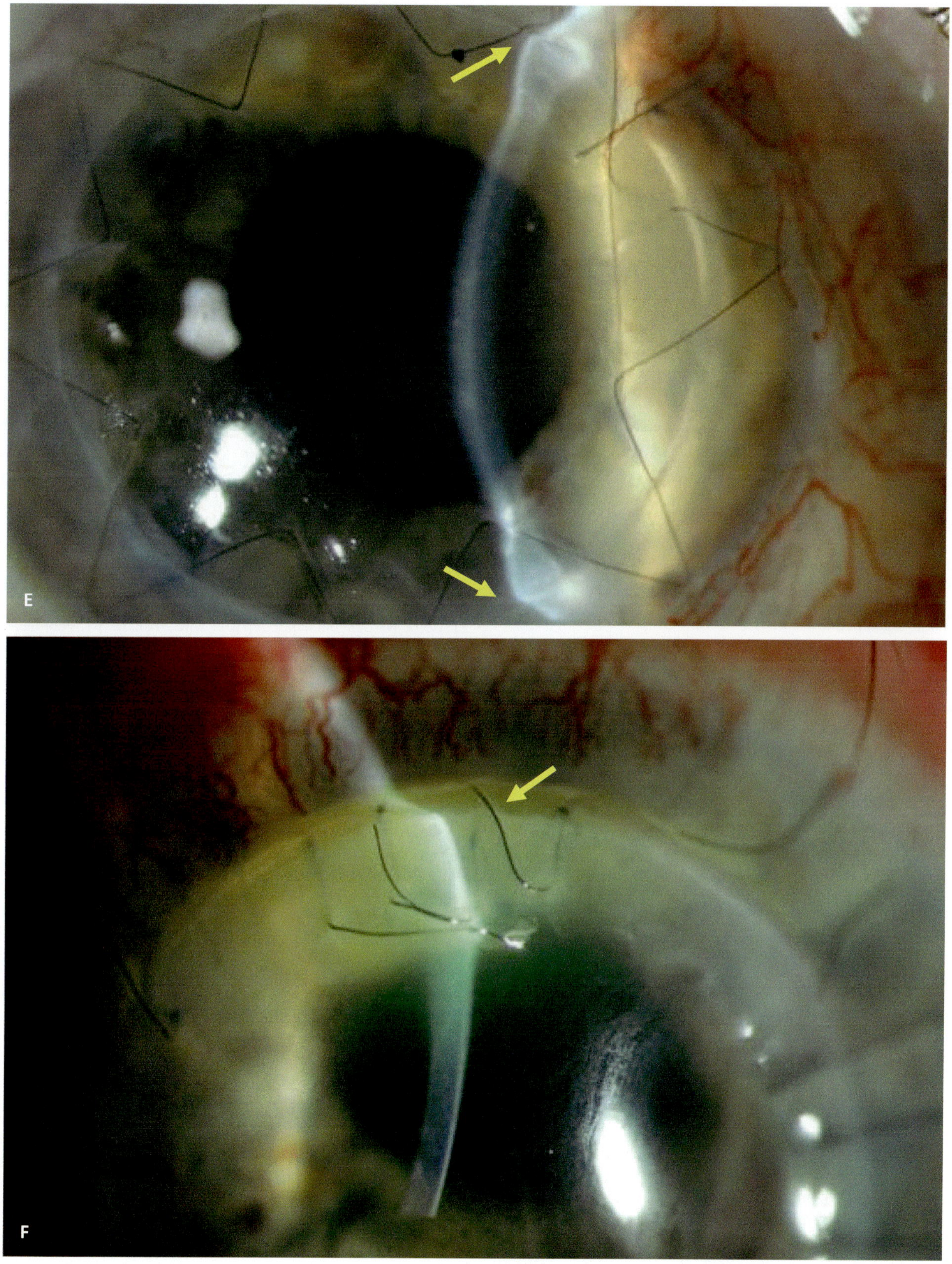

Fig. 9 (**F**) Traumatic graft dehiscence and step formation in a 61-year-old patient after penetrating keratoplasty caused by exposure keratitis secondary to facial nerve palsy after trauma. Notice the ruptured and loose sutures as well as the step formation in the slit light

5 Conclusion

The correct choice of suture technique is essential for optimal postoperative results in keratoplasty. The sutures are preferably removed sequentially 12 and 18 months postoperatively. A regular slit lamp examination with fluorescence staining under blue light is essential for early detection of suture-related complications. Loose and broken suture threads must be removed immediately to avoid the development of infectious keratitis.

If required, new sutures have to be placed in the operation theatre. For this reason, we plead to use at least 24 single sutures in regular PKP and 32 sutures in large-diameter emergency keratoplasty à chaud (i.e. diameter 9.0 mm or greater).

References

1. Zirm EK. A successful total keratoplasty. Graefes Arch Clin Exp Ophthalmol 1906;64:580–93.
2. Seitz B, El-Husseiny M, Langenbucher A, Szentmáry N. Prophylaxis and management of complications in penetrating keratoplasty. Ophthalmologe 2013;110:605–13.
3. F Hoffmann. Suture technique for penetrating keratoplasty. Klin Monbl Augenheilkd 1976;169:584–90.
4. Filatov V, Steinert RF, Talamo JH. Postkeratoplasty astigmatism with single running suture or interrupted sutures. Am J Ophthalmol 1993;115:715–21.
5. DoloricoAMT, Tayyani R, Ong HV, Gaster RN. Shortterm and longterm visual and astigmatic results of an opposing 10–0 nylon double running suture technique for penetrating keratoplasty. J Am Coll Surg 2003;197:991–9.
6. Behrens A, Seitz B, Langenbucher A, Kus MM, Küchle M, Naumann GO. Lens opacities after nonmechanical versus mechanical corneal trephination for keratoplasty in keratoconus J Cataract Refract Surg 2000;26(11):1605–11.
7. Birnbaum F, Wiggermann A, Maier PC, Böhringer D, Reinhard T. Clinical results of 123 femtosecond laser-assisted penetrating keratoplasties. Graefes Arch Clin Exp Ophthalmol 2013;251:95–103.
8. Frost NA, Wu J, Lai TF, Coster DJ. A review of randomized controlled trials of penetrating keratoplasty techniques. Ophthalmology 2006;113:942–9.
9. Kim SJ, Wee WR, Lee JH, Kim MK. The effect of different suturing techniques on astigmatism after penetrating keratoplasty. J Korean Med Sci 2008;23:1015–9.
10. Pagano L, Shah H, Al Ibrahim O, Gadhvi KA, Coco G, Lee JW, Kaye SB, Levis HJ, Hamill KJ, Semeraro F, Romano V. Update on suture techniques in corneal transplantation: a systematic review. J Clin Med 2022;11:1078.
11. Heinzelmann S, Böhringer D, Maier PC, Seitz B, Cursiefen C, Maier A-KB, Dietrich-Ntoukas T, Geerling G, Viestenz A, Pfeiffer N, Reinhard T. Survey of rejection prophylaxis following suture removal in penetrating keratoplasty in Germany. Klin Monbl Augenheilkd 2021;238:591–7.
12. Harris DJJ, Stulting RD, Waring GO 3rd, Wilson LA. Late bacterial and fungal keratitis after corneal transplantation. Spectrum of pathogens, graft survival, and visual prognosis. Ophthalmology 1988;95:1450–7.
13. Wagoner MD, Al-Swailem SA, Sutphin JE, Zimmerman MB. Bacterial keratitis after penetrating keratoplasty: incidence, microbiological profile, graft survival, and visual outcome. Ophthalmology 2007;114:1073–9.
14. Seitz B, Hager T, Szentmáry N, Langenbucher A, Naumann G. Keratoplasty in children-still a dilemma. Klin Monbl Augenheilkd 2013;230:587–94.
15. Sun J-P, Chen W-L, Huang J-Y, Hou Y-C, Wang I-J, Hu F-R. Microbial keratitis after penetrating Keratoplasty. Am J Ophthalmol 2017;178:150–6.
16. Christo CG, Rooij van J, Geerards AJ, Remeijer L, Beekhuis WH. Suture-related complications following keratoplasty: a 5-year retrospective study. Cornea 2001;20:816–9.
17. Hodge C, Chan C, Bali SJ, Sutton G. A review of corneal melting following kerato-refractive surgery. Clin Exp Optom [Internet]. 2013;96:14–9. https://doi.org/10.1111/j.1444-0938.2012.00759.x..
18. Szentmáry N, Seitz B, Langenbucher A, Naumann GOH. Repeat keratoplasty for correction of high or irregular postkeratoplasty astigmatism in clear corneal grafts. Am J Ophthalmol 2005;139:826–30.
19. Lang GK, Schroeder E, Koch JW, Yanoff M, Naumann GOH. Excimer laser keratoplasty. Part 2: Elliptical keratoplasty. Ophthalmic Surg 1989;20:342–6.
20. Langenbucher A, Seitz B, Kus MM, Vilchis E, Naumann GOH. Regularity of corneal topography after penetrating keratoplasty—nonmechanical trephination with the excimer laser 193 nm vs mechanical trephination. Klin Monbl Augenheilkd 1996;208:450–8.
21. Seitz B, Langenbucher A, Kus MM, Küchle M, Naumann GO. Nonmechanical corneal trephination with the excimer laser improves outcome after penetrating keratoplasty. Ophthalmology 1999;106:1156–64; discussion 1165.
22. Tóth G, Szentmáry N, Langenbucher A, Akhmedova E, El-Husseiny M, Seitz B. Comparison of excimer laser versus femtosecond laser assisted trephination in penetrating keratoplasty: a retrospective study. Adv Ther 2019;36:3471–82.
23. Seitz B, Daas L, Milioti G, Szentmàry N, Langenbucher A, Suffo S. Excimer laser-assisted penetrating keratoplasty : On 1 July 2019 excimer laser penetrating keratoplasty celebrates its 30th anniversary Video article. Ophthalmologe 2019;116(12)1221–30.
24. Seitz B, Langenbucher A, Küchle M, Naumann GOH. Impact of graft diameter on corneal power and the regularity of postkeratoplasty astigmatism before and after suture removal. Ophthalmology 2003;110;2162–7.
25. Seitz B, Hager T, Langenbucher A, Naumann GOH. Reconsidering sequential double running suture removal after penetrating keratoplasty: a prospective randomized study comparing excimer laser and motor trephination. Cornea 2018;37:301–6.
26. Behrens A, Seitz B, Küchle M, Langenbucher A, Kus MM, Rummelt C, Naumann GOH. Orientation teeth in non-mechanical laser corneal trephination for penetrating keratoplasty: 2.94 microm Er:YAG v 193 nm ArF excimer laser. Br J Ophthalmol 1999;83:1008–12.
27. Seitz B, Langenbucher A, Meiller R, Kus MM. Decentration of donor cornea in mechanical and excimer laser trephination for penetrating keratoplasty. Klin Monbl Augenheilkd 2000;217:144–51.
28. Szentmáry N, Langenbucher A, Naumann GOH, Seitz B. Intra-individual variability of penetrating keratoplasty outcome after

excimer laser versus motorized corneal trephination. J Refract Surg 2006;22:804–810.
29. Van Meter WS, Gussler JR, Soloman KD, Wood TO. Postkeratoplasty astigmatism control. Single continuous suture adjustment versus selective interrupted suture removal. Ophthalmology 1991;98:177–83.
30. Seitz B, Daas L, Wykrota AA, Flockerzi E, Suffo S. Graft Failure after PKP and DMEK: What is the Best Option? Klin Monbl Augenheilkd 2022;239:775–85.

Conjunctival Flap—Indications, Limitations and Re-opening

Yaser Abu Dail, Loay Daas, and Berthold Seitz

Abstract

This chapter provides an overview on conjunctival flaps and subsequent visual rehabilitation. Since its introduction in the late 1950s, the conjunctival flap has become a treatment of last resort in developed countries. The main indications include emergency coverage of almost penetrated corneal ulcers in areas where better surgical procedures are not available, and relief of eye pain in eyes with reduced visual potential. Visual rehabilitation can be partially achieved by excision of the conjunctival flap and penetrating keratoplasty even years after the original surgery, provided the ocular structures and function are still intact.

Keywords

Conjunctival flap · Optical perforating keratoplasty · Visual deprivation · Corneal ulcer · Visual rehabilitation

1 Introduction

The use of a thin conjunctival flap (CF) to treat chronic corneal ulceration was first introduced by Gundersen in 1958 [1, 2]. CF covers corneal ulcers, preventing stromal lysis mediated by proteolytic enzymes, tears and proinflammatory mediators [3, 4]. Thus, they prevent perforation of the cornea, promote corneal healing and reduce pain [5] (Fig. 1A). However, due to the development of other more effective procedures to treat corneal perforations and stabilize the corneal surface (tissue adhesive, amniotic membrane transplantation, lamellar and penetrating keratoplasty), the use of CF has recently declined in developed countries [4, 6–8]. Nevertheless, CF can still be considered as a therapeutic option in certain cases, especially in developing countries.

2 Indications, Limitations, and Disadvantages

CF was originally used to treat bullous keratopathy, herpetic keratitis, neurotrophic keratopathy and traumatic keratopathy [1, 4, 5]. Although newer medications and methods such as amniotic membrane transplantation, bandage contact lenses, and various forms of keratoplasty have largely replaced CF in the treatment of many corneal diseases, their limited availability in small hospitals as well as in developing countries still makes CF a viable option. A CF is to be considered under the following conditions:

- Corneal ulceration: corneal ulcers can be classified as non-infectious (neurotrophic keratopathy, lagophthalmos, autoimmune, advanced keratoconjunctivitis sicca, chemical and thermal burns) and infectious (bacterial, herpetic, mycotic, acanthamoeba) [9–12]. CF can be used as a temporary solution to treat deep or penetrating **non-infectious** ulcerations or as a permanent solution in eyes with reduced visual potential. For superficial, non-infectious ulcers, amniotic membrane grafts are preferred [2]. However, in autoimmune-related ulcerative keratitis (e.g., Mooren ulcer, peripheral ulcerative keratitis) the use of CF could lead to a rapid relapse, probably due to the increased blood circulation and the resulting increased exposure of stromal antigens to immune cells [13]. In case of infectious ulceration, the use of CF is also limited due to the risk of persisting infectious activity or perforation under CF.

Supplementary Information The online version contains supplementary material available at https://doi.org/10.1007/978-3-031-65422-0_61.

Y. Abu Dail (✉) · L. Daas · B. Seitz
Department of Ophthalmology, Saarland University Medical Center, Homburg, Germany
e-mail: yaser.abu-dail@uks.eu

B. Seitz et al. (eds.), *Atlas on Cornea*, https://doi.org/10.1007/978-3-031-65422-0_61

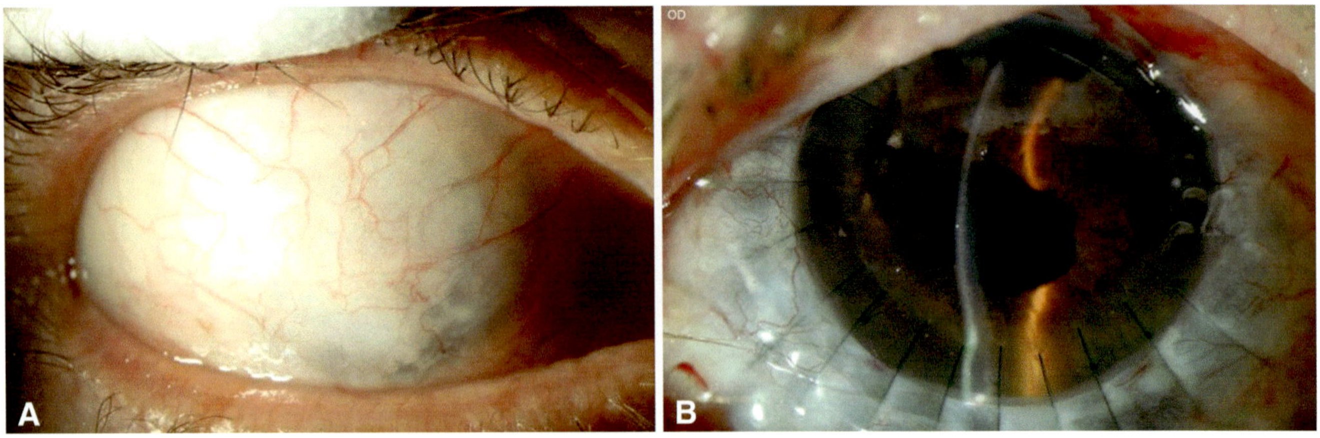

Fig. 1 (**A**) Total conjunctival flap in the right eye of a 66-year-old patient with conjunctivalisation and vascularisation of the cornea without intraocular visibility. The flap was used externally to cover a corneal ulcer 6 years before visual rehabilitation. Visual acuity preoperatively: light perception. (**B**) Clear corneal graft 4 weeks after removal of conjunctival flap and simultaneous keratoplasty. Visual acuity: 0.1 decimal

- Pain relief in eyes with bullous keratopathy and no visual potential: CF helps to cover the exposed corneal nerves with an even surface, reducing corneal pain [9].
- Preparation of a phthitic eye for a prosthetic shell (Fig. 2).

The disadvantages of CF include limited ability to assess underlying ocular structures or intraocular pressure beyond palpation, reduced visual acuity and loss of limbal stem cells resulting in corneal vascularization [4] (Fig. 1A).

3 Visual Rehabilitation After Conjunctival Flaps

Partial rehabilitation of vision after CF is possible even years after corneal blindness [12, 14]. The intervention includes removal of the CF and optical penetrating keratoplasty (Fig. 1B). The surgery should be preceded by a thorough assessment of the eye structures and function. If intraocular visibility is limited, ultrasound biomicroscopy (UBM) or anterior segment ocular coherence tomography are helpful to assess the integrity of the anterior chamber of the eye as well as the chamber angle and to determine the corneal thickness. It is important that the anterior chamber is present and that circular anterior synechiae are excluded [12] (Fig. 3). Adequate regulation of intraocular pressure (IOP) before surgery is also crucial. However, applanatory measurement of intraocular pressure is not possible in the presence of total CF. If an elevated IOP cannot be ruled out by palpation, a direct intracameral measurement may be done preoperatively. The retina can be partially examined using an A-scan and B-scan ultrasound. Eye function can be roughly assessed using Flash-visual evoked potentials (F-VEPs). Patients should be thoroughly informed about the reduced postoperative visual prognosis and the increased risk of graft rejection even after a technically successful operation.

The surgery includes a 360° peritomy with removal of the CF with scissors and forceps, followed by penetrating keratoplasty and simultaneous amniotic membrane transplantation (AMT) as a patch and temporal lateral tarsorrhaphy. The AMT patch is attached end-to-end to the peritomy with single sutures. AMT and lateral tarsorrhaphy are important to support healing of the epithelium and prevent lagophthalmos postoperatively [12, 15, 16]. A gentle anterior synechiolysis (avoid bleeding!) and cataract surgery can also be simultaneously performed (Video 1: Triple penetrating keratoplasty adhoc with simultaneous amniotic patch 6 years after total corneal conjunctival flap) [12].

Please scan to access video content

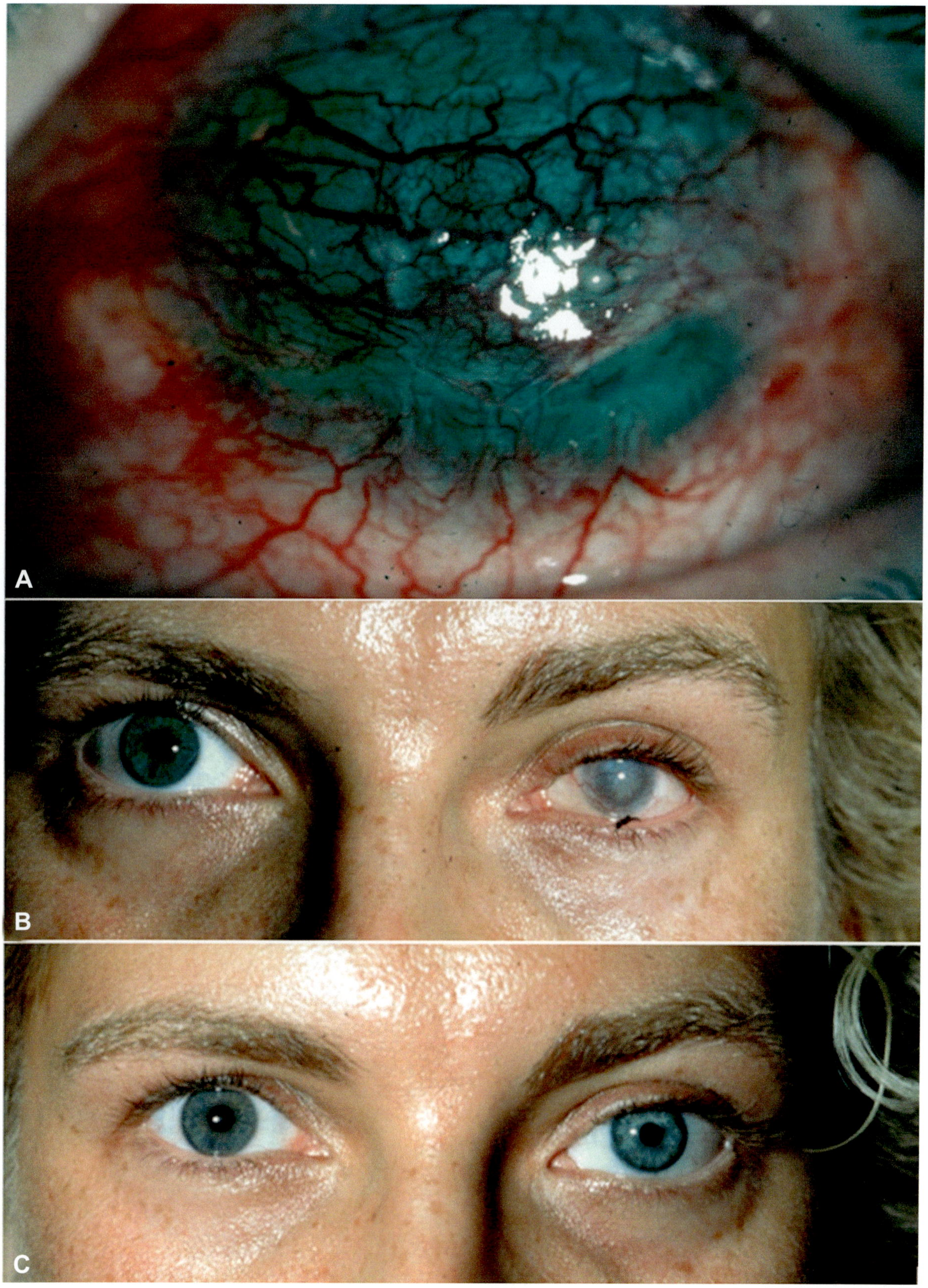

Fig. 2 (**A**, **B**) Total conjunctival flap in the left eye of a female patient with conjunctivalisation and vascularisation of the cornea. The eye has no visual potential. (**C**) The same eye after the application of a prosthetic shell. The photos were made available with the courtesy of Prof. Dr. Thomas Reinhard, Freiburg

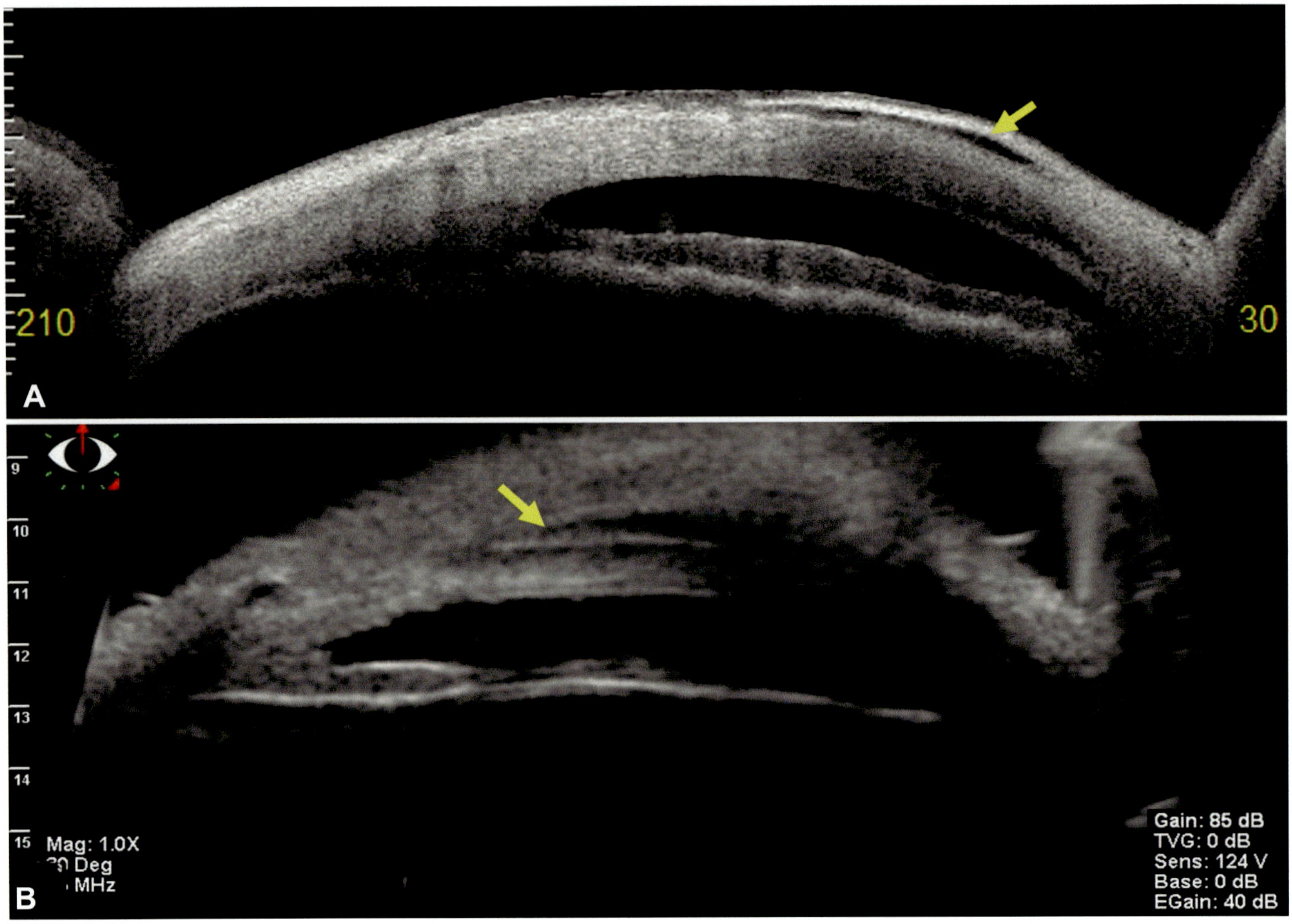

Fig. 3 (**A**) Anterior segment ocular coherence tomography (Casia 2®, Tomey, Nagoya, Japan) and (**B**) ultrasound microbioscopy from eyes with total conjunctival flaps. Mid-deep anterior chamber with anterior synechiae and total conjunctival flap (arrows)

4 Conclusion

Although less commonly used nowadays, conjunctival flaps are still an important and easily accessible procedure for stabilizing the ocular surface and relieving pain in situations where other, more appropriate therapeutic options are not available or when visual potential is severely reduced. Subsequent partial visual rehabilitation by removal of the conjunctival flap and penetrating keratoplasty (with/without lens surgery) is possible even years after corneal blindness, as long as the other eye structures are intact.

References

1. Gundersen T. Conjunctival flaps in the treatment of corneal disease with reference to a new technique of application. AMA Arch Ophthalmol. 1958;60(5):880–8.
2. Gao H, Jia Y, Li S, Wang T, Tan Y, Shi W. Conjunctival flap covering combined with antiviral and steroid therapy for severe herpes simplex virus necrotizing stromal keratitis. Sci World J. 2015:565964.
3. van Rij G, Rinkel-van Driel B, Beekhuis WH. Renardel de Lavalette JG. Conjunctival transplantation Doc Ophthalmol. 1987;67(1–2):145–50.
4. Zemba M, Stamate A-C, Tataru CP, Branisteanu DC, Balta F. Conjunctival flap surgery in the management of ocular surface disease (Review). Exp Ther Med. 2020;20(4):3412–6.
5. Gundersen T, Pearlson HR. Conjunctival flaps for corneal disease: their usefulness and complications. Trans Am Ophthalmol Soc. 1969;67:78–95.
6. Deshmukh R, Stevenson LJ, Vajpayee R. Management of corneal perforations: an update. Indian J Ophthalmol. 2020;68(1):7–14.
7. El Halabi M, Seitz B, Quintin A, Suffo S, Flockerzi F, Schlötzer-Schrehardt U, et al. Histoacryl adhesive for acute treatment of corneal penetration in necrotizing herpetic keratitis. Ophthalmologie. 2022;119(1):59–64.
8. Stamate A-C, Tătaru CP, Zemba M. Update on surgical management of corneal ulceration and perforation. Rom J Ophthalmol. 2019;63(2):166–73.
9. Lim LS, How AC, Ang LPK, Tan DTH. Gundersen flaps in the management of ocular surface disease in an Asian population. Cornea. 2009;28(7):747–51.
10. Ladas JG, Mondino BJ. Systemic disorders associated with peripheral corneal ulceration. Curr Opin Ophthalmol. 2000;11(6):468–71.
11. Farahani M, Patel R, Dwarakanathan S. Infectious corneal ulcers. Dis Mon. 2017;63(2):33–7.

12. Abu Dail Y, Daas L, Flockerzi FA, Seitz B. Partial visual rehabilitation 5 and 6 years after a Gundersen total conjunctival flap procedure. Ophthalmologie. 2022;119(2):203–8.
13. Chen K-H, Hsu W-M, Liang C-K. Relapsing Mooren's ulcer after amniotic membrane transplantation combined with conjunctival autografting. Ophthalmology. 2004;111(4):792–5.
14. Schoth F, Burgel U, Dorsch R, Reinges MHT, Krings T. Diffusion tensor imaging in acquired blind humans. Neurosci Lett. 2006;398(3):178–82.
15. Seitz B, El-Husseiny M, Langenbucher A, Szentmáry N. Prophylaxis and management of complications in penetrating keratoplasty. Ophthalmologe. 2013;110(7):605–13.
16. Dietrich T, Sauer R, Hofmann-Rummelt C, Langenbucher A, Seitz B. Simultaneous amniotic membrane transplantation in emergency penetrating keratoplasty: a therapeutic option for severe corneal ulcerations and melting disorders. Br J Ophthalmol. 2011;95(7):1034–5.

Small Incision Lenticule Extraction (SMILE): Standard Procedure, Intraoperative and Postoperative Complications

Dan Z. Reinstein and Timothy J. Archer

Abstract

Small incision lenticule extraction (SMILE) has become an established procedure for the correction of myopia. In this chapter, we describe the treatment parameters, protocol for docking and centration, and the standardized surgical technique for lenticule removal. The most relevant intraoperative and postoperative complications are also discussed including the management of suction loss, femtosecond energy settings and black spots, difficulty in identifying the cap and lenticule interfaces, management of lenticule remnants, sterile multifocal presentation of DLK unique to SMILE, and epithelial implantation (as opposed to classical epithelial ingrowth). SMILE can now be considered a mature procedure with over 6 million procedures having been performed, with a thorough understanding of surgical instruments, surgical technique and complication management.

Keywords

SMILE · Femtosecond laser · Lenticule · Cap · Small incision

Financial Disclosure: Dr Reinstein is a consultant for Carl Zeiss Meditec (Jena, Germany) and CSO Italia (Florence, Italy), and has a proprietary interest in the Artemis Insight 100 technology (ArcScan Inc, Morrison, Colorado) through patents administered by the Cornell Center for Technology Enterprise and Commercialization (CCTEC), Ithaca, New York. The remaining authors have no proprietary or financial interest in the materials presented herein.

Supplementary Information The online version contains supplementary material available at https://doi.org/10.1007/978-3-031-65422-0_62.

D. Z. Reinstein (✉) · T. J. Archer
London Vision Clinic, EuroEyes Group, London, UK
e-mail: dzr@reinsteinvision.com

D. Z. Reinstein
Columbia University Medical Center, New York, NY, USA

Biomedical Science Research Institute, Ulster University, Coleraine, UK

Sorbonne Université, Paris, France

1 Introduction

With the Introduction of the VisuMax (Carl Zeiss Meditec) came the re-emergence of the intrastromal lenticule method which had first been described in 1996 using a picosecond laser by Ito et al. [1]. The results of femtosecond lenticule extraction (FLEx) were first published in 2008, [2] followed by the first prospective trials for small incision lenticule extraction (SMILE) published in 2011 [3–5]. As of the end of June 2022 there have been over 6,000,000 procedures performed worldwide with more than 2,500 surgeons trained to perform SMILE. United States Food and Drug Administration (FDA) approval was obtained in October 2016 for spherical myopia [6] and in October 2018 for myopic astigmatism [7].

During SMILE, four interfaces are created within the stroma that delineates a lenticule, as shown in Fig. 1. The lenticule of tissue is then removed through a small incision to achieve the desired refractive correction. These interfaces are created from posterior to anterior because once an interface has been created it will obstruct the focus of the femtosecond laser.

(1) **Lenticule interface**; this interface defines the refractive power of the lenticule and is created from the periphery and moves towards the center.
(2) **Lenticule side cut**; this interface is created at the border of the lenticule to provide a clearly defined edge. This is also known, and programmed, as the minimum lenticule thickness.

B. Seitz et al. (eds.), *Atlas on Cornea*, https://doi.org/10.1007/978-3-031-65422-0_62

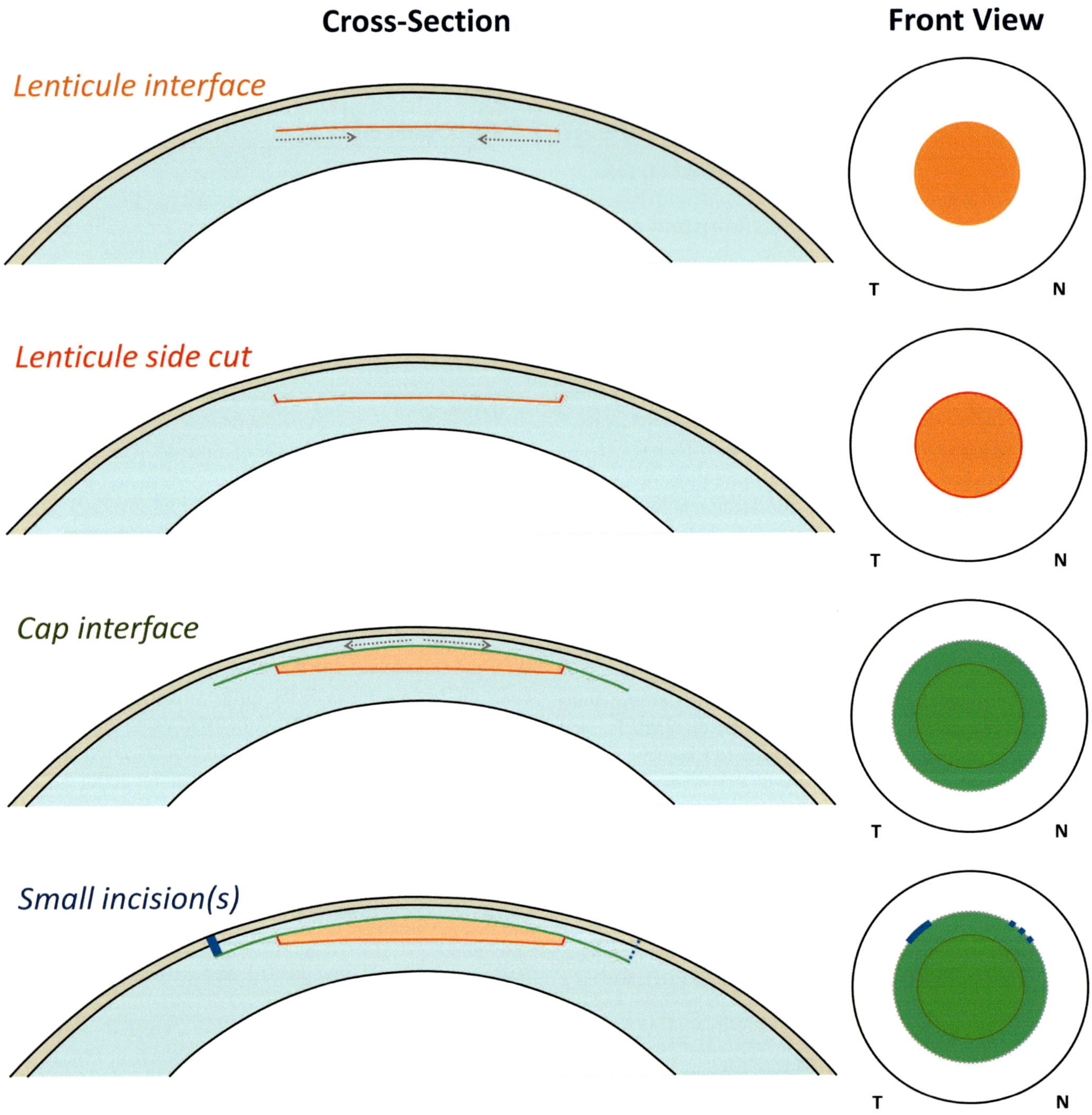

Fig. 1 Series of diagrams showing the femtosecond cutting sequence for a SMILE procedure; (1) lenticule interface from out-to-in, (2) lenticule side cut, (3) cap interface from in-to-out, and (4) the small incision(s). *Reprinted with permission from Reinstein DZ, Archer TJ, Carp GI. The Surgeon's Guide to Small Incision Lenticule Extraction (SMILE). Thorofare, New Jersey: SLACK Incorporated, 2018*

(3) **Cap interface**; this interface is created parallel to the corneal surface to delineate the upper surface of the lenticule, and extend further peripherally to provide access for the surgeon. The cap interface is created from the center towards the periphery.

(4) **Small incision (s)**; this interface creates a tunnel to link the cap interface to the corneal surface, created at the outside edge of the cap.

In this chapter we aim to describe the routine SMILE procedure as well as the most important intraoperative and postoperative complications.

2 Docking, Centration and Cyclotorsion

2.1 Cornea Preparation

The preferred method to wet the cornea is to use a single wipe, with a dripping wet BSS-soaked sponge, to create a homogenized fluid layer—the VisuMax is programmed to assume a tear film layer of 10 µm between the cornea and the contact glass. The goal is to use surface tension to draw the fluid layer across the cornea without the sponge actually touching the surface.

2.2 Routine Docking Process

The docking process is an extremely important part of the procedure as this is where the treatment centration is defined. It is highly recommended to prepare a centration guide prior to surgery.

Centration in SMILE is based on the patient essentially auto-centrating by looking at the fixation light. During the docking process, the surgeon needs to verify that centration is on the visual axis, using the position of the reflex from the green fixation light as a reference in relation to the pupil. To help this process, we prepare a printout (Fig. 2), including the topography eye image and the Hirschberg test, for the surgeon to compare to the intraoperative appearance (a template is available to download from www.londonvision-clinic.com/SMILECentrationTemplate). The aim is to center the treatment as close to the visual axis as possible. The Atlas eye images are rotated 180° in order to be in the same orientation as seen through the operating microscope.

The docking process, as seen in Fig. 3, is performed with the surgeon observing through the treatment microscope. The flashing green fixation light will be visible in the center of the view, and the white illuminated circular border of the contact glass reflected on the surface of the cornea will slowly start coming into focus as the patient bed is raised. Once it is possible to identify the blurred white circle, the surgeon can use the joystick to make small adjustments to place this light circle reflection to be concentric with the flashing green fixation light.

At the moment of contact between the curved contact glass and the cornea, a meniscus of fluid contact appears, at which point the green flashing fixation light will come into clear focus for the patient because the vergence of the beam is adjusted according the individual eye's sphero-cylindrical refraction as entered into the system for the refractive correction. Suction should be activated when approximately 80–90% of the accurvation of the cornea in the contact glass is achieved, which is visualized by the border of the meniscus. This will draw the cornea onto the contact glass, immobilizing it in the optimal position to begin the femtosecond cutting.

Femtosecond cutting should be started as soon as all final checks have been completed. If suction has been applied and you are not satisfied with the centration, you can simply turn off the suction and start the centration process again.

We conducted a matched-control study, using tangential topography difference maps, and found no statistically significant difference in centration between 100 SMILE eyes and 100 MEL 90 LASIK eyes ($p=0.082$); mean $\pm$ SD centration offset was 0.20 ± 0.11 mm (range: 0.00–0.50 mm)

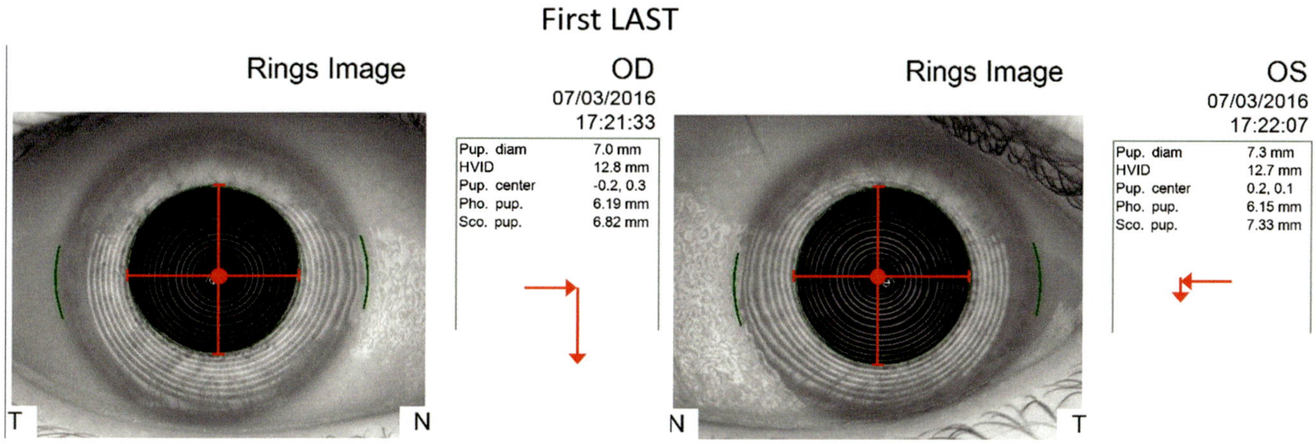

Fig. 2 Example of the printout used as a reference to the expected position of the corneal reflex during docking. The corneal vertex (center of the Mires rings) is indicated as a red dot, with red cross-hair guidelines overlaid to visualize the position relative to the pupil border. A further visual cue is included in the form of arrows representing the magnitude and direction of the corneal vertex relative to the center of the entrance pupil, as defined by the coordinates measured by the Atlas. *Reprinted with permission from Reinstein DZ, Archer TJ, Carp GI. The Surgeon's Guide to Small Incision Lenticule Extraction (SMILE). Thorofare, New Jersey: SLACK Incorporated, 2018*

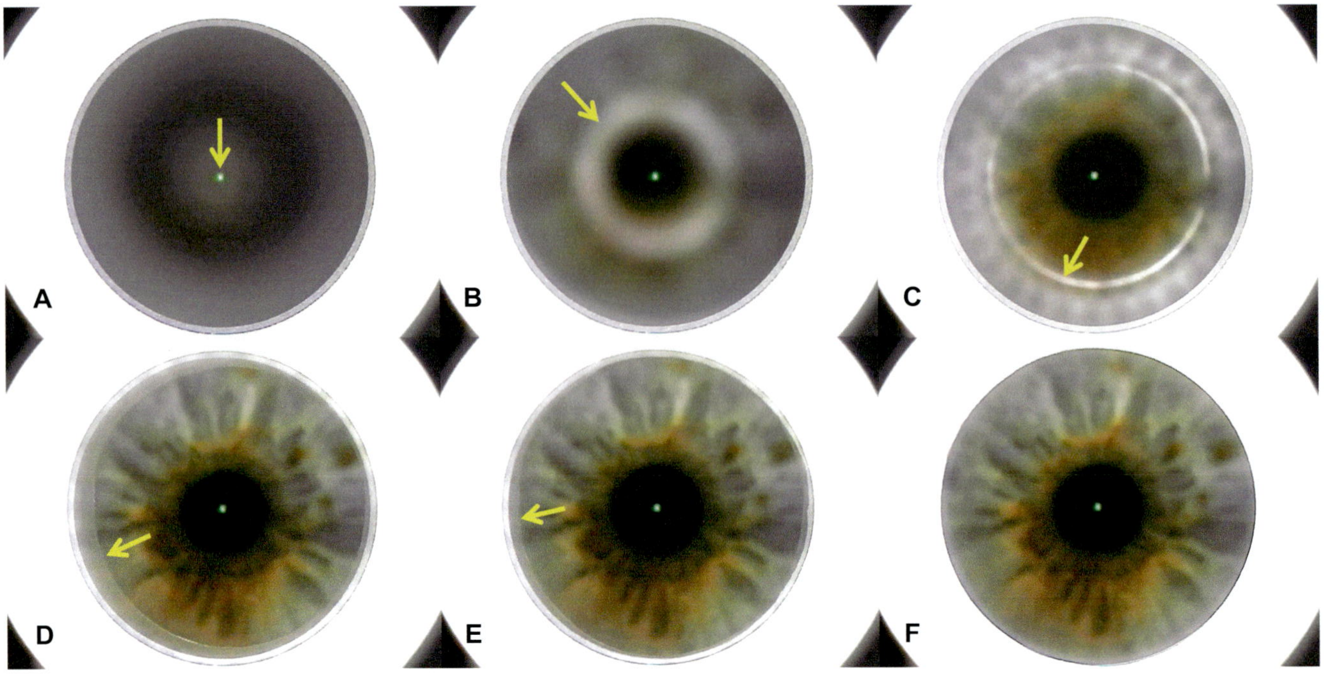

Fig. 3 Images showing the steps in the docking process and the features that should be monitored by the surgeon. (**A**) With the patient in position under the treatment cone, the reflection of the green fixation light will be visible on the cornea. (**B**) As the patient bed is raised, the reflection of the illuminated contact glass circumference will become visible, which can be used to start adjusting the centration. (**C**) At first contact with the contact glass, a tear film meniscus appears and the green fixation light will come into clear focus for the patient. (**D**) As the patient bed is slowly raised, the surgeon should continue to make small adjustments to the centration if necessary. (**E**) The patient bed should be raised until 80–90% of the accurvation of the cornea into the contact glass has been achieved, (**F**) at which point suction can be activated. *Reprinted with permission from Reinstein DZ, Archer TJ, Carp GI. The Surgeon's Guide to Small Incision Lenticule Extraction (SMILE). Thorofare, New Jersey: SLACK Incorporated, 2018*

for the SMILE group and 0.17 ± 0.10 mm (range: 0.00–0.53 mm) for the LASIK group [8]. Similar results were found in other studies [9–11].

3 Femtosecond Laser

The femtosecond cutting is the most critical part of the procedure. While a suction loss rarely leads to the patient not receiving a complete treatment, it is obviously better if these can be avoided.

In our experience, the most common reason for losing suction is a patient attempting to maintain fixation on the flashing green light; some patients can perceive the light as being slightly off to one side once suction immobilization has been achieved, and so try to turn their eye in order to look directly at the light. This however causes further displacement of the image of the light on the retina, so the patient will think the light has moved further away, which can result in a negative feedback loop leading to a shift in the corneal position or a suction loss. So the patient should be instructed *not* to follow the green light should it start moving.

The photodisruption process, as seen in Fig. 4, should be monitored through the surgical microscope, with the microscope focused at the plane of the femtosecond bubble formation within the cornea. The surgeon should be monitoring the following features:

- Monitor the sequence, size and position of the cuts (see Sect. 1.1)
- Total suction time
- Eye movements or torque—This may cause an irregularity in the lenticule, which could lead to a poor outcome if the lenticule is removed
- Edges of the contact glass—To evaluate the stability of the suction; a meniscus forming at the edge of the contact glass or intrusion of the conjunctiva into the diameter of the contact glass are early warning signs of potential suction loss.
- Quality of the femtosecond bubble interface—Noting areas of opaque bubble layer and dark spots. There are certain situations where the procedure should be aborted (see Sect. 5.3).

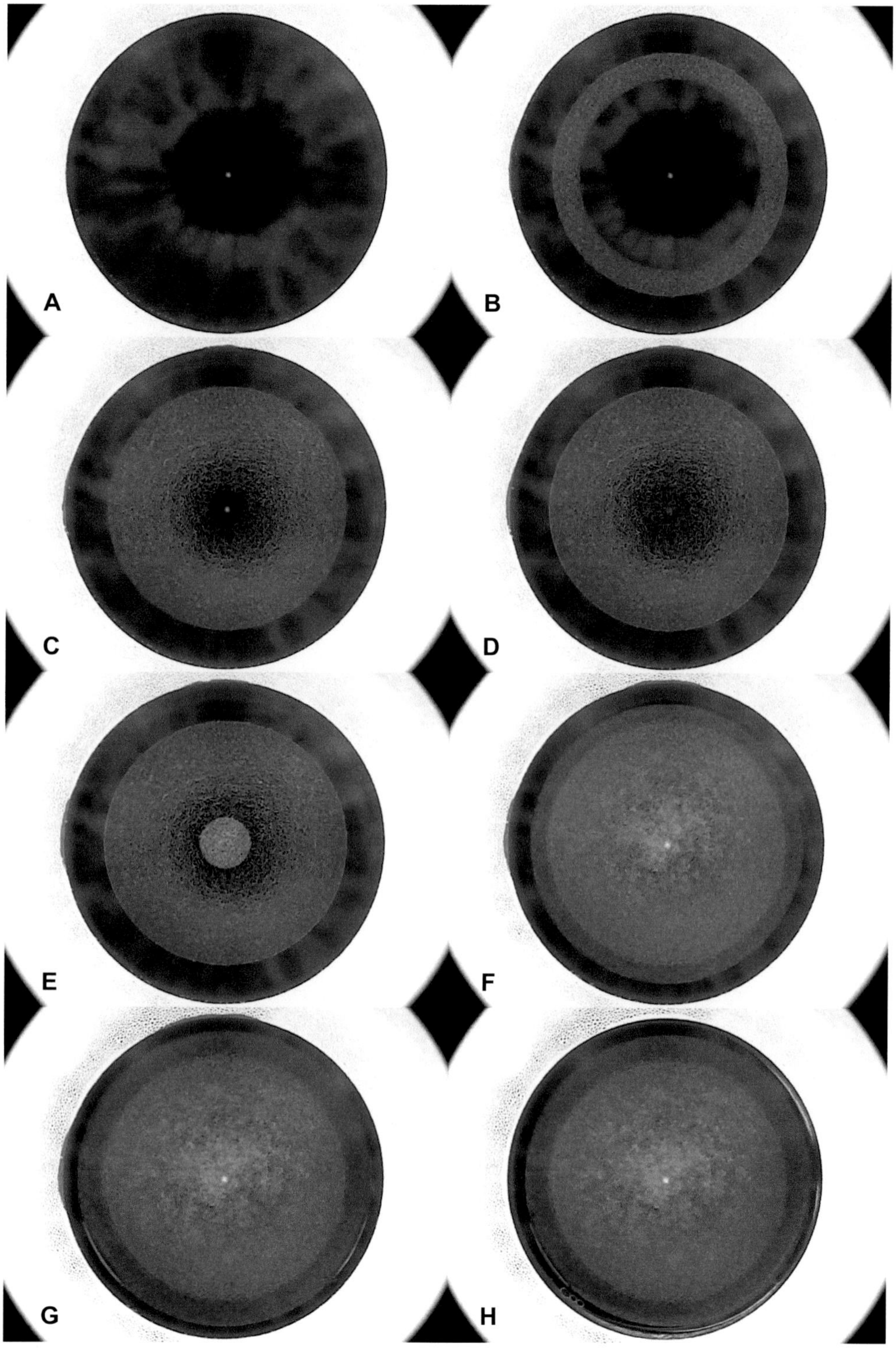

Fig. 4 Series of images showing the femtosecond cutting sequence. (**A**) After applying suction, the system takes a few seconds to confirm that adequate suction has been achieved before femtosecond cutting can begin. This time should be used to make a final confirmation of the centration. (**B**), (**C**) The lenticule interface is created first from out-to-in. (**D**) The lenticule side cut is created. (**E**), (**F**) The cap interface is created from in-to-out. (**G**) The small incisions are created. (**H**) Suction is automatically deactivated upon completion of the small incisions. *Reprinted with permission from Reinstein DZ, Archer TJ, Carp GI. The Surgeon's Guide to Small Incision Lenticule Extraction (SMILE). Thorofare, New Jersey: SLACK Incorporated, 2018*

4 Surgical Technique

After observing the completion of the femtosecond cutting, the cap and lenticule can be manually separated and the lenticule can be extracted. The following protocol describes the bimanual surgical technique we developed at London Vision Clinic (Reinstein, Carp) and Tilganga Institute of Ophthalmology (Pradhan) through our collective experience of over 7,500 procedures. For our SMILE surgical technique, we use two instruments: a fine toothed forceps to hold and immobilize the globe during interface separation and the Reinstein lenticule separator. The step-wise description of the technique is illustrated in Fig. 5 and can be seen in Video 1. A full detailed description has been previously published [12, 13].

Please scan to access video content

In brief, the Sinskey tip is used to score and open the superotemporal incision, followed by pocketing the cap interface across the whole diameter of the small incision. The Sinskey tip is then used to pocket the lenticule interface across one half of the small incision. The SMILE separator bulb is used to separate the cap interface, followed by separating the lenticule interface. The separator bulb can then be used to drag the lenticule out through the small incision.

As the cap in SMILE is fixed in place, there is no need for repositioning as for a LASIK flap. However, there is a need to redistribute the cap due to the mismatch in length between the cap and the bed. This mismatch comes from the difference between the lengths of the cap and the bed following the refractive lenticule removal (i.e. the bed is now a chord across the original curvature). Checking the cap is best done at the slit-lamp with heavy fluorescein staining using a dry microspear to distend the cap by centrifugal stroking. This process can also be repeated at the early postoperative visits if needed.

A similar cap repositioning technique has been described by Shetty et al., [14] who reported that quality of vision measures by HD Analyzer were better if intraoperative cap repositioning was performed compared to no repositioning.

5 Intraoperative Complications

Suction loss is the most obvious intraoperative complication of SMILE as this prevents the femtosecond cutting from completing. In almost all cases, a suction loss is caused by the patient moving their eye, so the management of eye movements and suction loss are closely connected. It is important to be aware that small, or even large, eye movements can occur without breaking suction. Fortunately, SMILE has matured to a point where the safety of the final outcome (loss of visual quality) should rarely be affected by eye movements or suction loss events. This requires an in-depth understanding of each step of the process and how to manage these appropriately [15, 16].

5.1 Suction Stability Management

Eye movements can present in the following ways: fixation light tracking, Bell's reflex, small saccades, large saccades, oscillations, anxiety/uncooperative patient, nociceptive reflex movement, false suction, and nystagmus.

Once the cause is determined, it is then important to grade the magnitude of the eye movement.

- **Type I**—small eye movements such as small saccades that shift the corneal position by a clinically negligible amount. A type I eye movement would not be large enough to create a visible discontinuity in the femtosecond bubble pattern. Therefore, it is not expected for a type I movement to induce a clinically significant irregularity in the lenticule surface.
- **Type II**—large eye movements, such as a Bell's reflex or tracking the green fixation light. Type II movements are visually obvious and require an immediate management action. The visual cues are a sudden relative shift in the bubble layer already created, a meniscus forming at the edge of the contact glass, intrusion of the conjunctiva within the contact glass, or a distortion or discontinuity in the femtosecond bubble pattern. It is possible for a large movement to occur, but for the eye to return to its original position, in which case the treatment can be continued. Alternatively, if the movement is such that the lenticule regularity or centration is deemed to have been compromised, the surgeon may well choose to release suction, i.e. a surgeon-initiated suction loss (SISL).
- **Type III**—an eye movement with sufficient force to break suction, i.e. a patient-generated suction loss (PGSL).

Early detection of eye movements acts as an early warning of a possible suction loss and provides an opportunity to control the patient. It is often useful to pause the femtosecond cutting in order to verbally control the patient to prevent small movements escalating to a suction loss. Once it has been confirmed that suction is stable, the surgeon can resume the femtosecond cutting. 'Pause, regain control, continue' (P/R/C) therefore becomes the first cornerstone of suction stability management.

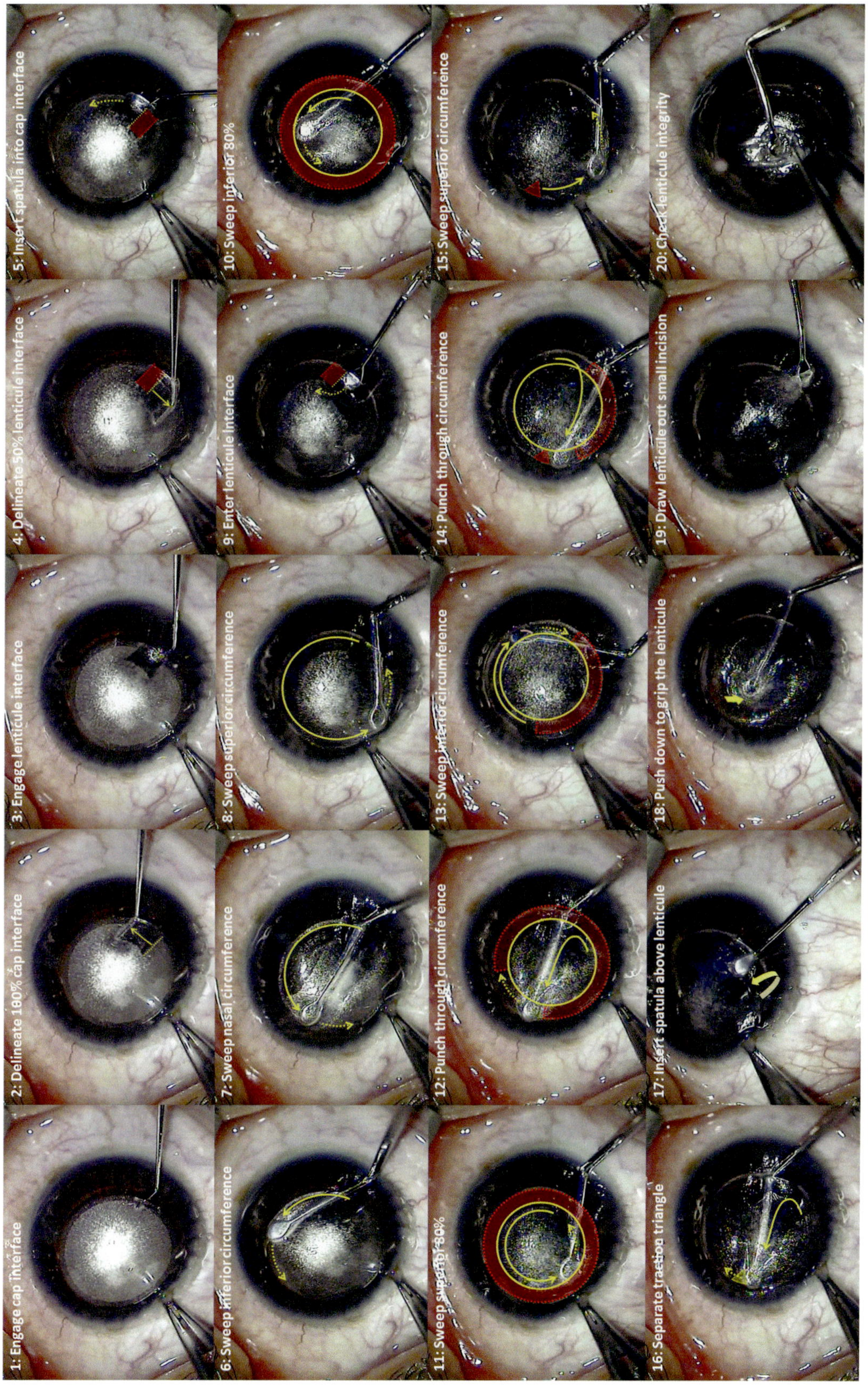

Fig. 5 Series of steps required to perform a routine SMILE procedure, including (1) opening the small incision and pocketing the interfaces (steps 1 to 4), (2) separating the cap interface (steps 5 to 8), (3) separating the lenticule interface (steps 9 to 16), (4) removing the lenticule (steps 17 to 19), and (5) checking the lenticule integrity (step 20). *Reprinted with permission from Reinstein DZ, Archer TJ, Carp GI. The Surgeon's Guide to Small Incision Lenticule Extraction (SMILE). Thorofare, New Jersey: SLACK Incorporated, 2018*

The VisuMax software is programmed to handle a suction loss—known as the *Restart treatment* module. This wizard-style software system will provide a recommendation for continuing the procedure following a suction loss.

The list below summarizes the procedure recommended by the *Restart treatment* module for suction loss during each interface. In cases of suction loss, the same contact glass can be used and only needs to be wiped to clear any visible debris or fibers. There are some situations where it may not be suitable to follow the treatment wizard. For example, if the interface had tracked upward as the cornea was released from the contact glass, it may be preferable to convert to LASIK.

- **Lenticule interface (first 10%)**—restart SMILE with the same settings.
- **Lenticule interface (10–100%)**—convert to LASIK with flap thickness equivalent to the planned cap thickness. Restarting SMILE is not advised as the lenticule interface is the refractive component.
- **Lenticule side cut**—restart SMILE from the lenticule side cut with the same settings.
- **Cap interface**—restart SMILE from the cap interface with the same cap thickness. The risk of an irregular lenticule is relatively low as the cap interface is parallel to the corneal surface.
- **Small incision**—restart SMILE from the small incision.

A more in-depth protocol which introduces further scenarios not discussed in this chapter can be found in *Reinstein DZ, Archer TJ, Carp GI. The Surgeon's Guide to Small Incision Lenticule Extraction (SMILE). Thorofare, New Jersey: SLACK Incorporated, 2018.*

There are four studies published to date that report the incidence of suction loss in large SMILE populations of more than 1,500 procedures, [17–20] ranging from 0.17 [20] to 0.41 [17] up to 0.78%, [19] and a highest value of 2.10%. [18] In our experience of 4,000 SMILE procedures to date, there have been 20 cases of suction loss, representing an incidence of 0.50% (1 in 200, confidence interval 0.32–0.77%). Referring to the suction loss cases reported in the smaller population studies, the overall impression is that a good result can be achieved either by restarting SMILE or converting the patient to LASIK [21]. In our experience, the outcomes of the suction loss cases were equivalent to the outcomes of the fellow eyes where SMILE was completed without a suction loss.

5.2 Femtosecond Energy and Opaque Bubble Layer (OBL)

The surgeon has some control over the performance of the femtosecond laser, and therefore the quality of the lenticule interfaces, by adjusting the energy and stop spacing settings. *Spot distance*, *Track distance*, *Energy offset*, *Scan direction* and *Scan mode* can be adjusted within a certain range. Each parameter can be set independently for each interface. These should initially be set and optimized with the help of a Carl Zeiss Meditec applications specialist, as there are usually small differences between laser systems. The effect of changing and finding the optimal balance between these parameters is summarized below:

- OBL is more likely to occur for higher energy levels because the bubbles are larger and therefore more likely to coalesce [22, 23].
- OBL is also more likely to occur if the bubbles are closer together (the spot and track distance is small).
- Interface separation is easier for higher energy and closer spot separation. However, both of these factors can also increase the incidence of OBL, which makes interface separation significantly more difficult.
- Interface separation becomes more difficult for very low energies and wide spot separation because more tissue bridges need to be broken.
- Reducing the spot separation distance increases the suction time and therefore the risk of suction loss.
- The lenticule surfaces are less regular for higher energy levels because larger bubbles create irregularities [22, 24].
- Studies have shown that visual recovery is optimized when using lower energy levels [22, 23, 25, 26].
- Therefore, an optimal energy is low enough to avoid OBL and lenticule surface irregularities, but high enough to ensure acceptable interface separation.

It is important to note that energy settings cannot simply be transferred between lasers as there are differences between individual units; there may be variations in the laser head or laser optics.

5.3 Dark Spots in Femtosecond Bubble Pattern

Dark spots represent areas where there may not have been effective femtosecond cutting, which can be more difficult to separate. Significant manual separation can lead to irregularities in the lenticule that manifest as irregular astigmatism after surgery.

The risk of dark spots is the downside to using very low energy levels, close to the plasma threshold. As with anything, there is some variation between treatments in the actual energy delivered, meaning that there are some rare outlier cases where the energy is sub-threshold in some areas. This risk offsets any additional gain in visual recovery for the slightly lower energy. Therefore, we and others have settled on an energy level 2–3 clicks up from the plasma threshold as the optimal energy. If any trace of dark spots is identified, the energy might be increased for the next eye treated (even the second eye of the same patient), in order to shift the energy further away from the plasma threshold for that patient.

Another possibility is that dark spots might sometimes be related to stromal geometry, stromal packing order, or intrastromal inflammation with lamellar remodeling (e.g. previous asymptomatic herpes simplex virus)—something that has caused stromal structural changes that leads to irregular forms of cutting. One example would be translucent lines in the cutting pattern (especially in the lenticule interface) as seen in Fig. 6. These lines can lead to an irregular lenticule which puts the patient at risk for losing lines of CDVA.

Another cause of dark spots is the presence of debris or fibers on the surface of the contact glass, or meibom in the tear film. Figure 7 demonstrates how debris and meibom can obstruct the femtosecond laser beam path and result in an area of no effective femtosecond cutting. Debris can be removed from the surface of the contact glass by using a surgical sponge which is dipped in BSS and dragged across the contact glass. Once cleaned, the surface should be inspected to ensure there is no remaining particles or meibom.

5.4 Identifying the Interface Edges

The most common difficulty faced by a novice SMILE surgeon is finding the edges of either the cap or lenticule interfaces. There are cases where, for no apparent reason, the lenticule interface edge is simply more difficult to access, although this is usually due to the shape of an astigmatic lenticule. Alternatively, the cap interface can appear difficult to identify if the lenticule interface was unintentionally separated first. This is why it is important to start the procedure by pocketing in each interface before proceeding to separate the cap interface so that you can be sure that both interfaces are accessible before starting the separation. However, there are techniques to find either interface in these situations meaning that it should be extremely rare to have to abort the lenticule extraction.

During the development of SMILE, many surgeons experienced difficulty identifying the cap interface if the lenticule interface was separated first, as the lenticule can become compacted against the anterior stromal surface. To solve this issue, we have developed a very simple and reliable technique for finding the cap interface using the Sinskey tip of the regular SMILE Separator [27].

In this technique, shown in Video 2, the Sinskey tip is inserted sideways into the small incision and moved across until the shaft reaches the superior limit of the incision. The tip is rotated upwards and around, tenting up the cap layer and engaging the lenticule edge in the process. This motion is successful first time in most cases, but sometimes it might take a few attempts. Once the cap interface has been pocketed, the separation can proceed as normal. Armed with this technique, separating the lenticule interface first can no longer be considered a complication of SMILE.

Please scan to access video content

Similar to finding the cap interface, if the lenticule interface was difficult to identify through the primary small incision, the reserve incision offers another area over which the lenticule interface might be identified. Almost all cases of difficulty finding the lenticule interface edge are eyes with high astigmatism. This is due to the geometry of an astigmatic lenticule where the side cut in the topographic flat axis is less well defined. Therefore, if the topographic flat axis is aligned with the small incision, the surgeon can expect the identification of the lenticule interface to be challenging.

If the lenticule interface cannot be identified even via the reserve small incision, the next step is to extend the 2 mm small incision to lift or even fold back the cap edge to gain access to a larger stromal area to aid in finding the interface edge.

5.5 Lenticule Remnants

Another possible complication of SMILE is leaving a lenticule remnant in the interface. A lenticule remnant is most likely to occur in cases where the separation was difficult, and is more likely when extracting thinner, more delicate lenticules. However, these can also occur after lenticule separations that had appeared routine. Lenticule remnants can cause distortions and irregular astigmatism on topography, and consequently cause issues with quality of vision. Therefore, every care should be taken during surgery to ensure the entire lenticule has been removed.

The first step in the process of managing lenticule remnants is to identify when they occur. This is why it is important to check the integrity of the lenticule for every eye treated, by placing it on top of the cornea immediately after removal. If the lenticule is found to be incomplete, there are a few techniques that can be used to help locate the residual piece:

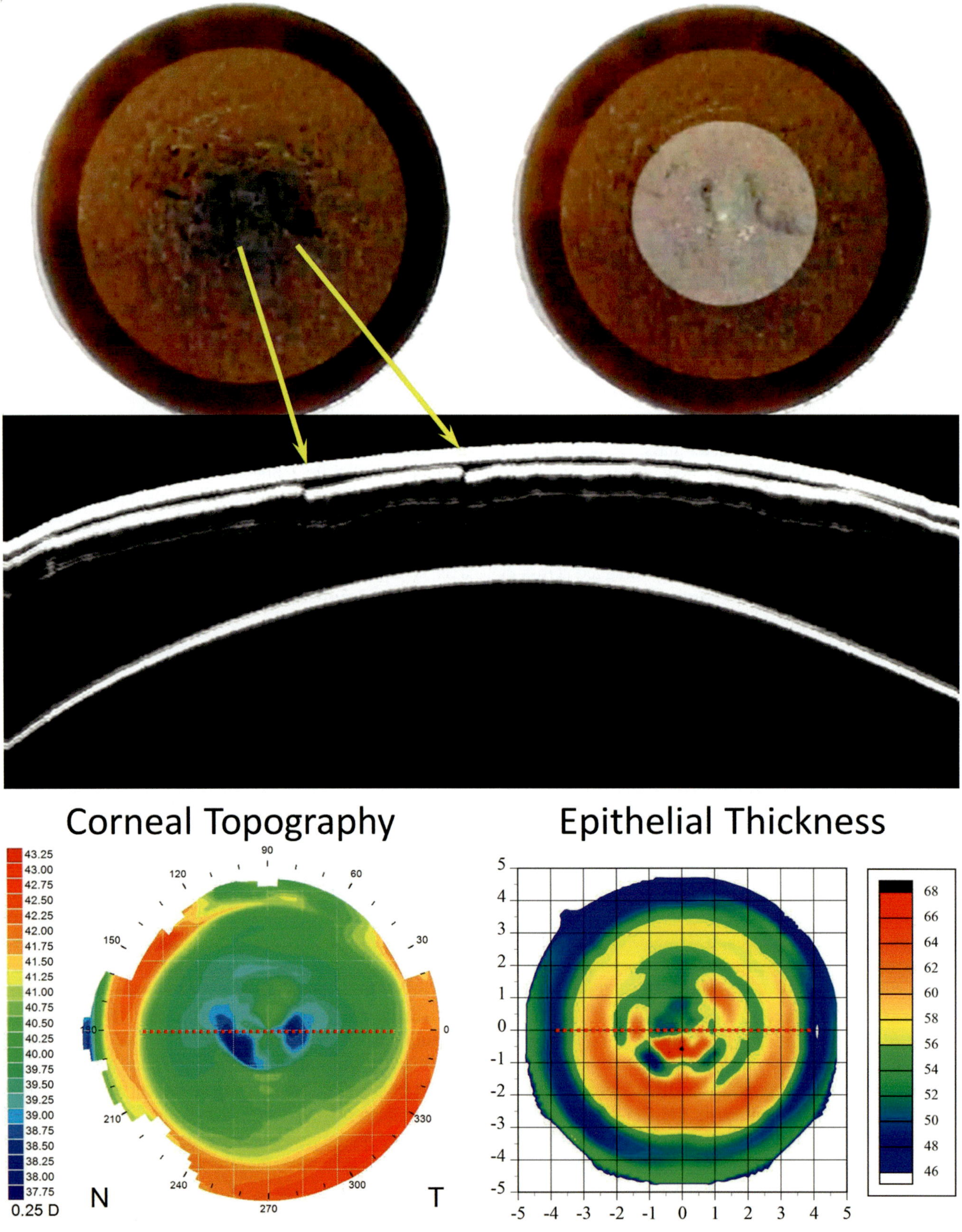
Corneal Topography
43.25
43.00
42.75
42.50
42.25
42.00
41.75
41.50
41.25
41.00
40.75
40.50
40.25
40.00
39.75
39.50
39.25
39.00
38.75
38.50
38.25
38.00
37.75
0.25 D
90
120
60
150
30
180
0
210
330
240
300
270
N
T
Epithelial Thickness
68
66
64
62
60
58
56
54
52
50
48
46
5
4
3
2
1
0
-1
-2
-3
-4
-5

◀ **Fig. 6** In this eye, transulcent lines were observed centrally in the femtosecond cutting of the lenticule interface (top), but the lenticule was extracted. Three months after surgery, an Artemis Insight 100 VHF digital ultrasound B-scan (middle) showed significant irregularities in the SMILE interface that were mirrored on Bowman layer. Although epithelial remodeling (bottom right) had partially smoothed the irregularities, the topography (bottom left) showed irregularly irregular astigmatism, which was causing visual disturbances and loss of contrast sensitivity for the patient. *Reprinted with permission from Reinstein DZ, Archer TJ, Carp GI. The Surgeon's Guide to Small Incision Lenticule Extraction (SMILE). Thorofare, New Jersey: SLACK Incorporated, 2018*

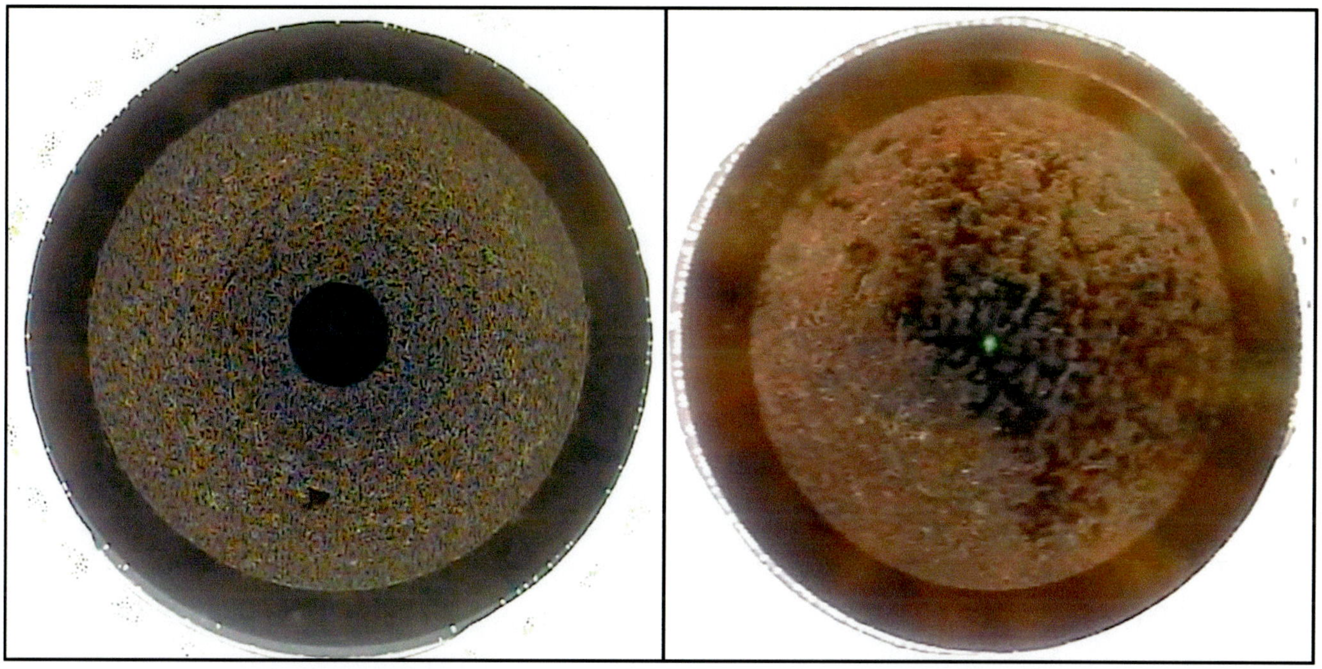

Fig. 7 Example of a small black spot created in the lenticule interface by a fiber on the surface of the contact glass (left) to severe disruption caused by the presence of meibom in the tear film (right). *Reprinted with permission from Reinstein DZ, Archer TJ, Carp GI. The Surgeon's Guide to Small Incision Lenticule Extraction (SMILE). Thorofare, New Jersey: SLACK Incorporated, 2018*

- The circumference of the lenticule border can be evaluated using the Separator bulb and the remnant may be large and obvious enough to be found simply by the feel of the instrument, akin to finding the end on a reel of sticky tape.
- The built-in slit-lamp feature within the operating microscope can be used to aid visualization of the edges of a lenticule remnant (Fig. 8).
- Lifting the instrument to raise the cap away from the stromal bed creates an air pocket that improves visibility of the stromal bed to identify the border of any unseparated areas (see Fig. 8).
- Using the reserve incision to improve instrument manipulation or change direction of force to help aid in removal (see Fig. 8).
- Flooding the interface with an opaque suspension (e.g. Kenalog-10 [triamcinolone acetonide, Bristol Myers Squibb]) can be used to demarcate the contours within the interface, such that the location of a lenticule remnant is outlined by the white liquid pooling in the relative trough created by the abrupt change in curvature (see Fig. 8).

Once the location of the lenticule remnant has been identified, it can sometimes be separated using the Separator bulb as for a normal lenticule, although an instrument with a sharper tip is often required if the area was unseparated by the Separator bulb the first time. In other cases where there is a thin strip remaining in situ, forceps can be used to circumferentially tear the strip of lenticule away from the border in a lenticulerhexis-type technique.

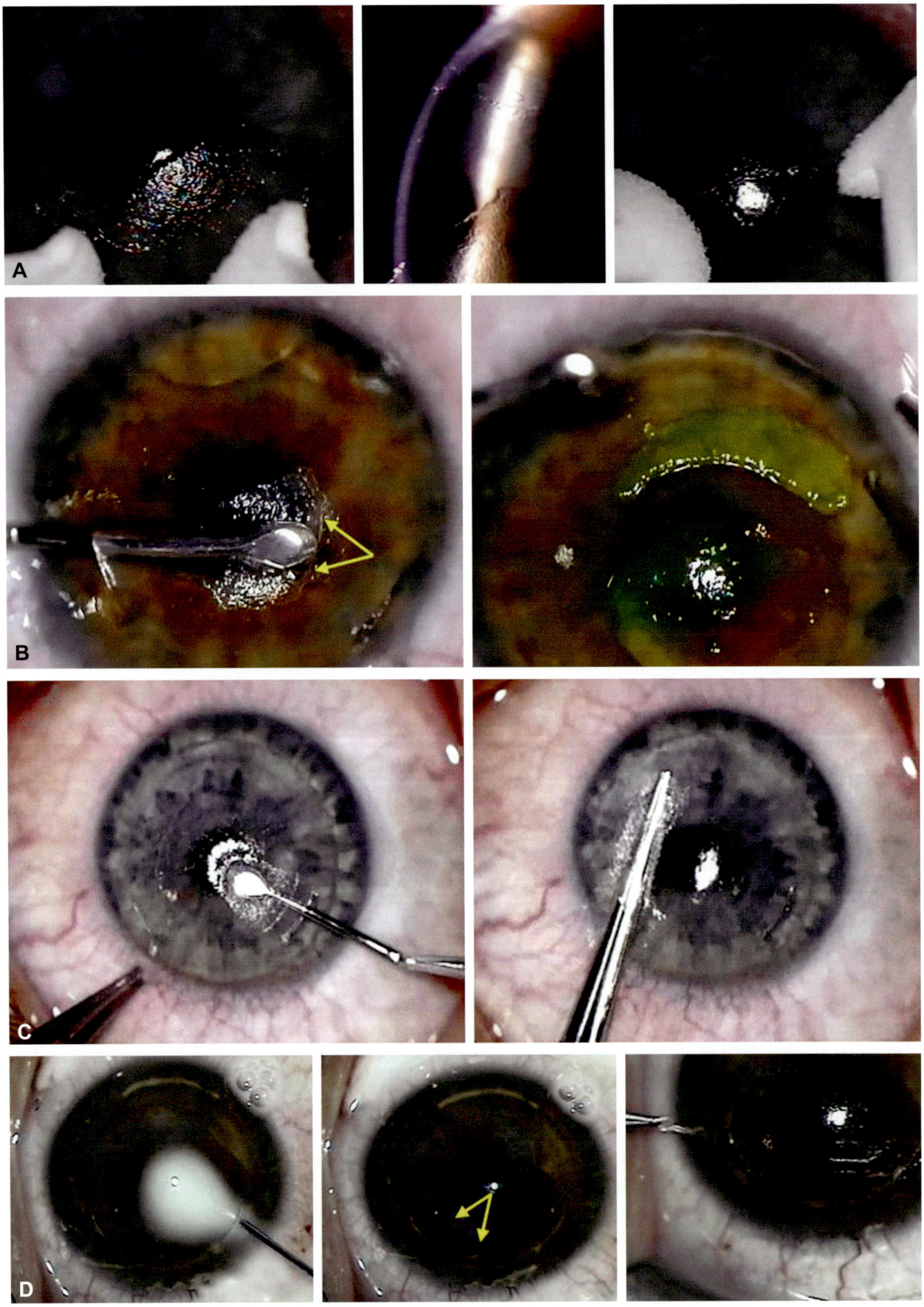

Fig. 8 A series of images identifying and removing a lenticule remnant via visualizing with the slit-lamp technique (**A**) visualizing with the air-pocket technique (**B**) using the reserve incision (**C**) and visualizing by injecting an opaque solution into the interface (**D**) *Reprinted with permission from Reinstein DZ, Archer TJ, Carp GI. The Surgeon's Guide to Small Incision Lenticule Extraction (SMILE). Thorofare, New Jersey: SLACK Incorporated, 2018*

Once removed, the lenticule should be placed on the cornea together with the main body of the lenticule to check if the pieces of the puzzle fit together. As before, by doing this on the cornea, the final lenticule is captured as part of the VisuMax video recording. If the pieces do not fit perfectly, then further investigation of the interface might be performed. The final lenticule can also be recorded with fluorescein staining after surgery.

The clinical significance of leaving a lenticule remnant in the interface depends on the size and location. In many cases, a small peripheral lenticule remnant will not be visually significant even if there is a noticeable irregularity on topography. In some cases, the lenticule remnant might not be picked up by the on-cornea lenticule review, but is only identified as part of a routine OCT or VHF digital ultrasound scan after surgery. There are other cases where a small lenticule edge truncation is identified when checking the lenticule. If the lenticule remnant is so small, it can be almost impossible to extract. There is almost no risk to the vision if a remnant is left, if it is small and in a peripheral location, and epithelial remodeling will mask the majority of the stromal irregularity [28].

A large lenticule remnant is obviously a different story and a topographic irregularity would be expected in such cases. An example of this has been reported by Dong and Zhou [29] who described a case of inferior steepening after SMILE that was found by OCT imaging 5 months after surgery to be due to a lenticule remnant. This was correlated to a large region of dense opaque bubble layer, although the lenticule had appeared complete after removal. However, if a visually significant lenticule remnant is found after surgery, this can be resolved by surgically removing the remnant. An example of this has been published by Ganesh et al. [30] who published a case series of lenticule fragment removal after failed primary SMILE.

6 Postoperative Complications

Many of the postoperative complications are the same as found in LASIK and can be managed the same way and so will not be described in this Chapter. These include epithelial defects, anterior basement membrane dystrophy, interface haze, interface debris, infection, and interface fluid syndrome. As with LASIK, dry eye symptoms are an expected side effect after SMILE albeit less severe and usually faster to recover. Additionally, epithelial ingrowth and diffuse lamellar keratitis (DLK) are also possible postoperative complications of SMILE. In many respects, the presentation and management of these two entities is equivalent between the two procedures. However, there are some differences to what is typically found after LASIK which are important to highlight. These will be discussed below.

6.1 Atypical DLK: Interface Focal Inflammatory Keratitis After SMILE

DLK can occur after SMILE with the same classical presentation as after LASIK and the management is the same [31]. Sterile lamellar inflammatory infiltration can also present after SMILE with a unique appearance not typically seen after LASIK, appearing as focal infiltrates scattered throughout the interface with or without a diffuse component (Fig. 9). This presentation is usually seen on day one after SMILE and can be alarming given the focal appearance, so the index of suspicion for infection needs to be very high and these cases need extremely close monitoring during the perioperative period. While the appearance is that of a multifocal infectious process, which if presenting 2–3 weeks later would need to include fungal and atypical mycobacteria in the differential, it is conceivable that staphylococcus and streptococcus could produce rapid multi-colony growth of this kind overnight, even though topical steroids have been used on the cornea. However, it is more likely to be a sterile inflammation such as staph marginal type from eyelid margin disease, from endotoxin or chemicals on the instruments, or due to autoimmune causes.

As described in a recent case report [32], the first time we saw this, we had to rule out every possibility, so Gram stain and cultures of the infiltrates were performed and sent for analysis. A comprehensive interface washout and scraping of the infiltrates was also performed. All of the culture results were returned as negative—no growth, and the patient responded to the washout and topical treatment. Since this early experience we have seen 5 other cases with a similar presentation and now manage this similar to a classical DLK case. However, focal infiltrates are still more likely to cause localized melting, thus the threshold

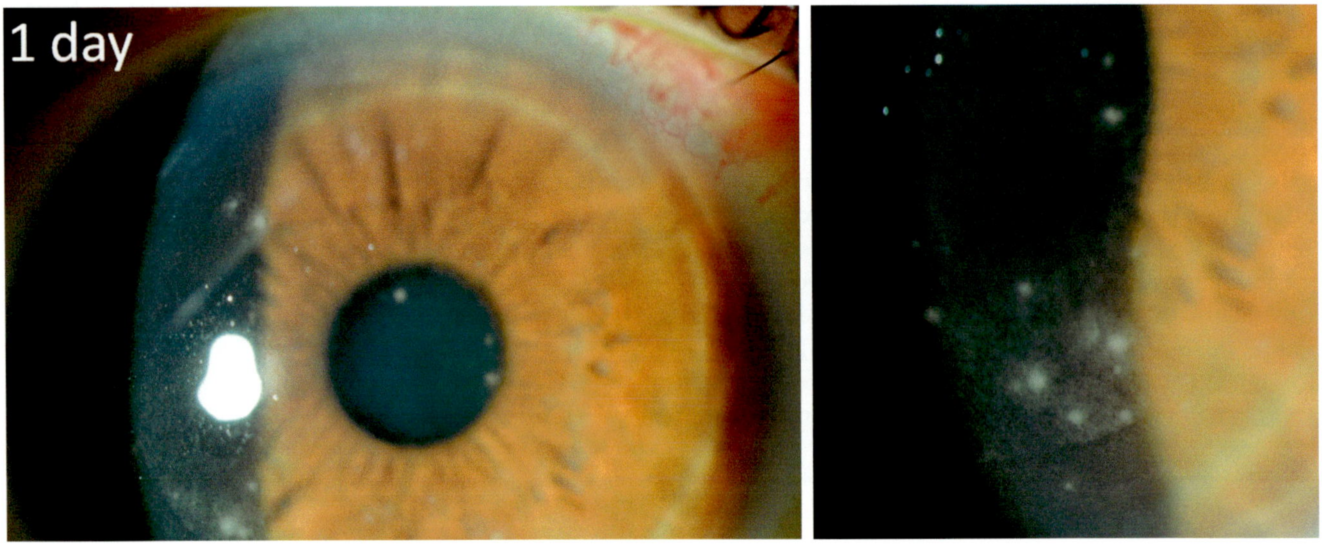

Fig. 9 Slit-lamp photographs of focal DLK, or focal keratitis, one day after SMILE. The infiltrates were dense and scattered diffusely throughout the cornea. *Reprinted with permission from Reinstein DZ, Archer TJ, Carp GI. The Surgeon's Guide to Small Incision Lenticule Extraction (SMILE). Thorofare, New Jersey: SLACK Incorporated, 2018*

for performing an interface washout should be much lower compared with classical DLK.

6.2 Epithelial Implant

Epithelial ingrowth after SMILE can sometimes present as an 'implant' rather than 'ingrowth', caused by stray epithelial cells being drawn into the interface by the surgical instrument. An example of this can be seen in Fig. 10. The UDVA was 20/25 the day after SMILE, and slit-lamp examination showed a mild epithelial implant near the visual axis in the left eye. The patient returned to the clinic 3 weeks later and UDVA had decreased to 20/50 with a manifest refraction of $+1.00$ -1.00×95 (20/20). An OCT scan showed the nest of cells causing a distortion in the stromal surface. Although epithelial thinning had partially compensated for the bump, an irregularity had also been induced on front surface corneal topography.

An epithelial scrape and washout was performed one week later without complications. The patient was seen over a 6-month period, at which time the UDVA was 20/50 with a manifest refraction of $+0.75$ -1.25×102 (20/20). Slit-lamp examination showed a smooth corneal surface with trace residual haze. Corneal mapping with OCT and topography showed essentially normal anatomy with no residual irregularity, mirrored by a regular epithelial thickness profile.

In this patient's case, a single scrape and washout was sufficient, however, there may be a need to further address recurrent ingrowth. Due to the small entrance point in SMILE, other methods might be considered to decrease the chance of further recurrence such as using Hydrogel Ocular Sealant to seal the wound and stop recalcitrant ingrowth [33]. For implanted islands that become elevated over time, focal Nd:YAG laser has been shown to speed absorption in 80% of cases, although 40% of the cases in this study required two or more sessions to entirely eliminate the areas of epithelial ingrowth [34].

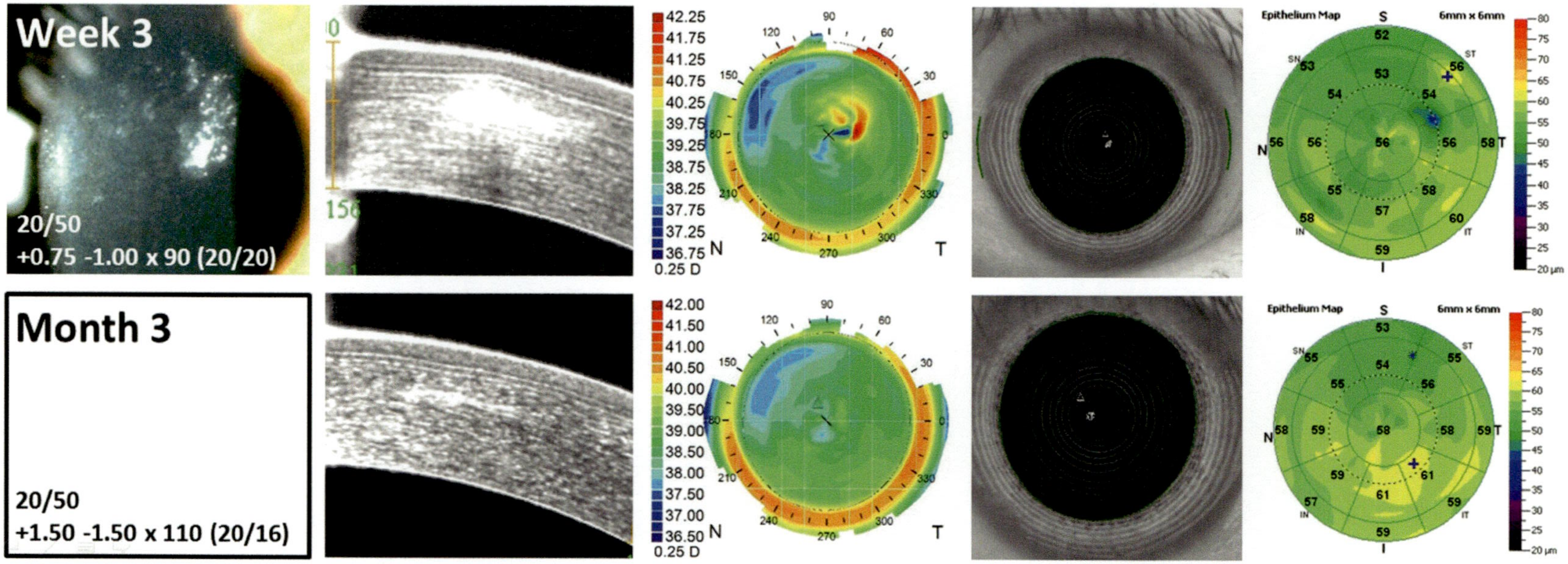

Fig. 10 Slit-lamp photography (first column), OCT B-scan (second column), topography (third column), topography eye image with Mires rings (fourth column), and RTVue OCT epithelial thickness map (fifth column). An epithelial implant associated with topographic elevation and irregularity, and compensatory epithelial thickness changes, was observed one day after SMILE. (Top row) OCT and topography 4 weeks later showed no improvement or reabsorption and continued elevation affecting surface regularity, so an interface washout was performed. (Bottom row) Three months later, OCT showed normal cellular structure and the central irregularity on topography was no longer evident, with the epithelial thickness also returning to a regular pattern. *Reprinted with permission from Reinstein DZ, Archer TJ, Carp GI. The Surgeon's Guide to Small Incision Lenticule Extraction (SMILE). Thorofare, New Jersey: SLACK Incorporated, 2018*

7 Conclusion

Since its introduction in 2011, SMILE has become an established procedure for the treatment of myopia up to −10.00 D [12] and recent studies indicate that this might be extended to −14.00 D [35, 36]. Almost every aspect of the SMILE procedure has now been standardized and protocolized, meaning that outcomes and safety are becoming more consistent between sites and easing the learning curve for surgeons new to SMILE [13]. The surgical instruments and surgical technique have been standardized as described here [13]. The process for optimizing energy and spot spacing settings has been established [13, 23, 25, 26] which has improved visual outcomes and recovery. Intraoperative and postoperative complications are well understood and protocols for the management of suction loss [15, 16] lenticule remnants, [30, 37] DLK, [38, 39] and epithelial implant [40] are in place. Therefore, SMILE can now be considered a mature procedure.

References

1. Intrastromal corneal ring implants for corneal thinning disorders: an evidence-based analysis. Ont Health Technol Assess Ser. 2009;9:1–90.
2. Sekundo W, Kunert K, Russmann C, Gille A, Bissmann W, Stobrawa G, Sticker M, Bischoff M, Blum M. First efficacy and safety study of femtosecond lenticule extraction for the correction of myopia: six-month results. J Cataract Refract Surg. 2008;34:1513–20.
3. Sekundo W, Kunert KS, Blum M. Small incision corneal refractive surgery using the small incision lenticule extraction (SMILE) procedure for the correction of myopia and myopic astigmatism: results of a 6 month prospective study. Br J Ophthalmol. 2011;95:335–9.
4. Shah R, Shah S, Sengupta S. Results of small incision lenticule extraction: all-in-one femtosecond laser refractive surgery. J Cataract Refract Surg. 2011;37:127–37.
5. Hjortdal JO, Vestergaard AH, Ivarsen A, Ragunathan S, Asp S. Predictors for the outcome of small-incision lenticule extraction for Myopia. J Refract Surg. 2012;28:865–71.
6. FDA. VisuMax femtosecond laser system for refractive correction (PMA), 2016.
7. FDA. VisuMax femtosecond laser PMA supplement for approval of myopia with and without astigmatism, 2018.
8. Reinstein DZ, Gobbe M, Gobbe L, Archer TJ, Carp GI. Optical zone centration accuracy using corneal fixation-based SMILE compared to eye tracker-based femtosecond laser-assisted LASIK for Myopia. J Refract Surg. 2015;31:586–92.
9. Li M, Zhao J, Miao H, Shen Y, Sun L, Tian M, Wadium E, Zhou X. Mild decentration measured by a Scheimpflug camera and its impact on visual quality following SMILE in the early learning curve. Invest Ophthalmol Vis Sci. 2014;55:3886–92.
10. Lazaridis A, Droutsas K, Sekundo W. Topographic analysis of the centration of the treatment zone after SMILE for Myopia and comparison to FS-LASIK: subjective versus objective alignment. J Refract Surg. 2014;30:680–6.
11. Liu M, Sun Y, Wang D, Zhang T, Zhou Y, Zheng H, Liu Q. Decentration of optical zone center and its impact on visual outcomes following SMILE. Cornea. 2015;34:392–7.
12. Reinstein DZ, Carp GI, Archer TJ, Vida RS, Yammouni R. Large population outcomes of small incision Lenticule extraction in Young Myopic Patients. J Refract Surg. 2022;38:488–96.
13. Reinstein DZ, Archer TJ, Carp GI. The Surgeon's Guide to Small Incision Lenticule Extraction (SMILE). Thorofare, New Jersey: SLACK Incorporated, 2018.
14. Shetty R, Shroff R, Kaweri L, Jayadev C, Kummelil MK, Sinha RA. Intra-operative cap repositioning in small incision lenticule extraction (SMILE) for enhanced visual recovery. Curr Eye Res. 2016;41:1532–8.
15. Reinstein DZ, Archer TJ, Vida RS, Carp GI. Suction stability management in small incision lenticule extraction: incidence and outcomes of suction loss in 4000 consecutive procedures. Acta Ophthalmol. 2020;98:e72–e80.
16. Reinstein DZ, Archer TJ, Vida RS, Carp GI. Suction stability management in SMILE: development of a decision tree for managing eye movements and suction loss. J Refract Surg. 2018;34:809–16.
17. Liu M, Wang J, Zhong W, Wang D, Zhou Y, Liu Q. Impact of suction loss during small incision Lenticule extraction (SMILE). J Refract Surg. 2016;32:686–92.
18. Osman IM, Awad R, Shi W, Abou SM. Suction loss during femtosecond laser-assisted small-incision lenticule extraction: incidence and analysis of risk factors. J Cataract Refract Surg. 2016;42:246–50.
19. Ivarsen A, Asp S, Hjortdal J. Safety and complications of more than 1500 small-incision lenticule extraction procedures. Ophthalmology. 2014;121:822–8.
20. Pradhan KR, Reinstein DZ, Carp GI, Archer TJ, Gobbe M, Dhungana P. Quality control outcomes analysis of small-incision lenticule extraction for myopia by a novice surgeon at the first refractive surgery unit in Nepal during the first 2 years of operation. J Cataract Refract Surg. 2016;42:267–74.
21. Qiu PJ, Yang YB. Analysis and management of intraoperative complications during small-incision lenticule extraction. Int J Ophthalmol. 2016;9:1697–700.
22. Ji YW, Kang DSY, Reinstein DZ, Archer TJ, Choi JY, Kim EK, Lee HK, Seo KY, Kim T. Effect of lowering laser energy on the surface roughness of human corneal lenticules in small-incision lenticule extraction. J Refract Surg. 2017;33:617–24.
23. Ji YW, Kim M, Yong Kang DS, Reinstein D, Archer T, Choi JY, Kim EK, Lee HK, Seo KY, Kim TI. Lower laser energy levels lead to better visual recovery after small-incision lenticule extraction: Prospective, randomized clinical trial. Am J Ophthalmol. 2017;179:159–70.
24. Kunert KS, Blum M, Duncker GI, Sietmann R, Heichel J. Surface quality of human corneal lenticules after femtosecond laser surgery for myopia comparing different laser parameters. Graefes Arch Clin Exp Ophthalmol. 2011;249:1417–24.
25. Donate D, Thaeron R. Lower Energy Levels Improve visual recovery in small incision Lenticule extraction (SMILE). J Refract Surg. 2016;32:636–42.
26. Li L, Schallhorn JM, Ma J, Cui T, Wang Y. Energy setting and visual outcomes in SMILE: a retrospective cohort study. J Refract Surg. 2018;34:11–6.
27. Carp GI, Reinstein DZ, Stuart A, Vida RS, Archer TJ, Finkel JN. Cap recovery technique and double-edge sign during small-incision lenticule extraction. J Cataract Refract Surg. 2021;47:1191–5.
28. Reinstein DZ, Archer TJ, Dickeson ZI, Gobbe M. Trans-epithelial phototherapeutic keratectomy protocol for treating irregular astigmatism based on population epithelial thickness measurements by Artemis very high-frequency digital ultrasound. J Refract Surg. 2014;30:380–7.
29. Dong Z, Zhou X. Irregular astigmatism after femtosecond laser refractive lenticule extraction. J Cataract Refract Surg. 2013;39:952–4.

30. Ganesh S, Brar S, Lazaridis A. Management and Outcomes of Retained Lenticules and Lenticule fragments removal after failed primary SMILE: a case series. J Refract Surg. 2017;33:848–53.
31. Linebarger EJ, Hardten DR, Lindstrom RL. Diffuse lamellar keratitis: diagnosis and management. J Cataract Refract Surg. 2000;26:1072–7.
32. Reinstein DZ, Stuart AJ, Vida RS, Archer TJ, Carp GI. Atypical presentation of diffuse lamellar keratitis after SMILE: sterile multifocal inflammatory keratitis. J Cataract Refract Surg. 2018;44(6):774–779.
33. Thulasi P, Kim SW, Shetty R, Randleman JB. Recalcitrant Epithelial Ingrowth After SMILE Treated With a Hydrogel Ocular Sealant. J Refract Surg. 2015;31:847–50.
34. Ayala MJ, Alio JL, Mulet ME, De La Hoz F. Treatment of laser in situ keratomileusis interface epithelial ingrowth with neodymium:ytrium-aluminum-garnet laser. Am J Ophthalmol. 2008;145:630–4.
35. Reinstein DZ, Archer TJ, Vida RS, Carp GI, Reinstein JFR, McChesney T, Potter JG. Small Incision Lenticule Extraction (SMILE) for the Correction of High Myopia With Astigmatism. J Refract Surg. 2022;38:262–71.
36. Reinstein DZ, Archer TJ, Vida RS, Carp GI, Reinstein JFR, McAlinden C. Objective and subjective quality of vision after SMILE for high Myopia and astigmatism. J Refract Surg. 2022;38:404–13.
37. Sachdev GS, Ramamurthy S, Dandapani R. Triamcinolone acetonide for remnant lenticule identification in small incision lenticule extraction. J Cataract Refract Surg. 2020;46:811–3.
38. Stuart A, Reinstein DZ, Vida RS, Archer TJ, Carp G. Atypical presentation of diffuse lamellar keratitis after small-incision lenticule extraction: Sterile multifocal inflammatory keratitis. J Cataract Refract Surg. 2018;44:774–9.
39. Reinstein DZ, Stuart AJ, Vida RS, Archer TJ, Carp GI. Incidence and outcomes of sterile multifocal inflammatory keratitis and diffuse Lamellar Keratitis after SMILE. J Refract Surg. 2018;34:751–9.
40. Piccinini P, Vida RS, Piccinini R, Maiore I, Archer TJ, Carp GI, Reinstein DZ. Epithelial implantation treatment after small-incision lenticule extraction. J Cataract Refract Surg. 2020;46:636–40.

LASIK with the Femtosecond Laser

Dan Z. Reinstein and Timothy J. Archer

Abstract

Laser in situ keratomileusis (LASIK) has become the most common corneal refractive surgery procedure since its introduction in the early 1990s. Improvements in ablation profile and optical zone design have significantly improved refractive stability and postoperative quality of vision, while the introduction of femtosecond lasers has improved the safety of flap creation and enabled thin-flap LASIK. In this chapter, we describe in detail the surgical protocol for performing a femtosecond LASIK procedure, with a particular focus on how to lift and replace a flap to minimize the formation of microfolds, or even nanofolds. Careful flap management enables optimal quality of vision for the patient and reduces the risk of epithelial ingrowth.

Keywords

LASIK · Excimer laser · Femtosecond laser · Flap · Ablation

Financial Disclosure: Dr Reinstein is a consultant for Carl Zeiss Meditec (Jena, Germany) and CSO Italia (Florence, Italy), and has a proprietary interest in the Artemis Insight 100 technology (ArcScan Inc, Morrison, Colorado) through patents administered by the Cornell Center for Technology Enterprise and Commercialization (CCTEC), Ithaca, New York. The remaining authors have no proprietary or financial interest in the materials presented herein.

Supplementary Information The online version contains supplementary material available at https://doi.org/10.1007/978-3-031-65422-0_63.

D. Z. Reinstein (✉) · T. J. Archer
London Vision Clinic, EuroEyes Group, London, UK
e-mail: dzr@reinsteinvision.com

D. Z. Reinstein
Columbia University Medical Center, New York, NY, USA

Biomedical Science Research Institute, Ulster University, Coleraine, UK

Sorbonne Université, Paris, France

1 Introduction

Laser in situ keratomileusis (LASIK) has become the most common corneal refractive surgery procedure since its introduction in the early 1990s. Initially performed using a manual microkeratome to create the flap, the advent of femtosecond lasers for flap creation made a significant impact during the 2000s. Femtosecond lasers greatly reduced the risk of some of the more significant flap complications, such as buttonhole, free cap, and irregular flaps, and also reduced the rate of epithelial ingrowth [1, 2]. However, probably the main benefit of femtosecond lasers was to improve the reproducibility of flap thickness and enable the use of thinner flaps, both of which improved the safety with respect to the risk of excessive keratectomy. Flap thickness reproducibility is the most important factor for residual stromal thickness (RST) safety planning as a thicker than intended flap can lead to a lower than predicted RST and possibly to ectasia.

Central flap thickness standard deviation of certain older mechanical microkeratomes was reported to be in the range of 20–40 μm [3–5]. With a flap thickness standard deviation of 30 μm, an RST error of over 90 μm is likely to occur in 0.15% of eyes. More recent mechanical microkeratomes have improved flap thickness standard deviation to between 10–20 μm, [6–8] with some studies reporting 7–10 μm [9, 10]. However, even with a reproducibility of 10 μm, the flap thickness can still be 30 μm thicker than intended.

When femtosecond lasers were first introduced in 2004, the flap thickness reproducibility was reported to be between 10–15 μm, which was about 5 μm lower than the reproducibility for microkeratomes at that time. Since then, there has been a similar trend for improving flap thickness reproducibility such that most published reports find this to be less than 5 μm for the current femtosecond laser systems [9, 11, 12].

Therefore, femtosecond lasers enabled an improvement in flap thickness reproducibility since their introduction,

B. Seitz et al. (eds.), *Atlas on Cornea*, https://doi.org/10.1007/978-3-031-65422-0_63

which has continued to improve over time, keeping ahead of the improvement in microkeratomes. In addition, femtosecond lasers have also been shown to create flaps that are more regular in thickness, which has consequently reduced the induced higher order aberrations. Finally, femtosecond lasers are associated with a faster learning curve, so provide a safer option for less experienced or lower volume surgeons [13].

In this chapter, we describe the treatment preparation and surgical technique for performing a femtosecond LASIK procedure. As our experience has been with the VisuMax femtosecond laser and MEL 90 excimer laser (both Carl Zeiss Meditec), the procedure will be described from this perspective.

2 Femtosecond Laser

The VisuMax femtosecond laser system obtained CE mark approval and was granted clearance to market by the US Food and Drug Administration (FDA) in January 2007. The VisuMax femtosecond laser system was conceived with intrastromal lenticule creation as the end goal—i.e. small incision lenticule extraction (SMILE) [14–18]. Therefore, it was designed to enable coupling of the femtosecond laser source to the cornea with minimal tissue distortion and rapid high precision femtosecond pulse placement. Elements of this system are summarized below:

1. The VisuMax coupling contact glass interface with the cornea is curved, thus leading to very little corneal distortion when securing full corneal surface contact (Fig. 1).
2. Corneal coupling of the contact glass is achieved with very low suction force [19, 20] applied through specifically designed suction ports that are applied to the peripheral cornea/limbus, but not the bulbar conjunctiva/sclera. This low suction coupling force minimizes corneal distortion. From the patient's point of view, the most remarkable feature of SMILE is that they literally feel nothing from start to finish, and the eye emerges white and comfortable after the procedure. In contrast, many other femtosecond lasers used for LASIK cause marked subconjunctival hemorrhage due to scleral suction.
3. Each contact glass is individually calibrated by a built-in confocal imaging system thus compensating for individual differences in contact glass geometry that are inevitable in serial production.
4. The optical beam path system coupled to the contact glass is suspended on a fulcrum. The fulcrum together with a continuous force-feedback servo control for patient bed height produces a system delivering a constant force of the contact glass onto the cornea. This constant force minimizes changes in corneal distortion that may occur with patient head movement in the z-axis during the femtosecond laser cutting process.
5. The optical system delivering the femtosecond laser beam is designed with very high numerical aperture optics thus allowing for very tight concentration of femtosecond energy, very little collateral energy dissipation and high femtosecond spot placement accuracy.
6. The laser–tissue interaction dynamics are optimized for speed with a repetition rate of 500 kHz which minimizes treatment time and achieves the critical refractive cuts in a short enough time to reduce the chances of eye or head movements during this phase of the cutting.

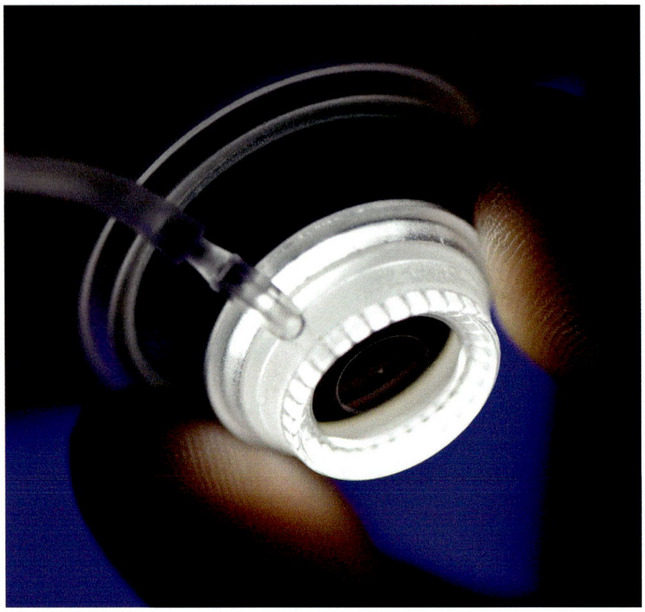

Fig. 1 A close-up view of the curved contact glass used with the VisuMax femtosecond laser. *Reprinted with permission from Reinstein DZ, Archer TJ, Carp GI. The Surgeon's Guide to Small Incision Lenticule Extraction (SMILE). Thorofare, New Jersey: SLACK Incorporated, 2018*

The overall efficacy of the device for flap creation and SMILE is dependent on the precision of these technical design elements. Numerous studies have evaluated LASIK flap or SMILE cap thickness with the VisuMax, reporting excellent reproducibility and accuracy (Table 1) [11, 21–30].

In our study using Artemis Insight 100 VHF digital ultrasound (ArcScan Inc), we also mapped the SMILE cap thickness accuracy over a 5 mm diameter (Fig. 2) [11]. The cap thickness was within 2 μm of the intended thickness across the horizontal meridian, demonstrating the uniform nature of the cap. There was a slight vertical asymmetry

Table 1 Accuracy and reproducibility of LASIK flap and SMILE cap thickness with the VisuMax femtosecond laser

Author	VisuMax (kHz)	LASIK/SMILE	Measurement method	Eyes	Accuracy (μm)	Reproducibility (μm)
Reinstein 2010 [21]	200	LASIK	Artemis Insight 100 VHF digital ultrasound	20	+2.3	7.9
Yu 2010 [22]	200	LASIK	AS-OCT	82	+12.7	5.1
Ju 2011 [23]	200	LASIK	Visante AS-OCT	87	+2.3	3.8
Yao 2011 [24]	200	LASIK	Visante AS-OCT	25	+0.2	7.9
Ahn 2011 [25]	200	LASIK	RTVue AS-OCT	40	+23.9	13.9
Issa 2011 [26]	200	LASIK	Intraop ultrasound pachymetry	55	+3.8	9.6
Tay 2012 [27]	500	SMILE	RTVue AS-OCT	95	+5.0	N/R
Reinstein 2013 [11]	500	SMILE	Artemis Insight 100 VHF digital ultrasound	70	–0.7	4.4
Zhao 2013 [28]	500	SMILE	RTVue AS-OCT	54	–1.2	5.1
Ozgurhan 2013 [29]	500	LASIK	Visante AS-OCT	33	+4.9	5.0
Ozgurhan 2013 [29]	500	SMILE	Visante AS-OCT	33	+4.6	5.2
Vestergaard 2014 [30]	500	SMILE	Heidelberg Spectralis AS-OCT	34	+4.0	9.0

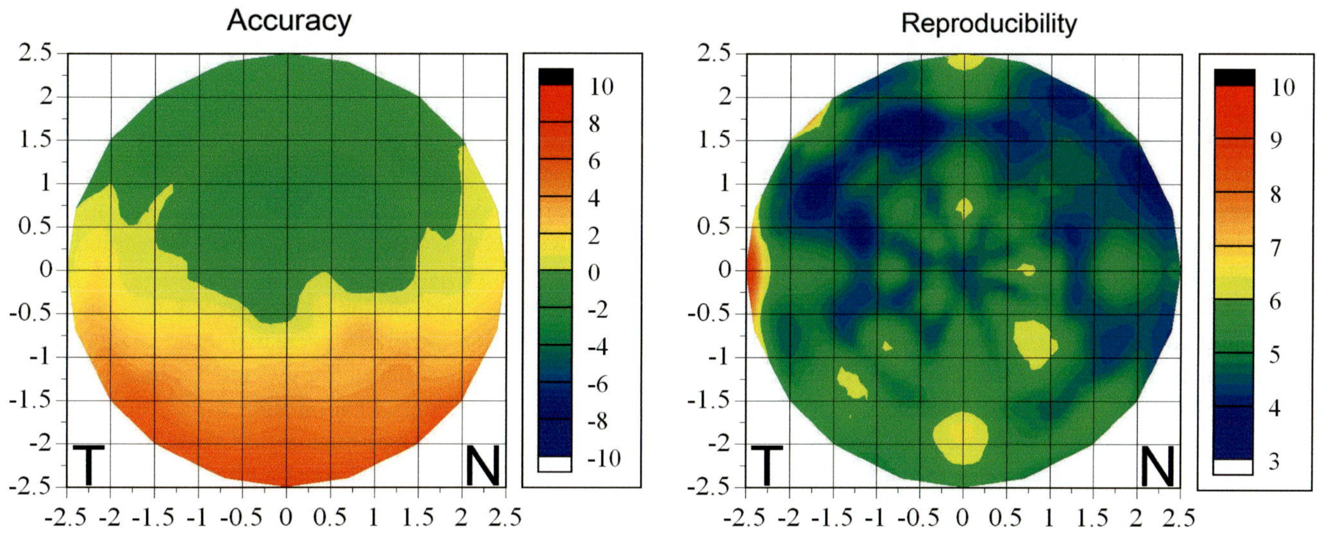

Fig. 2 Topographical map of the accuracy (left) and reproducibility (right) of cap thickness centered on the corneal vertex for the central 5 mm diameter zone for a population of 70 eyes. Cap thickness data were normalized to the intended cap thickness, which was 110, 120, or 130 μm for this population. All left eyes were mirrored so that positive x-values represent the nasal cornea and negative x-values represent the temporal cornea. A Cartesian 1-mm grid is superimposed with the origin at the corneal vertex. For the accuracy map, the break point is set to 0 so that positive values (yellow/red) represent areas where the cap was thicker than intended and negative values (green/blue) represent areas where the cap was thinner than intended. The color scale for the reproducibility map represents the standard deviation in μm. The break point is set to 6 μm so that all areas where the reproducibility was better than 6 μm are displayed in green or blue. *Reprinted with permission from Reinstein DZ, Archer TJ, Gobbe M. Accuracy and Reproducibility of Cap Thickness in Small Incision Lenticule Extraction. J Refract Surg. 2013;29:810–815*

with the cap 2.3 μm thinner than intended superiorly and 6.5 μm thicker than intended inferiorly. This small tilt has been determined to not be optically or clinically significant (personal communication, Carl Zeiss Meditec, December 19, 2007). The cap thickness was accurate with a central accuracy of –0.7 μm, with similar accuracy for cap thicknesses between 80–140 μm [11].

3 Settings

Within the VisuMax software, the following parameters are required when planning a LASIK flap:

- ***Corneal radius [mm]*** – the average simulated keratometry value can be entered within a range from 6.50 to

8.50 mm (39.7 to 51.9 D). This average keratometry is used to calculate the peripheral femtosecond laser focal depth to account for the accurvation of the cornea to the curved contact glass according to the curvature of each individual eye. The corneal curvature also impacts the maximum cap diameter that is allowed; the cap diameter can be larger for flatter corneas.

- ***Pachymetry [μm]*** – the pachymetry value is used to calculate the predicted residual stromal thickness (RST) for safety monitoring. A warning will be displayed within the software if the RST falls below the limit set by the user.
- ***Manifest refraction*** – the manifest refraction is entered, even for flap creation, as this is used to adjust the vergence of the beam and bring the green fixation light into sharp focus for each individual patient.
- ***Treatment pack size*** – the contact glass is available in three sizes: small (S), medium (M), and large (L). The size is selected according to the patient's white-to-white diameter, to ensure that suction is applied predominantly to the cornea. According to the VisuMax user manual, the minimum white-to-white is 11.2 mm for the 'S' contact glass, 11.7 mm for the 'M' contact glass, and 12.4 mm for the 'L' contact glass. The contact glass size is the major determinant for the maximum flap diameter.
- ***Diameter [mm]*** – this defines the flap diameter, which will usually be selected as the largest possible for the contact glass size being used. In general, the maximum flap diameter is 8.00 mm for a small contact glass and 8.80 mm for a medium contact glass. The maximum values are influenced slightly by the corneal radius and flap thickness; the maximum value decreases for steeper corneas and for thicker flaps. Finding the absolute maximum for an individual eye is best achieved by manually reducing the diameter in 0.01 mm increments. Best practice for flap diameter to minimize the incidence of OBL is described later.
- ***Thickness [μm]*** – flap thickness in the range 100–120 μm is commonly used, but flap thickness can be programmed with a thinnest flap of 80 μm, which is possible due to the accuracy and reproducibility (Table 1). In normal eyes, the epithelium is rarely thicker than 60 μm, [31] so the risk of a buttonhole is low given the flap thickness reproducibility of about 5 μm. An 80 μm intended flap thickness is 4 standard deviations away from the 60 μm. However, ideally an epithelial thickness measurement would be obtained to screen for eyes with abnormally thick epithelium if using an 80 μm flap.
- ***Side cut angle [°]*** – this defines the angle of the side cut around the flap border. Our standard protocol for VisuMax flaps is to use a side cut angle of 55°, so that the flap edge is slightly in-cut. This allows the flap border to fit in a lock-and-key fashion with the residual stromal bed under the hypothesis that this reduces the risk of epithelial ingrowth.
- ***Hinge position [°]*** – any hinge position can be selected, or one of the radio button presets can be used (superior, inferior, nasal, temporal). Our standard protocol is to use a superior hinge as this is ergonomically easier to handle for the surgeon and blinking naturally aids the flap repositioning.
- ***Hinge width [mm]*** – the width of the hinge can be set according to the surgeon's preference. Our standard protocol is to use a hinge width of 5.0 mm.
- ***Energy and spot spacing*** – these settings should be adjusted for each device to maximize the ease of interface separation and minimize the incidence of opaque bubble layer (OBL). This adjustment process is done by a Carl Zeiss Meditec applications specialist.

4 Docking and Femtosecond Cutting

The docking process is an important part of the procedure, although not as important as in SMILE, as there is some tolerance for flap centration. The docking process is the same as for SMILE, as described in Chap. 62. For this reason, it is recommended that a surgeon performs a series of LASIK procedures before starting SMILE in order to become accustomed to the docking process with the VisuMax.

The femtosecond cutting is performed in two stages. Firstly, the lamellar interface is created using a spiral in pattern (i.e. from the periphery to the center), which allows the patient to see the green fixation light for as long as possible (due to the low suction pressure). Once this is done, the side cut is created. The total suction time is about 25 s using the 500 kHz VisuMax, although the time varies slightly depending on the flap diameter.

The main intraoperative complication of flap creation using a femtosecond laser is suction loss. To date, we have had 86 cases of suction loss out of 17,243 LASIK procedures using the VisuMax, which gives an incidence of 0.50%. Suction loss during flap creation can be managed by redocking using the same contact glass and repeating the procedure with the same flap thickness. The contact glass will usually continue to slot into the same position when reapplied, as it is guided by the particular 'fit' of the cornea into the contact glass as well as indentations that will have been made by the suction ports in the limbal areas during the first attempt. When repeating the femtosecond cutting at the same thickness, the femtosecond laser energy will be blocked by the existing bubbles within the region that has already been treated, but will then continue the interface outside of this zone. More detailed discussion of suction loss during a SMILE procedure is included in Chap. 62.

5 Surgical Technique

5.1 Surgical Technique for Flap Lift and Repositioning

It has been shown that experience accumulated by surgeons as a group significantly improves outcomes compared with an individual surgeon [32]. Therefore, our philosophy has been to define and have all our surgeons strictly follow a standardized surgical treatment protocol. Prof Reinstein first developed a standardized surgical treatment protocol between 1998–2001 in a high-volume corporate practice (LASIK Vision Corp.) [33]. This surgical treatment protocol was refined and adopted as the recommended surgical treatment protocol for use with the MEL 80 excimer laser (Carl Zeiss Meditec) in 2003 and modified for incorporation of the VisuMax femtosecond laser in 2007. This was subsequently published in two studies demonstrating identical technique and outcomes achieved by two surgeons using this standardized technique [13, 34].

Before lifting the flap, the tear film is homogenized using balanced salt solution (BSS) in order to obtain a clear reflex from the aiming beam. The height of the patient bed is adjusted to bring the eye to the correct working distance for the laser. The eye tracker is then enabled and adjusted to be centered on the coaxially sighted corneal light reflex.

Video 1 and Video 2 show the bimanual flap lifting technique that we developed to manage VisuMax flaps as these require some separation of the interface, as opposed to the clean and complete cut produced by a microkeratome or some other higher energy femtosecond lasers. In this bimanual flap lifting technique, a flap lifter and McPherson's forceps are used. The flap border is scored from the inferotemporal region up to the hinge superiorly using the flap lifter, which is then inserted into the flap interface next to the hinge. The flap lifter is pushed across to the opposite side to create an opening for the McPherson's forceps to be inserted from the other side, also at the superior hinge. Either instrument can then be held at the hinge to maintain the eye in the primary position, while the other is used for separation (Video 1, Video 2).

Please scan to access video content

After lifting the flap, the stromal bed surface is homogenized by wiping with a surgical sponge. The time between lifting the flap and starting the ablation should be kept constant between patients as the excimer laser fluence can be affected by the hydration of the stroma. A surgical sponge should be used to protect the underside of the flap at the hinge. The excimer laser ablation is started by pressing the foot pedal. The duration of an excimer laser ablation depends on the magnitude of correction and the optical zone, as more pulses are required to remove more tissue. The time also depends on the laser head frequency. During the ablation, dynamic eye tracking corrects for the position of the eye for small movements, and passive eye tracking stops the ablation if the eye moves outside the permitted zone.

The most important part of a LASIK procedure from a surgical technique standpoint is the replacement of the flap, particularly with the goal of minimizing microfolds and epithelial ingrowth. The concept behind our technique [13, 34] (Video 1, Video 2) is to minimize the flap manipulation (especially to avoid bending, stretching or pulling of the flap) and irrigation. Irrigation is performed using a 27 gauge anterior chamber cannula to expel 1 ml of fluid in 1 s, so that there is a very high fluid pressure stream, which avoids hydrating the flap or bed while effectively 'blowing' particles from the interface. However, care should be taken to keep the tip of the cannula away from the small incisions, to avoid creating a tear in the flap. One or two wipes are usually all that is needed to return the flap to the exact anatomical position without microfolds.

When replacing the flap, the goal is to see a zero gutter appearance (i.e. no space between the flap and the bed). A gutter will often be left if extensive irrigation is performed as flap swelling due to hydration causes flap diameter retraction. Epithelial cells can then grow into the space left by the gutter meaning that there is not enough space for the flap to expand into as it dehydrates after the procedure, resulting in microfolds—a 'flap crunch' syndrome. Alternatively, hydration may cause the flap to swell asymmetrically. In that case, if the flap is repositioned such that the ink marks are aligned, there may not be sufficient space on one side of the flap to expand into as it dehydrates, again resulting in microfolds.

As after SMILE, micro-adjustments to the flap are made at the slit-lamp immediately after the procedure using a dry surgical microspear (Fig. 3). Visualization of even the finest microfolds (nanofolds) can be achieved by using heavy fluorescein staining and pressing down onto the cornea with the dry sponge. The microspear is used to distend the flap and smooth out any microfolds by stroking from the center towards the periphery.

The technique involves using the thumb of the opposite hand to raise the upper eyelid while the palm blocks the view of the contralateral eye. The patient is instructed to look directly into the blue light (coaxial slit-lamp). The ring finger of the temporal-side hand is placed on the patient's lower lid to achieve full exposure of the cornea. A dry

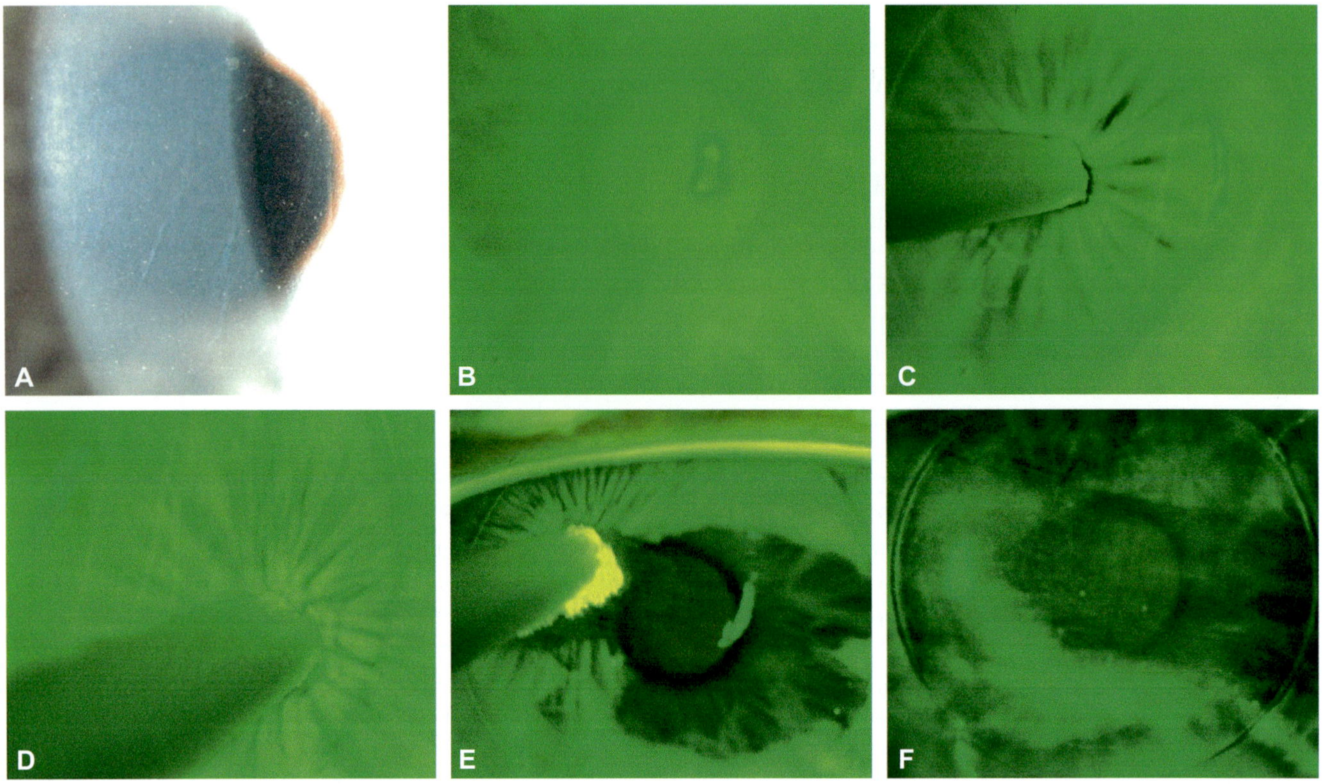

Fig. 3 Sequence of images showing smoothing of the flap at the slit-lamp immediately after surgery. (**A**) Some vertical microfolds are visible centrally. (**B**) Heavy fluorescein staining is introduced to optimize the visibility of even the finest nanofolds. (**C**), (**D**) A dry microspear is used to first identify the location of any microfolds by pressing on the corneal surface. (**E**) The microspear is used to distend the flap and smooth out any microfolds by stroking from the center towards the periphery. (**F**) The final appearance of the flap showing no signs of microfolds. *Reprinted with permission from Reinstein DZ, Archer TJ, Carp GI. The Surgeon's Guide to Small Incision Lenticule Extraction (SMILE). Thorofare, New Jersey: SLACK Incorporated, 2018*

sponge is held in this hand with the index finger, middle finder, and thumb to stroke the cap radially.

Further fine-tuning can be performed using the same technique at the 1-day, and even 1-month, postoperative appointments. In a retrospective analysis of 14,374 VisuMax LASIK procedures since January 2010, a slit-lamp adjustment was performed at day 1 in 983 eyes (6.84%). At 3 months after surgery, there were trace microfolds in 1.10%, grade 1 microfolds in 0.184%, and grade 2 microfolds in 0.016%. A flap lift for visually significant microfolds was required for only one eye (0.007%), performed at the day 1 visit to address a microfold that could not be managed at the slit-lamp.

5.2 Surgical Technique for LASIK Retreatment After SMILE

Retreatment after SMILE can be performed as PRK, [35, 36] by converting the existing cap into a flap by a side cut only [37] or Circle [38, 39] treatment, or using a thin-flap LASIK procedure (Circle and side cut only software options are not available in the US). A new technique has also recently been described, known as sub-cap-lenticule-extraction, that enables a retreatment to be performed as a SMILE using the small incision and cap from the primary procedure [40].

Many SMILE surgeons use a cap thickness of 135–145 μm [41] given the advantages of a thicker cap in preserving the anterior stroma in order to minimize the disturbance to the corneal nerve plexus [42–44] and take advantage of the stronger corneal lamellae in the anterior stroma [45–48]. Side cut only and Circle provide a good option for retreatment in cases where a thinner cap was used, but are less appropriate for thicker caps as the procedure forces the flap to be created at the same thickness as the original cap. Modern LASIK rarely involves intentionally creating a 145 μm flap. However, the consequence of using a thicker cap is this almost always leaves sufficient space anterior to the existing SMILE interface to safely create a thin LASIK flap if a retreatment is required.

A thin-flap LASIK procedure after SMILE is essentially the same as performing LASIK in an eye that has previously had LASIK, such as performing femto-LASIK with a thin flap for retreating an eye with a thick flap following primary microkeratome LASIK [49]. The safety of creating a new flap is related to the risk of the flap entering the epithelium (i.e. a cryptic buttonhole) or crossing the existing interface resulting in tissue slivers. Therefore, it is important to measure the epithelial thickness and cap thickness by VHF digital ultrasound or OCT in order to plan a safe flap thickness. The main point of differentiation with LASIK after SMILE is that the small incision(s) from the primary procedure will be within the diameter of the flap and therefore introduce the risk that the instruments might enter and tear the small incision or access the existing SMILE interface. Alternatively, if a superior small incision had been used, the small incision may compromise the integrity of the hinge if a superior-hinge flap is created.

As we use supero-temporal and superonasal small incisions for our SMILE patients, the small incisions are then located close to where we would like to push the instruments across the flap. In our early experience we found that the instruments can sometimes slip into the small incision creating a tear. There is also the potential for the instrument to actually go down the tunnel to the cap interface, rather than into the more anterior interface of the new flap.

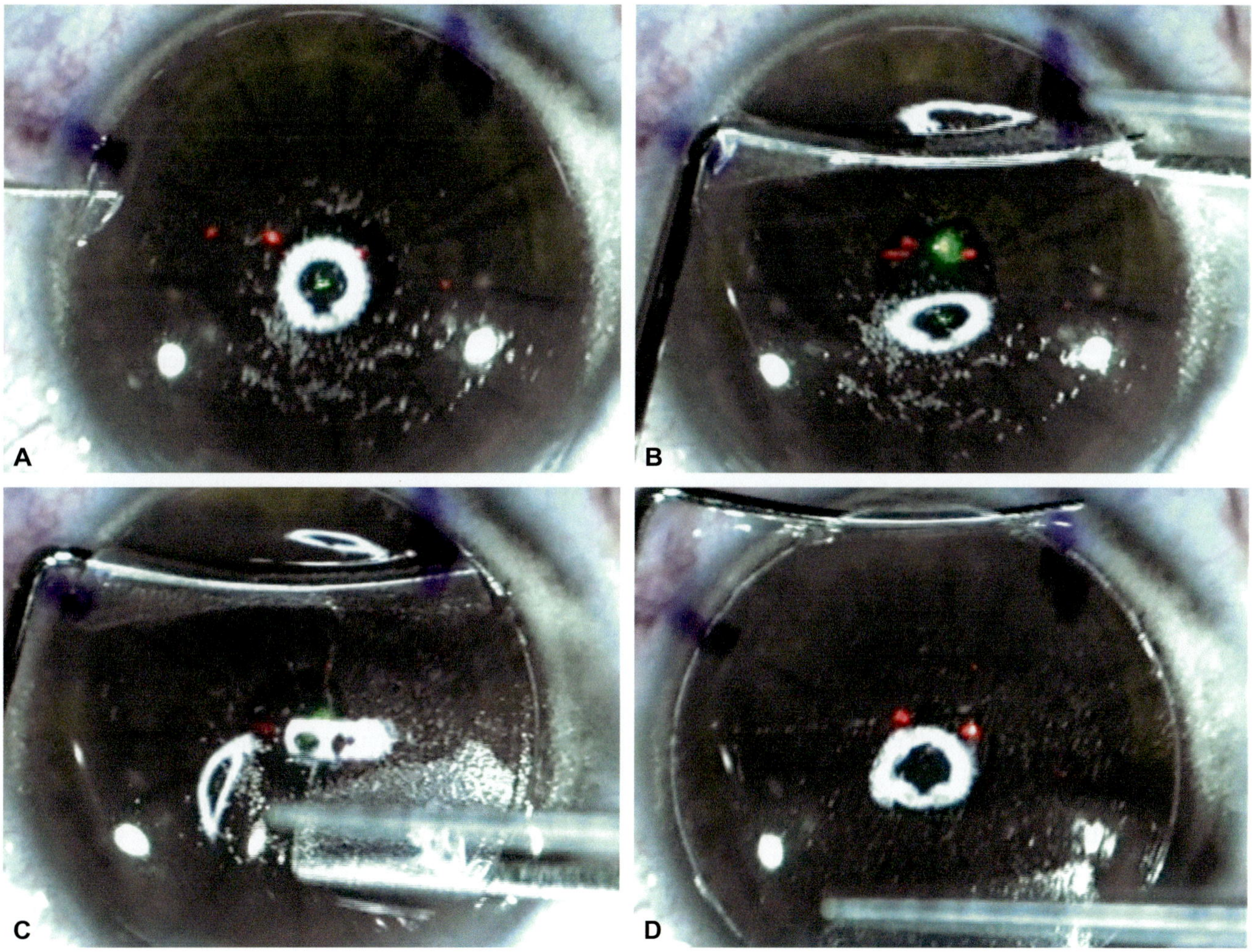

Fig. 4 Series of images describing the surgical technique for lifting a LASIK flap in an eye that has previously had SMILE. The aim of the technique is to avoid placing the tip of either instrument in the vicinity of either of the small incisions as this may tear the flap. (**A**) The flap lifter is used to open the flap side cut in the inferior third of the flap. (**B**) The flap lifter is pushed across the flap and used to open the flap side cut on the opposite side to create an access point for the McPherson's forceps. This motion is made with some upward force to avoid the instrument tip breaking through to the original SMILE interface. (**C**) The McPherson's forceps is inserted to the mid-point of the flap and swept superiorly, thereby separating the region of the small incision with the arm of the instrument and not the tip. The flap lifter is held in place using the inferior unseparated portion of the flap to provide counter-traction for the McPherson's forceps. A second sweep is made to separate the other half of the flap. (**D**) The McPherson's forceps is then placed against the superior hinge to provide counter-traction for the flap lifter to be used to separate the inferior portion of the flap in the usual manner. *Reprinted with permission from Reinstein DZ, Archer TJ, Carp GI. The Surgeon's Guide to Small Incision Lenticule Extraction (SMILE). Thorofare, New Jersey: SLACK Incorporated, 2018*

Therefore, we adapted our technique for LASIK after SMILE (Fig. 4) to first insert the instruments in the inferior third of the flap. The flap edge is opened in this region using the tip of the flap lifter as normal. The flap lifter is then inserted into the interface and pushed across to the other side; applying some upward pressure and 'tenting up' the flap avoids the risk of the instrument breaking through to the SMILE interface. The tip of the flap lifter is then used to open the opposite edge of the flap from the inside, thereby creating an access point for the second instrument, a McPherson's forceps, to be introduced into the flap interface through this opening until the mid-point of the flap. The McPherson's forceps can be pulled gently superiorly towards the hinge to separate the flap interface, with the flap lifter held in position by the unseparated inferior third of the flap to provide counter-traction. This process can then be repeated to separate the second half of the flap with a second sweep of the forceps. This method means that the superior small incision is approached with the whole arm of the instrument already inside the flap interface, virtually eliminating the possibility of the tip inadvertently entering and tearing the small incision.

With the superior portion of the flap separated, one instrument can then be placed in the standard position pressed against the hinge, allowing the inferior portion to be separated using the other instrument. If there is any resistance at the inferior side cut, this can be opened using a capsulorhexis-type technique; with the arm of the flap lifter placed against the inferior side cut from inside the flap, rotate the instrument using the tip as a fulcrum, thus raising the instrument shaft and causing the flap side cut to tear open.

During the learning curve of adapting to this technique, we experienced 10 instances of a tear at the small incision or an interaction with the SMILE interface in 10 of the first 55 cases. Since settling on this inferior pseudo-hinge fulcrum technique, we have not experienced any intraoperative complications in the last 84 consecutive treatments.

5.3 Opaque Bubble Layer (OBL)

Opaque bubble layer is relatively common when creating flaps with the VisuMax with an incidence of between about 5% and 20% [12, 50–53]. The femtosecond cutting starts in the periphery when making a flap interface, and there can be a jet of gas that escapes towards the center almost immediately after the first bubbles are created. This jet of gas moves ahead of the inward spiral of bubbles. It is thought that if the femtosecond laser energy is too high, the shock wave generated after optical breakdown of corneal tissue may force the collagen lamellae apart, thus forming a gas bubble [54, 55]. This then provides a weak point through which excess gas can escape, explaining why the OBL shoots out in front of the scanning pattern of the femtosecond laser.

OBL jets (also referred to as 'hard OBL') have been shown to have different appearance between femtosecond laser systems [56]. For the VisuMax, the OBL layer usually extends anterior to the flap interface up to Bowman layer, as demonstrated by Hurmeric et al. [56] using ultrahigh-resolution OCT. The presence of this OBL layer impedes the focusing of the laser pulses, resulting in either smaller bubbles or, in some cases, no bubble formation in the region of the OBL. The flap interface is then more difficult, but always possible, to separate in these areas; it is important to use very small and very gentle bites with the separating instrument.

OBL jets are more common when the interface is more superficial; Lim et al. [12] reported that the incidence of OBL increased from 8% for 120 μm flaps to 19% for 80 μm flaps. Incidence of OBL jets is also increased when using higher energies. However, using a higher energy also makes it easier to separate areas covered by an OBL jet. Therefore, it has been our routine protocol to increase the energy when making an ultra-thin flap of between 80–100 μm [57]. For deeper interfaces, OBL jets will only occur for extremely high energy levels.

It has recently been found by a number of groups that there is a simple adjustment that virtually eliminates the formation of OBL jets in VisuMax flaps [52, 53]. This technique involves planning the treatment having selected one contact glass size larger than the size that you intend to use. The flap diameter is then selected to be 0.1–0.2 mm larger than the maximum allowed for the smaller contact glass size. For example, the treatment would be planned for an 'M' contact glass with a flap diameter of 8.1–8.2 mm, but an 'S' contact glass is actually used for the treatment.

This acts to move the starting point of the femtosecond cutting closer to the edge of the contact glass, as long as the 'spiral in' scan direction is used that goes from the periphery to the center. It was found that this small 0.1–0.2 mm change effectively stopped any peripheral OBL from forming. For example, Fig. 5 shows two eyes of the same patient both treated with an 8.1 mm flap diameter. Significant OBL can be seen in the eye where an 'M' contact glass was used, whereas the bubble pattern was perfect in the eye where an 'S' contact glass was used.

This has been demonstrated in two large population studies. Using the VisuMax with the 'S' contact glass, Mastropasqua et al. [52] reported that the incidence of OBL was 23.6% with a mild/moderate presence for a 7.9 mm flap diameter, 20.8% with mild presence for an 8.0 mm flap diameter, but was significantly reduced to 4.1% with a minimal presence for an 8.2 mm flap diameter. Similarly, Wu et al. [53] found that the incidence of OBL reduced from

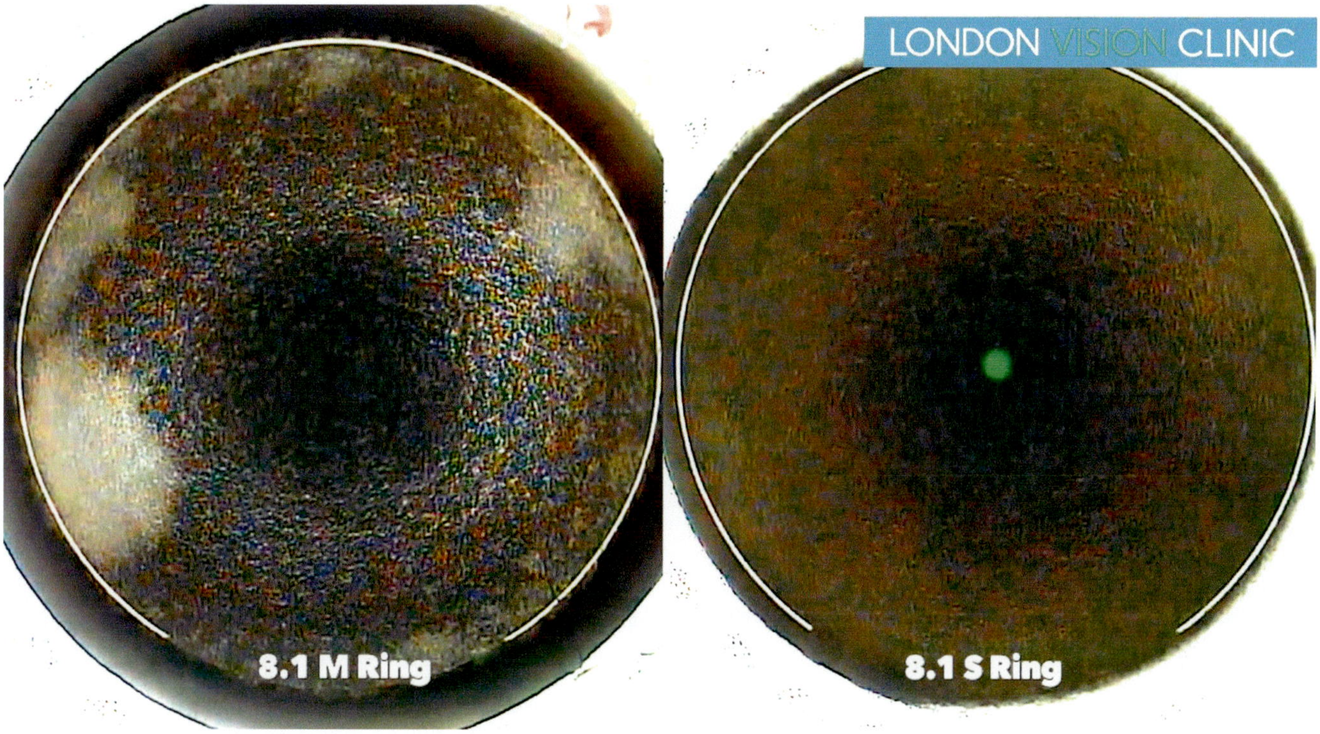

Fig. 5 Femtosecond bubble pattern for the right and left eyes of the same patient in which a 8.1 mm diameter flap was created in both eyes, but an 'S' contact glass was used for one eye and an 'M' contact glass for the other. There was obvious OBL in the eye treated with an 'M' contact glass, whereas there was no OBL when using an 'S' contact glass. This demonstrates the effectiveness of avoiding OBL by starting the femtosecond cutting closer to the edge of the contact glass to allow the gas to escape peripherally rather than be forced centrally. *Reprinted with permission from Reinstein DZ, Archer TJ, Carp GI. The Surgeon's Guide to Small Incision Lenticule Extraction (SMILE). Thorofare, New Jersey: SLACK Incorporated, 2018*

28.8% for a 7.9–8.0 mm flap diameter to 7.6% for a 8.1 mm flap diameter when using an S contact glass.

It is thought that having the flap diameter so close to the contact glass allows the gas to escape through the peripheral cornea underneath the rim of the contact glass, as this is the area of least resistance of the stromal lamellae. In contrast, when the femtosecond cutting starts further from the contact glass, the pressure of the contact glass onto the cornea is enough to compress the stromal lamellae and block the gas from escaping, hence forcing the gas to travel towards the center.

6 Conclusion

Corneal laser refractive surgery by femtosecond LASIK has been established as a safe and effective treatment for myopia up to –10.00 D [13, 58] and hyperopia up to + 3.00 D [59], while studies have also shown the range can be extended to –14.00 D [57] and + 6.50 D [60] under the right conditions. For myopia, outcomes have been optimized by the development of modern flying spot excimer lasers, advances in eye-tracking, and ablation profile design including the use of larger optical zones, wavefront-optimized aspheric profiles [61, 62], modern algorithms for compensation for fluence projection and reflection errors [63], biomechanical factors [64] and the availability of topography-guided ablation profiles [65]. For hyperopia, outcomes have been optimized by the same factors as for myopia, plus centration on the coaxially sighted corneal light reflex [66–68] and the use of epithelial thickness profiles for evaluating how much steepening can be safely achieved [60].

As described in this chapter, the surgical protocol for performing a femtosecond LASIK procedure has been standardized, which helps further to optimize outcomes and safety, as well as easing the learning curve for new refractive surgeons. In particular, the technique described of how to lift and replace a flap minimizes the formation of microfolds, or even nanofolds. Careful flap management enables optimal quality of vision for the patient and reduces the risk of epithelial ingrowth.

References

1. Santhiago MR, Kara-Junior N, Waring GOt. Microkeratome versus femtosecond flaps: accuracy and complications. Curr Opin Ophthalmol. 2014;25:270–274.
2. Farjo AA, Sugar A, Schallhorn SC, Majmudar PA, Tanzer DJ, Trattler WB, Cason JB, Donaldson KE, Kymionis GD. Femtosecond lasers for LASIK flap creation: a report by the American Academy of Ophthalmology. Ophthalmology. 2013;120:e5–20.
3. Arbelaez MC, Nidek MK. 2000 microkeratome clinical evaluation. J Refract Surg. 2002;18:S357–360.
4. Shemesh G, Dotan G, Lipshitz I. Predictability of corneal flap thickness in laser in situ keratomileusis using three different microkeratomes. J Refract Surg. 2002;18:S347–351.
5. Solomon KD, Donnenfeld E, Sandoval HP, Al Sarraf O, Kasper TJ, Holzer MP, Slate EH, Vroman DT. Flap thickness accuracy: comparison of 6 microkeratome models. J Cataract Refract Surg. 2004;30:964–77.
6. Li Y, Netto MV, Shekhar R, Krueger RR, Huang D. A longitudinal study of LASIK flap and stromal thickness with high-speed optical coherence tomography. Ophthalmology. 2007;114:1124–32.
7. Talamo JH, Meltzer J, Gardner J. Reproducibility of flap thickness with IntraLase FS and Moria LSK-1 and M2 microkeratomes. J Refract Surg. 2006;22:556–61.
8. Reinstein DZ, Srivannaboon S, Archer TJ, Silverman RH, Sutton H, Coleman DJ. Probability model of the inaccuracy of residual stromal thickness prediction to reduce the risk of ectasia after LASIK part II: quantifying population risk. J Refract Surg. 2006;22:861–70.
9. Zhai CB, Tian L, Zhou YH, Zhang QW, Zhang J. Comparison of the flaps made by femtosecond laser and automated keratomes for sub-bowman keratomileusis. Chin Med J (Engl). 2013;126:2440–4.
10. Lackerbauer CA, Kollias A, Kreutzer TC, Ulbig M, Kampik A, Grueterich M. Amadeus II microkeratome: optimizing microkeratome settings for high flap accuracy using optical low coherence reflectometry. Eur J Ophthalmol. 2010;20:41-7.
11. Reinstein DZ, Archer TJ, Gobbe M. Accuracy and reproducibility of cap thickness in small incision lenticule extraction. J Refract Surg. 2013;29:810–5.
12. Lim DH, Keum JE, Ju WK, Lee JH, Chung TY, Chung ES. Prospective contralateral eye study to compare 80- and 120-mum flap LASIK using the VisuMax femtosecond laser. J Refract Surg. 2013;29:462–8.
13. Reinstein DZ, Carp GI, Archer TJ, Gobbe M. Transitioning from mechanical microkeratome to femtosecond flap creation: comparing experienced vs novice LASIK surgeon visual outcomes for the first 200 myopic procedures. J Cataract Refract Surg. 2012;38:1788–95.
14. Sekundo W, Kunert K, Russmann C, Gille A, Bissmann W, Stobrawa G, Sticker M, Bischoff M, Blum M. First efficacy and safety study of femtosecond lenticule extraction for the correction of myopia: six-month results. J Cataract Refract Surg. 2008;34:1513–20.
15. Sekundo W, Kunert KS, Blum M. Small incision corneal refractive surgery using the small incision lenticule extraction (SMILE) procedure for the correction of myopia and myopic astigmatism: results of a 6 month prospective study. Br J Ophthalmol. 2011;95:335–9.
16. Shah R, Shah S, Sengupta S. Results of small incision lenticule extraction: all-in-one femtosecond laser refractive surgery. J Cataract Refract Surg. 2011;37:127–37.
17. Hjortdal JO, Vestergaard AH, Ivarsen A, Ragunathan S, Asp S. Predictors for the outcome of small-incision lenticule extraction for Myopia. J Refract Surg. 2012;28:865–71.
18. FDA. VisuMax femtosecond laser system for refractive correction (PMA), 2016.
19. Vetter JM, Faust M, Gericke A, Pfeiffer N, Weingartner WE, Sekundo W. Intraocular pressure measurements during flap preparation using 2 femtosecond lasers and 1 microkeratome in human donor eyes. J Cataract Refract Surg. 2012;38:2011–8.
20. Vetter JM, Holzer MP, Teping C, Weingartner WE, Gericke A, Stoffelns B, Pfeiffer N, Sekundo W. Intraocular pressure during corneal flap preparation: comparison among four femtosecond lasers in porcine eyes. J Refract Surg. 2011;27:427–33.
21. Reinstein DZ, Archer TJ, Gobbe M, Johnson N. Accuracy and reproducibility of Artemis central flap thickness and visual outcomes of LASIK With the Carl Zeiss Meditec VisuMax Femtosecond Laser and MEL 80 Excimer laser platforms. J Refract Surg. 2010;26:107–19.
22. Yu ZQ, Xu Y, Yao PJ, Qin B, Zhou XT. Chu RY Analysis of flap thickness by anterior segment optical coherence tomography in different flap preparation styles of excimer laser surgery. Zhonghua Yan Ke Za Zhi. 2010;46:203–8.
23. Ju WK, Lee JH, Chung TY, Chung ES. Reproducibility of LASIK flap thickness using the zeiss femtosecond laser measured postoperatively by optical coherence tomography. J Refract Surg. 2011;27:106–10.
24. Yao P, Xu Y, Zhou X. Comparison of the predictability, uniformity and stability of a laser in situ keratomileusis corneal flap created with a VisuMax femtosecond laser or a Moria microkeratome. J Int Med Res. 2011;39:748–58.
25. Ahn H, Kim JK, Kim CK, Han GH, Seo KY, Kim EK, Kim TI. Comparison of laser in situ keratomileusis flaps created by 3 femtosecond lasers and a microkeratome. J Cataract Refract Surg. 2011;37:349–57.
26. Issa A, Al HU. Femtosecond laser flap parameters and visual outcomes in laser in situ keratomileusis. J Cataract Refract Surg. 2011;37:665–74.
27. Tay E, Li X, Chan C, Tan DT, Mehta JS. Refractive lenticule extraction flap and stromal bed morphology assessment with anterior segment optical coherence tomography. J Cataract Refract Surg. 2012;38:1544–51.
28. Zhao J, Yao P, Li M, Chen Z, Shen Y, Zhao Z, Zhou Z, Zhou X. The morphology of corneal cap and its relation to refractive outcomes in femtosecond laser small incision lenticule extraction (SMILE) with anterior segment optical coherence tomography observation. PLoS ONE. 2013;8: e70208.
29. Ozgurhan EB, Agca A, Bozkurt E, Gencer B, Celik U, Cankaya KI, Demirok A, Yilmaz OF. Accuracy and precision of cap thickness in small incision lenticule extraction. Clin Ophthalmol. 2013;7:923–6.
30. Vestergaard AH, Grauslund J, Ivarsen AR, Hjortdal JO. Central corneal sublayer pachymetry and biomechanical properties after refractive femtosecond lenticule extraction. J Refract Surg. 2014;30:102–8.
31. Reinstein DZ, Archer TJ, Gobbe M, Silverman RH, Coleman DJ. Epithelial thickness in the normal cornea: three-dimensional display with Artemis very high-frequency digital ultrasound. J Refract Surg. 2008;24:571–81.
32. Contreras JM, Kim B, Tristao IM. Does doctors' experience matter in LASIK surgeries? Health Econ. 2011;20:699–722.
33. Reinstein DZ, Threlfall WB, Cook R, Cremonesi E, Sutton HF, Archer TJ, Gobbe M. Short term LASIK outcomes using the Technolas 217C excimer laser and Hansatome microkeratome in 46 708 eyes treated between 1998 and 2001. Br J Ophthalmol. 2012;96:1173–9.
34. Reinstein DZ, Carp GI, de Benedictis D, Archer TJ, Gobbe M, Khan R, von Borch M. Standardization of LASIK surgical technique evaluated by comparison of procedure time between two experienced surgeons. J Cataract Refract Surg. 2015;41:1004–8.

35. Siedlecki J, Luft N, Kook D, Wertheimer C, Mayer WJ, Bechmann M, Wiltfang R, Priglinger SG, Sekundo W, Dirisamer M. Enhancement after myopic small incision lenticule extraction (SMILE) using surface ablation. J Refract Surg. 2017;33:513–8.
36. Liu YC, Rosman M, Mehta JS. Enhancement after small-incision lenticule extraction: incidence, risk factors, and outcomes. Ophthalmology. 2017;124:813–21.
37. Vaddavalli PK, Yoo SH, Diakonis VF, Canto AP, Shah NV, Haddock LJ, Feuer WJ, Culbertson WW. Femtosecond laser-assisted retreatment for residual refractive errors after laser in situ keratomileusis. J Cataract Refract Surg. 2013;39:1241–7.
38. Riau AK, Ang HP, Lwin NC, Chaurasia SS, Tan DT, Mehta JS. Comparison of four different VisuMax circle patterns for flap creation after small incision lenticule extraction. J Refract Surg. 2013;29:236–44.
39. Chansue E, Tanehsakdi M, Swasdibutra S, McAlinden C. Safety and efficacy of VisuMax(R) circle patterns for flap creation and enhancement following small incision lenticule extraction. Eye Vis (Lond). 2015;2:21.
40. Donate D, Thaeron R. Preliminary evidence of successful enhancement after a primary SMILE procedure with the sub-cap-lenticule-extraction technique. J Refract Surg. 2015;31:708–10.
41. Reinstein DZ, Carp GI, Archer TJ, Gobbe M. Outcomes of small incision lenticule extraction (SMILE) in low myopia. J Refract Surg. 2014;30:812–8.
42. Tuisku IS, Lindbohm N, Wilson SE, Tervo TM. Dry eye and corneal sensitivity after high myopic LASIK. J Refract Surg. 2007;23:338–42.
43. Denoyer A, Landman E, Trinh L, Faure JF, Auclin F, Baudouin C. Dry eye disease after refractive surgery: comparative outcomes of small incision lenticule extraction versus LASIK. Ophthalmology. 2015;122:669–76.
44. Reinstein DZ, Archer TJ, Gobbe M, Bartoli E. Corneal sensitivity after small-incision lenticule extraction and laser in situ keratomileusis. J Cataract Refract Surg. 2015;41:1580–7.
45. Randleman JB, Dawson DG, Grossniklaus HE, McCarey BE, Edelhauser HF. Depth-dependent cohesive tensile strength in human donor corneas: implications for refractive surgery. J Refract Surg. 2008;24:S85–89.
46. Scarcelli G, Pineda R, Yun SH. Brillouin optical microscopy for corneal biomechanics. Invest Ophthalmol Vis Sci. 2012;53:185–90.
47. Reinstein DZ, Archer TJ, Randleman JB. Mathematical model to compare the relative tensile strength of the cornea after PRK, LASIK, and small incision lenticule extraction. J Refract Surg. 2013;29:454–60.
48. Spiru B, Kling S, Hafezi F, Sekundo W. Biomechanical differences between femtosecond lenticule extraction (FLEx) and small incision lenticule extraction (SMILE) Tested by 2D-Extensometry in Ex Vivo Porcine Eyes. Invest Ophthalmol Vis Sci. 2017;58:2591–5.
49. Reinstein DZ, Dickeson ZI, Archer TJ, Gobbe M. Artemis very high-frequency digital ultrasound guided femtosecond laser recut after flap complication. Digit J Ophth. 2014;20:1–5.
50. Luengo Gimeno F, Chan CM, Li L, Tan DT, Mehta JS. Comparison of eye-tracking success in laser in situ keratomileusis after flap creation with 2 femtosecond laser models. J Cataract Refract Surg. 2011;37:538–43.
51. Jung HG, Kim J, Lim TH. Possible risk factors and clinical effects of an opaque bubble layer created with femtosecond laser-assisted laser in situ keratomileusis. J Cataract Refract Surg. 2015;41:1393–9.
52. Mastropasqua L, Calienno R, Lanzini M, Salgari N, De Vecchi S, Mastropasqua R, Nubile M. Opaque bubble layer incidence in Femtosecond laser-assisted LASIK: comparison among different flap design parameters. Int Ophthalmol. 2017;37:635–41.
53. Wu N, Christenbury JG, Dishler JG, Bozkurt K, Duel D, Zhang L, Hamilton DR. A Technique to Reduce Incidence of Opaque Bubble Layer Formation during LASIK Flap Creation Using the VisuMax Femtosecond Laser. J Refract Surg. 2017;33:584–90.
54. Juhasz T, Kastis GA, Suarez C, Bor Z, Bron WE. Time-resolved observations of shock waves and cavitation bubbles generated by femtosecond laser pulses in corneal tissue and water. Lasers Surg Med. 1996;19:23–31.
55. Juhasz T, Hu XH, Turi L, Bor Z. Dynamics of shock waves and cavitation bubbles generated by picosecond laser pulses in corneal tissue and water. Lasers Surg Med. 1994;15:91–8.
56. Hurmeric V, Yoo SH, Fishler J, Chang VS, Wang J, Culbertson WW. In vivo structural characteristics of the femtosecond LASIK-induced opaque bubble layers with ultrahigh-resolution SD-OCT. Ophthalmic Surg Lasers Imaging. 2010;41(Suppl):S109–113.
57. Reinstein DZ, Carp GI, Archer TJ, Lewis TA, Gobbe M, Moore J, Moore T. Long-term visual and refractive outcomes after LASIK for high Myopia and Astigmatism From -8.00 to -14.25 D. J Refract Surg. 2016;32:290–297.
58. Reinstein DZ, Carp GI, Lewis TA, Archer TJ, Gobbe M. Outcomes for Myopic LASIK With the MEL 90 excimer laser. J Refract Surg. 2015;31:316–21.
59. Reinstein DZ, Carp GI, Archer TJ, Day AC, Vida RS. Outcomes for Hyperopic LASIK With the MEL 90((R)) Excimer Laser. J Refract Surg. 2018;34:799–808.
60. Reinstein DZ, Carp GI, Archer TJ, Buick T, Gobbe M, Rowe EL, Jukic M, Brandon E, Moore J, Moore T. LASIK for the correction of high Hyperopic Astigmatism with Epithelial thickness monitoring. J Refract Surg. 2017;33:314–21.
61. Reinstein DZ, Archer TJ, Gobbe M. LASIK for Myopic Astigmatism and Presbyopia Using Non-Linear Aspheric Micro-Monovision with the Carl Zeiss Meditec MEL 80 Platform. J Refract Surg. 2011;27:23–37.
62. Srivannaboon S, Reinstein DZ, Archer TJ, Chansue E. Spherical Aberration from Myopic Excimer Laser Ablation for Aspheric and Non-Aspheric Profiles. Optom Vis Sci. 2012;89:1211–8.
63. Mrochen M, Seiler T. Influence of corneal curvature on calculation of ablation patterns used in photorefractive laser surgery. J Refract Surg. 2001;17:S584-587.
64. Dupps WJ Jr, Roberts C. Effect of acute biomechanical changes on corneal curvature after photokeratectomy. J Refract Surg. 2001;17:658–69.
65. Reinstein DZ, Archer TJ, Gobbe M. Combined corneal topography and corneal wavefront data in the treatment of corneal irregularity and refractive error in LASIK or PRK using the Carl Zeiss Meditec MEL80 and CRS Master. J Refract Surg. 2009;25:503–15.
66. Reinstein DZ, Gobbe M, Archer TJ. Coaxially sighted corneal light reflex versus entrance pupil center centration of moderate to high hyperopic corneal ablations in eyes with small and large angle kappa. J Refract Surg. 2013;29:518–25.
67. Nepomuceno RL, Boxer BS, Wachler, Kim JM, Scruggs R, Sato M. Laser in situ keratomileusis for hyperopia with the LADARVision 4000 with centration on the coaxially sighted corneal light reflex. J Cataract Refract Surg. 2004;30:1281–1286.
68. Kanellopoulos AJ. Topography-guided hyperopic and hyperopic astigmatism femtosecond laser-assisted LASIK: long-term experience with the 400 Hz eye-Q excimer platform. Clin Ophthalmol. 2012;6:895–901.

Incisional Corneal Refractive Surgery

Tim Berger, Loay Daas, and Berthold Seitz

Abstract

Refractive surgery has developed into a highly specialized field of ophthalmology in recent years. Today, it offers a wide range of surgical methods for the individual correction of refractive errors. Following the introduction of laser-assisted corneal refractive surgery, incisional corneal procedures such as **arcuate keratotomy**, **peripheral corneal relaxing incisions** and **radial keratotomy** have become less popular due to their limited accuracy and predictability. Although the latter procedure is only of historical relevance, the other two options are used in selected cases.

Keywords

Radial keratotomy · Arcuate keratotomy · Peripheral corneal relaxing incisions · Incisional corneal surgery · Astigmatism

1 Radial Keratotomy

1.1 Surgical Principle and Technique

Radial keratotomy (RK) was a popular procedure for myopia correction [1]. Nowadays, it is considered obsolete, as other surgical methods have been introduced for correction of myopia with better accuracy and predictability. However, RK is still part of clinical practice today due to the management of late postoperative complications.

The principle of RK is based on a redistribution of corneal power from the center to the periphery by placing several radial incisions sparing the central optical zone. This procedure does not involve active tissue ablation, however the cuts cause disruption of the collagen fibrils in the periphery with structural weakening. Thus, steepening of the midperiphery/periphery results in compensatory flattening of the center ("coupling effect") with reduced refractive power (Fig. 1) [2].

Regarding the extent of the desired myopia correction, there are several modifications such as the number, the depth (usually in 90% corneal depth), and the length of the incisions (size of the optical zone). Especially the latter might be very variable and higher myopia correction might only be achieved if the incisions are closer to the optical center [3].

1.2 Complications

Intraoperative complications include corneal perforation (Fig. 2) and a decentered clear zone. Incisions across the visual axis might lead to corneal scarring with irregular astigmatism, which significantly affects vision, especially if the optical zone is small (Fig. 3) [4]. Incorrect simultaneous placement of transverse incisions for astigmatism reduction may result in undesirable refractive outcomes [5]. Intersecting incisions (Fig. 4) might lead to severe wound gapes, recurrent erosion and larger amount of scarring [5].

RK does not only alter the curvature of the central cornea, but also affect the entire corneal topography, which might increase spherical aberrations leading to reduced contrast sensitivity [6].

Further complications associated with corneal incisions include limbal scarring, corneal vascularization (Fig. 5), epithelial inclusions of debris and deposits or infectious keratitis [4, 5, 7].

Many patients (up to 60%) complain about diurnal fluctuations (caused by nocturnal flattening of the cornea), with

T. Berger (✉) · L. Daas · B. Seitz
Department of Ophthalmology, Saarland University Medical Center, Homburg, Germany
e-mail: tim.berger@uks.eu

B. Seitz et al. (eds.), *Atlas on Cornea*, https://doi.org/10.1007/978-3-031-65422-0_64

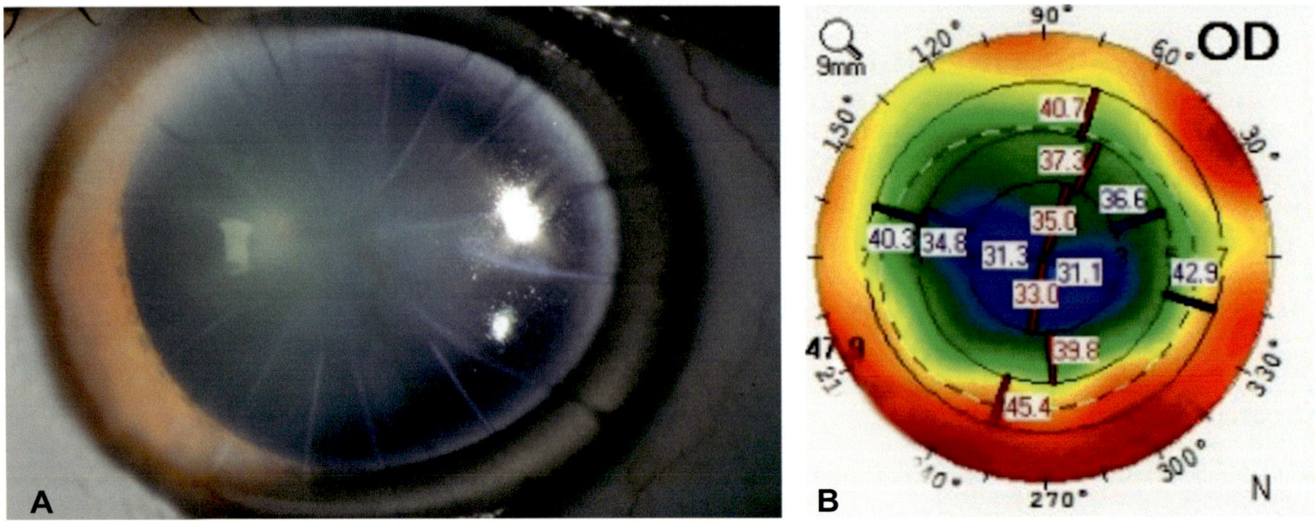

Fig. 1 Slit lamp photographs and corneal tomography of a cornea after radial keratotomy 30 years postoperatively. (**A**) Multiple incisions of a cornea after radial keratotomy. (**B**) Corneal tomography demonstrates a steepening of the periphery with compensatory flattening of the central cornea

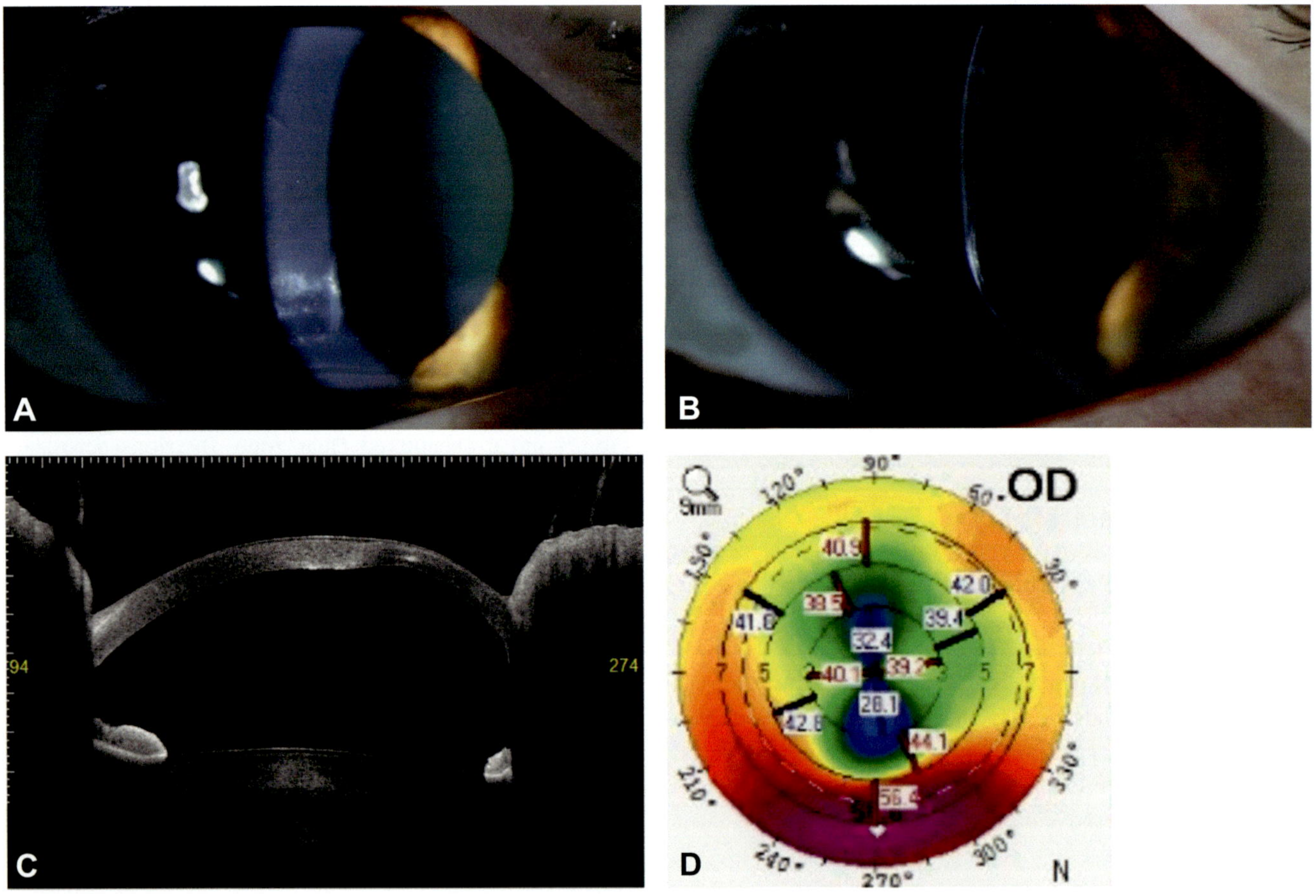

Fig. 2 Cornea after radial keratotomy with stromal scarring secondary to intraoperative perforation (**A**, **B**) Clinical examination shows midperipheral stromal scarring of the cornea at 6 o 'clock (**A**) moderate slit, (**B**) narrow slit. (**C**, **D**) Anterior segment optical coherence tomography (**C**) and Pentacam (**D**) demonstrate flattening of the corneal center with focal steepening of the inferior cornea due to corneal scarring

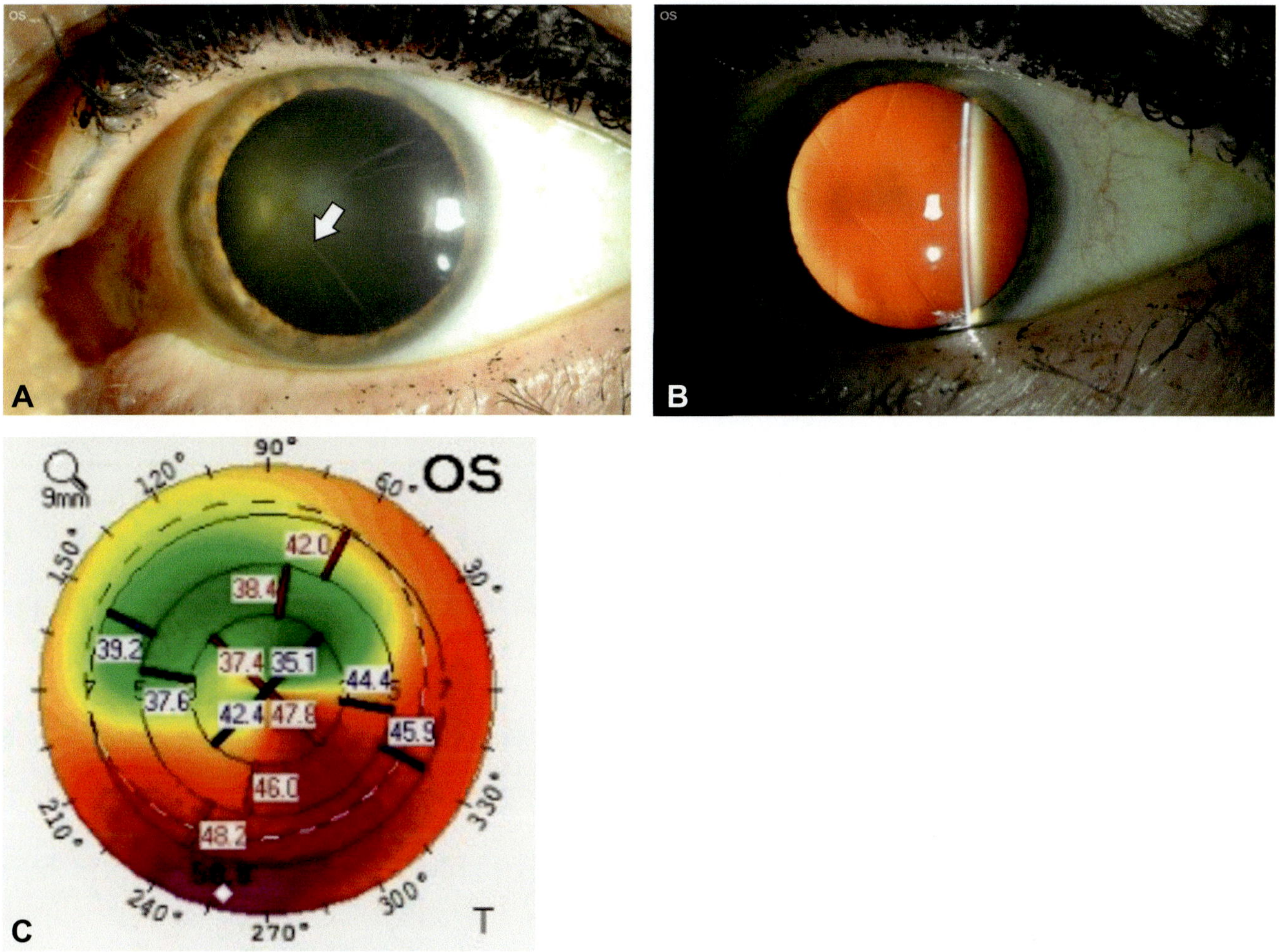

Fig. 3 Cornea after radial keratotomy with decentered incisions (**A**, **B**) The corneal incisions are incorrectly placed, decentered ((**A**): arrow) and partially reach the optical center. (**C**) Tomography shows asymmetric refractive power distribution of the cornea with inferior steepening and irregular astigmatism (pseudo-keratoconus-formation)

the greatest variability in visual acuity occurring in the first few hours after awakening as most corneas become steeper during the day [8].

Approximately 80% of patients suffered from undercorrection with regression of the intended effect between 0.5 Diopters and 4.25 Diopters [4]. In the past, surgical management of undercorrection included placement of additional incisions or deepening of pre-existing incisions [4, 5, 9]. Induced astigmatism may occur especially in cases of low incision number, asymmetrical incisions, variable depth or decentered optical zone. Irregular astigmatism is more common for repeated surgeries or for incisions that reach too far into the visual axis (smaller clear zone than 3.0 mm) [4, 10]. A very frequent complication is overcorrection and occurred mainly when the optical zone was too small, when the incisions were too deep, started at the corneal limbus, or the procedure was repeated. Furthermore, few patients complained about glare or halo at night (Fig. 6) [4, 5, 9].

Laser-in-situ-Keratomileusis (LASIK) (Fig. 7) or photorefractive keratectomy (PRK) are feasible treatment options for progressive hyperopia or myopia after RK, however surface ablation should be the preferred method after RK [11–13].

Flap creation carries the risk of irregular astigmatism, rupture of the incisions, or epithelial ingrowth. In case of PRK after RK, topical Mitomycin C application (0.02%) is recommended intraoperatively to prevent corneal haze [11]. In severe cases, penetrating keratoplasty is advised [14].

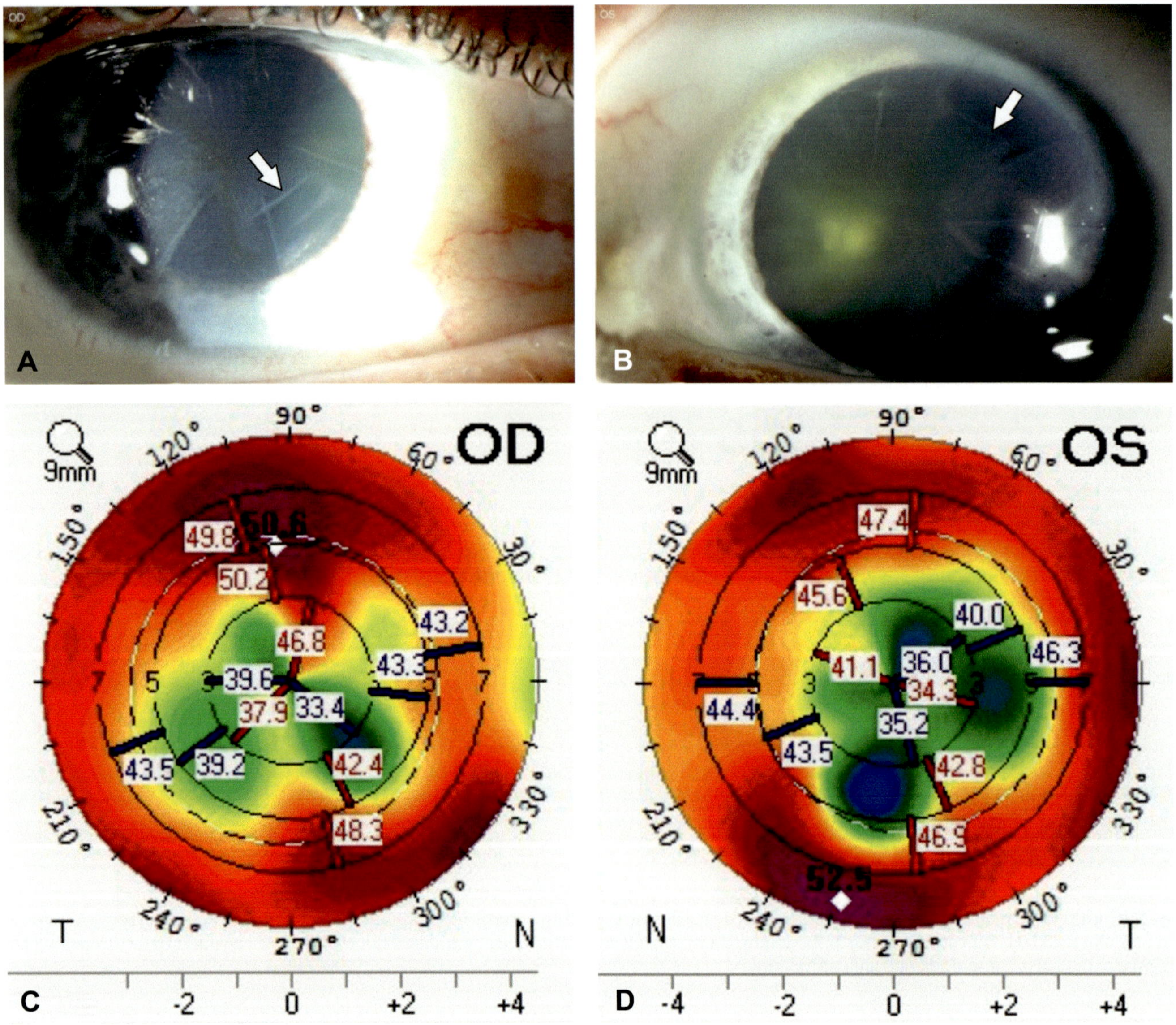

Fig. 4 Combined radial and transverse keratotomies. (**A**, **B**) Transverse keratotomies (arrow) overlap with radial keratotomies on the right (**B**) and left eye (**A**). (**C**, **D**) Tomography shows a central flattening with peripheral steepening and irregular astigmatism ("trefoil pattern") in the right (**C**) and left (**D**) eye

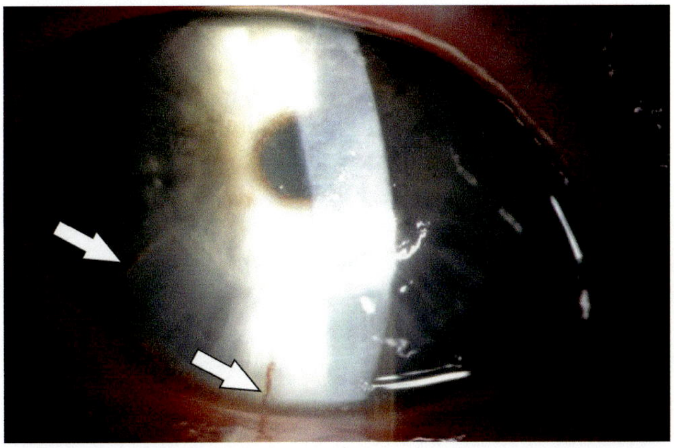

Fig. 5 Cornea after radial keratotomy and Laser-in-situ-Keratomileusis with corneal ulcer and vascularization along the incisions (arrows)

2 Arcuate Keratotomy

2.1 Surgical Principle and Technique

Arcuate keratotomy (AK, synonym: astigmatic keratotomy) is a well-established procedure for treating high postkeratoplasty astigmatism, which cannot be managed by spectacles or hard contact lenses [15, 16]. The principle of AK (Fig. 8) is based on paired corneal incisions perpendicular to the meridian with the steepest sagittal slope causing a decrease in corneal refractive power through tissue relaxation. These incisions lead to increase in corneal refractive power of the flat meridian, known as coupling effect [2]. The simultaneous use of compression sutures can further increase the corneal refractive power on the flat meridian, resulting in additional astigmatism reduction [16].

Mechanical (adjustable diamond blade) or laser-assisted (femtosecond laser) incisions are feasible. The correction of astigmatism can be adjusted by the number, the length and the depth of the incisions (typically 90% depth) [17]. Identification of the steep and flat meridian by preoperative corneal topography is necessary.

However, the first step of the procedure (Fig. 9) is to identify the flat and steep meridians, which is usually done by keratoscopy in the lying patient. Since placement of the arcuate incision in the area of the host cornea is associated with significantly poor effect, we usually use a uniform diameter of 6.0 mm [16]. To avoid halos, glares and aberrations, incisions should not be placed closer than 3.0 mm radial distance to the pupil center [18, 19].

Postoperatively, selective suture removal (Fig. 10) might help to achieve acceptable amount of astigmatism. It has also been observed that tightening of the compression sutures is associated with widening of the keratotomies and allows the formation of larger epithelial plugs in the incisions, maintaining the effect of the arcuate incisions even after removal of the sutures [20].

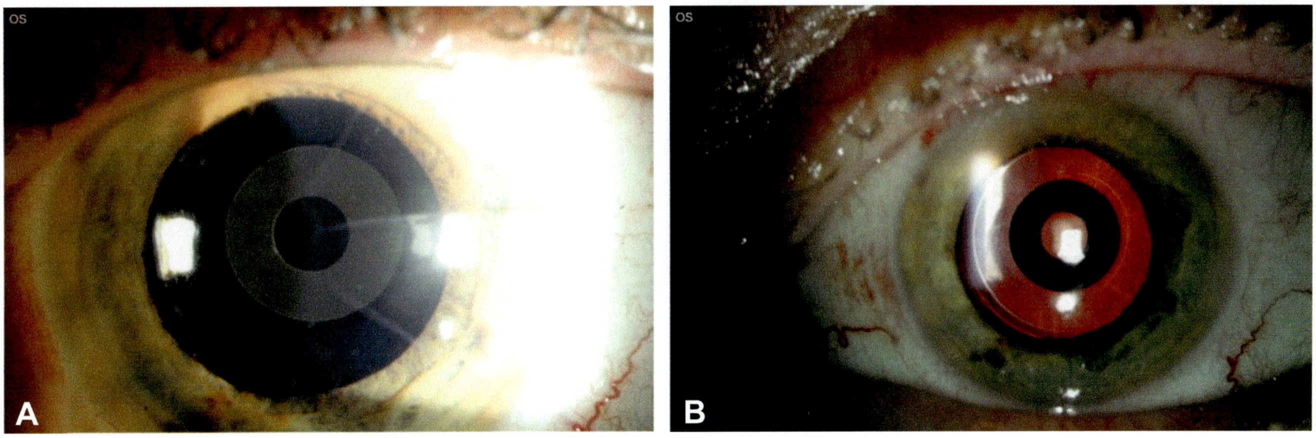

Fig. 6 Implantation of a small aperture intraocular lens due to increased light sensitivity after radial keratotomy ((**A**): overview, (**B**): retroillumination)

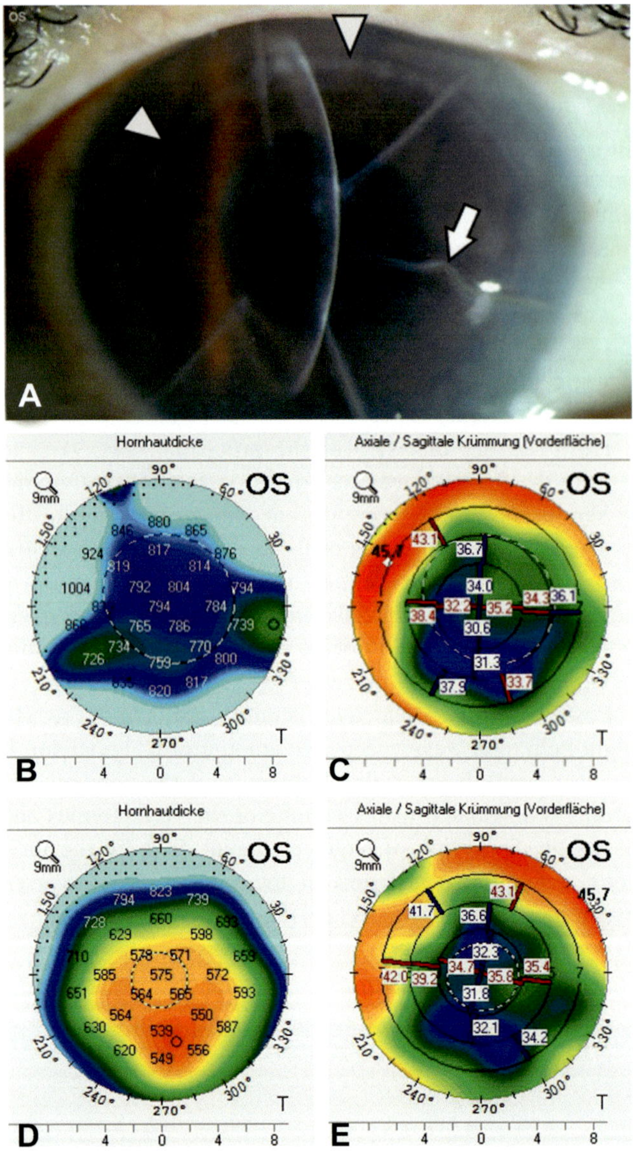

Fig. 7 Endothelial decompensation after cataract surgery in a cornea with previous radial keratotomies and LASIK. (**A**) Slit lamp photography showing corneal edema after previous radial keratotomies (arrow) and LASIK (flap margins: arrowheads). (**B**, **C**) Preoperative corneal pachymetry (**B**) and tomography (**C**) demonstrating increased corneal thickness and central regular astigmatism. (**D**, **E**) Postoperative corneal pachymetry (**D**) and tomography (**E**) after Descemet membrane endothelial keratoplasty. Normal corneal thickness is achieved without impairment of the preoperative refractive capabilities of the cornea

2.2 Complications

Common complications of AK include visual loss and irregular astigmatism. Incorrect alignment may result in undercorrection or worsening of existing astigmatism. Intraoperatively, there is a low risk of corneal perforation. In the early but also in the late postoperative course, infections of the incisions might occur (Fig. 11 A, B). Likewise, loose sutures must always be removed due to the risk of infectious keratitis (Fig. 11C) [17]. The risk of allograft rejection in case of previous penetrating keratoplasty was reported to be 2.2–4.8% [17]. Therefore, it is always recommended to apply systemic and local steroids after AK.

3 Peripheral Corneal Relaxing Incisions

3.1 Surgical Principle and Technique

Peripheral corneal relaxing incisions (formerly: Limbal relaxing incisions) are a surgical technique used to reduce small degrees of astigmatism in patients undergoing cataract surgery or other refractive procedures [21, 22].

The surgical principle of peripheral corneal relaxing incisions is to create one or more small incisions (manual, automated, or femtosecond laser-assisted) in the cornea of 1–2 mm in length that are located at the corneal limbus. The incisions are oriented along the steep axis of the cornea and are performed in a depth of 70–90% [23].

Compared to other methods for correcting astigmatism, peripheral corneal relaxing incisions are relatively easy to perform, generally less expensive and also have a lower risk of inducing higher-order aberrations [21, 22].

The achievable correction of astigmatism is up to 2.5 diopters (number, depth, length and placement of incision), however the implantation of a toric intraocular lens is generally recommended for astigmatism over 1.5 diopters due to greater predictability [23].

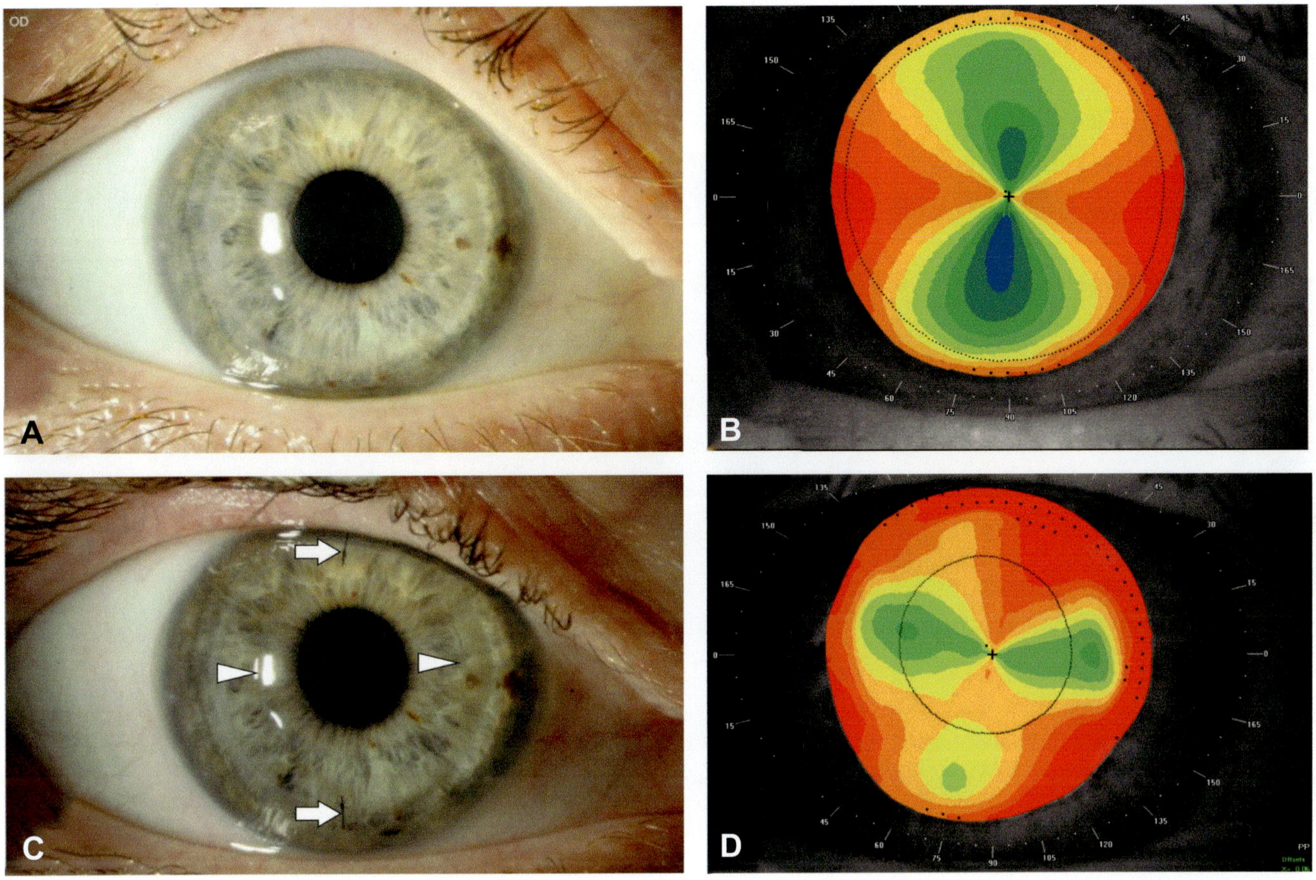

Fig. 8 Arcuate keratotomy for high postkeratoplasty astigmatism. (**A**, **B**) Clear corneal graft (**A**), but topography is demonstrating a high regular astigmatism (**B**). (**C**, **D**) Arcuate keratotomy (incision: arrowheads) with compression sutures (arrows) resulted in rotation of the steep axis by 90° with half of the amount of preoperative astigmatism. Removal of the compression sutures might decrease the refractive power of the steep meridian and thus result in additional astigmatism reduction

3.2 Complications

Complications are similar to other incisional procedures and include over– or undercorrection, infection and corneal perforation [24].

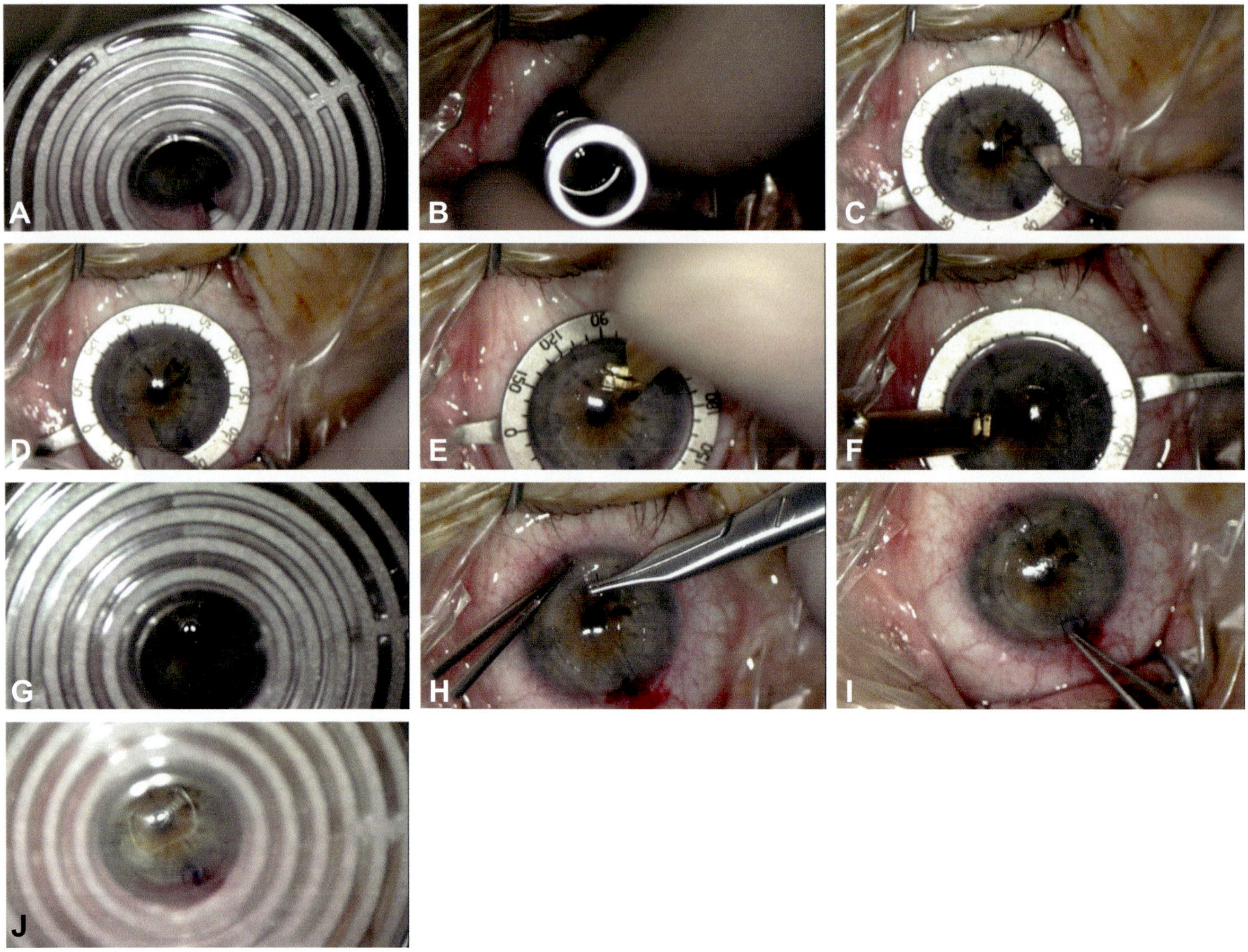

Fig. 9 Main surgical steps of arcuate keratotomy and compression sutures.(**A**) Identification and marking of the flat meridian by using a handheld keratoscope. (**B**) Marking of the incision diameter with a 6.0 mm trephine (pupil oriented). (**C**, **D**) Marking of the incision length at the steep axis on both hemimeridians by using the Gimbel/Mendez ring for orientation. (**E**, **F**) Performing the corneal incisions with a diamond knife at a depth of 90% (measured preoperatively with optical coherence tomography of the anterior segment). (**G**) Monitoring the effect with the keratoscope. (**H**, **I**) Placement of interrupted sutures in the area of the flat meridian for additional steepening and astigmatism reduction. (**J**) Further astigmatism control with a keratoscope at the end of the surgery

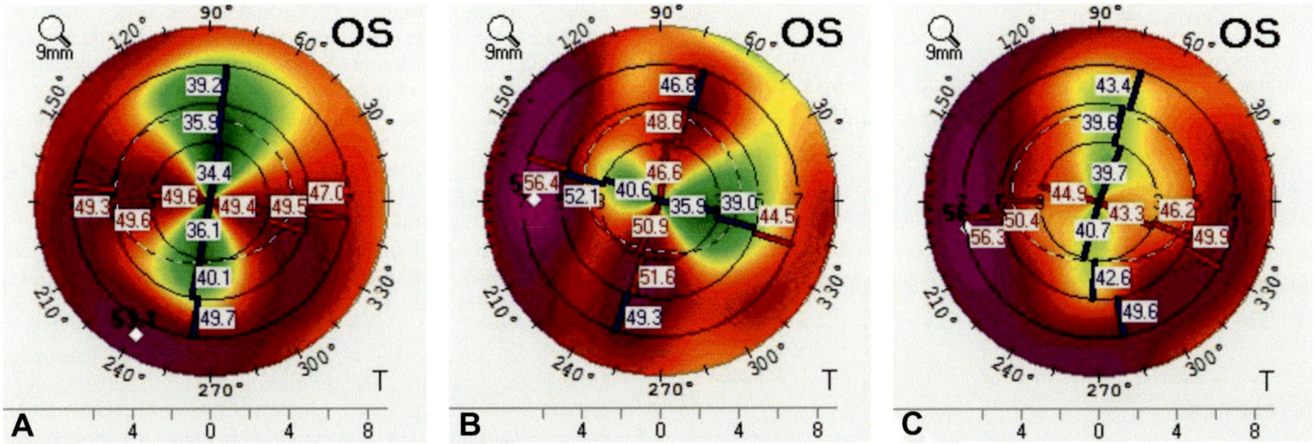

Fig. 10 Corneal tomography before and after arcuate keratotomy with compression sutures. (**A**) Preoperative tomography showing high regular postkeratoplasty astigmatism. (**B**) Tomography after arcuate keratotomy with compression sutures. Decrease of refractive power in the steep meridian with simultaneous increase in the flat meridian. (**C**) Removal of the compression sutures in the steep axis results in further astigmatism reduction (original axis is reachieved)

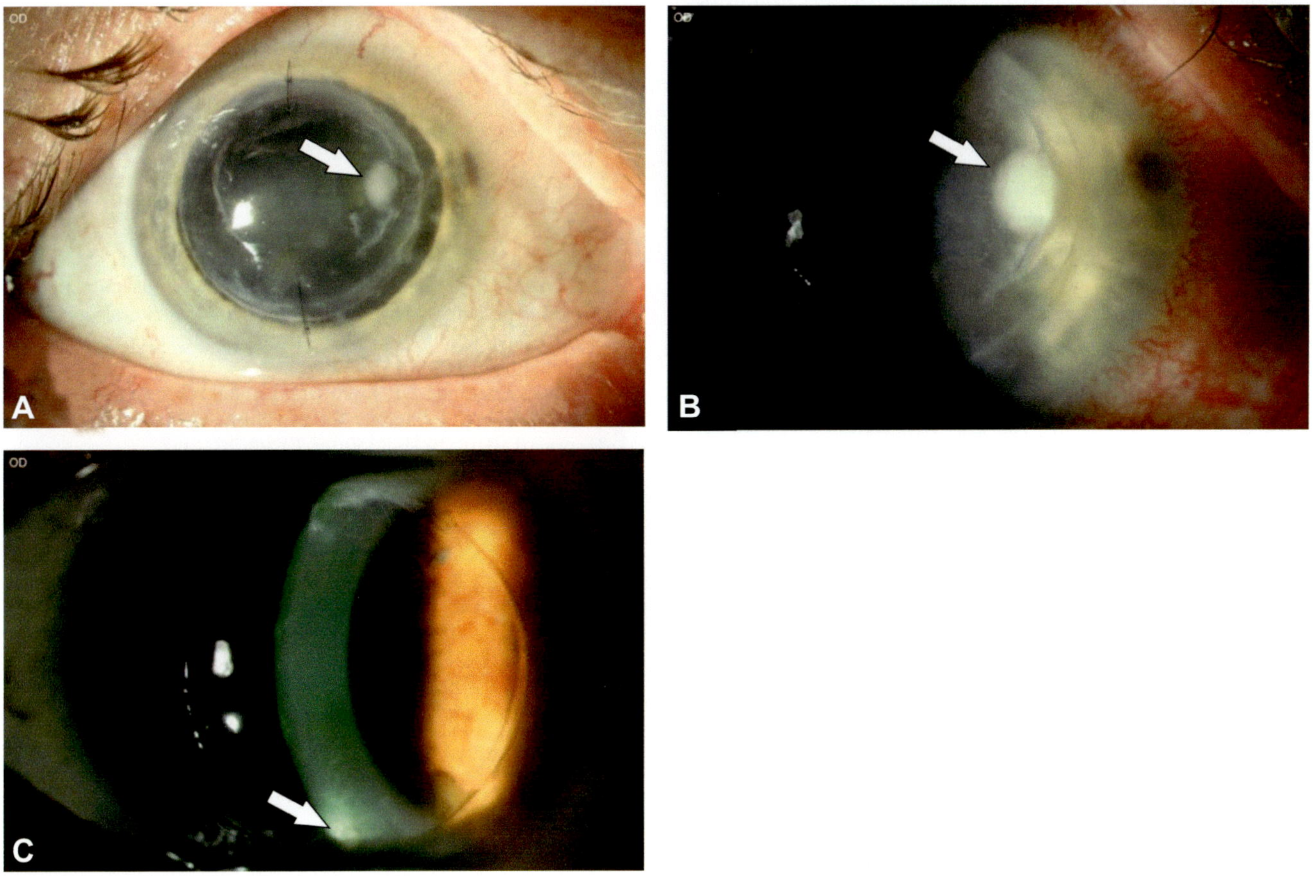

Fig. 11 Infectious keratitis after arcuate keratotomy with compression sutures. (**A**, **B**) Bacterial infiltrate at the arcuate incision (arrow, (**A**): overview, (**B**): magnification). (**C**) Other patient: Infectious keratitis (arrow) due to suture loosening

4 Conclusion

Incisional surgery is a useful method for the correction of moderate corneal astigmatism. Every surgeon must be aware of the indication, the technique and the intra– and postoperative complications. It is particularly important that the patient has realistic expectations.

Funding The authors have no funding or conflicts of interest to disclose.

References

1. Salamon SA, Hjortdal JØ, Ehlers N. Refractive results of radial keratotomy: a ten-year retrospective study. Acta Ophthalmol Scand. 2000;78:566–8. https://doi.org/10.1034/j.1600-0420.2000.078005566.x.
2. Alpins N, Ong JKY, Stamatelatos G. Corneal coupling of astigmatism applied to incisional and ablative surgery. J Cataract Refract Surg. 2014;40:1813–27. https://doi.org/10.1016/j.jcrs.2014.02.047.
3. Schwiegerling J, Greivekamp JE, Miller JM, Snyder RW, Palmer ML. Optical Modeling of Radial Keratotomy Incision Patterns. Am J Ophthalmol. 1996;122:808–17. https://doi.org/10.1016/S0002-9394(14)70377-0.
4. Waring GO III, Lynn MJ, McDonnell PJ. Results of the Prospective Evaluation of Radial Keratotomy (PERK) Study 10 Years After Surgery. Arch Ophthalmol. 1994;112:1298–308. https://doi.org/10.1001/archopht.1994.01090220048022.
5. Rashid ER, Waring GO. Complications of radial and transverse keratotomy. Surv Ophthalmol. 1989;34:73–106. https://doi.org/10.1016/0039-6257(89)90037-4.
6. Applegate RA, Howland HC, Sharp RP, Cottingham AJ, Yee RW. Corneal aberrations and visual performance after radial Keratotomy. J Refract Surg. 1998;14:397–407. https://doi.org/10.3928/1081-597X-19980701-05.
7. Nirankari VS, Katzen LE, Richards RD, Karesh JW, Lakhanpal V, Billings E. Prospective clinical study of Radial Keratotomy. Ophthalmology. 1982;89:677–83. https://doi.org/10.1016/S0161-6420(82)34739-9.
8. McDonnell PJ, Nizam A, Lynn MJ, Waring GO. Morning-to-evening Change in Refraction, Corneal Curvature, and Visual Acuity 11 Years after Radial Keratotomy in the Prospective Evaluation of Radial Keratotomy Study. Ophthalmology. 1996;103:233–9. https://doi.org/10.1016/S0161-6420(96)30711-2.
9. Lovisolo CF, Mularoni A, Calossi A, Stewart CW. Complications of Refractive Keratotomy. In: Management of Complications in Refractive Surgery, Springer Verlag, Heidelberg; 2008, p. 197–224. https://doi.org/10.1007/978-3-540-37584-5_12.
10. Jory WJ. Radial keratotomy: 500 consecutive cases. Eye. 1989;3:663–71. https://doi.org/10.1038/eye.1989.102.
11. Anbar R, Malta JB, Barbosa JB, Leoratti MC, Beer S, Campos M. Photorefractive Keratectomy with Mitomycin-C for consecutive hyperopia after radial Keratotomy. Cornea. 2009;28:371–4. https://doi.org/10.1097/ICO.0b013e31818c4d47.
12. Rush SW, Rush RB. One-Year Outcomes of Femtosecond Laser-Assisted LASIK following previous radial Keratotomy. J Refract Surg. 2016;32:15–9. https://doi.org/10.3928/1081597X-20151207-07.
13. Farah CJ, El HM, Daas L, Seitz B. Descemet membrane endothelial keratoplasty after sequential radial keratotomies, LASIK, and cataract surgery with endothelial decompensation. J Case Rep Images Opthalmol. 2020;3:1–6. https://doi.org/10.5348/100019Z17CF2021CR.
14. Parmley V, Ng J, Gee B, Rotkis W, Mader T. Penetrating Keratoplasty after radial Keratotomy. Ophthalmology. 1995;102:947–50. https://doi.org/10.1016/S0161-6420(95)30929-3.
15. Poole TRG, Ficker LA. Astigmatic keratotomy for post-keratoplasty astigmatism. J Cataract Refract Surg. 2006;32:1175–9. https://doi.org/10.1016/j.jcrs.2006.01.103.
16. Vilchis E, Seitz B, Langenbucher A, Küchle M, Kus M, Naumann GOH. Limbus-parallel keratotomies with compression sutures in treatment of high astigmatism after perforating keratoplasty: a vector analysis and topographic study. Klin Monbl Augenheilkd. 1997;211:151–8. https://doi.org/10.1055/s-2008-1035115.
17. Chang JSM. Femtosecond laser-assisted astigmatic keratotomy: a review. Eye Vis. 2018;5:6. https://doi.org/10.1186/s40662-018-0099-9.
18. Martínez CE. Effect of Pupillary Dilation on Corneal optical aberrations after Pshotorefractive Keratectomy. Arch Ophthalmol. 1998;116:1053. https://doi.org/10.1001/archopht.116.8.1053.
19. Tabernero J, Klyce SD, Sarver EJ, Artal P. Functional Optical Zone of the Cornea. Investig Opthalmology Vis Sci. 2007;48:1053. https://doi.org/10.1167/iovs.06-0867.
20. Fares U, Mokashi AA, Al-Aqaba MA, Otri AM, Miri A, Dua HS. Management of postkeratoplasty astigmatism by paired arcuate incisions with compression sutures. Br J Ophthalmol. 2013;97:438–43. https://doi.org/10.1136/bjophthalmol-2012-302128.
21. Budak K, Friedman NJ, Koch DD. Limbal relaxing incisions with cataract surgery. J Cataract Refract Surg. 1998;24:503–8. https://doi.org/10.1016/S0886-3350(98)80292-7.
22. Carvalho MJ, Suzuki SH, Freitas LL, Branco BC, Schor P, Lima ALH. Limbal Relaxing Incisions to Correct Corneal Astigmatism During Phacoemulsification. J Refract Surg. 2007;23:499–504. https://doi.org/10.3928/1081-597X-20070501-14.
23. Amesbury EC, Miller KM. Correction of astigmatism at the time of cataract surgery. Curr Opin Ophthalmol. 2009;20:19–24. https://doi.org/10.1097/ICU.0b013e328319c27a.
24. Zuberbuhler B, Tuft S, Gartry D, Spokes D. Refractive Corneal Surgery. In: Corneal Surgery. Springer Verlag, Heidelberg; 2013, p 91–134. https://doi.org/10.1007/978-3-642-12502-7_4.

Index

B. Seitz et al. (eds.), *Atlas on Cornea,* https://doi.org/10.1007/978-3-031-65422-0

D

GPSR Compliance

The European Union's (EU) General Product Safety Regulation (GPSR) is a set of rules that requires consumer products to be safe and our obligations to ensure this.

If you have any concerns about our products, you can contact us on ProductSafety@springernature.com

In case Publisher is established outside the EU, the EU authorized representative is:

Springer Nature Customer Service Center GmbH
Europaplatz 3
69115 Heidelberg, Germany

Batch number: 10529431

Printed by Printforce, the Netherlands

GPSR Compliance

The European Union's (EU) General Product Safety Regulation (GPSR) is a set of rules that requires consumer products to be safe and our obligations to ensure this.

If you have any concerns about our products, you can contact us on ProductSafety@springernature.com

In case Publisher is established outside the EU, the EU authorized representative is:

Springer Nature Customer Service Center GmbH
Europaplatz 3
69115 Heidelberg, Germany

Batch number: 10733514

Printed by Printforce, the Netherlands